ABNORMAL LABORATORY FINDINGS

Robert M. Dufort

Liver Failure
Hypoadrenocorticism

Cholinesterase
Decreased
Organophosphates
Carbamates

Cobalamin (B₁₂)
Decreased
Bacterial Overgrowth

Creatinine
Increased
Azotemia
  Prerenal
  Renal
  Postrenal
Decreased
Decrease Muscle Mass

Creatine Kinase (CK)
Increased
Muscle Inflammation
  Immune Mediated
    Eosinophilic Myositis
    Masticatory Muscle Myositis
    Endocarditis
    Infectious
      Toxoplasmosis
      Neosporum Caninum
Nutritional
  Hypokalemia (Polymyopathy)
  Taurine Deficiency
Trauma
Exertional Myositis
Surgical
Intramuscular Injections
Hypothermia
Pyrexia
Prolonged Recumbency
Post-Infarct Ischemia
  Cardiomyopathy
  Disseminated Intravascular
    Coagulation

Fibrinogen
Increased
Inflammation
Pregnancy
Decreased
Liver Failure
Coagulopathies
Primary Hypofibrinogenemia

Folate
Increased
Bacterial Overgrowth

Fructosamine
Increased
Diabetes Mellitus
Decreased
Spurious
Hypoproteinemia
Anemia (False)

Gamma Glutamyltransferase (GGT)
Increased
Cholestasis
  Intrahepatic
  Extrahepatic
Drugs (Canine)
  Glucocorticoids
Anticonvulsants
  Primadone
  Phenobarbital
Decreased
Spurious
Hemolysis

Globulin
Increased
Dehydration (Albumin and Total Protein)
Inflammation
Gammopathy
  Monoclonal
    Plasma Cell Myeloma
    Ehrlichia
    Dirofilariasis

Polyclonal
  Chronic Inflammatory Disease
  Feline Infectious Peritonitis
  Dental Disease
  Dermatitis
  Inflammatory Bowel Disease
  Parasitic Diseases
  Immune-Mediated Diseases
  Neoplasia
Decreased
Neonatal
Immunodeficiency
  Congenital
  Acquired
Blood Loss
Protein-Losing Enteropathy

Glucose
Increased
Endocrine
  Acromegaly
  Diabetes Mellitus
  Hyperadrenocorticism
Pancreatitis
Stress (Cats)
Drugs
  Intravenous Glucose
    Administration
  Glucocorticoids
  Xylazine
  Progestagens (Ovaban and Others)
Decreased
Liver Failure
Endocrine
  Hypoadrenocorticism
  Hypopituitarism
Starvation
Neoplasia
Hyperinsulinism
  Iatrogenic
  Insulinoma
Idiopathic
  Puppies
  Toy Breed Dogs
Septicemia
Polycythemia
Leukemia
Glycogen Storage Disease
Artifact
  Delayed Serum Separation

Iron
Increased
Hemolysis
Decreased
Chronic Blood Loss
Dietary Deficiency

Lactate Dehydrogenase (LDH)
Increased
Organ/Tissue Damage
Hemolysis
  In Vivo
  In Vitro
Hepatocytes
Muscle
Kidney
Spurious
  Failure to Separate Serum
    From Rbcs

Lipase
Increased
Pancreatic Disease
  Pancreatitis
    Necrosis
    Neoplasia
Enteritis
Renal Disease
Glucocorticoids

Magnesium
Decreased
Dietary
Diabetic Ketacidosis
Potential Causes:
  Gastrointestinal
    Malabsorption
    Chronic Diarrhea

Renal
  Glomerular Disease
  Tubular Disease
Drugs
  Diuretics
  Amphotericin B
Others

Phosphorus
Increased
Reduced GFR
  Renal
    Acute
    Chronic
  Postrenal
Hemolysis
Hyperthyroidism
Neonates
Intoxication
  Hypervitaminosis D
  Jasmine Ingestion
Dietary Excess
Iatrogenic
  Phosphate Enemas
  Intravenous Phosphate
    Administration
Osteolysis
Hypoparathyroidism
Spurious
  Delayed Serum Separation
Decreased
Hyperparathyroidism
  Primary
  Nutritional Secondary
Neoplasia
  PTH-Like Hormone
  C-Cell Thyroid Tumors
Insulin Therapy
Diabetic Ketoacidosis
Dietary Deficiency
Eclampsia
Hyperadrenocorticism

Potassium
Increased
Renal Failure
  Distal RTA
  Oliguric/Anuric
Postrenal
  Obstruction
  Ruptured Bladder
Spurious
  Breed Idiosyncracy (Akitas)
  Leukemias
  Thrombocytosis
  Collection In Potassium
    Heparin
  Collection in Potassium EDTA
Hypoadrenocorticism
Acidosis
  Diabetic Ketoacidosis
Diffuse Tissue Damage
  Massive Muscle Trauma
  Post-Ischemic Reperfusion
Dehydration
Hypoaldosterone
Drugs
  Propranolol
  Potassium-Sparing Diuretics
  Ace Inhibitors
Decreased
Alkalosis
Dietary Deficiency (Feline)
Potassium-Free Fluids
Bicarbonate Administration
Drugs
  Penicillins
  Amphotericin B
  Loop Diuretics
GI Fluid Loss (K⁺-Rich)
Hyperadrenocorticism
Hyperaldosterone
Insulin Therapy
Renal
  Postobstructive Diuresis
  Renal Tubular Acidosis
  Dialysis

Hypokalemic Periodic
  Paralysis
  Burmese
  Pit Bull
Renal Failure
  Chronic Polyuria

Protein, Total
Increased
Dehydration (Albumin and Globulin)
Hyperglobulinemia
Spurious
  Hemolysis
  Lipemia
Decreased
Hemorrhage
External Plasma Loss
GI Loss
Overhydration
Liver Failure
Glomerular Loss

Sodium
Increased
Hyperaldosterone
GI Fluid Loss (Na⁺-Poor)
  Vomiting
  Diarrhea
Diabetes Insipidus
Renal Failure
Dehydration
Insensible Fluid Loss
  Fever
  Panting
  High Ambient
    Temperature
Decreased Water Intake
  Limited Water Access
  Primary Adipsia
Increased Salt Intake
  Intravenous
  Oral
Spurious
  Serum Evaporation
Decreased
Hypoadrenocorticism
Diabetes Mellitus
GI Fluid Loss (Na⁺-Rich)
  Vomiting
  Diarrhea
Hookworms
Burns
Chronic Effusions
Excess Adh
Diuretics
Hypotonic Fluids
Diet (Severe Sodium Restriction)
Psychogenic Polydipsia
Renal Failure (Polyuric)
Spurious
  Hyperlipidemia

Thyroxine (T₄)
Increased
Hyperthyroidism
Anti-T₄ Autoantibodies
Decreased
Hypothyroidism
Nonthyroid Illness
Drugs
  Corticosteroids
  Phenobarbital

Triiodothyronine (T₃)
Increased
Hyperthyroidism
Anti-T₃ Autoantibodies
Decreased
Hypothyroidism

Trypsinogen-Like Immunoreactivity (TLI)
Increased
Pancreatitis
Postprandial
Decreased
Pancreatic Exocrine
  Insufficiency

TEXTBOOK *of*
Veterinary
Internal Medicine

Diseases of the Dog and Cat

TEXTBOOK *of*
Veterinary
Internal Medicine
Diseases of the Dog and Cat

SIXTH EDITION

VOLUME II

STEPHEN J. ETTINGER, DVM

California Animal Hospital
Los Angeles, California

EDWARD C. FELDMAN, DVM

University of California
Davis, California

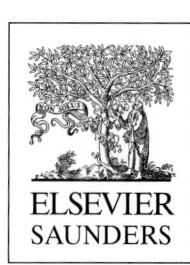

ELSEVIER
SAUNDERS

ELSEVIER
SAUNDERS

11830 Westline Industrial Drive
St. Louis, Missouri 63146

TEXTBOOK OF VETERINARY INTERNAL MEDICINE, SIXTH EDITION
Two-volume set   0-7216-0117-0
Two-volume e-dition 1-4160-0110-7
Copyright © 2005, Elsevier Inc.

NOTICE

Veterinary Medicine is an ever-changing field. Standard safety precautions must be followed, but as new research and clinical experience broaden our knowledge, changes in treatment and drug therapy may become necessary or appropriate. Readers are advised to check the most current product information provided by the manufacturer of each drug to be administered to verify the recommended dose, the method and duration of administration, and contraindications. It is the responsibility of the treating veterinarian, relying on experience and knowledge of the animal, to determine dosages and the best treatment for the animal. Neither the publisher nor the editors assume any liability for any injury and/or damage to animals or property arising from this publication.

The Publisher

Previous editions © 2000, 1995, 1989, 1983, 1975.
Cover image: *Livre de la Chasse*. Used by permission.
Ms. Francais 616, fol. 40". Bibliothèque Nationale, Paris.

Two-volume set ISBN-13: 978-0-7216-0117-5
Two-volume set ISBN-10: 0-7216-0117-0
Two-volume e-dition ISBN-13: 978-1-4160-0110-2
Two-volume e-dition ISBN-10: 1-4160-0110-7

Senior Editor: Liz Fathman
Senior Developmental Editor: Jolynn Gower
Publishing Services Manager: Linda McKinley
Senior Project Manager: Ellen Kunkelmann
Senior Book Designer: Julia Dummitt
Cover Art: Cliché Bibliothèque Nationale de France, Paris

Printed in the United States of America

Last digit is the print number: 9 8 7 6 5 4

CONTENTS

VOLUME I

Neurologic

Cardiorespiratory

Hematologic/Chemical

SECTION II
Toxicology

SECTION III
Techniques

SECTION IV
Critical Care

SECTION V
Blood Pressure

SECTION VI
Therapeutic Considerations in Medicine and Disease

SECTION VII
Dietary Considerations of Systemic Problems

SECTION VIII
Infectious Disease

SECTION IX
Cancer

REFERENCES AND CLIENT INFORMATION SHEETS

References and Client Information Sheets can be found on the CD bound in the book.

Abnormal Laboratory Findings, Conditions Associated with Hematologic Changes, and Urinalysis Abnormalities are located on the inside covers.
Robert M. DuFort

SECTION XI

Cardiovascular System

CHAPTER 197

Pathophysiology of Heart Failure

Helio Autran de Morais
Denise Saretta Schwartz

The heart, consequently, is the beginning of life; the sun of the microcosm, even as the sun in his turn might well be designated the heart of the world; for it is the heart by whose virtue and pulse the blood is moved, perfected, and made nutrient, and is preserved from corruption and coagulation; it is the household divinity which, discharging its function, nourishes, cherishes, quickens the whole body, and is indeed the foundation of life, the source of all action.

William Harvey (1628)

WHAT IS HEART FAILURE?

Heart failure is a clinical syndrome in which impaired pumping decreases ventricular ejection and impedes venous return. During heart failure the heart cannot pump blood at a rate adequate to maintain metabolizing tissue requirements, or it can do so only with elevated filling pressures.[1] However, this definition is not complete because it does not mention that heart failure is a progressive disease.[2] The hemodynamic abnormalities associated with heart failure are in many cases complicated by depressed myocardial contractility and relaxation, caused by biochemical and biophysical disorders in the myocardial cells. These cellular disorders, in turn, are partly the result of molecular abnormalities that not only impair the heart's performance, but also accelerate deterioration of the myocardium and hasten myocardial cell death.[3] *Circulatory failure* is a decrease in cardiac output caused by abnormalities in one or more components of the circulation (i.e., heart, blood volume, oxyhemoglobin concentration, vasculature). Heart failure therefore is one of the many causes of circulatory failure (Figure 197-1).

The heart, like any pump, has only two ways to fail: It either cannot pump enough blood into the aorta or pulmonary artery to maintain arterial pressure (low-output heart failure), or it cannot adequately empty the venous reservoirs (congestive heart failure [CHF]). Heart failure therefore can be recognized clinically by signs of low cardiac output (e.g., depression, lethargy, hypotension) or congestion (e.g., ascites, pleural effusion, pulmonary edema). Heart failure can also be classified, based on the side that is failing, as right, left, or bilateral heart failure. Right-sided heart failure is associated with signs of congestion in the systemic circulation (ascites, peripheral edema), whereas left-sided heart failure causes signs of congestion in the pulmonary circulation (pulmonary edema, dyspnea). Bilateral heart failure presents a combination of left- and right-side signs. In small animal practice, pleural effusion is usually associated with bilateral CHF. Both left- and right-sided heart failure can be associated with low-output signs.

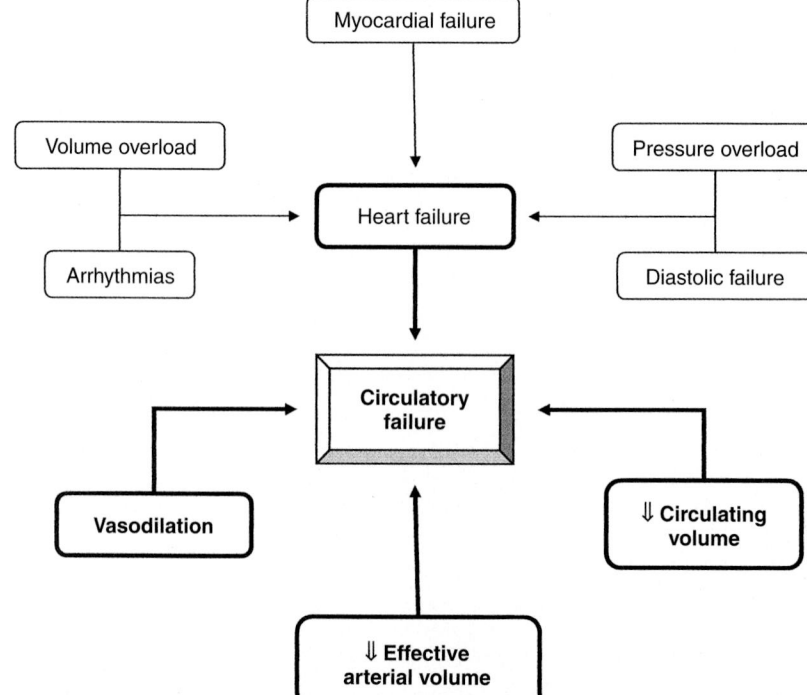

Figure 197-1 Causes of circulatory and heart failure.

WHY DO HEARTS FAIL?

Heart failure may result from inability by the heart to eject blood properly (systolic failure), from inadequate ventricular filling (diastolic failure), or both. The final result in all three cases is a reduction in stroke volume, leading to a decrease in cardiac output and a tendency toward decreased arterial pressure. Patients with severe heart failure have reduced or inadequate cardiac output even at rest, whereas patients with mild heart failure or diastolic failure have an inadequate increase in cardiac output with perturbation (e.g., exercise or stress).

Systolic Function and Dysfunction

Systemic arterial blood pressure (ABP) is a result of the interplay between the arterial system and the heart. Any pressure can be estimated as the product of flow × resistance. In the cardiovascular system, cardiac output (CO), or the amount of blood pumped at a given time, is the flow, and the aortic input impedance (Z), the opposition that the vasculature offers to the ejection of blood by the heart, is the resistance factor:

$$ABP \approx CO \times Z$$

Cardiac output (CO) is the product of the left ventricular stroke volume (SV) and the heart rate (HR):

$$CO = SV \times HR$$

The higher the stroke volume, the higher the cardiac output. Increases in the heart rate increase cardiac output linearly until a plateau is reached, at which point further increases in the heart rate do not affect cardiac output. This latter effect occurs because there is less diastolic time for ventricular filling, and increases in the heart rate are balanced by decreases in the stroke volume. With further increases in the heart rate, cardiac output starts to fall. Stroke volume is primarily determined by an intrinsic property of the myocardial cell, contractility, and two coupling factors, preload and afterload. Preload and afterload are considered coupling factors because they depend on vascular changes. Stroke volume increases with increases in preload and contractility and decreases in afterload. *Preload* is the force acting to stretch the ventricular fibers at the end of diastole and to determine the maximal resting length of the sarcomeres.[4] It reflects the degree of ventricular filling just before contraction. Clinically, preload is estimated as being the end-diastolic volume or, less precisely, the end-diastolic pressure. Substitution of pressure for volume in the estimation of preload is not accurate in all clinical situations (e.g., noncompliant or stiff ventricles). *Afterload* is the force opposing ventricular ejection. This opposition is presented by the vasculature to the ejecting ventricle and is best described by the aortic input impedance.[5-7] An increase in afterload communicates itself to the ventricles during systole by increasing wall stress. The end-systolic wall stress, therefore, can be used as an index of the afterload.[7] *Contractility* is a change in the heart's ability to do work when the preload, afterload, and heart rate are kept constant.[3,7] Stroke volume is also affected by ventricular filling during diastole, ventricular wall motion abnormalities, space-occupying lesions, and arrhythmias. All determinants of cardiac output are intertwined. Therefore as physiologic compensatory and reflex mechanisms affect one component, the other components may also change (Box 197-1).

In the estimation of blood pressure, the resistance factor is best represented by the arterial impedance, which is the aortic pressure divided by aortic flow at a given time. The properties of the arterial system can be described by the total arterial compliance, the peripheral resistance, and the characteristic impedance.[8] *Total arterial compliance* is the change in volume that results from a given change in pressure in the elastic arteries. *Peripheral resistance* is largely determined by small arteries and arterioles and represents the resistance to the steady (nonpulsatile) flow. *Aortic characteristic impedance*, the opposition to pulsatile flow, accounts for the elastic wall and blood mass properties in the proximal aorta.[8] Increases in peripheral resistance and characteristic impedance and decreases in compliance increase left ventricular afterload. With a decrease in compliance, the ventricle ejects into a stiff vasculature, increasing both the energetic cost to maintain blood flow and myocardial oxygen consumption (MVO_2). With decreased compliance, ventricles expend more energy to distend less compliant elastic arteries, making less energy available for tissue perfusion.[9,10] Characteristic impedance, a property of the proximal aorta, increases whenever the stiffness of the aorta increases or its radius becomes smaller. Increases in peripheral resistance (caused by decreases in the cross-sectional area of the arterioles) increase the mean aortic pressure and decrease the left ventricular stroke work and stroke volume.[11-13] Peripheral resistance has a greater effect on ventricular performance than does characteristic impedance or compliance.[9] However, it should be remembered that the left ventricle ejects blood into the proximal aorta and not into

---

Box • 197-1

Interrelation between Determinants of Cardiac Performance and Properties of the Heart

- **Preload and contractility** → Increases in the preload lead to increases in contractility as a result of optimum myocardial fiber length and greater interaction between actin and myosin.
- **Heart rate and preload** → Ventricular filling depends on the duration of the diastolic period. Decreases in the heart rate may increase preload by lengthening diastole. Excessive increases in the heart rate interfere with ventricular filling, decreasing preload.
- **Heart rate and contractility** → Excessive increases in the heart rate decrease the diastolic period, leading to a decrease in myocardial oxygen delivery, and might negatively affect contractility. Increases in the heart rate can also decrease contractility by decreasing preload.
- **Heart rate and myocardial relaxation (lusitropism)** → Decreased diastolic myocardial oxygen delivery during fast heart rates negatively affects relaxation, an energy-dependent process. Ventricular suction capacity is impaired, and ventricular compliance is decreased because of increased stiffness.
- **Heart rate and automatism** → Increases in the heart rate decrease oxygen offer to myocardial cells, changing membrane potential and favoring the development of arrhythmias.
- **Preload and afterload** → Excessive increases in preload increase wall tension. Increases in wall tension increase afterload, leading to increased myocardial oxygen consumption.

Figure 197-2 Determinants of arterial blood pressure. Arterial blood pressure is a function of cardiac output and arterial impedance. Contractility, preload, and afterload determine the stroke volume, which, multiplied by the heart rate, yields the cardiac output. Changes in arterioles, elastic arteries, and the aorta all influence the aortic input impedance (afterload). Increases in afterload increase arterial blood pressure but decrease cardiac output. (+), Increases in the parameter increase aortic input impedance, stroke volume, cardiac output, or arterial blood pressure; (−), increases in the parameter decrease aortic input impedance or stroke volume; (=), afterload and aortic input impedance are synonymous.

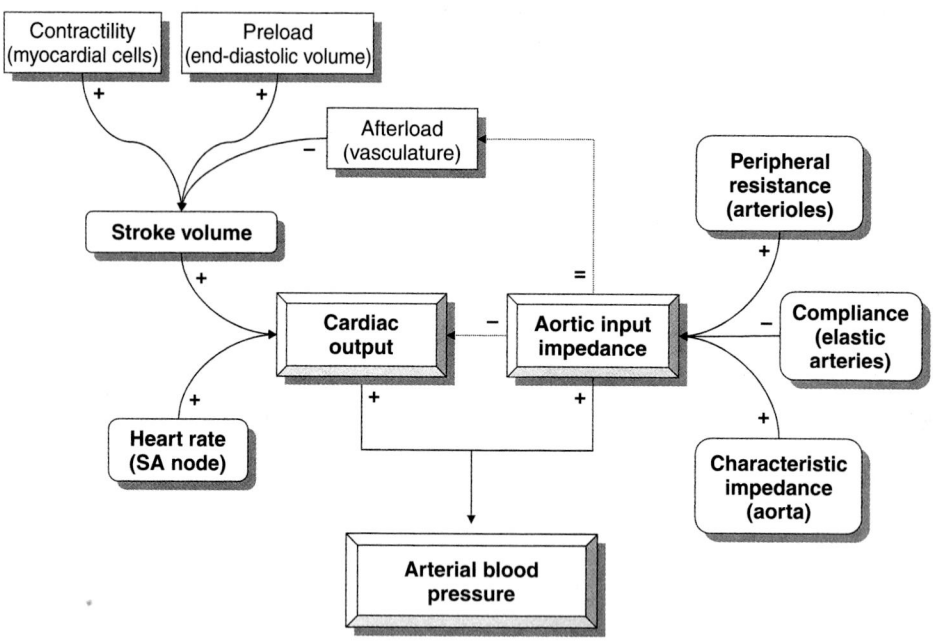

the arterioles. The principal factors involved in the determination of arterial pressure are shown in Figure 197-2.

Systolic failure is characterized by normal filling of the ventricle and a decrease in the forward stroke volume. The decrease in SV may stem from a decrease in contractility *(myocardial failure)* or from a primary increase in ventricular pressure *(pressure overload)* or volume *(volume overload)* (Box 197-2). Increases in volume are usually caused by a leaking valve or an abnormal communication between the systemic and pulmonary circulations.

Myocardial Failure

Myocardial failure may be primary (e.g., dilated cardiomyopathy) or may occur secondary to chronic volume or pressure overload. In patients with myocardial failure, a decrease in contractility lowers the stroke volume, cardiac output, and arterial blood pressure. Myocardial failure depresses the heart's ability to compensate for the decrease in cardiac output (Figure 197-3).

Pressure Overload

The most common reasons for pressure overload in small animal medicine are subaortic stenosis and systemic arterial hypertension on the left side of the heart and heartworm disease and pulmonic stenosis on the right side. In pressure overload states, the ventricles must overcome the increase in resistance to eject blood. The first response is to dilate, increasing the sarcomere length to the point where overlap between myofilaments is optimum (approximately 2.2 μm). Dilatation increases ventricular contractility and pressure through a length-dependent activation of contractility, which helps overcome the increased resistance and maintain stroke volume. However, this adaptation increases ventricular wall stress and consequently MVO₂.

Left ventricular wall stress can be approximated as the product of intraventricular pressure times the left ventricular radius divided by twice the left ventricular wall thickness (Figure 197-4). During the initial dilatation, the ventricular radius increases and wall thickness decreases; both of these factors increase ventricular wall stress. With a sustained pressure

Box • 197-2

Mechanisms Leading to Systolic Heart Failure*

Myocardial failure
    Dilated cardiomyopathy
    Infective myocarditis
    Doxorubicin toxicity
    Cardiomyopathy of overload
    Myocardial infarct
    Right ventricular cardiomyopathy
Volume overload
    Valvular diseases
        Endocardiosis
        Endocarditis
        Rupture of mitral chordae tendineae
        Valvular dysplasia
    Patent ductus arteriosus
    Ventricular septal defect
    Atrial septal defect
    Thyrotoxicosis
    Chronic anemia
    Peripheral arteriovenous fistula
Pressure overload
    Subaortic stenosis
    Pulmonic stenosis
    Systemic hypertension
    Pulmonary hypertension
        Primary
        Pulmonary embolism
        Heartworm disease

*Many disease are also associated with diastolic dysfunction.

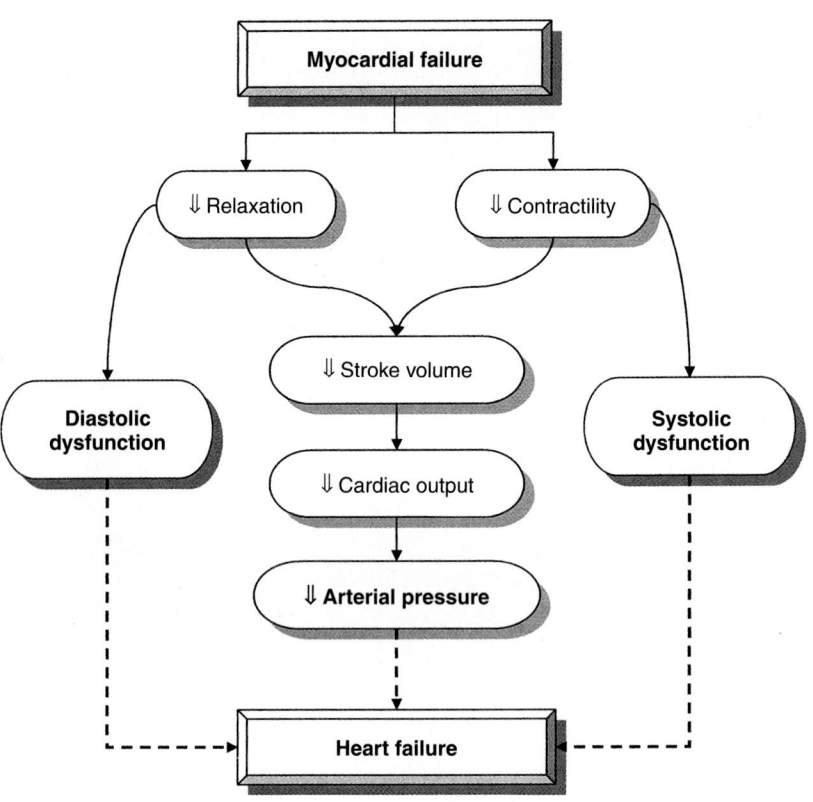

Figure 197-3 Progression from myocardial failure to heart failure.

overload, the ventricular muscle adapts by undergoing concentric hypertrophy (Figure 197-5). In this type of hypertrophy, an increase in wall thickness occurs at the expense of a decrease in chamber size (decrease in ventricular radius), returning ventricular wall stress toward normal and increasing contractility.

Myocardium that undergoes hypertrophy secondary to pressure overload is not normal. A close link exists between hypertrophy and systolic dysfunction. The hypertrophied ventricle is also prone to ischemia, which leads to fibrosis and an increase in collagen content. The early increase in collagen helps maintain systolic function, but it interferes with

diastolic function. With progression of the myocardial hypertrophy, perimuscular fibrosis impairs both systolic and diastolic function.[1] As secondary myocardial failure settles in, the ventricle again dilates. The sequence of events in heart failure secondary to pressure overload is shown in Figure 197-6.

Volume Overload
Volume overload may occur with valvular insufficiency, abnormal communications (e.g., patent ductus arteriosus, septal defects), and high-output states (e.g., hyperthyroidism). The initial event, an increase in chamber size, occurs as a result of the need to accommodate a large ventricular

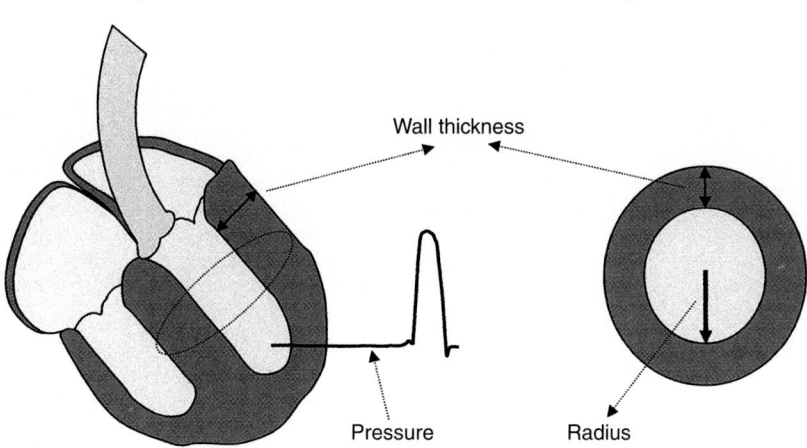

Figure 197-4 Determinants of left ventricular wall stress. *LV*, Left ventricle.

$$\text{LV wall stress} = \text{LV pressure} \times \frac{\text{LV radius}}{2 \times \text{LV wall thickness}}$$

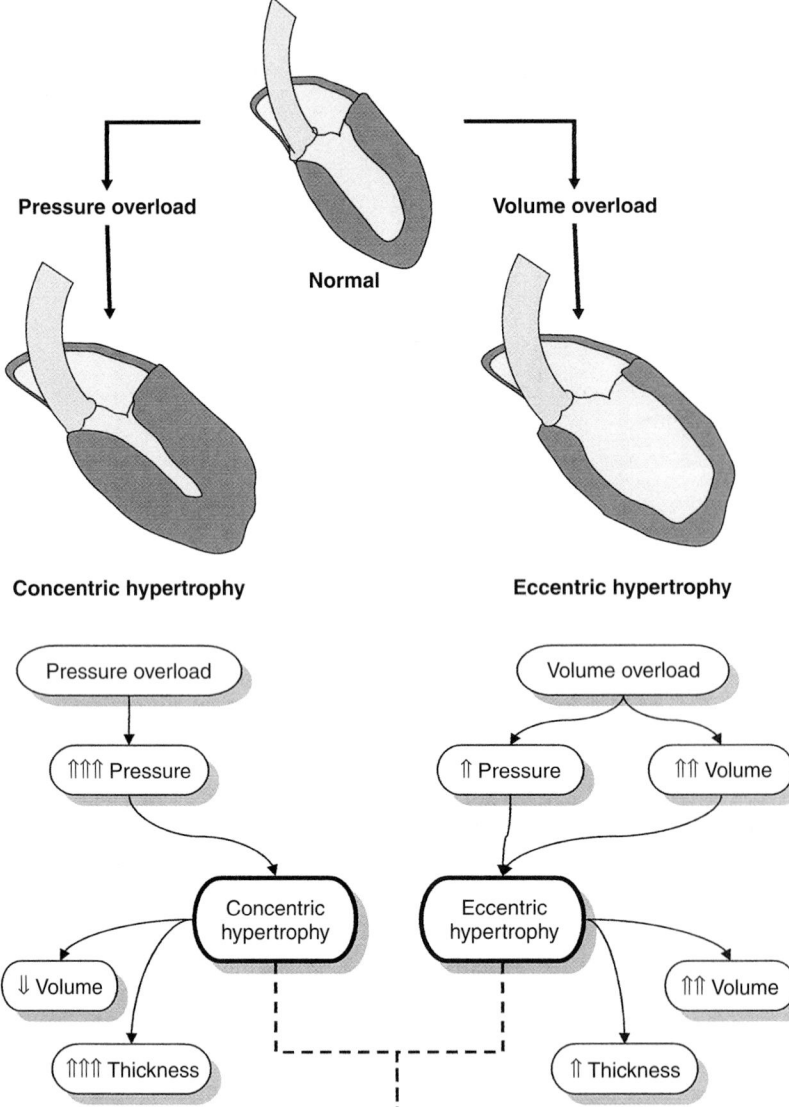

Figure 197-5 Types of ventricular hypertrophy. Increases in pressure lead to concentric hypertrophy (parallel addition of new sarcomeres), whereas increases in volume lead to eccentric hypertrophy (in-line addition of new sarcomeres).

end-diastolic volume; this increases the sarcomere length to the optimal 2.2 μm. Again, dilatation leads to an increase in wall stress, which in turn causes ventricular hypertrophy and normalizes wall stress. Volume overload is marked by an eccentric hypertrophy, with a mild increase in wall thickness and an increase in radius (see Figure 197-6). The degree of hypertrophy is not as severe as in pressure overload states because the primary event now is an increase in volume, which causes only a mild increase in ventricular pressure. The performance of each unit of myocardium in a chronically volume-overloaded heart is normal or near normal, allowing a greater than normal stroke volume. The ventricle responds to a volume overload situation by increasing size and also by changing its geometry. Contrary to what happens in the pressure-overloaded myocardium, collagen formation is not a problem in the early stages of volume overload. In fact, a loss of myocardial collagen occurs in volume-overloaded hearts. The loss of collagen causes the ventricle to dilate and increases ventricular compliance. Left ventricular dilatation and increased compliance do not occur in volume-overloaded hearts when

collagenase stimulation caused by mast cell degranulation is blocked.[14]

With progression of the disease, ventricular end-diastolic pressure again rises above the normal range, increasing resting tension and compromising the endocardial perfusion pressure.[15] The increase in tension that occurs in this setting is the result of slippage of fibers, with an excessive increase in chamber size. The mechanism for fiber slippage is poorly understood, but it is probably related to a disruption in normal collagen-myocyte interaction. If collagen fibers fail to support the myocytes, increases in intracavitary pressure may push the myocytes apart by means of fiber slippage.[16] Fiber slippage helps maintain stroke volume by an unknown mechanism, probably by improving diastolic function. The stretched collagen and the longer fiber length act in the diastole in the opposite way that hypertrophied myocardium does, thereby increasing diastolic compliance. Fiber slippage, on the other hand, sets the stage for progressive disease. The increase in chamber size increases wall stress and MVO_2, changes the ventricular geometry, and may cause pressure hypertrophy

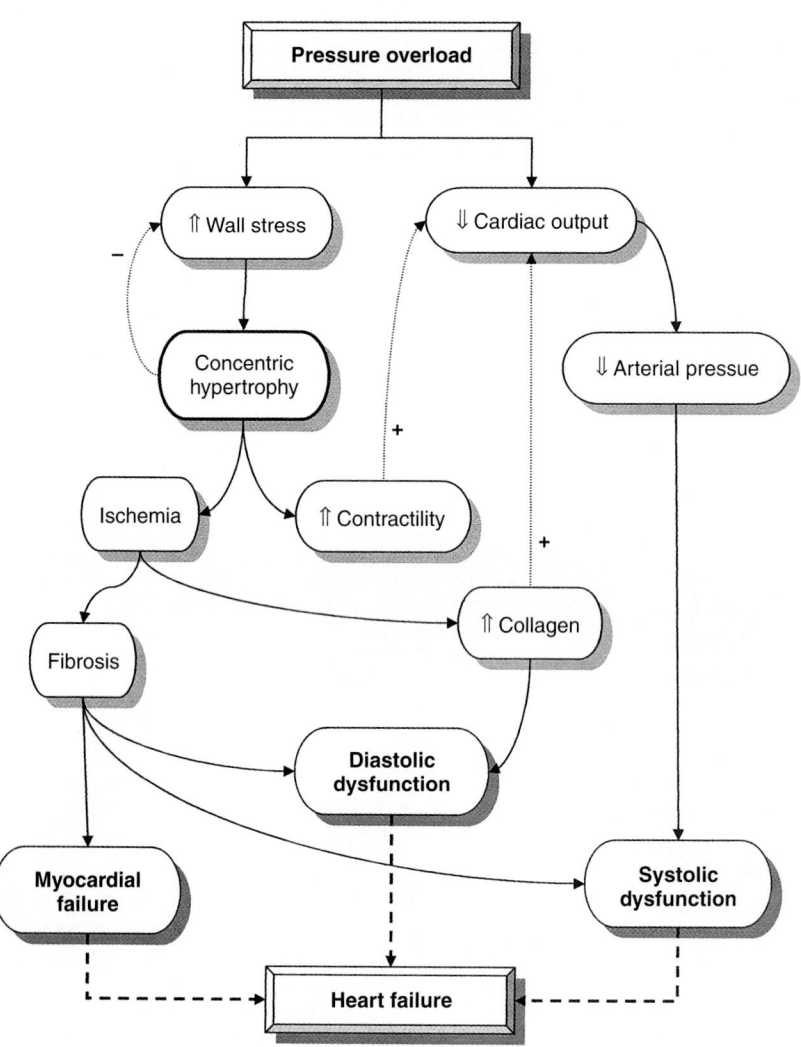

Figure 197-6 Progression from pressure overload to heart failure. Pressure overload states increase wall stress, leading to concentric hypertrophy. Hypertrophy increases contractility and decreases wall stress. Unfortunately, pressure hypertrophy leads to ischemia, fibrosis, and increased collagen formation. The end result is myocardial failure and diastolic dysfunction, leading to heart failure. *(−)*, Decreases wall stress; *(+)*, increases cardiac output.

and fibrosis. Stretch also stimulates the production of tumor necrosis factor alpha (TNF-alpha) in cardiac fibroblasts,[17] increasing protein synthesis and stimulating hypertrophy.[18] With progression of the disease, secondary myocardial failure may ensue, and the ventricle will undergo further dilatation. The sequence of events in heart failure secondary to volume overload is shown in Figure 197-7.

Diastolic Function and Dysfunction

Diastolic dysfunction results from impairment in ventricular filling. Diastolic heart failure exists when pulmonary venous congestion and resultant clinical signs occur in the presence of normal or near normal left ventricular (LV) systolic function.[19] Approximately one third of human patients with heart failure have diastolic failure, another one third have systolic failure, and the remaining one third have impairment of both systolic and diastolic function.[15] Mechanisms that lead to diastolic heart failure are listed in Box 197-3. Diastolic failure may result from abnormal relaxation (early diastole), abnormal compliance (early to late diastole), or external constraint by the pericardium. If diastole is defined as starting at the time of aortic valve closure (there are other definitions), it can be divided into four phases: (1) isovolumic relaxation (aortic valve closure to mitral valve opening); (2) rapid early mitral inflow (or the rapid filling phase, during which most of ventricular filling occurs); (3) diastasis (or the slow filling phase, during which little change occurs in ventricular volume and pressure);

and (4) atrial contraction (atrial systole and its contribution to ventricular filling). The second through fourth phases of diastole represent ventricular filling.

Relaxation is a dynamic, energy-dependent process that begins at the end of contraction and lasts throughout isovolumic relaxation and early ventricular filling. Beta-adrenergic stimulation improves relaxation, whereas ischemia, asynchrony of relaxation, an increase in afterload, ventricular hypertrophy, and abnormal calcium fluxes in the myocardial cells delay relaxation. Ventricular *compliance* is the ability of the heart to fill passively, and it is usually measured at the end of diastole, when the heart is relaxed. It is determined by volume, geometry, and the tissue characteristics of the ventricular wall. Compliance is an expression of the distensibility of a fluid-filled organ. The higher the compliance, the lower the pressure at a given volume. Ventricular compliance decreases with increases in filling pressures and intrinsic myocardial stiffness (e.g., infiltrative diseases, fibrosis, ischemia) and with hypertrophy and cardiac tamponade. *Lusitropy*, a measure of the global diastolic performance of the heart, comprises the relaxation and filling phases.[20]

Ventricular filling may be affected by several factors, including the atrioventricular pressure gradient, isovolumic relaxation rate, synchronized atrial kick and ventricular relaxation, and compliance. The driving force for ventricular filling is the pressure gradient between the left atrium and ventricle when the mitral valve opens. This gradient is affected mostly

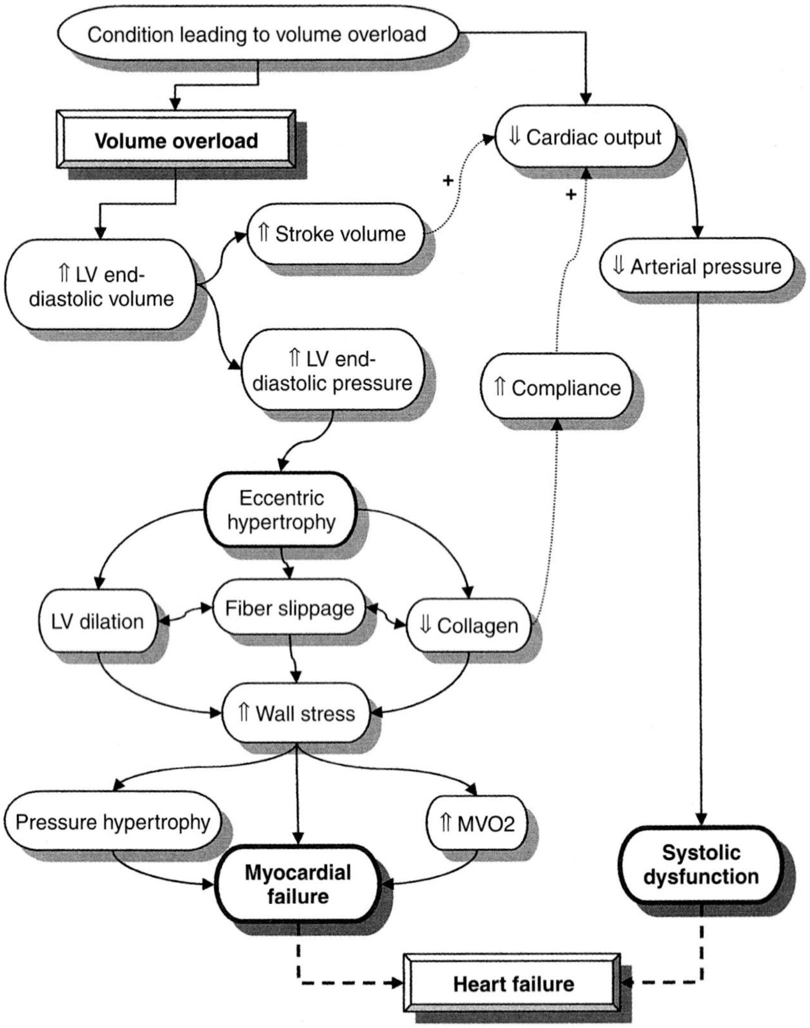

Figure 197-7 Progression from volume overload to heart failure. Volume overload states decrease forward stroke volume, leading to systolic dysfunction and an increased end-diastolic volume. The increase in the end-diastolic volume increases the stroke volume but also the end-diastolic pressure, leading to eccentric hypertrophy. Eccentric hypertrophy leads to a decrease in collagen content that helps diastolic function, but it also causes fiber slippage, thereby increasing wall stress and ultimately leading to myocardial failure. Patients with volume-over-loaded hearts usually develop congestive heart failure (CHF) secondary to a decrease in forward stroke volume, but in some patients CHF may occur secondary to myocardial failure. (+), Increases cardiac output.

Box • 197-3

Mechanisms Leading to Diastolic Heart Failure

Impaired energy-dependent ventricular relaxation or abnormal ventricular chamber or muscle properties
  Ventricular hypertrophy
    Hypertrophic cardiomyopathy
    Subaortic stenosis
    Pulmonic stenosis
    Heartworm disease
    Systemic hypertension
  Dilated cardiomyopathy
  Myocardial infarct
  Restrictive cardiomyopathy
Obstruction to ventricular filling at veins, atria, and atrioventricular valves
  Mitral stenosis
  Tricuspid stenosis
  Intracardiac neoplasia causing intracardiac obstruction
  Cor triatriatum
Pericardial abnormalities
  Constrictive disease
  Cardiac tamponade

---

by the intravascular volume and the degree of vasodilatation. The isovolumic relaxation rate is also an important determinant of early ventricular filling. Adrenergic stimulation increases the rate of relaxation, improving relaxation to a greater extent than it improves contractility. This makes evolutionary sense because during faster heart rates, diastole is shortened to a greater extent than is systole. Tachycardia shortens the duration of the diastasis. Incremental increases in the heart rate up to 180 beats/min in dogs progressively increase the rate of relaxation, improve left ventricular contractility, and decrease left ventricular end-diastolic pressure.[21,22] These changes allow increases in early filling when higher heart rates are needed (e.g., during exercise). Patients with ventricular hypertrophy that are ischemic, however, show a decrease in left ventricular distensibility with increases in the heart rate.

Normal diastolic filling also depends on synchronized contraction between the left ventricle and left atrium.[19] Loss of atrial contraction is one reason why dogs with dilated cardiomyopathy or mitral endocardiosis develop heart failure when the atria start to fibrillate. Asynchronous relaxation of the left ventricle may be observed in cats with restrictive cardiomyopathy. A decrease in the uniformity of relaxation reduces ventricular filling and may contribute to development of heart failure in these patients. Left ventricular compliance also affects ventricular filling. Patients with left ventricular hypertrophy have decreased left ventricular compliance and poor diastolic function as a result of the increases in cardiomyocyte size, collagen formation, and wall thickness.[19]

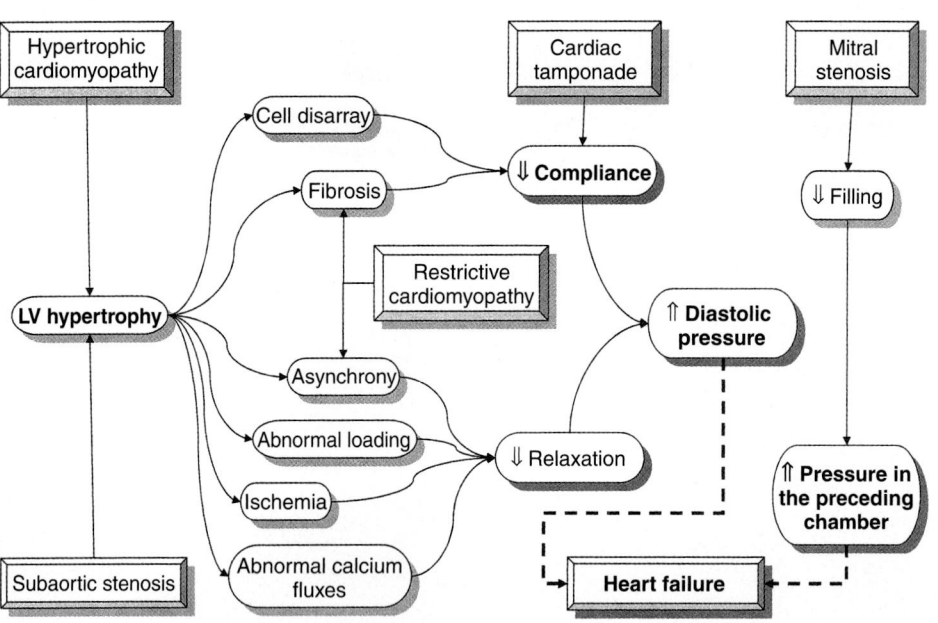

Figure 197-8 Sequence of events leading to diastolic heart failure. Most mechanisms leading to diastolic failure decrease lusitropy by reducing compliance (thus increasing stiffness) or relaxation, or both. Mitral stenosis leads to diastolic heart failure through interference with left ventricular filling.

The pericardium may also restrict ventricular filling in constrictive pericardial disease or cardiac tamponade. In these situations ventricular filling is abruptly halted in mid-diastole by the abnormal pericardium, which imposes its mechanical properties on those of the ventricle during the final phases of diastole. The mechanisms that lead to the development of congestive heart failure during diastolic dysfunction are shown schematically in Figure 197-8.

HOW DOES THE BODY REACT TO HEART FAILURE?

Many conditions and different heart diseases can progress into heart failure. Regardless of the cause, there is an initial fall in cardiac output that lowers arterial pressure. Clinical signs observed in heart failure are mainly the result of chronic activation of compensatory mechanisms to restore and maintain blood pressure. The cardiovascular system is part of a biologic control system that works in co-operation with the central nervous, renal, and endocrine systems to keep cardiovascular variables at physiologic levels. Maintenance of arterial blood pressure and effective plasma volume are the main priorities of this integrated system. Changes are sensed by high-pressure baroreceptors in the aortic arch and carotid sinus, by mechanoreceptors in the ventricular myocardium, by volume receptors in the atria and great veins, and by the juxtaglomerular apparatus in the kidneys. During episodes of low blood pressure, a reactive neuroendocrine activation occurs to re-establish normal blood pressure. The immediate response is a decrease in parasympathetic drive and an increase in sympathetic drive, causing vasoconstriction (increasing arterial impedance) and tachycardia (increasing cardiac output). Vagal responses tend to be immediate and short-lived, whereas sympathetic responses are slower but last longer. A decrease in renal blood flow causes the release of renin and activation of the renin-angiotensin-aldosterone system (RAS), contributing to vasoconstriction and causing sodium and water retention, which increases the circulating volume. Compensatory mechanisms are acute responses that evolved to maintain an animal's life during and immediately after an episode of bleeding. During heart failure, however, compensatory mechanisms are chronically activated (Figure 197-9). In an effort to maintain blood pressure, the cardiovascular system allows the venous pressure to increase and redistributes cardiac output, maintaining blood flow mostly to essential organs (Figure 197-10).

Compensation cannot be viewed as an isolated response of the circulation. The heart and the myocardial cells undergo changes to adapt to ventricular dysfunction. A common characteristic of all compensatory responses is that the short-term effects are helpful, but the long-term effects are deleterious. In acute injuries to the heart, cardiac output decreases and acute heart failure may occur; this phase, known as *transient breakdown*, initiates activation of the compensatory mechanisms.[23] In small animals, heart failure is usually a chronic problem, and the transient breakdown phase merges with the following phase. As compensation occurs, cardiac output and clinical signs steadily improve, because the heart and circulation are performing extra work; this compensated phase is known as *stable hyperfunction*. Chronic hyperfunction leads to progression of left ventricular dysfunction, myocardial cell death, the development of clinical signs, and death, the *exhaustion and progressive cardiosclerosis* phase. The chronic effects of the compensatory mechanisms that lead to progression of left ventricular dysfunction are shown in Figure 197-11.

Neuroendocrine Activation

Neuroendocrine activation in CHF is a result of the decrease in cardiac output and atrial hypertension. Neuroendocrine mechanisms include vasoconstrictive/sodium-retaining systems and vasodilator/natriuretic systems (Box 197-4). All neuroendocrine mechanisms are operating fully during severe CHF. The exact point at which each neuroendocrine mechanism is activated is the subject of debate. In a tachycardia-induced heart failure model, increases in neurohormones were detected within 3 weeks of pacing at 180 beats/min during early myocardial dysfunction, when the animals were still asymptomatic.[24] Clinical data are still lacking in small animals with naturally occurring CHF. The underlying cause of the ventricular dysfunction appears to play a role in the determination of when activation of a particular neuroendocrine mechanism starts. The net effect of neuroendocrine activation is vasoconstriction, sodium and water retention, and LV hypertrophy, leading to ventricular and peripheral vessel remodeling.

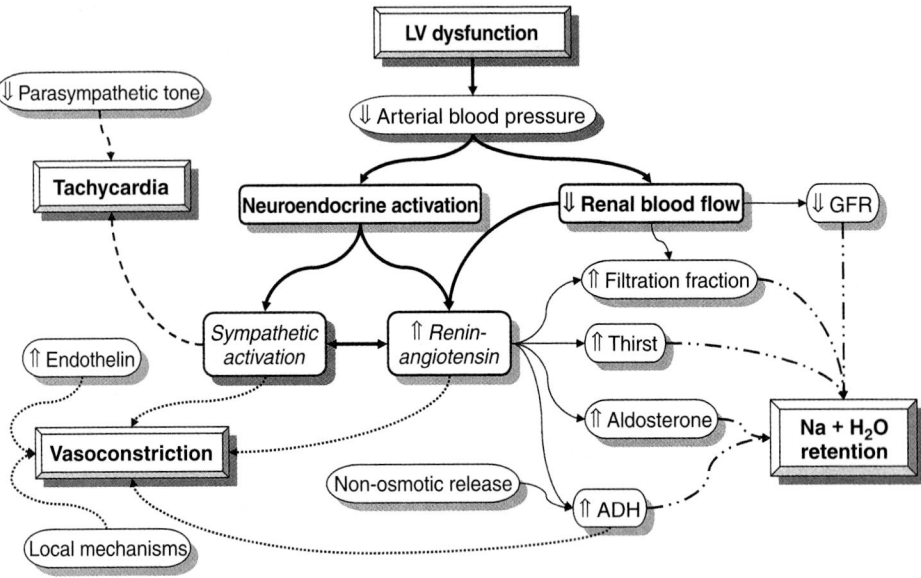

Figure 197-9 Compensation in congestive heart failure. Left ventricular (LV) dysfunction decreases cardiac output and arterial blood pressure. The decrease in renal blood flow and concomitant neuroendocrine activation set in motion compensatory mechanisms designed to restore blood pressure:sodium and water retention *(dash-and-dot line)*; vasoconstriction *(dotted line)*; and tachycardia *(dashed line)*. ADH, Vasopressin; GFR, glomerular filtration rate.

Autonomic Nervous System

CHF is accompanied by a generalized increase in sympathetic nerve activity and attenuation of parasympathetic tone. Dogs with naturally occurring CHF caused by dilated cardiomyopathy and mitral regurgitation have increased norepinephrine concentrations, a finding that correlates positively with the clinical severity of the CHF.[25] The increase in norepinephrine, however, does not correlate with the degree of myocardial dysfunction.[25,26] The norepinephrine concentration correlates with cardiac death in human patients with CHF. Increased release of norepinephrine from adrenergic endings and its "spillover" into plasma, as well as decreased uptake by adrenergic nerve endings, are responsible for the observed increase in the norepinephrine concentration during CHF. The decrease in left ventricular function leads to relative hypotension, which stimulates the baroreceptors to activate the sympathetic nervous system.[27] However, the precise mechanisms responsible for the persistent sympathetic overactivity and blunted baroreflex control seen in CHF remain obscure and cannot be explained solely by chronic withdrawal of baroreflex inhibition.[28] Augmented peripheral chemosensitivity also has been demonstrated in CHF.[29] A link between increased peripheral chemosensitivity and impaired autonomic control, including baroreflex inhibition, has been demonstrated in human patients with CHF.[30] Overactivity of muscle metaboreceptors (ergoreceptors) may also contribute to the autonomic imbalance,[31] because ergoreflexes from the ailing skeletal muscle may further promote adrenergic and RAS activation.[32]

Despite the increase in the plasma concentration of norepinephrine, patients with CHF have depletion of norepinephrine from the atria and ventricles, which blunts the

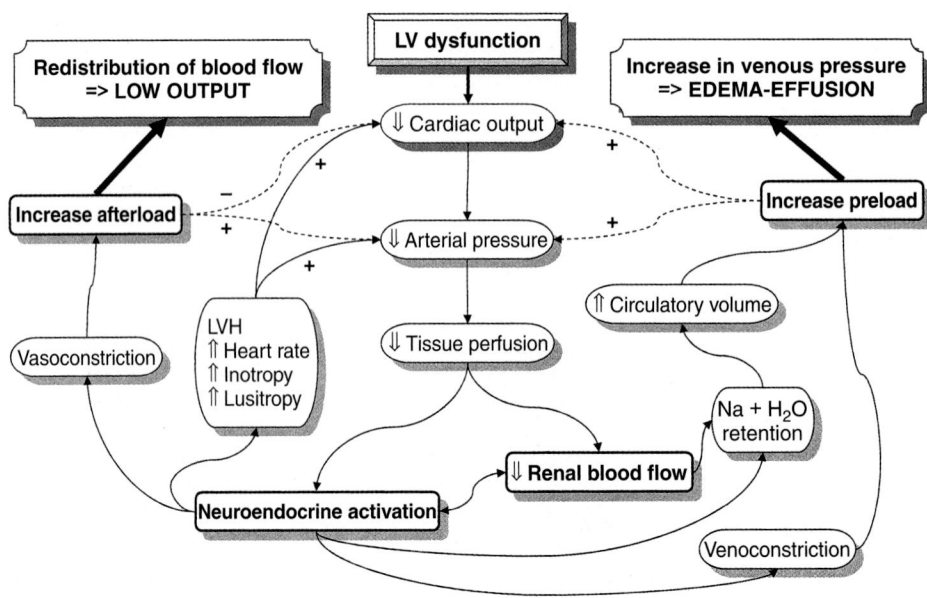

Figure 197-10 Compensation and clinical signs of congestive heart failure. The compensatory mechanisms activated to restore arterial blood pressure during heart failure are ultimately responsible for the clinical signs of the disorder. Retention of sodium and water leads to the formation of edema and effusions, and an increased afterload decreases cardiac output. *(+)*, Increases arterial pressure or cardiac output; *(−)*, decreases cardiac output; ADH, vasopressin; LV, left ventricle; LVH, left ventricular hypertrophy.

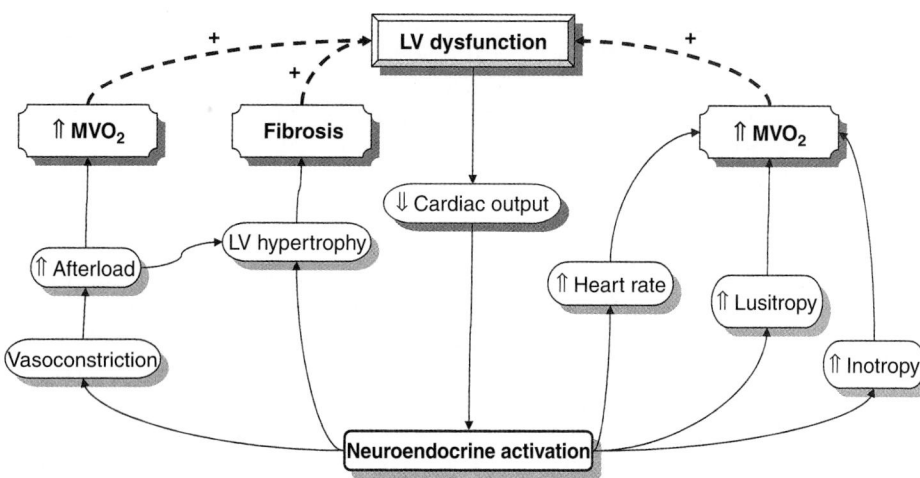

Figure 197-11 Compensation process and progression of left ventricular dysfunction. The compensatory mechanisms activated to restore arterial blood pressure during heart failure are ultimately responsible for progression of the disease. Increased afterload and increased cardiac activity increase myocardial oxygen consumption (MVO_2); left ventricular (LV) hypertrophy is associated with fibrosis. *(+)*, Causes further left ventricular dysfunction.

response to sympathetic activation. Increased levels of norepinephrine in the vicinity of beta adrenoreceptors leads to downregulation of these receptors. Downregulation of beta adrenoreceptors occurs in patients with severe cardiomyopathy and correlates with the severity of the heart disease. In normal hearts, the ratio of $beta_1$ to $beta_2$ receptors is approximately 80:20, whereas in failing hearts, it approaches 60:40.[33] In patients with dilated cardiomyopathy, downregulation is consistently shown in $beta_1$ adrenoreceptors but not in $beta_2$ adrenoreceptors, whereas in mitral disease and in ischemic cardiomyopathy, both subsets of beta adrenoreceptors are downregulated. The selective downregulation of $beta_1$ adrenoreceptors may occur because myocardial $beta_1$ adrenoreceptors are innervated and therefore are exposed to the increased norepinephrine released from the nerve endings, whereas myocardial $beta_2$ adrenoreceptors are not innervated. Postadrenoreceptor changes in the beta adrenoreceptor–adenylate cyclase complex can contribute to changes in adrenergic responsiveness.

The increase in sympathetic activity is partly responsible for the vasoconstriction and sodium and water retention, whereas the decrease in norepinephrine stores and the changes in adrenoreceptors lead to a decrease in the contractile response of the myocardial cells and in the chronotropic response of the sinoatrial node cells during exercise. Chronic adrenergic stimulation also leads to increases in afterload and MVO_2, as well as to ventricular arrhythmias, and it favors progression of left ventricular dysfunction (Figure 197-12). Remodeling of the heart and peripheral vessels, also stimulated by chronic sympathetic activation, further favors progression of left ventricular dysfunction. It is interesting to note that $beta_2$-adrenergic stimulation leads to vasodilatation and may be antiapoptotic and cardioprotective.[32]

Baroreflex control is altered during CHF, a circumstance that is partly responsible for the increased sympathetic activity and the blunted tachycardic response during exercise or hypotension. Abnormal baroreflexes also contribute to sodium and water retention. Normally, increases in atrial pressure stimulate atrial stretch receptors, inhibiting the release of antidiuretic hormone (ADH), decreasing sympathetic activity, and increasing renal blood flow and the glomerular filtration rate. During CHF atrial and arterial receptors show a decreased response to stimulation, and baroreceptor function is impaired. The mechanisms are not clear but appear to be related to increases in sodium-potassium adenosine triphosphatase (Na^+-K^+ ATPase) activity in the baroreceptors. The decrease in parasympathetic activity in CHF decreases the restraint of the sinoatrial (SA) node. The net result is a higher heart rate for a given arterial pressure and a decrease in heart rate variability. Decreases in heart rate variability have been observed in dogs with naturally occurring[34] and experimentally induced[35,36] heart failure (Figure 197-13). Impairment of the heart rate response to postural changes is an early finding in experimental heart failure progression in dogs,[37] which suggests that parasympathetic activity is reduced in the initial phases of heart failure (Figure 197-14). A decrease in parasympathetic tone in CHF carries a poor prognosis.

Renin-Angiotensin-Aldosterone System

Low cardiac output during CHF stimulates renin release through direct beta adrenoreceptor stimulation and a decrease in renal flow in the juxtaglomerular apparatus of the kidneys. Renin increases angiotension II concentration. An array of effects of angiotensin II initially brings the blood pressure toward the normal range, but perpetuation of its effects leads

---

Box • 197-4

Neuroendocrine Factors in Heart Failure

Vasoconstrictive or sodium-retaining factors
↑ Sympathetic nervous tone*
↑ Renin-angiotensin II-Aldosterone
↑ ADH (vasopressin)
↑ Endothelin-1
↑ Thromboxane
↑ Neuropeptide Y
↑ Tumor necrosis factor alpha
Vasodilatative or natriuretic factors
↑ Atrial natriuretic factor
↑ Nitric oxide (basal, decreased release upon stimulation)
↑ Prostaglandins (E_2, I_2)
↓ Kallikrein
↑ Dopamine
↓ Calcitonin gene-related peptide

*$Beta_2$-adrenergic stimulation causes vasodilatation and may be antiapoptotic and cardioprotective.

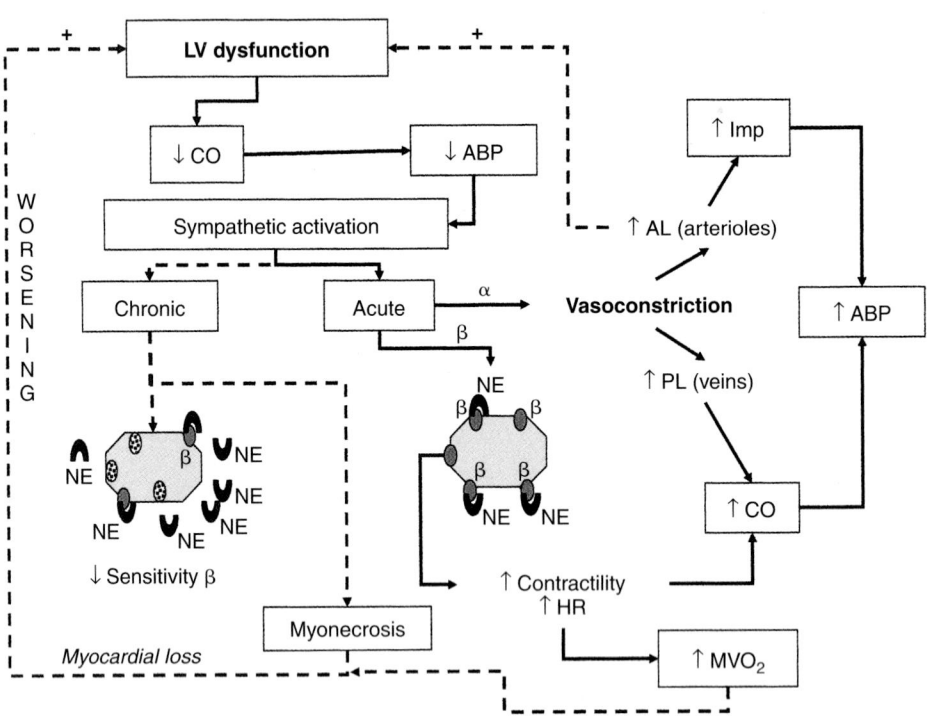

Figure 197-12   Beneficial and detrimental effects of sympathetic activation. Short-term sympathetic effects are beneficial, whereas chronic activation favors progression of left ventricular dysfunction. Dashed lines indicate long-term effects. *(+)*, Causes further left ventricular dysfunction; *CO*, cardiac output; *ABP*, arterial blood pressure; *HR*, heart rate; *AL*, afterload; *NE*, norepinephrine; *Imp*, arterial impedance; *PL*, preload.

to a vicious cycle that contributes to further declines in ventricular function. Angiotensin II is a potent vasoconstrictor. Vasoconstriction increases arteriolar resistance, which helps to normalize blood pressure but also increases afterload. The higher afterload increases MVO_2 and negatively affects cardiac output. On the venous side, angiotensin-induced venoconstriction decreases venous capacity, increasing venous return to the heart and cardiac output. Angiotensin II also stimulates the release of ADH and aldosterone. ADH causes vasoconstriction and stimulates water resorption in the renal distal tubules, whereas aldosterone causes sodium and water retention and contributes to baroreceptor dysfunction. Aldosterone increases total body

water and may contribute to increased tissue water content, increasing stiffness and decreasing compliance of the arterial system.[38] Aldosterone also increases potassium and magnesium excretion. Even in the absence of a low serum magnesium level, aldosterone decreases the cytosolic magnesium concentration by decreasing alpha[1] antiproteinase activity, a marker of oxidative stress.[39] Increases in plasma aldosterone are associated with an inflammatory response with evidence of oxidative stress and may lead to intramural coronary artery remodeling and fibrosis.[39] Angiotensin II also enhances sympathetic activity, constricts the efferent renal artery, and stimulates thirst.[38] Thus activation of the RAS contributes to

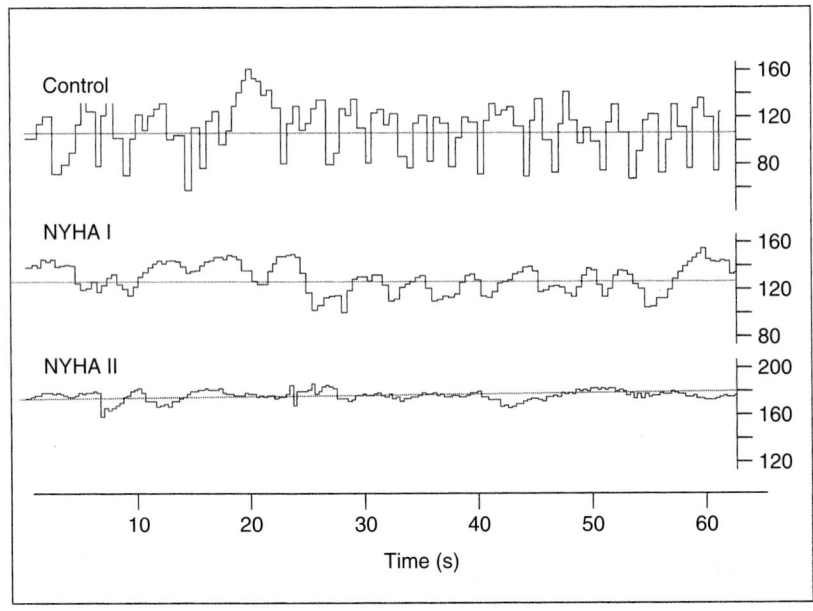

Figure 197-13   Heart rate variability over 1 minute in a dog before and after induction of progressive congestive heart failure. Heart rate variability is shown over time *(x axis)* as heart rate *(y axis)* fluctuation above and below the mean heart rate per minute *(horizontal line)*. With progression of the disease, the heart rate increases and heart rate variability decreases. (From Schwatrz DS: *Studies on baroreceptor function in dogs*, doctoral dissertation, Columbus, Ohio, 2000, Ohio State University.)

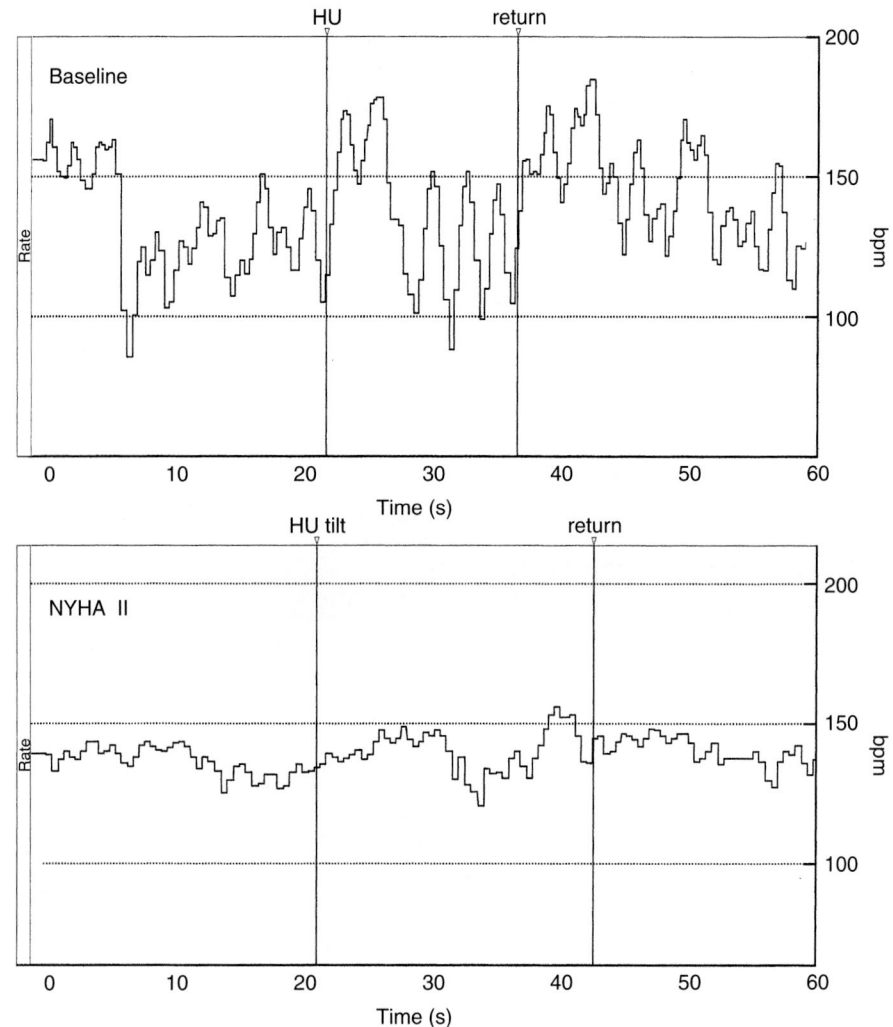

Figure 197-14 Lack of heart rate response to postural change (active head-up tilt, HU) in a dog with rapid pacing-induced heart failure (New York Heart Association [NYHA] class II) *(lower figure)*. Note that before induction of heart failure *(baseline)*, a rapid increase in the heart rate and large heart rate variability immediately after postural change are seen. (From Schwatrz DS: *Studies on baroreceptor function in dogs*, doctoral dissertation, Columbus, Ohio, 2000, Ohio State University.)

vasoconstriction with sodium and water retention during CHF. Sympathetic activation usually precedes RAS activation, although some of the sympathetic activation during CHF is caused by the increased activity of the RAS.

Angiotensin II stimulates growth factors, promoting remodeling in the vessels and myocardium. It may also stimulate vessel remodeling by reducing nitric oxide synthesis or by increasing local angiotensin-converting enzyme (ACE) breakdown of bradykinin. Vascular remodeling causes structural changes that further decrease the compliance of the arterial system. Angiotensin II stimulates smooth muscle cell growth, leading to cellular hyperplasia, hypertrophy, and apoptosis (programmed cell death).[38] An increased level of angiotensin II is associated with superoxide formation (oxidative stress), endothelin secretion, plasminogen activation, TNF-alpha production (inflammation), fibroblast hypertrophy, and increased production of collagen. The final result is myocyte and vascular wall fibrosis. Angiotensin II plays a key role in the development of pathologic hypertrophy, exerting cytotoxic effects on the myocardium, causing myocyte necrosis, and contributing to myocardial loss.[40] Stimulation of angiotensin receptors (AT_1) is responsible for altered gene expression and gene reprogramming of cardiac myocytes and fibroblasts, leading to increases in skeletal alpha actin, atrial natriuretic peptide, and beta myosin heavy chain, as well as increases in fibronectin, impairing diastolic and systolic function.[40] The beneficial and detrimental effects of angiotensin II during heart failure are presented in Figure 197-15.

Activation of the RAS contributes to vasoconstriction, increasing afterload and MVO_2 and causing the kidneys to retain sodium and water. Remodeling of the heart and peripheral vessels is also stimulated by the RAAS, conditions that favor progression of left ventricular dysfunction. Angiotensin II induces cardiac myocyte necrosis associated with increased apoptosis and contributes to myocardial loss, perpetuating the progression of left ventricular dysfunction.

Other Vasoconstrictive Agents

ADH levels are increased in patients with heart failure as a result of nonosmotic release, impairment in baroreceptor-mediated inhibition of brain stem centers, and an increase in circulating angiotensin II. ADH synthesis is substantially and chronically elevated in patients with heart failure despite the volume overload and reductions in plasma osmolality often observed in these patients. ADH levels may be increased even in patients with asymptomatic left ventricular dysfunction. The release of ADH leads to vasoconstriction and water resorption and favors the development of hyponatremia. ADH also appears to affect hemodynamics and cardiac remodeling adversely while potentiating the effects of norepinephrine and angiotensin II. Chronic ADH receptor blockade did not attenuate ventricular remodeling in at least one model of left ventricular dysfunction.[41] ADH, therefore, may not play a major role in the structural progression of heart failure.

Endothelin is the most potent vasoconstrictor known for vascular smooth muscle cells. It is elevated in a canine pacing

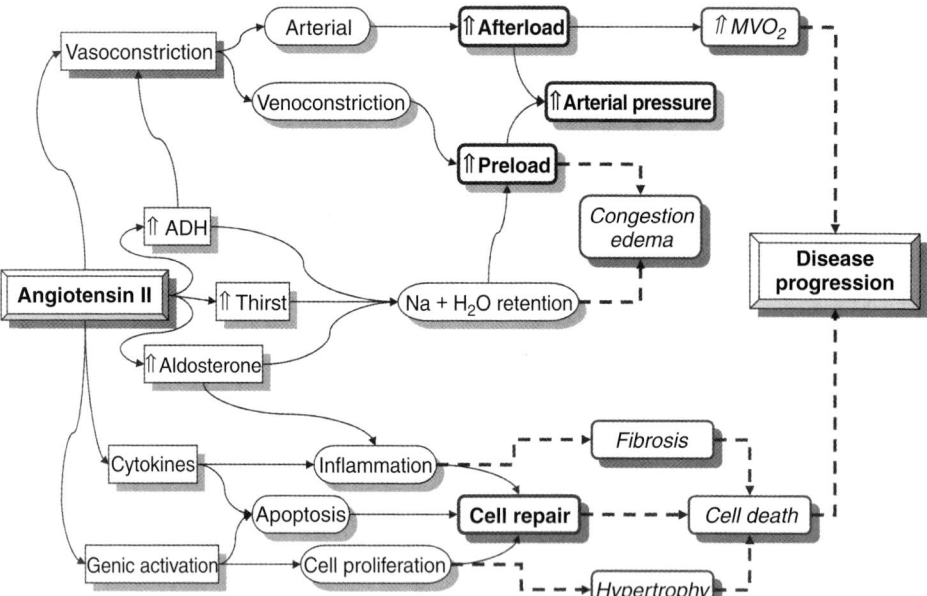

Figure 197-15 Beneficial (bold) and detrimental (italics) effects of angiotensin II during heart failure. The short-term effects of angiotensin II are beneficial, whereas chronic activation favors the appearance of clinical signs and progression of left ventricular dysfunction. Angiotensin II also participates in sympathetic activation. Dashed lines indicate long-term effects.

model of heart failure, and the increase correlates well with the right atrial or pulmonary capillary wedge pressure.[42] The increase in endothelin during heart failure is likely due to increased production and not decreased clearance.[43] It has been shown that cardiac overexpression of endothelin-1 (ET-1) is sufficient to increase inflammatory cytokines and cause an inflammatory cardiomyopathy that leads to heart failure and death.[44] Activation of myocardial and plasma ET-1 precedes activation of myocardial and plasma RAS in a canine model of CHF,[45] but angiotensin II further increases the ET-1 concentration. Endothelin plays an important role in the maintenance of blood pressure and blood flow during CHF.[46] Chronic blockage of endothelin receptors may prevent the progression of experimental heart failure in dogs,[47] and an endothelin-converting enzyme prevented vascular remodeling during experimental heart failure.[48] Unfortunately, clinical trials with chronic ET-receptor antagonism showed worsening of CHF symptoms.

Vasodilatory Agents

The natriuretic peptides are counter-regulatory hormones involved in volume homeostasis and cardiovascular remodeling. They consist of atrial natriuretic peptide (ANP), brain natriuretic peptide (BNP), C-type natriuretic peptide (CNP), dendroaspis natriuretic peptides (DNP), and urodilatin. The natriuretic peptides promote natriuresis, diuresis, peripheral vasodilatation, and inhibition of the RAS. ANP and BNP are elevated in patients with left ventricular dysfunction; the serum levels correlate with the severity of heart failure and appear to have prognostic value.[49] ANP is stored in the right atrium and released by increases in atrial distending pressures. This peptide causes arterial dilatation, venodilatation, natriuresis, and water diuresis, counteracting the effects of vasoconstrictory agents. It also inhibits renin and aldosterone secretion and reduces sympathetic vasoconstriction.[50] BNP is stored in the ventricular myocardium and also causes vasodilatation and natriuresis. Congestive heart failure is associated with an increase in ANP, and the changes are related to the fall in the ejection fraction and the increase in cardiac filling pressures. Despite the natriuretic peptides' beneficial effects during CHF, their release is over-ridden by the release of agents that cause vasoconstriction and sodium and water retention.

Nitric oxide (NO) is the major physiologic regulator of basal blood vessel tone. NO is produced by virtually all cell types that make up the myocardium, and it regulates cardiac function through both vascular-dependent and vascular-independent effects. Vascular-dependent factors include regulation of coronary vessel tone, thrombogenicity, and proliferative and inflammatory properties, and the cellular cross-talk that supports angiogenesis. Vascular-independent factors constitute the direct effects of NO on several aspects of cardiomyocyte contractility, from the fine regulation of excitation-contraction coupling to· modulation of autonomic signaling and mitochondrial respiration.[51] NO also plays a very important role in the maintenance of cardiac architecture and the prevention of pathologic hypertrophy. A dissociation of stimulated and basal release of NO appears to exist in patients with heart failure. The stimulated, endothelial-dependent dilatation exerted by acetylcholine in peripheral resistance vessels is blunted during heart failure, which suggests a reduced release of NO on stimulation. This defective mechanism may be involved in the impaired vasodilator capacity in the peripheral circulation (e.g., during exercise).[52] In contrast, basal release of NO from the endothelium of resistance vessels appears to be preserved and may even be enhanced; also, it may play an important compensatory role in CHF during resting conditions by antagonizing neuroendocrine vasoconstrictive forces.[52]

Peripheral Compensation

Peripheral compensation occurs outside the heart and is directed at normalization of the arterial blood pressure. The main mechanisms involved in peripheral compensation are vasoconstriction in addition to sodium and water retention (see Table 197-1).

Blood Vessels and Vasoconstriction

The mechanism responsible for the increased tone of the vascular smooth muscle in CHF is multifactorial but basically results from neuroendocrine activation and the interplay of local mechanisms. Decreased blood flow to muscles causes overactivity of muscle metaboreceptors (afferents sensitive to skeletal muscle work) and peripheral chemoreceptors, which contributes to the autonomic imbalance. An increase in efferent sympathetic neuron discharge causes vasoconstriction.

Table • 197-1

Peripheral Compensatory Mechanisms in Heart Failure

RESPONSE	MECHANISM	POTENTIAL BENEFIT	POTENTIAL HARM	MANIFESTATIONS	CORRELATES
Sympathetic activation	Decrease in arterial pressure; RAS activation	Inotropic support, tachycardia, RAS activation, vasoconstriction, venoconstriction	Increased MVO_2 and afterload, sympathetic desensitization, excessive preload	Tachycardia, arrhythmias, pale mucous membranes	Norepinephrine concentration correlates with mortality. Beta-adrenoreceptor blockade may improve survival time.
Vasoconstriction	Sympathetic and RAS activation, increase in ADH, local blood vessel mechanisms	Maintenance of arterial pressure and perfusion of "essential" organs	Increased MVO_2 and afterload, stimulation of LVH, decreased cardiac output, redirection of blood flow	Pale mucous membranes	Modulation of excessive arterial tone with vasodilators is beneficial during heart failure.
Activation of renin-angiotensin system	Sympathetic activation, decreased renal perfusion	Vasoconstriction, stimulation of thirst, release of ADH and aldosterone, increased sympathetic tone	Increased MVO_2 and afterload, stimulation of LVH and blood vessel remodeling, decreased cardiac output and tissue perfusion, potentiation of mitral regurgitation	Pale mucous membranes	Angiotensin-converting enzyme (ACE) blockade increases survival time in patients with heart failure
Sodium and water retention	Poor renal perfusion, increases in thirst, ADH, and aldosterone	Increased preload, improved LV function	Congestion; excessive preload, which increases wall stress; hypokalemia (aldosterone)	Edema and cavitary effusions, arrhythmias (hypokalemia)	Use of diuretics in CHF decreases sodium and water retention. Aldosterone inhibition reduces risk of hypokalemia. Aldosterone receptor blockade may improve survival time.
Venoconstriction	Sympathetic activation	Increased preload and ventricular function	Congestion; excessive preload, which increases wall stress	Edema and cavitary effusions, venous distention	Venodilators and nitrates can be used in the treatment of heart failure.

ADH, Antidiuretic hormone (vasopressin); *CHF*, congestive heart failure; *LV*, left ventricle; *LVH*, left ventricular hypertrophy; MVO_2, myocardial oxygen consumption; *RAS*, renin-angiotensin system.

Dogs with paced-induced CHF show an increase in aortic stiffness (characteristic impedance) and a decrease in the compliance of large arteries before vasoconstriction of the small arterioles (increase in peripheral resistance).[53] Sympathetic activation occurs even in patients with asymptomatic left ventricular dysfunction. Further increases in plasma norepinephrine appear to occur in these patients when signs of heart failure develop. The RAS is activated by the decrease in cardiac output, further increasing vascular tone as a direct effect of angiotensin II and indirectly through the facilitative effect of angiotensin II in the alpha-adrenergic neurons. Unlike the sympathetic system, the RAS normalizes as compensation returns cardiac output to normal. Whether dogs with asymptomatic mitral regurgitation or left ventricular dysfunction show activation of the RAS is still the subject of debate.[54-57] ADH may be increased even in patients with asymptomatic left ventricular dysfunction, and this contributes to the increase in peripheral vascular resistance in patients with heart failure.

Local vasoregulatory mechanisms are very important in the modulation of vascular tone during heart failure. In normal dogs, shear stress caused by pulsatile flow prompts the release of NO and prostacyclin and inhibits ET-1, leading to vasodilatation. During CHF, decreased shear stress secondary to decreased peripheral blood flow and neuroendocrine activation reduces the release of NO and increases ET-1, leading to vasoconstriction.[58] Endothelin is a potent vasoconstrictor that is overexpressed during CHF.

Vasoconstriction is primarily mediated by increased sympathetic tone, RAS activation, and an increased ET-1 concentration.[46,59] ADH becomes an important vasoconstrictive agent only in hyponatremic patients.[59] These mechanisms also lead to venoconstriction, which increases venous pressure and venous return to the heart. Vasoconstriction helps maintain arterial pressure, but the increase in afterload reduces the stroke volume. Failing ventricles are afterload dependent, and the stroke volume falls with any increase in afterload (Figure 197-16). When cardiac output is low, the cardiovascular system redistributes the cardiac output, reducing blood perfusion to "less essential" organs. Increases in afterload also increase MVO_2 by increasing wall stress. In patients with severe mitral regurgitation, the increase in opposition to ventricular ejection increases regurgitation; in patients with a left-to-right shunt, it increases the shunting fraction.

Skeletal Muscles

Left ventricular dysfunction leads to a decrease in blood flow to the periphery, causing vasomotor changes and muscle alterations. Mechanisms unrelated to the decrease in blood flow (e.g., decrease in activity, increase in catabolic factors, insulin resistance) also may play a role in muscle changes during CHF. Patients with CHF have substantial skeletal muscle atrophy, and the degree of atrophy correlates with muscle strength and peak oxygen consumption.[60] Skeletal muscles are morphologically and metabolically abnormal in CHF. Muscle apoptosis

is observed in a high percentage of heart failure patients but not in normal subjects. The presence of collagen, indicative of fibrosis, is also detected in some heart failure patients and is more pronounced in those with cachexia.[61] Atrophy; changes in muscle fiber type and the mitochondrial ultrastructure; and a decrease in oxidative enzymatic capacity, leading to an increased reliance on anaerobic metabolism and lactate production, all have been demonstrated in patients with CHF. An increase in lactate during exercise stimulates peripheral metaboreceptors (or serves as a marker for the presence of other stimulants). Patients with CHF, therefore, have a higher metaboreceptor stimulation for a given degree of exercise than normal subjects.[28,60] Metaboreceptor stimulation increases sympathetic outflow, which adds to vasoconstriction and reduces blood flow to exercising muscles, because alpha adrenergic–mediated vasoconstriction is not impaired during CHF. In patients with mild heart failure, exercise limitation correlates well with central hemodynamic factors (e.g., cardiac output), whereas in advanced heart failure, peripheral hemodynamic factors become more important (e.g., local blood flow, vascular resistance, and venous tone).[62]

Kidneys and Sodium and Water Retention

Several mechanisms are responsible for sodium and water retention in CHF. Competing vasodilator/natriuretic and vasoconstrictive/sodium-retaining mechanisms operate. A decrease in cardiac output decreases renal blood flow and increases sympathetic drive, which causes renal vasoconstriction and further decreases in renal blood flow. Renin is released through activation of the juxtaglomerular apparatus by beta-adrenoreceptor stimulation and decreases in renal blood flow. The end result of renin release is an increase in angiotensin II and aldosterone. Angiotensin II stimulates thirst and release of ADH, leading to water retention. Aldosterone causes sodium and water retention and potassium wasting by the kidneys. Decreases in renal perfusion are countered by the release of prostaglandin E, which dilates the afferent renal arteriole and constricts the efferent renal arteriole, a response mediated by angiotensin II. These alterations combine to increase the glomerular filtration pressure and the filtration fraction (the ratio of glomerular filtration to renal plasma flow) and to maintain the glomerular filtration rate despite the reduction in renal blood flow. Sodium and water retention increases the circulating volume and preload, helping to maintain cardiac filling pressures and increasing cardiac output. Retention of sodium and water, however, leads to an excessive increase in the venous filling pressure, resulting in the development of edema and cavitary effusions. It also increases afterload and favors progression of left ventricular dysfunction.

Central Compensation (the Heart)

The heart participates actively in the compensation for the decrease in cardiac output. Sympathetic activation leads to an increase in the heart rate, inotropy, and lusitropy, all of which increase cardiac output. In addition, hypertrophy helps normalize cardiac output by increasing the stroke volume. Compensatory mechanisms that act on the heart are shown in Table 197-2.

Tachycardia

During heart failure, sympathetic tone increases (increasing the heart rate) and parasympathetic tone decreases, a combination that leads to tachycardia. It is usually believed that sinus rates above 160 beats/min imply not only parasympathetic withdrawal but also sympathetic activation. The end result is an increase in the heart rate and a decrease in heart rate variability. The increase in the heart rate helps normalize arterial pressure, but at a high price: an increase in MVO_2.

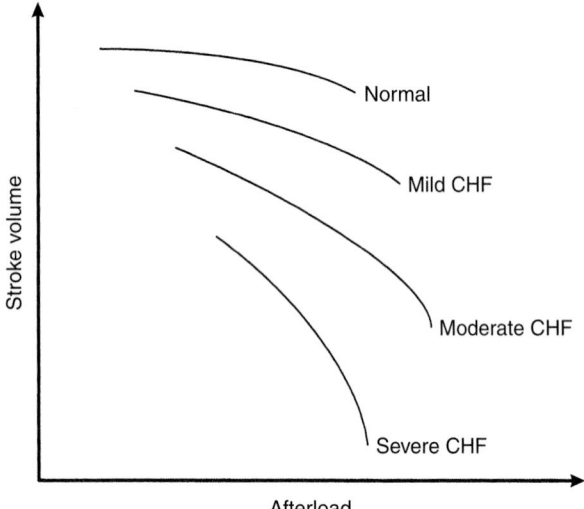

Figure 197-16 Effects of increasing afterload in left ventricular stroke volume in normal animals and in patients with congestive heart failure.

Table • 197-2

Central (Cardiac) Compensatory Mechanisms in Heart Failure

RESPONSE	MECHANISM	POTENTIAL BENEFIT	POTENTIAL HARM	MANIFESTATIONS	CORRELATES
Sympathetic desensitization	Downregulation of beta$_1$ adrenoreceptors, uncoupling of beta$_2$ adrenoreceptors, depletion of myocardial norepinephrine	Energy sparing	Decreased contractility	Low-output signs (e.g., depression, lethargy, hypotension)	Beta-adrenoreceptor blockade may reverse sympathetic desensitization.
Tachycardia	Sympathetic activation, parasympathetic withdrawal	Increased cardiac output	Increased MVO$_2$	Tachycardia, decreased heart rate variability	Decrease in heart rate variability correlates with mortality. Increase in heart rate correlates with sympathetic activation and severity of CHF.
Increased inotropy	Sympathetic activation	Increased stroke volume	Increased MVO$_2$	—	—
Increased relaxation	Sympathetic activation	Improved diastolic function (lusitropy)	Increased MVO$_2$	—	—
Appearance of slow myosin in the atria	Changes in isogene expression	Decreased cost to achieve normal tension, energy sparing, increased atrial kick	Atrial failure	—	Changes do not occur in the ventricles of dogs and cats.
Reduced myocardial ATPase activity	Unknown (altered isoenzymes?)	Facilitation of high-pressure, low-speed work; energy sparing	Slowed contraction rate, decreased contractility	Low-output signs	Myocardial ATPase activity is increased in high-output CHF (e.g., thyrotoxicosis).
Pressure overload (concentric hypertrophy)	Increased afterload, RAS activation, increased levels of TNF-alpha and other cytokines	Unloading of individual muscle fibers, decreased wall stress and MVO$_2$	Imbalance in energy demand and supply, focal necrosis, fibrosis, increased collagen formation, diastolic dysfunction	Cardiomegaly, increased diastolic dysfunction and venous congestion	Pressure overload induces cardiomyopathy of overload. Growth-inhibitory drugs (e.g., ACE inhibitors, nitrates) may delay development of cardiomyopathy of overload.
Volume overload (eccentric hypertrophy)	Fiber slippage, increased tension	Increased compliance(?); increased stroke volume with same ejection fraction (dilatation)	Increased wall stress and MVO$_2$; pressure hypertrophy	Cardiomegaly	Increased wall stress leads to pressure hypertrophy.

ACE, Angiotensin-converting enzyme; *ATPase,* adenosine triphosphatase; *CHF,* congestive heart failure; *MVO$_2$,* myocardial oxygen consumption; *TNF-alpha,* tumor necrosis factor alpha.

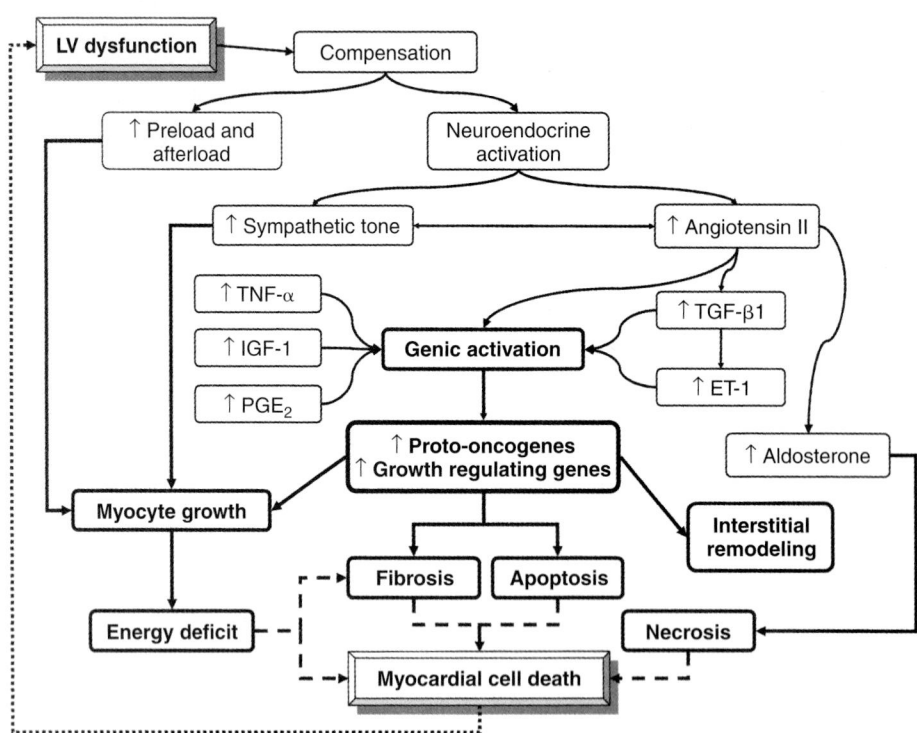

Figure 197-17 Mechanisms that lead to myocardial hypertrophy and remodeling. Increases in the load and activation of proto-oncogenes and growth-regulating genes lead to hypertrophy (myocyte growth) and remodeling. Short-term sympathetic effects are beneficial, but chronic activation favors progression of left ventricular dysfunction. Hypertrophy is beneficial because it decreases left ventricular wall stress and increases cardiac output. Unfortunately, chronic myocardial hypertrophy and remodeling are associated with myocardial cell death. Dashed lines indicate long-term effects. *TNF-alpha*, Tumor necrosis factor alpha; *IGF-1*, insulin-like growth factor-1; *PGE$_2$*, prostaglandin E$_2$; *TGF-beta$_1$*, transforming growth factor beta$_1$; *ET-1*, endothelin-1.

A decrease in heart rate variability is a negative prognostic factor for overall mortality in human patients with myocardial infarct. In dogs with chronic mitral valve disease, a decrease in heart rate variability correlates with the severity of congestive heart failure.[34] Patients with decreased heart rate variability are also less likely to respond to vasodilator infusion. The increase in the heart rate in patients with heart failure parallels sympathetic activation, which in turn correlates with the severity of the heart failure.

Increased Inotropy and Lusitropy

Beta-adrenergic stimulation caused by increased sympathetic tone during heart failure increases calcium entry in the atrial and ventricular cells, calcium release from the sarcoplasmic reticulum, and the interaction between contractile proteins. All these actions increase contractility. Beta-adrenergic stimulation also increases lusitropy by increasing calcium efflux from the cell and calcium uptake by the sarcoplasmic reticulum.[3] The increase in calcium entry is largely responsible for the positive inotropic effect; the facilitated dissociation from troponin and increased calcium uptake by the sarcoplasmic reticulum are the key factors in causing a positive lusitropic effect.[3] Beta-adrenergic stimulation increases cardiac output, but also increases MVO$_2$ and contributes to myocardial remodeling.

Myocardial Growth

Cardiac mass is increased in patients with heart failure, apparently as a result of a combination of reactive fibrosis and myocyte hypertrophy, along with alterations in the cytoskeletal structure in the myocyte. An increase in afterload and neuroendocrine activation lead to left ventricular hypertrophy. Hypertrophy reduces the load in individual cells and increases cardiac output. Hypertrophy causes growth of myocyte and nonmyocyte cells in the extracellular matrix of the myocardium. The growth of myocytes and nonmyocyte cells occurs independent of each other. Chronic anemia and thyrotoxicoses cause myocyte growth without the involvement of fibroblasts, whereas hypertrophy secondary to pressure overload is accompanied by reactive fibrosis that is not secondary to myocyte necrosis. Increases in preload, afterload, sympathetic activation, and growth hormone induce myocardial growth, whereas activation of the RAS, prostaglandin E$_2$, transforming growth factor-beta$_1$ (TGF-beta$_1$), and insulin-like growth factor-1 (IGF-1) induce remodeling of the cardiac interstitium (Figure 197-17).[63] All these substances induce expression of proto-oncogenes and growth-regulating genes that play an important role in the mediation of hypertrophy. Structural remodeling of myocardial collagen matrix contributes to the progression of heart failure.

Hypertrophy in patients with CHF results in a ventricle that is not normal. Morphologic, biochemical, and genetic changes cause ventricular remodeling, leading to progression of the left ventricular dysfunction. The appearance of a "slow" myosin, a more efficient myosin that spares energy in the heart, has been detected in the atria[64] but not the ventricles[65] of dogs with CHF. Pressure-induced hypertrophy unloads the individual myocardial cells and decreases wall stress and MVO$_2$. However, hypertrophied ventricles have a capillary deficit and a decreased number of mitochondria, leading to a state of energy starvation.[66] The chronic energy starvation leads to necrosis, fibrosis, an increase in the collagen concentration, and diastolic dysfunction. Volume-induced hypertrophy decreases wall stress and MVO$_2$ and helps maintain stroke volume, probably by increasing compliance. Fiber slippage, however, causes further dilatation of the heart, again increasing wall stress and MVO$_2$ and favoring progression of the left ventricular dysfunction.

WHAT IS THE ROLE OF INFLAMMATION IN HEART FAILURE?

Cytokines are highly potent, endogenous peptides with autocrine and paracrine actions; they are produced by a variety of cell types. Unlike hormones, cytokines are not stored but are secreted in response to specific stimuli. TNF-alpha, interleukin-1-alpha (IL-1α), interleukin-1-beta (IL-1β), and interleukin-6 (IL-6) are classified as proinflammatory cytokines.[2] These cytokines initiate both primary host responses and tissue repair. Interleukin-2 (IL-2) is a potent immunostimulatory polypeptide that amplifies the immune response to antigens. Evidence suggests that proinflammatory cytokines are capable of modulating cardiovascular function through a variety of mechanisms, such as promotion of left ventricular remodeling, induction of contractile dysfunction, and uncoupling of myocardial beta-adrenergic receptors (Table 197-3).[67] Several studies have shown that CHF is associated with increased circulating levels of proinflammatory cytokines. Short-term expression of cytokines in the heart may be an adaptive response to different forms of stress, whereas long-term expression may be maladaptive by producing cardiac decompensation. The cytokine hypothesis for heart failure does not imply that cytokines cause heart failure per se. However, they are potentially involved in the genesis of this pathology, and overexpression of cytokines contributes to the progression of heart failure once ventricular dysfunction ensues.[68] Chronic sympathetic activation[69] and increases in angiotensin II[70,71] and aldosterone[72] play a role in the overexpression of cytokines during CHF. Sustained hemodynamic overloading provokes a transient increase in proinflammatory cytokine and cytokine-receptor gene expression.[73]

The main stimulus for cytokine activation in CHF is not known.[74] The heart is primarily involved and could be the main source of proinflammatory cytokines, because the failing myocardium is capable of producing TNF-alpha.[75] It has also been demonstrated that pressure overload stimulates the synthesis of TNF-alpha messenger ribonucleic acid (mRNA). Myocardial stretch induces mRNA production by myocytes.[76] Another potential stimulus for an increase in the production of TNF-alpha by the failing heart is extramyocardial cytokine release caused by tissue hypoxia.[77] Tissue hypoxia and the production of free radicals are potent stimuli for the generation of cytokine release via nuclear factor-kappa-B (NF-kappa-B)–dependent pathways.[78] Cytokines are expressed in the myocardium in end-stage heart failure to a much greater degree than in patients with recent onset of symptoms. Plasma levels of TNF-alpha correlate with mRNA expression in the myocardium and thus may serve as an appropriate marker of myocardial cytokine activation. Whether the production of cytokines in the failing human heart precedes the elevation of cytokines in the plasma remains undefined.[79]

The bowel could also be a source of proinflammatory cytokines during CHF. The intestinal wall edema and ischemia that occur during CHF favor bacterial translocation and may cause the release of endotoxins, with subsequent immune activation.[80] It has been shown that during acute, edematous exacerbation of CHF, endotoxin and cytokine concentrations increase but can be normalized by diuretic therapy.[81]

Tumor Necrosis Factor Alpha

TNF-alpha is a proinflammatory cytokine that exerts negative inotropic effects *in vivo* and *in vitro*. Acute negative inotrope results from disruption of calcium transients, whereas chronic effects are associated with induction of inducible NO synthase (iNOS) and are due to NO-induced myofilament desensitization to calcium.[82] TNF-alpha also can produce left ventricular remodeling, hypertrophy and apoptosis, pulmonary edema, and cardiomyopathy.[83] It stimulates production of other endogenous pyrogens, such as IL-1β. The main known stimuli that prompt adult mammalian myocardial cells to produce TNF are endotoxins, hypoxia, and increased mechanical stress.[76,84] NF-kappa-B can also participate in the production of TNF-alpha. Oxidative stress activates NF-kappa-B, which binds to a TNF promoter, increasing TNF-alpha transcription.[85] Mild acute increases in TNF-alpha are an adaptive response to stress; they protect the heart during ischemia and favor remodeling during infarcts and adaptive growth during hemodynamic overload. Severe acute increases lead to myocarditis as a result of an exacerbated inflammatory response, and chronic increases are maladaptive, favoring cardiac decompensation and apoptosis.[86]

Table • 197-3

Effects of Chronic Proinflammatory Cytokine Activation in Heart Failure

EFFECT	MECHANISM	CLINICAL CORRELATE
Heart		
Myocyte hypertrophy	Generation of reactive oxygen intermediates in cardiac myocytes; activation of fetal gene programs	Cardiac hypertrophy
Left ventricular remodeling	Stimulation of production of extracellular matrix proteins and increased turnover of matrix	Cardiomyopathy of overload
Cardiomyocyte loss	Necrosis, apoptosis	Progression of heart failure
Depression of myocardial function	Nitric oxide dependent; sphingomyelinase pathway; uncoupling of beta adrenoreceptors; abnormal mitochondria energetics	Decreased contractility
Exacerbated inflammatory response	Cytokine cascade	Myocarditis
Skeletal Muscle		
Myopathy	Free radical and nitric oxide overproduction; endothelial dysfunction	Reduced blood flow in muscles, exercise intolerance
Decreased skeletal mass	Apoptosis	Cardiac cachexia
Other Effects		
Anorexia		Cardiac cachexia
Pulmonary edema		Dyspnea

Cats with naturally occurring CHF have increased concentrations of TNF-alpha.[87] Increases in the TNF-alpha concentration have been independently associated with a poorer prognosis for CHF. TNF-alpha is produced in the heart by cardiac myocytes and resident macrophages under conditions of cardiac stress. Normal hearts do not produce TNF-alpha, but failing human hearts make abundant quantities.[83] The source of cardiac TNF-alpha appears to be at least partly attributable to production by the cardiac myocyte.[75] TNF-alpha plays an important role in the development of heart failure. Administration of TNF-alpha to experimental animals and transgenic overexpression of TNF-alpha lead to CHF. Mice that overexpress TNF-alpha recapitulate heart failure and a dilated cardiomyopathy state in other species shows (1) four-chamber dilatation, (2) myocyte hypertrophy, (3) interstitial infiltrates, (4) extracellular matrix remodeling with fibrosis, (5) diminished beta-adrenergic responsiveness, and (6) premature death.[86] Attenuation of the biologic activity of TNF-alpha abrogates the development of CHF in experimental model systems. Unfortunately, anti-TNF strategies to date have not demonstrated salutary benefits in large, multicenter, randomized and placebo-controlled clinical trials in patients with symptomatic heart failure.[88]

Interleukins

Interleukin-1 (IL-1) mediates immune response and the production of inflammatory responses through an increase in prostaglandins, and it may be a basal part of the overactivated cytokine cascade during CHF.[2] IL-1 appears capable of modulating myocardial function. It exerts a potent antiproliferative effect on cardiac fibroblasts but induces cardiac myocyte hypertrophy. IL-1β is increased during CHF; it decreases myocardial contractility by stimulating iNOS, and it may uncouple beta adrenoreceptors from adenylate-cyclase, one of the mechanisms of heart failure progression.[89] The negative inotropic effect of IL-1 appears to be mediated, at least partly, by production of NO or by the activation and release of interleukin-18, a member of the IL-1 family.[88] IL-1 induces synthesis by T lymphocytes of interleukin-2 (IL-2), an endogenous T-cell mitogen that enhances T-cell proliferation. IL-2 thus amplifies the immune response and stimulates the production of interferon-gamma and the release of other inflammatory factors (e.g., TNF-alpha). IL-2 levels are increased in human patients with dilated cardiomyopathy and in their relatives, with left ventricular enlargement usually being higher in patients with CHF.[90] Interleukin-6 (IL-6) is a multifunctional cytokine that mediates both immune and inflammatory responses. It is also a promoter of cardiomyocyte hypertrophy and a negative inotrope that is elevated in patients with heart failure, especially those with cardiac cachexia or severe CHF.[91] In human patients with CHF, IL-6 is a predictor of mortality independent of etiology, the sodium concentration, the severity of heart failure, and the ejection fraction.[92]

Nuclear Factor—Kappa-B

During CHF, oxidative stress, increased expression of TNF-alpha, and an increase in the angiotensin II concentration serve to activate NF-kappa-B. NF-kappa-B is a redox-sensitive transcription factor that is critical to initiation of the co-ordinated expression of classic components of the myocardial inflammatory response, including increased expression of proinflammatory cytokines (e.g., TNF-alpha, IL-6), NO, chemokines, and adhesion molecules.[84,88] NF-kappa-B is an important player in inflammation during heart failure. Activation of NF-kappa-B initiates gene transcription of several substances that can lead to cardiovascular injury. NF-kappa-B signaling also plays an important role in myocardial growth, and its inhibition attenuates cardiomyocyte hypertrophy.[93,94] Myocardial cells from patients with heart failure exhibit activation of NF-kappa-B and increased expression of genes it regulates (e.g., TNF-alpha, iNOS). Elevation of NF-kappa-B seems to occur independent of the etiology of heart failure but appears to be related to the severity of CHF. NF-kappa-B can activate cell death pathways, and TNF-alpha–induced apoptosis is associated with an increase in NF-kappa-B. However, blocking of NF-kappa-B in this setting paradoxically exacerbates cell death.[85] It is not known if NF-kappa-B activates antiapoptotic factors. The paradoxical effect of activating detrimental molecules while protecting cells may be related to the inflammatory program mediated by NF-kappa-B; it generates toxic molecules that can kill invading micro-organisms without damaging host cells.[85]

Reactive Oxygen Species

Increases in angiotensin II induce production of reactive oxygen species. An important effect of angiotensin II is activation of the NAD(P)H oxidase, a major source of reactive oxygen species (ROS) production by vascular cells. Reactive oxygen species are the end result of univalent reductions in oxygen that produce superoxide anion, hydrogen peroxide, and water.[95] ROS influence both normal and abnormal cellular processes, including cellular growth, hypertrophy, remodeling, lipid oxidation, modulation of vascular tone, and inflammation. The increase in cellular ROS contributes to the pathogenesis of vascular disease by altering endothelial cell function; enhancing smooth muscle cell growth and proliferation; stimulating inflammatory proteins, including macrophage chemoattractant agents, growth factors and cytokines; and modulating matrix remodelling.[96] These ROS can be released from the cardiac myocyte mitochondria, and chronic release of ROS recently was linked to the development of left ventricular hypertrophy and progression of heart failure.[97] The release of ROS is required for the normal physiologic activity of cardiac cells, but abnormal activation of nonphagocytic NAD(P)H oxidase in response to neurohormones and cytokines (angiotensin II, norepinephrine, TNF-alpha) has been shown to contribute to cardiac myocyte hypertrophy. The fibrosis, collagen deposition, and metalloproteinase activation involved in the remodeling of a failing myocardium depend on ROS released during the phenotypic transformation of fibroblasts to myofibroblasts that is associated with progression of end-stage heart failure.[97] Studies of genetically altered mice have shown that activation of the NAD(P)H oxidase by angiotensin II contributes to hypertension and left ventricular hypertrophy.[98,99]

The *cytokine hypothesis*[2,100] for heart failure suggests that heart failure progresses because cytokine cascades that are activated after myocardial injury exert deleterious effects on the heart and circulation. This hypothesis does not imply that cytokines cause CHF, but rather that overexpression of cytokines contributes to the progression of heart failure once left ventricular dysfunction ensues.[101] TNF-alpha and IL-6 become activated after left ventricular injury or myocardial stretch. These stress-activated cytokines can exert autocrine and paracrine effects in the myocardium by binding to specific cytokine receptors. If cytokine expression is excessive, these molecules may produce left ventricular dysfunction and left ventricular dilatation. It is further postulated that cytokines, when overproduced, may spill over into the circulation, leading to secondary activation of the immune system, which is then capable of amplifying the cytokine signal in the periphery.[101] There is an easily recognizable overlap between the neurohormonal and cytokine hypothesis. However, there are likely to be important differences in the mechanisms that initiate overexpression of these molecules, as well as differences in the biologic effects that these molecules exert.

WHAT ARE THE CLINICAL MANIFESTATIONS OF HEART FAILURE?

Clinical signs in heart failure may result from accumulation of fluids, low cardiac output, or changes in the skeletal muscles (Box 197-5). Dogs with CHF are usually brought to the veterinarian because of a cough, dyspnea, exercise intolerance, abdominal enlargement, or syncope. Cats, on the other hand, are usually presented because they cannot breathe (pleural effusion or pulmonary edema) or cannot walk (aortic thromboembolism) properly.

Sodium and water retention increase the circulating volume and venous pressure, an effect that is potentiated by venous constriction. Venous hypertension and microcirculatory congestion lead to transudation of fluids in body cavities (effusion) or the interstitium (edema). These signs develop preferentially in the capillary beds drained by the failing ventricle.

Box • 197-5

Clinical Signs in Congestive Heart Failure

Low-Output Signs
  Complaints → Exercise intolerance, syncope
  Clinical signs → Weak arterial pulses, tachycardia, arrhythmias, cool extremities

Signs Related to Poor Skeletal Muscle Function
  Complaints → Loss of weight, exercise intolerance, dyspnea*
  Clinical signs → Decreased muscle bulk

Signs Related to Fluid Retention
Left side (pulmonary edema)
  Complaints → Dyspnea, orthopnea, exercise intolerance, cough†
  Clinical signs → Pulmonary crackles, tachypnea, gallop rhythm, functional mitral regurgitation, cyanosis caused by ventilation-perfusion inequality

Right side (systemic venous congestion)
  Complaints → Abdominal enlargement (ascites), subcutaneous edema
  Clinical signs → Jugular distention and pulsation, ascites, hepatomegaly, splenomegaly, hepatojugular reflux, gallop rhythm

Bilateral
  Complaints → Left side plus right side complaints, dyspnea caused by pleural effusion
  Clinical signs → Left side plus right side clinical signs, muffled heart and lung sounds with fluid line in the chest (pleural effusion)

Other Signs
  Arrhythmias
  Weight loss
  Cough

---

*Activation of metaboreceptors and peripheral chemoreceptors may contribute to dyspnea in patients without congestion.
†Cough may also occur in dogs without congestive heart failure because of left main stem bronchus compression.

Thus elevated pulmonary venous and capillary hydrostatic pressures in small animals lead to pulmonary edema and can be manifested as dyspnea, cough, pulmonary crackles, and exercise intolerance. Systemic venous hypertension causes jugular distention, hepatic congestion, ascites, and subcutaneous edema. In dogs, ascites always precedes subcutaneous edema in patients with right-sided CHF. Cats rarely develop ascites secondary to right-sided CHF. Biventricular failure shows a combination of left- and right-side signs and is often associated with accumulation of pleural fluid. Although cats may occasionally develop pleural effusion during experimentally induced right-sided CHF,[102] almost all cats with pleural effusion from CHF have bilateral disease or a disease of the left side, with pulmonary hypertension or atrial fibrillation. Pleural effusion in small animals usually accompanies biventricular failure, not isolated right-sided failure.[103] Dogs develop pleural effusion only during experimentally induced right-sided CHF, when large volumes of crystalloid are infused, leading to severe hypoproteinemia.[104] In this setting, pleural effusion correlates better with the pulmonary capillary wedge pressure than with the right atrial pressure, which suggests that right-sided CHF was not the main cause of the development of pleural effusion.

A decrease in cardiac output may lead to exercise intolerance, tiring, and fatigue. Because exercise intolerance can occur only in animals that exercise, it is not a prominent complaint of cat owners or of the owners of dogs that spend most of their life on the lap. Syncope may be due to low cardiac output of the failing heart or to concurrent arrhythmia. Low-output signs are nonspecific but, when due to CHF, tend to worsen with exercise.

Dyspnea is usually caused by pulmonary edema or pleural effusion, but it may also occur before the patient develops severe fluid retention. Dyspnea and exercise intolerance may be related to skeletal muscle changes that occur during CHF. Abnormal muscle function and increased fatigability during CHF have been linked to the decrease in muscle bulk, an increased reliance on anaerobic metabolism, decreased muscle blood flow, and metaboreceptor activation.[28] Normal animals become dyspneic during exercise in a manner similar to that which occurs in CHF. The main difference among a normal, fit animal, an untrained animal, and a patient with CHF is the amount of exercise that leads to dyspnea and fatigue. Muscle fatigue is an important determinant of exercise intolerance and dyspnea (fatigue of respiratory muscle) during CHF. In human beings, the same patient may complain of fatigue or dyspnea, depending on the type of exercise performed. It has been proposed that the sensation of fatigue during CHF is generated as a central mechanism to protect against hypoxic damage to essential organs. Ergoreceptors may be responsible for mediating both dyspnea and sensation of fatigue.[105] The muscle hypothesis for CHF states that abnormalities in skeletal muscle blood flow, bulk, and function are major determinants of clinical signs, leading to fatigue and increased ventilatory stimulus. Activation of ergoreceptors leads to persistent sympathetic activation, increasing afterload and reducing blood flow. As cardiac function deteriorates, a catabolic state exacerbates muscle wasting (cardiac cachexia), and patient inactivity leads to further deterioration of muscle function. Such a progression leads to a vicious cycle, in which muscle abnormalities cause clinical signs and favor progression of left ventricular dysfunction, worsening muscle abnormalities and increasing clinical signs.[28]

Cardiac cachexia is a common finding in CHF. It is usually more prominent in right-sided CHF and in giant breeds with dilated cardiomyopathy. In one study, more than half of the dogs with CHF secondary to dilated cardiomyopathy were cachectic.[106] It is very uncommon for an animal with overt

CHF to be obese. Obesity is usually associated with respiratory problems. When CHF develops rapidly (e.g., with rupture of a chorda tendineae or the development of atrial fibrillation, or in a few Dobermans with dilated cardiomyopathy), time may not be sufficient for cardiac cachexia to develop, and the animal may show a reasonably normal body condition. The cachectic state is a strong independent risk factor for mortality in patients with CHF.[107] Cachexia is more closely associated with hormonal changes in CHF than are conventional hemodynamic measures of the severity of CHF.[108] Neuroendocrine activation leads to increases in TNF-alpha, IL-1β, norepinephrine, and cortisol and to insulin resistance. All these factors appear to play a major role in the development of cardiac cachexia. An increase in TNF-alpha and its soluble receptors is seen in chronic heart failure. This increase is associated with a rise in the cortisol/dehydroepiandrosterone (catabolic/anabolic) ratio, suggesting that an increase in TNF-alpha is at least partly responsible for the cachexia.[109] In right-sided heart failure, interference with normal absorption of nutrients in the gastrointestinal tract, caused by intestinal and hepatic congestion, may also contribute to cachexia.

Cough is a common sign of heart disease in dogs but not in cats. Dogs with heart disease may cough because of left-sided CHF, compression of the left main stem bronchus without CHF, or a concurrent respiratory disease (e.g., collapsing trachea, chronic bronchitis). Dogs that cough from pulmonary edema are frequently thin, show severe weight loss, and have a more subtle cough that tends to worsen at night and may be accompanied by a pink nasal discharge or sputum. Dogs that cough because of left main stem bronchus compression or respiratory disease are more likely to be obese or of normal weight and tend to have dry, hacking coughs that are usually worse during the day. Dogs with left-sided CHF usually have fast heart rates caused by sympathetic activation, whereas dogs with left main stem bronchus compression or respiratory disease have normal heart rates with pronounced sinus arrhythmia due to high vagal tone.

Arrhythmias in patients with heart failure may be caused by the underlying disease or by the CHF itself. In addition, chronic, persistent tachycardia may cause left ventricular dysfunction and CHF. The enlargement, fibrosis, and hypertrophy that occur during left ventricular dysfunction lead to conduction abnormalities that predispose the animal to arrhythmias. A rise in cytosolic calcium, caused by sympathetic activation, may also cause arrhythmias. The presence of arrhythmias is an important negative prognostic factor in patients with CHF.

Clinical signs suggestive of heart disease (although not necessarily CHF) include a diastolic, continuous, or loud systolic murmur; arrhythmias with pulse deficit and gallop rhythms; and ascites with jugular distention and hepatojugular reflux. An aortic thromboembolism (saddle thrombus) in cats also suggests the presence of heart disease. Right-sided CHF is a clinical diagnosis in dogs. It is likely to be present in patients with ascites and jugular vein distention, hepatomegaly, and abnormal cardiac auscultation. Diagnosis of left-sided heart failure, however, requires a chest radiograph. Auscultative pulmonary abnormalities in pulmonary edema are neither sensitive nor specific. A patient with dyspnea, cough, or pulmonary crackles, even with abnormal heart ausculation, may have respiratory signs caused by a primary respiratory disease. In cats, chest radiographs are very useful for diagnosing both right- and left-sided CHF.

WHY DOES A PATIENT DEVELOP CLINICAL SIGNS OF CONGESTIVE HEART FAILURE?

CHF is a progressive disease, and systolic or diastolic function is eventually compromised to a degree that clinical signs are inevitable. One should not conclude, however, that recent development or worsening of clinical signs is due to disease progression. In many patients a precipitating factor for the CHF can be found, and it may not necessarily be related to the heart itself. Lack of client compliance is a common cause of treatment failure. Clients should be carefully questioned about medications used. Treatment of heart failure usually requires multiple drugs, and confusion about the proper use of the medications is not uncommon. The doses given, the frequency and route of administration, and use of the proper formulation should be verified. Furthermore, the possibility that a person other than the owner (e.g., a pet sitter) may have been temporarily responsible for the dog or cat should be investigated. Inappropriate reduction of therapy is the most common reason for sudden worsening of the clinical condition in human patients with CHF. In small animal practice, inappropriate therapy is more likely when a person who is not completely familiar with the patient's clinical condition is caring for the dog or cat or when the patient goes for a long period without clinical signs and is assumed to be "cured."

The development of complications is an important precipitating factor for CHF in small animal medicine. Extracardiac complications that impose an extra load on the cardiovascular system may induce CHF in patients with heart disease. Conditions that lead to a hyperdynamic circulation (e.g., anemia, hyperthyroidism, infection, fever) increase MVO_2 and sympathetic tone. Systemic arterial hypertension causes an increase in afterload, which has a devastating effect on a failing myocardium. Systemic hypertension also increases the regurgitant fraction in patients with aortic and mitral regurgitation. In addition, physical, environmental, and emotional stress may lead to CHF, and a second, unrelated disease may affect cardiac function indirectly. Renal failure can potentially cause hypertension and may interfere with sodium excretion, exacerbating the CHF.

A common cause of sudden decompensation of CHF is a cardiac complication. The two most common cardiac complications leading to CHF are the development of mitral regurgitation and arrhythmias. Mitral regurgitation may develop suddenly as a result of dilatation of the annulus valvulus in patients with dilated cardiomyopathy or as a result of the Venturi effect in cats with hypertrophic cardiomyopathy. However, the most devastating cause of acute worsening of mitral regurgitation that leads to CHF is the rupture of chordae tendineae, which occurs in dogs with mitral endocardiosis. The sudden appearance of atrial fibrillation is a common cause of the precipitation of CHF in dogs with dilated cardiomyopathy or mitral endocardiosis. Progression of the cardiac disease, usually with development of myocardial failure, eventually leads to the appearance of signs of CHF in patients with heart disease.

HOW CAN WE CLINICALLY EVALUATE HEART FUNCTION?

Is Heart Failure Present?

Heart disease is not synonymous with heart failure. A patient may be presented with a heart murmur or gallop and may even have myocardial failure, yet may not necessarily be in CHF. To facilitate characterization of the severity of heart failure, functional classifications based on clinical signs at rest are used (Box 197-6). The presence of heart failure may be suspected during the physical examination. Right-sided CHF is a clinical diagnosis based on jugular distention and pulsation, the presence of ascites (dogs) and pleural effusion (cats, usually indicating bilateral failure), and peripheral edema. The diagnosis is confirmed by showing elevation of the central venous pressure or, more loosely, by observing a large right

Box • 197-6

Functional Classification of Heart Failure

Modified from the New York Heart Association Classification*

I. Normal activity does not produce undue fatigue, dyspnea, or coughing.

II. The dog or cat is comfortable at rest, but ordinary physical activity causes fatigue, dyspnea, or coughing.

III. The dog or cat is comfortable at rest, but minimal exercise may produce fatigue, dyspnea, or coughing. Signs may also develop while the patient is in a recumbent position (orthopnea).

IV. Congestive heart failure, dyspnea, and coughing are present even when the dog or cat is at rest. Signs are exaggerated by any physical activity.

International Small Animal Cardiac Health Council†

I. Asymptomatic patient

   Ia. Signs of heart disease but no cardiomegaly

   Ib. Signs of heart disease and evidence of compensation (cardiomegaly)

II. Mild to moderate heart failure

   Clinical signs of heart failure are evident at rest or with mild exercise and adversely affect the quality of life.

III. Advanced heart failure

   Clinical signs of congestive heart failure are immediately obvious.

   IIIa. Home care is possible.

   IIIb. Hospitalization is recommended (cardiogenic shock, life-threatening edema, large pleural effusion, refractory ascites).

*Adapted from Ettinger SJ, Suter PF: The recognition of cardiac disease and congestive heart failure. *In* Ettinger SJ, Suter PF (eds): *Canine cardiology.* Philadelphia, WB Saunders, 1970, p 215.
†Adapted from International Small Animal Cardiac Health Council: Recommendations for the diagnosis of heart disease and the treatment of heart failure in small animals. *In* Miller MS, Tilley LP (eds): *Manual of canine and feline cardiology,* Philadelphia, WB Saunders, 1995, p 473.

heart on radiographs or echocardiography. Left-sided heart failure is a radiographic diagnosis that can be suspected in patients with dyspnea and abnormal respiratory sounds. It can be confirmed by showing elevation of the pulmonary capillary wedge pressure, but identification of pulmonary edema in association with left-heart enlargement would suffice from a clinical standpoint.

Some clinical findings may be helpful, providing indications of cardiovascular function. Gallop rhythms suggest the presence of ventricular dysfunction. The fourth heart sound (S_4 gallop) occurs during late diastole and represents atrial contraction. An S_4 gallop is associated with elevated ventricular end-diastolic pressure related to a decrease in ventricular compliance. An early diastolic filling sound (S_3 gallop) may occur during ventricular dysfunction of any cause and is a very sensitive indicator of ventricular dysfunction. Increased loudness and splitting of the second heart sound suggest the presence of pulmonary hypertension. A distended and sometimes pulsating jugular vein suggests that the right atrial pressure is elevated and the patient is in right-sided heart failure.

What Tests Should Be Performed?

Laboratory tests are used to confirm the presence and cause of the heart disease, the presence and severity of the CHF and ventricular dysfunction, and the presence of complications. Some tests are useful for diagnosing specific conditions and may offer no information about cardiovascular function, whereas others may assess only function or may offer a combination of functional and diagnostic information. In addition to the physical examination, confirmation of the exact cause of CHF usually requires a combination of radiographic, electrocardiographic, echocardiographic, and laboratory assessment techniques. Echocardiography is very helpful in determining the disease leading to the CHF.

Electrocardiography can be used to evaluate the heart rhythm, but it provides only indirect information about cardiovascular function. Arrhythmias may be due to heart disease, but they also can arise from noncardiac causes. The electrocardiogram provides no definitive criteria for diagnosing heart failure. However, it may contribute to the diagnosis (e.g., showing a decrease in QRS voltage and electrical alternans with pericardial effusion). One should bear in mind that a normal electrocardiogram does not rule out CHF or heart disease.

Chest radiographs are very important for patients suspected of having heart disease. Changes in cardiac size and shape may show the compensation effects in the heart (cardiomegaly) and can be very helpful in determining the cause of CHF in dogs. Unfortunately, in cats, chest radiographs do not discriminate among the different myocardial diseases that may lead to heart failure, and echocardiography is usually necessary. Chest radiographs are of paramount importance in the detection of left-sided CHF (pulmonary venous congestion, pulmonary interstitial or alveolar edema). They are also useful for visualization of pleural effusion in patients with CHF.

Echocardiographic examination is extremely helpful for determining the cause of CHF. There are no echocardiographic criteria for diagnosing CHF, but it is uncommon to see left-sided CHF without echocardiographic abnormalities, such as left atrial enlargement; and right atrial enlargement or pericardial effusion, in right-sided CHF.

Echocardiography, measurement of the arterial blood pressure, and cardiac catheterization may all provide useful information about cardiovascular function. Cardiac catheterization has been used less and less, because most of the information provided by cardiac catheterization can now be obtained noninvasively and without the need to anesthetize the patient. Pressures behind the pumping chambers are useful for estimating ventricular filling pressures. The central venous pressure can be measured with a water- or saline-filled catheter placed in the cranial vena cava or right atrium. The central venous pressure provides an estimation of the right ventricular end-diastolic pressure. The pulmonary capillary wedge pressure is obtained by placing a balloon-tipped (Swan-Ganz) catheter in the pulmonary artery, inflating the balloon to wedge the catheter tip, and then recording the pressure. The pulmonary capillary wedge pressure provides an estimate of the left ventricular end-diastolic pressure. Clinically speaking, congestive heart failure is evidenced by increased ventricular filling (end-diastolic) pressures.[110]

The arterial blood pressure should be measured in all patients with heart disease or CHF. Arterial hypertension can lead to left ventricular hypertrophy and dysfunction and eventually to CHF. CHF secondary to systemic hypertension appears not to be as common in dogs and cats as it is human beings. However, hypertension is a potentially controllable reason for heart disease. In addition, systemic hypertension in a patient with any left ventricular dysfunction increases left ventricular afterload and decreases cardiac output. It also favors progression of left ventricular dysfunction. Hypertension increases valvular regurgitation in patients with mitral or aortic insufficiency and the shunt fraction in dogs and cats with left-to-right shunts.

Measurement of biochemical markers that are increased during heart disease or CHF can provide information about the disease and in some cases may have prognostic value. The most commonly used markers in small animals are cardiac troponin I, cardiac troponin T, ANP, and BNP. Cardiac troponins are leakage markers that are released into the circulation when cardiac cell membrane integrity has been compromised; they therefore indicate myocardial damage. Any myocardial injury, including CHF, can increase cardiac troponins; a correlation exists between the magnitude of myocardial damage and the degree of elevation of cardiac troponins only in acute states.[111] ANP and BNP are functional markers that increase with an increase in circulating volume (e.g., CHF) or during left ventricular hypertrophy. ANP and BNP tend to increase regardless of the underlying heart disease, but their levels correlate well with the degree of left ventricular dysfunction. They can potentially be used to assess cardiac function, to monitor therapy, and to help determine the prognosis.[49,112] Unfortunately, few clinical studies have highlighted the indications, usefulness, and limitations of different biochemical markers in heart disease in dogs and cats, which limits the use of these markers. As more information becomes available, clinical use of biochemical markers likely will increase.

Several indices are available to aid the evaluation of systolic and diastolic function in intact animals. The large number of indices (Box 197-7 presents a partial list) probably reflects the fact that no single index meets all needs. Only indices that are clinically useful are discussed here.

Systolic function   Systolic function is assessed by evaluation of the determinants of stroke volume (preload, afterload, and contractility) and by use of indices of global ventricular systolic performance. For evaluation of cardiac function, many indices require a knowledge of the left ventricular volume or stroke volume. The left ventricular volume can be estimated echocardiographically or by angiography. An echocardiogram provides a good estimation of left ventricular volume noninvasively in dogs and is economically feasible. Two-dimensional echocardiography is superior to M-mode echocardiography in the estimation of left ventricular volume in dogs. The stroke volume can also be obtained by two-dimensional echocardiography (end-diastolic volume/end-systolic volume) or preferentially by Doppler echocardiography. Using Doppler echocardiography, the stroke volume can be determined from the integrated velocity of blood flow across the aorta or pulmonary artery, multiplied by the cross-sectional area of the respective valve orifice.

Preload   Left ventricular end-diastolic volume is the best clinical approximation of preload. M-mode–based models for evaluation of the left ventricular volume are associated with unacceptably high variation, especially for the end-diastolic volume. Whenever possible, left ventricular volume should be estimated with two-dimensional echocardiography, using the Simpson's rule or the cylinder-truncated-cone-cone method.[113] Alternatively, preload can be estimated as being equal to the left ventricular end-diastolic pressure based on the relationship between left ventricular pressure and volume. Pressure, rather than volume, cannot be used to estimate preload in stiff or noncompliant ventricles.

Afterload   Ideally, afterload should be measured as the aortic input impedance, but this is not clinically feasible. An alternative is to use the effective arterial elastance (Ea). The Ea is a steady-state arterial parameter that incorporates the principal elements of vascular load and is obtained from the ratio of end-systolic pressure to stroke volume.[10] To avoid the

---

Box • **197-7**

Some Hemodynamic Indices Used to Evaluate Cardiovascular Function

- Pressure behind the pumping chamber
  - Left or right ventricular end-diastolic pressure*
  - Pulmonary capillary wedge pressure* (left side)
  - Central venous pressure (right side)
- Systolic function
  - Preload
    - Left ventricular (LV) volume
    - LV end-diastolic pressure*
  - Afterload
    - Aortic input impedance*
    - Effective arterial elastance
    - Systemic vascular resistance
    - Arterial blood pressure
  - Contractility
    - Isovolumic indices
      - dP/dt_{max} and derived indices*
    - Pressure-volume indices
      - Preload recruitable stroke work*
      - dP/dt-SdPV*
      - End-systolic elastance*
    - Integrated systolic function
      - Systolic time intervals
      - Ejection fraction
      - Fractional shortening
      - End-systolic volume index
      - Mean normalized systolic ejection rate
      - Mean velocity of circumferential fiber shortening
      - Stroke work*
- Diastolic function
  - Diastolic time intervals
    - Isovolumic relaxation time
  - Flow and volume measurements
    - Transmitral valve flow profile
    - Transmitral filling fractions
    - Pulmonary venous flow systolic fraction
    - LV flow propagation velocity
    - Filling fraction
    - Peak filling rate
    - dV/dt
  - Other echocardiographically derived indices
    - Rate of change in wall thickness
    - Rate of wall relaxation
    - Relaxation half-time
  - Pressure-derived isovolumic relaxation
    - dP/dt_{min}*
    - Time constant of relaxation* (τ)
  - Pressure-volume indices
    - End-diastolic pressure-volume relationship*
    - Chamber stiffness*

*Requires cardiac catheterization for proper measurement. dP/dt_{max}, maximum rate of increase in pressure; dP/dt-$SdPV$, end-diastolic volume relation; dV/dt, rate of change in volume; dP/dt_{min}, maximum rate of fall in pressure.

need for cardiac catheterization, the mean femoral artery pressure can be used as an estimation of the left ventricular end-systolic pressure.[114] Changes in the Ea show a high correlation with changes in input impedance. Peripheral resistance is another option for estimating left ventricular afterload, but it accounts only for the opposition to steady flow and not for the opposition to pulsatile flow. Peripheral (systemic) vascular resistance (SVR) can be calculated using cardiac output (CO), mean aortic pressure (MAP), and venous pressure (VP) as follows:

$$SVR = 80 \times (MAP - VP)/CO$$

The arterial blood pressure can be used as a simple, noninvasive means of assessing the opposition to left ventricular ejection. CHF, however, involves a combination of decreased cardiac output and increased afterload. Because the arterial blood pressure depends on both these factors, it does not provide an adequate evaluation of left ventricular afterload.[115] Nevertheless, it is important to know whether a patient with CHF also has systemic hypertension. The arterial blood pressure may also be important for monitoring vasodilator therapy during CHF.

Contractility Contractility is difficult to define and even more difficult to measure without interference from preload and afterload. Ventricular contraction has an isovolumic phase and an ejection phase. Isovolumic indices evaluate only the isovolumic contraction phase but are less affected by load changes. Ejection phase indices are so affected by changes in afterload and preload that they reflect not the contractility but the integrated systolic function. Indices based on the pressure-volume relationship are relatively load independent and are probably the best indices for evaluating contractility in intact animals. However, they are not routinely used clinically and are beyond the scope of this chapter.

The isovolumic index most commonly used in the evaluation of cardiac contractility is the maximum rate of pressure rise (dP/dt_{max}). dP/dt_{max} is the tangent to the maximum slope of the ascending portion of the left ventricular pressure curve, therefore it can be obtained only with left ventricular catheterization. dP/dt_{max} is influenced by preload (and to a lesser extent by afterload) and cannot be used in presence of valvular regurgitation. It is a sensitive index of contractility but is not specific because of its load dependence. Many other indices based on dP/dt have been developed, but they have roughly the same limitations as the dP/dt_{max}.

Integrated left ventricular systolic function Indices of left ventricular function that evaluate global systolic function can be based on systolic time intervals or on left ventricular volume, diameter, or flow characteristics. The most commonly used systolic time intervals are the left ventricular ejection time (LVET) and the pre-ejection period (PEP). The PEP corresponds to the electric-mechanic interval plus the pressure rise time (onset of QRS to the opening of the aortic valve); it is influenced by changes in afterload, preload, and contractility. The LVET (opening to closing of the aortic valve) is affected by the heart rate and contractility and only mildly by preload and afterload. The information necessary to determine the PEP and LVET can be obtained with an electrocardiogram, a phonocardiogram, and an arterial pressure curve or M-mode echocardiogram of the aortic valve. The PEP/LVET ratio is independent of the heart rate and inversely related to systolic function.[116]

The ejection fraction (stroke volume/end-diastolic volume) and fractional shortening ([end-diastolic dimension – end-systolic dimension]/end-diastolic dimension) are two indices of systolic function expressed as a percentage. They are very sensitive and easy to measure using echocardiography, but they are influenced by changes in load. In addition, the low correlation

between M-mode–derived volumes and the true left ventricular end-diastolic volume[113] probably renders an ejection fraction obtained with M-mode echocardiography inaccurate. The left ventricle also must be contracting uniformly, and the ultrasound beam must be parallel to the short axis of the ventricle for an M-mode–derived volume to be representative of global ventricular function.

M-mode imaging of the left ventricle may be performed using short or long axis views of the heart. Left ventricular dimensions obtained from short axis views tend to be higher than those obtained from long axis views, and there may be a lack of agreement between short and long axis views in dogs with heart disease.[117] Fortunately, fractional shortening values obtained from short axis views have shown good agreement with those obtained from long axis images in normal dogs and in dogs with heart disease.[117] When an M-mode of the left ventricle is recorded, it is important to be in the center of the left ventricle, perpendicular to the left ventricular wall, and with the ultrasound beam just below the mitral valve. The short axis view allows better centering of the beam in the heart, whereas the long axis view is preferred for assuring that the beam is perpendicular to the wall. Either plan can be used to place the beam below the mitral valve. The choice of view (short axis, long axis, or both) for obtaining M-mode measurement of fractional shortening in dogs and cats remains a matter of the examiner's personal preference. Fractional shortening in dogs is also affected by body size, being smaller in giant breed dogs. The end-systolic volume index, left ventricular end-systolic volume obtained by M-mode indexed to body surface. It has been used in dogs,[118] but it is also dependent on afterload and in M-mode estimation of left ventricular volume. The end-systolic volume index may be more accurate than other volume-based indices because only one volume must be estimated, which avoids compounding error from multiple measurements. In addition, measurement of the end-systolic volume improves precision because of the better correlation between M-mode–derived volumes and true ventricular volume at smaller volumes.[113] The time to aortic peak velocity, which can be obtained by Doppler echocardiography, correlates well with global systolic function. Like all ejection indices, it is affected by changes in afterload.

Diastolic Function

Diastolic function is harder to evaluate noninvasively than systolic function. Doppler echocardiography remains the primary technique for assessing diastolic function noninvasively. Some indices of diastolic function assess ventricular function during a specific phase, whereas others evaluate global performance during diastole.

Diastolic time intervals can be used to evaluate diastolic properties. The most commonly used diastolic time interval is the isovolumic relaxation time, which is the time from aortic valve closure to mitral valve opening, when the left ventricular volume is constant. It is a relaxation index and can be obtained from phonocardiography (for aortic closure) and M-mode echocardiography (to mitral opening) or from Doppler echocardiography (the time from cessation of aortic flow to commencement of transmitral flow). An isovolumic relaxation time obtained echocardiographically correlated well with the time constant of isovolumic relaxation (τ) in anesthetized cats.[119] Unfortunately, the rate of decline in left ventricular pressure is only one of several factors that determine the isovolumic relaxation period. The aortic diastolic pressure and left atrial pressure affect the length of this period. The isovolumic relaxation time cannot be used in patients with aortic or mitral regurgitation because there is no true isovolumic period.

Doppler echocardiogram–derived changes in blood flow can be used to evaluate diastolic function. Many indices have been proposed, but the ones based on the transmitral valve flow profile (E and A waves) are more commonly used. The E wave represents early ventricular filling and precedes the A wave (atrial filling wave). The E wave is normally larger than the A wave (E/A ratio usually greater than 1). During fast heart rates, especially in cats, E and A waves are often fused, and the E/A ratio cannot be evaluated. An increase in the size of the A wave and a decrease in the E wave occur in patients with relaxation abnormalities. Unfortunately, with progression of the disease and an increase in the left ventricular end-diastolic pressure, the presence of mitral regurgitation, and an increase in the left atrial pressure, pseudonormalization of the E and A waves occurs. Patients with restrictive diseases tend to have smaller A waves and larger E waves.

M-mode echocardiography can also be used to evaluate diastolic function. The rate of change in wall thickness, the rate of wall relaxation, and the relaxation half time can be obtained with an M-mode echocardiogram (ideally a digitized echocardiogram). The peak rate of posterior wall motion has also been used, but this measurement is susceptible to distortion because of translational motion.

Hemodynamic indices that use pressure rather than volume have been used to evaluate diastolic function. These all require cardiac catheterization. The peak negative dP/dt measures the maximal rate of decline of left ventricular pressure during relaxation and is usually taken as the lowest value of the first derivative of this pressure. It usually occurs around the time of aortic closure. It should be remembered that the peak negative dP/dt occurs at one point in time and does not represent the totality of events, even during relaxation only. In addition, the peak minimum dP/dt is highly dependent on the left ventricular and the aortic systolic pressures.

Integrated Function
Cardiac output is considered a measure of integrated cardiovascular performance. Cardiac output is usually measured by thermodilution, a technique based on the indicator-dilution method. Thermodilution offers advantages because it does not require arterial puncture or the withdrawal of blood, and an inert and inexpensive indicator (e.g., cold saline or 5% dextrose in water) is used with virtually no recirculation. However, all indicator techniques require placement of a catheter in the pulmonary artery, which makes these techniques impractical for routine use in clinical veterinary medicine outside critical care units. Doppler echocardiography can also be used to estimate cardiac output. The stroke volume can be determined from the integrated velocity of blood flow across the aorta or pulmonary artery multiplied by the cross-sectional area of the respective valve orifice.[120] Doppler determination of blood flow velocity is a noninvasive method that can be performed in awake, untrained, dogs.[121] It is useful for documenting beat-to-beat variation in the stroke volume in dogs[122] and can be used to determine the cardiac output when the stroke volume is multiplied by the heart rate. As with thermodilution determination of cardiac output, Doppler-derived values for cardiac outputs are variable.[123] Cardiac outputs obtained by Doppler echocardiography and thermodilution show an excellent correlation[124]; however, the technique for obtaining cardiac output by echocardiography appears to be quite operator dependent. It should be remembered that cardiac output at rest is not a sensitive indicator of heart function during CHF because all compensatory mechanisms act to increase cardiac output.

What Tests Should I Use in a Clinical Patient?
Of all the tests available for the evaluation of cardiovascular function, a few are routinely used. Chest radiographs and echocardiography are performed in virtually all patients with CHF. Measurement of the arterial blood pressure and central venous pressure can be easily performed and provides important information about cardiovascular status. Not surprisingly, the most commonly used tests of cardiovascular function are based on echocardiography, whereas chest radiographs are used to confirm left-sided CHF. In the majority of patients, systolic performance is assessed by fractional shortening, the ejection fraction, or the end-systolic volume index. No clinical comparison of these indices has been performed in small animals, therefore the choice of index is a matter of personal preference. In selected patients the aortic velocity, time to peak aortic velocity, and cardiac output can be measured using Doppler echocardiography. Diastolic performance is usually assessed by Doppler evaluation of transmitral flow. In patients undergoing cardiac catheterization, pressure traces, dP/dt$_{max}$, cardiac output, and estimated systemic vascular resistance, among other measurements, can be obtained.

HOW DOES HEART FAILURE BECOME A PROGRESSIVE DISEASE?

Vicious Cycles in Congestive Heart Failure
Compensatory mechanisms activated during heart failure paradoxically serve simultaneously as adaptive, compensatory changes and, by causing myocardial cell death, as major contributing elements in the progression of CHF. Cell death in an already overloaded heart adds to the overload on survival myocytes in a vicious cycle. Three primary, interlocked vicious cycles ultimately result in myocardial cell death (Figure 197-18).

Increased Left Ventricular Afterload and Myocardial Oxygen Consumption (Cycle 1)
Vasoconstriction and increases in cardiac contractility and the heart rate help maintain blood pressure but also increase MVO$_2$. Increasing cardiac MVO$_2$ accelerates myocardial cell death. Wall stress (a function of afterload), contractility, and the heart rate are the main determinants of MVO$_2$. Myocardial hypertrophy reduces oxygen consumption by decreasing wall stress during ejection. Hypertrophy caused by increases in load, however, does not yield a normal heart. Load-induced hypertrophy sets the stage for myocardial death. An increase in afterload leads to further left ventricular dysfunction, and the patient spirals down until a new, decreased steady-state level is reached, where cardiac output is lower and vasoconstriction is higher than is optimal for the patient.

Sodium and Water Retention and Increased Left Atrial Pressure (Cycle 2)
Sodium and water retention increase the circulating volume, resulting in increases in preload and the left atrial pressure. An increase in preload increases cardiac output and helps maintain filling pressures but also leads to signs of congestion and edema. An excessive preload increases ventricular pressures, volume, and wall stress, further adding to the deterioration of left ventricular function.

Left Ventricular and Vascular Remodeling (Cycle 3)
Stretching of myocardium as a result of overload seems to be the initiating signal for adaptive processes to begin in the myocardium. This leads to hypertrophy as a result of growth factor and proto-oncogene stimulation.[66] Hypertrophy unloads the cells of the failing heart by adding new sarcomeres and also increases contractility and cardiac output. Unfortunately, hypertrophy ultimately leads to cellular abnormalities that result in mitochondrial deoxyribonucleic acid (DNA) abnormalities and apoptosis (programmed cell death), which hasten myocardial cell death.[66] Chronic neuro-endocrine activation, especially increases in angiotensin II and norepinephrine, and increases in afterload lead to left ventricular and vascular remodeling. Globally, the remodeling process in the ventricle is characterized by progressive left ventricular enlargement and

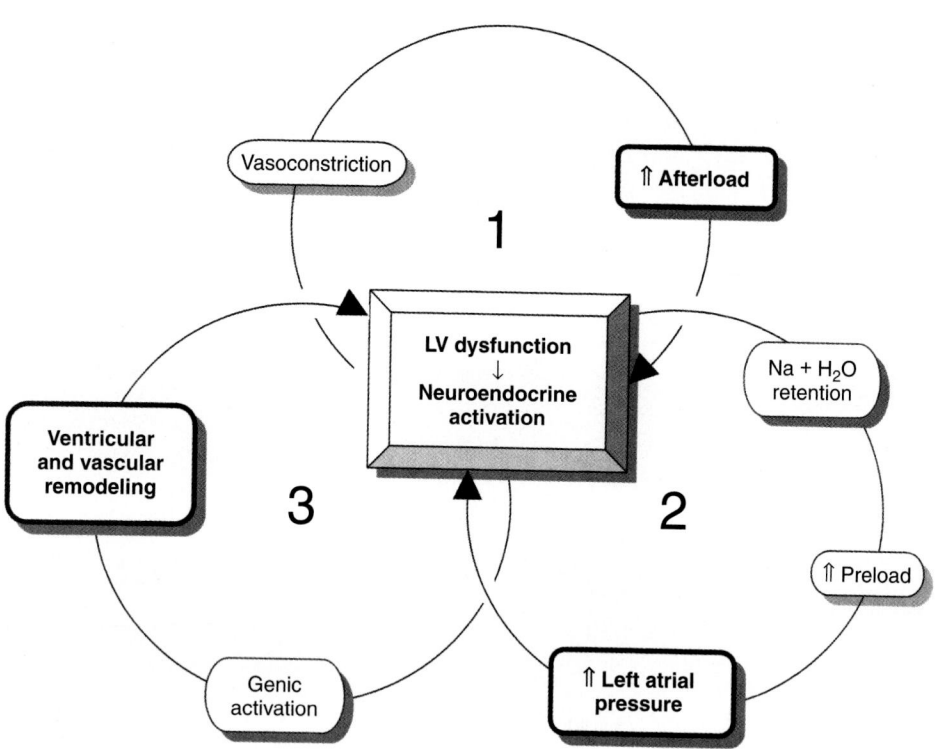

Figure 197-18 Interlocked vicious cycles that lead to progression of congestive heart failure: increased afterload (cycle 1), increased left atrial pressure (cycle 2), and ventricular and vascular remodeling (cycle 3). *LV,* Left ventricle.

increased chamber sphericity. At the cellular level, the remodeling process is associated with myocyte slippage, hypertrophy, and accumulation of collagen in the interstitial compartment. The final result of this process is the so-called cardiomyopathy of overload. Angiotensin II also causes vascular remodeling, which leads to hypertrophy of smooth muscle cells of the vessel walls.[125] Vascular remodeling decreases vessel compliance, thereby increasing ventricular afterload.

Cardiomyopathy of Overload

Long-term overload-induce hypertrophy in the heart is accompanied by myocardial cell death and cardiac fibrosis. This progressive and eventually lethal growth abnormality has been called cardiomyopathy of overload.[23,66] In embryonic hearts, growth factors induce protein synthesis, leading to normal cell division. Soon after an animal is born, cardiac myocytes withdraw from the cell cycle and are no longer able to divide, and protein synthesis slows to rates appropriate for maintaining and repairing the cells. Stimulation of growth factors by chronic overload leads to an increase in protein synthesis. The cell cycle, however, remains blocked, and the end result is not normal cell division but abnormal hypertrophy. Increases in angiotensin II, a peptide that is not only a vasoconstrictor but also a mitogen, appear to be an important mediator of the reversal of protein synthesis inhibition in the adult heart.

Overload-induced hypertrophy leads to a state of chronic energy starvation in the heart. Because the increase in cardiac mass is not accompanied by an increase in capillary vessels, the hypertrophied ventricle outstrips its blood supply. The cell volume occupied by sarcomeres increases, leading to an increased ratio of mitochondria to myofibrils, which can exacerbate the energy deficit. The net result is a decrease in capillary density and coronary reserve, with the myocardium becoming prone to ischemia, especially in the subendocardium. The relative decrease in oxygen delivery complicates the failing heart's increased need for oxygen, which is already increased by vasoconstriction and sympathetic activation.

Hypertrophy and increasing systolic dysfunction are closely linked. The ischemia resulting from hypertrophy leads to the development of focal fibrosis, which increases the myocardial collagen content. The early increase in collagen helps maintain systolic function, but it also interferes with diastolic function. With progression of the myocardial hypertrophy, the early interstitial fibrosis progresses to perimuscular fibrosis, impairing both systolic and diastolic function. Myocardial cell necrosis occurs in overloaded hearts in the transition to heart failure. Myocyte cell death results not only from necrosis (accidental cell death) but also from apoptosis (programmed cell death). The activation of proto-oncogenes and the increased concentrations of TGF-1α that occur in CHF may induce apoptosis. Regardless of the cause, myocardial cell death occurs in overload-induced hypertrophy, increasing the overload in the surviving myocytes in a vicious cycle. Cardiomyopathy of overload, therefore, represents an unnatural growth of the adult heart that leads to myocardial cell death, progression of myocardial failure, and death.

SUMMARY

Heart failure is a state in which cardiac output is inadequate to meet the perfusion needs of the metabolizing tissues and exercise capacity is limited. It may be the result of inability of the heart to eject blood properly (systolic failure) or of inadequate ventricular filling (diastolic failure). Correct identification of the cause of heart disease and of the mechanism leading to heart failure allows the clinician to choose the appropriate therapy, thereby improving the prognosis.

Regardless of the mechanism, CHF is associated with a fall in blood pressure and activation of compensatory mechanisms aimed at restoring normal arterial blood pressure. These mechanisms include neuroendocrine activation and renal retention of sodium and water. Vasoconstriction, tachycardia, and volume retention are the initial responses of the circulation to the fall in blood pressure. Excessive compensatory response may lead to overcompensation, and compensatory mechanisms that are beneficial in the beginning become responsible for the development of clinical signs.

Therapy is aimed at modulating the excessively activated compensatory mechanisms. The inciting cause of the cardiac dysfunction and neuroendocrine activation also stimulates myocardial compensation, leading to increased contractility and relaxation, sympathetic desensitization, and unnatural growth (hypertrophy). Modulation of the unnatural growth response with drugs that have growth-inhibitory as well as vasodilative properties (e.g., ACE inhibitors and nitrates) may delay the appearance of cardiomyopathy of overload and improve the prognosis for patients with CHF. Myocyte changes determined by overload-induced hypertrophy ultimately lead to myocardial cell death, which further compromises myocardial function. Thus once a certain point of myocardial dysfunction is reached, CHF becomes a progressive, irreversible disease.

CHAPTER • 198

Biochemical Markers of Cardiovascular Disease

Karsten E. Schober

During the past decade, considerable research has been conducted into the use of circulating markers of myocardial cell integrity (leakage markers) and of specific proteins of cardiac function (functional markers), their diagnostic capability, and their potential to aid therapeutic decisions and allow prognostic risk assessment in patients with cardiovascular abnormalities (Box 198-1). Biochemical screening for heart disease or for definition of the functional status of the heart in certain pet populations based on readily available circulating marker proteins such as cardiac troponins, natriuretic peptides, or endothelin is an attractive hypothesis. Moreover, the prospect of identifying dogs and cats with early asymptomatic or minimally symptomatic congestive heart failure (CHF) or patients at risk for sudden deterioration of ongoing disease processes via biochemical testing is exciting from several perspectives. For example, it would allow individuals without extensive training in cardiology to detect animals with cardiac abnormalities more accurately and at an earlier point in time. This would permit early therapeutic intervention and potentially reduce the morbidity and mortality associated with advanced stages of heart disease, while avoiding unnecessary treatment of unaffected or mildly affected animals. In addition, conditions that currently are still difficult to identify clearly with conventional diagnostic methods (e.g., myocarditis, ischemic heart disease, and pulmonary hypertension) could be detected more specifically.

Biochemical testing might also help clarify the status of animals with equivocal results from other diagnostic modalities, such as for dogs with borderline systolic function on echocardiography, animals with arrhythmias of unknown origin, or dogs with questionable cardiomegaly on thoracic radiographs. Other applications might include monitoring of the effects of potentially cardiotoxic drugs or of extracardiac disease on myocardial integrity and function.

The advent of biochemical markers also opens a category of the pathophysiologic aspect of nonischemic cardiac damage that is not yet fully understood or verified. It likely will provide important prognostic information and may prove useful for monitoring the success of treatment or for determining the need to change treatment protocols. Screening of certain breeding populations for asymptomatic myocardial diseases, such as hypertrophic cardiomyopathy (HCM) and dilated cardiomyopathy (DCM), may be another possibility.

LEAKAGE MARKERS

Circulating markers of myocardial integrity provide evidence of cell degradation, supplying the rationale for diagnosis of a disease process using such markers. That is, detection of intracellular constituents released into the blood when a cell either ruptures or loses membrane integrity allows identification of the damaged target tissue. Measurable changes in the serum concentration of these markers are determined primarily by the markers' molecular mass, intracellular compartmentalization, solubility, release kinetics, post-translational modifications, and assay characteristics; by local blood and lymphatic flow; and by the route by which the markers are cleared from the circulation.

Myocardial cell injury is a common event in the pathogenesis of heart failure in dogs and cats.[1,2] Pressure and volume overload, hypoxia and ischemia, abnormal neurohormonal stimulation, toxins, and cytokines all may cause myocardial remodeling, characterized by hypertrophy and dilatation or, at the cellular level, by oxidative and mechanical stress, degeneration, inflammation, fiber slippage, apoptosis, necrosis, and fibrosis of myocardial tissue that finally results in cardiac functional abnormalities.

Analysis of cardiac leakage markers has progressed from measurement of enzymes (e.g., plasma aspartate transaminase) to measurement of structural proteins, including cardiac troponins (see Box 198-1; Table 198-1). Although commonly used diagnostic procedures can serve as the current gold standard for the assessment of cardiac anatomy and function in clinical practice, they most often are inadequate for detecting and quantifying minor myocardial cell injury or active myocardial damage.

ALPHA-HYDROXYBUTYRATE DEHYDROGENASE (ALPHA-HBDH)

Lactate dehydrogenase (LD) is a tetrameric enzyme with M (muscle) and H (heart) subunits that is responsible for the interconversion of pyruvate and lactate as the final step in glycolysis. The two subunits are encoded by different genes and give rise to five distinct isoenzymes that provide LD with an element of tissue specificity. LD-1 has four H subunits, and

Box • 198-1

Biochemical Markers of Cardiac Disease

Leakage Markers

Cardiac troponin I*
Cardiac troponin T*
Myoglobin
Creatine kinase isoenzyme MB
Creatine kinase
Lactate dehydrogenase isoenzymes 1 and 2
Aspartate transaminase
Heart fatty acid-binding proteins
Glycogenphosphorylase isoenzyme BB
Myosin light chain
Myosin heavy chain
Plasma oxidase

Functional Markers

Brain natriuretic peptide
Atrial natriuretic peptide*
Endothelin-1
Epinephrine
Norepinephrine
Renin
Angiotensin II
Aldosterone
Arginine vasopressin
Tumor necrosis factor-alpha
Adrenomedullin
C-reactive protein

*Currently one of the most commonly used markers in companion animals.

LD-2 has three H subunits and one M subunit. LD-1 and LD-2 form alpha-HBDH, which has some cardiac specificity. However, because other sources of LD-1 and LD-2 exist (i.e., erythrocytes, as well as the brain, kidneys, pancreas, and stomach), tissue specificity for the detection of myocardial injury is rather poor. Reference values for alpha-HBDH in dogs and cats have been published (see Table 198-1),[3,4] but because more specific serum markers of myocardial cell damage are available, analysis of alpha-HBDH is no longer recommended for the diagnosis of myocardial injury in dogs and cats.

MYOGLOBIN (Mb)

Myoglobin is a low-molecular-weight heme protein that is abundant in cardiac and skeletal muscle but not smooth muscle. It is found predominantly in the cytosol of the cell.[5] Because of its high sensitivity and rapid release after myocardial injury, it has drawn considerable attention in the early diagnosis of acute myocardial infarction (AMI) in humans. It may be less clinically useful in animals, however, because of its low cardiac specificity and rapid clearance after injury, and because, compared with humans, dogs and cats have a low incidence of ischemic heart disease.

CREATINE KINASE ISOENZYME MB (CK-MB)

Creatine kinase (CK) is a dimeric enzyme with M (muscle) and B (brain) subunits, each having 381 amino acids.[5] CK catalyzes the transfer of a high-energy phosphate from adenosine triphosphate (ATP) to creatine, producing creatine phosphate. CK isoenzymes consist of CK-MM, CK-MB, or CK-BB. A unique dimeric mitochondrial form not composed of either M or B subunits also exists. Each subunit of CK is regulated by a distinct gene and is expressed in a tissue-specific manner. CK-MB is functionally unbound and cytosolically dissolved and is found predominantly in the myocardium[6] in concentration ranges of 1% to 42% of total CK activity of the heart. There is a significant difference in the concentration of CK-MB between normal and diseased myocardium,[6] depending on the disease state, the patient's age, the chronicity of

Table • 198-1

Characteristics and Reference Values* of Circulating Myocardial Leakage Markers in Dogs and Cats

MARKER	MOLECULAR WEIGHT (kDa)	SERUM HALF-LIFE (h)	TIME TO INITIAL ELEVATION (h)†	TIME TO PEAK (h)†	TIME TO RETURN TO BASELINE (d)†	CATS (n = 28)	DOGS (n = 40)
AST (U/L)	93	20	6-12	18-36	3-6	20 (12-36)	26 (14-63)
Alpha-HBDH (U/L)	135	10	6-12	24-48	7-10	30 (20-44)	26 (3-52)
Mb (ng/mL)	17,8	0.25	1-4	6-8	1	0 (0-1.86)	0 (0)
CK-MB (ng/mL)	86	2	3-6	12-24	3-4	0 (0-1.30)	0 (0-2.48)
cTnT (ng/mL)	37	2	3-8	12-96	5-14	0 (0-0.01)	0 (0)
cTnI (ng/mL)	22,5	2-4	3-8	12-24	5-10	0 (0)	0 (0-0.93)

*From Kirbach B et al: Diagnostik von Herzmuskelschäden bei Katzen mit stumpfen Thoraxtraumen über biochemische Parameter im Blut. Tierärztl Prax 28 (K):25, 2000; and Schober K et al: Noninvasive assessment of myocardial cell injury in dogs with suspected cardiac contusion. J Vet Cardiol 1:17, 1999.

†After acute ischemic myocardial damage. "0" refers to the lower limit of detection of the assay used (1.0 ng/mL for Mb, 0.5 ng/mL for CK-MB, 0.1 ng/mL for cTnI [OPUS Troponin I; Dade-Behring Diagnostics, Westwood, Massachusetts], and 0.01 ng/mL for cTnT [ELECSYS 1010 Troponin T STAT; Boehringer, Mannheim, Germany]).

AST, Aspartate transaminase; *alpha-HBDH*, alpha-hydroxybutyrate dehydrogenase; *CK*, creatine kinase; *Mb*, myoglobin, *CK-MB*, CK isoenzyme MB (mass determination); *cTnT*, cardiac troponin T; *cTnI*, cardiac troponin I.
Median (2.5th to 97.5th percentile).

myocardial stress, and the severity and duration of ischemia. Marked upregulation of CK-MB synthesis in cardiomyocytes may be seen after myocardial injury despite a decrease in absolute CK concentrations. Such dynamic CK-MB alterations may cause a significant elevation of the relative amount of CK-MB in ventricular myocardium within several weeks of the onset of disease. Circulating CK-MB is not 100% specific for cardiac muscle tissue, because a significant portion of CK-MB may be expressed in skeletal muscle, the lungs, intestines, and spleen. Moreover, CK-MB immunoreactivity is not well conserved across species,[7] and species-specific immunoassays for CK-MB are not commercially available for use in dogs and cats. CK-MB is released early after acute myocardial cell damage (see Table 198-1), is inactivated by proteolysis in lymph, and is rapidly cleared by the reticuloendothelial system. In normal dogs and cats, CK-MB in serum is not detectable.[3,4]

CARDIAC TROPONIN (cTn)

Since the descriptions of the measurement of cardiac troponin T (cTnT) in 1989 and cardiac troponin I (cTnI) in 1992, analysis of circulating cTn has revolutionized the noninvasive diagnosis of acute coronary syndromes in human beings. Cardiac troponin levels allow more specific detection of myocardial damage than do traditional "cardiac enzymes" such as LD and CK-MB. A series of landmark clinical studies has defined cTn measurement as the gold standard test for AMI in humans. The advantage of cTn lies in its ability to provide an early, highly cardiac specific diagnosis of even micronecrotic pathology and prognostic risk assessment and to guide therapy. Despite the obvious lack of importance of ischemic heart disease in small animals compared with humans, studies performed in dogs and cats have suggested similar findings indicating superior efficacy of cTnI and cTnT in the diagnosis of myocardial injury in a variety of clinical conditions.[1-17]

Structure and Function

The troponin complex is made up of three structurally and functionally different proteins (TnI, TnT, and TnC), which exist in different isoforms in both skeletal and cardiac muscle but not in smooth muscle. It is located on the thin filament of the contractile apparatus that regulates the calcium-mediated interaction of myosin and actin. Although both TnI and TnT are present in skeletal muscle (in slow- and fast-twitch fibers) and cardiac muscle, they are encoded by individual genes, yielding proteins that are immunologically distinct. Cardiac troponin T has 276 amino acids and is a structural protein that binds the troponin-tropomyosin complex to the actin filament. Cardiac troponin I is a linear protein with five alpha-helices; it has 211 amino acids[18] and is an inhibitory protein that regulates muscle contraction. Its phosphorylation causes a decrease in the affinity of Ca^{2+} for the calcium-binding TnC, leading to inhibition of actomyosin ATPase activity. Cardiac TnI is uniquely specific to the heart, containing an additional 31-amino-acid sequence on its N-terminal region. The remaining amino acid sequence shows approximately 40% dissimilarity from skeletal muscle forms. In the cardiomyocyte, the troponins are compartmentalized into a major, structurally bound pool and a minor, free cytosolic pool, estimated at 6% to 8% for cTnT and 2% to 6% for cTnI. This cellular distribution determines release kinetics, with free cytosolic proteins released earlier. The third protein of the troponin-tropomyosin complex, TnC, has only two isoforms (160 and 161 amino acids) and is an 18 kDa protein with calcium-binding properties. The complete homology between the cardiac and the skeletal muscle isoforms of TnC has limited its diagnostic value.

Release, Degradation, and Clearance

Both loss of membrane integrity and cell necrosis cause the release of cTn from damaged cardiomyocytes. Two basic cTn release patterns have been postulated, depending on the type of underlying disease, the time to peak damage, and the severity of cell injury. In cases of slow disintegration of myofibrils, the release pattern may be biphasic, with the cytosolic pool released first. If the insult is more severe, a more protracted, persistent release from structurally bound stores may occur, representing irreversible cell damage. An important question is whether cTnI and cTnT leaks across the myocardial cell membrane in reversible injury, such as transient ischemia (reversible injury concept), as postulated by some investigators. In such cases, only mild cTn elevations and a temporary, monophasic release pattern would be expected.

Early work revealed that cTn first is released as a ternary complex of cTnT-I-C, which subsequently degrades into binary complexes of cTnI-C, free cTnT (with little or no free cTnI), and smaller immunologic fragments. However, more recent data suggest that troponin may already be degraded into small fragments within the myocyte. Once released into circulation, N- and C-terminal regions of cTn are particularly vulnerable to additional, progressive, and highly variable biochemical modifications, including phosphorylation, complex formation, and proteolytic cleavage. The newly formed degradation products may alter their recognition by monoclonal antibodies, affecting assay performance. Furthermore, different pathologic states (e.g., ischemia, inflammation, toxic injury) result in different post-translational profiles of cTn, with cTnI being more susceptible to postrelease modifications and less stable than cTnT.

Clearance of cTn is not well documented. As with most marker proteins with molecular weights above 20 kDa, cTn appears to be catabolized in organs with a high metabolic rate, such as the liver and pancreas, and the reticuloendothelial system. The serum half-life of cTnT is approximately 120 minutes, with a prolonged window of detection due to continuous release of cTnT from the myofibrillar pool during the myocyte degradation processes.

Analysis

Clinicians must be aware of several analytic issues. Investigations in animals have demonstrated that both cTnI and cTnT immunoassays designed for use in humans can be used reliably and specifically to detect myocardial injury in dogs and cats, because cTn immunoreactivity has been highly conserved across species.[19] The monoclonal antibodies used in second- and third-generation assays for cTn analysis have no known species specificity and no detectable cross-reactivity with skeletal muscle isoforms.

Due to patent restrictions, assays for cTnT are available from only one manufacturer; they therefore are relatively uniform with regard to cutoff concentrations and precision. In contrast, at least 16 different assays for cTnI have been approved by the U.S. Food and Drug Administration (FDA). Because of the lack of standardization in cTnI assays, significant variability exists in the assay methods and cutoff values used. Up to 100-fold differences in absolute concentrations of cTnI for a given patient sample have been observed. With so much variation, attention must be paid to the assay used when the data and results of troponin I measurements are interpreted. Sample requirements for the different assays also may vary. The optimal sample material for most systems seems to be serum clotted adequately. The cTnT molecule is stable at a room temperature of 4° C and when frozen. Cardiac TnI is more susceptible to early epitope degradation; however, serum samples may be stored at room temperature for 4 days without clinically relevant reduction of detectable cTnI concentrations.[2,8,20] In terms of substate stability for analyns, differences between different CTnI assays may, however, exist.

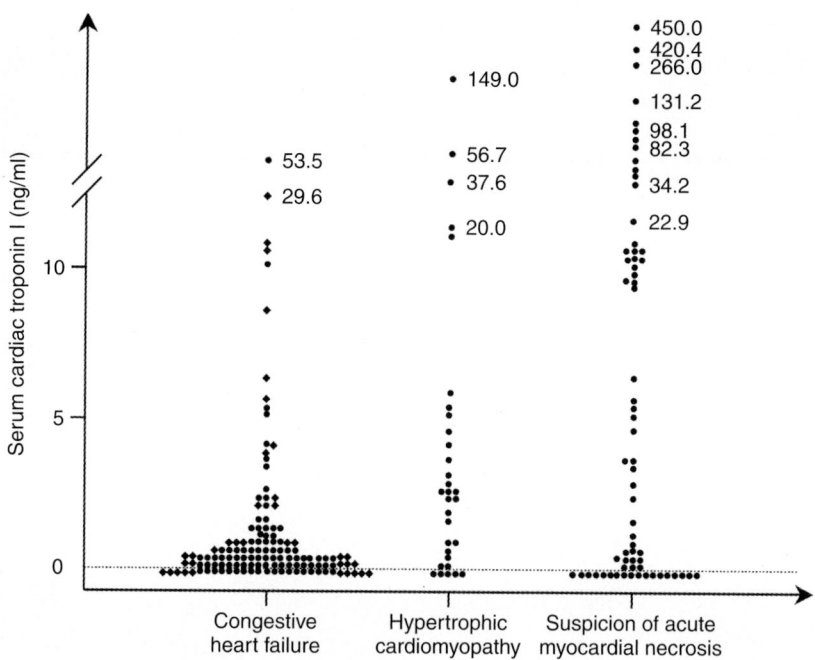

Figure 198-1 Serum cardiac troponin I concentrations in 129 dogs with congestive heart failure (•, dilated cardiomyopathy; ♦, congestive heart failure of other cause), 31 cats with hypertrophic cardiomyopathy, and 67 dogs with the clinical suspicion of acute myocardial necrosis of noncardiomyopathic origin based on the occurence of venticular arrhythmia. Zero CTnI refers to the lower limit of detection of the immunoassay used (0.1 ng/ml; OPUS® Troponin I, Dade-Behring Diagnostics Inc., Westwood, MA). From the veterinary medical database of the Department of Small Animal Medicine, University of Leip zig and reference 2 with permission.

Reference Intervals and Clinical Cutoff Values

In healthy dogs and cats, the background level of cTn in the circulation appears to be undetectable (see Table 198-1). Several clinical studies, involving more than 331 dogs[4,9,15-17,21] and 150 cats,[3,10,17,21-23] have shown that both cTnI and cTnT are below the detection limit of the assay used or occur only in trace amounts in the peripheral circulation. However, because of the very high sensitivity of second- and third-generation immunoassays, minimal elevations of cTn may occur in obviously healthy animals as a result of strenuous exercise or noncardiac disease. This is particularly true for cTnI. To distinguish between minor myocardial cell damage (so-called micronecrosis) and major myocardial injury, two cutoff points were suggested for clinical use in humans: the upper reference limit, defined as the 97.5th percentile of the values measured in the normal control population, and a higher limit, indicating clinically relevant myocardial damage. Given the difficulties in objectively defining the latter value and the currently used, rather liberal thresholds, it is not clear whether the exact magnitude of troponin elevation is indeed essential for clinical decision making. From the clinician's point of view, it appears that characterizing patients as "troponin negative/mildly elevated" or "troponin positive/moderately to severely elevated" and dynamic monitoring of cTn concentrations are most useful for diagnosing and semiquantifying myocardial necrosis and for making a subsequent risk assessment.

Sensitivity and Specificity

When the most current assays are used, cTnI is elevated earlier and more frequently than cTnT in a variety of clinical conditions in dogs and cats, as confirmed by meta-analysis using 500 simultaneously measured serum samples.[2] Circulating cTn is highly specific for myocardial cell injury. Correlation of histopathologic findings with biochemistry results showed that elevated cTn values can be directly related to evidence of cardiac myonecrosis in dogs.*

Comparative values for differences in the level of cardiac specificity between cTnI and cTnT have not yet been defined in animals. In humans, however, both markers demonstrated

equivalent specificity for myocardial damage. The author believes that cTnI has some advantage in terms of sensitivity, whereas cTnT appears to have a stronger association with the patient's outcome.

Circulating Cardiac Troponin in Disease

The diagnostic benefit of assessing myocardial injury in dogs and cats through cTn analysis has been shown in numerous studies (Figure 198-1).[2-5,7-12,15,16,23] Circulating cTn levels are frequently above normal in different clinical settings (Box 198-2), even in disease states in which acute myocardial necrosis is not a prominent aspect, such as dilated cardiomyopathy, chronic CHF, cardiac contusion, pericardial disease, or cardiac injury in critically ill patients. In general, increased concentrations of cTnI or cTnT in circulation reflect myocardial damage; thus cTn serves as a means to detect both major and minor injury. An association exists between the magnitude of myocardial damage and serum concentrations of cTn in acute situations; this has been verified by histopathologic testing in canine myocardial infarction,[5,7,11,12,16] gastric dilatation-volvulus syndrome (GDV),[8] canine myocarditis,[2,15,16] and dogs with sepsis.[2] In chronic myocardial disease, however, this relationship is not as obvious, for several reasons. Only minor myocardial injury may be present at the time of cTn determination; also, permanent leakage of cTn leads to a significant reduction in the tissue concentration of cTn over time.[13] Therefore absolute levels of circulating cTn do not necessarily represent the amount of irreversibly damaged myocardium in chronic situations.

In symptomatic canine DCM,[2,9,16] circulating cTn is increased in a significant number of patients (see Figure 198-1), with rather minor elevations being the most common finding.[2,9,16,21] Serial monitoring of cTn has revealed different release patterns (Figure 198-2) that not only define the status of the failing heart with regard to acute myocyte damage, but also provide prognostic information. Progressive left ventricular (LV) remodeling, a hallmark of DCM, leads to intermittent or permanent leakage of cTn into the circulation. In addition, the presence of coronary artery disease with small myocardial infarctions, focal myocarditis, and increased wall strain may contribute to cTn release in heart failure. Elevated concentrations of circulating cTn in such patients reflect ongoing degradation of the contractile apparatus. Presumably, continuous loss

---

*References 2, 5, 7, 8, 12-14, and 16.

Box • 198-2

Clinical Conditions Associated with Elevated Circulating Markers of Myocardial Leakage Recently Reported in Dogs and Cats

Primary Myocardial Disease
Idiopathic dilated cardiomyopathy
Hypertrophic cardiomyopathy
Myocardial contusion

Ischemic Myocardial Disease
Myocarditis/endomyocarditis/
    endocarditis

Congenital Heart Disease
Patent ductus arteriosus
Subaortic stenosis

**Degenerative Cardiac
    Valve Disease**
Mitral valve endocardiosis

Pericardial Disease
Pericarditis
Pericardial effusion

Systemic Disease
Gastric dilatation-volvulus syndrome
Sepsis
Renal failure/uremia
Babesiosis
Body trauma
Hyperthermia

Neurologic Disease
Subarachnoid hemorrhage
Steroid responsive meningoencephalitis
Epilepsy

Endocrine Disease
Hyperthyroidism

Neoplasia
Splenic mass
Lymphosarcoma
Doxorubicin chemotherapy

of cTn facilitates the process of myocyte dysfunction that accompanies the spontaneous progression of heart failure. In humans, an inverse relationship between peak cTn values and LV function, as assessed by echocardiography, has been reported, and detectable cTn was associated with an adverse prognosis. A similar situation may be expected in animals. Clinical improvement in signs of CHF is associated with normalization of cTn levels, which may serve as a biochemical target in the management of DCM. Therefore dynamic monitoring of serum cTn is recommended in animals with heart failure.

Detectable cTn concentrations in blood with asymptomatic DCM is a rare event that recently was described in only one of 28 affected dogs.[2,9,16] For this reason, screening of selected populations of dogs for DCM based on cTn analysis does not seem to provide any advantage over commonly used diagnostic methods. However, with further improvement of

test sensitivities and with large-scale clinical trials in affected breeds, more promising findings may be anticipated.

Analysis of cTn may also be useful in cats with HCM, primarily to identify animals suspected of having inflammatory myocardial lesions or ischemic heart disease as a result of microvessel pathology or intramural coronary artery embolism. Circulating cTn is detectable in almost all cats with HCM, regardless of whether heart failure is present.[2,10,19,21,23] Cats with CHF have higher cTn levels than cats with no clinical signs or those with a history of heart failure.[10] Further studies are needed to determine whether serum cTn levels may be used to differentiate HCM from other types of cardiomyopathy in cats and to obtain reliable prognostic information.

Monitoring of animals undergoing chemotherapy for signs of cardiotoxicity of antineoplastic drugs may be another promising application of cTn analysis. A small-scale clinical trial in dogs

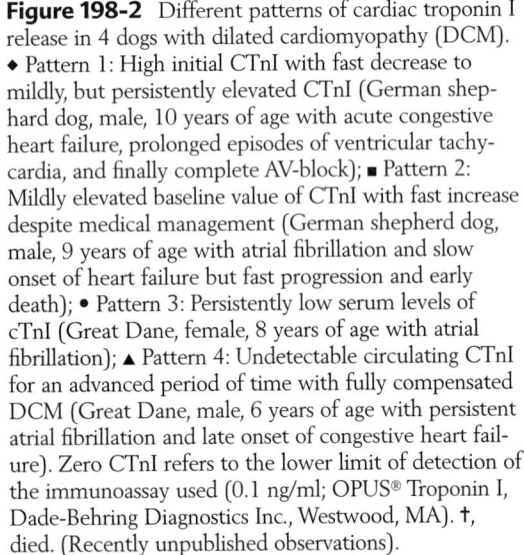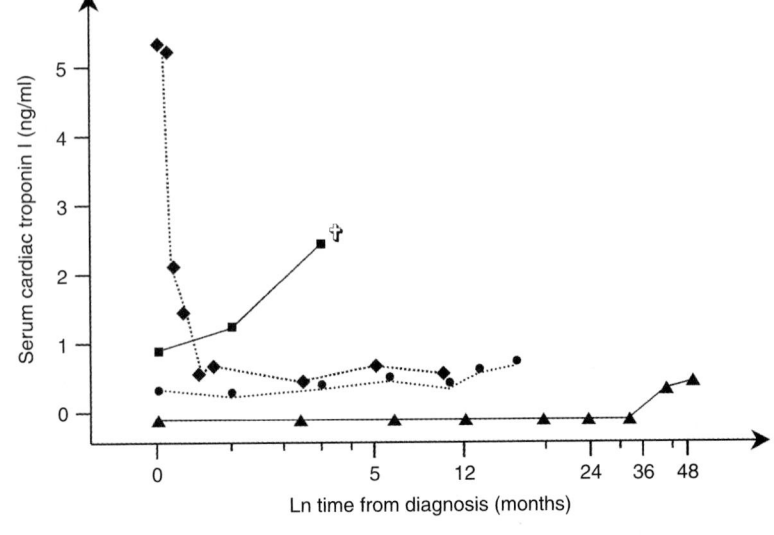

Figure 198-2 Different patterns of cardiac troponin I release in 4 dogs with dilated cardiomyopathy (DCM). ◆ Pattern 1: High initial CTnI with fast decrease to mildly, but persistently elevated CTnI (German shephard dog, male, 10 years of age with acute congestive heart failure, prolonged episodes of ventricular tachycardia, and finally complete AV-block); ■ Pattern 2: Mildly elevated baseline value of CTnI with fast increase despite medical management (German shepherd dog, male, 9 years of age with atrial fibrillation and slow onset of heart failure but fast progression and early death); ● Pattern 3: Persistently low serum levels of cTnI (Great Dane, female, 8 years of age with atrial fibrillation); ▲ Pattern 4: Undetectable circulating CTnI for an advanced period of time with fully compensated DCM (Great Dane, male, 6 years of age with persistent atrial fibrillation and late onset of congestive heart failure). Zero CTnI refers to the lower limit of detection of the immunoassay used (0.1 ng/ml; OPUS® Troponin I, Dade-Behring Diagnostics Inc., Westwood, MA). †, died. (Recently unpublished observations).

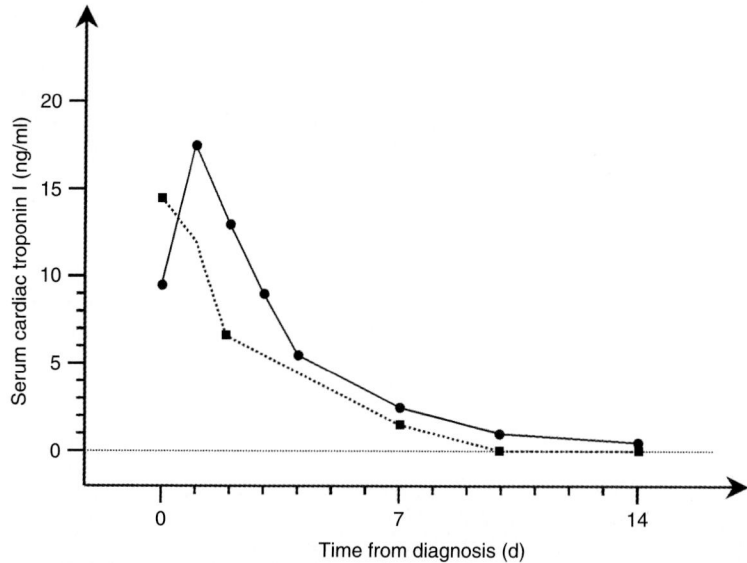

Figure 198-3 Cardiac troponin I release in 2 dogs with suspected acute myocardial necrosis. •, Bobtail, male, 9 years of age with a splenic mass and polymorphic ventricular arrhythmia on days 0, 1, and 2. Splenectomy was done on day 1. ■, Doberman pinscher, female, 2 years old with acute spinal cord trauma on the day before admission and ventricular arrhythmia prior to and after surgery done on day 0. Zero CTnI refers to the lower limit of detection of the immunoassay used (0.1 ng/ml; OPUS® Troponin I, Dade-Behring Diagnostics Inc., Westwood, MA). (Recently unpublished observations).

with lymphosarcoma has provided evidence of detectable myocardial injury at cumulative doses of doxorubicin of at least 150 mg/m².[6] It has been recommended that serum cTnT levels be analyzed 2 to 3 weeks after each dose of doxorubicin beyond a 90 mg/m² cumulative dose. Elevations of cTn may accurately predict the future development of LV systolic dysfunction and ventricular arrhythmias in dogs with anthracycline chemotherapy.

Subendocardial injury caused by increased myocardial stress can induce a rise in cTn in patients with arterial hypertension, tachycardia, aortic and pulmonic stenosis,[2] volume overload, or pulmonary embolism. Alternatively, increased serum concentrations of cTn may occur after severe blunt trauma to the thorax that causes myocardial contusion[3,4,9] or in response to severe hypotension or the release of endogenous substances in critically ill patients (e.g., in animals with multiple organ dysfunction syndrome in GDV or after septic shock).[2,8] The clinical usefulness of serial cTn analyses in detecting myocardial cell injury, predicting electrocardiographic abnormalities, and identifying patients at high risk for a fatal outcome has previously been reported in dogs with GDV.[8] In those studies, the predictive abilities of cTnI and cTnT for an adverse outcome were comparable. Furthermore, increased levels of cTn were observed in dogs with pericardial disease,[2,16,24] suggesting involvement of the myocardium in ischemic, degenerative, or inflammatory processes, and in animals with cerebrovascular events and splenic masses (Figure 198-3), most likely due to myocardial necrosis secondary to abnormal catecholamine release.

Monitoring of circulating cTn may also be useful for assessing myocardial cell damage caused by DC cardioversion or interventional cardiac procedures. In addition, cTn analysis has been used to detect myocyte injury in clinically suspected myocarditis and endomyocarditis in dogs[2] and in experimental myocarditis in laboratory animals. However, the diagnosis of myocarditis can be confirmed only by immune histochemical techniques using tissue samples, which makes unambiguous clinical diagnosis based on elevated cTn concentrations difficult. The extent to which knowledge of the troponin status could affect medical care under these conditions deserves further investigation.

FUNCTIONAL MARKERS

Since the discovery of atrial natriuretic peptide more than 20 years ago, it has been apparent that the heart is not only a simple pump, but also a true endocrine organ that releases specific hormones in response to defined stimuli. Recent studies in humans and preliminary findings in dogs[25-34] and cats[35-37] with heart disease indicate that biochemical markers of cardiovascular function, such as natriuretic peptides (NPs) and endothelin (ET), as well as circulating catecholamines, vasopressin, aldosterone, and cytokines, including tumor necrosis factor-alpha (TNF-alpha), can be used to identify patients with heart disease, to predict disease severity, to monitor therapy, and to obtain prognostic information. In the near future, routine immunoassays for functional marker proteins may provide a preliminary test of cardiac performance and may permit clinicians to more carefully select patients for further investigation and treatment.

Natriuretic Peptides

Natriuretic peptides belong to a unique family of naturally occurring, structurally similar, but genetically distinct hormones that share a central loop containing 17 amino acids closed by a disulfide bond between 2 cysteine residues, with variable carboxy-terminal and amino-terminal tails. The NPs include atrial natriuretic peptides (ANP), brain natriuretic peptides (BNP), C-type natriuretic peptides (CNP), dendroaspis natriuretic peptides (DNP), and urodilatin. The NPs act as key regulators of salt and water homeostasis and blood pressure control. They have potential value as diagnostic and prognostic markers and as therapeutic tools for several clinical conditions associated with expanded fluid volume, such as CHF.

Atrial Natriuretic Peptides and Brain Natriuretic Peptides

Structure ANP is typically produced by the left and right atrium but may also be expressed in the ventricular myocardium, particularly with ventricular hypertrophy or myocardial ischemia. ANP transcripts also may be present in noncardiac tissues. ANP is synthesized as pre-proANP, which contains 153 amino acids in cats.[38] After cleavage of a 25-amino-acid signal peptide, the precursor proANP, consisting of 128 amino acids, is stored in atrial myocyte granules. In response to an adequate stimulus, proANP is split by a membrane-bound protease into inactive 98-amino-acid N-terminal (NT)-proANP and biologically active 30-amino-acid C-terminal ANP on an equimolar basis and released into the blood. NT-proANP may be further cleaved into smaller, endocrinologically active fragments.[38] The amino acid sequences of ANP and CNP have been highly conserved across species. Canine and human mature ANP are structurally very similar.

Under normal conditions, BNP is produced primarily in the cardiac atria, with very little synthesis in the ventricles. In cardiac pathologies with chronic pressure or volume overload or ventricular hypertrophy, ventricular myocytes become the major source of BNP. Minor extracardiac BNP production has also been reported. Unlike with ANP, regulation of BNP synthesis and excretion occurs mainly at the level of gene expression. Cardiac BNP is stored to a much smaller extent than ANP (coexisting with ANP in granules of atrial and ventricular myocardium), therefore increased BNP release requires increased synthesis. BNP arises from a single precursor pre-proBNP molecule containing 132 amino acids in cats.[39] The signal peptide has 26 amino acid residues, followed by 106 amino acids of proBNP. This peptide is further processed into mature, active BNP that has 35 amino acid residues at the C-terminus, with likely 26 and 29 amino acid isomers. The biologically inactive peptide, NT-proBNP, has 71 amino acids in cats.[39] BNP and NT-proBNP are secreted into the circulation in equimolar quantities. Mature BNP in dogs and humans has only 32 amino acid residues. In contrast to ANP, there is much variability in the length and structure of BNP across species, and the predominant forms differ considerably, resulting in variations in cross-species actions.

Physiologic actions   The principal function of NPs is to protect the cardiovascular system from volume overload. The major biologic effects of ANP and BNP are qualitatively similar and include potent natriuresis, diuresis, and balanced vasodilatation. Both NPs antagonize the renin-angiotensin-aldosterone system (RAAS) and the sympathetic nervous system (SNS), inhibit the release and action of vasopressin, prevent myocardial fibrosis, and modulate cell growth and myocardial hypertrophy. In addition to the many other important actions of natriuretic peptides, ANP, in particular, enhances vascular permeability, causing redistribution of plasma volume to the extravascular space. The biologic actions of NPs are mediated by two specific receptors, natriuretic peptide receptor type A (NPR-A) and natriuretic peptide receptor type B (NPR-B). A third natriuretic peptide receptor, NPR-C, mainly acts as a clearance receptor. NPRs are widely distributed throughout the body and can be found in the heart, kidneys, vascular endothelium and smooth muscle, adrenals, and central nervous system.

Release, metabolism, and clearance   ANP secretion is controlled by immediate release from previously synthesized atrial storage granules in direct proportion to atrial stretch,[25,26,29,31,35] which occurs during intravascular volume expansion. Only a minor part is derived from newly synthesized hormone. A second stimulus for ANP secretion is an increase in the heart rate.[26,31,35] The plasma concentration of ANP therefore can change rapidly in response to acute alterations in posture, volume loading, or tachycardia. Thus ANP is a good marker of acute volume overload or of rapid hemodynamic changes. Release of BNP is chiefly controlled at the transcription level, with increased secretion preceded by an increase in messenger ribonucleic acid (mRNA) production. Therefore, in contrast to ANP, a longer term stimulus is required to increase plasma BNP concentrations; this makes BNP blood levels less susceptible to wide fluctuation in response to short-term external stimuli. The production and secretion of BNP are regulated by myocardial stretch and wall tension, primarily that induced by volume load. Circulating BNP is also increased in ventricular dysfunction and in states of ventricular hypertrophy (even in the absence of elevated intraventricular pressure). Atrial production of BNP occurs within 60 minutes of stretch, whereas ventricular production of BNP is stimulated within a few hours. In humans, the plasma half-life of ANP and BNP is approximately 1 to 3 minutes and 20 to 22 minutes, respectively, and that of both N-terminal peptides is 60 to 120 minutes.

Clearance of NPs occurs through two major mechanisms: first, binding to NPR-C, which is followed by endocytosis and subsequent lysosomal degradation, and second, degradation by the nonspecific membrane-bound enzyme neutral

endopeptidase 24.11 (NEP), in a competitive fashion. However, enzymatic degradation via NEP does not seem to be as important for N-terminal fragments, resulting in longer half-lives. A small amount of the NPs is accounted for by renal elimination (less than 15%) and other nonspecific degradative enzymes. The liver, lungs, and especially the kidneys are major sites of extraction of the NPs.

Analysis, storage, and reference intervals   Currently, no consensus exists on the best procedure for measuring NPs in humans and animals, because determination by different immunoassay methods is affected by several analytic problems concerning a lack of sensitivity, specificity, and precision. Commercial assays are not yet standardized, and the results obtained with assays from different manufacturers may differ markedly, affecting reference intervals and decision limits. Commonly used assays for measuring NPs are either competitive immunoassays (radioimmunoassay [RIA] and electroimmunoassay [EIA]) or noncompetitive sandwich immunoassays (IRMA and EIMA). RIA methods use radiolabeled tracers and usually require a time-consuming extraction step before NPs can be measured. In addition, the detection limit of RIA tends to be higher than that of IRMA. IRMA methods are generally highly sensitive and more specific, and extraction and purification of plasma samples are not required. NT-proANP and NT-proBNP are larger molecules than the C-terminal biologically active peptides, which makes it easier to use immunometric assay design to measure them. In addition, much higher plasma concentrations of the N-terminal fragments (20 to 50 times) and longer plasma half-lives lead to high analytic precision. Unlike the universal nature of ANP antibodies, antibodies for BNP are species specific. Therefore, in contrast to assays for ANP and NT-proANP, C- or N-terminal human BNP assays cannot be used in dogs and cats.

The *in vitro* stability of BNP, NT-proBNP, and proANP in ethylenediamine tetra-acetic acid (EDTA) in whole blood at room temperature is sufficient for routine use. BNP is stable for up to 72 hours, even in the absence of aprotinin. NT-proBNP and proANP appear to be stable for up to 48 hours, and NT-proANP for 6 hours, in whole blood. ANP is stable only for 2 to 3 hours in blood at room temperature, it is stable for up to several months in plasma frozen at −80° C.

Because of the lack of assay standardization and the differences in methodology, no generally applicable reference intervals for NPs and their N-terminal prohormone fragments can be defined. In addition, normal plasma concentrations of NPs have been shown to increase with age[27] and to be dependent on gender and body weight.[27] Thus reference limits vary, depending on the nature of the control population and the assay used. In general, circulating ANP and BNP concentrations in normal subjects are very low, ranging from 3 to 15 pmol/L* for different assays, with plasma BNP being lower than ANP. Unlike ANP, circulating BNP does not generally show rapid and wide fluctuations in healthy subjects. A cutoff point for BNP (23 pmol/L) for the detection of heart failure in humans more than 55 years of age was recently suggested (BNP-Triage; Biosite Diagnostics, San Diego, California). Small-scale clinical trials in healthy dogs reported similar values for plasma ANP[25,29,31] using a human RIA (means between 10 and 22 pmol/L) and for plasma BNP using a porcine RIA[25,27] (means of 7.0 and 13.6 pmol/L). Preliminary RIA studies in healthy cats revealed a normal BNP range of 1.6 to 8.3 pmol/L (mean, 3.3 pmol/L).[35] As mentioned earlier, the plasma concentrations of N-terminal NPs are much

*Equivalent units of measurement can be determined as follows: 1 pmol/L of ANP = 3.1 pg/mL; 1 pmol/L of BNP = 3.5 pg/mL; 1 pmol/L of NT-proANP = 10.5 pg/mL; and 1 pmol/L of NT-proBNP = 8.6 pg/mL.

higher than those of ANP[25] and BNP. The NT-proANP concentration has been reported in normal pets (mean, less than 500 pmol/L in dogs[25-27]; and 540 pmol/L in cats),[35] and an optimal cutoff point for cardiac decompensation in Cavalier King Charles spaniels with chronic mitral valve disease (MVD) has been suggested (700 pmol/L).[25]

Circulating Natriuretic Peptides in Disease

In general, the plasma concentrations of the NPs are increased in disease states characterized by an expanded fluid volume, reduced renal clearance of the peptides, and stimulation of peptide production (e.g., disease states caused by ventricular hypertrophy or myocardial strain, tachycardia, hypoxia, ectopic production from tumor, or excessive circulating glucocorticoid or thyroid hormones). However, the most promising use of NPs may be in their diagnostic potential as functional markers of cardiac disease. As with increased levels of circulating cTn, ANP and BNP are not specific for a particular cardiac pathology. Plasma levels of NPs are increased in many disease states, including chronic MVD, DCM, pacing-induced heart failure, aortic stenosis, congenital heart disease, and dirofilariasis in dogs[25,26,29,31-34] and in different types of cardiomyopathy in cats.[35] In addition, elevated concentrations of NPs have been demonstrated in humans with AMI, hypertension, supraventricular tachycardia, cardiac amyloidosis, myocarditis, right ventricular dysfunction and hypertrophy due to chronic respiratory disease, renal failure, and severe LV diastolic dysfunction.

Considering that ANP originates primarily from the atria and BNP from the ventricles, increased circulating levels of these peptides may reflect different abnormalities. Thus, depending on the underlying disease process in heart failure patients, the secretion pattern of ANP and BNP may vary. ANP and NT-proANP have been shown to be more useful than BNP in the overall assessment of disease severity in chronic MVD[25] and cardiac abnormalities characterized by acute volume overload. In addition, particularly high concentrations of NT-proANP have been reported in patients with DCM and atrial fibrillation compared with DCM and sinus rhythm.[26] However, BNP is more sensitive than ANP in detecting chronic LV systolic and diastolic dysfunction and ventricular hypertrophy of any cause. BNP secretion increases in proportion to the severity of LV dysfunction.[32] The negative predictive value is the strongest feature of this peptide in humans (more than 90%); however, the reverse is not true, because the positive predictive value is only 30% to 40% in people. BNP analysis may be used as a screening tool, with a value in the normal range virtually excluding LV systolic dysfunction. However, analysis of BNP is not a stand-alone test. An increase in BNP would always warrant follow-up examinations, such as echocardiography, to identify the underlying cardiac pathology. NT-proBNP and BNP appear to be equivalent markers for the detection of LV dysfunction, but the N-terminus has some clinical advantage with respect to plasma concentration, half-life, and stability.

In contrast to humans, there is limited evidence in dogs and cats suggesting that plasma NPs are useful markers for the detection of LV dysfunction in asymptomatic patients.[32] NT-proANP has been found elevated in only a subset of dogs with asymptomatic chronic MVD[25] or DCM[26] despite significant cardiac enlargement. However, in cats with hypertrophic, restrictive, or unclassified cardiomyopathy and no clinical signs, proANP, NT-proANP and, in particular, BNP were raised. If BNP or its N-terminal fragment emerge as a superior diagnostic marker of LV dysfunction in companion animals with asymptomatic heart disease, it may also be used for routine screening for DCM and HCM in selected, high-risk populations; however, this requires further confirmation. In humans, for the time being, analysis of circulating BNP is the most promising biochemical marker for the diagnosis of CHF and has shown the best characteristics for a screening test.

Circulating NP levels have been shown to correlate with the class of heart failure in dogs,[25,26,29,31-33] and their measurement may allow veterinarians to offer pet owners a more accurate long-term prognosis. Elevated concentrations of BNP and NT-proBNP were found to be independent predictors of increased mortality in humans with CHF and both systolic and diastolic dysfunction. In addition, BNP correlates with right and left ventricular mass and may potentially be used as a marker for ventricular remodeling in hypertension and HCM. ANP as well as BNP may also be clinically useful as a biochemical discriminators of cardiogenic and noncardiogenic cough and dyspnea.

As congestion in heart failure is relieved, the levels of ANP and BNP rapidly regress,[29] thus serial analyses of plasma NPs might also prove useful as a guide to therapy in chronic CHF. Moreover, determination of circulating NPs may be used to identify patients that would likely benefit from therapeutic angiotensin-converting enzyme (ACE) inhibition or beta-receptor blockade. In the future, the treatment of patients with CHF may be tailored by neurohormonal profiling.

Other Natriuretic Peptides

C-type natriuretic peptide is primarily secreted by vascular endothelial cells and has local vasodilatatory and antiproliferative effects. It is usually undetectable in cardiac tissue. DNP was first isolated from the venom of the green mamba snake but has also been found in human plasma. Its importance in small animal cardiology has not yet been determined. Urodilatin (ANP 95-126) is localized in the kidney and secreted into the urine. It is a paracrine factor involved in the local regulation of body fluid volume and water and electrolyte excretion.

ENDOTHELIN

Endothelin (ET) belongs to a family of vasoactive peptides, including ET-1, ET-2, ET-3, and ET-4, that are genetically distinct. ET is composed of 21 amino acids in humans, dogs, and cats and is derived from precursors known as pre-proET, which has 212 amino acid residues. The large precursors undergo intermediate cleavage by endopeptidases to form the biologically inactive proET, also called big ET. Big ET is converted to active ET by endothelin-converting enzyme (ECE), which exerts its effects either locally or after release into the circulation. The predominant form of ET produced by endothelial cells and cardiac myocytes is ET-1. It has a wide spectrum of biologic actions, which are mediated by three receptor subtypes: ET_A, ET_B, and ET_C. ET_A is selective for ET-1, but the other receptor types are considered nonselective. ET-1 is a strong, long-lasting, balanced vasoconstrictive agent with inotropic and mitogenic actions; it is a potent stimulus for activation of the RAAS and SNS and plays an important role in the regulation of vascular tone and blood pressure.

Release of ET is regulated at the level of gene expression and peptide synthesis because cells do not store ET. The ET system is activated and synthesis of ET-1 is induced within minutes in response to a variety of factors, including pulsatile stretch, low shear stress, hypoxia, angiotensin II, epinephrine, cytokines, and growth factors. Most ET-1 (about 90%) is released from endothelial cells abluminally, where it acts on endothelial and smooth muscle cells as an autocrine and paracrine mediator. The concentration of ET in vascular tissue is approximately 100 times higher than in plasma. The plasma half-life of ET-1 in healthy humans is only 1 to 4 minutes because it is rapidly cleared from the circulation by ET_B receptors, the kidneys, and NEP. The plasma ET-1 level therefore may not accurately reflect the synthesis of ET-1. The plasma big ET-1 level has been proposed as a more reliable measure of ET-1 synthesis because its removal from the circulation is slower and less variable.

Plasma ET currently is analyzed either by RIA or by enzyme-linked immunosorbent assay (ELISA). In healthy humans, the plasma ET-1 concentration ranges from 1 to 5 pg/mL. Preliminary results from small scale clinical studies in healthy dogs[40] and cats[37] reported mean (±SD) plasma ET-1 concentrations of 2.07 ± 0.15 pg/mL and 0.805 ± 0.230 fmol/mL, respectively. However, many problems are still associated with the measurement and interpretation of plasma ET-1 concentrations, because the assays available are not yet standardized. In dogs, plasma ET immunoreactivity can be broken down as about 60% big ET-1, 30% ET-1, and 10% ET-3.[30] Because of marked cross-reactivity of the ET antibodies used in current assays, the more realistic term *ET-like immunoreactivity* should be used, rather than "ET-1 concentration."

There is compelling evidence that the ET system is activated in CHF in people, dogs[33-40], and cats[37] and therefore may be diagnostically useful. Plasma ET–like immunoreactivity is increased twofold to tenfold in CHF compared with controls, regardless of disease etiology, and the magnitude of elevation correlates with hemodynamic compromise and functional class in people and small animals.[37,40] The plasma level of ET appears to be a less powerful discriminator between patients with asymptomatic or mild CHF and control subjects with normal function compared with BNP, NT-proBNP, and NT-proANP but is equally sensitive for predicting short-term mortality. An alternative approach may be measurement of the salivary ET concentration. In addition, ET seems to be important in the pathogenesis of primary and secondary pulmonary hypertension, and a close correlation between plasma ET-1 levels and the extent of pulmonary circulatory abnormalities has been identified in dogs[40] and people. This relationship is unique and deserves further attention with regard to the diagnostic and therapeutic potential of ET-1 and ET-1 antagonists in pulmonary hypertension.

OTHER MARKERS OF CARDIOVASCULAR FUNCTION

TNF-alpha is a proinflammatory cytokine that seems to be involved in the pathophysiology of CHF. It is produced mainly by activated macrophages but is also expressed in failing cardiac tissue. TNF-alpha has a variety of biologic effects, including induction of cachexia, ventricular systolic dysfunction, pulmonary edema, and direct myocardial cytotoxicity. Moreover, it may play a role in apoptosis, cell dropout, and myocardial fibrosis associated with ventricular remodeling, leading to progression of heart failure. The bioactivity of TNF-alpha and its soluble receptors in serum is likely to be increased in patients with chronic CHF,[36] particularly in association with increased severity of disease. As such, TNF-alpha may be used as a marker of disease progression. In addition, increased circulating concentrations of TNF-alpha may provide a potential target for therapeutic interventions.

Considerable evidence in humans indicates the presence of abnormal endothelial function in patients with CHF, resulting in impaired tissue perfusion, myocardial ischemia, and vascular remodeling. Elevated levels of proinflammatory cytokines, increased vasomotor tone, and reduced vasodilator response to exercise may be responsible for the impairment of endothelium-dependent vasodilatation. Nitric oxide (NO), also called *endothelium-derived relaxing factor (EDRF)*, has important regulatory functions in the cardiovascular system. As with NPs, NO is a functional antagonist of ET and angiotensin II. It is expressed in the vascular endothelium and the myocardium. In heart failure, endothelial release of NO is impaired and myocardial NO synthesis is increased, leading to reduced vasodilatation, negative inotropic and chronotropic effects, and loss of cardiomyocytes. Circulating NO has previously been used as a functional marker of cardiovascular disease in humans. Prospective studies in dogs and cats are needed to determine the exact role of NO as a circulating biomarker of disease.[41,42]

Adrenomedullin is another vasodilating and natriuretic peptide that shows increased plasma concentrations with heart failure. The blood levels of adrenomedullin correlate with the pulmonary artery and pulmonary wedge pressures in patients with CHF and therefore may be used as a marker of pulmonary hypertension. However, its diagnostic importance has not yet been elucidated in companion animals.

CHAPTER • 199

Therapy of Heart Failure

Barret J. Bulmer
D. David Sisson

Heart failure may be recognized as a clinical end-point in nearly all cardiac diseases. Because the underlying cause of the development of heart failure varies significantly between species and disease conditions, it is often difficult to define heart failure accurately and concisely. In 1994, a panel of the National Heart, Lung and Blood Institute concluded:

Heart failure occurs when an abnormality of cardiac function causes the heart to fail to pump blood at a rate required by the metabolizing tissues or when the heart can do so only with an elevated filling pressure. The heart's inability to pump a sufficient amount of blood to meet the needs of the body tissues may be due to insufficient or defective cardiac filling and/or impaired contraction and emptying. Compensatory mechanisms increase blood volume and raise cardiac filling pressures, heart rate, and cardiac muscle mass to maintain the heart's pumping function and cause redistribution of blood flow. Eventually, however, despite these compensatory mechanisms, the ability of the heart to contract and relax declines progressively, and the heart failure worsens.[1]

Because all cardiac diseases have the potential to produce heart failure through similar mechanisms, we frequently view their pathophysiology and therapy from a unified perspective. Agents that promote preload and afterload reduction are used to control the clinical signs associated with elevated filling pressures, and neurohormonal modulators are prescribed to blunt the progressive nature of heart disease. This approach allows clinical experience and research to be extrapolated across a wide range of diseases. Although the remainder of this chapter is written primarily from a unified perspective, caution must be exercised to ensure that the variations within cardiovascular diseases are not forgotten.

PHASES OF HEART FAILURE

Currently, three distinct phases of heart failure are recognized. Phase 1 constitutes the initial cardiac injury. This phase most frequently passes silently, without detectable clinical signs, because compensatory mechanisms (phase 2) are quickly activated (Figure 199-1). Ultimately, myocardial hypertrophy accounts for the long-term stabilization of cardiac output and the normalization of afterload. Unfortunately, the natural history of cardiac disease often is progressive, and the heart's ability to hypertrophy is overwhelmed. The previously beneficial short-term compensatory mechanisms now serve only to increase both preload (contributing to the development of congestion) and afterload (increasing myocardial work and oxygen demand). Often a heart murmur, gallop rhythm, cardiac arrhythmia, or cardiomegaly may be identified during this second phase despite the absence of significant or activity-limiting clinical signs. Phase 3 of heart failure is recognized by the emergence of clinical signs (e.g., exercise intolerance, lethargy, coughing, tachypnea) at rest or with minimal activity. Veterinary patients apparently do not show clinical signs that

are recognized by their owners until very late in the disease process. Presumably this may skew our understanding of the natural history of canine and feline cardiovascular disease. This understanding of disease progression is further clouded by the recognition that, depending on the disease process, the first clinical event may be the development of systemic thromboembolism, syncopal episodes, or possibly sudden death.

NATURAL HISTORY OF CARDIOVASCULAR DISEASE

Despite decades of treatment of cardiovascular disease in companion animals, relatively few studies have reported on the survival characteristics of patients afflicted with dilated cardiomyopathy,[2-4] mitral insufficiency,[5] and hypertrophic cardiomyopathy.[6] The spectrum of clinical signs, therapeutic strategies, breed differences, and disease sequelae hampers the formation of any sweeping conclusions regarding the natural history of these cardiovascular diseases; however, some generalities may be recognized. After dilated cardiomyopathy has been diagnosed, the survival curve drops precipitously for the first 3 months, with median survival times from two retrospective studies reported as 27 days and 65 days.[2,3] Months 3 through 6 continue to see a large number of dropouts, although interestingly, the curves appear to flatten markedly at approximately 6 months after the initial diagnosis (Figure 199-2). Whether this represents differences in individual responses to therapy or in the severity of disease at the time of diagnosis is difficult to ascertain.

Analysis of the survival curves for cats with hypertrophic cardiomyopathy presenting with congestive heart failure (CHF) or aortic thromboembolism (ATE) that lived for greater than 24 hours initially showed a steep slope similar to that seen in dogs with dilated cardiomyopathy (Figure 199-3).[6] Approximately 25% of the CHF group and 40% of the ATE group died within 3 months of diagnosis. After 3 months, cats presenting for congestive heart failure began to display a less

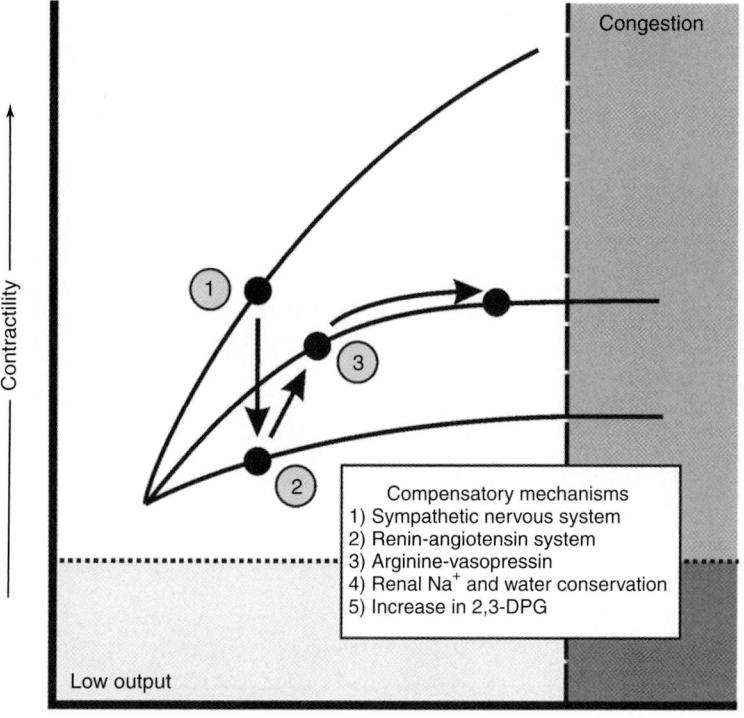

Figure 199-1 The short-term compensatory mechanisms that help normalize cardiac output during the initial injury often prove detrimental in the face of long-standing cardiac disease.

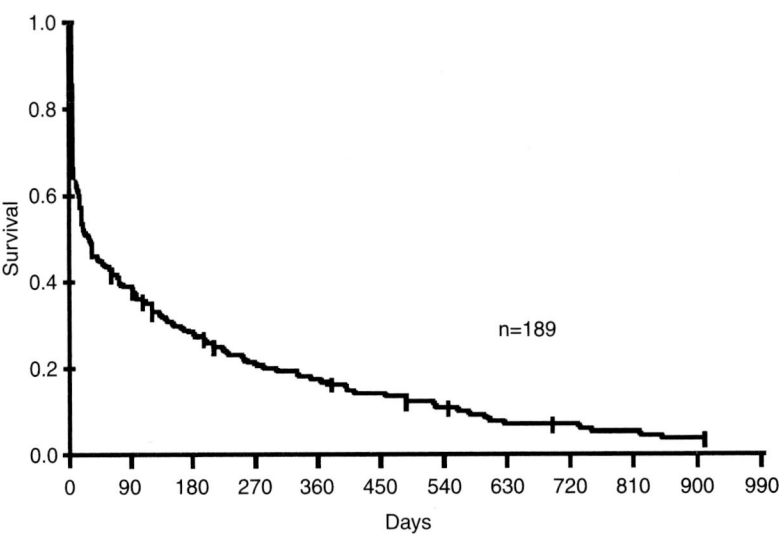

Figure 199-2 Historically the survival of dogs with dilated cardiomyopathy has been poor, presumably because the disease is significantly advanced at the time of diagnosis. Whether earlier identification of occult DCM, with subsequent administration of neurohormonal antagonists (beta blockers, aldosterone antagonists, ACE inhibitors) or potent positive inotropes (pimobendan), could alter this disease course is uncertain. (From Tidholm A: Survival and prognostic factors in 189 dogs with dilated cardiomyopathy. *J Am Anim Hosp Assoc* 33:4, 1997.)

steep, linear survival curve that concluded in a plateau several years after the diagnosis. The survival curve for cats with ATE also displayed some flattening after the first 3 months, although it ultimately remained linear for the rest of the study period. The median survival times were 563 days and 184 days, respectively, for cats with congestive heart failure and those with aortic thromboembolism.[6] Cats with subclinical hypertrophic cardiomyopathy were significantly more likely to die of noncardiac disease (P <0.001) and displayed a linear mortality curve for the first 4 years, followed by a prolonged plateau for an additional 4 years.[6]

Interestingly, although mitral insufficiency is the most commonly recognized cardiovascular condition in dogs, the natural history and mortality characteristics after the development of

congestive heart failure have received little attention. Investigators for the Long-Term Investigation of Veterinary Enalapril (LIVE) study evaluated the time to treatment failure for dogs with congestive heart failure treated with enalapril and standard medical therapy (furosemide with or without digoxin) versus those treated with placebo and standard medical therapy.[5] In the mitral insufficiency subgroup, the number of dogs remaining in the study randomized to placebo mimicked the survival curve of dogs with dilated cardiomyopathy. A relatively high dropout rate was seen over the first 50 days, followed by a prolonged period of stability. The data for dogs randomized to enalapril did not display this steep dropout rate, but rather formed a linear curve from the time of enrollment until completion of the study.[5]

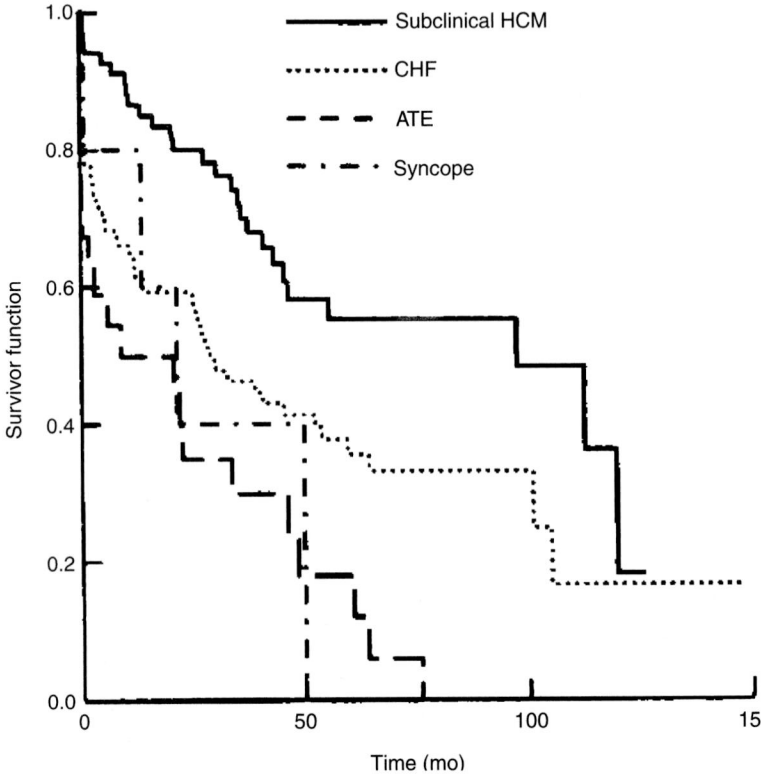

Figure 199-3 The variable presentation and treatment regimens associated with feline hypertrophic cardiomyopathy make evaluation of survival curves difficult. Not surprisingly, symptomatic cats appear to fare worse than those without clinical signs, many of which eventually died of noncardiac disease. (From Rush JE: Population and survival characteristics of cats with hypertrophic cardiomyopathy: 260 cases [1990-1999]. *J Am Vet Med Assoc* 220:2, 2002.)

INFLUENCES ON THE NATURAL HISTORY

Unlike in the management of heart disease in humans, veterinary medicine has the profound ability to influence the natural history of cardiovascular disease in companion animals through the use of euthanasia. The ready access to euthanasia in veterinary medicine not only influences patients' survival times, but also may alter the clinician's responsibilities in treating the heart failure. A study by Mallery et al.[7] evaluated the factors that contributed to clients' decision for euthanasia for 38 dogs with congestive heart failure. The most important factors cited were a perceived poor prognosis (37%), recurrent signs of congestive heart failure (26%), and poor quality of life (13%).[7] Common contributing factors included weakness (76%), anorexia (68%), recurrent clinical signs of congestive heart failure (55%), and a poor prognosis (42%).[7] These findings suggest that the goals of the practitioner should include careful client education before and after initiation of medical therapy, along with efforts to improve the patient's strength, appetite, and quality of life, possibly at the expense of prolonged survival.

CLASSIFICATION OF HEART FAILURE

Some measure of subjective criteria must be used to classify the degree of disability in veterinary patients in order to optimize the management and understanding of heart failure. Because the human classification system is based on signs and symptoms evident at rest and during exercise, it does not easily correlate with disease in often sedentary veterinary patients. The International Small Animal Cardiac Health Council has devised a classification scheme based on anatomic diagnosis and the severity of clinical signs at rest.

Asymptomatic Patient

Heart disease is detectable, but the patient is not overtly affected and does not demonstrate clinical signs of heart failure. Diagnostic findings could include a cardiac murmur, arrhythmia, or cardiac chamber enlargement detected by radiography or echocardiography. The subcategories of this stage are:
- No signs of compensation (e.g., volume or pressure overload ventricular hypertrophy) are evident.
- Radiographic or echocardiographic evidence of compensation (e.g., volume or pressure overload ventricular hypertrophy) is present.

Mild to Moderate Heart Failure

Clinical signs of heart failure are evident at rest or with mild exercise and adversely affect the quality of life. Typical signs of heart failure include exercise intolerance, cough, tachypnea, mild respiratory distress (dyspnea), and mild to moderate ascites. Hypoperfusion at rest generally is not present.

Advanced Heart Failure

Clinical signs of advanced congestive heart failure are immediately obvious. These include respiratory distress (dyspnea), marked ascites, profound exercise intolerance, and hypoperfusion at rest. In the most severe cases, the patient is moribund and suffers from cardiogenic shock. Death or severe debilitation is likely without therapy.

Many patients present acutely for respiratory distress despite the absence of significant clinical signs before the "inciting" event. Owners may report one to several days of tachypnea with or without coughing, nocturnal dyspnea, lethargy, weakness, and inappetence. Cats with congestive heart failure may present acutely for severe respiratory distress because they were able to hide successfully for several days before the owner could detect a problem. Astute owners may present patients with mild to moderate heart failure for evaluation of exercise intolerance or subtle changes in the respiratory pattern. Patients with right-sided heart failure may be presented for evaluation of unexplained weight gain. At the far end of the spectrum from acute heart failure are patients that are re-evaluated for refractory congestive heart failure despite aggressive medical management. These patients may be re-evaluated for recurrent signs of congestive heart failure (i.e., pulmonary edema, pleural effusion, or ascites), weight loss and inappetence, or profound exercise intolerance and malaise. Effective management of acute, chronic, and refractory heart failure requires specific aims and strategies that target the appropriate mechanisms.

TREATMENT STRATEGIES

Management of Acute Decompensated Congestive Heart Failure

Dogs with dilated cardiomyopathy or mitral regurgitation often present with acute onset of coughing, dyspnea, restlessness, orthopnea, and weakness subsequent to the development of severe pulmonary edema and/or low cardiac output. The immediate priorities in these patients are resolution of the pulmonary edema, maintenance of adequate tissue perfusion pressure, and adequate delivery of blood flow to vital tissues. These goals must be achieved quickly, therefore it is important that the practitioner use drugs with proven hemodynamic benefits and a rapid onset of action.

Oxygen Supplementation

As left atrial and pulmonary capillary pressures increase and the lymphatics' capacity to remove fluid is overwhelmed, the interstitial space and alveoli become flooded. Because these flooded alveoli lack ventilation and represent areas of functional shunting, oxygen administration must be combined with agents that effectively lower pulmonary venous pressure. Oxygen can easily be administered to compromised patients by provision of an oxygen-enriched environment (i.e., oxygen cage) or by use of nasal insufflation, achieving maximal inspired oxygen concentrations of 40% to 90%, respectively.

Reduction of Pulmonary Venous Pressure

Rapid reduction of pulmonary venous pressure is most readily achieved through use of a combination of intravenous (IV) drugs that lower the circulating plasma volume and redistribute the intravascular volume. Intravenous furosemide (2 to 8 mg/kg) should be administered to dogs with severe pulmonary edema to promote natriuresis and diuresis quickly. These large doses may be repeated (initially every 1 to 2 hours) until the respiratory rate and dyspnea start to decline. After stabilization, the dose should be reduced (2 to 4 mg/kg every 8 to 12 hours), because excessive administration may lead to profound dehydration, electrolyte depletion, renal failure, low cardiac output, and circulatory collapse.

Drugs that decrease preload (to combat congestion) and afterload (to decrease myocardial work) are administered concurrently with furosemide. Intravenous sodium nitroprusside is a potent, ultrarapid, balanced vasodilator that seems to reduce pulmonary venous pressure quickly and effectively. When used in animals with congestive heart failure, nitroprusside decreases right atrial and pulmonary capillary wedge pressures and systemic vascular resistance and increases cardiac output.[8] Although hypotension and tachycardia are reported side effects, the reduction in systemic vascular resistance (SVR) is theoretically associated with an increase in cardiac output (CO) that serves to maintain systemic arterial blood pressure (BP = SVR × CO). Nausea, vomiting, and cyanide toxicity during prolonged administration are other reported side effects. Because of its short half-life, nitroprusside, mixed with 5% dextrose, must be administered by constant-rate infusion (CRI). After institution of an initial dose of 1 µg/kg/min, the rate is slowly titrated upward while the blood pressure is monitored. An infusion rate of 2 to 5 µg/kg/min usually is sufficient to decrease afterload, although rarely doses as high as 10 µg/kg/min may be required. If significant hypotension is encountered after administration of nitroprusside, slowing the infusion rate generally is effective at raising the blood pressure to acceptable levels.

Sodium nitroprusside Nitroprusside is an intravenous preparation with potent arteriolar and venous vasodilative properties mediated by the formation of nitric oxide and subsequently the second messenger cyclic guanosine monophosphate (cGMP). To some degree, the combination of nitroprusside and dobutamine can be considered short-term "cardiac life support," used primarily during an attempt to rescue dogs with severe, life-threatening pulmonary edema subsequent to dilated cardiomyopathy. This drug combination's ability to reduce afterload quickly appears to be beneficial also in patients with chronic degenerative valvular disease and pulmonary edema, although management of these cases often can be accomplished less intensively.

Unfortunately, the beneficial hemodynamic profile of nitroprusside is accompanied by a difficult administration protocol that requires intensive monitoring. Because nitroprusside produces an almost immediate and often profound reduction in systemic vascular resistance, continuous blood pressure monitoring throughout administration is recommended. The drug is light sensitive, is given by constant-rate infusion (typically 2 to 5 µg/kg/min), and should not be infused with another agent, which necessitates placement of a second intravenous catheter for administration of dobutamine. These stringent requirements may provide cause for more frequent use of intravenous bipyridines to combat life-threatening heart failure, at least until studies are able to elucidate whether either method produces better results.

If nitroprusside is unavailable, balanced vasodilatation may be attempted through administration of an arterial vasodilator (hydralazine, 0.5 to 2 mg/kg given orally) in combination with a venodilator (nitroglycerin ointment, ¼- to ¾-inch applied cutaneously every 8 to 12 hours; or isosorbide dinitrate, 0.5 to 2 mg/kg given orally every 8 hours). Although easier to administer, this therapy seems to be less effective at quickly reducing pulmonary venous pressure compared with nitroprusside.

Potent afterload reduction in patients with severe mitral insufficiency and large regurgitant volumes serves to decrease the left ventricular to left atrial pressure gradient and hence the volume of insufficiency. Nitroprusside, or possibly hydralazine, can effectively decrease the volume of mitral regurgitation and lower left atrial pressure in cases of severe CHF subsequent to rupture of the chordae tendineae or the onset of atrial fibrillation. Despite this obvious theoretical advantage, a recent human study showed that mitral regurgitation worsened in four of nine patients with mitral valve prolapse during nitroprusside infusion.[9] This finding highlights the point that adjustments in the therapeutic regimen may be required and should be based on patient response rather than physiologic principles.

Augmentation of Systolic Performance

Preload reducing agents, such as furosemide, cannot enhance systolic function and in fact at high doses serve only to decrease cardiac output. Therefore the use of a rapid-acting, intravenous inotropic agent is vital to the management of acute decompensated congestive heart failure in dogs with dilated cardiomyopathy. Although there is debate over whether dogs with mitral valve insufficiency have systolic dysfunction, acutely positive inotropic agents may serve to decrease the regurgitant orifice area and hence the volume of insufficiency.

The short-acting, positive inotropic agents most commonly used to manage decompensated heart failure increase cyclic adenosine monophosphate (cAMP). Dobutamine and dopamine are sympathomimetic agents that bind to beta$_1$ receptors, thereby stimulating adenylyl cyclase activity and production of cAMP. The bipyridines amrinone and milrinone increase cAMP by preventing its degradation by phosphodiesterase. Both drug classes are capable of rapidly augmenting systolic function during constant-rate intravenous infusions. By increasing cytosolic cAMP, these agents enhance (1) calcium entry into the cell, promoting ventricular contraction; (2) diastolic calcium uptake by the sarcoplasmic reticulum, promoting ventricular relaxation; and (3) peripheral vasodilatation, reducing afterload. It should be remembered that the sympathomimetics also have alpha-agonistic properties that promote vasoconstriction. Unfortunately, both the sympathomimetics and the bipyridines may promote tachycardia and undesirable ventricular arrhythmias. Therefore careful electrocardiographic (ECG) monitoring is required during administration of these drugs, and significant or worsening ventricular arrhythmias may warrant discontinuation of the infusion and institution of antiarrhythmic therapy.

Sympathomimetics The sympathomimetics enhance cardiac contractility by complexing with myocardial beta receptors. After substrate binding to an unoccupied beta receptor, a coupled G-protein stimulates the enzyme cyclase to produce cAMP. This second-messenger "effector" system acts by means of protein kinase A to phosphorylate intracellular proteins, including the L-type calcium channel, phospholamban, and troponin I, thereby enhancing ventricular contraction and relaxation. Despite the sympathomimetics' ability to increase cardiac contractility approximately 100% above baseline, not all drugs in this class are suitable for the management of heart failure. The specificity for beta receptor binding depends on the specific agent and dose administered. Sympathomimetics inappropriate for the management of heart failure include the pure beta agonist isoproterenol and the naturally occurring catecholamines norepinephrine and epinephrine. These agents tend to promote tachycardia, arrhythmias, and untoward alterations in systemic vascular resistance.

Dobutamine and dopamine are more appropriate sympathomimetics for the management of heart failure. Although both drugs can enhance cardiac contractility, several drawbacks discourage long-term use: (1) they must be given intravenously, because successful oral administration is precluded by extensive first-pass hepatic metabolism; (2) because of their extremely short half-lives (approximately 1 to 2 minutes), they must be administered by constant-rate infusion; (3) almost any positive inotropic response tends to increase myocardial work and thus the propensity for ventricular arrhythmias; and (4) after 24 to 48 hours of constant-rate infusion, their positive inotropic response is limited by beta receptor downregulation and uncoupling. The tendency for long-term sympathomimetic administration to increase mortality, as documented in humans, appears to relegate these agents to short-term management of acute, life-threatening heart failure.

Dobutamine Dobutamine is a synthetic analog of dopamine that displays predominately beta$_1$ receptor binding (beta$_1$ > beta$_2$ > alpha). Dobutamine is able to increase cardiac contractility and thus cardiac output without causing a profound, concomitant increase in the heart rate. The mechanism underlying the lack of a positive chronotropic response is not well understood, but this characteristic tends to make dobutamine the most appropriate agent for short-term treatment of heart failure. It appears that complexing with vasodilative beta receptors and vasoconstrictive alpha receptors, combined with an increase in cardiac output, maintains arterial blood pressure at near baseline values. If the systolic blood pressure is normal to elevated, dobutamine infusion (slow titration up to

5 to 15 µg/kg/min in 5% dextrose) can be combined with the potent vasodilator nitroprusside in an attempt to decrease internal cardiac work and further enhance forward blood flow. Continuous ECG and blood pressure monitoring is recommended during this treatment regimen, and exacerbation of tachycardia or ventricular arrhythmias may necessitate discontinuation of dobutamine.

Dopamine   A precursor of norepinephrine, dopamine can bind myocardial beta receptors in addition to peripherally located dopaminergic, beta$_2$, and alpha receptors. Within the renal, mesenteric, coronary, and cerebral vascular beds, these dopaminergic DA$_2$ receptors are able to promote vasodilation at low infusion rates of dopamine (1 to 2 µg/kg/min). However, at higher infusion rates (10 to 20 µg/kg/min), these vasodilative properties are over-ridden by an undesirable, alpha-mediated vasoconstrictive response. Also, high doses are accompanied by increases in the heart rate, the likelihood of arrhythmogenesis, the release of norepinephrine, and the myocardial oxygen demand. Dopamine (slow titration up to 1 to 10 µg/kg/min) may be used in situations similar to those in which dobutamine is appropriate (e.g., profound myocardial failure) and may further enhance renal blood flow. For the authors, an increased propensity for the development of tachycardia relegates dopamine to the role of second-choice drug. As with dobutamine, careful ECG and blood pressure monitoring is indicated during dopamine administration.

Bipyridines   Similar to the sympathomimetics, the bipyridines promote an increase in cardiac contractility by increasing cytosolic cAMP levels. However, rather than directly enhancing the production of cAMP, they increase circulating levels by inhibiting phosphodiesterase III, the enzyme responsible for cAMP inactivation. Unlike the sympathomimetics, the bipyridines do not rely on beta-adrenergic receptors and therefore are less affected by downregulation and uncoupling. Furthermore, because phosphodiesterase inhibitors increase vascular smooth muscle cAMP without displaying affinity for alpha receptors, they are also vasodilators. Because of the bipyridines' combination of positive inotropic and vasodilative properties, the term *inodilators* has come into use for these agents. Because they increase cytosolic calcium and myocardial work, they inherently carry the caveats of tachycardia and ventricular arrhythmias. In fact, the 28% increase in all-cause mortality identified in humans randomized to oral milrinone versus placebo has severely limited further attempts to evaluate agents that act via cAMP-dependent mechanisms.[10]

Milrinone   The phosphodiesterase inhibitor milrinone is substantially more potent than amrinone and is available in an intravenous preparation. Because of its combined positive inotropic and vasodilative properties, milrinone may be used as a substitute for the dobutamine/nitroprusside combination in the management of acute life-threatening heart failure. Despite milrinone's ability to increase measures of fractional shortening after oral administration in dogs, this formulation is no longer available for prescription.[11]

There are no published reports regarding the hemodynamic effects of intravenous milrinone administered to dogs with acute myocardial failure. When administered to normal dogs at an infusion rate of 1 to 10 µg/kg/min, milrinone increased cardiac contractility 50% to 140%.[12] Whether similar doses are efficacious in dogs with heart failure is uncertain, and dosing recommendations currently are difficult to propose. Because CRI milrinone requires 10 to 30 minutes to reach maximal peak effects in normal dogs, it may be prudent to administer a loading dose, followed by constant-rate infusion. Theoretical administration guidelines after the bolus would be to titrate the infusion rate upward slowly while monitoring the systemic blood pressure and a continuous electrocardiogram. Efficacy may be monitored clinically (e.g., reduction in the respiratory rate, alleviation of orthopnea) or echocardiographically with periodic measures of systolic function.

Amrinone   The effects of amrinone are almost identical to those of milrinone except that it does not appear to be as potent. Although there are no reports of its large-scale use in the management of acute decompensated congestive heart failure, treatment recommendations have been extrapolated from studies of normal dogs. Constant-rate infusions of 10 to 100 µg/kg/min appear to be capable of increasing cardiac contractility by 10% to 80% in awake, normal dogs.[12] Anesthetized dogs showed a 15% increase in the heart rate at an infusion rate of 30 µg/kg/min and a 20% increase at 100 µg/kg/min.[12] This tachycardia may have been induced either directly, through cAMP stimulation, or indirectly, in response to a decrease in blood pressure. The 30 µg/kg/min infusion rate was associated with a 10% decrease in blood pressure, whereas the 100 µg/kg/min rate reduced blood pressure by 30%.[12] After institution of a CRI, amrinone requires approximately 45 minutes to reach peak effect. Therefore, similar to milrinone, it appears most appropriate to administer a slow IV bolus of 1 to 3 mg/kg, followed by a slowly up-titrated CRI of 10 to 100 µg/kg/min. Continuous ECG monitoring should be instituted to allow evaluation for excessive tachycardia or arrhythmogenesis, and the systemic blood pressure should be monitored to avoid hypotension.

Management of Acute Heart Failure Secondary to Diastolic Dysfunction

Cats with hypertrophic cardiomyopathy (HCM) often present with signs of respiratory distress subsequent to the development of pulmonary edema or pleural effusion. Impaired ventricular relaxation produces elevated atrial and venous pressures, with eventual fluid exudation into the alveoli or pleural space. The treatment goals for cats with HCM and heart failure focus on relieving congestion through preload reduction rather than augmenting systolic function or decreasing afterload.

PROGRESSION OF HEART FAILURE (THE HUMAN EXPERIENCE)

Traditionally heart failure has been perceived as a hemodynamic disorder that promotes weakness, the development of debilitating congestive signs, deterioration of cardiac function, and ultimately death. Although the initial cardiac insult varies, it was historically rationalized that ventricular remodeling and disease progression occur as consequences of the compensatory mechanisms that promote vasoconstriction and fluid retention. It was recognized that diseased hearts operate on a depressed and flattened Frank-Starling curve, such that volume retention and vasoconstriction, rather than promoting cardiac output, merely exacerbated congestive heart failure. The symptoms of heart failure developed as venous pressures breached the lymphatics' ability to remove edema or as blood flow to exercising muscles was severely limited.

If disease progression were solely mediated by hemodynamic alterations, it was hypothesized, drugs capable of "unloading" the heart (e.g., vasodilators and positive inotropes) would retard this progression and improve survival. In the first Veterans Affairs Heart Failure Trial (V-HeFT) completed in 1985, prazosin or a combination of hydralazine and isosorbide dinitrate was used to decrease preload and afterload.[13] Although prazosin was more effective at reducing blood pressure, only the hydralazine/isosorbide dinitrate combination reduced mortality compared with placebo. The discordance between the hemodynamic and prognostic findings could not be explained by the traditional perception of heart failure. Support for the hemodynamic hypothesis was further undermined by the Prospective Randomized Amlodipine Survival Evaluation (PRAISE) trial completed in December of 1994, which found that administration of amlodipine to patients with severe chronic heart failure had no significant effect on mortality.[14]

Similar to the use of vasodilators to decrease ventricular wall stress and increase cardiac output, potent inotropic drugs capable of increasing cAMP levels were developed with the intent to improve survival. If poor pump performance were responsible for the progressive nature of heart failure, it was hypothesized, these positive inotropes should alter the natural course of cardiovascular disease. The phosphodiesterase inhibitor milrinone, which has potent inotropic and vasodilative properties, in fact was found to alter the course of heart failure but in a fashion opposite that expected. In October of 1990, the Prospective Randomized Milrinone Survival Evaluation (PROMISE) trial was stopped 5 months prior to its scheduled completion date because administration of oral milrinone was found to increase all-cause mortality by 28%.[10] Patients with the severest symptoms (i.e., New York Heart Association [NYHA] class IV), who therefore would be the most likely to receive additional medical therapy, showed a 53% increase in mortality. Administration of the partial beta-agonist xamoterol also failed to improve survival in a study of 516 patients.[15]

These drug trial failures were accompanied in the late 1980s and early 1990s by an evolution in the understanding of the traditional hemodynamic model of heart failure. It still was recognized that hemodynamic alterations accounted for the symptomatic manifestations of cardiac disease, but a new understanding of the condition resulted in the conclusion that the body's compensatory neurohormonal mechanisms contributed to the dilemma of disease progression. Activation of the sympathetic nervous system (SNS) and the renin-angiotensin system (RAS) was found to promote both adverse hemodynamic consequences and direct toxic effects on the myocardium. Cultured mammalian cardiomyocytes exposed to norepinephrine displayed a concentration-dependent decrease in viability that was attenuated significantly by beta-receptor blockade.[16] In addition, norepinephrine was implicated in the provocation of ventricular arrhythmias and the impairment of sodium excretion by the kidneys.[17] Pathophysiologic levels of angiotensin II were found to promote myocytolysis with subsequent fibroblast proliferation, and aldosterone was implicated in the process of myocardial extracellular matrix remodeling.[18,19] These findings established a connection between hemodynamic mechanisms and neurohormonal consequences, which mutually promote a cycle of disease progression. The initial cardiac insult is followed by activation of neurohormonal compensatory mechanisms that produce further hemodynamic alterations and myocardial fibrosis. Cardiac output continues to decline, the compensatory mechanisms continue to be activated, and the disease process proceeds unabated.

This more complete understanding of the neurohormonal systems led to the development and use of drugs designed to antagonize the RAS. A breakthrough in the management of cardiovascular disease came with the utilization of angiotensin-converting enzyme (ACE) inhibitors in the mid to late 1980's. Angiotensin-converting enzyme is capable of degrading vasodilative bradykinin and is responsible for cleaving relatively inactive angiotensin I to the potent vasoconstrictor angiotensin II (AT II). Indirectly ACE is responsible for aldosterone production, because AT II is a primary stimulus for adrenal gland production of mineralocorticoids. Given angiotensin-converting enzyme's critical position in the RAS, it was proposed that ACE inhibition may promote beneficial hemodynamic and neurohormonal antagonistic and antifibrotic actions.

The ACE inhibitor enalapril has been extensively studied in humans with varying stages of heart failure. In three studies,[20-22] compared with placebo or the combination of hydralazine and isosorbide dinitrate, enalapril reduced all-cause mortality in humans with a reduced ejection fraction and heart failure.

In another study,[23] compared with placebo, enalapril did not reduce the mortality rate in asymptomatic patients with reduced ejection fraction, although it delayed the onset of heart failure. Because ACE inhibitors have been shown to alleviate symptoms, improve patients' clinical status, and decrease mortality, the current recommendation is that all humans with heart failure due to left ventricular systolic dysfunction receive an ACE inhibitor.[17] The mortality reductions associated with administration of ACE inhibitors lends support to the theory that disease progression is mediated by factors other than hemodynamics alone.

Management of Stable Compensated Congestive Heart Failure

After stabilization of the acute crisis, during which hemodynamic support is the goal, long-term management of heart failure ensues. The goals for this stage are to combat congestion, improve exercise capacity and quality of life, blunt adverse neurohormonal sequelae, and prolong survival time. Drugs can be administered to promote pump function (positive inotropes), to alter hemodynamics (preload and afterload reducers), and to blunt the adverse sequelae mediated by the body's compensatory mechanisms (neurohormonal antagonists). Numerous studies have been performed in humans to evaluate the benefits or limitations of drugs used to combat congestive heart failure, but the cost of well-designed, multi-institutional studies has precluded large-scale investigation in companion animals. For this reason, theoretical benefit often is extrapolated to dogs and cats; however, the practitioner should exercise caution in making these assumptions.

Triple drug therapy using furosemide and an ACE inhibitor, frequently combined with digoxin, serves as the mainstay of treatment for dogs with congestive heart failure secondary to degenerative valve disease and dilated cardiomyopathy.

Diuretics

The importance of appropriate administration of diuretics in the management of heart failure should not be underestimated. Diuretics play a pivotal role because they are the most effective agents for promoting rapid symptomatic benefits, and they are the only agents capable of controlling the fluid retention of heart failure. Although no large-scale trials have been done to evaluate the effect of diuretics on morbidity and mortality, there is little debate that they are a vital class of drug in both the acute and the long-term management of patients with congestive heart failure. Trials that would withhold a diuretic in heart failure would be immoral.

The kidney represents a major target organ for the neurohormonal and hemodynamic alterations that occur with a failing heart. Activation of the sympathetic nervous system, stimulation of the RAS, and intrarenal hemodynamic alterations all contribute to an avid state of sodium and water retention. Dogs with severe heart failure have had a 24% increase in plasma volume.[24] Unfortunately, these dogs are existing on the plateau of a depressed Frank-Starling curve, meaning the increased plasma volume is unable to enhance cardiac output. The premise behind administration of a diuretic, therefore, is to control congestion while maintaining optimal cardiac output. The three primary classes of diuretics are the loop, the thiazide, and the potassium-sparing diuretics. Each acts at a different site in the nephron.

Loop diuretics The loop diuretics (furosemide, torsemide, bumetanide, and ethacrynic acid) constitute the drug class most commonly used to treat heart failure. They inhibit the sodium, potassium, chloride ($Na^+/K^+/2Cl^-$) cotransporter on the luminal surface of the ascending limb of the loop of Henle. This inhibition markedly increases the fractional excretion of Na^+ and Cl^- and prevents establishment of the normal medullary concentration gradient, thereby promoting diuresis. In addition to promoting natriuresis and diuresis, furosemide, the most frequently used loop diuretic, appears capable of decreasing pulmonary capillary wedge pressure and promoting venodilatation, prior to the onset of diuresis, through local vascular prostaglandin synthesis.[25,26] The loop diuretics are the most effective agents for controlling the fluid retention of heart failure, and their proven safety, combined with their low cost, makes them a crucial therapeutic weapon.

Furosemide is available in formulations for enteral and parenteral administration. When it is administered intravenously, the onset of action is 5 minutes, the peak diuretic effect occurs within 30 minutes, and the duration of effect is 2 hours. After oral administration, the onset of action occurs within 60 minutes and the peak effect and duration of effect are 1 to 2 hours and 6 hours, respectively.

Furosemide's rapid onset of action explains its presence in most emergency crash carts. Severe pulmonary edema requires intravenous furosemide administration (2 to 8 mg/kg in dogs every 1 to 2 hours; 1 to 2 mg/kg in cats every 1 to 4 hours) to reduce preload rapidly. Although mild electrolyte abnormalities and dehydration may result with high doses, these conditions generally resolve when the pet resumes eating and drinking. After alleviation of the acute crisis, it is best to decrease the furosemide dose to the lowest capable of eliminating congestive signs. The authors have found that most dogs with a previous history of heart failure require 1 to 2 mg/kg given orally once or twice daily. Initially some dogs may be managed with as little as every-other-day therapy; however, as the disease process continues, cardiac output declines and diuretic resistance develops, extremely high doses of furosemide may be required to fend off congestive signs (4 mg/kg given orally three times daily). Periodic evaluation of electrolyte and renal parameters should be performed, especially when furosemide is administered concurrently with an ACE inhibitor and digoxin. It is well recognized that hypokalemia may contribute to ventricular arrhythmias and increase the likelihood of digoxin toxicity.

Bumetanide and torsemide have been reported to have more consistent oral bioavailability than furosemide (ranges of 80% to 100% and 10% to 100%, respectively).[27] The diuretic response occurs more slowly with intravenous torsemide than with furosemide, but torsemide promotes diuresis for a longer period.[28] Whether use of bumetanide or torsemide could allow for a more predictable diuretic response has not been evaluated.

Thiazide diuretics The thiazides were among the first effective oral diuretic classes that developed widespread use in clinical practice. They block resorption of Na^+ in the distal convoluted tubule by inhibiting the Na^+/Cl^- cotransporter. The increased delivery of Na^+ to the collecting duct enhances potassium (K^+) and hydrogen (H^+) secretion and may promote the development of hypokalemia and metabolic alkalosis. Compared with loop diuretics, the thiazides are relatively weak; they increase renal sodium excretion from a normal value of about 1% to 5% to 8% of the filtered load. Nonetheless, they appear to promote a synergistic effect when administered with a loop diuretic. Although the combination of loop and thiazide diuretics appears effective at combating refractory pulmonary edema, caution must be exercised to avoid hypokalemia. One strategy to prevent excessive potassium loss is to administer the thiazide every second or third day while continuing daily treatment with furosemide. The two most frequently used thiazide diuretics are chlorothiazide and hydrochlorothiazide. Both drugs show good oral absorption and a relatively rapid onset of action. Chlorothiazide (20 to 40 mg/kg given orally twice daily) promotes diuresis within 1 hour, reaches peak activity at 4 hours, and has a duration of effect of 6 to 12 hours. For hydrochlorothiazide (*dogs:* 2 to

4 mg/kg given orally twice daily; *cats:* 1 to 2 mg/kg given orally twice daily), onset of action occurs within 2 hours, activity peaks at 4 hours, and the effect lasts 12 hours.

Potassium-sparing diuretics Potassium-sparing diuretics formerly were allocated solely to the late stages of heart failure or to patients with hypokalemia, but they recently have come to the forefront in the battle against neurohormonally mediated progression of cardiac disease. This class of diuretics (spironolactone, eplerenone, and triamterene) recently has gained prominence because evidence suggests the presence of "aldosterone escape" in approximately one third of humans treated with ACE inhibitors.[29] The precise mechanisms behind this RAS-independent increase in aldosterone are unknown, although increased potassium levels induced by ACE inhibitors and decreased hepatic clearance may be contributing factors. Tissue pathways for the production of aldosterone have also been identified, although their role in the progression of heart failure is uncertain.

Aldosterone promotes the production of Na^+/K^+ exchangers along the luminal surface of the distal tubule and collecting ducts. In addition to its ability to increase sodium resorption, aldosterone now is recognized to contribute to myocardial fibrosis, augmentation of sympathetic tone, and possibly diuretic resistance. It has been postulated that spironolactone's ability to decrease collagen turnover, and presumably myocardial fibrosis, is responsible for the marked mortality benefits recognized in the Randomized Aldactone Evaluation Study (RALES) trial. Whether dogs and cats will benefit similarly has yet to be determined, but more frequent use of spironolactone in companion animals may be warranted.

Spironolactone is well absorbed from the gastrointestinal tract but has a relatively slow onset of action, peaking at 2 to 3 days after administration. It undergoes rapid hepatic metabolism to pharmacologically active canrenone. Spironolactone is administered to dogs and cats at a dosage of 1 to 2 mg/kg given orally every 12 hours, in conjunction with an ACE inhibitor and a loop diuretic, to combat congestive heart failure.

Angiotensin-Converting Enzyme (ACE) Inhibitors
Despite their symptomatic benefits, diuretics should not be used as monotherapy in the management of congestive heart failure because they further activate the renin-angiotensin system.[30,31] Drugs designed to inhibit angiotensin-converting enzyme block the formation of AT II, promote an increase in the circulating levels of bradykinin, and may temporarily reduce circulating aldosterone levels. Although ACE inhibitors are frequently categorized as balanced vasodilators, it appears likely that their beneficial effect on mortality is not mediated purely by hemodynamic alterations.[22] They are relatively weak vasodilators compared with direct-acting arterial vasodilators such as hydralazine, and their ability to promote diuresis is much overshadowed by the less expensive loop diuretics. Rather, it is believed that ACE inhibitors reduce mortality through their ability to blunt the detrimental consequences associated with long-standing activation of the RAS. Their early success has helped spearhead the current pharmacologic trend toward neurohormonal antagonism.

Activation of the neurohormonal cascade often begins with detection of arterial underfilling by mechanoreceptors in the carotid sinus and kidney (Figure 199-4). Regardless of whether this relative "hypotension" occurs secondary to low-output heart failure, severe mitral insufficiency, or profound hypovolemia, the common end-point is activation of the sympathetic nervous system and RAS. Additional activators of the RAS are reduced sodium delivery to the macula densa and sympathetic stimulation. Release of the protease renin from the juxtaglomerular apparatus promotes conversion of angiotensinogen to angiotensin I. Angiotensin-converting

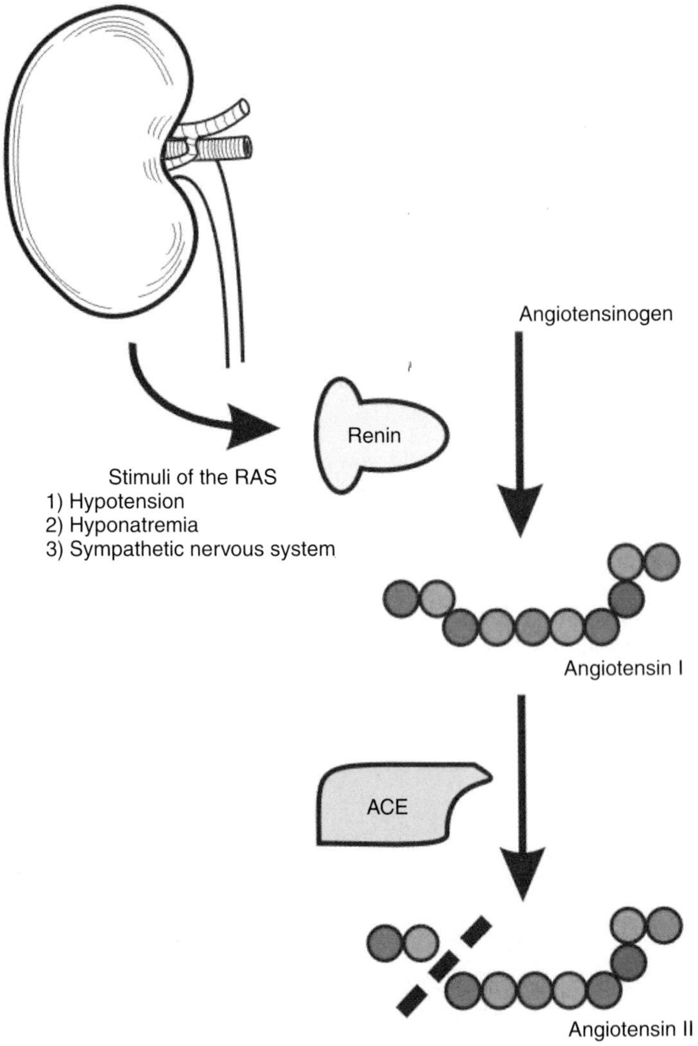

Figure 199-4 After the release of renin, angiotensinogen is cleaved to form angiotensin I, which is subsequently cleaved by angiotensin-converting enzyme (ACE) to form angiotensin II. Angiotensin II promotes numerous physiologic actions, including activation of the sympathetic nervous system and production of aldosterone (see Figure 199-12).

enzyme cleaves the C-terminal dipeptide from angiotensin I, thereby forming the octapeptide angiotensin II. In addition to being a potent vasoconstrictor, AT II has several other properties: (1) it is a primary secretagogue for aldosterone; (2) it potentiates presynaptic norepinephrine release; (3) it stimulates the release of antidiuretic hormone (vasopressin); (4) it promotes renal tubular sodium resorption; and (5) it has been linked to cardiomyocyte necrosis, apoptosis, and progression of ventricular fibrosis.[18,32,33] Angiotensin-converting enzyme is also capable of cleaving the C-terminal dipeptide from bradykinin, therefore it appears to be a regulator of vasoconstrictive/ sodium retentive and vasodilative/natriuretic mechanisms. Although tissue ACE and additional enzymatic pathways (e.g., chymase, cathepsin G, tonin, and tissue plasminogen activator) capable of producing AT II have been identified, their significance is unknown at this time.[32]

ACE-inhibiting compounds are numerous and vary in their chemical structure, potency, bioavailability, and route of elimination. Most ACE inhibitors, excluding captopril and lisinopril, are administered in the form of prodrugs that require conversion to their active form by hepatic metabolism. Enalapril requires conversion to enalaprilat, and benazepril is metabolized to benazeprilat. Although claims have been made that some formulations produce more profound ACE inhibition, prolonged periods of efficacy, or superior tissue ACE inhibition, the importance of these characteristics is unclear in naturally occurring heart failure.

The degree of ACE inhibition and the duration of action of several agents, including benazepril, captopril, enalapril, lisinopril, and ramipril, have been evaluated in normal dogs.[34] Hamlin and Nakayama[34] documented that benazepril, enalapril, lisinopril, and ramipril were able to achieve similar degrees of ACE inhibition after drug administration (about 75% inhibition at 1.5 hours and about 50% inhibition through 12 hours). Enalapril, lisinopril, and ramipril continued to display significant activity (about 25% inhibition) beyond 24 hours. These researchers also found that captopril was unable to reduce ACE activity substantially, compared with control, beyond the 1.5-hour sample. Whether captopril's inability to suppress ACE activity was a consequence of sample handling or merely an inability to suppress circulating versus tissue ACE is uncertain.[35] Evaluations of enalapril and benazepril in normal cats have identified maximal ACE inhibition of 48% and 98%, respectively, after single-dose administration.[36,37] Benazepril was reported to show greater than 90% ACE inhibition beyond 24 hours.[37]

Excretion of the ACE inhibitors is primarily via the kidneys, although benazepril appears to undergo significant biliary excretion in companion animals (about 50% in dogs and about 85% in cats).[38] When ACE inhibitors have been prescribed for patients with mild renal insufficiency, the recommendation historically has been to reduce both the dosage and frequency interval by approximately 50%. Administration of enalapril to dogs with experimental mild renal insufficiency is associated with a significant increase in the area under the curve (AUC) for the active metabolite enalaprilat.[39] After benazepril was administered to the same dogs, no significant increase was seen in the AUC for benazeprilat. Whether concurrent cardiac disease, with its relatively depressed cardiac output, would be associated with impaired benazeprilat excretion is unclear. Current trends using "standard" doses of enalapril to treat glomerulonephritis and renal insufficiency are difficult to extrapolate to patients with heart failure and renal insufficiency because of their limited ability to increase cardiac output in the face of a reduced rate of glomerular filtration.[40]

In summary, the merits and limitations of the different formulations are unknown, and only the ACE inhibitor enalapril has been specifically approved in the United States for the treatment of heart failure in dogs. The hypothesized improved safety of using benazepril rather than enalapril in patients with renal insufficiency has not been clinically evaluated in companion animals with cardiac disease.

Enalapril   Enalapril is one of the few drugs that has been closely evaluated in dogs with naturally occurring congestive heart failure. The first reported placebo-controlled studies in dogs were short-term investigations, the Invasive Multicenter Prospective Veterinary Evaluation of Enalapril study (IMPROVE; 21 days) and the Cooperative Veterinary Enalapril study (COVE; 28 days), both published in 1995.[41,42] These studies enrolled dogs with mitral valve insufficiency or dilated cardiomyopathy (DCM) to evaluate the hemodynamic (IMPROVE) and clinical (COVE) benefits of enalapril. The drug decreased pulmonary capillary wedge pressures in dogs with DCM and improved the heart failure class, pulmonary edema scores, and overall evaluation for both groups of dogs with heart failure. The benefits of these short-term studies were more pronounced for dogs with DCM than for those with mitral valve insufficiency. The COVE investigators found that twice daily oral administration of enalapril (0.5 mg/kg) appeared to promote more significant improvements than once daily therapy.[42] The LIVE study group followed a subpopulation of dogs from the two short-term studies to evaluate the long-term effects of enalapril administration.[5] These researchers found that dogs treated with enalapril were able to continue the study for longer than those receiving placebo (157.5 versus 77 days, P = 0.006). In contrast to the results of the short-term studies, the beneficial effect was more prominent in dogs with mitral valve insufficiency (P = 0.041) than in those with dilated cardiomyopathy (P = 0.06). An additional study supporting the benefits of ACE inhibitor administration to dogs with heart failure found that enalapril significantly increased the exercise tolerance of dogs with experimentally created mitral insufficiency.[43]

Despite these symptomatic benefits, the hope that early institution of ACE inhibition will delay the onset of heart failure may go unfulfilled. To date, enalapril has been unable to delay the onset of heart failure in asymptomatic cases of mitral insufficiency.[44] Whether ACE inhibitors can reduce mortality in dogs or cats with heart failure has yet to be determined; even so, preliminary evidence reported in 2003 looks supportive, although not conclusive, for cats with diastolic dysfunction.[45]

Benazepril   Similar to enalapril, benazepril is a prodrug that must undergo hepatic metabolism to produce the active compound, benazeprilat. Oral administration of benazepril has produced variable and conflicting degrees of ACE inhibition. An initial study reported that peak plasma benazeprilat concentrations were achieved 2 hours after oral administration.[46] The percentage of ACE inhibition after a single dose of 0.5 mg/kg of benazepril administered to normal dogs was 99.7% after 2 hours, 95.2% after 12 hours, and 87.3% after 24 hours. Similar results were found for the same intervals at doses of 0.25 mg/kg (97.8%, 89.2%, and 75.7%) and 1 mg/kg (99.1%, 94.0%, and 83.1%). Maximal ACE inhibition after

15 doses was attained in dogs receiving 0.25 mg/kg of benazepril once daily (96.9% at 2 hours, 92.5% at 12 hours, and 83.6% at 24 hours). A second study, which also evaluated a single dose of 0.5 mg/kg of benazepril in normal dogs, showed ACE inhibition of 81% at 1.5 hours, 37% at 12 hours, and 10.3% at 24 hours.[34] Prolonged administration of benazepril was not evaluated. A final study, in which 0.5 mg/kg of benazepril was administered orally once daily to dogs with mitral insufficiency, showed ACE inhibition to be 33.3% at 1 week, 28% at 2 weeks, and 42.7% at 4 weeks.[47]

Based on these conflicting results, the current dosing recommendations are broad (0.25 to 0.5 mg/kg given orally once or twice daily). Whether benazepril is clinically more effective or safer than enalapril for dogs and cats with congestive heart failure remains unclear.

Adverse effects   The mechanism by which ACE inhibitors exert their beneficial properties (e.g., inhibition of angiotensin II production) also lends to the potential for adverse consequences. Although infrequently encountered, complications may include systemic hypotension, azotemia, and hyperkalemia.

ACE inhibitors reduce systemic vascular resistance by decreasing circulating levels of angiotensin II and increasing circulating levels of bradykinin. In patients with severe heart failure in which an increase in cardiac output is unable to sustain systemic blood pressure, symptomatic hypotension may develop. Although this complication is infrequent, its likelihood increases with concomitant overzealous use of diuretics. Unfortunately, the clinical signs associated with severe low-output heart failure and systemic hypotension are very similar (e.g., weakness, exercise intolerance, and possibly stupor), a fact that lends emphasis to an important point: if a patient appears refractory to medical management, the blood pressure should be evaluated before more aggressive measures to combat heart failure are instituted.

A second adverse effect attributed to ACE inhibitors' unique ability to decrease angiotensin II production is a reduction in the glomerular filtration rate (GFR) and the development of azotemia. The GFR is determined by the glomerular capillary pressure (GC_P). Based on the knowledge that pressure is equal to the product of flow and resistance ($P = Q \times R$), it can be ascertained that the GFR ultimately is determined by renal plasma flow and the degree of efferent arteriolar vasoconstriction (Figure 199-5). In cases of heart failure in which renal plasma flow is diminished, the glomerular filtration rate is supported by the ability of ATII to constrict the efferent renal arteriole. ACE inhibitors' ability to depress production of AT II promotes efferent renal arteriolar vasodilatation and hence a reduction in the GFR. The failing heart cannot further increase cardiac output, and an acute bout of azotemia may subsequently develop. A recent study evaluating early institution of enalapril therapy in dogs with compensated mitral valve insufficiency found that dogs allocated to an ACE inhibitor were not at a more significant risk of developing azotemia compared with dogs receiving placebo.[48] In the authors' experience, mild increases in blood urea nitrogen (BUN) and creatinine occur frequently after institution of therapy with an ACE inhibitor and furosemide. However, the development of severe azotemia, necessitating discontinuation of the ACE inhibitor or a reduction in its dosage, occurs infrequently. This complication seems to occur most often in patients with severe heart failure that require aggressive diuretic administration to control congestive signs. Prior to institution of enalapril therapy, the authors evaluate the baseline biochemical parameters and perform a second measurement of the BUN, creatinine, and electrolytes 5 to 7 days after the start of treatment. If patients become anorectic or develop gastrointestinal signs during this time, we instruct the owners to discontinue all drugs and immediately present the animal for veterinary attention.

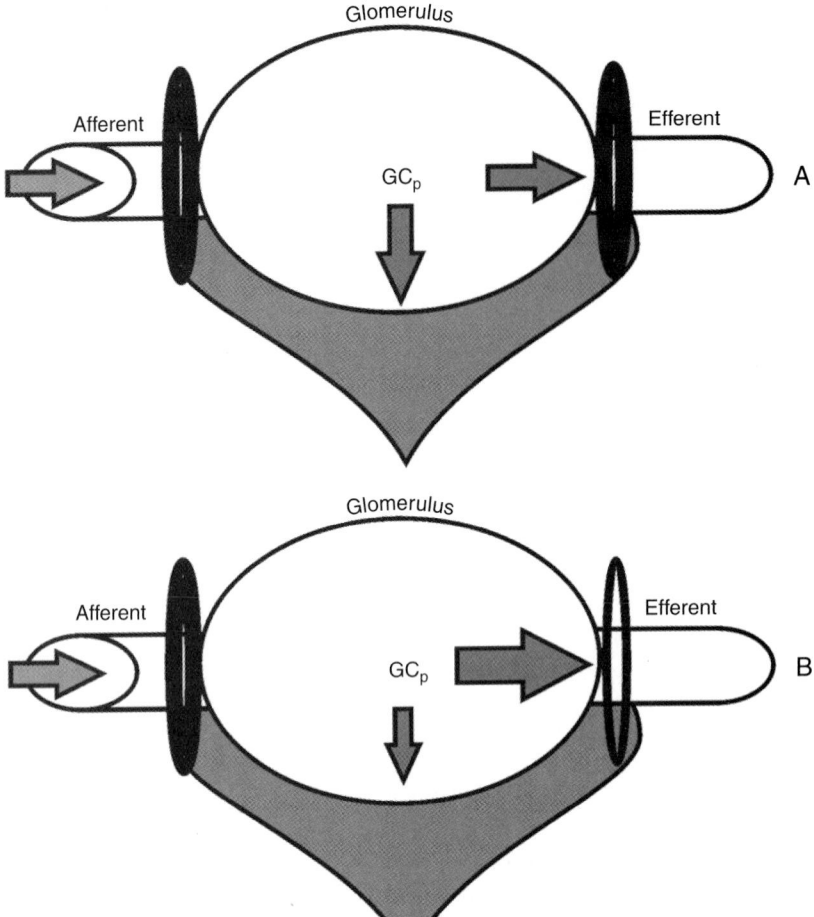

Figure 199-5 Glomerular capillary pressure (GC$_p$), and therefore the glomerular filtration rate (GFR), is determined by cardiac output and the relative resistances imparted by the afferent and efferent renal arterioles. Compared with normal (**A**), ACE inhibitors preferentially dilate the efferent renal arteriole (**B**) and may therefore decrease the GFR and promote the development of azotemia. It appears this consequence is most frequent in patients with low output heart failure that require large doses of diuretics to control their congestive signs.

Hyperkalemia may be encountered during therapy with ACE inhibitors as the result of a reduction in the GFR and a decline in circulating aldosterone levels. In the absence of aldosterone, sodium loss is favored and potassium levels rise. This complication appears to occur infrequently, presumably because most of the potent diuretics have potassium-wasting properties and tend to prevent the development of hyperkalemia. The authors have rarely encountered an increase in potassium that necessitated a dosage reduction for or discontinuation of an ACE inhibitor. There is concern that the addition of spironolactone may potentiate hyperkalemia, therefore periodic electrolyte monitoring is prudent in patients receiving an ACE inhibitor and a potassium-sparing diuretic.

Drug interactions   Because aspirin inhibits cyclo-oxygenase and decreases prostaglandin formation, some have questioned whether administration of aspirin may negate some of the beneficial vasodilative properties exerted by ACE inhibitors.[49] An additional concern is that aspirin's ability to reduce renal prostaglandin formation may worsen the ACE inhibitor–induced reduction in the GFR.[50] A recent retrospective analysis of six long-term, randomized trials of ACE inhibitors found that aspirin did not significantly alter the beneficial effects of ACE inhibitors in CHF.[50] Whether other commonly prescribed, nonsteroidal anti-inflammatory agents blunt the potentially beneficial vasodilative properties of ACE inhibitors is uncertain.

Positive Inotropes
Agents capable of increasing cardiac contractility can improve a patient's strength and exercise capacity, thereby potentially enhancing the pet's quality of life. Ideally, these compounds

would concurrently promote mortality benefits by improving cardiac efficiency and limiting the activation of endogenous compensatory mechanisms (with their detrimental long-term consequences). Unfortunately, to date most of the potent agents available to augment systolic function act by means of "upstream," cAMP-dependent mechanisms that have shown negative effects on survival.

Membrane-associated adenylate cyclase is the enzyme responsible for cAMP production, and phosphodiesterase III is responsible for its degradation. Therefore mechanisms to increase cAMP concentrations may take one of two pathways (Figure 199-6): beta agonists increase production of cAMP, and phosphodiesterase inhibitors increase cytosolic cAMP by inhibiting its breakdown. Acting through protein kinase A, cAMP promotes phosphorylation of the L-type calcium channel to increase calcium release from the sarcoplasmic reticulum (SR). The increased systolic Ca^{2+} concentration (1) deinhibits the troponin complex to promote actin and myosin interaction and (2) increases the activity of myosin ATPase.[51] These mechanisms serve to increase both the total force developed and the rate at which the force is developed. Protein kinase A also exerts beneficial lusitropic effects by promoting phosphorylation of (1) the regulatory SR membrane phosphoprotein, phospholamban, to enhance diastolic calcium uptake and (2) troponin I, to increase the rate of cross-bridge detachment and relaxation.[51] Paradoxically, despite these beneficial properties, long-term administration of agents capable of increasing cAMP has been linked to increased mortality rates in patients with heart failure.[10] The increased Ca^{2+} concentrations are believed to contribute to the development of arrhythmias and to increase myocardial energy consumption and oxygen demand,

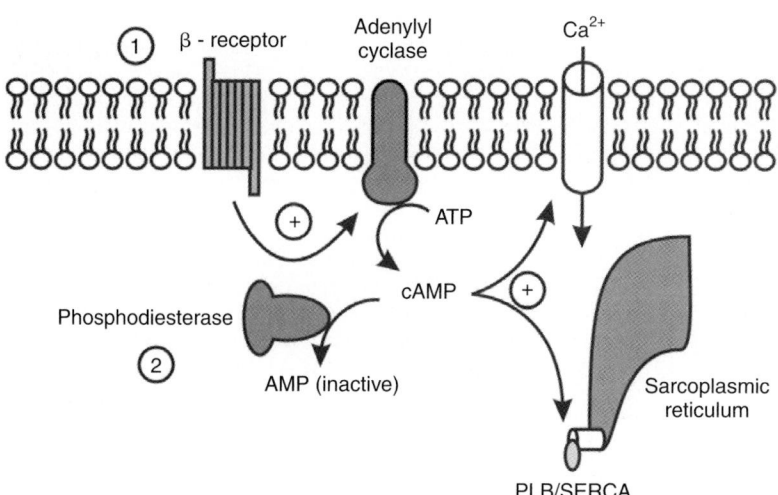

Figure 199-6 The beta-agonists (*1*) dobutamine and dopamine promote their positive inotropic and lusitropic effects through activation of adenylyl cyclase, with a subsequent amplification of cAMP production. The phosphodiesterase inhibitors (*2*) amrinone, milrinone and, to some degree, pimobendan blunt the degradation of cAMP, thereby promoting similar positive inotropic and lusitropic effects that should not be blunted by beta-receptor downregulation. Phosphorylation of the sarcolemmal L-type calcium channel is responsible for the positive inotropic action, whereas phosphorylation of phospholamban (PLB), with ensuing deinhibition of the sarcoplasmic reticulum calcium ATPase (SERCA), accounts for the enhanced diastolic function. Phosphorylation of troponin I (not shown) further enhances diastolic function by altering the cross-bridge kinetics between actin and myosin.

thereby worsening the outcome. These findings lend support to the premise that downregulation and uncoupling of beta receptors, along with upregulation of adenylate cyclase inhibitory proteins, serve as compensatory protective mechanisms rather than primary biochemical abnormalities. Current investigations are evaluating agents capable of enhancing systolic performance "downstream" from cytosolic Ca^{2+} in the hopes of avoiding excessive mortality.

Digitalis glycosides The digitalis glycosides are the only readily available class of inotropic agents that act independently of the cAMP second-messenger system. This characteristic imparts a degree of safety to the glycosides, with regard to their neutral effect on mortality, but simultaneously limits their inotropic potency.[52] Because of digoxin's potential positive inotropic effects and rate-controlling properties for atrial fibrillation, there is little debate that it is indicated in the treatment of dilated cardiomyopathy; however, there is substantial debate over its role in the management of mitral valve insufficiency. The authors' rationale for the use of digoxin (0.003 mg/kg given orally twice daily) in dogs with mitral valve insufficiency is primarily its neurohormonal antagonism effect rather than pump support. Inhibition of the Na^+/K^+ ATPase pump in the vagal afferents sensitizes the baroreceptors to the prevailing blood pressure, which may decrease sympathetic outflow and renin-angiotensin activity.[17] Although the findings are purely anecdotal, the authors have had and continue to have cases in which the addition of digoxin to background therapy of furosemide and enalapril has produced clear symptomatic improvement.

The cardiac glycosides inhibit the action of the Na^+/K^+ ATPase pump by competitively binding to the extracellular potassium site (Figure 199-7). This antagonism promotes an increase in the intracellular sodium concentration, with its subsequent exchange for calcium via the reversible Na^+/Ca^{2+} pump. The net result is an increase in cytosolic calcium levels and enhanced cardiac contractility. Inhibition of the Na^+/K^+ ATPase pump further sensitizes the baroreceptors (blunting sympathetic discharge), inhibits renal tubular resorption of sodium (promoting mild diuresis), and increases the delivery of sodium to the distal tubules (inhibiting renin release).[17]

Despite these theoretical benefits, digitalis has been unable to alter the natural course of heart failure.[52] The Digitalis Investigation Group (DIG) enrolled 6800 human patients in a placebo-controlled study to evaluate whether digoxin administration affected mortality or morbidity.[52] Digoxin did not reduce overall mortality but did reduce the rate of hospitalization for worsening heart failure (26.8% versus 34.7%, $P < 0.001$). Subgroup analysis revealed that patients in class III or class IV heart failure showed the greatest benefit from digoxin administration. Compared with results from agents not related to glycosides, including dobutamine and milrinone, the findings of this investigation did not demonstrate excess mortality. It is unlikely that a similar study evaluating the efficacy of digoxin will ever be performed in dogs because of the extreme sample size needed to detect these small differences. One study reported that four of 10 dogs with dilated cardiomyopathy showed echocardiographically identifiable improvements in cardiac contractility after treatment with digoxin.[53] Whether the 7% increase in fractional shortening was a true increase in contractility or merely occurred subsequent to rate control (250 beats per minute [bpm] pretreatment versus 145 bpm post-treatment) is uncertain, but

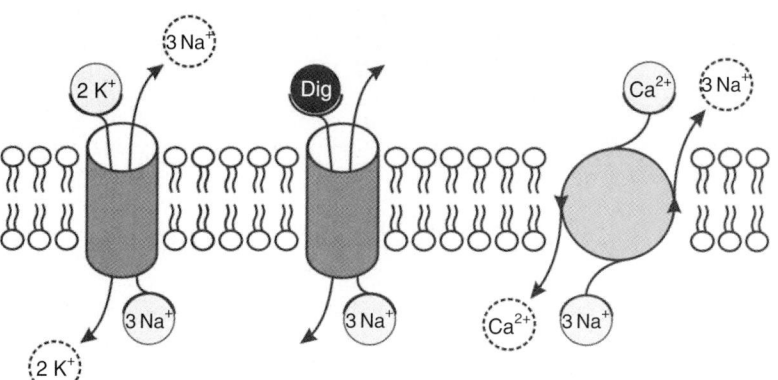

Figure 199-7 The Na^+/K^+ ATPase pump contributes to maintenance of the resting membrane potential by actively pumping three Na^+ ions out across the sarcolemmal membrane and two K^+ ions into the cell. The pump therefore is capable of maintaining both an electrical and a chemical gradient. Digoxin competitively binds the K^+ binding site on the extracellular surface, thereby inhibiting sodium efflux by means of this mechanism. The excessive intracellular Na^+ reverses the Na^+/Ca^{2+} exchanger and ultimately promotes an influx of Ca^{2+} and efflux of Na^+. The increased calcium transport augments calcium-induced calcium release from the sarcoplasmic reticulum, enhancing contractility.

digoxin appears to be a relatively weak inotropic agent in dogs with heart failure. Nonetheless, it is the only oral inotropic agent that is readily available in the United States.

Therapeutic levels of digitalis increase parasympathetic tone, while blunting sympathetic activation, to promote slowing of the sinus node and increased atrioventricular (AV) node refractoriness with decreased conduction velocity. This property makes them useful in the management of DCM complicated by atrial fibrillation, because the other negative chronotropes (e.g., beta blockers, Ca^{2+} channel blockers) acutely depress systolic function. Digitalis is further indicated for the management of symptomatic DCM with sinus rhythm or left to right shunting lesions complicated by myocardial failure. Although digoxin is not always considered a mainstay of therapy for the management of mitral insufficiency, the authors continue to use it in cases of heart failure subsequent to chronic degenerative valve disease (CDVD). Although some of these mitral insufficiency patients fail to attain symptomatic benefit from digoxin therapy, the drug's low cost and safety when used appropriately continue to make it a useful agent. Digoxin is an inappropriate agent to use for rate control in cases of hypertrophic cardiomyopathy in which the primary abnormality is diastolic rather than systolic dysfunction. Any positive inotropic response predisposes HCM patients to the development or worsening of systolic anterior motion of the mitral valve.

Digoxin Digoxin is the digitalis glycoside most commonly used in dogs, and it appears to be the most suitable glycoside for cats with systolic dysfunction. The bioavailability of digoxin after oral administration of the tablet form is approximately 60%.[12] The digoxin elixir shows better bioavailability after oral administration (about 75%) and is easier to dose appropriately for small dogs. After absorption, digoxin has a relatively long and variable serum half-life in dogs, with reports ranging from 23 to 39 hours.[12] In cats the duration is even more uncertain, with reports of mean half-lives ranging from 33.5 hours to 57.8 hours, with even longer half-lives during prolonged administration. Because approximately five half-lives are required to attain steady-state concentrations of a drug, digoxin cannot be expected to produce rapid symptomatic or rate-controlling benefits. Digoxin predominately undergoes renal excretion, although a small amount (approximately 15%) is metabolized by the liver. Renal failure significantly reduces the clearance of digoxin and profoundly increases the serum concentration, often to the point of intoxication. Patients with renal failure that require a cardiac glycoside should be given *digitoxin* because it undergoes hepatic elimination.

Determining the appropriate dose of digoxin to attain therapeutic levels yet avoid digitalis intoxication can be a frustrating endeavor. Traditionally, small dogs (less than 20 kg) have been treated with 0.005 to 0.008 mg/kg given orally twice daily, and larger dogs have been treated based on body surface area, with 0.22 mg/m² given orally twice daily. The intent with these doses was to attain a therapeutic digoxin level of 1 to 2 ng/mL. The DIG trial found that human mortality varied directly with serum digoxin levels, even within this "therapeutic" range. A new trend has emerged from that data whereby the human medical profession has aimed to keep trough levels of digoxin at 0.5 to 1 ng/ml. Whether these recommendations hold true for dogs is uncertain, but aiming for the low end of the reference range appears to be appropriate. The authors currently institute digoxin therapy at a dosage of 0.003 mg/kg given orally twice daily. If the digoxin level is subtherapeutic 5 to 7 days after initiation of therapy, the dosage is increased by 25%, and the serum level is rechecked a week later. This regimen is continued until therapeutic levels have been attained.

A number of factors may influence the distribution of digoxin, creating a need for special consideration and monitoring. The principal reservoir for digoxin is skeletal muscle, therefore dosing recommendations should be based on lean body mass. Obese dogs require lower doses of digoxin than

thin dogs, and the dosing requirement for dogs that experience marked muscle loss tends to decline. Patients with right-sided heart failure and large volumes of ascites need dosage reductions because digoxin does not distribute into free abdominal fluid.[12] After institution of digoxin therapy, it is most appropriate to alter the dosing scheme based on the serum digoxin level, the response to therapy, and evidence of intoxication.

A number of drug interactions also are possible with digoxin. The best recognized interaction is between digoxin and the class Ia antiarrhythmic quinidine. When these drugs are combined, serum digoxin levels increase because quinidine displaces digoxin from the Na^+/K^+ ATPase pump and reduces its renal clearance through inhibition of P-glycoprotein. The binding of digoxin with myocardial Na^+/K^+ ATPase is "tighter" than that with skeletal muscle, therefore the net effect of this drug combination is an increase in the likelihood of digitalis intoxication. It is recommended that these agents not be used together. Fortunately, no interactions have been reported between digoxin and the more frequently used class I anti-arrhythmics procainamide and mexiletine. Most of the other reported drug interactions, with amiodarone, verapamil, nifedipine, propafenone and, to a lesser extent diltiazem, occur because of inhibition of P-glycoprotein. Any agent that alters renal blood flow or hepatic microsomal enzymes has the potential to disturb digoxin's pharmacokinetics.

Similar to quinidine, the extracellular potassium concentration can influence digoxin binding to the Na^+/K^+ ATPase pump. The hypokalemia often associated with anorexia or large doses of a diuretic leaves more receptors exposed for digoxin attachment, thereby increasing the likelihood of digitalis intoxication. With hyperkalemia, more receptors are bound, and digoxin is displaced from the Na^+/K^+ ATPase. Hypercalcemia and hypernatremia promote digoxin's inotropic and toxic properties, whereas decreased calcium and sodium concentrations have the opposite effects.

Since it was recognized that taurine deficiency was responsible for most cases of feline DCM, the number of cats receiving digoxin has declined over the past decade. The authors still encounter an infrequent case of DCM unrelated to taurine deficiency, and some cases of restrictive cardiomyopathy have such poor systolic function that digoxin is indicated. Cats appear to tolerate the tablet form of digoxin better than the alcohol-based elixir. The recommended dose is one fourth of a 0.125 mg tablet given orally. Dosing intervals are as follows: (1) cats weighing 3 kg or less: every 48 hours; (2) cats weighing 4 to 5 kg: every 24 to 48 hours; (3) cats weighing 6 kg or greater: every 24 hours. Because of the variable half-life of digoxin in cats, the authors typically monitor serum levels 7 to 10 days after initiation of therapy.

Digitalis toxicity Without a doubt, digoxin is a toxic substance when excessive amounts accumulate. This narrow therapeutic index highlights the need for careful client and veterinary attention when digoxin is part of a treatment regimen. In the authors' experience, when digoxin therapy is instituted at a dosage of 0.003 mg/kg given orally twice daily, with uptitration based on serum digoxin concentrations, the incidence of digitalis toxicity is low both clinically and biochemically.

Clients should be informed of the most common manifestations of digoxin intoxication and given concise instructions on what to do if clinical signs develop. Continuing drug administration and waiting until the next recheck is not an appropriate step; the authors recommend discontinuation of all drugs followed by an immediate veterinary evaluation. It should be emphasized that the three regions frequently affected by excessive digoxin accumulation are the myocardial, gastrointestinal, and central nervous systems. Gastrointestinal manifestations, which often precede central nervous system (CNS) and myocardial toxicity, commonly include anorexia and vomiting, presumably from a direct chemoreceptor triggering effect exerted by digoxin. The serum concentration at which gastrointestinal signs develop is extremely variable. Some dogs have digoxin-associated anorexia at subtherapeutic drug concentrations, whereas others do not show any evidence of toxicity even with serum concentrations well above the therapeutic range. It can be difficult to determine whether the anorexia is associated with digoxin administration, azotemia secondary to a decreased GFR or renal insufficiency, poor diet palatability, or worsening heart failure. A biochemical profile, serum digoxin determination, and thoracic radiographs should be obtained in any digoxin-treated dog with heart failure that suddenly develops anorexia. In the absence of complicating factors such as azotemia or pulmonary edema, the authors temporarily discontinue digoxin administration even if the serum level is within the therapeutic range. If the pet's appetite returns (suggesting digoxin-associated anorexia), a lower digoxin dose may be instituted or the drug may be discontinued all together. Digoxin does not provide enough mortality benefit or positive inotropic response to warrant administration in the face of profound anorexia or other complications.

Although the myocardial complications may be more difficult for owners to recognize, they often are the most serious. Digoxin toxicity may induce almost every known cardiac arrhythmia, including both bradyarrhythmias and tachyarrhythmias. First- and second-degree AV block, sinus bradycardia, and sinus arrest are presumably influenced by digoxin's parasympathomimetic properties. Life-threatening ventricular tachyarrhythmias may develop as a consequence of cellular calcium overload. Excessive calcium precipitates late afterdepolarizations, whereby oscillations within the diastolic membrane potential periodically reach threshold and produce a premature complex. The slowed conduction and altered refractory period may then precipitate re-entry, yielding ventricular tachycardia. Obviously, determining whether the ventricular arrhythmia is associated with digoxin administration or is a manifestation of the underlying disease process may be difficult, but in general, discontinuation of digitalis is indicated.

The CNS alterations mediated by digoxin toxicity may include depression, disorientation, or delirium. Again, determining whether such clinical signs are attributable to digitalis intoxication or progression of the underlying disease process often is difficult. These patients should be evaluated for hypotension, in addition to having their serum digoxin levels measured.

Treatment of digitalis toxicity   The aggressiveness with which digoxin toxicity is treated depends on the manifestation of intoxication rather than the serum digoxin level. Gastrointestinal disturbances can frequently be managed by discontinuation of the drug. Dogs with bradyarrhythmias are often asymptomatic, and withdrawal of digoxin is the only therapeutic alteration required. In the rare case of symptomatic patients, short-term administration of atropine may be required while the toxic digoxin concentrations expire. The most aggressively managed complication of digitalis intoxication is ventricular tachyarrhythmias.

The class Ib antiarrhythmic drug lidocaine is the first-choice agent for acute management of digitalis-induced ventricular tachycardia. It is effective at targeting late afterdepolarizations without substantially affecting the sinus rate or AV nodal conduction. An initial bolus of 2 to 4 mg/kg is administered intravenously over 1 to 2 minutes, followed by a constant-rate infusion to suppress the arrhythmias. Lidocaine should be administered conservatively to cats because they are more sensitive to the neurotoxic side effects. Although infrequently used, phenytoin also appears efficacious for the treatment of digoxin-induced arrhythmias.

Because hypokalemia may precipitate digoxin toxicity and limit the efficacy of antiarrhythmic agents, it is important to evaluate the serum potassium concentration and to correct underlying deficits. Because of its ability to bind competitively the Na^+/K^+ ATPase pump, potassium can displace digoxin from the myocardium, thereby decreasing the likelihood of toxicity.

The development of a specific antibody fragment for cardiac glycosides has enabled production of an "antidote" for severe digoxin intoxication. Digibind® (GlaxoSmith Kline, Durham NC) complexes with the digoxin molecule and inhibits binding to the Na^+/K^+ ATPase pump, quickly resolving drug intoxication. Unfortunately, this drug is expensive, and its use in clinical practice therefore is limited.

Deficiencies of the Triple Drug Regimen
Early Institution of Therapy

Despite the relative safety and symptomatic benefit of triple drug therapy (i.e., furosemide, enalapril, and digoxin), this regimen has limitations. A possible ineptitude of this combination for the early treatment of cardiac disease is the mechanism by which ACE inhibitors promote their beneficial response. It is logical that, for these drugs to blunt the adverse consequences of the renin-angiotensin system, the system must be activated. In response to RAS activation after cardiac injury, the heart hypertrophies to normalize cardiac output and wall stress. Within physiologic limits, this hypertrophy, possibly combined with the inhibitory effects of circulating atrial natriuretic peptide, may be able to restore the renin-angiotensin system to resting levels.

Studies that have evaluated activation of the RAS in normal dogs, in dogs with asymptomatic dilated cardiomyopathy, and in dogs with symptomatic dilated cardiomyopathy lend support to this hypothesis.[54,55] In a study by Koch et al.,[54] 23 dogs were evaluated; nine dogs had asymptomatic DCM, eight had symptomatic DCM, and six had severe congestive heart failure subsequent to DCM. Sixteen giant breed dogs without evidence of cardiac disease were used to establish the neuroendocrine control values. In dogs with asymptomatic dilated cardiomyopathy, the plasma renin activity and aldosterone concentrations were not significantly different from those in control dogs (1.48 versus 0.89 and 35 versus 61, respectively). In dogs with symptomatic DCM and congestive heart failure, significant activation of the neurohormonal axis was seen compared with normal dogs and those with asymptomatic DCM. Plasma renin activity and aldosterone concentrations increased substantially between dogs with functional class III and class IV heart failure (3.8 versus 30.8 and 123 versus 600, respectively). Tidholm et al.[55] further evaluated activation of the neurohormonal systems of 45 dogs: 15 dogs with DCM and radiographic evidence of heart failure, 15 dogs with DCM without evidence of heart failure, and 15 age-, breed-, and gender-matched control dogs. They, too, found that in dogs with asymptomatic DCM, plasma renin activity, aldosterone concentrations, and N-terminal (NT)-pro atrial natriuretic peptide levels were not significantly different from those in control dogs. Dogs with DCM and congestive heart failure showed significant differences in all three variables compared with normal dogs and those with asymptomatic DCM.

Investigation of the effects of mitral valve insufficiency on the circulating neurohormonal system has also proved interesting, with some conflicting results. Pedersen et al.[56] evaluated the plasma renin and aldosterone concentrations of 18 Cavalier King Charles spaniels with asymptomatic or mildly symptomatic mitral insufficiency. Compared with 18 Cavalier King Charles spaniels without signs of heart disease, the plasma renin levels (median 3.44 versus 2.51, P = 0.03) and aldosterone concentrations (median 53 versus 27, P = 0.03) were significantly higher in dogs with valvular insufficiency. Haggstrom et al.[57] repeatedly evaluated 11 Cavalier King Charles spaniels with mitral insufficiency at 6-month intervals until signs of decompensation developed. The dogs did not receive cardiac medications during the study, and their diets remained the same throughout. The time of decompensation was considered the end-point of the study (situation 2), and the two most recent study periods (at 4.6 ± 2.2 months [situation 1] and 11.7 ± 1.8 months [situation 0]) prior to decompensation completed the three periods analyzed. The investigators found that N-terminal atrial natriuretic peptide (ANP) concentrations increased significantly from situation 0 to situation 1 and were further increased from situation 1 until the time of decompensation (situation 2). Plasma aldosterone concentrations were not significantly different from situation 0 to situation 1 but were found to decrease significantly at the time of decompensation (P < 0.01). Plasma angiotensin II concentrations were not significantly different between situation 0 and situation 1 or between the beginning of the study and the end of the study, but similar to the aldosterone levels, angiotensin II was significantly decreased between situation 1 and situation 2 (P < 0.05). The investigators concluded that the reductions in circulating angiotensin II and aldosterone at the onset of decompensation likely occurred subsequent to the elevation in ANP levels. Atrial natriuretic peptide has been reported to directly inhibit the release of renin and aldosterone and to promote a reduction in intravascular volume, thereby limiting RAS activation in the early stages of decompensation.[57] However, significant, long-term elevation of ANP in cases of severe heart failure may promote receptor downregulation, attenuating the inhibitory activity on the renin-angiotensin system.[58] Renal hypoperfusion and enhanced elimination of ANP may further blunt the counterbalancing activity of ANP, possibly allowing the RAS to accelerate the progression of heart failure unabated.[58]

Although it was determined that systemic, circulating RAS is not activated at the onset of heart failure in Cavalier King Charles spaniels or in asymptomatic dogs with DCM, recognition that local tissue pathways exist for the RAS may still support early institution of ACE inhibition. Canine ventricular myocytes have been recognized locally to contain the constituents of the RAS that may promote ventricular remodeling in an autocrine fashion.[59] Dogs subjected to rapid ventricular pacing to induce heart failure were compared with control dogs that were instrumented but not paced. Using reverse-transcriptase polymerase chain reaction (RT-PCR) and Western blot testing, Barlucchi et al.[59] found significant differences in canine myocyte RAS activity between control and failing hearts. Angiotensinogen expression was increased 2.5-fold (P < 0.001), renin was increased 3.6-fold (P < 0.001), the two forms of ACE identified at 134 and 170 kDa were increased 1.45-fold (P < 0.005) and 1.44-fold (P < 0.002), respectively, and the AT_1 receptor subtype of angiotensin II was increased 1.7-fold (P < 0.001) after 4 weeks of pacing. Angiotensin II levels measured by enzyme-linked immunosorbent assay (ELISA) were increased 2.2-fold (P < 0.004) in dogs subjected to pacing, whereas no significant differences were seen in chymase expression (P = 0.28) or the expression of the myocyte AT_2 receptor subtype of angiotensin II (P < 0.06).[59]

These findings point out one of the most challenging questions in the treatment of cardiac disease in companion animals: when is the appropriate time to initiate therapy? Although ACE inhibitors have proved efficacious at delaying the onset of heart failure in humans with asymptomatic left ventricular dysfunction, no similar published studies exist to support this conclusion in dogs and cats.[23] A double-blind, placebo-controlled study of 229 Cavalier King Charles spaniels with asymptomatic mitral regurgitation found that enalapril was unable to delay the onset of heart failure (Figure 199-8).[44] Although this study has been criticized on some counts (e.g., inadequate dose of ACE inhibitor [0.25 to 0.5 mg/kg daily], use of a single breed with a disease course that may not be representative of all dogs, and insufficient statistical power), it nonetheless was a 4.5-year endeavor that remains the largest published evaluation of therapy aimed at delaying the onset of heart failure in dogs with asymptomatic mitral regurgitation. These findings cannot completely exclude the potential for other ACE inhibitors to delay the onset of heart failure in cases of mitral insufficiency or the possible benefit of early institution of ACE inhibition in dogs with DCM or cats with HCM; however, while awaiting study findings on those questions, the authors will continue to delay institution of ACE inhibitor therapy until cardiac disease has progressed to a point where diuretics are needed to control congestion.

Therapeutic Efficacy in Dilated Cardiomyopathy versus Mitral Insufficiency

Activation of the renin-angiotensin system occurs subsequent to one of three major stimuli: decreased renal perfusion pressure, reduced sodium delivery to the macula densa, or sympathetic activation.[60] Therefore many cardiovascular and systemic disease processes may promote renin release, with eventual production of angiotensin II. Despite the potential for ACE inhibitors to blunt angiotensin II formation, they may have variable efficacy in alleviating the clinical signs of heart failure, depending on the underlying disease process.

The potential for discrepancies in response to ACE inhibitor therapy seemed apparent in the IMPROVE and COVE studies, which evaluated enalapril in the management of heart failure subsequent to dilated cardiomyopathy or mitral regurgitation (MR).[41,42] In both studies, dogs with DCM appeared to show a more dramatic response compared with those that had MR. After 28 days of enalapril therapy, the dogs with DCM showed significant improvement, compared with animals receiving placebo, in the class of heart failure, pulmonary edema scores, overall evaluation, mobility, attitude, activity, demeanor, cough (total, night, normal activity, and exercise), and appetite scores.[42] Dogs with MR allocated to enalapril showed significant improvement only in overall evaluation, mobility, activity, and cough (total).[42] It was noted that a longer study may have identified further significant improvements in patients with mitral regurgitation.

Figure 199-8 Early institution of enalapril therapy was unable to delay the onset of congestive heart failure in a study of 229 asymptomatic Cavalier King Charles spaniels. (From Kvart C: Efficacy of enalapril for prevention of congestive heart failure in a study of 229 cases of asymptomatic myxomatous valve disease and asymptomatic mitral regurgitation. *J Vet Intern Med* 16:1, 2002.)

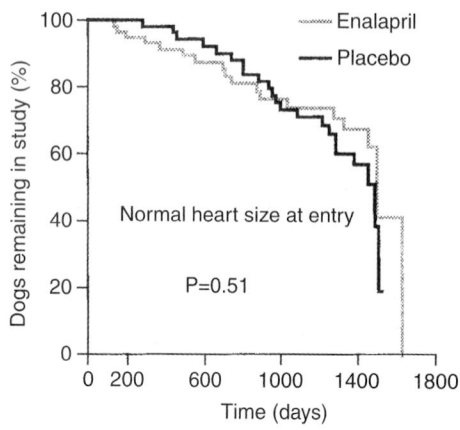

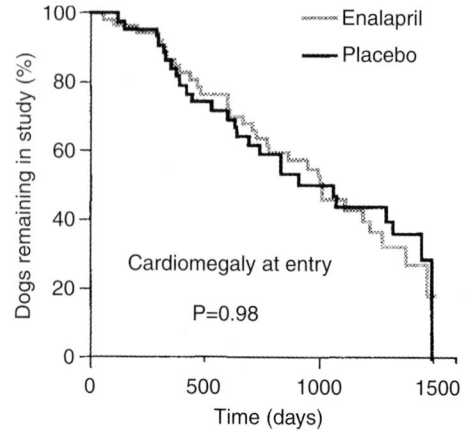

Subsequently, a longer term study was performed in an effort to determine the effects of enalapril on the survival of dogs with heart failure.[5] Dogs with DCM or MR that had developed congestive heart failure were enrolled and randomly allocated to enalapril or placebo in addition to receiving standard medical therapy. The dogs were followed until death, treatment failure (defined as deterioration of condition requiring additional medications), or termination of the study. In contrast to the short-term investigations, dogs with mitral insufficiency randomized to enalapril remained in this study significantly longer than those randomized to placebo (mean, 159.5 days versus 86.6 days, P = 0.041), whereas the DCM subgroup showed no significant differences (mean, 142.8 days versus 56.5 days, P = 0.06).[5]

Although no steadfast conclusions can be drawn from the differences between the short- and long-term studies, these findings highlight the difficulty in extrapolating across disease conditions. Furthermore, they should show the pitfalls of extrapolating results from human studies, in which the vast majority of patients have left ventricular dysfunction secondary to coronary artery disease or myocardial infarction. Until further studies can better elucidate the benefits or detriments of current veterinary medical management, practitioners must continue to rely on anecdotal evidence, presumption, and clinical judgment.

Failure to Target Other Neurohormonal Pathways

An additional limitation of triple drug therapy is the failure to target two of the neurohormonal modulators that perpetuate cardiomyocyte necrosis and ventricular fibrosis. Studies have shown that adrenergic stimulation decreases cardiomyocyte viability by means of cAMP-mediated calcium overload and that aldosterone promotes myocardial hypertrophy and fibrosis, autonomic imbalance, and electrolyte imbalances that may precipitate arrhythmias.[16,61]

Potential therapeutic strategies

Aldosterone antagonists   The neurohormonal hypothesis of heart failure gains further support from the fact that the aldosterone antagonist spironolactone has proved efficacious in the management of severe heart failure in humans. Studies have recognized that small concentrations of aldosterone can stimulate cardiac fibroblast expression of type I and type III collagen, thereby promoting myocardial fibrosis.[19] Although ACE inhibitors are considered effective at reducing aldosterone levels by inhibiting the formation of aldosterone's primary secretagogue, angiotensin II, there is mounting evidence of a phenomenon called *aldosterone escape*.[29] Increased potassium levels induced by ACE inhibitors and decreased hepatic clearance may contribute to this RAS-independent increase in aldosterone.[19] It also has become apparent that local tissue pathways for the production of aldosterone exist in extra-adrenal sites, although the importance of these tissue pathways has not been clarified.[19] Because aldosterone impairs normal vasodilative responses, promotes myocardial fibrosis, potentiates the sympathetic nervous system, and influences electrolyte transport, a recent strategy to target heart failure has been the administration of aldosterone antagonists.[61]

Addition of the aldosterone antagonist spironolactone to the baseline therapy of patients with severe heart failure produced a 30% reduction in mortality and a 35% reduction in the frequency of hospitalization for worsening heart failure.[62] Although identification of the mechanism by which spironolactone exerts its beneficial effects was not the aim of the Randomized Aldactone Evaluation Study (RALES) group, a small substudy of 261 participants suggests that limitation of aldosterone-stimulated collagen synthesis is the major contributor.[63] In a recent model of experimental heart failure created in dogs, the aldosterone antagonist eplerenone was able to

attenuate the development of interstitial fibrosis and cardiomyocyte hypertrophy while increasing capillary density.[64] Although the frequency and likelihood of aldosterone escape are unknown in dogs treated with ACE inhibitors, it seems prudent to consider spironolactone administration for patients treated with enalapril. Currently the optimal dosing scheme for dogs is unknown; however, the authors combine spironolactone (2 mg/kg given orally twice daily) with their standard therapy (furosemide and enalapril with or without digoxin) to further combat the detrimental consequences of aldosterone. Whether this is the optimal regimen or whether spironolactone promotes symptomatic or survival benefit in dogs with heart failure is unknown at this time.

Beta-blockers   Similar to what happens in humans, in dogs with congestive heart failure the body activates the sympathetic nervous system and RAS in an effort to maintain homeostasis. Unfortunately these short-term compensatory mechanisms promote adverse hemodynamic and biochemical alterations that ultimately contribute to weakness, debilitating congestive signs, deterioration of cardiac function, and ultimately death. The IMPROVE and COVE investigators identified the short-term utility of enalapril in combating dilated cardiomyopathy, and since then ACE inhibition has become routine therapy.[41,42] Although it has not been evaluated in controlled clinical trials, the loop diuretic furosemide appears to have a potent effect in alleviating the congestive clinical signs that frequently accompany heart failure. The efficacy, safety, and affordability of furosemide have made it a mainstay in the management of heart failure. Because systolic dysfunction is the primary phenotypic manifestation of dilated cardiomyopathy, the authors' ideal therapy would further use an agent that augments systolic performance without promoting adverse events. In humans, long-term administration of beta agonists and phosphodiesterase inhibitors is marred by the resultant increase in mortality and in hospitalizations for heart failure. Whether these findings would also be reflected in large-scale canine trials is unknown, but the historical adverse events have caused pharmaceutical companies to abandon their marketing in the United States. Thus digoxin is the primary positive inotrope available to improve systolic function. Although it has been reported to produce echocardiographically identifiable improvements in fractional shortening in some dogs, it remains a relatively weak positive inotrope.[53]

Just when some investigators had given up on the search for a safe positive inotropic agent, new investigations have identified a drug class that increased measures of systolic performance while decreasing mortality and hospitalizations. Surprisingly, this class of drugs is the beta blockers.

Agents that antagonize beta receptors act by interfering with the endogenous neurohormonal system. The primary integrator of the neurohormonal response to arterial underfilling appears to be the sympathetic nervous system.[19] Excessive catecholamine levels promote a daunting number of detrimental effects: peripheral vasoconstriction, impaired sodium excretion by the kidneys, myocardial hypertrophy with impaired coronary flow, provocation of arrhythmias, apoptosis, and myocytolysis.[17] Some researchers suggested that blockade of this primary integrator may retard the unrelenting nature of heart failure, whereas others were reluctant to blunt the effects (e.g., positive inotropic and chronotropic) of this potentially beneficial system. The proponents of beta blockade contended that these potential benefits are already self-limited by internalization and degradation of beta receptors in response to elevated circulating levels of norepinephrine. To settle the controversy, large-scale, placebo-controlled trials were conducted to identify the potential benefits of antiadrenergic therapy. In these studies, the second-generation beta blockers bisoprolol and metoprolol and the third-generation beta blocker carvedilol were shown to reduce mortality substantially in patients with a reduced ejection fraction.[65-67] Because the study protocols included stringent observation, slow upward drug titration, and recruitment of patients with stable rather than decompensated heart failure, most of the patients enrolled in these trials were able to tolerate the short-term negative inotropic effects associated with beta blocker administration. With long-term administration, at 4 to 12 months of treatment beta blockers were found to induce a time-dependent process of reverse remodeling in which systolic function improved as myocardial hypertrophy regressed and the ventricular geometry normalized.[68] Among the medications used to treat heart failure, this improvement in intrinsic systolic function appears to be unique to beta blockers. Based on these results, beta blocker administration currently is recommended for humans with stable heart failure secondary to systolic dysfunction.[17]

The primary types of beta blockers evaluated thus far have been those that selectively inhibit the beta$_1$ receptor (metoprolol and bisoprolol) and that antagonize beta$_1$, beta$_2$, and alpha$_1$-adrenergic receptors (carvedilol). Although carvedilol blocks peripheral vasodilative beta$_2$ receptors, it concurrently blocks vasoconstrictive alpha$_1$-adrenergic receptors, thereby enhancing its tolerance in patients afflicted with systolic dysfunction. In patients with mild to moderate heart failure, the reported tolerance for beta$_1$-selective antagonists ranges from 79% to 100%, whereas carvedilol is tolerated by approximately 92% of patients.[68] The most recent carvedilol study was performed in patients with stable NYHA class IV heart failure and an ejection fraction of less than 25%. Despite the severity of their disease, at 4 months 65% of patients assigned to carvedilol were receiving the target dose of their assigned medication.[67]

The safety and efficacy of beta blockers in the management of heart failure have been more critically evaluated in controlled drug trials than has any other class of drugs. A meta-analysis of 18 published double-blind, placebo-controlled trials involving primarily NYHA class II and class III heart failure that were conducted through 1998 revealed persuasive positive effects on mortality, hospitalization, and the ejection fraction. Beta blockers reduced the risk of death by 32% and the risk of hospitalization for heart failure by 41% while increasing the ejection fraction by 29%.[69] Patients assigned to beta blockers were 32% more likely to show improvement in their heart failure class and 30% less likely to experience worsening heart failure.[69] Large-scale trials of bisoprolol, metoprolol, and carvedilol have been reported since 1998, in which mortality reductions of 34%, 34%, and 35%, respectively, were identified.[65-67] These impressive findings have led to small-scale investigations into the management of canine heart failure with carvedilol. While the results of those trials are awaited, new treatment strategies for the management of canine dilated cardiomyopathy and degenerative mitral valve disease can be hypothesized.

Beta-blockers for the management of DCM
The management of canine dilated cardiomyopathy is often frustrating and unrewarding. Two retrospective analyses have shown median survival times of 65 days and 27 days, and 1-year survival probabilities of 37.5% and 17.5% have been reported.[2,3] The prognosis for Doberman pinschers appears even worse, with a reported median survival time of 6.5 weeks and a 1-year survival probability of 3%.[4] Survival times may since have improved with more robust use of ACE inhibitors, but dilated cardiomyopathy seems to progress much more rapidly in dogs than in humans. Approximately 25% of human patients referred to major medical centers with newly diagnosed dilated cardiomyopathy die within 1 year, and the 5-year survival rate is 50%.[70]

This discrepancy between humans and dogs in the rate of disease progression poses a problem for the management of DCM in dogs. As previously described, beta blockers have proved to be one of the most effective agents for combating heart failure, because their antiadrenergic properties offset the toxic and hemodynamic derangements induced by norepinephrine. Unfortunately, therapy for 1 to 3 months appears to be necessary before any improvement in systolic function is recognized, and administration for up to 18 months is needed for reversal of maladaptive remodeling with reduction in left ventricular volumes.[71] It therefore seems that many dogs with dilated cardiomyopathy would not live long enough to reap the beneficial effects of beta blockers. The percentage of dogs that would tolerate the short-term negative inotropic effects induced by beta blockade also is uncertain.

A potential remedy for this situation may be concurrent, low-dose administration of a positive inotropic agent during the uptitration and early target phases of beta blocker therapy. The phosphodiesterase inhibitor and calcium sensitizer pimobendan may satisfactorily fulfill this role. A study evaluating the effectiveness of carvedilol therapy compared with a combination of carvedilol and pimobendan found that withdrawal of therapy because of worsening of heart failure occurred less often in the combination group.[72]

Similar to amrinone and milrinone, pimobendan is able to improve cardiac contractility, promote ventricular relaxation, and induce vasodilatation by increasing cAMP levels. However, pimobendan also has calcium-sensitizing properties that increase contractility by enhancing the interaction between troponin C and the prevailing cytosolic calcium level. Compared with agents that increase cAMP, a calcium sensitizer has several benefits: (1) it lowers the risk of induction of arrhythmias; (2) it reduces cell injury and death caused by calcium overload; (3) it exerts its effects without increasing energy demands; and (4) it has the potential to reverse systolic dysfunction in the face of acidosis and myocardial stunning.[73] In a study of humans with heart failure, pimobendan was able to increase exercise capacity significantly without increasing oxygen consumption.[74] Proarrhythmic effects were not identified during 24-hour electrocardiography, but a trend toward increased mortality was seen in the patients assigned to pimobendan. Enrollment criteria excluded any patients treated with beta blockers, therefore whether combination therapy may have reduced the trend toward increased mortality is speculative. Nonetheless, the concept of combining a novel positive inotropic agent with a slowly titrated beta blocker may very well deserve attention. Unfortunately, pimobendan currently is not available in the United States, and the use of beta blockers in the management of DCM should be considered purely investigational.

Beta-blockers for the management of chronic degenerative valve disease
The authors currently manage CDVD with furosemide, an ACE inhibitor, and digoxin, with the addition of spironolactone in moderate to severe cases. This combination directly targets excessive plasma volume and the renin-angiotensin system while indirectly combating activation of the sympathetic nervous system. A new concept may include the addition of a beta blocker to antagonize directly the detrimental consequences of adrenergic activation. A recent study evaluated the hemodynamic effects of the ACE inhibitor lisinopril versus a combination of lisinopril and the beta blocker atenolol in the treatment of experimental mitral regurgitation.[75] Lisinopril was found to reduce significantly left ventricular end-diastolic pressure, pulmonary capillary wedge pressure, and end-diastolic stress, but it had no marked effect on forward stroke volume or left ventricular contractility. Three months after the addition of atenolol to this regimen, forward stroke volume and left ventricular contractility had returned to normal. Whether this effect occurred subsequent to an additional 3 months of ACE inhibition or was mediated by the beta blockade is uncertain. Regardless, this study suggests that direct adrenergic antagonism may prove beneficial in the management of CDVD, and further studies may be warranted.

Management of Refractory Congestive Heart Failure

Over time, many patients become refractory to standard medical therapy as disease progression continues or if a concurrent systemic disease process develops that exerts detrimental effects on the cardiovascular system (e.g., hyperadrenocorticism, hypothyroidism, renal failure, systemic hypertension, neoplasia, anemia, pneumonia, or pulmonary thromboembolism). Infrequent causes of an acute bout of decompensation include the development of hemodynamically important arrhythmias, sudden rupture of chordae tendineae, or splitting of the left atrial wall subsequent to severe mitral insufficiency and elevated left atrial pressure. For these reasons, any patient that continues to show clinical signs of congestion or low cardiac output despite appropriate medical therapy should be closely re-evaluated. After determining whether the owner is administering the prescribed drugs at the appropriate intervals, the practitioner should obtain an ECG, thoracic radiographs, complete blood count, biochemical profile, and blood pressure measurement. Echocardiography often is warranted to characterize the severity of valvular insufficiency, the extent of chamber enlargement, and the degree of systolic dysfunction.

If an underlying disease process is identified, it should be managed appropriately before institution of therapy with new cardiac drugs. Attempts should be made to suppress significant ventricular arrhythmias; agents capable of slowing conduction through the atrioventricular node (e.g., calcium channel blockers or beta blockers) may be required to help control the ventricular response rate in the face of atrial fibrillation. Potent afterload reduction with nitroprusside or hydralazine often is required to combat the effects of ruptured chordae tendineae. Left atrial tears are difficult to manage.

If no underlying disease process is identified, several strategies may be used to manage these refractory patients (Figure 199-9). Afterload reduction using arterial vasodilators, preload reduction using additional diuretics or venodilators, or additional neurohormonal blockade using beta blockers or spironolactone may be warranted. The route of diuretic administration may be modified, or positive inotropic agents periodically may be given intravenously. The inherent risks and complications of treatment are greatest in patients with refractory heart failure, and referral to a specialist is wiser than embarking on an unconventional treatment protocol.

Vasodilators

Vasodilators promote smooth muscle relaxation of the arterioles (arterial vasodilators), veins (venodilators), or arteries and veins (balanced vasodilators). Although these drug classes promote a similar therapeutic end-point, vasodilatation, a variety of mechanisms are involved in achieving their effect.

Heart failure is associated with activation of the sympathetic nervous system and renin-angiotensin system. In the face of decreased cardiac output, these systems promote arteriolar vasoconstriction to maintain adequate perfusion pressure and venoconstriction to enhance venous return to the heart. Unfortunately, the arteriolar vasoconstriction further increases the workload of the failing heart; more energy must be expended to overcome high systemic vascular resistance, and less energy is available to expel blood into the aorta. Stroke volume (and hence cardiac output [CO]) decreases, but systemic vascular resistance (SVR) continues to increase in an effort to maintain blood pressure (BP = CO × SVR). The increase in preload promoted by venoconstriction also proves detrimental because the diseased heart, operating on the plateau of the Frank-Starling curve, is unable to further hypertrophy or increase its contractility. Ventricular end-diastolic pressures begin to rise, leading to the eventual formation of edema.

Based on these hemodynamic sequelae, it seemed apparent that a reduction in afterload and/or preload ultimately would reduce mortality. Interestingly, the first V-HeFT study found that prazosin, the agent most capable of reducing blood pressure, was unable to reduce mortality compared with placebo.[13] The combination of hydralazine and isosorbide dinitrate reduced mortality, but in the V-HeFT II trial, enalapril was more effective than the combined vasodilators at preventing death.[22] This beneficial effect was seen despite the inability of the ACE inhibitor to reduce blood pressure. Obviously blood pressure and systemic vascular resistance are not synonymous, but these findings have detracted from the use of potent afterload reducers in the routine management of heart failure. Venodilators may still be effective at reducing the development of edema, but the problem of drug tolerance has limited their use to animals with refractory heart failure.

Amlodipine Amlodipine is a second-generation, dihydropyridine (DHP) calcium channel blocker that primarily produces arteriolar vasodilatation and is used in the treatment of systemic hypertension. Unlike the non-DHPs diltiazem and verapamil, amlodipine has little effect on conduction through the atrioventricular node, and its negative inotropic properties appear to be offset by a reduction in afterload. Although amlodipine was unable to reduce mortality in an evaluation of 1153 patients with left ventricular dysfunction and severe

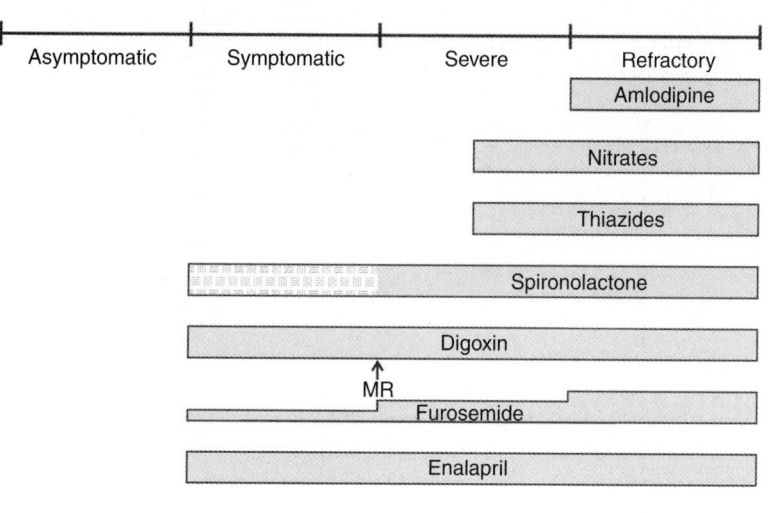

Figure 199-9 Although therapy must be tailored on a case-by-case basis, the authors traditionally do not start medical therapy in asymptomatic patients. As the disease progresses over time and compensatory mechanisms overwhelm traditional ACE inhibitor, diuretic, and digoxin therapy, other strategies must be used to combat congestive and low-output signs. Currently the optimal time for institution of therapy with aldosterone antagonists is uncertain.

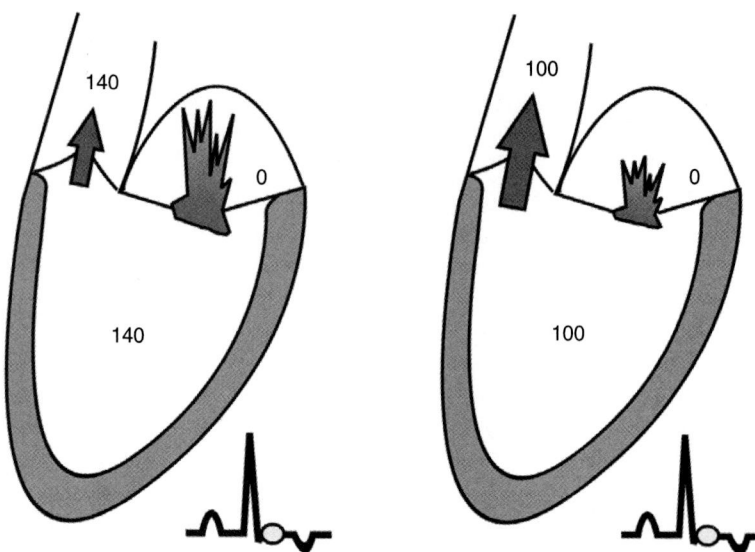

Figure 199-10 Left ventricular systolic pressure is influenced by the systemic vascular resistance, therefore agents capable of reducing afterload have the potential to decrease the volume of mitral insufficiency while increasing the effective forward stroke volume.

heart failure (P = 0.07), it did reduce the mortality rate by 31% (P = 0.04) in the subgroup of patients with nonischemic DCM.[14] Despite this mortality benefit, 14 of the 209 patients with DCM assigned to amlodipine developed pulmonary edema (compared with 2 of 212 patients assigned to placebo). The mechanism involved in this development was uncertain.

An interesting application of amlodipine therapy may be for severe mitral valve insufficiency. A reduction in systemic vascular resistance (and hence the systolic left ventricular to left atrial pressure gradient) may serve to decrease the volume of mitral valve insufficiency (Figures 199-10 and 199-11). Potential benefits of amlodipine are its 30-hour half-life and peak effect in 4 to 7 days after institution of therapy to dogs. This slow onset of action may give the baroreceptors time to reset, thereby avoiding sympathetic activation and reflex tachycardia. The effective dose of amlodipine seems to vary; a common strategy is to institute therapy at a low dose (0.05 mg/kg given orally once daily), followed by slow titration up to 0.2 mg/kg until a reduction in blood pressure is achieved. Because of the drug's long half-life, the authors typically monitor blood pressure weekly, using uptitration until the target blood pressure is attained.

Hydralazine Hydralazine is a direct-acting arterial vasodilator that promotes vasodilatation through an unknown mechanism. It was studied in the 1980s for the management of CDVD in dogs and was found to produce substantial decreases in mean arterial blood pressure, total systemic resistance index, and

pulmonary capillary wedge pressure.[76] Since that time, hydralazine appears to have been pushed aside by the ACE inhibitors in the management of uncomplicated heart failure. This trend likely resulted from the commonly encountered side effects of hydralazine (i.e., symptomatic hypotension, anorexia, vomiting, and diarrhea), the presence of elevated aldosterone levels seen after hydralazine therapy compared with captopril, and the significant results of the V-HeFT II trial.[77]

Hydralazine is still used in the acute management of decompensated heart failure when nitroprusside is unavailable (or impractical to use) because of its rapid onset of action. Similar to amlodipine, the reduction in systemic vascular resistance may reduce the volume of mitral insufficiency and promote an increase in the forward stroke volume. In contrast to amlodipine, the peak vasodilative effect of hydralazine occurs within 3 hours and subsides within 12 hours. Unfortunately, this same characteristic may result in reflex tachycardia and further stimulation of the sympathetic nervous system and RAS. A study by Haggstrom et al.[31] identified significant increases in heart rate and plasma aldosterone and angiotensin II concentrations, as well as evidence of fluid retention, in Cavalier King Charles spaniels with mitral insufficiency that were treated with hydralazine monotherapy for 3 weeks. These findings suggest that ACE inhibitors should be used concurrently with hydralazine if chronic afterload reduction is warranted.

For the management of fulminant congestive heart failure, hydralazine may be administered at a dosage of 2 mg/kg given

Figure 199-11 After administration of the calcium channel blocker amlodipine, the regurgitant stroke volume in dogs with mitral insufficiency was significantly reduced (by 18.9%). Although these data look promising, it should be noted that this study had no control population, the echocardiographer was not blinded, and no data evaluation of the neurohormonal consequences of afterload reduction was performed. (Courtesy Dr. Mark Oyama, University of Illinois College of Veterinary Medicine, Urbana-Champaign.)

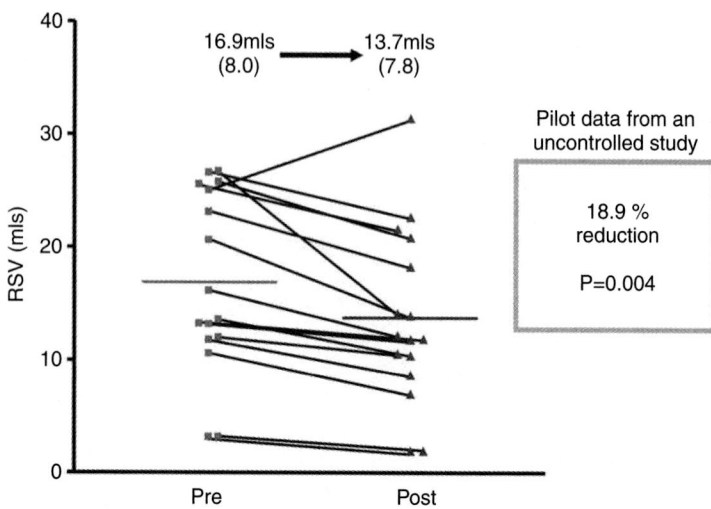

orally twice daily to dogs with a systolic blood pressure above 100 mm Hg. The authors recommend blood pressure monitoring, with the twin goals of avoiding hypotension and monitoring therapeutic efficacy. Ideally the increase in effective cardiac output will counterbalance the hydralazine-mediated reduction in systemic vascular resistance, preventing the development of symptomatic hypotension.

Nitrates The nitrates, which include nitroglycerin, isosorbide dinitrate and isosorbide mononitrate, and nitroprusside, are a class of vasodilators that promote the formation of nitric oxide. Although nitroprusside administered intravenously is a potent balanced vasodilator, topical and oral administration of nitroglycerin and oral administration of isosorbide dinitrate and isosorbide mononitrate appear to promote primarily venodilatation. The premise behind venodilatation is to promote redistribution of the circulating blood volume from the heart and pulmonary vasculature to the systemic venous circulation. This reduction in preload should decrease ventricular end-diastolic, atrial, and pulmonary capillary pressures, shifting the Frank-Starling curve to the left and alleviating pulmonary edema. Currently the efficacy of nitrates in the management of chronic heart failure is uncertain and may be limited by *nitrate tolerance*, the phenomenon in which continued drug exposure reduces the agent's effectiveness.

Nitroglycerin A 2% topical formulation of nitroglycerin combined with furosemide and oxygen (with or without hydralazine) is frequently used in the management of acute heart failure. Anecdotal recommendations have called for application of nitroglycerin cream to a clipped or hairless region ($\frac{1}{2}$ to 2 inches every 6 to 8 hours for dogs; $\frac{1}{4}$-inch every 6 to 8 hours for cats) to promote continuous transdermal absorption and venodilatation. Studies evaluating the absorption of cutaneously applied nitroglycerin, the optimal site for topical administration, and the efficacy of this therapy for dogs or cats with heart failure have not been reported. There is a report that nitroglycerin applied to the auricular pinna promotes splenic vasodilatation in normal anesthetized dogs, but by no means should nitroglycerin replace furosemide as the primary agent for reducing preload and alleviating pulmonary edema.[78]

Isosorbide dinitrate and isosorbide mononitrate Isosorbide dinitrate and its major metabolite, mononitrate, are orally administered venodilators that may help reduce preload and hence pulmonary edema. Similar to nitroglycerin, the orally administered nitrates have not been extensively studied in naturally occurring heart failure. However, Adin et al.[79] were unable to document circulatory redistribution after a single dose of isosorbide mononitrate in normal dogs or in those with heart failure. Whether nitrates can regress cardiac remodeling in naturally occurring heart failure remains to be investigated.[80]

Although their efficacy is unknown, isosorbide dinitrate (0.5 to 2 mg/kg given orally twice daily) and isosorbide mononitrate (0.25 to 2 mg/kg given orally twice daily) occasionally are used in the management of refractory heart failure or in combination with hydralazine or amlodipine for patients unable to tolerate ACE inhibitors. Whether dosing-free intervals are required to combat the development of nitrate tolerance for dogs and cats is unknown.

Triple Diuretic Therapy

Although twice-daily administration of a loop diuretic appears to be the regimen most frequently used to manage congestive heart failure, there are physiologic benefits to altering the dosing frequency or combining agents from different classes. Although not a true component of diuretic resistance, the activity of the nephron in the absence of therapeutic diuretic concentrations must be kept in mind. The loop diuretics currently available are not long-acting formulations. Therefore the original diuretic effects have dissipated well before the administration of a second daily dose. During this time, when

it is not inhibited, the $Na^+/K^+/2Cl^-$ pump promotes avid sodium resorption, possibly to a degree that negates any previous natriuretic effect.[27] This highlights the point that, in cases of worsening heart failure, three times daily dosing of furosemide may be more beneficial than merely increasing the twice daily dose. In cases of right-sided heart failure, in which oral drug absorption may be impaired, changing the type of administration to the subcutaneous or intramuscular route may prove beneficial. Administration of a diuretic by means of a constant-rate infusion may prove the most beneficial during emergency treatment of heart failure, although frequent, moderate doses likely achieve a similar end-point.

No matter the dosing interval or the route of administration, the segments of the nephron distal to the loop of Henle are capable of producing diuretic resistance. Increased solute exposure to the distal nephron promotes hypertrophy and increased resorptive capacity of the early distal tubule, the connecting tubule, and the cortical collecting duct.[81] Although the exact mechanisms are unclear, aldosterone has been implicated as promoting this process.[81] Strategies to combat diuretic resistance associated with long-standing administration of a loop diuretic include (1) addition of a thiazide diuretic to encourage diuresis in the hypertrophied region and/or (2) addition of an aldosterone antagonist to target the proposed hypertrophic mechanism. This synergistic nephron blockade, using multiple agents with activity in different regions of the nephron, may allow a reduction in the dose of furosemide required to control the patient's congestive signs. In the authors' experience, furosemide and spironolactone, combined with conservative doses of hydrochlorothiazide, have palliated the congestive signs of many heart failure patients. However, this more aggressive diuretic management predisposes the patient to the development of electrolyte abnormalities and a reduction in cardiac output and the GFR unless care is taken to avoid overzealous volume contraction. Outpatients should be carefully and periodically evaluated through biochemical profiles to make sure that adverse effects are avoided.

Additional factors that can contribute to diuretic resistance include (1) poor cardiac output, which impairs delivery of the diuretic to its site of action; (2) prominent activation of the renin-angiotensin system; and (3) hypokalemia, which may impair the efficacy of the diuretic. If concern exists about diuretic resistance, care should be taken to optimize the ACE inhibitor dose, to correct electrolyte imbalances, and to combat low-output conditions.

Dietary Sodium Restriction

Historically, sodium restriction has been recommended for patients with cardiovascular disease to decrease the delivery of sodium to and its resorption in the distal tubule.[82] This recommendation was in place well before any of the current understanding of the renin-angiotensin system developed, and it therefore may need to be reevaluated.

It currently is recognized that reduced sodium concentrations at the macula densa serve as a stimulus for renin release and subsequent production of angiotensin. A study of Cavalier King Charles spaniels with mild asymptomatic mitral valve insufficiency showed that a low-sodium diet (17 mg/kg/day) was associated with higher plasma renin activity and aldosterone concentrations than a control diet (96 mg/kg/day).[83] In light of the concern that activation of neurohormonal pathways promotes the progressive nature of cardiovascular disease, the authors currently do not use sodium restriction in asymptomatic patients. Whether symptomatic patients receive clinical benefit from sodium restriction is uncertain, but one study found that dogs with mitral valve insufficiency that were fed a low-sodium diet (24 mg/kg/day) had significantly smaller left atrial and left ventricular dimensions than they did when fed a moderate-sodium diet (42 mg/kg/day).[84] Only a small number of dogs with dilated cardiomyopathy were enrolled in the study, but no significant differences in their echocardiographic parameters were seen between the two diets. Despite ACE inhibitor therapy, greater than 70% of the dogs enrolled in the study had increased baseline concentrations of ANP and increased plasma renin activity and aldosterone concentrations; however, the dietary modifications were not associated with significant alterations from baseline.[84]

Whether exclusively feeding a low-sodium diet to patients with heart failure is feasible often hinges on the palatability of the diet and the willingness of the owner to abandon treats and table scraps. Although uncertain of its clinical benefit or potential detriment, the authors often recommend a low- to moderate-sodium diet for patients with refractory heart failure. As evidenced by the study by Mallery et al.,[7] anorexia is a large contributing factor (68%) in the decision for euthanasia; therefore caution, education, and a willingness to abandon the regimen must accompany the prescription of a potentially less palatable, sodium-restricted diet.

Management of Heart Failure Secondary to Diastolic Dysfunction

Maintenance Therapy

After stabilization, furosemide is switched to oral administration and the dose is decreased (6.25 mg given twice daily) to prevent excessive preload reduction, dehydration, and hypokalemia. In cases of hypertrophic cardiomyopathy, additional drugs may be instituted to reduce the heart rate and improve diastolic filling. Drugs frequently used in the management of HCM include the beta blocker atenolol and the calcium channel blocker diltiazem. Calcium channel blockers theoretically can exert a beneficial effect in the management of HCM by modestly reducing the heart rate and contractility, thereby diminishing myocardial oxygen demand. Diltiazem may promote a direct positive lusitropic effect, and verapamil may partially reduce coronary endothelial dysfunction compared with propranolol.[85,86] Atenolol (6.25 to 12.5 mg given orally every 12 to 24 hours) appears to exert better rate control and more consistently alleviates left ventricular outflow tract obstruction compared with diltiazem. Beta-adrenergic blockade may also prevent myocardial fibrosis by inhibiting catecholamine-induced cardiotoxicity and may combat ventricular arrhythmias by decreasing myocardial oxygen consumption. One theoretical disadvantage of the use of beta blockers in the management of diastolic dysfunction is that phospholamban is an inhibitory protein that controls the rate of diastolic calcium uptake into the sarcoplasmic reticulum. Beta-adrenergic stimulation phosphorylates phospholamban and removes this inhibitory effect. Beta blockade may prevent this phosphorylation (and therefore decrease diastolic calcium uptake) and further impair the active process of ventricular relaxation.

Similar to beta blockers, with their proposed neurohormonal benefits, ACE inhibitors likely are beneficial in the management of feline HCM. The authors have seen cats with symptomatic cardiomyopathy show marked neurohormonal activation.[87] With this finding, and with the frequent requirement for furosemide to control pulmonary edema, it appears prudent to use enalapril (1.25 to 2.5 mg given orally every 12 to 24 hours) in the management of diastolic dysfunction. Although there is concern that afterload reduction may precipitate dynamic left ventricular outflow tract obstruction, recent data suggest that ACE inhibitors can be used safely in cats with systolic anterior motion of the mitral valve.[88]

FUTURE PROSPECTS CURRENTLY UNDER INVESTIGATION

Medical Therapy

Search for a Safe Positive Inotropic Agent

A class of drugs currently receiving attention in the management of congestive heart failure is the calcium sensitizers. These agents can augment systolic performance by enhancing calcium binding to troponin C or by affecting the cross-bridge turnover kinetics without increasing cytosolic calcium levels.[89] A potential drawback to clinical use of pure calcium sensitizers would be the enhanced reactivity of troponin C with diastolic cytosolic calcium levels, which would slow the process of myocardial relaxation.[73] In an attempt to avoid this potential diastolic dysfunction, most of the agents under investigation today use a combination of phosphodiesterase (PDE) inhibition and calcium sensitization. Because these drugs produce both calcium sensitization and PDE inhibition, it becomes difficult to determine whether the positive inotropic action stems from enhanced reactivity of troponin C and Ca^{2+} or cAMP-mediated phosphorylation of phosphoproteins, or a combination of the two.

In an effort to elucidate the mechanisms of the positive inotropic effects of pimobendan, EMD 53998, levosimendan, and OR-1896, a group of investigators sought to determine whether these drugs were capable of increasing left ventricular contractility (+dP/dt) without altering the myoplasmic Ca^{2+} transient.[90] Each agent was administered at variable concentrations, and subsequently +dP/dt, myocardial calcium transients, phosphorylation of key intracellular phosphoproteins, and myocardial cAMP levels were measured. The investigators found that low concentrations of levosimendan and OR-1896 were capable of increasing left ventricular contractility without affecting Ca^{2+} transients or myocardial cAMP levels and without promoting significant phosphorylation of troponin I and C proteins.[90] Administration of low concentrations of pimobendan or EMD 53998 produced more pronounced increases in Ca^{2+} transients compared with increases in left ventricular contractility. As the administration dose increased, all of the agents caused an increase in +dP/dt that was associated with further increases in myocardial cAMP levels and phosphorylation of intracellular phosphoproteins.[90] The investigators therefore concluded that pimobendan, EMD 53998, and higher doses of levosimendan and OR-1896 exerted positive inotropic properties through PDE inhibition–mediated responses rather than through calcium sensitization.[90] These researchers felt that their results lent support to the premise that low-dose levosimendan and OR-1896 were capable of augmenting left ventricular contractility by increasing the response of the myofilaments to the prevailing calcium concentrations.[90]

It should be noted that these conclusions are far from universally accepted. Other investigators, including Endoh,[73] have found that pimobendan can elicit a positive inotropic effect even in the presence of carbachol, a muscarinic receptor agonist that is useful for differentiating cAMP-mediated effects from those classified as calcium sensitization. Endoh's report[73] found that although levosimendan appears to have calcium-sensitizing properties, it must rely on simultaneous activation of cAMP-mediated signaling processes.[73]

The varying results of these studies show that the precise mechanisms by which the calcium sensitizers exert a positive inotropic effect is uncertain and that long-term controlled studies are required to evaluate the effects of these drugs on the heart rate, arrhythmogenesis, and sudden death.

Pimobendan Despite its questionable calcium-sensitizing properties, pimobendan currently is the most investigated agent in this drug class. Similar to other agents in this class, pimobendan combines calcium sensitization and PDE inhibition to circumvent any diastolic dysfunction. However, this same property carries the potential for cAMP-dependent increases in arrhythmogenesis. Despite its predominantly cAMP-mediated inotropic effect, pimobendan can increase cardiac contractility to a degree similar to that of dobutamine but at a lower oxygen cost for contractility.[91] Although pimobendan appears to lower myocardial oxygen consumption, the stigma associated with positive inotropic agents, especially those that increase cAMP concentrations, may have doused early enthusiasm for pimobendan in the United States. Although not available in the United States, pimobendan currently is available in Canada, Europe, and Japan and has undergone several small to medium-sized investigations in humans and dogs.

Multiple pimobendan trials have been completed in humans with heart failure.[74,92] The results of these trials have been variable, pointing out both apparent beneficial effects and questionable, undesirable side effects.

A recent placebo-controlled study has been published that evaluated pimobendan therapy (0.3 to 0.6 mg/kg/day) in a small number of Doberman pinschers and cocker spaniels with dilated cardiomyopathy.[93] The addition of pimobendan to standard therapy with digoxin, enalapril, and furosemide was associated with a significant improvement in the heart failure class. The cocker spaniels allocated to placebo and to pimobendan showed statistically similar median survival times (537 days versus 1037 days, P = 0.77), whereas the Doberman pinschers allocated to placebo had significantly shorter median survival times than those given pimobendan (50 days versus 329 days, P < 0.02).[93]

This small study highlighted several findings. The first interesting finding is that cocker spaniels with dilated cardiomyopathy appear to have the potential for long-term survival. At the conclusion of the 4-year study, six of the 10 cocker spaniels were still alive (two in the pimobendan group and four in the placebo group). Three of the four dogs that had died (one in the placebo group and two in the pimobendan group) were euthanized for noncardiac disease; the fourth dog, allocated to pimobendan, died suddenly within 1 month of diagnosis. The study was too small to allow assessment of the propensity of pimobendan to exacerbate arrhythmias, but the drug may have contributed to the cocker spaniel's sudden death.

Another interesting aspect of this study is that although positive inotropic therapy may prolong survival in Doberman pinschers with DCM, it may be prudent to randomize patients with atrial fibrillation (AF) separately from those without this condition. Historically Doberman pinschers with atrial fibrillation have had an abysmal 2.9-week median survival time.[4] The pimobendan randomization happened to allocate three Doberman pinschers with AF into the placebo group and only one into the pimobendan group. This may have negatively affected survival in the placebo group, but it should be noted that the Doberman with atrial fibrillation that was treated with pimobendan survived for 37 weeks.[93]

The observed reduction in heart failure class associated with pimobendan therapy likely will prompt further investigations into this agent. Whether pimobendan administration to dogs produces a trend toward increased mortality, as identified in the Pimobendan in Congestive Heart Failure (PICO) trial, is uncertain.[74] Whether the combination of low-dose pimobendan and a beta blocker would have synergistic properties in dogs with dilated cardiomyopathy is uncertain but is an interesting concept. The study by Mallery et al.[7] continues to pose the question of whether a small but significantly increased incidence of sudden death in dogs should preclude the availability of an agent with the potential to enhance their quality of life.

Angiotensin II Receptor Antagonists

The beneficial effects of ACE inhibitors have largely been attributed to these drugs' ability to decrease the formation of angiotensin II and increase circulating levels of bradykinin. However, alternative, ACE-independent pathways for the production of angiotensin II, including tissue plasminogen activator, cathepsin G, tonin, and chymase, may enable AT II "escape" even with administration of ACE inhibitors.[32] A study of patients treated with a variety of ACE inhibitors identified angiotensin II "reactivation" in 15% of patients.[29] This process occurred in the face of both high and low levels of ACE activity, which suggests that alternate pathways were responsible for the production of angiotensin II. As a potential strategy for offsetting these alternate angiotensin II–generating pathways, agents capable of directly antagonizing the AT II receptors were developed.

Two subtypes of angiotensin II receptors have been identified in humans: angiotensin II type 1 (AT_1) and angiotensin II type 2 (AT_2). Although these receptors belong to the same family, some researchers have suggested that their biologic activities differ markedly (Figure 199-12).[32] AT_1 receptors are found primarily in the adrenal glands, vascular smooth muscle cells, kidney, and heart, where they mediate almost exclusively all the known actions of angiotensin II on blood pressure and osmoregulation.[32] AT_2 receptors are expressed in high density during fetal development; in adults they are found less abundantly in the adrenal medulla, uterus, ovary, and vascular endothelium and in areas of the brain. AT_2 receptors appear to mediate biologic processes that counteract the trophic, AT_1-mediated responses.[32] Agents capable of blocking the AT_1 receptor subtype were developed with the aim of achieving more complete angiotensin II antagonism than is obtained with ACE inhibitors. Also, selectively targeting the AT_1 receptor subtype would still allow for the potentially beneficial actions mediated by the AT_2 receptors and avoid common side effects, predominantly coughing, associated with ACE inhibitor therapy in humans. It is believed that the increased circulating levels of bradykinin promoted by ACE inhibitors contribute to these drugs' side effects, but it must be noted that this same property, which is lacking in AT II receptor antagonists, may contribute to the ACE inhibitors' success in the management of heart failure.

Efforts to determine whether ACE inhibitors or angiotensin II receptor antagonists were superior or noninferior quickly followed the development of the latter agents. An early study, the Evaluation of Losartan in the Elderly (ELITE) trial, lent support to the premise that ATII receptor blockade may yield mortality benefits compared with ACE inhibitors.[94] Other studies that examined various subgroups followed. Mortality and morbidity end-points were examined to determine whether AT II inhibitors are preferable to ACE inhibitors.[94-96]

The results of ELITE II and the Valsartan Heart Failure Trial (Val-HeFT) suggest better tolerability of AT II inhibitors compared with ACE inhibitors, but these studies provide no data to support the superiority of AT II inhibitors in the management of heart failure subsequent to systolic dysfunction. The proposed significant benefit behind combination therapy with AT II inhibitors and ACE inhibitors identified in Val-HeFT is limited after the ACE inhibitor–naïve subgroup is removed from the analysis.[97] Of additional concern was the fact that valsartan, compared to placebo, had an adverse effect on mortality (P = 0.009) in patients previously treated with ACE inhibitors and beta blockers.[96] Although these results cannot be extrapolated to veterinary medicine and because clinical trials have not been performed in dogs or cats with naturally occurring heart failure, the current utility of angiotensin II receptor antagonists appears limited.

Neutral Endopeptidase Inhibitors

With the success of the ACE inhibitors established, research interests quickly shifted to additional, potentially beneficial neurohormonal pathways. Based on the recognition that ANP can promote natriuresis and diuresis and can directly inhibit the release of renin and aldosterone, new agents were developed in an effort to increase ANP's circulating concentration. Neutral endopeptidase (NEP) is an enzyme that inactivates several substrates, including natriuretic peptides, angiotensins, and bradykinins.[98] It was hypothesized that drugs capable of inhibiting NEP may prove beneficial in the management of congestive heart failure as single agents or in combination therapy. Early studies of the NEP inhibitor ecadotril given to dogs with pacing-induced heart failure showed increased urine output, sodium clearance, and renal sodium excretion compared with dogs given placebo.[98] Another short-term study of ecadotril identified a dose- and time-dependent reduction in left ventricular

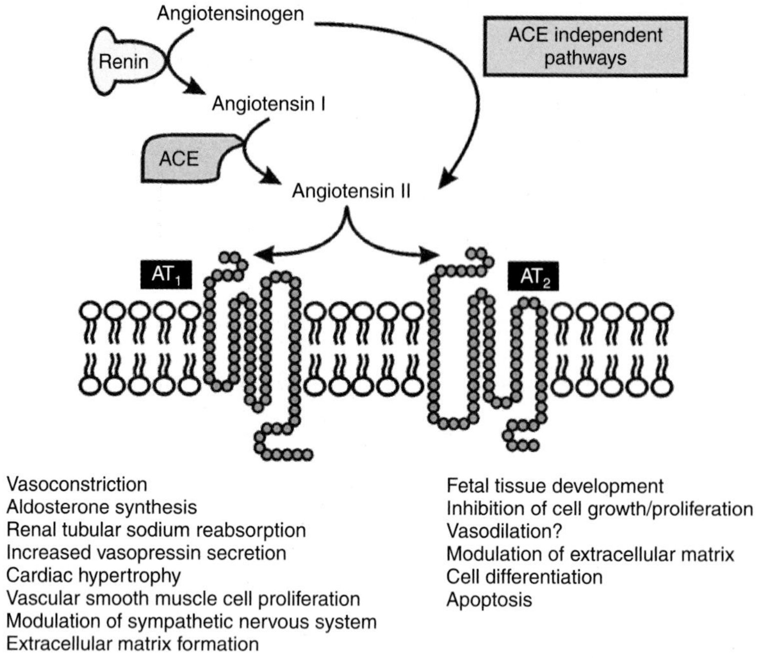

Figure 199-12 The formation of angiotensin II may follow ACE-dependent or ACE-independent pathways. Despite the potential for angiotensin II receptor blockers to promote more complete antagonism, current studies in humans have found them no better than traditional ACE inhibitors at combating heart failure.

end-diastolic pressures in dogs with experimental heart failure produced by repeated coronary embolization.[99] Long-term administration of ecadotril (3 months) in dogs with left ventricular dysfunction produced by sequential intracoronary microembolizations was recently reported to attenuate left ventricular remodeling and progressive left ventricular dysfunction compared with dogs receiving placebo.[100]

Despite these findings, NEP inhibitors administered as single agents appear to have fallen out of the research arena. A communication on behalf of the International Ecadotril Multi-Centre Dose-Ranging Study reported findings from a study of 279 patients with chronic heart failure randomized to placebo or one of four doses of ecadotril.[101] The study's primary aim was to evaluate the safety and tolerability of ecadotril at doses of 50-400 mg twice daily. Two patients randomized to the highest dose of ecadotril developed pancytopenia at 47 and 53 days, and died rapidly of sepsis. The presence of a thioester group within the compound suggested an idiosyncratic ecadotril-induced aplastic anemia that was potentially dose related.[101] Lower doses of ecadotril were not associated with adverse reactions. Although the study was not powered to exclude symptomatic benefit, patient-reported symptoms and quality of life-scores were unable to reveal any overall symptomatic benefit during the administration of ecadotril.[101] A similar, smaller pilot study from the United States evaluating 50 patients randomized to placebo or ecadotril, 50 to 400 mg twice daily, did not identify any adverse sequela but again there were no changes identified in signs and symptoms of heart failure, NYHA class, or patient self-assessment of symptoms.[102]

Vasopeptidase Inhibitors

Although it is difficult to determine the reasons for the relative lack of efficacy seen in the small pilot studies of ecadotril, the problem may have been that the drug increased not only natriuretic peptide levels but also the levels of circulating angiotensin II. More recently a group of drugs that can inhibit NEP and ACE, the so-called *vasopeptidase inhibitors*, has been developed.

Omapatrilat has been the most rigorously evaluated vasopeptidase inhibitor in several trials for the management of congestive heart failure. No significant difference was seen in the primary end-point of combined risk of death or hospitalization for heart failure requiring intravenous treatment (P = 0.187)

between omapatrilat and ACE inhibitors.[104] To date, the inability of vasopeptidase inhibitors to provide substantial benefit compared with the proven efficacy of ACE inhibitors may limit their clinical utility.

Endothelin Antagonists

Endothelin, a peptide released from endothelial cells, has powerful vasoconstrictive activity. Currently three peptides, endothelin-1, endothelin-2, and endothelin-3, and two receptor subtypes, ET_A and ET_B, have been identified. In principle, endothelin-1 promotes vasoconstriction by complexing with the ET_A receptor and vasodilatation by binding to the ET_B receptor, but this is somewhat species dependent. In addition to its vasodilative properties, the ET_B receptor may promote vasoconstriction in some regional blood vessels, including the mesenteric and coronary vasculature.[105]

Although endothelin's name suggests that it is produced only in vascular endothelial cells, the genes that encode the three peptides have been identified in varying patterns in vascular smooth muscle cells, cardiac myocytes, renal tubular epithelial cells, bronchial epithelial cells, glial cells, pituitary cells, macrophages, and mast cells.[105] Therefore the importance of endothelin may extend well beyond simple vasoconstriction and include additional pleiotropic effects on many nonvascular tissues. Although endothelin is suspected of being linked to systemic hypertension, pulmonary hypertension, vascular remodeling, and acute renal failure, the emphasis of this discussion is on potential applications of endothelin to the progression of heart failure.[105]

Heart failure, through increased filling pressures and decreased peripheral perfusion, promotes activation of numerous neurohormonal reflexes to maintain cardiac output and circulatory homeostasis. Activation of the RAS and SNS and the release of arginine vasopressin are recognized to increase the concentration of circulating vasoconstrictors (i.e., angiotensin II, norepinephrine, and vasopressin) and to promote maladaptive remodeling. Furthermore, it has been shown that these compensatory mechanisms enhance the production of endothelin.[105] Increased endothelin binding to the ET_A receptors promotes vasoconstriction and smooth muscle cell proliferation, thereby further diminishing cardiac performance through afterload mismatch. Studies have also shown that the ET_B receptors become upregulated and can promote vasoconstriction and cardiac fibrosis in the presence of heart failure.[106] These findings have raised the possibility of administration of ET_A receptor antagonists or a combination of ET_A/ET_B receptor antagonists to combat heart failure.

Chronic administration of endothelin antagonists to laboratory animals with experimental heart failure and acute administration to humans with heart failure resulted in beneficial hemodynamic profiles. In rats with heart failure induced by coronary artery ligation, the combination of an ACE inhibitor and an endothelin (ET_A) antagonist lowered the systolic blood pressure and the left ventricular end-systolic and left ventricular end-diastolic pressures significantly more than the ACE inhibitor or endothelin antagonist alone.[107] However, the drug combination did not significantly improve survival or reduce left ventricular weight and collagen density compared with rats randomized to an ACE inhibitor alone. Endothelin antagonism without the benefit of ACE inhibition did not result in a survival benefit compared with untreated rats with heart failure.

Despite these promising hemodynamic profiles, early evidence suggests that chronic nonselective and ET_A-selective antagonism of endothelin receptors is of limited benefit in patients with severe heart failure. The Endothelin Antagonist Bosentan for Lowering Cardiac Events in Heart Failure (ENABLE) trial evaluated the nonselective endothelin antagonist bosentan, which has proved beneficial in pulmonary hypertension, for the management of humans with NYHA class IIIb-IV heart failure and an ejection fraction of less than 35%. The patients randomized to Bosentan appeared to have an increased early risk of worsening heart failure requiring hospitalization.[108]

These studies appear to highlight the fact that hemodynamic benefit may not equate with clinical benefit. Whether lower doses of the endothelin antagonists and slow uptitration might prove beneficial is unresolved at this time; however, the results of studies to date may have curtailed the momentum for the use of endothelin antagonists in the management of chronic heart failure.

Interventional Therapy
Passive Ventricular Constraint
In the early 1990s an experimental "ventricular assist" technique was developed in which a patient's native skeletal muscle was wrapped around the failing ventricles to provide cardiac support. The latissimus dorsi, connected to a synchronizable burst stimulator, was used in an effort to increase cardiac contractility and hence functional status.[110] The utility of dynamic cardiomyoplasty held promise because it alleviated the need for cardiac bypass, donor organs, and immunosuppression, which are required for cardiac transplantation. The feasibility of dynamic cardiomyoplasty in dogs was subsequently documented, and researchers found a potential for improved contractile function even during contractions that were not assisted by myostimulation of the latissimus dorsi.[111]

Although dynamic cardiomyoplasty has failed to gain prominence in the management of heart failure, the potential for limiting ventricular dilatation by means of passive constraint has prompted further study. The premise is that passive ventricular constraint may significantly slow or stabilize the remodeling process that accompanies heart failure. Because the constraint is passive and does not require myostimulation, a synthetic wrap could be used, simplifying the surgical procedure.[112,113]

Despite the potential benefit of passive ventricular constraint in these models, the fact remains that veterinary patients tend to be presented for evaluation after severe cardiac dysfunction has already developed. New diagnostic modalities may allow for earlier detection of occult cardiac disease, but the variable nature of disease progression could still complicate the determination of which patients should be fitted with a cardiac support device. At this time, further studies are required to evaluate the efficacy of passive ventricular constraint in severe cardiac dysfunction, and diagnostic tests allowing early detection of cardiac disease must be developed.

Ventricular Resynchronization
Although systolic dysfunction classically is believed to be a myocardial phenomenon, the important role the cardiac conduction system plays in maintaining optimal cardiac performance is often forgotten. The normal conduction pathway modulates the contraction rate, the mechanical efficacy of atrial systole, and the co-ordination of the ventricular chambers.[114] In humans the presence of an intraventricular conduction delay, typically in a left bundle branch block pattern, promotes disco-ordinate contraction, with early activation of the septal wall followed by delayed lateral contraction at higher stress.[114] The presence of this conduction defect has been associated with a 60% to 70% higher risk of all-cause mortality and has remained an independent risk factor after adjustment for age, underlying cardiac disease, severity of heart failure, and treatment with ACE inhibitors or beta blockers.[115] The problem of ventricular discordance has long been recognized in patients with artificial ventricular pacemakers, and efforts to approximate the ventricular activation sequence more closely (i.e., by pacing the right ventricular outflow tract rather than the apex) have been shown to increase cardiac output.[116-118]

Recently a similar approach, called *cardiac resynchronization therapy* (CRT), has been used in patients with congestive heart failure and intraventricular conduction delay. Biventricular pacing or univentricular pacing of the left ventricular free wall has improved the contractile index $+dP/dT_{max}$ and arterial pulse pressure within a single beat of commencement of pacing.[114] The proposed benefits of CRT include a reduction in end-systolic and end-diastolic volumes and the ability to promote reverse remodeling. Ventricular resynchronization has been associated with increased systolic function despite a decline in myocardial oxygen consumption.[114] This contrasts with traditional cAMP-dependent inotropic therapy and may explain the ability of biventricular pacing to improve functional patient status while promoting mortality benefits. Unfortunately, the ability of CRT to improve heart failure class and reduce mortality in veterinary medicine may be limited by the low prevalence of intraventricular conduction disturbances in dogs with dilated cardiomyopathy.

Stem Cells and Cellular Transplantation
Historically it has been recognized that cardiac and neural tissues lack the large postnatal regenerative capacity seen in the epithelial layers of the skin, intestinal and pulmonary mucosal linings, and connective tissues. Therefore the ability to repopulate areas of ischemic myocardium with cells capable of promoting angiogenesis or areas of fibrosis with cells that contribute to contractile function could prove curative.

Numerous cell types have been identified that may serve as potential sources for tissue grafting, including skeletal myoblasts, fetal cardiomyocytes, smooth muscle cells, embryonic stem cells and bone marrow–derived stromal and hematopoietic stem cells.[120] Because of the complex electrophysiologic, structural, and contractile properties of myocardial cells, cardiomyocytes appear to be the ideal donor cells. The difficulty lies in harvesting and transplanting enough cells to mitigate the degree of cardiac dysfunction. The isolation of pluripotent stem cells from mouse blastocysts in 1981 may have provided the key to an endless vault of viable, transplantable cardiomyocytes.[120]

The promise of stem cells lies in their capacity for prolonged self-renewal and their potential to differentiate into one or more cell types. Embryonic stem (ES) cells display wide-ranging plasticity, which allows them to form derivatives of all three germ layers. Their ability to undergo near endless cell doublings while retaining the capacity to differentiate into various cell types further advances their therapeutic potential. However, beyond the ethical considerations involved in the use of human embryonic stem cells (which veterinary practitioners may not face), many other hurdles must be overcome. One of the most important obstacles is defining a methodology to generate reproducible, spontaneous cardiomyocyte-differentiating stem cells with sufficient purity for clinical purposes.[120] Emerging evidence suggests that an unknown combination of growth factors, transcription factors, feeder layers, and physical properties is involved in early cardiomyocyte differentiation.[120] Delivery systems such as intracoronary catheterization techniques, intramyocardial injection, transendocardial delivery by means of catheter-based systems, and intravenous administration are currently being evaluated and refined to optimize the long-term survival of the grafted cells, to ensure the delivery of a critical mass of viable cells, and to promote the appropriate alignment with the host cells.[120] These steps are vital to the functional and structural integration of stem cells in the host tissue.[120] The immunogenicity of embryonic stem cells poses yet another challenge.

Stem cells are not confined to embryos; rather, small numbers of stem cells can be harvested from adult bone marrow. These adult mesenchymal stem (MS) cells maintain an undifferentiated phenotype in culture and appear to have the capacity for multilineage differentiation.[121] The potential benefits of autologous adult MS cells, including ease of attainability, lack of immunogenicity, and absence of ethical objections, have prompted widespread research into their use in the management of cardiovascular disease. It remains to be seen whether repopulation of the myocardium with these cells is feasible in veterinary medicine and whether a sufficient number of viable cells to enhance systolic function can be delivered.

CHAPTER • 200

Congenital Heart Disease

Mark A. Oyama
D. David Sisson
William P. Thomas
John D. Bonagura

DEFINITION

The term *congenital heart disease* includes morphologic and functional abnormalities of the heart and adjacent great vessels that are present at birth. These abnormalities are defined as congenital even if they are not discovered until much later in life. Congenital heart disease arises from altered or arrested embryonic development of the rudimentary heart. The eventual consequences of such a failure can include gross anatomic alterations and/or inability of the heart to perform its normal functions of maintaining normal venous and arterial pressures and providing adequate perfusion of the tissues with oxygenated blood.

CLINICAL APPROACH TO CONGENITAL HEART DISEASE

Malformations of the heart and great vessels constitute a relatively small but clinically important percentage of cardiovascular disorders in dogs and cats.[1a,14a]* The types of defects, pathogenesis, and etiology of disease that afflict animals and humans are remarkably similar, and most of the diagnostic and therapeutic methods used in veterinary cardiology have been adapted from those used in the management of children and adults with congenital heart disease. Although absolute diagnosis and evaluation of congenital heart disease may require echocardiography or cardiac catheterization, a complete physical examination, electrocardiography, and chest radiographs provide a wealth of information that can be used to make a provisional diagnosis and to guide the formulation of an appropriate treatment plan. To this end, every veterinarian should be familiar with the most common congenital diseases and should be able to counsel owners regarding the prognosis, the treatment options, and the impact on breeding programs.

HISTORY AND PHYSICAL EXAMINATION

The diagnostic approach for animals with congenital heart disease is similar to that used to evaluate animals with acquired disease. In this regard, the evaluation should always include a careful history and complete physical examination. When assembling the history, the clinician should take care to note the breed of the patient, because many congenital diseases have a suspected or proven genetic basis, and most have breed predilections. Whenever possible, the health records of the sire, dam, and any siblings should be reviewed. Additional testing (e.g., electrocardiography, radiography, and echocardiography) usually is advisable, depending on the client's expectations, the nature and severity of the disease, and the medical or surgical treatment options available.

History

The breed and age should always be considered in the evaluation of animals suspected of having congenital heart disease. Table 200-1 shows the breed predilections reported for canine cardiac defects in North America and Europe.[1c-6c] These associations support the suspected genetic basis of many malformations. Gender predispositions to congenital heart disease are weak or poorly established in dogs except for the higher prevalence of patent ductus arteriosus in females.[1a,4a,8a] In cats, Siamese, Burmese, and Asian shorthair breeds may be predisposed to

---

*References with a superscript (a) correspond to the reference from the third edition with the same number; those with a superscript (b) correspond to the reference from the fourth edition with the same number; and those with a superscript (c) correspond to the reference from the fifth edition with the same number.

Table • 200-1

Canine Breed Predilections for Congenital Heart Disease

BREED	DEFECTS
Basset hound	PS
Beagle	PS
Bichon frise	PDA
Boxer	SAS, PS, ASD
Boykin spaniel	PS
Bull terrier	MVD, AS
Chihuahua	PDA, PS
Chow chow	PS, CTD
Cocker spaniel	PDA, PS
Collie	PDA
Doberman pinscher	ASD
English bulldog	PS, VSD, TOF
English springer spaniel	PDA, VSD
German shepherd	SAS, PDA, TVD, MVD
German shorthair pointer	SAS
Golden retriever	SAS, TVD, MVD
Great Dane	TVD, MVD, SAS
Keeshond	TOF, PDA
Labrador retriever	TVD, PDA, PS
Maltese	PDA
Mastiff	PS, MVD
Newfoundland	SAS, MVD, PS
Pomeranian	PDA
Poodle	PDA
Rottweiler	SAS
Samoyed	PS, SAS, ASD
Schnauzer	PS
Shetland sheepdog	PDA
Terrier breeds	PS
Weimaraner	TVD, PPDH
Welsh corgi	PDA
West Highland white terrier	PS, VSD
Yorkshire terrier	PDA

AS, Aortic stenosis; ASD, atrial septal defect; CTD, cor triatriatum dexter; MVD, mitral valve dysplasia; PDA, patent ductus arteriosus; PPDH, peritoneopericardial diaphragmatic hernia; PS, pulmonic stenosis; SAS, subaortic stenosis; TOF, tetralogy of Fallot; TVD, tricuspid valve dysplasia; VSD, ventral septal defect.

some defects, and male kittens seem to be affected more often than females.[2c,36a] Consideration of gender predilection, however, has little influence on the evaluation of individual patients. Age may be an important factor in the interpretation of the results of initial examinations. Most defects are detectable shortly after birth, but the severity of the hemodynamic abnormalities may change significantly during the first 6 to 12 months of life. For example, the lesion of congenital subaortic stenosis may not be present at birth, but it can develop during the first 2 months of life and can increase in severity during the first year of life.[2a,9a] Similarly, the consequences of left-to-right shunting defects may not be fully manifested until pulmonary vascular resistance and right heart pressures decrease to the low levels of a normal adult, several weeks after birth. Some defects appear to be severe in the very young but have relatively modest consequences in adulthood.

Most animals with congenital heart defects are asymptomatic when first examined; these patients are recognized when a heart murmur is detected during a routine examination. Dogs and cats with hemodynamically severe regurgitant, obstructive, or shunting defects may appear completely normal to the owner during the first 6 to 12 months of life, therefore it should not necessarily be concluded from an unremarkable history that the underlying defect is mild. For instance, dogs with severe subaortic stenosis may not demonstrate any clinical signs prior to sudden and unexpected death. Similarly, young animals with patent ductus arteriosus and imminent cardiac failure often appear normal to the owner until pulmonary edema becomes life-threatening and causes dyspnea. Additional clinical signs that may develop with severe defects include failure to grow at a normal rate or to a normal size, exertional fatigue, abdominal distention (ascites), episodic weakness or syncope, or cyanosis.

Physical Examination

The ability to detect and decipher heart murmurs and abnormal transient heart sounds is an invaluable skill that cannot be overemphasized in the evaluation of patients with congenital heart disease. The typical characteristics of the heart murmurs associated with the most common congenital defects are listed in Table 200-2. Descriptions of the acoustic properties of the various murmurs and an algorithm for differentiating their causes are presented in Chapter 55. When a heart murmur is first detected, the examiner must determine whether it is pathologic or innocent, because normal puppies and kittens often have benign heart murmurs. Innocent murmurs are usually of low intensity (grade I-II/VI), protosystolic or midsystolic in timing, and best heard at the left heart base. They often vary in intensity according to changes in the heart rate or body position. Innocent murmurs usually but not invariably diminish or resolve by 6 months of age; however, soft systolic innocent murmurs can persist well into adulthood, especially in large-breed dogs.

Cardiac murmurs caused by congenital disease are typically louder (grade III-VI/VI) and of longer duration than innocent murmurs, often obscuring the normal heart sounds. Murmurs of this description are unlikely to be innocent, and additional diagnostics are warranted; however, the examiner is cautioned not to correlate the intensity of the murmur with the severity of the suspected underlying defect. The murmur associated with patent ductus arteriosus or a small ventral septal defect is often very intense, even when the volume of the shunted blood is relatively modest. The murmurs of some lesions, notably atrial septal defects and mild subvalvular aortic stenosis, are easily misinterpreted as innocent. In animals with large septal defects, including severe atrioventricular valve dysplasia and some forms of serious cyanotic heart disease, the heart murmur may be soft or even inaudible. Although a cardiac murmur of any grade indicates the possibility of congenital heart disease, common sense, guided by the patient's clinical circumstances and the owner's wishes, should dictate the vigor of the diagnostic evaluation.

Abnormalities of the arterial pulse, mucous membranes, jugular veins, or precordial impulse may support a suspicion of congenital heart disease. Hyperkinetic and bounding ("waterhammer") arterial pulses are characteristic of lesions that cause abnormal diastolic runoff of aortic blood and low arterial diastolic pressure, such as patent ductus arteriosus or severe aortic regurgitation. Hypokinetic pulses are typical of moderate to severe left ventricular outflow obstruction (i.e., subaortic stenosis) or of other severe defects accompanied by low left ventricular output. Visible cyanosis develops when the partial pressure of arterial oxygen falls below 45 mm Hg and reduced (unoxygenated) arterial hemoglobin reaches 5 g/dL. Cyanosis in animals with congenital heart disease is usually caused by a systemic to pulmonary (right-to-left) shunt at the level of the heart or great vessels. Distended jugular

Table • 200-2

Auscultatory Findings in Congenital Heart Disease

LESION	TIMING	FEATURES	POINT OF MAXIMUM INTENSITY	COMMENTS
Atrial septal defect	Systolic (diastolic)	Ejection (diastolic rumble)	Left base	Systolic murmur ends prior to S_2, which is usually split; murmur (or murmurs) due to relative pulmonic (tricuspid) stenosis
(Sub)aortic stenosis	Systolic*	Ejection (crescendo-decrescendo)	Left base	Often nearly as loud at the right base; diastolic murmur of aortic regurgitation may also occur
Mitral valve dysplasia†	Systolic	Regurgitant (holosystolic)	Left apex	May radiate widely
Patent ductus arteriosus	Continuous	Machinery	Left base	Murmur peaks at S_2, often radiates to right base and thoracic inlet
Pulmonary hypertension (Eisenmenger's syndrome)	None (systolic)	Split S_2 (ejection)	Left base	Accentuated and split S_2; systolic murmur of tricuspid regurgitation or blowing, decrescendo diastolic murmur of pulmonic regurgitation may also occur
Pulmonic stenosis	Systolic	Ejection (crescendo-decrescendo)	Left base	Occasional systolic ejection sound; blowing, decrescendo diastolic murmur of pulmonic regurgitation may occur
Tetralogy of Fallot	Systolic	Ejection (crescendo-decrescendo)	Left base	Murmur due to pulmonic stenosis; may be soft or absent with pulmonary artery hypoplasia
Tricuspid valve dysplasia†	Systolic	Regurgitant (holosystolic)	Right midprecordium	Often low pitched and rumbling
Ventricular septal defect	Systolic*	Regurgitant (holosystolic)	Right base	Often higher pitched and more cranially located than tricuspid regurgitation; may also be loud at left base

*At time a diastolic murmur of aortic regurgitation may also be present.
†Mitral stenosis and tricuspid stenosis are rare but may cause diastolic murmurs over the affected valve and ventricle.
PMI, Point of maximum intensity.

veins indicate elevated central venous pressure, which is usually caused by an abnormality of the right side of the heart, such as tricuspid valve dysplasia or pulmonic stenosis. A precordial impulse of increased strength or area often indicates enlargement of the underlying ventricle or ventricles. The presence of a precordial thrill defines the most intense cardiac murmurs (grade V-VI/VI). The focus of this vibration is synonymous with the point of maximal acoustical intensity and is characteristic of the associated underlying defect.

LABORATORY TESTS

Even though a strong clinical suspicion of congenital heart disease may arise based on the history and physical examination, definitive diagnosis of an animal with a cardiac murmur usually requires additional studies. In this regard, an electrocardiogram, thoracic radiographs, and echocardiography are usually required. The results of these studies often dictate the performance of subsequent diagnostic procedures, such as blood gas determinations, cardiac catheterization, and angiography. Distinctive laboratory abnormalities may occur in animals with cyanotic heart disease (i.e., tetralogy of Fallot, reversed

patent ductus arteriosus) and may include arterial hypoxemia, hypocarbia, metabolic acidosis, and erythrocytosis. However, in most cases hematologic testing is not an important part of the evaluation for congenital heart disease. Although serum biochemical test results may be abnormal in the presence of congestive heart failure or concurrent organ disease, the biochemical profile and urinalysis results typically are normal.

ELECTROCARDIOGRAPHY

In most animals with congenital heart disease, an electrocardiogram (ECG) can provide helpful information, mainly through its ability to detect cardiac chamber enlargement. Although a normal ECG does not rule out heart disease, an abnormal ECG indicating left- or right-sided enlargement in a young animal can strongly suggest a short list of likely cardiac defects. For instance, an ECG indicating a rightward shift in the mean electrical axis and right ventricular hypertrophy immediately suggests the possibilities of pulmonic stenosis, tetralogy of Fallot, or tricuspid valve dysplasia. Such an ECG would be rare in dogs with predominantly left-sided disease, such as mitral dysplasia or subaortic stenosis.

Conduction delay with right mean electrical axis deviation and widening of the QRS complex (partial or complete right bundle branch block) can indicate pronounced right ventricular enlargement, congenital right bundle branch block, or the presence of both abnormalities. An ECG should be recorded whenever a rhythm disorder is suspected. Serious congenital heart defects often result in cardiac arrhythmias, some of which require specific treatment or some modification of diagnostic or therapeutic plans. Supraventricular arrhythmias, such as atrial tachycardia and atrial fibrillation, are prone to occur in animals with congenital defects that cause marked atrial enlargement, such as mitral or tricuspid valve dysplasia. Ventricular arrhythmias are common in disorders resulting in arterial hypoxemia, extreme hypertrophy of the ventricular myocardium, or reduced myocardial perfusion. Relevant examples include pups with tetralogy of Fallot or subvalvular aortic stenosis. Rhythm disorders with a genetic basis are being recognized with increasing frequency in juvenile and adult cats and dogs (see Chapter 202).

CARDIAC IMAGING

Radiography

Radiographs of the thorax assist in the determination of cardiac size, identification of chamber or great vessel enlargement, assessment of the pulmonary circulation, and detection of congestive heart failure. Much of radiographic interpretation is subjective in nature, and distinguishing left heart, right heart, or bilateral enlargement in young animals is relatively difficult.[1] There is a general tendency to overinterpret the size of the right heart in neonates because of normal right ventricular prominence. This can lead to the erroneous diagnosis of pulmonic stenosis in a young animal with an innocent heart murmur. Further confusing the examiner, the ventricular apex can be shifted rightward on the dorsoventral or ventrodorsal view, contributing to the illusion of right heart enlargement in a normal animal. Despite these pitfalls, thoracic radiographs provide a reasonably sensitive and specific indication of heart size and the severity of disease, especially when the underlying disease is one of volume overload (i.e., patent ductus arteriosus, tricuspid dysplasia). This is not the case for congenital diseases characterized by pressure overload (i.e., pulmonic stenosis, subvalvular aortic stenosis), in which concentric hypertrophy is better appreciated with echocardiography. Measurement of the radiographic cardiac silhouette, using a vertebral heart scoring system similar to that used in adult dogs, provides objective criteria for the interpretation of heart size. In one study, using the lateral radiographic projection, the sum of the long and short axis cardiac dimensions averaged 10 ± 0.5 vertebrae (as measured caudally from the fourth thoracic vertebra) in healthy 3-month-old pups and did not change significantly as the dogs reached 6, 12, and 36 months of age.[2]

Inspection of the great vessels often provides additional information about the underlying cardiac defect. Aneurysmal dilatation of the proximal ascending aorta is typical for subvalvular aortic stenosis and aortic insufficiency, whereas dilatation of the proximal descending aorta is typical of patent ductus arteriosus. Dilatation of the main pulmonary artery can develop as a consequence of pulmonic stenosis or insufficiency, increased pulmonary blood flow caused by a left-to-right shunt, or pulmonary hypertension. Assessment of the size and symmetry of more peripheral pulmonary arteries and veins can help identify pulmonary overcirculation or undercirculation, as well as pulmonary venous congestion. Left-to-right shunts potentiate pulmonary blood flow, increasing the number, diameter, and prominence of the pulmonary arteries and veins, whereas right-to-left shunts reduce pulmonary flow, resulting in diminished prominence and reduced diameters of the pulmonary arteries and veins. Animals with decompensated or impending congestive heart failure may show selective widening of the caudal vena cava (right heart failure) or pulmonary veins (left heart failure). The typical radiographic findings of the common congenital heart defects are specifically addressed in their respective sections of this chapter.

Echocardiography

Echocardiography is an extremely powerful noninvasive diagnostic tool and has reduced the need for invasive cardiac catheterization and angiography to establish a definitive diagnosis of congenital heart disease. The various congenital heart diseases exert excessive pressure or volume loads (or both) on specific chambers of the heart, resulting in concentric or eccentric hypertrophy, respectively (or both). These patterns of hypertrophy can be easily recognized and quantified by two-dimensional and M-mode echocardiography.[3] Doppler echocardiography can be used to examine cardiac blood flow, which is often disturbed by the presence of congenital disease.[3] By relying on the shift of ultrasound frequencies reflected by moving objects (e.g., red blood cells), Doppler ultrasound allows the examiner to measure the velocity and direction of blood flow and to distinguish turbulent from laminar flow. Doppler ultrasound information can be viewed as a spectral display or can be superimposed on two-dimensional images as a color flow map. Spectral Doppler is used primarily to quantify the velocity of blood flow. An electronic cursor is positioned parallel to the direction of flow, and the resulting Doppler study displays blood flow velocity in a graphic format. Blood flow toward or away from the transducer location is displayed above and below the baseline, respectively. Maximal velocity of flow is measured from the peak of the Doppler signal and can be converted to units of pressure (mm Hg) using the modified Bernoulli equation:

Pressure gradient between two
    cardiac chambers (mm Hg) = 4 × Maximal velocity $(m/s)^2$

The Bernoulli equation allows the examiner to estimate the hydrostatic (blood) pressure difference between individual cardiac chambers. This information is particularly important for quantifying the severity of disease with obstructive lesions (e.g., subaortic stenosis). As the severity of a lesion worsens, pressure in the ventricle increases to produce the required cardiac output. This increase in pressure translates into a higher blood flow velocity across the area of obstruction. Proper alignment of the cursor with respect to the direction of flow is crucial to the accuracy of spectral Doppler studies. The cursor must be positioned within 20 degrees of parallel along the main direction of blood flow to ensure accurate measurements.[4]

Range-gated or *pulsed wave Doppler* allows interrogation of blood cell velocities in specific locations by having the operator direct a depth-range "gate" (which is superimposed over a two-dimensional image) to the region of interest. This mode provides accurate information about the exact anatomic site of the abnormal flow and the relative direction of flow. It is limited to the measurement of relatively low velocities because of a sampling phenomenon called *aliasing* (related mainly to the sampling rate), in which velocities greater than a known limit (the *Nyquist limit*) appear to reverse direction and cause an ambiguous display. *Continuous wave Doppler* uses two crystals (a constant transmitter and a constant receiver) to achieve very high sampling rates and to allow recording and measurement of very high velocities along the directed ultrasound beam. The velocities of all cells along the beam line are recorded and displayed, a technique that allows the high flow velocities across stenotic or insufficient valves to be displayed and measured but prevents precise localization of the abnormal flow. Pulsed wave and continuous wave Doppler are therefore complementary; the pulsed wave mode is used to identify and localize a lesion, and the continuous wave mode is used to measure any high velocities.

Color flow Doppler images consist of range-gaited, color-encoded velocity data that are superimposed on two-dimensional images. Laminar flow toward or away from the transducer is displayed as red or blue, respectively, with lighter hues of each color representing higher velocities. Turbulent flow is often displayed as a mosaic pattern of green, light blue, or yellow, but different color patterns can be selected by the user as a matter of personal preference. Color flow Doppler is conveniently used to identify and localize areas of high velocity and turbulent blood flow, which allows the operator to survey the heart quickly and identify regional flow disturbances. When areas of high velocity or turbulent flow are discovered, the examiner can focus attention on the two-dimensional anatomy of that region and perform more detailed, quantitative Doppler interrogations of blood flow in that area.

Echocardiographic contrast agents, composed of highly reflective air-agitated saline or other gas-containing microbubbles, can be used to enhance Doppler studies by amplifying weak signals from small jets that are otherwise difficult to interrogate. When Doppler technology is not available, contrast agents are used as sonographic targets to improve the detection of shunting lesions (especially right-to-left shunts) and other cardiac defects. Contrast echocardiography is a useful tool when Doppler technology is not available, and it can also enhance Doppler studies.

Experienced examiners have found that evaluation of patients suspected of having congenital disease is facilitated if the echocardiographic study is performed in a stepwise fashion, with particular attention paid to the pattern of cardiac hypertrophy, the identification and quantification of high-velocity and turbulent blood flow, and the detection of anatomic lesions particular to each type of congenital disease.[3]

OTHER IMAGING MODALITIES

Single-pass or blood pool radionuclide scanning studies can also be used to detect and quantify congenital shunts, but such methods are generally limited to university teaching hospitals. Computed tomography (CT) and magnetic resonance imaging (MRI) offer particular advantages in the evaluation of specific congenital heart diseases. MRI, for example, is an effective method of evaluating the aortic arch and related vascular anomalies in humans. However, because of their expense and limited availability to veterinarians, these modalities are infrequently used to evaluate animals with congenital heart disease.

CARDIAC CATHETERIZATION AND ANGIOGRAPHY

Cardiac catheterization is an invasive hemodynamic and angiographic procedure performed for diagnostic or therapeutic reasons. Prior to the widespread use of echocardiography, cardiac catheterization was considered the gold standard for diagnosis and evaluation of congenital heart disease. Much of the anatomic and hemodynamic information gathered during cardiac catheterization can now be obtained noninvasively with two-dimensional and Doppler echocardiography. For this reason, cardiac catheterization is reserved mainly for attempts to repair certain congenital defects (e.g., balloon valvuloplasty for pulmonic stenosis and device occlusion of patent ductus arteriosus) or to clarify ambiguous anatomic lesions when surgery is contemplated. In selected cases, diagnostic cardiac catheterization is warranted to verify pressure estimates derived from Doppler echocardiographic studies, to collect blood for oximetry, to measure cardiac output, or to examine structures not accessible to echocardiographic interrogation, such as the peripheral pulmonary or systemic vasculature.

Hemodynamic Measurements

For selective catheterization of the heart, the operator introduces specially designed catheters into a peripheral vessel and guides them into specific cardiac chambers or great vessels to measure intracardiac and vascular pressures, cardiac output, and oxygen content (oximetry). Such studies are performed before angiographic imaging, because all radiopaque contrast agents can alter vascular tone and cardiac performance. Vascular and intracardiac pressures are measured either by attaching the proximal end of fluid-filled catheters to a pressure-sensing transducer or by using specially designed catheters with microtransducers incorporated into the distal end. Pressures are displayed and saved with a digital or an analog physiologic recorder.

The peak systolic pressure in the left ventricle and aorta is approximately four times that in the right ventricle and pulmonary artery. Because the systemic and pulmonary circulations are connected in series and cardiac output from the left and right ventricles is balanced, it can be appreciated that pulmonary vascular resistance is much lower than systemic vascular resistance. Blood flowing through the heart moves from areas of high to low resistance and therefore from areas of high to low pressure. For instance, left ventricular systole produces a small, instantaneous pressure gradient between the left ventricle and the aorta, causing opening of the aortic valve and commencement of left ventricular outflow. It is important to note, however, that once the aortic valve is open, the pressures in the ventricle and aorta quickly equalize. In contrast, a pressure gradient during systole is maintained between the left ventricle and left atrium because of the intervening and closed mitral valve. Should the aortic valve not open completely, pressure between the left ventricle and the aorta does not equalize, and a pressure gradient (increased pressure proximal to the obstruction, relative to the pressure distal to the obstruction) is maintained during the entirety of systole. This pressure gradient is needed to maintain normal flow through the stenotic aortic valve. Thus an intracardiac pressure gradient is indicative of an obstructive lesion, and its severity correlates with the magnitude of the obstruction. A systolic pressure gradient between the right ventricle and main pulmonary artery, consistent with pulmonic stenosis, is shown in Figure 200-1. Pressure, resistance, and flow (cardiac output) are interrelated so that the magnitude of a pressure gradient across obstruction varies with flow; it can be diminished by heart failure, anesthesia, or hypovolemia and can be increased by exercise, anemia, or excitement. The configuration of the pressure waveforms is also altered in predictable ways by congenital heart defects. In dogs with severe subvalvular aortic stenosis, the slope of the aortic pressure rise and the peak systolic pressure are decreased. In cases of patent ductus arteriosus, diastolic runoff of aortic blood into the pulmonary artery reduces the systemic diastolic pressure, and the pulse pressure (the difference between the peak systolic and diastolic pressures) increases.

Elevation of end-diastolic pressure is a subtle but important abnormality that can be identified by a ventricular pressure recording. This important abnormality may be caused by volume overloading from regurgitant valvular lesions or left-to-right shunts, by increased diastolic ventricular stiffness associated with ventricular concentric hypertrophy or myocardial fibrosis, or by pericardial disease. Substantial increases in ventricular end-diastolic pressures (i.e., greater than 15 to 20 mm Hg) herald the development of overt congestive heart failure (i.e., edema, effusion, ascites). Pressures in the right atrium (measured directly) and left atrium (estimated by measuring pulmonary wedge pressure) increase as an unavoidable consequence of high ventricular end-diastolic pressure. Stenosis of the atrioventricular (AV) valves is characterized by elevated atrial and normal ventricular diastolic pressure, which produces a measurable diastolic pressure gradient across the affected valve. Transmission of ventricular systolic pressure to the atria across

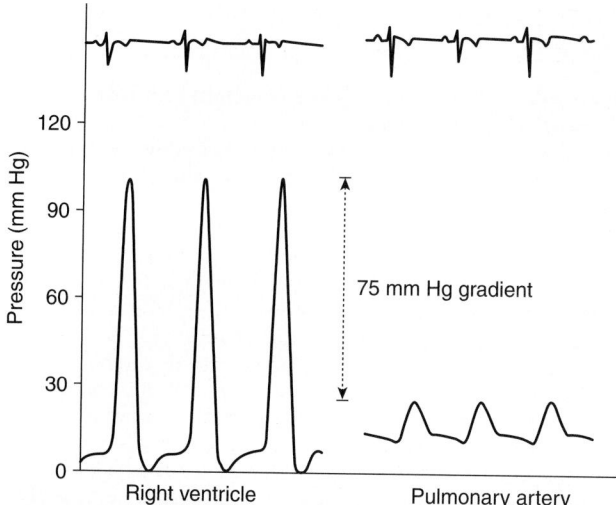

Figure 200-1 Intracardiac pressure tracing from a 1-year-old mixed breed dog made during catheterization of the right heart and pulmonary artery. The pulmonary artery pressures are normal. A systolic pressure gradient of 75 mm Hg exists between the right ventricle and pulmonary artery, indicating the presence of an obstruction to right ventricular outflow (in this case, valvular pulmonic stenosis). A small diastolic pressure gradient also exists between the pulmonary artery and right ventricle; this is caused by diastolic closure of the pulmonic valve and is a normal finding. The ECG displays a deep S wave, which is often found in animals with pulmonic stenosis and secondary right ventricular hypertrophy.

an incompetent AV valve results in ventricularization of the atrial pressure tracing and elevated mean atrial pressure.

Flow through the heart (cardiac output) can be measured by means of cardiac catheterization using a variety of indicator-dilution techniques or by combining measurements of the oxygen content of arterial and mixed-venous blood (oximetry) and oxygen consumption in respiratory gases. The most commonly performed technique, thermodilution, involves injection of an indicator (temperature, in the form of cold saline solution) and subsequent downstream measurement of its dilution over time (the change in the temperature of the blood). Cardiac output measurements are used to quantify cardiac performance, to calculate the pulmonary or systemic vascular resistance (R = Pressure/Flow), and to help define the severity of obstructing lesions. *Oximetry*, the measurement of blood oxygen content or saturation, is used mainly to detect and quantify cardiac shunts. Blood samples are sequentially drawn from the great vessels and right and left cardiac chambers and processed through a blood gas analyzer. The oxygen content in chambers and vessels on the ipsilateral sides of the heart should be roughly equivalent. A substantial change in oxygen content indicates mixing of blood from the two sides of the heart and the presence of a shunt. For instance, when oxygen saturations are recorded from the right atrium, ventricle, and pulmonary artery, a significant increase between chambers (usually greater than 5%) indicates the presence of a left-to-right shunt just proximal to the site of the step-up. Conversely, when oxygen saturations are recorded from the left side of the heart, a significant decrease indicates the presence of a right-to-left shunt. The magnitude of change in oxygen saturation directly correlates with the degree of cardiac shunting, and the severity of the shunt lesion can be calculated.

Angiography

For selective angiographic studies of animals with congenital heart disease, a bolus of radiopaque contrast solution is injected into a specific location in the heart or vessels, and its transit through the circulation is visualized by fluoroscopy. This allows identification of any anatomic abnormalities and alterations in the normal pattern of blood flow. Multiple injection sites are often used to define a lesion completely. In some instances angiograms are performed with the patient in both lateral and sternal or dorsal recumbence to provide images from multiple orientations. For shunts and obstructive lesions, contrast is injected into the chamber just proximal to (upstream from) the site of the suspected defect, whereas for valvular insufficiency lesions, the contrast is injected into the chamber just distal to (downstream from) the lesion. Commonly performed injections include those made into (1) the right ventricle, to identify pulmonic stenosis, tricuspid dysplasia, right-to-left shunting ventricular septal defects, tetralogy of Fallot, transposition of the great vessels, (pseudo)truncus arteriosus, right-to-left shunting patent ductus arteriosus, and abnormalities of the pulmonary vascular tree; (2) the left ventricle, to identify subaortic stenosis, mitral dysplasia, left-to-right shunting ventricular septal defects, transposition of the great vessels, aorticopulmonary windows, and left-to-right shunting patent ductus arteriosus; (3) the main pulmonary artery, to identify anomalous pulmonary venous drainage, aorticopulmonary windows, left-to-right shunting atrial septal defects, and mitral valve stenosis; and (4) the aortic root, to identify aortic insufficiency, aorticopulmonary windows, anomalous coronary arteries, aortic coarctation, left-to-right shunting patent ductus arteriosus, and bronchoesophageal or other collateral pulmonary vessels. Angiograms can be recorded on videotape or multiple radiographic plates, or they can be stored digitally to optical or magnetic media.

Therapeutic Procedures

In the current era, cardiac catheterization plays an important role in the treatment of several types of congenital heart disease. Specialized catheters with inflatable balloons on the distal tip can be used to dilate stenotic valves or narrowed vessels. Catheters can also be used to deliver embolization devices to close shunting defects, such as patent ductus arteriosus. The electrical activity of the heart can be mapped and arrhythmias can be abolished using radiofrequency waves generated from an appropriately positioned catheter (see Treatment of Arrhythmias.)

A primary advantage of catheter-based therapy over traditional surgical approaches (thoracotomy) is the minimally invasive nature of cardiac catheterization. The evolution and clinical application of specific therapies are discussed further in later sections of this chapter.

ETIOLOGY AND PREVALENCE OF CONGENITAL HEART DISEASE

Etiology

Congenital cardiac malformations may be caused by a large number of genetic and environmental factors, and in most cases a single causative agent cannot be conclusively proven. The possible interaction of the potential toxicologic, nutritional, infectious, and genetic factors makes it difficult to answer the question posed by many clients, "Why did my pet get this congenital disease?" The observation that certain congenital defects display a species and/or breed predilection suggests that many defects have a heritable basis (see Table 200-1). This hypothesis has been unequivocally demonstrated for several specific defects in certain dog breeds.[5-7] Most of these studies indicate a simple mendelian basis for transmission, indicating that identifiable genetic factors contribute to malformations during development of the embryonic heart, giving rise to each specific type of congenital heart disease. Additional genes with additive effects may produce a discrete phenotype once a mendelian trait has been inherited.[8-11] Regrettably, the complexity and uncertainty surrounding the exact mode of inheritance of many defects makes it difficult to counsel breeders about the breeding of individual dogs. Although recent attempts have been made to identify dogs with congenital heart disease before breeding, these efforts are often confounded by the limited sensitivity and specificity of currently available screening methods. A normal physical examination does not equate with genetic normalcy, soft murmurs are difficult to interpret, and echocardiographic screenings often yield similarly equivocal findings. Even with careful attention to pedigree and the results of breeding trials, it can be very difficult to affect the overall prevalence of a specific defect in a large population. Progress in this regard hinges on the development of economical tests that can detect the genes responsible for the congenital defect.

Prevalence

Surveys in North America indicate that the overall prevalence of congenital heart disease in dogs is 0.46% to 0.85% of hospital admissions. For 40 years, patent ductus arteriosus (PDA), subvalvular aortic stenosis (SAS), and pulmonic stenosis (PS) have topped the list of most commonly reported congenital defects in dogs. Hospital surveys of congenital heart defects in the United States have been reported by Patterson and Detweiler in dogs and by Liu and by Harpster in cats.[2a,12a,14a,36a] In the largest survey of dogs from the 1960s, 325 malformations were detected in 290 dogs, and the overall prevalence in a university hospital population was 6.8 per 1000 dogs.[1a,2a,14a] The frequency of diagnosis was approximately 28% for PDA, 20% for PS, 14% for aortic stenosis, 8% for persistent right aortic arch, 7% for ventricular septal defect, and less than 5% for tetralogy of Fallot, persistent left cranial vena cava, and atrial septal defects. In a 1989 survey of 339 cases of congenital cardiac defects in dogs in the United Kingdom, the most common diagnoses were subaortic stenosis (32%), PDA (20%), mitral valve dysplasia (14%), PS (12%), and ventricular septal defect (8%). A more recent report by Buchanan[1c,9b] that includes prevalence information from a North American database of more than 1300 cases indicates that patent ductus arteriosus is still most frequently reported (31.7% of cases), but subaortic stenosis (22.1%) now exceeds pulmonic stenosis (18.3%) in prevalence.

The shifting popularity of some dog breeds over time influences the regional or global prevalence of a particular defect. For example, the growing popularity of golden retrievers may increase the number of dogs diagnosed with subvalvular aortic stenosis. Harpster's review of congenital heart disease in cats summarizes data from the literature, from Angell Memorial Animal Hospital (Boston), and from the Animal Medical Center (New York City). The prevalence of congenital heart defects in cats was 0.2% to 1% of hospital admissions. Of the reported diagnoses, the most commonly diagnosed defects included atrioventricular septal defects (24%, including ventricular septal defect, atrial septal defect, and endocardial cushion defect), atrioventricular valve dysplasia (17%), endocardial fibroelastosis (11.5%), PDA (11%), aortic stenosis (6%), and tetralogy of Fallot (6%). Males were affected nearly twice as often as females.[36a]

CLASSIFICATION OF CONGENITAL HEART DISEASE

A number of schemes have been devised for classifying congenital heart defects. The system presented in Box 200-1 emphasizes the nature of the cardiac overload and the physiologic consequences rather than the embryologic basis for maldevelopment. It should be apparent that some lesions fit into more than one category. Some of the lesions listed are very rare, and some have been reported only in conjunction with other defects.

DEFECTS THAT CAUSE PRIMARILY VOLUME OVERLOAD

Systemic to Pulmonary (Left-to-Right) Shunts
Patent Ductus Arteriosus

The circulation in the fetus differs from that in the adult. In fetal animals the ductus arteriosus develops from the left sixth embryonic arch and extends from the pulmonary artery to the descending aorta, where it diverts blood from the nonfunctional fetal lungs back into the systemic circulation. Prior to birth, the ductus diverts approximately 80% to 90% of the right ventricular output back to the left side of the circulation. After parturition and the onset of breathing, pulmonary vascular resistance falls, flow in the ductus reverses, and the resulting rise in arterial oxygen tension inhibits local prostaglandin release, causing constriction of the vascular smooth muscle in the vessel wall and functional closure of the ductus arteriosus. Although the ductus may be probe patent in puppies less than 4 days of age, it usually is closed securely 7 to 10 days after birth.[4a,41a,42a] Persistence of a PDA beyond the early neonatal period is the first or second most commonly diagnosed congenital cardiac defect in dogs.[37a,61a] Cats are also affected but much less commonly than dogs.

Pathogenesis   Failed ductal closure in dogs is characterized by distinct histologic abnormalities in the ductal wall. The normal fetal ductal wall contains a loose, branching pattern of circumferential smooth muscle throughout its length. In prenatal puppies bred to have a high probability of PDA, varying portions of the ductal wall are comprised of elastic fibers rather than contractile smooth muscle fibers. According to the work of Patterson et al., increasing genetic liability to PDA results in "extension of the noncontractile wall structure of the aorta to an increasing segment of the ductus arteriosus, progressively impairing its capacity to undergo physiologic closure."[4a] It is tempting to speculate that some defect prevents one or more of the series of processes that permits smooth muscle cells to proliferate in the wall of the ductus prior to birth. In the defect's mildest form, the ductus closes at the pulmonary arterial end only and a blind, funnel-shaped outpouching of the ventral aspect of the aorta, called a *ductus diverticulum*, results. This hidden form *(forme fruste)* of incomplete ductal closure can be diagnosed only by angiography or necropsy, but it indicates that the dog possesses genes for this defect.[4a,39a,40a] Increasing genetic liability results in a tapering, funnel-shaped ductus arteriosus that remains patent after the early natal period and that allows blood to flow from the high-pressure aorta to the low-pressure pulmonary artery (Figure 200-2), thereby creating varying amounts of left-to-right shunting. The most severe but least common form is the cylindrical, nontapering ductus with persistent, postnatal pulmonary hypertension (Eisenmenger's syndrome) and bidirectional or right-to-left shunting (see Figure 200-2). Based on the breeding studies of poodle-type dogs, Patterson et al. concluded that the mode of transmission of PDA in dogs is most likely polygenic, but other mechanisms of inheritance are possible. For additional information on the morphology and pathogenesis of PDA, the reader is referred to several outstanding reviews of the subject.[12-14]

Pathophysiology   The direction of flow through the PDA is determined by the relative resistances of the pulmonary and systemic vascular beds; in the vast majority of cases, it is directed from left to right (from the aorta to pulmonary artery). This results in a continuous cardiac murmur, increased pulmonary blood flow, and volume overloading of the left atrium and left ventricle. Because of the relatively high resistance of the systemic circulation after birth, aortic blood pressure is greater than pulmonary pressure, and blood shunts continuously across the PDA during both systole and diastole. For a given pressure gradient, the magnitude of shunting is determined by the morphology (effective resistance) of the ductus arteriosus. In most cases the ductus is widest at the aortic end and tapers to its

Box • 200-1

Classification of Congenital Defects According to Pathophysiology

Canine	**Feline**

Defects primarily causing volume overload
Systemic to pulmonary (left-to-right) shunting

Canine	**Feline**
Common	Common
Patent ductus arteriosus	Ventricular septal defect
Ventricular septal defect	Patent ductus arteriosus
Uncommon	Atrial septal defect
Atrial septal defect	Endocardial cushion defect
Endocardial cushion defect	Uncommon
(Pseudo) truncus arteriosus	Truncus arteriosus
Valvular regurgitation	Valvular regurgitation
Common	Common
Mitral dysplasia	Mitral dysplasia
Tricuspid dysplasia	Tricuspid dysplasia
Uncommon	
Pulmonic insufficiency	
Aortic insufficiency	

Defects primarily causing pressure overload

Canine	**Feline**
Common	Common
Pulmonic stenosis	Dynamic subaortic stenosis
Subaortic stenosis	Uncommon
Uncommon	Pulmonic stenosis
Valvular aortic stenosis	Pulmonary artery branch stenosis
Coarctation and interruption of	Fixed subaortic stenosis
the aorta	Valvular aortic stenosis
Cor triatriatum dexter	Cor triatriatum dexter
	Cor triatriatum sinister

Defects primarily causing cyanosis

Canine	**Feline**
Common	Common
Tetralogy of Fallot	Tetralogy of Fallot
Uncommon	Endocardial cushion defect
Pulmonary to systemic shunting (ventral septal defect [VSD])	Uncommon
Pulmonary to systemic shunting (patent ductus arteriosus [PDA])	Pulmonary to systemic shunting (VSD)
Tricuspid atresia/right ventricular hypoplasia	Pulmonary to systemic shunting (PDA)
Double outlet right ventricle	Double outlet right ventricle
Transposition of the great vessels	Truncus arteriosus
Truncus arteriosus	
Aorticopulmonary window	

Miscellaneous cardiac and vascular defects

Canine	**Feline**
Common	Common
Peritoneopericardial diaphragmatic hernia	Peritoneopericardial diaphragmatic hernia
Persistent right aortic arch	Endocardial fibroelastosis
Persistent left cranial vena cava	Uncommon
Uncommon	Persistent right aortic arch
Endocardial fibroelastosis	Anomalous right atrium
Pericardial defects	
Anomalous pulmonary venous return	
Double aortic arch	
Retroesophageal left subclavian artery	
Situs inversus	

narrowest (flow limiting) region at the point of attachment to the pulmonary artery. Increased left ventricular stroke volume and rapid runoff of blood from the aorta to the low pressure pulmonary circulation via the PDA causes increased aortic systolic and decreased aortic diastolic pressures. The resulting widened arterial pulse pressure offers a hemodynamic explanation for the bounding or hyperkinetic (waterhammer, Corrigan's) arterial pulse detected in dogs with substantial shunts.

All vascular structures involved in the transport of the shunted blood enlarge to accommodate the extra volume flow.

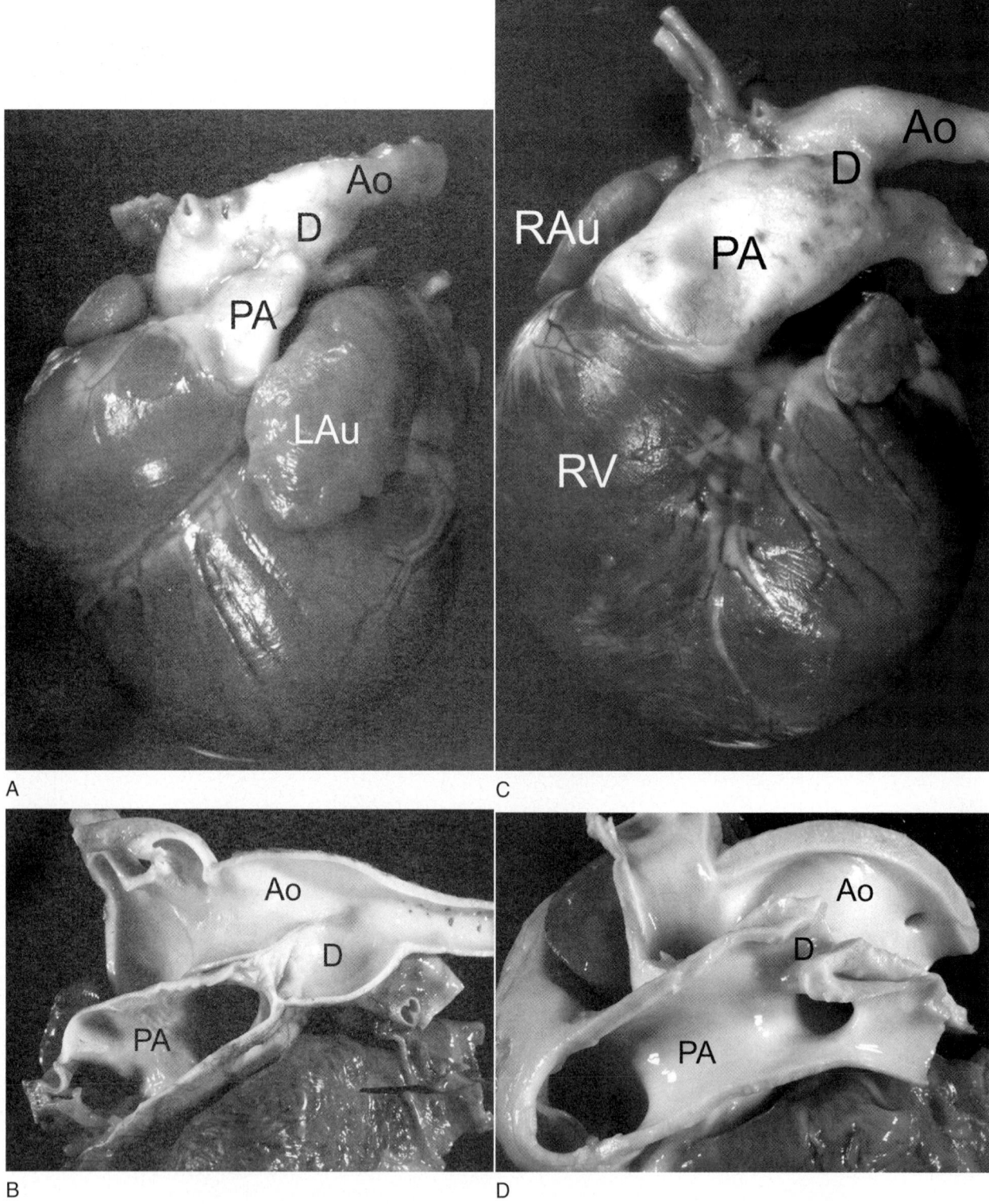

Figure 200-2   Gross pathology of patent ductus arteriosus (PDA). **A,** Left-sided view of the heart of a 9-week-old Australian shepherd with a left-to-right PDA, demonstrating the anatomic location of the ductus *(D)* between the descending aorta *(Ao)* and the main pulmonary artery *(PA)*. The left auricle *(LAu)* is enlarged. **B,** Cutaway view of a left-to-right PDA in a dog. The ductus is funnel shaped, tapering toward the PA end. **C,** Left-sided view of the heart of a dog with a right-to-left shunting PDA. Note the enlargement of the right ventricle *(RV)* and right auricle *(RAu)*. The pulmonary artery *(PA)* is enlarged. **D,** Cutaway view of a right-to-left shunting PDA in a dog. Note the cylindrical nature of the ductus *(D)* and the fact that the anatomic location of the ductus is distal to the aortic branches that supply the cranial portion of the body.

Increased volume flow causes dilatation of the proximal aorta and main pulmonary artery and overcirculation of the pulmonary vascular bed. Dilatation of the left atrium and eccentric hypertrophy of the left ventricle develop in proportion to the volume flow of the shunt. This mechanism permits compensation for a variable period, but if the shunt is large, myocardial failure (cardiomyopathy of volume overload) develops, together with progressive elevation of left ventricular end-diastolic pressure and overt pulmonary edema. Because the left-to-right shunt occurs at the level of the great vessels, the right ventricle and atrium never handle the shunted blood, and these structures remain normal unless pulmonary vascular resistance and pulmonary arterial pressure increase.

In a small percentage of cases, the lumen of the PDA remains wide open after birth. The absence of a restrictive ductal orifice allows aortic pressure to be transmitted to the pulmonary circulation, precluding the normal postnatal decline in pulmonary vascular resistance. In this circumstance the aortic and pulmonary artery pressures equilibrate, and the right ventricle remains concentrically hypertrophied after birth. In Patterson's colony of dogs, this pattern of pulmonary hypertension and reversed (right-to-left) shunting developed within the first few weeks of life.[39a] These observations fit the usual clinical presentation of most dogs diagnosed with a *reversed PDA*, in which the animal usually has no history of a continuous murmur and no evidence of left ventricular enlargement or a large left-to-right shunt earlier in life. Most dogs with reversed PDA flow have diminished pulmonary blood flow, a normal to small left ventricle, and marked concentric hypertrophy of the right ventricle. On rare occasions, dogs with a moderate to large left-to-right shunting PDA experience a gradual increase in pulmonary resistance and gradual reversal of the direction of shunting, typically at several months to several years of age. These dogs often have a history of prior left heart failure. Substantial residual left ventricular (LV) enlargement is evident on thoracic radiographs and by echocardiography. Pulmonary blood flow is reduced, but right ventricular hypertrophy is less pronounced than in dogs in which the direction of shunting is reversed at an early age. The precise pathogenesis of pulmonary hypertension is not completely understood, but anatomic descriptions of the pulmonary vasculature are similar in humans and animals. Histologic changes within small pulmonary arteries include hypertrophy of the media, thickening of the intima and reduction of lumen dimensions, and development of plexiform lesions of the vessel wall.[60a,61a,15] Most of these changes are considered to be irreversible, precluding surgical correction of the reversed PDA.

Clinical findings The clinical features of PDA have been thoroughly characterized in both a breeding colony and in clinic populations.[1a,4a,10c,16,37a-53a] Compared with male dogs, female dogs have a substantially greater risk of developing a PDA (2.49 per 1000 versus 1.45 per 1000).[2a] The Chihuahua, collie, Maltese, poodle, Pomeranian, English springer spaniel, keeshond, bichon frise, and Shetland sheepdog are most frequently affected, although other breeds, such as the Cavalier King Charles spaniel, may also be predisposed. Many other breeds, including larger dogs, such as the German shepherd, Newfoundland, and Labrador retriever, may also be prone to PDA in some regions. Although severely affected pups and kittens may appear stunted, thin, or tachypneic from left heart failure, most are reported to be asymptomatic and developing normally at the time the condition is discovered. Clinical signs are rarely recognized within the first few weeks of life, and most dogs are not diagnosed until the initial examination at 6 to 8 weeks of age.

Left-to-right shunting patent ductus arteriosus A thorough physical examination and chest radiographs usually suffice to suggest the diagnosis. Mucous membranes are pink in the

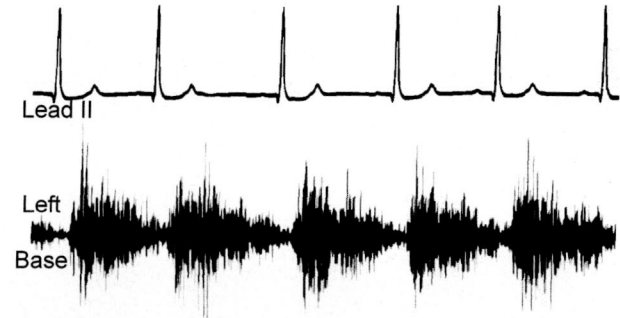

Figure 200-3 Phonocardiogram recorded at the left heart base from a dog with left-to-right patent ductus arteriosus. The lead II ECG is recorded simultaneously for timing purposes (ventricular mechanical systole is approximately the period from the middle of the QRS complex to the end of the T wave; the remainder of the time is diastole). The recorded murmur is continuous, increasing in intensity during systole, peaking near the end of systole, and decreasing in intensity during diastole.

absence of heart failure. The precordial impulse is often exaggerated and more diffuse than normal as a result of left ventricular enlargement. A thrill may be palpated at the heart base, and a continuous murmur is best heard in the same location (Figure 200-3). The murmur's point of maximum intensity is located over the main pulmonary artery at the dorsocranial left heart base and may radiate cranially to the thoracic inlet and to the right base, where it is almost always softer.[5a,16,39a,47a] Often only a systolic murmur is audible over the mitral area. This murmur may simply represent radiation of the loudest portion of the continuous murmur from the heart base to this location, or it may indicate that secondary mitral regurgitation has developed as a consequence of severe left ventricular dilatation. In cats, the continuous murmur of a PDA may be heard best somewhat more caudoventrally than in affected dogs. Increased LV stroke volume and rapid diastolic runoff through the PDA combine to produce peripheral arterial pulses that are hyperkinetic (bounding).

Electrocardiography typically indicates left ventricular enlargement (increased R-wave voltages in leads II, III, and aVF and in the left chest leads, V_2 and V_4) and normal mean electrical axis (Figure 200-4). Widened P waves may also be found,

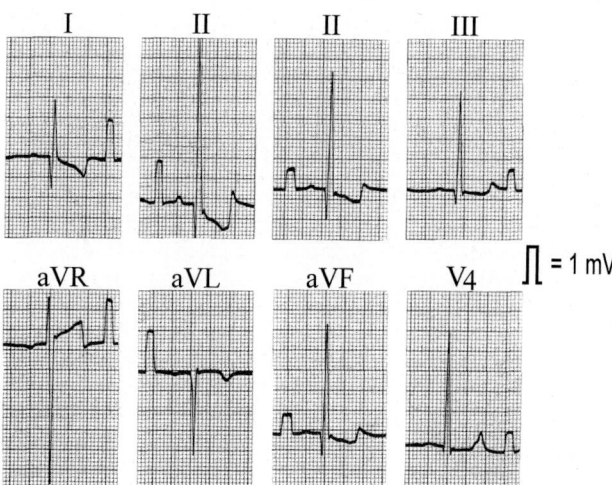

Figure 200-4 Electrocardiogram from a dog with left-to-right patent ductus arteriosus. The mean QRS axis is normal (+80%), but the QRS voltage (amplitude) is increased in several leads, including leads II, III, aVF, and V_4, consistent with left ventricular enlargement. (The square waves in each lead are 1 mV standardization impulses). Paper speed = 50 mm/s.

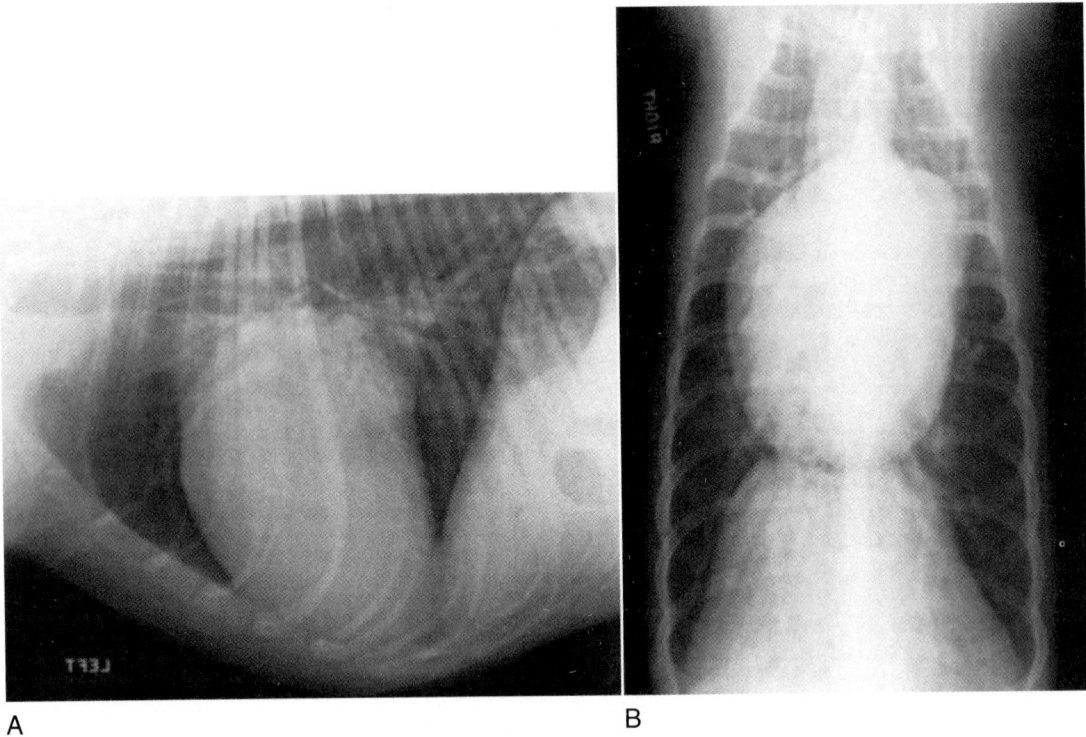

Figure 200-5   Thoracic radiographs from a dog with a left-to-right shunting PDA. **A,** Lateral projection shows left atrial enlargement and enlarged cranial pulmonary arteries and veins. **B,** Dorsoventral projection shows moderate cardiomegaly, a characteristic bulge in the descending aorta, dilatation of the main pulmonary artery, and left auricular enlargement. The pulmonary vasculature is prominent.

indicating left atrial enlargement. Chest radiographs indicate left atrial and left ventricular enlargement and pulmonary hypervascularity in proportion to the magnitude of the left-to-right shunt (Figure 200-5). On the dorsoventral (DV) projection, the aortic arch, left auricle, and main pulmonary artery may be abnormally prominent. The most specific radiographic finding is the appearance of an aortic bulge ("ductus bump") near the origin of the ductus, which is caused by abrupt narrowing of the descending aorta just caudal to the origin of the ductus (see Figure 200-5). Moderate to severe LV enlargement sometimes causes the cardiac apex to shift to the right (common in cats).

The diagnosis of a PDA can be confirmed by echocardiography in almost all cases. Two-dimensional and M-mode echocardiography demonstrate eccentric LV hypertrophy and dilatation of the left atrium, ascending aorta, and pulmonary artery (Figure 200-6).[11c] Reduced myocardial contractility is often observed and is reflected by reduced fractional shortening and/or increased LV end-systolic dimension and e-point to septal separation (EPSS) measurements. The ductus usually can be imaged from the left cranial parasternal window (see Figure 200-6). Doppler interrogation of the pulmonary artery consistently demonstrates high-velocity continuous ductal flow directed toward the pulmonic valve (see Figure 200-6). In the typical case, the peak velocity of this jet is about 4.5 to 5 m/s and occurs at end-systole. Other common echocardiographic findings include a mildly increased LV outflow velocity (1.8 to 2.3 m/s) and modest secondary mitral and pulmonary valve insufficiency. In dogs with PDA, associated cardiac defects are uncommon; nonetheless, a careful echocardiographic examination is worthwhile to exclude the concurrent presence of other common congenital defects, such as subaortic stenosis.[4a,44a] Cardiac catheterization and angiocardiography are usually not needed to confirm a diagnosis of PDA and are not advised unless the Doppler echocardiographic evaluation is ambiguous or additional congenital malformations are suspected.[12c,13c]

Patent ductus arteriosus with pulmonary hypertension (right-to-left shunting PDA)   High pulmonary vascular resistance that causes right-to-left shunting through a PDA defines the clinical syndrome commonly referred to as a reversed PDA.* Right-to-left shunting is observed in a very small minority of dogs with a PDA, but the prevalence of this phenomenon is probably underestimated and may be greater in dogs living at altitudes higher than 5000 feet above sea level.[16c] Obvious clinical signs are usually evident during the first year of life, but many owners do not recognize clinical signs in their pet during the first 6 to 12 months of life, and some animals are not diagnosed until 3 to 4 years of age or later. Reported signs include exertional fatigue, hindlimb weakness, shortness of breath, hyperpnea, differential cyanosis and, more rarely, seizures.

The clinical examination findings are very different from those in the more common left-to-right PDA. Right-to-left flow through a widely patent ductus arteriosus exhibits little turbulence, and the physical examination reveals either no murmur or only a soft, systolic murmur at the left base. The most common auscultatory finding is an accentuated and split second heart sound. Differential cyanosis (cyanosis of the caudal mucous membranes with pink cranial membranes) may be observed, but recognition may require examination after exercise. Differential cyanosis is caused by the location of the PDA, which shunts right to left from the pulmonary artery into the descending aorta (see Figure 200-2) but spares the proximal branches of the aorta, which provide normal oxygen delivery to the cranial portion of the body. Perfusion of the kidneys with hypoxemic blood triggers elaboration of erythropoietin and secondary polycythemia and hyperviscosity as the packed cell volume (PCV) gradually increases

---

*References 5a, 8a, 9a, 16c., 39a, 46a, 59a, and 61a.

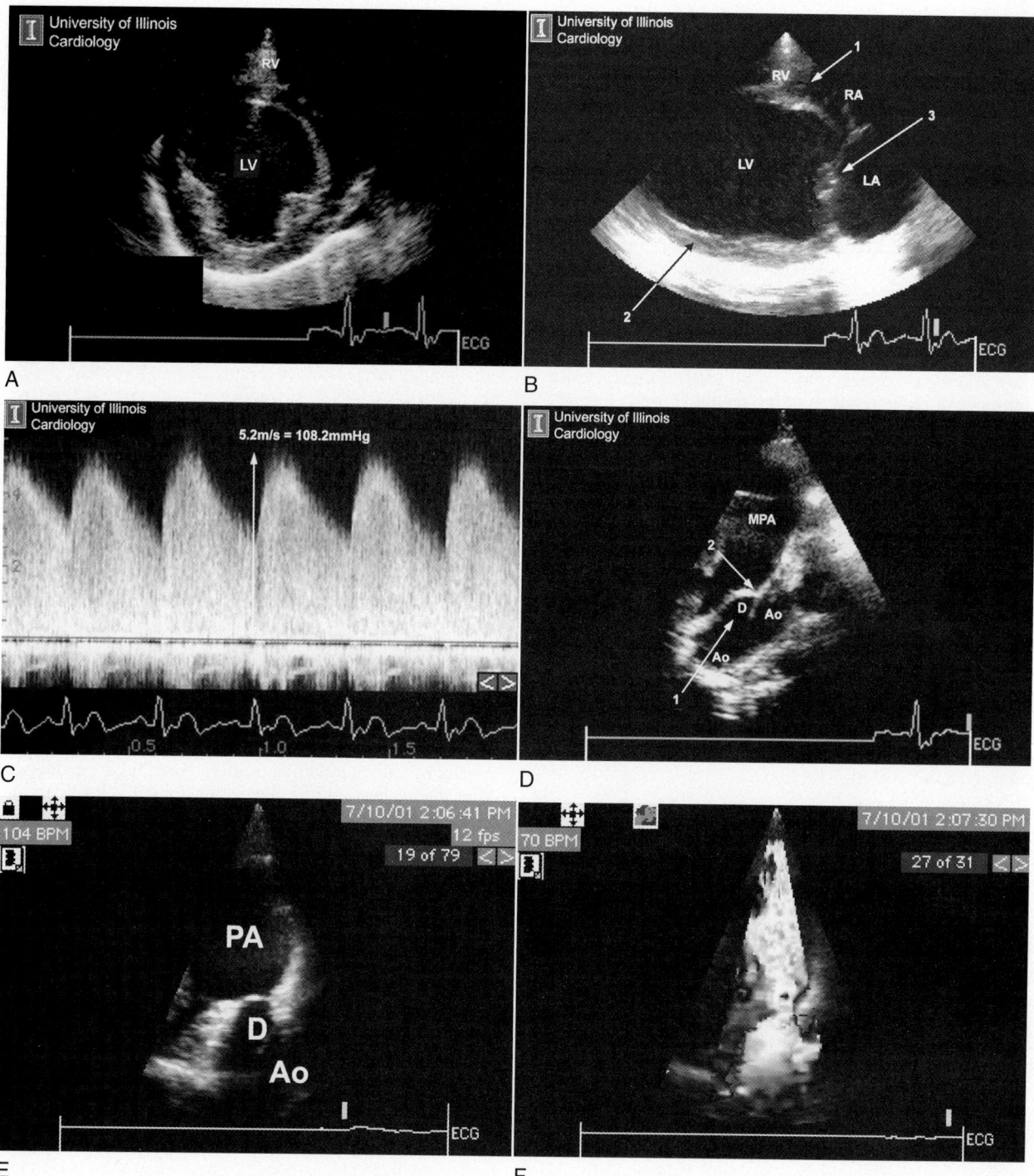

Figure 200-6 Echocardiography of left-to-right PDA. **A,** Right short axis view shows eccentric dilatation of the left ventricular cavity *(LV)* compared with the right ventricle *(RV)*. **B,** Right long axis view from the same dog reveals eccentric dilatation of the left ventricle *(LV)* and left atrium *(LA)*. The interventricular septum *(1)* and left ventricular posterior wall *(2)* appear relatively thin compared with the dilated left ventricle. The mitral valve *(3)* is in the closed position. The right ventricle *(RV)* and right atrium *(RA)* are normal. **C,** Continuous wave Doppler tracing of the PDA jet obtained from the left heart base, demonstrating continuous flow and a peak velocity of 5.2 m/s, which is converted to units of pressure (108 mm Hg) using the modified Bernoulli equation. **D,** View of the ductus *(D)* imaged from the left heart base. The typical left-to-right ductus is widest at the aortic *(Ao)* end *(1)* and tapers near the main pulmonary artery *(MPA) (2)*. **E,** Close-up view of the ductus *(D)*, pulmonary artery *(PA)*, and aorta *(Ao)*. **F,** Color flow Doppler imaging applied to the echocardiographic view in **E,** demonstrating turbulent left-to-right blood flow through the ductus.

to 65% or greater.[59a] Polycythemia may occur during the first year of life, but it often does not become severe until 18 to 24 months of age.

The electrocardiogram of dogs with a reversed PDA almost always reveals evidence of right ventricular hypertrophy (i.e., right axis deviation and increased S-wave amplitude in leads I, II, and III and in the left precordial chest leads V_2, and V_4) (see Chapter 202). Thoracic radiographs indicate right heart enlargement, dilatation of the main pulmonary artery, a visible ductus bump, and variable appearance of the lobar and peripheral arteries. Echocardiography demonstrates right ventricular concentric hypertrophy and a dilated main pulmonary artery. In some cases a wide, cylindrical ductus may be imaged (Figure 200-7). Pulmonary hypertension can be verified in some cases by Doppler interrogation of tricuspid or pulmonic insufficiency jets. Contrast echocardiography, nuclear scintigraphy, oximetry, or angiography can be used to demonstrate the presence of right-to-left shunting should Doppler interrogation prove inadequate. Contrast echocardiography is performed by injecting air-agitated saline into a cephalic or saphenous vein, thereby opacifying the right heart, pulmonary artery, and descending aorta (best observed by imaging of the abdominal aorta dorsal to the bladder). Cardiac catheterization can demonstrate pulmonary artery hypertension with equilibration of right and left ventricular and aortic systolic pressures. Oximetry verifies decreased oxygen saturation distal to the entrance of the PDA in the descending aorta. Right ventricular angiography demonstrates right ventricular hypertrophy and usually outlines a wide PDA that appears to continue distally as the descending aorta (Figure 200-8). The lobar pulmonary arteries may appear normal, especially during the first year of life, or may show increased tortuosity. Aortic or left ventricular contrast injections permit visualization of an often extensive bronchoesophageal collateral circulation (see Figure 200-8).

Natural history of patent ductus arteriosus

Eyster[53a] reported that approximately 64% of dogs diagnosed with a left-to-right shunting PDA die of complications within 1 year of diagnosis if the condition is not surgically corrected. Complications include left heart failure with pulmonary edema, atrial fibrillation, pulmonary hypertension secondary to left heart failure, and mitral regurgitation secondary to left ventricular dilatation.[53a,58a] Dogs and cats with PDA and more modest shunts often survive to maturity, and some live beyond 10 years of age.[10c] In humans with an uncorrected PDA, the gradual development of pulmonary hypertension and shunt reversal is a significant risk, but this gradual transition to right-to-left shunting is uncommon in dogs. When persistent pulmonary hypertension in the neonate leads to reversed shunting, clinical signs result from hypoxemia, polycythemia, hyperviscosity, and cardiac arrhythmias. Congestive heart failure almost never develops, but sudden death and complications from hyperviscosity are common. Animals with reversed PDA often live 3 to 5 years, and some survive beyond 7 years if the PCV is kept below 65%.

Clinical management

Surgical correction is recommended in virtually all young dogs and cats with a left-to-right shunting PDA. Correction may not be warranted in older pets if the shunt volume is small and cardiomegaly is minimal or absent. Consultation with a specialist may be helpful in borderline circumstances. Recommended preoperative studies include ECG and chest radiographs to help assess the severity of the shunt and to determine whether congestive heart failure is present. An echocardiogram should always be performed to verify the diagnosis and to rule out additional defects. The timing of surgery is debatable, but PDA correction is typically recommended at an early age or as soon as the

diagnosis is made, especially if congestive heart failure appears imminent. If pulmonary edema is found on the chest radiograph, the patient should be treated medically for heart failure (furosemide, angiotensin-converting enzyme [ACE] inhibitors) prior to surgery. Positive inotropic support should also be considered. Treatment with prostaglandin inhibitors such as indomethacin (often used in premature human infants to assist closure of a structurally normal but functionally immature PDA) is not effective in dogs and cats, most likely because of the absence of smooth muscle in the ductal wall.

Two approaches to PDA correction are currently available. For many years, left thoracotomy and surgical closure, typically by ligation, was the only available treatment.[15c] Other surgical methods of repair include suture occlusion with metallic clips and surgical division. These techniques and their results have been described in detail in several reports, indicating high surgical success rates and an excellent prognosis after repair.[10b-12b,48a-54a] Complications of surgical PDA repair in dogs most often include hemorrhage, infection, pneumothorax, cardiac arrhythmias, cardiac arrest, and heart failure. Surgical mortality should be less than 3% in uncomplicated cases.[10b-12b,53a] Pre-existing congestive heart failure (CHF) dramatically increases the risk of anesthetic or operative death and the rate of serious complications, underscoring the necessity of resolving pulmonary congestion prior to surgery. Positive inotropic support provided through a dobutamine infusion should also be considered for patients in this circumstance. Most dogs experience an uneventful recovery after surgery, and overall cardiac size gradually decreases toward normal, although the heart and great vessels often retain an abnormal shape.[44a] Postoperative Doppler examination may indicate a small residual shunt, although the continuous murmur is usually absent and the clinical outcomes are good. A soft left apical systolic murmur, usually from residual secondary mitral regurgitation, is often heard for a variable period after ductus ligation.[47a] Echocardiographic LV fractional shortening declines sharply immediately after surgery as a result of diminished preload and increased afterload. Medical therapy is not usually needed if signs of heart failure were not evident preoperatively. Medical therapies required prior to surgery for CHF are often required for several months after repair. Postoperative ductal recanalization has been reported but is uncommon, occurring in less than 2% of cases, and it most commonly is associated with infection.[15c] Postoperative fever and pulmonary infiltrates may indicate infection at the surgical site and hematogenous pneumonia.[57a] The owner should be informed of the suspected heritable nature of the defect and should be advised not to use the animal for breeding.

Less invasive alternative techniques for PDA occlusion are gaining popularity.[17-20,17c-21c] Percutaneous embolization of the ductus using expandable metal devices imbedded with thrombogenic Dacron strands can be accomplished in most small animals with a PDA, avoiding the morbidity of surgical thoracotomy (see Fig. 200-9 A and B). The most commonly used embolization device is a helical metal coil that is delivered through a small catheter via the femoral artery or other peripheral vessel. After the device has been deployed in the ductus arteriosus, the attached Dacron feathers induce thrombus formation, thereby occluding the PDA. The purported advantages of PDA coil embolization over thoracotomy and surgical ligation include lower morbidity, shorter hospitalization, and faster recovery. To date the success rate of this technique has been promising and the major complication rate has been acceptably low, consisting mainly of residual shunting and pulmonary embolization of a coil.[17,19,17c-21c] Coils that embolize to the lungs can be ignored, pushed to a peripheral location, or removed. The authors prefer to remove dislodged coils, which can be quite easily accomplished using heartworm extraction forceps or other retrieval devices. Because device retention within the PDA is

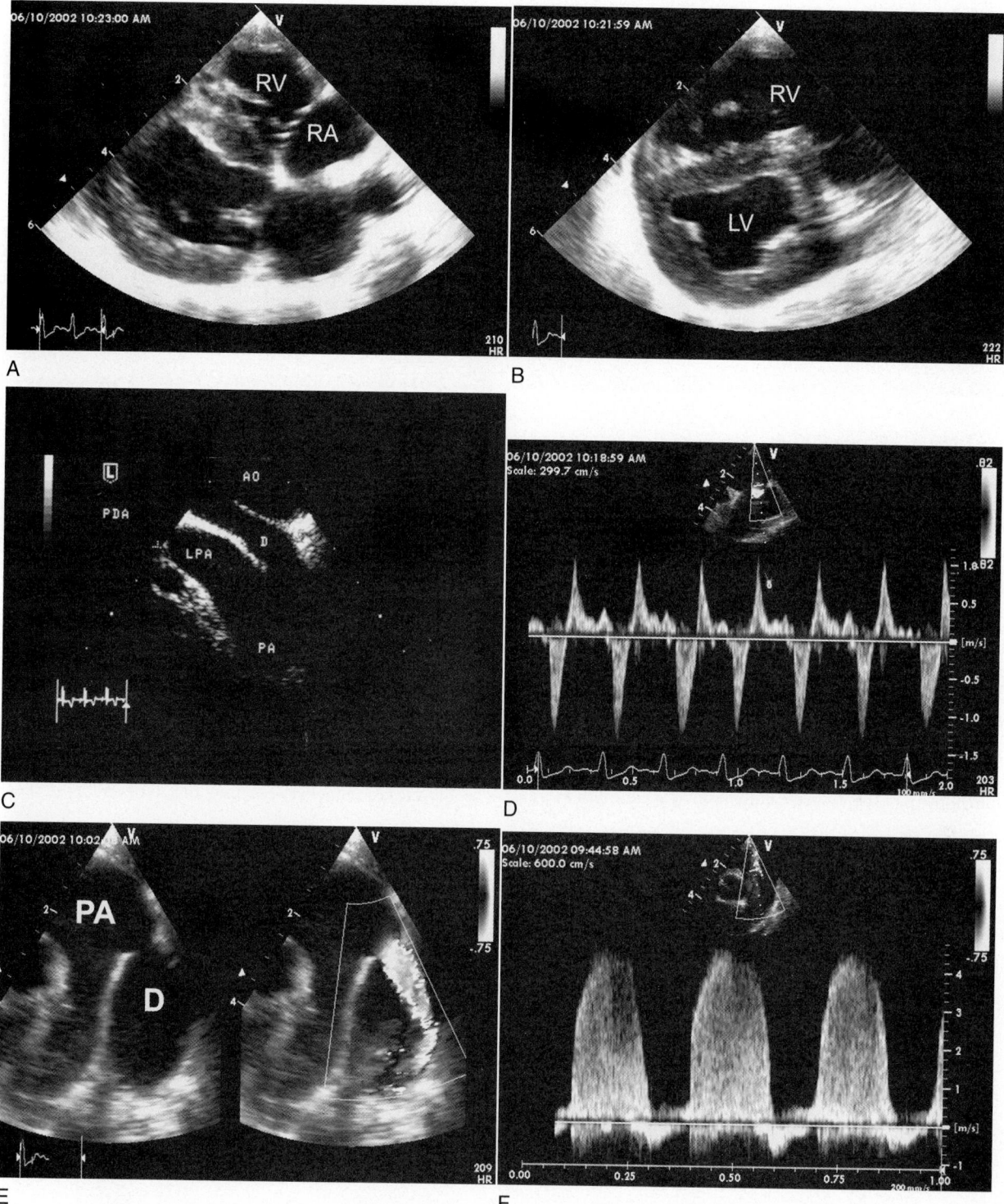

Figure 200-7 Echocardiography in right-to-left PDA. **A,** Right long axis view from an American Eskimo dog shows enlargement of the right ventricle *(RV)* and atrium *(RA)*. **B,** Right short axis view shows enlargement of the right ventricle and flattening of the interventricular septum toward the left ventricle. This finding is highly suspicious for pressure overload of the right ventricle. **C,** Transesophageal echocardiogram of a dog with a right-to-left PDA. The ductus *(D)* connects the aorta *(Ao)* with the pulmonary artery *(PA)* and is wide and cylindrical in shape. Both the pulmonary artery and the left pulmonary artery *(LPA)* are enlarged. **D,** Continuous wave Doppler study of the dog in **A** showing bidirectional flow through the ductus. Right-to-left flow (below the baseline) occurs during systole, and left-to-right flow (above the baseline) occurs during diastole. **E,** Simultaneous two-dimensional and color flow Doppler study of the dog in **A.** Flow from the pulmonary artery *(PA)* can be seen moving right-to-left into the large ductus *(D)*. **F,** Continuous wave Doppler study of pulmonic insufficiency in the dog in **A.** The peak velocity of insufficiency is 4.5 m/s, indicating a pulmonary artery diastolic pressure of approximately 80 mm Hg. This finding is consistent with a diagnosis of pulmonary arterial hypertension and the presence of a right-to-left shunt.

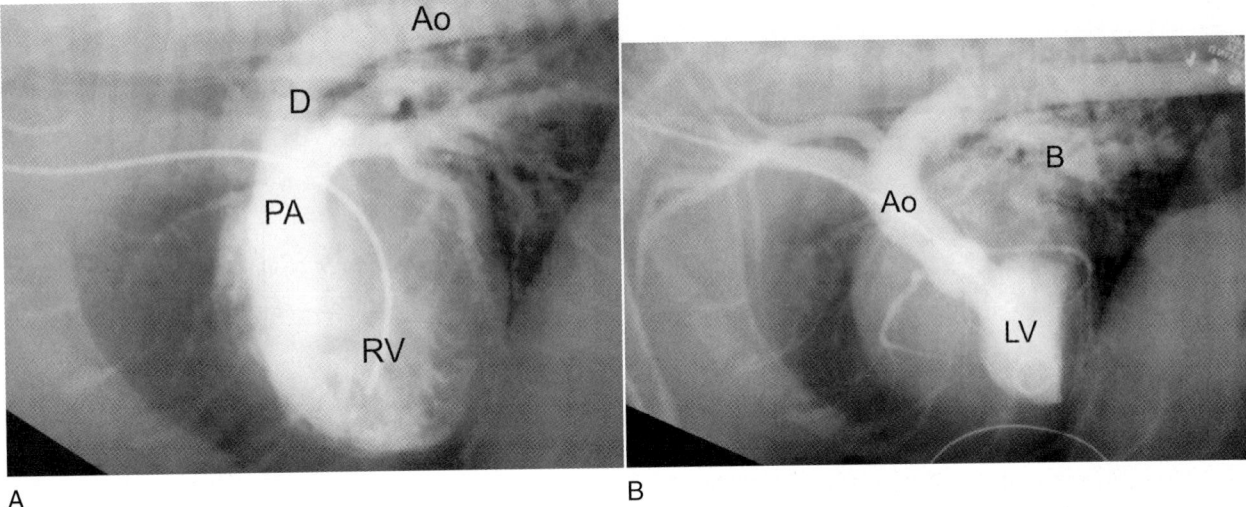

A   B

Figure 200-8   Angiographic diagnosis of right-to-left PDA in a dog. **A,** Right ventricular injection opacifies the right ventricle *(RV)*, pulmonary artery *(PA)*, ductus *(D)*, and descending aorta *(Ao)*. Note that the systemic arteries to the cranial portion of the dog are not opacified. **B,** Left ventricular injection of the same dog opacifies the left ventricle *(LV)*, the aorta *(Ao)*, and prominent collateral bronchoesophageal circulation *(B)*.

required for successful closure, the ideal candidates for coil occlusion should have a relatively small, funnel-shaped PDA that tapers to a diameter of 2 or 3 mm at the pulmonary artery end.[20]

Occlusion of large-diameter PDAs (4 mm or greater) can be attempted by deploying multiple coils into the ductal ampulla, but coil dislodgment and residual shunting are more problematic in this circumstance (Figure 200-9).[19] Mushroom-shaped, self-expanding, occluding stents (Amplatzer) developed for human use have been successfully used to accomplish PDA

closure in dogs (Figure 200-10).[18] Advantages of this technique include secure retention of the device in the ductus with a correspondingly low rate of dislodgment, ease of delivery through the femoral vein, and suitability for closing large-diameter PDAs with a single implant. The need for specialized equipment (i.e., coils, occluding stents, catheters, fluoroscopy) and an operator experienced in performing cardiac catheterization limits the application of transcatheter PDA closure techniques to university teaching hospitals and large specialty

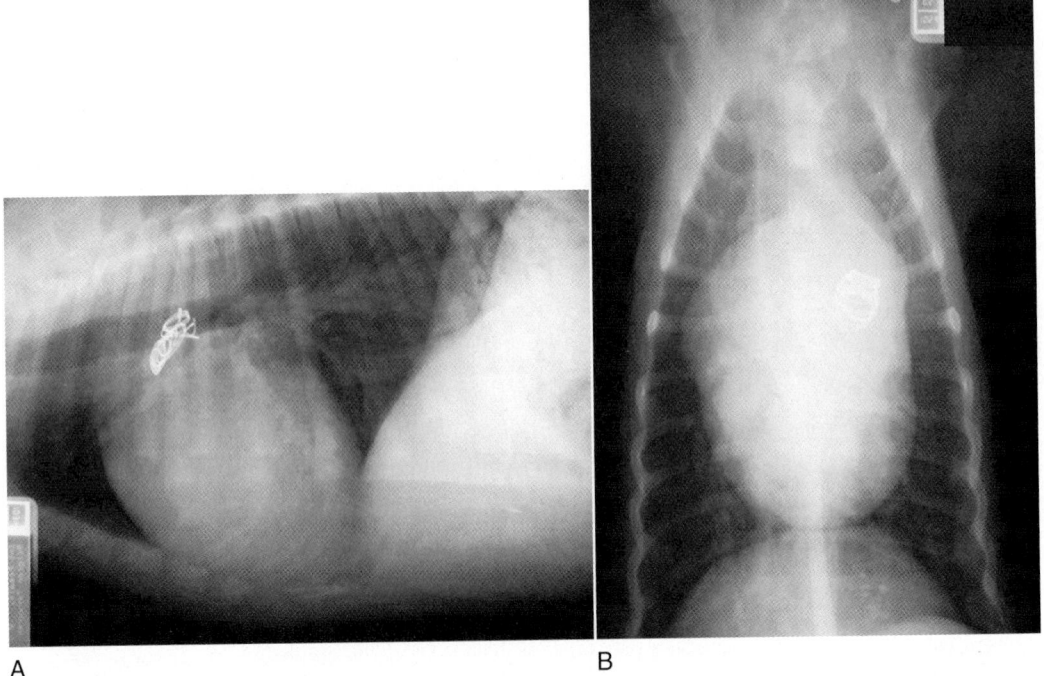

A   B

Figure 200-9   Thoracic radiographs from a dog after coil embolization of a left-to-right PDA. **A,** Lateral view shows multiple coils in the ductus. **B,** Dorsoventral view shows multiple coils in the ductus near the bulge in the descending aorta.

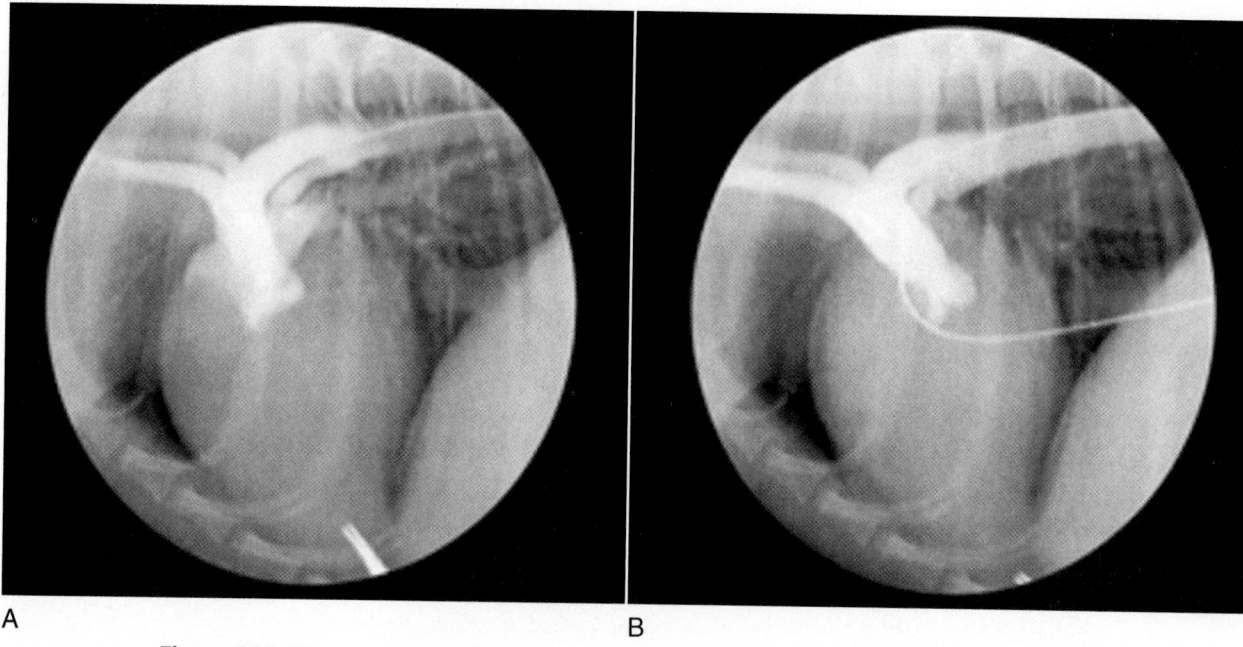

Figure 200-10 Aortic angiograms prior to and 15 minutes after deployment of an Amplatzer duct occluder into a patent ductus arteriosus (PDA). **A,** Contrast agent injected into the aorta before deployment of the duct occluder is seen flowing through the PDA into the pulmonary circulation. **B,** Contrast agent stops in the proximal PDA at the level of the Amplatzer occluder because of thrombus formation in the device.

referral centers. The historical success of the traditional PDA surgery makes thoracotomy and ligation a perfectly acceptable and, in some circumstances, a preferable alternative to transcatheter closure.

Animals with reversed PDA have irreversible obstructive pulmonary vascular disease. Morbidity and mortality is usually due to complications related to polycythemia and chronic hypoxemia rather than congestive heart failure. Treatment of these patients consists of exercise restriction, avoidance of stress, and maintenance of the PCV between 58% and 65% by periodic phlebotomy.[14] Long-term management by these techniques is possible.[21] Phlebotomy should be performed cautiously to avoid weakness or collapse, and intravascular volume may be supported during phlebotomy by administration of crystalloid solutions. Attempts to reduce the red cell volume of reversed PDA cases using drug therapy (e.g., hydroxyurea) have been reported and may be an alternative to repeated phlebotomy.[22] Activity restriction is usually advised, because exercise-induced systemic vasodilatation increases the degree of right-to-left shunting and predisposes to posterior paresis or collapse and cyanosis. Closure of reversed PDA is strongly contraindicated, because it invariably leads to late operative or early postoperative acute right heart failure and death.

Atrial and Ventricular Septal Defects

During cardiac embryonic development, the atria and ventricles begin as a common chamber. The heart is subsequently partitioned into the normal four-chambered heart by the growth of cardiac septa.[15a] The atria are partitioned by a wall formed mainly from two septa, the septum primum, which forms first, and the septum secundum, which develops to the right of the septum primum. The foramen ovale, a slitlike passageway that persists between these septa, permits right-to-left atrial shunting in the fetus, but functionally and anatomically closes in the neonate when left atrial pressure rises. The major portion of the ventricular septum forms by inward growth from the ventricular walls. The area of atrioventricular confluence, including the upper ventricular septum, lower atrial septum,

and atrioventricular valves, is formed primarily by growth and differentiation of the endocardial cushions. Defects in the development of the embryonic ventricular septum, the primum or secundum atrial septa, or the endocardial cushions may result in atrial or ventricular septal defects, or both. Congenital septal defects are common in both dogs and cats as isolated lesions and as components of more complex lesions, such as tetralogy of Fallot.[4a,13a,62a-79a]

Pathogenesis Except for the proven genetic basis of ventricular septal defect in keeshonden with conotruncal malformation,[124a] no data are available on the cause or causes of spontaneous septal defects in dogs or cats.[4a] Atrial septal defects (ASDs) are usually classified based on the anatomic region of the malformation.[15a,16a] Defects at or near the foramen ovale are referred to as *ostium* (or *septum*) *secundum defects*, and defects of the lower atrial septum are called *ostium primum defects* (Figure 200-11). Rarely observed sinus venosus atrial septal defects are found dorsocranial to the fossa ovalis near the entrance of the cranial vena cava.[65a] Because the endocardial cushions are responsible for partitioning the lowermost atrial septum, defects in the region immediately adjacent to the AV valves (septum primum) are often included in the term *endocardial cushion defects*. A defect in this area may also include anomalous development of the atrioventricular valves, such as a "cleft" in the septal leaflet of the mitral valve. A complete endocardial cushion defect is a large defect of the lower atrial septum and upper ventricular septum with fusion of the septal leaflets of both AV valves. This is also referred to as an *AV canal defect*, because the embryonic atrioventricular canal area never partitions, and communication exists between all four cardiac chambers. Patent foramen ovale is not a true ASD inasmuch as the atrial septum forms normally but the walls of the foramen are pushed apart, usually by conditions that increase right atrial pressure.[62a] A patent foramen ovale achieves clinical significance when it allows right-to-left shunting, as may occur with severe pulmonic stenosis or tricuspid valve dysplasia.

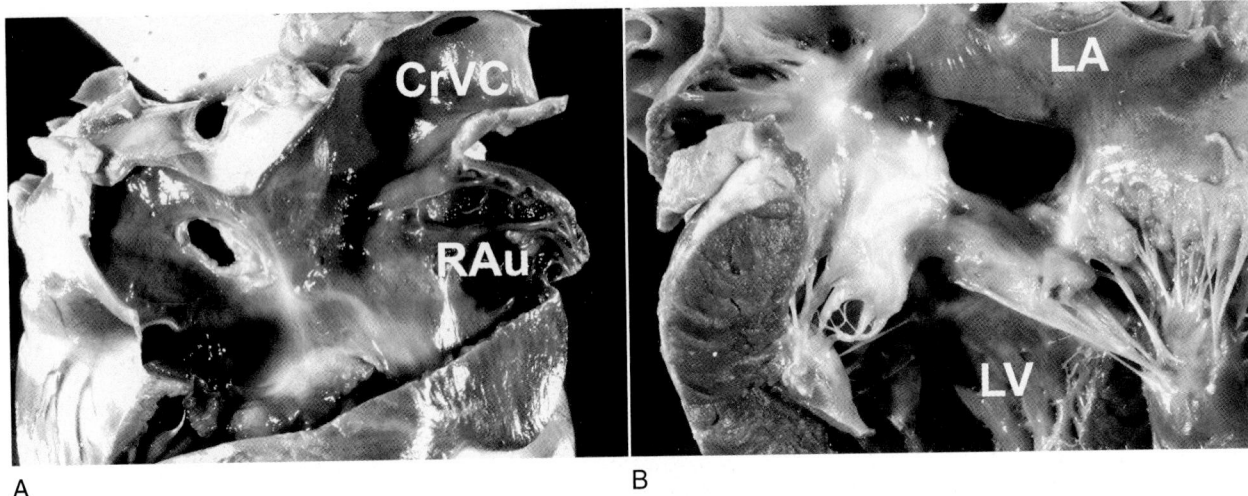

Figure 200-11 Gross pathology of atrial septal defects (ASDs). **A,** Right atrial view in an 18-year-old dachshund with a secundum ASD. Location of the ASD at the site of the fetal foramen ovale and relative to the cranial vena cava *(CrVC)* and right auricle *(RAu)* is shown. **B,** Left-sided view in a 12-year-old Brittany spaniel with a primum ASD. Location of the ASD, low in the left atrium *(LA)* and near the mitral valve, can be appreciated. A prominent cleft in the mitral valve just below the ASD is also present. *LV,* Left ventricle.

Most ventricular septal defects (VSDs) are located in the upper ventricular septum (Figure 200-12).[68a] Muscular apical or midventricular septal defects are uncommon in small animals. On the left side, the typical location of a VSD is just below the aortic valve, most often centered between the right coronary and non-coronary cusps. On the right side, the opening is often described by its position relative to the crista supraventricularis muscular ridge.[15a] A subcristal (infracristal) VSD is located proximal to the crista supraventricularis near the cranial aspect of the septal leaflet of the tricuspid valve, which may partially cover it. A supracristal VSD is located distal to the crista supraventricularis just below the pulmonic valve. Large defects may obliterate the crista and are usually associated with additional defects, as in tetralogy of Fallot (see Figure 200-12).[2a,4a] The right side of the root of the aorta, including the right coronary and noncoronary cusps, may be displaced to the right so that the aorta straddles the defect. The altered geometry of the aortic root that accompanies many VSDs sometimes results in substantial aortic valve regurgitation.[17b]

Pathophysiology Shunting across small (resistive) defects depends primarily on the size of the communication and the pressure difference between the two chambers, whereas shunting across large (nonresistive) defects depends primarily on the relative resistances of the systemic and

Figure 200-12 Pathology of ventricular septal defect (VSD). **A,** Small, restrictive VSD in a young cat, viewed from the left ventricle *(LV)*. The defect is located in the upper septum, just beneath the aortic valve *(Ao)*. **B,** Large, unrestricted VSD in a young dog with tetralogy of Fallot, viewed from the right ventricle. The large defect is located just cranial to the tricuspid valve *(arrow)*. The right ventricle *(RV)* is markedly thickened, and a narrow, fibrous ring of subvalvular pulmonic stenosis *(PS)* is present where the pulmonic valve should be seen.

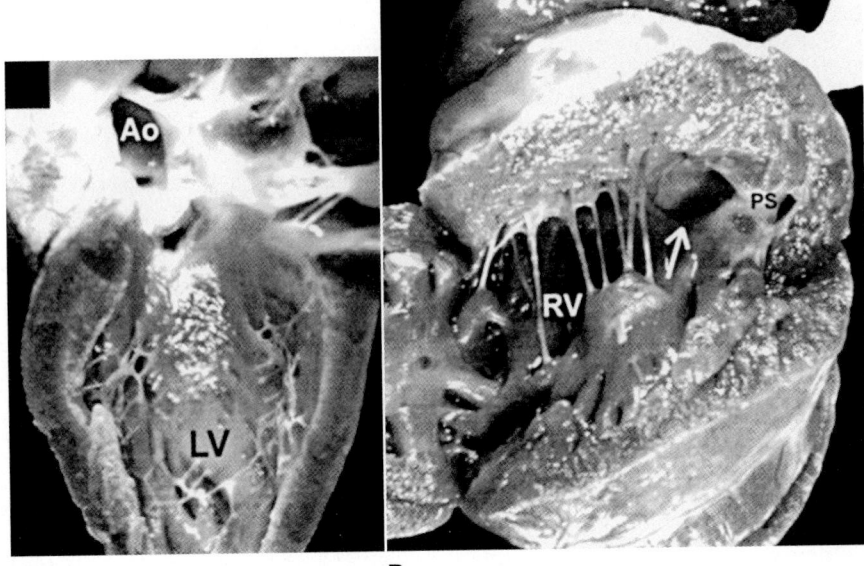

pulmonary circulations.[15a,62a,68a,72a,73a] In the absence of other abnormalities, left heart pressures exceed those on the right, and the direction of shunting is left to right. Cardiac chambers in the circuit of the shunt enlarge to accommodate the excess blood volume, and the pulmonary vasculature is overcirculated. Large-volume left-to-right shunts eventually result in myocardial failure, elevated filling pressures, and the development of overt congestive heart failure. Right-to-left shunting occurs via a septal defect when pulmonic stenosis, tricuspid dysplasia, or pulmonary arterial hypertension raise pressures on the right side of the heart. The consequences of reversed shunting include cyanosis from arterial hypoxemia, polycythemia, hyperviscosity, and sudden death.

Atrial septal defect Flow across an atrial septal defect occurs primarily during diastole. The pressure difference across the defect is low, and the direction and magnitude of the shunt are determined mainly by the relative diastolic resistance to inflow for each ventricle.[15a,65a] Normally, the right ventricle is more compliant than the left and offers little resistance to filling, causing blood preferentially to shunt from the left atrium into the right atrium and ventricle. The result is dilatation of the right atrium, eccentric hypertrophy of the right ventricle, and pulmonary overcirculation. Oxygen saturation in the right heart and pulmonary arteries is increased. The left atrium receives the shunted blood, but most of the increased pulmonary venous return is shunted immediately into the right atrium, resulting in minimal left atrial dilatation. If considerable left atrial enlargement is observed in an animal with an ASD, an additional defect, such as an endocardial cushion defect with mitral regurgitation, should be suspected. Endocardial cushion defects are more commonly detected in cats and may cause left-sided or bilateral congestive heart failure. Endocardial cushion defects are reported in dogs but are rare.[23]

The flow across an ASD does not usually generate an audible heart murmur because the pressure gradient and flow velocity across the defect are low. When the shunted blood joins blood entering from the vena cava, the volume and velocity of flow through the right heart are increased, resulting a murmur of relative pulmonic stenosis (common) or tricuspid stenosis (uncommon). Delayed closure of the pulmonic valve (and early closure of the aortic valve) causes splitting of the second heart sound.[62a,63a] Because the volume overload affects the right ventricle and not the left, large shunts culminate in the development of right heart failure.

Ventricular septal defect Flow across ventricular septal defects occurs primarily during ventricular systole. In the absence of other cardiovascular defects, LV systolic pressure is four to five times that of the right ventricle, and flow proceeds from the left to the right ventricle. The magnitude of left-to-right shunting with small (resistive) defects is mainly determined by the diameter of the defect and the systolic pressure difference (gradient) between the ventricles. The peak pressure difference across the defect can be estimated noninvasively by Doppler echocardiography. Using the peak flow velocity (in meters per second) of the blood flow passing through the defect, the pressure gradient is calculated using the simplified Bernoulli equation ($\Delta P = 4V^2$). A resistive defect with normal right and left ventricular pressures (approximately 20 mm Hg and 100 mm Hg, respectively) would be expected to have a peak jet velocity equal to or greater than 4.5 m/s, corresponding with a peak pressure gradient across the defect equal to or greater than 80 mm Hg. If the peak velocity is lower than predicted, right ventricular systolic pressure is most likely increased, due either to the presence of pulmonic stenosis or to increased pulmonary vascular resistance (pulmonary arterial hypertension).

When a small VSD is located high in the membranous septum, blood is ejected by the left ventricle directly into the

right ventricular (RV) outflow tract and out the main pulmonary artery; the right heart experiences only a very modest volume load, and right heart enlargement is minimal. Right heart enlargement is more prominent when the VSD is large or located in the muscular region of the interventricular septum. With a typical, small, high VSD, oxygen saturation in the right ventricular outflow tract and pulmonary artery is higher than in the right atrium or apex of the right ventricle. Large shunts (those with a pulmonary to systemic flow ratio greater than 3:1) may overload the left and/or right heart enough to increase ventricular diastolic pressures and cause signs of left, right, or biventricular failure. Very large, nonresistive VSDs cause the pressures in both ventricles to equilibrate, and the two ventricles behave as a common pumping chamber. Unless the pulmonary circulation is protected by a stenotic pulmonic valve, the development of pulmonary hypertension is unavoidable.

Eisenmenger's syndrome In newborn animals with a large VSD, pulmonary vascular resistance may not decline after birth, resulting in sustained pulmonary arterial hypertension.[13b,14b] If right ventricular systolic and diastolic pressures equilibrate at or above systemic (left ventricular) levels, bidirectional or right-to-left shunting may occur. The development of pulmonary hypertension associated with a shunting cardiac defect is known as *Eisenmenger's physiology* (or *syndrome*). When the defect is a VSD, the term *Eisenmenger's complex* often is used. Sustained pulmonary hypertension is characterized by progressive and irreversible changes in the pulmonary arteries similar to those mentioned in the section on reversed PDA. As in dogs with a PDA, reversed (right to left) shunting through a ventral septal defect is usually established prior to 6 months of age. In contrast to human patients, gradual development of pulmonary vascular disease and progressive pulmonary hypertension is relatively common in dogs and cats.

Clinical findings Breed predispositions for atrial and ventricular septal defects are presented in Table 200-1. Clinical findings of the typical left-to-right ASD include a soft, grade II-III/VI, systolic ejection murmur over the left heart base and splitting of the second heart sound (Figure 200-13).[23c-25c,24]

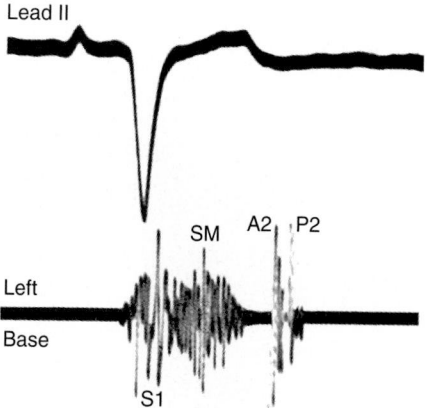

Figure 200-13 Phonocardiogram recorded at the left heart base from a dog with a primum atrial septal defect. The lead II ECG has a negative, slightly prolonged QRS complex, which is indicative of a right ventricular conduction disorder (partial or incomplete right bundle branch block). The phonocardiogram shows a systolic ejection murmur *(SM)* that ends well before the second heart sound, which is widely split. S_1, First heart sound; A_2, aortic component of the second heart sound; P_2, pulmonic component of the second heart sound.

The murmur is often misinterpreted as mild pulmonic stenosis or as an innocent murmur. A low-pitched, right-sided diastolic murmur of relative tricuspid stenosis may occur, but it is usually not audible, especially in smaller patients. Cyanosis is absent unless an additional defect (e.g., pulmonic stenosis or tricuspid valve dysplasia)[15b] or the infrequent complication of pulmonary hypertension is present.[26c] Signs of right heart failure develop in dogs or cats with large defects. The differential diagnosis is anomalous pulmonary venous return, which is an extremely rare anomaly in dogs and cats.[80a]

The main cardiac structural changes caused by an ASD include dilatation of the right atrium and eccentric hypertrophy of the right ventricle. The electrocardiogram may indicate right ventricular enlargement (i.e., right axis shift, increased S-wave depth in leads I, II, and III). Intraventricular conduction disturbances, especially partial or complete right bundle branch block (Figure 200-14), are also common, especially with atrial ostium primum or atrioventricular septal defects.[4a,64a,66a] Thoracic radiographs show enlargement of the right heart and main pulmonary artery, as well as pulmonary hypervascularity proportional to the magnitude of the shunt (Figure 200-15). The left atrium is only modestly enlarged unless concurrent mitral regurgitation from a cleft mitral valve or a more extensive endocardial cushion defect is present. Echocardiography permits direct imaging of atrial septal defects, but false-positive impressions of an ASD are common due to imaging artifacts caused by beam orientation and the thinness of some portions of the normal interatrial septum. Doppler evidence of transatrial shunting is more reliable and typically shows laminar or mildly turbulent diastolic flow through the ASD (Figure 200-16) and increased RV outflow and pulmonary artery velocities. Doppler studies are also helpful for demonstrating associated problems such as mitral regurgitation or other associated defects.[16b,24] Contrast echocardiography is helpful, particularly when the defect is large or when

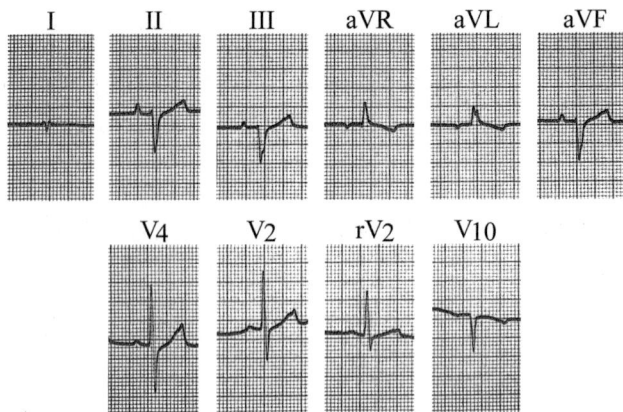

Figure 200-14 Electrocardiogram from a dog with a primum atrial septal defect. The QRS axis is shifted to the right and cranially (+265 degrees), and the last two thirds of the complex is prolonged, as shown by widened and notched S waves in leads III and aVF. A prominent S wave is also present in lead V4. These changes are consistent with a right ventricular conduction disorder, often referred to as a partial or incomplete right bundle branch block. Paper speed = 50 mm/s, 10 mm = 1 mV.

elevated right heart pressures cause reversed flow across the defect (see Figure 200-16).

Cardiac catheterization of animals with an ASD is helpful in the evaluation of the magnitude and direction of shunting. In cases of left-to-right shunting, oximetry samples from the venae cavae, right atrium, and right ventricle indicate an increase in oxygen saturation between the venae cavae and the atrium and/or ventricle, and the magnitude of systemic to

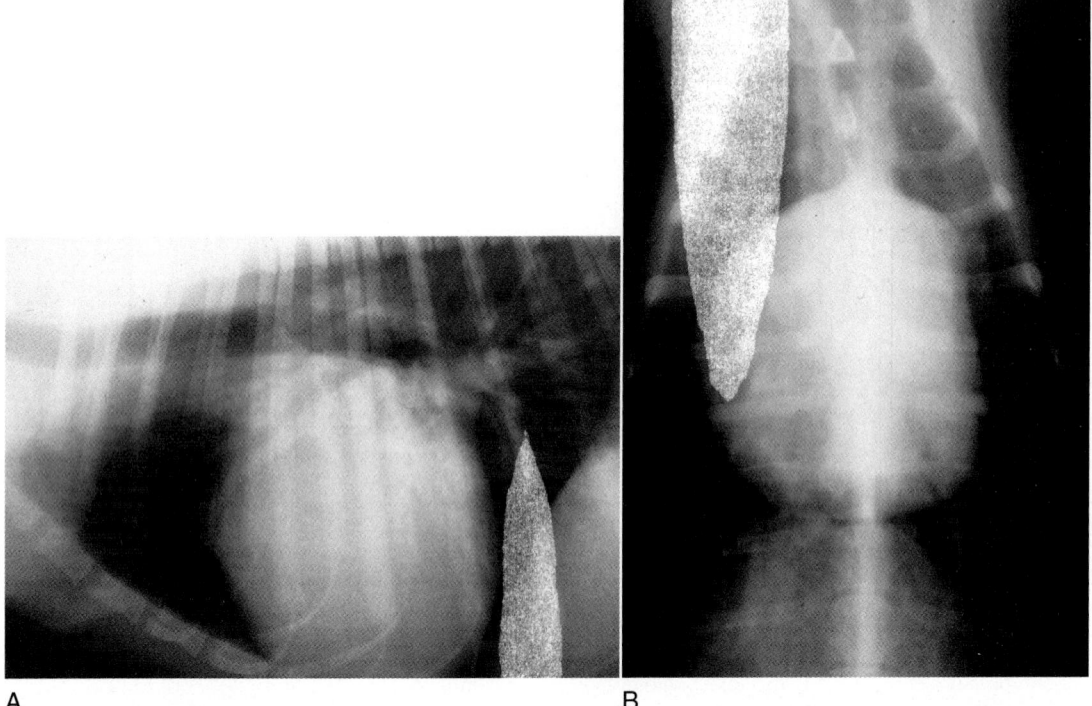

A   B

Figure 200-15 Lateral (**A**) and dorsoventral (**B**) radiographs from a standard poodle with an atrial septal defect. The cardiac silhouette is enlarged, with prominence of the right atrium, right ventricle, and pulmonary vessels.

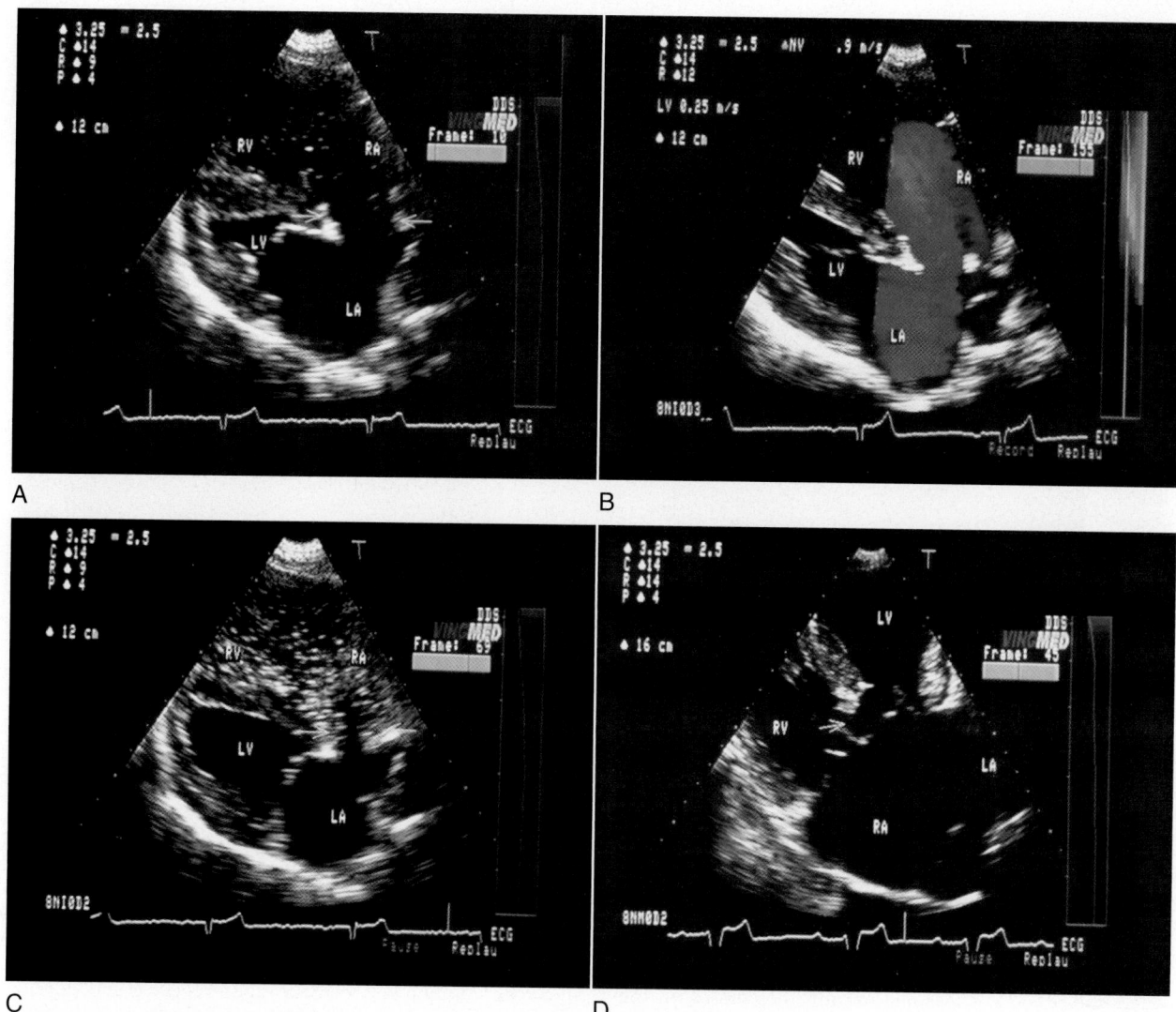

Figure 200-16 Echocardiography of atrial septal defect (ASD) and endocardial cushion defect. **A,** Right long axis view from a standard poodle with a secundum ASD. Color flow Doppler **(B)** and contrast echocardiography **(C)** studies indicate left-to-right flow through the ASD. **D,** Right long axis view from a dog with an endocardial cushion defect. A large ASD, a ventricular septal defect, and a single atrioventricular valve override the interventricular septum. Both the left and right atria are enlarged. *RA,* Right atrium; *RV,* right ventricle; *LA,* left atrium; *LV,* left ventricle.

pulmonary shunting can be estimated.[25] Central venous and right ventricular diastolic pressures are elevated when congestive heart failure is present or imminent. Increased systolic flow across the pulmonic valve may result in "relative" pulmonic stenosis, identified by a mild systolic pressure gradient (5 to 15 mm Hg) between the right ventricle and pulmonary artery.[63a] Flow through the atrial septal defect can be demonstrated by angiocardiography. When introduced via a femoral vein, a catheter often can be easily passed from the right atrium through an ASD or patent foramen ovale into the left atrium, allowing injection of a contrast medium and visualization of the left-to-right shunting. Alternatively, injection of the contrast material into the pulmonary artery outlines left-to-right shunting defects during the left-sided phase of the study. After pulmonary venous return, the atrial septum usually can be seen between the left atrium and the aorta on the lateral projection. Passage of dye from the left atrium into the

right atrium and vena cavae confirms the presence of the defect. With more extensive endocardial cushion defects, a left ventricular injection can be performed to demonstrate the VSD, mitral regurgitation, and occasionally left ventricular-to-right atrial shunting.

The clinical features of a VSD depend on the magnitude of the shunt and whether complications or other defects are present. In animals with a typical small, subcristal VSD, a harsh, holosystolic murmur is heard best over the right midprecordium to cranial precordium.* In rare cases of supracristal VSD, the defect opens just under the pulmonic valve, and the systolic murmur may be heard best at the left base. Splitting of the second heart sound can occur, but it often is not recognized because of the imposition of the murmur on the second

---

*References 5a, 10a, 23c, 27c, 28c, and 68a.

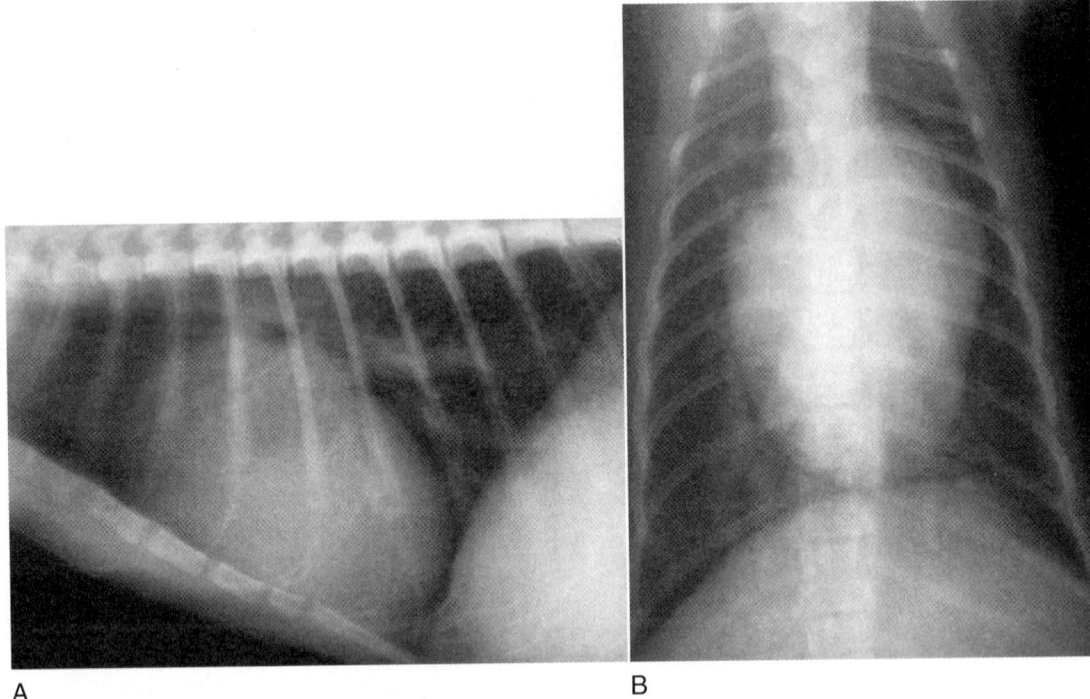

A   B

Figure 200-17 Lateral **(A)** and dorsoventral **(B)** thoracic radiographs of a cat with a ventricular septal defect and a large left-to-right shunt. Cardiac silhouette is enlarged, and rounding of the cranial border of the heart can be seen on the lateral view. The main pulmonary artery and left atrium are enlarged on the dorsoventral view. The pulmonary vasculature is prominent.

heart sound. If distortion of the aortic root causes significant aortic regurgitation, a blowing, decrescendo diastolic murmur is audible over the left ventricular outflow area. These combined systolic and diastolic murmurs are sometimes described as a *to-and-fro murmur*. Aortic regurgitation flow into the right ventricle can produce a diastolic murmur best heard on the right hemithorax.[17b] Systolic murmurs over the atrioventricular valves may also be detected if the defect is part of a more extensive endocardial cushion defect.

Electrocardiographic findings in animals with a VSD are variable. With moderate or large left-to-right shunts, there is often evidence of left atrial or ventricular enlargement, but right ventricular conduction defects also occur. Frontal plane leads may demonstrate a subtle abnormality in early ventricular septal activation, characterized by a Q wave that is wide or contains high-frequency notching.[69a] Right axis deviation and a narrow QRS complex in a dog with VSD usually indicates right ventricular hypertrophy and a more complex lesion, such as VSD with pulmonic stenosis or pulmonary hypertension. Thoracic radiographs are very useful in assessing the magnitude of left-to-right shunting VSDs. Pulmonary hypervascularity and left atrial and ventricular enlargement are observed in proportion to the magnitude of the shunt (Figure 200-17).[22a,24a] The main, lobar, and peripheral pulmonary arteries are usually prominent. In animals with small defects, thoracic radiographs may appear entirely normal. With large defects, the right ventricle may also enlarge. A large pulmonary artery segment, underperfused lungs, and small peripheral pulmonary vasculature suggest the possibility of pulmonic stenosis or pulmonary hypertension and right-to-left shunting. Two-dimensional color flow Doppler echocardiography usually identifies all but the smallest VSDs (Figure 200-18). Spectral Doppler studies are useful for quantifying the high-velocity jet through small, resistive VSDs, as previously mentioned. Contrast echocardiography may also be used to identify flow through the defect,

but it is usually not necessary if a careful echocardiographic examination is performed.

Cardiac catheterization in animals with a VSD allows identification of the anatomic defect and estimation of the degree of shunting.[27c] Oximetry samples demonstrate a "step-up" in oxygen content between the right ventricle and pulmonary artery. Intracardiac pressures are usually normal in dogs and cats with a small VSD. Right ventricular pressures are often elevated 5 to 15 mm Hg above the pressure in the pulmonary artery, a reflection of increased transvalvular flow and relative pulmonic stenosis. More dramatic increases in right ventricular systolic pressure indicate pulmonary hypertension or concurrent pulmonic stenosis, and the development of elevated end-diastolic ventricular pressures and central venous pressure herald the onset of heart failure. In uncomplicated cases, left ventricular angiocardiography can outline the VSD (Figure 200-19). Bidirectional or right-to-left shunting is observed when RV systolic pressure reaches and exceeds LV systolic pressure. Anatomic changes of the semilunar valves or great vessels, especially of the aortic root, are best visualized by injection of contrast in the proximal aorta, which is also the preferred location for determining the presence and severity of aortic regurgitation.[17b]

Natural history The morbidity and mortality associated with atrioventricular septal defects depend on the size and location of the defect, the magnitude and direction of shunt flow, and whether additional lesions are present. Spontaneous closure of small VSDs often occurs in children, but this is an uncommon occurrence in cats and dogs.[71a] Animals with uncomplicated small defects (ASDs and VSDs) and modest shunts usually live a normal life span without ever developing recognizable clinical signs. Large shunts that cause moderate to severe cardiomegaly often lead to intractable congestive heart failure. Moderate to severe aortic regurgitation, an

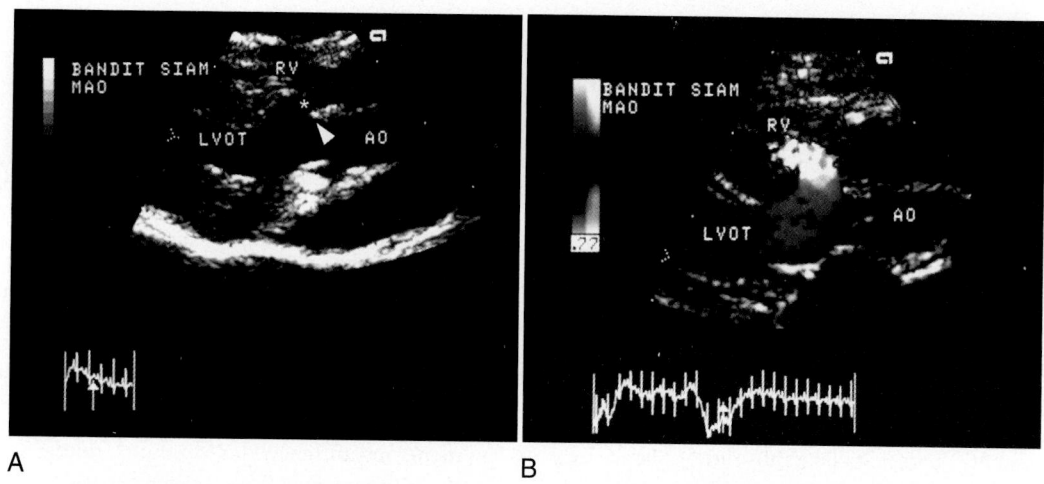

Figure 200-18 Echocardiography of a Siamese cat with a ventricular septal defect (VSD). **A,** Right long axis view shows the VSD (*) between the left ventricular outflow tract *(LVOT)* and aorta *(Ao)* and opening into the right ventricle *(RV)*. Note the proximity of the VSD to the root of the aorta and the origin of the aortic valve *(arrowhead)*. **B,** Right long axis color flow Doppler study reveals systolic left-to-right shunting across the VSD into the right ventricle.

uncommon complication of VSD, presents a very substantial risk of left heart failure and shortened survival.[17b] It is often difficult to predict the outcome in very young animals with a VSD; this is more easily done when they grow closer to adult size at 6 to 12 months of age. Animals that develop pulmonary hypertension (Eisenmenger's syndrome) have a guarded short-term prognosis and a very guarded to poor long-term prognosis, although survival beyond 7 years is possible. Cats with severe endocardial cushion defects often develop marked cardiomegaly and biventricular congestive heart failure at an early age (less than 2 years), warranting a very guarded to poor prognosis.

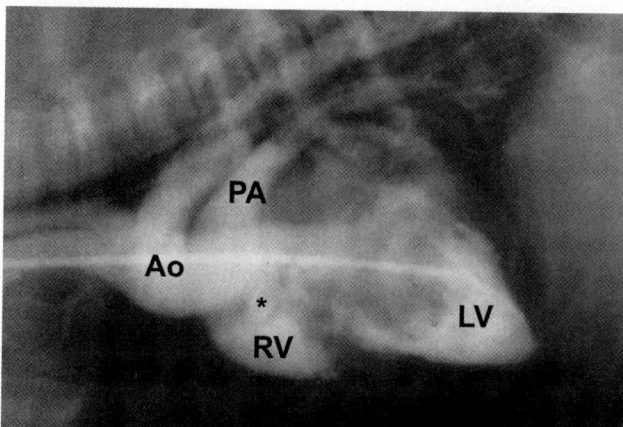

Figure 200-19 Angiogram of a 6-month-old Welsh corgi with a ventricular septal defect (VSD). An injection into the left ventricle *(LV)* outlines the aorta *(Ao)*. Contrast can be seen shunting across the VSD into the right ventricle *(RV)* and the pulmonary artery *(PA)*. The left ventricle is mildly enlarged. A portion of an aortic valve leaflet (*) appears to prolapse into the VSD.

Clinical management Surgical closure is the definitive treatment for all atrioventricular septal defects, but open-heart correction is uncommonly attempted in animals because of the usual requirement for cardiopulmonary bypass or other techniques to arrest the heart.[29c-31c,76a,77a] Palliative treatment of a VSD may be accomplished without bypass by applying a constrictive band around the main pulmonary artery. This technique creates supravalvular pulmonic stenosis and increases the right ventricular systolic pressure, thereby reducing the magnitude of left-to-right shunting.[75a] This procedure is recommended for dogs and cats showing signs of rapidly progressive cardiomegaly and overt or impending congestive heart failure. Overaggressive banding should be avoided, because it can result in pressure overload, acute right heart failure or, in surviving animals, right-to-left shunting. Alternatively, systemic arterial vasodilators can be administered to reduce systemic vascular resistance and the magnitude of left-to-right shunting.[79a] As noted for reversed PDA, surgical correction should not be attempted in animals with Eisenmenger's syndrome. Restricted physical activity is probably the most prudent and effective strategy, and periodic phlebotomy may be useful in some patients that develop extreme polycythemia. The PCV should be maintained at 58% to 65%.

Valvular Regurgitation
Pulmonic and Aortic Valve Insufficiency
Pulmonic insufficiency Primary congenital pulmonic insufficiency (PI) is an uncommon abnormality that results from abnormal development of valve leaflets or dilatation of the pulmonary artery annulus.[95a,96a] Pulmonic valve insufficiency causes volume overload and eccentric hypertrophy of the right ventricle. The main and proximal branches of the right and left pulmonary arteries enlarge to accommodate the concomitant increase in RV stroke volume. Isolated pulmonic valve insufficiency is often well tolerated, but heart failure can develop when severe PI is induced experimentally in dogs. Congenital pulmonic insufficiency is more likely to cause

heart failure if pulmonary vascular resistance subsequently increases as a result of severe pulmonary parenchymal or vascular disease. Trivial pulmonic insufficiency is often observed in dogs with a PDA, presumably from dilatation of the main pulmonary artery. Most dogs with pulmonic valve stenosis have mild valvular insufficiency, but severe concurrent PI is sometimes seen. Pulmonic insufficiency of varying degrees of severity may also develop as a result of surgery or balloon dilatation to relieve PS. Pulmonic insufficiency is a potential consequence of any disorder that prompts the development of pulmonary hypertension.

Clinical features of PI include variable systolic (due to increased flow) and diastolic murmurs best heard at the left heart base. This to-and-fro murmur should not be confused with the continuous murmur of PDA. Electrocardiograms from dogs with congenital PI may be normal or may reflect right ventricular enlargement. Thoracic radiographs show enlargement of the main pulmonary artery and right ventricle, giving the erroneous impression of PS to the unaware (Figure 200-20). Injection of a contrast medium into the main pulmonary artery using a small-diameter catheter documents valvular insufficiency (Figure 200-21). Slow clearance of contrast from the dilated and thin-walled right ventricle also supports a diagnosis of PI. Color flow Doppler echocardiography elegantly demonstrates these same features and permits visualization of the rudimentary or misshapen valve leaflets (see Figure 200-21). Doppler studies also aid the recognition of pulmonary arterial hypertension. When the velocity of the pulmonary regurgitant jet exceeds 3 m/s, pulmonary hypertension is the likely cause of the pulmonary artery dilatation and valvular insufficiency. Treatment for congenital PI has not been described in companion animals. In dogs suffering from heart failure, conventional medical therapy with diuretics and ACE inhibitors is a reasonable palliative approach.

Aortic insufficiency   Isolated congenital aortic insufficiency (AI) is a rare disorder. It occasionally is detected in young or older dogs with idiopathic dilatation of the aorta *(annuloaortic ectasia)*. Mild to moderate aortic insufficiency has also been reported in a boxer and a hound with quadricuspid aortic valves.[26] With the increasing application of Doppler echocardiography, aortic regurgitation is recognized with increasing frequency as a complication of other cardiac malformations.[108a,109a] Aortic insufficiency often accompanies subvalvular aortic stenosis and has been observed with ventricular septal defects and tetralogy of Fallot and after balloon catheter dilatation for SAS. The potential mechanisms for aortic valvular insufficiency in these conditions have been reviewed.[108a] As in congenital pulmonic insufficiency, the murmur resulting from AI can be both systolic and diastolic (to-and-fro murmur) and is best heard over the left hemithorax. Many dogs with mild AI do not evidence an audible murmur. The diagnosis of AI is supported by palpation of a hyperkinetic arterial pulse resulting from the increased stroke volume and diastolic runoff of aortic blood back into the left ventricle. Left ventricular eccentric hypertrophy develops in proportion to the severity of the insufficiency. Severe AI commonly results in left-sided congestive heart failure. Documentation of AI and estimation of its severity requires angiocardiography or Doppler echocardiography. Definitive repair requires cardiac bypass surgery and valve replacement, an unlikely proposition. Use of arterial vasodilators can reduce the regurgitant volume and may delay the onset of heart failure. Treatment with diuretics, ACE inhibitors, and positive inotropic drugs are indicated if heart failure is present.

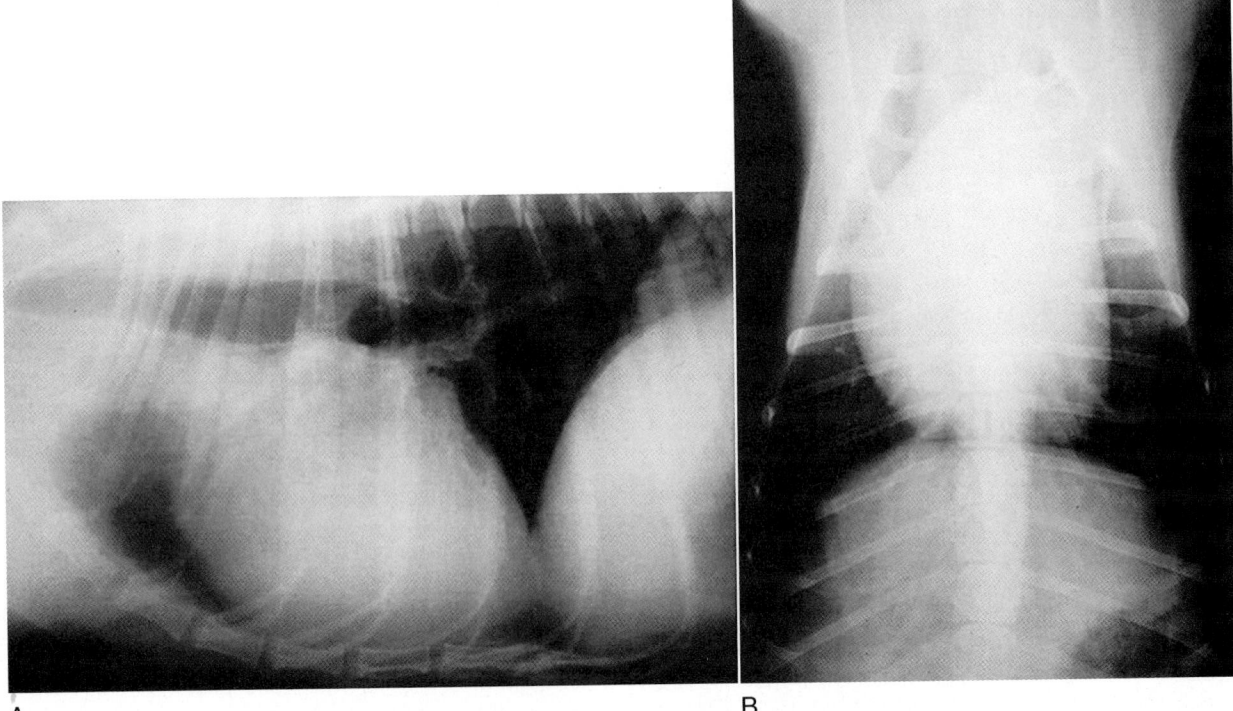

A   B

Figure 200-20 Radiographs from a Cavalier King Charles spaniel with congenital pulmonic valve insufficiency, showing convincing evidence of right ventricular enlargement in the lateral **(A)** and dorsoventral **(B)** projections. The pulmonary artery segment is markedly enlarged (see text for discussion).

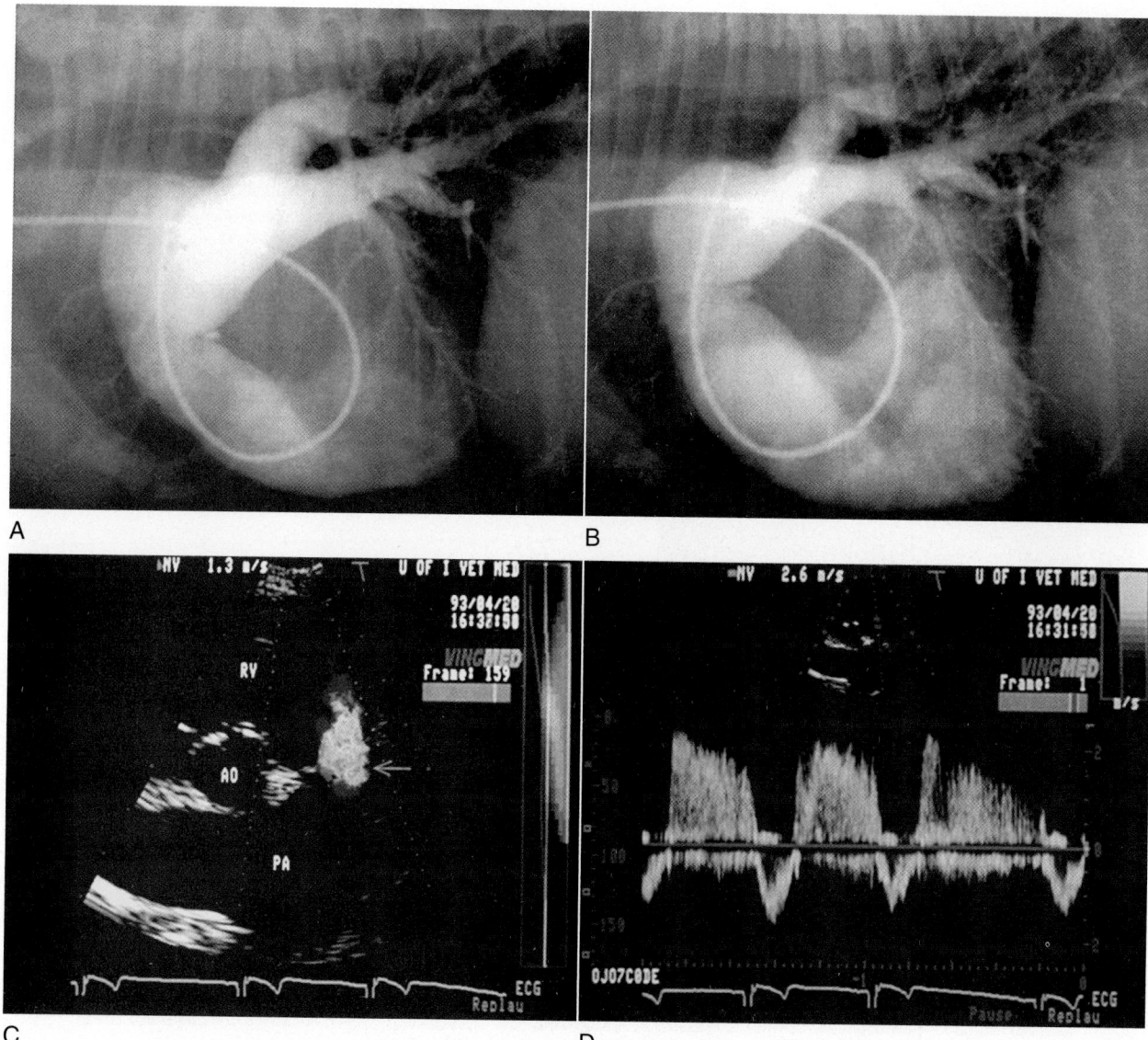

Figure 200-21 Angiocardiogram recorded from the same dog as in Figure 200-20. **A,** Contrast material injected into the pulmonary artery leaks immediately back into the right ventricle through the incompetent pulmonic valve. **B,** Several frames later, the right ventricle has filled with contrast, establishing substantial pulmonic valve incompetence. A dysplastic valve remnant is also visible. **C,** A color flow Doppler study was performed several years later in the same dog. Disturbed flow entering the right ventricle *(RV)* from the pulmonary artery is shown on this black and white rendition of a color study. Note the very dilated main pulmonary artery. *Ao,* aorta. **D,** Pulsed wave Doppler study shows that the diastolic flow is moving at a relatively low velocity (just over 2 m/s), excluding the possibility of pulmonary hypertension.

Atrioventricular Valve Dysplasia

Congenital malformations of the mitral and tricuspid valves are reported in both cats and dogs.[1-5c,12a,58-62c,110a-121a] Consequences of these malformations include mitral and tricuspid regurgitation, inflow obstruction (i.e., mitral or tricuspid valve stenosis), and dynamic obstruction of the left ventricular outflow tract. The most common physiologic consequence of atrioventricular valve malformation is valvular insufficiency. The pathophysiology and clinical course of congenital mitral regurgitation are similar to acquired degenerative valvular disease in the dog. For this reason, only the salient features of these conditions are reviewed, and the reader is directed to Chapter 201 for greater detail. Congenital stenoses of the atrioventricular valves, as well as other interatrial obstructs, are recognized more frequently in dogs and cats, presumably because of the increased use of Doppler echocardiography. Systolic anterior motion (SAM) of the mitral valve apparatus and dynamic LV outflow obstruction in cats and dogs, long regarded solely as a manifestation of hypertrophic cardiomyopathy (see Chapter 203; 204), may be caused solely by architectural changes in the mitral valve apparatus in some animals. When the primary disorder is valve dysplasia, concentric left ventricular hypertrophy resolves if the obstruction is abolished by treatment (beta-receptor blocking drugs).

Pathology and pathogenesis Tricuspid valve dysplasia has been shown to have a genetic basis in the most commonly afflicted breed, Labrador retrievers.[6,7] A heritable basis for mitral valve dysplasia in cats and some breeds of dogs is suspected, but convincing evidence has not yet been reported. A wide spectrum of morphologic abnormalities of the mitral and tricuspid valves have been described, including shortening, rolling, notching, and thickening of the valve leaflets; incomplete separation of valve components from the ventricular wall; elongation, shortening, fusion, and thickening of the chordae tendineae; direct insertion of the valve edge into a papillary muscle; and atrophy, hypertrophy, fusion, and malpositioning of the papillary muscles and chordae

tendineae.[27,113a,120a] The usual consequence of these changes is valvular insufficiency. Examples of tricuspid and mitral valve dysplasia are shown in Figures 200-22 and 200-23. In dogs, mitral valve stenosis is common only in bull terriers, often occurring along with valvular aortic stenosis.[40b] Some dogs and cats with mitral or tricuspid dysplasia evidence a patent foramen ovale or a concurrent ASD, resulting in left-to-right or right-to-left shunting. Supravalvular mitral stenosis is discussed in a later section of this chapter, together with cor triatriatum.

Pathophysiology The fundamental pathophysiologic abnormalities of atrioventricular valve malformations are

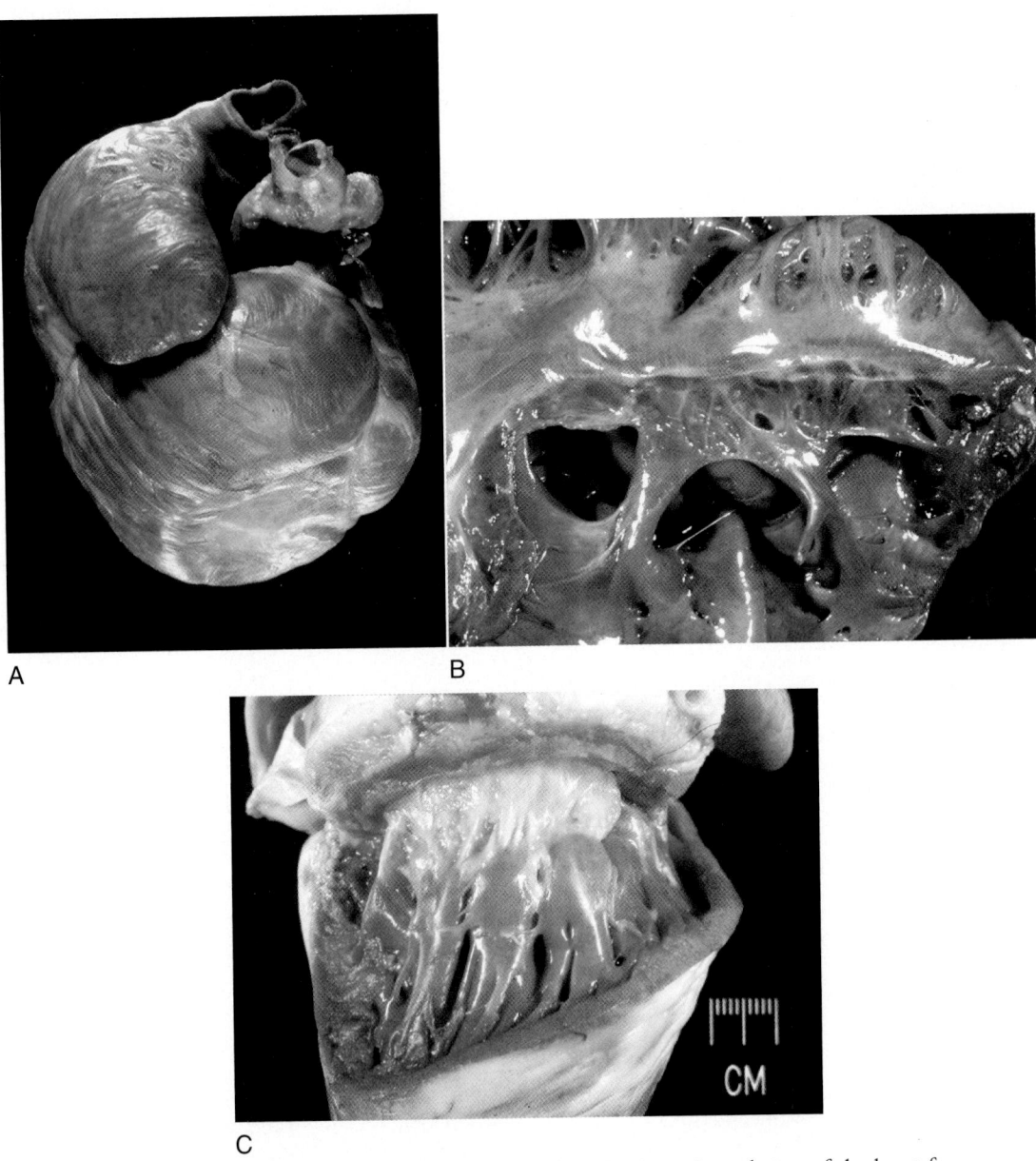

A

B

C

Figure 200-22 Gross pathology of tricuspid dysplasia (TD). **A,** Cranial view of the heart from a patient with severe right atrial, auricular, and ventricular enlargement caused by TD. **B,** Tricuspid valve from a 2-year-old Labrador with severe TD. The edges of the valve leaflets insert directly into the papillary muscles, and conspicuous absence and shortening of the chordae tendineae are seen. The right atrium and ventricle are dilated. **C,** Curtainlike deformity of the tricuspid valve from a 2-year-old Samoyed with TD and tricuspid stenosis. The tricuspid valve is thickened and opaque. Multiple large, fused papillary muscles with short chordae tendineae are present.

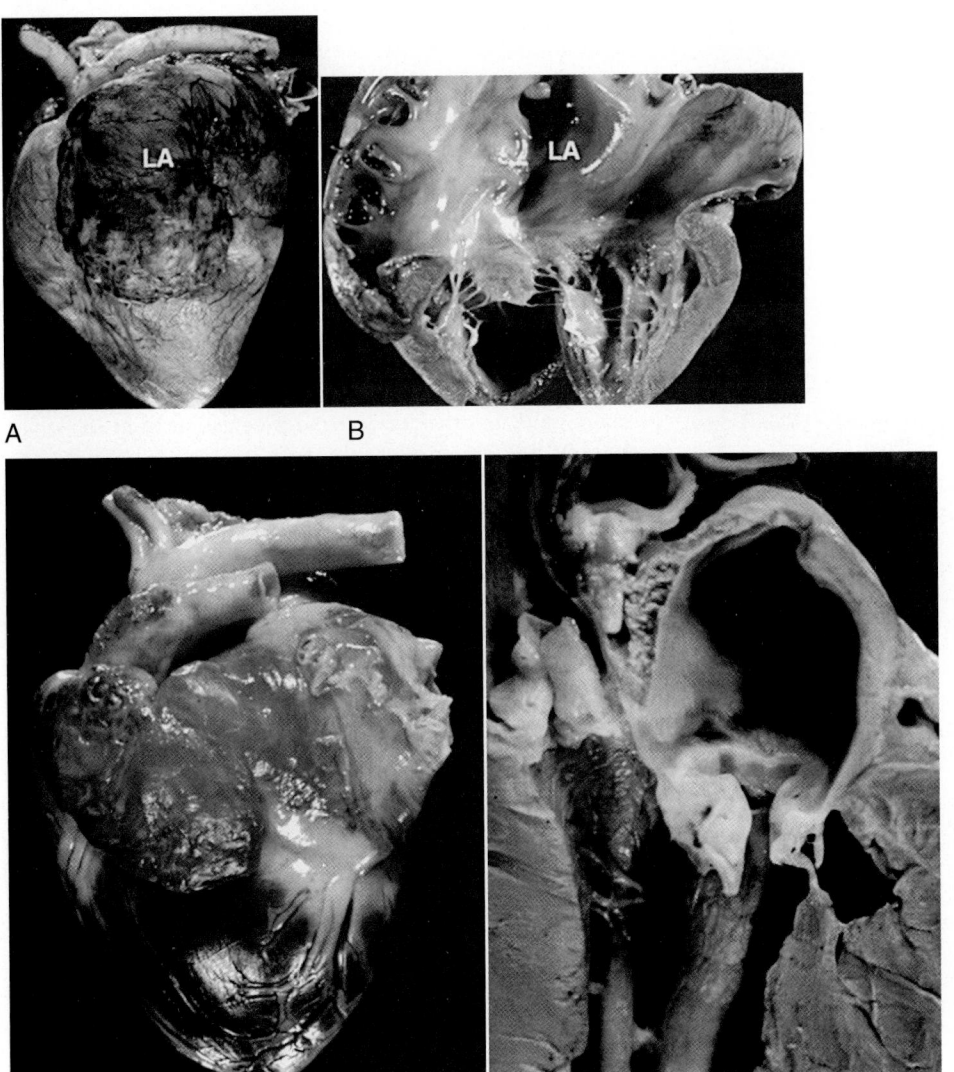

Figure 200-23 Gross pathology of mitral valve dysplasia. **A,** Marked left atrial dilatation in a cat with mitral valve dysplasia. **B,** Mitral valve in this cat shows a bizarre malformation of the anterior (cranioventral) leaflet. Also, the posterior (caudodorsal) papillary muscle is abnormally located, and it attaches directly to the leaflet with no intervening chordae. **C,** Marked dilatation of the left atrium is seen as a result of obstructed flow into the left ventricle. **D,** Grossly distorted mitral valve from a bull terrier with concurrent stenosis and insufficiency of the mitral valve. A thickened aortic valve, which caused mild aortic stenosis, is just visible on the left side of the picture. *LA,* left atrium.

briefly presented. Valvular insufficiency produces volume overloading, manifested as atrial dilatation and eccentric hypertrophy of the affected ventricle. Congestive heart failure often develops at a young age but occasionally does not develop until adulthood. In some dogs and cats with tricuspid dysplasia, cyanosis can be observed as a consequence of right-to-left shunting across a patent foramen ovale or ASD. Malformations that cause valve stenosis obstruct ventricular filling, resulting in increased atrial pressures and signs of congestive heart failure. Severe stenosis limits cardiac output such that hypotension, syncope, or collapse with exertion may be observed. Pulmonary hypertension and right heart failure frequently develop secondary to severe mitral stenosis as a consequence of chronically elevated left atrial pressure. As a result, some dogs that initially present with signs of pulmonary congestion from mitral stenosis can present again months later with signs of right heart failure. Dogs and cats with severe congenital valvular stenosis or regurgitation are predisposed to atrial fibrillation and paroxysmal or sustained supraventricular tachycardia; these conditions typically result in sudden clinical deterioration.

Clinical findings Cats of all breeds, Great Danes, German shepherds, bull terriers, golden retrievers, Newfoundland retrievers, Dalmatians, and mastiffs are predisposed to mitral dysplasia.[30b,111a,114a] Tricuspid dysplasia occurs in cats but seems to be most common in large male dogs, particularly Labrador retrievers.[9a,28] Clinical signs are referable to exertional fatigue or to right ventricular, left ventricular, or biventricular congestive heart failure. The hallmark of valvular insufficiency is a holosystolic murmur heard best over the affected valve area. A loud gallop may also be detected.[111a] A soft, late diastolic murmur and opening snap are sometimes auscultated in dogs or cats with valvular stenosis, but these findings are often absent or missed (Figure 200-24). In severe cases of tricuspid dysplasia, a murmur may not be present because the valve offers no resistance to regurgitant blood flow (Figure 200-25). Jugular venous distension and pulses are common findings in cases of tricuspid dysplasia.

Splintered QRS complexes (Rr', RR', rR', rr') are a distinctive and common ECG finding in dogs and cats with tricuspid dysplasia.[64c] Right heart enlargement patterns are also manifest. Tall or wide P waves are observed with all types of valvular dysplasia, but ventricular enlargement patterns are mainly limited to animals with regurgitant physiology and are not observed with isolated valve stenosis except when pulmonary hypertension develops secondary to mitral stenosis. Atrial arrhythmias, especially atrial fibrillation, are often recorded.

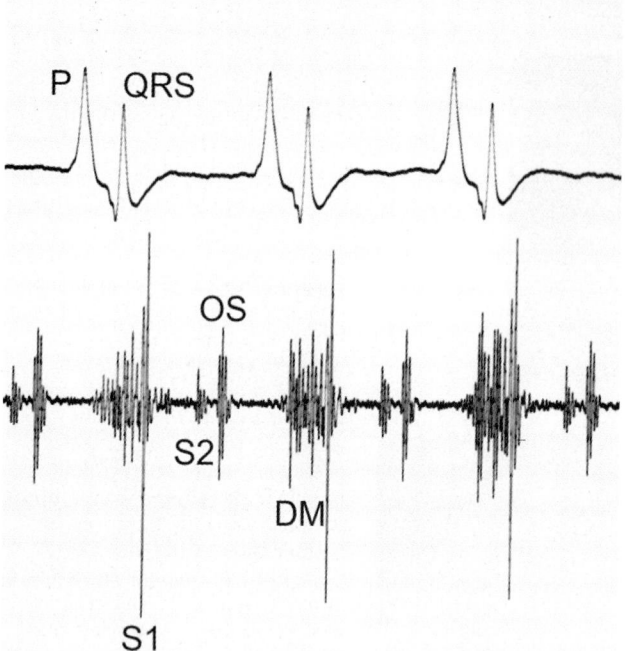

Figure 200-24 Phonocardiogram from the right apex in a 2-year-old Samoyed with tricuspid dysplasia and tricuspid stenosis. The ECG shows markedly elevated P waves consistent with right atrial enlargement. An early diastolic opening snap (OS) is present, followed by a late diastolic (presystolic) murmur (DM) that coincides with the P wave and atrial systole. S_1, First heart sound; S_2, second heart sound.

The pattern of chamber enlargement on the thoracic radiographs generally reflects the involvement of the affected valve and resulting physiologic consequences (Figure 200-26). In cases of tricuspid dysplasia the degree of cardiomegaly is often impressive, and the heart may have a globoid appearance resembling that produced by pericardial effusion. The possibility of valvular stenosis should be considered whenever the atrium is markedly dilated without enlargement of the ipsilateral ventricle.

Definitive diagnosis of atrioventricular valve malformation requires echocardiography or cardiac catheterization and angiocardiography. Abnormal location, shape, motion, or attachment of the valve apparatus is easily observed by echocardiography (see Figure 200-25). With valve stenosis, color flow Doppler studies show a prolonged high-velocity jet (often greater than 2 m/s) entering the left or right ventricle during diastole, indicating the presence of a diastolic pressure gradient. With valve insufficiency, Doppler studies demonstrate regurgitant jets streaming from the ventricle into the atrium through the incompetent valve. Diastolic pressure gradients (valve stenosis) and varying degrees of ventricularization of atrial wave forms (valve insufficiency) can be recorded during cardiac catheterization. Angiographic visualization of valvular insufficiency is best appreciated by ventricular injections of contrast material, whereas valve stenosis is best demonstrated after an atrial injection (transseptal catheterization is required to accomplish left atrial injection).

Clinical management   Repair of the affected valve can be attempted, and surgical replacement of dysplastic atrioventricular valves has been successfully accomplished in a small number of animals.[65c-67c] Cardiac bypass is required for these

infrequently performed procedures. Balloon valvuloplasty, with limited success, has been described in dogs with tricuspid stenosis.[68c,29] In most affected animals, medical treatment is instituted only if heart failure develops. Treatment of valvular insufficiency largely consists of diuretics, ACE inhibitors, and digoxin.[28] In dogs with tricuspid dysplasia and refractory heart failure, periodic thoracocentesis or abdominocentesis is often needed. In patients with valve stenosis, diuretics are used to control congestion. Inasmuch as tachycardia is poorly tolerated in patients with stenosis, every effort should be made to prevent stress and to restrict exercise. Administration of beta blockers, calcium channel blockers, and/or digoxin is helpful in some cases for the management of atrial fibrillation or other supraventricular tachyarrhythmias. Some patients tolerate serious defects surprisingly well for many years. In other cases, rapid progression to heart failure and death occur.

DEFECTS THAT CAUSE PRIMARILY PRESSURE OVERLOAD

Ventricular Outflow Obstructions
Pulmonic Stenosis
Pulmonic stenosis (PS) is the third most common congenital heart defect in dogs,[5c,30] and it is occasionally recognized in cats.[2c,32c,89a] In most cases pulmonic stenosis occurs as an isolated heart defect, but it frequently is accompanied by other cardiac anomalies, such as tricuspid dysplasia. Congenital outflow tract obstructions of the right heart can develop in the subvalvular and supravalvular regions, but primary malformation of the pulmonary valve (dysplasia) is the most frequently observed defect in dogs. Patterson et al.,[86a] who studied the heritability and pathology of pulmonic valve dysplasia in the beagle, initially suggested a polygenic mode of transmission for this defect. However, these breeding studies did not exclude the possibility of a single-gene mechanism with variable penetrance. The pattern of inheritance of PS has not been studied in other predisposed dog breeds or in cats.

Pathology   Valvular lesions consist of varying degrees of valve thickening, leaflet fusion, and/or hypoplasia of the valve annulus. Although some dogs manifest a thin, dome-shaped valve with a central orifice (Figure 200-27), many dogs have more complicated lesions that resemble atypical PS in children.[15a,86a,88a] The valve leaflets are often thickened, misshapen, and/or fused (see Figure 200-27). The annulus of the pulmonic valve is hypoplastic in some dogs, which further narrows the area available for right ventricular ejection. Histologic abnormalities include thickening of the valve spongiosa and the presence of bands of fusiform cells in a dense collagen network. These changes are thought to represent overproduction of normal valve elements or failure of conversion of the cushionlike embryonic valve primordia. Some dogs with valve dysplasia have a fibrous ring just below the valve leaflets in addition to the valvular changes. In other dogs, the obstructive lesion occurs in the infundibular region of the right ventricular outflow tract (RVOT). On occasion the RVOT is partitioned from the body (inflow region) of the right ventricle by a well-developed, fibromuscular ridge, resulting in an anomaly referred to as double- or dual-chambered right ventricle.[31] Supravalvular PS is uncommon and in the authors' experience has been most often observed in giant schnauzers. A unique form of subvalvular PS caused by anomalous development of the coronary arteries has been described in English bulldogs and in boxers.[32,33] In this condition, the left and right coronary arteries branch from a single large coronary artery, which originates from the right aortic sinus

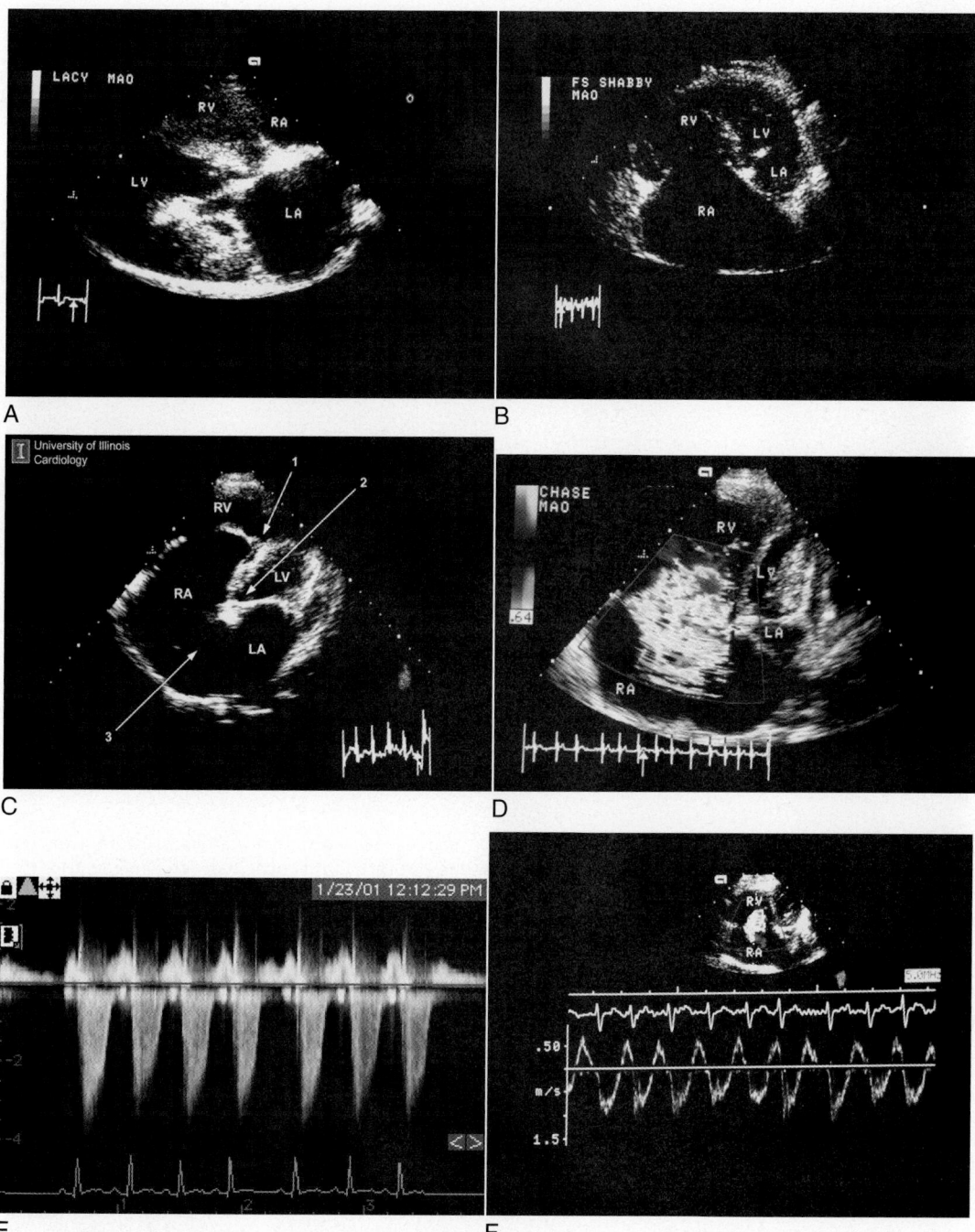

Figure 200-25 Echocardiography of mitral dysplasia (MD) and tricuspid dysplasia (TD). **A,** Right axis view from a 4-month-old pit bull with MD and aortic stenosis. The mitral valve leaflets are markedly thickened, and the chordae tendineae are shortened. The left atrium *(LA)* is enlarged, and the left ventricle *(LV)* is hypertrophied. **B,** Left apical view from a cat with TD, showing severe right atrial *(RA)* and right ventricular *(RV)* enlargement. **C,** Left apical view from a dog with an Ebstein-like abnormality. The origin of the tricuspid valve is displaced apically, and the septal leaflet is fused to the interventricular septum *(1)*. The origin of the mitral valve leaflet *(2)* is shown for comparison. The near-parallel orientation of the ultrasound beam gives the false impression of a large atrial septal defect *(3)*. **D,** Left apical color flow Doppler study from a 2-year-old Labrador retriever with severe tricuspid regurgitation caused by TD. **E,** Continuous wave Doppler tracing of tricuspid regurgitation from a dog with TD. The maximal velocity of the regurgitant jet is 3.5 m/s, suggesting a moderate increase in right ventricular systolic pressure. **F,** Pulsed wave Doppler study from a 7-year-old cat with severe TD demonstrates low velocity and laminar tricuspid regurgitation, indicating that the defect is very large and offers little resistance to regurgitant flow. No murmur was ausculted in this patient.

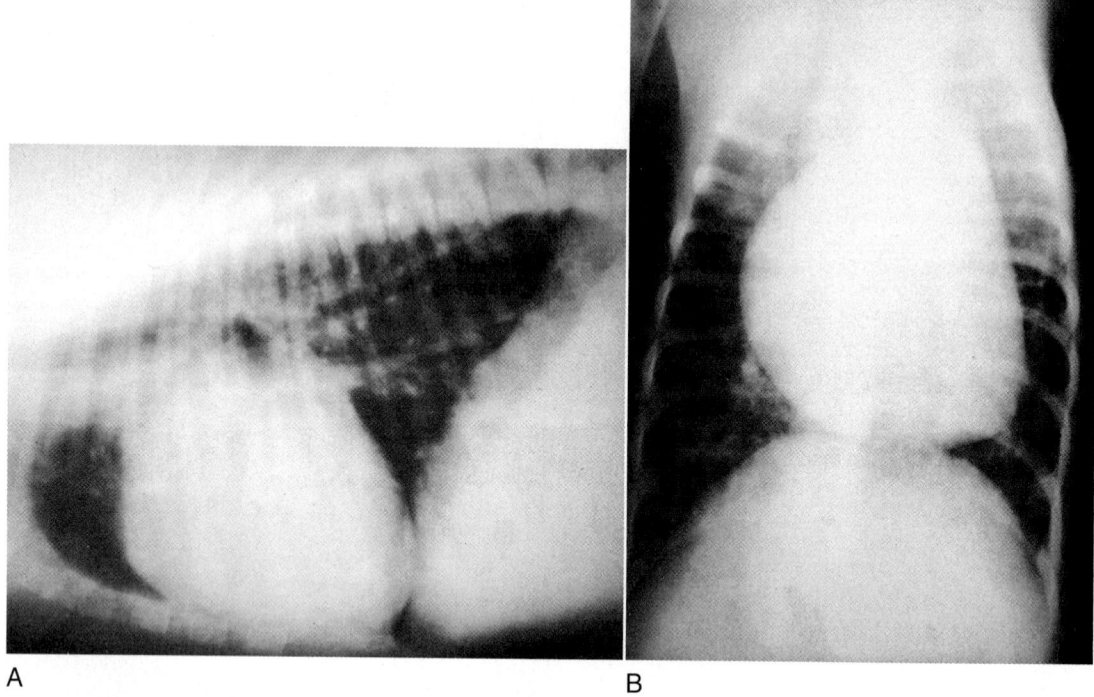

A   B

Figure 200-26 Lateral (**A**) and dorsoventral (**B**) thoracic radiographs from a dog with tricuspid dysplasia (TD). Right atrial and ventricular enlargement is seen in both views. The lateral film demonstrates a bulge in the cranial waist, most likely due to right auricular enlargement.

of Valsalva (Figure 200-28). From this location the anomalous left coronary artery encircles the RVOT just below the pulmonary valve, contributing to the subvalvular component of this complex malformation (see Figure 200-28).

Increased resistance to systolic ejection results in concentric right ventricular hypertrophy, which generally develops in proportion to the severity of the obstructing defect. Although this compensatory response serves to normalize wall stress, it can have deleterious effects. In some dogs with PS, secondary hypertrophy of the infundibular region of the RVOT contributes to outflow tract obstruction, particularly during exercise or stress. The existence of this additional mechanism of obstruction can complicate the clinical outcome of surgical valvotomy or interventional balloon valvuloplasty. Other cardiac defects can complicate the physiology and alter the clinical presentation and prognosis of patients with PS. Pulmonic stenosis and tricuspid valve dysplasia can be a particularly injurious combination. Insofar as the volume of tricuspid regurgitation is a function of the size of the regurgitant orifice (the severity of dysplasia) and the systolic pressure gradient (the severity of PS), severe tricuspid regurgitation tends to develop in affected dogs, leading to intractable right-sided heart failure.

Meticulous ultrasonic examination, often using contrast echocardiography, reveals that patent connections between the right and left heart occur in a substantial percentage of dogs with PS, and some dogs with severe PS become cyanotic as a result of right-to-left shunting through an ASD, patent foramen ovale, or VSD. Many of these abnormalities have a common origin in the maldevelopment of the embryonic conotruncal septum. These types of defects are discussed more thoroughly in the section on tetralogy of Fallot.

Pathophysiology Obstruction to right ventricular outflow increases resistance to ejection, causing a proportional increase in ventricular systolic pressure. Concentric hypertrophy of the right ventricle develops in an attempt to normalize wall stress. During systole, blood ejected from the right ventricle accelerates as it traverses the obstructive orifice. Blood flow velocity increases and becomes turbulent distal to the obstruction. A poststenotic dilatation develops in the main pulmonary artery as the turbulent jet of blood decelerates and expends some of its kinetic energy against the vessel wall.

Concentric hypertrophy reduces right ventricular diastolic compliance, impairs ventricular filling, and often results in elevated right atrial pressure. Tricuspid regurgitation from progressive ventricular dilatation, valvular dysplasia, or a combination of these factors can contribute to further increases in atrial pressure. As right atrial pressure approaches 15 mm Hg, jugular distension, ascites, pleural effusion, and other signs of right-sided congestive heart failure develop. Syncope and sudden death are uncommon in dogs with PS. The physiologic mechanisms responsible have not been elucidated. Hypotension is presumed to develop as a consequence of reduced cardiac output (secondary to bradycardia or worsening of a dynamic infundibular obstruction) and in combination with peripheral arteriolar vasodilatation (with or in anticipation of exercise). Stimulation of mechanoreceptors in the pressure overloaded right ventricle may trigger the reflex bradycardia and vasodilatation. Reduced right coronary blood flow has been documented in some dogs with pulmonic stenosis and may contribute to the development of syncope, exercise intolerance, and myocardial failure. On rare occasion, severe septal hypertrophy due to PS results in dynamic left ventricular outflow tract (LVOT) obstruction.

Clinical findings Pulmonic stenosis is common in certain breeds, including beagles, Samoyeds, Chihuahuas, English bulldogs, miniature schnauzers, cocker spaniels, Boykin spaniels, Labrador retrievers, mastiffs, chow chows, Newfoundland

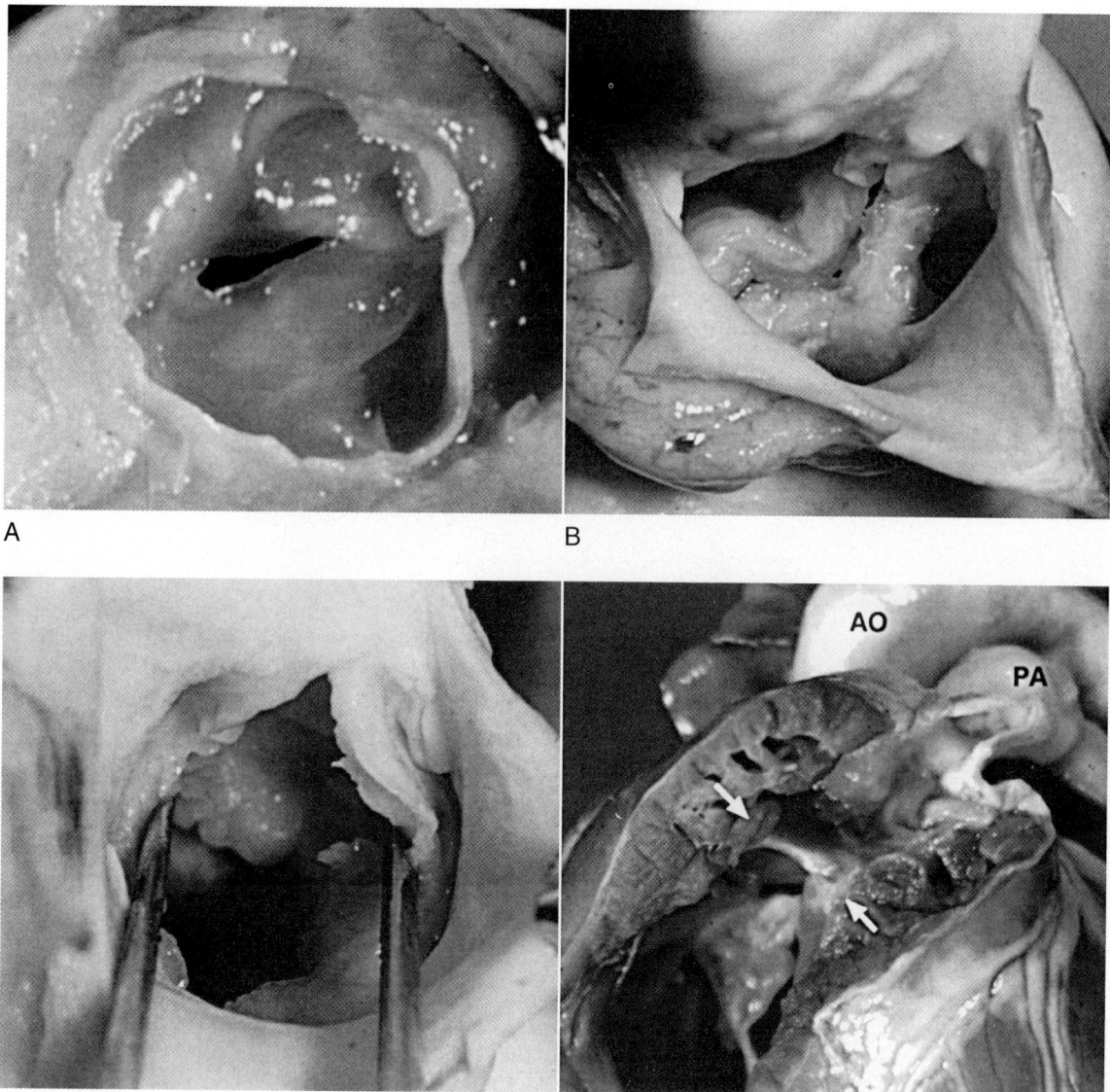

Figure 200-27 Pathology specimens from dogs with pulmonic stenosis (PS). **A,** Pulmonic valve leaflets are thin but fused with a central orifice in this 1-year-old Labrador retriever; they are similar to the domed valves of children with PS. **B,** Very thick (dysplastic) and bicuspid pulmonic valve from a Staffordshire terrier. **C,** Same dog as in **B;** the leaflets have been distracted to show a small subvalvular ridge. **D,** Fibromuscular ring *(arrows)* in the right ventricular infundibulum several centimeters below the pulmonic valve.

retrievers, basset hounds, and other terrier and spaniel breeds.[8a,9a,9b,19b] Miniature Doberman pinschers also seem predisposed. Most dogs with PS are asymptomatic in the first year of life, during which the condition usually is discovered through detection of a heart murmur. Approximately 35% of dogs with severe disease demonstrate clinical signs, which can include exertional fatigue, syncope, or ascites.[34] Signs of congestive right heart failure (e.g., ascites) are most often reported in older dogs.[88a] Cyanosis may be noted when PS is complicated by right-to-left shunting across a patent foramen ovale or coexisting atrial or ventricular septal defect.

The most prominent physical examination finding is a systolic ejection murmur that is best heard over the left heart base and that often radiates dorsally. In some cases the murmur is heard equally well on the right cranial thorax.

In dogs with concurrent severe pulmonic valvular insufficiency, the systolic ejection murmur is accompanied by a soft decrescendo diastolic murmur, which is heard best just ventral to the pulmonic valve region. A holosystolic murmur of tricuspid regurgitation may be noted over the right hemithorax as well. Large-amplitude jugular pulses may result either from a giant *a wave* caused by atrial contraction into the stiff right ventricle or from *cv waves*, which indicate significant tricuspid regurgitation. Jugular venous distension and prominent jugular pulses are evident in most dogs with right heart failure and ascites. Peripheral arterial pulses are usually normal.

Right ventricular enlargement is usually present on the electrocardiogram unless the lesion is very mild.[31a,32a,90a] Right axis deviation and deep S waves in leads I, II, and III and in the left precordial chest leads (V_2 and V_4) are common indicators

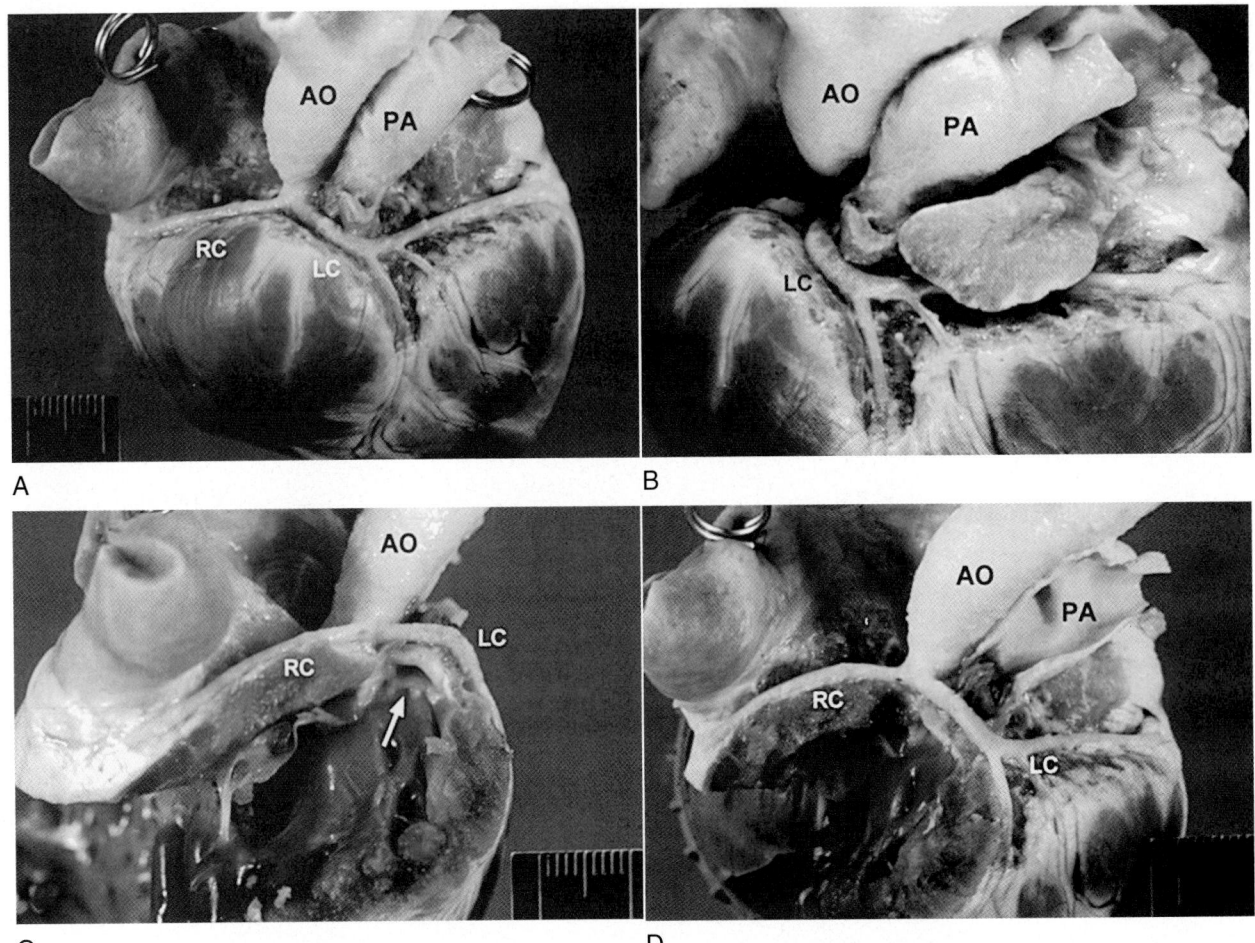

Figure 200-28 Coronary artery anomaly seen in some English bulldogs with pulmonic stenosis. **A,** Left and right coronary arteries are seen to branch from a single large coronary artery that originates from the right aortic sinus of Valsalva. From this location, the left coronary artery encircles the right ventricular outflow tract just below the pulmonary valve **(B),** thereby contributing to the subvalvular component of this complex malformation **(C and D). C,** Left coronary artery courses over the right ventricular outflow tract just below the annulus of the pulmonic valve *(arrow).* **D,** Anterior wall of the pulmonary artery *(PA)* has been removed to show the hypoplastic pulmonic annulus, the diminutive proximal PA, and the crowded and thickened valve leaflets.

of right heart enlargement (Figure 200-29). Thoracic radiographs typically show a prominent right heart and poststenotic dilatation of the main pulmonary artery (Figure 200-30).[8a,22a,24a,88a] These changes are usually most evident on the dorsoventral view. Additional and more variable findings include dilatation of the proximal left pulmonary artery, diminished size of the pulmonary vasculature, and enlargement of the caudal vena cava.

Echocardiography is the technique most commonly used to confirm a diagnosis of PS. M-mode and two-dimensional imaging typically show concentric hypertrophy of the right ventricle, increased prominence of the papillary muscles, deformity in the region of the obstruction or obstructions, narrowing of the RVOT, varying degrees of right atrial enlargement, and poststenotic dilatation of the main pulmonary artery (Figure 200-31).[3,35] Of the four cardiac valves, the pulmonic valve is often the most difficult to visualize clearly by transthoracic echocardiography. Thus it is impossible to visualize the exact location and nature of the obstruction in some dogs. It is often particularly difficult to identify a discrete subvalvular obstruction close to the pulmonary valve. The pulmonic valve leaflets are typically thickened and often fused, and they

appear to dome upwards into the pulmonary artery during systole (see Figure 200-31). Hypoplasia of the pulmonic valve annulus further obscures the valve anatomy and confounds consideration of treatment. Color flow Doppler echocardiography is useful for establishing the anatomic location of the obstruction, because the turbulent, high-velocity jet can usually be seen emerging just distal to the obstructive orifice (see Figure 200-31). Mild to moderate pulmonic valve insufficiency is also apparent in many dogs with valvular PS.

For accurate quantification of the severity of the obstruction, the peak velocity of the blood flow jet must be recorded on a spectral Doppler tracing acquired with the continuous wave Doppler beam in parallel alignment with the direction of flow (see Figure 200-31). This usually is accomplished from either the right or left cranial parasternal windows. The modified Bernoulli equation ($\Delta P = 4V^2$) is applied to relate the instantaneous pressure gradient across an obstruction (ΔP, in mm Hg) to the peak velocity of the jet distal to the obstruction (V, in m/s). As a general rule, Doppler-derived gradients are 40% to 50% higher than the gradient measured during cardiac catheterization in an individual dog.[20b] Such discrepancies are attributed in part to the fact that Doppler studies

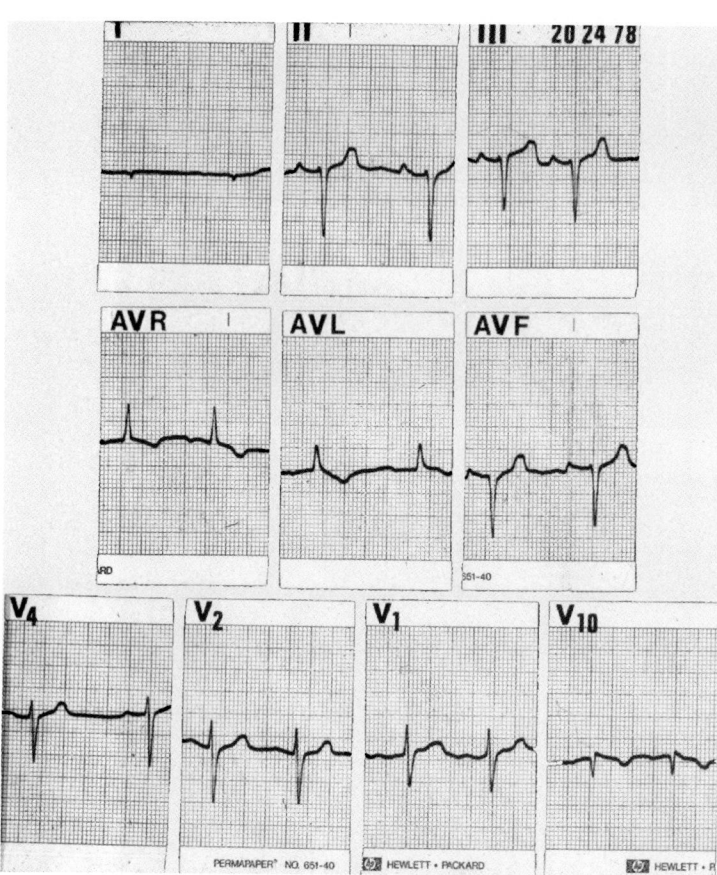

Figure 200-29 Electrocardiogram from a dog with pulmonic stenosis, showing a typical right ventricular enlargement pattern. The mean electrical axis is shifted to the right (–100 degrees), and prominent S waves are seen in leads II, III, aVF, V_2, and V_4.

are performed in awake animals, and transvalvular flow is considerably higher under these circumstances than in dogs that have been anesthetized for cardiac catheterization. In addition, hemodynamic studies typically indicate the severity of obstruction as a peak-to-peak pressure gradient, and such measures are almost always lower than the instantaneous peak pressure gradient calculated from Doppler measures of peak flow velocity.[36] Doppler interrogation of the right heart is also particularly helpful for identifying and assessing the severity of coexisting tricuspid valve insufficiency. Measurement of the

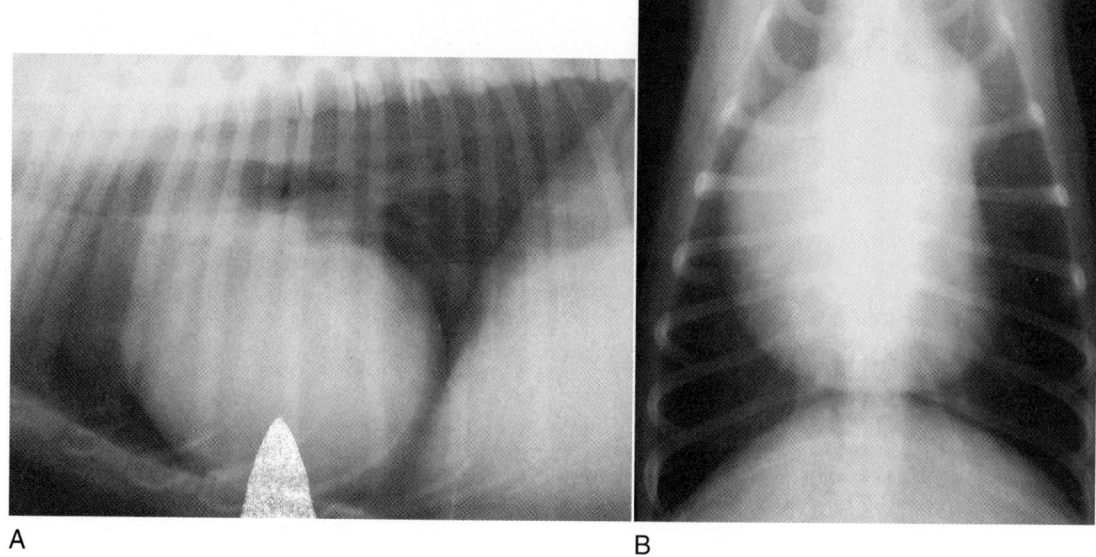

A B

Figure 200-30 Lateral (**A**) and dorsoventral (**B**) thoracic radiographs from a dog with pulmonic stenosis. Rounding of the sternal border and a bulge in the cranial waist of the heart can be seen in the lateral view. Right heart enlargement and a bulge in the main pulmonary artery segment are seen in the dorsoventral view. Pulmonary vessels are diminished even in the absence of a right-to-left shunt.

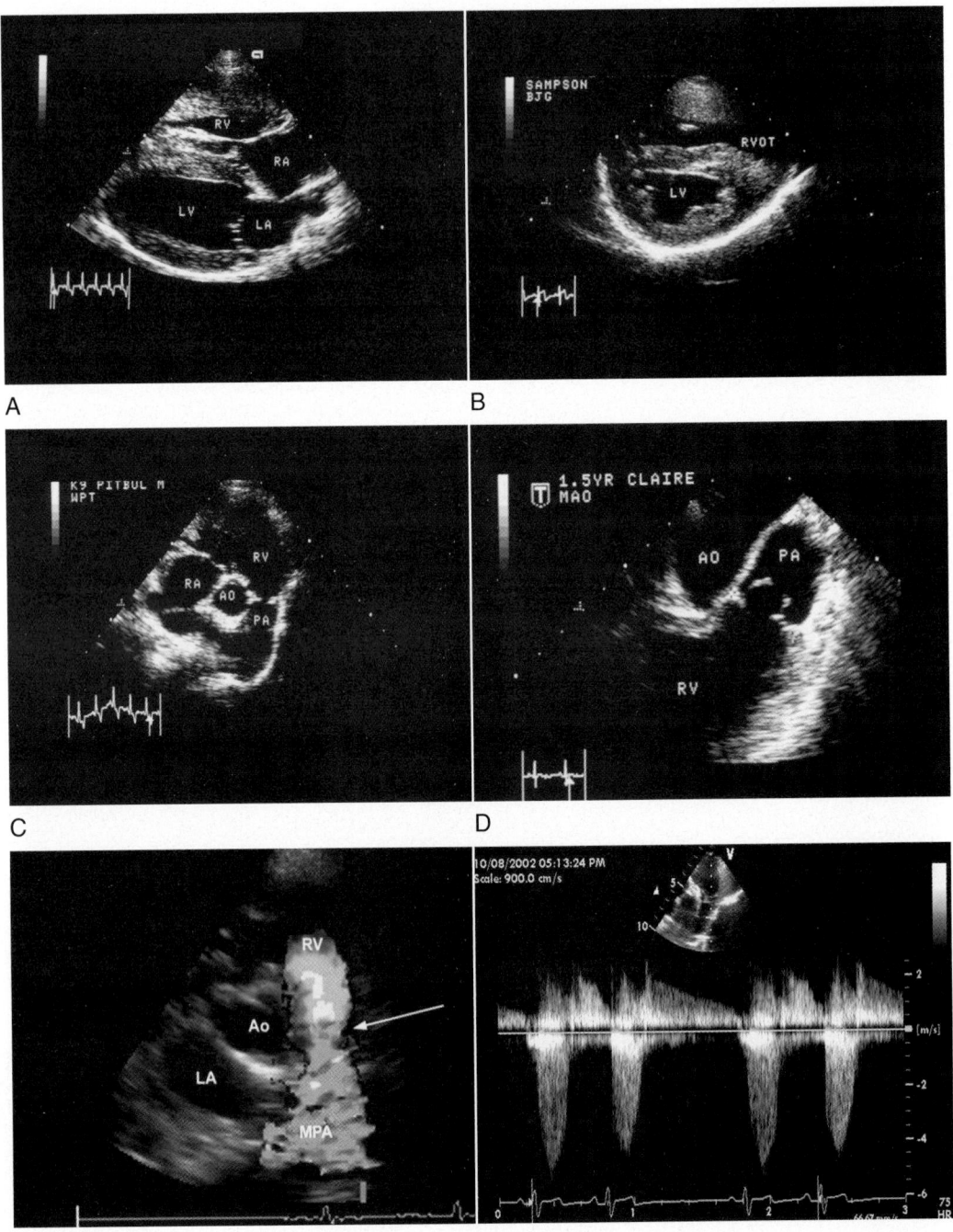

Figure 200-31 Echocardiography of pulmonic stenosis (PS). **A,** Right long axis view from a dog reveals severe concentric hypertrophy of the right ventricle *(RV)*. Right atrium *(RA)* is dilated. **B,** Right short axis view from a dog shows flattening of the interventricular septum and right ventricular concentric hypertrophy caused by pressure overload. **C,** Right short axis view of the heart base from a dog with valvular PS shows thickened pulmonic valves. Poststenotic dilatation of the PA can be seen (PA, pulmonary artery). **D,** Transesophageal ultrasound study of a young rottweiler with valvular PS. The pulmonic valve leaflets can be seen doming into the pulmonary artery *(PA)* during systole. **E,** Color flow Doppler study in a dog shows high velocity and turbulent blood flow moving from the right ventricle *(RV)* through the stenosis *(arrow)* and into the main pulmonary artery *(MPA)*. **F,** Continuous wave Doppler tracing obtained from a view similar to **E** shows high-velocity systolic flow (5 m/s) through the obstruction. Pulmonic insufficiency is also noted during diastole. *LA,* Left atrium; *LV,* left ventricle; *RVOT,* right ventricular outflow tract.

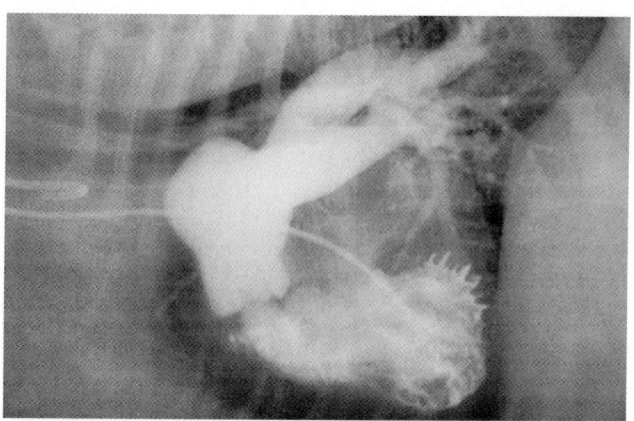

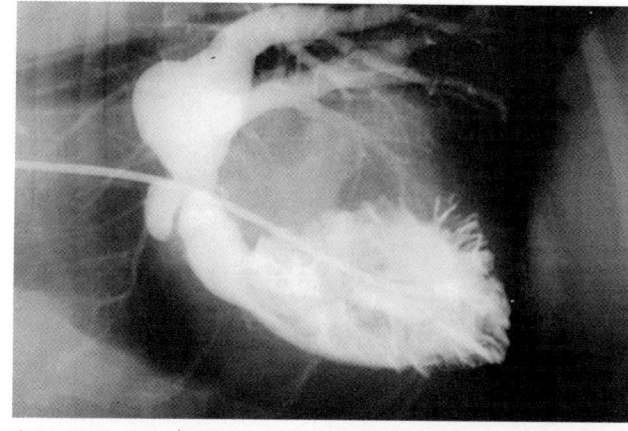

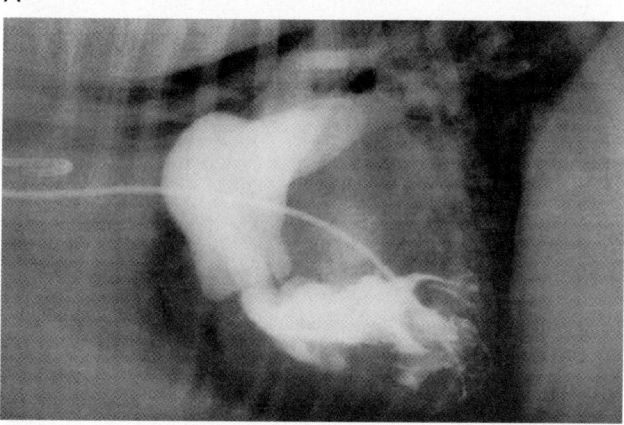

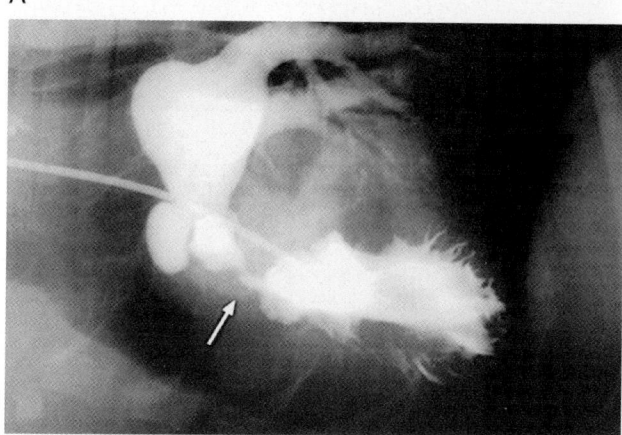

Figure 200-32 Diastolic (**A**) and systolic (**B**) frames of a right ventricular angiogram in a dog with pulmonic stenosis. Note the narrow jet of contrast as it passes through the pulmonic orifice. Poststenotic dilatation of the pulmonary artery is visible in both frames, as is hypertrophy of the RV wall and papillary muscles.

Figure 200-33 Right ventricular angiocardiogram from a dog with severe pulmonic stenosis. Comparison of the diastolic (**A**) and systolic (**B**) frames shows complete obliteration of the outflow tract due to vigorous contraction of the hypertrophied infundibulum. Compare with Figure 200-32. Also note the distortion of the pulmonic valve sinuses *(arrow)*.

velocity of this regurgitant jet is particularly helpful for assessing the severity of the PS obstruction when proper alignment with flow through the outflow tract cannot be obtained. In dogs with both dynamic (infundibular) and fixed (valvular) stenosis, Doppler interrogation of the outflow tract and pulmonary artery can produce a tracing that displays the temporal and velocity relationship between the two components of the stenosis.

Angiocardiography is often performed just prior to balloon valvuloplasty or to clarify right heart anatomy in anticipation of surgery. Such studies clearly demonstrate the anatomic location of the obstruction or obstructions, the degree of right ventricular hypertrophy, whether tricuspid regurgitation is present, and poststenotic dilatation of the pulmonary artery. The angiographic features of valvular stenosis consist of any combination of the following: narrowing at the immediate base of the valve sinuses; asymmetric valve sinuses; hypoplasia of the annulus or of a valve sinus; thickening of individual valve leaflets, producing a lucent filling defect; narrowing of the dye column, with a central or asymmetric jet of contrast medium observed within a narrowed valve orifice; or systolic doming of the valve (indicating fusion of the commissures) (Figure 200-32).[86a,88a] Dynamic muscular obstruction of the right ventricular infundibulum is often visible in dogs with PS (Figure 200-33). The term *double-chambered right ventricle* is used when the right ventricle is divided into a low-pressure region (the infundibulum) and a high-pressure region (the apex and inlet portion of the RV) by a muscular or fibromuscular

ridge deep in the infundibulum (Figure 200-34). Left ventricular angiography or coronary arteriography should be performed when abnormalities of the left heart or coronary circulation are suspected. Such studies must be performed whenever surgery or balloon valvuloplasty is contemplated in an English bulldog or a boxer. Enlargement of the right coronary artery is an expected finding in all dogs with PS, as is well-developed right ventricular hypertrophy.

Hemodynamic confirmation of outflow tract obstruction is accomplished by measurement of a systolic pressure gradient across the lesion (see Figure 200-1). The severity of the obstruction usually is defined as the difference in peak systolic pressures measured above and below the obstruction (peak-to-peak pressure gradient). Inasmuch as the recorded gradient varies with the rate of flow across the obstruction, this measurement is greatly affected by myocardial contractility and the anesthetic regimen selected. Despite these limitations, the systolic pressure gradient has been used to categorize patients with pulmonic stenosis as having mild (less than 50 mm Hg), moderate (50 to 80 mm Hg), or severe (greater than 80 mm Hg) disease.[87a,88a,93a] A more accurate approach requires the measurement of cardiac output and calculation of the functional area of the constricted orifice.

Natural history Precise criteria for establishing an accurate prognosis have not been developed for dogs and cats with PS. Clinical experience indicates that most dogs with mild and even

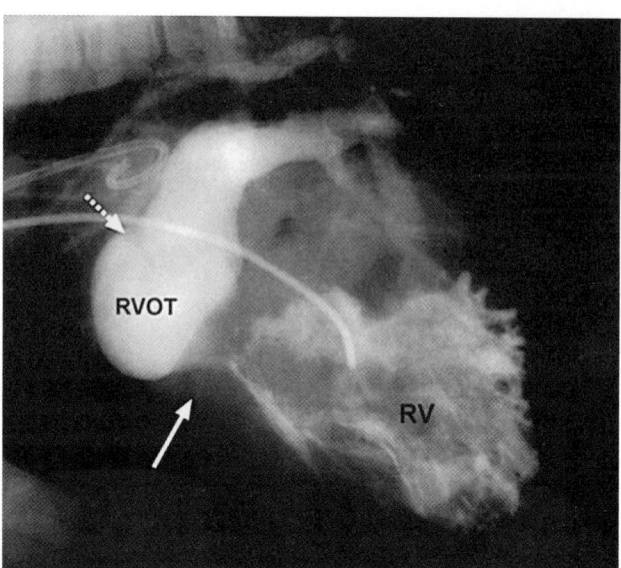

Figure 200-34 Right ventricular angiocardiogram recorded from a rottweiler with an unusual form of subvalvular muscular pulmonic stenosis. Some refer to this lesion as a "double-chambered right ventricle" to distinguish it from dynamic collapse of the hypertrophied infundibulum (see Figure 200-32). Others use the term only when the lesion is deeper within the right ventricle, and some avoid the term altogether. Solid arrow indicates the muscular obstructing lesion in the right ventricular outflow tract. Dashed arrow indicates the location of the pulmonic valve.

moderate PS (Doppler-derived gradient less than 80 mm Hg) usually live normal or nearly normal lives. This generalization does not include dogs with other complicating defects. The problem of concurrent tricuspid valve dysplasia and its relation to developing heart failure has already been discussed. Although systolic pressure gradients are not always predictive of clinical outcome, a general correlation between pressure gradient and survival appears to exist. Dogs with Doppler-derived gradients greater than 125 mm Hg frequently develop secondary tricuspid regurgitation, heart failure, exertional syncope, or a serious cardiac arrhythmia (e.g., atrial fibrillation). When an ASD, patent foramen ovale, or VSD coexists with PS, the potential for right-to-left shunting exists. If the right-to-left shunting is pronounced, the consequences include arterial hypoxemia, polycythemia, and serious debilitation. Sudden death occurs in some dogs with severe PS, but this is uncommon.

Clinical management Patients with uncomplicated PS of mild or moderate severity usually do not require treatment. Serial echocardiographic examinations can be performed to monitor the degree of ventricular hypertrophy and to determine whether secondary infundibular stenosis or tricuspid regurgitation has developed. Exercise restriction is usually unnecessary. Some dogs develop more severe obstruction over time. Dogs with severe or symptomatic disease are candidates for surgery or balloon valvuloplasty. The exact pressure gradient warranting intervention cannot be stated with certainty. Dogs with a Doppler gradient exceeding 100 to 125 mm Hg should be considered candidates for balloon valvuloplasty or surgery. Dogs with lesser gradients are also candidates for these procedures if they are symptomatic or have a large amount of tricuspid regurgitation. Intervention at a young age should be encouraged, because the development of overt congestive heart failure substantially lessens the chance for a successful outcome, regardless of the method of repair. Due to a high likelihood of heritability, even mildly affected dogs should not be bred.

The goals of intervention in dogs with severe PS are to abolish or reduce the systolic pressure gradient to the mild range and to provide symptomatic relief in dogs experiencing clinical signs. The effect of intervention on survival time in dogs or cats is not known. For many years surgery was the only available option for treating PS, and a number of surgical techniques have been advocated, including valve dilatation, patch grafting, or the placement of a conduit from the right ventricle to the pulmonary artery.* The open patch-graft technique is a particularly versatile and cost-effective method of treating dogs with PS, particularly cases involving a substantial subvalvular obstruction.[22b,34c,35c] The technique is well-suited to the treatment of some defects not amenable to balloon valvuloplasty (e.g., muscular RVOT obstruction, double-chambered right ventricle, or severe hypoplasia of the pulmonic annulus). The patch-graft technique should not be performed in dogs with subvalvular PS caused by anomalous coronary artery development, because severing of the artery and death will result.

Catheter-based percutaneous balloon valvuloplasty is a preferred alternative to surgery in many dogs with valvular PS.*,† A dilatation catheter tipped with an inflatable balloon is placed across the obstructing orifice and repeatedly inflated (Figure 200-35). Successful reduction of the obstructive gradient by 50% or more has been reported in 75% to 80% of dogs treated with this technique.[34,38-40] Improvements in the design of the balloon catheter and refinements in the technique have expanded the application of this procedure to dogs weighing as little as 2 kg.[40c] Balloon valvuloplasty is most successful when the pulmonary annulus is normally developed and the valves are relatively thin and fused. More variable results are obtained in dogs with complex lesions and hypoplasia of the pulmonary annulus.[38c,41c] In the authors' experience, balloon dilatation has been of dubious value in dogs with severe muscular RVOT obstruction or double-chamber-type defects. Although balloon valvuloplasty is generally regarded as a safe procedure with a low complication rate, life-threatening problems such as hemorrhage, cardiac puncture, and arrhythmias do occur. Dogs with hypoplasia of the pulmonary annulus or anomalous development of the coronary arteries are at particular risk for serious complications, including avulsion of the coronary artery or rupture of the pulmonary annulus.[36c] Delayed restenosis can occur, but this is not thought to be an important problem.[39] When CHF or atrial fibrillation develops secondary to PS, the prognosis is poor. If medical stabilization can be achieved, balloon valvuloplasty or surgery can be attempted.

Aortic Stenosis
Subvalvular aortic stenosis is the most common congenital cardiac malformation in large-breed dogs.[1c-5c,42c,97a,109a] Most cases of SAS result from a fixed ridge or ring of fibrous tissue located in the left ventricular outflow tract just below the aortic valve. Subvalvular aortic stenosis is a problematic disorder for several reasons. It is very difficult to diagnose in mildly affected dogs, and when the condition is severe, it is difficult to treat. The phenomenon of dynamic SAS is also being recognized with increasing frequency in dogs and cats with a variety of cardiac disorders, including fixed SAS, mitral valve dysplasia, hypertrophic cardiomyopathy, and other conditions that cause hypertrophy of the interventricular septum (i.e., PS, tetralogy of Fallot).[26b] Bull terriers are predisposed to valvular aortic stenosis in which the leaflets are thickened and the aortic valve annulus is mildly hypoplastic. Mild aortic stenosis (AS) caused by

---

*References 21b, 22b, 34c, 35c, 37, 87a, 91a, and 94a.
†References 20b, 23b, 24b, 35c-39c, 38, and 94a.

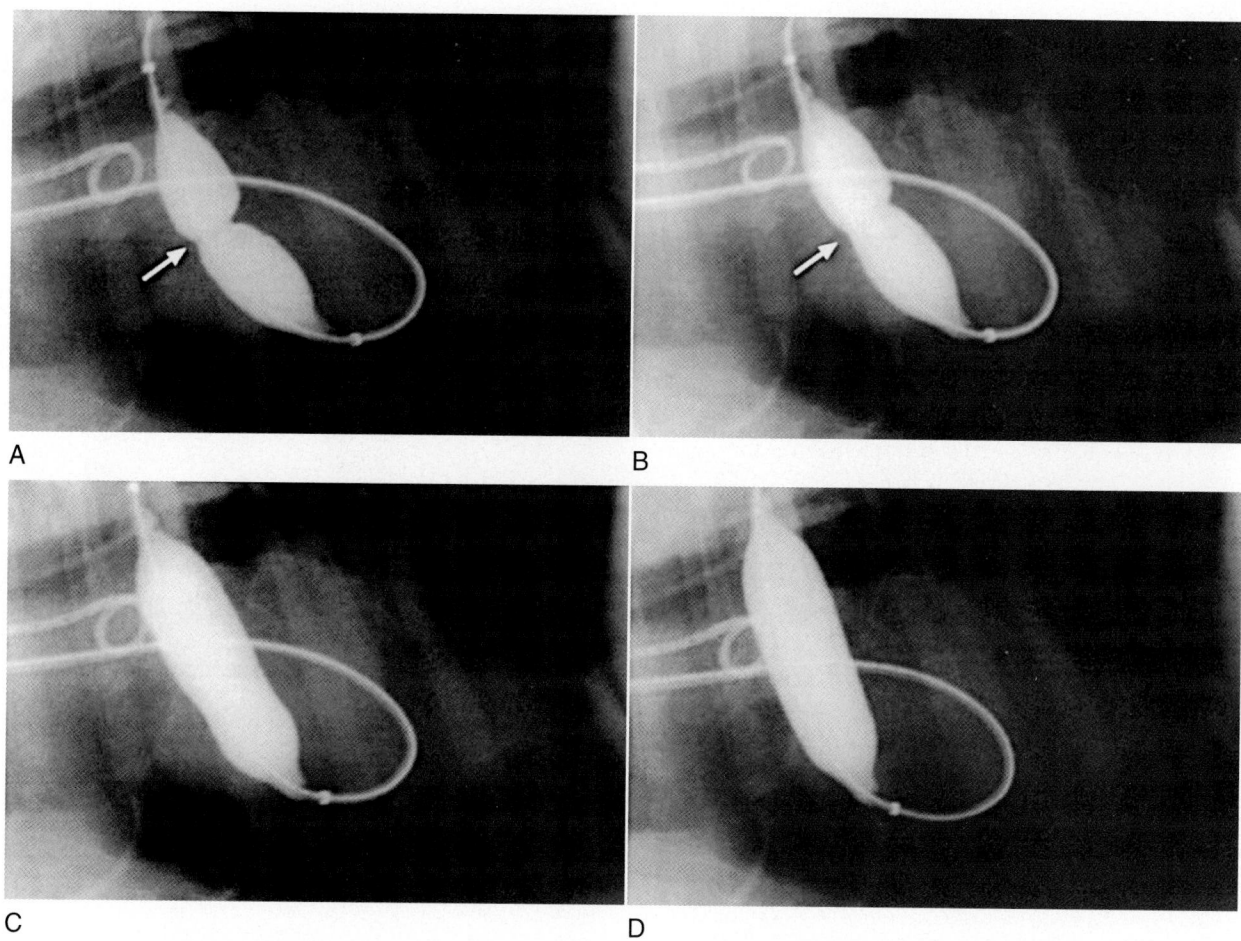

Figure 200-35 Sequence of radiographs taken during balloon dilatation in a dog with valvular pulmonic stenosis. The balloon catheter is seen to traverse the cranial vena cava, right atrium and ventricle, and pulmonary artery. Radiopaque markers on the catheter are used to help position the balloon across the valve. Prominent stenotic lesion (*arrow*) is seen on inflation of the balloon (**A**); it becomes less obvious as the lesion is stretched or torn open (**B**) and (**C**); and it is no longer evident when the balloon is fully inflated (**D**).

a bicuspid valve occurs on rare occasion. Fixed aortic stenosis has been described in a small number of cats,[12a,13a,25b,36a] including one case of supravalvular stenosis.[101a]

Pathology and pathogenesis Subvalvular aortic stenosis has been extensively studied in Newfoundlands, for which breeding studies have established a genetic basis for the perpetuation of SAS.[4a,100a] The pattern of inheritance is most compatible with an autosomal dominant mode of transmission with modifying genes; however, a polygenic mechanism cannot be excluded. The breeding colony studies of Pyle and Patterson further indicate that the obstruction may not be present at birth but rather may develop during the first 4 to 8 weeks of life.[4a,99a,100a,103a,104a] This progression is particularly significant with regard to identification of cardiac murmurs in pups of breeds known to be at risk for SAS.

The lesions of SAS in Newfoundlands have been described in postmortem studies as mild (grade 1), consisting of "small, whitish, slightly raised nodules on the endocardial surface of the ventricular septum immediately below the aortic valve"; moderate (grade 2), consisting of a "narrow ridge of whitish, thickened endocardium" extending partly about the LVOT; and severe (grade 3), consisting of "a fibrous band, ridge, or collar completely encircling the left ventricular outflow tract just below the aortic valve".[4a,100a] This ring is raised above the endocardium, extends

to, and may involve the cranioventral leaflet of the mitral valve and the base of the aortic valves (Figure 200-36). The stenotic ring consists of loosely arranged reticular fibers, mucopolysaccharide ground substance, and elastic fibers. Discrete bundles of collagen and even cartilage are found in advanced lesions.[100a] Cardiac catheterization of dogs with grade 1 lesions failed to reliably detect the postmortem lesion, whereas grade 2 lesions often were associated with soft cardiac murmurs and minimal systolic pressure gradients. As evidenced by these studies, clinical detection of mild SAS can be quite difficult and genetic counseling can be fraught with error. A variety of cardiac abnormalities can accompany SAS, most notably mitral valve dysplasia, PDA, and a host of aortic arch abnormalities. The valvular lesions seen in bull terriers, including myxomatous degeneration and cartilaginous metaplasia of the valve leaflets, resemble those in humans with calcific valvular stenosis.[41]

In some affected dogs, the pathologic findings diverge from the classical description. The anterior mitral valve leaflet is thickened in apposition to a septal plaque of endocardial fibrosis where the mitral leaflets impact the interventricular septum as a consequence of dynamic obstruction. Instead of a fibrous collar, the septum is uniformly hypertrophied, or a broad, fibromuscular ridge that arises from the base of the interventricular septum protrudes into the LVOT. Malformed, malpositioned, or malaligned papillary muscles, thickened

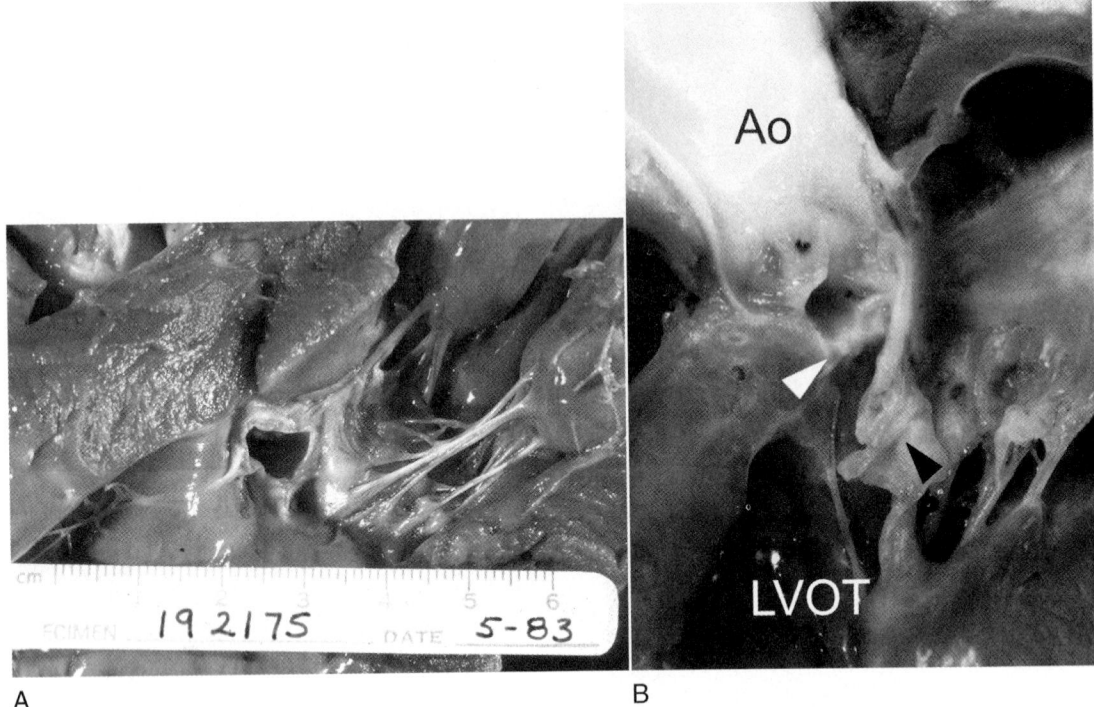

A   **B**

Figure 200-36 Gross pathology of subaortic stenosis (SAS). **A,** Left ventricular outflow tract in a dog, as viewed from the apex of the left ventricle, shows a circumferential ring of fibrous tissue. The anterior mitral valve leaflet and associated chordae tendineae are seen to the right of the lesion. **B,** Cutaway view of the left ventricular outflow tract *(LVOT)* and aorta *(Ao)* in a dog with fixed, dynamic SAS. A ridge of thick, fibrous tissue *(white arrowhead)* is seen just below the aortic valve. The anterior leaflet of the mitral valve *(black arrowhead)* is thickened and elongated.

chordae tendineae, and elongated or distorted mitral leaflets contribute to the development of obstruction.[42,43]

Concentric hypertrophy of the left ventricle develops in dogs with valvular, fixed, or dynamic SAS more or less in proportion to the severity of the outflow obstruction, although the correlation between wall thickness and the magnitude of the measured gradient is often poor.[44] Structural and functional abnormalities of the left ventricle[45] and coronary circulation are well documented in dogs with SAS.[103a,104a] Abnormal coronary flow has also been measured in the larger, extramural arteries, with diminished baseline diastolic flow and reversal of coronary flow during systole.[8a,104a] Focal areas of myocardial infarction and fibrosis are commonly observed in the papillary muscles and subendocardium of dogs with severe SAS, often in association with abnormal intramural coronary arteries. Histologic changes of the intramural coronary arteries in these locations include intimal proliferation of connective tissue and smooth muscle, and medial degeneration. These changes are presumably related to the high wall tension found in this condition, and their genesis may be related to the elaboration of angiotensin II or other biochemical mediators of hypertrophy and remodeling.[46-48] Moreover, these arterial lesions may be important in the genesis of malignant ventricular arrhythmias and sudden death.

Pathophysiology   Obstruction to left ventricular outflow causes an increase in left ventricular systolic pressure and concentric hypertrophy. Consequent to fixed obstruction, left ventricular ejection is delayed, causing a diminished and late rising arterial pulse *(parvus et tardus)*. High-velocity and turbulent flow across the stenotic area produces the systolic ejection murmur and results in poststenotic dilatation of the

ascending aorta, aortic arch, and brachiocephalic trunk. Left atrial hypertrophy develops as a consequence of the reduced compliance of the hypertrophied left ventricle. Mild aortic regurgitation is commonly present, presumably due to thickening of the valve leaflets or dilatation of the ascending aorta. Damage to the aortic valvular endothelium (jet lesions) predisposes dogs with SAS to bacterial endocarditis. Dogs with severe SAS can develop left-sided congestive heart failure from myocardial failure, diastolic pump failure due to increased ventricular stiffness, mitral regurgitation, atrial fibrillation, or a combination of these factors. More often, exertional syncope or sudden death is reported, presumably as a result of myocardial ischemia and the development of malignant ventricular arrhythmias. In some dogs, exertional collapse may be due to hypotension precipitated by exercise-induced increases in left ventricular pressure, activation of ventricular mechanoreceptors, and inappropriate bradycardia or vasodilatation.[49]

Clinical findings   Congenital SAS is most common in Newfoundland retrievers, boxers, rottweilers, golden retrievers, and German shepherds.[30,50] Valvular AS is common only in bull terriers. The clinical findings of SAS vary with the severity of the obstruction and the presence of concurrent cardiac defects. Clinical findings in pups with mild SAS are often subtle and easily overlooked.[5a,9a,98a,100a] Asymptomatic dogs have a soft to moderately intense ejection murmur that can easily be confused with an innocent or functional heart murmur.[51] Insofar as the lesions of SAS can develop during the postnatal period, the murmur may become increasingly prominent during the first 6 months of life. Severely affected dogs may present with exertional fatigue, syncope, or left-sided congestive heart failure, but the vast majority of dogs are asymptomatic. In dogs with severe

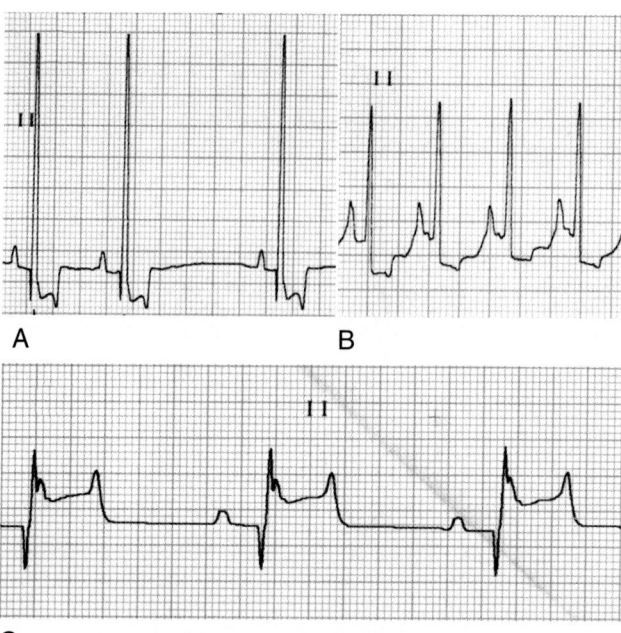

Figure 200-37 Electrocardiograms demonstrating ST segment depression (**A** and **B**) and elevation (**C**) in three dogs with severe SAS. These results are suggestive of myocardial ischemia. (Sensitivity = 10 mm/mV.) **A,** Tracing from a 1-year-old golden retriever (25 mm/s). **B,** Tracing from a 6-month-old Newfoundland retriever that collapsed and died suddenly 1 hour after the ECG was performed (25 mm/s). **C,** Tracing from a 1-year-old golden retriever (50 mm/s).

disease, a common client observation is that the affected dog is smaller than healthy littermates. Sudden death, without premonitory signs, is common in dogs 1 to 3 years of age.[50c]

Recognition of severe SAS is not difficult, because the murmur generally becomes louder and longer when the obstruction

is more severe.[46c] The murmur of severe SAS is usually best heard at the left heart base, recognizing that in some dogs, the systolic murmur is equally loud or louder at the right cardiac base, presumably from radiation into the ascending aorta. The murmur of aortic stenosis often radiates up the carotid arteries and can be ausculted over the ventral cervical region. In some affected dogs, a soft diastolic murmur secondary to aortic valve insufficiency is also detected. A substantial percentage of dogs with SAS have mitral regurgitation, but these murmurs are usually difficult to separate, given their similar timing and overlapping areas of maximal intensity. Other physical abnormalities detected in moderate to severely affected dogs include a diminished and late-rising arterial pulse and a prominent left ventricular heave arising from the hypertrophied left ventricle.

The electrocardiogram is often normal but in severe cases may indicate left ventricular hypertrophy (increased R wave amplitude in leads II, III, aVF, V_2, and V_4). Depression of the ST segment and T-wave changes suggest myocardial ischemia, particularly when these alterations are precipitated by exercise or occur in the company of ventricular ectopia (Figure 200-37). Compared with the resting electrocardiogram, 24-hour ambulatory (Holter) ECG recordings offer a more sensitive method of detecting ventricular arrhythmia and ST-segment changes, particularly when such changes are precipitated only by exercise. The severity of arrhythmias detected in this fashion often corresponds to the severity of disease.[52]

Thoracic radiographs may be normal or may indicate left ventricular hypertrophy.[8a,22a-24a] Poststenotic dilatation of the horizontally inclined ascending aorta causes loss of the cranial waist on the lateral radiograph and widening of the mediastinum on the dorsoventral radiograph (Figure 200-38). Mild left atrial enlargement is common in dogs with moderate or severe SAS, but marked left atrial enlargement suggests concurrent mitral regurgitation. Angiocardiography is useful for delineating the site and geometry of obstruction, which is usually most evident in the ventral aspect of the outflow tract when viewed on the lateral projection (Figure 200-39). Other angiographic findings include poststenotic dilatation of the ascending aorta, enlargement of the left coronary artery and its extramural branches, a small left ventricular cavity, and hypertrophy of the papillary muscles and left

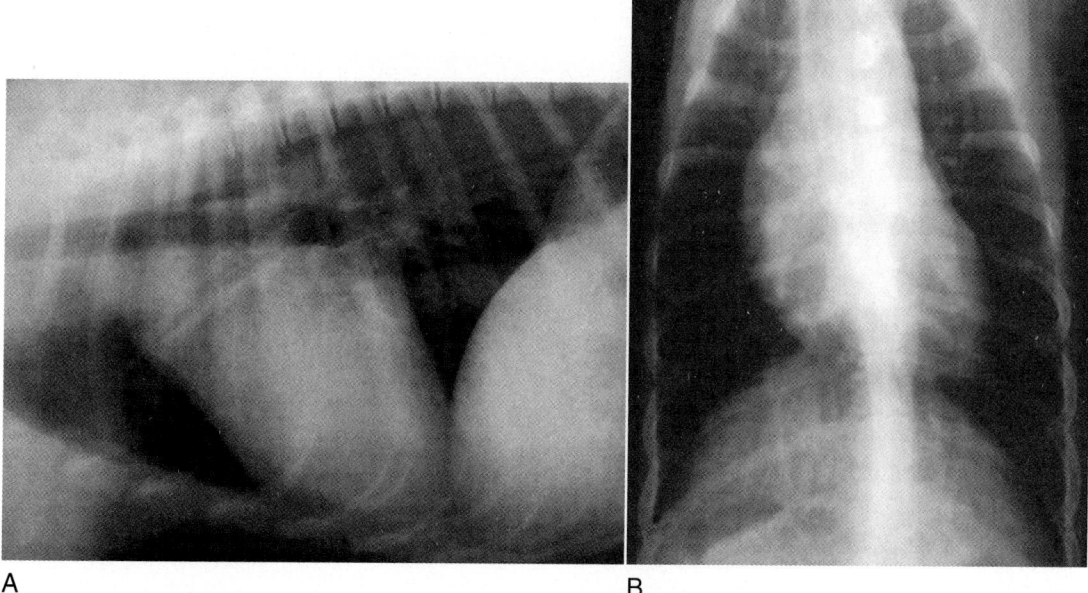

Figure 200-38 Lateral (**A**) and dorsoventral (**B**) radiographs from a young dog with subaortic stenosis. Prominent bulge in the cranial waist on the lateral view and widening of the cranial mediastinum on the dorsoventral view are consistent with poststenotic dilatation of the ascending aorta.

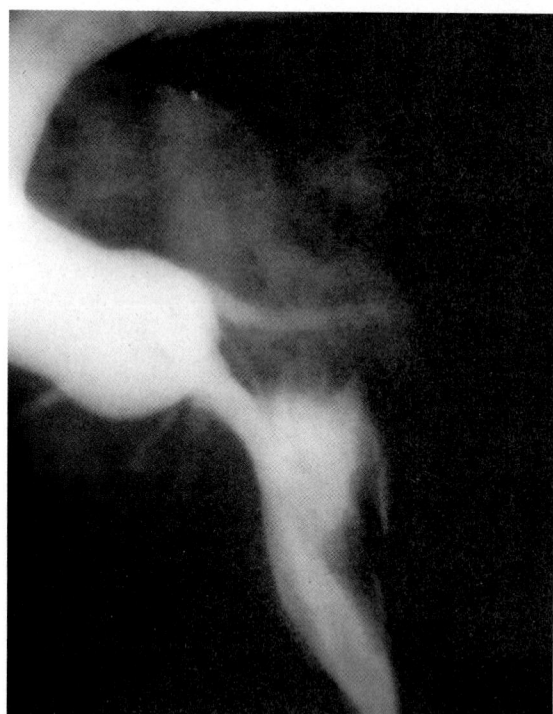

Figure 200-39 Angiogram from a dog with subaortic stenosis. Left ventricular injection opacifies the left ventricle and aorta. Tunnel-like narrowing of the contrast column is seen in the left ventricular outflow tract; a prominent left circumflex coronary artery is also seen.

ventricular wall. Supravalvular aortic injections can be performed to identify insufficiency of the aortic valve, but Doppler echocardiography is a more sensitive technique. Hemodynamic recordings are made to document the presence and severity of a systolic pressure gradient across the obstruction (Figure 200-40). Such recordings are also useful for detecting elevated left ventricular end-diastolic pressure and impending congestive heart failure.[8a,105a] As a result of diminished flow (cardiac output), pressure gradients recorded from dogs with SAS are depressed

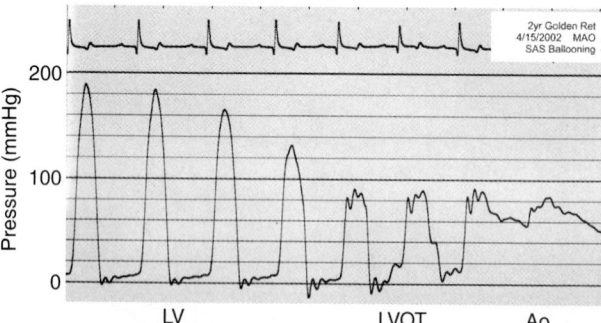

Figure 200-40 Intracardiac and aortic pressures from a 2-year-old golden retriever with subaortic stenosis obtained through cardiac catheterization. The catheter is withdrawn from the left ventricle (LV) into the left ventricular outflow tract (LVOT) and the ascending aorta (Ao). A 100 mm Hg systolic pressure gradient is demonstrated between the LV and LVOT, indicating the subvalvular location of the obstruction.

by general anesthesia to approximately 40% to 50% of those measured in the unanesthetized state.[47c]

Moderate to severe SAS is easily confirmed by two-dimensional and Doppler echocardiography. Typical findings include concentric left ventricular hypertrophy, a subvalvular obstructing lesion, and poststenotic dilatation of the aorta (Figure 200-41).[3,27a,35,106a] The papillary muscles and endocardial surface of the ventricular myocardium often appear hyperechoic, presumably as a result of myocardial ischemia and replacement fibrosis or calcification. Structural changes in the mitral valve can often be appreciated and abnormal motion of the mitral valve (systolic anterior motion) can be detected in dogs with coexisting mitral valve dysplasia and dynamic obstruction.[43] Spectral Doppler interrogation of the left ventricular outflow tract is used to assess the severity of disease through measurement of the peak velocity of flow in the LVOT.[48c] Such measurements show excellent correlation with invasive measurements (see Figure 200-41).[49c] Doppler measurements can be made from a variety of parasternal or subcostal imaging windows, although velocities obtained from the subcostal position generally display the highest values.[27b] Doppler-estimated pressure gradients between 80 and 100 mm Hg (peak flow velocities ranging from 4.5 to 5 m/s) are used to indicate moderate LVOT obstruction, and higher velocities are used to indicate severe obstruction, but these designations are somewhat arbitrary. Doppler-derived pressure gradients are affected by the amount of flow (cardiac output) through the obstructive orifice and may either overestimate the severity of obstruction if cardiac output is high (e.g., in dogs that are stressed or excited) or underestimate severity if flow is subnormal (e.g., in dogs with concurrent myocardial failure). In these cases, indexing the gradient to stroke volume or some related measure or simple estimation of the two-dimensional orifice area may provide a better estimate of disease severity.[44,53] Color flow Doppler recordings are valuable for detecting and estimating the severity of coexisting aortic or mitral valve insufficiency.

Antemortem detection of the mildest forms of SAS by echocardiography is often not possible. Dogs with subtle abnormalities (i.e., grade 1 lesions as described previously) escape detection by even the most accomplished examiners. Even with dogs that have grade 2 lesions, segregation from normal dogs on the basis of left ventricular velocities is problematic. An upper limit for aortic velocity in normal dogs has been reported but is not well established for differing breeds and examination conditions.[54] The maximum normal aortic velocity in the authors' laboratory is 1.7 m/s (upper limit of the 95% confidence interval); however, velocities in excess of this value are sometimes recorded in completely normal dogs or in dogs with no evidence of a discrete outflow obstruction but that have slightly diminished outflow tract dimensions (boxers, bull terriers, golden retrievers). A diagnosis of mild SAS is more secure when mildly elevated velocity measurements are accompanied by disturbed flow, when an anatomic lesion is visible, and when velocity flow suddenly accelerates over a discrete region in the LVOT. Inability to reliably detect mild SAS is a great source of frustration with regard to efforts to provide genetic counseling to breeders, who are interested in reducing the incidence of disease.

Natural history Severe SAS is a discouraging condition, because many affected dogs die prematurely. In a retrospective survey of 96 dogs with SAS, 21 died suddenly, most often during the first 3 years of life.[50c] Eleven dogs developed endocarditis or left heart failure and 32 dogs showed evidence of exercise intolerance or syncope. Dogs with minimal ventricular hypertrophy, mild ventricular outflow obstruction, and a maximal Doppler pressure gradient of less than 50 mm Hg

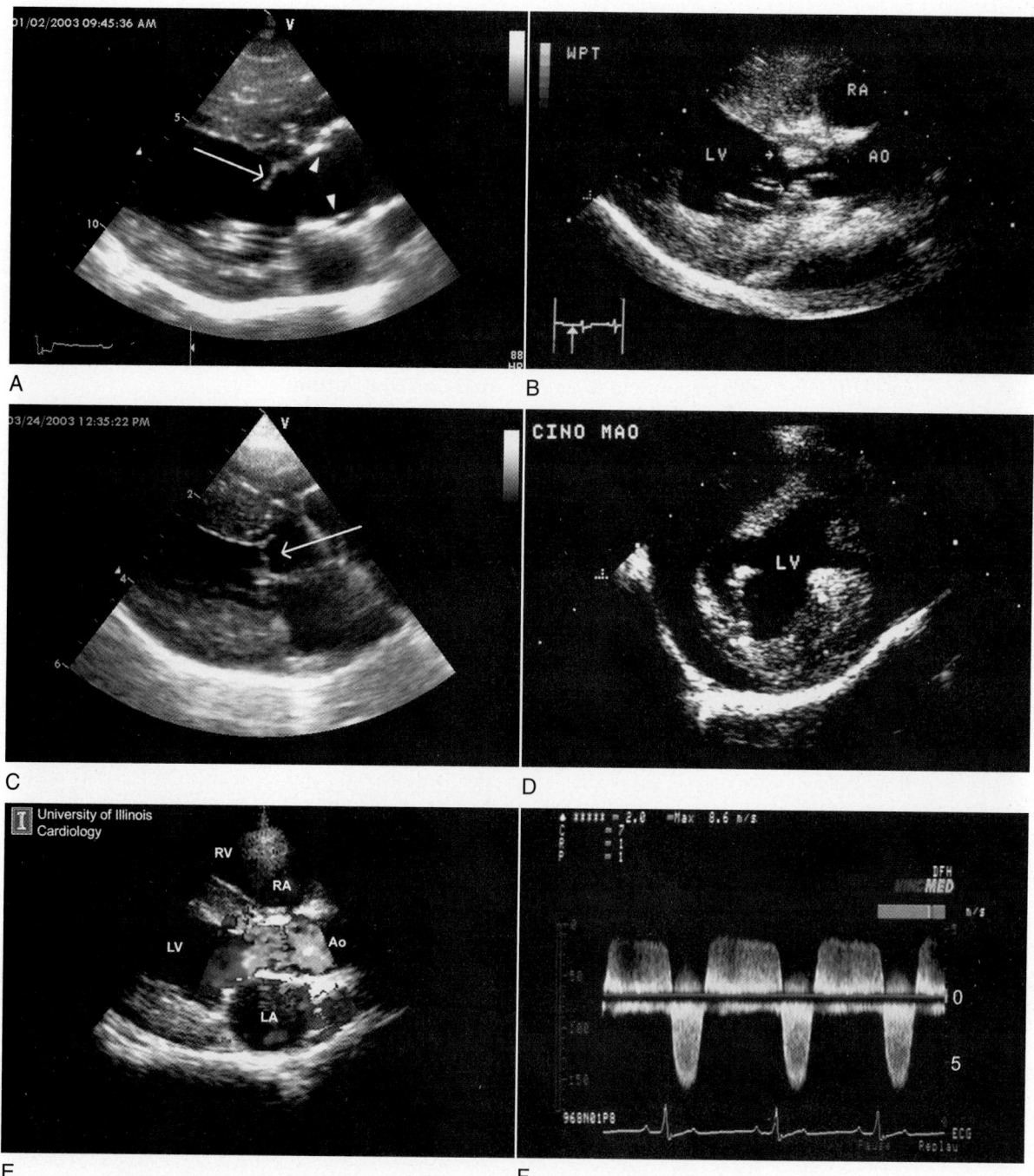

Figure 200-41 Echocardiography of subaortic stenosis (SAS). **A, B,** and **C** are right long axis views showing the various morphologic forms of obstruction in the left ventricular outflow tract in dogs with SAS. **A,** Mild membranous SAS in a 5-year-old rottweiler. A thin, membranous flap of tissue extends from the interventricular septum. No appreciable left ventricular concentric hypertrophy is noted. The open aortic valve leaflets are indicated by the arrowheads. **B,** Severe, tunnel-like SAS in a 4-year-old golden retriever. Two ridges of hyperechoic tissue are present at the base of the aortic valve *(arrows)*. The left ventricle is hypertrophied and has a hyperechoic endocardial surface. **C,** Dynamic SAS in a poodle. Systolic anterior motion of the mitral valve is seen projecting into the left ventricular outflow tract *(arrow)*. The left ventricle shows concentric hypertrophy. The blood flow velocity across the obstruction exceeded 5.5 m/s, indicating a severe degree of pressure overload to the left ventricle. **D,** Right short axis view from a 3-month-old mixed breed dog shows left ventricular concentric hypertrophy and marked hyperechogenicity of the subendocardial tissue and papillary muscles. This finding is thought to represent areas of myocardial ischemia and replacement fibrosis. **E,** Right long axis color flow Doppler study from a dog with SAS shows high-velocity, turbulent blood flow in the left ventricular outflow tract and aorta. **F,** Continuous wave Doppler tracing from the left apical view in a dog with severe SAS shows a peak systolic velocity of 6.5 m/s, indicating a pressure gradient of 169 mm Hg across the obstruction. Aortic insufficiency is also detected.

are more likely to live normal lives, whereas dogs with pressure gradients in excess of 125 mm Hg are very likely to develop serious complications or to experience sudden death. Complicating factors that contribute to an adverse outcome include: mitral regurgitation, aortic regurgitation, aortic valve endocarditis, and atrial fibrillation.[51c-53c] Sudden death is most likely to occur during or shortly after vigorous activity.

Clinical management Dogs with mild SAS are not treated other than with administration of prophylactic antibiotics during periods of anticipated bacteremia, such as during dental procedures, surgery, or whenever a concurrent infectious disease is suspected. This practice remains common despite the fact that the efficacy of prophylactic antibiotics for reducing the risk of bacterial endocarditis in dogs with SAS has not been definitively established.[53c] A number of treatment options can be considered for dogs with moderate to severe SAS, but most are of uncertain value. Open resection of the obstructing lesion during cardiopulmonary bypass clearly offers the best opportunity to reduce the systolic pressure gradient substantially and permanently[54c,55c]; however, an otherwise successful procedure does appear to alter the prevalence of sudden death significantly.[55c] Other surgical procedures for dilating or bypassing the obstruction have either failed to achieve sustained reduction of the systolic pressure gradient or have entailed an unacceptable risk of complications.[56c,57c] Moreover, these remedies are usually limited in their availability and are prohibitively expensive.

Balloon dilatation of SAS has been attempted in dogs as an alternative to surgery. On average, catheter-based balloon dilatation can reduce the severity of SAS obstruction in dogs by 50%.[29b] This benefit is attenuated in some (and perhaps a majority) of dogs over time.[48c] Balloon dilatation of SAS is more challenging than balloon valvuloplasty of pulmonic stenosis. Life-threatening complications of SAS include fatal arrhythmia, the development of aortic valve endocarditis, rupture of the aortic annulus, and avulsion of the brachiocephalic artery during balloon withdrawal. Moreover, the inability of surgical resection to prevent sudden death suggests that effective treatment requires more than reduction of the pressure gradient.

The authors typically recommend avoidance of prolonged, vigorous exercise, recognizing that in young and otherwise healthy dogs, even this conservative recommendation is not always practical. Based on clinical and pathologic evidence of myocardial ischemia, the authors also advise administration of beta-adrenergic receptor blockers to dogs with high gradients or a history of syncope. Beta blockers (e.g., atenolol) reduce the maximal heart rate, decrease myocardial oxygen consumption, and improve diastolic coronary artery flow, thereby exerting a protective effect on the myocardium against ischemia and the development of arrhythmias. Moreover, dogs on high doses of beta blockers seem less willing (or are less able) to indulge in prolonged, vigorous exercise. In theory, treatment with calcium channel blockers or ACE inhibitors may also be of value in dogs with SAS; however, none of the medical strategies have been evaluated in placebo-controlled clinical trials.

Anomalous Development of the Atria and Cor Triatriatum

Cor triatriatum (sinister and/or dexter) has been reported in both cats and dogs.[33b,69c-72c,156a,158a] With these defects, the atrium is partitioned into an accessory atrial chamber, which receives venous return, and is separated from the true atrium by a perforate membrane. The suffix, *sinister* or *dexter*, is used to indicate whether the left or right atrium is abnormally partitioned; the term *cor triatriatum* alone usually refers to a left-sided lesion. If the partitioning membrane causes obstruction, dilatation of the venous chamber and the entering veins is evident and congestion develops. In contrast to mitral or tricuspid valve stenosis, blood flows through the stenotic orifice during both systole and diastole; however, the functional consequences of these defects are very similar. From a clinical perspective, supravalvular mitral stenosis (SMS) often closely resembles cor triatriatum (sinister); however, SMS is frequently accompanied by additional mitral valve abnormalities. The primary distinction between SMS and cor triatriatum (sinister) relates to the location of the obstructing membrane. In animals with SMS, the obstructing membrane is located ventral (distal) to the foramen ovale, and the left auricle is functionally part of the proximal chamber and dilates as pressure in this chamber rises (Figure 200-42).[55] In animals with true cor triatriatum (sinister), the obstructing membrane is located dorsal (proximal) to the foramen ovale; the left auricle lies downstream from the obstruction and is not enlarged. If the foramen ovale is closed,

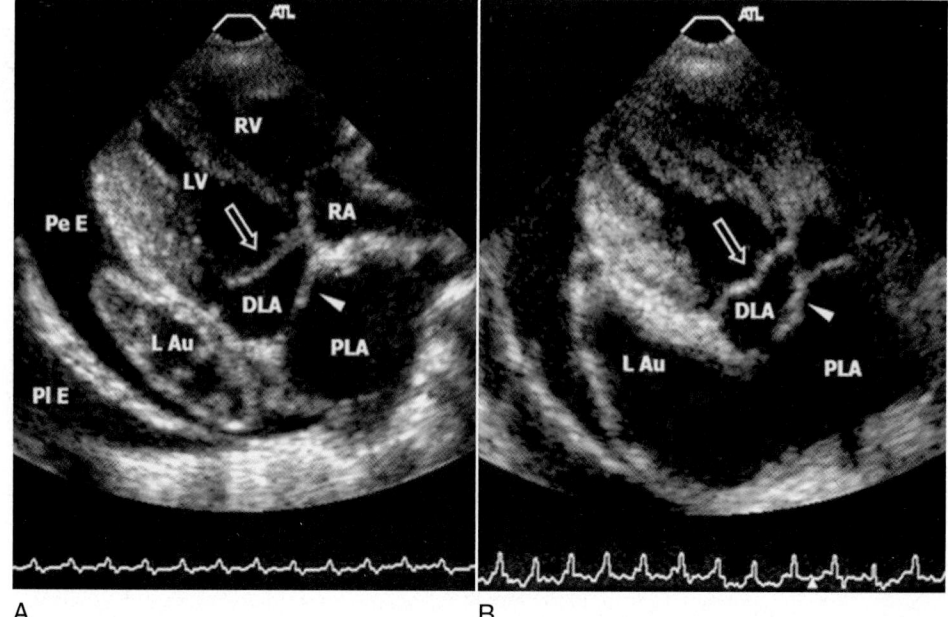

Figure 200-42 Long-axis, four-chamber, two-dimensional echocardiograms of a cat with supravalvular mitral stenosis. **A,** Clearly visible membrane *(solid arrow)* is located above the mitral valve *(open arrow)* that partitions the left atrium into proximal (PLA) and distal (DLA) compartments. **B,** Left auricle (LAu) communicates with the proximal left atrial compartment, and the membrane is located distally. This feature distinguishes supraventricular mitral stenosis from cor triatriatum (sinister), in which the partitioning membrane is proximal to the auricle. *RV,* Right ventricle; *RA,* right atrium; *Pe E,* pericardial effusion; *Pl E,* pleural effusion. (Fine DM, Tobias AH, Jacob KA: Supravalvular mitral stenosis in a cat. *J Am Anim Hosp Assoc* 38:403-406, 2002.)

A

B

there is little difference between these defects. Affected cats typically present with signs of pulmonary congestion, but pulmonary hypertension and right heart failure are also seen.

Cor triatriatum dexter results from persistence of the embryologic right sinus venosus valve.[71c] In dogs with this malformation, the right atrium is partitioned by a diaphragm located caudal to the tricuspid valve and foramen ovale. Affected dogs usually evidence congestion in the caudal half of the body (ascites) but fail to demonstrate jugular distension or an audible murmur. Other clinical findings include prominence of the cutaneous abdominal veins, hepatomegaly, and diarrhea from malabsorption. Dogs with congenital or acquired obstruction of the caudal vena cava (Budd-Chiari syndrome) present with similar clinical findings. In most affected dogs, the electrocardiogram and thoracic radiographs, with the notable exception of caudal vena cava enlargement, are unremarkable. Diagnosis can be accomplished by echocardiography or angiography.[56] Treatment for cor triatriatum generally requires surgical resection or bypass of the obstruction,[57,73c,74c] Balloon dilatation of the obstructing membrane can also be attempted.[58,59]

LESIONS THAT CAUSE RIGHT-TO-LEFT SHUNTING: CYANOTIC HEART DISEASE

The term *cyanotic congenital heart disease* is used to categorize congenital defects that cause admixture of venous and arterial blood, such as tetralogy of Fallot. Because the pathophysiology and clinical signs of these conditions are similar, they are considered as a group. Only the most important defects are discussed to illustrate the clinical syndrome common to these conditions. The reader is also directed to the previous sections on PDA and VSD, which comment on the complicating conditions promoting right-to-left shunting.

Pathophysiology
Mechanisms of Right-to-Left Shunting
For desaturated blood to shunt into the systemic arteries, a defect must exist that allows admixture of unsaturated and saturated blood, as occurs with transposition of the great vessels, or a communicating defect that connects the two sides of the circulation and some mechanism elevating pressures on the right. Reversed shunting has been observed with PDA, aorticopulmonary window, ventricular septal defect, and atrial septal defect. The term *Eisenmenger's syndrome* is invoked to describe circumstances in which increased pulmonary vascular resistance causes reversal of a left-to-right shunt and cyanotic heart disease.[148a-150a] The factors underlying the development Eisenmenger's syndrome are incompletely understood but are most likely related to shear stresses caused by the high flow rates in the pulmonary vasculature and proliferative changes in the vessel wall.[15a,49a,60a,148a,150a] Eisenmenger's syndrome usually develops rapidly in small animals and almost always before 6 months of age.

Intimal thickening, medial hypertrophy, and plexiform lesions of dogs and cats with Eisenmenger's physiology are similar to those of humans as described by Edwards and Heath and amended by Roberts.[15] These plexiform lesions are considered irreversible; consequently, neither medical therapy nor closure of the shunt effectively improves the condition once these changes have developed. In fact, surgical closure of the shunt pathway forces the right ventricle to work solely against a tremendous resistance, resulting in right ventricular failure, circulatory collapse, and death.

Effects of Hypoxemia
Systemic response to arterial hypoxemia includes an increase in red blood cell mass in an attempt to improve systemic oxygen transport. Hypoxia of the renal tissue incites erythropoietin release and induces secondary polycythemia. When the PCV exceeds 65% to 68%, the high viscosity of the blood predisposes the patient to thrombosis and microvascular complications.[15a,148a] This hyperviscosity syndrome is the primary cause of morbidity and mortality in affected animals. Clinical manifestations include weakness, hemostatic deficiencies, renal dysfunction, metabolic acidosis, iron deficiency, cerebrovascular events, syncope, and seizures.[59a,60,137a,139a]

Ratio of Systemic to Pulmonary Resistance
The magnitude of right-to-left shunting fluctuates with the relative resistances of the systemic and pulmonary circulations. Exercise promotes systemic arteriolar vasodilatation and decreases systemic resistance, thereby increasing the magnitude of right-to-left shunting. In cases of right ventricular hypertrophy and VSD, tachycardia or elevated sympathetic tone can increase the magnitude of right-to-left shunting by exacerbating dynamic infundibular obstruction and increasing resistance to right ventricular ejection.[60] Beta-adrenergic blocking drugs are sometimes used to blunt or prevent this phenomenon, particularly in patients with tetralogy of Fallot.[139a,140a] Beta blockers also tend to limit exercise, offering another explanation for their efficacy in some patients. Anemia, absolute or relative, reduces the ratio of systemic to pulmonary resistance when pulmonary resistance is fixed.[138a] By this mechanism, overzealous phlebotomy can increase the severity of arterial hypoxemia as it decreases the oxygen-carrying capacity of blood.

Additional Circulatory Factors
Right-to-left shunting leads to compensatory increases in nutritive blood flow to the lung via the bronchial arteries. These systemic collateral vessels are easily recognized at angiography. Although the phenomenon is uncommon, these vessels can rupture, leading to hemoptysis. Paradoxical embolization is another potential complication of right-to-left shunting defects. Normally, the pulmonary vasculature filters systemic venous emboli before they can reach the left side of the circulation. With reversed shunting, the possibility of a venous embolus reaching the coronary, cerebral, or other systemic arteries must be considered, particularly when intravenous catheters are used. By this mechanism, a thrombus, infectious agents, or air may gain access to vital systemic organs. Animals with cyanotic heart disease sometimes experience adverse reactions (particularly bradycardia) to sedatives and tranquilizers.

Clinical Evaluation of the Patient with Cyanotic Heart Disease
Common causes of cyanotic heart disease in companion animals include septal defects in association with tricuspid valve disease (ASD + TVD) or pulmonic stenosis (ASD or VSD + PS); and patent ductus arteriosus or septal defects complicated by pulmonary hypertension (PHT + ASD or VSD or PDA). Presenting signs include failure to grow, shortness of breath, exertional fatigue, weakness, syncope, and seizures. Affected animals evidence dyspnea when stressed. Systemic hypoxemia is best confirmed by measurement of the oxygen content of an arterial blood sample obtained while the animal breathes room air. It is important to realize that providing 100% oxygen does not significantly improve the hypoxemia caused by right-to-left shunting.[61] Administration of 100% oxygen raises the concentration of dissolved oxygen but does not substantially raise the amount of oxygen bound to hemoglobin, which represents the primary reservoir of oxygen in the blood. Animals with cyanotic heart disease are usually polycythemic. This phenomenon is most obvious when the hemoglobin concentration of young animals with cyanotic heart disease is compared to age-matched normal animals.[128a]

Clinically detectable peripheral cyanosis of the mucous membranes or skin occurs when the amount of reduced (unoxygenated) hemoglobin is greater than 3 g/dL. If this condition is suspected, the mucous membranes of both the cranial and caudal portions of the patient should be examined and compared, preferably both before and after exercise. A finding of cyanosis limited to the caudal tissues is known as *differential cyanosis* and suggests the presence of a right-to-left shunting PDA.

Cardiac auscultation of cyanotic patients varies in accordance with the underlying defects. Dogs and cats with tetralogy of Fallot usually evidence the typical systolic murmur of pulmonic stenosis. In contrast, most animals with Eisenmenger's physiology lack a prominent murmur but often display a loud or split second heart sound due to pulmonary hypertension and asynchronous semilunar valve closure.[8a,9a,128a] On occasion, an ejection sound with a soft, short, systolic murmur may be evident at the left heart base.

Cyanotic heart disease, with rare exceptions (i.e., tricuspid atresia and anomalous systemic venous return), is characterized by right ventricular hypertrophy, which is usually evident on ECG recordings, thoracic radiographs, and echocardiograms. As a general rule, the pulmonary arteries and veins are diminished in size and the lungs appear underperfused (hyperlucent) on survey chest films.[24a] The main pulmonary artery and proximal lobar arteries are usually visibly dilated when Eisenmenger's syndrome is the basis for reversed shunting, but these structures are not enlarged with pulmonary or tricuspid atresia. In dogs with classic tetralogy of Fallot with a muscular infundibular obstruction, the pulmonary artery is hypoplastic, and poststenotic dilatation of the main pulmonary artery is not prominent on the dorsoventral radiograph. Dogs and cats with valvular pulmonic stenosis and a restrictive VSD demonstrate more prominent enlargement of the pulmonary artery segment and proximal lobar arteries. These seemingly trivial distinctions often become important when surgical repair is contemplated.

Echocardiography

The echocardiogram is particularly helpful in the assessment of the cyanotic patient, because most defects can be easily visualized. Careful evaluation of the right ventricular inflow and outflow tracts usually reveals the site of shunting, and the direction of blood flow can be easily ascertained by Doppler or contrast imaging.[3] Detailed ultrasound studies often render cardiac catheterization unnecessary unless surgery is contemplated and pulmonary hypertension (as opposed to pulmonic stenosis) cannot be otherwise ruled out. The pulmonary vascular and right ventricular pressures can often be estimated noninvasively by measuring the peak velocity of even a small jet of pulmonic or tricuspid valve insufficiency and applying the Bernoulli equation (see Cardiac Imaging). Echocardiographic contrast agents can be used to amplify weak signals from small jets, permitting more accurate assessment of jet peak velocity and cardiac pressures.

Cardiac Catheterization

Cardiac catheterization and angiocardiography are advisable whenever uncommon or complex defects are suspected or when surgical repair is contemplated. In addition to showing the location and severity of the shunt, angiography outlines the anatomy of the defect (e.g., pulmonic, tricuspid dysplasia) and permits visualization of the pulmonary vasculature. Direct measurements of intravascular pressure are useful for assessing the severity of pulmonary hypertension and for confirming the presence of unusual or easily overlooked defects, such as tricuspid valve stenosis. The measurement of pulmonary artery pressure is essential when cardiac or vascular surgery is contemplated for a patient with cyanotic heart disease. If pulmonary vascular resistance is normal, pulmonary flow can be augmented and systemic hypoxemia improved by the creation of an artificial left-to-right shunt between a systemic and a pulmonary artery distal to the site of the cyanotic defect (e.g., Blalock-Taussig shunt).[61,128a,136a,141a]

Tetralogy of Fallot

The defining anatomic features of tetralogy of Fallot include right ventricular outflow obstruction (pulmonic stenosis), secondary right ventricular hypertrophy, a subaortic ventricular septal defect, and a rightward-positioned aorta (Figure 200-43). Pulmonic stenosis that occurs in combination with an isolated VSD produces similar findings, but the infundibular septum is not malaligned, the aorta is normal in size, and the infundibulum of the right ventricle is not narrowed.[75c] These distinctions are

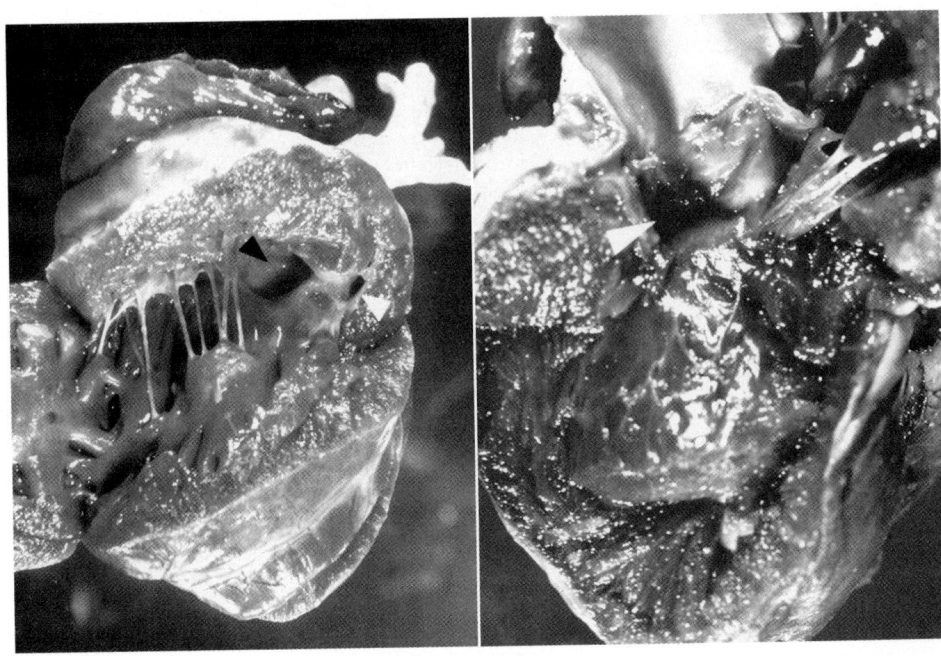

Figure 200-43 Gross pathology of tetralogy of Fallot. **A,** Right-sided view of a dog with tetralogy of Fallot shows concentric hypertrophy of the right ventricular wall, a markedly narrowed and hypoplastic right ventricular outflow tract *(white arrowhead)*, and a large ventricular septal defect (VSD) *(black arrowhead)*. **B,** Left-sided view of a large, nonresistive VSD *(white arrowhead)* in a patient with tetralogy of Fallot. Note the proximity to the root of the aorta and the possibility for prolapse of an aortic valve leaflet into the VSD.

A   B

commonly ignored in veterinary patients because corrective surgery is rarely performed.

Pathogenesis

Tetralogy of Fallot has been extensively studied in keeshond breeding colonies, and a spectrum of lesions ranging from the subclinical to the clinically complicated has been identified.[31b,124a,127a] Patterson et al.[124a] graded the conotruncal defects as follows:

- *Grade 1:* Subclinical malformations involving persistence of the conus septum fusion line, aneurysm of the ventricular septum, and absence of the papillary muscle of the conus.
- *Grade 2:* Pulmonic stenosis or ventricular septal defect in addition to the grade 1 lesions.
- *Grade 3:* Tetralogy of Fallot—pulmonic stenosis, ventricular septal defect, and dextropositioned aorta (with secondary right ventricular hypertrophy.

Additional abnormalities found in some dogs included a dilated and tortuous ascending aorta, pulmonary atresia, hypoplasia of the supraventricular crest, and anomalies of the aortic arch system. Based on extensive breeding studies and sophisticated genetic analysis, conotruncal defects have been shown to be an inherited autosomal recessive trait with variable expression.[76c]

Pathophysiology

The essential components of tetralogy of Fallot are severe right ventricular outflow tract obstruction and a ventricular septal defect. As a result of the outflow obstruction and elevated right ventricular pressure, desaturated blood shunts from the right heart through the septal defect to mix with oxygenated blood coming from the left ventricle.[122a-123a] Pulmonary arterial blood flow and pulmonary venous return are scant, and the left atrium and left ventricle are small (underdeveloped). The addition of unoxygenated blood from the right ventricle to the systemic side of the circulation causes arterial hypoxemia, decreased hemoglobin oxygen saturation, cyanosis, and secondary polycythemia. Systemic collateral circulation to the lung increases via the bronchial arterial system. These vessels supply blood to the capillaries of the pulmonary parenchyma either directly or via anastomosing connections with a larger pulmonary artery. A substantial portion of this blood can participate in pulmonary gas exchange. Other aspects of clinical pathophysiology have been previously described (see Clinical Evaluation of the Patient with Cyanotic Heart Disease, above).

Clinical Findings

Tetralogy of Fallot is common in the keeshond and English bulldog and in some families of other breeds.[30] It has also been recognized in the cat.[9a] Presenting complaints and clinical signs are as previously described for cyanotic heart disease. In most cases, the murmur of tetralogy of Fallot is produced by blood flowing through the stenotic pulmonic valve.[75c] A right-sided murmur, resulting from blood flow through the VSD, may predominate when PS is mild and left-to-right shunting occurs across a restrictive VSD (i.e., an acyanotic defect). The absence of an obvious murmur suggests pulmonary atresia and/or polycythemia with hyperviscosity (which reduces blood flow turbulence) and ejection across a large, nonrestrictive VSD. Exercise or excitement may induce or enhance detection of peripheral cyanosis by accentuating right-to-left shunting by mechanisms previously described.

Radiography usually reveals a small or normal-sized heart with rounding of the right ventricular border (Figure 200-44). The main pulmonary artery is not always visibly enlarged, in

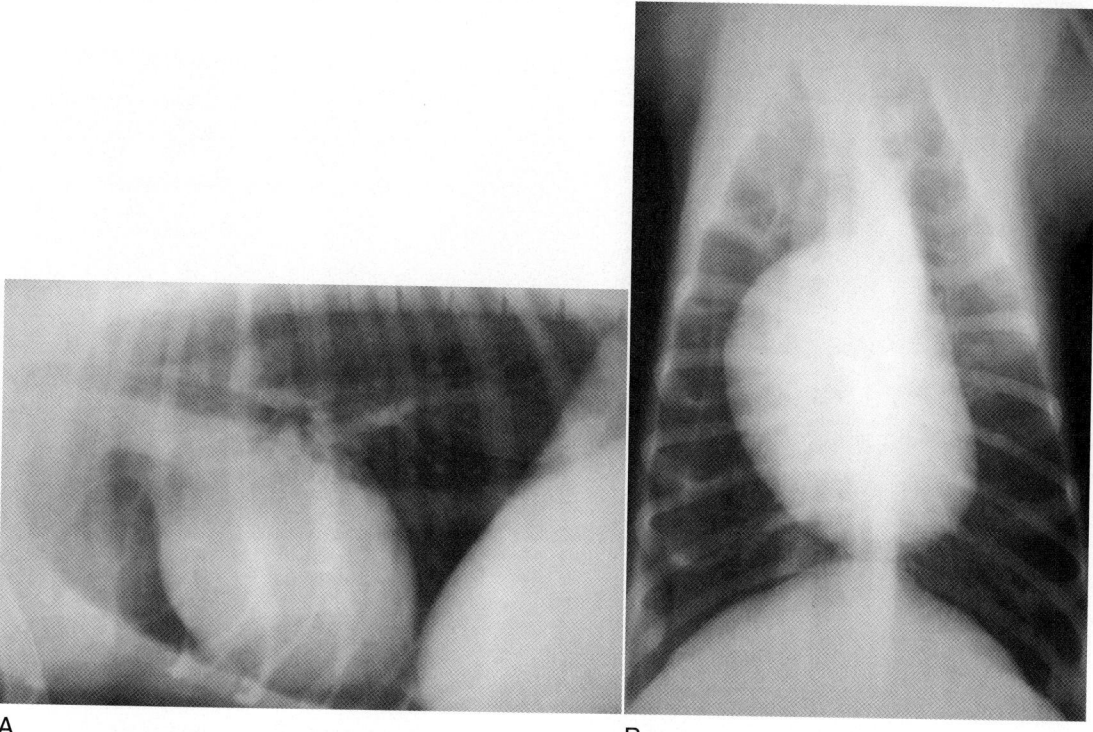

A   B

Figure 200-44 Lateral (**A**) and dorsoventral (**B**) radiographs of a dog with tetralogy of Fallot. Right heart enlargement is suggested by the rounding of the sternal border on the lateral view and the reverse D appearance on the dorsoventral view. The main pulmonary artery and peripheral pulmonary vessels are diminished. The appearance of the heart on the dorsoventral view is classically described as "boot shaped" *(coeur en sabot)* but is often difficult to reconcile.

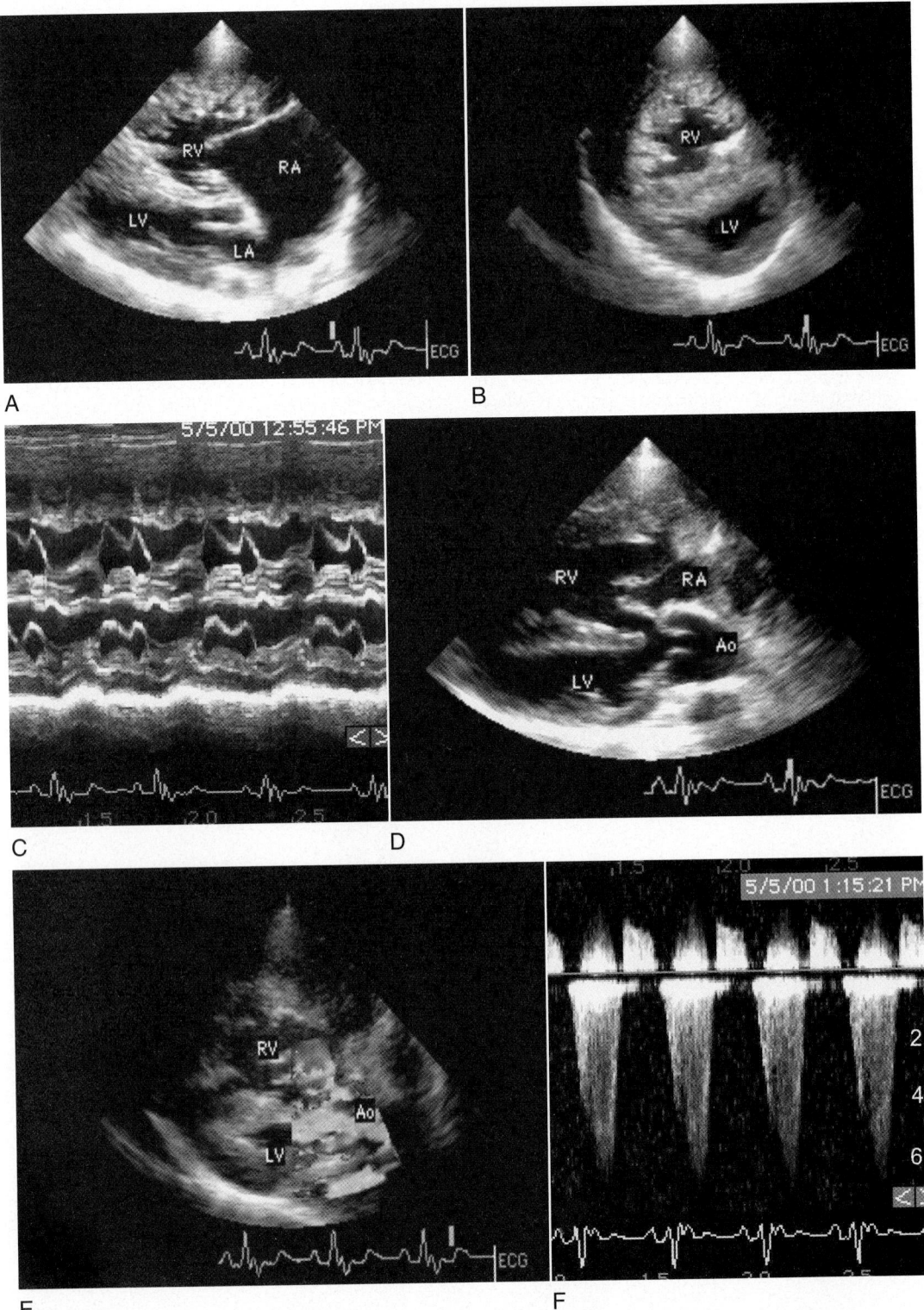

Figure 200-45 Echocardiography of tetralogy of Fallot in a keeshond puppy. **A,** Right long axis view shows severe right ventricular (RV) concentric hypertrophy and right atrial enlargement. **B,** Right short axis view shows severe RV concentric hypertrophy, flattening of the interventricular septum, a small, underloaded left ventricle (LV), and hyperechogenicity of the RV subendocardium. **C,** M-mode study shows enlargement of the RV compared with the LV. The tricuspid and mitral valves are seen moving in the center of their respective ventricles. Paradoxical septal motion toward the RV during systole appears to occur. **D,** Right long axis view shows the ventricular septal defect (VSD) and rightward (dextropositioned) displacement of the aortic root and aorta (Ao). **E,** Color flow Doppler study of an image similar to that in **D** shows right-to-left shunting of blood from the right ventricle, across the VSD, and into the aorta. **F,** Continuous wave Doppler study from the left heart base across the pulmonic valve indicates the presence of high-velocity blood flow and pulmonic stenosis.

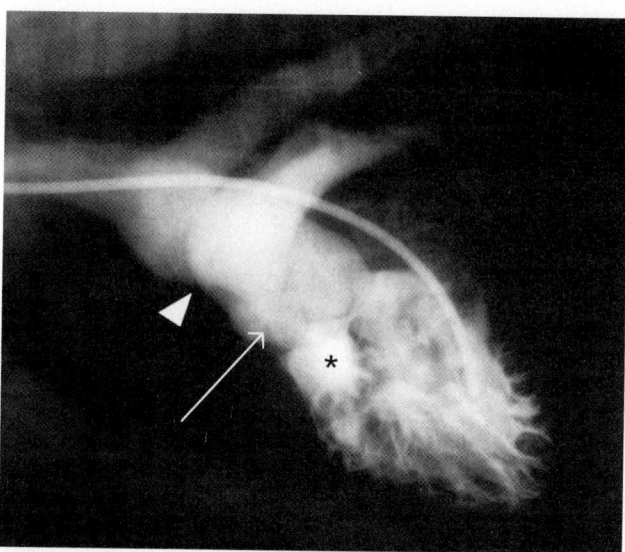

Figure 200-46 Angiogram from a keeshond with tetralogy of Fallot. The right ventricular injection opacifies the right ventricle, pulmonary artery, and aorta. Contrast can be seen in the region of the suspected ventral septal defect (*). The contrast column narrows in the right ventricular outflow tract and the region of the pulmonic valve (*arrow*). A large, poststenotic dilatation of the main pulmonary artery (*arrowhead*) is present. A wide, rightward-positioned aorta can be appreciated.

contrast to the usual case of pulmonic stenosis with intact ventricular septum. The pulmonary vasculature is diminished, and the left auricle may be inconspicuous as a consequence of decreased venous return. The ECG typically exhibits criteria for right heart enlargement, including right axis deviation, although left or cranially directed vectors may be found in some cats.[129a] Echocardiographic findings include right ventricular hypertrophy, increased right ventricular chamber dimensions, reduced left atrial (LA) and LV dimensions, a large subaortic VSD, and right ventricular outflow obstruction (Figure 200-45). Doppler or contrast studies can be used to document right-to-left shunting at the ventricular outflow level (Figure 200-46).[3,130a]

Cardiac catheterization demonstrates equilibration of left and right ventricular systolic pressures, compatible with a large, nonrestrictive VSD.[128a] Oximetry samples reveal a step-down at the left ventricular outflow level, and the aortic blood is relatively desaturated. Angiocardiography reveals right ventricular hypertrophy, narrowing of the right ventricular infundibulum, pulmonic stenosis with minimal poststenotic dilatation, varying degrees of pulmonary artery hypoplasia, a large subaortic VSD, a small, dorsally displaced left ventricle, an enlarged and rightward-positioned aorta, and prominent bronchial circulation (Figure 200-46).[124a,128a] Bidirectional shunting across the VSD is common in anesthetized animals. Anticoagulation therapy (e.g., heparin) should be considered to prevent cerebral embolization during and immediately after cardiac catheterization.

Clinical Management
The natural history and survival times of dogs and cats with tetralogy of Fallot are not well characterized. Like other cyanotic heart diseases, tetralogy of Fallot can be tolerated for years if pulmonary blood flow is maintained and hyperviscosity is controlled.[21] Most affected animals have severely limited exercise capacity. In cases of pulmonary atresia, pulmonary blood flow must be derived from a patent ductus arteriosus, the bronchial artery, or an elaborate network of systemic collaterals.

Sudden death is common due to the combined consequences of hypoxia, hyperviscosity, or cardiac arrhythmia. Unlike with pulmonic stenosis with intact ventricular septum, congestive heart failure is an unusual outcome.

Options for treating animals with tetralogy of Fallot include medical and surgical approaches. Definitive correction of the defect (i.e., closure of the VSD and removal or bypass of the stenosis) can be done under cardiopulmonary bypass, but such surgery is rarely performed in animals.[62,77c] As a general rule, the stenosis should not be relieved if the VSD cannot be closed because the loss of right ventricular pressure results in marked left-to-right shunting with subsequent left-sided congestive heart failure.[63,128a] As an alternative to definitive correction, surgical palliation through the creation of a systemic to pulmonary shunt can be quite rewarding.[64,78c,128a,141a] Subclavian to pulmonary artery (Blalock-Taussig), ascending aorta to pulmonary artery (Potts), and aorta to right pulmonary artery (Waterston-Cooley) connections have been made in dogs and cats. Creation of a left-to-right shunt distal to the cyanotic defect increases pulmonary perfusion and allows a greater contribution of oxygenated blood to the systemic circulation. The size of the accessory shunt must be controlled to prevent overloading of the diminutive left ventricle and subsequent pulmonary edema. The extent to which these shunts remain patent over long periods in veterinary patients has not been reported.

Periodic phlebotomy, performed to maintain the PCV between 62% and 68%, produces a satisfactory result in many cases.[21] Excessive bleeding should be avoided, and the blood that is withdrawn is replaced with crystalloid fluids to maintain cardiac output and tissue oxygen delivery.[138a] Some children with tetralogy of Fallot benefit from beta blockade with propranolol; however, controlled studies of the clinical efficacy of this treatment in animals are lacking.[139a,140a] Severe hypoxic spells should be treated with cage rest, oxygen, and sodium bicarbonate (if metabolic acidosis is evident). Treatment with vasoconstrictive agents such as phenylephrine can also help reduce the amount of right-to-left shunting. Drugs with marked systemic vasodilating properties should be avoided.

Other Causes of Cyanotic Congenital Heart Disease
Valvular Atresia
Pulmonary atresia with a ventricular septal defect is essentially an exaggerated form of tetralogy of Fallot (Figure 200-47). All the blood ejected from the right heart is shunted right-to-left across a large VSD and into an enlarged aorta. The tricuspid valve is usually normal. The term *pseudotruncus arteriosus* has been used to describe this defect, which differs from a true truncus arteriosus because careful dissection reveals an imperforate pulmonic valve and a vestigial cord representing the main pulmonary trunk. On occasion, both the pulmonic and tricuspid valves are atretic (see Figure 200-47). The right ventricle is small or hypoplastic, and blood returning to the right atrium shunts through a patent foramen ovale or ASD to produce cyanosis. The lungs are supplied via a PDA or an extensive bronchoesophageal collateral circulation.

Aortic atresia with a hypoplastic left heart is a rare form of cyanotic heart disease in dogs. The aortic orifice is often imperforate, the ascending aorta is hypoplastic, and the mitral valve is usually atretic or hypoplastic. In the absence of a VSD, the left ventricle is very small; when a VSD is present, the left ventricle is better developed. The right heart supplies the entire pulmonary and systemic circulations, resulting in profound cyanosis and, in most cases, early death.

Double outlet right ventricle   Double outlet right ventricle (DORV), in which both great vessels exit from the right ventricle, has been reported in dogs and cats (Figure 200-48).[146a,147a] A VSD provides the left ventricle with an avenue for outflow

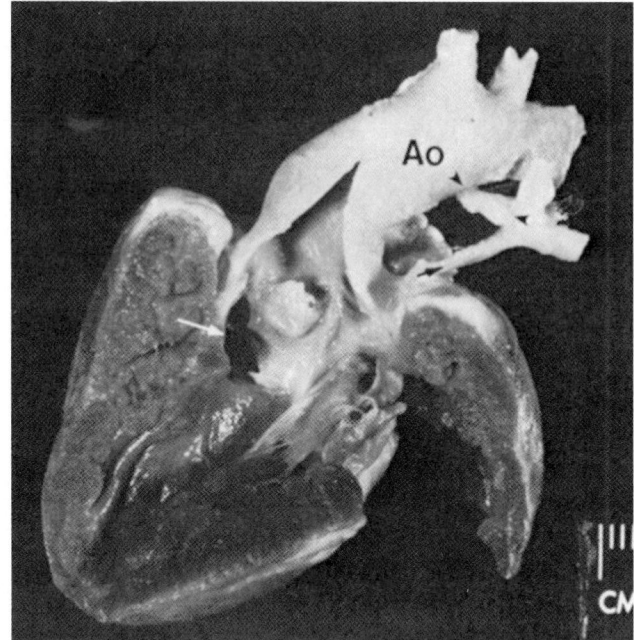

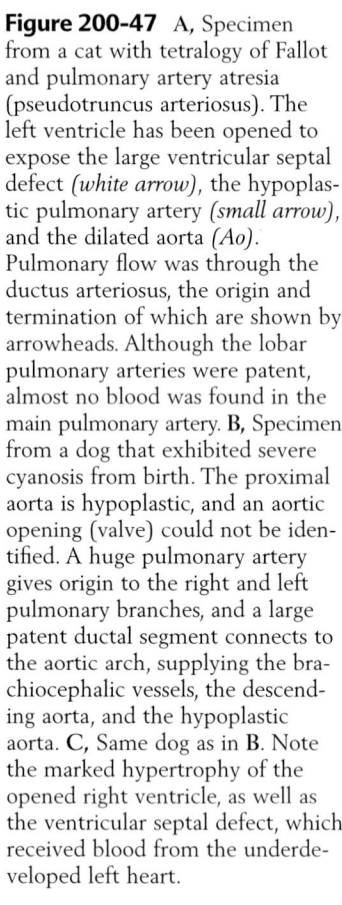

Figure 200-47 **A,** Specimen from a cat with tetralogy of Fallot and pulmonary artery atresia (pseudotruncus arteriosus). The left ventricle has been opened to expose the large ventricular septal defect *(white arrow),* the hypoplastic pulmonary artery *(small arrow),* and the dilated aorta *(Ao).* Pulmonary flow was through the ductus arteriosus, the origin and termination of which are shown by arrowheads. Although the lobar pulmonary arteries were patent, almost no blood was found in the main pulmonary artery. **B,** Specimen from a dog that exhibited severe cyanosis from birth. The proximal aorta is hypoplastic, and an aortic opening (valve) could not be identified. A huge pulmonary artery gives origin to the right and left pulmonary branches, and a large patent ductal segment connects to the aortic arch, supplying the brachiocephalic vessels, the descending aorta, and the hypoplastic aorta. **C,** Same dog as in **B.** Note the marked hypertrophy of the opened right ventricle, as well as the ventricular septal defect, which received blood from the underdeveloped left heart.

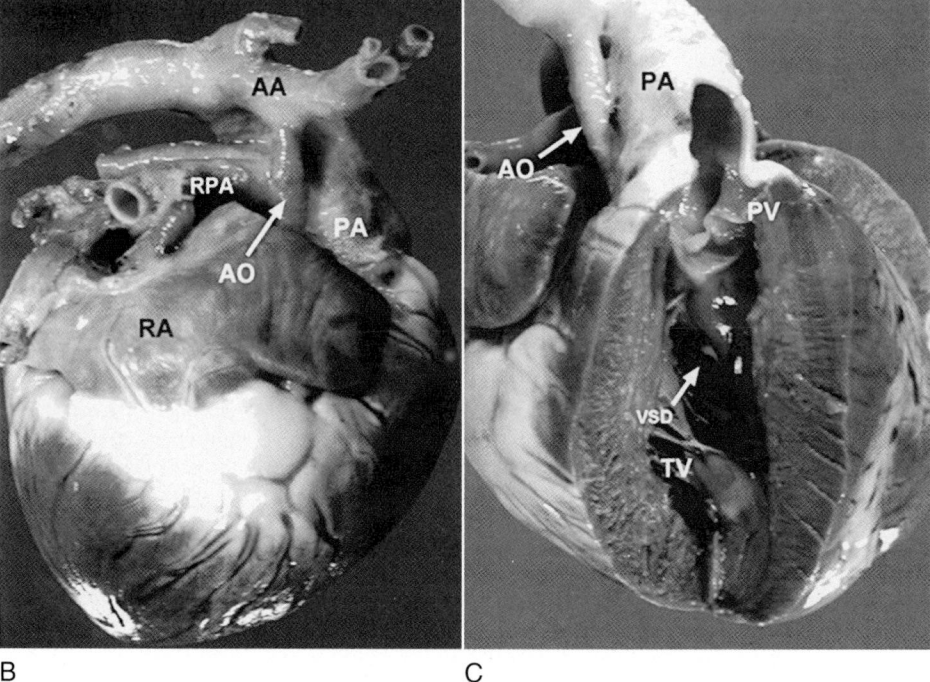

into the great vessels. Depending on the location of the VSD in relation to the origin of the great vessels, DORV can manifest as either pulmonary overcirculation or cyanosis. Concurrent abnormalities such as pulmonic stenosis, pulmonary hypertension, and coarctation of the aorta can also affect the development of clinical signs. Cyanosis is likely if the VSD lies under the pulmonary artery. Surgical correction of this condition in dogs has been reported.[31]

Transposition of the great arteries   In D-transposition of the great arteries, the aorta originates from the right ventricle and the pulmonary trunk from the left ventricle.[15a,145a] In the pure and fatal case, two independent circulations exist, and the systemic arteries never receive oxygenated blood.

Survival of an animal with D-transposition depends on the presence (or production) of shunts between the two circulations to allow for mixing of blood to prevent fatal hypoxemia. These defects are complex, generally lethal, and most likely underdiagnosed in animals, relative to children, because most animals probably die at a very young age undiagnosed.

Miscellaneous Cardiac Defects
The potential for anatomic and physiologic variants of congenital heart disease is tremendous, and it is beyond the scope of this chapter to discuss the entire spectrum of malformations. The following descriptions summarize clinically relevant aspects of rarely encountered cardiac and pericardial defects.

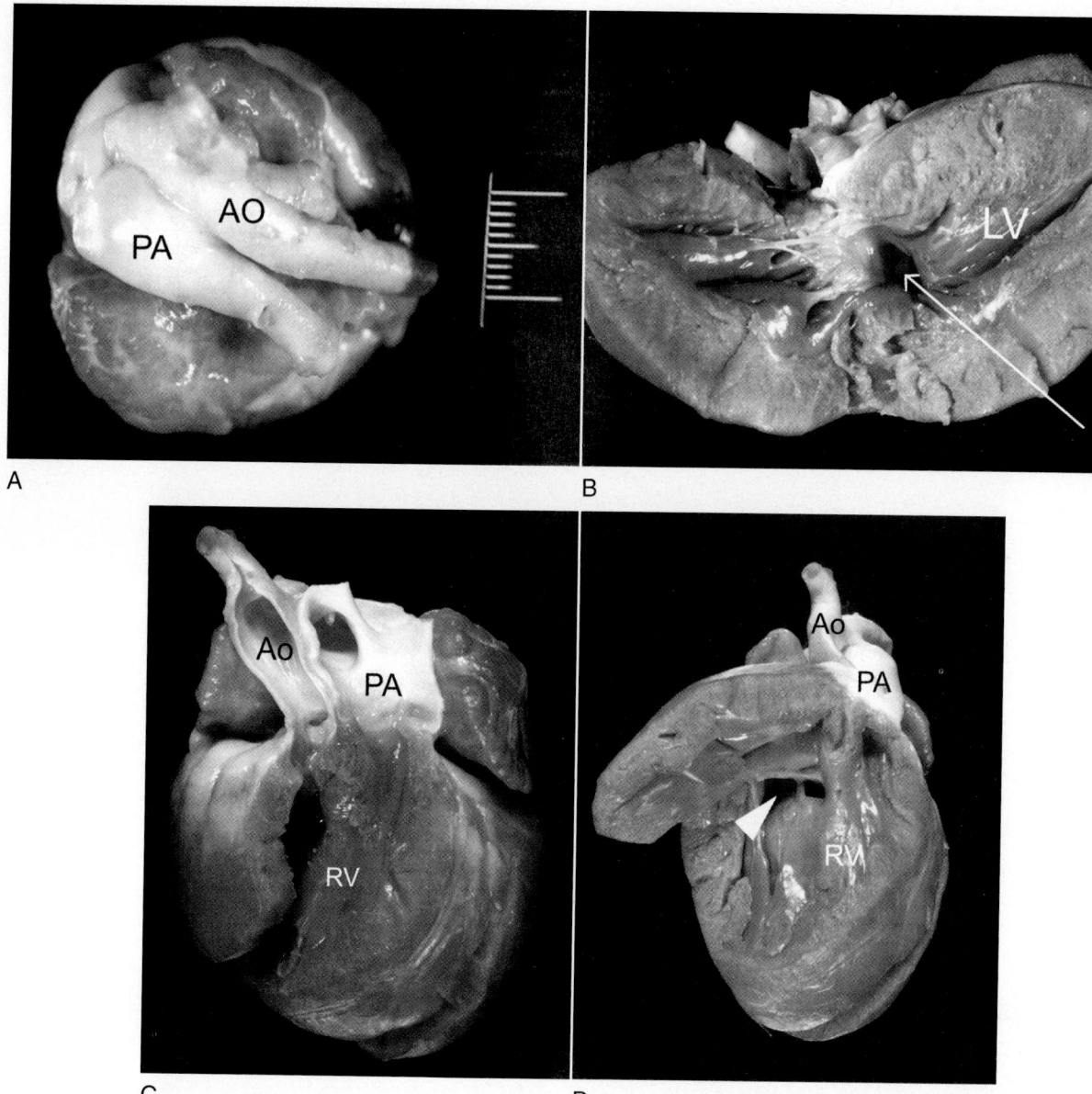

Figure 200-48 Pathology of a double outlet right ventricle (DORV) in a 6-month-old domestic shorthair cat. **A,** Dorsal view of the heart showing the side-by-side positioning of the aorta *(Ao)* and pulmonary artery *(PA)* at the cranial right edge of the heart. **B,** View of the ventricular septal defect *(arrow)* from the left ventricular *(LV)* side. Note the absence of a left ventricular outflow tract and aorta originating from the LV and the discontinuity between the mitral valve apparatus and the missing aorta. **C,** View from the right cranial aspect showing the origin of the aorta and pulmonary artery from the right ventricle. The opening of the VSD into the right ventricle is below the crista supraventricularis and is not easily seen in this view. **D,** View of the right side of the interventricular septum reveals the location of the VSD *(arrowhead)* near the origin of the aorta (aortic-committed DORV) (Courtesy Dr. Richard Kienle, Gilroy, CA.)

Endocardial fibroelastosis has been reported in dogs[65,151a,154a,155a] and cats and is probably familial in some lines of Burmese and Siamese cats.[12a,79c,151a-153a] The gross anatomic findings include left ventricular and left atrial dilatation with severe endocardial thickening, characterized grossly by diffuse, white, opaque thickening of the luminal surface (Figure 200-49). Histologic lesions in the cat include diffuse hypocellular, fibroelastic thickening of the endocardium with layering of thin, randomly organized collagen and elastic fibers.[151a,153a] Edema of the endocardium with dilatation of

lymphatics is prominent, and there is no evidence of myocardial inflammation or necrosis. The clinical features of endocardial fibroelastosis include early development of left or biventricular failure, generally before 6 months of age. Mitral regurgitation may be detected. Left ventricular and atrial dilatation are evident on radiographs and on the ECG. The limited echocardiographic studies performed to date suggest reduction of left ventricular myocardial function as opposed to pure valvular disease in which shortening fraction tends to be normal or increased.[155a] The diagnosis of primary endocardial

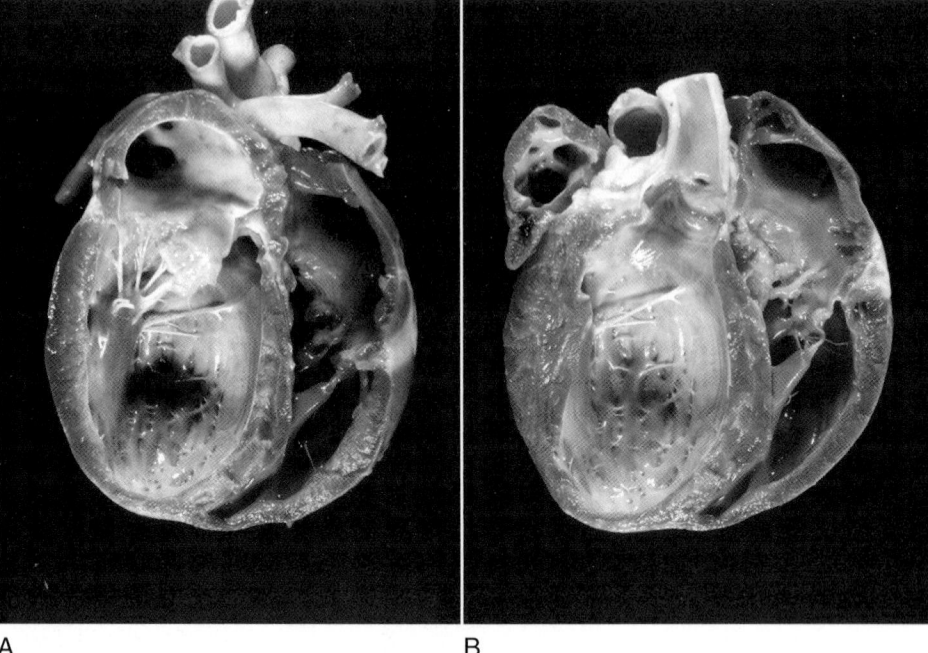

A   B

Figure 200-49 Gross pathology of a cat with endomyocardial fibrosis. Cutaway views of the left ventricular inflow tract **(A)** and the left ventricular outflow tract **(B)** show diffuse fibrosis of the endomyocardial surface of both the atrium and ventricle.

fibroelastosis is at times tenuous, inasmuch as chronic left ventricular dilatation may lead to similar changes, particularly in the setting of mitral dysplasia, aortic stenosis, restrictive and dilated cardiomyopathy, or myocarditis. Dogs with endocardial fibroelastosis often have thickening of the mitral valve leaflets and mitral regurgitation.[154a,155a] Affected animals fail to thrive. Medical treatment of congestive heart failure may be effective in prolonging life, but recovery is unlikely.

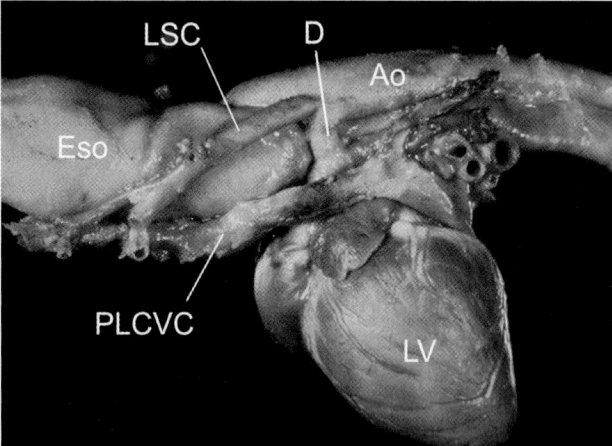

Figure 200-50 Gross pathology from a dog with persistent right aortic arch, patent ductus arteriosus *(D)*, anomalous origin of the left subclavian artery *(LSC)*, and persistent left cranial vena cava *(PLCVC)*. The left-sided view of the heart, great vessels, and esophagus *(Eso)* shows the entrapment and cranial dilatation of the esophagus by the patent ductus arteriosus. The origin of the left subclavian artery is moved distal from its usual location and is behind the esophagus. The persistent left cranial vena cava can be seen extending laterally alongside the esophagus and left heart base and coursing around the caudal waist of the heart.

Peritoneal-pericardial diaphragmatic hernia (PPDH) is a relatively common developmental anomaly of dogs and cats.[163a,170a] This condition is not a true cardiac anomaly, but it can be confused with other congenital and acquired conditions. For further information, the reader is referred to Chapter 205.

Vascular Anomalies

Vascular anomalies can be classified based on their location in the vascular system. A number of vascular malformations have been reported.[49a,50a,66-68,171a-196a] Patent ductus arteriosus, discussed previously, is the most important of the vascular malformations. Peripheral vascular disorders, including abnormal abdominal and hepatic venous drainage and arteriovenous fistulas,[37b] are detailed in their respective chapters. Unilateral atresia of a pulmonary artery has been described in a cat with respiratory difficulty.[185a] Coronary arteries can develop anomalously but rarely cause documented clinical disease except when associated with pulmonic stenosis.[33] Other major vascular defects center about the aorta and the systemic venous drainage, and the salient features of these disorders are briefly addressed.

Aortic Anomalies

Persistence of the right aortic arch, as opposed to the left fourth aortic arch, causes regurgitation in weanlings due to constriction of the esophagus.[49a,50a,171a-183a] Vascular ring anomalies include this common malformation and other total or partial ring anomalies, such as those formed by retroesophageal subclavian arteries, double aortic arch, or left aortic arch with right-sided ligamentum arteriosum.[177a,179a,180a,184a] The condition is quite common in German shepherds and has been recognized in many other canine breeds, including Irish setters and Great Danes. The condition is uncommon in cats. Occasionally, other cardiac defects are present, including PDA (Figure 200-50 and Figure 200-51). This condition is described more fully in Chapter 208.

Aorticopulmonary septal defect (window) is caused by failure of the truncus arteriosus to differentiate; this results in

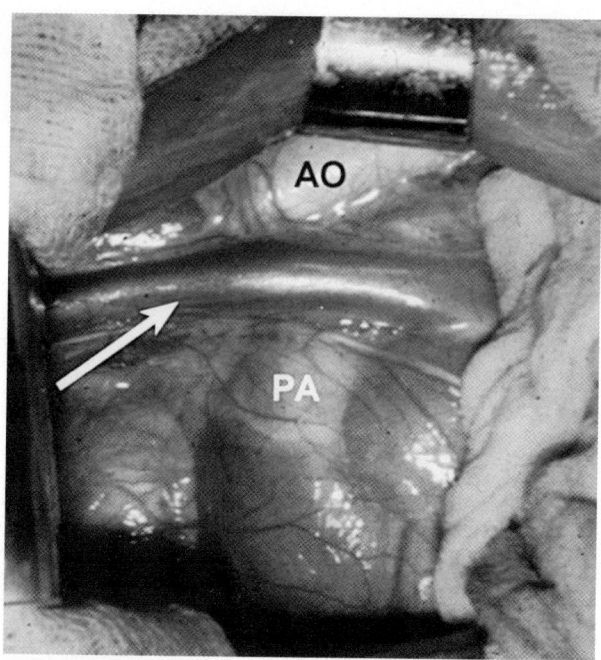

Figure 200-51 Surgeon's view of a persistent left cranial vena cava. This venous anomaly is often encountered during the approach to a patent ductus arteriosus. No hemodynamic consequences result from this anomaly.

a common opening between the aorta and the pulmonary artery, and shunting develops between the left and right sides of the circulation. Although a clinical condition similar to PDA can develop, some reports suggest that in most cases, pulmonary hypertension develops during the first year of life and that clinical signs are similar to those in dogs that develop Eisenmenger's syndrome due to other defects.[68,188a,191a] Management is similar to that for a reversed PDA. Surgery is difficult without cardiopulmonary bypass and should not

be attempted if pulmonary vascular resistance is markedly elevated.

Coarctation and interruption of the aorta is a rare defect in dogs that is characterized by narrowing of the aorta distal to the subclavian artery, adjacent to the ductus arteriosus. A case reported by Eyster[193a] demonstrated systolic and diastolic murmurs and left ventricular failure. The clinical features of coarctation in children are well described and in many ways are similar to this case.[15a] Aortic interruption has been reported in two dogs,[80c,193a] and a case of tubular hypoplasia of the ascending aorta in a dog has also been described.[194a] Although these lesions differ from coarctation, they are additional examples of malformation of the aorta in small animals. Definitive diagnosis usually requires angiography, although MRI and CT are effective methods of evaluating lesions of the aortic arch. Surgical correction has been successful in affected dogs.

Venous Anomalies

Thoracic venous anomalies rarely cause cardiac problems in small animals. Total or partial anomalous pulmonary venous return, which has been reported in a dog, behaves functionally as a left-to-right shunt at the atrial level.[80a] Abnormalities of abdominal venous drainage, such as patent ductus venosus, can induce hepatic encephalopathy. A relatively common venous abnormality of clinical significance during thoracic surgery or cardiac catheterization is the persistent left cranial vena cava.[69,81c,195a] This structure, normally present in the fetus as part of the left cardinal venous system, may persist and drain into the embryologically related coronary sinus in the caudal aspect of the right atrium. Persistent left cranial vena cava may interfere with surgical exposure, particularly during surgical treatment of persistent right fourth aortic arch, or may confound cardiac catheterization, but otherwise it is of no known functional significance. As with persistence of the right fourth aortic arch, this vascular anomaly is common in German shepherds and has been reported in other canine breeds and in cats.[133a,195a] Division of this vessel generally poses no clinical problem provided the normal right cranial vena cava is also present. Venous aneurysms or related anomalies are extremely rare.[38b]

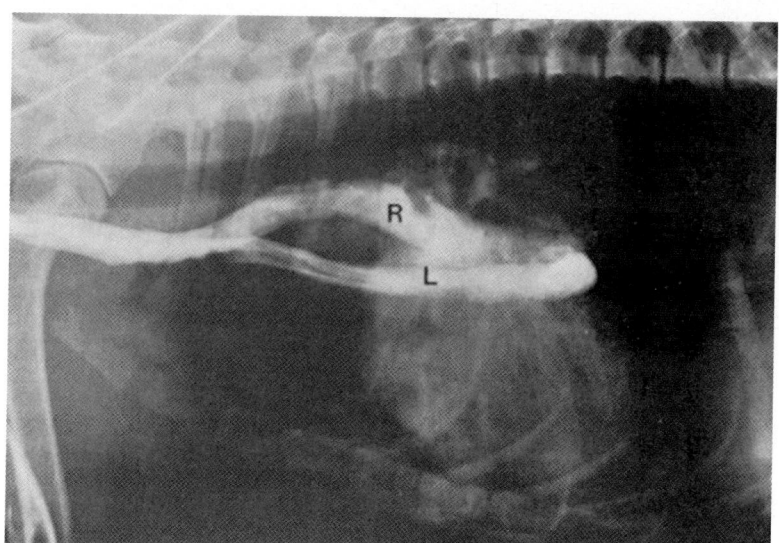

Figure 200-52 Persistent left cranial vena cava in a dog. Contrast was injected simultaneously into the right and left jugular veins. The normal right cranial vena cava is evident (*R*), as is the persistent left vena cava (*L*). Note that the left vena cava enters the caudal portion of the right atrium and empties into the coronary sinus.

CHAPTER 201

Acquired Valvular Heart Disease

Jens Häggström
Clarence Kvart
Henrik D. Pedersen

CHRONIC MITRAL VALVE INSUFFICIENCY

Chronic mitral valve insufficiency (CMVI) in dogs is usually caused by a progressive myxomatous degeneration of the atrioventricular valves. The disease has been given many names in the veterinary literature, including endocardiosis and chronic valvular disease. Similar changes of the mitral valve are also seen in humans, horses, and pigs.[1-3]

Occurrence

CMVI is common in the dog and has been estimated to account for 75% to 80% of canine cardiac diseases.[4-7] The prevalence of CMVI is strongly age dependent: from only a few percent in young dogs to approximately 75% in dogs older than 16 years.[4,5,7,8] CMVI is encountered in all breeds, but the prevalence of the disease varies greatly: dogs of small- to medium-size breeds, such as the Papillon, Poodle, Chihuahua, Dachshund, and Cavalier King Charles spaniel, are most commonly affected.[9-12] The prevalence of CMVI in cats without primary myocardial disease is unknown but seems to be low.

Significance and Progression

CMVI is characterized by slow progression. Risk factors for progression of CMVI from mild to severe in small dogs include severity of valve lesion, age, and gender.[13-17] The disease progresses into moderate and severe CMVI at a lower age in males than in females.[13,14,18,19] Whether or not these risk factors apply in large dogs is unknown. Typically, it takes several years for the disease to evolve from mild, clinically silent CMVI to severe disease with signs of heart failure.[14,15,19] Many affected dogs will therefore not develop clinical signs from the disease during their lifetime. The most severely affected dogs, however, will end up needing therapy for heart failure, and, in the end, die or be euthanized due to refractory cardiac failure (Figure 201-1). CMVI has been reported to account for 75% of the cases of congestive heart failure in dogs[7,20], a proportion which is considerably higher in affected breeds.[10,13,21] Furthermore, the presence of CMVI and ongoing medical treatment for heart failure may complicate medical treatment for other conditons and decisions for surgical procedures or anesthesia.

Pathology

Macroscopic appearance of myxomatous degeneration depends on at which stage of disease the valve is examined. Macroscopic findings in cases of mild myxomatous degeneration may not be apparent and may be overlooked, especially in dogs without evidence of valvular insufficiency. Common findings at early stages include elongated chordae tendineae and enlarged, thickened leaflets with areas showing bulging/ballooning/prolapse towards the atrial side (Figure 201-2, *A*).[6,22,23] The changes begin in the area of apposition of the leaflets and are usually most pronounced in sections where chordae tendineae inserts.

The bulging of such areas towards the atrial side of the leaflets has been described as rolling of the edges. With progression, the bulging becomes worse and the free edge becomes thickened and irregular and the lesions spread into other parts of the leaflets. Within the same valve leaflet one section may look relatively normal while another, neighboring section is moderately or severely diseased. In late stages, secondary fibrosis can cause marked thickening and contraction of leaflets and chordae tendineae. The chordae tendineae may rupture[23], which leads to an unattached free edge, that is, a flail leaflet.[24] Ultrastructurally, there is myxomatous proliferation of the valve, in which the spongiosa component of the valve is unusually prominent and the quantity of acid-staining glucosaminoglycans (GAGs) is increased (Figure 201-2, *B*).[6,22,23] The valvular interstitial cells in affected areas often have morphologic changes of the nucleus, a localized concentration of abnormally shaped mitochondria and rough endoplasmic reticulum,

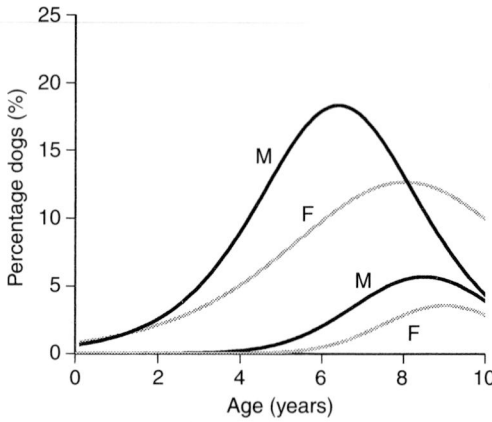

Figure 201-1 Proposed model for progression of CMVI in the Cavalier King Charles Spaniel population. The effect of age on the annual percentage of new cases of heart murmurs attributable to CMVI out of the total population in male (thin black line) and female dogs (thin gray line), and on the annual percentage deaths/euthanasias caused by heart failure (thick black or gray lines). Note that both curves resemble a distribution of a random variable with a means of approximately 6 to 7 years (heart murmurs) and 9 to 10 years (deaths/euthanasias), respectively. The male and female populations differ in their epidemiology concerning age of onset of MR and mortality attributable to CMVI. Initiated breeding programs aim at pushing the curve of new cases of CMVI to higher age to reduce the number of cases of congestive heart failure. (From Häggström J: Chronic valvular disease in Cavalier King Charles Spaniels—epidemiology, inheritance and pathophysiology. Thesis, Swedish University of Agricultural Sciences, Uppsala, 1996.)

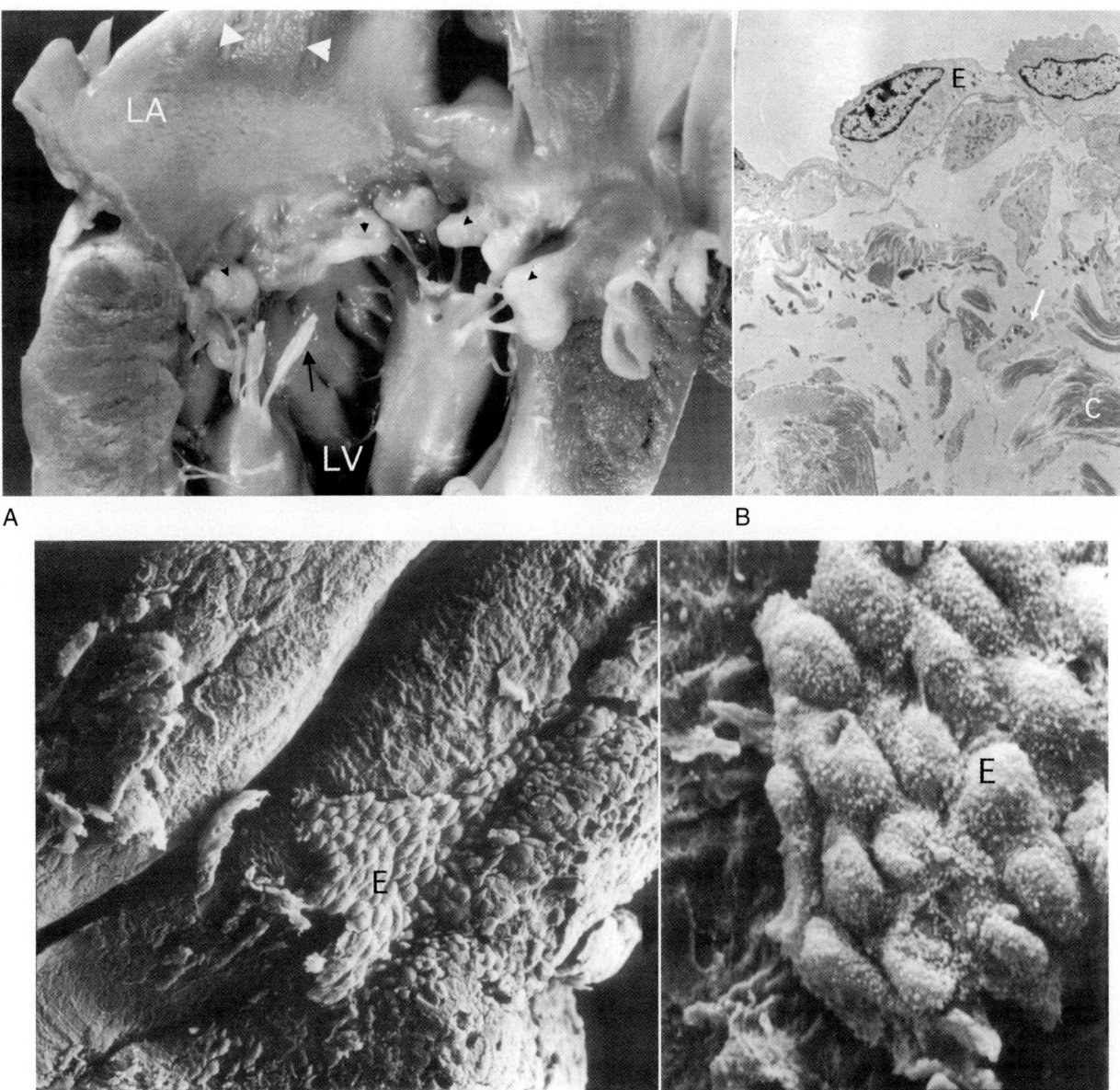

Figure 201-2 **A,** Postmortem specimen of an opened left ventricle (LV) and left atrium (LA) from a dog that suffered from CMVI. The left ventricle and atrium are dilated, and the mitral valve leaflets are thickened and contracted, with nodules rolling in the free edges *(arrowheads)*. Evidence of chordal involvement present in the form of ruptured chordae tendinae *(arrow)*. Jet lesion is present on the atrial wall *(between white arrowheads)* result when the regurgitant streams of blood from the left ventricle strike the atrial wall. **B,** Transmission electron micrograph demonstrating loss of collagen in the subendothelial layer of the mitral valve of a dog with CMVI due to myxomatous degeneration. Fragments of valvular interstitial cells *(white arrow)* are visible interspersed between disrupted bundles of collagen (C). There is obvious variation in the appearance of the endothelial cells (E). **C,** Scanning electron micrograph of the surface of the distal zone of a diseased mitral valve. The triangular area of endothelium in the middle of the picture (E) is the only endothelium left in this area; the remaining area is completely denuded. Underlying collagen has been revealed, which indicates the absence of basement membrane remnants. **D,** Higher magnification of the triangular "endothelial island *(E)*" in Figure **C,** shows that these cells are somewhat clumped, with a very dense microappendage population, considerably more dense than is seen in the normal state with the entire cell surface covered. (**A,** From Pedersen HD, Häggström J: Mitral valve prolapse in the dog: a model of mitral valve prolapse in man, *J Cardiovasc Res* 47:234, 2000. **B, C,** and **D,** Courtesy Brendan Corcoran, Alexander Black, Joanna Dukes-McEwan, Anne French, University of Edinburgh, Scotland and University College Galway, Ireland.)

disorganized cytoskeleton, and lack of secretory vesicles.[25] There is haphazard arrangement, disruption and fragmentation of the collagen fibrils surrounding the interstitial cells (see Figure 201-2, *B*). The endothelial cells covering affected areas become polymorphic and some areas completely loose the endothelium, exposing the underlying extracellular matrix (Figure 201-2, *C*, and 201-2, *D*).[25] Exposure of collagen and other matrix components to the blood is expected to promote thrombosis. Although thrombosis may develop as a complication in CMVI dogs, thrombus formation on the mitral valve is uncommon. Why it is absent in the presence of endothelial damage is currently not known. Inflammation is not an apparent part of the degenerative changes.

The valvular regurgitation leads to secondary changes including dilation of the left atrium, mitral annulus, and left ventricle (eccentric hypertrophy), atrial endocardial lesions (fibrosis) opposite the mitral orifice (i.e., "jet lesions"), and, in severe cases, varying degrees of atrial rupture, such as endomyocardial splits, ruptured pectinate muscles in the atrial appendage, acquired atrial septal defect, and hemopericardium.[6] Myxomatous degeneration is not restricted to the mitral valve and it may be detected in any of the four intracardiac valves. The incidence of valve involvement in dogs was reported as follows: mitral valve alone 62%; mitral and tricuspid valve 32.5%; tricuspid valve alone 1.3%.[6] The pulmonary and aortic valves are less commonly affected. Interstingly, lesions similar to myxomatous degeneration of the atrioventricular valves have been described in the main pulmonary artery in Cavalier King Charles spaniels.[26] Other findings in dogs with advanced stages of CMVI include intramural arteriosclerosis and multiple small myocardial infarcts.[27-29] In contrast to humans with mitral valve prolapse, infectious endocarditis affecting the damaged leaflet is a rare complication in dogs.[1]

Inheritance and Breeding

The etiology of CMVI has not been ascertained but heredity has long been suspected to play a major role, owing to the strong association of this disease with certain small to medium-sized breeds. Two recent studies of families of Cavalier King Charles spaniels and families of Dachshunds provide evidence that genetic factors play a large role in the etiology.[17,18] The disease seems to have a polygenic inheritance; that is, multiple genes influence the trait and a certain threshold has to be reached before CMVI develops.[17,18] Males have a lower threshold than females, which means that males will develop the disease at younger age than females within a family of dogs in which the offspring on average have the same genotype. The polygenic mode of inheritance means that a combination of a sire and a dam that both have an early onset of CMVI will give offspring that have, on average, an early onset of CMVI (and heart failure). A combination of dogs with late onset will give offspring that manifest the disease at old age or never. The major role played by genetic factors implies that other factors, such as level of exercise, degree of obesity, and diet, play a relatively minor role in the etiology. Likely because of this, very little is known about the influence of such factors on the disease. Breeding programs aimed at reducing the prevalence of CMVI have been launched in Europe and North America and elsewhere for Cavalier King Charles spaniels and Dachshunds. These breeding programs use auscultation to identify the presence of a heart murmur or echocardiography to detect and quantify mitral valve prolapse or regurgitation. Dogs that are under a specific age and have developed a heart murmur or echocardiographic findings consistent with CMVI are not allowed to breed. Likewise, offspring from parents that have developed a heart murmur or echocardiographic evidence of early CMVI under a certain age limit are excuded from breeding in some programs. The age limit for potential breeding dogs and parents is very important. It should be set at an age at which dogs with an early onset of CMVI are excluded, but not too high because this may impoverish the breeding population to unacceptable low numbers.[13]

Etiology and Pathogenesis

Little is known about the pathogenesis of the progressive thickening and degeneration of the leaflets. An old theory is that the changes are response-to-injury type lesions, such as that repeated impact to the leaflets (especially the areas of apposition) results in slowly progressing changes.[30] Probably, one or more primary inciting factors increase the risk of disease in predisposed animals as not all dogs develop atrioventricular valve myxomatous degeneration. The nature of these primary initiating factors are currently not known, although certain abnormalities of collagen and other extracellular matrix components have been suggested.[13] It has been suggested that a primary defect leads to abnormal valve motion, that is, prolapse of the leaflets, which in turn increase the shear stress imposed on them, both directly through the abnormal leaflet apposition and indirectly through the increased regurgitant flow.[15,19] It likely plays an important role for the progression of the disease that the endothelium is damaged or even missing in diseased areas[25,31], because endothelial cells are known to communicate extensively with subendothelial cells (e.g., valvular interstitial cells). Specifically, endothelial damage may lead to an imbalance in local concentrations of growth-promoting and growth-inhibiting substances produced by endothelial cells. For instance, associations have been found between disease severity and the expression of endothelin receptors and nitric oxide synthase.[32,33] Future research into local disease mechanisms may suggest ways of treating the actual disease rather than merely the resulting circulatory disturbances.

Pathophysiology

Proper mitral valve closure requires an anatomically and functionally intact valve apparatus. Mitral regurgitation (MR) can be due to alterations of the valve leaflets, dilatation of the atrioventricular annulus, rupture of chordae tendineae, or inappropriate contraction of the papillary muscles. More than one of these factors can usually be identified when CMVI is present. The consequences of CMVI depend on several factors[34]: the reduction in forward flow, the regurgitant volume, the size and compliance of the left atrium and the pulmonary vascular bed, the development of tachyarrhythmias (atrial or ventricular) or thromboembolism, and rupture of the left atrial wall.

Primary MR of lesser degree does not induce any apparent change in indices of cardiac size or function. The forward stroke volume is maintained, and the small regurgitant volume is easily accepted by the left atrium. With progression of the valve lesions, the regurgitant part of the total left ventricular stroke volume increases, but several cardiac and non-cardiac (e.g., renal, neurohumoral, and vascular) compensatory mechanisms contribute to maintain the forward stroke volume.[13,34] The left ventricle compensates for the loss of forward stroke volume by increasing the end diastolic volume (preload) and, to some extent by increased heart rate.[35,36] However, the heart rate is usually not significantly changed until advanced stages of CMVI, when it increases.[34,36] The increased preload causes an increased force of contraction according to the Frank-Starling mechanism.[37] The resistance to ventricular emptying is reduced in the first stages of ejection because the regurgitant volume is ejected into the left atrium at low pressure, before sufficient pressure is generated at lower volume to open the aortic valve and cause forward ejection into the aorta. These mechanisms lead to exaggerated motion of the left ventricle (hyperkinesia). Myocardial systolic function is relatively well preserved because the ejection into the left atrium at low pressure require relatively little work by the left ventricle.

Patients may tolerate even severe CMVI for years.[7,34] Nevertheless, because of chronic volume overload and the fact that the hypertrophy, while necessary, is a pathologic remodeling, myocardial contractility decreases slowly, even in clinically compensated dogs, but progressively and inexorably.[7,35,38] Arteriosclerosis may complicate the condition by being the cause for multiple small myocardial infarctions, further decreases in contractility, and increased risk of congestive heart failure or sudden death.[28,29]

The left atrium has an important function by allowing the regurgitant volume to be absorbed within the atrial cavity, and it protects the pulmonary vascular bed from hypertension.[39] Increased left atrial pressure results in pulmonary venous congestion and edema. The effect of regurgitant volume on left atrial pressure and volume and consequently pulmonary capillary pressure, depends on the left atrial size, as well as on the compliance of the left atrial wall. Consequently, left atrial compliance is determined by the rate of increase in regurgitant volume, which itself is determined by the rate of progression of CMVI, and by remodeling in response to the volume overload. Maintained left ventricular compliance allows filling at low pressures with the large volume overload of MR, and is a result of the remodeling that is inherent in eccentric hypertrophy. In cases with slowly progressing CMVI, there is often a drastic enlargement of the left atrium, whereas pulmonary congestion and pulmonary edema develop late. The edema is also delayed by the development of a more effective lymphatic drainage of the pulmonary interstitium in chronic pulmonary venous hypertension.[40] The enlarged left atrium may induce coughing by compression of the left main stem bronchus that lies dorsal to the left atrium. In cases with acutely increased MR, as in rupture of a tendinous cord, the left atrium is unable to adapt, which results in a rapid elevation of left atrial pressure. Pulmonary capillary pressure subsequently increases, which leads to pulmonary congestion and edema.

Advanced cases of CMVI may be complicated by processes that are related to increased left atrial size and pressure.[7,41] The left atrium may rupture and cause cardiac tamponade; right-sided heart failure may develop as a consequence of concurrent tricuspid valve insufficiency and/or pulmonary artery hypertension; and tachyarrhythmias may develop as a consequence of ultrastructural changes in the myocardium. These complications are discussed later.

Clinical Signs

The progress of CMVI from the detection of a soft heart murmur to end-stage is often a matter of years in small dogs. Some large dogs appear to be less tolerant to CMVI. In these dogs, the disease has a more drastic progression with more severe clinical signs than in small dogs. The first clinical signs of decompensation are usually mild but may be aggravated within days or sometimes weeks. Since these signs are vague and not specific for decompensated heart failure, the differential diagnostic challenge in CMVI is often not if the disease is present, but whether or not CMVI is responsible for the clinical signs. The signs relate to the presence and degree of one or several of the following pathophysiologic events, listed in order of their relative importance: (1) elevated left atrial and pulmonary venous pressure, which results in respiratory distress and cough due to pulmonary edema and main-stem bronchial compression; (2) reduced left ventricular or right ventricular forward flow, which results in weakness and reduced stamina; (3) right-sided heart failure, which results in pleural effusion and ascites; (4) acute decompensation with fulminant pulmonary edema or ventricular fibrillation, which causes sudden death.

Mild to moderate CMVI is usually not associated with any signs of disease. Most dogs with CMVI are free of clinical signs for most of the time they have a murmur, although exercise intolerance might be noted. Cough is the most common presenting complaint in CMVI. Although this sign is not specific for heart disease or heart failure, it should merit further evaluation. In the case of advanced CMVI, the cough may be caused by pressure of the left atrium on the left mainstem bronchus, by pulmonary congestion and edema or, most commonly, a combination.[20] With pulmonary edema present, other common clinical signs are tachypnea and dyspnea. The dogs are often anxious and restless during the night while they lie in lateral recumbency (orthopnea) and prefer sternal positioning. In more advanced cases respiratory sounds, often wheezes, may be audible. These dogs are often inactive and have varying degrees of inappetence. Cardiac cachexia may develop, although loss of body weight may be masked by concurrent fluid retention and edema. Dogs with left mainstem bronchial compression but without pulmonary congestion or edema may have coughing spells at any time during the day, especially during physical exercise or excitement. Otherwise they do not demonstrate clinical signs.

Syncope is encountered in some dogs with CMVI. Syncope may be associated with a tachyarrhythmia, but the course of events often resembles that which is described in vasovagal syncope.[42] The frequency of the syncope vary from occasional spells to several attacks per day. Other causes of syncope include tussive fainting that may occur in conjunction with paroxysm of coughing or exercise in the presence of pulmonary hypertension.[20]

Physical Examination

A mid-systolic click is frequently encountered in early stages of CMVI (Figure 201-3, A),[43,44] although it may be difficult to detect by auscultation. The presence of this sound is dependent on heart rate and body position.[43] A systolic click may be accompanied by a low-intensity systolic murmur. The murmur is most frequently early systolic but may be late systolic or may in some dogs vary between the two. With progression, the most prominent clinical finding is a holosystolic heart murmur. The sound begins as a soft apical systolic murmur on the left side of the thorax and may be intermittent and sometimes audible only during inspiration (Figure 201-3, B). In the early stages of CMVI, the murmur can often be augmented by physical maneuvers, such as a short run.[43] With further progression, the sound becomes holosystolic and more intense (Figures 201-3, C, and 201-3, D)[13,15,43-45] and may radiate over to the right side of the thorax. A thrill may be palpated over the left thoracic wall (cardiac apical area) and the apical beat may be pronounced. Musical murmurs (whoop sounds) of high intensity occur less frequently. This murmur does not indicate the severity of CMVI (Figure 201-3, E).[44] There is usually a shift in the relative intensity of S1 and S2 (see Figure 201-3, D).[45] In the absence of significant myocardial failure, the first heart sound is usually enhanced, whereas the second heart sound becomes less intense.[20,44,45] A low-intensity third heart sound is often present, but this sound is often difficult to detect by auscultation (see Figure 201-3, D).[44,45] The presence of a clearly audible third (gallop) sound is a strong indicator for myocardial failure.[44] In cases of severe heart failure, the heart sounds and murmurs may be muffled by pleural effusion or cardiac tamponade. Thus even though auscultatory findings may be suggestive, the clinician must rely on the supporting historical, clinical, echocardiographic, and radiographic data to determine the hemodynamic significance of the insufficiency.

The presence of sinus arrhythmia in advanced CMVI indicates that decompensated heart failure is absent.[36] The heart rate increases in response to decreased forward cardiac output as decompensation develops, and the heart rate becomes more regular. A rapid and irregular heart rate is indicative of arrhythmia. The most common form of ectopy is atrial premature contractions. In more advanced CMVI, supraventricular

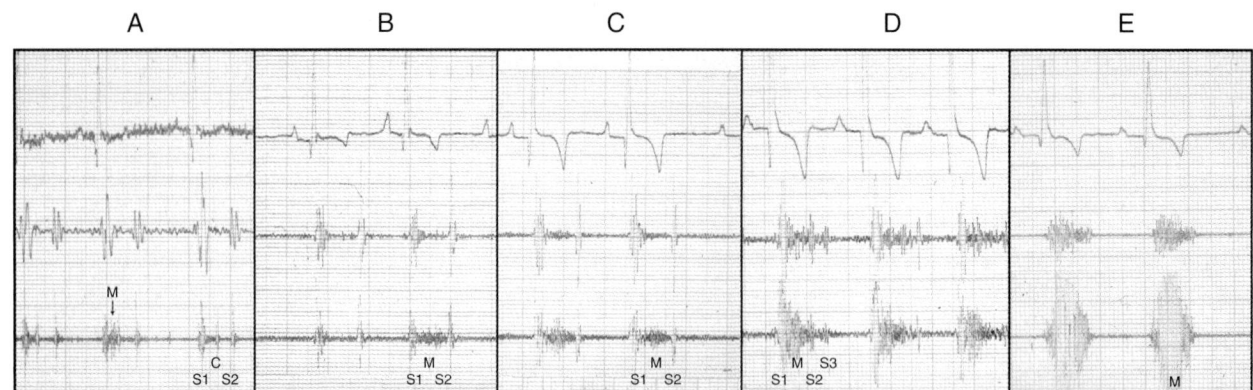

Figure 201-3 ECG lead II (upper registration) and phonocardiograms (middle and lower registrations) in dogs with different stages of CMVI. Recordings were obtained from the following dogs: **(A)** a dog with a systolic click (C) and an intermittent early systolic murmur (M), **(B)** a dog with an intermittent systolic murmur (M), **(C)** a dog with a continuous holosystolic murmur (M), **(D)** a dog in end-stage MR with a loud first heart sound (S1), a dampened second heart sound (S2), a systolic murmur (M) and a prominent third heart sound (S3), **(E)** a dog with a comparably uncommon high intensity musical murmur (M) where the intensity of the murmur does not reflect the severity of MR. (**A, B, C,** and **D** From Häggström J: Chronic valvular disease in Cavalier King Charles spaniels—epidemiology, inheritance and pathophysiology, thesis, Swedish University of Agricultural Sciences, Uppsala, 1996. **E** from Kvart C, Häggström J: Cardiac auscultation and phonocardiography in dogs, horses and cats, Uppsala, 2002.)

tachycardia, atrial fibrillation, and ventricular premature contractions may be encountered.

With sinus rhythm the femoral arterial pulse is usually normal. Weak pulses may be noted in heart failure. Weak and variable pulses with deficits can also be observed with rhythm disturbances. If tamponade occurs, owing to a tear in the left atrium and pericardial hemorrhage, the femoral pulse will be weak. Jugular venous distention may be present in severe heart failure, pulmonary hypertension, or pericardial effusion.

In cases of CMVI without signs of heart failure, the lung sounds are expected to be normal. Crackles, snaps, and popping sounds, best heard at end of inspiration, may be detected in advanced CMVI with pulmonary interstitial edema. Similar findings are common in dogs with small airway disease,[46] and if concurrent it may be a diagnostic challenge to determine the cause of the clinical signs. In more severe cases with alveolar edema, the pulmonary sounds are usually more pronounced and they may be auscultated even without a stethoscope.

Mucous membranes are usually normal, even in cases with pulmonary edema but may be cyanotic, grayish, or ashen in advanced cases of heart failure. Ascites in isolated CMVI is uncommon, but progressed CMVI often tends to involve the right side of the heart as a consequence of pulmonary hypertension or development of a tachyarrhythmia. In these dogs, ascites, hepatic, and splenic enlargement are common.

Electrocardiographic Findings
Electrocardiographic findings in CMVI vary from normal tracings to marked abnormalities in rate, rhythm, or configuration of complexes. With the exception to document and classify a certain arrhythmia, the ECG is of limited use in the diagnosis or management of CMVI. ECG is an insensitive indicator of cardiac enlargement and cannot detect heart failure or pulmonary edema.

Sinus arrhythmia is usually preserved during the early course of CMVI. In heart failure, sinus tachycardia and a loss of sinus arrhythmia are common.[36] Decompensated heart failure from CMVI should be questioned in a coughing patient with sinus arrhythmia. Cats with MR usually maintain sinus rhythm, although atrial fibrillation and/or ventricular ectopy may develop.

Most ECG abnormalities associated with CMVI are the result of accentuations of the normal ECG. The mean electrical axis in the frontal plane often remains within the normal range throughout the progression of the disease. In cases with significant left atrial enlargement, the P-wave may be prolonged. In cases of significant left ventricular enlargement, the QRS complex may be prolonged and the R wave amplitude in lead II increased,[47] but the former is generally a more reliable criteria to detect left ventricular enlargement.

Supraventricular premature beats are common in CMVI. In most cases, this finding is of little hemodynamic significance. Atrial fibrillation, paroxysmal supraventricular tachycardia, atrioventricular dissociation, ventricular premature beats, and ventricular tachycardia are less common. These arrhythmias are most often encountered in progressed cases and hence often indicate a poor prognosis.

Radiographic Findings
The value of radiography is in assessment of the hemodynamic consequences of CMVI (global cardiac size and presence of pulmomary congestion and edema). It helps to exclude other possible causes for the clinical signs: presence of pulmonary congestion and edema is of particular interest in geriatric dogs. Two orthogonal projections should be obtained: lateral and dorsoventral or ventrodorsal. Absolute straight positioning is essential for accurate evaluation of heart size and shape and position of the main bronchi. In dogs with CMVI, important structures to evaluate are the left atrium, the left ventricle, the mainstem bronchi, the pulmonary vessels, and the lungfield. Dogs with a low degree of CMVI usually have a normal heart size, normal lung fields, and normal vascular markings.

Left atrial enlargement is one of the earliest and most consistent radiologic features of CMVI. The left atrium and left ventricle continue to enlarge with progression of the disease. Signs of left atrial and left ventricular enlargement in lateral projection include dorsal elevation of the caudal portion of the trachea and carina; dorsal displacement of the left mainstem bronchus; visible prominence of the left atrium causing the caudal border of the heart to appear straight or bulge dorsocaudally (Figure 201-4). In the dorsoventral (or ventrodorsal) projection, the enlarged left atrial appendage may

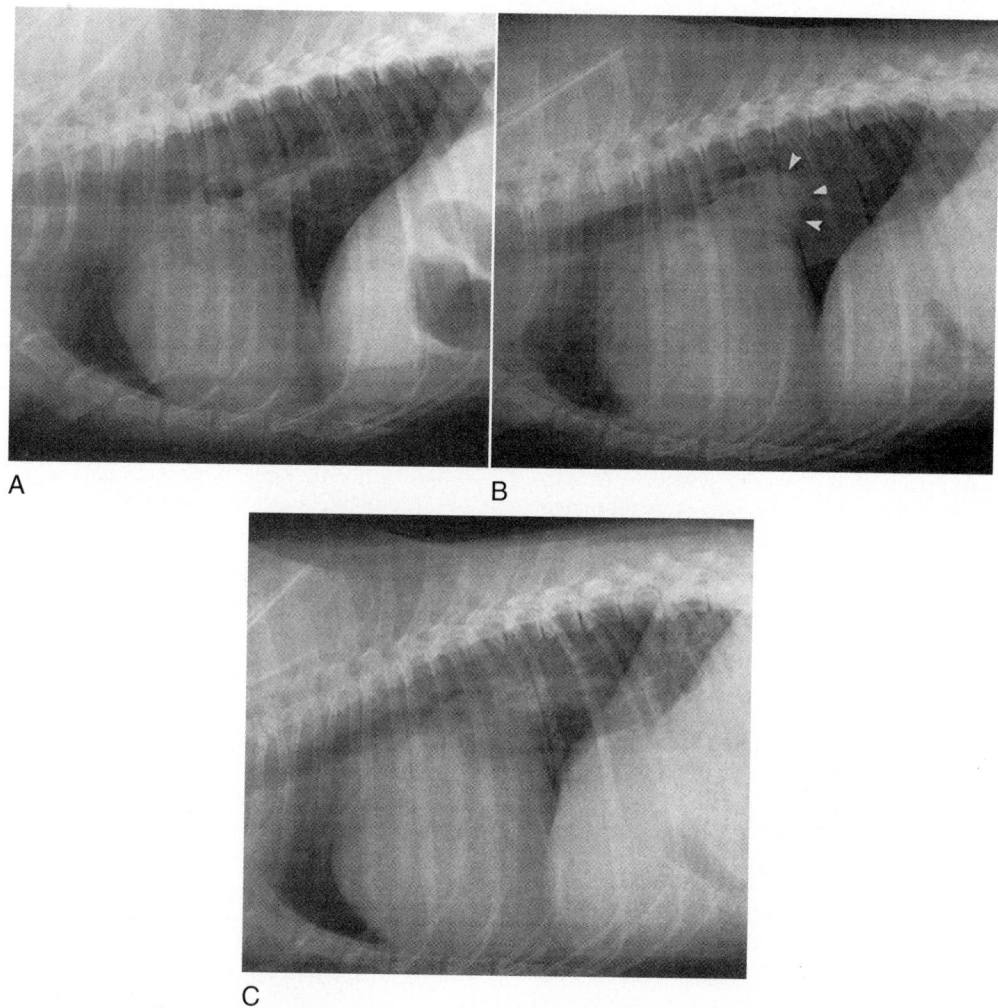

Figure 201-4 Radiographs in left lateral projection of a dog with CMVI: **(A)** The dog was at this time asymptomatic, and the radiograph shows a slight left atrial enlargement and normal vascular perfusion. **B,** Radiograph of the same dog 4 years later. The dog had developed exercise intolerance and persistent cough. Visible are marked left atrial *(white arrows)* and left ventricular enlargement and elevation and slight compression of the left mainstem bronchus, whereas the vascular markings are within normal limits. **C,** Six months later the dog had also developed dyspnea and had suffered episodes of syncope. In addition to the findings in previous radiograph **(B),** there is a more obvious compression of the left mainstem bronchus and evidence of pulmonary congestion and interstitial edema. (Courtesy Kerstin Hansson, Uppsala, Sweden.)

be identified as a bulge in the left cranial part of the cardiac border (between the 2 and 3 o'clock positions). The border of the enlarged left ventricle appears rounded and there may be a shift of the cardiac apex to the left or right. In advanced cases of decompensated CMVI, pleural effusion, ascites, and enlargement of the liver and spleen are commonly identified as signs of associated right heart failure.

During the progression of CMVI, radiographic signs of pulmonary congestion and edema usually develop. Pulmonary edema and congestion is more likely to be present in a dog with significant heart enlargement (indicating advanced CMVI) than in a dog with normal or slightly increased heart size. However, the degree of cardiac enlargement is poorly related to the severity of pulmonary congestion and edema (see Pathophysiology). Because many dogs with significant CMVI and enlarged hearts have not developed decompensated heart failure, therapy should be based primarily on clinical signs and the presence of pulmonary edema and congestion, not the degree of cardiac enlargement. Pulmonary venous distension,

when present, is an early indication of pulmonary congestion; the diameter of the veins is greater than that of the corresponding pulmonary arteries and they often become tortuous (especially in cats). However, venous distention is not a consistent finding even in dogs with pulmonary edema, and in some dogs, the outlining of the distended vein is indistinct as interstitial edema partially obscures the pulmonary vessels. With progression, interstitial and alveolar edema develop. In dogs, alveolar edema is often first detected in the perihilar region and the dorsal parts of the caudal lung lobes, sometimes more prominent on the right side, but acute edema may involve the cranial lobes. In cats, the location of a cardiogenic pulmonary edema is not as predictable as in dogs. It commonly has an ill-defined, patchy appearance.

Pulmonary findings may be inconclusive, since early radiographic changes of pulmonary interstitial edema and bronchial pattern resemble the radiographic appearance of chronic airway disease. The tendency is to overdiagnose pulmonary edema of heart failure. It is therefore important, if possible, to have series of radiographs and evaluate other evidence of left-sided heart failure that should be present by the time pulmonary edema has developed, such as venous distention, before diagnosis is determined.

Echocardiographic Findings

Echocardiography is useful for obtaining a diagnosis of CMVI, and thereafter to monitor the condition, although it cannot diagnose the presence of heart failure. Two-dimensional echocardiography allows the ultrasonographer to evaluate the anatomy of the mitral valve and to identify leaflet thickening and leaflet protrusion into the left atrium. A systolic bulging of one or both leaflets to the atrial side of the mitral annulus is an early indication of affected valves and it may be present in dogs with or without mitral regurgitation (MR).[15,48] The presence and severity of protrusion of the leaflets may be measured in the right parasternal long axis view.[16,48]

In cases with insufficient valves, the degree of displacement is reported to relate well with the severity of MR.[15,16,48] With progression, the degenerative changes become more prominent and the leaflets often have an irregular "club-like" appearance with greatest thickening at the tip (Figure 201-5, *B*). The gross pathologic changes of the two leaflets (anterior and posterior) are often equally severe at postmortem examination, but the degenerative changes commonly appear more prominent on the anterior leaflet in the right parasternal long axis view on the echocardiogram.

It is important to examine the entire valve as the lesions are often quite unevenly distributed. Chordal thickening may be identified and systolic displacement (prolapse) of the leaflets or a valve flail may be evident (Figure 201-5, *C*). Valve flail is when the edge of a leaflet or, in severe cases, a complete leaflet moves into the left atrium in systole. The finding of a valve flail leads to the suspicion of chordal rupture, which may occasionally be identified in the left atrium or in the left ventricle.[24]

The left atrium is an important structure to evaluate with MR because its size reflects disease severity. The general "rule of thumb" is that the larger the left atrium, the greater is the degree of MR present, but there are exceptions (see Pathophysiology).

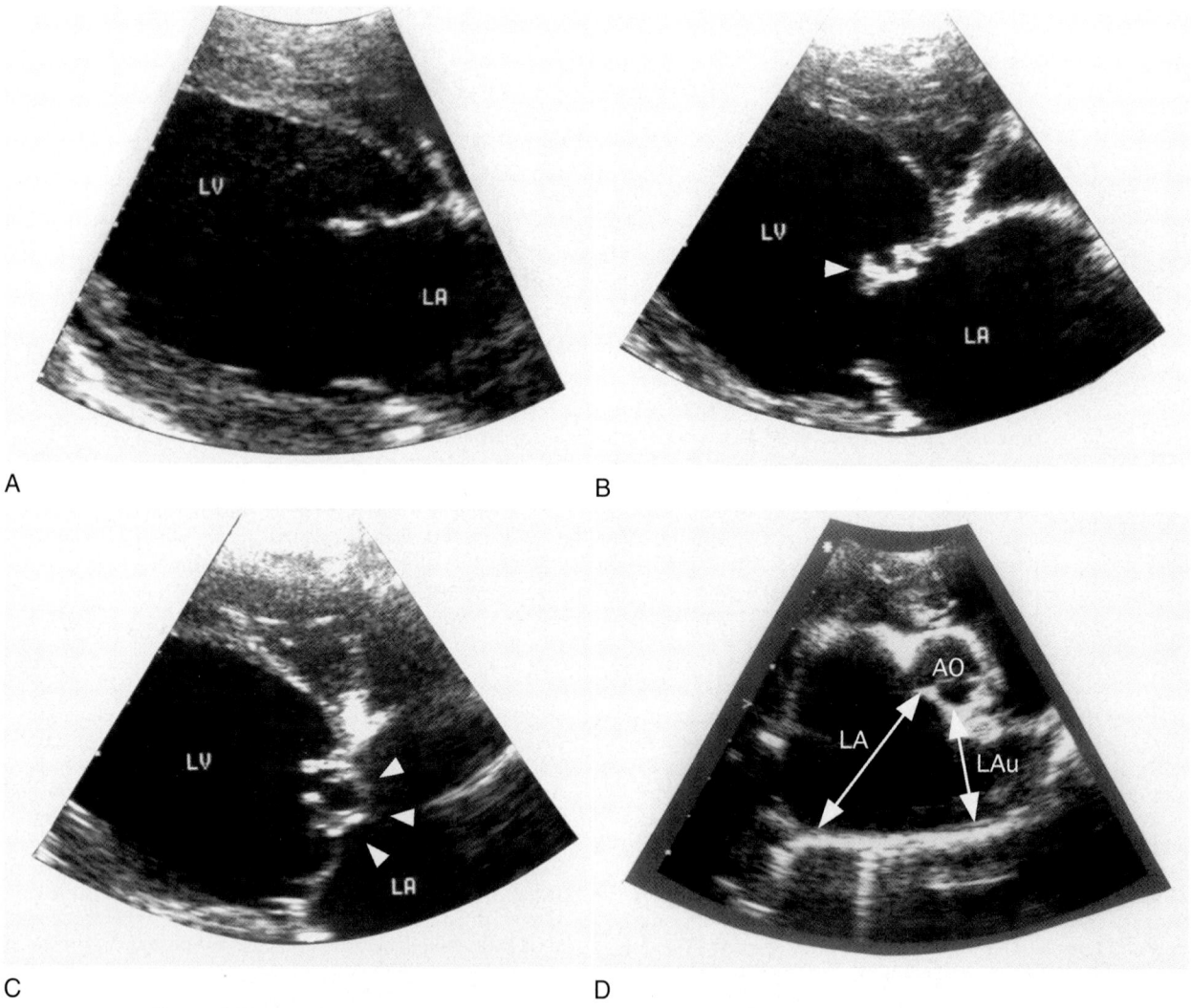

Figure 201-5 Echocardiographic right parasternal long-axis views of the left atrium *(LA)* and left ventricle *(LV)* during diastole (**A** and **B**) and systole (**C**), in a normal dog (**A**), and in the same dog with CMVI (**B** and **C**). The mitral valve appears thickened (**B**) *(arrowhead)*, and there is systolic displacement of both leaflets to the atrial side of the mitral annulus (**C**). Figure **D** shows the left atrium in a right parasternal short axis view at the aortic valve *(AO)* level of a dog with severely enlarged left atrium. The *arrows* demonstrate the difference in LA diameter obtained by measuring the greatest diameter and the diameter often used in M-mode. *Lau,* Left auricle.

Although the left atrium may be examined from a right parasternal long axis view and a left apical four chamber view, the best view is the the right parasternal short axis view with the aortic root, the left atrial body and the auricle in view (Figure 201-5, D). The most useful information from this view is the left atrial size because it can be compared with the size of the aortic root, which is relatively constant for a given dog size. The normal ratio of the left atrial diameter to the aortic root (LA/Ao) in M-mode is reported to be between 0.8 to 1.2.[49] With the more traditional M-mode method, however, the left atrial dimension measured is not the largest that can be obtained, as it measures the diameter of the left atrial appendage or underestimates the diameter of the left atrial body. In dogs with MR, the diameter of the left atrial body may be considerably greater than that of the left atrial appendage (see Figure 201-5, D).[50] The normal range for 2D La/Ao values is reported to be 0.84 to 1.27 in Cavalier King Charles spaniels and 0.86 to 1.59 in a mixture of breeds.[50,51] In the authors' experience, a 2D La/Ao greater than 1.5 represents an enlarged left atrium in all breeds. This limit is presumably lower in specific breeds. Early cases of CMVI with a small degree of MR have no echocardiographic signs of left atrial enlargement. With progression of CMVI the left atrial dimension increases and dogs in congestive heart failure often have a left atrial to aortic root ratio of 2 or greater.[52]

Evaluation of left ventricular size and motion is important in MR and measurements are often obtained in the M-mode. Mild MR usually does not lead to abnormal dimensions. With progression, the left ventricular-end-diastolic short axis dimension increases, whereas the end-systolic dimension does not increase at the same rate. The left ventricular wall thickness is usually within normal limits. The increased size of the left ventricle combined with a normal wall thickness indicates that volume overload and eccentric hypertrophy are present. An increase in left ventricular end-diastolic dimension in the presence of normal or minimally increased left ventricular end-systolic dimension is a consequence of increased preload and rapid left ventricular emptying into the low-pressure left atrium.[7,53] In MR, values of ejection phase indices (e.g., left ventricular fractional shortening, ejection fraction, and mean velocity of circumferential shortening) are often normal (mild MR) or greater than normal (moderate to severe MR). Therefore in the setting of moderate or severe MR, a normal fractional shortening represents a significant reduction of myocardial contractility. End-systolic volume indices (e.g., left ventricular end-systolic short axis dimension or end-systolic volume index) more accurately estimate myocardial contractility in MR.[7,53] However, when heart failure is present and the sympathetic nervous system is activated to increase apparent contractility, even these measurements overestimate intrinsic myocardial contractility.[38]

End-systolic dimension may increase in small dogs with end-stage CMVI, but increase appears to be more common in large dogs that present with heart failure and severe MR but with a fractional shortening in the normal range or slightly increased. In these dogs, the mitral valve leaflets may or may not look as severely affected as in small dogs. Often, they look less affected, and it is currently an enigma why these dogs present with severe MR and prominent myocardial failure. The large dogs with MR and myocardial failure may be confused with DCM, but DCM may be questioned in a dog with normal or slightly depressed fractional shortening. It has been suggested that these dogs may actually suffer from congenital mitral dysplasia rather than myxomatous degeneration.[54] Mild pericardial effusion may be present in dogs with heart failure, whereas significant pericardial effusion should raise the suspicion of another disease or of a complication of CMVI such as left atrial rupture. Mild pleural effusion may also be evident in dogs with heart failure.

It is rare, even in severe cases of CMVI, to detect incomplete closure of the leaflets as means of confirmation of the presence of MR. Instead, the valvular insufficiency may be detected and quantified by spectral or color-flow Doppler.[43] Ideally, the regurgitant flow should be aligned with the ultrasound beam and this is most often acheived in the left apical four-chamber view. As the flow direction depends on the orientation of the regurgitant orifice, which, in turn depends on the leaflet morphology, other views may also give good alignment. Spectral Doppler may be used to identify the regurgitant jet when color-Doppler mapping is not available. Furthermore, spectral Doppler gives information of the velocity of the regurgitant jet and velocity time tracings may help in estimating regurgitant volume (see below). Typically, dogs with CMVI without myocardial failure have a velocity of the regurgitant jet of 5 to 6 m/sec.[54] However, the velocity may be increased in individuals with systemic hypertension and decreased in individuals with hypotension, significantly increased left atrial pressure or myocardial failure.

Color-flow echocardiography confirms the presence of a regurgitant jet and the size of the jet can be compared with the size of the left atrium. This measurement is semiquantitative in dogs and cats. A small jet rules out moderate to severe MR, but it is difficult to discriminate between moderate and severe regurgitation from the jet size. Small jets in the vicinity of the mitral valve should not be overinterpreted in dogs without any other valve abnormality, as trivial regurgitation may often be detected in normal dogs.[55] Recently, it was demonstrated that the regurgitant fraction may be quantified with use of the proximal isovelocity surface area (PISA) color-flow method in dogs with MR (Figure 201-6).[56,57] In MR, blood

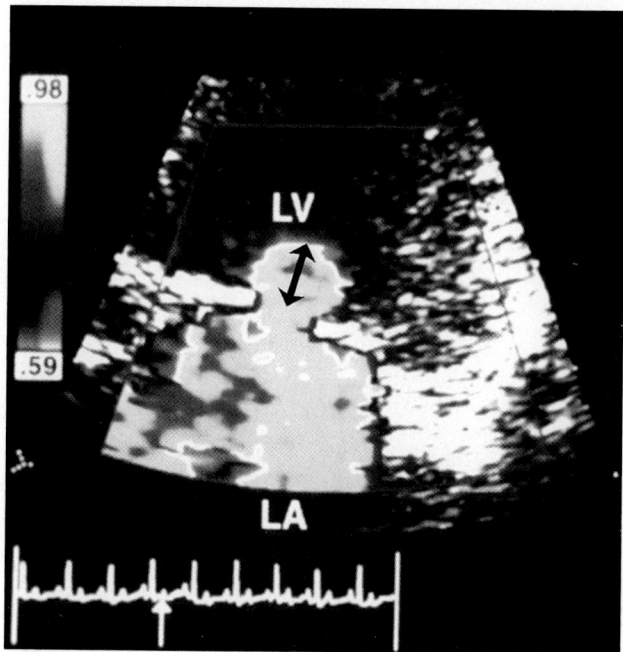

Figure 201-6 Zoomed color-flow Doppler image of the mitral valve in a left apical 4-chamber view showing the hemicircle of the flow convergence on the ventricular side of the mitral valve. The radius of the proximal isovelocity region is measured from the ventricular side of the mitral valve leaflets to the edge of the hemisphere (*double-sided arrow*). The radius of the hemisphere is used to calculate the regurgitant fraction of the total stroke volume. There is also evidence of significant regurgitation into the left atrium. *LV*, left ventricular chamber; *LA*, left atrial chamber. (From Kittleson MD, Brown WA: Regurgitant fraction measured by using the proximal isovelocity surface area in dogs with chronic myxomatous mitral valve disease, *J Vet Intern Med* 17:84, 2003.)

flow converges on the ventricular side of the mitral valve orifice before it passes the regurgitant orifice, and this area is characterized on the color-Doppler echocardiogram as a hemisphere. Based on the values of the radius of this hemisphere, the aliasing velocity, the maximal velocity of the regurgitant jet, and the velocity time integral of the regurgitant flow (the latter two are obtained from spectral Doppler measurements), the regurgitant stroke volume may be calculated. The regurgitant fraction is obtained by dividing the regurgitant volume with the sum of the forward and regurgitant stroke volumes. Although this method has significant advantages compared to other methods of measuring regurgitant fraction, it has several practical limitations and may not be readily applicable in all cases of MR.

The mitral regurgitant stroke volume may also be estimated indirectly using the difference between total stroke volume and forward stroke volume into the aorta. The total stroke volume may be estimated using M-mode measurements of left ventricular size, and the forward stroke volume may be estimated by multiplying the aortic cross sectional area with the velocity time integral obtained from the spectral Doppler tracing of the aortic flow. Alternatively, the total stroke volume may be estimated by multiplying the annular cross-sectional area of the mitral valve obtained from the two-dimensional mode with the velocity time integral obtained from the spectral Doppler tracing of the diastolic flow over the valve. Both these methods involve multiple measurements, each with its own errors, which means that they will only provide estimates of regurgitant volume. Measurements of regurgitant fraction in dogs with moderate to severe MR indicate that they can eject more than 75% of the total stroke volume into the left atrium, which is remarkable.

At present, none of the Doppler methods (subjective estimation of jet size, spectral Doppler methods, and the PISA method) have been shown to be more reliable indicators of disease severity than left atrial size in dogs and cats with MR. Spectral Doppler may be used to study the transmitral flow during diastole. Significant mitral regurgitation is usually associated with increased diastolic filling velocities as a consequence of increased diastolic transmitral flow.[58] Furthermore, abnormal diastolic ventricular function as a consequence of severe volume overload may be detected. It is important to time the events when evaluating the transmitral flow to separate systolic regurgitation from diastolic to avoid a false-positive diagnosis of clinically significant mitral regurgitation. Diastolic regurgitation is common in cases with bradycardia or arrhythmias and probably indicates small reverse pressure gradients during cardiac filling.[59]

Differential Diagnosis

The signalment, clinical signs, and physical examination findings are often such that they strongly suggest CMVI. Although the usual cause for MR is myxomatous degeneration, other causes are noteworthy: dilated and hypertrophic cardiomyopathy; widespread arteriosclerosis with myocardial infarcts; bacterial endocarditis of the mitral valve; undiscovered congenital heart disease, such as mitral valve dysplasia and patent ductus arteriosus (PDA). Early cases of CMVI may have an early systolic heart murmur that may be confused with slight aortic or pulmonic stenosis or physiologic flow murmur. Often the early or late systolic murmur due to MR is accompanied by a systolic click, which is an indicator for early myxomatous degeneration and mitral valve prolapse. The signalment, point of maximal intensity of the murmur, and echocardiography are distinctions between slight MR and slight aortic or pulmonic stenosis and physiologic flow murmurs. Furthermore, dogs with slight MR are usually old and the murmur has maximal intensity over the mitral area, whereas dogs with physiologic flow murmurs or aortic or pulmonic

stenosis are usually young and have a murmur with maximal intensity over the heart base. The exclusion of dilated cardiomyopathy and hypertrophic cardiomyopathy requires echocardiographic examination. However, it may not be possible to discriminate CMVI from DCM in some medium- and large-sized dogs, such as Cocker spaniels, which present with valvular abnormalities, significant MR, left ventricular and left atrial enlargement and a normal to subnormal fractional shortening. Measurement of biochemical markers of myocardial damage, such as Troponins, may aid in diagnosing myocardial infarcts, provided that the myocardial damage was recent and significant.[60]

The echocardiographic appearance of a mitral valve affected with endocarditis may appear very similar to nodular thickening of valve leaflets characteristic for myxomatous degeneration. However, lesions of endocarditis may be more echogenic and more isolated. The signalment usually helps to distinguish between these two diseases. Bacterial endocarditis occurs most frequently in large dogs; CMVI is more common in small dogs; dogs with bacterial endocarditis often have a history of fever, arthritis, systemic disease, a recently developed heart murmur, and clinical signs that may indicate thromboembolic disease. Dogs with CMVI are usually older, often have had a heart murmur for years, and do not have fever or signs of systemic disease. Bilateral regurgitation is commonly encountered, but isolated tricuspid regurgitation does occur. In these cases, the heart murmur may radiate to the left side of the thorax.

Although CMVI may readily be diagnosed in a patient with clinical signs, the true diagnostic challenge lies in determining if decompensated heart failure is the underlying cause. Most dogs with CMVI are older, small to medium-sized dogs, and many of these dogs exercise little. Thus exercise intolerance may be difficult to identify and, if present, difficult to attribute to the heart condition as obesity, chronic joint disease, and other disease may be present. Furthermore, the hallmark of left side heart failure, coughing and dyspnea, may be caused by several conditions, such as small airway disease, tracheal instability, pulmonary fibrosis, neoplasia, heartworm disease, and pneumonia. Many of these differential diagnoses can be excluded by different clinical tests, particularly radiography, but in some cases, the results may be inclusive. In these cases, a 48- to 72-hour trial diuretic therapy with repeat radiographs may help to identify the underlying etiology. In addition, "bedside" assays of natriuretic peptides (ANP and BNP) will soon be available to aid in diagnosis of such cases.

Management

Ideally, therapy of CMVI would halt the progression of the valvular degeneration. Improvement of valvular function by surgical repair or valve replacement would likewise stop further deterioration. However, no therapy is currently known to inhibit or prevent the valvular degeneration, and surgery is usually not technically, economically, or ethically possible in canine and feline patients. The management of CMVI is therefore concerned with improving quality of life, by ameliorating the clinical signs and improving survival. This usually means that therapy is tailored for the individual patient, owner, and practitioner and often involves concurrent treatment with two or more drugs once signs of heart failure are evident. Management of CMVI will be discussed in five groups of patients: those without overt signs of heart failure (asymptomatic), those with left mainstem bronchial compression, those with syncope, those with mild to moderate heart failure, those with recurrent heart failure, and those with severe and fulminant heart failure. Possible complications are discussed separately. It is unusual to treat cases of isolated CMVI in cats and details of drug dosages for cats are therefore not included in this section.

Asymptomatic Disease

The stage when a patient starts to show clinical signs of CMVI, that is, have developed decompensated heart failure, is the end of a process started much earlier with the onset of valve leakage. The valvular leakage was compensated through a variety of mechanisms but as the leakage increases the valves eventually became incapable of preventing pulmonary capillary pressures from exceeding the threshold for pulmonary edema, and of maintaining forward cardiac output. It is likely that minor signs of reduced activity and mobility are present even before overt signs of heart failure develop. However, it is very difficult to objectively evaluate the presence of slight to moderately reduced exercise capacity in most dogs with CMVI, as they are often old small companion dogs, which if obese, have little, if any, demand on their exercise capacity. Furthermore, other concurrent diseases in the locomotor system or elsewhere are common and restrict exercise. Thus vague clinical signs such as slightly reduced exercise capacity in a typical dog with progressed CMVI may or may not be attributable to CMVI.

This dilemma leads to the questions of when to start therapy, and if therapy before the onset of decompensated heart failure is beneficial, ineffective, or harmful. ACE-inhibitors are frequently prescribed to dogs with CMVI before the onset on heart failure. At present, however, there is no evidence that administration of any medication to a patient with asymptomatic CMVI has a preventive effect on development and progression of clinical signs of heart failure or improves survival. Two large placebo-controlled multicenter trials, the SVEP and the VetProof trials,[14,61] have been conducted to study the effect of monotherapy of the ACE-inhibitor enalapril on the progression of clinical signs in asymptomatic CMVI in dogs. Both failed to show a significant difference between the placebo and the treatment groups in time from onset of therapy to confirmed congestive heart failure (Figure 201-7).[14,61] The two trials differ in the following features: the SVEP trial included only dogs of one breed (Cavalier King Charles spaniels) whereas the VetProof trial included a variety of breeds. The dogs in the VetProof trial were more frequently progressed cases of CMVI than the dogs in the SVEP trial, and the SVEP trial comprised more dogs than the VetProof trial (229 versus 139 dogs). Suggested reasons for the non-significant findings in these trials include lack of activation of circulating RAAS activity in asymptomatic animals,[62] low concentration of angiotensin II receptors in the canine mitral valve,[63] or lack of effect of ACE-inhibitors on myocardial remodeling and progressive ventricular dilatation in MR.[64]

Owners of dogs with progressed asymptomatic CMVI should be instructed about signs of developing heart failure and, in case of breeding, about the fact that the disease is significantly influenced by genetic factors. The disease may be monitored at regular intervals of 3 to 12 months if significant cardiomegaly is present. Milder cases do not warrant frequent monitoring (see Significance and Progression). Frequently asked questions from owners of dogs with asymptomatic CMVI are if exercise should be restricted and if dietary measures should be instituted. At present there is little evidence-based information concerning the effects of exercise or diet on the progression of CMVI in dogs. Dogs with mild CMVI do not need any dietary or exercise restriction. However, from the pathophysiologic standpoint, strenuous exercise or diets with high sodium content should be avoided in progressed CMVI as this may promote pulmonary edema. Furthermore, it is the authors' experience that dogs with advanced asymptomatic CMVI usually tolerate comparably long walks at their own pace and do better if obesity is avoided.

Patients with Left Mainstem Bronchial Compression Without Pulmonary Congestion and Edema

Severe left atrial enlargement may produce coughing even in the absence of pulmonary congestion and edema by compression of the left mainstem bronchi, which may be identified on the lateral radiograph. With significant coughing, therapy is aimed at suppression of the cough reflex or reduction of the influence of the underlying cause for the compression, the left atrial enlargement. Cough suppressants such as butorphanol (0.55 to 1.1 mg/kg q6-12h PO), hydrocodone bitartrate (0.22 mg/kg q4-8h PO), or dextromethorphan (0.5 to 2 mg/kg q6-8h PO) may alleviate the coughing in some cases. Dogs with evidence of concurrent tracheal instability or chronic small airway disease may improve with a bronchodilator, or a brief course of glucocorticoids. Different xanthine derivatives, such as aminophylline (8 to 11 mg/kg q6-8h) and theophylline (Theo-Dur (sustained duration) 20 mg/kg q12h PO, Detriphylline (Choledyl) (sustained action) 25 to 30 mg/kg q12h PO), are commonly used bronchodilators, although the efficacy of these drugs varies considerably between individuals. Beta 2-receptor agonists such as terbutaline and albuterol should be used with caution in CMVI dogs, as these drugs may produce unwanted elevation in heart rate and contractility as a consequence of myocardial beta 2-receptor stimulation. A reduction of left atrial size may be obtained either by reduction of the regurgitation or by reduction of pulmonary venous pressure. Regurgitation can be decreased by reducing aortic impedance with an arterial dilator or by contracting blood volume with a diuretic.

ACE-inhibitors or a directly acting arterial vasodilator, such as hydralazine, may reduce systemic arterial resistance.[65] The ACE-inhibitors are substantially weaker arterial vasodilators than hydralazine.[65] Side effects of ACE-inhibitors are infrequent, but monitoring of renal function and serum electrolytes, particularly potassium, may be indicated.

Hydralazine has been widely used in patients with CMVI at an initial dosage of 0.5 mg/kg every 12 hours PO. The dosage is increased at daily to weekly intervals to an appropriate maintenance dose of 1 to 2 mg/kg every 12 hours PO, or until

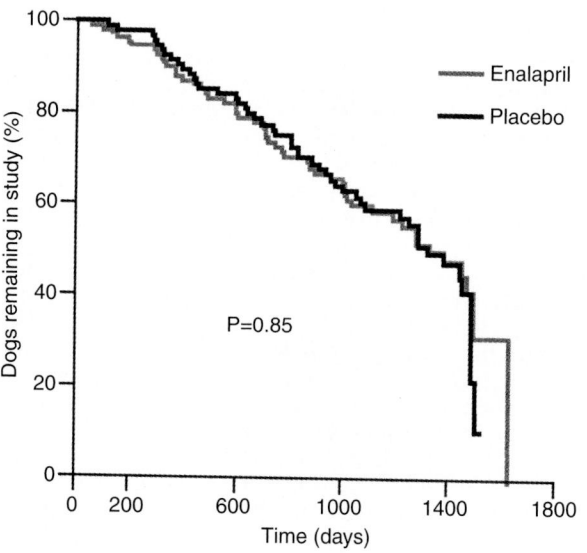

Figure 201-7 The SVEP study investigated the effect of enalapril on preventing decompensated heart failure in dogs with asymptomatic CMVI. The graph shows the percentage of dogs included in the enalapril and the placebo groups, respectively, versus time. The difference in number of days in the study between placebo- and enalapril treated dogs was not significant. (From Kvart C et al: Efficacy of enalapril for prevention of congestive heart failure in dogs with myxomatous valve disease and asymptomatic mitral regurgitation, *J Vet Intern Med* 16:80, 2002.)

hypotension develops, detected either by blood pressure measurements or by clinical signs. Clinical hypotension is defined as a mean arterial blood pressure of less than 50 to 60 mm Hg or a systolic blood pressure below 90 mm Hg.[54] Reflex tachycardia may develop in response to hypotension, and gastrointestinal problems are sometimes observed. In tachycardia, digoxin may be considered in order to limit the resting heart rate. As a consequence of hypotension, hydralazine may induce fluid retention and thereby is needed in the form of a diuretic.[66] Patients that receive hydralazine should routinely be monitored, including having the owner check the heart rate at home and having renal function assessed periodically. Diuretic monotherapy may be considered to decrease the MR by contracting the blood volume and thereby the left ventricular size. However, diuretics activate the renin-angiotensin-aldosterone system (RAAS),[66] and in the long term may cause electrolyte disturbances. Accordingly, these drugs are often reserved for patients with signs of pulmonary congestion and edema or patients in which cough suppressants, glucocortocoids, and vasodilators have failed to alleviate clinical signs.

Patients with Syncopes but Without Pulmonary Congestion and Edema

With advancing CMVI it is not uncommon that episodes of syncope develop in otherwise asymptomatic dogs (see Clinical Signs). These episodes vary in frequency from isolated to multiple events every day. In dogs with CMVI with syncope, it is important to ascertain that the patient is actually fainting and not suffering from neurologic or metabolic disease. Furthermore, it is important to rule out the presence of congestive heart failure or a bradyarrhythmia such as third degree AV-block or a tachyarrhythmia such as atrial fibrillation. Although ventricular tachyarrhythmias do occur in dogs with advanced CMVI, supraventricular tachyarrhythmia is far more common. Typically, the 24-hour (Holter) ECG shows episodes of a rapid supraventricular rhythm immediately followed by a bradycardia during which the dog faints. Management of these dogs often includes digoxin to control the supraventricular tachyarrhythmia. In fact, the frequency of syncopes may often be controlled at lower doses, such as 50%, of digoxin than the recommended dose (which is 0.22 mg/m2 q12h PO). The place for beta-blockers in controlling episodes of fainting in CMVI dogs is not clear. Reports indicate positive results of carvedilol in some dogs.[67] However, beta-blockers may reduce myocardial performance and some CMVI dogs do not tolerate this type of therapy.

Patients with Pulmonary Edema Secondary to CMVI

Considering the pathophysiology of CMVI, therapy should be directed toward (1) reduction of the venous pressures to alleviate edema and effusions, (2) maintainance of adequate cardiac output to prevent signs of weakness, lethargy and prerenal azotemia, (3) reduction of the cardiac workload and regurgitation, and (4) protection of the heart from negative long-term effects of neurohormones. Cases with mild pulmonary edema may be managed on an outpatient basis with regular re-examinations. Cases with moderate to severe pulmonary edema may need intensive care, including cage-rest and sometimes oxygen supplementation.

Mild to Moderate Heart Failure

Patients with mild to moderate heart failure usually present with cough, tachypnea, and dyspnea. It is not common for an untreated dog in congestive heart failure to present initially with isolated significant ascites. Signs of congestive heart failure are usually present on thoracic radiographs as pulmonary venous congestion and increased pulmonary opacity. In some cases, it may be difficult to appreciate mild edema owing to obesity, chest conformation, underinflated lungs, or presence of age-related changes. Radiographs from the patient obtained

before the onset of clinical signs may be helpful for comparison. Dogs with mild to moderate heart failure should be treated. Treatment can often be managed on an outpatient basis and should include a diuretic, such as furosemide, and an ACE-inhibitor. The place of digoxin and other positive inotropes are more controversial for treating dogs with mild to moderate heart failure (see below). The dosage of furosemide should preferably be based on clinical signs rather than radiographic findings. A patient may breathe with ease even in the presence of radiologic signs of interstitial edema, or vice versa. The usual course of treatment of a case with mild to moderate heart failure is an initial intensive treatment with furosemide (2 to 4 mg/kg q8-12h) for 2 to 3 days, after which the dosage of the diuretic is decreased to a maintenance level, such as 1 to 2 mg/kg every 12 to 48 hours or lower. More severe cases of heart failure may require higher dosages. It is important to use an appropriate dosage of diuretic to relieve clinical signs but to avoid an unnecessarily high maintenance dosage. Overzealous use of diuretics may lead to weakness, hypotension, syncope, aggravation of prerenal azotemia, and acid-base and electrolyte imbalances. Often the owner can be instructed to vary the dosage, within a fixed dose range, according to the need of the dog.

The dosage of ACE-inhibitor (e.g., enalapril, benazepril, lisinopril, ramipril, and imidapril) is usually fixed and depends on the specific ACE-inhibitor used. ACE-inhibitors are indicated in advanced CMVI with heart failure in combination with diuretics, because dogs in large placebo-controlled clinical trials receiving an ACE-inhibitor have been shown to have less severe clinical signs of disease, better exercise tolerance,[68-70] and live longer than those not receiving an ACE-inhibitor.[68-70] In the dose range that is recommended for use in dogs and cats, the vasodilating actions of the drugs are not prominent and side effects associated with hypotension, such as fainting and syncope, are rare.[14,65,69,70] A reason for this may be that the short-term effects of ACE-inhibitors on the circulation are dependent on the activity of the RAAS prior to administration of the drug, the higher activity the more pronounced effect of the drug.[62] In combination with diuretics, such as furosemide, the ACE-inhibitors have synergistic effect with the diuretic by counteracting the reflectory stimulation of RAAS that occurs in diuretic therapy. Thus they decrease the tendency for fluid retention and counteract a peripheral vasoconstriction and other negative effects on the heart.

Digoxin is controversial in treating dogs with CMVI. There is generally a lack of scientific evidence supporting the use of digoxin. Many cardiologists, however, initiate digoxin therapy when signs of heart failure first appear. Although digoxin is a comparably weak positive inotrope and myocardial failure may not be a prominent feature of CMVI until progressed stages, digoxin has a place in heart failure therapy by reducing reflex tachycardia, by normalizing baroreceptor activity and by reducing central sympathetic activity.[71] Thus digoxin may be useful to reduce the heart rate, such as when hydralazine is administered, or in supraventricular tachycardia such as atrial fibrillation, and to abolish or limit the frequency of syncope (see above).

The place for a positive inotrope in the management of CMVI is controversial, since in small dogs signs of left-side heart failure usually precede overt myocardial failure. Nevertheless, the combined calcium sensitizer/PDE III inhibitor pimobendan is now approved for veterinary use in dogs with DCM and CMVI in many European countries, Canada, and Australia at a dose of 0.25 mg/kg every 12 hours PO. Data from controlled clinical trials of pimobendan in veterinary patients is available, although its efficacy is less documented in CMVI than in DCM. Recently, two controlled clinical trials (the PITCH trial and a recently completed study from UK) were presented (unpublished).[72,73] The results indicate that dogs with CMVI receiving pimobendan as adjunct therapy to diuretics show less severe signs of heart failure and are less likely to die or reach the treatment failure end-point than those receiving an ACE-inhibitor and diuretics. Many practitioners using pimobendan have experienced a dramatic improvement in overall clinical status in some CVMI dogs, even in dogs without overt myocardial failure. The reason for this may be that pimobendan, in addition to being a positive inotrope, has arterial vasodilating properties and differs from the pure PDE III antagonists (such as milrinone) in that it increases myocardial contractility with minimal increase in myocardial energy consumption. Furthermore, positive inotropes may theoretically reduce the MR by decreasing the size of the left ventricle and the mitral valve annulus through a more complete emptying of the left ventricle. However, the increased contractility may also theoretically lead to an increased systolic pressure gradient across the mitral valve and thereby generate increased regurgitation in some cases with high peripheral vascular resistance and increase the risk for chordal rupture in affected dogs. Therefore some cardiologists initiate pimobendan as adjunct therapy to other heart failure treatment in CMVI dogs only when echocardiographic evidence of reduced myocardial performance (increased left ventricular end-systolic dimension) is evident. Whether or not this treatment strategy is the optimal use of calcium sensitizers has not been evaluated. Some cases of CMVI with evidence of myocardial failure have evidence of disseminated myocardial micro-infarctions, most commonly as a consequence of widespread arteriosclerosis.[28,29] Some of these patients might benefit from prophylactic antithrombotic and antiplatelelet therapy, although this has not been evaluated in veterinary medicine.

The way dogs with mild to moderate heart failure are managed after initiation of therapy varies. Typically, the dog is re-examined after 1 to 2 weeks of therapy, if the dog is managed on an outpatient basis, to monitor therapeutic outcome and to establish a suitable maintenance dosage of diuretic. Should the treatment response be satisfactory after this visit, dogs may often be managed by phone contacts and re-examinations every 3 to 6 months. More severe cases may require more frequent monitoring of the disease. In areas with a seasonal climate it may be valuable to re-examine the dog before the temperature increases and instruct the owner to avoid high ambient temperatures. The use of low-sodium diets as complementary therapy in heart failure is controversial. Currently, there are no clinical studies to support that they are beneficial in managing heart failure in dogs and cats. However, dogs with symptomatic CMVI should avoid excessive intake of sodium. Dogs that are stable on their heart failure therapy usually tolerate walks at their own pace, but strenuous exercise should be avoided.

Recurrent Heart Failure

Once an appropriate maintenance dosage of furosemide has been set in a CMVI patient with decompensated heart failure, the dosage has to be gradually increased, often over weeks or years. Reasons for increasing the dosage often include recurrent dyspnea caused by pulmonary edema or the development of ascites. Severe ascites, which compromises respiration, may require abdominocentesis. Many CMVI cases with less severe ascites respond to an increased dose of diuretics. Even in case of abdominocentesis, the diuretic dosage should be increased as the ascites will re-occur without changed medication after evacuation. When the dosage of furosemide has reached a level of approximately 4 to 5 mg/kg every 8 to 12 hours, sequential blocking of the nephron should be considered by adding another diuretic. The drug of choice is spironolactone (1 to 3 mg q12-24h PO) which is an aldosterone antagonist and a potassium-sparing diuretic. A thiazide, such as hydrochlorothiazide (2 to 4 mg/kg q12h PO), or triamterene (1 to 2 mg/kg q12h PO) or amiloride (0.1 to 0.3 mg/kg q24h PO), may also be considered. The documentation of triamterene and amiloride in veterinary medicine is limited.

Because the furosemide treatment precedes and is used concomitantly with these drugs, the risk of hyperkalemia is low, even when they are added to a patient that is currently treated with an ACE-inhibitor. The risk of inducing prerenal azotemia, hypotension, and acid-base and electrolyte imbalances increases with the intensity of the diuretic treatment. However, the practitioner usually has to accept some degree of these disturbances when treating a patient with heart failure and, although common, they seldom result in clinical problems. A calcium senzitizer (pimobendan) is often introduced in cases with recurrent heart failure, as echocardiographic evidence of systolic dysfunction often has developed (see above).

Severe and Life-Threatening (Fulminant) Heart Failure

The causes of acute severe heart failure are often a ruptured major tendinous chord, development of atrial fibrillation, undertreatment of existing heart failure, or intense physical activity, such as chasing birds or cats, in the presence of significant CMVI. Patients with severe heart failure have radiographic evidence of severe interstitial or alveolar edema and have significant clinical signs of heart failure at rest. They are often severely dyspneic and tachypneic and have respiratory rates in the range of 40 to 90. They may cough white or pink froth, which is edema fluid. These dogs require immediate hospitalization and aggressive treatment. However, euthanasia should also be considered, if the dog is already on high doses of diuretics and other heart failure therapy, owing to the poor long-term prognosis. It is important not to stress dogs with severe or fulminant heart failure as stress may lead to death. Therefore thoracic radiographs and other diagnostic procedures may have to wait until the dog has been stabilized.

Dogs with significant dyspnea benefit from intravenous injections of furosemide at a relatively high dose (4 to 6 mg/kg q2-6h IV). The furosemide may be administered intramuscularly should placement of an intravenous catheter not be possible. Dogs with fulminant pulmonary edema may require Herculean furosemide doses at 6 to 8 mg/kg every 2 to 8 hours IV over the first 24 hours. The exact dosage of furosemide depends not only on severity of clinical signs but also on whether or not the dog is already on oral furosemide treatment. Oxygen therapy is always beneficial in hypoxemic patients and it can preferably be administered using an oxygen cage provided that the temperature can be controlled inside the cage. Nasal inflation or a facial mask may also be used provided that the animal accepts them without struggle. Once the dog has received furosemide and oxygen treatment, an arterial vasodilator and a positive inotrope may be considered to stabilize the patient.

Commonly used vasodilating agents are hydralazine per os or intravenous nitroprusside (2.0-10 mg/kg/min). Of these two vasodilators, hydralazine is most commonly used. Owing to the severity of heart failure, dogs without previous vasodilating therapy may receive an initial dose of hydralazine of 1 to 2 mg/kg PO. Titration of the hydralazine dosage as described above is indicated in dogs already on an ACE-inhibitor and blood pressure should be monitored to detect hypotension. Nitroprusside can only be administered as an intravenous infusion, which requires an intravenous catheter. This potent vasodilator has actions on both the venous and arterial circulation. However, it is not easy to control the effects of nitroprusside and the dosage has to be titrated under careful blood-pressure monitoring to avoid serious hypotension and to ensure efficacy. These disadvantages have prevented nitroprusside from being a commonly used arterial vasodilator.

A positive inotrope such as dobutamine, or more commonly the calcium-sensitizer pimobendan (0.25 mg/kg q12h PO), may be considered to stabilize the patient with fulminant heart failure. Pimobendan may be administered together with furosemide without any arterial vasodilator as the drug has vasodilating properties itself. The dose of any concurrently administered arterial vasodilator has to be adjusted. Dobutamine is administered as a constant infusion usually in combination with nitroprusside. One problem with dobutamine that limits its use is that the patient needs to be weaned from IV to oral therapy within 1 to 2 days.

Patients with severe or fulminant heart failure need frequent initial monitoring of the respiratory rate because it reflects the clinical response to the furosemide treatment. Significantly decreased respiratory rate within the first hours indicates successful therapy, whereas absence of change indicate that furosemide is required at a higher dose or more frequently. Once the respiratory rate has decreased, the dose of furosemide may be reduced according to the status of the animal and clinical judgment. Abnormal laboratory findings such as pre-renal azotemia, electrolyte imbalances and dehydration are common after high doses of furosemide. Again, these abnormalities are seldom a clinical problem and the laboratory values often tend to shift towards normal with clinical improvement and as the dog starts to eat and drink. Dehydration is usually not severe even after intensive furosemide treatment and intravenous rehydration should be performed slowly and with caution in cases where it is needed, as the volume challenge may produce pulmonary edema.

Complications

Acute Exacerbation of Pulmonary Congestion and Edema due to Ruptured Chordae Tendineae

Ruptured chordae tendineae (RCT) may be suspected in all dogs that suffer from CMVI with drastic aggravation of pulmonary congestion and edema, whereas RCT is a rare finding in cats. It is not unusual for the RCT to be a result of extraordinary stress or exercise (e.g., chasing cats or birds). The most important ruptures involve those of first order chordae that are attached to the septal leaflet, and these patients are expected to die rapidly from acute volume overload and fulminant pulmonary edema. Ruptures of lesser order chordae or perhaps first order chordae that are attached to the free wall leaflet may result in minor clinical signs or none at all. Significant RCT causes acutely increased MR, and the clinical findings may differ from those encountered in chronic MR. Due to the acute increase in MR, there may be a marked increase in left atrial and pulmonary venous pressures leading to acute pulmonary edema, pulmonary artery hypertension and right heart failure.[34,39,41]

The physical examination of these patients often reveals a heart murmur of lower intensity than that of chronic MR, an S3 gallop is more likely to be present, and jugular venous distention is more likely to be present with pulsations. The radiographic and echocardiographic findings of cardiac size vary, depending on how far the CMVI had progressed before the onset of RCT. Doppler echocardiography shows severe MR, and a flail segment of the mitral valve leaflet may be detected using two-dimensional views. Thoracic radiographs show a markedly increased interstitial and alveolar pattern with distention of the pulmonary veins. These patients require intensive care to stabilize the condition, and thereafter maintainance therapy for CMVI (see under Management section). As long as a first order chordae attaching to the septal leaflet has not occurred, many of these cases may sustain with the aid of appropriate medication.

Right-Sided Heart Failure due to Pulmonary Hypertension

Many patients with long-standing history of CMVI develop right-sided heart failure. It is presumed that this condition develops as a consequence of concurrent chronic tricuspid insufficiency attributable to myxomatous degeneration, or the development pulmonary hypertension, or a combination of both. In CMVI, the pulmonary hypertension is believed to develop secondary to the persistent elevation of the left atrial and pulmonary venous pressures, but concurrent chronic airway disease may also contribute. Because the right ventricle is thinner and more compliant than the left ventricle, it can accept relatively large increases in volume but not in pressure.[74] Even small increases in pulmonary artery pressure cause sharp decreases in right ventricular stroke volume.[74] Individuals with pulmonary hypertension are sensitive to exercise, with signs of weakness or collapse, even at mild exercise. A physical examination may reveal evidence of right heart failure, such as ascites, pleural effusion, hepatic and splenic congestion, and distention of the jugular veins with abnormal pulsations. The presence and degree of pulmonary hypertension may be indirectly quantitated by Doppler echocardiography (see later section on TVI).

Individuals with pulmonary hypertension may be difficult to manage. The goal of therapy is to eliminate contributing factors and restrict even mild exercise. Oxygen supplementation is indicated in cases of acute collapse. Since persistently increased left atrial and pulmonary vein pressures are in large part responsible for the condition, therapy should be directed as for CMVI with pulmonary congestion (see Management). At present, there is no vasodilator available that specifically acts on the pulmonary artery, but it appears that hydralazine may be one of the better drugs in this aspect.[41] In humans, several endothelin-receptor antagonists are either launched or in Phase II or III clinical trials for treatment of pulmonary hypertension. So far, the experiences with these drugs in dogs are limited. Bronchodilator therapy may also be indicated, and methylxanthines and beta 2-selective agonists may be considered in these cases. Aggressive diuretic treatment may be required to resolve ascites, if present.

Acute Exacerbation of Pulmonary Congestion due to Tachyarrhythmia

An enlarged left atrium predisposes to supraventricular premature beats, atrial fibrillation, and supraventricular tachycardia. Ventricular arrhythmias are less common but may occur in progressed cases. A tachycardia with a ventricular rate greater than 180 bpm is of hemodynamic significance. These patients often have a long-standing history of CMVI, with an acute onset of pulmonary edema. In addition to other findings characteristic of CMVI, these cases have a change in cardiac rhythm. The goal of therapy is to relieve the pulmonary edema, as described earlier under management, and to reduce heart rate to an acceptable rate for improving cardiac output. Digoxin is the drug of choice in cases with supraventricular tachycardia. Should this fail to control heart rate, diltiazem (0.5 to 1.5 mg/kg q8h PO) or a beta1-receptor antagonist such as, atenolol (6.25 to 12.5 mg/kg q12h PO) or metoprolol (0.5 to 1 mg/kg q8-12h PO), could be added. It should be noted that some individuals with CMVI are highly dependent on sympathetic drive so that these drugs may not be well tolerated in the recommended dose range. Therefore both types of drugs should be initiated at the lowest possible dose and then gradually increased with careful monitoring.

Left Atrial Rupture and Cardiac Tamponade

As a consequence of the left atrial dilatation in CMVI the left atrium becomes thin walled and more vulnerable to increases in pressure, such as in the case of a ruptured tendinous chord or trauma. Endocardial splitting is a frequent postmortem finding in dogs with a history of long-standing CMVI.[7] The significance of this finding is that it may progress to rupture of the left atrium with the sudden development of hemopericardium, cardiac tamponade, and sudden death. Most cases with atrial rupture and cardiac tamponade are expected to die suddenly. There is often a history of trauma, excitement, or physical exercise, preceding the atrial rupture and sudden death. For those dogs that survive the initial event, clinical signs of cardiac tamponade together with signs of CMVI can be found. Thus acute development of ascites, collapse, or marked exercise intolerance are to be expected. The physical examination may reveal signs of pericardial effusion (see separate chapter) together with evidence of CMVI. Echocardiography is often required for definite diagnosis by identifying the presence of significant pericardial effusion, whereas the left atrial tear is often difficult to detect. Treatment of atrial rupture with hemopericardium and cardiac tamponade is usually futile. Immediate pericardiocentesis is indicated, and pericardial fluid should be removed to alleviate the tamponade without removing so much that further bleeding is stimulated. If the bleeding continues after pericardiocentesis, the final option is emergency thoracotomy with pericardiectomy and closure of the tear, but the prognosis for this procedure is poor to grave.

TRICUSPID VALVE INSUFFICIENCY

Since the advent of Doppler echocardiography, tricuspid valve insufficiency (TVI) has been recognized as a common incidental finding in dogs and cats.[75] TVI of clinical significance most often occurs concomitantly with chronic CMVI as a consequence of primary valvular changes, secondary right ventricular enlargement, or both.[7] In these circumstances, the degenerative changes of the tricuspid valve apparatus are identical to those found in CMVI (see Pathology section).[7] Other conditions that may affect the tricuspid valve apparatus itself include infective endocarditis and, more seldom, chordal rupture.[7,44,54] Secondary or functional TVI may occur as a consequence of right ventricular dilatation in all conditions associated with an acquired increase in right ventricular pressure. These include heartworm disease, pulmonary thromboembolism, pulmonary hypertension secondary to left heart disease, and idiopathic pulmonary hypertension. In addition, secondary TVI occurs in biventricular or right ventricular dilated cardiomyopathy and in congenital pulmonic stenosis. TVI occurs in cats with cardiomyopathy and hyperthyroidism.[76]

Consequences (Pathophysiology)

TVI, in the absence of concurrent obstruction of the pulmonary valve or pulmonary artery hypertension, is comparably well tolerated.[77] However, because the right ventricle is designed to contract against a low-pressure artery, it is vulnerable to increases in pressure. It responds poorly to the increased work; even relatively small acute increases in pulmonary artery pressure cause sharp decreases in right ventricular stroke volume.[74] Thus TVI is of significance if pulmonary hypertension is present. In addition to the right ventricular dilatation, right atrial enlargement develops and adds to the tricuspid annular dilatation and TVI. Enlargement of this chamber may result in atrial tachyarrhythmias, such as atrial fibrillation and supraventricular tachycardia. As a consequence of increased right atrial pressure, ascites, pleural effusion (especially in cats), pericardial effusion, hepatomegaly, and splenomegaly may develop.

Clinical Signs

Isolated TVI does not commonly result in clinical signs of disease.[7,41,54] Evidence of reduced exercise tolerance, weakness, or syncope occur mainly in instances with pulmonary hypertension, such as secondary to CMVI or tachyarrhythmia. It is common for these animals to show signs of right heart failure that may include respiratory distress due to pleural effusion; abdominal distention due to ascites, hepatomegaly, or splenomegaly; or gastrointestinal signs such as diarrhea, vomiting, and anorexia.

Physical Examination

Significant TVI is characterized by a holosystolic murmur with varying intensity and with the point of maximal intensity over the tricuspid area, and, in some cases, by the presence of venous distention and pulsations in the jugular veins. The heart sounds may be muffled by pleural effusion. Abdominal distention may be present with ascites, hepatomegaly, or splenomegaly. A rapid irregular heart rhythm and femoral artery pulse are observed in the presence of tachyarrhythmia, and pulse deficits may be detected. A weak femoral artery pulse may be found in cases with pulmonary hypertension or left-side heart failure.

Electrocardiographic Findings

ECG has a low sensitivity in detecting right atrial and right ventricular enlargement secondary to primary TVI.[7] In significant TVI with pulmonary hypertension, the ECG changes may include evidence of right atrial enlargement (tall P wave), a right ventricular enlargement pattern, and a right deviation of the mean electrical axis.[47] However, even in severe cases of TVI and pulmonary hypertension secondary to CMVI, these signs may not be obvious because of the concurrent changes to the left cardiac side. In these cases, the recording may only show evidence of left side involvement.[7,41] Arrhythmias, such as supraventricular premature beats, atrial fibrillation, and ventricular premature beats, may be noted.

Radiographic Findings

Mild right atrial and ventricular enlargement are usually not associated with detectable radiologic signs. Signs of moderate to severe right atrial enlargement in lateral projection include bulging of the right atrium in the craniodorsal direction. This causes the cranial border of the heart to appear straight rather than convex and elevates the trachea as it courses dorsally over the right atrium. In addition to elevations of the trachea and caudal vena cava, signs of right ventricular enlargement include increased sternal contact and rounding of the right heart border. In the dorsoventral (or ventrodorsal) projection, the enlarged right atrium may be identified as a bulge in the right cranial part of the cardiac border (in the 9 to 12 o'clock position). The border of the enlarged right ventricle appears rounded and, in severe enlargement, it may resemble an inverted "D" sign. There is a shift of the cardiac apex to the left. Signs of right heart failure may be observed including pleural effusion, abdominal effusion, hepatomegaly, and splenomegaly. If biventricular failure occurs, the global cardiac size will be increased and signs of left heart failure may be present.

Echocardiographic Findings

Echocardiography is useful to detect increased right atrial and right ventricular size and for evaluation of tricuspid valve morphology. Thus it is an important tool to rule out differential diagnoses, such as an undiscovered congenital heart defect. The echocardiographic appearance of the tricuspid valve with myxomatous degeneration is similar in two-dimensional mode to myxomatous lesions on the mitral valve already described (see CMVI Echocardiography section). With the use of color-flow Doppler, TVI may be detected and semiquantified. The right atrium is, however, not as easily accessible as the left atrium owing to the anatomy, and the orientation of TVI jets is not consistent. The Doppler echocardiographic findings in TVI are similar to those of MR with a few exceptions. Trivial, physiologic TVI is common in dogs and this regurgitation is usually silent to auscultation. Spectral Doppler may be used to estimate right ventricular stroke volume and to identify pulmonary hypertension by estimation of right ventricular systolic pressure and pulmonary arterial systolic and diastolic pressures.[54] The right ventricular pressure is estimated by finding a tricuspid regurgitant jet and measure its peak velocity by continuous-wave Doppler. TVI jet velocities generally peaks at approximately 2.6 m/sec, unless there is elevation of right ventricular pressure that forces blood at a higher velocity, usually above 3 m/sec.[58] The pressure gradient between the right atrium and ventricle may be calculated with use of the peak velocity of the regurgitant jet and the modified Bernouilli equation.[78] The right ventricular pressure is obtained by adding an estimate of the right atrial pressure to the pressure gradient over the AV-valve. It has been suggested that appropriate estimates of right atrial pressure is 5 mm Hg in patients without right heart failure and 10 to 15 mm Hg in patients with right heart failure.[54] Similarly, the peak velocity of a pulmonic valve regurgitation and an estimate of right ventricular diastolic pressure may be used to predict pulmonary artery diastolic pressure.[79]

Management

Because primary TVI is usually relatively benign, patients with clinical signs of right-sided heart failure with suspected TVI must be thoroughly evaluated for concurrent conditions that may mimic or exaggerate TVI. Examples of these include congenital heart defects, heartworm disease, CMVI, pulmonary hypertension, pericardial effusion, restrictive pericarditis, and mitral valve stenosis. The signs of right heart failure, that is, abdominal and pleural effusions, may be alleviated with diuretic treatment and often involves two or more drugs to obtain sequential blocking of the nephron (see CMVI under Management), but abdominocentesis may be required. If tachyarrhythmia is present, successful management depends on controlling the increased heart rate or preferably abolishing the tachyarrhythmia.

SEMILUNAR VALVE INSUFFICIENCY

With the advent of color flow echocardiography, a low degree of aortic and, more commonly, pulmonic valve insufficiency are frequently detected.[75] This finding may be of no clinical significance but in others it occurs with different types of congenital heart disease. Aortic valve insufficiency (AVI) occurs most often in dogs as a consequence of subaortic stenosis and pulmonic valve insufficiency (PVI) of pulmonic valve stenosis.[7,41,54] Acquired AVI of clinical significance, except in association with bacterial endocarditis (see Infective Endocarditis), is a rare disorder in dogs and cats. PVI is observed in the majority of cases with pulmonary artery hypertension, and secondary to pulmonary artery dilatation, such as in PDA and severe heartworm disease. Isolated PVI as cause of clinical signs is extremely rare. Although myxomatous degeneration is sometimes evident at postmortem on one or both semilunar valves,[7,41,54] it is not expected to have caused significant insufficiency associated with clinical signs.

INFECTIVE ENDOCARDITIS

Infective endocarditis (IE) is a life-threatening disorder that results from microorganisms that colonize the cardiac endocardium, which commonly causes destruction of valves or other structures within the heart. Bacteremia is by far the most common etiology, with the mitral and aortic valve most frequently affected.[80] Vegetation may cause thromboembolism or metastatic infections, which involve multiple body organs and produce a large variety of clinical signs which makes diagnosis difficult. The incidence of infective endocarditis in necropsied dogs has been reported to range from 0.06% to 6.6%.[41,81] Evaluation of clinical data from university animal hospitals points to IE as a comparably rare condition with incidences ranging from 0.04% to 0.13%.[82] Medium to large

breed, mainly purebred, middle-aged male dogs are reported to be predisposed.[80] The incidence in cats, based on clinical experience, is considered to be 7 to 10 times lower than in dogs.[82,23] Animals with congenital heart disease have a low incidence of IE[41,80], but associations have been reported with subaortic stenosis[84] and occasionally with PDA.[85] IE has not been found to have any association with CMVI in dogs.[13,41,81]

Pathology

Vegetation associated with by IE mainly affects the left heart with the highest incidence involving the mitral valve.[86] Involvement of the right heart or mural endocardium is uncommon.[86] Pathologic findings vary and depend on the virulence of the infecting organism, the duration of infection, and the immunologic response. Intracardiac vegetation consists of different layers of fibrin, platelets, bacteria, red and white cells, and is often covered by an intact endothelium. Bacteria may continue to grow despite antibiotic therapy owing to the location deep within the vegetation and a slow metabolic rate (Figure 201-8).[87] Necrosis and destruction of the valve stroma or chordae tendineae proceed rapidly in peracute or acute IE, which causes valvular insufficiency and cardiac failure.

Etiology and Pathogenesis

Transient or persistent bacteremia is a prerequisite for the development of IE. A large number of bacteria have been associated with bacteremia[88] (see section on Blood Culture below) and some are known to cause IE.[86,88] Most bacteria require predisposing factors to cause IE, such as depression of the immunosystem or endothelial damage, sometimes with depositions of platelet-fibrin complexes, to adhere to the valve and create IE.[87] The origin of the bacteremia may be active infection localized somewhere within the body.[88] A proportion of cases with IE has no clinically detectable source of infection.[86,88] Possible routes for bacteria to reach and infect the endocardium are by direct contact with the surface endothelium via the bloodstream or from capillaries within the valve (vasculitis).[89]

The consequences of IE depend on several factors: virulence of the infective agent; site of infection; degree of valvular destruction; influence of vegetation on valvular function; production of exo- or endotoxins; interaction with the immunosystem with the formation of immunocomplexes[90]; and development of thromboembolism and metastatic infections. Gram-negative bacteremia results often in a peracute or acute clinical manifestation, whereas gram-positive bacteremia typically results in a subacute or chronic condition. The vegetation may cause valvular insufficiency or obstruction. The destruction of valvular tissue is caused by the action of bacteria or the cellular response from the immunologic system. Deposition of immunocomplexes in different organs may cause glomerulonephritis, myositis, or polyarthritis.[90] Septic embolization that produces clinical signs is uncommon but 84% of affected dogs had evidence of systemic embolization at necropsy and glomerulonephritis was reported in 16% of 44 dogs with IE.[80]

Case History and Clinical Signs

The diagnosis of IE can easily be overlooked because the case history and clinical signs are not specific and there may be an absence of predisposing factors to raise the suspicion of IE. Clinical signs are variable and occur in different combinations. Commonly reported signs include lethargy, weakness, fever (sometimes recurrent), anorexia, weight loss, GI disturbances, and lameness.[80,90] Stiffness and pain originating from joints or muscles may be caused by immunomediated responses and abdominal pain may be caused by secondary renal or splenic infarction, septic embolization, or abscess formation. If the condition leads to severe valvular damage, especially of the

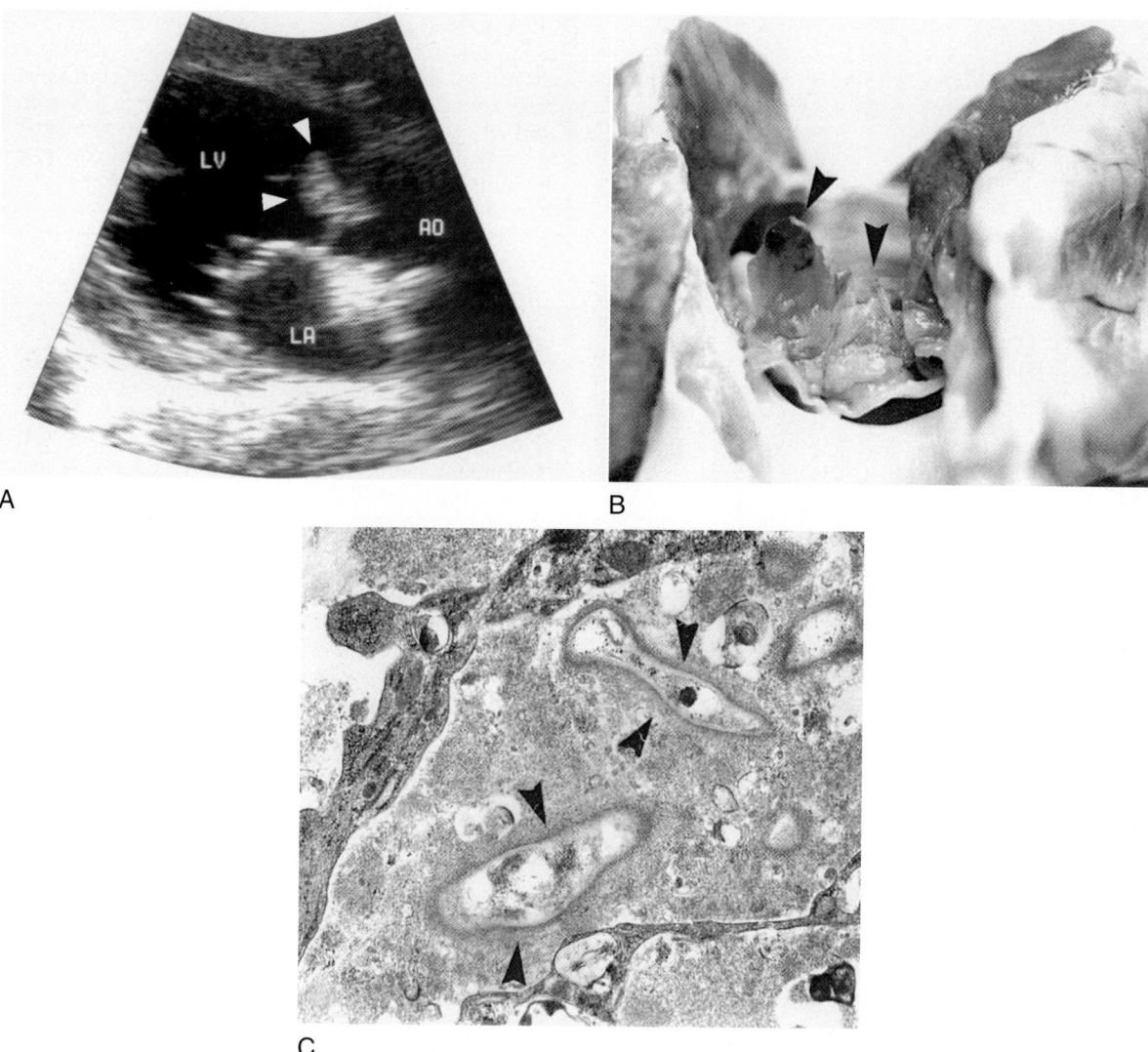

Figure 201-8 **A,** Echocardiographic long axis view from a 3-year-old male boxer. The dog had previously been diagnosed with slight aortic stenosis but had recently suffered recurrent episodes of fewer and lethargy. An irregular-shaped echogenic mass was attached to the aortic valve *(white arrowheads).* **B,** A valvular vegetation *(arrowheads)* localized to the base of the aortic valve leaflet was evident at postmortem examination. **C,** Electron micrograph showing two rod-shaped bacteria *(arrowheads)* about 1μ in diameter located intracellularly in a phagocytic cell found within the vegetation (original magnification ×35000). (Courtesy L. Jönsson and T. Nikkile, Upsala, Sweden.)

aortic valve, signs of cardiac failure and syncope from arrhythmias may occur. Predisposing factors that in combination with the clinical signs above, should raise the suspicion of IE are immunosuppressive drug therapy, such as corticosteroids[88,91]; aortic stenosis[84]; recent surgery, especially in conjunction with trauma to mucosal surfaces in the oral or genital tract and infections in these body regions, especially prostatitis; indwelling catheters, infected wounds, abscesses, or pyoderma.[88]

Physical Examination

Most clinical signs lack specificity for IE. However, fever, heart murmur (particularly if newly developed), and lameness are considered classical signs. Fever is reported to occur in 80% to 90% in dogs with IE.[80] Absence of fever is reported to be more common in cases with aortic valve involvement[86] but may also be attributed to treatment with antibiotics or corticosteroids.

Since aortic insufficiency is otherwise uncommon in dogs, the finding of a diastolic murmur (Figure 201-9) and bounding peripheral pulse should raise the suspicion of IE of the aortic valve. Systolic murmurs may be caused by destruction of the mitral valve, which results in MR or vegetations that obstruct the aortic outflow tract, which leads to stenosis.[80] These murmurs are, in contrast to diastolic murmurs, poor indicators of IE since they frequently occur in dogs with other conditions, such as CMVI and aortic stenosis. It should be noted that 26% of dogs with IE are reported to lack audible murmurs.[80] Lameness is also an inconsistent finding in IE with an incidence of 34% in one study.[81] A range of other physical findings may be present, depending on which organs are affected by circulating immunocomplexes or septic embolization. Possible findings are pain reactions from muscles or abdomen (spleen, intestines, or kidneys), cold extremities, cyanosis, and skin necrosis from severe embolization and

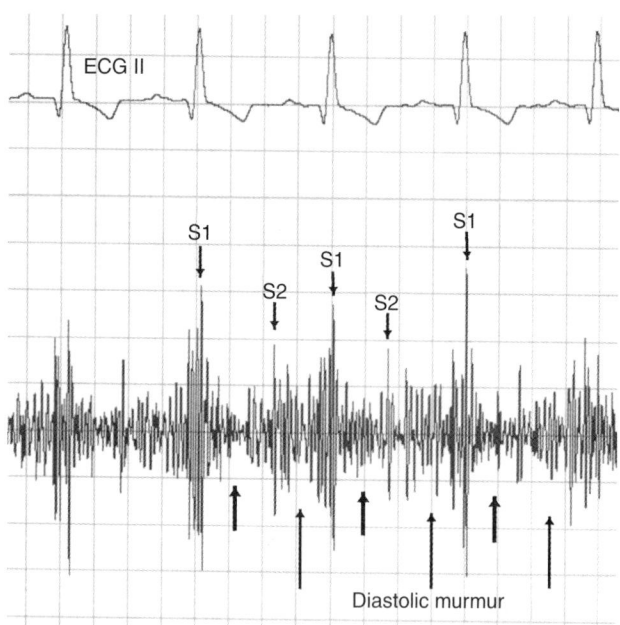

Figure 201-9 Phonocardiogram (PCG) and ECG lead II recorded from a dog with a diastolic murmur from aortic regurgitation caused by IE. A systolic murmur from mitral regurgitation is also present *(thick arrows)*, which in combination with the diastolic murmur from aortic regurgitation causes the auscultatory finding of a continuous murmur easily be misinterpreted to be caused by PDA. The PCG rules out the diagnosis of PDA as the lowest murmur intensity recorded is around the second heart sound (S2). Continous murmurs caused by PDA usually has maximal intensity at the location for S2.[44] The PCG is filtered with a nominal frequency of 100 Hz. *S1,* First heart sound; *S2,* second heart sound.

a variety of neurologic disturbances if the central nervous system is affected.

Blood Culture

Positive blood cultures are crucial evidence of IE. The theory that bacteremia from IE is intermittent has changed in recent years to the opinion that, if existent, it is continuous.[87] Thus negative or intermittent positive cultures are unusual when collection and handling of samples is conducted properly.[87] The time for sampling is probably not critical, but a constant finding through repeat samplings is valuable to exclude sample contamination. The technique for obtaining samples aseptically and anaerobically is important and described in detail below. In cases of positive blood culture, it is important to evaluate if the microorganism is consistent with the diagnosis of IE.

Microorganisms known to cause IE in dogs are, in order of reported incidence, *Staphylococcus aureus*, *E. coli*, betahemolytic streptococci, *Pseudomonas aeroginosa*, *Corynebacterium* spp., *Erysipelothrix rhusiopathiae (tonsillarium)*[86], and *Bartonella vinsonii*.[92] *B. vinsonii* and related proteobacteria has recently been recognized as a potential cause for endocarditis in dogs. They have been found in dogs with cardiac arrhythmias, endocarditis, or myocarditis.[93] *Bartonella* spp. are also a potential cause for IE in cats.[94] Furthermore, *Bartonella* spp. have been reported to occasionally cause IE in immunocompromised (but also immunocompetent) humans, with the cat serving as the major reservoir (cat scratch disease). The recommended antibiotic therapy when the resistance is unknown is erythromycin or doxycycline. Immediate antibiotic therapy of humans after significant dog or cat bites may furthermore be

motivated as commensals, such as *Capnocytophaga canimorsus*, in the saliva of dogs and cats have been reported to occasionally cause septicemia with a mortality as high as 30%.[95,96] Negative blood cultures are fairly common and may be due to antibiotic therapy, chronic situations with "incapsulated" infections, noninfective IE (only platelets and fibrin in vegetation), or failure to grow organisms from samples. Some bacteria may grow slowly and samples should not be regarded as definitely negative until they have been incubated for 10 days. More common is a rapid growth of microorganisms with 90% of cultures positive within 72 hours of incubation.[97]

Obtaining Blood Cultures

The referral laboratory should be contacted concerning the preferred type of preprepared vials before obtaining a sample; special additives are available if the patient has been on antibiotics. Pediatric vials are useful because less blood is required but volumes in the range of 20 to 30 mL increase the chance for growth. To avoid contamination, strictly aseptic sampling should be observed which includes thorough shaving and disinfection of the sampling site and strict use of sterile gloves. Three samples with adequately filled vials from different puncture sites should be collected. If samples are collected with a syringe, suction should cease before withdrawal of the needle from the patient to avoid contamination with skin bacteria and a new sterile needle should be used for the transfer of blood into the bottles. The bottles should be prewarmed to 37° C and, after sampling, incubated at the same temperature. Sampling through indwelling catheters should be avoided but may be used as a second choice. The former recommendation to draw samples over 24-hour periods has changed, since multiple simultaneously drawn samples in humans have been shown to be equally sensitive.[87]

Electrocardiographic Findings

Arrhythmia is reported to occur in 50% to 75% of dogs with IE.[80,86] Ventricular premature beats and tachyarrhythmias are the most commonly encountered arrhythmias, but they are usually not life threatening. Deviation in the ST-segment suggests myocardial hypoxia and may indicate coronary artery embolism or ischemia from heart failure. Evidence of chamber enlargement may occur in chronic IE. All the mentioned ECG abnormalities are, however, nonspecific.

Radiographic Findings

Radiography often does not add any information specific for IE. In cases of chronic IE with aortic or mitral insufficiency, left-sided cardiac enlargement may be detected. Calcified deposits on the valve leaflets are occasionally observed in chronic cases.

Echocardiographic Findings

Echocardiography has significantly improved the possibility of diagnosis and monitoring of animals with IE.[88] Valvular vegetations may be detected using two-dimensional echocardiography, although minor lesions may be difficult to distinguish from myxomatous lesions. M-mode can be used to measure secondary changes in cardiac size and to detect abnormal mitral valve motion such as fluttering from aortic regurgitation. Mitral or aortic regurgitation may be detected using continous or color-flow Doppler echocardiography.

Other Laboratory Findings

Mild anemia is found in 50% to 60% of cases with IE.[80,86] The anemia is similar to those from other infections, usually being normocytic and normochromic. Leukocytosis is found in about 80% of dogs with IE, usually due to neutrophilia and monocytosis (left shift). Other findings that may be encountered include elevated blood urea nitrogen (BUN) due to embolization, metastatic infection, heart failure, or immune-mediated disease.

Urine analysis may reveal pyuria, bacteriuria, or proteinuria. Elevated serum alkaline phosphatase may be found, probably caused by circulating endotoxins[88] and reduced hepatic function, which may cause hypoalbuminemia.[81] The serum glucose concentration may be decreased and serologic tests for immuno-mediated disease, such as Coombs test, may be positive.[88]

Diagnosis

Since the clinical signs of IE are often a result of complications, rather than reflecting the intracardiac infection, the diagnosis may easily be overlooked. Major criteria for IE are positive blood cultures with typical microorganisms for IE from two separate samples plus evidence of cardiac involvement.[87] The localization and severity of cardiac lesions is confirmed by echocardiographic visualization of vegetations. In the absence of positive cultures, a tentative diagnosis of IE can be made if there is clinical and laboratory evidence of systemic infection, such as fever and leukocytosis plus cardiac involvement and possibly signs of embolization.

Management

The goal of therapy is to eradicate the infective microorganism and to treat all secondary complications. A successful outcome of the therapy is based on early diagnosis and immediate and aggressive treatment. Only bactericidal antibiotics capable of penetrating fibrin should be considered. The antibiotic concentration in serum and deep within vegetations should exceed the organisms minimal inhibitory concentration (MIC), but preferably also the minimum bactericidal concentration (MBC), continuously or throughout most of the interval between doses. Treatment should continue for at least 6 weeks to eradicate dormant microorganisms.[87]

Management of Cases with Tentative Diagnosis of IE

A blood culture (see section above) and an antibiotic sensitivity profile should be obtained. While results from cultures and sensitivity tests are awaited, intravenous treatment with a high dosage of bactericidal antibiotic IV, such as cephalosporins (second generation), should be initiated. Alternatives to cephalosporins are combinations of ampicillin or amoxicillin for gram-positive organisms and gentamicin or amikacin for gram-negative organisms. An alternative to gentamicin and amikacin, which are potentially toxic and only recommended to be used for at most one week, is enrofloxacin for suspected gram-negative IE. Enrofloxacin is bactericidal and may penetrate myocardium and heart valves and is also indicated for treating *Bartonella* infections. Choice of antibiotic should preferably depend on the suspected source of

infection and the estimated resistance pattern for the primary infection. Practitioners should try to identify the source of infection and treat it as aggressively as possible, such as use of surgical drainage or debridement.[98] Possible secondary problems should be identified, such as heart or renal failure that need therapy or may impair the prognosis.

For dogs with heart failure from aortic regurgitation, hydralazine titered to an adequate reduction of arterial blood pressure is effective and should be considered as a part of medical therapy. When results are available from blood cultures, appropriate antibiotics are selected and aggressive IV treatment continued for 5 to 10 days while renal function is monitored. If results from cultures are negative, the decision to continue antibiotic therapy should be based on clinical improvement. Depending on the early outcome of therapy, subcutaneous administration may substitute a 5 to 10 days IV treatment, and later be superseded by oral preparations. The duration of therapy should be at least 6 weeks on the effective antibiotic. Frequent clinical examinations, blood screening, and urine analyses should be performed during that period.

Prognosis

Factors that indicate a poor prognosis include late diagnosis and late start of therapy; vegetations on valves (especially the aortic)[86]; gram-negative infections, heart or renal failure that do not respond to therapy; septic embolization or metastatic infection; elevation of serum alkaline phosphatase and hypoalbuminemia (70% mortality is reported if this is found in cases with IE)[81]; concurrent treatment with corticosteroids, regardless if antibiotics are given simultaneously[80,91]; treatment with bacteriostatic antibiotics or premature termination of antibiotic therapy. Factors that indicate a more favorable prognosis include only mitral valve involvement (47% of dogs are reported to survive)[80]; gram-positive infections, origin of infection being the skin, abscesses, cellulitis, or wound infections.[88]

Prevention

Prophylactic antibiotics may be indicated 1 to 2 hours before and 12 to 24 hours after diagnostic or surgical procedures when turbulent blood flow is suspected to have damaged the endocardium, such as aortic stenosis, PDA, or VSD. In these cases, early treatment of all manifest infections is important to avoid bacteremia and reduce the risk for IE, and caution should be observed when bleeding or infection is anticipated or evident in the oral, urogenital, intestinal, or respiratory tract. Amoxicillin may be the first choice, but other antibiotics, such as clindamycin or cephalosporins, may also be considered depending on the organ system involved and site of infection.[87]

CHAPTER 202

Electrocardiography and Cardiac Arrhythmias

Etienne Côté
Stephen J. Ettinger

The diagnostic test of choice for clinical evaluation of cardiac arrhythmias is the electrocardiogram (ECG).[1-5] The ECG also has invaluable applications in monitoring patients with systemic abnormalities, including electrolyte disturbances and hypoxia. Additionally, abnormalities in the dimensions of various components of the ECG may serve as a rough guide for evaluating structural heart disease. These ECG morphologic criteria are rarely based on controlled studies identifying specificity and sensitivity, however, and ECG parameters for dogs or cats by breed, body type, age, and sex are not comprehensively established. An abnormal heart may have a normal ECG and vice versa. Therefore the ECG, like a blood count, is not an absolute indicator of normalcy or disease, and deviations from normal suggest but do not identify structural cardiac abnormalities (Boxes 202-1 and 202-2).

CARDIAC CONDUCTION SYSTEM AND ELECTROCARDIOGRAPHY

Each component of an ECG tracing reflects an electrical event occurring in a specific part of the heart.[1,2,5,6] The sequence of electrical events follows specific anatomic pathways within the heart, and in health, does so precisely and consistently (Figure 202-1).

Initiation of the normal heartbeat occurs in the *sinoatrial (SA) node*, located in the dorsolateral right atrium (RA), and spreads through both atria, forming the *P wave* on the ECG (Figure 202-2). Specifically, part of the electrical spread from the SA node travels along three sets of specialized fibers in the atria, the internodal pathways,[7] which converge on the *atrioventricular (AV) node* in the floor of the RA. Thus the outward movement of electrical activity from the SA node both activates the muscular contraction of the atria and carries a sequence of electrical impulses to be transmitted to the ventricles.

At the level of the AV node, the electrical impulse depolarizing the heart is purposefully delayed, allowing the atria to finish contracting. The period of relative electrical quiescence during which the impulse slowly passes through the AV node is reflected on the ECG as a flat segment between the P wave and QRS complex. In addition to transmitting impulses from the atria to the ventricles, the healthy AV node acts as a *gatekeeper*, blocking unwanted atrial impulses from crossing to and activating the ventricles, such as when these impulses are

---

Box • 202-1

*Criteria for the Normal Canine Electrocardiogram (ECG)** (Note: Patient in right lateral recumbency; no ECG filtering†)

Heart rate: 70 to 160 beats per minute (bpm) in adult dogs; 60 to 140 bpm in giant breeds; up to 180 bpm in toy breeds; up to 220 bpm in puppies

Heart rhythm: normal sinus rhythm (NSR); respiratory sinus arrhythmia (RSA); wandering SA pacemaker common (cyclic changes in the R-R interval can be associated with cyclic alterations in P-wave amplitude)

P wave: up to 0.4 mV in amplitude; up to 0.04 sec duration (0.05 sec in large breeds); positive in leads II and aVF; positive or isoelectric in lead I

P-R interval: 0.06 to 0.13 sec (inversely related to heart rate)

QRS complex: ‡positive in leads II and aVF, negative in lead V_{10}; mean electrical axis (MEA), frontal plane: +40° to +100°

Amplitude: maximum R wave 2.5 to 3.0 mV in leads II, III, and aVF (dogs > 2 years of age); R in rV_2 or V_{10} < 3 mV; V_2 and V_4 < 5.0 mV; minimum amplitude R wave leads II, III, and aVF is 0.5 mV; duration: up to 0.05 sec (0.06 sec in large breeds) S in V_4 not deeper than 0.7 mV; QRS negative in V_{10}

Q-T segment: 0.15 to 0.25 sec; varies with heart rate

S-T segment and T wave: S-T segment free of marked coving (repolarization changes); S-T segment depression not > 0.2 mV in limb leads and not > 0.25 mV in chest leads; S-T segment elevation not > 0.15 mV in leads II and III; T wave positive in lead V_1 (rV_2) and negative in V_{10} (except in the Chihuahua); T wave amplitude not > 25% of amplitude of the R wave; T waves may be positive, negative, or biphasic

---

*Represents commonly encountered values for dogs and cats. The ECG is extremely variable; serial ECGs are recommended. Measurements outside these ranges suggest but do not identify cardiac disease. Values from references 1, 2, 5, and personal experience.

†Dvir E, Lobetti R: Effect of electrocardiographic filters on the R-amplitude of canine electrocardiograms. *Vet Rec* 150:171-176, 2002.

‡Detweiler DK: The dog electrocardiogram: a critical review. *In* MacFarlane PW, Veitch Lawrie TD (eds): Comprehensive Electrocardiology: Theory and Practice in Health and Disease. Oxford, UK, Pergamon Press, 1989, pp 1267-1329; Hurst JW: Naming of the waves in the ECG, with a brief account of their genesis. *Circulation* 98:1937-1942, 1998.

Box • 202-2

Criteria for the Normal Feline Electrocardiogram (ECG)* (Note: Patient in right lateral recumbency; no ECG filtering†)

Heart rate: up to 240 beats per minute (bpm) (usually 140-180 bpm)

Heart rhythm: normal sinus rhythm (NSR) or physiologic sinus tachycardia (STach)

P wave: positive and up to 0.2 mV in leads II and aVF; may be positive or isoelectric in lead I; should not exceed 0.04 sec (rate dependent) in duration

P-R interval: 0.04 to 0.09 sec duration (inversely related to heart rate)

QRS complex: †more variable than in the canine; the mean electrical axis (MEA) in the frontal plane is often irrelevant and may be isoelectric in all frontal plane limb leads; MEA most commonly from 0° to +160° (frontal plane); amplitude of the R wave is usually low; maximum is 0.9 mV; duration: under 0.04 sec

Q-T segment: 0.12-0.18 sec duration; varies inversely with heart rate

S-T segment and T wave: S-T segment and T wave should be small and free of repolarization changes, marked depression, or elevation; T waves usually positive, occasionally negative or biphasic; up to 0.3 mV height

Precordial leads: few established rules exist for the V leads in cats; R in V_4 should not exceed 1.0 mV

---

*Represents commonly encountered numbers for dogs and cats. The ECG is extremely variable; serial ECGs are recommended. Measurements outside these ranges suggest but do not identify cardiac disease. Values from references 3, 5, 10, 14, and personal experience.
†Schrope DP et al: Effects of electrocardiograph frequency filters on P-QRS-T amplitudes of the feline electrocardiogram. *Am J Vet Res* 56:1534-1540, 1995.

---

premature or excessive (e.g., atrial fibrillation [AFib]). In normal individuals, the unidirectionally conducting fibers of the AV node-His bundle complex make up the only electrical connection between the atria and the ventricles.

Having crossed through the AV node, the electrical impulse of a normal heartbeat travels rapidly and uniformly through the ventricles via the *His-Purkinje* system.[8] This network of conductive fibers ensures that the impulse is carried quickly and distributed uniformly, such that the ventricles depolarize in a synchronized fashion. The fibers begin as a thick shaft, the *His bundle*, that accepts transmission from the AV node and crosses through the endocardial cushion to the ventricles. The His bundle quickly divides into *right and left bundle branches* (RBB and LBB), directed to their respective ventricles, and the left bundle in turn divides into *left anterior, left posterior, and septal fascicles*. The clinical relevance of this division relates to interruptions of electrical conduction through these bundles, which can occur under various pathologic, and occasionally normal, conditions (see Bundle Branch Blocks, following). Overall, depolarization of the ventricles is apparent on the ECG as the *QRS complex*. When the ventricles have completely finished depolarizing, a sequence of repolarization returns the myocardial cells to their resting state. This repolarization sequence, which follows in the wake of the depolarization sequence, is seen as the *T wave* on the ECG.

CLINICAL USE OF ELECTROCARDIOGRAPHIC LEADS AND MEAN ELECTRICAL AXIS

Electrocardiographic Leads

In practical terms, an ECG lead is nothing more than one perspective on the electrical activity of the heart. That is, different leads offer different vantage points on the same electrical events that take place during a heartbeat.[9] Therefore an ECG showing multiple leads can be thought of as an ECG with multiple observers reporting the electrical activity of the heart from different positions (Figures 202-3 to 202-5).

Having multiple observation points (multiple leads) is important because all cardiac electrical events are not always

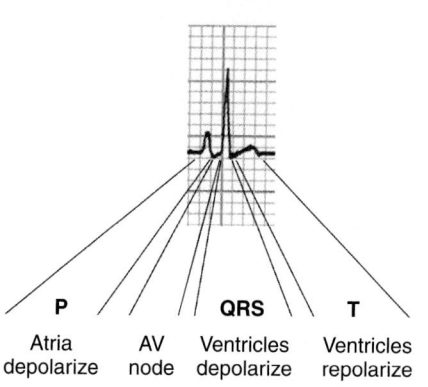

Figure 202-1 A heartbeat on the electrocardiogram (ECG). Correlation with electrical activity in anatomic regions of the heart.

P — Atria depolarize
AV node
QRS — Ventricles depolarize
T — Ventricles repolarize

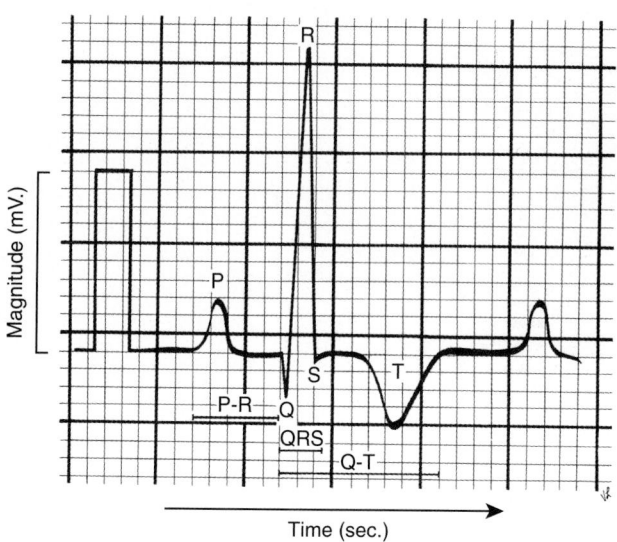

Figure 202-2 Electrocardiogram (ECG) dimensions and nomenclature for a normal heartbeat.

Magnitude (mV.)

Time (sec.)

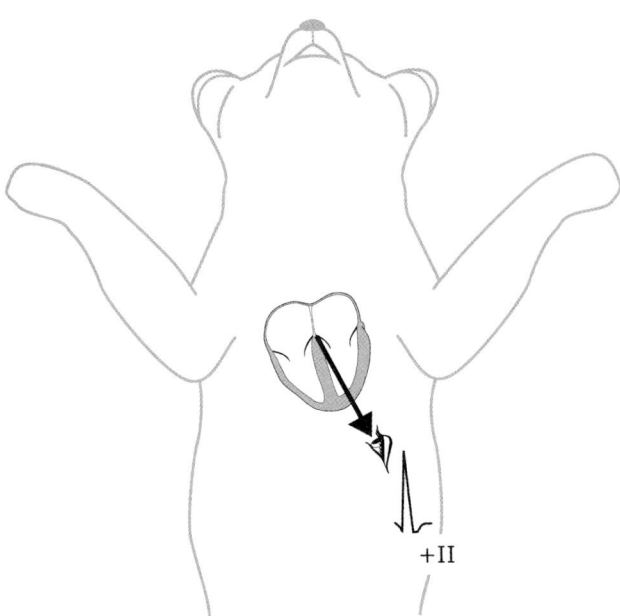

Figure 202-3 The positive pole of an electrocardiogram (ECG) lead as observer. The overall thrust of electrical energy for one beat of the ventricles is oriented caudally and slightly leftward (i.e., directly toward the positive pole of lead II [eye]) in the normal dog. Therefore a large, positive QRS complex is registered in that lead.

apparent in all leads. Indeed, important information about the heartbeat is often visible in some ECG leads but not in others. This is because any ECG lead is characterized by the ability to sense only electrical activity traveling toward or away from it. The drawback of this characteristic is that electrical activity coursing through a three-dimensional structure like the heart often occurs in a direction that is neither toward nor away

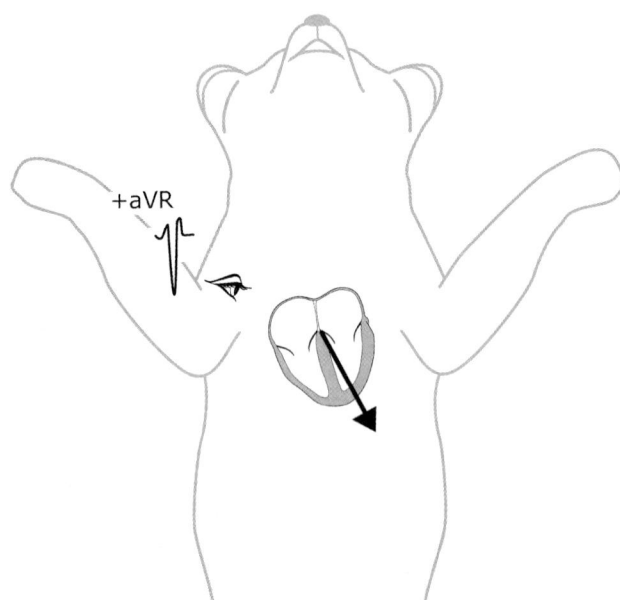

Figure 202-4 Same normal heart as in Figure 202-3. The observer at the positive pole of lead aVR registers an overall thrust of electrical energy directed away from it. Therefore lead aVR displays a large (deep) negative QRS complex.

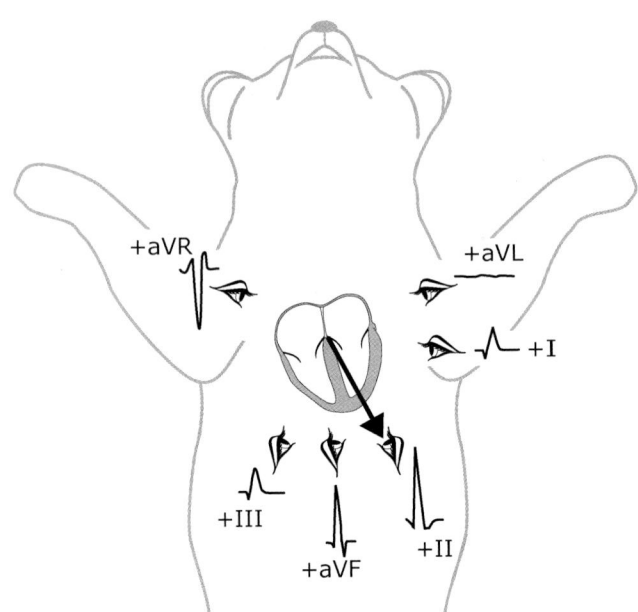

Figure 202-5 Typical appearance of QRS complexes in the six limb leads when the mean electrical axis (MEA) is in the normal range for dogs (here: +60 degrees). The reader should note that the overall size and polarity of each QRS reflects the amount and direction of electrical energy detected by the positive pole (observer) of each lead. This is the basic principle that allows the clinician to understand the overall direction of electrical thrust (MEA) based on observing QRS complexes in all leads of a patient's electrocardiogram (ECG).[9]

from a particular lead and therefore is perceived partially, or suboptimally, in any one lead alone. At an extreme, electrical activity that occurs exactly perpendicular to a lead (i.e., the electrical activity moves in a direction that is in no way toward or away from the lead) registers nothing (isoelectric ECG) for that lead, regardless of how normal or strong the electrical activity.

Electrical activity that travels directly toward the positive pole of a lead creates a strong positive deflection (wave) above the baseline on the ECG for that lead (see Figure 202-3). Similarly, electrical activity that travels directly away from the positive pole of a lead registers a strong negative ECG wave, below the baseline (see Figure 202-4). Intermediate orientations of electrical activity create waves that are of intermediate degrees of positivity or negativity, depending on the magnitude of the positive or negative component of the electrical activity that is detectable on that lead. For example, an impulse traveling *almost* directly toward the positive pole of a lead will create a large positive wave (see Figure 202-5, lead aVF) but not quite as tall as when the energy is traveling fully toward the positive pole of the lead (see Figure 202-5, lead II). All leads register the amount of positivity or negativity generated by that impulse relative to their positive pole and record a wave in proportion to that. The lead that is almost 90 degrees away from the direction of the electrical activity will record little to no activity (i.e., almost isoelectric line; see Figure 202-5, lead [aVL]), and the positive pole of the lead that is closest to 180 degrees away from the direction of electrical activity will register a very large, negative complex (see Figure 202-5, lead [aVR]).

Therefore it can be seen that using multiple leads for an ECG has two major advantages (Figure 202-6). First, the leads directly and proportionally perceive the amount of energy (i.e., number of cells depolarizing, the smoothness of conduction) involved in depolarization. Thus left ventricular (LV) hypertrophy may

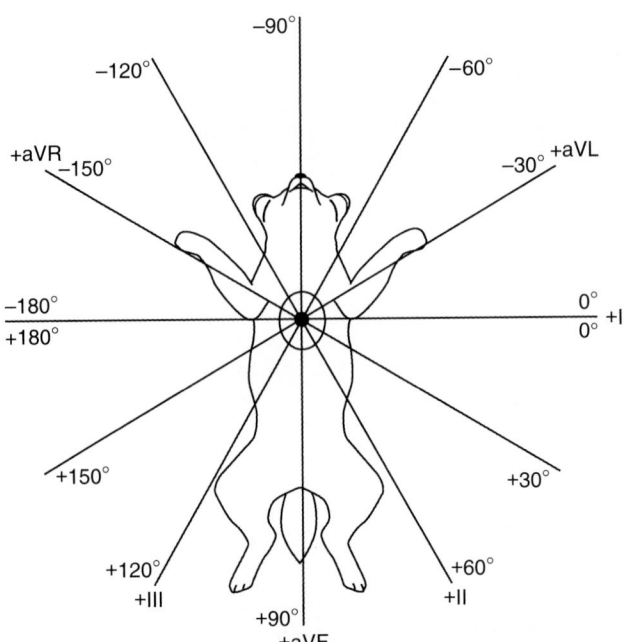

Figure 202-6 Location and names of electrocardiogram (ECG) limb leads in the standard hexaxial system (frontal plane).

be suspected when QRS complexes are abnormally tall in lead II, for example, because the amount of energy transmitted in the normal direction (toward the LV) is greater due to the increased myocardial mass. Right ventricular (RV) hypertrophy can be suspected when the bulk of ventricular electrical activity is directed abnormally toward the right heart (see discussion of right axis deviation, following). Second, having multiple leads solves the problem of any single lead's "blindness" to perpendicularity. Posting numerous observers at regular stations around the heart (i.e., having multiple leads) ensures that some leads inevitably will perceive the heart's electrical energy better than others and therefore will show larger, more easily interpreted waves and complexes (see Figure 202-5). Therefore on any ECG that shows multiple leads, the clinician will usually find it easiest to interpret the rhythm by first scanning the different leads to see which ones offer the clearest (i.e., largest and with the least artifact) P waves, QRS complexes, and T waves.

It is worth noting that by convention the diagram that shows the position of the 6 standard ECG limb leads is visualized in a ventral-dorsal orientation—or seen from above when the patient is in dorsal recumbency (see Figure 202-6). Each lead is named according to the location of its positive pole. The points around the circumference of the map, unfortunately, are named in a confusing manner. The change from +180 degrees to −180 degrees at the 9 o'clock position is a meaningless designation that has no implication regarding the positivity or negativity of the electrical energy or leads in the upper (cranial) half of the circle, and a much less confusing approach would have been simply to continue numbering the points from +180 degrees to +359 degrees. A more detailed description of this basic series of concepts may be found in most comprehensive books on electrocardiography.[2,4,5,9,10]

Mean Electrical Axis

As the ventricles depolarize, the sequential activation of the cardiomyocytes creates an overall direction or thrust of electrical activity in the ventricles. This electrical activity is best detected by an ECG lead most closely oriented with the direction of the electrical activity, as described previously.

The sum total of electrical energy for all the depolarizations in one beat of the ventricles represents the final tally of individual depolarizations, with impulses headed in the same direction adding to each other and impulses headed away from each other canceling each other out. Therefore in a normal heart, the sum total of electrical energy expended for one beat of the ventricles has an overall thrust that is leftward (because the left ventricle [LV] is larger than the right) and caudal (because more energy is directed toward the apex of the heart during initial activation than travels back toward the base at the end of ventricular activation). This sum total, or overall thrust, of electrical energy, is also called the *mean electrical axis* (MEA) (see Figures 202-3 to 202-6).

The direction and thrust of electrical energy (MEA) is characteristic for an individual and, barring an intermittent intraventricular conduction abnormality, is constant from beat to beat on an ECG tracing. In normal individuals, the MEA, as just mentioned, points leftward and caudally because that is the overall direction in which the normal ventricles point (see Figure 202-5). However, the sum total of electrical energy for one beat of the ventricles (the MEA) may change if the heart changes in shape. For example, if a patient's RV becomes pathologically enlarged to a sufficient degree, the bulk of electrical energy for ventricular depolarization may be directed more towards the right instead of the left. This is called a *right axis shift* or *right-axis deviation*. In such a case an ECG with multiple leads in a clinical patient could show QRS complexes that were more positive than usual in the right-sided lead (aVR) and QRS complexes that were more negative than usual in the left-sided leads (aVL, I, and II) (Figures 202-7 and 202-8). This simple ECG finding would increase the suspicion of disorders that cause RV enlargement. As a second example, conduction

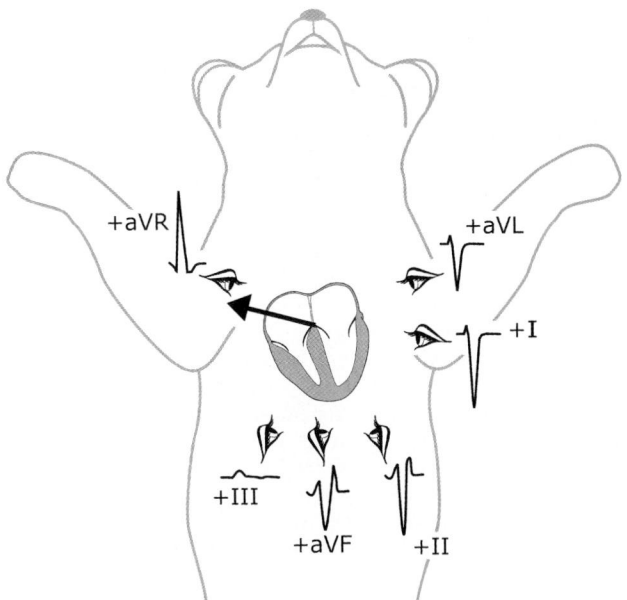

Figure 202-7 In this heart, marked right ventricular (RV) hypertrophy is present. The greater myocardial mass directs the overall thrust of ventricular activity rightward. This physiologic phenomenon is revealed on a standard electrocardiogram (ECG): the positive pole of a lead aVR registers more electrical energy directed toward it, and its QRS complex is markedly more positive than normal, whereas leads aVL, I, II, and aVF are more negative than normal because the thrust of energy travels away from them. These findings represent a right-axis deviation.

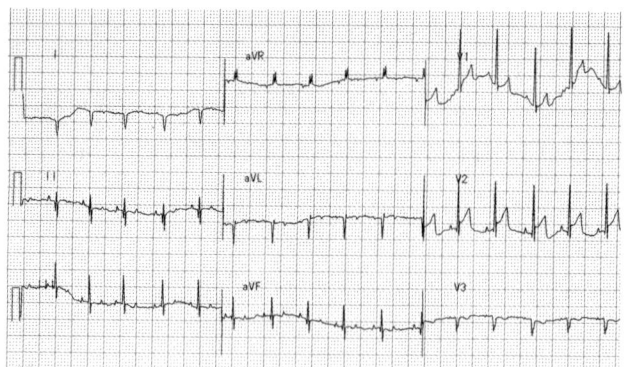

Figure 202-8 Right axis deviation. The mean electrical axis (MEA) is +150 degrees. Precordial leads also indicate a predominance of electrical activity to the right (rV2, marked "V1"; V_4 marked "V3"). Right ventricular (RV) hypertrophy was confirmed echocardiographically in this young miniature Schnauzer dog with severe pulmonic stenosis (25 mm/sec, 1 cm = 1 mV).

through the RV involves passage of the electrical impulse along the right bundle branch (RBB) for rapid spread through the RV. Hampered conduction through the RBB, a phenomenon called *RBB block*, redirects the electrical impulse, a variation that is visible on the ECG (see Bundle Branch Blocks, following; see Figure 202-45).[11] As a result of RBB block, the incompletely depolarized RV is depolarized late, and slightly less efficiently, by impulses redirected from the LV. This "swing" of electrical energy reorients the overall thrust of electrical energy for that beat of the ventricles toward the right, creating a right axis deviation. Therefore the two main differential diagnoses for right axis deviation in a patient with sinus rhythm are (1) RV hypertrophy and (2) RBB block. Left axis deviations occur uncommonly because the bulk of electrical activity already is directed toward the left in the normal heart. LV hypertrophy does not alter the direction of thrust of overall electrical activity from the left-caudal direction but often will increase its magnitude (e.g., taller R waves in lead II). Left anterior fascicular (LAF) block is an example of a conduction abnormality within the ventricles that is compensated for with a thrust of energy in the left dorsal direction, which can cause a left axis shift (see Figure 202-46 for an example).[12]

The concept of using the polarity and size of ECG deflections to infer the orientation of electrical thrust applies to the atria (P waves) and to the ventricles. Variations in atrial MEA have been associated with atrial enlargement or intra-atrial conduction abnormalities, yet as with the ventricles, MEA is at best a rough index, and its accuracy for assessing morphology appears to have been widely surpassed by that of other diagnostic modalities such as echocardiography.

Using vectorial enhancement, the ECG machine uses the three electrode wires connected to patients undergoing an ECG (the fourth is an electrical ground) to assess electrical activity from three additional perspectives (aVR, aVL, and aVF) in addition to I, II, and III, for a total of six different perspectives. The six positions, or leads, are evenly spaced 30 degrees apart and are called the *limb leads* (see Figure 202-6).

MEA can be calculated on an ECG in several ways, allowing the clinician to understand the overall direction of electrical thrust in the ventricles. Probably the simplest is to look for the lead with the most positive QRS complex. This represents the lead toward which the bulk of electrical activity is most directly oriented (i.e., the MEA). An equally effective, converse approach is to find the most isoelectric lead, namely the lead that perceives the least electrical energy. Because the isoelectric lead is the lead that is least aligned with the thrust of electrical activity,

then the lead 90 degrees to it must be the lead with the most electrical activity. The MEA is therefore the positive pole of the lead perpendicular to the isoelectric lead, in the direction that corresponds to positive QRS complexes. Finally, the classic way of determining MEA consists of calculating the surface area of the QRS complexes of two ECG leads (as the number of small boxes within the complexes). On the ECG axis map (see Figure 202-6), one then places a marker on the lines of each of the two leads examined. The distance of the two markers away from the center of the diagram is the number of small boxes that made up the surface area of each of the two examined leads. From the markers on each of these two leads' lines, a perpendicular line is drawn such that the two perpendiculars meet. A line from the center of the axis map to the point where the perpendiculars cross indicates the MEA. When MEA is correctly determined by any technique, all leads "agree" and are consistent with one direction of thrust of electrical activity, because the leads are only offering different perspectives on the same cardiac electrical activity. Any contradictory, nonsensical information in this regard is usually explained by erroneous connection of the electrode wires (ECG lead-patient limb mismatch).

Determining which is the "most positive QRS complex" or "most isoelectric lead" must take into account that the negative elements of a QRS complex cancel out an equivalent amount of the positive elements on the ECG tracing. Therefore it is a QRS complex's net positivity or negativity that is assessed. For instance, if lead II shows the tallest R wave and no Q or S wave, and lead aVF shows an identically tall R wave but some small Q and/or S waves as well, then the QRS is considered to be smaller in lead aVF; therefore the MEA is closer to +60 degrees than to +90 degrees (see Figure 202-5). By the same principle, a QRS complex that is wide is considered "bigger" (greater surface area) than a narrow QRS complex of the same height.

On an ECG, the cardiac rhythm is not affected by a patient's posture. However, the MEA is markedly altered by the position of the limbs, and a consistent approach to patient restraint is essential (by convention: right lateral recumbency, with limbs held perpendicular to the long axis of the patient's body). Changes in recumbency or in limb position can markedly and misleadingly alter the MEA.[6,14,15] This artifact was nicely illustrated in an experiment in which dogs in right lateral recumbency had an ECG done with one forelimb held forward and the other drawn back, and then the leg positions were reversed. A marked, but artifactual, change in MEA was observed.[15] Therefore in the ambulatory patient, no information can be inferred regarding MEA (see Ambulatory Electrocardiogram, following).

Precordial Leads

The concept of designing ECG leads to "survey" the electrical activity of the heart from multiple angles is a sound one, but even with a lead at every 30 degrees, a major shortcoming still exists. The six limb leads (I, II, III, aVR, aVL, aVF) may cover the entire frontal plane of the body (see Figure 202-6), but electrical energy traveling through a three-dimensional structure like the heart may travel "outward" or "inward" (i.e., in a dorsal or ventral direction). In such a situation, none of the six leads perceives the electrical activity as going clearly toward or away from any positive pole; electrical activity is perpendicular to all of them and therefore is invisible to all. The solution to this problem is the precordial leads (chest leads, thoracic leads, V leads). With precordial leads the ability to perceive electrical activity of the heart extends to three dimensions, because the ECG clips for precordial leads are placed circumferentially around the chest. Thus the precordial leads (rV_2, V_2, V_4, and V_{10}) assess electrical activity in the transverse (lateral and ventral-dorsal) plane (Figure 202-9). Precordial leads provide essential

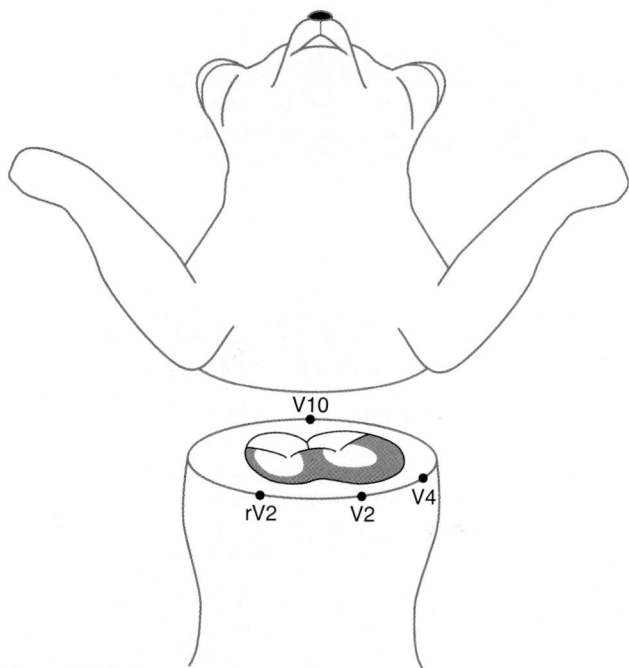

Figure 202-9 Precordial leads. Using the summation of limb leads as one "virtual" pole in the center of the chest, the positive poles of precordial leads are positioned to register electrical energy in the transverse plane as follows: right fifth intercostal space, just lateral to the sternum (rV2, or CV5RL), left sixth intercostal space, just lateral to the sternum (V2, or CV6LL), left sixth costochondral junction (V4, or CV6LU), and dorsal midline directly dorsal to lead V4 (V10), approximately over the seventh thoracic vertebra.[9]

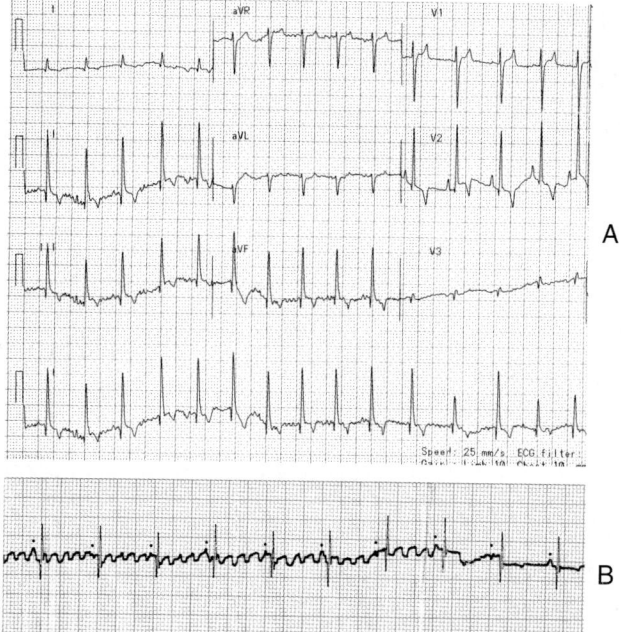

Figure 202-10 Deficiencies of limb leads and utility of precordial leads. **A,** This electrocardiogram (ECG) from an adult male Doberman dog with a chief complaint of dyspnea could be misinterpreted as indicating atrial fibrillation (AFib) because no P waves are seen in the limb leads and a fine, undulating baseline is present. However, P waves are clearly present, as seen in lead V2. This ECG shows normal sinus rhythm (NSR), not AFib. The P waves are isoelectric to the limb leads, indicating that the overall thrust of atrial electrical activity was oriented ventrally, toward lead V2 (Figure 202-9). The fine baseline undulations are motion artifact. The erroneous suspicion of AFib also was at odds with the regular rhythm and pulse noted on physical examination. Mild variation in R wave amplitude, as seen toward the end of the lead II rhythm strip at bottom, can occur with aberrant ventricular conduction or as an artifact of ECG filtration. Simultaneously recorded nine-lead tracing and rhythm strip (25 mm/sec, 1 cm = 1 mV). **B,** Sinus rhythm with motion artifact mimicking atrial flutter or fibrillation. Unlike true atrial flutter or fibrillation, the QRS complexes occur at regular intervals. P waves *(dots)* are seen, especially when the dog stops shivering at the end of the tracing (lead I, 25 mm/sec, 1 cm = 1 mV). (*B,* tracing courtesy of Sophia David, AHT.)

information that may not be apparent in the limb leads (frontal plane) (Figure 202-10) but they are more susceptible to artifact caused by chest wall motion (Figure 202-11).

Combining Mean Electrical Axis and Electrocardiographic Leads: Understanding the Direction and Force of Electrical Activity in a Heartbeat

From the explanations given previously, it should be seen as logical that lead II is routinely used for evaluating the ECG in small animals. This is because the positive pole of lead II (i.e., the point from which a lead II "observer" detects electrical activity) is at + 60 degrees, or in the left caudal region (see Figures 202-5 and 202-6). This is in the middle of the normal range of MEA for healthy dogs and cats.[2,5] The LV receives more energy than the right, and the overall thrust of electrical energy is caudal, so the positive pole of lead II is likely to perceive a large thrust of electrical energy toward it in normal small animals and thus display a clear ECG with large, visible QRS complexes (see Figure 202-3). The same can be said for atrial activity and the P waves. However, interindividual variation reveals the limitation of using only lead II. Certain patients may fail to provide the desired information in a specific lead (see Figure 202-10).

Deviation of the QRS MEA denotes an abnormal orientation of the sum total of ventricular electrical energy.[1,2,5] Normal MEA is +30 degrees clockwise to +110 degrees for the dog, and zero degrees clockwise to +160 degrees for the cat. The most common causes of right axis deviation (MEA to the right of normal [from +110 degrees clockwise to –90 degrees in the dog]) are RV hypertrophy and enlargement (see Figure 202-7 and 202-8), RBB block (see Figure 202-45), and ventricular

ectopy of LV origin (see Figure 202-32)—all conditions in which the bulk of ventricular electrical activity travels toward the RV. Left axis deviation (MEA to the left of normal [from +30 degrees clockwise to –90 degrees in the dog]) is rare and can be caused by LAF block (see Figure 202-46) or experimental transection of the left bundle branch. In cats the wide range of normal for MEA and the substantial overlap between normal and abnormal limits the usefulness of MEA, and some cardiologists omit it altogether. It can also be seen that a premature ventricular complex (PVC, VPC) originating from the LV, for example, will spread outward (i.e., toward the right) and thus presents a thrust of energy that is directed rightward. This radical difference in orientation of electrical thrust explains why classic PVCs of LV origin are commonly *bizarre looking:* they are oriented away from the positive pole of lead II, so are predominantly negative in that lead (i.e., bizarre in shape). PVCs also are usually wider than sinus beats because they spread from an ectopic focus through ventricular myocardium, not

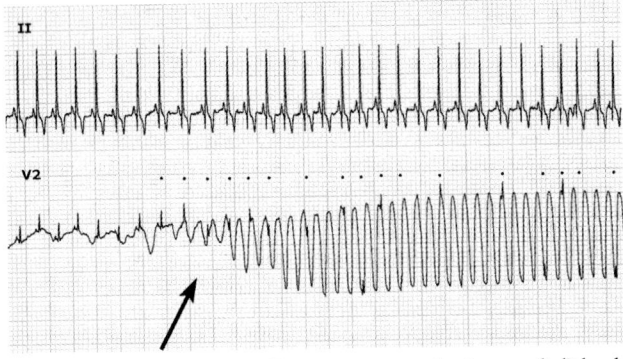

Figure 202-11 Artifact affecting a ventricular (precordial) lead; leads II and V₂ recorded simultaneously. In this dog, the cyclical chest excursions of panting *(onset: arrow)* can disrupt the ECG similar to ventricular arrhythmias. A closer inspection of lead V₂ reveals the persistence of superimposed, normally timed QRS complexes *(dots)*, many of which can be seen and none of which would occur if the rhythm were VT. This artifact is absent in the limb leads, which do not move with panting as does the chest wall. Speed: 5 mm/sec; scale: 10 mm/mV.

along the rapidly conductive fibers of the His-Purkinje system as normal beats would. This slower conduction means the QRS complex will be wider on the ECG (takes longer to be traced). Because the His-Purkinje system is more widely developed in the LV, PVCs of RV origin are more apt to propagate along on it and thus RV PVCs often are only slightly different from normal sinus QRS complexes.

Despite the incontestable superiority of echocardiography over ECG for assessing cardiac size and structure, the ECG continues to provide clues about abnormal heart size or shape. It can increase the index of suspicion for cardiac disease or can help to refine the differential diagnosis before an echocardiogram is performed. For example, heart diseases causing RV enlargement continue to be noted as causing a right axis deviation in many or most affected patients, including those with pulmonic stenosis (right axis deviation in 19 of 21 patients [90%][16]), right-to-left patent ductus arteriosus (right axis deviation in eight of eight patients [100%][17,18]), and cor pulmonale.[19]

Confounding Factors

Sources of error may alter the apparent MEA and result in an erroneous diagnosis. Changes in position of the limbs[14,15] and of the position of the heart within the chest (e.g., pericardial effusion [see Figure 202-17], peritoneopericardial diaphragmatic hernia, intrapericardial mass, or body motion in ambulatory ECG) change the perspective from which ECG leads perceive the heart's electrical activity, often causing the false appearance of changes in the MEA.

NORMAL ELECTROCARDIOGRAM

Extremely fit dogs with athletic hearts, such as Alaskan sled dogs, deviate substantially from the "normal" ranges listed at the beginning of the chapter (see Box 202-1).[20] In most normal dogs, heart rates range between 60 and 160/min. Rates above these limits are classified as *tachycardias*, and below 70 beats per minute (bpm) are *bradycardias*. Bursts of sinus tachycardia (STach) of up to 300 bpm have been identified for brief periods in normal dogs.[1] In healthy cats in the hospital setting, the normal heart rate extends up to 260 bpm, with a median of 180 bpm.[21] The low limit of normal varies, depending on whether the patient is at home or in the hospital. Generally 130 to 150 bpm would be considered low-normal for a healthy

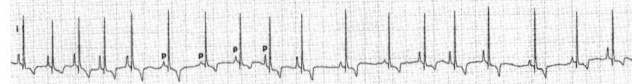

Figure 202-12 Respiratory sinus arrhythmia (RSA) and wandering pacemaker (WP). Lead II, 25 mm/sec, 1 cm = 1 mV.

cat in a clinical environment.[21] Ambulatory electrocardiographic testing provides an excellent opportunity to evaluate the real heart rate across the species and identifies a higher prevalence of arrhythmias than conventional monitoring.[22-25]

The *P wave* is the first deflection on the ECG after isoelectric diastole (baseline after T wave) (see Figures 202-1 and 202-2).[13] It should be positive in leads II and aVF, and isoelectric or positive in lead I. It may be negative in leads III, aVR, aVL, V₂, and V₁₀. The first half of the P wave represents RA activation, and the second half represents left atrial (LA) activation. The spread of atrial excitation begins in the upper portion of the RA at the SA node and spreads across the atrium, depolarizing the LA. The maximum normal amplitude of the P wave in any limb lead is 0.4 mV in the dog and 0.2 mV in the cat. The amplitude of the P wave may increase during inspiration and with increased heart rate. High vagal tone also allows the exact pacemaking site within the SA node to change. Higher centers are responsible for early activation, and lower centers closer to the AV node produce lower rates and lower amplitude P waves.[1] This vagally mediated change in the origin of the pacemaking site in the SA node is a normal feature of canine ECGs and is called a *wandering pacemaker* (WP) (Figure 202-12). The amplitude of the P wave may also vary between tracings due to changes in the position of the heart and of the ECG clips.

The duration of the P wave should not exceed 0.04 second in the dog (0.05 second in larger breeds) and 0.04 second in the cat. Notching of the P wave is not significant unless the duration of the wave exceeds stated limits, in which case it may indicate LA enlargement *(P mitrale)* (Figure 202-13). Conversely, P waves of increased amplitude, especially with a peaked shape, have been associated with enlargement or hypoxia of the RA *(P pulmonale)* (see Figure 202-13).

The morphology and amplitude of the canine P wave are more variable than in other animals, especially in the limb leads. The mean P wave MEA in normal dogs is within 90 degrees of the ventricular MEA in the frontal plane.

The *P-R segment* is the isoelectric period that follows the P wave on the ECG (see Figures 202-1 and 202-2). It is measured from the end of the P wave to the beginning of the first deflection away from the baseline, indicating ventricular activity. During the P-R segment, the electrical impulse is being conducted slowly through the AV node. Atrial repolarization

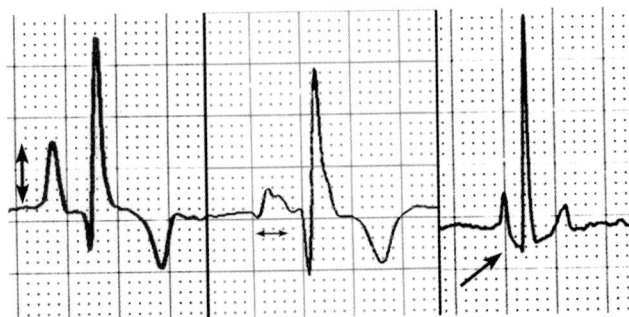

Figure 202-13 P wave abnormalities. Lead II, 25 mm/sec, 1 cm = 1 mV. A tall P wave (P pulmonale) is seen in the left panel, a wide P wave (P mitrale) is seen in the middle panel, and a Tₐ wave is seen in the right panel.

occurs during this period and into the QRS; atrial repolarization generally is too low in amplitude (or occurs too far into the QRS complex) to be detected on surface recordings, except in rare cases in which an atrial repolarization wave, or T_a wave, is seen within the PR segment (see Figure 202-13).[26] T_a waves distort the baseline of the PR segment and usually are indicative of atrial enlargement, hypoxia, or electrolyte changes.

The period from the onset of the P wave to the onset of the QRS complex is the *P-R interval* (see Figure 202-2). The duration of the P-R interval varies inversely with the heart rate. With rapid heart rates it may be 0.04 second but usually varies from 0.06 second to 0.14 second (dog) and from 0.04 to 0.09 second (cat). Normal dogs vary considerably. Prolongation of the PR interval is first-degree heart block, an electrocardiographic—but not hemodynamically important—term (see Atrioventricular Block, following). Short P-R intervals suggest rapid heart rates or accessory pathways that bypass normal A-V conduction (see Pre-Excitation Syndromes, following).

The *QRS complex* is the ECG representation of ventricular depolarization (see Figures 202-1 and 202-2).[13] It occurs immediately after the P-R interval. The components of the QRS complex are named for their sequence of occurrence, not for correlations with activation of specific parts of the ventricles. The Q wave is the first negative deflection occurring before a positive wave after the isoelectric P-R segment. The R wave is the first positive deflection after the P-R segment, regardless of whether or not a Q wave precedes it. The S wave is a negative deflection occurring after a (Q) or (R) deflection (or both). If no positive waves are present, the negative deflection is called a *QS complex* (e.g., lead I in Figure 202-8). Additional positive or negative deflections that occur in the QRS complex after the R or S wave has returned to the baseline (producing "splintered" QRS complexes) are called *prime (R'; S') waves* (Figure 202-14).[13] Any of the following ventricular patterns may arise: QR, QS, RS, R, QRS, plus prime deflections. If the wave amplitude is small (i.e., < 0.5 mV), it is written as a small letter (e.g., *q*); if it is greater than 0.5 mV,

a capital letter is used (e.g., Q).[1,13] These types of complexes occur under various conditions. For example, an association with congenital tricuspid valve malformations in Labrador retrievers is known to exist.[27]

The size of QRS complexes (and P waves) is significantly affected by the presence or absence of filters on the ECG machine. Use of routine ECG filtration in one canine study produced a median 51% reduction in QRS amplitude,[28] with the greatest amount of artifactual attenuation noted in smaller dogs and in tracings with narrower QRS complexes. Marked filtration effects also have been noted in feline ECGs.[29] Therefore the presence or absence of filtration should be recorded on ECG tracings whenever possible.

LV muscle mass normally exceeds RV mass. Depolarization of the LV overwhelmingly controls the magnitude and direction of the forces of the QRS complex in the dog and the cat. Ventricular activation occurs in three smooth, transitional phases: (1) initial, (2) main, and (3) terminal. The interventricular septum, except for the basilar region, is depolarized first, followed by bilateral apical and central endocardial to epicardial activation until a single cone of depolarized muscle surrounds each cavity. Terminal electrical activity proceeds from apex to base, exciting the basal septum and basal and lateral LV. The electrical thrust (vector) is directed from left to right in the interventricular septum, then endocardium to the epicardium, depolarizing the free (lateral) ventricular walls, and finally basally in the upper walls and septum (ventricular outflow tracts).[1,2,5,30] The durations of these phases are normally 0.01 second, 0.025 to 0.035 second, and 0.01 second, respectively, in the dog.[30,31] They are proportionate but shorter in the cat, where the entire QRS complex duration is usually between 0.02 and 0.03 second.

Prolongation of the QRS complex beyond 0.05 second (0.06 second in large breeds) indicates delayed ventricular depolarization. In cats, durations exceeding 0.04 second are unusual. Ventricular hypertrophy, bundle branch block (BBB), electrolyte disorders, formation of ventricular ectopic beats (either premature or escape rhythms; see discussion of premature ventricular complexes and conduction disorders, following), and aberrantly conducted beats (e.g., RBB block) can result in prolonged complexes.

More specifically, the initial ventricular electrical thrust, or vector, when the impulse first emerges from the AV node and begins to travel in the His bundle, is oriented rightward, craniad, and ventrad. Leads I and V_{10} should therefore each have a Q wave, indicating an initial rightward (lead I) and ventrad (lead V_{10}) force. The Q wave in canine leads II and aVF represent cranially directed initial forces (duration under 0.01 second). The initial vector is directed cranially for only a short period prior to turning caudad. If a Q wave is present in older dogs in leads I, II, III, and aVF, and if its amplitude is greater than −0.5 mV in lead II, it is probably abnormal and specifically suggests the possibilities of RV enlargement or RBB block.

The main portion of the QRS complex reflects depolarization of the LV and RV free walls. The main ECG deflection is formed by depolarization of the LV wall directed to the left, caudad, and ventrad, producing an R wave in leads I, II, III, and aVF (leftward and caudad) and a Q wave in lead V_{10} (ventrad).

The terminal force of the QRS complex represents dorsal basal (apicobasilar) depolarization. The force is either rightward or leftward, depending on the extent to which the basal region of the LV lies to one side of the midline. If part of the dorsal basal region lies electrically to the right side of the thorax, then the terminal electrical forces will be directed cranially and to the right, producing a small S wave in leads I, II, III, and aVF. This $S_1S_2S_3$ pattern sometimes is noted with severe heartworm disease and other causes of marked RV hypertrophy (Figure 202-15). Normally no S wave occurs in lead I and it may also be absent in lead II. Lead V_{10} should always have

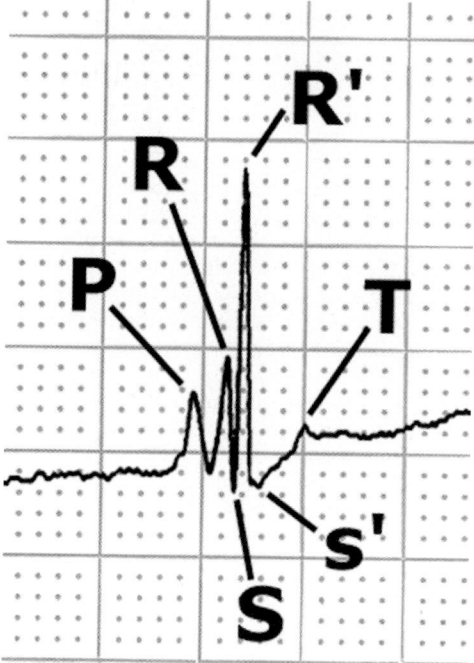

Figure 202-14 Example of a splintered QRS complex. The exact description is an RSR's' complex. The short P-R interval also suggests pre-excitation. Lead II, 25 mm/sec, 1 cm = 1 mV.

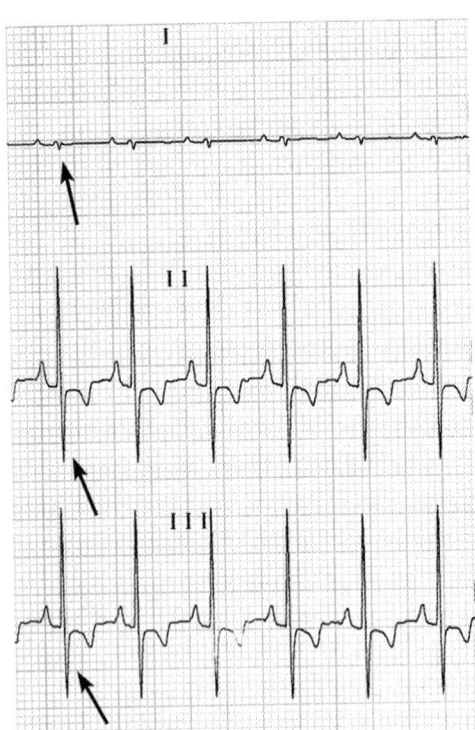

Figure 202-15 S waves *(arrows)* seen in leads I, II, and III (S₁S₂S₃ pattern). This is a manifestation of the final forces of ventricular depolarization being directed cranially (S waves in leads II and III) and to the right (S waves in leads I and II). Classically it has been associated with right ventricular (RV) hypertrophy, as in this 6-year-old Husky dog with severe heartworm disease (25 mm/sec, 1 cm = 1 mV).

a Qr complex, the small *r* wave representing the terminal dorsal basal depolarization of the ventricles.

The upper-normal limit of amplitude of the canine R wave is 2.5 mV; above 3.0 mV is virtually always abnormal except in some young dogs. Abnormally tall R waves in lead II suggest LV enlargement. R waves of amplitude less than 0.5 mV in leads I, II, and III are small.[1] Consistently diminished R wave amplitude suggests pericardial or pleural effusion (or both), intrathoracic mass, severe pulmonary disease, hypovolemia, hypothyroidism, hypothermia, acute hemorrhage,[32] or obesity.

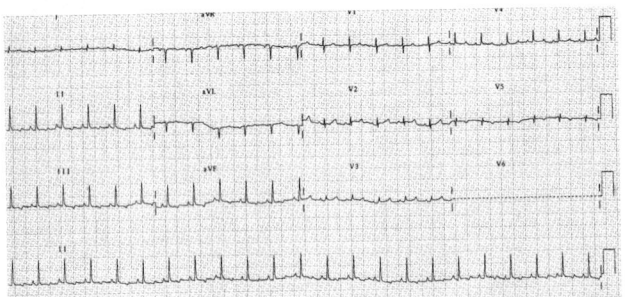

Figure 202-16 Normal sinus rhythm (NSR) in a cat. Heart rate: 140 beats per minute (bpm). Mean electrical axis (MEA): +85 degrees. Left ventricular (LV) hypertrophy is also suspected based on the tall R Waves in lead II and was confirmed echocardiographically. The fifth precordial lead is inserted between V₂ and V₄ as described by Harpster[10] (25 mm/sec, 1 cm = 1 mV).

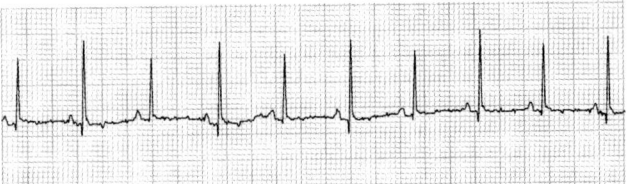

Figure 202-17 Electrical alternans. Lead II, 25 mm/sec, 1 cm = 1 mV.

These associations are true only if QRS complexes are diminished in all leads, including the V leads. Otherwise, QRS complexes may simply be small in one lead because they are larger in other leads (i.e., the MEA is directed elsewhere; see Mean Electrical Axis). Cyclic changes in heart rate may cause cyclic variations in QRS complex size. A pattern of alternating change in R-wave height from beat to beat is seen in some dogs with pericardial effusion (Figure 202-17). This finding, called *electrical alternans*, results from the swinging motion of the beating heart within a distended, fluid-filled pericardial sac.

Occasionally the QRS complex is nearly isoelectric in all six limb leads, a variation of normal referred to as a *horizontal heart*. The MEA is indeterminate in the frontal plane, and normal MEA parameters cannot be used; however, the precordial leads often still give useful information regarding left-right and dorsal-ventral orientation of the electrical thrust. The rhythm durations of waves, complexes, and intervals are not altered by the horizontal heart situation.

The Q-T interval begins with the onset of the QRS complex, ends when the T wave returns to baseline, and denotes the entire period of ventricular electrical activity (see Figure 202-2).[2,13] The duration of the Q-T interval varies directly with the preceding RR interval. Nevertheless, and despite wide variations in heart rate in the dog, the Q-T interval does not vary during respiratory sinus arrhythmia (RSA).[33] Measurements of the Q-T interval have traditionally been corrected (Q-T_c) for the effect of heart rate using the Bazett formula:

$$\text{Q-T}_c = \text{Q-T interval/square root of R-R interval}$$

This formula may overcorrect at rapid heart rates and undercorrect at lower heart rates and is dependent on identification of the exact duration of the T wave, which may be challenging in some ECGs. Clinically the Q-T interval may be assessed routinely without correction and, when that is required, the formula is the simplest adequate method. In small animal practice, Q-T interval prolongation is usually associated with certain medications[34] specific medical conditions[34,35] but not the arrhythmogenic cardiomyopathy of boxer dogs.[36] Amiodarone, a class III antiarrhythmic agent (see Therapy of Arrhythmias, following) is known in human beings and in dogs to prolong the Q-T interval when administered over long periods of time.[37] This effect is due to its effect on potassium ion channels (I_to transient outward K+ current and others). Such electrocardiographic changes have been linked to proarrhythmia in humans, although this association has not been clearly demonstrated clinically in dogs or cats. Some veterinarians are called upon to evaluate Q-T intervals critically because their work involves research laboratory studies that test the effects of drugs on such ECG changes as Q-T interval prolongation. In this instance the reader may wish to pursue specific information on Q-T interval corrections and nonclinical electrocardiology.[1,34,38,39] Regardless of context, marked prolongation of the Q-T interval can be an issue of concern; it raises the possibility of such acute, "malignant" arrhythmias as torsades de pointes (TdP, see Figure 202-38) and ventricular fibrillation (VF, see Figure 202-37).

The S-T segment and T wave represent ventricular repolarization (see Figures 202-1 and 202-2).[13] The S-T segment, which represents the slower phase of repolarization and its predominance of slow calcium channel activity, begins with the end of the QRS complex (i.e., the J or junctional point or wave) and ends with the first deflection of the T wave.[2,34] The T wave represents the most rapid period of ventricular repolarization, during which potassium briskly leaks out of the cell. It ends when the wave returns to the isoelectric baseline. The S-T segment and T wave should be examined for depression or elevation from the baseline, either of which may be associated with myocardial hypoxia, nonspecific electrolyte changes, or cardiac hypertrophy (Figure 202-18). The degree of ST deviation appears to vary cyclically with the R-R interval, and deviation increases with shorter preceding R-R intervals.[1] Abnormal deviations of the S-T segment are defined as a depression of 0.2 mV or elevation of 0.15 mV in leads II and III, or they are defined as a depression or elevation of 0.3 mV in lead V_4. A subjective appearance of a delayed return to baseline in the S-T segment (i.e., an S wave that has an oblique or curved terminal upstroke) is referred to as *S-T segment slurring* or *coving* (see Figure 202-18). Like S-T elevation or depression, S-T slurring most often suggests myocardial hypoxia, particularly when it is new (e.g., intraoperative ECG demonstrating its sudden onset). In a study comparing normal and sick cats, S-T changes were frequently reported in cats with identifiable cardiac disease. Abnormal S-T segments occurred in 70% of cats with congenital heart disease, in 43% to 47% of cats with cardiomyopathy, and only in 10% of normal cats.[40,41]

The T wave may be concordant or discordant in normal dogs, meaning that its polarity may be in the same direction or in the opposite direction, respectively, compared with the QRS complex. The polarity of the T wave depends on the direction of repolarization within the ventricular wall (from epicardium to endocardium, or vice versa) and is of no known clinical importance in small animals at this time. In healthy human beings, the QRS complex and T wave are usually concordant, and this important interspecies difference has led physicians and nurses to misinterpret canine ECGs with QRS-T discordance as abnormal (because QRS-T discordance is sometimes a feature of myocardial infarction in people). Normally the T wave is positive in lead V_2 and negative in V_{10} or else RV hypertrophy is suggested (exception: Chihuahua). If the amplitude of the T wave is greater than 25% of that of the R wave (Q wave if it is deeper), LV enlargement may be suspected. These links between T wave morphology and cardiac structure appear to be fairly insensitive and nonspecific, and their utility has been essentially replaced by echocardiography.

Technical Aspects of the Electrocardiograph

Techniques for obtaining the ECG are discussed in Chapter 90. By convention, paper speed is 50 mm/sec in small animals, although the paper speed commonly used in human cardiology, 25 mm/sec, may be used in veterinary medicine if the heart rate is 120 bpm or lower. The usual amplitude setting is 1 cm = 1 mV, and this is halved or doubled if the patient's tracing shows unusually large or small deflections, respectively.

Evolution of the Electrocardiograph

At birth the MEA of the normal canine ECG is directed rightward, cranially, and ventrally. Over the first 3 months of life this orientation slowly changes in the normal dog to leftward, caudal, and ventrad. A similar pattern of evolution exists for kittens.[42] The criteria used for establishing a "normal" ECG are not the same for a dog less than 12 weeks of age as they are for an older dog.[43] In a study of normal dogs raised on regular or calorie-restricted diets from adulthood until death, no changes were observed with advancing age on the annual ECGs of dogs in either group during the dogs' lifetimes.[44]

DIAGNOSTIC MANIPULATIONS WITH ELECTROCARDIOGRAPHY

Vagal Maneuver

Artificially increasing a patient's vagal tone has potential value both diagnostically and therapeutically. Diagnostically, slowing the heart rate and increasing AV nodal refractoriness through vagal maneuvers may slow a rapid tachycardia, allowing some of its features to be more apparent and facilitating the ECG diagnosis (Figure 202-19). Therapeutically, an increase in vagal tone that interrupts macro re-entrant circuits can briefly reduce an excessively high ventricular rate through AV block (as described for atrial flutter later in the chapter) or can terminate such arrhythmias as AV nodal re-entrant tachycardia and orthodromic AV reciprocating tachycardia (see Pre-Excitation Syndromes, following).

Carotid sinus massage (gentle, sustained compression of the carotid sinuses, located just caudal to the dorsal aspect of the larynx, often to the point of eliciting a gag reflex) can be applied for 5 to 10 seconds and should be tolerated by the patient (signs of discomfort, resentment, or a marked change in heart rate warrant immediate termination of the vagal maneuver). Because dogs and cats very rarely suffer from carotid artery atherosclerosis, concern for thromboembolic consequences of carotid sinus massage as expressed in human cardiology is unlikely to be relevant to small animal practice. Ocular pressure over closed eyelids is another form of vagal maneuver, but it is contraindicated in patients with ocular problems and subjectively appears to be less effective than carotid sinus massage.

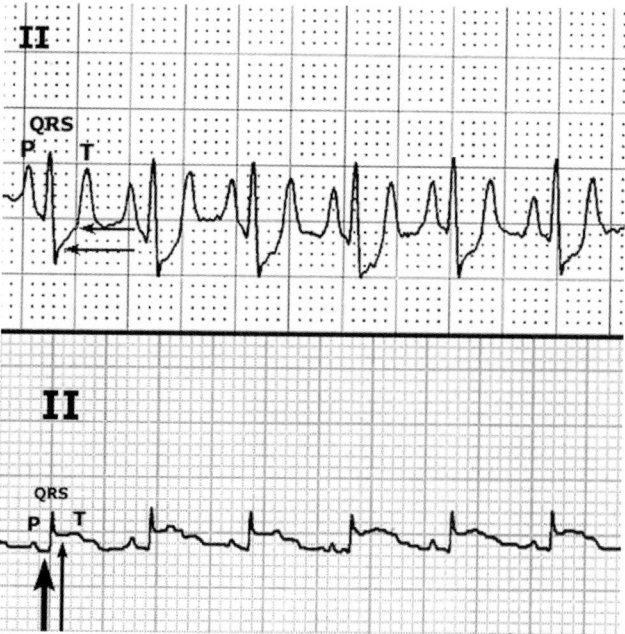

Figure 202-18 ST segment changes in two cats. *Upper panel,* ST segment depression. The two arrows should completely overlap. ST segment coving, or slurring, also is present (50 mm/sec, 2 cm = 1 mV). *Lower panel,* ST segment elevation. The height of the ST segment *(small arrow)* should be the same as the baseline *(large arrow).* Lead II, 25 mm/sec, 1 cm = 0.5 mV.

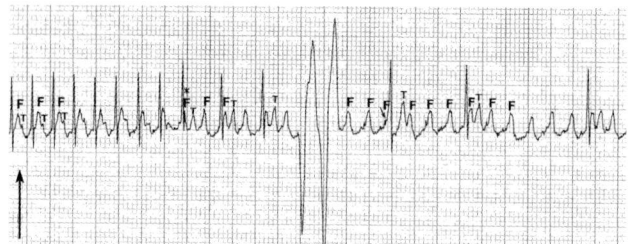

Figure 202-19 Atrial flutter. The diagnosis of atrial flutter is made easier by the initiation of carotid sinus massage *(arrow)*. This vagal maneuver was applied because this dog had a persistently high heart rate in the absence of an identifiable cause (320 beats per minute [bpm], first part of tracing). Carotid sinus massage induces second-degree AV block beginning after the ninth QRS complex *(small asterisk)*. As a result the flutter waves *(F)* are seen more distinctly as separate from the T waves and QRS complexes. Two premature ventricular complexes (PVCs) also are seen in the middle of the tracing. After the AV node has increased in refractoriness, the flutter waves *(F)* are much more clearly seen as distinct from the QRS complexes and T waves and are always evenly spaced, even when buried in a QRS complex *(small arrow)*. Lead aVF, 25 mm/sec, 1 cm = 1 mV.

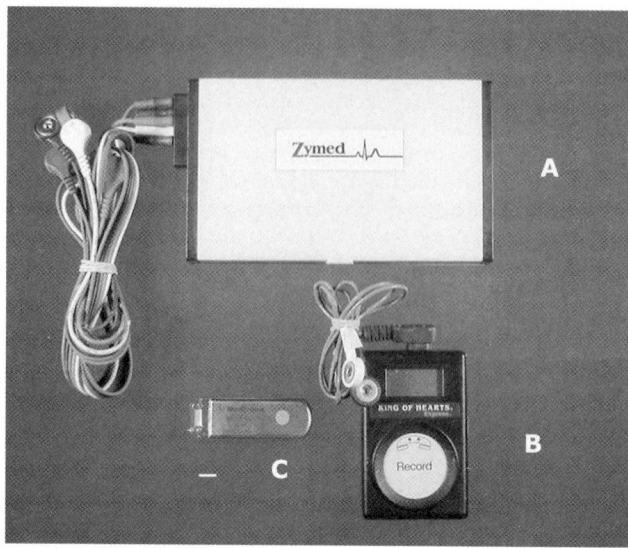

Figure 202-20 Ambulatory heart monitors. **A,** 24-hour (Holter) monitor. **B,** External event monitor. **C,** Implantable event monitor. Scale: white bar = 1 cm.

Atropine Response Test

Administration of atropine sulfate 0.02 mg/lb (0.04 mg/kg) intravenously can be used diagnostically to evaluate bradycardias.[3] It allows the differentiation between bradycardias purely of vagal origin (atropine increases the heart rate) and bradycardias caused by intrinsic disturbances of impulse formation or conduction (atropine has no effect). The response occurs within seconds to minutes (always within 15 minutes) after injection.[3] Unfortunately, a positive response to atropine is poorly predictive of response to oral vagolytic drugs such as propantheline bromide in dogs with sick sinus syndrome (SSS).

AMBULATORY ELECTROCARDIOGRAPHY

In a patient with clinical signs caused by an intermittent cardiac arrhythmia, an ECG performed in the veterinary hospital may or may not be abnormal. Ambulatory ECG offers the possibility of correlating the ECG to the overt clinical manifestations observed by the owner. As a result, ambulatory ECG is valuable for evaluation of patients with episodic clinical signs because it can either rule in an arrhythmic problem (arrhythmia is diagnosed) or rule it out (normal rhythm occurs throughout the episode).[23-25,45-48]

Three types of ambulatory ECG monitors are available (Figure 202-20). Dr. Norman Holter developed the continuous monitor that now bears his name in the 1950s, when the earliest models weighed some 80 lbs (36 kg). Currently, Holter monitors are approximately the size and weight of a VHS videocassette, and they record the ECG continuously for 24 or 48 hours, usually on multiple leads simultaneously.[49,50] An audiocassette inside the monitor typically is used for storing the information during the recording period and must be decoded afterwards in an analyzer machine. Veterinarians can rent Holter monitors from various suppliers, including such on-line sources as www.labcorp.com, www.vetheart.com, www.idexx.com, and www.pdsheart.com. Holter monitor leads are placed on dogs as shown in Figure 202-21. Owners need to maintain a diary of the patient's activities—and lack thereof—during the entire monitoring period to provide a context for analysis of the tracing. For example, a heart rate of 40 bpm may not be unusual for a sleeping dog, but it would be an important

finding if it occurred during brisk exercise. A veterinary patient's Holter report, if produced through human cardiology software, should be reviewed carefully.[49] Over- and underinterpretation are common, because software for automated Holter analysis is designed only for human ECGs at this time. Common sources of error from human Holter interpretation programs include inaccurate heart rate counting (undercounting QRS complexes that are too small during body movement or overcounting such as interpreting T waves as QRS complexes) and inaccurate arrhythmia diagnosis (over- or underinterpretation). It remains the veterinarian's obligation to assess the abnormal ECG segments shown in the Holter report and to decide whether the interpretation correlates well with the rest of the patient's information. Continuous in-hospital monitoring systems similarly allow long-term cardiac rhythm monitoring and manual analysis of tracings, and they offer the advantage of immediately displaying ECG information during patient observation and treatment.

The second and third types of ambulatory ECG monitors are event monitors (see Figure 202-20). They continuously receive ECG information into a loop memory system, which can usually only retain the information temporarily. When an episode of clinical signs is observed, however, the owner needs to trigger the event monitor. Doing so saves an exact

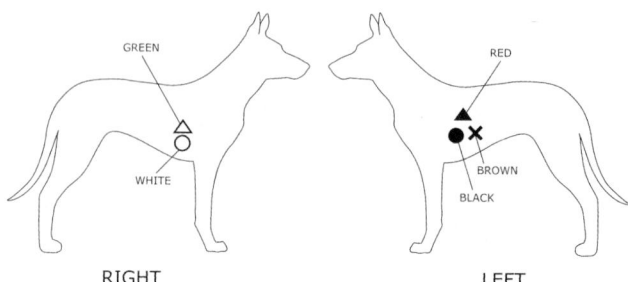

Figure 202-21 Electrode patch placement for Holter monitor. Colors correspond to the colors of the connecting tips on the ends of the Holter monitor wires.

segment of ECG information in the monitor's permanent memory. Several episodes can thus be recorded over a number of days and then decoded either at the veterinary hospital or transtelephonically. Event monitors usually record only one lead, although newer models may record two leads. The difference between the two types of event monitors is that one is external, whereas the other is implanted subcutaneously. External event monitors are approximately the size of a deck of cards and require standard commercial (e.g., AA) batteries that provide 5 to 7 days of monitoring time.[47,48] If the batteries run out, all acquired episodes are deleted. External event monitors are connected to patients using two or three wires attached to cutaneous ECG patches, one on each side of the chest over the heart (modified precordial lead). The memory capacity of external event monitors ranges from 5 to 18 minutes, and the monitors are programmed beforehand to save a selected amount of ECG information (e.g., 45 seconds preceding the push of the button and 15 seconds after it for each triggered episode). They are available for use from various sources, including many of those listed previously for Holter monitors. Internal event monitors are implanted subcutaneously.[51,52] They measure $0.5 \times 2 \times 7$ cm, about the size of a man's thumb, have a battery life of 1 year or more, and have a memory capacity of about 1 hour of ECG recording. The information they capture is retrieved after the episode is over, using a handheld unit placed over the area of skin where the monitor is located. The use of both types of event monitors is of proven diagnostic value in humans; both external, and to a much lesser extent so far, internal, monitors are in use in small animal patients.[23-25,47,48,51-53]

Each form of ambulatory ECG monitoring has its relative merits.[47] Holter monitors are superior for screening the number of abnormal heartbeats on the ECG in a fixed 24- or 48-hour period, such as for assessing boxers for familial arrhythmic heart disease or for the evaluation of animals receiving systemic experimental drugs.[23,25,39,45,54] Holter monitors are also superior for therapeutic monitoring of antiarrhythmic drug effects[46] and recently have been shown to provide predictive information regarding the future development of dilated cardiomyopathy in Doberman pinschers, often before the earliest echocardiographic changes.[55,56] Conversely, external event monitors also have a number of advantages: they are smaller and lighter (3.5 oz [100 g], compared with 14 oz [400 g] for a Holter monitor), making them practical for cats and small dogs; they have a longer memory (up to 1 week), which is useful for episodes occurring less frequently; they eliminate some uncertainty of interpretation by directly associating the ECG information with an observed event; and they can transmit information transtelephonically, allowing the monitor to be reset and a new monitoring period to begin without a return visit to the hospital. Both Holter and external event monitors are costly electronic devices carried by patients that can damage them, and owners must be instructed to avoid their pets' exposure to moisture, extremes of temperature, and rough handling of the monitors.

CLASSIFICATION OF CARDIAC RHYTHM DISTURBANCES

A useful and practical classification scheme is one that separates cardiac arrhythmias into three groups: (1) disturbances of impulse formation (cardiac excitability), (2) disturbances of impulse transmission (cardiac conduction), and (3) complex disturbances involving abnormalities both of excitation and conduction. Some rhythm disturbances fit poorly into any category. Some disturbances of cardiac excitability are secondary to conduction disturbances (e.g., junctional or ventricular escape rhythms). Disturbances are listed according to the anatomic level of their origin (i.e., atrial, junctional, or ventricular).

Excitation disturbances can cause either excessive or inadequate contraction of the heart or its parts. Increased excitability produces extrasystoles (if intermittent) and tachycardia (if sustained). *Ectopy* is the term that describes spontaneous production of impulses anywhere in the heart. Decreased excitability leads to loss of impulse formation with electrical quiescence, resulting in bradycardia or asystole.

Conduction disturbances within the heart are all called *blocks*. Their categorization depends on the anatomic location of the block and its extent or degree. *First-degree block* refers to a slowing of conduction, *second-degree block* implies complete but intermittent interruption, and *third-degree block* involves complete and sustained interruption of conduction. Block can occur at the SA node (rarely identified), the AV node, or in branches of the His bundle (BBBs).

Finally, two disturbances combining excitability and conduction abnormalities are discussed. In pre-excitation, accessory conduction pathways bypass part of the normal A-V conduction pathway. Sick sinus syndrome (SSS) generally involves periods of bradycardia and tachycardia caused by dysfunction of the sinus node and supraventricular and ventricular conductive tissues.

Clinical Impact of Rhythm Disturbances

The rhythm disturbances mentioned previously do not all carry the same clinical importance. Furthermore, interspecies differences are marked. Some are commonly encountered, whereas others are extremely rare. Their clinical impact may range from harmless (some are benign variations of normal) to severely detrimental (potentially life-threatening arrhythmias). In cats, pre-excitation and isorhythmic AV dissociation have been associated with feline cardiomyopathies. In the dog, disturbances of excitability, especially extrasystoles and AFib, are more common than are disturbances of conduction, the majority of which are AV blocks.[1,2,57]

The hemodynamic consequences of cardiac arrhythmias depend on at least eight factors: (1) the ventricular rate, (2) the duration of the abnormal rhythm, (3) the temporal relationship between the atria and ventricles, (4) the sequence of ventricular activation, (5) inherent myocardial and valvular function, (6) cycle length irregularity, (7) drug therapy, and (8) extracardiac influences.[1-3] Ultimately, the sum of these factors—not just the appearance of the ECG—determines the impact of the arrhythmia on the patient. This is the reason that some animals with ventricular tachycardia (VT) are asymptomatic, whereas others are moribund.

Identification of Rhythm Disturbances

Today most clinical electrocardiography in veterinary medicine relies on single-lead, in-hospital ECGs. Multilead ECGs provide an additional level of information that is sometimes indispensable (see Figure 202-10). Ambulatory ECG is an effective and increasingly popular method for detecting intermittent rhythm disturbances or identifying the frequency of arrhythmias over a period of time (see previous discussion).

Rhythm disturbances are identified on the ECG using a methodical four-point examination. First, a rapid, cursory evaluation from left to right of the entire tracing gives a general idea of the cardiac rhythm and an initial diagnostic orientation. This step reveals whether a single rhythm or many rhythms exist. (Are all QRS complexes of the same morphology? Are the R-R intervals the same, or do they vary? If so, does the variation occur in a predictable manner?) One grossly assesses the heart rate (slow, normal, or fast), whether the rhythm is regular or irregular, and detects premature or delayed complexes.

Second, the R-R intervals are evaluated in representative sections of the entire tracing (Figure 202-22). In cats, variability of the R-R interval is not normally seen and is

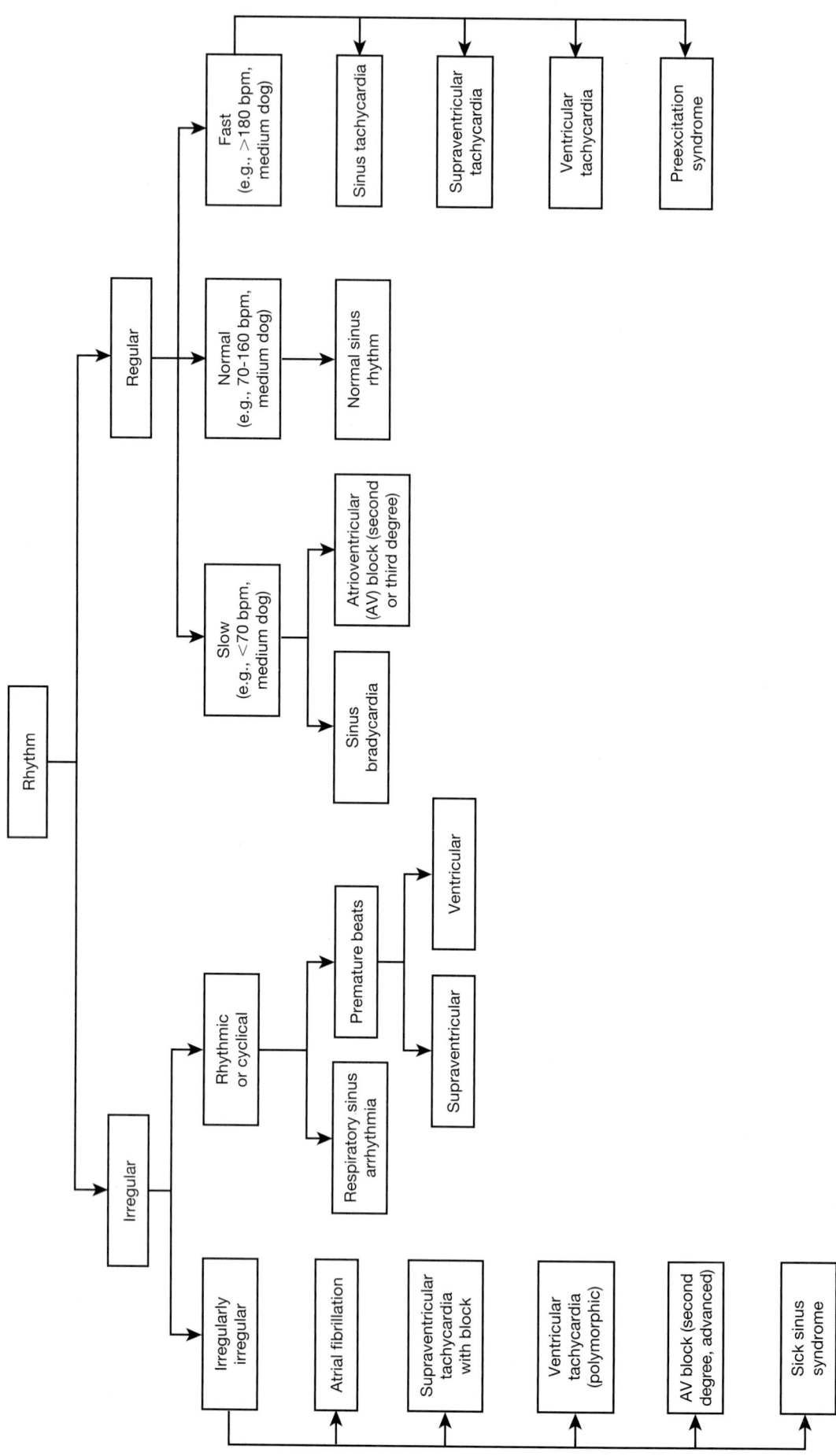

Figure 202-22 Approach to the recognition of cardiac rhythm disturbances.

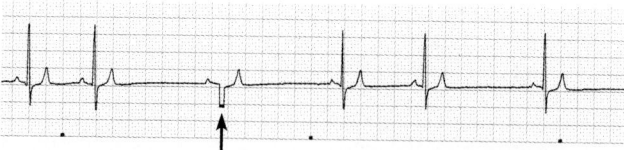

Figure 202-23 Artifact producing a wide, bizarre deflection in a dog. This is not an abnormal depolarization of the ventricles because the T wave is normal. Abnormal depolarization would invariably be followed by different or "abnormal" waves of repolarization (see Figures 202-32, 202-33, 202-35, and 202-36). Lead V$_2$, 25 mm/sec, 1 cm = 1 mV.

considered pathologic.[58] In dogs, a cyclical (i.e., rhythmic, patterned) variation of the R-R interval, respiratory sinus arrhythmia (RSA), is normal (see Figures 202-12 and 202-22). Irregularly irregular R-R variations are always abnormal in both species (see Figure 202-22).

Third, the examination of individual QRS complexes consists of determining whether they are narrow or wide. Narrow QRSs generally identify ventricular depolarization of supraventricular origin (e.g., Figure 202-16). Wide QRSs represent the asynchronous depolarization of the two ventricles, which may be due to the ventricular origin of a depolarization, to BBB, or to pre-excitation (see following). Because repolarization follows directly in the wake of the wave of depolarization, then a QRS complex of abnormal shape should also have a T wave of abnormal or different shape. If the T wave is normal, the possibility of artifact, rather than a truly abnormal QRS, should be considered (Figure 202-23).

Fourth, examination of the P waves (present, absent; positive, negative; see Figure 202-13) provides information on the depolarization of the atria. Examination of the PR interval (1) determines if a P wave exists for every QRS complex and a QRS complex for every P wave (to assess A-V synchrony) and (2) assesses AV nodal conduction (PR interval duration) (see Figure 202-2).

Finally, the basic underlying rhythm and any additional or secondary rhythms that are superimposed are identified. Normally a P wave exists for every QRS complex (an atrial depolarization for every ventricular depolarization). Abnormalities causing more than one P wave for each QRS complex include second- and third-degree AV blocks, and abnormalities producing QRS complexes without P waves include ventricular arrhythmias, AFib, and atrial standstill.

Disturbances of Excitability

An important subdivision involves classifying disturbances of excitability,[59,60] including STach, atrial extrasystoles (premature atrial complexes [PACs]), atrial tachycardias, atrial flutter, and AFib; or as disturbances of ventricular excitability, including ventricular extrasystoles (PVCs, VPCs), VT, TdP, ventricular flutter, and VF. The inciting factors that produce the arrhythmias in these two subgroups are often specific to the subgroup, and antiarrhythmic treatment is also sharply different between the two subgroups.

Disturbances and Alterations of Sinus Excitability
These arrhythmias are variations of sinus rhythm (see Figure 202-16), and are most commonly linked to normal, autonomic inputs. They may sometimes be abnormal and then are potentially detrimental. For example, STach is a normal and appropriate physiologic phenomenon during exercise, but it is commonly encountered in heart failure where, pathologically, it occurs even at rest.

Respiratory (normal) sinus arrhythmia (RSA)
In the dog the balance between the sympathetic and parasympathetic inputs to the heart generally tilts in favor of the parasympathetic system. This characteristic is in contrast to the average adult human or cat. This vagal predominance in the dog produces two particular features of sinus rhythm on the canine ECG: (1) RSA and (2) wandering pacemaker (WP).

RSA is the result of vagal effects that occur within the thorax during each respiratory cycle (see Figure 202-12). In dogs it is a normal physiologic phenomenon requiring no treatment. The result is a correlation between heart rate and respiratory rate, with slowing of the heart rate during expiration and acceleration of the heart rate during inspiration. The repeating cyclic nature of this arrhythmia is its hallmark. RSA is first noted in the puppy after 4 weeks of age,[1] generally disappears when the heart rate exceeds 150 bpm,[1,2] and often is enhanced when severe dyspnea is present (pneumothorax, fibrosis, emphysema) due to exaggerated changes in intrathoracic pressure.[1] Interestingly, the presence of RSA may constitute a valuable diagnostic clue in a common clinical situation, namely in the coughing, small- to medium-breed adult dog. It is common for these dogs to have concurrent mitral valvular heart disease (typical murmur is auscultated) and a primary respiratory disorder such as collapsing trachea or chronic bronchitis. It may be difficult to pinpoint whether congestive heart failure (CHF) or a primary respiratory problem is responsible for the animal's cough, yet the need for immediate and long-term treatment and the prognosis both depend on knowing which disease process is the cause of the cough. The presence of RSA makes decompensated mitral valvular disease as the sole cause of the cough highly unlikely, because the cardiogenic pulmonary edema of CHF would almost invariably bring on increased sympathetic tone and loss of RSA. In cats in the hospital setting, RSA generally is considered pathologic.[58]

In the treatment of CHF with tachycardia (sinus or other supraventricular), successful digitalization may bring about the reappearance of RSA. This return of RSA is due to the reactivation of baroreceptors, which had been downregulated ("exhausted") by the ongoing sympathetic stimulation of heart failure.

Wandering pacemaker
WP is a normal, physiologic phenomenon in dogs that is not associated with pathologic conditions and requires no treatment (see Figure 202-12). In the dog the origin of depolarization in the heart is not fixed but may move within the RA, between the SA node and the AV node. On the ECG the result is variation in the P wave amplitude, with QRS complexes that retain a normal, supraventricular appearance. This variability in the P wave is often cyclic and often associated with RSA (see Figure 202-12). In this situation the amplitude of the P wave increases with an increased heart rate (inspiration) and decreases with decreased heart rate (expiration), sometimes to the point of disappearance (isoelectric P wave) or, rarely, negativity in leads II, III, and aVF.[1,2] The ECG differential diagnosis for WP includes morphologic abnormalities (e.g., P pulmonale) and supraventricular extrasystoles. In some individuals with marked resting vagal tone (e.g., brachycephalic dogs), an exaggerated but normal RSA and WP may be difficult to distinguish from a pathologic arrhythmia, namely PACs (supraventricular extrasystoles). Both PACs and the combination of WP and RSA produce a P wave of different morphology, a shorter R-R interval, and QRS complexes of normal morphology. Differentiation rests on the degree of prematurity (WP and RSA should not occur so prematurely as to produce a P wave inside the preceding T wave), and the appearance of a series or "paroxysm" of such beats closely coupled to each other (corresponding to multiple supraventricular extrasystoles [i.e., supraventricular tachycardia], not RSA). If neither characteristic is apparent, a Holter monitor can be used for assessing a large number of heartbeats (see previous discussion), or an atropine response test (see previous discussion) can be performed to

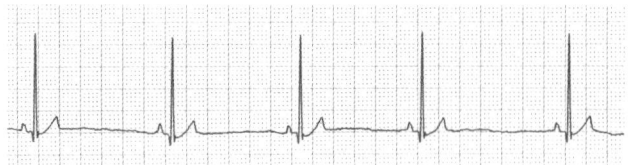

Figure 202-24 Sinus bradycardia (SB) in a dog. The heart rate is 50/min. Lead II, 25 mm/sec, 1 cm = 1 mV.

abolish the vagal effect and seek out persistently premature heartbeats with a different P wave morphology and normal QRS complexes (i.e., PACs, in the absence of vagal tone).

Sinus bradycardia Sinus bradycardia (SB) is a sinus rhythm in which the heart rate is abnormally low (see Boxes 202-1 and 202-2; Figure 202-24). A 1:1 ratio of normal-appearing QRS complexes and P waves exists. Although some approximate normal ranges of heart rate exist for dogs and cats (see Boxes 202-1 and 202-2), the notion of bradycardia varies according to species, body weight, age, and breed, with larger, older, or brachycephalic dogs tending to have slower heart rates than average, and cats having normal heart rates that are markedly influenced by environmental stimuli.

SB generally indicates the physiologic (e.g., brachycephalic, athletic individual) or pathologic (e.g., systemic intoxication) predominance of the parasympathetic system. A diagnostic aid is the response to an intravenous injection of atropine (see previous discussion).[61] In general, only severe bradycardias directly linked to overt clinical signs (syncope, malaise, seizures) warrant specific treatment with drugs or pacemaker implantation, and SB is rarely the primary cause of such clinical manifestations. One exception is the instantaneous transition from a tachycardia to SB (or other bradycardia [e.g., ventricular escape rhythm]; see following) in a debilitated, unstable, often unconscious patient. Such a rapid change may herald an upcoming cardiac arrest and should be addressed with assessment of the patient for underlying causes and preparation for cardiopulmonary resuscitation.[62] (Antiarrhythmic drugs to consider: none; parasympatholytics; sympathomimetics; rarely pacemaker.)

Sinus tachycardia STach is a sinus rhythm that occurs at an elevated rate (see Boxes 202-1 and 202-2; Figure 202-25). The wide range of resting heart rates in normal cats and dogs makes the cut-off between NSR and STach an approximate one. In dogs, STach exists when the increase in heart rate (P-QRS-T complexes of normal sinus origin) gives rise to the loss of RSA, the latter being a normal physiologic phenomenon in the dog (see previous discussion; see also Figure 202-12). Diagnosing this arrhythmia on the ECG can be difficult when the heart rate is extremely elevated, causing T and P waves to blend together. Carotid sinus massage, which temporarily slows the heart rate, separates the P and T waves, and clarifies that the tachycardia is of sinus origin (see previous discussion).

The causes of STach are diverse and are all marked by sympathetic predominance over parasympathetic inputs. Treatment of this arrhythmia is therefore aimed at the underlying cause when one exists. To slow a STach is only indicated if the tachycardia itself is producing clinical signs and is poorly controlled with treatment of the underlying disorder. For example, in hyperthyroidism, a beta-blocker may be given concurrently with antithyroid treatment. (Antiarrhythmic drugs to consider: class II.)

Disturbances of Atrial Excitability Disturbances of atrial excitability are common, especially in the dog. Indeed, in the most common forms of heart disease in dogs (endocardiosis, cardiomyopathy, many congenital malformations), atrial distension leads to pathologic disorganization of the atrial tissue, which can then generate atrial hyperexcitability (and possibly conduction disturbances as well).

Atrial extrasystoles Atrial extrasystoles (synonyms: PACs or premature atrial contractions, atrial premature complexes or contractions (APCs), atrial premature depolarizations) are premature depolarizations that originate in an ectopic atrial focus (Figure 202-26). Identification of atrial extrasystoles is based on a combination of two or more of the following five abnormalities but always must include the first two points: (1) prematurity of the P-QRS-T sequence; (2) QRS complexes that have a supraventricular appearance, in that they are narrow and comparable in shape to the sinus QRS complexes (rarely, QRS complexes may be absent or widened in cases of atrial extrasystoles that are exceptionally early and thus occur during the total or partial refractory period, respectively); (3) a P wave of different amplitude than sinus P waves, including negative, biphasic, or positive P waves, but always preceding the QRS complexes; (4) a P-R interval that is often different from the sinus PR interval, be it shorter or longer,[2] and (5) a postextrasystolic pause that most often is noncompensatory (Figure 202-27). The pathogenesis of atrial extrasystoles is most commonly related to a structural cardiac (atrial) lesion. Distension of the atria is the main cause of these ectopic foci, but atrial tumors (hemangiosarcoma), hyperthyroidism in the cat, digitalis toxicity, and other systemic disturbances also are recognized causes.[3] Clinical repercussions of atrial extrasystoles are minor, except in cases of multiple repeated bursts (Atrial Tachycardias, following), and the main interest in identifying atrial extrasystoles on an ECG is to add weight to a suspicion of atrial disease. Treatment for atrial extrasystoles is therefore first aimed at addressing the underlying cause rather than resorting to antiarrhythmic drugs specifically.

Atrial tachycardias An atrial tachycardia (supraventricular tachycardia) is a series of atrial extrasystoles occurring at a rate greater than sinus rhythm (Figure 202-28). It may be intermittent or continuous, and the impulses may all be transmitted

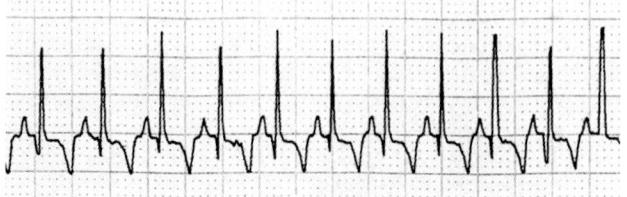

Figure 202-25 Sinus tachycardia (STach). The heart rate is 200/min in this dog with chocolate (theobromine) toxicity. Lead II, 25 mm/sec, 1 cm = 1 mV.

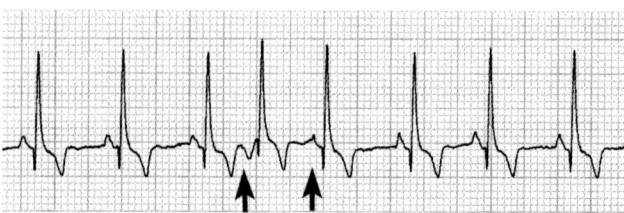

Figure 202-26 Premature atrial complexes (PACs) in a dog. Two PACs are seen in the middle of this lead II strip; the first is more premature than the second one (25 mm/sec; 1 cm = 1 mV). Premature P waves (*arrows*) of a different morphology than the sinus P waves and QRS complexes of the same shape as sinus QRS complexes are noted.

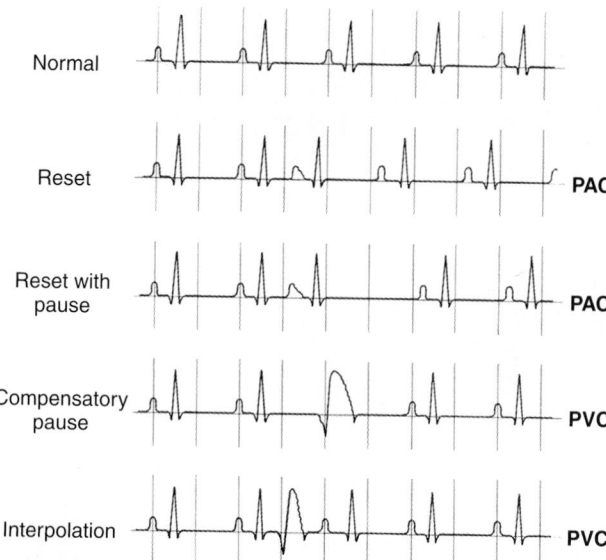

Normal

Reset — PAC

Reset with pause — PAC

Compensatory pause — PVC

Interpolation — PVC

Figure 202-27 Schematic representations of normal sinus rhythm (NSR) and premature complexes. *NSR:* The heart rate remains constant, and the interval from P to P or from R to R does not change. *Resetting:* A premature atrial complex (PAC; beat 3) resets the sinus rhythm so that the period from the beginning of the premature P waves to the next normal P wave is equal to exactly one P-P interval. *Resetting with pause:* The PAC (beat 3) is followed by a pause greater than one P-P interval but less than two P-P intervals. Both resetting and resetting with pause are examples of noncompensatory pauses (the rhythm of the *SA* node is affected by the premature beat, which alters the SA node's ability to provide a normally-timed, "compensatory" beat after the premature beat). *Compensatory pause:* The premature ventricular complex (PVC, beat 3) is followed by a compensatory pause; that is, the period from the normal P wave in the beat preceding the PVC to the normal P wave of the beat after the PVC is equivalent to exactly two P-P intervals. The sinus P wave occurs on time, but it is not conducted through the atrioventricular (AV) node to the ventricles, which are in a refractory state due to the PVC. *Interpolation:* A PVC (beat 3) occurs between two normal sinus complexes without disrupting normal rhythm. Because of concealed conduction into the AV node, interpolated PVCs commonly delay AV nodal transmission of the next beat, which manifests as prolongation of the PR interval for the heartbeat that follows the interpolated PVC (see also Figure 202-32). This characteristic is useful for differentiating interpolated PVCs from motion artifact.

to the ventricles or AV block may be noted in some instances. The exact mechanism of atrial tachycardias can involve micro re-entry (intra-atrial re-entrant tachycardia) or spontaneous automaticity of an ectopic atrial focus (automatic atrial tachycardia).[59,63] Identifying intermittent atrial tachycardias is usually straightforward: the ECG shows a burst of atrial extrasystoles. Establishing a diagnosis of sustained atrial tachycardia may be difficult, however, because P waves may not be clearly evident, each one potentially being buried within the previous QRS complex. Differentiation between sustained atrial tachycardia and "high" ventricular (i.e., originating near the AV node) tachycardia can therefore be helped by exteriorizing the P waves, which can be elicited with a vagal maneuver (see previous discussion) and subsequent slowing of the tachycardia or even sinus capture (resumption of sinus rhythm). The same goal may also be reached pharmacologically using graded doses of such intravenous agents as propranolol, esmolol, edrophonium, or phenylephrine (Table 202-1). Intravenous adenosine used for this

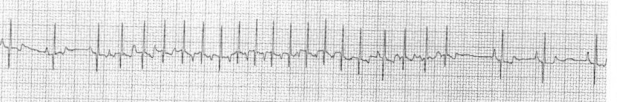

Figure 202-28 Supraventricular tachycardia. A burst of premature (rapid) QRS complexes is seen in the middle of the tracing. The QRS complexes are of the same shape as sinus QRS complexes. No clinical signs were present in this older Golden retriever dog, either at admission or during follow-up, and an echocardiogram was unremarkable. Lead II, 25 mm/sec, 1 cm = 1 mV.

purpose subjectively appears to be much less effective in dogs than in humans. Causes for atrial tachycardias are the same as those listed for atrial extrasystoles (see previous discussion). The clinical impact of an atrial tachycardia depends on its duration, rate, and underlying cardiac lesions. Intermittent AV block can limit the ventricular rate and may lessen clinical impact in cases of rapid atrial tachycardias. Atrial tachycardias often precede the development of AFib. Treatment of the underlying disease is an essential part of managing these arrhythmias. (Antiarrhythmic drugs to consider: digoxin, class II, IV.)

Atrial flutter Atrial flutter is characterized by a rapid and regular series of atrial depolarizations, without a rest phase between atrial depolarizations (see Figure 202-19). Identification of this arrhythmia is therefore based on the occurrence of (1) rapid, rhythmic waves of atrial electrical activity referred to as *flutter (F) waves*, usually occurring at a very high rate (often > 300/min); (2) absence of a return to baseline of the F waves (giving a "saw tooth" baseline appearance); (3) QRS complexes of a supraventricular appearance; and (4) a variable, irregularly irregular R-R interval. Atrial flutter is different from other atrial tachycardias in that no return to the isoelectric baseline occurs after each atrial depolarization in atrial flutter. This diagnosis may be very challenging when each flutter wave is transmitted through the AV node to the ventricles. Such 1:1 conduction leaves the F waves buried in the preceding QRS complexes, which complicates the diagnosis (see Figure 202-19). Atrial flutter occurs as a result of a macro re-entrant circuit within one atrium—an abnormal, self-perpetuating cyclical electrical loop in the atrium in which an endless circle of electrical conduction can be initiated through atrial stretch, for example. Termination of atrial flutter can occur spontaneously, but treatment is necessary when a persistently high ventricular rate occurs. Treatment most commonly aims to control ventricular rate (see Atrial Fibrillation, following). Permanent abolition of atrial flutter is achieved with radiofrequency catheter-based interruption of the flutter circuit (see Radiofrequency Ablation, following).[59]

Atrial fibrillation AFib is a common and important arrhythmia. It represents 14% of all canine arrhythmias, including a 50% incidence in cases of dilated cardiomyopathy in dogs, and it can bring on clinically overt hemodynamic changes requiring specific treatment.[64] A prevalence of AFib in up to 2% of the human population is estimated,[59,65,66] but a similar statistic is not available in veterinary medicine. AFib is characterized by complete electrical disorganization at the atrial level, leading to a chaotic, rapid series of atrial depolarizations (400 to 1200 per minute) (Figure 202-29). In AFib, the AV node acts as a "gatekeeper" for this chaotic electrical activity, allowing only those electrical depolarizations with optimal intensity, timing, and orientation to pass through to the ventricles and thus controlling the ventricular rate to some extent.

The three ECG characteristics of AFib are (1) supraventricular-appearing QRS complexes (narrow, upright, and of only slightly variable amplitude in lead II, unless ventricular aberrancy/BBBs are concurrent); (2) an irregularly irregular

Text continued on p. 1059

Table • 202-1

Drugs Used for the Treatment of Cardiac Arrhythmias

GENERIC NAME	TRADE NAME	ADMINISTRATION ROUTE	COMMON INDICATIONS	DOSE	COMMENTS
Adenosine	Adenocard	IV	Terminates acute paroxysmal supraventricular tachycardia	1.5-3.0 mg/dose; repeat in 1 min to maximum of 6-12 mg	Side effects: sinus arrest, sinus bradycardia (SB), and atrioventricular (AV) block; often ineffective in dogs and cats
Amiodarone	Cordarone	Oral	Recurrent ventricular fibrillation; recurrent hemodynamically unstable or malignant ventricular tachycardia (VT); atrial fibrillation (AFib)	4.5 mg/lb bid PO × 1 week, then 2.2-3.8 mg/lb PO sid; if IV, give in graded dose to 5 mg/lb; in sick dogs dose is unknown; serum levels is 1-2 μg/mL	Side effects include proarrhythmia, Coombs' positive test result, pulmonary fibrosis, hypothyroidism, liver necrosis, photosensitivity, and gastrointestinal (GI) toxicity
Atenolol	Tenormin	Oral	Same as propranolol	0.15-0.5 mg/lb bid in the dog; 0.5-1.4 mg/lb sid to bid in the cat	Weakness, depression, hypotension, bradycardia, inappetence
Atropine Tablets Injectable		Oral IV, IM, SQ	1. Test responsiveness of sinus node 2. Hyperactive carotid sinus reflex (SA arrest) 3. AV block (second and third degree)	0.01-0.03 mg/lb IV	1. Do not use in states of heart failure 2. Do not administer when bronchial tree secretions a problem
Digoxin Tablets Elixir Injectable	Lanoxin Cardoxin	Oral Oral IV	1. Supraventricular premature contractions and tachyarrhythmias 2. Right heart failure 3. Pump dysfunction	0.22 mg/m² bid PO as maintenance dose; double dose initially first 24 h for rapid effect; lower dose in large (>30 lb) and giant breeds of dogs 0.0312 mg per cat eod PO in cats—not for use in restrictive disease states	1. Digitalize cautiously 2. Monitor with ECG 3. All doses approximate and must be titrated based on patient response 4. Side effects: malaise, anorexia, vomiting, diarrhea
Diltiazem	Cardizem (not sustained-release form)	Oral IV	Supraventricular tachyarrhythmias; feline hypertrophic cardiomyopathy used orally and chronically	0.2-0.7 mg/lb q8h PO in dogs 0.7 mg/lb q8h PO in cats IV: 0.02-0.03 mg/lb; repeat every 2 min to effect—max dose 2 mg/lb IV	Side effects include bradycardia, hypotension, collapse, and severe weakness; if SUT is physiologic response to systemic problem, correct the problem first (or risk of cardiac arrest)
Esmolol	Brevibloc	IV	Supraventricular tachycardia	0.025-0.1 mg/lb/min (25-100 μg/lb/min) 0.05-0.22 mg/lb IV Effects occur within 2 min	Short-term IV agent; used to control ventricular rate while agents are given for long-term effects; used for AFib, atrial flutter, supraventricular tachycardia; side effect is rapid, severe hypotension; do not use in congestive heart failure (CHF)-compromised patient

CARDIOVASCULAR SYSTEM

Drug	Trade Name	Route	Indications	Dosage	Comments
Isoproterenol Injectable	Isuprel Injectable	IM, IV, SC	1. Advanced second-degree and third-degree heart block 2. SA arrest 3. SB (?)	For bradyarrhythmias: one 1-ml vial (0.2 mg) in 250 D5W IV to increase heart rate, use to effect (0.5-1 mL/min) 0.1-0.2 mg SQ or IM q4h for heart block (variable efficacy by these routes)	May be used on temporary basis parentally until conduction improves or pacemaker is implanted
Lidocaine 2% without epinephrine	Xylocaine	IV only	Ventricular tachyarrhythmias causing hemodynamic disturbances or malignant arrhythmias; do not use for occasional VPC or hemodynamically stable multiform beats	1. 1-2 mg/lb IV slow bolus over 2 min or until arrhythmia controlled 2. 1 mg/lb IV slowly, then 10-40 µ/lb/min continuous infusion or 1 mg up to 4 times over 5 minutes to effect 3. For cats, 0.25-0.5 mg/lb IV bolus, then 5-20 µ/lb/min (0.005-0.02 mg/lb/min) CRI	1. Reserve for serious arrhythmias 2. Toxicity includes convulsions and respiratory arrest 3. Single IV dose lasts 15-20 min only 4. Excretion is hepatic
Metoprolol	Lopressor Toprol XL	Oral	Hypertension, beta-blockade	0.2-0.5 mg/lb sid or divided in multiple doses bid-tid depending on product used	Used for hypertension, beta-blockade, CHF arrhythmias (both supraventricular and ventricular)
Mexiletine	Mexitil	Oral	Ventricular tachyarrhythmias	2-5 mg/lb q8-12h (dogs)	Few side effects; may be used with digoxin and class I and II antiarrhythmic agents; hepatic excretion
Phenytoin Capsules Injectable	Dilantin	Oral IV	1. Some ventricular tachyarrhythmias 2. May be useful in treating arrhythmias caused by digitalis overdose	7-14 mg/lb q8h orally 2.24-4.5 mg/lb IV	Infrequently used as an antiarrhythmic drug; hepatic excretion
Procainamide Capsules Tablets Injectable	Pronestyl Pronestyl-SR Procan SR	Oral IV	1. Ventricular premature contractions 2. VT	1. 3-10 mg/lb q2-6h (to 8h sustained release form) 2. Dogs: 1-10 mg/lb IV over 30 min, then infuse 10-20 µg/lb/min (0.01-0.02 mg/lb/min) CRI 3. Cats: 0.5-1.0 mg/lb IV bolus, then 5-10 µg/lb/min CRI	1. IV effect is brief, and oral maintenance dose must be given q4h 2. Oral forms available in sustained release tablets may not be absorbed 3. Hepatic excretion
Propafenone	Rhythmol	Oral IV (?)	(a) Supraventricular tachyarrhythmias (b) Accessory conduction arrhythmias (c) VT	Unknown; begin in medium- to large-size dogs with 75-125 mg orally tid	May be proarrhythmic with structural heart disease; do not use if Q-T is prolonged

Continued

Table • 202-1

Drugs Used for the Treatment of Cardiac Arrhythmias—cont'd

GENERIC NAME	TRADE NAME	ADMINISTRATION ROUTE	COMMON INDICATIONS	DOSE	COMMENTS
Propranolol Tablets Injectable	Inderal	Oral IV	1. Supraventricular tachyarrhythmias 2. To slow ventricular rate in atrial fibrillation or to distinguish the latter from VT 3. Arrhythmias of digitalis intoxication 4. Pre-excitation syndromes 5. Some ventricular arrhythmias, when other agents fail	Oral: general 0.2-0.5 mg/lb q8h: 2.5-20 mg q8-12h small dogs; 10-40 mg q8-12h medium and large dogs; 40-80 mg q8-12h large and giant dogs; 2.5 mg q12-24h cats; 0.1-0.5 mg IV no more frequently than q1-3 min to 5 mg maximum; administer until rate slows or toxicity occurs Cats: 0.1-0.5 mg IV boluses, 2.5-5 mg/cat PO sid-bid	1. Use with caution: as a negative inotropic agent, it may induce CHF 2. Excessive dose causes reduction in cardiac rate and prolongation of PR and QT intervals
1. Quinidine sulfate (tablets)	Quinidine sulfate	Oral	1. Ventricular premature contractions 2. VT	3-10 mg/lb (of base) IM or PO q6-8h; may be given q2h until loading dose controls arrhythmia or induces toxicity	1. Do not use in presence of CHF unless this is being treated simultaneously 2. Toxicity results in increased heart rate and prolongation of the PR, QRS, and QT intervals
2. Gluconate (long-acting tablets)		Oral	Sustained release forms given 8.8-12h PO		3. Often effective in lower doses when used with procainamide, mexiletine, or a beta-blocking agent 4. Hepatic excretion
3. Gluconate (injection)		IM		3-10 mg/lb (of base) q2-4h IM, PO; sustained-release forms: 4-10 mg/lb PO q8h	5. IV use may cause hypotension 6. Injectable product is not used IV—only IM (epaxial) 7. Competitive with digoxin; do not use together
Sotalol	Betapace	Oral	Class II and III for ventricular arrhythmias	Canine: 0.44-2.8 mg/lb bid-tid Feline: 10-20 mg/cat bid	GI disturbances; hepatotoxicity; decreased HR; P-R prolongation
Tocainide	Tonocard	Oral	Ventricular tachyarrhythmias	7-11 mg/lb q8-12h (dogs)	May need to use with other class Ia antiarrhythmic agents for better effect; hepatic excretion
Verapamil	Isoptin	Oral IV	Supraventricular tachycardia	Oral: 0.2-1.0 mg/lb bid-tid IV: 0.01 mg/lb IV to maximum of 0.07 mg/lb	Side effects: weakness, collapse, bradycardia; contraindicated in shock, heart block, sick sinus syndrome (SSS), CHF, VT

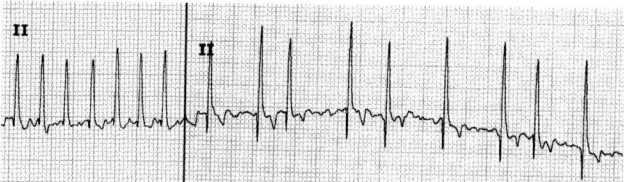

Figure 202-29 Atrial fibrillation (AFib). The irregularity of the rhythm is less apparent when the ventricular rate is fast, as when this dog with dilated cardiomyopathy and congestive heart failure (CHF) was first evaluated (*left panel*, ventricular rate = 280/min). Diuretics, digoxin, and eventually beta-blocking therapy led to good rate control and a clearer electrocardiogram (ECG) diagnosis (*right panel*, ventricular rate = 135/min). Lead II, 25 mm/sec, 1 cm = 1 mV.

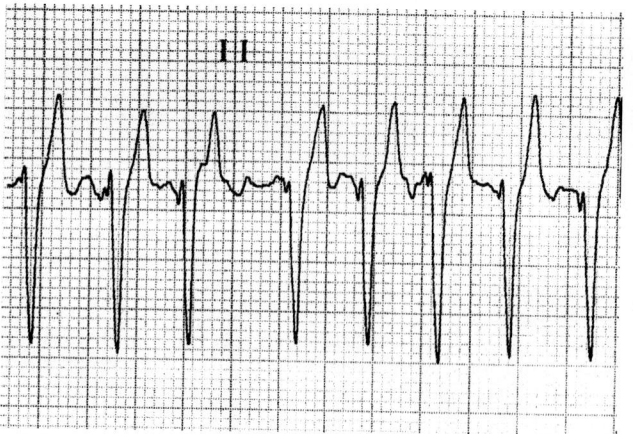

Figure 202-30 Atrial fibrillation (AFib) with right bundle branch block (RBBB). This impostor for ventricular arrhythmia is distinctive in its irregular R-R interval and its response to vagal maneuvers. Lead II, 25 mm/sec, 1 cm = 1 mV.

rhythm, with ventricular rates that may be low, normal, or most commonly without treatment, high; and (3) no visible P waves (replaced by a fine undulation of the isoelectric line, termed *f waves*). The absence of organized atrial depolarizations can have hemodynamic, and therefore clinical, consequences during physical activity or in patients with advanced stages of structural heart disease. During diastole, active filling is associated with the P wave (i.e., atrial contraction), which can account for up to 30% of total ventricular filling. Its absence therefore can reduce ventricular volume to suboptimal levels, producing overt clinical signs during exertion. Furthermore, the rapid overall ventricular rate, as well as the premature occurrence of some individual QRS complexes, bring about poor diastolic filling. For these reasons, some contractions may be ineffective intermittently and one or more auscultated heartbeat, may be without a corresponding palpable arterial pulse (i.e., pulse deficit). AFib is one of the few arrhythmias that may be suspected from the moment of auscultation and palpation during the physical examination, based on the chaotic irregularity of the cardiac rhythm on auscultation and palpation of the chest, together with pulse deficits. Polymorphic VT and frequent PVCs, however, should be included in the differential diagnosis of this physical exam finding (see following). Counterintuitively, high vagal tone (e.g., from concurrent gastrointestinal [GI] disease) predisposes to AFib, because parasympathetic stimulation of atrial myocytes accelerates their repolarization in a heterogeneous fashion, which increases the likelihood of the initiation of arrhythmia.

A major diagnostic impostor on ECG is the combination of AFib and BBB (Figure 202-30), which produces wide QRS complexes and therefore can appear to mimic VT, but without P waves to conclusively indicate AV association (BBB) or dissociation (VT). In such a situation, a vagal maneuver can be performed, and its effect on the AV node could reduce the ventricular rate with AFib + right bundle branch block (RBBB) but not with VT. In addition, sustained, monomorphic VT is generally characterized by regular R-R intervals, whereas AFib with BBB is not.

AFib in dogs most often is caused by primary, underlying cardiac disease. However, AFib may also occur in individuals with structurally normal hearts (e.g., anesthesia, hypothyroidism, rapid, large-volume pericardiocentesis, GI disease, volume overload causing atrial stretch) if those hearts contain sufficient atrial myocardial mass to permit fibrillation (i.e., medium to large breed dogs).[67] In giant breed dogs, particularly the Irish wolfhound, AFib commonly occurs in otherwise healthy dogs with grossly normal atria (i.e., lone AFib).[67,68] It remains to be determined whether those patients with AFib and structurally normal hearts that progress to dilated cardiomyopathy do so because of their arrhythmia, or whether, conversely, AFib is only the arrhythmic prelude to a disease that later causes dilation and systolic dysfunction.

In cats, AFib occurs uncommonly and is virtually always associated with structural heart disease causing atrial enlargement.[69] Most cats have clinical signs suggesting heart failure (e.g., dyspnea) or thromboembolism at the time of diagnosis of AFib, but 20% to 25% of cases of AFib in cats are discovered incidentally (e.g., during a routine annual examination) and as such, this arrhythmia may be an early manifestation of

Table • 202-2

Comparison of Ectopic Beats of Supraventricular or Ventricular Origin

FEATURE	SUPRAVENTRICULAR	VENTRICULAR
Wide, bizarre QRS complexes	Very rare	Common
QRS complex shape	Same as sinus QRS	>10% different from sinus QRS
P wave for every QRS	Yes; often of different shape	No; Ps occur regularly throughout tracing, but independently of QRSs
T wave	Same as sinus T wave	Different from sinus T wave
Postextrasystolic pause (see Figure 202-27)	Usually noncompensatory	Usually compensatory
QRS fusion beats as hallmark	No	Yes
Positive response to vagal maneuver	Possible	Virtually never

heart disease in some cats. AFib does not clearly influence survival negatively in cats compared with the prognosis associated with the underlying heart diseases proper. In a subgroup of 24 cats with AFib and known survival statistics, 21% lived between 6 and 12 months after the diagnosis of AFib and 33% survived 1 year or more.[69]

AFib usually is a persistent, permanent arrhythmia. It does occur paroxysmally in the dog[70] and very rarely so in the cat. Paroxysmal AFib usually is of short duration and in most cases progresses to persistent AFib because of severe underlying cardiac disease (usually atrial enlargement).

In most cases of AFib, two goals of treatment exist: (1) managing the underlying heart disease and (2) maximizing cardiac output by controlling (slowing) the rate of conduction through the AV node if needed (see Figures 202-29 and 202-31). The approach of letting the atria fibrillate and concentrating on ventricular rate control, rather than attempting to convert the AFib to sinus rhythm, was recently supported by the results of a prospective study of 4000 human AFib patients. It was found that converting the AFib back to sinus rhythm brought no significant benefit in terms of survival, and that conversion carried a higher risk of adverse effects.[71] As a rule, beta-blockers, calcium channel blockers, or both are given in low initial doses and up-titrated to effect, typically over a period of days to a few weeks, based on heart rate. Subsequently, even once an acceptable range of heart rates has been reached, periodic drug dose adjustments (e.g., re-evaluation every 3 to 6 months, sooner if problems occur) are usually necessary to maintain good rate control.

In small animal medicine, the ideal ventricular rate varies for each patient depending on many factors, including stage of CHF and body weight. One substantiated guideline suggests a target ventricular rate for dogs with AFib weighing 20 to 25 kg of approximately 130 to 145 bpm.[72] A recent study compared ventricular rates in canine AFib obtained on careful physical examination by trained persons including cardiologists to the rate obtained simultaneously by ECG. The level of accuracy ranged from 64% to as low as 12% for veterinary students and some veterinarians.[73] Follow-up monitoring of ventricular rate control relies on repeated ECGs rather than physical exams alone. (Antiarrhythmic drugs to consider: digoxin; class II or class IV agents; combination therapy is often most successful and produces fewer adverse effects than high doses of a single drug.)

Disturbances of Ventricular Excitability Disturbances of ventricular excitability are important because they involve the main element in the cardiac pump, and may therefore have very severe hemodynamic and clinical repercussions. However, it must be recognized that ventricular arrhythmias have very diverse mechanisms and causes (especially noncardiac), such that severity, treatment, and prognosis depend on more than ECG findings alone.

Ventricular Ectopy: Premature Ventricular Complexes, Accelerated Idioventricular Rhythm, and Ventricular Tachycardia

Ventricular extrasystoles or premature ventricular complexes Ventricular extrasystoles (synonyms: premature ventricular contractions, beats, or depolarizations [PVC; VPB, VPC, VPD, ventricular ectopy]) are premature depolarizations generated by an ectopic focus located in the ventricular tissue.[1,2,23,45,74] These arrhythmias are the most common of all rhythm disturbances.[64] Their identification often is simplified by the wide QRS complexes they generate, which have a different morphology (shape) than normal sinus QRS complexes. Most ventricular extrasystoles have a wide, often bizarre-appearing QRS complex (>0.07 second in dogs), without an associated P wave, and a different (often very large) associated T wave (Figures 202-32 and 202-33). Single PVCs are usually followed by a compensatory pause (see Figures 202-27 and 202-33) but may be interpolated instead (see Figures 202-27 and 202-32). Multiples of two PVCs are referred to as *a pair*; 1:1 alternation between sinus beats and PVCs is referred to as *bigeminy;* and three or more PVCs in a row constitutes ventricular tachycardia (VT; see following). *Trigeminy* describes a repeating pattern of either 2:1 PVCs:sinus beat, or 2:1 sinus beats:PVC.

For purposes of identifying an underlying cause and for accurate therapy, it is important to differentiate ventricular extrasystoles from PACs (see Table 202-1). It is also essential to differentiate ventricular extrasystoles from the other major causes of widened QRS complexes: (1) morphologic changes due to cardiomegaly and axis shift (see Figure 202-8); (2) intraventricular conduction disturbances within the bundle branches (see Figures 202-44 and 202-45); (3) abrupt motion or other artifact (see Figure 202-23); and (4) the wide but nonpremature QRS complexes of ventricular escape beats (see Figure 202-42, *a*). These four causes for wide QRSs are not ventricular arrhythmias, do not involve a pathologic focus in the ventricle, are not associated with a disproportionately high occurrence of VT/VF, and therefore are not treated with antiarrhythmic drugs.

Causes of ventricular extrasystoles include virtually any cardiac or systemic disorder,[75] with the most common of these including such primary cardiac diseases as cardiomyopathy,[55,56,76] valvular heart disease, congenital heart disease, and endocarditis[77] and such systemic problems as hypokalemia, anemia, hypoxia, blunt trauma,[78] gastric dilatation-volvulus,[79,80] abdominal masses (commonly splenic or hepatic)[81-83] intoxication, and acidosis. Normal dogs will commonly have up to 24 PVCs daily as recorded on Holter studies.[22,23] In cats, ventricular extrasystoles seem to be associated predominantly with cardiomyopathy rather than extracardiac causes. The most challenging aspect of managing ventricular extrasystoles remains the evaluation of their severity and the assessment of the need for treatment (see Ventricular Tachycardia and treatment discussions, following). Evaluation of causes and whether to treat ventricular ectopy are discussed under Ventricular Tachycardia, following.

Two specific diseases of dogs are almost exclusively arrhythmogenic, producing PVCs and VT, and often overt clinical manifestations of acute arrhythmia (malaise, syncope, Stokes-Adams seizures, or sudden death) as the chief abnormality. Familial ventricular arrhythmia of Boxer dogs (Boxer cardiomyopathy, arrhythmogenic RV cardiomyopathy and dysplasia) causes ventricular extrasystoles and VT.[84,85] Initially no thoracic radiographic or echocardiographic changes are seen, although individuals with disease that is more advanced may have dilated cardiomyopathy (see Chapter 203, Canine Myocardial Diseases). No sex predilection has been found, and it is suspected that the syndrome is inherited as an autosomal dominant trait (no carriers).[45] The causative lesion is a degeneration of myocytes in the outflow tract region of the RV, as supported by histopathologic studies[84] and the typical, left BBB-like appearance of the PVCs indicating their RV origin.[74] In many cases the ventricular arrhythmia is an incidental finding in Boxer dogs that otherwise appear normal. These occult, latent cases are predisposed to developing clinical signs later in life, having offspring with the disease, or both. Also commonly, familial ventricular arrhythmia of Boxers produces overt clinical signs that are the patient's chief complaint. Overt arrhythmic manifestations range from aborted syncope (episodes of stumbling or "drunken" appearance) to true syncope, sudden cardiac death, or both.[46,84] These events may be triggered in some cases by intense sympathetic activity, including excitement and physical exertion, and thus are managed by avoiding circumstances that trigger such behavior. Since its original description,[84] the disease seems to coexist less commonly with grossly dilated ventricles, poor contractility, or

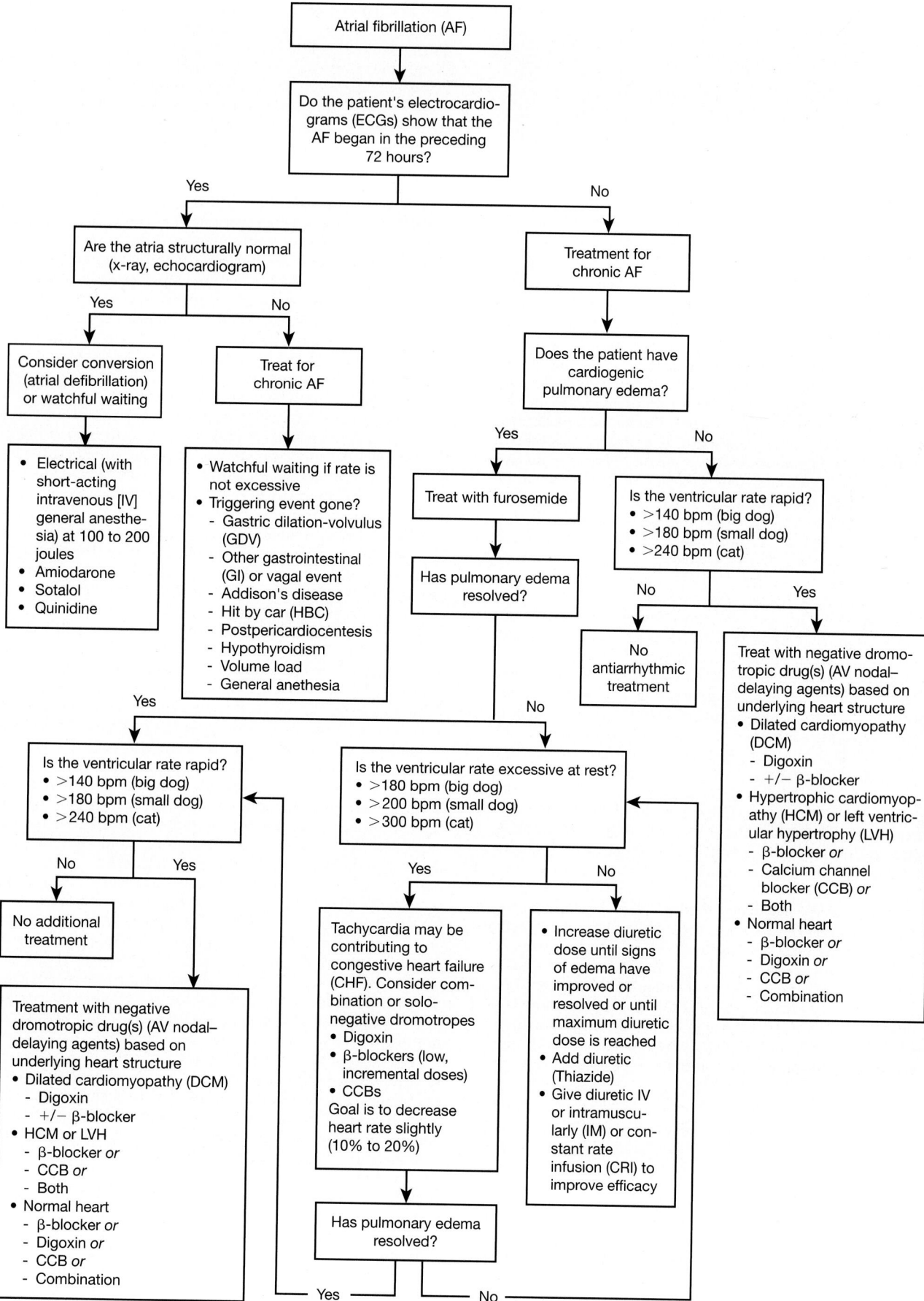

Figure 202-31 Therapeutic approach to atrial fibrillation (AFib).

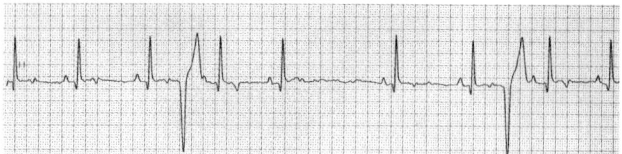

Figure 202-32 Premature ventricular complex (PVC). The classic, wide and bizarre appearance of a prematurely occurring heartbeat is seen. These PVCs are interpolated between normal QRS complexes (see also Figure 202-27). Lead II, 50 mm/sec, 1 cm = 1 mV.

both, whereas overt manifestations due to severe ventricular extrasystoles are now a common problem in the breed. This change may simply reflect increased awareness of the problem and early screening. Clinical confirmation of the diagnosis begins with identification of the signalment and chief complaints as described previously and ultimately rests on the demonstration of ventricular extrasystoles on ECG in the absence of any other inciting cause (diagnosis of exclusion). Frequently, serial Holter monitoring is necessary to evaluate potential breeding individuals, because affected dogs may have only a few PVCs per hour. The presence of PVC pairs, or of VT, strongly supports the diagnosis.[24,85] Treatment involves management of arrhythmias (see Ventricular Tachycardia, following) and prevention of transmission of the disease through screening and not breeding affected individuals.

Inherited sudden cardiac death of German shepherd dogs may similarly exist in a latent state or may produce overt clinical signs.[86,87] The disease occurs rarely but is international in distribution and has affected several generations.[87] The predominant abnormality is paroxysmal, rapid VT. Dogs with this disease often develop clinical signs early in life, and these include both syncope and a high prevalence of sudden death. Therefore the disease causes clinical manifestations mainly in puppies or young adult dogs (mean age: approximately 1 year; age range: 4 to 30 months). As a rule the arrhythmia does not coexist with structural cardiac changes, such that thoracic radiographs and echocardiograms generally are normal. A myocardial repolarization defect appears to be the cause of the arrhythmia.[88] Although treatments that limit bradycardia (e.g., vagolytic drugs, ventricular pacing) reduce the occurrence of arrhythmia, no definitive treatment exists for the disorder at this time.

Accelerated idioventricular rhythm Accelerated idioventricular rhythm (AIVRs) has been identified as a specific subset of ventricular tachycardia (VT) for the last 30 years (and was given the clear but oxymoronic name *slow VT* at first). AIVRs have the same ECG characteristics as VT, except rate. AV dissociation, wide and bizarre QRS complexes, and the possibility of capture beats and fusion beats are seen. In medium-sized dogs, the rate of AIVRs is between 70 and 160 bpm, which places it between idioventricular (i.e., escape) rhythms

(<70 bpm) and true VT in terms of rate. The causes of AIVRs are similar to those of ventricular extrasystoles, but the lower ventricular rate is less compromising of diastolic ventricular filling time; as a result, AIVRs generally are well-tolerated.[89] Treatment therefore is directed at the underlying cause; antiarrhythmic medications are not considered unless management of the underlying cause is ineffective at abolishing the arrhythmia and the rate increases to the point that the criteria for VT are met (Figure 202-34).

Ventricular tachycardia VT is a series of three or more ventricular extrasystoles occurring at a high rate (Figures 202-35 and 202-36). It may be continuous (sustained) or intermittent (paroxysmal). Causes are the same as those listed for ventricular premature complexes (see previous discussion). Clinical manifestations are frequent (weakness, syncope, Stokes-Adams-type seizures) but their occurrence depends directly on the hemodynamic consequences of the rhythm (see Clinical Impact of Rhythm Disturbances). An increasingly rapid tachycardia, for example, will cross a threshold of ventricular rate beyond which a greater number of beats will not translate into greater cardiac output. This "point of diminishing returns," which is highly individual and varies according to the variables described previously, exists because diastolic filling time is most compromised at high heart rates. Thus very rapid VT, like any other very rapid tachycardia, can produce overt clinical signs of reduced cardiac output. At a lesser extreme, Doppler echocardiography has shown that VT may be asymptomatic because VT has been demonstrated in conjunction with an adequate cardiac output. This situation is particularly true in cases of VT at slower rates (approaching AIVR; see previous discussion).

The identification of VT is easier when it is paroxysmal. The typical appearance is one or several series of QRS complexes that are widened (>0.07 second in the dog), do not resemble the sinus QRS complexes, are associated with giant T waves, are not linked to P waves, and may include capture beats (sinus P-QRS complexes after the paroxysm of VT) and fusion beats (QRS complexes with a morphology that is intermediate, between sinus QRS complexes and ectopic QRS complexes) (see Figure 202-35). Capture beats and fusion beats are pathognomonic for VT. In VT, P waves are present (the atria depolarize, but the impulse is blocked at [or just after] the AV node because the more rapid rhythm [VT] dominates the ventricles) but are often masked by QRS complexes. Thus the presence of P waves at regular intervals but not fixedly associated with QRS complexes is consistent with VT (see Figure 202-36). The ECG diagnosis can become more challenging when VT is continuous, particularly if it is of septal or RV origin and thus produces QRS complexes that are fairly narrow and that may resemble supraventricular complexes. Wide QRS complexes caused by other factors (see previous discussion of ventricular extrasystoles) must not be mistaken for VT.

The goals of treatment of VT are, in order: (1) to accurately identify the arrhythmia, (2) to eliminate or palliate predisposing factors that may be responsible for the arrhythmia, (3) to control the rhythm and rate so as to optimize cardiac output, and (4) to avoid detrimental side effects of antiarrhythmic treatment (see Figure 202-34). The desire to suppress VT to reduce the risk of progression to lethal arrhythmias is not sound. Although it is known that ventricular arrhythmias can degenerate into increasingly unstable rhythms, no drug has ever been shown to delay this progression (see Therapy of Arrhythmias, following). Prophylactic treatment of asymptomatic ventricular arrhythmias is detrimental in human medicine and therefore is not recommended in human or veterinary medicine. (Antiarrhythmics drugs to consider for VT: none or class I, II, or III antiarrhythmics.)

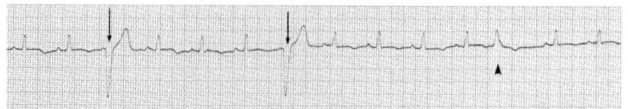

Figure 202-33 Three premature ventricular complexes (PVCs). This cat with hypertrophic cardiomyopathy developed PVCs both of the classic wide and bizarre appearance *(arrows)* and of a more subtly different morphology *(arrowhead)*. In all cases, PVCs are premature, not associated with a P wave, different in morphology from sinus QRS complexes, and have a T wave that is different from sinus T waves. Lead II, 50 mm/sec, 1 cm = 1 mV.

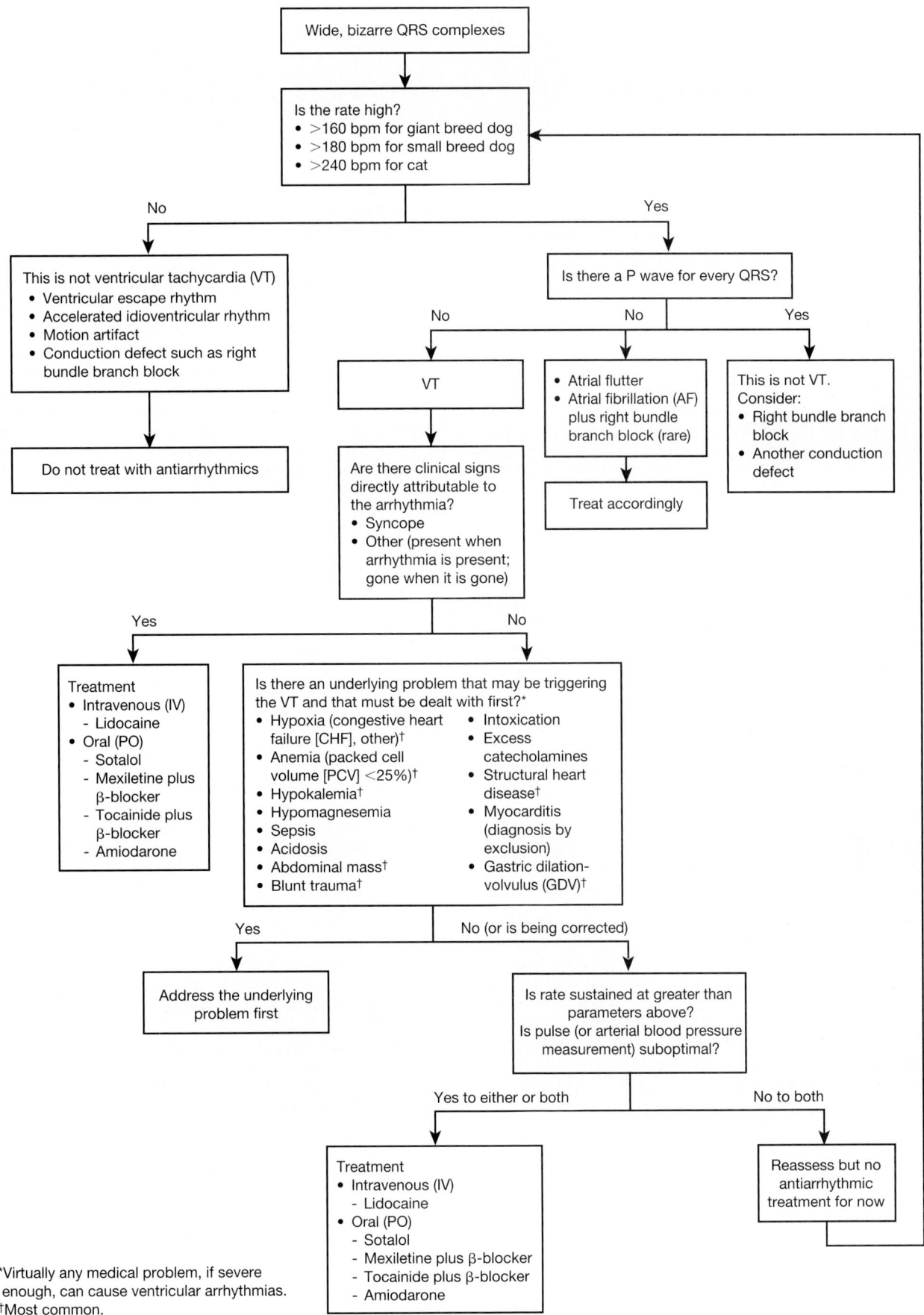

Figure 202-34 Approach to patients with a rhythm consisting entirely of wide, bizarre QRS complexes.

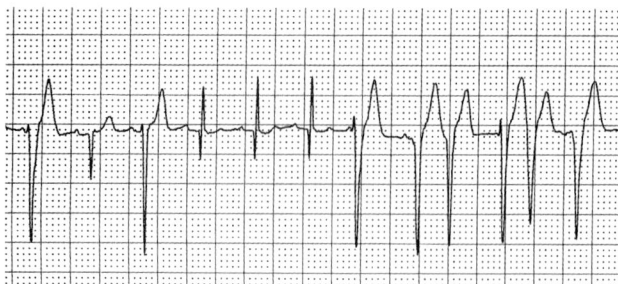

Figure 202-35 Ventricular ectopy in a dog. Premature ventricular complexes (PVCs) (first and third beats) and ventricular tachycardia (VT) (from seventh beat to end of tracing). This tracing presents many hallmark findings of ventricular ectopy. A *fusion beat* (beat 2) is an electrical hybrid formed by the collision of a PVC and a sinus beat. The reader should note its characteristically normal PR interval and QRS morphology that is intermediate between a PVC and a sinus beat. A *capture beat* is the term given to the sinus beat that resumes normal sinus rhythm (NSR) after ventricular ectopy (beat 4). In this case the sinus rhythm lasts for only three beats. The next-to-last beat occurs very prematurely and thus demonstrates the R-on-T phenomenon. Lead II, 25 mm/sec, 1 cm = 1 mV.

Ventricular flutter Ventricular flutter is a rapid and prefibrillatory stage of VT. The ECG appearance of this rhythm is a tight, tall sinusoidal wave in which it is impossible to separate QRS complexes and T waves and in which neither capture nor fusion beats are seen. This intermediate stage between VT and VF is rare, brief, and precedes cardiac arrest. It must be differentiated from motion artifact. Artifact masquerading as ventricular flutter still shows evidence of coordinated ventricular activity (normal QRS complexes within the "flutter" impostors) on close inspection (see Figure 202-11). Ventricular flutter is considered a severe ventricular arrhythmia and warrants immediate correction of predisposing causes, intravenous antiarrhythmic treatment, and possibly electrical defibrillation.

Ventricular fibrillation VF is a disorganized, chaotic pattern of ventricular depolarizations involving complete desynchronization of ventricular electrical activity. Hemodynamically, it produces circulatory collapse and arrest. Therefore it is a preagonal state leading to death within minutes. Indeed, the cardiac rhythms that are defined as producing cardiac arrest include VF, asystole, and pulseless electrical activity (pulseless VT, electromechanical dissociation [EMD]).[90] The ECG appearance of VF consists of erratic, patternless waves of variable morphology, amplitude, and frequency (Figure 202-37). The underlying cause is generally a severe disorder, such as myocardial trauma, anoxia, severe electrolyte disturbance, and advanced states of shock. If VF is suspected on ECG, artifact must

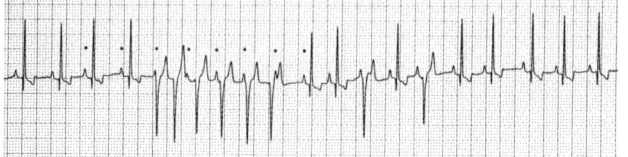

Figure 202-36 Ventricular tachycardia (VT) in a dog. With ventricular arrhythmias, the sinus node and atria continue to function, as evidenced by P waves *(dots)*. Atrial activity occurs regularly but independently of the QRS complexes (AV dissociation). Lead II, 25 mm/sec, 1 cm = 1 mV.

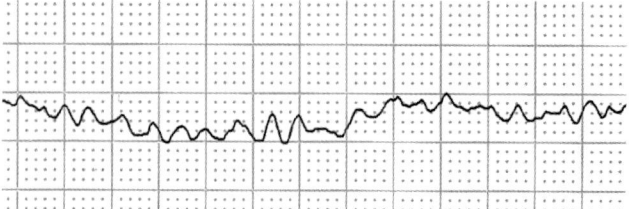

Figure 202-37 Ventricular fibrillation (VF) in a dog. An important differential diagnosis is technical error (poor electrical connection between patient and ECG machine). Lead I, 25 mm/sec, 1 cm = 1 mV.

immediately be ruled out; poor electrical connection between the patient and the ECG leads can mimic VF. Rapid confirmation of VF consists of (1) applying isopropyl alcohol to the skin-ECG lead interface to improve conductivity; (2) assessing that the arrhythmia is present in multiple leads, not just lead II; and (3) noting that the patient is unconscious, because VF is inconsistent with adequate cerebral perfusion. VF is often preceded, and therefore heralded, by ventricular extrasystoles (possibly demonstrating the R on T phenomenon), then sustained VT, then ventricular flutter.[2] When the rhythm has reached VF, treatment (cardiopulmonary resuscitation), though often unrewarding, must be instituted immediately and generally involves electrical defibrillation if available. (Antiarrhythmic treatments to consider: electrical defibrillation, precordial thump, KCl and $CaCl_2$, Class III).

Torsade de pointes TdP is a ventricular arrhythmia that arises from prolongation of the QT interval.[91,92] The rotation of the peaks of the QRS complexes on the horizontal axis of the ECG is due to the ever-changing geometry of the re-entry circuit, which oscillates within the ventricles. The diagnosis of TdP is based on the following criteria: (1) the rhythm immediately prior to onset of TdP is slow, and the QT interval is prolonged (>0.25 second in the dog); (2) the onset of TdP involves an R on T ventricular extrasystole (e.g., depolarization [R wave] occurs during the vulnerable part of the T wave); (3) the ensuing rapid (>180 bpm) ventricular rhythm has QRS complexes that are more regular than in VF but that are continuously changing in amplitude and polarity (Figure 202-38). The total duration of a self-resolving paroxysm of TdP is usually very brief (5 to 10 seconds), but it may persist for longer; in those instances it often evolves lethally into VF. TdP is not commonly recognized in the dog but may be caused by any disorder that prolongs the QT interval:[92] congenital long QT syndrome (Dalmatian), hypokalemia, hypocalcemia, and overdose or toxicity due to antiarrhythmic drugs, particularly class 1A antiarrhythmics such as quinidine. The treatment is highly specific and requires discontinuation of all antiarrhythmic drugs and institution of intravenous magnesium sulfate (10 to 30 mg/lb slow intravenous administration).[92]

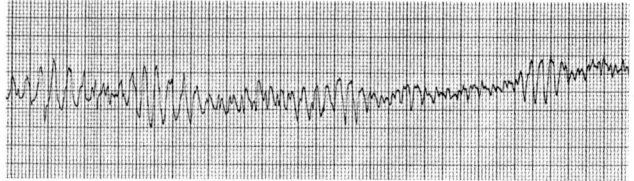

Figure 202-38 Torsade de pointes (TdP) in a dog. Lead II, 25 mm/sec, 1 cm = 1 mV. (Tracing courtesy of Dr. Michael B. Lesser, Lawndale, Calif.)

Ventricular parasystole Ventricular parasystole ("one heart beats as two") is a complex arrhythmia that results from the concurrent and independent activity of two pacemakers, one being a normal supraventricular pacemaker and the other existing in a protected site in a ventricle.[93] By definition, parasystole has (1) a ventricular focus with independent, abnormal automaticity and that has a rate that is greater than an escape focus and (2) a unidirectional (entry) block that shields this focus from sinus depolarizations. Parasystole is most often benign, does not warrant antiarrhythmic treatment, and regardless is usually refractory to antiarrhythmic therapy.

Disorders of Conduction

Disorders arising from faulty intracardiac electrical conduction are simply referred to as *blocks*. Blocks are grouped according to anatomic and functional criteria. Anatomic criteria separate them depending on their level of physical location: SA blocks, AV blocks, BBBs, and fascicular blocks.

Functional criteria characterize blocks according to their degree of severity. First-degree block produces a delay in conduction; second-degree block causes complete but intermittent block; and third-degree block causes complete, sustained block.

Atrioventricular Block   AV blocks are defined as delays or stoppages of conduction between the atria and the ventricles (specifically, between the upper part of the AV node and the His bundle prior to its trifurcation). First-degree AV block simply is a delay in AV conduction. Conduction through the AV node is slower than normal, but every impulse crosses the node successfully (Figure 202-39). It may be permanent or transient and may arise from a structural lesion or simply be functional. The ECG diagnosis is based on normal, sinus-appearing QRS complexes and a prolonged PR interval. The clinical manifestations are nil; first-degree AV block is an ECG finding only and does not warrant treatment. Its importance is at best diagnostic, drawing the clinician's attention to possible causes of delayed conduction, which include AV nodal damage in the major forms of heart disease and iatrogenic problems including excessive administration of such cardiac glycosides as digitalis or other antiarrhythmic therapy. Most commonly it is normal and is due only to high vagal tone. First-degree AV block does not progress to second- or third-degree AV block except in cases of drug toxicity.

Second-degree AV blocks involve the complete (but transient) interruption of AV conduction. Therefore a P wave exists for every QRS complex, but a QRS complex does not exist for every P wave. Two important subtypes of second-degree AV block exist. The first, Mobitz type I second-degree AV block, is characterized by a progressive lengthening of the PR interval until ultimately a P wave is blocked (P wave without QRS complex), known as the *Wenckebach phenomenon*. Anatomically, Mobitz type I second-degree AV block originates high in the AV node and is said to carry a good prognosis because it is closely related to first-degree AV block, and

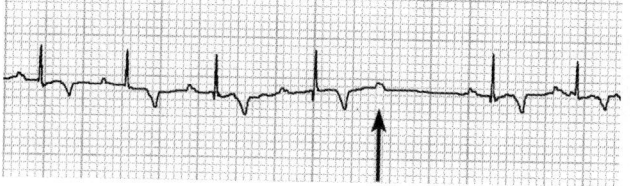

Figure 202-40 Second-degree AV block, Mobitz type I (Wenckebach phenomenon). Gradual prolongation of the PR interval occurs until a P wave is completely blocked *(arrow)*. Lead II, 25 mm/sec, 1 cm = 1 mV.

virtually never causes clinical signs (Figure 202-40). The second, Mobitz type II second-degree AV block, by contrast, demonstrates perfectly regular PR intervals for all QRS complexes, but one or more P wave or waves is or are blocked (Figure 202-41). Mobitz type II second-degree AV block arises from the AV bundle and is said to carry a more guarded to poor prognosis because it more closely resembles third-degree AV block; however, objective evidence to support this extrapolation from human cardiology in veterinary patients is lacking. In *simple* Mobitz type II second-degree AV block, more conducted P waves occur than blocked P waves, whereas in *advanced* Mobitz type II second-degree AV block (as in Figure 202-41), more blocked P waves occur than conducted P waves. The presence or absence of clinical signs appears to be related to the overall ventricular rate. Therefore simple Mobitz type II second-degree AV blocks rarely produce clinical manifestations such as exercise intolerance, whereas the more advanced Mobitz type II second-degree AV blocks commonly produce clinical signs that are similar to third-degree AV block: weakness, lethargy, syncope, and Stokes-Adams seizures (true convulsions caused by critical, arrhythmia-induced cerebral hypoperfusion) even with minimal exertion.

Third-degree AV block is a complete and sustained interruption of AV conduction. The ventricles depolarize according to a slow, regular, autonomic rhythm, called an *escape rhythm* (junctional or ventricular; see following) (Figure 202-42). It is essential to recognize the lifesaving *salvage* function of a ventricular escape rhythm, because it prevents asystole. Therefore even though ventricular escape QRS complexes are wide and bizarre, ventricular antiarrhythmic therapy is absolutely contraindicated.

In third-degree AV block, communication between the atria and ventricles is nonexistent (complete AV dissociation). Therefore the ECG diagnosis is based on the complete absence of P wave conduction (P waves without QRS complexes; no consistent PR interval) and on slow ventricular QRS complexes, which are usually of a uniform, but wide, bizarre morphology (shape) and that usually occur with near-perfect regularity. Third-degree AV blocks typically produce marked exercise intolerance, weakness, and syncope. Even so, it is possible

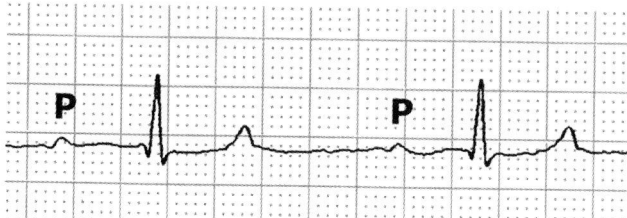

Figure 202-39 First-degree AV block. The interval between each P wave and the following QRS complex is markedly prolonged in this extreme example (PR interval = 0.18 second). Lead II, 50 mm/sec, 1 cm = 1 mV.

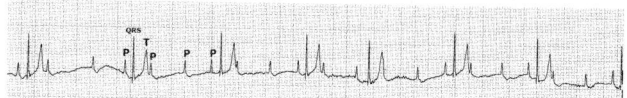

Figure 202-41 Second-degree AV block, Mobitz type II. P waves are blocked without a gradual lengthening of the preceding P-R interval, in contrast to Mobitz type I second-degree AV block. For most of the tracing, only every third atrial impulse crosses the AV node and activates the ventricles, as evidenced by the fixed P-R interval for every third P wave (3:1 block). Lead II, 25 mm/sec, 1 cm = 1 mV.

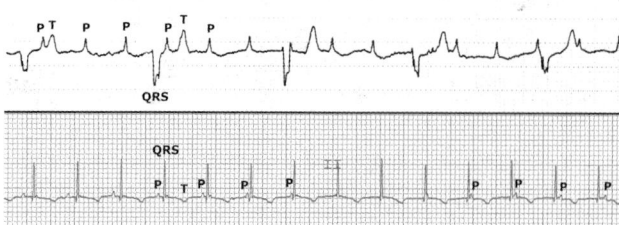

Figure 202-42 Third-degree AV block. No connection occurs between P waves and QRS complexes. Lead II, 25 mm/sec, 1 cm = 1 mV. In the upper panel, the escape rhythm is clearly ventricular because the QRS complexes are wide and bizarre in lead II and are slow to occur (rate = 55/min). This cat had clinical signs caused by the arrhythmia (lethargy) and required implantation of a pacemaker. In the lower panel, the escape rhythm is likely junctional (supraventricular), because the QRS complexes are narrow and upright in lead II, and they occur at a near-normal (near-sinus) rate (150/minute). That is, AV block is present in the proximal part of the AV nodal-His complex, and the escape rhythm originates in the distal part. This arrhythmia was an incidental finding in an otherwise normal cat.

to encounter older animals, not very active by nature, who have "asymptomatic" third-degree AV blocks, or individuals (especially cats) with third-degree AV block and a rapid escape rhythm in which the block is an incidental finding (see Figure 202-42).[1,3] The asymptomatic situation also is likely in cases of *isorhythmic AV dissociation*, a situation in which third-degree AV block occurs but the atrial rate and ventricular rate are nearly identical (see Figure 202-42).

The causes of AV blocks are diverse. First-degree AV and Mobitz type I second-degree AV blocks often are functional (high vagal tone in healthy individuals, negative dromotropic effects of digitalis, antiarrhythmics, or alpha 2-stimulating anesthetics). Less commonly, cardiac disease with atrial dilation and AV nodal lesions may be present. Mobitz type II second-degree AV block and third-degree AV block are sometimes functional (hyperkalemia, digitalis toxicity, alpha 2-stimulating anesthetics), but are commonly associated with a structural lesion, be it inflammatory (endocarditis, Lyme myocarditis, traumatic myocarditis) or degenerative (physical disruption arising from cardiomyopathy, endocardiosis, or fibrosis).[94,95] Treatment is therefore aimed at the underlying cause when possible. In clinically overt, advanced, Mobitz type II second-degree AV blocks or third-degree AV blocks, response to parasympatholytic or sympathomimetic drugs tends to be fairly disappointing and potentially dangerous. Pacemaker implantation is a better choice (Figure 202-43).

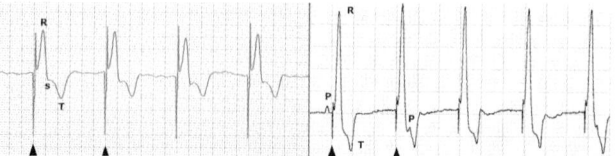

Figure 202-43 Normal pacemaker function. Electrical activity generated by pacemakers appears as spikes on the electrocardiogram (ECG) (*arrowheads*). The spikes are larger for unipolar pacemakers (left panel) than for bipolar pacemakers (right panel). No atrial activity was present in the dog in the left panel. No association exists between atrial activity (P waves) and paced activity in the right panel because the pacemaker activates only the ventricles (VVI mode). Lead II, 25 mm/sec, 1 cm = 1 mV.

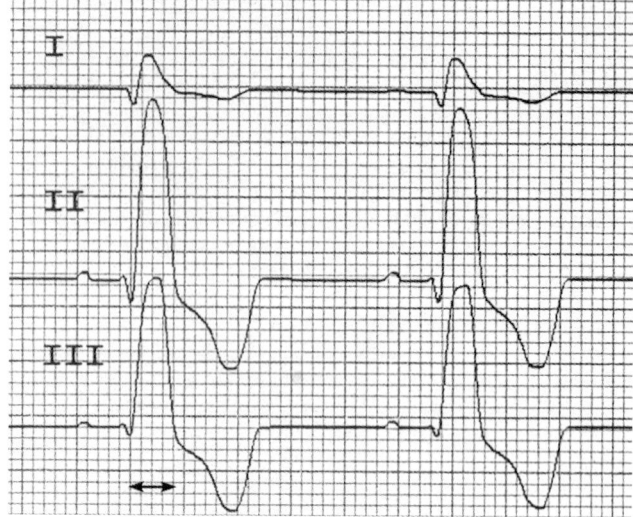

Figure 202-44 Left bundle branch block (LBBB) in a dog. The QRS complexes are very wide (0.10 second, *small double arrow*) but of otherwise normal configuration. Normal sinus rhythm. Simultaneous leads I, II, and III, 50 mm/sec, 1 cm = 1 mV.

Bundle Branch Blocks   BBBs are slowings or interruptions of conduction involving one or more of the ventricular branches of the His bundle. Blocks may be functional (transient interruptions due to the depolarizations occurring during the refractory period) or structural (permanent interruptions due to a physical disturbance). The ECG diagnosis of BBBs is based on the abnormal shape of the QRS complexes, which become widened due to the desynchronization of the two ventricles. The duration of the QRS complexes is greater than 0.07 second in dogs with BBB, and the polarity is positive in lead II for left BBBs and negative in lead II for RBB blocks (Figure 202-44 and 202-45). If BBBs occur during sinus rhythm, the ECG diagnosis is straightforward, because other than the very abnormal appearance of the QRS complexes, the P-QRS-T sequence throughout the ECG is normal: a P wave occurs before each QRS and the PR interval is fixed and normal. If the block occurs concurrently with a nonsinus rhythm, such as AFib, however, establishing a diagnosis in BBB can be much more challenging (see Figure 202-30).

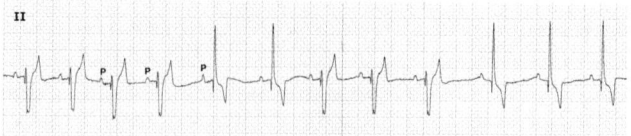

Figure 202-45 Intermittent right bundle branch block (RBBB) in a dog. Each QRS complex is preceded by a P wave. This important finding indicates that this is a supraventricular rhythm and not a ventricular arrhythmia. The cyclical increasing-decreasing heart rate, constant PR interval, and similar appearance of all P waves indicate that this rhythm is respiratory sinus arrhythmia (RSA). The wide, bizarre QRS complexes occur when the sinus rhythm is slightly faster (shorter R-R intervals), indicating a rate-dependent form of intraventricular conduction disturbance. The wide, bizarre appearance of QRS complexes in this lead II tracing indicates that this disturbance is a block of the RBB. RBB block generally is a normal or inconsequential finding in dogs and has no hemodynamic repercussions in the patient. The main significance of RBB block lies in how easily it can be mistaken for a ventricular arrhythmia. Lead II, 25 mm/sec, 1 cm = 1 mV.

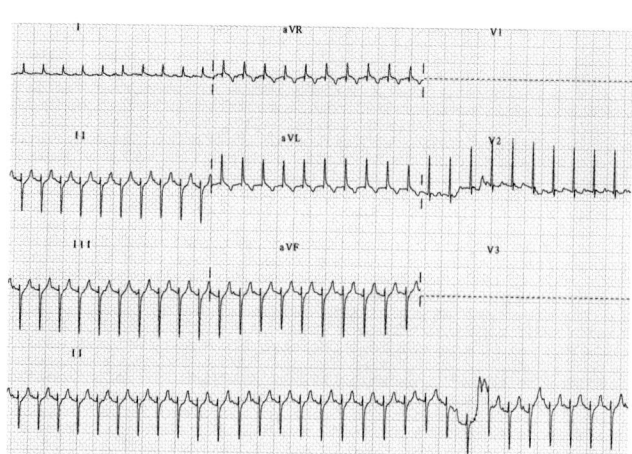

Figure 202-46 Left anterior fascicular (LAF) block. Prominent S waves occur in leads II, III, and aVF, indicating a leftward mean electrical axis (MEA) deviation (–75 degrees). Motion artifact is noted in the last quarter of the rhythm strip *(lower-right corner)*. This adult cat had moderate left ventricular (LV) hypertrophy echocardiographically, as suspected from the large (deep) QRS complexes. Seven-lead electrocardiogram (ECG) and simultaneous rhythm strip; 25 mm/sec, 1 cm = 1 mV.

A BBB together with AFib mimics ventricular extrasystoles or VT, which may misdirect therapeutic decisions, (see previous discussion of atrial fibrillation). Cats with heart disease (especially cardiomyopathy) are classically described as being prone to developing block in a subdivision of the LBB known as the *left anterior fascicle* (or LAF).[5] LAF block produces a tall R wave in leads I and aVL, and a deep S wave in leads II, III, and aVF, and therefore a left-axis deviation (see Figure 202-6; Figure 202-46).[12]

The causes of BBB are many, because they may be due to a variety of pathologic changes including hypertrophy (as in feline hypertrophic cardiomyopathy), dilation (as seen in dilated cardiomyopathy), and inflammation (endocarditis, traumatic myocarditis). In the dog, RBB block is often a completely normal, unnecessarily worrisome ECG finding (see Figures 202-30, 202-45). Clinical manifestations of BBBs alone generally do not occur.[11,12] These disturbances therefore do not warrant specific treatment beyond that of their underlying cause. The importance of recognizing BBB lies in the fact that they could be the first indicators of underlying cardiac disease, which itself warrants further diagnosis and treatment, and that they can be misinterpreted as ventricular arrhythmias.

Atrial Standstill (*Silent Atrium*)

This rhythm disturbance does not truly fall into the category of blocks. It is an arrhythmia characterized by the total absence of atrial depolarization (Figure 202-47). A sinus impulse may nevertheless be properly formed and conducted to the AV node if the internodal pathways remain functional. In this situation, common with hyperkalemia, the rhythm is referred to as *sinoventricular*. Otherwise, if no sinus impulse arises and the atria are electrically silent, then a junctional or ventricular escape rhythm must emerge to avoid asystole. The three differential diagnoses for atrial standstill are (1) moderate to marked hyperkalemia (K+ > 7.5 mEq/L), (2) atrial myopathy, and (3) ECG artifact (P waves too small, or isoelectric, preventing them from being seen properly on a chosen ECG lead). Perhaps the most easily identified initial change of moderate hyperkalemia on ECG is disappearance of the P waves; this change follows mild tenting of the T waves (often imperceptible) and precedes ventricular flutter and cardiac arrest. Alternatively, atrial

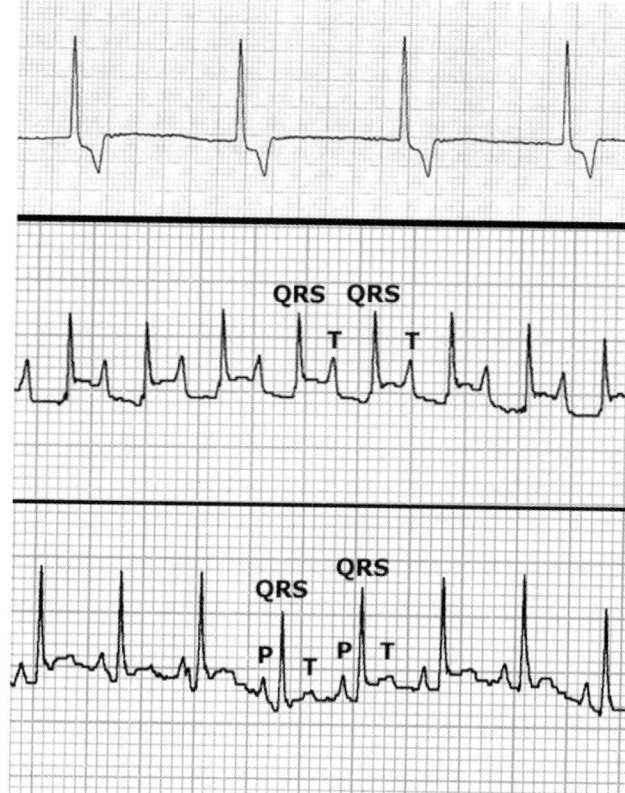

Figure 202-47 Atrial standstill. In the upper panel, a primary atrial myopathy was responsible for the lack of atrial activity seen in this dog's tracing. Serum [K+] = 4.3 mEq/L (within normal limits). Lead II, 25 mm/sec, 1 cm = 1 mV. In the middle and lower panels, presence (middle) and absence (lower) of atrial standstill in a cat with urinary obstruction before and after correction of severe hyperkalemia, respectively. The reader should note the rapid ventricular rate in the middle panel (220/min) despite an elevated serum [K+] (8.4 mEq/L). In contrast to dogs, severely hyperkalemic cats often are tachycardic. Lead II, 25 mm/sec, 1 cm = 0.5 mV.

standstill may occur due to marked atrial stretch,[96] as occurs particularly in cats with various forms of cardiomyopathy, or atrial parenchymal hypoplasia, as is seen in association with a dystrophic form of neuromyopathy, particularly in the Springer spaniel. Either way, the ECG appearance is therefore of a regular rhythm, usually with QRS complexes that are of a supraventricular appearance, and with a normal rate but without detectable P waves in any lead on the ECG. Differentiating between the two main causes of this rhythm using the ECG alone is difficult, and immediate measurement of serum electrolytes is warranted.

Electromechanical Dissociation

EMD is not, strictly speaking, an abnormality of cardiac rhythm. *EMD* refers to the absence of conversion of an electrical rhythm into a mechanical force of contractility.[97,98] The ECG therefore may show virtually any rhythm, and the diagnosis rests on the combination of a hemodynamically collapsed patient with an ECG that shows any rhythm but asystole. The pulse is usually barely perceptible or absent, the patient typically is unconscious, and EMD most commonly is a prearrest or terminal condition (Figure 202-48). Treatment requires correction of underlying causes if possible and then is aimed at increasing circulation to improve myocardial perfusion. Because EMD generally indicates profound myocardial hypoxia, the prognosis is poor even with treatment.

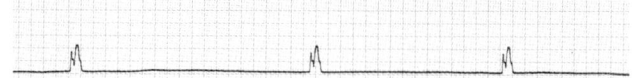

Figure 202-48 Electromechanical dissociation (EMD). By definition, pulselessness was present during this ECG. Lead II, 25 mm/sec, 1 cm = 1 mV.

Complex Disorders Involving Abnormalities of Both Excitability and Conduction

Of the multiple rhythm disturbances described previously, many can occur jointly on the same ECG tracing, producing mixed disturbances of excitability and of conduction. This next section will discuss examples of disturbances of excitability and of conduction that produce specific clinical syndromes.

Pre-Excitation Syndromes In pre-excitation, the normal impulse originating from the SA node is split at the end of atrial depolarization, with part of the impulse traveling normally through the AV node and another part of the impulse traveling simultaneously through an abnormal shaft of rapidly conductive fibers that links the atria and the ventricles, (also called an *accessory pathway* or *bypass tract*) thus bypassing the AV node. The result is partial, premature, immediate activation of the ventricles through the bypass tract, without the benefit of a pause in the AV node; hence the term *pre-excitation*. With one major exception (see following), the effect of this abnormal pattern of activation is minimal, because only a part of the atrial contribution to ventricular filling is lost. The ECG demonstrates that the normal delay through the AV node was pre-empted by conduction through the bypass tract (i.e., no segment separates the P wave from the QRS complex) and that conduction through the bypass tract caused asynchronous activation of the ventricles (the bypass tract and the normal AV nodal conduction ultimately each activate their share of the ventricles), resulting in a notched QRS complex. The size and location of the QRS complex's notch, the *delta wave*, depends on the distance that separates the bypass tract and the AV node in the individual's heart (i.e., on the amount of myocardium that the His bundle and the bypass tract can each depolarize before the impulses collide with each other; Figure 202-49).

Under usual circumstances, pre-excitation is an incidental, clinically silent finding. However, in individuals with pre-excitation, a premature atrial depolarization may initiate a type of re-entry cycle that can produce extreme tachycardias. Although bypass tracts conduct impulses rapidly, their refractory period typically is longer than that of the AV node. Therefore the timing of a premature supraventricular depolarization may fail to conduct through the bypass tract but be able to conduct through the AV node, depolarizing the ventricles normally. As the impulse completes the depolarization of the ventricles, the bypass tract has repolarized and is able to conduct. Bypass tracts can often conduct impulses in either direction, such that the ventricular impulse conducts retrograde through the bypass tract to the atria, initiating an endless loop of conduction. This type of self-perpetuating circuit is a type of *macrore-entry circuit*, and it may produce a potentially very rapid and clinically overt (apparent discomfort, exercise intolerance, lethargy, syncope) tachycardia called *orthodromic* [the impulse travels in a normal direction through the AV node] *AV re-entrant tachycardia*, or the *Wolff-Parkinson-White* (WPW) syndrome.[59,63,99] Dogs with this syndrome may have unrelenting heart rates above 300 bpm. Initial treatment can involve vagal maneuvers that, through slowing of AV conduction (i.e., negative dromotropic action), break the cycle of re-entry. Amiodarone or procainamide may be used in the

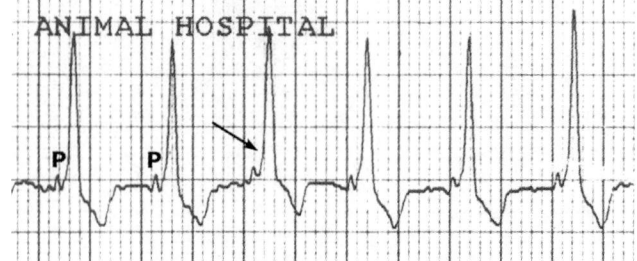

Figure 202-49 Pre-excitation. The P-R interval is the same as the duration of the P wave (i.e., no P-R segment is seen). This finding indicates pre-excitation of the ventricles through an accessory bypass tract. The asynchronous activation of the ventricles is demonstrated through the presence of a subtle notch in the QRS complex, the delta wave *(arrow)*. Lead I, 25 mm/sec, 1 cm = 1 mV.

management of such tachyarrhythmias in dogs. Conversely, digoxin is contraindicated because it decreases the refractory period of the bypass tract. Many drug therapies or combinations thereof have been used to reduce the occurrence of WPW episodes in pets with *symptomatic* re-entrant tachycardias caused by pre-excitation. Frequently in these cases, no drug therapy is entirely successful, and the clearest and most successful form of treatment involves referral to a specialized center for intracardiac catheter-based radiofrequency interruption (ablation) of the re-entrant pathway, which permanently abolishes pre-excitation and all future risk of recurrence of the WPW syndrome.[63,100]

Sick Sinus Syndrome SSS (bradycardia-tachycardia syndrome, sinus node dysfunction) involves a complex disturbance of the cardiac conductive tissues, producing simultaneous defects in sinus activity (SB and sinus arrest), AV conduction disturbances (first-degree and second-degree AV blocks) and disturbances in supraventricular and ventricular excitability (Figure 202-50). Therefore the disturbance is not a problem involving only the SA node, as the name *SSS* suggests, but rather is an illness that affects cardiac tissue at all levels.

The cause of SSS is unknown. Some human beings with SSS have autoantibodies directed at SA nodal tissue or at cholinergic receptors,[101,102] but these mechanisms have not been described in dogs with SSS. Certain epidemiologic features stand out from cases reported in the veterinary literature. The disease is recognized almost exclusively in dogs, and the stereotypical breed predilection for female miniature Schnauzers is far from exclusive, many other breeds, notably Cocker spaniels,[103,104] West Highland white terriers,[103,105] and mixed breed dogs represent an ever-increasing proportion of patients with this disorder. The spectrum of disease described as SSS likely regroups more than one distinct disorder that future research will categorize into separate entities.

The age of onset typically is mid to late adulthood (6 to 10 years), and the association with chronic mitral valvular disease is common but not obligatory. Histopathologically, nodal

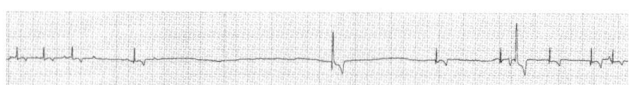

Figure 202-50 Sick sinus syndrome (SSS). Second-degree AV block followed by an extremely long sinus pause, an escape beat, sinus bradycardia or a supraventricular escape rhythm, and one premature ventricular complex, are seen. Lead II, 25 mm/sec, 1 cm = 1 mV.

tissue fibrosis is seen, associated with vascular disturbances (microcoronary arteritis). The ECG diagnosis often requires repeated and sufficiently long (2 to 3 minute) tracings, to convincingly demonstrate some or all of the aspects of SSS: SB (often with first- or second-degree AV block), prolonged sinus pauses with variable escape beats and bursts of supraventricular tachycardia or ventricular extrasystoles at various rates (see Figure 202-50). In some cases only SB occurs. Because these features occur intermittently, the diagnosis often is only made by obtaining an ECG during an episode of syncope, stumbling, or ataxia (near syncope), which are the most common overt clinical manifestations of this arrhythmia. Ambulatory ECG, especially cardiac event recording, is ideally suited for establishing the diagnosis of SSS when the in-hospital ECG is unhelpful (see Ambulatory Electrocardiography). Such technology has identified that episodes occur during bradycardia rather than tachycardia. Vagolytic drugs may acutely improve the situation by reducing the impact of bradycardia episodes and pauses, but definitive treatment when episodes are recurrent generally requires the implantation of a pacemaker (see following). Digitalis glycosides are usually contraindicated, including in the CHF patient, because of the risk of furthering AV block and thus decreasing ventricular rate. If CHF is present, diuretics (e.g., furosemide) and angiotensin-converting enzyme (ACE) inhibitors are typically used, with or without spironolactone. Correction of bradycardia through pacemaker implantation occasionally improves cardiac output sufficiently to eliminate CHF and allow the gradual reduction, and possibly discontinuation, of diuretics.

THERAPY OF ARRHYTHMIAS (Table 202-1)

First and foremost, any underlying or predisposing factors involved in the precipitation of arrhythmias need to be identified and resolved when possible (see Figure 202-34). For example, attempting to treat VT with antiarrhythmic drugs when a patient is hypokalemic is counterproductive and probably dangerous. Hypokalemia can both make ventricular arrhythmias more likely to occur and, through effects on myocardial sodium channels, hypokalemia makes the arrhythmia refractory to the more commonly used intravenous antiarrhythmics including lidocaine.

Overall, a practical approach to choosing antiarrhythmic therapy incorporates known clinical efficacy, adverse drug reactions, pharmacokinetic effects, and results of administration. Substantial changes in the approach to antiarrhythmic therapy have evolved since the publication of the 1991 Cardiac Arrhythmia Suppression Trial (CAST) in human beings with myocardial infarction. In this multigroup, placebo-controlled, double-blinded study, researchers unexpectedly found an increased rather than decreased risk of death when certain type IC antiarrhythmic agents were administered. Although ambient ventricular arrhythmias are still regarded as a risk factor for adverse cardiovascular events, these arrhythmias are increasingly perceived as *messengers* of myocardial disturbance rather than primary problems needing to be quelled. Accordingly, the rush to treat asymptomatic ventricular arrhythmias has been markedly reduced.[106,107] By contrast, the general approach to the treatment of supraventricular tachyarrhythmias, whether latent or responsible for clinical signs, has remained the same or become more aggressive in small animal medicine (Figure 202-51).[63,100]

The decision to treat ventricular arrhythmias in veterinary medicine should be based on the functional effects of the rhythm, not the frequency ("more than x PVCs/min") or morphologic complexity (monomorphic versus polymorphic) of the abnormal beats.[89,106] Expressions of the functional effects of arrhythmias that can be assessed clinically include the presence of clinical signs (e.g., lethargy, syncope, Stokes-Adams seizures)

and perfusion during the arrhythmia (pulse quality, mentation, and if available, short-term trends in blood pressure parameters).

Ventricular tachyarrhythmias may be progressive and can compromise cardiac output. However, even complex ventricular arrhythmias, when they are asymptomatic, do not necessarily represent a target for attempting to reduce the risk of sudden death.[107] In human medicine, from which the overwhelming majority of veterinary clinical cardiac arrhythmia information is extrapolated, "rendering treatment to suppress a risk factor because of the temptation to equate causality with association between the risk factor and a putative clinical outcome has never been more misguided than with nonsustained ventricular tachycardia."[107]

"When to treat?" probably remains the single most important and unresolved question in veterinary cardiology. The veterinary experience may or may not be substantively different from the human. Therapy based on human medical recommendations may be inappropriate considering the principal differences in causes of disease between the species (e.g., coronary versus noncoronary heart diseases). Clinicians do not know what happens to dogs or cats with arrhythmias of differing causes, nor are we generally able to compare arrhythmias of different causes regarding outcome or specific drug therapies. Survival and efficacy studies for complex arrhythmias in veterinary medicine are few, and, with one exception, none has been double-blinded or controlled. The exception is a prospective study of 49 Boxer dogs with familial ventricular arrhythmia *(Boxer cardiomyopathy)* that were randomized to receive one of four antiarrhythmic medication strategies. Results of the study showed that some antiarrhythmics were better than others for reducing the occurrence of arrhythmia, but none of the four significantly decreased the extent of clinical manifestations of the arrhythmias (syncope).[46] Otherwise, experience-based generalizations may be made, including the observation that dogs with mitral endocardiosis are not likely to die suddenly of arrhythmic causes, whereas cardiomyopathic Doberman pinschers and dogs with advanced subaortic stenosis have a greater risk of sudden death when they reach a stage of disease associated with ventricular ectopy. When overt clinical signs such as syncope or aborted syncope are present, it is difficult to argue with therapeutic efforts to contain the arrhythmia. When clinical signs are absent, however, it is relevant to compare the potential side effects of therapy, including proarrhythmia, to the potential and difficult-to-prove benefit of a stabilized or normalized rhythm. Proarrhythmic effects of cardiac drugs aside, Calvert[108] has shown the adverse effects of routine anesthesia and surgery in Doberman pinschers with occult cardiomyopathy, thereby reminding the clinician to consider the dangers of medical procedures that may exacerbate uncontrolled arrhythmias.

Classification Systems for Antiarrhythmic Agents
Antiarrhythmic drugs have traditionally been classified into one of four groups according to their predominant effect on the action potential. Dissatisfaction with the shortcomings of the Vaughn-Williams (V-W) classification scheme for antiarrhythmic drugs resulted in the creation of a competing classification system[109] correlating antiarrhythmic drugs with the mechanism of the arrhythmia and vulnerable parameters, as well as actions of the drug.[110] The scheme, known as the *Sicilian gambit* (SG), is based on the actions of drugs on arrhythmogenic mechanisms and was another attempt to provide a rational basis for therapy. Regrettably, although academically reasonable, it has not improved the clinical approach to arrhythmia therapy in human or veterinary medicine.

Limitations of the traditional V-W system include its incomplete classification, crossover within the system among specific drugs, and its discussion principally of blocking mechanisms,

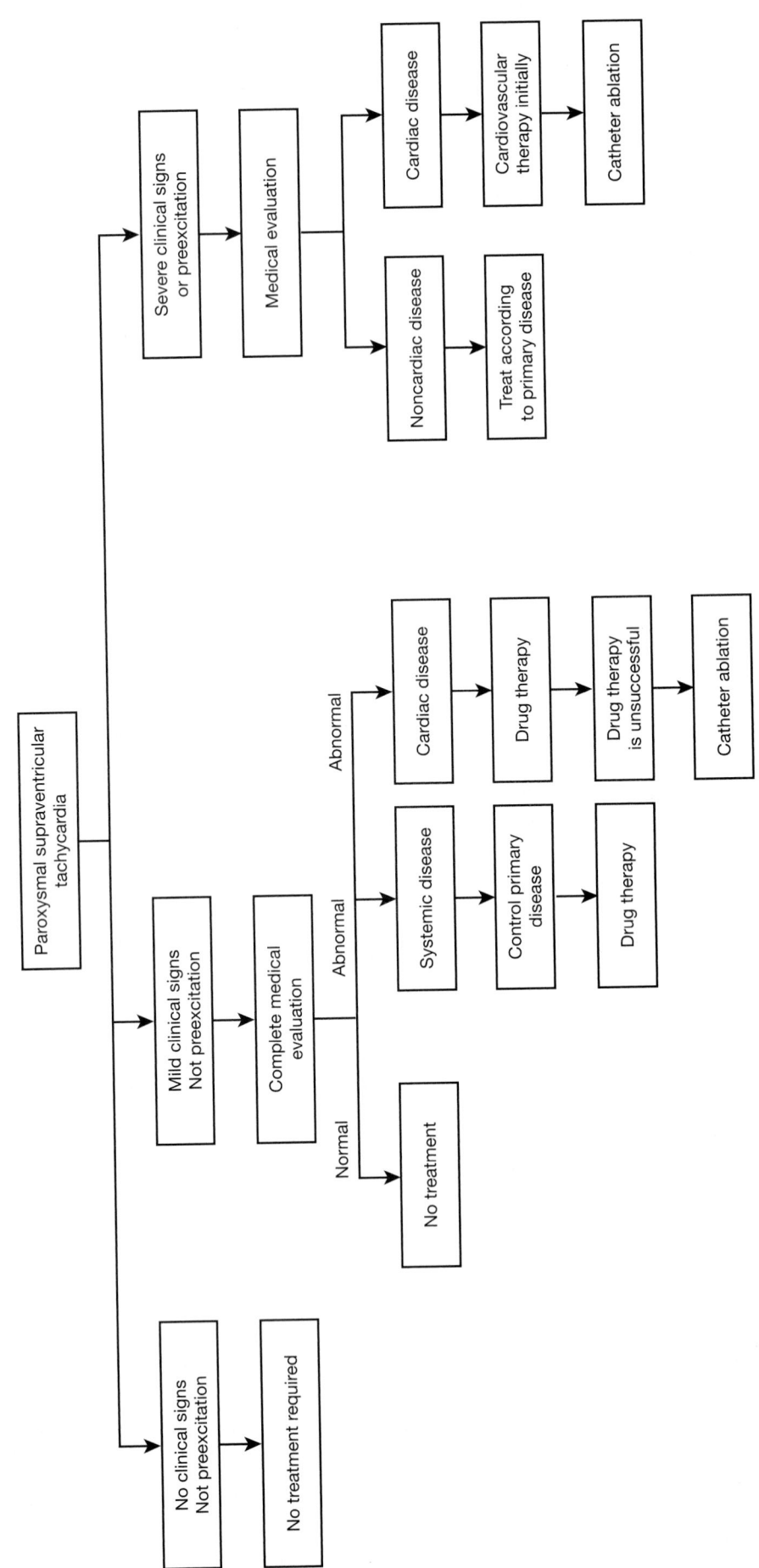

Figure 202-51 Approach to management of supraventricular arrhythmias.

whereas activation of channels, receptors, or both are down-played. Antiarrhythmic agents may be effective in a number of ways: slowing tachycardias, terminating arrhythmias, making them tolerable, or preventing their initiation.[109] The V-W classification is based only on the electrophysiologic drug effects of isolated, normal cardiac tissue (except for class II agents), which is different from the diseased state. The classification excludes compounds such as digitalis, adenosine, and alpha-adrenergic-blocking agents. The V-W classification system assumes that we know more than we really do. Not all drugs within a class have the same physiologic or clinical effects. The danger in using only the V-W scheme is that most drugs have more than one mode of action, and all the drugs within a category clearly are not always the same.

Antiarrhythmic therapy for the practicing veterinarian with access to ECG monitoring, ambulatory ECG (available at most referral veterinary centers or via on-line rental [see previous discussion]), and echocardiography (available at many referral facilities) is described later in this chapter. Electrophysiologic testing and terminology, although desirable, are (with few exceptions) not practiced. Therefore the discussion of these techniques is limited to what is required to make knowledgeable medical decisions in practice. Only commonly used drugs or those likely to be useful in canine or feline heart disease are discussed. New drugs are identified, as are new uses for older drugs.

CLASS I ANTIARRHYTHMICS (Table 202-1)

Class I drugs selectively block the fast sodium channels, decreasing sodium influx during phase zero of depolarization. A reduced slope of phase zero is the manifestation of decreased conduction velocity. Slowed conduction velocity can interrupt a reentrant pattern.[3] These drugs work best in cells dependent on the fast sodium channel for their action potential, such as normal and ischemic Purkinje cells and ventricular myocardial cells. Within this class are three subgroups, distinguished by their electrophysiologic and antiarrhythmic differences. Most of the compounds within this class fail to perform adequately in the presence of hypokalemia.

Class IA Drugs

Class IA antiarrhythmic drugs are intermediate sodium channel blockers that markedly depress phase zero action potential, depress conduction of electrical impulses through the heart, and slow cardiac repolarization by lengthening the effective refractory period.[3] By depressing the conduction velocity and prolonging the refractory period, arrhythmias dependent on re-entry may be interrupted. Drugs in this class include quinidine (prototype IA drug), procainamide, and disopyramide (Table 202-1). Quinidine decreases the rate of spontaneous depolarization in pacemaker fibers, prolongs anterograde refractoriness accessory pathways, and can suppress or trigger delayed afterdepolarizations. Quinidine may prolong the PR interval, widen the QRS complex, and lengthen the QT interval, and it was originally indicated for the control of supraventricular and ventricular arrhythmias. Today it and the other class IA drugs have very limited usefulness in clinical antiarrhythmic therapy of small animals. Proarrhythmic and other side effects make quinidine an agent that is now rarely used.

Procainamide has cardiac effects similar to those of quinidine. However, its propensity for inducing hypotension with intravenous use or increasing ventricular rates from enhanced AV conduction is less than that of quinidine. Procainamide specifically has been demonstrated to prolong the effective refractory period and slow conduction in the accessory pathway of dogs with orthodromic AV reciprocating tachycardia.[111]

Procainamide is metabolized by the liver and eliminated by the kidneys. The sustained release formulations may be poorly absorbed and even eliminated as intact tablets in the feces of dogs. Procainamide may be used in conjunction with other class I agents and beta-blockers for refractory arrhythmias. Oral administration of the drug at higher than usually recommended doses to achieve trough serum concentrations of 10 to 12 μg/mL were successful in controlling some supraventricular tachyarrhythmias.[111,112] Side effects are infrequent and include anorexia, nausea, vomiting, fever, proarrhythmia, and agranulocytosis. In a four-way trial of antiarrhythmic drugs in boxer dogs with ventricular arrhythmias, procainamide (10 to 12 mg/lb orally, three times a day) successfully reduced the frequency of ventricular ectopy. However, the frequency of syncope was unaffected, and there were substantial side effects.[46]

Class IB Drugs

Class IB agents block fast sodium channels, which decreases the slope of phase zero, depresses automaticity, and increases the threshold for VF. These drugs have an affinity for binding with inactivated sodium channels, thereby acting selectively on diseased or ischemic tissue. Minimal effects are seen on the sinus node, AV node, and atrial muscle or on inotropy. Lidocaine, phenytoin, tocainide, and mexiletine are examples of drugs in this class (Table 202-1).

Lidocaine is used for acute control of life-threatening ventricular arrhythmias. In usual doses it is not likely to affect myocardial contractility, systemic arterial blood pressure, the QRS complex, or AV conduction time,[3] although extremely high doses have been shown to decrease ventricular contractility. Lidocaine suppresses automaticity and conduction velocity and prolongs refractoriness in ischemic cardiac cells.

Lidocaine is most effective when used intravenously, owing to first-pass hepatic metabolism. It is less than 10% protein bound. Hepatic disease, chloramphenicol, propranolol, halothane, cimetidine, and norepinephrine may all delay hepatic metabolism of lidocaine. Hepatic microenzyme inducers enhance degradation.

Lidocaine intoxication results in ataxia, mental depression, and seizures. These signs usually subside within minutes after lidocaine infusion is discontinued. Diazepam or a short-acting barbiturate may be necessary to control seizures. Lidocaine may be administered by slow (2 to 5 minute) intravenous loading bolus (1 to 2 mg/lb) followed by a continuous rate infusion (CRI) of 10 to 30 μg/lb/min in dogs. Alternatively, after the initial bolus, an additional amount can be given at half the dose every 10 minutes to maintain the rhythm. Caution is recommended when using lidocaine in cats because of historical reports of bradyarrhythmias and sudden death. Lower bolus doses of 0.25 to 0.5 mg/lb slowly followed by 5 to 10 μg/lb/min CRI are recommended for cats. Intramuscular lidocaine is less efficacious and is rarely used.

Tocainide and mexiletine are structurally analogous to lidocaine but have oral bioavailability. Response to lidocaine may not be a predictor of response to these oral agents, however.

Tocainide is orally absorbed and undergoes hepatic metabolism and renal excretion. It may be used after lidocaine or as initial treatment in a hemodynamically stable patient. At 6.8 to 11.4 mg/lb orally every 8 hours, peak levels were reached in cardiomyopathic Doberman pinscher dogs after 2 hours and began to diminish by 8 hours. Fifteen of 23 (70%) dogs experienced a 90% diminution of VT, and there was a 70% reduction of all PVCs in 80% of the cardiomyopathic dogs. Although there was no relationship between dose and serum concentration, dogs without signs of toxicity had serum levels under 11 mg/L and all those with toxic signs exceeded 14 mg/L.[113] Side effects observed within 8 days are weakness, head tremor, ataxia, and head bobbing. Long-term side effects, including corneal dystrophy, corneal edema, and renal failure, were observed in more than 50% of dogs.[113,114]

Mexiletine is absorbed orally and undergoes less than 10% first-pass hepatic elimination. It is 70% protein bound. The drug is eliminated by renal excretion, and its half-life varies depending on urine pH. Side effects are infrequent in the dog but can include nausea, inappetence, and tremor.[115] Sinus bradycardia, ataxia, dizziness, and thrombocytopenia are other potential problems. No data exist regarding its use in cats. In a group of Boxers with familial arrhythmia, mexiletine was given jointly with the beta-blocker atenolol as one of four forms of therapy being tested. This antiarrhythmic therapy reduced the frequency and "grade" of ventricular arrhythmia, and there was a reduction in peak heart rate. However, the frequency of syncope was not reduced with this form of treatment or with any other in the study.[46] Mexiletine is only available in the oral formulation in North America. Both mexiletine and tocainide appear to have synergistic properties when combined with class IA or class II agents.[46]

Class IC Drugs

Class IC drugs are blockers of slow sodium channels and are strong depressants of phase zero and conduction velocity. They exert a minimal effect on refractoriness or action potential duration. They are indicated for supraventricular and some ventricular arrhythmias and arrhythmias involving accessory pathways. They are notorious in humans for their proarrhythmic tendencies when given in patients with coronary artery disease. They depress contractility, cardiac output, and systemic blood pressure. These drugs are contraindicated in the presence of AV block, BBB, and myocardial depression. Flecainide and propafenone are class IC agents.

Flecainide is indicated for paroxysmal supraventricular tachycardia (SVT) and paroxysmal AFib but not for chronic AFib or in patients with ventricular dysfunction, ventricular hypertrophy, ischemic heart disease, or valvular heart disease. It has not been studied in clinical small animal medicine. This drug may induce or aggravate congestive heart failure.

Propafenone has local anesthetic effects and a direct stabilizing action on myocardial tissue, as well as weak beta-adrenergic–blocking activity. It prolongs A-V nodal conduction (A-H and H-V) and has negative inotropic action. It is effective against many SVT and accessory pathway arrhythmias but has not performed as well as had been hoped in the context of treating ventricular arrhythmias.[116] In structurally normal hearts, proarrhythmia is unlikely in humans. Propafenone is only available in the oral form in North America.

CLASS II ANTIARRHYTHMICS

Class II antiarrhythmics (beta-blockers) decrease or nullify the electrophysiologic and arrhythmogenic effects of beta-adrenergic sympathetic stimulation.[117-119] The magnitude of the beta-blockade effect is dependent on the prevailing level of sympathetic tone. Sympathetic stimulation increases the likelihood of slow calcium channels opening and increases the rate of pacemaker discharge. Overall, beta-blockers depress the slope of phase 4 depolarization and minimally raise the threshold for activation in sinus and AV nodal cells, thereby suppressing automaticity. The effect of beta-blockers on normal cell refractoriness and conduction is modest, and it is unlikely that they influence cardiac repolarization. As a result of the negative inotropic (contractility), chronotropic (rate), and dromotropic (AV node clearance time) effects, cardiac output is reduced and myocardial oxygen requirements and LV work are decreased in normal tissue. In the past several years the beneficial effects of beta-blockers have become increasingly recognized in the setting of severe myocardial disease, where initiation of treatment at extremely low doses and careful up-titration appear to provide a long-term cardioprotective effect.

Beta-blockade is indicated for supraventricular tachycardias, including atrial flutter, AFib, and pre-excitation tachyarrhythmias. It is more effective in controlling the ventricular rate response to AFib when combined with digitalis. Beta-blockade should be helpful in ventricular arrhythmias induced by sympathetic stimulation.[120] It may be used in combination with a class I agent for refractory ventricular tachyarrhythmias in the dog[46] or alone as the primary agent in the cat. Beta-blockade traditionally has been useful in the treatment of systemic hypertension, obstructive heart disease,[121] thyrotoxicosis, and digitalis toxicity. Elimination of propranolol paradoxically is longer in hyperthyroid cats than in euthyroid cats. Additional roles in the management of pheochromocytoma, theobromine intoxication (see Figure 202-25), dilated cardiomyopathy, and portal hypertension are possible.[119]

Contraindications include AV block and SSS (unless a functional artificial pacemaker is in place). Many beta-blockers are not cardioselective (i.e., they exert their effects on both beta$_1$ and beta$_2$ receptors), resulting in bronchial smooth muscle constriction. Nonselective beta-blockers are contraindicated in patients with dynamic bronchial disease. Beta-blockers, especially nonselective types, may interfere with the compensatory response to hypoglycemia and exercise.[119]

Since the publication of the last edition of this textbook, a number of clinical studies involving thousands of human patients have been conducted, and they have demonstrated conclusively that when properly initiated and titrated, some specific beta-blockers are of benefit in patients being treated for CHF (see Chapter 199).[117, 122-125] Of specific interest in CHF, carvedilol has both beta-adrenergic and alpha$_1$-blocking activity, which provides additional vasodilation. These effects appear to be unrelated to the drug's antiarrhythmic action. However, other beta-blockers that do not also possess alpha$_1$-blocking properties are also similarly effective in treating heart failure patients.[124] When administered correctly, beta-blocking drugs improve long-term myocardial function through a number of mechanisms.[117,118,125,126] Because of the potential for adverse effects from excess beta-blockade, the dose rate must be individually titrated.[127] Side effects of beta-blockade therapy include lethargy, fatigue, depression, anorexia, vomiting, and diarrhea. Adverse reactions might include hypotension, onset or recurrence of CHF, AV block, bronchospasm, or hypoglycemia. Myocardial depression may be addressed with carefully titrated isoproterenol or dobutamine infusions, and sinus bradycardia with atropine or glycopyrrolate administration, but prevention of these effects through slow, meticulous up-titration and regular monitoring is the preferred course. After chronic oral use, drug withdrawal should be gradual to prevent acute arrhythmia induction or systemic hypertension.

When a beta-blocker is given to patients with CHF, they must be euvolemic. That is, patients receiving beta-blockers under any circumstance should not have pulmonary edema or other form of critical fluid retention. The slight decrease in heart rate and ventricular contractility that may occur with even small doses of these agents may mean the difference between survival and decompensation in a patient with fulminant pulmonary edema, for example. Other contraindications for beta-blockers include systemic hypotension and peripheral vascular disease.

Cardioselective (beta$_1$-blocking) agents exert their primary effect on cardiac beta$_1$ receptors, especially at lower doses. This property is helpful in patients with asthma, chronic bronchial disease, hypoglycemia, peripheral vascular disease, or thrombosis. Atenolol, esmolol, and metoprolol are examples of beta$_1$-selective blockers. Other beta-blockers possess mild intrinsic sympathomimetic activity (ISA) that provides some protection for patients with underlying myocardial failure or those dependent on high sympathetic tone to maintain cardiac output.

As with all beta-blockers, dose must be titrated individually. Published doses are target doses, and initiation of therapy often begins at one eighth, one quarter, or one half of these doses, with the lowest fraction used when the myocardium is most dyskinetic (hypocontractile).[127] For example, in healthy dogs, acute carvedilol doses of 1.5 mg/kg orally, twice a day are tolerated and effective at preventing STach.[128] However, in dogs with experimentally induced mitral regurgitation, a target dose of 0.4 mg/kg once daily of carvedilol should be reached via initiating the drug at a dose of 0.2 mg/kg or less, because a small but significant, acute decrease in systemic blood pressure is seen with the 0.4 mg/kg dose.[127] In general with beta-blockers, careful up-titration from small initial doses is the rule, especially with a history of CHF. Retitration is also required when switching to sustained release formulations. Intravenous therapy is reserved for acute arrhythmias, especially anesthetic- or pre-excitation related supraventricular tachycardias (see Class IV Antiarrhythmics, following).

Propranolol was the standard beta-blocker used in veterinary medicine for years, and it remains the drug against which newer agents are compared. It blocks both beta₁ and beta₂ receptors. It is well absorbed orally, experiences large and variable first-pass hepatic and portal elimination, and has variable plasma protein binding. The half-life is 3 to 6 hours in dogs, but effects may persist long enough to require only twice-daily dosing after prolonged use. Lethargy in cats is a prominent side effect. Beta-blocking agents with longer durations of action are often used in place of propranolol.

Atenolol is a beta₁-selective agent with the advantage of requiring once or twice daily dosing in cats. In nine normal cats, atenolol reduced heart rates for 12 hours or more; β-blockade was not evident at 24 hours using an oral dose of 1.4 mg/lb.[129] A practical approach for determining whether once daily or twice daily atenolol dosing is best for a particular cat consists of initiating the medication to be given once daily in the evening. A daytime recheck visit is scheduled for 7 to 14 days after initiation of treatment, and if an exam room heart rate is superior to the desired maximum with beta-blockade (e.g., maximum 180 bpm in a chronic heart failure patient; maximum 160/min in a compensated patient never having been in heart failure), then the dose is increased to twice a day. In a four-way drug study involving boxer dogs with familial arrhythmia, atenolol alone at 0.17 to 0.27 mg/lb did not change the frequency or "grade" of ventricular ectopy or the heart rate, and there was no reduction in the frequency of syncope.[46] When atenolol was combined with mexiletine, results were slightly more positive (see previous discussion).

Another longer-acting drug, metoprolol, is effective in dogs requiring beta-blockade and in those with CHF associated with MVD or DCM. Studies of induced CHF in dogs indicate efficacy of a sustained release human formulation for the dog, and suggest a possible beneficial increase in ejection fraction when beta-blocking agents are added.[130]

Esmolol is an ultrashort-acting (9 minutes), rapid onset (2 minutes), cardioselective beta-blocker. It has been used as a trial agent (initial dose of 0.05 mg/lb intravenously; may increase to dose of 0.22 mg/lb [0.5 mg/kg] given intravenously over 1 minute) to transiently block AV nodal conduction in supraventricular arrhythmias[63] and at a similar dose over a period of 6 minutes to reduce LV outflow tract gradients in cats with obstructive hypertrophic cardiomyopathy.[131] It may also be given at the lower dose to temporarily slow a supraventricular tachycardia, which can assist in identifying its ECG features for an accurate diagnosis or may terminate the arrhythmia.

CLASS III ANTIARRHYTHMICS

Class III drugs specifically prolong the action potential duration and the refractory period, principally by inhibiting the repolarizing potassium channel (I_K). This class of drugs reduces the myocardium's ability to generate a new action potential before repolarizing, and thus these drugs slow or terminate tachycardia. These effects are most pronounced at higher heart rates. These drugs lengthen the action potential duration in a tachycardia,[132] but they should have few effects at normal heart rates. They are noted for increasing the threshold for AFib and VF. Each drug in this class also frequently displays properties of other antiarrhythmic classes. This drug group includes amiodarone, sotalol, bretylium, ibutilide, and dofetilide (Table 202-1). Only the first three agents are used in small animal medicine, and bretylium is expected soon to be unavailable because of the exhaustion of the world supply of bretylium.[90]

Amiodarone is one of the drugs of choice for many supraventricular and malignant ventricular tachyarrhythmias in humans. It exhibits properties of all four classes of antiarrhythmic agents and thus is considered a "broad-spectrum" antiarrhythmic. Unlike many antiarrhythmics, amiodarone has not been linked to increased mortality in large clinical trials in human cardiology, and it is second only to automated internal defibrillators in terms of beneficial outcomes in human patients with severe ventricular arrhythmia.[116] It may be useful in dogs with LV systolic dysfunction and to offer rate control, as well as for converting acute AFib to sinus rhythm. Amiodarone relaxes vascular smooth muscle, resulting in a decreased afterload that also may be beneficial. Amiodarone increases serum digoxin levels so that the dose of digoxin should be halved. Quinidine and procainamide levels are also elevated.[133] Side effects reported in humans include liver damage, photosensitization, thyroid derangements, ocular lesions, and irreversible pulmonary fibrosis. In dogs, neutropenia and hepatopathy have been reported with amiodarone treatment,[134] as have anorexia, GI disturbances, hepatopathy, and positive Coombs' testing.[135] These signs resolved with discontinuation of treatment. Anecdotal reports of acute hypersensitivity, hyper- or hypothyroidism, likewise have surfaced but are not conclusively attributable to the drug. In an experimental study, normal dogs given amiodarone 12 mg/lb orally, twice a day for 3.5 weeks, followed by 12 to 14 mg/lb orally, once a day as maintenance, had serum amiodarone concentrations considered to be therapeutic (1 to 2.5 µg/mL) within 4 days, but these levels only reached a steady state after 11 weeks of treatment.[37] However, several anecdotal reports have surfaced indicating that adverse effects occur at this dose and that a lower dose may be preferable, such as 4.5 mg/lb orally, twice a day for 1 week and 2.2 to 3.8 mg/lb orally, once a day subsequently for maintenance.[136] No clinical reports exist in veterinary medicine that address hemodynamic or electrophysiologic effects that could indicate proarrhythmia—a major concern in humans with the long QT syndrome. Despite the clear benefits of amiodarone in human cardiology, acceptance in veterinary medicine is compromised by these descriptions of adverse effects and the lack of reports indicating a benefit of amiodarone therapy over other antiarrhythmic agents. Amiodarone use has not been described in cats.

Sotalol provides both class III (higher dose) and class II (l-isomer, lower dose) effects. It is not a negative inotrope and thus does not decrease LV contractility. It induces systolic and diastolic hypotension and is considered to have ~30% beta-blocking potency compared with propranolol. It is considered to be protective against proarrhythmia, particularly life-threatening ventricular arrhythmias. Currently, only dl-sotalol, which combines the class III and class II effects, is used (d-sotalol caused increased mortality in human clinical trials and is not advocated).

In the first reported veterinary study using sotalol, three classes of Boxer dogs with familial ventricular arrhythmia were identified: asymptomatic, syncopal, and CHF. Slowing of the heart rate and first-degree AV block were the only side effects observed, although proarrhythmic effects have been suspected in other cardiomyopathic dogs with sotalol. The dose of sotalol administered to these dogs was 0.44 to 2.8 mg/lb/day twice a day orally, titrated to effect. The heart failure dogs received less medication, up to 104 mg/day average versus the syncopal group at 183 mg/day. Syncopal signs were diminished on sotalol therapy, and dogs with markedly diminished shortening fraction did not appear to exhibit untoward drug effects.[139] In a second study comparing four types of treatment for familial ventricular arrhythmia of Boxers, sotalol 0.68 mg/lb to 1.6 mg/lb orally twice a day significantly reduced the number of PVCs, arrhythmia grade, and maximum and minimum heart rates. However, there was no significant change in the occurrence of syncope for sotalol or for any of the other three treatments studied.[46] Sotalol has been effectively administered to cats with severe ventricular arrhythmias at 10 to 20 mg orally every 8 to 12 hours.[138] It is thought that class II effects are predominant at lower doses and class III effects are predominant only at higher doses (>160 mg in humans).

Sotalol's good oral absorption is reduced when given with food. Steady state is reached within 2 to 3 days. It is indicated for life-threatening ventricular arrhythmias, may be used with caution in CHF, and should not be abruptly discontinued. Sotalol is used cautiously with other drugs that decrease blood pressure, as well as other antiarrhythmics, specifically those that prolong the Q-T interval. The authors of this chapter have observed prolongation of the P-R interval with sotalol treatment in dogs, as has been reported anecdotally. No overt problems or progression occurred, and it was not necessary to discontinue the drug concurrent with this finding.

CLASS IV ANTIARRHYTHMICS

Class IV drugs, known as the *calcium channel blockers*, selectively inhibit slow inward calcium current channels (L-type) during the action potential. Calcium channel blockers interrupt arrhythmias resulting from abnormal automaticity and triggered mechanisms and inhibit re-entry. They slow the sinus rate and, more profoundly, AV conduction by blocking the inward calcium current carried by the L- (and probably T-) type channels.[140] By decreasing sarcoplasmic reticulum release of Ca^{++}, they also decrease the force of contraction. Decreasing the amount of calcium into the myocyte may help to decrease myocardial protein synthesis and thus attenuate the pathologic process of hypertrophy. They have indications for the control of most supraventricular tachycardias. Contraindications include SB, AV block, myocardial failure, SSS, and digoxin toxicity. Calcium channel blockers are classified as either dihydropyridines, which do not affect conduction and act principally on the vasculature (e.g., nifedipine, amlodipine), or nondihydropyridines, which have SA and AV nodal (but minimum vascular) effects (e.g., verapamil, diltiazem) (see Table 202-1).

Verapamil has potent negative inotropic effects, offers moderate rate control, and has minimal peripheral vascular effects. In dogs it may slow the sinus rate, increase AV conduction time, or decrease the ventricular response. In acute supraventricular tachycardias, it is given in 0.01 mg/lb intravenously in increments to a maximum of 0.07 mg/lb. Acute hypotension, AV block, collapse, or hypocalcemia may result from overly zealous up-titration. Judicious calcium chloride administration may correct iatrogenic disturbances.

Diltiazem's effective antiarrhythmic properties, combined with minimal inotropic depressive actions, have caused it to be used widely in cats with hypertrophic cardiomyopathy. Its frequency-dependent channel blockade in the AV node makes it effective in slowing supraventricular arrhythmias as has been shown in experimental dogs.[141] It is usually used in combination with digoxin to effectively slow the ventricular rate

in AFib, except if LV thickening is present. Comparison studies in dogs between diltiazem and beta-blockade, with or without digoxin, are not available. Diltiazem-induced vasodilation may create a reduction in afterload that is of chronic benefit to the patient with systolic heart failure.[140] Regular (not sustained release) diltiazem has been administered to cats with hypertrophic cardiomyopathy in a nonplacebo-controlled study. Over 6 months there was a reduction in LV and septal wall thickness and a reduction in LA size.[142] The dose of diltiazem for dogs and cats is 0.2 to 0.7 mg/lb three times a day. However, because three-times-daily dosing of a lifelong drug can be extremely challenging for many cat owners, sustained release formulations of diltiazem (e.g., Dilacor®, Cardizem-CD®), which carry the advantage of once daily administration, have been used extensively. Evidence has shown that cats receiving 4.4 mg/lb oral sustained release diltiazem CD have plasma concentrations of the drug that are similar to cats receiving 0.44 mg/lb regular diltiazem orally, three times a day.[143] However, sustained release diltiazem is hampered by its apparently lower efficacy at preventing STach when compared with the beta-blocker atenolol, as well as a significant occurrence of reversible but severe adverse effects including anorexia, vomiting, lethargy, and evidence of hepatopathy in a substantial proportion of treated cats in one large prospective, placebo-controlled study.[144] For these reasons, sustained release diltiazem is used cautiously or not at all in cats with hypertrophic cardiomyopathy.

For intravenous treatment of supraventricular tachycardias, diltiazem has been recommended at 0.2 to 0.44 mg/lb[141] or 0.12 mg/lb over 2 minutes and repeating until conversion or a maximal dose of 2.2 mg/lb has been reached. These high doses are reserved for patients with tachycardia and a structurally normal heart. Patients with a structurally compromised heart (e.g., cardiomyopathy) should be given one-sixth to one-quarter of the starting dose (i.e., 0.02 to 0.03 mg/lb) initially, and then the dose should be titrated upwards to effect. If the tachycardia is a physiologic response to a systemic problem (e.g., hypovolemia, CHF), it is essential to treat the underlying problem first. Administration of intravenous drugs to suppress an appropriate physiologic tachycardic response can be fatal. Intravenous rate-suppressing drugs such as the calcium channel blockers are given when, despite treating systemic problems that could trigger high heart rates (e.g., CHF), an extreme tachycardia persists and is felt to compromise cardiac output. An example is a dog with dyspnea and weakness caused by dilated cardiomyopathy, cardiogenic pulmonary edema, and AFib with a ventricular rate of 310 bpm. If vigorous diuretic treatment, oxygen therapy, thoracentesis (if necessary), calming, and possibly mild sedation do not reduce the ventricular rate, the tachycardia itself may be compromising cardiac output and intravenous calcium channel–blocking (or beta-blocking) treatment meant to acutely and *slightly* lower the ventricular rate (e.g., to 260 bpm initally) should be considered. Continuous ECG and blood pressure monitoring are essential with all IV calcium channel–blocking agents.

Amlodipine and nifedipine are potent vasodilators that produce a marked decline in arterial blood pressure through calcium channel blockade. They have minimal effect on AV nodal tissue and are not used as antiarrhythmic agents. Instead they are used for treating systemic hypertension (see Chapter 130).

Digitalis Glycosides

Digitalis glycosides (digoxin) have multiple effects on cardiac muscle and conductive tissues. Their predominant antiarrhythmic properties result from neuroendocrine and baroreceptor effects and parasympathomimetic action on the SA and AV nodes and atrial muscle.[145] AV nodal conduction is slowed, AV nodal refractoriness is increased, and vagal tone to ventricular muscle is increased. Digitalis glycosides are the only antiarrhythmic agents that produce a positive inotropic effect, although this effect may be limited in degree and real benefit. Their primary indications for use are treatment of supraventricular tachycardias, which they accomplish by slowing the ventricular rate response. Often a second agent in combination, such as a beta-blocker or calcium channel blocker, is needed to attain adequate rate control. Combination therapy of this sort is particularly beneficial because both products are then administered at lower doses and thus are less likely to induce toxic reactions. A recent, intriguing finding is an endogenous cardiac glycoside deficiency that appears to exist in some dogs with naturally occurring CHF and AFib.[146]

They are contraindicated in pre-excitation, because they may speed conduction through the accessory pathway and thus promote VF. Caution should be exercised with the use of digoxin in the face of existing ventricular arrhythmias. Dosing and pharmacokinetics are discussed in Chapter 199.

Digitalis intoxication is a serious, potentially life-threatening event. GI signs may be the first symptoms observed. Myocardial poisoning may take one of several forms, all of which culminate in cardiac arrhythmias. Increased sympathetic tone may result in increased automaticity. Slowed conduction and altered refractoriness may precipitate re-entry. Increased intracellular calcium levels predispose the cell to delayed after depolarizations. Any of these changes can be the source of arrhythmogenesis. Electrocardiographically, VT, supraventricular tachycardia, junctional escape complexes, SA arrest, Wenckebach or other forms of AV block, and tachycardias with aberrant conduction may be seen. The cornerstone of treatment is to stop the drug immediately and completely. Supportive fluid and electrolyte therapy should be provided as necessary. Hypokalemia exacerbates digitalis intoxication. Specific treatment for VTs may be needed. Lidocaine and beta-blockers may be considered, as well as many other drugs, depending on the predominant arrhythmia. Atropine may help patients that are symptomatic from bradyarrhythmias. Acute ingestion may be treated with cholestyramine or activated charcoal to reduce absorption. Soluble, intravenously administered digitalis neutralizing antibodies (Fab fragments) bind serum digitalis molecules and are the treatment of choice for life-threatening digitalis (or oleander) poisoning,[147] although high cost limits the use of this treatment. After resolution of clinical signs of intoxication and a minimum of 48 hours without receiving a dose, the digoxin may be restarted at half the dose.

One must be aware of numerous potential drug interactions when using digitalis glycosides. Kaolin-pectin, metoclopramide, neomycin, antacids, and bran decrease oral absorption, and quinidine and verapamil may increase serum digoxin levels substantially. Decreased excretion may result with captopril, verapamil, and spironolactone,[3] although newer protocols incorporating spironolactone therapy in the standardized treatment of CHF have not demonstrated this interaction to be a problem.

Adenosine, Edrophonium, Phenylephrine
Adenosine is an endogenous nucleoside occurring in all cells of the body. Therapeutically, when given intravenously, it slows AV nodal conduction and restores sinus rhythm in patients with paroxysmal supraventricular tachycardia. Adenosine is indicated as the drug of choice in human patients with acute paroxysmal supraventricular tachycardia, including those caused by the WPW syndrome (see previous discussion). Suggested total doses for a human adult are 1.5 to 3.0 mg initially, repeated to a maximum of 6 to 12 mg.[120] In dogs, doses corresponding to two or more times this amount on a body weight basis have been ineffective in abolishing supraventricular tachycardias,[63] and adenosine is considered much less effective in veterinary patients. In small animal medicine, adenosine's lack of a convincing advantage over intravenous

diltiazem or esmolol and its high cost make it a second- or third-line treatment agent.

Edrophonium is an anticholinesterase agent with both nicotinic and muscarinic side effects. This drug classically has been used for the diagnosis of myasthenia gravis (MG) and may be useful to treat SVT acutely. The dose is 0.05 mg/lb intravenously. Side effects include vomiting and muscular twitching.[3,120]

Phenylephrine, an alpha-adrenergic agonist, slows AV nodal conduction and induces vasoconstriction and hypertension. A baroreceptor-mediated reflex is thought to be the mode of slowing SVT. It is given at 0.002 to 0.004 mg/lb intravenously.[120]

Radiofrequency Ablation
In human medicine, cardiac catheter-based electrophysiologic testing followed by radiofrequency ablation of re-entrant circuits has become the treatment of choice for intra-atrial re-entry (e.g., atrial flutter) and AV reciprocating tachycardias such as WPW. This type of treatment can permanently interrupt the pathways and terminate the arrhythmia. Radiofrequency ablation thus offers the possibility of a permanent cure for certain arrhythmias including WPW and atrial flutter.

The high rate of success, low morbidity and mortality, and cost-effectiveness of this technique have resulted in an entirely new subspecialty of human medicine dedicated to the study and treatment of specific electrophysiologic dysfunctions of the heart. In veterinary medicine, radiofrequency ablation has received limited attention.[100,111,148] In addition to eliminating the subsequent need for antiarrhythmic medications, radiofrequency ablation of arrhythmia pathways prevents, and can even reverse and eliminate, structural changes such as ventricular dilation caused by a persistent arrhythmia (tachycardiomyopathy).[100] Although radiofrequency ablation therapy has clear indications and applications in small animal medicine, the cost, need for specialized equipment, required skills, and limited demand restrict its use to a small number of highly specialized cardiac institutions at this time.

Pacemaker Therapy
Implantable cardiac pacemakers were first placed in human beings in 1958.[149] During the intervening period there has been a revolution in the understanding and treatment of bradyarrhythmias, as well as pacemaker and electrode technology.[149] Whereas over one-half million pacemakers are now placed annually by physicians, only several thousand have been implanted clinically in dogs and cats during the past four decades.[95] Internal cardioverter-defibrillator-pacemaker implants increasingly are the treatment of choice for ventricular arrhythmias in humans.[116] Their clinical use in dogs previously has met with problems, and such treatment remains under development.[150]

In small animal medicine, pacemakers are used predominantly for bradyarrhythmia therapy, including sinus node dysfunction (SSS), AV block, and atrial standstill.[103,104,151,152] In human beings, implantable electrical devices are used for pacing and cardioversion, defibrillation, and specific forms of heart failure.[149]

Costs, availability of pacemaker generators and pacing leads, the age and debilitated state of some candidate dogs or cats, and concerns regarding complications, aftercare, and general philosophy continue to restrict the availability of this technique to a limited number of patients. Whereas the human literature is replete with articles and current recommendations, such as dual-chamber versus single-chamber ventricular pacing, the balance of this section identifies current veterinary techniques and experiences with pacemaker implantation in North America. Although veterinary pacemaker techniques are not up to those used in humans, current treatment options for animals are discussed.

Reported methodology, problems, side effects, and expectations are addressed in three large cases series totaling some 300 dogs[3,103,104] and reports of fewer than 10 cats.[3,94,153] Pacemakers were originally implanted transdiaphragmatically using epicardial leads,[95] but now most are implanted in the dog transvenously through the jugular vein and attached internally to the RV wall. This is accomplished either with a "tined" lead or a lead that is screwed into the ventricular endocardium and myocardium.[151,152] In cats such adverse reactions to transvenous leads as chylothorax have been observed anecdotally and in at least one report.[94] The trend today is to implant epicardial leads in cats requiring pacemaker treatment. The permanent pacemaker generator is usually buried in a subcutaneous pocket of the neck, lateral thorax under the cutaneous trunci muscle,[104] or cranial abdomen and is connected to the pacing lead through a subcutaneous tunnel. Anesthesia has used a balanced formula avoiding barbiturates,[151] and temporary pacing during the initial part of pacemaker implantation is recommended. Traditionally, temporary pacing was achieved transvenously,[151] but a recent evaluation of transthoracic pacing, a function found in many modern defibrillators in veterinary intensive care units, has demonstrated that this completely noninvasive form of temporary cardiac pacing is effective and safe in canine patients.[154]

Pacemakers are usually identified via a three-letter code.[3,149,152] The first letters identify the chamber or chambers paced, sensed, and the response to sensing. Whereas the DDD mode is the preferred pacemaker for most humans, the VVI mode is used most often in dogs and cats. It is essential to ensure that the pacemaker generator's polarity and the pacing lead polarity are compatible. Unipolar generators may be used with any pacing lead that fits, but bipolar generators must only be used with bipolar pacing leads.[151] The pacemaker's program, the fit between generator and pacing lead, and the length of the lead must all be confirmed prior to beginning implantation.

Most veterinary cardiologists and internists secure their pacemakers from private sources, morgues, or from the ACVIM Cardiology Specialty group. With limited equipment availability, especially pacing lead wires, clinicians must be gracious about the gifts they receive. New pacemakers and wires individually would otherwise cost tens of thousands of dollars for each unit.

Perhaps a perfect pacemaker candidate does not exist. Patients are often older, and the pacemaker does not provide a cardiac panacea. Nevertheless, some stratification of prognosis is possible. Some dogs requiring a pacemaker are in CHF when the need for a pacemaker is identified. These dogs generally experience a marked improvement in, or resolution of, heart failure with pacing, but overall still have a prognosis that is less favorable than dogs without CHF. In one study the 1-year mortality rate after pacemaker implantation was 60% if there was pre-existing CHF and 25% if there was not.[103] Evidence of renal failure (azotemia with isosthenuria) or opportunistic infection (e.g. pneumonia) has resolved with pacing, and such findings at the time of initial diagnosis should not be considered absolute contraindications to pacemaker implantation.

New developments in cardiac pacing include the single-lead AV mode of pacing and alternate sites of generator and lead placement. Using a specific type of single RV pacing lead, it is possible to pace both the atria (through a nexus in the lead that transmits impulses at the level of the RA) and the ventricles (at the distal tip of the lead). This approach offers several advantages, including the use of only one pacing lead to activate both the atria and the ventricles, and preservation of AV synchrony, resulting in superior hemodynamics.[155] In terms of placement of the pacing lead and generator, two reports address the high complication rate (10% overall[103] and up to 35% in large breed dogs[156]) of lead dislodgement. An alternative approach uses thoracotomy and passage of the pacing lead through the costocervical vein instead of the external jugular vein. This approach was successful, with none of six large dogs undergoing pacemaker implantation in this manner sustaining dislodgement of the lead.[156] A drawback is the need for concurrent thoracotomy and fluoroscopic guidance. A second approach consists of routine transvenous jugular implantation but with placement of the generator under the cutaneous trunci muscle instead of between muscles of the lateral neck. This modification was associated with a complication rate of only 6.7% in terms of lead dislodgement.[104]

Overall, pacemaker implantation is an effective form of cardiac therapy in dogs. Prolonged survival routinely is documented, reported complications continue to be addressed via refinements of technique, and in the largest retrospective study of dogs with pacemakers, 80% of owners described a high degree of satisfaction with the procedure.[103]

CHAPTER • 203

Primary Myocardial Disease in the Dog

Kathryn M. Meurs

Canine myocardial disease is one of the most common forms of acquired heart disease in the dog.[1] The most common form of myocardial disease in the dog is dilated cardiomyopathy, but arrhythmogenic right ventricular cardiomyopathy, hypertrophic cardiomyopathy and myocarditis, among others, are also reported.

CANINE DILATED CARDIOMYOPATHY

Dilated cardiomyopathy (DCM) is a primary myocardial disease characterized by cardiac enlargement and impaired systolic function of one or both ventricles (Figure 203-1). Diastolic dysfunction may also be observed.[2] An increased understanding of the etiology of both the human and canine disease has lead to the development of the theory that DCM is the final result of a variety of myocardial insults including viral, nutritional, toxic, and genetic.[3] In human beings, the disease has been shown to be familial in almost 50% of the cases, caused by mutations in nine different genes.[4] The etiology in many cases is never determined and they are considered idiopathic.

Although canine DCM is described as one disease, significant variation in the presenting complaint, clinical evaluation, and rate of progression has been observed depending on the breed of dog.[5-11]

Generally DCM is a disease of large and medium-sized dog breeds. Some breeds are clearly overrepresented, particularly in specific geographic regions. Surveys in North American publications find an increased incidence in the Doberman pinscher, Irish wolfhound, Great Dane, and Cocker spaniels.[12,13] European sources suggest an increased incidence of the Airedale terrier, Doberman pinscher, Newfoundland, and English cocker spaniel.[14] This difference may suggest an influence of environmental factors on the development of DCM, but more likely it is related to the strong genetic influences of certain popular dogs within an area.

Clinical Presentation

Dilated cardiomyopathy is an adult onset disease, with the exception of the Portuguese water dog.[11] The clinical presentation may be subtle and include the gradual development of exercise intolerance and weight loss.[15] However more commonly, early indications of disease may be overlooked. A diagnosis is not made until CHF develops and the patient is presented for coughing, dyspnea, tachypnea, and occasionally, ascites.

Physical Examination

A soft systolic murmur consistent with mitral valve regurgitation and/or a gallop rhythm (S_3) may be ausculted at the left apex. A tachyarrhythmia may be noted. In some cases, these may be the first signs of the disease in an otherwise healthy dog. Since primary valvular disease is relatively uncommon in large breed dogs, and the detection of DCM before the development of CHF may be beneficial in the long-term management of the case, identification of a new murmur, gallop or tachyarrhythmia in suspect breeds may warrant a thorough cardiac work-up. Although canine DCM is predominantly a left ventricular disease, biventricular involvement and heart failure with jugular venous distension and ascites is frequently noted, particularly in the giant breeds.

Electrocardiography

Left atrial and ventricular enlargement and sinus tachycardia, atrial fibrillation, or ventricular tachyarrhythmias are common.

Radiography

Left atrial and ventricular enlargement with or without pulmonary venous distension and pulmonary edema may be observed. In some cases, biatrial and biventricular enlargement may be noted. If the disease is diagnosed in the early stages, radiographic findings may be subtle.

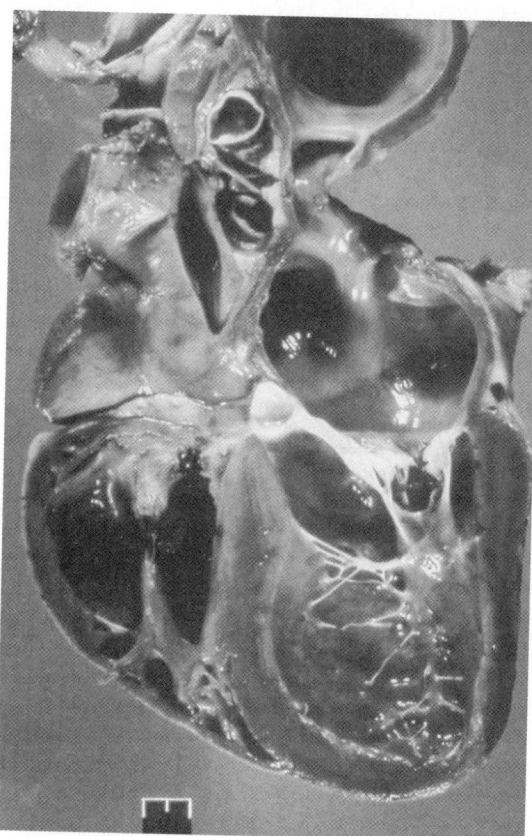

Figure 203-1   Heart from a Doberman pinscher with dilated cardiomyopathy. The left ventricle and left atrium are grossly dilated. (Courtesy Bruce Keene.)

Echocardiography

Echocardiography is the diagnostic test of choice for canine DCM and is also an important part of detection of occult disease. Echocardiographic findings in the symptomatic patient should include left and sometimes right atrial and ventricular dilation as quantified by M-mode and two-dimensional measurements (Figure 203-2). The measurements should be compared with the normal values for that particular breed or size (body surface area) of dog. In some cases, the ventricular wall thickness may appear thin during diastole, but more often it is within normal limits. An important part of the diagnosis is usually concurrent left ventricular systolic dysfunction based upon decreased fractional shortening, ejection fraction, or shortening area and increased end-systolic volume.[16] Doppler echocardiography may be used to document a central jet of mitral regurgitation that may be associated with dilation of the ventricle.

A differential diagnosis for DCM is severe atrioventricular (AV) valve disease since severe ventricular dilation and systolic dysfunction may be observed. Consideration of the breed of dog may be helpful in differentiation between DCM and AV valve disease since it is uncommon for many of the large breed dogs to develop primary valve disease. An exception to this may be the Cocker spaniel, a breed that has a high incidence of primary valve disease and also is at increased risk of DCM.

Unfortunately, the diagnosis of the affected dog in the occult (asymptomatic) stage is much more difficult. In some cases, dilation of the ventricle precedes the development of systolic dysfunction and is an early indicator of DCM.[17] However, this is not always the case and systolic dysfunction may precede dilation. Annual two-dimensional and M-mode echocardiography is recommended for adult dogs of at risk breeds or if early signs (e.g., heart murmur, gallop, tachyarrhythmias) are detected. Suggested additional studies for additive information when evaluation of borderline cases include measurement of the mitral valve annulus motion, systolic time intervals, systolic and diastolic performance index, and stress echocardiography.[18-20]

BREED VARIATIONS

There is an increasing amount of breed specific information about canine DCM. Because of differences the specific breed should be considered when considering etiology, developing treatment plans, and providing prognostic information.

Occasionally, atypical breeds of dogs develop DCM. The etiology of the disease in these cases is unknown.

Cocker Spaniels

Dilated cardiomyopathy has been reported in both American and English cocker spaniels; however, DCM occurs less commonly in this breed than valvular endocardiosis.[5,21,22]

An association between the development of DCM and low plasma taurine levels has been reported in some American cocker spaniels.[5] Dogs provided taurine and L-carnitine supplementation showed an increase in FS% and a decrease in LVEDD and LVESD over a 4-month period, although myocardial function did not return to normal.[23] This study suggests that at least some Cocker spaniels with DCM may benefit from supplementation with taurine and, perhaps L-carnitine. The current recommendations for American cocker spaniels with DCM are to measure plasma taurine levels (normal >50 ng/ml) and to treat with 500 mg of taurine orally every 12 hours and 1.0 gram of L-carnitine orally every 12 hours.[23] Additional treatment should be given as needed to address such conditions as CHF and arrhythmias. The investigators suggest that supportive cardiovascular medications can be gradually withdrawn after the FS% increases to more than 20% (usually 3 to 4 months of supplementation). Supplementation with taurine, and L-carnitine if possible, should be continued for life. If taurine deficiency is not identified the prognosis is poorer.

English cocker spaniels also get a form of DCM but a relationship to taurine or carnitine levels has not been well studied. Many reported dogs were from the same kennel, which may suggest a heritable component.[24,25] Profound evidence of left ventricular enlargement on the electrocardiogram with R wave amplitudes more than 3.0 mV in lead II was frequently observed.[22,26] Some of the reported dogs died suddenly, but many have had a prolonged, fairly asymptomatic course of disease, or a long survival (years) with medical management.[24-26]

Dalmatians

Male dogs appear to be over represented in Dalmatian DCM, although large studies have not been performed.[6] All dogs had adult onset disease and presented for signs consistent with left heart failure (cough, dyspnea) or syncope. None of the dogs had evidence of biventricular heart failure. Electrocardiography frequently demonstrated sinus rhythm or sinus tachycardia with occasional ventricular ectopy. Atrial fibrillation was not observed in any of the dogs. Duration of survival ranged from 1.5 to 30 months with euthanasia due to refractory CHF. None of the dogs died suddenly. Interestingly, the majority (8/9) of reported dogs had been fed a low protein diet for all or part of their lives for prevention or treatment of urate stones. The cause and effect of these diets on the development of DCM is not known, but Dalmatians that develop DCM that are being fed a low protein diet should be switched to a more balanced diet if possible.

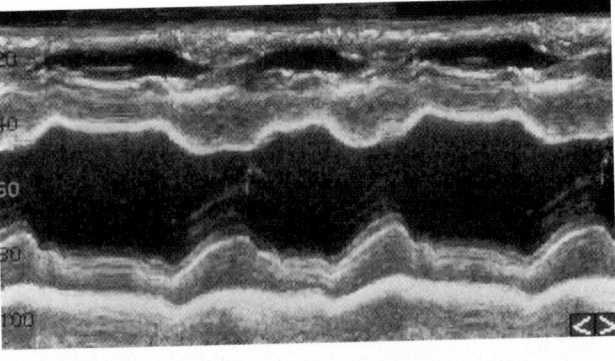

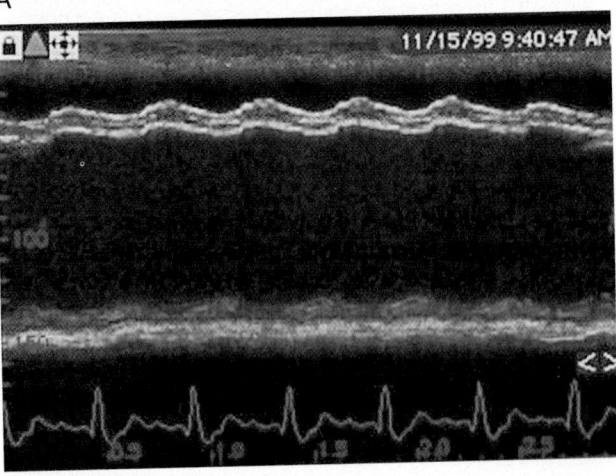

Figure 203-2 A, M-mode echocardiogram from a normal dog with adequate contractility. B, M-mode echocardiogram from a Great Dane with a dilated left ventricle with a markedly decreased systolic function.

Occasionally Dalmatians develop acquired AV valve disease, so this should be considered as an important differential diagnosis.

Doberman Pinschers

The Doberman pinscher is one of the most commonly reported breeds of dogs to be affected with DCM in North America.[7,13,27] It is characterized as an adult disease that results in the development of left and/or biventricular failure, often with atrial fibrillation. However, about 30% of the dogs develop ventricular tachyarrhythmias and may present for syncope or die of sudden death before the development of heart failure, and in some cases, before the development of ventricular dilation and systolic dysfunction.[28,29]

Dilated cardiomyopathy in this breed is believed to be familial, although the pattern of inheritance is not well documented.[30]

The clinical stage of DCM in the Doberman pinscher appears to be malignant in comparison to the disease in other breeds. The median survival time for dogs once heart failure has developed is 9.6 weeks. Atrial fibrillation and bilateral CHF are poor prognostic signs.[7] However, the occult stage appears to be slowly progressive (2 to 3 years), and some affected dogs die from noncardiac disease before they become symptomatic from DCM. Although there is only a small amount of evidence, there may be some benefit to early diagnosis and initiation of treatment in the occult stage (as discussed below).[31]

Some Doberman pinschers develop syncope or die suddenly before left ventricular dilation or systolic dysfunction ever develops. In most cases, these symptoms are associated with the presence of ventricular tachyarrhythmias. However, bradycardia-associated episodic weakness and syncope has also been observed in cardiomyopathic Doberman pinschers. Therefore Holter monitoring should be performed on the syncopal dog to document the causative arrhythmia before treatment is initiated.[32]

The timing and procedure for treatment of ventricular arrhythmias in the affected dog is not clear cut. Rapid ventricular tachycardia, complex ventricular arrhythmias, or the combination of ventricular arrhythmias, ventricular dilation, and systolic dysfunction is thought to be associated with a higher risk of sudden cardiac death and to be indications for treatment, but this has not been well documented. Additionally, some dogs die suddenly without having any of these arrhythmias documented. If treatment is warranted, consideration might be given to the use of one of several ventricular antiarrhythmics. Sotalol, a combination beta-blocker and potassium channel blocker, may be beneficial in some cases but should be used with caution if systolic dysfunction is present. Amiodarone has been studied in the affected Doberman pinscher at a dose of 10.0 mg/kg orally every 12 hours for 1 week, followed by 8.0 mg/kg every 24 hours.[28] After 6 months the dose may be reduced to 5.0 mg/kg every 24 hours. Careful evaluation of serum concentrations, complete blood counts (neutropenia has been reported), and liver enzymes monthly is suggested.[28] Although the goals of treatment include decreasing the number of VPCs, decreasing symptoms, and decreasing the risk of sudden death. The ability of any antiarrhythmic to reach these goals for these cases has not been proven.

Evidence that the disease is familial and that early intervention may increase survival has lead to significant interest in screening asymptomatic dogs for signs of early disease. Annual echocardiography and ambulatory electrocardiography (Holter monitoring) are believed to be the best predictors of early DCM.[33,34] Criteria that are believed to be indicators of occult disease include an echocardiographically determined LVEDD more than 4.6 cm and a LVESD more than 3.8 cm, even in the absence of systolic dysfunction.[17] These numbers are based on average sized dogs and may not be valid for very

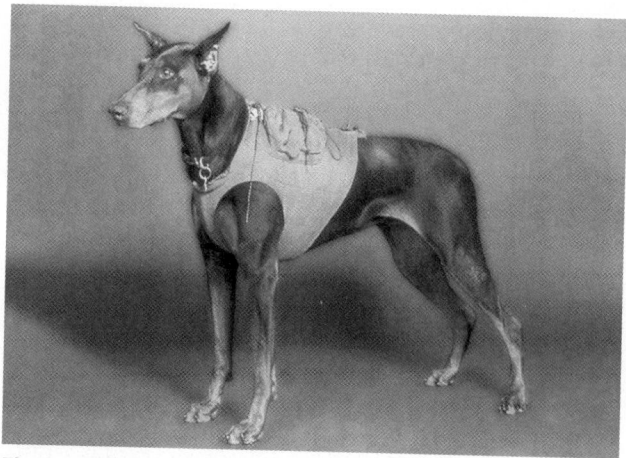

Figure 203-3 Adult Doberman pinscher with a Holter monitor used for screening for occult disease.

large dogs. Annual Holter monitoring has also been recommended to detect Doberman pinschers that may develop ventricular arrhythmias before ventricular dilation and systolic dysfunction (Figure 203-3). Adult Doberman pinschers with greater than 50 ventricular premature complexes (VPCs) per 24 hours, or with couplets or triplets are suspect for the development of DCM.[34] Owners should be advised that since this is an adult onset disease with variability in the age of onset, screening tests should be performed annually.

Great Danes

Dilated cardiomyopathy in the Great Dane appears to be a familial disease.[8] Affected male dogs were overrepresented, which suggests an X-linked pattern of inheritance in at least some families. If this is true, sons of affected females are at high risk of developing the disease; daughters of affected fathers are likely to be silent carriers.

Affected Great Danes presented most commonly for weight loss and/or coughing. Left-sided heart murmurs, gallops, and ascites were frequently observed. The most common electrocardiographic findings included atrial fibrillation with occasional ventricular premature complexes. In some cases, atrial fibrillation may develop before any other evidence of underlying myocardial disease (chamber enlargement or systolic dysfunction). These dogs should be carefully followed for the possible development of DCM.

Irish Wolfhounds

Atrial fibrillation frequently preceded the development of a heart murmur, clinical signs, and CHF in the Irish wolfhound with DCM and was present in the majority of dogs by the time they developed DCM.[9,35] The progression of the disease is not well understood but appears to be slow, with the development of atrial fibrillation preceding the development of CHF by an average of 24 months.[9] Occasionally, additional electrocardiographic abnormalities have been described, which include ventricular premature complexes and left anterior fascicular block patterns. Echocardiography is useful for separation of normal dogs, dogs with occult disease, and dogs with clinical evidence of heart failure.[36] Affected Irish wolfhounds occasionally died suddenly but more commonly were euthanized due to heart failure, most commonly biventricular and sometimes with chylothorax.[35,36]

Newfoundlands

Adult-onset DCM without a gender predisposition has been reported in the Newfoundland.[10,20] Clinical presentation included dyspnea, cough, inappetence, and ascites with left or biventricular heart failure. Interestingly a heart murmur was auscultable in a very small percentage of the dogs (4 out of 37).[10]

The most common electrical abnormality was atrial fibrillation, but isolated ventricular premature complexes were also observed.

Portuguese Water Dogs

A juvenile form of familial DCM has been reported in the Portuguese water dog.[11,15] Affected puppies were from apparently unaffected parents. Puppies died from CHF at an average age of 13 weeks after a very rapid course of disease.

Treatment of the Dog with Occult Dilated Cardiomyopathy

Administration of angiotensin converting enzyme (ACE) inhibitors may have some benefit for the dog with early ventricular dilation, with or without systolic dysfunction. Specifically, the use of ACE inhibitors (enalapril, lisinopril, captopril) in the Doberman pinscher with ventricular dilation was found to prolong the amount of time before the onset of CHF.[31] Although this study was limited to evaluation of Doberman pinschers, the use of ACE inhibitors for other breeds of dogs with occult DCM may be considered. This information provides additional support for the practice of screening adult dogs that are at increased risk of developing DCM because of their breed, and perhaps a family history, to allow early medical intervention.

Administration of beta-blockers at this stage is still being evaluated. The addition of low-dose beta-blockers to the treatment of human patients with DCM and stable heart failure has demonstrated a reduction in both mortality and morbidity.[37] However, many human patients with DCM cannot tolerate even very low doses of beta-blockers and demonstrate rapid cardiac decompensation. The use of beta-blockers for the canine patient with DCM has not yet been well studied and a consensus opinion on use of these drugs for patients is not yet available.

Beta-blockers might be considered for the patient with occult disease, but they should be very carefully monitored and should not be given once there is evidence of fluid retention and heart failure until it is very well stabilized. The optimal beta-blocker for this purpose appears to be carvedilol because of its effects on both alpha and beta-receptors. It cannot be overemphasized that the addition of beta-blockers in canine DCM patients should be done very cautiously with gradual increases in dosing after a 2-week period and careful monitoring of heart rate, blood pressure, and symptomology.

Treatment of the Dog with Dilated Cardiomyopathy and CHF

There are no specific therapeutic recommendations for the treatment of DCM other than those mentioned above. Nonspecific treatments, including surgery and nutritional supplementation, have been reported but have not yet been shown to have significant long-term benefits for most dogs.[38-40] As discussed above, early diagnosis and intervention may be of the most benefit. A thorough discussion of treatment of the dog with CHF is provided elsewhere in this textbook.

ARRHYTHMOGENIC RIGHT VENTRICULAR CARDIOMYOPATHY IN THE BOXER

Since the early 1980s, the term *boxer cardiomyopathy* has been used to describe adult boxer dogs that present with ventricular arrhythmias, and sometimes, syncope.[41] Recent studies have demonstrated that the disease has many similarities to a human disease called *arrhythmogenic right ventricular cardiomyopathy* (ARVC). The similarities between the diseases include clinical presentation, etiology, and a fairly unique histopathology that includes a fibrous fatty infiltrate of the right ventricular free wall.[42] The disease is most commonly characterized by ventricular arrhythmias, syncope, and sudden death. However, systolic dysfunction and ventricular dilation are seen in a small percentage of cases.

Arrhythmogenic right ventricular cardiomyopathy is a familial disease in the boxer and appears to be inherited as an autosomal dominant trait.[43] Unfortunately, the disease also appears to be a disease of variable genetic penetrance and affected dogs can have many different presentations including asymptomatic, syncope, sudden death, and systolic dysfunction with CHF.

The most common presenting complaint is syncope. Episodes of syncope may be but are not always associated with a period of exercise or excitement. Some dogs present for exercise intolerance or lethargy and others die suddenly without ever developing symptoms. Infrequently (approximately 10% of affected dogs), a dog may present with signs of left or biventricular heart failure.

Most affected Boxers have a completely normal physical examination. However, a tachyarrhythmia may be ausculted. In the small percentage of cases with ventricular dilation and systolic dysfunction, a systolic murmur and/or gallop (S₃) may be ausculted at the left apex. Infrequently, signs of right heart failure (ascites and jugular venous distension) may be observed. The Boxer breed also has a very high incidence of left basilar systolic murmurs. These murmurs may be associated with aortic stenosis, or potentially may be physiologic. Many boxers with ARVC have these murmurs in addition to their arrhythmic disease, but left basilar systolic heart murmurs are not an indication of boxer ARVC.

A 2- to 5-minute electrocardiogram is frequently normal in the affected Boxer. However, ventricular premature complexes (VPCs) may be present singly, in pairs, and in runs of paroxysmal ventricular tachycardia (Figure 203-4). The VPCs typically have a left bundle branch block morphology in leads I, II, III, and AVF, consistent with the right ventricular origin of this arrhythmia.[44] In some cases, the ventricular arrhythmias that cause syncope may not be observed on the electrocardiogram and a 24-hour Holter monitor should be performed to evaluate for arrhythmias. Interpretation of the Holter results can sometimes be challenging because strict criteria for this diagnosis do not exist. However, since it is unusual for a normal dog to have any VPCs in a 24-hour period, the observation of more than 100 VPCs, or periods of couplets, triplets, or runs of ventricular tachycardia are abnormal and may be diagnostic in a dog with clinical signs.[45] Supraventricular premature

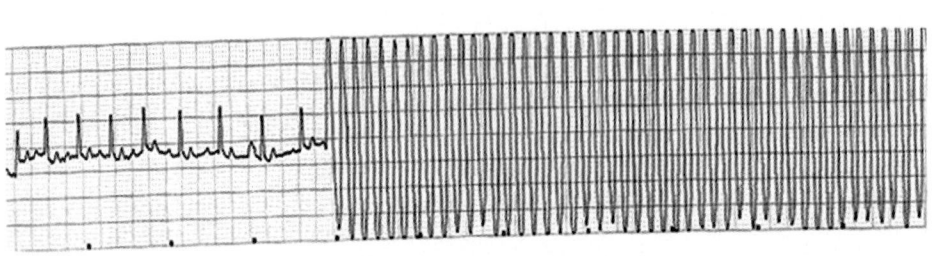

Figure 203-4 An electrocardiogram from a syncopal Boxer with ARVC. Sinus rhythm with a sudden onset of ventricular tachycardia is present. (Courtesy Alan Spier.)

complexes may also be observed, particularly in boxers with ventricular dilation and systolic dysfunction.

Thoracic radiographs are usually within normal limits. However, in the small number of cases with left ventricular dilation and systolic dysfunction, generalized cardiomegaly with pulmonary edema and/or pleural effusion may be noted.

Echocardiography is an important part of the evaluation because ventricular dilation and systolic dysfunction may occur, but in most cases affected dogs have normal chamber sizes and systolic function. In some cases, careful evaluation will allow the identification of right ventricular enlargement.

The familial etiology of ARVC has led to a widespread interest in screening dogs before selection of them as breeding animals. Since ARVC presents as an electrical abnormality more often than one of myocardial dysfunction, screening efforts should be based on annual Holter monitoring as well as annual echocardiography. Unfortunately, clear criteria for the diagnosis of occult ARVC do not exist. However, dogs that are symptomatic (syncope, heart failure) or have evidence of ventricular tachycardia on a Holter should not be used for breeding. Additionally, dogs that have over 100 left bundle branch block morphology VPCs in 24 hours are probably highly suspicious of being affected. However, not all affected dogs will ever develop clinical signs and many may live a normal lifespan.

It is likely that there are multiple factors that may influence which dogs become symptomatic for the disease. To help decrease the risk of making an error when adding or removing a dog from a breeding program, owners should be encouraged to screen annually rather than putting significant emphasis on a single Holter monitor reading. Since the disease is adult onset and an increase in VPCs has been observed with age in affected animals, an animal that is clear at the age of 2 is not guaranteed to stay clear. Additionally, an animal with a few hundred VPCs at the age of 2 years may have more, less, or the same number the next year. Until a greater understanding of disease inheritance and disease progression exists, caution should be used when advising breeders to remove dogs from breeding programs. Overzealous removal of animals based on the results of a single Holter monitor may have a significant negative impact on the breed.

At this time, there is no evidence that treatment will significantly alter the outcome for affected dogs. However, treatment has been shown to decrease the number of syncopal episodes.[46]

If an arrhythmia is detected on routine examination in an asymptomatic dog a Holter monitor should be performed to evaluate for the frequency and complexity of the arrhythmia. Although a strict relationship between the development of symptoms and the number of VPCs does not exist, treatment is generally started if more than 1000 VPCs occur in 24 hours, runs of ventricular tachycardia occur, or evidence of the R on T phenomenon exist. Owners should be advised that ventricular antiarrhythmics have the potential for proarrhythmic effects and that treatment is not known to decrease risk of sudden death.

Dogs with syncope and ventricular arrhythmias are generally started on treatment. There are two choices for treatment that are well tolerated and have been shown to decrease VPC number and complexity: sotalol at a dose of 1.5 to 3.5 mg/kg, every 12 hours, orally or the combination of mexiletine at a dose of 5 to 8 mg/kg, every 8 hours, orally and atenolol at a dose of 12.5 mg/DOG, every 12 hours, orally.[46] It is likely that there is individual variation for drug response and if a poor response is observed with one drug, a different one may prove to more effective. Ideally, a Holter monitor would be placed before starting therapy and repeated 2 to 3 weeks after starting therapy to prove that the therapy is helping. Significant day-to-day variation in VPC number exists and a therapeutic effect is likely to exist if at least an 85% reduction in VPC number while on medication is observed.[47]

If echocardiography demonstrates systolic dysfunction and ventricular dilation treatment for DCM (ACE inhibitors, etc.) may be warranted. Additionally, supplementation with L-carnitine might be considered at a dose of 50 mg/kg, every 8 to 12 hours, orally since a small number of affected Boxers have demonstrated improvement in systolic function and prognosis after supplementation.[48]

Dogs with ARVC are always at risk of developing sudden death. However, many dogs may live for years on antiarrhythmics without symptoms, some of these may eventually develop ventricular dilation and systolic dysfunction.

MYOCARDITIS

Myocarditis is defined by the presence of myocardial necrosis or degeneration and inflammation.[49] A variety of physical, chemical, and infectious agents can damage the myocardial tissue and evoke an inflammatory response. In the dog, protozoal and viral organisms are reported most commonly.

Chagas' disease, caused by the protozoan parasite *Trypanosoma cruzi*, has been reported in the dog, particularly in the southern part of North America. Three stages of infection have been described: acute, latent, and chronic. The acute stage is characterized by lethargy, generalized lymphadenopathy, pale mucous membranes, increased capillary refill time, and hepato-splenomegaly.[50] This stage is associated with a variety of electrocardiographic (ECG) abnormalities, including sinus tachycardia, prolonged PR interval, decreased R wave amplitude, axis shifts, and conduction disturbances.[51] Sudden death may be observed. Dogs that survive the acute stage may enter a prolonged latent period during which the clinical signs appear to regress.[50] The chronic stage of Chagas' disease is associated with signs of progressive right-sided cardiac dysfunction, ascites, pleural effusion, hepatomegaly, and jugular venous distention.[50] Occasional ventricular tachycardias have been reported.[51] Diagnosis is most commonly performed by serology, although the acute form can sometimes be diagnosed by the presence of circulating trypomastigotes on thick blood smears. In general, treatment of Chagas disease is directed at palliation since destruction of the intracellular form of the parasite may result in severe exacerbation of the host inflammatory response.

Additional protozoan parasites that have been associated with the development of myocarditis include *Neopsora caninum* and *Toxoplasmosis gondii*.[52,53]

Parvovirus myocarditis is an uncommon form of myocardial disease. It may present with a peracute form that affects puppies between 3 and 8 weeks of age. Puppies present with acute dyspnea consistent with severe left heart failure and die within hours.[54] At necropsy, the hearts are found to be dilated with multifocal myofiber necrosis, mononuclear cell infiltrate, and intranuclear inclusion bodies in the myocardial nuclei.[54,55] A second form of the disease in juvenile dogs (generally less than 1 year of age) may be very similar to DCM.[54,56]

Infrequently, infectious organisms including bacteria *Bacillus piliformis*, *Citrobacter koseri*, and the spirochete *Borrelia burgdorferi* have been associated with the development of myocarditis.[57,58]

HYPERTROPHIC CARDIOMYOPATHY

Hypertrophic cardiomyopathy is a primary myocardial disease characterized by concentric hypertrophy of the IVS and LV free wall. Hypertrophic cardiomyopathy (HCM) and the variant hypertrophic obstructive cardiomyopathy (HOCM) are infrequent forms of canine myocardial disease. There appear to be significant differences between the canine disease and the disease more commonly observed in cats and human beings with regard to etiology and pathologic findings.[59,60] An inheritable form of hypertrophic obstructive cardiomyopathy has been observed in the Pointer dog, but most canine cases appear to be sporadic.[59-62] Because of the relative infrequency that hypertrophic and hypertrophic obstructive cardiomyopathy is observed in the dog, suspect patients should be carefully evaluated for other reasons that might result in concentric hypertrophy of the LV, including the much more common left ventricular outflow tract obstruction observed with subvalvular and valvular aortic stenosis.

HYPOTHYROIDISM

Some dogs with hypothyroidism have been observed to have a reduction in fractional shortening % and an increase in LVESD; however, the values had significant overlap with normal dogs.[63]

Thus, although evaluation of thyroid levels might be considered in dogs that have minor echocardiographic changes in addition to other signs of hypothyroidism, it should not be considered a common cause of myocardial dysfunction nor ventricular dilation.[64]

MYOCARDIAL INFARCTION

Acute myocardial infarctions are an uncommon form of myocardial disease and appear to be most commonly associated with concurrent systemic or cardiac disease that has lead to a thromboembolic state. These conditions might include endocarditis, neoplasia, renal disease, immune mediated hemolytic anemia, and pancreatic disease. Dogs with infarcts were very rarely diagnosed with atherosclerosis as opposed to human beings who have a high incidence of infarcts associated with atherosclerosis.[65]

CHAPTER • 204

Feline Myocardial Disease

Mark D. Kittleson

CLASSIFICATION

Primary myocardial diseases are generally classified under the general heading of cardiomyopathy. *Primary* indicates the myocardial disease is not secondary to valvular disease, pericardial disease coronary vascular disease, systemic or pulmonary hypertension, congenital abnormalities other than those of the myocardium itself, and myocardial changes due to systemic disease such as hyperthyroidism. The World Health Organization (WHO) has categorized the types of cardiomyopathies and based the categorization scheme primarily on the dominant pathophysiology produced by the myocardial disease.[1] Historically, cardiomyopathy was defined as a myocardial disease of unknown cause, whereas a myocardial disease with a known cause was given a specific name. Over the past 15 years the causes of many of the idiopathic myocardial diseases have been identified in human medicine. Consequently, many of the classic "idiopathic" cardiomyopathies now include groups of patients with a known cause and other groups of patients without a known cause—blurring all lines between idiopathic and specific myocardial diseases. However, the original names of the diseases persist and are useful because they still describe the dominant pathophysiologic process produced by the abnormality in the myocardium.

Cardiomyopathies are the dominant form of cardiac disease in domestic cats. Because there has been only one cause identified for a feline cardiomyopathy (i.e., taurine deficiency in dilated cardiomyopathy [DCM]), no pressure exists to rename the cardiomyopathies from a causative standpoint. Although the WHO classification of cardiomyopathies includes identification of cardiac dysfunction in the definition, this portion of the definition is certainly outdated in human medicine because many patients are now identified as having genetic mutations that produce abnormalities in the myocardium that are not severe enough or are too early to cause cardiac dysfunction.

Therefore feline cardiomyopathy is still defined simply as a primary disease of the myocardium. Cardiomyopathies are classified as (1) DCM, (2) hypertrophic cardiomyopathy (HCM), (3) restrictive cardiomyopathy (RCM), (4) arrhythmogenic right ventricular cardiomyopathy (ARVC) (dysplasia), (5) unclassified cardiomyopathy, and (6) specific cardiomyopathies. Myocarditis is commonly placed in the specific category, although it is also frequently classified separately. In general this classification scheme works reasonably well for cats, and all categories have been identified in cats. However, in individual cats it may be difficult or impossible to comfortably place a cat's myocardial disease into one of these categories. In addition, because cardiomyopathies are so prevalent in cats, it is common for other forms of cardiac disease to be misidentified as one of the forms of cardiomyopathy. For example, mitral valve degeneration is uncommon in cats, and when it is present the cardiac changes are frequently thought to be due to some form of cardiomyopathy.

Is categorization important? In some cases it is extremely important, whereas in other situations the importance is more academic than it is practical. For example, correctly identifying DCM in a cat is essential because DCM may be caused by taurine deficiency, and this form of DCM can be cured using taurine supplementation. HCM is inherited in some cat breeds. Correctly identifying this form of cardiomyopathy is often important to breeding programs.

DILATED CARDIOMYOPATHY

Myocardial contractility and myocardial contraction are not the same. *Myocardial contractility* is the inherent capability of the myocardium to contract without any forces acting on it. *Myocardial contraction* is how much the myocardium moves and thickens from end-diastole to end-systole (the amount of wall motion and thickening usually observed on an echocardiogram) and is determined by myocardial contractility, preload, afterload, and other variables. It is commonly calculated as the shortening fraction. *Myocardial failure* is defined as a decrease in myocardial contractility and is most commonly manifested as an increase in end-systolic diameter on an echocardiogram. DCM is the name given to diseases in which myocardial failure is present due to primary myocardial disease. Myocardial failure can occur secondary to nonprimary myocardial disease processes.

DCM is characterized on echocardiography by a primary increase in left ventricular (LV) end-systolic diameter and volume (and usually by a compensatory increase in LV end-diastolic diameter and volume). Because end-diastolic diameter and volume do not need to increase as much as end-systolic diameter and volume to maintain a normal stroke volume, shortening fraction (one measure of the amount of wall motion) decreases.

Although most of the cats that are diagnosed with DCM have clinical signs, the diagnosis of DCM may be made in the absence of heart failure, arrhythmia, or sudden death. DCM has a long subclinical phase during which myocardial function, along with cardiac compensatory mechanisms, are adequate to maintain normal hemodynamics.[2] This phase of the disease, during which echocardiographic or electrocardiographic evidence (or both) of the disease is present but clinical signs of the disease are not present, is often termed *occult* in the literature. A patient with DCM may spend most of its life in a subclinical phase and only a short time during which it has clinical signs.

Incidence
Because of the discovery of taurine deficiency as the major cause of feline DCM and the subsequent increase in taurine content in all cat foods, the current incidence of DCM is rare.[3,4] From 1993 to 2003, only 24 cases of feline DCM were diagnosed at the University of California, Davis Veterinary Medical Teaching Hospital (UCD-VMTH). Eight had DCM due to taurine deficiency, whereas 13 were idiopathic. The other three died before a plasma sample could be obtained.

Cause
Taurine deficiency was identified as the primary cause of DCM in cats in 1986 to 1987.[3] Taurine is a sulfur-containing amino acid. One of its functions is to conjugate bile acids.[5] Although some species can also conjugate bile acids with glycine, cats lack this ability and therefore have an obligate loss of taurine through the bile. In addition, they have very limited ability to synthesize taurine in the liver because of the lack of key enzymes. Taurine's definitive role in cellular function is not known, but it is concentrated in the cytoplasm of excitable cells up to 250 times that in plasma.[6] In the heart, taurine has been postulated to help modulate intracellular osmolality, calcium concentration, and transmembrane ion fluxes.[7]

The cause of taurine deficiency in cats is primarily nutritional, although a genetic factor may also be involved.[8] Prior to 1987, dry cat foods contained too little taurine, whereas the taurine in canned foods was not biologically available in adequate amounts, probably because of bacterial overgrowth in the intestinal tract.[9]

Feline DCM due to taurine deficiency has not totally disappeared. It can still occur with the exclusive feeding of one canned food diet. More frequently, taurine deficiency is caused by feeding the cat a home-cooked diet, most commonly one including chicken. One study has documented that cooking meat reduces the taurine content, especially when the meat is constantly surrounded by water during the cooking process.[10] The classic method of producing taurine deficiency is to feed dog food to a cat. Because no taurine is found in vegetables, vegetarian diets also produce taurine deficiency.

Idiopathic feline DCM is now the predominant form of DCM seen in cats. In humans, it is estimated that 30% to 40% of DCM is hereditary, and numerous mutations in a relatively large number of genes have now been identified as causing DCM in people (these include mutations in the genes that encode for cardiac dystrophin, δ-sarcoglycan, actin, α-tropomyosin, β-myosin heavy chain, troponin T, titin, adhalin, lamin A/C, tafazzin, and emerin).[11] It is likely that some cats with idiopathic DCM have a mutational cause for their disease, either because they inherited a mutation from a parent or because they developed a de novo mutation in utero. The latter may be more likely because no cat breeds are known to have feline DCM as a problem.

Pathophysiology
DCM is caused by a myocardial disease that results in a progressive decrease in myocardial contractility, either because of global myocyte dysfunction or because of myocyte death (necrosis or apoptosis). Contractility is mildly decreased initially, which may progress over months to years to a severe decrease in contractility.[12] The decrease in contractility results in an increase in end-systolic diameter and end-systolic volume, which results in a decrease in stroke volume. Chronically the heart compensates for this decreased function by growing larger ventricular chambers through eccentric (volume overload) hypertrophy. This growth is also commonly referred to as *ventricular remodeling* and occurs primarily due to renal sodium and water retention leading to an increase in blood volume that leads to an increase in venous return to the heart. This places stretch on the myocardium that stimulates the myocytes to grow longer and the chambers to grow larger (increased end-diastolic diameter and end-diastolic volume). The increased chamber size allows stroke volume to return to normal when the disease is mild to moderate. At some stage the myocardial failure becomes so severe that the ability of the cardiovascular system to compensate for the disease is overwhelmed. At this stage, LV end-diastolic pressure increases as renal sodium and water retention continues to increase blood volume, resulting in congestive heart failure (CHF).

Myocardial diseases that cause DCM may also cause concurrent diastolic dysfunction, primarily reduced ventricular compliance. A stiffer or less compliant LV results in a higher diastolic pressure for any given diastolic volume, causing pulmonary edema, pleural effusion, or both. Decreased LV compliance has not been documented in cats with DCM but has been in dogs.[13]

Secondary mitral regurgitation is commonly present in DCM. In DCM the atrioventricular (AV) annulus dilates as the LV enlarges, and the papillary muscles are displaced laterally and apically as the ventricular chamber enlarges.[14-16] Both result in the leaflets failing to close completely during systole (incomplete valve closure). The regurgitation is usually mild, however, and so its contribution to the production of heart failure is probably minimal.

Pathology
In cats with severe DCM, the most striking gross pathologic finding is moderate to marked enlargement of all four cardiac chambers. Often the left heart appears more affected. The walls of the LV may appear thin but when measured may be normal or thin. The papillary muscles often appear flattened. Heart weight is greater than normal, indicating the presence of hypertrophy.[17] On cut-section, the LV myocardium often appears remarkably normal, especially in cats with DCM due to taurine deficiency. In other cases, pale regions may be noted. In DCM due to taurine deficiency, histologic findings primarily reveal hypertrophy. In cats with idiopathic DCM, histologically there may be evidence of myocytolysis, myofibril fragmentation, abnormal mitochondria, vacuolization, and fibrosis.

Natural History and Prognosis
Only about 30% of cats that are taurine deficient develop echocardiographic evidence of myocardial failure.[18] Of the cats

with myocardial failure, about 30% develop severe myocardial failure (shortening fraction < 20%). Some cats have severe myocardial failure for months to years prior to heart failure, yet many cats appear to develop heart failure suddenly.

The short-term prognosis for survival in cats with DCM due to taurine deficiency is guarded. They usually have severe CHF (often with low-output heart failure) and require intensive therapy. Taurine supplementation does not help clinically during this phase. Almost all cats that live longer than 2 to 3 weeks survive. Within 2 to 4 weeks they appear to improve clinically, although no apparent change occurs echocardiographically. Their myocardial function then normalizes over the ensuing 3 to 5 months. Consequently, their long-term prognosis is excellent. In cats with DCM that is not due to taurine deficiency, the long-term prognosis is usually grave (the median survival time [MST] is 2 weeks).[19]

Clinical Manifestations

History   Because cats are relatively sedentary, they often hide the signs of their disease until they are in severe distress. Cats most commonly present in acute respiratory distress from pulmonary edema, pleural effusion, or both. Some cats will cough. This is frequently thought to be vomiting by the owner because vomiting and coughing in cats appear very similar. Distinguishing the two may be possible in the exam room by palpating the trachea vigorously enough to produce a cough while the owners witness the event. A thorough diet history should be obtained on any cat with DCM.

Physical Examination   Many cats are tachypneic and dyspneic upon presentation. They may also be lethargic, dehydrated, or hypothermic (or a combination of these symptoms).

Auscultation often reveals a soft to moderately loud systolic heart murmur (usually heard best over the sternum, just medial to the left apex beat). A gallop sound may also be heard if the disease is severe. Most cats with DCM have an elevated heart rate so that atrial systole occurs immediately after rapid ventricular filling, making it impossible to distinguish a third from a fourth heart sound. Auscultation of the lungs is often normal except for increased airway sounds due to hyperpnea. If pleural effusion is present, lung sounds may be absent ventrally when the cat is upright. The ears and feet are commonly cold because of intense peripheral vasoconstriction.

The retinas should be examined in all cats suspected of having feline DCM for the presence of feline central retinal degeneration (FCRD). If it is present the cat is most likely taurine deficient. However, many cats with taurine deficiency do not have FCRD.[20]

If the cat is severely dyspneic, pleurocentesis using a butterfly catheter should be part of the examination process to determine if pleural effusion is the cause of the dyspnea. If pleural effusion is the cause, one should be able to remove 150 to 250 mL of fluid from the pleural space.

Radiography   Radiographs cannot be used to distinguish feline DCM from other forms of feline cardiomyopathy. They should primarily be used initially to determine if a dyspneic cat is in heart failure (cardiomegaly plus pleural effusion, pulmonary edema, or both). Radiographs should not be attempted in a severely dyspneic cat if the process is stressful to the cat because this will often result in death. In cases of severe feline DCM, the cardiac silhouette is markedly enlarged, often especially in the area of the left auricle on the dorsoventral (DV) or ventrodorsal (VD) view (Figure 204-1).

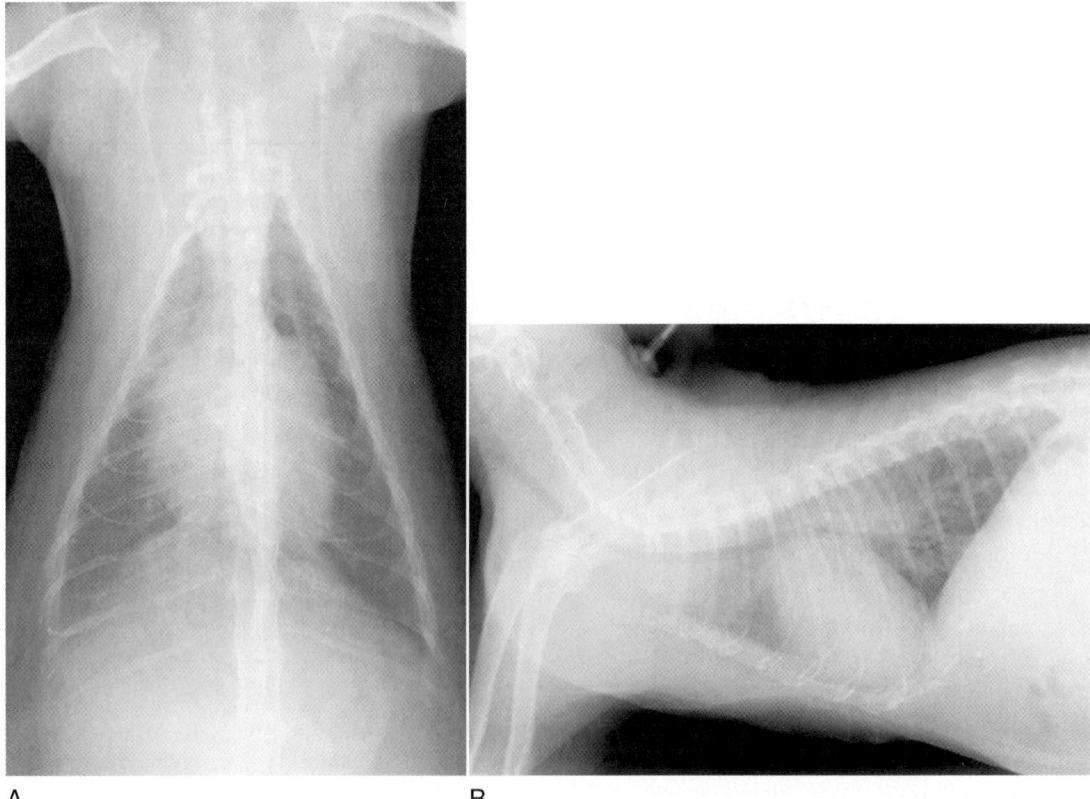

A   B

Figure 204-1   **A,** Dorsoventral (DV) radiograph from a cat with dilated cardiomyopathy (DCM) due to taurine deficiency. The cardiac silhouette is grossly enlarged. **B,** Lateral radiograph from the same cat. The cardiac silhouette again is grossly enlarged and pulmonary edema is present.

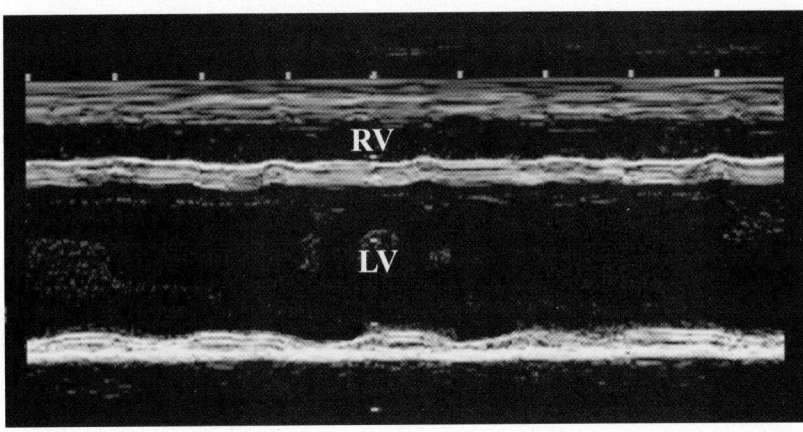

Figure 204-2 M-mode echocardiogram from a cat with severe dilated cardiomyopathy (DCM). The motion of the interventricular septum (IVS) (between the right ventricle [*RV*] and left ventricle [*LV*]) and the left ventricular free wall (below the LV chamber) are markedly reduced.

Left atrial enlargement generally cannot be appreciated on the lateral view. If pleural effusion is present, it often becomes impossible to identify pulmonary edema. Pulmonary edema in cats can be caudodorsal in distribution (as in the dog) but is more commonly patchy, is often more ventrally distributed, and may involve the accessory lung lobe.

Echocardiography Echocardiography is the diagnostic test of choice for identifying DCM. The striking feature of severe DCM is the remarkable lack of LV wall motion (Figure 204-2). The end-systolic diameter is increased to a value over 10 mm (usually over 12 mm and often in the 15 to 20 mm range when severe), whereas the end-diastolic diameter is also increased but to a lesser degree (usually in the 18 to 23 mm range). In cats with severe DCM, the shortening fraction is commonly less than 20%. Both the left ventricular free wall and the interventricular septal motion are reduced, although one may be more reduced than the other. Neither wall is hyperdynamic. Cats that have severely reduced free wall motion and a hyperdynamic interventricular septum (IVS) most commonly have primary mitral valve degeneration or dysplasia rather than DCM. Rarely a cat will have one region of the LV myocardium that is hypokinetic, akinetic, or even dyskinetic and may also be thinner than the rest of the myocardium. Although this may be due to a primary regional myocardial disease, it may also be due to a thrombus or a thromboembolus that has produced an infarct in that region. This pattern of motion may or may not be categorized as DCM, depending on one's viewpoint.

Color flow Doppler echocardiography often reveals the presence of mild mitral regurgitation. Spontaneous echo contrast due to red cell aggregation may be present, especially in the left atrium.

Electrocardiography Electrocardiography rarely reveals clinically significant information unless an arrhythmia is ausculted. Abnormalities in QRS morphology and an axis deviation may be noted but are nonspecific findings.

Clinical Pathology Any cat with DCM should have a plasma and whole blood taurine concentration measured. The sample must be anticoagulated with heparin, placed on ice, and a portion centrifuged within 15 minutes. Platelets contain a large concentration of taurine, which is released upon platelet activation during the clotting process, so any thrombotic activity in the tube will result in a falsely high plasma taurine concentration. Taurine will also leach out of platelets and white cells into plasma if the sample is left standing, especially at room temperature. Taurine is a very stable compound, but plasma and whole blood samples should generally be frozen to prevent bacterial growth because bacteria will destroy taurine. Normal cats have a plasma taurine concentration greater than 60 nmol and mL and a whole blood taurine concentration greater than 250 nmol/mL. Most, but not all, cats with DCM due to taurine deficiency have a plasma taurine concentration less than 20 nmol/mL and a whole blood taurine concentration less than 100 nmol/mL. Fasting can lower the plasma taurine concentration in cats. Fasting does not alter whole blood taurine concentration.[21] Thromboembolism of skeletal muscle will cause skeletal muscle necrosis and the release of taurine into the circulation, causing a false elevation in a cat that is taurine deficient.

Prerenal azotemia due to low cardiac output is common in cats with severe DCM, cats with dehydration, cats that are not eating or drinking, or cats receiving a high dose of a diuretic. If the azotemia is mild to moderate and the cat feels good enough to eat and drink, the azotemia can safely be ignored. If the azotemia is severe, diuretic therapy must be discontinued and judicious fluid therapy administered. Electrolyte abnormalities occur more frequently in cats on diuretic therapy than in dogs, probably because cats tend to become anorexic more easily when they are dehydrated. Electrolyte levels below the reference range for a laboratory do not mean that this decrease is clinically significant.

Differential Diagnoses

Rarely HCM will progress to severe myocardial failure. Some cases of regional myocardial failure appear to be due to myocardial infarction.[22] Myocardial failure can occur secondary to chronic, severe volume overload, such as primary mitral regurgitation. Sustained tachycardia can also produce myocardial failure, although the rate to produce this phenomenon is not known in cats.

Cats with DCM commonly have pleural effusion. This effusion may be a modified transudate, pseudochylous, or chylous and may change from a modified transudate to a chylous effusion over time. Heart failure is the most common cause of chylous pleural effusion in cats.

Acute Therapy

Treatment Goals The treatment goals depend on the type and severity of the clinical signs. If severely dyspneic the initial goal is to make it easier for the cat to breathe by removing pleural effusion, by reducing pulmonary edema pharmacologically, or by administering oxygen. If the primary problem is a marked reduction in perfusion leading to hypothermia, the goal is to increase cardiac output, if possible, via the administration of an intravenous positive inotropic agent, such as dobutamine, and possibly the judicious use of intravenous fluid administration, especially if the cat is severely dehydrated.

Pleurocentesis Pleurocentesis is often life saving in the severely dyspneic cat that has a large amount of pleural effusion. Thoracocentesis is described in Chapter 103.

Diuretic Therapy Diuretic administration is the only reliable way to reduce pulmonary edema formation in a cat with severe DCM. Furosemide is used almost exclusively. The dose depends on the severity of the pulmonary edema, on whether the cat is currently on furosemide for heart failure, and whether the situation is acute or chronic. Cats in severe respiratory distress may need an initial dose as high as 2 mg/lb parenterally. Intravenous administration is preferred, but the drug should be administered intramuscularly if restraint for intravenous administration produces stress. Absorption half-life after intramuscular administration is around 5 minutes, so the entire dose is fully absorbed within 20 to 25 minutes. The duration of effect of furosemide after parenteral administration is probably 1 to 2 hours in a cat in heart failure. Consequently, another dose should be administered within that period if the cat is still in respiratory distress and is not severely dehydrated. A cat with a lesser amount of pulmonary edema and less respiratory distress needs a smaller dose of furosemide parenterally in the acute setting. Respiratory rate and character should be monitored carefully after diuretic administration with the cat in an oxygen-enriched environment.

Oxygen Increasing the percent concentration of oxygen delivered to the alveoli is critical in cats in respiratory distress. This can be accomplished using a face mask, standard oxygen cage, a pediatric incubator, or nasal insufflation. Generally the goal is to increase fraction of inspired oxygen (FIO_2) to at least 40% (normal is 21%). If the cat resists a face mask, it should not be used. When placed in a confined space, especially a small space like an incubator, it is mandatory to keep the environmental temperature and the carbon dioxide concentration within reasonable levels. Failure to do so can cause death. A canister containing sodium lime or barium hydroxide lime controls carbon dioxide level in an oxygen cage, and a refrigeration unit controls temperature. Carbon dioxide concentration is usually controlled in an incubator by maximizing the flow rate of oxygen (and therefore flushing out the carbon dioxide).

Inotropic Support Beta-adrenergic agonists, usually dobutamine or dopamine, can be used for acute inotropic support in a cat with severe DCM and severe heart failure. However, conscious cats have more side effects with these drugs than do dogs. They often appear agitated and may even seizure. The half-life of these drugs is around 1 minute, so stopping the drug infusion results in rapid cessation of adverse effects. The infusion rate for dobutamine and dopamine in a cat is less than that used in a dog and is generally in the range of 1 to 2.5 µg/lb/min.

Nitroprusside Nitroprusside is a potent dilator (i.e., smooth muscle relaxant) of systemic arterioles and systemic veins. It can only be used in cats with DCM that are not in cardiogenic shock (systolic systemic arterial blood pressure over 100 mm Hg). If systemic pressure is adequate, the drug can be used in one of two ways: (1) empirically at a dose of 2 µg/lb/min or (2) titrated using blood pressure starting at a dose of 1 µg/lb/min and increased until the systolic pressure has decreased by at least 10 to 15 mm Hg. (See Systolic Blood Pressure Monitoring and Techniques in Chapter 128.)[23]

General Supportive Measures Although dogs commonly start to drink water and eat once they are no longer in respiratory distress, cats may not. Dehydration is a common side effect of aggressive diuretic therapy, and some cats are dehydrated at presentation. Generally cats do better if they are sent home as soon as possible. However, if hospitalization is required after the edema and effusion are controlled, judicious use of fluid therapy may be needed. Electrolyte disturbances, most commonly hyponatremia, hypokalemia, and hypochloremia, are also more frequent in cats than in dogs in this acute setting. Consequently, serum electrolyte concentrations should be monitored.

Chronic Therapy

Diuretic Therapy Diuretics are the only drugs that can routinely control the clinical signs referable to congestion and edema due to heart failure. Consequently, it is mandatory for cats with CHF to be on a diuretic, usually furosemide. The chronic orally administered dose for furosemide in cats is wide and ranges from 0.5 mg/lb a day to 2 mg/lb every 8 hours. The most common doses are 6.25 to 12.5 mg per cat every 8 to 12 hours, orally. In general, cats need a lower dose of furosemide when compared with dogs, although the upper end of the dose range can be similar. The goal of diuretic therapy is to keep pulmonary edema and pleural effusion controlled. This should be done with the lowest possible furosemide dose, although in the author's experience, underdosing appears to be a more frequent problem than does overdosing. Every owner should be instructed to count his or her cat's respiratory rate at home when the cat is sleeping or resting quietly in a cool environment and to keep a written log. The normal respiratory rate for a cat is in the 20 to 40 breaths per minute range. If the rate is greater than 40 breaths per minute or the owner notes that the character of breathing is more labored, these are signals that an increased dose of furosemide, pleurocentesis, or both are needed. Changes in furosemide dose should be done in consultation with a veterinarian during the initial stages of management. Some owners will require continued contact with a veterinarian to manage dose changes, whereas others will reach a point where they feel comfortable doing this on their own. Cats with severe disease that require a maximum dose of furosemide are often mildly to moderately dehydrated and mildly to moderately azotemic. As long as they continue to eat, drink, and appear comfortable, the dose of furosemide should not be decreased. If the dehydration or azotemia becomes severe enough to cause anorexia, the furosemide administration must be discontinued as long as the cat is not taking in fluid. Owners must be warned that continued use of high-dose furosemide administration in a cat that is not drinking or eating can result in severe, life-threatening dehydration. Judicious use of parenteral fluid administration may be required. These, of course, are poor prognostic signs. Cats that are refractory to the maximum dose of furosemide may need to have another diuretic administered along with the same maximum dose of furosemide. Choices include a thiazide diuretic and possibly spironolactone. (See Therapy in Chapter 199.) Parenteral administration of furosemide may also be beneficial because the oral bioavailability of the drug is only around 50%.

Pleurocentesis Repeated pleurocentesis is often required in cats with pleural effusion. Pleurocentesis may need to be done as infrequently as once a month or as frequently as every 4 or 5 days. As much fluid as possible should be removed at each visit. Ultrasound guidance often helps identify regions where fluid has pocketed. Chylothorax secondary to heart failure can result in chylofibrosis, making it very difficult to remove as much fluid as one would like. Risks of repeated pleurocentesis include infection, pneumothorax, and bleeding, but all are rare.

Angiotensin-Converting Enzyme Inhibitors Any cat with idiopathic DCM should be on an angiotensin-converting enzyme (ACE) inhibitor for long-term management unless they have an adverse reaction to the drug. Enalapril is most commonly used at a dose of 1.25 to 2.5 mg per cat orally every 24 hours. ACE inhibitors can almost never be used on their own to control signs of heart failure and are not effective for controlling heart failure in the acute care setting. Rather they must be administered in concert with a diuretic and help in the long-term control of the disease. Generally, ACE inhibitor therapy should be started when the cat is reasonably stable and not dehydrated.

Digoxin Digoxin, in theory, may be administered to cats with DCM. However, in the initial trial that identified taurine deficiency as a cause of feline DCM, digoxin was not administered and most of those cats survived; therefore clearly in cats with DCM due to taurine deficiency, no clear mandate exists to administer digoxin.[3]

Dietary Modifications Any cat with DCM should be supplemented with 250 mg taurine orally every 12 hours until the results of the plasma and whole blood taurine concentration analysis are evaluated. Taurine is inexpensive and can be purchased from health food stores or chemical supply houses. Cats that are taurine deficient should be continued on taurine supplementation, whereas those that are not may be taken off or left on at the discretion of the owner. Sodium-restricted diets may be useful, particularly in cats that are refractory to drug therapy. However, it is more important to keep the cat eating than it is to force sodium restriction.

HYPERTROPHIC CARDIOMYOPATHY

HCM is a disease of the ventricular (primarily LV) myocardium characterized by mild to severe thickening of the papillary muscles and wall (Figure 204-3). The word *primary* means the hypertrophy is due to an inherent myocardial problem, not secondary to a pressure overload or to hormonal stimulation. Concentric hypertrophy (a thickened wall with a normal to small chamber size) of the LV has several possible secondary causes, including aortic stenosis, systemic arterial hypertension, and hyperthyroidism. When any of these diseases are present, the diagnosis of HCM is in doubt and the cardiac abnormality should not be called *HCM* if one is convinced the primary

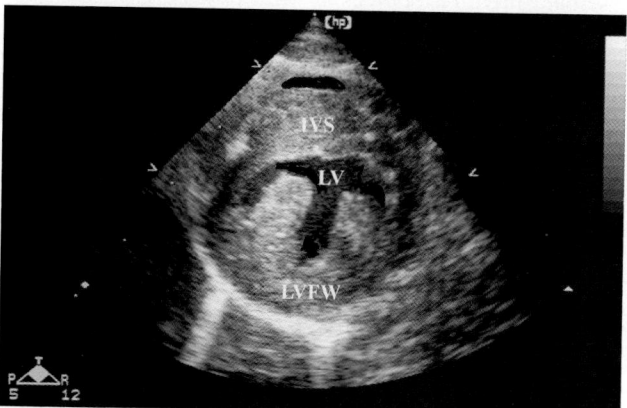

Figure 204-3 A cross-sectional view of a two-dimensional echocardiogram from a cat with severe hypertrophic cardiomyopathy (HCM). The interventricular septum *(IVS)* is markedly thickened and thicker than the left ventricular free wall *(LVFW)*. The two papillary muscles in the left ventricular chamber *(LV)* are also markedly enlarged.

cause of the hypertrophy is the other disease process. Instead it should be called *concentric hypertrophy secondary to the primary abnormality* (e.g., concentric hypertrophy secondary to hyperthyroidism). Besides concentric hypertrophy, the myocardium can also thicken due to infiltration (e.g., with lymphoma).[24]

Incidence

HCM is the most commonly diagnosed cardiac disease in cats, and its prevalence appears to be increasing. However, echocardiographic screening for the disease has also become more prevalent over the past 10 years, so increased awareness and ease of diagnosis may also be major contributing factors to this increase. During a recent 10-year period, the author's cardiology service diagnosed moderate to severe HCM in 447 cats. This is almost twice as many cases as during a previous 10-year period when the incidence was similar to another report in which 46 cats were diagnosed with HCM during a 2-year period at the Animal Medical Center in New York City.[25]

A male predisposition for HCM is commonly reported in clinical studies, although in a study of Maine coon cats the incidence was the same in males and females. However, males often develop the disease at an earlier age and often develop more severe disease. Consequently, it is likely that the male predominance seen clinically is purely because males develop worse disease, not because they are more predisposed to the disease.

Cause

Sarcomeric Gene Mutations in Humans with Hypertrophic Cardiomyopathy The exact cause of feline HCM is unknown, although the disease is known to be heritable in some breeds. In humans the familial nature of the disease was first reported in 1958.[26] It has been demonstrated that approximately 50% of the human cases of HCM are inherited in an autosomal dominant pattern, with the other cases being sporadic (although often still genetic in origin). Since 1989 over 150 mutations in 10 genes that encode for sarcomeric proteins have been identified in human families with HCM.[27-31] They include the β-myosin heavy chain; α-tropomyosin; cardiac troponins I, C, and T; myosin-binding protein C; essential and regulatory light chains; titin; and actin genes.[27,32-36] Several families with HCM have also been shown to have mutations in the gene that codes for LIM protein.[37] Another set of families has been identified with mutations in the gene coding for AMP-activated kinase that produces glycogen accumulation in the myocardium, mimicking HCM.[38] Interestingly, mutations in β-myosin heavy chain, α-tropomyosin, titin, and troponin T genes also cause DCM in humans (although the mutations are at different sites than those that cause HCM) and mutations in the LIM protein gene cause DCM in mice.[39] It is now known that sarcomeric gene mutations actually cause HCM because several mutations that have been identified in human families with HCM have been placed in transgenic mice, and the disease has been reproduced—thus fulfilling Koch's postulates.[40-42]

The pathophysiology of HCM production by sarcomeric mutations is controversial.[43] One theory is that the abnormal protein produced by a mutated gene results in dysfunctional sarcomeres that forces the functional sarcomeres to bear a larger load. The myocardium compensates by replacing the dysfunctional sarcomeres with additional functional and dysfunctional sarcomeres.[33,44-46] The net result is that the heart has twice as many sarcomeres as it should have. Because sarcomeres make up a large part of the heart muscle, the heart muscle ultimately almost doubles in thickness in severe cases.

Familial Feline Hypertrophic Cardiomyopathy The first "family" of cats with an inherited form of HCM was identified in Maine coon cats in 1992 and reported in 1999.[47] The disease is inherited as a simple autosomal dominant trait in this breed and is 100% expressed in experimental cats. However, in non-experimental Maine coon cats, it appears that the disease is not 100% expressed because both parents of an affected cat may have no echocardiographic evidence of the disease. This phenomenon is common in human families with HCM with a variety of gene mutations.[27] The disease has been reproduced in Maine coon cats by mating affected to unaffected and affected to affected cats, as well as by breeding affected Maine coon male cats to domestic shorthair female cats. The course of the disease is accelerated in affected cats produced by mating affected to affected cats. The disease is progressive. In most affected Maine coon cats, HCM is not apparent during the first year of life but becomes apparent by 2 years of age in males.[48] Females tend to get the disease later, with most manifesting the disease by 3 years of age but some not showing evidence of the disease until 6 or 7 years of age. When both parents have HCM, an affected Maine coon kitten may have echocardiographic evidence of the disease as early as 6 months of age and have severe disease by 1 year of age, whether male or female.

The most consistent feature of the disease in Maine coon cats and in most cats with HCM is papillary muscle hypertrophy. It is often present before wall thickening is evident. Systolic anterior motion (SAM) of the mitral valve is common. Studies are currently in progress to determine if a specific sarcomeric gene abnormality exists in this family of Maine coon cats.

A family of American shorthair cats, primarily with SAM of the mitral valve but with other evidence of HCM as well, has also been identified.[49] The disease in this breed also appears to be inherited as an autosomal dominant trait. In addition to these breeds, anecdotal evidence exists of HCM being inherited in numerous other breeds, including Persian, British shorthair, Norwegian forest cats, ragdoll, Turkish van, and Scottish fold cats, along with others. HCM is most likely inherited when it is identified in a specific breed. However, HCM is most commonly identified in domestic (mixed breed) cats. Whether the disease is inherited in these cats, is due to a de novo mutation, or is associated with a different disease process is unknown, although suspicion of inheritance has been reported in mixed breed cats.[50-52] Because the disease is inherited as an autosomal dominant trait in some purebred cats, it is not hard to imagine how these mutations could disseminate into the mixed breed population.

Some mutations in humans produce malignant disease in which survival time is short, whereas other mutations produce benign disease with little change in survival.[53,54] Although the Maine coon breed has a malignant disease, the American shorthair usually has a more benign disease. Ragdoll cats, on the other hand, have a particularly malignant form of the disease and often die before reaching 1 year of age.

Other Causes of Concentric Left Ventricular Hypertrophy
Congenital valvular or subvalvular aortic stenosis is a rare cause of concentric LV hypertrophy in cats. Certain systemic diseases, especially hyperthyroidism and systemic hypertension, can induce the LV myocardium to thicken.[55] Acromegaly is rare and usually does not produce concentric LV hypertrophy in the author's experience. At least in theory, each of these diseases should be ruled out before making a definitive diagnosis of HCM. However, in general, none of these diseases causes severe LV wall thickening on their own; therefore if severe hypertrophy is present, it is very unlikely that one of these diseases is the sole cause. Rather it is more likely the cat has severe HCM or the cat has had mild to moderate HCM most of its life and then developed one of these complicating diseases at an older age. This event then stimulates further hypertrophy, leading to severe HCM. The primary reasons for this belief are the documentation of this occurrence in a limited number of cases and the logic that HCM and these other diseases are prevalent in the domestic cat population (making it likely that some cats will have HCM in combination with a potentially exacerbating disease, especially when these cats are older). Consequently, cats with significant LV concentric hypertrophy, especially ones that are geriatric or have a disease that causes systemic hypertension, must be screened for hyperthyroidism and systemic hypertension.

PATHOPHYSIOLOGY

Hypertrophy, Diastolic Dysfunction, and Congestive Heart Failure
Enlarged papillary muscles and a thick LV myocardium with a normal to small LV chamber characterize HCM (see Figure 204-3). HCM may be mild, moderate, or severe. Severe concentric hypertrophy by itself increases chamber stiffness. In addition, blood flow and especially blood flow reserve to severely thickened myocardium is compromised, which causes myocardial ischemia, cell death, and replacement fibrosis.[56] This has been documented in cats by showing that cardiac troponin I concentration, a protein released into the systemic circulation after cell necrosis, is increased in cats with severe HCM.[57] Increased concentrations of circulating neurohormones may also stimulate interstitial fibrosis.[58] Fibrosis increases chamber stiffness (increased pressure for any given volume) further and is probably the primary reason for the marked diastolic dysfunction seen in this disease. The stiff ventricular chamber causes a greater increase in pressure for any given increase in volume when the ventricle fills in diastole. This produces CHF (i.e., pulmonary edema and pleural effusion). The myocardium from cats with HCM also takes a longer time to relax in early diastole, although the clinical significance of this is unknown.[59]

When LV hypertrophy is severe, it is common for the LV wall thickness to be twice the normal thickness. Consequently, LV wall thickness is commonly in the 7 to 10 mm range when HCM is severe in cats. This severe concentric hypertrophy may encroach on the LV cavity in diastole, decreasing its size, although LV diastolic diameter is commonly within the normal range. The end-systolic volume and diameter are almost always reduced, often to zero (end-systolic cavity obliteration; Figure 204-4). Global myocardial contractility is normal in humans with HCM, and the reduction in end-systolic volume is due to a decrease in afterload (wall stress) brought on by the increase in wall thickness.[60]

Systolic Anterior Motion of the Mitral Valve A phenomenon called systolic anterior motion (SAM) of the mitral valve is common in cats with HCM (Figures 204-5 and 204-6).

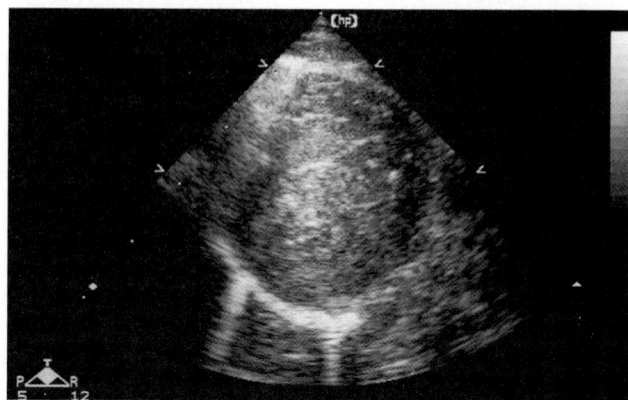

Figure 204-4 The same view as in Figure 204-3 but at the end of systole. End-systolic cavity obliteration occurs.

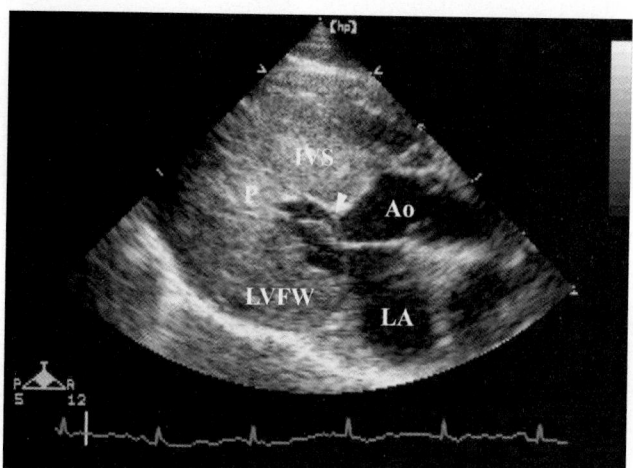

Figure 204-5 A long-axis view of a two-dimensional echocardiogram taken in late systole (same cat as in Figure 204-3). Systolic anterior motion (SAM) of the mitral valve *(arrowhead)*. The enlarged papillary muscle *(P)* is pulling the chordal structures and a portion of the tip of the anterior mitral valve leaflet into the left ventricular (LV) outflow tract, where it is contacting the interventricular septum *(IVS)* and creating an obstruction between the outflow tract and the aorta *(Ao)*. End-systolic cavity obliteration is again present. *LVFW*, Left ventricular free wall; *LA*, left atrium.

Cats with HCM and SAM are commonly said to have the obstructive type of HCM or hypertrophic obstructive cardiomyopathy (HOCM). In one survey of 46 cats, SAM was present in 67%.[25] SAM of the mitral valve is the process of the septal (anterior) mitral valve leaflet or the chordal structures

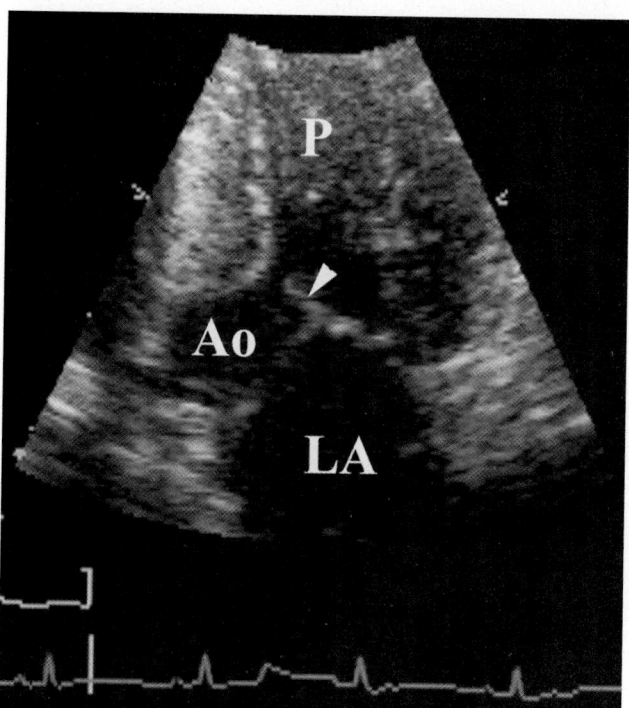

Figure 204-6 A left apical four-chamber view from the cat in Figure 204-4 showing systolic anterior motion (SAM) of the mitral valve. The portion of the mitral valve apparatus causing the dynamic obstruction is aligned with the caudal papillary muscle *(P)*. *LA*, Left atrium; *Ao*, aorta.

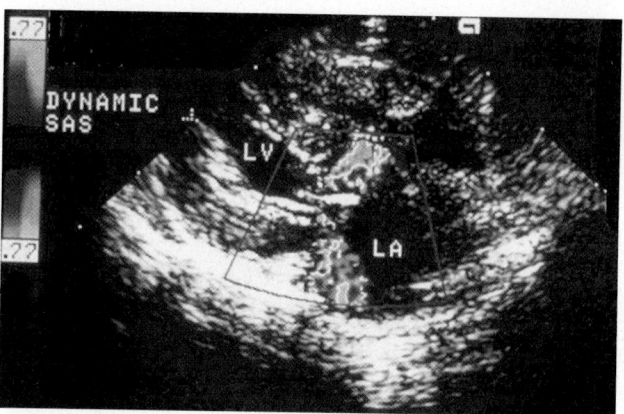

Figure 204-7 A black-and-white rendition of the color flow Doppler signal seen with systolic anterior motion (SAM) of the mitral valve. A bilobed jet—both originating from the left ventricular outflow tract region of the left ventricle *(LV)*. The top jet is created by the dynamic subaortic stenosis (SAS). The lower jet that extends into the left atrium *(LA)* is due to mitral regurgitation, created when the anterior mitral valve leaflet is displaced.

inserting on this leaflet being pulled into the LV outflow tract during systole. Here it is caught in the blood flow and pushed toward (and often ultimately against) the IVS. The initial pulling of the mitral valve leaflet toward the LV outflow tract in systole can clearly be seen on many echocardiograms from cats with HCM. The grossly enlarged papillary muscles encroach on the LV outflow tract (the region of the LV between the anterior leaflet of the mitral valve and the IVS in diastole) and pull the mitral apparatus structures into the basilar region of the outflow tract. This situation has been reproduced experimentally in dogs by surgically displacing the papillary muscles cranially.[61] SAM of the mitral valve produces a dynamic subaortic stenosis that increases systolic intraventricular pressure in mid- to late systole. The dynamic subaortic stenosis increases the velocity of blood flow through the subaortic region and often produces turbulence (Figure 204-7). Simultaneously, when the septal leaflet is pulled toward the IVS, this produces a gap in the mitral valve, creating mitral regurgitation. These abnormalities are by far the most common cause of the heart murmur heard in cats with HCM. The process of SAM is dynamic—worsening when contractility increases and lessening when contractility decreases. This also makes the murmur dynamic—increasing in intensity with increasing excitement and softening when the cat becomes calmer.

Pleural Effusion Along with pulmonary edema, pleural effusion is common in cats with heart failure. It can be a modified transudate, pseudochylous or true chylous in nature. The most common cause of chylothorax in cats is heart failure.[62] It is unknown exactly why pleural effusion develops in these cats. Two possibilities exist: The first is that left heart failure results in pulmonary hypertension severe enough to cause right heart failure. This does not appear to occur very frequently in cats because it is unusual to identify echocardiographic right heart enlargement, jugular and hepatic vein distension, or ascites in these cases. The second possibility is that feline visceral pleural veins drain into the pulmonary veins such that elevated pulmonary vein pressure (congestive left heart failure) causes the formation of pleural effusion. In the dog the visceral pleura is supplied by pulmonary arteries and drained by pulmonary veins.[63] The dog, the cat, and the monkey have type II lungs.[64] One characteristic of type II lungs is that the visceral pleura is supplied not by bronchial arteries but by pulmonary arteries.

Presumably this means that the cat visceral pleura is also drained by pulmonary veins. This means that pulmonary venous hypertension secondary to left heart failure could cause pleural effusion in cats as it does in humans.[65]

Pathology

Gross Pathology   Cats with severe HCM have severe thickening of the LV myocardium (the IVS and free wall), with the LV wall commonly being 7 to 10 mm thick (Figures 204-8 and 204-9). The hypertrophy may be symmetrical, involving the entire circumference of the LV, but it may also be asymmetrical. In some cats the IVS is significantly thicker than the free wall, whereas in others the free wall is thicker (asymmetrical hypertrophy).[25,66,67] In those cats with primarily septal hypertrophy, the hypertrophy may be confined to the basilar region of the septum, and in others may be apical. Isolated free wall hypertrophy most commonly occurs in the region between the papillary muscles. As in many pathologic specimens, hearts from cats with HCM may undergo contraction (rigor) after death, resulting in a wall thickness that is closer to the end-systolic wall thickness in life rather than the end-diastolic thickness. Consequently, heart weight must be combined with subjective or objective evidence of LV wall thickening to make the diagnosis of HCM postmortem. To weigh a cat heart the pericardium should be removed and the aorta and pulmonary artery transected so that no more than 2 to 4 cm are left. Normal heart weight-to-body weight ratio has been reported to be 10.6 +/– 4 g/lb, with cats with HCM having a ratio of 13.2 +/– 3.1 g/lb.[25] This results in a large overlap between the two groups. In the author's experience, most normal-sized cats (6 to 12 lb) have a heart that weighs less than 20 g and most cats in this size range with HCM have a heart that weighs more than 20 g. Cats with severe HCM almost always have a heart that weighs more than 25 g, usually over 30 g, and can be as heavy as 38 g.

The left atrium is often enlarged in cats with severe HCM, often markedly so (Figure 204-10). However, with early, severe disease, the author has identified normal left atrial size in some Maine coon cats. Occasionally a thrombus is present in the body of the left atrium or within the left auricle.

Cats with milder forms of the disease (mild to moderate HCM) have lesser wall thickening and a more normal-sized LV chamber. The left atrium may be normal in size or may be enlarged. Papillary muscle hypertrophy may be the predominant lesion.

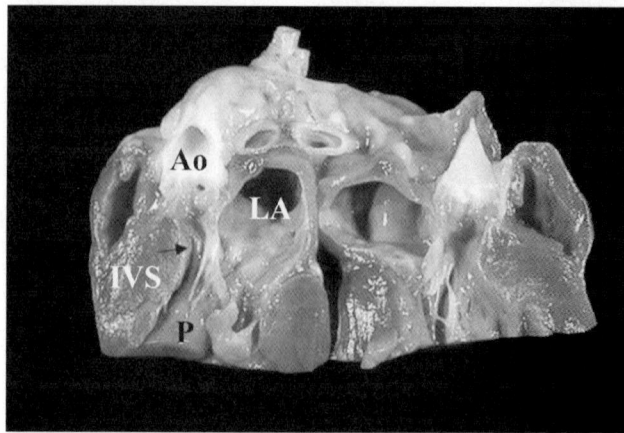

Figure 204-9   Gross pathologic cardiac specimen from a cat with severe hypertrophic cardiomyopathy (HCM). The left ventricular (LV) outflow tract *(arrow)* is narrowed as one papillary is pulling the anterior leaflet of the mitral valve into the outflow tract. *IVS*, Interventricular septum; *LA*, left atrium; *Ao*, aorta.

Histopathology   Histopathologically, a wide range of abnormalities exist. In some hearts, only myocyte hypertrophy is evident. On the other end of the spectrum, some cats have moderate to severe interstitial and replacement fibrosis and dystrophic mineralization (20% to 40% of cases).[66,68] Intramural coronary arteriosclerosis is present in approximately 75% of cats with HCM.[25,66] Intramyocardial small artery disease is not specific for HCM because it is also identified in cats and dogs with many cardiac diseases.[69]

In humans, myocardial fiber disarray that involves at least 5% of the myocardium in the IVS is found in 90% of patients

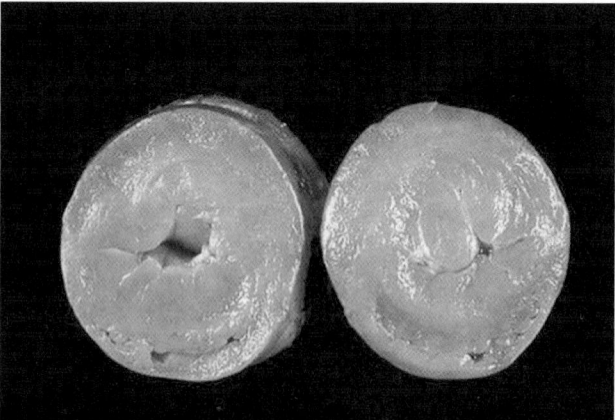

Figure 204-8   Gross pathologic cardiac specimen from a cat with severe hypertrophic cardiomyopathy (HCM). The heart has undergone rigor postmortem, causing end-systolic cavity obliteration. Heart weight must be obtained to confirm that the HCM is present (see text).

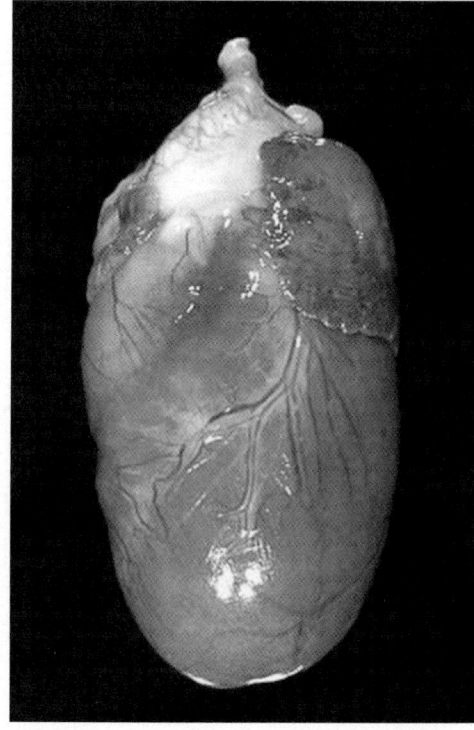

Figure 204-10   A view of the cranial aspect of a heart from a cat with severe hypertrophic cardiomyopathy (HCM). The left auricle *(top, right)* is markedly enlarged.

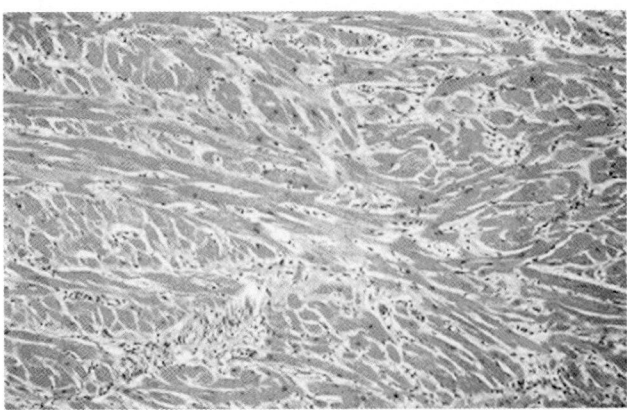

Figure 204-11 Histopathology from a Maine coon cat with severe hypertrophic cardiomyopathy (HCM) showing myocardial fiber disarray.

with familial HCM.[70,71] Other diseases that produce concentric hypertrophy can also cause myocardial fiber disarray, but this almost always involves less than 1% of the myocardium. In cats with HCM, myocardial fiber disarray in the IVS of the same magnitude observed in humans is only identified in 30% to 60% of cases.[66,68,72] However, myocardial fiber disarray is a consistent feature of HCM in Maine coon cats (Figure 204-11).[47] Sarcomeres also have disarray in human patients with HCM. Interestingly, infecting isolated feline cardiocytes with an adenoviral vector containing a full-length mutated human β-myosin heavy chain gene causes sarcomere disruption.[73]

Natural History and Prognosis

The prognosis, as with most cardiac diseases, is highly variable for HCM. Some of it is determined by clinical presentation and echocardiographic severity of the disease. Adult cats that are asymptomatic and have mild to moderate disease and no to mild left atrial enlargement have a good short-term (and possibly a good long-term) prognosis. Some, however, may progress to more severe disease and some may die suddenly. Asymptomatic cats with severe wall thickening and mild to moderate left atrial enlargement have a guarded prognosis for developing heart failure in the future. They probably have some risk for developing thromboembolism and may be at risk for sudden death.[74] Cats with no clinical signs but with severe wall thickening and moderate to severe left atrial enlargement are at risk for developing heart failure or often already have mild to moderate heart failure that has gone undetected. These cats are at risk for developing systemic thromboembolic disease and sudden death, although both of these risks appear to be relatively small.[74] Cats presented in heart failure usually have a poor prognosis, but survival time is highly variable. Most die of intractable heart failure. Some develop thromboembolism, and some die suddenly. In one study a MST of 3 months was reported yet some cats (about 20% in one study) in this class stabilize and do well for prolonged periods. The author and colleagues have seen some cats with severe HCM live as long as 2.5 years after the diagnosis of heart failure (see www.vmth.ucdavis.edu/cardio/cases/case5/case5.htm).[75] Some of these cats may develop heart failure when they are stressed and become severely tachycardic and then stabilize after that time. Cats with severe HCM and aortic thromboembolism in the aforementioned study had a very poor prognosis with a MST of 2 months.

Clinical Manifestations

Development In humans, familial HCM develops in most individuals over the first 2 decades of life.[76] HCM is a progressive

disease in Maine coon cats and likely in other purebred and mixed breed cats. When a veterinarian examines an older cat with HCM, the disease may have been present for most of the cat's life.

History Cats with HCM may have no clinical signs. Many have a heart murmur; some are brought to a veterinarian with subtle, moderate, or severe heart failure; and some are presented because of thromboembolic disease. Cats with no clinical signs can have mild to severe LV thickening; however, those with severe thickening usually go on to develop heart failure. Cats with severe disease that appear to have no clinical signs may show subtle signs of heart failure (e.g., tachypnea) that may be detected by an observant owner but more often goes undetected. The respiratory rate is often increased in these cats at rest, and they may become more tachypneic or even dyspneic if stressed. Stressed cats with severe HCM may recover quickly after stress or may go on to develop fulminant heart failure. Cats with mild to moderate thickening may never develop clinical signs referable to their disease and may live normal lives. In others, the LV wall may thicken further, and complications may develop when they are older and develop a complicating disease such as systemic hypertension or hyperthyroidism.

Cats with severe HCM and moderate to severe heart failure are usually presented to a veterinarian because of respiratory abnormalities (tachypnea, dyspnea, or both) due to pulmonary edema, pleural effusion, or both. Because household cats are generally sedentary, owners usually do not notice that they are having respiratory difficulty until the dyspnea is advanced. At that time the onset of the disease commonly appears to be acute or peracute to the owner; however, in reality the disease has been present for years, and the heart failure probably has been gradually worsening over weeks to months.

Cats with HCM may develop systemic thromboembolism (see the last section of this chapter). This markedly worsens their prognosis.

Cats with HCM may die suddenly, often with no prior clinical signs referable to heart disease or failure.[74] The cause of the sudden death in these cats is unknown. In humans, sudden death appears to be either due to arrhythmic or hemodynamic causes.[77] The hemodynamic cause is usually an acutely worsening outflow tract obstruction associated with strenuous exercise (which probably ultimately leads to a terminal arrhythmia). This can, in theory, occur with extreme excitement (e.g., being chased by a dog) in a cat with HCM. A large thrombus occluding flow in the left heart is another possible cause of sudden death. However, in the family of Maine coon cats studied by the author and colleagues, sudden death is usually not associated with physical stress or with thromboembolic disease. These cats likely die of an acute ventricular tachyarrhythmia that degenerates into ventricular fibrillation or of a bradyarrhythmia. The incidence of sudden death in feline HCM is probably underrepresented in the veterinary literature because cats that die suddenly are usually not presented or reported to veterinarians.

Physical Examination Cats with severe HCM commonly have auscultatory abnormalities. A systolic murmur, heard best over the midsternum or left apex beat is common and is usually due to SAM of the mitral valve. The murmur is often dynamic, increasing in intensity when the cat becomes excited and heart rate and myocardial contractility, especially contractility of the papillary muscles, increase and decreasing in intensity or disappearing when the cat is calm. A gallop sound may be present in cats with severe HCM. It should be noted that not all three heart sound rhythms are due to gallop sounds. In the author's experience, using an electronic stethoscope, systolic clicks also occur with some frequency in cats. Systolic clicks tend to wax and wane in intensity more than do gallop sounds and are more frequently present in cats with mild or no apparent cardiac disease.

Radiography HCM cannot be distinguished from the other forms of cardiomyopathy using plain radiography. In a cat in CHF the left atrium is almost always enlarged and usually severely enlarged. Pulmonary edema is commonly present, but its pattern is often different from dogs, being patchy or more ventrally distributed. Pleural effusion is also common. Angiography to diagnose HCM has been supplanted by echocardiography.

Echocardiography The diagnosis of HCM is almost always made using echocardiography. Cats with severe HCM have severe papillary muscle hypertrophy, markedly thickened LV walls (7 to 10 mm), and usually an enlarged left atrium (see Figure 204-3). The hypertrophy can be global, affecting all areas of the LV wall, or it can be regional or segmental.[25] Segmental forms can primarily affect the entire (or one region of) IVS or the free wall, the apex, or the papillary muscles (and often the adjacent free wall). Because of these forms, HCM is a diagnosis that should be made by examining several different two-dimensional echocardiographic views and measuring wall thickness in diastole from the thickest region or regions on the two-dimensional images. M-mode echocardiography may miss regional thickening unless it is guided by the two-dimensional view. End-systolic cavity obliteration is commonly present in cats with severe HCM, although this phenomenon can occasionally occur in cats without HCM (see Figure 204-4).

Systolic anterior motion of the mitral valve Mitral valve SAM can often be most easily identified using two-dimensional echocardiography, either in real time or in slow motion of a cine loop (see www.vmth.ucdavis.edu/cardio/cases/case5/echodopp.htm and Figures 204-5 and 204-6). Color flow Doppler echocardiography can be used to demonstrate the hemodynamic abnormalities associated with SAM (see Figure 204-7). With this modality, one observes two turbulent jets originating from the LV outflow tract: one regurgitating back into the left atrium and the other projecting into the aorta. Spectral Doppler can be used to determine the pressure gradient across the region of dynamic subaortic stenosis produced by the SAM. The pressure gradient roughly correlates with the severity of the SAM, although it can be quite labile, changing with the cat's level of excitement. Care must be taken not to record the high-velocity mitral regurgitation jet that is positioned close to the dynamic subaortic stenosis jet. Usually, the dynamic subaortic stenosis jet is narrower (shorter period of systole) on spectral Doppler than the mitral regurgitation jet, often becoming even narrower in mid- to late systole. SAM can also be seen with M-mode echocardiography but is usually more difficult to perform because cats' hearts are small.

SAM is not present in all cats with HCM. Although most cats with SAM have severe HCM, some cats develop SAM before they have any evidence of wall thickening, when their papillary muscles are thickened or long. Although the basilar region of the IVS is often thickened during diastole in cats with HCM, the basilar LV outflow tract does not need to be narrowed for SAM to occur.

Diastolic dysfunction Diastolic dysfunction in cats with severe HCM has been documented using Doppler tissue imaging (DTI) and measures of transmitral flow and relaxation time. Cats with severe HCM routinely have a decrease in early diastolic wall motion of the left ventricular free wall and mitral valve annulus using DTI (Figure 204-12).[78] In addition, on pulsed wave Doppler echocardiography, peak E wave velocity may be reduced, peak A wave velocity increased, isovolumic relaxation time prolonged, and rate of deceleration of early

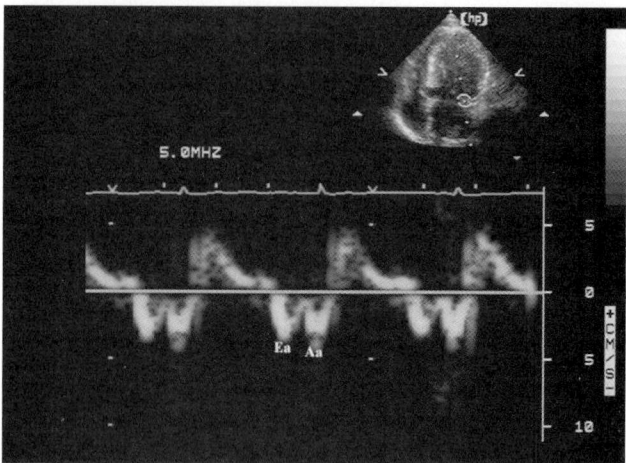

Figure 204-12 A Doppler tissue image (DTI) tracing taken from a cat with severe hypertrophic cardiomyopathy (HCM). The DTI is taken from the lateral mitral valve annulus. The early diastolic wave velocity *(Ea)* is markedly reduced to approximately 4 cm/sec. *Aa,* Annular velocity during atrial systole.

inflow reduced in cats with severe HCM when the heart rate is slow enough that E and A wave velocities can be identified (Figure 204-13).[79]

Mild to moderate hypertrophic cardiomyopathy The diagnosis of HCM is much more difficult and controversial in cats that do not have severe HCM or that only have regional wall thickening on an echocardiogram. In human families with HCM associated with specific gene abnormalities, varying degrees of severity have been noted within the affected family members.[80] Echocardiographic findings in family members with the same mutation range from no abnormalities to severe HCM.

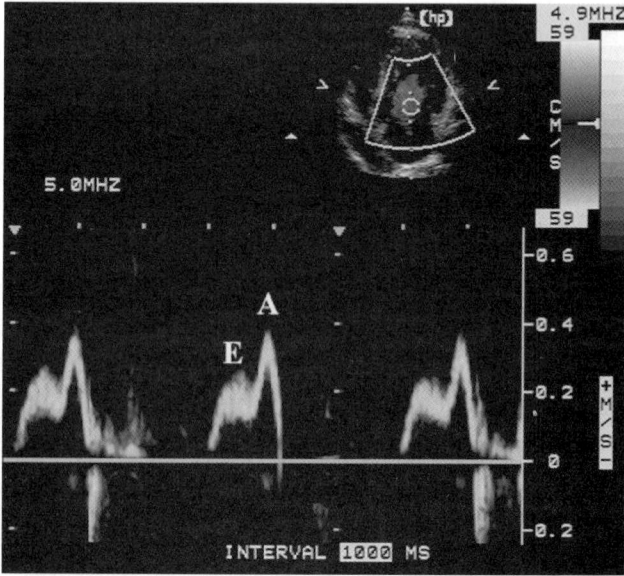

Figure 204-13 A pulsed wave blood flow Doppler tracing taken from just below the mitral valve leaflets during diastole from a cat with severe hypertrophic cardiomyopathy (HCM). Normally the early ventricular diastolic filling velocity *(E)* is faster than the ventricular filling velocity in late diastole, during atrial systole *(A)*. In this cat the relative waveform velocities are reversed.

This may also be true in cats. Distinguishing mild disease from normal or distinguishing mild to moderate HCM from hypertrophy secondary to other abnormalities is not easy in individual cases. In a clinical situation where one is examining an older cat with what appears to be mild to moderate concentric hypertrophy, one must first decide whether hypertrophy is present or not. Then one must determine if another disease is present and may be causing the hypertrophy before one can really make the diagnosis of feline HCM.

The upper limit for normal LV wall thickness is generally considered to be 5.0 to 5.5 mm in the cat, although normal ranges that have been generated in cats may be contaminated by cats with mild HCM because of the disease's prevalence. In most normal Maine coon cats the LV wall thickness is in the 3 to 4 mm range. Certainly any cat with a LV wall thickness greater than or equal to 6 mm is abnormal.

Magnetic Resonance Imaging
Magnetic resonance imaging (MRI) is a new modality that has been used primarily in humans to assess cardiac anatomy and function. It is more accurate than echocardiography in quantitating LV mass in patients with HCM.[81] It can also be used to quantitate diastolic function.[82] The technique is feasible in cats and may become a useful tool for identifying mild disease and assessing response to therapy (Figure 204-14).

Differential Diagnoses
Hyperthyroidism and systemic hypertension need to be ruled out as either primary or complicating factors. Hyperthyroidism is usually easy to rule out. Devices to measure blood pressure in the cat, however, are not always readily available, and the technique requires some practice to acquire accurate values. In addition, systolic systemic arterial blood pressure may be increased in a normal cat that is stressed, so repeat measurements of increased blood pressure are preferred before a diagnosis of systemic hypertension is made. If systemic arterial blood pressure cannot be measured, one should at least rule out the common causes of systemic hypertension in a cat with LV concentric hypertrophy (i.e., hyperthyroidism, renal failure).

Rarely, infiltrative disease such as lymphoma will produce hypertrophy that is indistinguishable from HCM on an echocardiogram. One such case has been reported.[24] Cats that are homozygous for the dystrophin deficiency seen in hypertrophic

feline muscular dystrophy also have thickened but hypoechoic myocardium with hyperechoic foci in the LV myocardium and papillary muscles.[83] The myocardium contains foci of mineralization and no dystrophin.

Precipitating Factors
Certain factors may precipitate heart failure or sudden death in a cat with HCM. Stress (cat fight), anesthesia (especially with ketamine), and surgery appear to be factors.[74] The administration of a long-acting corticosteroid also appears to be a factor that either produces or worsens heart failure in cats, presumably through the mineralocorticoid effects of these drugs.

Therapy of Cats with No Clinical Signs
No evidence exists to show that any drug alters the natural history of HCM in domestic cats until they are in heart failure. Diltiazem, atenolol, or enalapril are commonly administered to cats with mild to severe HCM that are not in heart failure on an empiric basis. Whenever HCM is diagnosed in a cat, the veterinarian should explain the situation to owners and try to let them make informed decisions based on their wishes and life styles. Because no intervention is known to change the course of the disease, treatment at this stage is not mandated.

Treatment Goals and General Therapy of Cats in Heart Failure
Cats that present in heart failure have clinical signs referable to pulmonary edema, pleural effusion, or both. Consequently, therapy is generally aimed at decreasing left atrial and pulmonary venous pressures in these cats and physically removing the effusion. In some cats with severe heart failure, clinical evidence of hypoperfusion (low-output heart failure) may be apparent in addition to the signs of CHF. The signs may be manifested primarily as cold extremities.

Pulmonary edema is primarily treated with diuretics (almost exclusively with furosemide) acutely and chronically and an ACE enzyme inhibitor chronically, although recent evidence suggests that ACE inhibition may not be that helpful in prolonging survival in cats with HCM.[84] Diltiazem and beta-adrenergic blockers, usually atenolol, have been commonly used as adjunctive agents. Recent evidence suggests that diltiazem is not helpful in prolonging survival in cats with heart failure due to severe HCM and that atenolol may actually shorten survival time.[84] Pleurocentesis is most effective for treating cats with severe pleural effusion. Furosemide is helpful for preventing or slowing recurrent effusion.

Acute Therapy
Just as with DCM, cats that have respiratory distress suspected of having heart failure secondary to HCM may need to be placed in an oxygen-enriched environment as soon as possible. If possible the cat should be initially evaluated by doing a cursory physical examination, taking care not to stress the patient during this or any other procedure, because stress exacerbates dyspnea and arrhythmias and often leads to death. Most, but not all, cats with severe HCM that are in heart failure will have a heart murmur and gallop rhythm. A butterfly catheter should be used to perform thoracentesis on both sides of the chest to look for pleural effusion as soon as possible. Generally this should be done with the cat in a sternal position so that it does not become stressed during the procedure. Clipping of the hair is not needed. If fluid is identified, it should be removed. Most cats that are dyspneic due to pleural effusion have 150 to 250 mL of fluid in their pleural space. If none is identified, a lateral thoracic radiograph to identify pulmonary edema may be taken with the veterinarian present to ensure that the cat is not stressed (e.g., the clinician should make sure no one stretches the cat out or in any way interferes with its ability to breathe). If the patient struggles or appears to be stressed or fractious during or before radiographic examination, the procedure

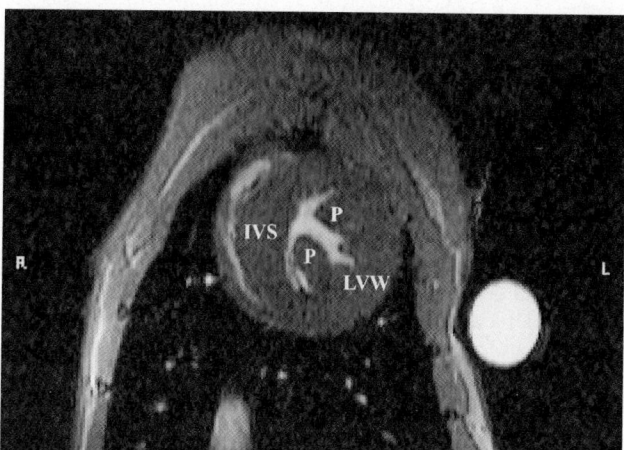

Figure 204-14 Cross-sectional view of the heart taken using magnetic resonance imaging (MRI) from a cat with severe HCM. The papillary muscles *(P)*, left ventricular free wall *(LVW)*, and interventricular septum *(IVS)* are all markedly thickened. (Picture courtesy of Dr. Kristin MacDonald.)

should be canceled and the patient placed into an oxygen-enriched environment. A preferable alternative to blind tapping is to perform a superficial ultrasonographic examination to identify and locate fluid accumulation.

Furosemide Furosemide should initially be administered intravenously or intramuscularly to the cat in severe respiratory distress. The route of administration depends on the stress level of the patient. Furosemide should be administered intramuscularly to cats that are very distressed and cannot tolerate restraint for an intravenous injection. Cats that can tolerate an intravenous injection may benefit from the more rapid onset of action (within 5 minutes of an intravenous injection versus 30 minutes for an intramuscular injection). The initial furosemide dose to a cat in distress should generally be in the 1 to 2 mg/lb range, intramuscularly or intravenously. This dose may be repeated within 1 hour to 2 hours (see Chapter 199).

High-dose parenteral furosemide therapy commonly produces electrolyte disturbances and dehydration in cats. Cats with severe heart failure that require intensive therapy are often precarious. They may be presented dehydrated and electrolyte-depleted because of anorexia. They may remain anorexic and consequently dehydrated and depleted of electrolytes once the edema, the effusion, or both are lessened. Judicious intravenous or subcutaneous fluid administration may be required to improve these cats clinically. Overzealous fluid administration will result in the return of CHF. If fluid administration is required, the furosemide administration must be discontinued for that time.

Nitroprusside Anecdotally, nitroprusside may be beneficial in cats with severe pulmonary edema due to HCM. As with DCM, it may be administered empirically at 2 µg/lb/min or titrated, using blood pressure measurement to document efficacy, starting at a dose of 1 to 2 µg/lb/min. Nitroprusside has a very short half-life. Consequently, if clinically significant systemic hypotension is produced (e.g., weakness, collapse, poor capillary refill time) cessation of the infusion will result in the systemic blood pressure returning to normal within several minutes.

Nitroglycerin Nitroglycerin cream may be beneficial in cats with severe edema formation secondary to feline cardiomyopathy. However, no studies have examined effects or efficacy. Nitroglycerin is safe and some benefit may occur with its administration in some cats. Consequently, one-eighth inch to one-fourth inch of a 2% cream may be administered to the inside of an ear every 4 to 6 hours for the first 24 hours as long as furosemide is being administered concomitantly. Nitroglycerin is not a primary drug. Tolerance develops rapidly in other species, and prolonged administration is probably of even lesser benefit.

Once drug administration is complete, the cat should be left to rest quietly in an oxygen-enriched environment. Care should be taken not to distress the cat. A baseline measurement of the respiratory rate and assessment of respiratory character should be taken when the cat is resting. This should be followed at 30-minute intervals and furosemide administration continued until the respiratory rate starts to decrease (a consistent decrease of the respiratory rate from 70 to 90 breaths per minute into the 50 to 60 breaths per minute range is a general guide), the character of the cat's respiratory effort improves, or both occur. When this happens, the furosemide dose and dose frequency should be curtailed sharply.

Sedation or Anesthesia In some cats, sedation with acepromazine (0.02 to 0.5 mg/lb intramuscularly or intravenously) may help by producing anxiolysis. Oxymorphone (0.02 to 0.04 mg/lb every 6 hours intramuscularly, intravenously, or subcutaneously) or butorphanol tartrate (0.04 mg/lb intravenously or 0.18 mg/lb every 4 hours subcutaneously) may also be used but are secondary choices because they can produce respiratory depression. Oxymorphone may produce excitement in some cats.

In some cats with fulminant heart failure, anesthesia, intubation, and ventilation are required to control the respiratory failure. Although this method is not preferred for most severely dyspneic cats, it can be life saving in some. This procedure has the advantage of being able to administer 100% oxygen and to be able to drain or suction fluid from the large airways in a controlled environment. The disadvantage is the administration of anesthetic agents to a cat that has cardiovascular compromise.

Chronic Therapy
Many aspects of chronic therapy of HCM are controversial. All therapy is palliative. Furosemide is the only drug that has a clearly beneficial effect chronically on survival in cats with HCM.[84]

Pleurocentesis Many cats with HCM are dyspneic because of pleural effusion that reaccumulates despite appropriate medical therapy. These cats need periodic pleurocentesis (see Chapter 103).

Furosemide In cats with CHF due to HCM, furosemide administration, once initiated, should usually be maintained for the rest of the cat's life. In a few cases, furosemide can be discontinued gradually once the cat has been stabilized. This usually only occurs in a cat that has had a precipitating stressful event.

As for DCM, the maintenance dose of furosemide in cats usually ranges from 6.25 (one half of a 12.5 mg tablet) once a day to 12.5 mg orally every 8 hours, although the dose may be increased further if the cat is not responding to a conventional dose. The author and colleagues have administered higher doses (up to 37.5 mg every 12 hours) than commonly recommended to a few cats with severe heart failure without identifying severe consequences as long as the cats were eating and drinking. Cats on high-dose furosemide therapy are commonly mildly dehydrated and mildly to moderately azotemic. However, they often continue to maintain a reasonable quality of life.

The furosemide dose needs to be titrated carefully in each patient. The owner should be taught how to count the resting respiratory rate at home and instructed to keep a daily written log of the respiratory rate as outlined previously under DCM. This is highly beneficial for making decisions regarding dose adjustment in individual patients.

Angiotensin-Converting Enzyme Inhibitors Although furosemide has been used to treat heart failure secondary to feline HCM for decades, the use of ACE inhibitors in cats with HCM is relatively recent, because veterinarians, like their colleagues who treat humans, feared that the use of ACE inhibitors would worsen SAM in their patients. Over the past 10 years it has become obvious to most veterinary cardiologists that ACE inhibitors do not worsen the clinical signs referable to HCM, and a recent study has documented that SAM is not worsened by enalapril administration in cats.[85] Many have believed and one study has suggested that ACE inhibitors improve the quality and quantity of life of cats with HCM.[86] Preliminary evidence from a recent placebo-controlled and blinded clinical trial suggests that enalapril produces little to no benefit when compared with furosemide alone in cats with heart failure due to HCM.[84] However, this study also included cats with unclassified (restrictive) cardiomyopathy and both cats with and without SAM. Subgroup analysis failed to change the conclusions of the study but the subgroups were small. Consequently, it is the recommendation of this author to continue to use an ACE inhibitor in cats in heart failure due to HCM at a dose of 1.25 to 2.5 mg orally every 24 hours.

Diltiazem In cats with severe HCM that have or have had evidence of CHF, diltiazem or a beta-adrenergic blocking agent are often administered. Both provide symptomatic benefit in human patients. Their use in cats with HCM is controversial; however, little doubt exists that neither drugs produces dramatic benefits. Diltiazem, however, appears to produce no harm.[84]

Diltiazem is a calcium channel blocker previously reported to produce beneficial effects in cats with HCM when dosed at 7.5 mg every 8 hours.[87,88] Beneficial effects that have been reported include lessened edema formation and decreased wall thickness in some cats. In the author's experience only a few cats appear to experience a clinically significant decrease in wall thickness, and it is impossible to tell if this is due to drug effect or time. Rarely does it appear clinically that diltiazem controls CHF on its own or helps control pulmonary edema or pleural effusion when added on to furosemide therapy. Diltiazem does improve the early diastolic relaxation abnormalities seen in feline HCM.[59,88] Whether this helps decrease diastolic intraventricular pressure and so decrease edema formation is unknown. Theoretically it should have little benefit in the resting cat with a slow heart rate. Slower myocardial relaxation during rapid heart rates may not allow the myocardium enough time to relax, resulting in increased diastolic intraventricular pressure. Diltiazem may help protect a cat that undergoes a stressful event. Incomplete relaxation and decreased compliance, however, are more plausible explanations for increased diastolic pressure due to diastolic dysfunction in feline HCM. In humans, diltiazem does not change LV chamber stiffness and so does not alter passive diastolic function.[89] In cats it also appears not to alter late diastolic filling properties.[90] Diltiazem decreases SAM, which may decrease the amount of mitral regurgitation, but beta blockers generally produce a greater decrease in the amount of SAM.[91] Recent evidence suggests that diltiazem has no effect on survival time in cats with severe HCM and heart failure.[84]

Dilacor XR is dosed at 30 mg per cat orally every 12 hours and produces a significant decrease in heart rate and blood pressure in cats with HCM for 12 to 14 hours.[92]

Beta-Adrenergic Receptor Blockers Beta blockers are primarily used to reduce SAM and heart rate in cats with HCM. At this stage, beta blockers should probably be reserved for cats with severe SAM at rest or with tachyarrhythmias and not routinely administered to the affected population as a whole, because a recent study has suggested that atenolol shortens the survival of cats with diastolic dysfunction, including cats with HCM.[84] Beta blockade is questionable for SAM and tachycardia observed in a clinical situation. Cats spend 85% of their life asleep, and sleep probably reduces sympathetic activity better than a beta-adrenergic blocking drug. Consequently, many cats with mild to moderate SAM in a veterinary clinic probably have no or milder SAM at home, and the same can be said for tachycardia. Beta blockers are effective for reducing SAM. Two studies have examined the effects of esmolol, a short-acting β_1-adrenergic blocking drug, in cats with HCM and obstruction to LV outflow due to SAM; both showed a reduction in the pressure gradient across the outflow tract.[91,93] In both studies the degree of outflow tract obstruction decreased and the heart rate slowed, and in one esmolol was more effective than diltiazem.[91] If the data on esmolol can be translated to atenolol's effects in cats (which seems reasonable), one would predict that atenolol would decrease SAM.

Atenolol is a specific β_1-adrenergic blocking drug that needs to be administered twice a day, usually at a total dose of 6.25 to 12.5 mg orally every 12 hours.[92,94] In the cat, atenolol has a half-life of 3.5 hours. When administered to cats at a dose of 1.4 mg/lb, atenolol attenuates the increase in heart rate produced by isoproterenol for 12 but not for 24 hours.

Refractory Heart Failure

Heart failure that is refractory to furosemide and an ACE inhibitor portends a poor prognosis. Another diuretic may be added to the therapeutic regimen. A thiazide diuretic is generally the most rewarding but is also more likely to cause complications, such as dehydration and electrolyte (sodium, potassium, chloride, magnesium) depletion. Spironolactone, in theory, may have some beneficial effects related to blocking aldosterone's actions; however, clinically it rarely results in noticeable improvement, and its efficacy is unproven. A low sodium diet may be helpful, if palatable. This diet can be a commercial one or one that is devised by a nutritional service. Home-cooked diets formulated by the owner are discouraged unless the owner is counseled. If severe SAM is present and atenolol is not already part of the therapeutic regimen, it may be added at this stage.

FELINE UNCLASSIFIED CARDIOMYOPATHY

A relatively common echocardiographic finding in cats with heart disease and heart failure is normal to mildly abnormal ventricular chamber size, wall thickness, and wall motion with atrial enlargement (Figure 204-15). The left heart is most commonly affected, but there may also be concurrent right heart changes. It is commonly believed that because no evidence of systolic dysfunction, left-to-right shunting, or obvious valvular regurgitation exists, these cats must have diastolic dysfunction. Consequently, these cats are often assumed to have RCM. One study has suggested that this is not the case.[78] In this study, diastolic function was examined in nine cats with the aforementioned findings using DTI. DTI is a pulsed Doppler technique that measures the velocity of ventricular or annular wall motion and is an accurate means of detecting RCM in humans.[95]

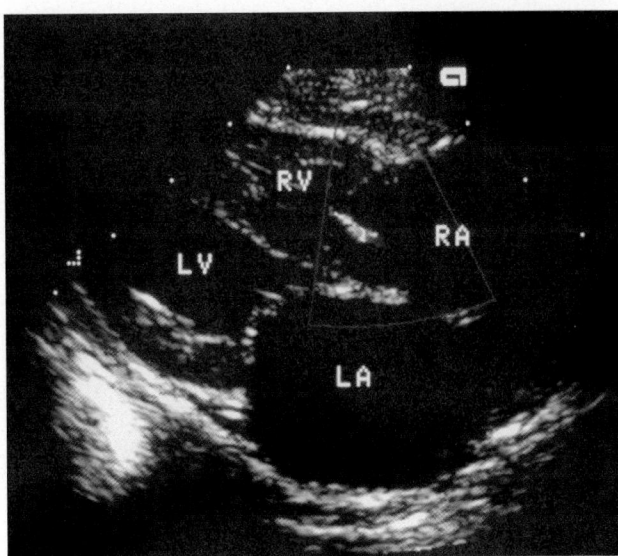

Figure 204-15 Two-dimensional echocardiogram from a cat with unclassified cardiomyopathy. The left ventricle *(LV)* appears normal and the left atrium *(LA)* is enlarged. A small color flow Doppler jet of tricuspid regurgitation in the right atrium *(RA)*, which is also enlarged but not to the same degree as the LA. *RV,* Right ventricular chamber.

Six of the cats in the study had clear evidence of diastolic dysfunction (i.e., lower than normal early diastolic wall velocity). Three cats clearly had normal diastolic function on DTI and therefore did not have RCM. Consequently, not all cats with the echocardiographic findings described previously have RCM. Therefore the author feels that the more appropriate term for this disease is *unclassified cardiomyopathy* unless it can be documented that diastolic dysfunction exists. In this scheme, RCM then is often a subclassification of unclassified cardiomyopathy, whereas the other subclass is unknown or idiopathic.

What could cause this echocardiographic pattern other than RCM? Some form of atrial myopathy is one possibility, and atrial standstill is occasionally identified in these cats (see www.vmth.ucdavis.edu/cardio/cases/case18/case18.htm). Misdiagnosis is another possibility. In the author's clinic, many cats arriving with a diagnosis of primary mitral regurgitation, mitral and tricuspid valve dysplasia, and hyperthyroidism have been placed into this category (called either *unclassified* or *RCM*), probably because it was convenient and gave the clinician a false sense of security of making a "definitive" diagnosis. Significant mitral regurgitation is most often missed when only a high-frequency ultrasound probe is used. A lower-frequency transducer and several views are recommended. Some ultrasound machines do not have a frame rate high enough to adequately detect apparent severe mitral regurgitation in cats.

In some cats, evidence of endocardial scarring can be seen on the echocardiogram, either as a discrete lesion most commonly at the level of the mid-LV or as diffuse scarring of the endocardium. In these cases the diagnosis of RCM may be made echocardiographically.

The terms *intermediate* and *intergrade cardiomyopathy* have been used previously to describe this class of cardiac disease in cats. They are probably inappropriate because they suggest that the characteristic changes seen in these cats share clinical and echocardiographic features of both dilated and HCM.

FELINE RESTRICTIVE CARDIOMYOPATHY

Although listed as a separate entity in this chapter, in most situations RCM is a subclassification of unclassified cardiomyopathy. Feline RCM is a diverse group of myocardial conditions characterized by abnormal diastolic function, normal to mildly increased LV wall thickness, and normal to mildly reduced systolic function. RCM occurs when ventricular diastolic compliance is impaired (i.e., stiffness is increased) by infiltration of the endocardium, subendocardium, or myocardium by fibrous tissue or another component. In contrast to human medicine where specific causes, such as amyloidosis and eosinophilic infiltration are causes of RCM, specific causes for RCM have not been clearly defined in the cat. Without the use of invasive diagnostic procedures to directly measure LV diastolic function, DTI, other indirect measures of diastolic function, or necropsy examination, it is often impossible to distinguish this disorder from the form or forms of unclassified cardiomyopathy that are idiopathic.

Incidence

The exact incidence of RCM is unknown. Unclassified cardiomyopathy is the second most common feline cardiomyopathy, of which RCM is a component.

Cause

The precise cause of feline RCM is unknown. Some evidence indicates that it may be inflammatory in nature. Endomyocarditis has been recognized in cats at postmortem examination for over 25 years.[96] Endomyocarditis in cats is characterized by focal or diffuse infiltration of the endocardium by lymphocytes,

plasma cells, histiocytes, and a lesser number of neutrophils. The inflammatory component of endomyocarditis may be infectious, immune-mediated, or toxic. An interstitial pneumonia may also be common in this group. Within the past 10 years a study documented endomyocarditis in 37 cats at necropsy over a 7-year period.[97] Over this same 7-year span, 25 cats with endocardial fibrosis were identified at the same institution. Four of these 62 cats had features of both diseases. This study and previous findings from Dr. Sam Liu have lead to the speculation that chronic endomyocarditis leads to endocardial fibrosis, a pathologic disease that leads to the physiologic entity termed *RCM*. However, unless an agent that causes endomyocarditis in cats is identified, the theory that endomyocarditis leads to endocardial fibrosis will remain unproven.

In addition to the previous findings and speculation, one study has identified a transmissible myocarditis-diaphragmitis in young cats.[98] The disease is generally self-limiting and causes a transient fever and depression. The investigators were unable to isolate a causative agent in these cats.

Eosinophilic endocardial inflammation is common in humans, more commonly in tropical climates. RCM has been reported in several cats with hypereosinophilic syndrome, although it is impossible to determine if the hypereosinophilia in this small number of cats caused RCM or the two diseases happened to occur together.[99,100]

Pathophysiology

In its classic form, endocardial, subendocardial, or myocardial fibrosis impede ventricular diastolic filling and so impair diastolic function. These disorders are generally and primarily characterized by decreased compliance leading to an elevated LV diastolic pressure with a normal LV filling volume. The elevation in diastolic ventricular pressure results in atrial enlargement and the formation of pulmonary edema and pleural effusion. The lesions are generally confined to the LV in humans and left CHF predominates the clinical presentation.[101] In cats, right atrial enlargement is also common. In some cats the LV is perfectly normal in appearance, whereas in others the LV may be misshapen and may have additional false tendons traversing the ventricle.

Pathology

The postmortem changes are unique to this form of cardiomyopathy and may be used to differentiate it from other disorders. Patchy or diffuse endocardial, subendocardial, or myocardial depositions of fibrous tissue are characteristic necropsy findings. The endocardium may appear whitish-gray, opaque, and thickened when endocardial or endomyocardial fibrosis is present (Figure 204-16). Fibrous adhesions between papillary muscles and the myocardium with distortion and fusion of the chordae tendineae and mitral valve leaflets may also be noted in RCM.[96] In extreme cases a portion of the LV cavity, most commonly the mid-LV, may be obliterated. As with most cardiomyopathies, the LV appears to be most severely affected, although other cardiac chambers may exhibit similar pathologic findings. Extreme left atrial and auricular enlargement is common. Other cats demonstrate apparently earlier stages of the disease in which microscopic evidence of myocarditis is evident without gross pathologic abnormalities. The lesions suggest an inflammatory response; however causative factors have not been identified. Systemic thromboembolism is prevalent.[102]

Histologic features of endocardial fibrosis include extreme endocardial thickening by hyaline, fibrous, and granulation tissue.[96] Chondroid metaplasia is occasionally exhibited by the surface layer of hyaline tissue. A layer of loose fibrous tissue lies beneath this layer with a layer of granulation tissue adjacent to the myocardium. These changes are similar but not identical to those seen in humans with RCM.

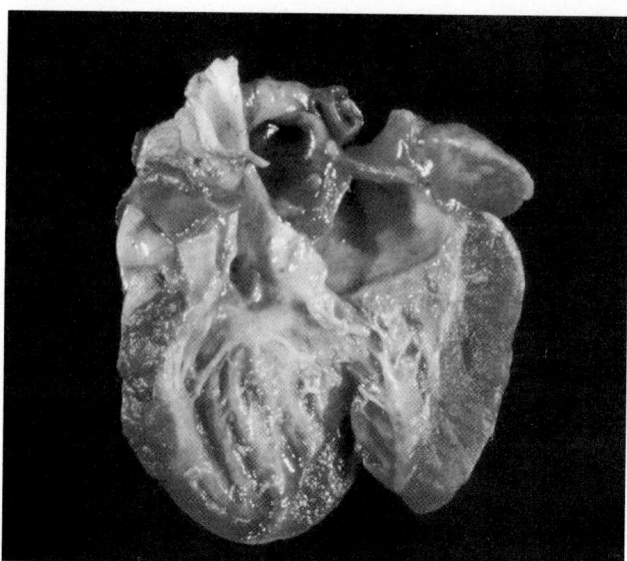

Figure 204-16 Postmortem specimen showing the left ventricle *(LV)* and left atrium from a cat with endomyocardial fibrosis producing restrictive cardiomyopathy (RCM). The endocardium of the LV is white and thickened by fibrotic tissue.

Natural History and Prognosis

As with other forms of cardiomyopathy, prognosis is difficult to predict for individual cases, especially prior to observing the initial response to therapy. A high incidence of serious arrhythmias, systemic thromboembolism, and refractory CHF is often present. In the author's experience, cats with RCM, on average, have a poor long-term prognosis. Although an initial response to standard therapy is often possible, progressive and refractory heart failure develops in the majority of cases.

Clinical Manifestations

History Signalment is difficult to accurately report, because little agreement exist among veterinary cardiologists as to which cases fall within this classification. From a series of pathologic studies in cats, Liu reported an age range of 8 months to 19 years.[103] No breed predisposition has been reported. There may be a male predominance, or it may be that males develop more severe disease, as in HCM. Most cats are middle-aged or older. Presenting complaints and clinical signs are similar to other forms of myocardial disease and include dyspnea and tachypnea, poor general condition, weakness, lethargy or rarely exercise intolerance, and anorexia. In one report, 45% had evidence of systemic thromboembolism at necropsy.[102]

Physical Examination A heart murmur heard best on the sternum, just medial to the left apex beat, is common. An arrhythmia may be ausculted. Many cats are dyspneic.

Radiographs No specific findings exist for unclassified or RCM. Pulmonary edema and pleural effusion are common.

Echocardiography The echocardiographic findings in RCM are variable. Left atrial dilation is the common feature, and the LV internal dimensions are typically normal but may be mildly to moderately reduced or mildly increased. Most commonly the LV looks normal. However, two-dimensional echocardiography may demonstrate loss of normal LV symmetry, distorted or fused papillary muscles, mild LV concentric hypertrophy, mild wall thickening, a mild reduction in shortening fraction, and a mild increase in chamber diameter. Some cats may have

evidence of more pronounced endocardial scarring. In these cases the endocardium may be notably thickened and irregular with an increased echogenicity. Others have evidence of cavity obliteration. Mild mitral regurgitation may be detectable with color flow Doppler. A large color flow Doppler jet suggests that the primary problem is primary mitral valve disease rather than unclassified cardiomyopathy. A left atrial thrombus may be identified.

Doppler echocardiography may be abnormal in cats with RCM. However, this remains to be proven. As noted previously, the early diastolic waveform on DTI is reduced in cats with RCM, whereas it is normal in cats with the idiopathic form of unclassified cardiomyopathy.

Electrocardiography No specific findings appear on electrocardiogram (ECG). Supraventricular and ventricular arrhythmias may be present, but sinus tachycardia is most commonly present in the clinic. Shifts in the mean electrical axis and evidence of chamber enlargement may occur.

Clinical Pathology No specific clinical pathologic findings exist. Azotemia due to reduced cardiac output, either from CHF or dehydration caused by diuretic therapy, is the most common abnormality. Elevated liver enzymes may be encountered.

Differential Diagnosis The primary differential diagnoses for RCM are unclassified cardiomyopathy not due to RCM, mitral regurgitation due to primary mitral valve disease, and myocardial infarction. Chronic myocardial infarction usually results in a region of akinetic or hypokinetic myocardium. Often the region of affected myocardium is thinner than normal. With severe mitral regurgitation due to primary mitral valve disease, a large jet is seen with color flow Doppler (although it may take a lower-frequency transducer and various views, including the left apical four-chamber view, to identify it). The IVS is commonly hyperdynamic, whereas the left ventricular free wall commonly moves less than normal. The LV chamber is usually larger than normal in diastole.

Therapy

Therapy of restrictive and unclassified cardiomyopathy is the same. It is palliative and consists primarily of the administration of furosemide and an ACE inhibitor as outlined in the two previous sections of this chapter. Diltiazem is not indicated because a calcium channel blocker is not able to help to relax scar (i.e., fibrous) tissue. A recent study suggests that atenolol may decrease the survival time in patients with diastolic dysfunction.[84] However, if the cat is persistently tachycardic at home, diltiazem or atenolol may be indicated in an attempt to slow the heart rate.

ARRHYTHMOGENIC RIGHT VENTRICULAR CARDIOMYOPATHY

ARVC is a recently reported and rare form of feline cardiomyopathy.[104] It has been identified in humans, dogs (boxer dogs), and cats. It is characterized by fibrofatty or fatty infiltration of primarily the right ventricular free wall. The right ventricular wall is commonly thinned in humans and cats with the disease. Ventricular tachyarrhythmias are common in all three species, and sudden death is a common feature of the disease in humans and boxer dogs.[105] The disease is also commonly known as arrhythmogenic right ventricular dysplasia (ARVD).

Cause

The cause of ARVC is unknown in cats. In humans at least six forms of the disease (ARVD 1 to 6) are inherited as an autosomal dominant trait, and one (Naxos syndrome) is inherited as an autosomal recessive trait.[105] The cause of ARVD 2 has been recently identified as several mutations in the gene that encodes for the calcium release channel (also known as the *ryanodine receptor*) on the myocardial sarcoplasmic reticulum.[106] Ryanodine receptor dysfunction has been identified in boxer dogs with ARVC.[107]

Pathophysiology

In cats, ARVC most commonly (8 of 12 cats in the one study reported to date) produces right heart failure, presumably through the destruction of right ventricular myocardium resulting in right ventricular systolic and, possibly, diastolic dysfunction along with secondary tricuspid regurgitation.[104] The changes in the right ventricular free wall also commonly produce ventricular tachyarrhythmias (9 of 12 cats) and supraventricular tachyarrhythmias (5 of 12 cats). Tumor necrosis factor (TNF) is commonly increased in cats with right heart failure, which may contribute to the systemic effects of the disease.[108]

Pathology

The right ventricular and atrial chambers are markedly enlarged in cats that die of the disease.[104] Thinning of the right ventricular free wall is a consistent feature of the disease and may be focal or diffuse. Aneurysms of the wall may occur, especially at the apex of the right ventricle (RV). The wall is often so thin that light can be seen through it. Histopathologically either fibrofatty or fatty replacement of myocardium exists. Inflammatory cells are commonly present, especially in regions of fibrofatty replacement. Although most prominent in the right ventricular free wall, these changes are also commonly present in the LV and occasionally identified in the left atrium. Apoptosis is common.

Clinical Manifestations

Evidence of right heart failure, including ascites, pleural and pericardial effusions, and jugular vein distension, is common. The pleural effusion may be severe enough to cause tachypnea and dyspnea. A heart murmur secondary to tricuspid regurgitation is common. Arrhythmias are also commonly heard on auscultation, and ECG evidence of a ventricular arrhythmia may be one clue that one is dealing with ARVC and not tricuspid valve dysplasia. Supraventricular tachyarrhythmias, including atrial fibrillation, may also occur. In the severe stage, echocardiography reveals marked enlargement of the right ventricular and right atrial chambers. The right ventricular chamber enlargement may be segmental. Tricuspid regurgitation is usually present on color flow Doppler. Careful echocardiographic interrogation may reveal localized regions of right ventricular wall thinning or regions of aneurysmal dilation. The right ventricular trabeculae may appear abnormal, especially at the apex. The disease may not be confined to the right heart, which means the left atrial and ventricular chambers may also be enlarged. Syncope due to ventricular tachycardia may be present.

Differential Diagnosis

Cats with severe ARVC are commonly misdiagnosed as having tricuspid valve dysplasia because tricuspid regurgitation is a common sequel to the disease. Cats from 1 to 20 years of age have been diagnosed with the disease.

Therapy

Right heart failure is treated with furosemide and an ACE inhibitor. Digoxin combined with either diltiazem or atenolol may be used to control supraventricular tachycardia or the ventricular rate in cats with atrial fibrillation. Malignant ventricular tachycardia or ventricular tachycardia that causes clinical signs (e.g., syncope) can be managed acutely with lidocaine (5 to 20 µg/lb/min) and chronically with sotalol (1 to 2 mg/lb every 12 hours orally).[109]

SECONDARY MYOCARDIAL DISEASES

Hyperthyroidism

Hyperthyroidism commonly produces echocardiographic changes, although the changes are usually relatively mild. Changes can include an increase in LV wall thickness, left atrial size, and LV diastolic diameter. Shortening fraction may also be increased.[110,111] Often these changes regress over months once the hyperthyroidism is successfully controlled. These changes are physiologic in response to the direct effects of the excess thyroid hormone on the cardiac myocytes, the increase in metabolic rate, and systemic hypertension. Consequently hyperthyroidism is not a form of cardiomyopathy (i.e., primary myocardial disease). However, some cats with hyperthyroidism will have the classic features of severe HCM, including SAM in some, and a few may experience heart failure. Although unproven, the author theorizes that some of these cats may have had mild to moderate HCM all their lives and that the hyperthyroidism has exacerbated the hypertrophy.

Systemic Hypertension

Systemic arterial hypertension causes a pressure overload of the LV and leads to concentric hypertrophy. This hypertrophy is generally mild, however, with the average increase in wall thickness being approximately 1 mm.[112] As with hyperthyroidism, the author theorizes that some cats with mild to moderate HCM have an exacerbation of their concentric hypertrophy when they develop systemic arterial hypertension. In addition to the LV wall becoming thicker, the proximal aorta also increases in size with systemic arterial hypertension.

Acromegaly

Acromegaly has been reported to increase LV wall thickness severe enough to produce heart failure in cats. In one study, significant wall thickening was identified in seven of 14 cats with acromegaly and six developed heart failure.[55] However, in six cats examined echocardiographically by the author, no evidence of cardiac change was found.

SYSTEMIC ARTERIAL THROMBOEMBOLISM

A thrombus is a blood clot. Thrombi are usually formed (to prevent hemorrhage) when a blood vessel is traumatized. They can also form spontaneously within the cardiovascular system. A systemic thrombus becomes a systemic thromboembolus when it dislodges from the primary site where it forms in the cardiovascular system and is pushed by blood flow to a distal site where it lodges, partially or completely occluding blood flow distal to the thromboembolus. Most clots that occlude systemic arterial blood vessels are thromboemboli. Spontaneous formation of a clot in a systemic arterial vessel causing occlusion of a systemic artery is an unusual event and requires a predisposing factor (e.g., trauma) to allow it to occur. Most systemic thrombi that form and cause thromboemboli in cats appear to form in the left atrium, most commonly in the left auricle, as they do in humans (Figure 204-17).[113]

Systemic arterial thromboembolism (STE) is most commonly observed in cats with any form of cardiomyopathy, most frequently in those with severe left atrial enlargement, although they also have been reported to occur in cats with hyperthyroidism.[114-116] However, it is unknown if cases of hyperthyroidism have confounding HCM or not. Left atrial chamber enlargement in the absence of mitral regurgitation causes blood flow stasis, especially in the left auricle, allowing red cells to aggregate and thrombus formation to occur. Although STE can occur in cats that do not have cardiac disease, more than 70% of cases seen in veterinary small animal practice are in cats with cardiomyopathy.[115,116]

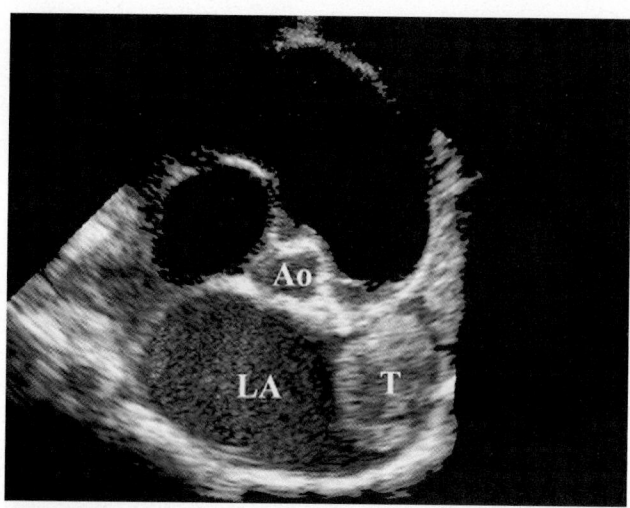

Figure 204-17 A two-dimensional echocardiogram from a cat with hypertrophic cardiomyopathy (HCM), showing a large thrombus *(T)* in the left atrium *(LA)*, specifically the left auricle, and spontaneous echocardiographic contrast in the left atrium. *Ao,* Aorta.

Most cats (approximately 90%) with STE have the thromboembolus lodge at the terminal abdominal aorta (the aortic trifurcation). The thromboembolus commonly extends down the external iliac arteries, giving it the appearance of a saddle. Consequently, it is commonly called a *saddle thromboembolus.* Thromboembolism of the terminal aorta causes acute cessation of blood flow to the caudal limbs, producing acute caudal limb paresis and paralysis and pain with a loss of the femoral pulses, cold extremities, and pale or cyanotic pads (pain, poikilothermia, paralysis, pulselessness, and pallor). Some cats have a smaller thromboembolus lodge in one femoral artery, a brachial artery, or another smaller artery. Occasionally, a large thromboembolus lodges more proximally in the aorta, above the renal arteries, resulting in acute renal failure. In other cats, a very large thromboembolus lodges in the mitral valve orifice, the LV, or the proximal aorta at the region of the brachiocephalic trunk, causing sudden death.[117]

Pathophysiology

In fast-flowing blood, as occurs with injury to a systemic blood vessel, the principal elements forming a thrombus are platelets, which form a white clot.[118] As blood flow slows due to the clot formation, red cells are incorporated in the clot to form a red thrombus. On the other hand, in slow-flowing blood, coagulation enzymes play the major role in thrombus formation. Here red cells entrapped in a fibrin network result in the formation of a red thrombus. Although no one has examined the composition of left atrial thrombi in cats, in humans they are composed of red cell aggregates within a fibrin meshwork.[118]

The most plausible explanation for thrombus formation in the left atrium of cats with STE is sluggish blood flow. At a postmortem examination, atria from cats with cardiac disease and thromboembolism are often very large and may be fibrotic. In one study the left atrium was severely enlarged in 57%, moderately enlarged in 14%, and mildly enlarged in 22% of cats with STE.[115] Only 5% had a normal left atrial size. The amount of blood that flows through an enlarged left atrium of a cat with cardiomyopathy is normal to low unless significant mitral regurgitation is present, resulting in a lower than normal blood flow velocity within the chamber. When blood flow slows to a certain velocity, red cells and other blood factors

clump together (see www.vmth.ucdavis.edu/cardio/cases/case18/echo.htm).[119] In vitro this occurs when blood flow velocity decreases below 10 cm/sec, whereas in humans with atrial fibrillation it occurs when the velocity from the left auricle to the left atrium slows to less than 35 cm/sec.[119,120] Increasing plasma fibrinogen concentration also increases red cell aggregation, whereas red cell aggregation is not altered by the absence of platelets, stimulation of platelet aggregation with ADP, or inhibition of platelet aggregation with aspirin.[119]

Red cell aggregation can be observed with ultrasound and is termed *spontaneous echocardiographic contrast* (SEC), also known euphemistically as "smoke." SEC is often observed swirling in the enlarged left atrium of a cat with severe cardiomyopathy. In humans, SEC is associated with increased left atrial size and with reduced left atrial blood flow velocity.[120] It is the factor most strongly associated with left auricular thrombus formation and with systemic embolic events. No studies on this subject have been performed in veterinary medicine. However, it is common to see spontaneous contrast in the left atrium of a cat with severe cardiomyopathy and an STE. If low blood flow velocity is such an important factor, one might also expect dogs with DCM to be prone to left atrial thrombus formation. Systemic thromboembolism is rare in dogs with DCM. The reason for this discrepancy may be due to species differences in erythrocyte aggregability. One study has documented that normal cat red cells are more aggregable than those of dogs, rats, rabbits, humans, and gerbils.[121] Although platelets are not necessary for thrombus formation in the left atrium and auricle, cat's platelets are also more reactive than other species. Feline platelets undergo spontaneous aggregation in vitro and are more responsive to serotonin-induced aggregation than are platelets from other species.[122,123] Cats also have a greater volume of platelets per body weight than other species.[122] One study has documented increased platelet aggregability in some cats with cardiomyopathy.[124]

In humans, hyperhomocysteinemia has been associated with venous thrombosis, atherosclerosis, and arterial occlusive disease.[125] Consequently, hyperhomocysteinemia is thought to be associated with atherogenesis and thrombogenesis. Homocysteine is an amino acid metabolically converted from methionine. This conversion is dependent on folic acid and vitamins B_6 and B_{12}, acting as cofactors. The resting plasma concentrations of vitamins B_6 and B_{12} are lower in cats with cardiomyopathy and in cats with STE than control cats, but resting plasma homocysteine concentration is not lower.[126] However, when challenged with methionine, some normal cats show a clear abnormality in their ability to produce homocysteine, showing a marked elevation in plasma homocysteine concentration after oral methionine administration.[127] This may suggest that some cats have an abnormality in their homocysteine metabolic pathway that could make them more susceptible to thrombosis.

Thromboembolism Once a left atrial thrombus has formed, it can do one of four things: (1) it can remain static, especially if it is lodged in the left auricle; (2) it can dislodge and become an STE; (3) it can grow very large and occlude intracardiac blood flow; or (4) it can be dissolved by the body's thrombolytic system. The incidence of the first and fourth outcomes is unknown, because if a thrombus causes no clinical abnormalities, the thrombus usually goes undetected. If it occludes intracardiac flow, it causes death, and if a postmortem examination is not done, the cause of death is never known. Only the second scenario results in clinical signs for which owners commonly seek medical attention for their pets.

The clinical signs produced depend primarily on the site occluded by the thromboembolus, whether the occlusion is total or partial, and the amount of collateral circulation.

Before they dislodge, most left atrial thrombi apparently become larger than any artery exiting off the aorta. Consequently, blood flow pushes them the length of the aorta to lodge at the aortic trifurcation, where the aorta divides into the two external iliac arteries and the common origin of the internal iliac arteries. Here they obstruct blood flow to the caudal limbs.

Physical obstruction is only a part of the pathophysiology. Experimentally, the terminal aorta has been ligated in an attempt to reproduce the disease.[128,129] Surprisingly, cats with aortic ligation exhibit no pain and walk after surgery, although the femoral pulses are absent and caudal limb blood flow is only 30% of baseline.[130] Slight weakness and hyporeflexia are present, but even these resolve within 72 hours when caudal limb blood flow returns to 90% of baseline. Aortograms in these cats confirm the presence of collateral blood flow through the lumbar vertebral arteries and the cranial and caudal epigastric arteries. The disease can be reproduced, however, if a thrombus is created within the terminal aorta.[129,130] Aortograms from these experimental cats are identical to those from spontaneous clinical cases; both demonstrate very poor collateral flow beyond the region of the thromboembolus. Pretreatment with an anti-serotoninergic agent or with indomethacin prevents the loss of collateral circulation, and serotonin or thromboxane A_2 injection reproduces the clinical situation when injected into a caudal aortic segment.[128,131-133] It is hypothesized that thromboemboli release serotonin and thromboxane A_2, agents present in platelets and known to produce intense vasoconstriction, and disrupt collateral flow.[134] Administering antiserotonin agents (e.g., cyproheptadine) and indomethacin after a thromboembolus is present apparently has no effect.

Clinical Manifestations

History   The majority of cats seen with STE are mixed breed cats.[115,135] Because more severe HCM is seen in males and HCM is the most common feline cardiomyopathy, more male cats are seen with STE. Most cats with STE have heart disease, but up to 90% have no evidence of heart disease prior to developing STE.[115] Consequently, owners often think that their cat has experienced an acute traumatic event. At the onset of STE, the cat may fall off a structure on which it was lying. Often the cat is found unable to walk and vocalizing because of pain.

Physical Examination   Auscultation often reveals a heart murmur or a gallop sound (or both) at presentation.[115] Many cats are in heart failure and so are tachypneic and dyspneic. The rectal temperature is usually reduced.

In cats with a large thromboembolus at the aortic trifurcation, the femoral artery pulses are absent to very weak. Once a thromboembolus lodges in the terminal aorta, ischemic damage to the skeletal muscles and peripheral nerves occurs. The cranial tibial and gastrocnemius muscles are most severely affected and are commonly swollen, turgid, and painful, especially when palpated and the animal has loss of neural reflexes and motor function to the hind limbs (paresis and paralysis). Initially, the ischemic damage to the muscles of the caudal legs results in intense pain. The pain usually subsides as sensory nervous input is lost. The distal portions of the legs are cool and the nail beds are pale or very dark (purple to black). Femoral artery pulses in most cats with STE (78% in one study) are absent upon presentation.[115] In some cats a smaller thromboembolus may lodge in one external iliac artery, resulting in cessation of blood flow to only one leg. In other cats the femoral artery pulses may be weakly present because of recanalization of the aorta. In some cats it is difficult to determine if a pulse is present or not and a false diagnosis of thromboembolism in a cat with neurologic disease is common.[136] A Doppler blood flow detection device is helpful to identify the presence or absence of blood flow. In cats that have no sensation in their distal limbs, a nail can be cut back to the "quick" to determine if active bleeding occurs.

Most aortic thromboemboli lodge terminally in the aorta where they disrupt blood flow to the spinal canal beyond L_5, meaning blood supply to the spinal cord is not disrupted. Instead, perfusion is lost to the cauda equina and the peripheral nerves that originate from this area. Consequently, loss of motor function is due to lower motor neuron disease. Motor function loss to the caudal body is variable. Many cats retain the ability to move their tails. Some cats lose the ability to move their caudal legs starting at the hip, whereas others only lose the ability to move the limbs distal to the stifles or distal to the hock. These latter cats can extend and flex their hips and so "walk" on their stifles. Loss of cutaneous sensation occurs relatively early and follows the pattern of motor loss. The patellar reflex is lost in many cats but remains intact in others. Anal tone and the anal reflex are usually normal. Bladder function is often normal. Some cats may have urine retention, but the bladder can usually be easily emptied by external manual compression. In cats with experimental thrombosis of the terminal aorta, neurologic function (patellar reflex, withdrawal reflex, thigh adduction, digit extension, caudal limb weight bearing, locomotive ability, and cutaneous sensation) to the caudal limbs is completely lost in 80% of cases.[130] The remaining cats have very little residual neurologic function. Presumably the cats seen clinically with some remaining neurologic function must have some collateral flow to explain their neurologic findings. Acute ligation of the aorta in experimental cats, prior to collateral circulation becoming fully developed, produces cessation of blood flow to the distal portion of the caudal limbs, although proximal flow remains apparently normal.[130] This mimics the situation observed in some feline patients that have function remaining in the proximal portion of their caudal limbs.

After the acute embolic event, thrombolysis starts as plasmin is activated. In some cats with a small thromboembolus, thrombolysis is rapid and complete, allowing function to return within hours. In other cats the thromboembolus is large and the thrombolytic activity of the cat is low, resulting in permanent loss of perfusion to the caudal limbs and permanent paralysis. Regions of necrotic skin and muscle (most commonly dry gangrene) often develop, and muscle contracture takes place over time. Between these two extremes are cats that recover function over time with no untoward events and cats that partially recover function but have skin and muscle necrosis develop. The latter cats may require surgery to débride open wounds or amputate toes or parts of limbs. Cats that have complete and lasting occlusion of blood supply to only one limb do very well after limb amputation.

Coagulopathies can occur in cats with STE, although they are usually not severe enough to produce clinical signs.[137] The platelet count is generally within the normal range, and no evidence of fibrin degradation products is seen. Individual clotting factors, however, may be low in certain cases.

Cats with thromboemboli commonly have severe underlying cardiac disease. Acute terminal aortic blockade by the thromboembolus increases afterload to the LV. This can increase left heart filling pressures and resultant pulmonary edema and respiratory distress.[116] The heart failure must be treated appropriately. If pulmonary edema is severe, it worsens the short-term prognosis.

Diagnosis

The diagnosis of STE in cats is usually based on the presence of typical clinical signs described previously in this chapter. However 20% to 30% of cases referred for STE have primary neurologic disease, so it does not appear that a diagnosis based only on clinical signs is accurate. Consequently, some effort should be placed into doing more definitive diagnostic tests in these cats. In most cases, simply cutting a nail back to the "quick" is adequate. Cats without blood flow to the caudal limbs will not have any bleeding from a cut nail, or very dark blood will ooze from the site. A Doppler device can also be used to determine if blood flow to affected limbs is present and if flow is returning to a limb. Imaging of the affected regional vessels by intravenous or intraarterial angiography or nuclear tracers is the definitive diagnostic procedure for thromboembolic disease. Risks to the patient must be considered when contemplating angiography. Stabilizing the patient is the primary consideration before attempting invasive diagnostic procedures. Color flow Doppler imaging of the area may demonstrate lack of or severely compromised flow.

Radiographs reveal cardiomegaly in almost 90% of cats with STE and evidence of heart failure in approximately 50% to 70%.[115,116,135] Most cats (85% in one study) have ECG abnormalities[115] (LV enlargement, conduction system abnormalities, and sinus tachycardia).

Echocardiography is used to identify the underlying cardiac disease. In one study, about 60% of cats had HCM and 25% had unclassified cardiomyopathy, whereas in another study unclassified cardiomyopathy predominated.[115,116]

Clinical Pathology Laboratory abnormalities are common in cats with STE.[115] Most have increases in serum aspartate aminotransferase and alanine aminotransferase concentrations due to muscle necrosis, and serum glucose concentration (stress). Severe increases in serum urea nitrogen and creatinine concentrations may suggest the thromboembolus has lodged in the region of the renal arteries.

Treatment

Euthanasia In cats that are in acute pain that have a poor prognosis due to severe cardiomyopathy, euthanasia is a humane means of dealing with the problem. Systemic thromboembolism is often a horrible complication of cardiomyopathy, the treatment options are all relatively poor, and rethrombosis is common. Consequently, although one should not automatically give up on a patient, one should not give false hope either.

Pain Control Cats that present in pain must be treated appropriately for their pain. Appropriate drugs include a fentanyl patch, oxymorphone (intramuscularly, intravenously, or subcutaneously) and butorphanol tartrate (subcutaneously). Aspirin does not produce adequate pain control. Oxymorphone may produce excitement in some cats. The analgesic properties of butorphanol are five times that of morphine, and it remains a nonscheduled drug by the Food and Drug Administration. Its respiratory depressant effects equal that of morphine. Consequently, one must be careful when administering this drug to a patient with dyspnea. Acepromazine may be administered intravenously in addition as an anxiolytic agent to cats that still appear distressed after the administration of the analgesic or to cats that become agitated after oxymorphone administration. The pain abates with time (usually hours) as sensory nerves undergo necrosis.

Palliative Therapy Beyond pain control, many cats with STE receive only supportive care or the administration of drugs with no proven benefit. The primary outcome of arterial occlusion depends upon the extent of occlusion and the time to spontaneous reperfusion. Poor prognostic factors for short-term survival include worsening azotemia, moderate to severe pulmonary edema or pleural effusion, malignant arrhythmias, severe hypothermia, disseminated intravascular coagulation, and evidence of multiorgan embolization. Long-term, cats may lose an affected leg because of ischemic necrosis, die of toxemia, remain paralyzed from peripheral nerve damage, or

regain full or partial function of their legs. About 50% of cats that are not treated definitively will regain all or most caudal limb motor function within 1 to 6 weeks.[116,138] Return of function presumably is due to the cat's own thrombolytic system (e.g., plasmin) disrupting the thromboembolus. The degree and rapidity of the dissolution depend on the activity of a particular cat's thrombolytic system and the size and quality of the thromboembolus. Usually, cats that have some evidence of caudal limb flow recover more rapidly than do cats with no evidence of flow. Presumably this is because the size of the thromboembolus in cats with some flow is smaller. With total occlusion, some cats recanalize within days (others never recanalize). This extreme variability makes it very difficult to render a prognosis for a particular patient at presentation.

Palliative therapy may be only cage rest and pain control or can include administering drugs such as heparin, aspirin, or arteriolar dilators along with the cage rest. No drugs administered for palliation have any proven benefit over cage rest alone.

Heparin is commonly administered in the hopes of preventing new thrombus formation on top of the existing thromboembolus or in the hope of preventing a new thrombus from forming in the left atrium. However, no evidence indicates that heparin is of benefit in cats with STE. Heparin does not aid in thrombolysis. Heparin can be administered at an initial dose of 100 U/lb intravenously followed by a maintenance dose of 30 to 100 U/lb subcutaneously every 6 hours. The dose should be tailored to each individual cat to increase the activated partial thromboplastin time (aPTT) to at least 1.5 times baseline.

Indomethacin is effective at preventing vasoconstriction distal to the thromboembolus when administered to experimental cats prior to creating an aortic thrombus.[139] Theoretically aspirin could do the same thing. However, no evidence indicates that it improves collateral blood flow.

The administration of drugs that dilate systemic arterioles (e.g., hydralazine, acepromazine) has been advocated. These drugs act by relaxing the smooth muscle in systemic arterioles. The exact anatomy of collateral vessels is not well described, but they are probably larger vessels than arterioles. They contain smooth muscle, because they can open and close. The ability of arteriolar dilators to counteract serotonin and thromboxane A_2-induced vasoconstriction is unknown.

Definitive Therapy Definitive treatments for STE in cats include administration of exogenous fibrinolytic agents, balloon embolectomy, rheolytic thrombectomy, and surgery. All definitive procedures are associated with high mortality and common recurrence of the thromboembolus days to months after the initial removal.

Surgery Surgical removal of systemic thromboemboli is generally thought to be associated with high mortality and is not frequently performed. Cats with STE commonly have underlying cardiac disease, and many are in heart failure. They are poor anesthetic risks, and reperfusion syndrome may be produced. In reperfusion syndrome the muscles of the legs prior to removal of the STE undergo necrosis, cellular breakdown, and the release of potassium and hydrogen ions from the cells into the interstitial spaces. Sudden reperfusion carries these ions into the systemic circulation, causing acute and often severe hyperkalemia and metabolic acidosis. Surgical intervention may be a viable option if careful monitoring and treatment for reperfusion syndrome with insulin and glucose, sodium bicarbonate, or calcium (or a combination of these therapies) can be initiated immediately if it occurs.

Balloon embolectomy The procedure of choice in human medicine is balloon embolectomy.[140] The author has had limited experience with balloon embolectomy. In this procedure the femoral arteries are isolated and a small balloon embolectomy catheter is passed from one femoral artery into the aorta. The femoral arteries are not extremely difficult to isolate. The catheter is pushed past the thromboembolus, and the balloon is then inflated and the catheter withdrawn, along with thromboembolic material. The catheter is passed sequentially, first in one artery and then in the other. Usually this sequence must be repeated several times. Reperfusion syndrome may occur with balloon embolectomy.

Thrombolytic therapy   Thrombolytic therapy is a possible means of dealing with cats with STE using fibrinolytic agents. Thromboemboli in cats are composed of red cells, strands of fibrin, and possibly platelets. Fibrinolytic agents cleave plasminogen to plasmin. Plasmin hydrolyzes fibrin, resulting in thrombolysis. Different agents vary in their ability to bind specifically to fibrin-bound plasminogen and in their half-lives. Efficacy and complication rates appear to be very similar in humans.[141] Complications consist primarily of hemorrhage due to fibrinolysis and rethrombosis. Fibrinolytic agents can be very effective at lysing systemic thromboemboli. However, the author and colleagues currently treat few cats with STE with these agents because reperfusion syndrome and rethrombosis are common.

Tissue plasminogen activator (t-PA) and streptokinase have been used in cats. Tissue plasminogen activator is an intrinsic protein present in all mammals. Numerous reports exist of the use of t-PA for the lysis of thrombi as therapy for acute myocardial infarction, pulmonary thromboembolism, and peripheral vascular obstruction in humans and experimental animals.[141] The activity of genetically engineered t-PA in feline plasma is 90% to 100% of that seen in human plasma. The half-life of t-PA is quite short. Heparin must be administered concomitantly to prevent acute rethrombosis but does not need to be administered with streptokinase because it has a longer half-life. A clinical trial with t-PA in cats with aortic thromboemboli has shown acute thrombolytic efficacy (shortened time to reperfusion and ambulation) associated with the administration of t-PA at a rate of 0.1 mg to 0.4 mg/lb/hr for a total dose of 0.4 to 4 mg/lb intravenously.[142] Forty three percent of cats treated survived therapy and were walking within 48 hours of presentation. Post-t-PA angiograms demonstrated resolution of the primary vascular occlusion. Thus acutely, t-PA effectively decreases the time to reperfusion and return to function in cats with aortic thromboemboli. However, 50% of the cats died during therapy in this clinical trial, which raises extreme concerns regarding acute thrombolysis. Fatalities resulted from reperfusion syndrome (70%), CHF (15%), and sudden arrhythmic death, presumably the result of embolization of a small thrombus to a coronary artery (15%). Severe hemorrhage into the region distal to the STE causing anemia was also a common complication. The cats that successfully completed t-PA therapy exhibited signs of increasing neuromuscular function and ambulatory ability within 2 days of presentation. This contrasts with 1 to 6 weeks before seeing similar signs of improvement in most cats exhibiting spontaneous resolution.

Mortality due to reperfusion syndrome can be reduced if the patient can be observed continuously by an individual trained to identify clinical and electrocardiographic evidence of hyperkalemia, if intensive monitoring of electrolytes and blood pH can be performed, and if aggressive medical therapy for hyperkalemia and metabolic acidosis can be initiated very quickly. This means dedicated care 24 hours a day until the thromboembolus is lysed. Thrombolysis may occur within 3 hours or take as long as 48 hours.

If reperfusion syndrome was the only major complicating factor in cats treated with thrombolytic agents, continued use in selected patients might be warranted. However, 90% of the cats that were successfully treated in the aforementioned clinical trial

had another STE within 1 to 3 months. Rethromboembolism occurred despite aspirin, warfarin, or heparin administration. In addition, t-PA is expensive. Consequently, the author does not currently use t-PA for STE in cats.

Streptokinase has clinical efficacy very similar to t-PA in human patients with coronary artery thrombosis.[143] Streptokinase is less expensive. No controlled clinical trials of streptokinase use for STE in cats are available, and the author's clinical experience with the drug has been generally negative. There has been one small experimental study in which thrombin was injected between two ligatures placed at the terminal aorta to create a soft thrombus, followed by removal of the ligatures.[144] Streptokinase was administered as a loading dose at 90,000 IU followed by 45,000 IU/hr for 3 hours. This dose produced evidence of systemic fibrinolysis in a separate group of normal cats but without evidence of severe fibrinolysis or bleeding. In most cats there was no angiographic change and no improvement in limb temperature. There was a tendency for the thrombus weight to be lower in the treated cats when compared with control cats at postmortem examination. However, lysis of a fresh thrombus created with thrombin is probably much different from trying to lyse an established thromboembolus. Streptokinase is usually unsuccessful, may hasten the death of some cats through bleeding complications, and should not be routinely used.

Rheolytic thrombectomy   Rheolytic thrombectomy is an experimental catheter-based system used for the dissolution of the thromboembolus using a high-velocity water jet at the end of the catheter that breaks up the thromboembolus and sucks it back into the system using the Venturi effect. Anesthesia is required and blood transfusion is almost always needed. The catheter is passed from the carotid artery to the region of the thromboembolus. The author and colleagues have used it in six cats. The procedure successfully removed the thromboembolus in five cats but only three left the hospital (Figure 204-18). Time from onset of clinical signs to thrombectomy was several hours to 8 days. The cat that had the procedure 8 days after the event had residual neurologic deficits but was the longest survivor. Interestingly, reperfusion syndrome has not been a common complication.

Adjunctive therapy   Cats with STE are commonly in heart failure at the time of presentation.[116] Medical therapy with furosemide and an ACE inhibitor is often indicated. Cats that are in pain usually do not eat or drink. Fluid therapy is warranted but must not aggravate or produce heart failure.

Cats that take a long time to recover caudal limb function or that only attain partial function may develop regions of skin and muscle necrosis, especially on the distal limbs. These regions may need to be débrided surgically. Cats that lose the function of only one leg or that do not regain function of one leg benefit from amputating that leg. Cats that have permanently lost muscle function distal to the hock may benefit from arthrodesis.

Prognosis   The short-term prognosis for life is guarded in cats without heart failure. Cats with a rectal temperature lower than 98.9° F had a worse prognosis in one study.[116] The long-term prognosis is highly variable and depends on the ability to control the heart failure and the events surrounding the STE. One of the most common causes of death within the first 24 hours is euthanasia.[135] In one study, cats lived between 3 and 30 months after the initial episode.[115] The average survival time was about 10 to 12 months. In another study, MST for cats that recovered and were discharged from the hospital was approximately 4 months but was only about 2.5 months in cats that were also being treated for heart failure.[116] The long-term prognosis for limb function depends on the ability

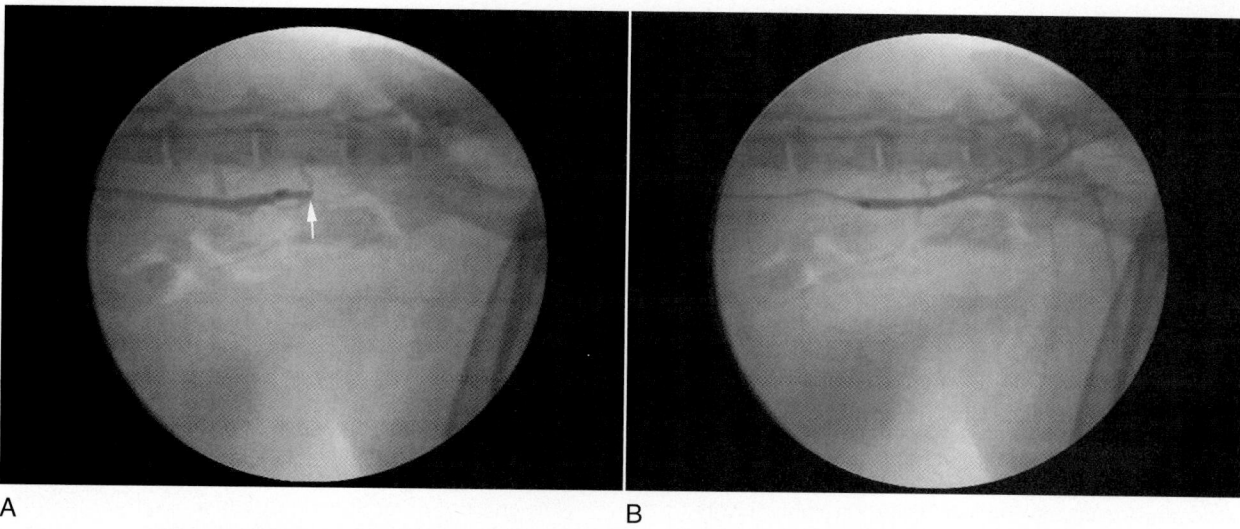

A   B

Figure 204-18 **A,** Angiogram of the aorta from a cat with a thromboembolus lodged in its terminal aorta. Contrast can be visualized in the aorta to the level of middle of the sixth lumbar vertebra where it abruptly terminates *(arrow)*. No blood flow is demonstrated past that point. **B,** An angiogram from the same cat after rheolytic thrombectomy. The thromboembolus has been removed. The tip of a catheter can be seen at the junction of the fifth and sixth lumbar vertebrae. Beyond that point the contrast agent outlines the normal blood flow pattern to the caudal limbs.

of the cat to lyse its own clot or on the success of intervention. Many biologic variables determine whether or not reperfusion will spontaneously occur. A significant percentage of cats will develop a new thromboembolus, days to months after recovery.

Prophylaxis Feline patients with myocardial disease, especially those with an enlarged left atrium, should be considered at risk for developing intracardiac thrombi and signs of peripheral arterial thromboembolism, although the incidence appears to be low. Preventing peripheral thrombosis is, in theory, one of the most important therapeutic objectives for the veterinarian managing cats with severe myocardial disease. The ideal means of preventing thrombosis is resolution of the underlying myocardial disease. This is usually only possible in a cat with DCM secondary to taurine deficiency.

At present, the only option available is to manipulate the patient's coagulation system in an attempt to alter the delicate balance between the pathways that promote clotting and those that inhibit thrombus formation to reduce the patient's thrombogenic potential. At this time, antiplatelet and anticoagulant therapies are the only means of preventing thrombus formation in cats with myocardial disease. Unfortunately, they are often ineffective and, in the case of warfarin, can produce serious side effects.[145] Experience is similar in human medicine.[146]

Antiplatelet therapy Prostaglandins enhance platelet aggregation via activation of cyclic adenosine monophosphate (cAMP). Aspirin (acetylsalicylic acid) acetylates platelet cyclooxygenase, preventing the formation of thromboxane A_2, a potent prostaglandin-like platelet aggregating substance.[147] The inhibition of platelet cyclooxygenase is irreversible, and bleeding time is restored to normal only after the production of new platelets. The inhibition of endothelial cyclooxygenase is reversible. The dose of aspirin recommended in cats is 10 mg/lb every third day. Whether or not this dose allows endothelial cyclooxygenase to recover or not in cats is undetermined. At this dose, aspirin has a half-life of 45 hours in the cat. In humans, doses as low as 20 to 100 mg/day inhibit platelet cyclooxygenase; however, no evidence suggests that this low

dose has any more benefit than conventional daily doses of 625 to 1250 mg. In one study in cats, no difference was seen in thromboembolus recurrence between cats on low dose (5 mg/cat every 72 hours) and high dose (greater than or equal to 40 mg/cat every 72 hours).[116] No evidence indicates that any dose of aspirin is effective at preventing the formation of an intracardiac thrombus in cats with myocardial disease. Clinical impression of aspirin's efficacy varies between clinicians. Cats that have already experienced one STE are the only appropriate population in which to study the efficacy of an agent meant to prevent STE. Aspirin does not prevent recurrence of peripheral thromboembolism in this population.

Glycoprotein IIb and IIIa, an integrin present on platelet surfaces, is a receptor for fibrinogen, fibronectin, and von Willebrand factor. It mediates aggregation, adhesion, and spreading of platelets. The binding of prothrombin to glycoprotein IIb and IIIa also enhances the conversion of prothrombin to thrombin. Glycoprotein IIb and IIIa antagonists have been developed, and one (abciximab) increased mucosal bleeding time and reduced thrombus area when combined with aspirin (when compared with aspirin and placebo).[148]

Anticoagulant therapy Available anticoagulants include heparin, the low molecular weight heparins, and warfarin. Heparin binds to a lysine site on AT, producing a conformational change at the arginine-reactive site that converts AT from a slow, progressive thrombin inhibitor to a very rapid inhibitor of thrombin and factor Xa. AT binds covalently to the active serine centers of coagulation enzymes.[150] Factor Xa bound to platelets and thrombin bound to fibrin are protected from activation by the heparin-antithrombin III complex.[147] Heparin may be administered intravenously or subcutaneously. Repeated intramuscular injection is discouraged because local hemorrhage may result. Some owners can administer heparin subcutaneously at home but the method is not ideal. The author and colleagues have noted rethrombosis with heparin therapy in some cats with cardiac disease. The dose of heparin for preventing thrombosis in cats is unknown.

Low molecular weight heparins include nadroparin calcium, enoxaparin sodium, dalteparin, ardeparin, tinzaparin, reviparin, and danaparoid sodium. The low molecular weight heparins have fewer bleeding complications in experimental animals, improved pharmacokinetics over heparin, are administered subcutaneously, and do not require monitoring in most situations.[150] Although heparin does not reduce red cell aggregation in slow-moving blood, heparin and low molecular weight heparins are effective at preventing deep vein thrombosis in humans. Consequently, they may be beneficial in preventing intracardiac thrombus formation in cats with cardiomyopathy. No controlled studies are available. The author empirically uses enoxaparin sodium at a dose of 2.2 mg/lb every 12 hours subcutaneously in cats that have recovered from an STE or that have a severely enlarged left atrium and SEC.

Warfarin sodium is an oral anticoagulant (see Chapter 199).[147] Warfarin exerts no anticoagulant effect in vitro. In vivo, inhibitory effects on synthesis of clotting factors begin immediately. However, clotting is unaffected until already existing clotting factors decline. Therefore a delay occurs between initial administration and effect on the prothrombin time (PT). Historically, oral warfarin therapy has been monitored with the PT. This test measures the activity of factors II, VII, and X. The factor depressed most quickly and profoundly (usually factor VII) determines the PT during the initial days of therapy. The PT is performed by measuring the clotting time of platelet-poor plasma after the addition of thromboplastin and calcium, a combination of tissue factor and phospholipid.[151] Intra- and interlaboratory variation in the PT was a significant problem for laboratories in the past, when crude extracts of human placenta or rabbit brain were the only source of thromboplastin. The international normalized ratio (INR), developed by the WHO in the early 1980s, is designed to eliminate problems in oral anticoagulant therapy caused by variability in the sensitivity of different commercial sources and different lots of thromboplastin. The INR is used worldwide by most laboratories performing oral anticoagulation monitoring and is routinely incorporated into dose planning for human patients receiving warfarin. When the anticoagulant effect is excessive, it can be counteracted by administering vitamin K_1. However, once synthesis of factors II, VII, IX, and X is reinstituted, time must elapse before factors achieve concentrations in the plasma that will adequately reverse the bleeding tendency. If serious bleeding occurs during therapy with warfarin, it may be stopped immediately by administering fresh blood or plasma that contains the missing clotting factors. Other drugs can modify the anticoagulant actions of warfarin by altering the bioavailability of vitamin K by altering the absorption, distribution, or elimination of the coumarins; by affecting synthesis or degradation of clotting factors; or by altering protein binding of the warfarin.[152] The maintenance dose should be evaluated daily during the initial titration (3 days), then every other day (twice), and then weekly until a safe and stable dose regimen is determined. The therapeutic effect should be reevaluated periodically (at least once per month). The recommended initial dose is 0.1 to 0.2 mg per cat every 24 hours orally to a 6 to 10 lb/cat. The dose may then be increased to maintain an INR of 2.0 to 3.0. It can take up to 1 week for new steady state conditions to be achieved.

The efficacy of warfarin at preventing recurrent thrombosis in cats with cardiac disease has been reported.[114,115] In one report, out of 23 cats examined retrospectively, 10 experienced a new thromboembolic episode while being administered warfarin. Two of these cats had at least two new episodes. In the other report, eight of 18 cats on warfarin experienced a new thromboembolic episode. This may be some improvement over the 75% recurrence rate reported for aspirin alone after t-PA therapy, but these results are still disappointing.[136] In the first report, four cases also died suddenly (which could have been caused by thromboembolism). Three of these cats did not have postmortem examinations. The one cat that did have a postmortem examination had a thrombus present in its left atrium. One cat also died of a renal infarct that produced renal failure. Four cats appeared to have bleeding complications. In the second report, one cat died of a hemoabdomen and one was suspected to have an acute intracranial hemorrhage resulting in death. Consequently, it appears that warfarin therapy can produce fatal complications. However, it should be noted that these studies were performed without using the INR for monitoring.

CHAPTER • 205

Pericardial Disorders

Anthony H. Tobias

Pericardial disorders have previously been reported to account for approximately 1% of cardiac disease in small animals.[1] More recent reports estimate that pericardial disorders comprise approximately 8% of the canine cardiology caseload at referral institutions. Pericardial disorders occur slightly less frequently in cats, but the prevalence remains fairly high at 6% of the feline cardiology caseload. In contrast to dogs, pericardial disorders in cats are usually found as incidental manifestations of underlying disease, rather than as the primary cause for the presenting signs.[2]

Pericardial disorders are emerging as increasingly common and important in small animal practice. The presenting signs associated with pericardial disorders are diverse, and the clinical findings are often subtle. Consequently the prevalence of pericardial disorders may previously have been underestimated, especially before the widespread use of echocardiography. Alternately or coincidentally the increased prevalence may reflect a change in the epidemiology of pericardial disorders over time, possibly associated with increased popularity of breeds that are predisposed to pericardial disorders, such as the golden retriever.

STRUCTURE AND FUNCTION

The pericardium is the fibroserous envelope of the heart. It is divided into an outer fibrous and inner serous part. The serous pericardium consists of a parietal and visceral layer.[3]

The fibrous pericardium is a thin tough sac that contains the heart, serous pericardium, and a small amount of fluid. The base of the fibrous pericardium is continued on the great arteries and veins that leave and enter the heart and blends with the adventitia of these vessels. The apex of the fibrous pericardium is continued to the ventral part of the diaphragm as the phrenico- or sternopericardical ligament.[3]

The serous pericardium is a closed sac, approximately half of which is invaginated by the heart. The invaginated portion forms the visceral layer of the serous pericardium or the epicardium. It is firmly attached to the heart muscle, except along the grooves that contain fat and the coronary vessels. The epicardium has a smooth mesothelial surface that is underlaid by a stroma containing elastic fibers. The noninvaginated part or parietal layer of the serous pericardium forms the inner surface of the fibrous pericardium. It is composed of interlacing collagen fibers that blend with the tissue of the fibrous pericardium on one side and a layer of mesothelium on the other. The pericardial space that occurs between the two layers of the serous pericardium contains a small amount of clear light-yellow fluid. The normal amount of pericardial fluid in the dog has been reported as 0.3 to 1.0 mL, and 0.25 ± 0.15 mL per kg.[3,4]

The vagus, recurrent laryngeal, and phrenic nerves pass over the outer surface of the pericardium. The pericardium is innervated by fibers from the vagus, recurrent laryngeal nerve, and various intrathoracic ganglia and plexi. Blood supply is derived from the pericardial branches of the aorta and internal thoracic and musculophrenic arteries.[5] Lymphatic drainage of the pericardial space occurs via the coronary lymphatic ducts to the cardiac and mediastinal lymph nodes and via the left and right parasternal lymphatic ducts to the cranial sternal lymph node.[6]

The physiologic significance of the pericardium remains speculative. Functions attributed to the pericardium include preventing overdilation of the heart, protecting the heart from infection and forming adhesions to surrounding tissue, maintaining the heart in a fixed position within the chest, regulating the interrelationship between stroke volumes of the two ventricles, and preventing tricuspid regurgitation when ventricular diastolic pressures are increased. In addition, the lubricant effect of pericardial fluid allows the heart to move easily within the pericardial sac during systole and diastole.[5] However, it is clear that the pericardium serves no vital function because it can be removed surgically when diseased without untoward effect.

CONGENITAL PERICARDIAL DISORDERS

Congenital pericardial disorders include pericardioperitoneal diaphragmatic hernia (PPDH), benign intrapericardial cysts, and pericardial defects. Congenital pericardial disorders are much less common than those that are acquired. However, they represent an important group because they are frequently amendable to surgical correction and, consequently, generally confer an excellent prognosis.

Pericardioperitoneal Diaphragmatic Hernia

A PPDH exists when a defect in the ventral diaphragm and pericardium allows abdominal contents to enter the pericardial space. Herniated structures include liver, gall bladder, spleen, stomach, small intestine, omentum, and falciform ligament. In the dog and cat the defect is congenital, whereas in humans, the diaphragm forms one wall of the pericardial sac and PPDH can be traumatic. The diaphragm does not form part of the pericardium in small animals, and traumatic PPDH has not been reported in either the dog or cat.[7,8]

Pathophysiology In the developing embryo, the diaphragm forms from four structures: (1) the septum transversum, (2) the mesesophagus (or caudal mediastinum), (3) a pair of pleuroperitoneal folds or membranes, and (4) tissue from the body wall (Figure 205-1). The septum transversum, a thick plate of ventrally located mesodermal tissue, partially separates the thoracic and abdominal cavities. It fuses with the mesesophagus, which is located dorsomedially. The aorta, esophagus, and the caudal vena cava pass through the mesesophagus. The pleural and peritoneal cavities communicate on either side of the mesesophagus via the right and left pleuroperitoneal canals. Closure of the pleuroperitoneal canals occurs via formation of the pleuroperitoneal folds or membranes, which expand and fuse with the septum transversum ventrally and with the mesesophagus medially. Finally, as the thoracic cage enlarges during fetal growth, tissue from the body wall becomes incorporated circumferentially into the diaphragm.[9-11]

Several theories for the formation of PPDH have been proposed, including failure of complete fusion of the pleuroperitoneal membranes with the septum transversum or mesesophagus.[12] However, defects in that location result in congenital diaphragmatic hernias or communications between the pleural and peritoneal spaces. Congenital diaphragmatic

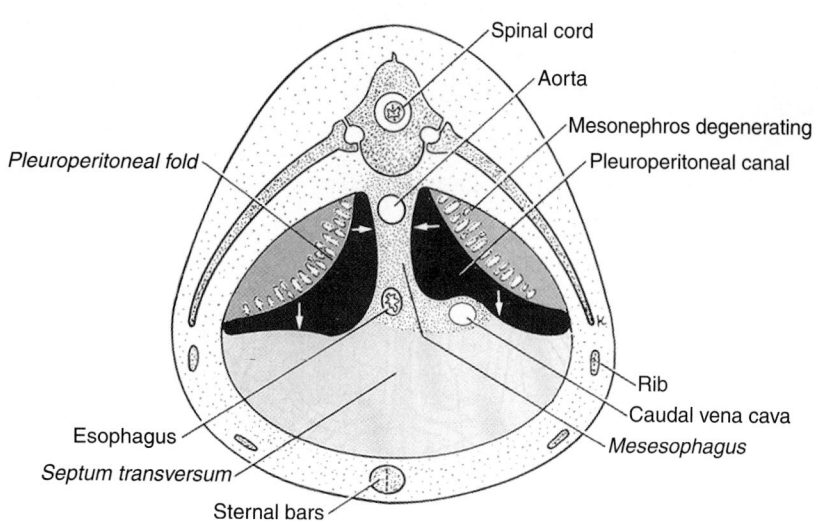

Figure 205-1 Diagram of the caudal surface of the developing diaphragm. Major structures involved in the formation of the diaphragm are in italics. *Septum transversum* forms the ventral half of the diaphragm and fuses dorsomedially with the *mesesophagus. Pleuroperitoneal folds* or membranes extend ventrally and medially *(arrows)* to close pleuroperitoneal canals by fusing with septum transversum and mesesophagus. A pericardioperitoneal diaphragmatic hernia develops as a result of a defect in the ventral portion of the septum transversum. (From King AS: The Cardiorespiratory System. Integration of Normal and Pathological Structure and Function. Oxford, Blackwell Science, 1999, pp 178-217. With permission.)

Labels in figure: Spinal cord; Aorta; Mesonephros degenerating; Pleuroperitoneal canal; Rib; Caudal vena cava; *Mesesophagus*; Sternal bars; *Septum transversum*; Esophagus; *Pleuroperitoneal fold*

hernias are among the most common congenital malformations in humans,[11] but they are rare in small animals.[9,10] In small animals with PPDH, communication between the peritoneal and pericardial space occurs via the ventral portion of the diaphragm, and the following pathogenesis has been proposed: the liver arises as a large ventral outgrowth from the foregut ectoderm, and it grows cranioventrally and penetrates the septum transversum.[9-11] Hematopoietic cells, Kupffer cells, and connective tissue of the liver are all derived from the septum transversum.[13] As the liver develops, it distracts from the septum transversum, forming the ventral mesentery that eventually becomes the falciform ligament. If separation between the developing liver and septum transversum is defective, an opening in the ventral part of the diaphragm may occur or the tissue may be so thin that it ruptures, allowing the peritoneal and pericardial cavities to communicate. Abdominal organs may then pass through the defect directly into the pericardial, space resulting in a PPDH.[9,10]

Epidemiology Whereas PPDH is the most common congenital pericardial anomaly in small animals, it is an uncommon diagnosis. The veterinary medical data base (VMDB) at Purdue University from January 1992 to April 2003 included 62 cats with PPDH among 114,826 new cases, giving a prevalence rate of 0.054%, or one case for every 1852 cats in the data base. Fifty three percent were diagnosed in cats 4 years of age or less, and 16% were first diagnosed in cats 10 years of age or older. The cases in the VMDB disclosed no apparent sex predisposition (35 males:27 females). The majority of affected cases were domestic long- or shorthairs (n = 35). The most commonly affected purebred cats were Himalayans (n = 11). Persians were the second most common purebred cats in the data base (n = 7), and this breed may be predisposed to PPDH.[8] A pattern of inheritance of PPDH in cats has not been established, but congenital agenesis of all or part of the diaphragm in cats is reported to have an autosomal recessive mode of inheritance.[14]

PPDH is less prevalent among dogs than cats. The VMDB from January 1992 to April 2003 included 76 dogs with a PPDH among 399,195 new cases, giving a prevalence rate of 0.019%, or one case for every 5263 dogs in the data base. The diagnosis was most common in younger dogs, with 65% of cases diagnosed in dogs 4 years of age or younger. As in cats, no sex predisposition was apparent (40 males:33 females [the sex of three dogs was not reported]). Most cases were in mixed breed dogs (n = 12). Among purebred dogs, weimaraners were most commonly affected (n = 7), and this breed appears to be predisposed.[12]

Presenting and Clinical Signs Presenting and clinical signs vary depending on the herniated organ, organs, or tissue. Some affected animals show no clinical signs, and PPDH is an incidental finding. In symptomatic animals, signs referable to the respiratory and gastrointestinal (GI) systems predominate. Tachypnea, respiratory distress, vomiting, and anorexia are common.[8,15] Other presenting complaints include lethargy, weight loss, diarrhea, and coughing. On physical examination, the apex beat may be absent or displaced, and heart sounds are frequently muffled. Some cases have a fever. Additional associated abnormalities in dogs are commonly reported and include sternal malformations (incomplete xiphoid; pectus excavatum; and absent, deformed, and fused sternebrae), ventral abdominal hernias, and other congenital heart defects (pulmonic stenosis, ventricular septal defect).[12,16] Associated abnormalities in cats are less common and are usually limited to sternal malformations and ventral abdominal hernias.[8,12,17] A PPDH should be suspected in any animal with a large umbilical or cranial abdominal hernia, sternal malformation, or history of abdominal hernia repair.[18,19]

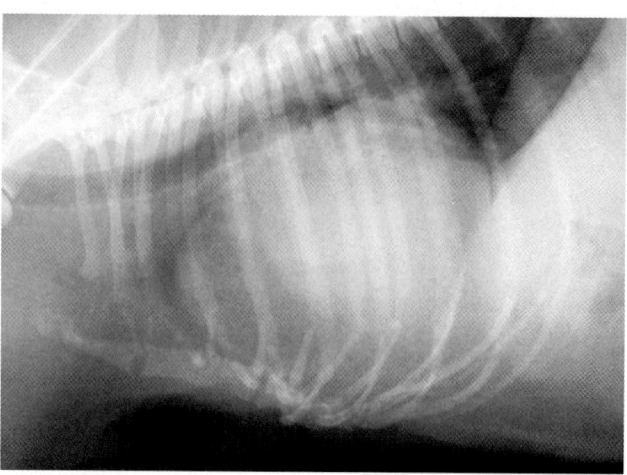

Figure 205-2 Lateral thoracic radiograph of a dog with a pericardioperitoneal diaphragmatic hernia showing an enlarged cardiac silhouette that contains differential opacities and missing and deformed sternebrae.

Diagnosis Radiographic findings that support a diagnosis of PPDH include enlargement of the cardiac silhouette with dorsal displacement of trachea, overlapping of the diaphragmatic and caudal cardiac silhouette borders, and sternal malformations. Signs of left-sided congestive heart failure (CHF) are absent. The cardiac silhouette often contains differential opacities and gas-filled bowel loops (Figure 205-2). A radiographic feature of PPDH that has been described in cats is the presence of a dorsal peritoneopericardial mesothelial remnant. The dorsal peritoneopericardial mesothelial remnant represents the dorsal border of the hernia, and it is recognized in the lateral view as a curvilinear opacity between the cardiac silhouette and the diaphragm ventral to or superimposed over the caudal vena cava. The hepatic silhouette may be smaller than normal or absent in the anterior abdomen (Figure 205-3).[12,17] Positive and negative contrast peritoneography and GI contrast studies are occasionally necessary to confirm the presence of a PPDH.

Electrocardiograms in cases with PPDH may be normal or show low-voltage complexes and abnormal orientation of the mean electrical axis.[8] Echocardiography readily discloses the presence of abdominal viscera within the pericardial sac.[7] Pericardial effusion is present in some cases.[7,8] In cats the liver is the most commonly herniated organ, and focal hyperechoic areas are frequently seen within the herniated liver lobe or lobes (Figure 205-4). Myelolipomas, nodules composed of mature adipose tissue and bone marrow elements, have been reported within herniated liver in cats. These nodules originate as metaplastic change resulting from chronic hypoxia caused by incarceration of liver.[7,20,21] The presence of myelolipomas, or nodular myelomatosis, probably accounts for the focal areas of hyperechogenicity seen within herniated liver lobes.[7]

Treatment Surgical repair is necessary for all cases with PPDH that show clinical signs ascribable to the defect. Repair is also recommended in all young animals with PPDH, whether symptomatic or not. Resection of devitalized herniated tissue is frequently necessary. The prognosis with surgery is generally excellent. In older animals, adhesions between herniated organs and the pericardium that complicate or preclude reduction of the hernia may be present.[15] Consequently, in an asymptomatic older animal in which PPDH is detected as an incidental finding, and especially in those cases where the hernia includes

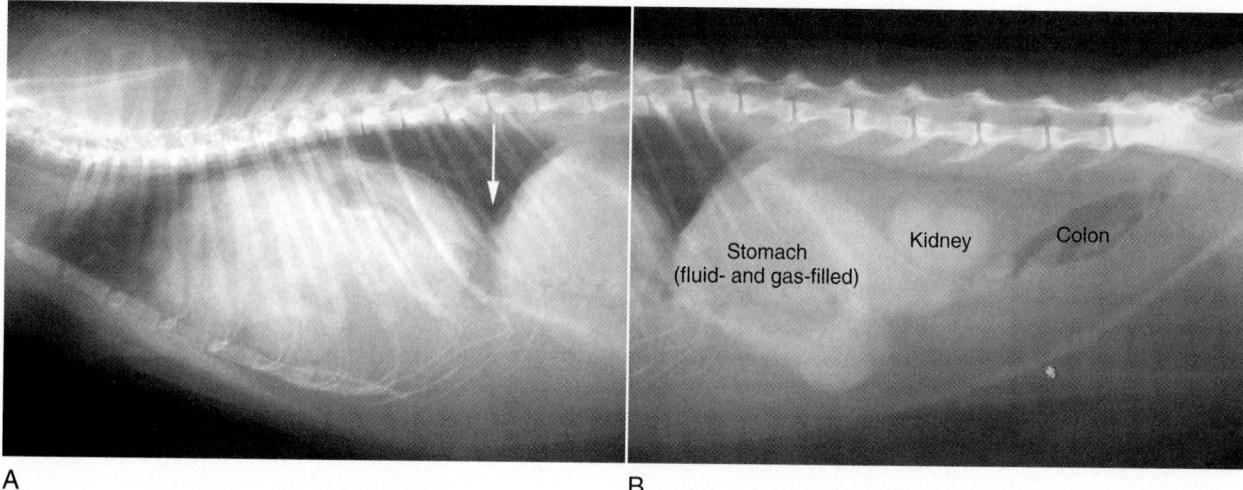

Figure 205-3 Lateral thoracic and abdominal radiographs of a cat with a pericardioperitoneal diaphragmatic hernia. **A,** Markedly enlarged cardiac silhouette that contains differential opacities and gas-filled bowel loops. The curvilinear opacity between the diaphragm and cardiac silhouette *(arrow)* is the dorsal margin of the hernia or the dorsal pericardioperitoneal mesothelial remnant. **B,** Most of the abdominal contents, including the liver and small intestines, are displaced into the pericardial sac.

only omentum or falciform fat, it may be prudent to recommend observation rather than surgical repair.

Benign Intrapericardial Cysts

Large benign intrapericardial cysts occur occasionally in dogs. In virtually all cases, histopathology discloses that the cysts are encapsulated adipose tissue (with extensive hemorrhage and necrosis) or organizing cystic hematomas. True congenital pericardial cysts in humans are endothelium-, epithelium-, or mesothelium-lined, depending on their origin. These are extremely rare in dogs[22,23] and have not been described in cats. Clinical signs in affected dogs include abdominal distention, exercise intolerance, anorexia, and labored breathing.

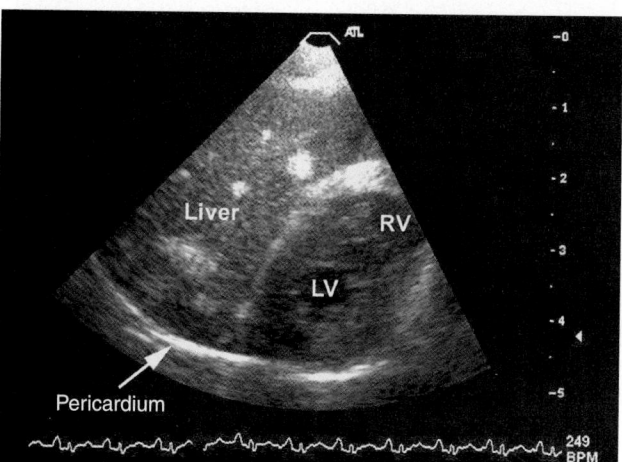

Figure 205-4 Echocardiogram (short axis view from the right parasternal location) from cat with a pericardioperitoneal diaphragmatic hernia. Liver is present within pericardial sac adjacent to caudal aspect and right side of heart. The focal areas of hyperechogenicity within the liver parenchyma are probably due to myelolipomas. *LV,* Left ventricle; *RV,* right ventricle.

The intrapericardial cysts are demonstrated by echocardiography, and most cases have concomitant pericardial effusion. In some cases, benign intrapericardial cysts are associated with a small PPDH. In others the cyst is attached by a pedicle to the apex of the pericardium. In such cases the cyst is thought to represent prenatal herniation of omentum or falciform fat from the peritoneum into the pericardium and subsequent closure of a PPDH. Cyst formation probably results from vascular obstruction of the herniated tissue or repeated trauma from the beating heart.[19,22] Intrapericardial hepatic cysts have been described in cats with PPDH as a result of incarceration of portions of the liver.[24,25] Benign intrapericardial cysts are treated by surgical removal of the cyst and its associated pedicle, pericardiectomy, and PPDH repair when necessary.

Pericardial Defects

Pericardial defects are very rare in dogs and are usually found incidentally on postmortem examination. Some of these defects are thought to be congenital. In a series of eight cases, single defects were present in four dogs, with up to four defects in the remaining dogs. The defects ranged in size from a single 10×5 mm hole to total absence of one side of the pericardium. The defects were on the left side in four dogs, on the right side in two, and on both sides in two.[26] Herniation and incarceration of cardiac chambers through pericardial defects has been reported.[26-28]

ACQUIRED PERICARDIAL DISORDERS

Pericardial Effusion

The most common pericardial disorders in small animals are associated with abnormal accumulations of pericardial fluid or pericardial effusions. At the Veterinary Hospital, University of Pennsylvania from 1990 to 1993, pericardial effusion was present in 7% of dogs with reliable signs of heart disease.[29] At the University of Minnesota Veterinary Medical Center (UMVMC) from January 1999 to December 2001, pericardial effusion was confirmed as the primary cause for clinical signs in 87 of 20,282 new canine cases that were presented to the small animal hospital. This reflects a prevalence rate of 0.43%, or one dog with clinically significant pericardial effusion among every 233 new hospital cases. Thus pericardial effusion is fairly common in the canine patient population at referral hospitals.

Pathophysiology of Pericardial Effusion: Cardiac Tamponade

Cardiac tamponade is defined as significant compression of the heart by accumulating pericardial contents. *Significant compression* depends on whether tamponade is approached from a physiologic or clinical standpoint. Tamponade is a pathophysiologic continuum, not an all-or-none phenomenon. Physiologic abnormalities can be detected with very small amounts of pericardial effusion, although affected cases may show only mild clinical signs (mild tamponade). At the opposite end of the spectrum, acute accumulations of even small amounts of effusion can result in life-threatening hemodynamic compromise (florid tamponade).[30] The classic clinical hemodynamic profile of tamponade includes pulsus paradoxus, elevation and equilibration of right and left ventricular diastolic pressure with pericardial pressure, and depressed cardiac output.[31]

The major pathophysiologic abnormality associated with increased intrapericardial pressure is impaired ventricular filling in diastole, resulting inevitably in diminished stroke volume. For each cardiac chamber, transmural pressure (intracardiac pressure minus intrapericardial pressure) is a principle determinant of its filling. Mean atrial pressure and ventricular diastolic pressure is normally higher than intrapericardial pressure, resulting in positive transmural or filling pressure. In tamponade, rising intrapericardial pressure progressively reduces and can eventually make the transmural pressures of first the right- and then the left-sided cardiac chambers phasically negative. In addition to the deleterious effects on diastolic function, pericardial effusion results in decreased systolic performance because the compressed and underfilled chambers operate at the lower end of their respective Frank-Starling curves.[30]

Figure 205-5 shows the results of an experiment in which intrapericardial volume was increased by infusing 10 mL of warm saline per minute in a dog. Cardiac output and stroke volume steadily decreased with increasing intrapericardial volume and pressure. Mean arterial pressure (MAP) was maintained until intrapericardial volume had increased to approximately 100 mL, and intrapericardial pressure was approximately 10 mm Hg. MAP then dropped sharply as intrapericardial volume was further increased.[32] As illustrated by this experiment, acute accumulations of relatively small amounts of pericardial effusion can result in profound hemodynamic compromise with a clinical picture that is dominated by signs of low cardiac output.

With more chronic accumulations of pericardial effusion, the volume of the pericardial space increases with concomitant expansion of the pericardial sac. The precise mechanisms of pericardial expansion are uncertain and may include fibroblast proliferation with new connective tissue deposition, remodeling of the pre-existent connective tissue, or both.[33] In addition, a variety of compensatory mechanisms increase preload or filling pressure in an effort to restore cardiac output. The compensatory mechanisms are similar to the various neurohormonal changes that accompany other forms of cardiac disease. Activation of the renin-angiotensin-aldosterone system leads to increased angiotensin II, aldosterone, vasopressin, and sympathetic nervous stimulation, which result in fluid retention and increased heart rate. However, unlike other forms of cardiac disease that result in increased preload, atrial natriuretic peptide does not increase. Despite increased venous pressure, atrial distention, the primary stimulus for secretion of atrial natriuretic peptide, does not occur because of external compression of the heart. Thus tamponade prevents this mechanism for increased

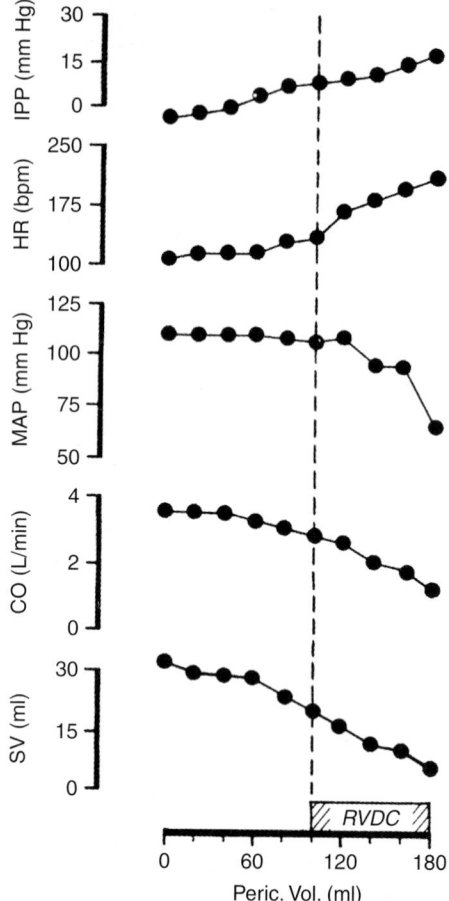

Figure 205-5 Hemodynamic effects of intrapericardial saline infusion in a dog. Cardiac output *(CO)* and stroke volume *(SV)* decrease as soon as intrapericardial volume begins to increase. Mean arterial pressure *(MAP)* is maintained until intrapericardial volume *(Peric. Vol.)* has increased to 100 mL and intrapericardial pressure *(IPP)* is approximately 10 mm Hg. MAP then drops rapidly with any further increases in intrapericardial volume and pressure. Echocardiography performed during experiment showed that right ventricular diastolic collapse *(RVDC)* first develops when intrapericardial pressure reaches approximately 10 mm Hg. *HR,* Heart rate. (From Leimgruber PP et al: The hemodynamic derangement associated with right ventricular diastolic collapse in cardiac tamponade: an experimental echocardiographic study. *Circulation* 68:612, 1983. With permission.)

renal natriuresis, and this, together with the various other compensatory mechanisms, contributes to increased blood volume and venous pressure.[34,35] Consequently, with chronic pericardial effusion, signs of increased systemic venous pressure predominate and manifest as right-sided CHF.

Pulsus paradoxus was first described by Kussmaul in 1873 as the apparent paradox of a disappearing pulse during inspiration despite persistence of the heartbeat in patients with pericardial disease.[36] It is defined as a decrease ($\geq$10 mm Hg) in systolic arterial blood pressure with inspiration during normal breathing (Figure 205-6).[37] Pulsus paradoxus is an accentuation of the normal small decline of left ventricular stroke volume and systemic arterial blood pressure that occurs with inspiration. During inspiration, intrathoracic pressure decreases and blood flows preferentially into the pulmonary veins, right atrium, and ventricle, because these are the most compliant intrathoracic blood vessels and cardiac chambers.

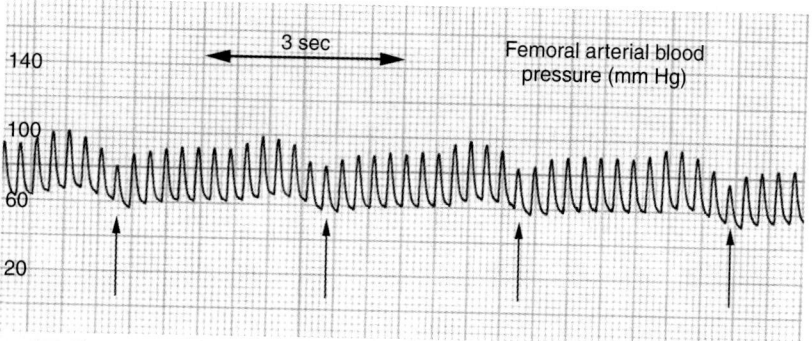

Figure 205-6 Femoral arterial blood pressure showing pulsus paradoxus in a dog with pericardial effusion. At end-inspiration *(arrows)*, systolic blood pressure decreases by more than 10 mm Hg and pulse pressure narrows.

Blood pooling in the pulmonary veins reduces preload to the left heart and consequently reduces left ventricular stroke volume. In humans, left ventricular stroke volume normally decreases by an average of 7% during inspiration, and this is associated with a 3% drop in systolic arterial blood pressure. Right ventricular stroke volume, on the other hand, increases during inspiration due to increased right-sided filling. With a normal pericardium, the phasic variations in right ventricular volume have little effect on the left ventricle, and pooling of blood in the pulmonary veins is the most important contributor to decreased left ventricular stroke volume during inspiration.[38]

Reciprocal and phasic changes with respiration in left and right ventricular filling and stroke volume are exaggerated in the presence of pericardial effusion. Outward expansion of the ventricles is limited, and any increase in the volume of one ventricle can only occur at the expense of the other. Thus greater right ventricular filling during inspiration increases the pressure within the pericardial sac. This, in turn, further compresses the left ventricle. In addition, increased right ventricular filling causes the interventricular septum to deviate toward the left ventricle, further compromising left ventricular volume.[36] This interaction between the ventricles is superimposed upon the normal decrease in left ventricular stroke volume that occurs during inspiration and leads to pulsus paradoxus. The inspiratory increase in right ventricular filling is indispensable for pulsus paradoxus. When systemic venous return is held constant, tamponade does not result in pulsus paradoxus.[39]

Epidemiology Pericardial disorders resulting in effusion occur primarily in older, large breed dogs. No apparent sex predisposition exists. At the UMVMC from January 1999 to December 2001, the average age among 87 dogs with pericardial effusion was 9.7 years (±2.2 years), average weight was 31.2 kg (±12.6 kg), and males and females were nearly equally represented (46 males:41 females). Pericardial effusion occurred most frequently in golden retrievers, and its prevalence in this breed was striking. Of the 87 affected dogs, 23 (26%) were golden retrievers. The breed was significantly over-represented when compared with the general hospital population (odds ratio, 4.4; 95% confidence interval, 2.7 to 7.0). Golden retrievers were also the most common breed among dogs with pericardial effusion at the Veterinary Hospital, University of Pennsylvania from 1990 to 1993.[29]

Information regarding the epidemiology of pericardial effusions in cats is limited. One study reported 66 cases with pericardial disease among 2852 feline necropsies. Pericardial effusion was present in 58 cases, and eight had pericardial pathology but no significant effusion. In virtually all cases the pericardial disorder formed part of a more generalized disease, most commonly CHF and feline infectious peritonitis (FIP). Pericardial pathology appears to attend many feline diseases, but symptomatic pericardial effusion in the cat is uncommon.[40]

Presenting and Clinical Signs The presenting signs among dogs with pericardial effusion are remarkably diverse and include lethargy, respiratory distress, reduced appetite, episodic collapse, vomiting, and abdominal distention. Polydipsia, weakness, and coughing are also occasionally reported. Common physical examination findings are muffled heart sounds, weak pulses, pale mucous membranes, and abdominal distention with a fluid wave. Thorough examination reveals jugular distention in most cases. Pulsus paradoxus is usually subtle, but careful pulse palpation may disclose variations in pulse quality associated with phase of respiration.

Diagnostic Procedures
Radiology Thoracic radiographs in cases with pericardial effusion are frequently described as showing an enlarged and globoid cardiac silhouette, with tracheal elevation and widening of the caudal vena cava. The cardiac silhouette and diaphragm overlap, and in the dorsoventral or ventrodorsal projection, the pericardial sac may touch the costal margins bilaterally. The edge of the distended pericardial sac is often distinct because it undergoes little, if any, motion during systole and diastole. The lung fields are clear of any infiltrate to indicate the presence of left-sided CHF (Figure 205-7).

These radiographic findings, when present, strongly support the presence of a pericardial effusion. However, such "typical" findings are only present in more chronic cases with

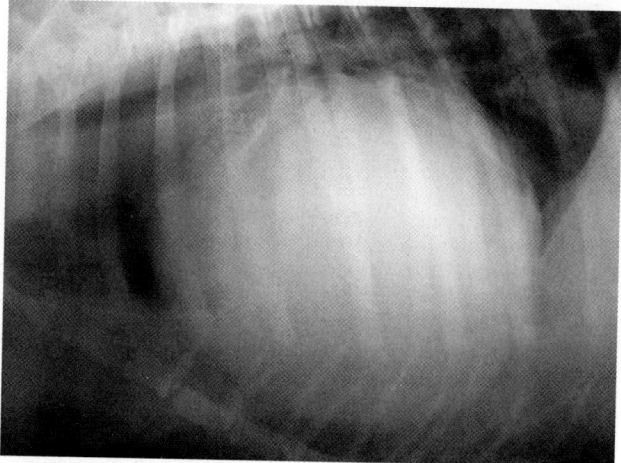

Figure 205-7 Lateral thoracic radiograph of a dog with severe, chronic pericardial effusion. Cardiac silhouette is globoid and overlaps diaphragm, and trachea is elevated. A total of 1600 mL of pericardial effusion was removed by pericardiocentesis. Histopathology of the pericardium disclosed pericardial mesothelioma.

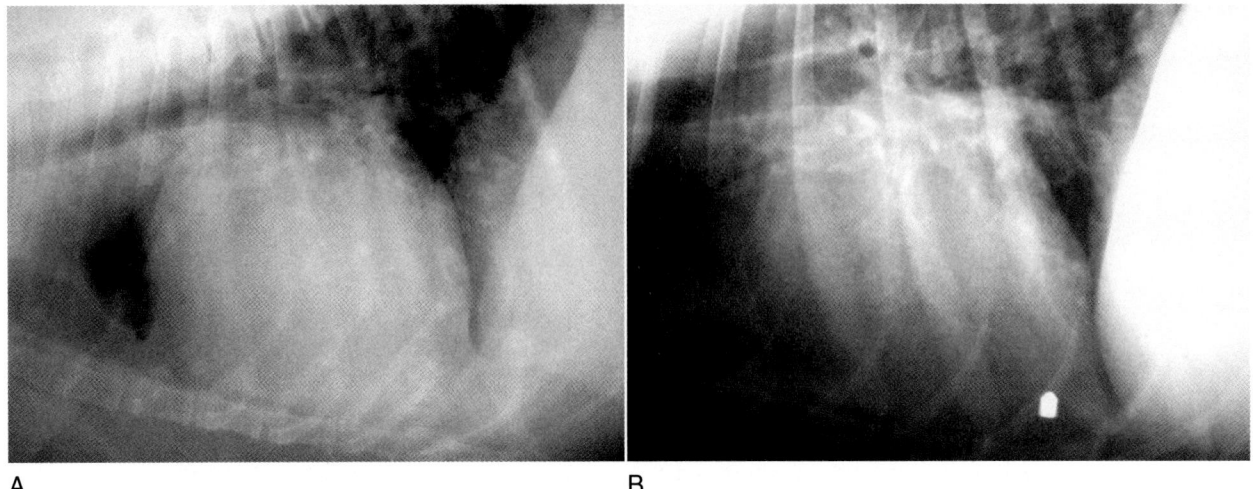

A   B

Figure 205-8 Lateral thoracic radiographs of two dogs with pericardial effusions. In both cases, volume of effusion was considerably less than in dog in Figure 205-7, and cardiac silhouettes are consequently much smaller and less globoid. **A,** Focal disseminate pulmonary metastases. The final diagnosis was metastatic cardiac hemangiosarcoma. **B,** A radiopaque foreign body due to an intrapericardial metal pellet.

large volume pericardial effusions. In cases with accumulations of smaller amounts of pericardial effusion, findings on thoracic radiography are much more subtle. In these cases the cardiac silhouette is enlarged but it is not necessarily globoid, suggesting additional differential diagnoses such as dilated cardiomyopathy. Some pleural effusion is frequently present in dogs with pericardial effusion and may obscure the cardiac silhouette.

Despite the various limitations, thoracic radiography is an important component of the diagnostic evaluation of cases with suspected pericardial effusion. In addition to facilitating a diagnosis of pericardial effusion in many cases, thoracic radiographs may demonstrate the presence of other abnormalities, such as pulmonary metastases (Figure 205-8, *A*), or radiopaque intrapericardial foreign bodies (Figure 205-8, *B*).

Electrocardiography   In most dogs with pericardial effusion, electrocardiography discloses either a normal sinus rhythm or a sinus tachycardia. Ventricular arrhythmias are fairly common, and supraventricular arrhythmias occasionally occur. Low-voltage QRS complexes (<1 mV in all limb leads) are present in approximately half of the cases with pericardial effusion in which electrocardiography is performed (Figure 205-9, *A*). Other differential diagnoses that result in low-voltage electrocardiographic complexes include pleural effusion, obesity, and hypothyroidism.

Electrical alternans, a beat-to-beat variation in the contour and amplitude of the QRS and ST-T complexes (Figure 205-9, *B*), is strongly suggestive of a pericardial effusion.[41] Electrical alternans results from 2:1 swinging of the heart, or swinging once every other heartbeat in large pericardial effusions. In humans, clinical data and mathematic modeling show that electrical alternans is a rate-dependant phenomenon that occurs at heart rates of between 90 and 144 beats per minute.[42]

In the original report of electrical alternans in dogs, the electrocardiographic feature was present in seven of 11 dogs (64%) with pericardial effusion, and it was more prone to occur in cases with larger effusions.[41] However, subsequent reports indicate that electrical alternans among dogs with pericardial effusion occurs relatively infrequently. In two studies in dogs with confirmed pericardial effusions, electrical alternans was present in only two of 33 (6.4%) and two of 10 cases (20%).[43,44] Electrical alternans is a similarly insensitive indicator of pericardial effusion in humans, and it occasionally occurs with disorders other than pericardial effusion in both humans and dogs.[41,45,46] Electrical alternans has been reported in cats with pericardial effusion.[40]

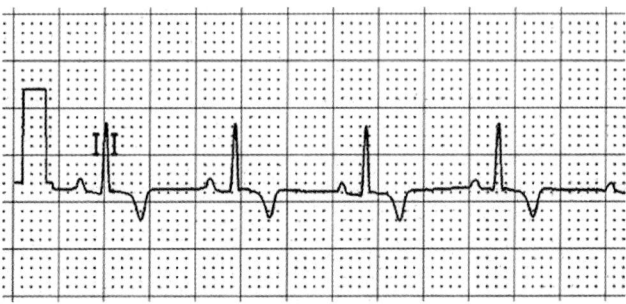

A

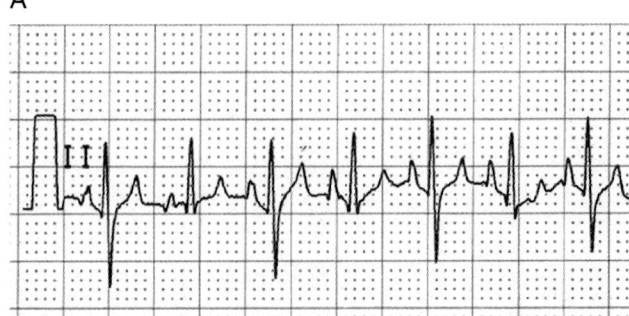

B

Figure 205-9 Electrocardiograms (lead *II*) from two dogs with pericardial effusions. Calibration square wave is 1 mV in amplitude. **A,** Low-voltage (<1 mV) complexes. **B,** Beat-to-beat variations in amplitude and contour of QRS and ST-T complexes that characterize electrical alternans.

Electrocardiographic findings are generally too few, subtle, and insensitive to be considered particularly useful as an indicator of the presence of pericardial effusion. However, electrocardiography is indicated in patients with signs of low cardiac output, when arrhythmias are detected on physical examination, and when thoracic radiographs demonstrate enlargement of the cardiac silhouette. Under these circumstances, an electrocardiogram that shows changes consistent with a pericardial effusion will facilitate the diagnosis.

Pericardial Fluid Analysis   The diagnostic value of pericardial fluid analysis is limited. In dogs, the gross appearance of pericardial effusions is virtually always sanguineous or serosanguineous irrespective of cause, and they are usually classified as hemorrhagic effusions or sterile inflammatory exudates. Total nucleated cell counts, red cell counts, and protein concentrations of pericardial fluid overlap extensively between the various neoplastic and non-neoplastic causes.[47] The pH of pericardial fluid has been reported to distinguish between neoplastic and non-neoplastic effusions.[48] However, considerable overlap in pH values exists between the various causes of pericardial effusion, and pH measurements of pericardial fluid have little clinical use.[49] Hemangiosarcoma and aortic body tumors, the most common tumors associated with pericardial effusions in dogs, are rarely identified on cytologic evaluation of pericardial fluid, presumably because they do not readily exfoliate. Further, pericardial diseases that lead to effusion result in dramatic mesothelial proliferation, and exfoliated mesothelial cells often have characteristics that mimic malignancy. Consequently, pericardial fluid analysis is associated with a high incidence of false-negative and false-positive cytologic diagnoses of neoplasia.[47,50,51]

Despite these limitations, pericardial effusion cytology does occasionally provide crucial information, and pericardial effusion analysis is especially important for those cases in which no intrapericardial masses suggestive of hemangiosarcoma or aortic body tumor are detected on echocardiography. Some of the less common causes of pericardial effusion, such as infective pericarditis and lymphosarcoma, are diagnosed primarily based on pericardial fluid cytology. Consequently, pericardial fluid analysis is an important component of the evaluation in cases with pericardial effusion, but the results must be interpreted with appropriate care and understanding of the limitations of the test.

Additional Laboratory Tests   Dogs with hemangiosarcoma are frequently anemic and may have nucleated red blood cells (RBCs), schistocytes, acanthocytes, and thrombocytopenia. Mild to moderate elevations in liver enzymes are frequently present as a result of hepatic congestion. Analysis of ascitic fluid is consistent with a modified transudate. Mild azotemia, which is usually prerenal, may be present. Cats with FIP may have a neutrophilia, lymphocytopenia, and hyperglobulinemia. *Coccidioides immitis* serology should be performed in cases with pericardial disease from endemic areas. Some assessment of coagulation (e.g., activated coagulation time [ACT]) should be performed prior to pericardiocentesis, especially if a coagulopathy is suspected clinically.

Echocardiography   Echocardiography is the most sensitive and specific noninvasive method to confirm the presence of pericardial effusion, and it has replaced many of the radiographic procedures (fluoroscopy, angiography, and pneumopericardiography) that were previously used to identify the presence and causes of pericardial effusions. With two-dimensional echocardiography, pericardial effusion appears as an anechoic space surrounding the heart. In cases with concurrent pleural effusion, the pericardium is well visualized with anechoic fluid on either side. The heart may show swinging motions within the

pericardial fluid. The various heart chambers may appear small, and the walls may show thickening or pseudohypertrophy due to compression.[52]

Pericardial fluid is usually readily distinguishable from pleural effusion, although this is not invariably the case. Pericardial effusion is contained within a circular region around the heart, where it provides contrast for various cardiac chambers, such as the walls of right atrium and auricle and the proximal aorta. Pleural effusion is more diffuse and contains the edges of lung lobes and mediastinum.

The changes in transmural pressure and intracardiac flow with pericardial effusion are reflected in several useful and readily detectable echocardiographic findings. These include inversion or collapse of the right atrial and ventricular free walls resulting from reversal of transmural pressure, as well as exaggerated respiratory variation in blood flow through the right and left heart.

The right atrial free wall is normally rounded throughout the cardiac cycle, reflecting the normal positive right atrial transmural pressure. Any inversion of the right atrial free wall is therefore indirect evidence of elevated intrapericardial pressure and transient reversal of transmural pressure. Right atrial inversion occurs in late diastole and continues into ventricular systole for a variable period before normalizing. Right ventricular diastolic collapse is characterized by inward motion of the right ventricular free wall during diastole. With mild tamponade, this inward movement produces a localized concavity of the right ventricular free wall. With severe cardiac tamponade, right ventricular diastolic collapse persists throughout diastole, and the right ventricular chamber is almost completely obliterated (Figure 205-10).[53]

Doppler studies of normal hearts demonstrate slightly decreased flow velocity across the mitral valve and slightly increased flow velocity across the tricuspid valve during inspiration. The changes in aortic and pulmonic flow velocity are smaller; however, aortic flow velocity decreases slightly during inspiration, and pulmonic flow velocity increases. In humans, these respiratory changes in flow velocity become markedly accentuated with pericardial effusion, even in the absence of clinical signs of cardiac tamponade.[53] These Doppler indicators are present in dogs with experimentally induced tamponade.[54]

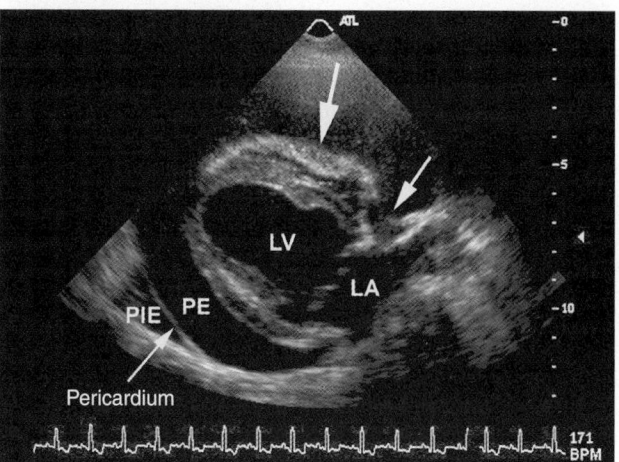

Figure 205-10 Echocardiogram (long axis four-chamber view from the right parasternal location) from dog with pericardial effusion *(PE)* and echocardiographic evidence of tamponade. Right atrial inversion is apparent *(small arrow)*, and right ventricular collapse *(large arrow)* results in virtually complete obliteration of right ventricular chamber. *LA,* Left atrium; *LV,* left ventricle; *PlE,* pleural effusion.

However, the clinical use of Doppler studies in the evaluation of small animals with pericardial effusion has yet to be determined. In addition to confirming the presence of a pericardial effusion and providing evidence of tamponade, echocardiography is the noninvasive procedure of choice to detect intrapericardial masses such as hemangiosarcoma and heart base tumors. Although histopathology is necessary to confirm and definitively identify a tumor, the location and characteristics of an intrapericardial or myocardial mass demonstrated during echocardiography provides important information about the probable tumor type.[55,56]

Hemangiosarcoma, a highly malignant neoplasm of vascular endothelium, is the most commonly diagnosed cardiac tumor in dogs. It occurs with an approximately tenfold greater prevalence than the second most common cardiac tumor—aortic body tumors.[57] Primary and metastatic cardiac hemangiosarcoma in the cat has been reported, but it is rare.[58] Hemangiosarcoma most commonly arises from the wall of the right atrium or auricle, protrudes into the pericardial space, and moves with the right auricle or atrium (Figures 205-11, A and B). These tumors may also protrude into the right atrial chamber, spread to involve other areas of the heart base and pericardium, and involve the right atrioventricular (AV) junction (Figure 205-11, C). Hemangiosarcoma involving the wall of the left ventricle has been described.[59] Hemangiosarcoma typically contains small hypoechoic spaces, giving the tumor a mottled or cavitary appearance, and the tumors are occasionally cystic. Hemangiosarcoma, when present, is usually demonstrated while imaging from the right parasternal long and short axis views. However, these tumors may be small and elusive. Imaging from the left caudal parasternal location to obtain a four-chamber view and from the left cranial parasternal location to provide alternate imaging planes, especially of the right auricle, is necessary to demonstrate the presence of hemangiosarcoma in some cases.

The term *heart base tumor* is used to designate any mass located at the base of the heart in association with the ascending aorta and main pulmonary artery. The most common heart

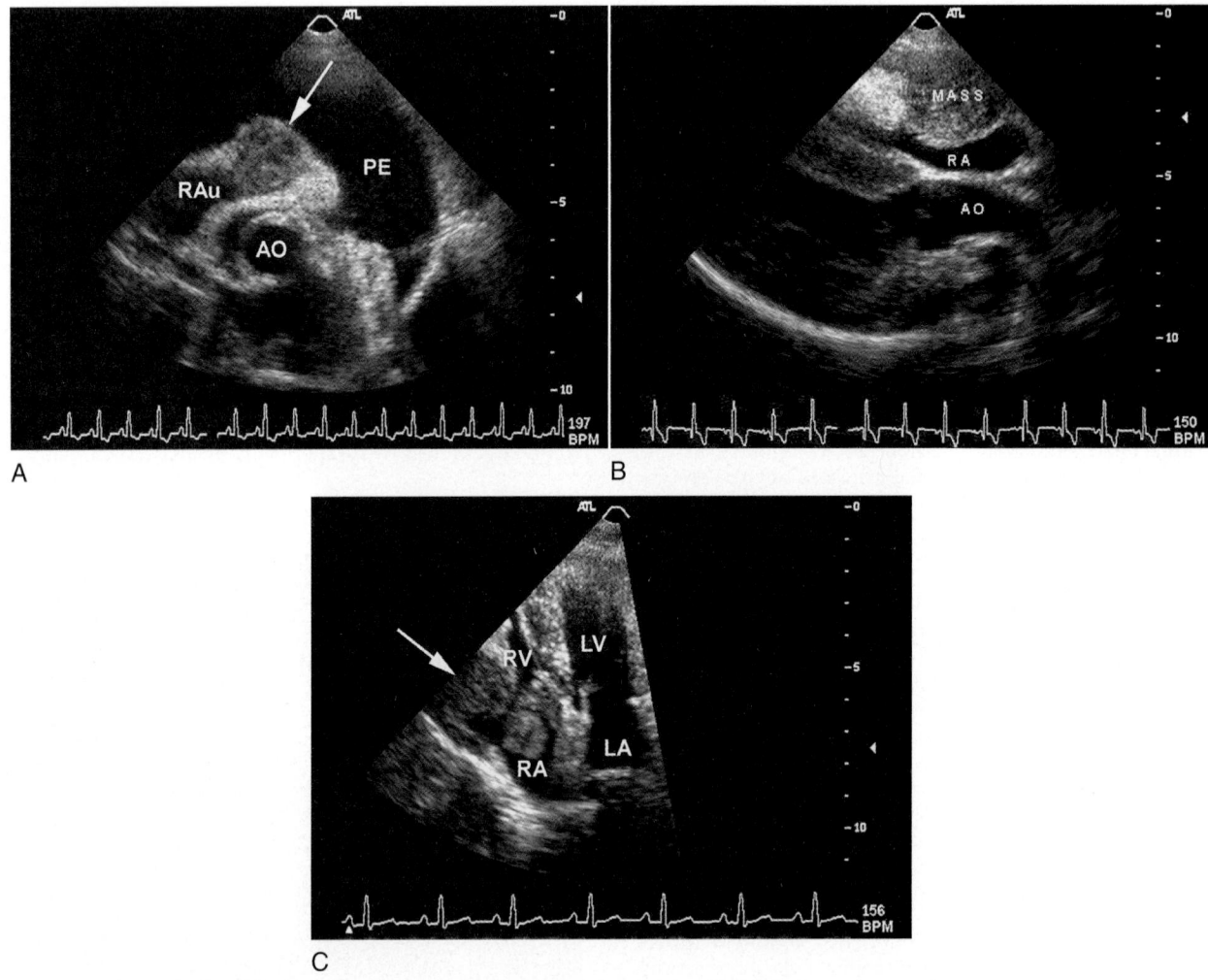

Figure 205-11 Echocardiograms from dogs with cardiac hemangiosarcoma. **A,** Short axis view from right parasternal location, shows a round, cavitary, transmural tumor *(arrow)* near tip of right auricle *(RAu)*. **B,** Long axis left ventricular outflow view from right parasternal location, shows tumor *(MASS)* that involves wall of the right atrium *(RA)*. **C,** Four-chamber (inflow) view from the left caudal parasternal location, shows cavitary tumor *(arrow)* that extensively involves right atrioventricular junction. Part of the tumor protrudes into the right atrium *(RA)* and partially occludes tricuspid valve. *AO,* Aorta; *PE,* pericardial effusion; *RV,* right ventricle; *LA,* left atrium; *LV,* left ventricle.

base tumors in dogs are aortic body tumors, which arise from specialized neuroepithelial cells that reside within the adventitia of the aortic arch. The specialized neuroepithelial cells or chemoreceptors serve to detect minute changes in blood oxygen and carbon dioxide tensions, pH, and temperature. Tumors of chemoreceptors are termed *chemodectomas*. They comprise a subgroup of tumors referred to as *paragangliomas*, all of which arise from cells that share a common embryologic origin from the neural crest. Chemoreceptors occur in a variety of locations in the body, including the aortic body, carotid body, nodose ganglion of the vagus nerve, ciliary ganglion in the orbit, pancreas, internal jugular vein below the middle ear, and glomus jugulare along the recurrent branch of the glossopharyngeal nerve.[60,61] Owing to the location of the aortic chemoreceptors, only aortic body chemodectomas are associated with pericardial effusion.[61] In addition to aortic body tumors, between 5% and 10% of heart base tumors in dogs are thyroid tumors (both adenomas and adenocarcinomas) that arise from ectopic thyroid tissue at the base of the heart.[62-66] Aortic body tumors have occasionally been reported in cats.[67-70]

Heart base tumors are usually associated with the ascending aorta. They vary from small ovoid structures attached to the cranial aspect of the ascending aorta to very extensive masses that surround the aorta and main pulmonary artery (Figure 205-12). Tumor indentation or invasion of the atria may be seen. Heart base tumors tend to have a more homogenous appearance than the mottled or cavitary appearance of hemangiosarcoma. They are usually (but not invariably) associated with pericardial effusions.

Echocardiography may also demonstrate other cardiac tumors, the presence of abdominal viscera within the pericardial sac in cases with PPDH, benign intrapericardial cysts, and intrapericardial thrombi associated with left atrial rupture. Left atrial rupture is suspected when signs of acute tamponade develop in smaller breed dogs with significant mitral regurgitation.

Confirming the presence of pericardial effusion with echocardiography is rapid, straightforward, and accurate. However, echocardiography is also crucial for determining the presence or absence of intrapericardial masses, and it provides important information about the size and location of tumors and their accessibility for surgical resection. Identification of intrapericardial tumors is frequently challenging, and transthoracic imaging in multiple planes from both left and right-sided locations may be necessary. The presence of pericardial fluid greatly facilitates the detection of intrapericardial masses, and this is particularly relevant to the diagnosis and delineation of hemangiosarcoma and heart base tumors. Pericardial fluid forms an echolucent zone around the right atrium and auricle and the ascending aorta, the locations at which these tumors most commonly occur. In the absence of pericardial fluid, these locations are obscured by lung interference. Consequently, whenever the clinical condition of the patient permits, pericardiocentesis should be deferred until a thorough echocardiographic examination has been completed.

Acquired Pericardial Effusions: Specific Causes, Epidemiology, Treatment, and Prognosis

Idiopathic Pericardial Effusion Idiopathic pericardial effusion is a diagnosis of exclusion. It is made in cases with pericardial effusion where no intrapericardial masses are identified after thorough echocardiographic evaluation and the results of ancillary tests, such as pericardial fluid analysis, fail to disclose a cause. Pericardial histopathology and immunohistochemistry from dogs with idiopathic pericardial effusion demonstrate extensive pericardial fibrosis and a mixed inflammatory response of greatest intensity at the cardiac surface of the tissue. Perivascular lymphoplasmacytic aggregates are present at the pleural surface within the fibrosed pericardium. No vascular pathology or deposition of immunoglobulin or complement within the vessel wall exists, suggesting that the pericarditis is not due to a vasculitis. Immunohistochemistry findings are consistent with a predominantly humoral immune response, but they do not support a primary immune-mediated pathogenesis. The factor or factors that initiate idiopathic pericarditis remain unknown.[71]

As with any diagnoses of exclusion, a diagnosis of idiopathic pericardial effusion should be made with appropriate caution. Small intrapericardial tumors may elude detection, especially in

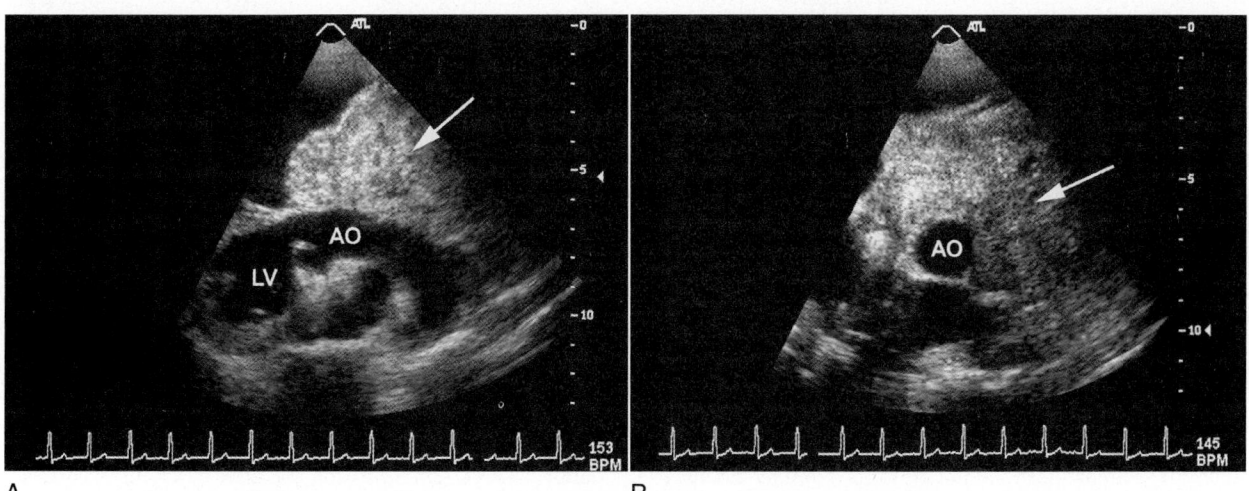

A   B

Figure 205-12 Echocardiogram from dog with a heart base tumor. **A,** Long axis left ventricular outflow view obtained from the right parasternal location, shows a large tumor *(arrow)* attached to cranial aspect of ascending aorta *(AO)*. **B,** Short axis view obtained from right parasternal location, shows that tumor *(arrow)* virtually completely encircles the aorta. Histopathologic diagnosis was ectopic thyroid adenocarcinoma. *LV,* Left ventricle.

cases where echocardiography is performed after pericardiocentesis. In addition, mesothelioma is a diffuse neoplasm of the pericardium and other serosal surfaces, and it does not result in appreciable thickening of the pericardium on echocardiography. Cytology of pericardial effusion cannot distinguish between idiopathic pericardial effusion and mesothelioma.[51] Consequently, mesothelioma should always be considered as an important differential diagnosis for idiopathic pericardial effusion. Idiopathic pericardial effusion has not been reported in cats.

Idiopathic pericardial effusion was diagnosed in eight of 42 dogs (19%) with pericardial effusion in a retrospective study from the Veterinary Teaching Hospital, Colorado State University.[43] Idiopathic pericardial effusion was provisionally diagnosed in 24 of 87 dogs with pericardial effusion at the UMVMC from January 1999 to December 2001, but mesothelioma was eventually confirmed in four of these cases. Consequently, 20 of 87 cases (23%) with pericardial effusion in the UMVMC study population were finally diagnosed as having idiopathic pericardial effusion, which is similar to the data from Colorado State University. Average age among the cases with idiopathic pericardial effusion in the UMVMC study population was 9.4 years (±2.2 years), average weight was 28.9 kg (±14.5 kg), and there was no apparent sex predisposition (11 males:9 females). Five of the 20 dogs (25%) were golden retrievers, and the breed was over-represented (odds ratio, 4.2; 95% confidence interval, 1.6 to 11.2).

The initial treatment for idiopathic pericardial effusion is pericardiocentesis to remove as much pericardial fluid as possible. The author's preferred approach is to restrain the animal in left lateral recumbency and to approach the pericardium from the right side (See Chapter 103).

The gross appearance of pericardial fluid is usually indistinguishable from blood. To confirm that the catheter is in the pericardial space, an aliquot of fluid is placed in an ACT tube. Blood will normally clot in an ACT tube within 60 to 90 seconds. In contrast, sanguineous effusions in body cavities are rapidly depleted of clotting factors and thrombocytes, and pericardial fluid will consequently not clot. If no clots form within the activated clotting tube after 3 to 5 minutes, all of pericardial fluid is aspirated and samples are collected for fluid analysis and culture. The catheter is then removed.

In virtually all cases with pericardial effusion, pericardiocentesis results in rapid and marked hemodynamic improvement. Clinical signs, pulse quality, and mucous membrane perfusion improve, and heart rate decreases. However, ventricular and supraventricular arrhythmias (including atrial fibrillation) are common after pericardiocentesis. These arrhythmias seldom require therapy and usually resolve spontaneously. The author prefers to hospitalize and monitor cases for 12 to 24 hours after pericardiocentesis.

The author usually treats an initial episode of idiopathic pericardial effusion by pericardiocentesis alone, followed by pericardiectomy in cases that develop recurrent effusions. Recurrent effusions, effusive-constrictive, and constrictive pericarditis are well-recognized complications after pericardiocentesis in cases with idiopathic pericardial effusion.[72-75] Among the 20 cases diagnosed with idiopathic pericardial effusion in the UMVMC study population, six died or were euthanized after developing recurrent effusions with tamponade within 44 days of their initial episode. Cardiac tamponade with pulmonary thromboembolism was the cause of death in one dog. Postmortem examinations were not performed in the remaining five cases, and the possibility that some dogs might have had cardiac tumors that eluded detection during echocardiography cannot be excluded. Among the remaining 14 dogs, four developed recurrent effusions necessitating pericardiectomy, and a further six developed effusive-constrictive pericarditis

between 3 months and 3 years after their initial episode. Median survival time (MST) among the 20 cases was 663 days, indicating a generally good prognosis in cases with idiopathic pericardial effusion. However, the complication rate among these cases was high, and this is consistent with the results of others.[73,74]

The complication rate among cases with idiopathic pericardial effusion would probably be lower if pericardiectomy was performed at the time of the initial episode rather than after recurrent effusion. Pericardiectomy would avoid the risk of recurrent life-threatening cardiac tamponade and the potential for developing effusive-constrictive and constrictive pericarditis. In addition, surgery permits examination of thoracic and intrapericardial structures to rule out other causes of pericardial effusion, including tumors and foreign bodies. Although pericardiectomy is by no means devoid of morbidity and mortality, it is an extremely successful procedure for idiopathic pericardial effusion.[76-79] Consequently, it is likely that pericardiectomy will increasingly form part of the initial treatment for cases with idiopathic pericardial effusion, especially as minimally invasive methods for the procedure become more widespread.[80,81]

Colchicine, nonsteroidal anti-inflammatories, and corticosteroids are prescribed for humans with recurrent idiopathic pericarditis. Colchicine and nonsteroidal anti-inflammatories are recommended in most cases, and the use of corticosteroids is limited to very severe cases. Colchicine for the treatment of recurrent pericarditis in humans is promising, although data from large controlled prospective studies are lacking.[82,83] The safety and efficacy of colchicine, nonsteroidal anti-inflammatories, corticosteroids, and any other medical therapies in the management of idiopathic pericardial effusion in small animals have yet to be established.

Mesothelioma Mesothelioma is emerging as an increasingly important cause of pericardial effusion. Mesothelioma was confirmed in four of 87 dogs (5%) in the UMVMC study population of dogs with pericardial effusion. Average age among the affected cases at time of presentation was 9.5 years (±2.2 years), average weight was 37.5 kg (±11.1 kg), and males and females were equally represented. No breed predisposition has been reported, and affected breeds in the UMVMC population were Akita, golden retriever, Labrador retriever, and springer spaniel. Mesothelioma causing pericardial effusion has been described in a cat,[84] but pericardial mesothelioma is rare in this species.

The clinical course of pericardial effusion due to mesothelioma in the UMVMC study population followed a characteristic pattern. Presenting and clinical signs were no different from other cause of pericardial effusion. In all four cases, a provisional diagnosis of idiopathic pericardial effusion was made after various diagnostic procedures, including echocardiography and pericardial fluid analysis failed to disclose a cause for the pericardial effusion. Pericardiocentesis was performed, and this was repeated at 77 days (± 46 days) when the dogs developed recurrent effusions with tamponade. Pericardiectomies were then performed in all cases; histopathology of the excised pericardia was consistent with idiopathic pericarditis in three cases, and mesothelioma in one. Severe and unremitting pleural effusions requiring repeated thoracocentesis began at 103 days (±44 days) after pericardiectomy. Intracavitary cisplatin was administered in two dogs, but this did not appear to significantly change the course of the disease. Thoracocentesis was necessary every 2 to 3 weeks until death or euthanasia, and MST from the initial episode of pericardial effusion was 312 days (range, 206 to 352). In all cases, mesothelioma that had spread throughout the thoracic cavity was confirmed on postmortem examination.

The signalment and clinical course among cases with pericardial effusion due to mesothelioma in the UMVMC study population are strikingly similar to those described by others.[77,85-87] It is extremely difficult to distinguish between idiopathic pericardial effusion and pericardial effusion due to mesothelioma, even with pericardial histopathology and immunohistochemistry.[87,88] The clinical course of the disease is suggestive, and accumulation of significant amounts of pleural effusion within 120 days of pericardiectomy increases the index of suspicion for mesothelioma.[87] In addition to being a diagnostic challenge, mesothelioma is difficult to treat. However, long-term survival has been reported in a dog in which a histopathologic diagnosis of pericardial mesothelioma was made after pericardiectomy for recurrent pericardial effusion. Treatment in that case was initiated 48 hours after surgery with intracavitary cisplatin and intravenous doxorubicin, and the dog was free of disease 27 months later.[89] Intracavitary cisplatin has successfully resolved pleural effusions in some dogs with pleural mesothelioma.[90]

Cardiac Hemangiosarcoma In a retrospective study from the Veterinary Teaching Hospital, Colorado State University, cardiac hemangiosarcoma was diagnosed in 14 of 42 dogs (33%) with pericardial effusion.[43] At the UMVMC, cardiac hemangiosarcoma was diagnosed either by echocardiography or echocardiography and histopathology in 53 of 87 dogs (61%) in the study population with pericardial effusion. Cardiac hemangiosarcoma with pericardial effusion was nearly three times more prevalent than the second most common form of pericardial effusion, idiopathic pericardial effusion. Average age among the affected dogs was 9.8 years (±2.1 years), and their average weight was 32.0 kg (±12.2 kg). Males slightly outnumbered females (31 males:22 females), but the difference was not statistically significant when compared with the general hospital population. Sixteen of the 57 dogs (28%) were golden retrievers and the breed was over-represented (odds ratio, 5.3; 95% confidence interval, 2.9 to 9.4).

Two features of these data suggest that important changes have occurred in the epidemiology of cardiac hemangiosarcoma. First, the prevalence of cardiac hemangiosarcoma in the UMVMC study population was nearly twice that of the Colorado State University study population. The reasons for this are not clear; however, regional differences in the epidemiology of cardiac hemangiosarcoma may exist, or the prevalence of the disease may have increased over time. Second, the golden retriever was the only over-represented breed among the cases with cardiac hemangiosarcoma in the UMVMC study population. Cardiac hemangiosarcoma has previously been recognized most frequently in German shepherds.[43,91,92] More recently, cardiac hemangiosarcoma has also been seen commonly in golden retrievers at the Veterinary Hospital, University of Pennsylvania.[93]

Treatment for all forms of hemangiosarcoma is challenging, and a diagnosis of cardiac hemangiosarcoma confers a grave prognosis. By the time of diagnosis, cardiac hemangiosarcoma usually has metastasized and should be considered a systemic disease.[77] At the UMVMC, the majority of owners of dogs with cardiac hemangiosarcoma elect to have their dogs treated by pericardiocentesis alone on one or more occasions. Pericardiocentesis is predictably associated with marked clinical improvement, but clinical signs of tamponade typically recur within a few days, often resulting in death or prompting euthanasia. In the UMVMC study population, MST among dogs with cardiac hemangiosarcoma treated by pericardiocentesis alone (n = 30) was just 11 days (range, 0 to 208). Percutaneous balloon pericardiotomy has been described in the dog,[94,95] and the procedure may provide longer periods of palliation in cases with cardiac hemangiosarcoma.

More aggressive approaches to the treatment of cardiac hemangiosarcoma include various combinations of pericardiectomy, tumor resection, splenectomy in cases with splenic metastases, and chemotherapy.[91,96-100] Survival data for cases managed in this manner are limited. In a case report of right atrial hemangiosarcoma treated with chemotherapy alone, survival time was 20 weeks.[98] In dogs treated by surgery alone (tumor resection and pericardiectomy or creation of a pericardial window, or pericardiectomy alone), reported survival times range from 2 days to 8 months.[91,99,100] No survival data are available that compare surgery alone, with surgery and chemotherapy for dogs with cardiac hemangiosarcoma. Further, no compelling evidence suggests that survival times in dogs with either splenic or cardiac hemangiosarcoma can be significantly prolonged with adjuvant chemotherapy. Nevertheless, the management of cardiac hemangiosarcoma should always involve consultation with an oncologist to take advantage of continually emerging modalities for the treatment of this highly malignant tumor.[101]

Heart Base Tumors The majority of heart base tumors in dogs are aortic body tumors. English bulldogs, boxers, and Boston terriers are predisposed, although aortic body tumors also occur in nonbrachycephalic breeds. In various studies, brachycephalic breeds have accounted for between 39% and 85% of dogs with aortic body tumors.[70,102,103] Chronic hypoxia induces hyperplasia and neoplasia of chemoreceptors, which may explain the predisposition of brachycephalic breeds to aortic body tumors.[102] Among the predisposed breeds, males may be at increased risk for developing aortic body tumors, but differences in sex predisposition are not statistically significant in all studies.[70,102,103] The age range at time of diagnosis of aortic body tumors is 6 to 15 years with an average of 10 years.[61,70] Between 5% and 10% of tumors at the heart base are ectopic thyroid tumors.[62] Aortic body tumors are reported in cats, but they are rare in this species.[67-70]

Most aortic body tumors are benign and locally expansive, although local invasiveness and metastases occur in both dogs and cats.[61,67-69,104,105] Two studies report metastases mostly to the lungs and liver in approximately 10% to 12% of dogs with aortic body tumors.[102,103] In a third study, 58% (14 of 24) of aortic body tumors were benign, 25% (6 of 24) were locally invasive, and 21% (5 of 24) were metastatic. Sites of metastases included the lungs, left atrium, pericardium, and kidneys.[70] The biologic behavior of ectopic thyroid tumors at the heart base is less well described, and both ectopic thyroid adenomas and adenocarcinomas with metastases have been reported.[63-66]

Heart base tumors were diagnosed either by echocardiography or echocardiography and histopathology in six dogs among the 87 cases (7%) with pericardial effusion in the UMVMC study population. Affected breeds were Great Dane, Labrador retriever, German shorthaired pointer, boxer, English springer spaniel, and Old English sheepdog. Average age was 11.1 years (±2.2 years), and average weight was 31.4 kg (±13.0 kg). One dog was male and five were female. The number of dogs with heart base tumors in the UMVMC study population is small, but the epidemiologic data are reasonably in accord with those of others, with the exception of sex distribution. The prevalence of heart base tumors is consistent with a recent review of the epidemiology of cardiac tumors in dogs. In that study, aortic body tumors were approximately tenfold less common than cardiac hemangiosarcoma.[57]

Complete surgical resection of heart base tumors is seldom possible because the tumors are highly vascular, located close to major blood vessels, and usually extensive by the time of diagnosis. However, palliation with pericardiectomy either alone or in combination with tumor resection often results in prolonged survival with an excellent quality of life.[106,107]

No evidence indicates that adjuvant chemotherapy improves the prognosis for dogs with heart base tumors. In a recent retrospective study in dogs with aortic body tumors in which surgery was performed, the following factors were evaluated for effect on survival time: sex; breed; presence or absence of respiratory distress; the presence of an arrhythmia other than respiratory sinus arrhythmia; the presence of pleural, pericardial, or peritoneal effusion; evidence of pulmonary metastases; treatment with pericardiectomy; and treatment with chemotherapy. No attempt was made to achieve tumorfree margins in the dogs in that study. Among the various factors evaluated, only treatment with pericardiectomy had a significant effect on survival, and the survival advantage was remarkable. MST among dogs after pericardiectomy was 730 days, whereas those that did not have a pericardiectomy had a MST of only 42 days.[106]

Other Causes of Acquired Pericardial Effusion

Bacterial, fungal, and viral infections are occasionally associated with pericardial effusions in small animals. Most cases of pericardial effusions due to bacterial infections are thought to arise as a consequence of intrapericardial foreign body penetration, usually by migrating foxtails (*Hordeum* spp.). Foxtail migration is a common and often serious problem in the western United States.[108,109] Bacterial pericarditis has also been described in a puppy after a dog bite and in a young adult dog after thoracic trauma.[110,111] In contrast to most other causes of pericardial effusion, pericardial fluid cytology and culture is crucial in the diagnosis of septic cases. In the largest series of infectious pericardial effusion reported in dogs (five cases), treatment involved pericardiectomy and removal of any foreign bodies, chest drainage, and antibiotic therapy for up to 6 months. All dogs recovered without complications, suggesting that dogs with bacterial pericarditis have a good prognosis when treated aggressively with a combination of surgical and medical therapy.[108]

Systemic coccidioidomycosis in dogs has been associated with pericardial disease. In most cases the fungal infection results in effusive-constrictive or constrictive pericarditis. Coccidioidomycosis should be considered, especially in dogs with pericardial disease that reside in or have a travel history that includes areas where the soil fungus *Coccidioides immitis* is endemic, such as the Southwestern United States.[75,112] Treatment involves pericardiectomy, chest drainage, and antifungal therapy (usually beginning with Amphotericin B). Based on limited published information and experience, the prognosis for cases of coccidioidomycosis with pericardial involvement is poor.[112] A case of effusive-constrictive pericarditis due to *Aspergillus niger* has been reported in a dog.[113]

FIP is one of the more common diseases associated with pericardial effusion in the cat.[40] Pericardial effusions that are occasionally voluminous are present in some cats suffering from this systemic and invariably fatal viral disease.

Left atrial rupture is an uncommon cause of pericardial effusion that occurs in smaller breed dogs with chronic degenerative disease of the mitral valve. Affected cases show clinical signs of acute tamponade, and a loud left apical murmur is usually apparent despite muffling of the heart sounds. Echocardiography discloses intrapericardial fluid, a mass caudal to the left ventricle due to thrombus formation, and substantial mitral regurgitation. Pericardiocentesis is immediately necessary in most cases. Further, the possibility of continued hemorrhage exists, necessitating blood transfusion and emergency thoracotomy to remove larger clots from the pericardial space and to repair the left atrium. The prognosis in such cases is grave.[114,115]

Cardiac lymphosarcoma and rhabdomyosarcoma with pericardial effusion have been reported in both dogs and cats, but these are rare.[40,116-118] Among the various cardiac tumors,

cardiac lymphosarcoma is unique because cytology of the pericardial fluid establishes the diagnosis in many cases, and the tumor is amenable to combination chemotherapy.[117,119]

Pericardial effusions secondary to coagulation disorders rarely result in clinically significant tamponade. However, a case of pericardial effusion and cardiac tamponade secondary to anticoagulant rodenticide toxicity has been reported in a dog.[120] Pericardial effusions secondary to disseminated intravascular coagulation, warfarin toxicity, and other coagulopathies have been reported in cats.[40]

Pericardial effusion is frequently detected in cases with CHF in small animals, but usually not in sufficient quantity to cause significant hemodynamic compromise. Pericardial effusion secondary to uremia has been recognized in both dogs and cats.[40,43]

Constrictive and Effusive-Constrictive Pericarditis

In cases with constrictive and effusive-constrictive pericarditis, cardiac filling is compromised by a nondistensible, thickened, fibrotic pericardium. In human medicine, these diseases are defined as follows: constrictive pericarditis consists of fibrotic fusion of visceral and parietal pericardial layers. Effusive-constrictive pericarditis is an unusual variant of constrictive pericarditis. It describes a condition in which constriction of the heart by the visceral pericardium or epicardium exists, and a tense effusion also occurs within the pericardial space. In cases with effusive-constrictive pericarditis, elevated right atrial pressure persists after pericardiocentesis because of the unyielding epicardium.[121,122]

Several reports exist of tamponade in dogs resulting from relatively small amounts of effusion contained within a fibrotic and nondistensible fibrous and parietal pericardium. The visceral pericardium or epicardium is usually spared or only mildly affected in these cases. Many cases are idiopathic, or develop months or years after an episode of idiopathic pericardial effusion. Other causes include metallic foreign bodies, *Coccidioides immitis*, *Aspergillus niger*, actinomycosis, and osseous metaplasia of the pericardium.[75,113,123,124] Some authors define effusive-constrictive pericarditis more liberally to include this combination of relatively little pericardial effusion with constriction due primarily to an unyielding parietal and fibrous pericardium.[37]

Dogs with effusive-constrictive pericarditis typically present with signs of right-sided CHF. Common complaints are abdominal distention and muscle wasting. Findings on physical examination include abdominal distention with a fluid wave, jugular distention, and muffled heart sounds. These presenting and clinical signs are essentially identical to dogs with chronic tamponade due to pericardial effusion. The similarities extend to electrocardiography where normal sinus rhythm or sinus tachycardia and low-voltage QRS complexes are commonly found. The appearance of the cardiac silhouette on thoracic radiography ranges from normal to moderately enlarged and rounded, and the caudal vena cava may appear wide. The presence of pleural effusion in some cases may complicate evaluation of the size and shape of the cardiac silhouette. Radiopaque intrapericardial foreign bodies may be detected. Echocardiography discloses pericardial effusion that separates the myocardium and fibrous pericardium by just a few millimeters (Figure 205-13, *A*). Echocardiographic signs of tamponade (late diastolic to systolic inversion of the right atrium and diastolic collapse of the right ventricle) are usually present (Figure 205-13, *B*). Pericardial thickness cannot be accurately assessed except in extreme cases.

A diagnosis of effusive-constrictive pericarditis can usually be established with confidence based on the previously mentioned constellation of findings. Treatment involves pericardiectomy, and clinicians at the UMVMC have found that the prognosis after pericardiectomy is excellent for idiopathic cases.

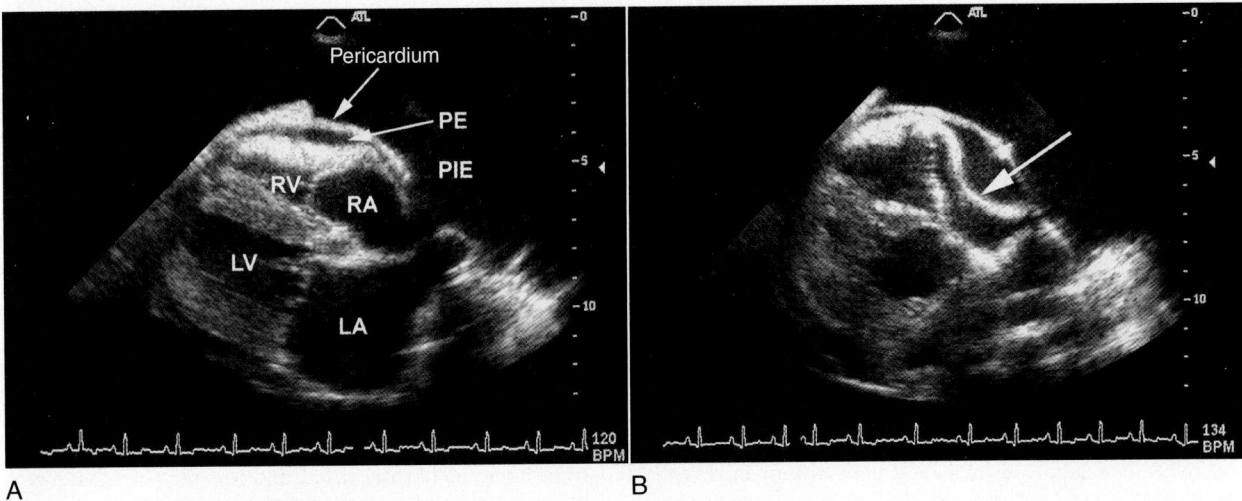

Figure 205-13 Echocardiogram from a dog with effusive-constrictive pericarditis. Dog had signs of right-sided congestive heart failure 25 months after pericardiocentesis had been performed for idiopathic pericardial effusion. **A,** Long axis four-chamber view from right parasternal location, shows small amount of pericardial effusion *(PE)* that separates fibrous pericardium from myocardium by just a few millimeters (reader should compare with centimeter scale on right side of echocardiogram). **B,** Late diastolic to systolic inversion of right atrium *(arrow)*, confirming the presence of tamponade. *PIE,* Pleural effusion; *RA,* right atrium; *RV,* right ventricle; *LA,* left atrium; *LV,* left ventricle.

Slight epicardial fibrosis and roughness that does not require any surgical intervention is present in most cases. Adhesions between the visceral and parietal pericardium are extremely uncommon. Severe involvement of the epicardium and adhesions between the parietal and visceral pericardium confer a much poorer prognosis. Cases with fungal pericarditis caused by *Coccidioides immitis* appear particularly prone to develop extensive involvement of both the visceral and parietal pericardium.

Epicardial stripping is necessary in such cases, and the procedure is associated with high perioperative morbidity and mortality.

Constrictive pericarditis is both rare and difficult to diagnose in small animals. In this disease, a stiff fibrotic pericardium encases the heart. Presenting and clinical signs, thoracic radiographs, and electrocardiography are similar to other causes of chronic tamponade and effusive-constrictive pericarditis.

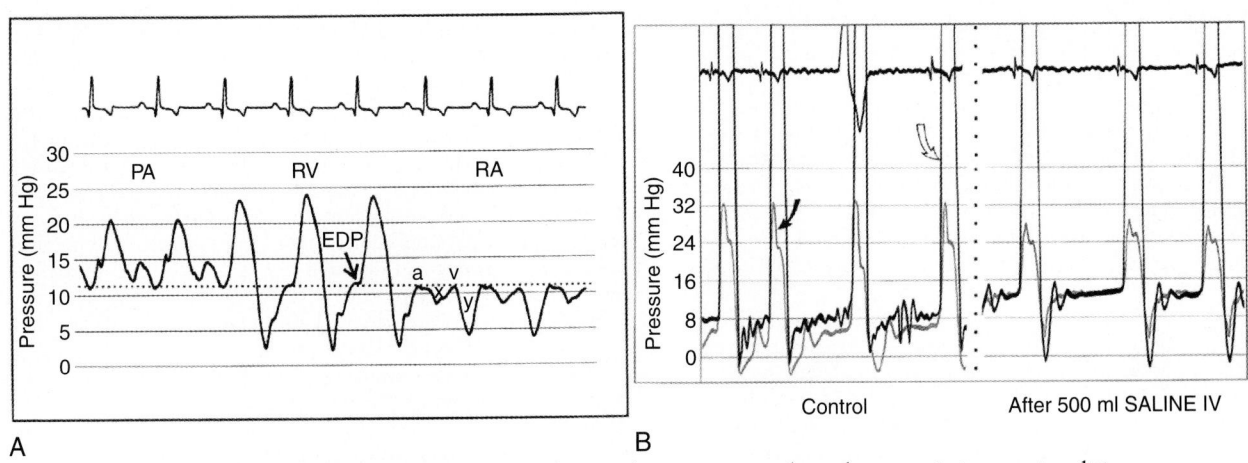

Figure 205-14 Hemodynamic abnormalities associated with constrictive pericarditis. **A,** Elevation and equilibration of end-diastolic pressure *(EDP)* in pulmonary artery *(PA)*, right ventricle *(RV)*, and right atrium *(RA)*. Right atrial pressure waveform has a *M*-shaped pattern due to reduced X descent and a prominent Y descent. **B,** Simultaneous recordings of left ventricular *(open arrow)* and right ventricular *(solid arrow)* pressures before and after saline infusion. Under control conditions, pressure waveforms show slight elevations in end-diastolic pressures. However, true circumstances of the case become apparent with rapid intravenous infusion of 500 mL saline. This procedure results in elevation and equilibration of left and right ventricular diastolic pressure, and a dip-and-plateau pattern in diastole emerges. (From Sisson D, Thomas WP: Pericardial diseases and cardiac tumors. In Fox PR et al (eds): Textbook of Canine and Feline Cardiology, 2nd ed. Philadelphia, WB Saunders Co, 1999, p 679. With permission.)

However, echocardiography demonstrates neither pericardial effusion nor right atrial and ventricular collapse. Constrictive pericarditis in dogs can develop as a consequence of any form of chronic pericarditis. However, it appears to occur most frequently as a severe complication of systemic coccidioidomycosis.

Certain echocardiographic findings that are suggestive of constrictive pericarditis have been described in humans. M-mode echocardiography may demonstrate abrupt flattening of mid-to-late diastolic movement of the left ventricular posterior wall, reflecting a sudden decline in diastolic filling. Rapid early closure of the mitral valve may be detected, as well as premature pulmonary valve opening because of increased right-sided diastolic pressure. Several other echocardiographic features have been described including a diastolic septal bounce; mild atrial enlargement and vena cava dilation; and alterations in the flow characteristics in pulmonary veins, vena cava, hepatic vein, and across the mitral valve. Transthoracic echocardiography may demonstrate a thickened pericardium in severe cases. However, transesophageal echocardiography, magnetic resonance imaging, and computer tomography scanning are superior to transthoracic echocardiography to detect pericardial thickening.[125] None of the echocardiographic or other imaging modalities for the diagnosis of constrictive pericarditis have been evaluated in small animals.

Hemodynamic data obtained by cardiac catheterization are generally necessary to establish a diagnosis of constrictive pericarditis in small animals. Usually elevation and equilibration (or near equilibration) of the diastolic pressures of all cardiac chambers occurs. The right atrial pressure trace is often described as having an *M* or *W* pattern. This pattern arises because the A and V waves are separated by a reduced X descent, whereas the Y descent is prominent (Figure 205-14, *A*). The ventricular pressure trace shows a dip-and-plateau pattern (or "square-root" sign) in diastole. A rapid intravenous fluid infusion may be necessary to fully reveal the characteristic hemodynamic features of constrictive pericarditis (Figure 205-14, *B*).[27,75,125]

Treatment for constrictive pericarditis involves surgical stripping of the fibrotic, fused, and adherent pericardium from the underlying myocardium (epicardial decortication). This technically difficult procedure is associated with high perioperative morbidity and mortality.

CHAPTER • 206

Canine Heartworm Disease

Clarke Atkins

Heartworm infection (HWI) (dirofilariasis), caused by *Dirofilaria immitis*, primarily affects members of the family Canidae. Dirofilariasis is widely distributed, being recognized in northern and southern temperate zones, in the tropics, and in the subtropics. Infections are recognized in most of the United States, although the distribution favors the Southeast and Mississippi River Valley (Figure 206-1). In some endemic areas in the United States, infection rates approach 45%, and in some hyperendemic tropical regions, virtually all dogs are infected. Dirofilariasis is generally infrequent in Canada. A recent survey of veterinarians indicated that in 2001 there were approximately 240,000 cases diagnosed in the United States.[1]

Species known to have been infected with *D. immitis* include the domestic dog, wolves, foxes, coyotes, domestic cats, ferrets, muskrats, sea lions, nondomestic cats, coatimundi, and humans. The species of greatest interest to the practicing veterinarian include the dog and domestic cat. Because the consequences, treatment, and prognoses differ between the two species, clinical aspects of canine and feline heartworm disease (HWD) will be discussed separately.

When HWI is severe or prolonged, it may result in the pathologic process, called *HWD*. HWD may vary from asymptomatic (radiographic lesions only) to severe, life-threatening, chronic pulmonary artery, lung, and cardiac disease. In chronic HWI, glomerulonephritis, anemia, and thrombocytopenia may also be recognized. Severe dirofilariasis may, in addition, produce acute and fulminant multisystemic presentations, such as caval syndrome (CS) and disseminated intravascular coagulation (DIC).

LIFE CYCLE

D. immitis is transmitted by over sixty species of mosquitoes, although important mosquito vectors probably number less than 12. Understanding the complex life cycle of *D. immitis* is imperative for veterinary practitioners in heartworm endemic areas (Figure 206-2). Adult heartworms (L5) reside in the pulmonary arteries and, to a lesser extent in heavy infections, the right ventricle. After mating, microfilariae (L1) are produced by mature adult female heartworms (L5) and are released into the circulation. These L1 are ingested by feeding female mosquitoes and undergo two moults (L1 to L2 to L3) over an 8- to 17-day period. It is important to note that this process is temperature dependent; in times of the year when insufficient numbers of days occur in which the ambient temperature is adequate, moulting in the mosquito does not occur during the lifetime of the female mosquito and transmission cannot occur.[2,3] The resultant L3 is infective and is transmitted by the feeding mosquito to the original or another host, most often a male dog. Another moult occurs in the subcutaneous, adipose, and skeletal muscular tissues shortly after infection (1 to 12 days), with a final moult to L5 3 months (50 to 68 days) after infection. This immature adult (1 to 2 cm in length) soon enters the vascular system, migrating to the heart and lungs, where final maturation (mature male adults range from 15 to 18 cm and females from 25 to 30 cm) and mating occur. Under optimum conditions, completion of the life cycle takes 184 to 210 days. The canine host typically becomes microfilaremic 6 to 7 months after infection. Microfilariae (L1), which are variably present in infected dogs, show both seasonal and diurnal

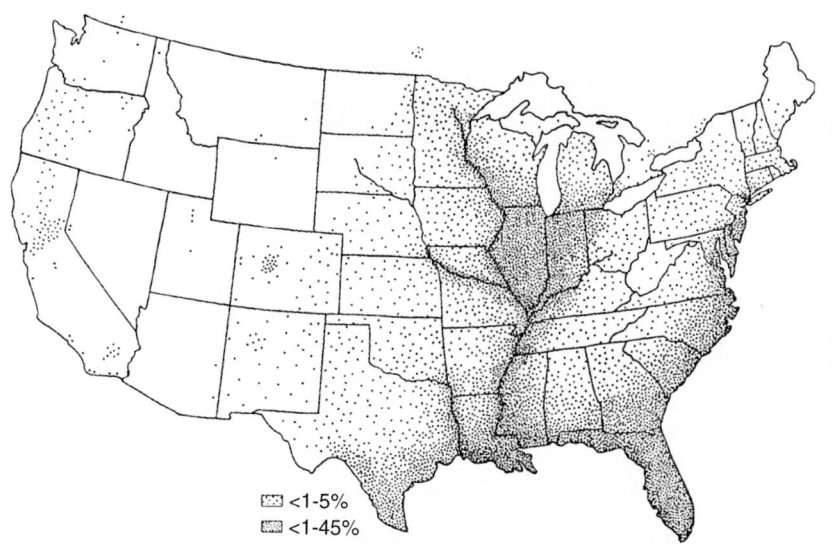

Figure 206-1 American Heartworm Society map, demonstrating relative prevalence of heartworm infection (HWI) in the United States and Canada in 1998. (From Seward L [ed]: Proceedings of the American Heartworm Symposium '98. Batavia, Ill., The American Heartworm Society, 1990.)

periodicity, with greatest numbers appearing in the peripheral blood during the evening hours and during the summer. Adult heartworms in dogs are known to live up to 5 years and microfilariae up to 30 months. Dillon has recently emphasized that the disease process in HWD begins with the moult to L5 (as soon as 2 to 3 months postinfection), at which time immature adults (L5) enter the vascular system, initiating vascular and possibly lung disease, with eosinophilia and eosinophilic infiltrates and signs of respiratory disease.[4] It is important to note that this antedates the profession's current ability to diagnose HWI.

PATHOPHYSIOLOGY

Heartworm is a misnomer because the adult actually resides in the pulmonary arterial system for the most part, and the primary insult to the health of the host is a manifestation of damage to the pulmonary arteries and lung. The severity of the lesions and hence clinical ramifications are related to the relative number of worms (ranging from one to over 250), the duration of infection, and the host and parasite interaction. Immature and mature adult heartworms reside primarily in the caudal pulmonary vascular tree, occasionally migrating

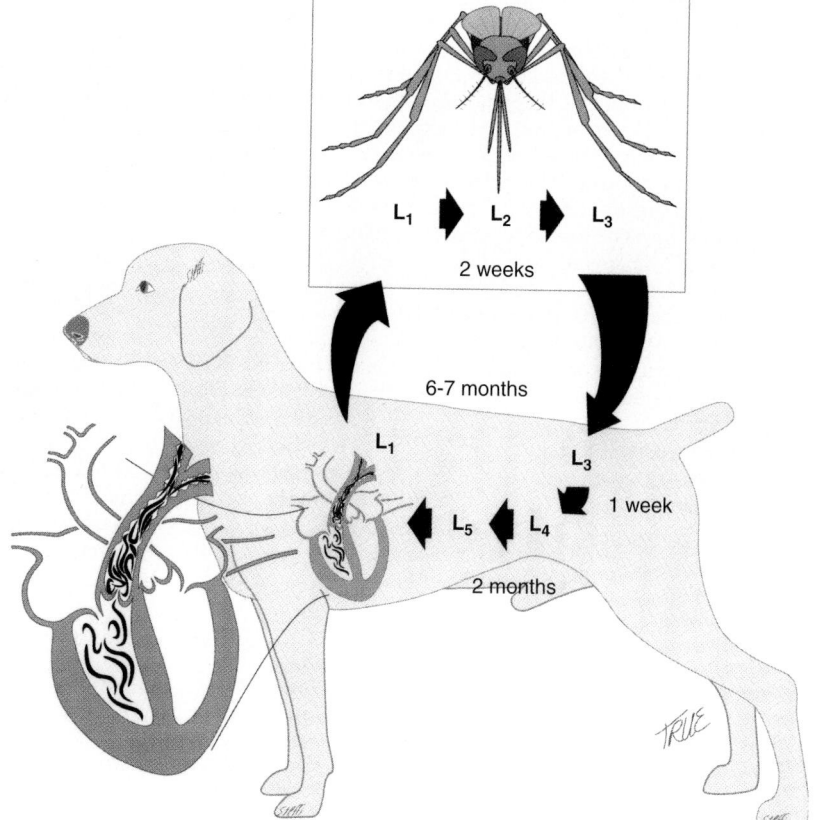

Figure 206-2 Life cycle of *Dirofilaria immitis* in the dog. (From Atkins CE: Heartworm disease. *In* Allen DG [ed]: Small Animal Medicine. Philadelphia, JB Lippincott Co, 1991, pp 341-363.)

into the main pulmonary arteries, the right heart, and even the great veins in heavy infections.

Obstruction of pulmonary vessels by living worms is of little clinical significance, unless worm burdens are extremely high. The major effect on the pulmonary arteries is produced by worm-induced (toxic substances, immune mechanisms, and trauma) villous myointimal proliferation, inflammation, pulmonary hypertension (PHT), disruption of vascular integrity, and fibrosis. This may be complicated by arterial obstruction and vasoconstriction caused by dead worm thromboemboli and their products. Pulmonary vascular lesions begin to develop within days of worm arrival (as early as 3 months postinfection), with endothelial damage and sloughing, villous proliferation, and activation and attraction of leucocytes and platelets. The immigration of such cells and the release of trophic factors induce smooth muscle cell proliferation and migration with collagen accumulation and eventual fibrosis. Proliferative lesions eventually encroach upon and even occlude vascular lumina. Endothelial swelling with altered intracellular junctions increases the permeability of the pulmonary vasculature. Worms, which have died naturally or have been killed, elicit an even more severe reaction, inciting thrombosis, granulomatous inflammation, and rugous villous inflammation. Grossly, the pulmonary arteries are enlarged, thick-walled, and tortuous, with roughened endothelial surfaces. These changes are only partially reversible.[5]

Although the role of exercise in exacerbation of the signs of thromboembolic HWD is accepted, its role in the development of pulmonary vascular disease and PHT is less clear. Although Rawlings[6] was unable to show an effect of 2.5 months' controlled treadmill exercise on PHT in heavily infected dogs, Dillon[7] showed more severe PHT in lightly infected, mildly exercised dogs than in more heavily infected but unexercised dogs receiving no exercise at 6 months postinfection.

Diseased pulmonary arteries are thrombosed, thickened, dilated, tortuous, noncompliant, and functionally incompetent, thereby resisting recruitment during increased demand; hence exercise capacity is diminished. Vessels to the caudal lung lobes are most severely affected. Pulmonary vasoconstriction results secondary to vasoactive substances released from heartworms. Furthermore, hypoxia (induced by ventilation-perfusion mismatching secondary to eosinophilic pneumonitis, pulmonary consolidation, or both), further contributes to vasoconstriction. The result is PHT and compromised cardiac output.[8] Pulmonary hypertension is exacerbated with exercise or other states of increased cardiac output. The right heart, which is an efficient volume pump but does not withstand pressure overload, first compensates by eccentric hypertrophy (dilatation and wall thickening) and, in severe infections, ultimately decompensation (right heart failure). In addition, hemodynamic stresses, geometric changes, and cardiac remodeling may contribute to secondary tricuspid insufficiency, thereby complicating or precipitating cardiac decompensation. Pulmonary infarction is uncommon because of the extensive collateral circulation provided the lung and because of the gradual nature of vascular occlusion. Because of increased pulmonary vascular permeability, perivascular edema may develop. Although, along with an inflammatory infiltrate, this may be evident radiographically as increased interstitial and even alveolar density, in and of itself, it is seemingly of minimal clinical significance and does not indicate left heart failure (in other words, furosemide is not indicated).

Spontaneous or postadulticidal thromboembolization (PTE) with dead worms may precipitate or worsen clinical signs, producing or aggravating PHT, right heart failure or, in rare instances, pulmonary infarction. Dying and disintegrating worms worsen vascular damage and enhance coagulation. Pulmonary blood flow is further compromised and consolidation of affected lung lobes may occur. With acute and massive worm death, this insult may be profound, particularly if associated with exercise. Exacerbation by exercise likely reflects increased pulmonary artery flow with escape of inflammatory mediators into the lung parenchyma through badly damaged and permeable pulmonary arteries (see Figure 207-7). Dillon has suggested that the lung injury is similar to that seen in adult respiratory distress syndrome (ARDS).[4]

Pulmonary parenchymal lesions also result by mechanisms other than post-thromboembolic consolidation. Eosinophilic pneumonitis is most often reported in true occult HWD, when immune-mediated destruction of microfilariae in the pulmonary microcirculation produces amicrofilaremia. This syndrome results when antibody-coated microfilariae, entrapped in the pulmonary circulation, incite an inflammatory reaction (eosinophilic pneumonitis).[9] A more sinister but uncommon form of parenchymal lung disease, termed *pulmonary eosinophilic granulomatosis*, has been associated with HWD. The exact cause and pathogenesis are unknown, but it is felt to be similar to HWD-related allergic pneumonitis.[10] It is postulated that microfilariae trapped in the lungs are surrounded by neutrophils and eosinophils, eventually forming granulomas and associated bronchial lymphadenopathy.

Antigen-antibody complexes, formed in response to heartworm antigens, commonly produce glomerulonephritis in heartworm-infected dogs.[11] The result is proteinuria (albuminuria) but uncommonly renal failure. Heartworms may also produce disease by aberrant migration. This uncommon phenomenon has been associated with neuromuscular and ocular manifestations, because worms have been described in tissues such as muscle, brain, spinal cord, and anterior chamber of the eye. In addition, arterial thrombosis with L5 has been observed when worms migrate aberrantly to the aortic bifurcation or more distally in the digital arteries.[12] Adult heartworms may also migrate in a retrograde manner from the pulmonary arteries to the right heart and venae cavae, producing CS, a devastating process, described following.[13]

CLINICAL SIGNS

The clinical signs of chronic HWD depend on the severity and duration of infection and, in most chronic cases, reflect the effects of the parasite on the pulmonary arteries and lungs, and secondarily, the heart. It is important to point out that the vast majority of dogs with HWI are asymptomatic. Historical findings in affected dogs variably include weight loss, diminished exercise tolerance, lethargy, poor condition, cough, dyspnea, syncope, and abdominal distension (ascites). Physical examination may reveal evidence of weight loss, split second heart sound (13%), right-sided heart murmur of tricuspid insufficiency (13%), and cardiac gallop.[14] If right heart failure is present, jugular venous distension and pulsation typically accompanies hepatosplenomegaly and ascites. Cardiac arrhythmias and conduction disturbances are uncommon in chronic HWD (<10%). With pulmonary parenchymal manifestations of HWD, cough and pulmonary crackles may be noted and, with granulomatosis (a rare occurrence), muffled lung sounds, dyspnea, and cyanosis are also reported. When massive pulmonary thromboembolization occurs, the additional signs of fever and hemoptysis may be noted.

DIAGNOSIS

Microfilarial Detection

Ideally the diagnosis is made by routine evaluation prior to the onset of symptoms (i.e., HWD). Dogs in areas in which heartworms are endemic should undergo a heartworm test yearly, particularly if on no heartworm preventative or if diethylcarbamazine is used (see discussion of controversies, following).

Table • 206-1

Differentiating Characteristics of Dipetalonema Reconditum and Dirofilaria Immitis

	NUMBER IN BLOOD	MOTION	SHAPE	LENGTH (MODIFIED KNOTT TEST)
D. reconditum	Usually few	Progressive	Curved body Blunt head Curved or "buttonhook" tail	263 U (250-288 U)
D. immitis	Usually many	Stationary	Straight body and tail Tapered head	308 U (295-325 U)

This was accomplished most commonly in the past by the microscopic identification of microfilariae on a direct blood smear, above the buffy coat in a microhematocrit tube, using the modified Knott test, or after millipore filtration. The accuracy of these tests, typically used for routine screening and for the diagnosis of suspected HWI, is improved by multiple testing. The modified Knott test and millipore filtration are more sensitive because they concentrate microfilariae, improving chances of diagnosis. The direct smear technique allows examination of larval motion, helping in the distinction of D. immitis from Dipetalonema reconditum (now termed Acanthocheilonema reconditum); other useful diagnostic criteria are included in Table 206-1. This distinction is important because the presence of the latter parasite does not require expensive and potentially harmful arsenical therapy, as does D. immitis. None of these tests can rule out HWI conclusively because of the potential for amicrofilarremic infections (5% to 67%) and the fact that false-negative results may occur, particularly if microfilarial numbers are small, a small amount of blood is collected, or direct smears are relied upon. The number of circulating microfilariae in the peripheral blood do not correlate well with the number of adult heartworms and therefore cannot be used to determine the severity of infection. In the most practices, microfilarial testing has been largely supplanted by (or supplemented with) immunodiagnositic antigen testing (i.e., enzyme-linked immunosorbent assay [ELISA]). The modified Knott test should always be performed, however, in antigen-positive dogs

to determine microfilarial status and in instances when owners continue to use diethylcarbamazine as a preventative. Some veterinarians choose to combine the antigen and microfilarial tests. This practice is most useful in dogs receiving diethylcarbamazine or no preventative (macrolides typically render the dog amicrofilaremic). Up to 1% of infected dogs are microfilaria positive and antigen negative.[15]

Immunodiagnostic Tests

In dogs not having received macrolide preventative therapies, the prevalence of amicrofilaremic infections is 5% to 67% (typically 10% to 20%).[16] This may be observed in prepatent (young) infections, in single-sex infections, with immune-mediated destruction of microfilaria, and with drug-induced amicrofilaremia. Dogs receiving macrolide preventatives are typically amicrofilaremic. Hence immunodiagnostic tests (heartworm ELISA antigen tests) are now regularly used for both screening and in cases suspected of having HWI. These tests have rapidly gained popularity because of their high sensitivity and specificity and ease of performance (Table 206-2).[17-20] The weakness of these tests is that they detect antigen from adult female heartworms and hence will produce negative results during the first ~6 (5 to 8) months of any infection, in all-male infections and in infections, with low female worm burdens. In fact, a recent study of the performance of three commercial test kits in detecting low worm burden (<4), naturally acquired infections demonstrated an overall (median for three test kits)

Table • 206-2

Commercial Antigen and Antibody Test Kits for Heartworm Diagnosis in Dogs and Cats*

MANUFACTURER	PRODUCT	TEST TYPE	FORMAT	SPECIES	SAMPLE	RUN TIME	STEPS
Heska	Solo Step™ CH	M	IMC	P,S,WB	Canine	10 (WB) 5 (S, P)	1
Heska	Solo Step™ CH Test Strips	M	IMC	P,S	Canine	5	1
Heska	Solo Step™ FH (antibody)	M	IMC	Feline	10 (WB) 5 (S, P)	1
IDEXX	PetCheck® Heartworm Antigen PF	MW	E	P,S,WB	Canine & feline	20	9 or 10
IDEXX	SNAP™ RT Heartworm Antigen Kit	M	E	P,S,WB	Canine	8	4
IDEXX	SNAP™ 3Dx	M	E	P,S,WB	Canine	8	4
IDEXX	SNAP™ Feline Heartworm Antigen Kit	M	E	P,S,WB	Feline	10	4
Synbiotics	Witness® HW	M	IMC	P,S,WB	Canine	10	4
Synbiotics	Witness® FHW (antibody)	M	IMC	P,S,WB	Feline	10	4
Synbiotics	Assure™ FH (antibody)	W (C)	E	P,S	Feline	15	6
Synbiotics	DiroCHEK® HW	MW	E	P,S	Canine & feline	20	8

*Tests listed in alphabetic order by manufacturer.
M, Membrane; MW, microwell; W, well; C, card; IMC, immunochromatographic; E, ELISA; P, plasma; S, serum; WB, whole blood.

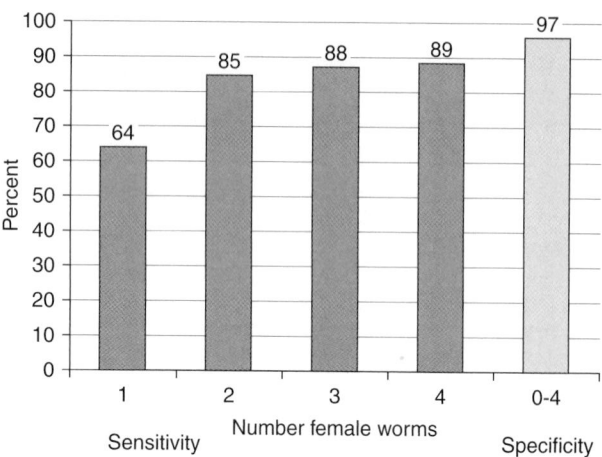

Figure 206-3 Comparison of sensitivity and specificity of three commercial heartworm test kits on known sera from naturally infected dogs with low worm burdens (zero to four adult female heartworms). Black bars represent median sensitivity of the three tests for sera of dogs with one, two, three, and four adult female heartworms. Grey bar represents the median specificity of the three tests for sera from dogs infected with zero to four adult female heartworms. (From Atkins CE: Comparison of results of 3 commercial heartworm antigen tests in dogs with low heartworm burdens. *J Am Vet Med Assoc*, 2003:222, 1221.)

sensitivity of 79% and a median specificity of 97%.[21] The sensitivity was relatively low (64%) for infections of only one female worm but improved with increasing female worm burden (median of 85%, 88%, and 89% for two, three, and four female worms, respectively for the three test kits evaluated). Of course with higher worm burdens, better sensitivity is experienced. Nevertheless, despite overall excellent results in detection of small worm burdens, false-negative results do occur (Figure 206-3).[21]

Certain ELISA antigen tests are designed to quantitatively predict worm burdens, based on antigen concentrations. Semiquantitative ELISA (Snap™ Canine Heartworm PF) has been used to successfully predict antigen load and hence approximate worm burden. Rawlings and colleagues[22] have shown this to be useful in predicting thromboembolic complications, with dogs bearing greater worm burdens being more likely to experience such complications after adulticide. This application is most useful, however, in instances of low antigen concentration (suggesting low worm burden), because high antigen concentrations might be recognized when all or most worms are dead, having released a large amount of antigen into the circulation. ELISA technology also allows determination of the efficacy of adulticide therapy. ELISA antigen concentration typically falls to undetectable levels 8 to 12 weeks after successful adulticide therapy, so a positive test persisting beyond 12 weeks post-therapy has been suggested to indicate persistent infection.[23] However, antigen tests may remain positive for longer periods, and this author does not assume a failure in adulticidal therapy unless the antigen test is positive 6 months after adulticidal therapy.

As previously suggested, macrolide therapy with ivermectin, milbemycin oxime, moxidectin, and selamectin results in clearance of microfilaria within 6 to 8 months.[23-25] In addition, embryostasis may be permanent. Thus the use of direct smears, the Knott test, and the millipore filter (microfilarial tests) in dogs receiving monthly heartworm preventatives (macrolides) is inappropriate. Therefore the only effective testing modality in the ever-increasing number of dogs receiving monthly preventative is the use of antigen assays.

A general approach to the diagnosis of HWI is demonstrated in Figure 206-4.

Radiography

Although not an effective screening test for HWI, thoracic radiography offers an excellent method for detecting HWD, for determining its severity, and for evaluating pulmonary parenchymal changes. Radiographic abnormalities, which develop relatively early in the disease course, are present in approximately 85% of cases. According to the study of 200 heartworm-infected dogs by Losonsky and colleagues,[26] radiographic features (Figure 206-5) include right ventricular enlargement (60%), increased prominence of the main pulmonary artery segment (70%), increased size and density of the pulmonary arteries (50%), and pulmonary artery tortuousity and "pruning" (50%). If heart failure is present, enlargement of the caudal vena cava, liver, and spleen, as well as pleural effusion, ascites, or both, may be evident. Thrall and Calvert[27] suggested that pleural effusion is uncommon in heart failure due to HWD, demonstrating that marked enlargement of the cranial lobar pulmonary artery was a more sensitive indicator of HWD-associated heart failure than is enlargement of the caudal vena cava.

Thoracic radiographs obtained in the ventrodorsal projection are preferable for cardiac silhouette evaluation, ease, and often minimizing patient stress. However, the dorsoventral projection is superior for the evaluation of the caudal lobar pulmonary vessels that are considered abnormal if larger than the diameter of the ninth rib where the rib and artery intersect (Figure 206-6). The cranial pulmonary artery is best evaluated in the lateral projection and should normally not be larger than its accompanying vein or the proximal one third of the fourth rib (Figure 206-7).

The pulmonary parenchyma can best be evaluated radiographically. With pneumonitis, the findings include a mixed interstitial to alveolar density, which is typically most severe in the caudal lung lobes (Figure 206-8). In eosinophilic nodular pulmonary granulomatosis, the inflammatory process is arranged into the interstitial nodules, associated with bronchial lymphadenopathy and, occasionally, pleural effusion. With pulmonary thromboembolism, the radiographic findings of coalescing interstitial and alveolar infiltrates, particularly in the caudal lung lobes, reflect the increased pulmonary vascular permeability and inflammation described previously (see Figure 206-13). Consolidation may accompany massive embolization, pulmonary infarction, or both.

Electrocardiography

Electrocardiography is useful in detecting arrhythmias but is generally insensitive in detection of cardiac chamber enlargement in HWD when compared with radiography and echocardiography. If radiography does not suggest HWD, it is unlikely that the electrocardiogram (ECG) will be useful in the absence of arrhythmias. With the exception of CS and heart failure, arrhythmias are rare (2% to 4%).[28] Nevertheless, the finding of a right ventricular enlargement pattern (Chapter 202) is supportive evidence for HWD. Lombard and Ackerman[28] demonstrated that ECG abnormalities were present in 38% to 62% of dogs with moderate and severe echocardiographic changes of HWD, while Calvert and Rawlings[29] found that only 6% of 276 dogs with dirofilariasis had ECG changes of right ventricular enlargement. Calvert and Rawlings[30] also showed that the most sensitive ECG parameters for detection of HWD are lead II S waves deeper than 0.8 mv, mean electrical axis greater than 103 degrees, and greater than three ECG parameters of right heart enlargement. The latter ECG finding (> three criteria) is considered to be the most accurate. P-pulmonale (tall P waves, indicative of right atrial enlargement) is unusual in HWD.

Diagnosis of Heartworm Infection in Dogs

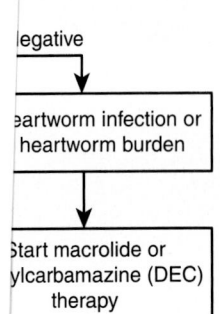

Perform an antigen test

negative

...eartworm infection or
...heartworm burden

Start macrolide or
...ylcarbamazine (DEC)
therapy

10-14 MF → infective stage.

Earliest detection is 5-6.5 mo post inf.
→ of MF or Antigen.

Antigen test is most sensitive

Smear: stationary - ~~straight~~ straight tail + body - tapered head

ML: MF 3rd + 4th larvae H-Adults.

Stage: XRAY
u/s.

TE: fever, cough, hemoptysis.
RHF
usually in 7-10d.
but up to 4 weeks later.

Caval Syndrome:

...nfection (HWI) in the dog.

vascular dz + severity of inf have most influence
on probability of TE + outcome of tx.

Tx - low TE Risk: 2 inj 24 hr apart.

- ↑ risk = 1 dose   1 mo later 2 inj 24 hr apart.

- start on ML right away

- re test 6 mo post tx

MF - live 2 yr
Adult - 5 yr

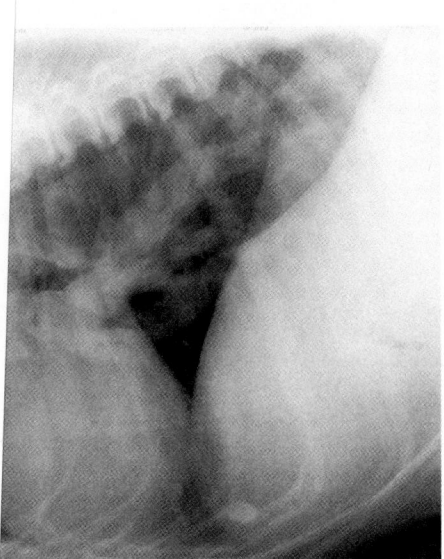

...ateral thoracic radiograph obtained from a dog
with chronic heartworm disease (HWD). Reader should note
right ventricular enlargement (evident in the apex having been
lifted from the sternum), enlarged apical pulmonary artery, and
an interstitial infiltrate in the caudal lung lobes.

Figure 206-5 The relative frequency of cardiovascular radiographic findings of heartworm disease (HWD). (Losonsky JM,
Thrall DE, Lewis RE: Thoracic radiographic abnormalities in
200 dogs with heartworm infestation. *Vet Radiol* 24:120, 1983.)

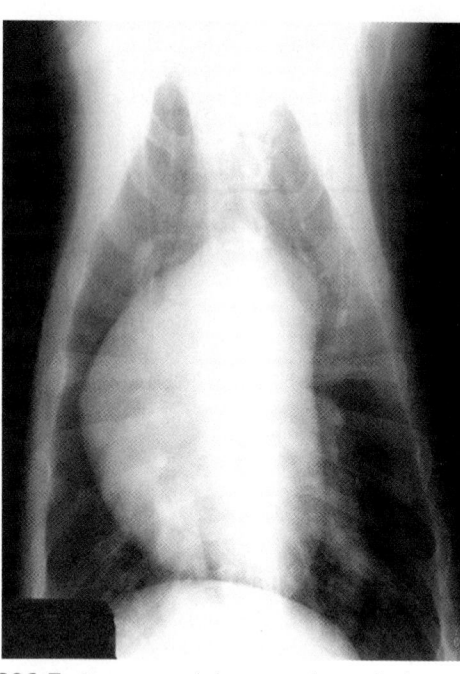

Figure 206-7 Dorsoventral thoracic radiograph obtained from a dog with chronic heartworm disease (HWD). Reader should note the enlarged main pulmonary artery, right ventricular enlargement, and enlarged, tortuous caudal lobar pulmonary arteries. (See Figure 206-5 for schematic of radiographic abnormalities.)

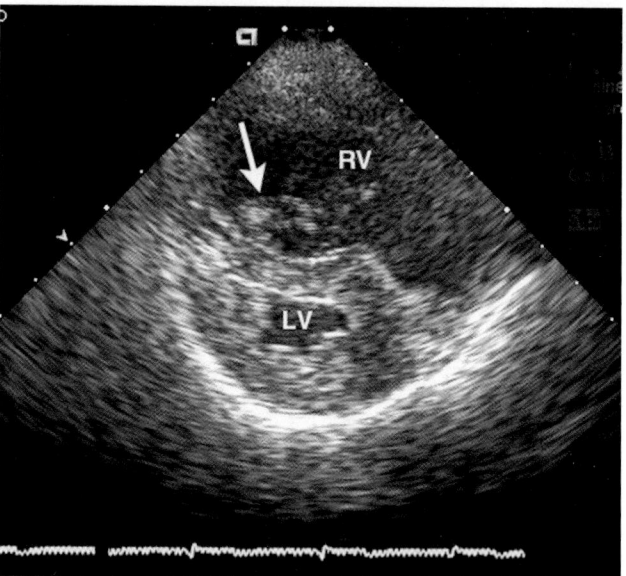

Figure 206-9 A short-axis, two-dimensional echocardiogram obtained from a dog with chronic heartworm disease (HWD). Reader should note the enlarged right ventricular lumen *(RV)* and right ventricular papillary muscle *(arrow)*. The septum is flattened and bows toward the small left ventricle *(LV)*. The electrocardiogram (ECG) at the bottom of the figure demonstrates that this is a diastolic frame.

Echocardiography

Echocardiography is relatively sensitive in the detection of right heart enlargement, because the right ventricular end diastolic dimension and septal and right ventricular free wall thickness are all increased (Figure 206-9). Lombard reported abnormal (paradoxical) septal motion in four of 10 dogs with HWD. The ratio of left to right ventricular internal dimensions is a useful calculation, being reduced from a normal

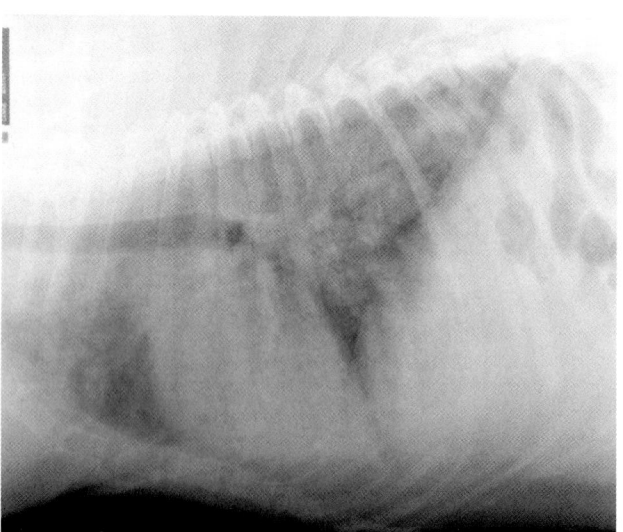

Figure 206-8 Lateral thoracic radiograph obtained from a coughing dog with chronic heartworm disease (HWD). The diffuse interstitial to alveolar infiltrate is severe and represents eosinophilic pneumonitis. Cardiac and pulmonary arterial changes are less severe than seen in Figures 206-6, 206-7, and 206-13.

value of 3 to 4 to a mean value of 0.7 in dogs with HWD. In some instances, two-dimensional echocardiography can be used to demonstrate worms in the pulmonary artery (see Chapter 207). Although heartworms can occasionally be demonstrated in the right ventricle, this method is insensitive except in dogs with CS or very heavy worm burdens, because the worms infrequently inhabit this location.[31]

Clinical Pathology

Hematological and serum chemical abnormalities, although of limited use in making a diagnosis of HWD, are frequently useful in providing supportive evidence and for evaluating concurrent disease processes that may or may not be related to HWD. Calvert and Rawlings[30] report that the dog with HWD in Georgia typically is found to have a low-grade, nonregenerative anemia (present in 10% of mildly to moderately affected dogs and up to 60% of severely affected dogs), neutrophilia (20% to 80% of cases), eosinophilia (~ 85% of cases), and basophilia (~ 60% of cases). Thrombocytopenia, which may be noted in chronic HWD, CS, and DIC, is most common 1 to 2 weeks after adulticidal therapy. In severe HWD, especially if heart failure is present, liver enzyme activities may be increased (10% of cases), and occasionally hyperbilirubinemia is noted. Azotemia, seen in only 5% of cases, may be prerenal in origin if dehydration or heart failure are present or may be secondary to glomerulonephritis. In 10% to 30% of cases, albuminuria is noted. If glomerular disease is severe, hypoproteinemia (hypoalbuminemia) has the potential to complicate the clinical picture. Not surprisingly, the most severe clinicopathologic findings are associated with the most severe clinical findings.

Evaluation of tracheobronchial cytology is at times useful, particularly in the coughing dog with eosinophilic pneumonitis, occult HWD, and minimal radiographic evidence of HWD. Microscopic examination reveals evidence of an eosinophilic infiltrate. In microfilaremic dogs, L1 may occasionally be detected in this manner. Abdominal fluid analysis in cases of congestive heart failure (CHF) typically reveals a modified transudate. Dogs with HWD and right heart failure have central venous pressure (CVP) that ranges from 12 to more than 20 cm H$_2$O, but ascites develop at lower CVPs if hypoalbuminemia is present.

MEDICAL MANAGEMENT

The medical management of HWI is complex because of the complicated parasite life cycle, the marked variability in clinical manifestations and severity of HWD, prophylactic considerations, adulticidal and microfilaricidal considerations, and the relative toxicity and complications associated with adulticidal therapy. For these reasons, the diagnosis, prevention, and treatment of HWI remains a challenge.

Prophylaxis

Prevention of HWI is an obvious and attainable goal for the veterinary profession. Prevention failure results from ignorance on the part of owners as to the presence or potential severity of HWI, lack of owner compliance, or from inadequate instruction on preventative measures by the attending veterinarian.[1,32-34] Studies of owner compliance have revealed that approximately 55% of dog owners that use veterinary care purchase heartworm preventative, and enough medication is dispensed only to meet the needs of approximately 56% of those dogs. Hence the proportion of "cared for" dogs in the population that receive adequate heartworm prophylaxis is less than one third.[33] If one takes into consideration doses purchased but not administered and dogs that are never taken to a veterinarian, the percentage of protected dogs falls drastically. This was emphasized in North Carolina in 1999, when Hurricane Floyd caused extensive flooding and disruption in the poorest part of the state. Of dogs rescued from the floodwaters, 67% were infected with heartworms (personal communication, Dr. Kelli Ferris, North Carolina State University, 2003). In addition, evidence suggests that the veterinary profession is failing in its education of clients. New and colleagues,[35] upon questioning veterinary clients purchasing macrolide preventatives, found that 38% did not realize that their prescribed drug's spectrum was broader than solely preventing HWI.

Diethylcarbamazine

Diethylcarbamazine (DEC), which long enjoyed popularity as the preventative of choice, has now been largely replaced by the safer and more convenient macrolide preventatives. This product is safe (only in *amicrofilaremic* dogs) and effective; however, it must be given daily, making owner compliance problematic. Diethylcarbamazine is thought to kill L3 and early L4 tissue migrating larvae but only has a small temporal window of therapeutic efficacy, thus explaining the need for frequent administration. Preventative should be administered daily from the onset of mosquito season, continuously until 1 to 2 months after a killing frost. In some geographic regions, the persistence of mosquitoes dictates yearlong prophylaxis, although this is controversial for much of the United States (see discussion of controversies, following).

Diethylcarbamazine must only be administered to dogs free of microfilariae, thus dictating a yearly heartworm test prior to reinstitution of preventative therapy. Inadvertent administration of diethylcarbamazine to microfilaremic dogs produces an adverse, possibly immune-mediated reaction in approximately 30%.[36] Signs associated with this adverse drug reaction usually occur within 1 hour of medication and include depression, ptyalism, vomiting, diarrhea, weak pulse, pale mucous membranes with poor capillary refill time, and bradycardia. Subsequently some dogs may become recumbent, dyspneic,

and tachycardic, and 18% of reactors succumb. Restated, 6% of microfilaremic dogs to which diethylcarbamazine is administered will die due an adverse reaction.

Not infrequently, owners inadvertently miss one or more doses of DEC preventative. If 1 day of therapy is omitted, no problem exists and drug administration should continue. In the event of a more prolonged lapse in diethylcarbamazine treatment, reinstitution of medication should be advised, with the realization that infection may have occurred during the prophylactic hiatus.

These dogs should be reevaluated in 6 to 7 months to determine if infection has resulted. If a dog is found to be microfilaremic when receiving diethylcarbamazine, prophylaxis should be continued; however, if inadvertently stopped, reinstitution may result in the aforementioned adverse reaction.

Macrolide Antibiotics

The introduction of the macrolide agents (macrocyclic lactones) ivermectin (Heartgard®), milbemycin oxime (Interceptor®), moxidectin (ProHeart® and ProHeart® 6), and selamectin (Revolution™) has provided the veterinary profession with effective heartworm preventatives in a variety of formulations. These agents, because they interrupt larval development during the first 2 months after infection, have a large window of efficacy and are administered monthly or less frequently. Macrolide agents are superior to DEC in convenience. They produce less severe reactions when inadvertently given to microfilaremic dogs, allow a grace period for inadvertent lapses in administration, are more effective with treatment lapses of up to 2 to 3 months when used continuously for the next 12 months,[37] and have a dual role as microfilaricides.[20,37-39] Recently it has been shown that some macrolides have adulticidal activity, if used continuously for prolonged periods.[39-41] (NOTE: ProHeart® 6 is no longer on the market.)

Ivermectin

Ivermectin, a chemical derivative of avermectin B$_1$ that is obtained from *Streptomyces* spp., is effective against a range of endo- and ectoparasites and is marketed as a once-monthly heartworm preventative. It is also marketed in a form with pyrantel pamoate to improve efficacy against intestinal parasites (Table 206-3). Macrolides provide a wide window of efficacy and provide some protection when lapses in therapy occur. Ivermectin is effective as a prophylactic with lapses of up to 2 months. Protection is extended, with continuous 12-month administration postexposure, with lapses of 3 months (98% efficacy) and of 4 months (95% efficacy).[37] As stated previously, ivermectin is microfilaricidal at preventative doses (6 to 12 μg/kg/month), resulting in a gradual decline in microfilarial numbers. Despite this gradual microfilarial destruction, generally mild, adverse reactions (transient diarrhea) can occur if administered to microfilaremic dogs.[37] Some breeds (collies and Shetland sheep dogs) are susceptible to ivermectin (and other macrolide) toxicosis at high doses, suffering neurologic signs. This has typically resulted with the use of concentrated livestock preparations, with clinical signs recognized with doses greater than 16 times the recommended dose.[25] For this reason, only preparations designed for pet use should be administered to dogs. When used appropriately, ivermectin is virtually 100% effective in preventing HWI. Additionally, recent studies have shown ivermectin to have partial adulticidal properties when used continuously for 16 months[40] and virtually 100% effective with continuous administration for 30 months.[41] (See discussion of controversies, following.)

Milbemycin

Milbemycin oxime is a member of a family of milbemycin macrolide antibiotics derived from a species of *Streptomyces*. At 500 to 999 μg/kg, it has efficacy against developing filarial

Table • 206-3

Comparison Clinical Spectrum of Commercially Available Macrolides

DRUG	HW	MICROFILARIAE	ADULTICIDE	HOOKWORMS	WHIPWORMS	ROUNDWORMS	TAPEWORMS	FLEAS & EGGS	TICKS
Ivermectin (chewable)	+	+	+	+*		+*			
Milbemycin (flavored tablet)	+	++		+	+	+		−/+†	
Moxidectin (tablet or injectable)	+	+		+‡					
Selamectin (topical)	+	+	(+)	+				+/+	+

For adulticidal effects, assumes 31 months' continuous therapy for ivermectin and 18 months' continuous therapy for selamectin.
HW, Heartworm preventative; ( ), partially effective or incompletely studied.
*Ivermectin/pyrantel pamoate.
†Milbemycin/lufenuron.
‡Injectable formulation (removed from the market in late 2004).

larvae, arresting development in the first 6 weeks. It can therefore be given at monthly intervals with a *reachback effect* of 2 months when doses are inadvertently delayed. With 12 months' continuous treatment postexposure, this "safety net" can be extended to 3 months (97% efficacy), falling to 41% with lapses of 4 months.[37] At the preventative dose, milbemycin is a broad-spectrum parasiticide, being also effective against certain hookworms, roundworms, and whipworms (see Table 206-3). In microfilaremic dogs, milbemycin has greater potential for adverse reactions than do other macrolides, because it is a potent microfilaricide at preventative doses.[20] Adverse reactions, similar to those observed with ivermectin at microfilaricidal doses, may be observed in microfilaremic dogs receiving milbemycin at preventative doses.[42] As with microfilaricidal doses (50 μg/kg) of ivermectin, Benadryl (2 mg/kg intramuscularly) and dexamethasone (0.25 mg/kg intravenously) may be administered prior to milbemycin to prevent adverse reactions, particularly in dogs with high microfilarial counts. Milbemycin is also safe for use in collies at the preventative dose. With appropriate use, milbemycin is virtually 100% efficacious as a heartworm prophylactic.

Moxidectin

The macrolide preventative, moxidectin, has been more recently marketed as a narrow-spectrum heartworm preventative (see Table 206-3) and shown to be safe and virtually 100% effective at 3 μg/kg orally, given monthly or bimonthly up to 2 months postinfection.[43] Moxidectin, at this dose, is gradually microfilaricidal and did not produce adverse reactions in a small number of microfilaremic dogs treated with the prophylactic dose.[38] At 15 μg/kg, 98% reduction in microfilarial numbers was documented 2 months post-treatment. Lastly, moxidectin appears to be safe in collies.[44] A new liposomal formulation of moxidectin, which provides the potential to improve owner compliance, gives 6 months' protection with one subcutaneous injection. With 12 months' (two injections) continuous treatment, injectable moxidectin is 97% effective at preventing infection after a 4-month lapse in preventative therapy.[45] (This product was removed from the market in late 2004 pending further study.)

Selamectin

Selamectin is a semisynthetic macrolide. It is unique in its broad spectrum and in the fact that it is applied topically once monthly (see Table 206-3). Its efficacy is similar to that of other macrolides (virtually 100%, when used as directed).[46] At 6 to 12 mg/kg topically, this preventative is effective at preventing heartworms infection and kills fleas and flea eggs, sarcoptic mange mites, ticks, and ear mites.[46] Bathing and swimming, as soon as 2 hours after application, does not alter efficacy. Safety has been shown at tenfold topical doses, with oral consumption of single doses and, in ivermectin-sensitive collies, at recommended doses and fivefold overdoses for 3 months.[47] Like other macrolides, selamectin has at least a 2-month *reachback* effect and with 12 months' continuous administration is 99% protective after 3-month lapses in prophylaxis.[46,48] Selamectin has microfilaricidal activity similar to other macrolides.[48] Chronic, continuous selamectin administration has adulticidal efficacy, although no published data indicate it is as effective in this role as ivermectin.

In summary, the macrolides offer a convenient, effective, and safe method of heartworm prophylaxis with varying spectra and methods of administration (see Table 206-1). They each have microfilaricidal efficacy and render female heartworms sterile. Hence microfilarial tests for HWI cannot be reliably used in dogs receiving these products. Prophylaxis should be commenced at 6 to 8 weeks of age in endemic areas or as soon thereafter as climatic conditions dictate.[19,49] Although safer than DEC in microfilaremic dogs, before first-time administration any dog over 6 months of age and at risk of infection should be tested (antigen test, followed by a microfilaria test, if antigen positive). Additionally, even though protective for at least 8 weeks postexposure, macrolides should be administered precisely as indicated by the manufacturer. If accidental lapses of more than 10 weeks occur, the preventative should be reinstituted at recommended doses and maintained for 12 consecutive months.[25] Macrolides can also be used to "rescue" dogs that have lapsed in their DEC daily therapy for up to 60 to 90 days.[19,49] In the event of a lapse in preventative administration during a time of known exposure risk, an antigen heartworm test should be performed 7 months after the last possible exposure to determine if infection has occurred.

The necessary duration of protection is controversial. The American Heartworm Society indicates that in colder climates, yearlong prevention is not necessary, advocating beginning macrolides within 1 month of the anticipation of transmission season[25] and continuing 1 month beyond the transmission season.[19,49] On the other hand, some experts

Table • 206-4

Manufacturer's Recommendations for the Use of Melarsomine Dihydrochloride, Based on Patient Status

CLASS 1 HEARTWORM INFECTION (ASYMPTOMATIC, NO RADIOGRAPHIC LESIONS)	CLASS 2 SYMPTOMATIC HEARTWORM DISEASE (MILD TO MODERATE SIGNS)	CLASS 3 SYMPTOMATIC HEARTWORM DISEASE (SEVERE SIGNS)	CLASS 4 CAVAL SYNDROME
Two doses melarsomine 24 hours apart (2.5 mg/kg IM)	Two doses melarsomine 24 hours apart (2.5 mg/kg IM)	One dose melarsomine (2.5 mg/kg IM), followed in approximately 1 month with 2 injections 24 hours apart	Melarsomine not indicated for acute care

believe that yearlong prevention should be embraced, regardless of geographic location.[50] This author advocates yearlong prevention, at least below the Mason-Dixon line in North America.

THERAPY

Melarsomine

In most cases of HWD, it is imperative to rid the patient of the offending parasite. Thiacetarsemide, for decades the only drug approved for this purpose, is no longer available. It has been replaced by melarsomine (Immiticide®), an organoarsenic superior in safety and efficacy to thiacetarsemide.[1] With two doses (2.5 mg/kg intramuscularly every 24 hours), the efficacy is over 96%. Melarsomine has a mean retention time five times longer than thiacetarsemide, and its metabolites are free in the plasma (on which heartworms feed).[51,52] In a study of 382 dogs with HWI receiving melarsomine, none required cessation of therapy due to hepatorenal toxicity (as compared with 15% to 30% with thiacetarsemide), and no case of severe PTE was observed.[53]

Despite the enhanced safety of this product, adverse reactions are still noted.[14,16,54] In fact, successful pharmacologic adulticidal therapy, by definition, dictates thromboembolic events. The clinician can diminish the severity of this complication by restricting exercise after melarsomine administration. Perhaps the drug's biggest asset is the possibility of flexible dosing ("split-dose"— three injections over 1 month or longer), allowing the potential for a safer 50% initial worm kill, followed by subsequent injections to approach 100% efficacy. Studies have shown that patients treated with the split-dose regimen have a higher seroconversion to a negative antigen status than patients treated with either caparsolate or the standard melarsomine dosing regimen.[55,56]

A split-dose protocol can be used in severely afflicted individuals or in those in which pulmonary thromboembolism is anticipated (Table 206-4). This method allows for destruction of only one half the worms initially (one intramuscular injection of 2.5 mg/kg), thereby lessening the chance for embolic complications. This single dose is followed by a two-dose regimen in 1 to 3 months, if clinical conditions permit. Although the manufacturer recommends this protocol for severely affected dogs, the author uses it for all cases unless financial constraint or underlying concern for arsenic toxicity exists (e.g., pre-existent severe renal or hepatic disease; Figure 206-10).[54] Disadvantages to the split-dose method include additional expense, increased total arsenic dose, and the need for 2 months' exercise restriction.

In 55 dogs with severe HWD that were treated in this manner, 96% had a good or very good outcome with more than 98% negative for antigenemia 90 days post-therapy.[53] Of the 55 severely affected dogs, 31% had "mild or moderate PTE," but no fatalities resulted. The most common sign was fever, cough, and anorexia 5 to 7 days post-treatment. This was associated with mild perivascular caudal lobar pulmonary radiographic densities and subsided spontaneously or after corticosteroid therapy.

Microfilaricidal and Preventative Therapy in Heartworm-Positive Dogs

At the time of diagnosis (usually by a positive heartworm antigen test) a minimum data base is completed. This includes a microfilaria test, chemistry panel, complete blood count (CBC), urinalysis, and thoracic radiographic evaluation. If liver disease is suspected from clinical and laboratory findings, serum bile acid evaluation may be useful in evaluating

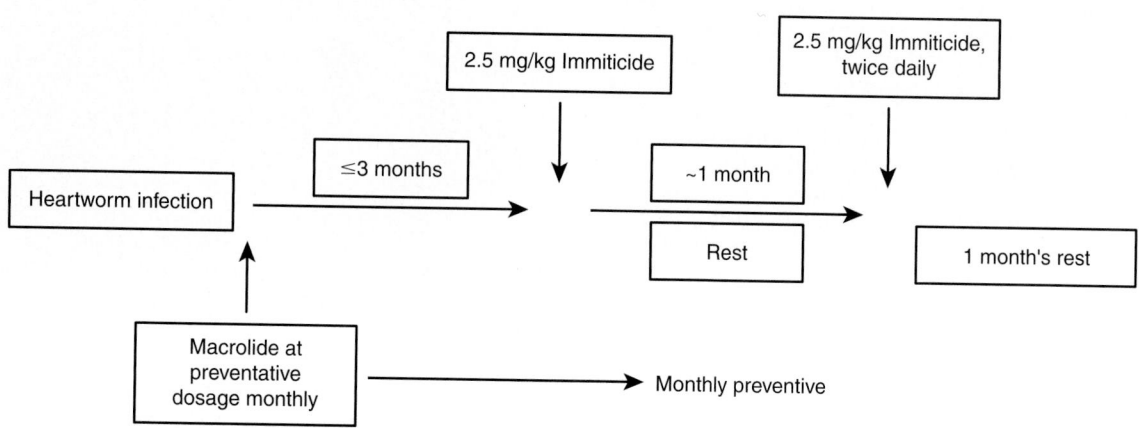

Figure 206-10 An algorithmic approach to the management of heartworm infection (HWI) in the dog. (Atkins CE, Miller M: Is there a better way to administer heartworm adulticidal therapy? *Vet Med*, April 310-317, 2003.)

liver function. At this time, monthly macrolide preventative is prescribed (see Figure 206-10). This approach, which differs from the recommendations of the American Heartworm Society, is used to prevent further infection, to eliminate microfilariae (chronic therapy renders the dog of no further risk to infect itself or other dogs and cats), and to destroy developing L4 (not yet susceptible to adulticidal therapy). In microfilaremic dogs, the first macrolide dose is administered in the hospital or at home, with observation, so an adverse reaction might be recognized and treated promptly.

Corticosteroids with or without antihistamines (dexamethasone at 0.25 mg/kg intravenously and Benadryl at 2 mg/kg intramuscularly or 1 mg/kg of prednisolone orally 1 hour before +/− 6 hours after administration of the first dose of preventative) may be administered to reduce the potential for adverse reaction in highly microfilaremic patients. It is important to emphasize that adverse reactions are unusual with macrolides at preventative doses.

Depending on the time of year, up to 2 to 3 months might be allowed to lapse before adulticidal therapy is administered. Although monthly macrolide administration prevents further infection, this delay allows larval maturation to adulthood, ensuring that the only stage of the life cycle present is the adult, which is vulnerable to melarsomine therapy. This is more important if the diagnosis is made during or at the end of a mosquito exposure season. If the diagnosis is made in the spring or late winter, when infective larvae have matured, adulticidal therapy may be immediately administered (see Figure 206-10).

Procedure

The first injection of Melarsomine is administered by deep intramuscular injection (2.5 mg/kg) in the lumbar musculature (as described in the package insert) and the injection site recorded. Before injection, the needle is changed and care is taken to inject deep into the muscle and nowhere else. Patients are typically, but not necessarily, hospitalized for the day. The need for exercise restriction for 1 month is emphasized, and sedation is provided if necessary. Owners are also advised as to adverse reactions (fever, local inflammation, lassitude, inappetence, cough, dyspnea, collapse), to call if they have concerns, and to return for a second series of two injections in approximately 1 month.

If serious systemic reaction results, the second stage of the adulticidal treatment is delayed or, occasionally, even canceled. Typically, however, even with severe reactions, the entire treatment protocol is completed within 2 to 3 months (see Figure 206-10). After a minimum of 1 month, the melarsomine injection procedure is repeated, again with a record of the injection site. If significant local reaction was noted after the first injection, subsequent injections are accompanied by dexamethasone or oral nonsteroidal anti-inflammatory drugs (NSAIDs) to minimize pain at the injection site. The next day (approximately 24 hours after the first injection) the process is repeated with melarsomine injection into the opposite lumbar area. Client instructions are similar to those previously given, with reemphasis of the need for 1 months' strict restriction of exercise. Antigen testing is repeated 6 months after the second series of injections, with a positive test result indicating incomplete adulticidal efficacy. It is emphasized that despite the proven efficacy of melarsomine, not all worms are killed in every patient. The worm burden is typically markedly reduced, but if as few as one to three adult female worms remain, positive antigen tests are likely. Whether to repeat adulticidal therapy, under these circumstances is decided on a case-by-case basis with input from the owners.

Macrolides

It is now known that certain macrolides have adulticidal properties.[39-41] Ivermectin, when administered monthly for 31 consecutive months, has nearly 100% adulticidal efficacy in young HWIs.[41] Selamectin, when administered continuously for 18 months, killed approximately 40% of transplanted worms.[39] Milbemycin and sustained release moxidectin appear to have minimal adulticidal efficacy.[39,40] Although there may be a role for this therapeutic strategy in cases in which financial constraints or concurrent medical problems prohibit melarsomine therapy, the current recommendations are that macrolides not be adapted as the primary adulticidal approach (see discussion of controversies, following).

Exercise Restriction

Cage rest is an important aspect of the management of HWD after adulticidal therapy, after PTE, or during therapy of heart failure. This can often be best, or only, accomplished in the veterinary clinic. If financial constraints preclude this, crating or housing in the bathroom or garage at home, tranquilization, or both, with only gentle leash walks are useful alternatives. Nevertheless, some owners do not or cannot restrict exercise, resulting in or worsening thromboembolic complications.

Surgical Therapy

Sasaki, Kitagawa, and Ishihara[57] have described a method of mechanical worm removal using a flexible alligator forceps (Figure 206-11). This method was 90% effective in 36 dogs with mild and severe HWD. Only two of the severely affected dogs (n = 9) died of heart and renal failure over 90 days postoperatively. These data suggest that, in skilled hands, the technique is safe. Subsequent studies by Morini and colleagues[58] demonstrated superior results as compared with melarsomine, producing less PTE and CS. It is important to note that the majority of dogs treated surgically required subsequent melarsomine administration for adequate worm destruction. Advantages to this technique include its diminished potential arsenic toxicity (subsequent adulticidal therapy would be administered to an asymptomatic dog) and relative freedom from thromboembolic complication. Disadvantages include the need for general anesthesia, a degree of operator skill, fluoroscopy, and subsequent arsenic administration. Nevertheless, it remains a potential alternative for the management of high-risk patients.

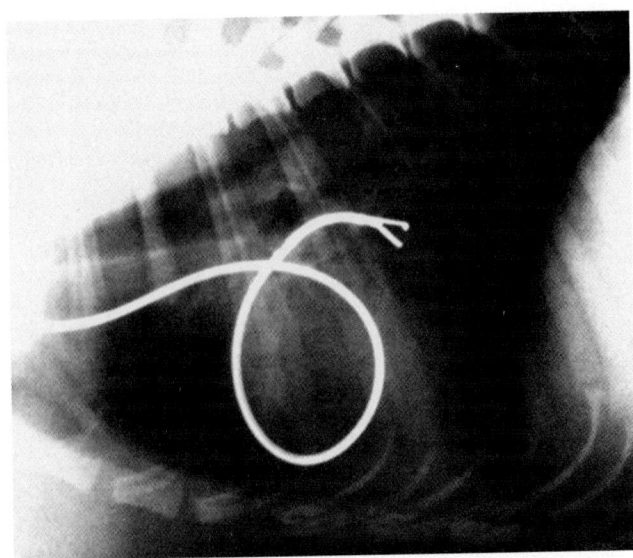

Figure 206-11 Heartworm retrieval using the flexible alligator forceps. (From Sasaki Y, Kitagawa H, Ishihara K: Clinical and pathological effects of heartworm removal from the pulmonary arteries using flexible alligator forceps. *In* Otto GF (ed): Proc Amer Heartworm Symposium '89. Batavia, Ill., American Heartworm Society, 1990, p 45.)

ANCILLARY THERAPY

Corticosteroids

The anti-inflammatory and immunosuppressive effects inherent to corticosteroids are useful for treatment of some aspects of HWD. Prednisone, the steroid most often advocated, reduces pulmonary arteritis but actually worsens the proliferative vascular lesions of HWD, diminishes pulmonary arterial flow, and reduces the effectiveness of thiacetarsemide. For these reasons, corticosteroids are indicated in HWD only in the face of pulmonary parenchymal complications (eosinophilic pneumonitis, eosinophilic granulomas, and PTE), to treat or prevent adverse reactions to microfilaricides, and possibly to minimize tissue reaction to melarsomine. For allergic pneumonitis, prednisone (1 mg/kg/day) is administered for 3 to 5 days and discontinued or tapered as indicated.[9,16] The response is generally favorable. Prednisone has also been advocated, along with cage rest, for the management of PTE at 1 to 2 mg/kg per day, continued until radiographic and clinical improvement is noted.[16] Because of the potential for steroid-induced fluid retention, such therapy should be used cautiously in the face of heart failure. In addition, caution is warranted because early studies demonstrated that postadulticidal corticosteroid therapy reduced pulmonary blood flow and worsened intimal disease in a model of HWI[59]; corticosteroids are also procoagulant.[16] As mentioned with adulticidal (previously discussed) and microfilaricidal (discussed following) therapies, corticosteroids may be used to minimize potential adverse reactions to melarsomine and to macrolides given to rapidly kill microfilariae.

Aspirin

Antithrombotic agents have received a good deal of attention in the management of HWD.[59-63] Potential benefits include reduction in severity of vascular lesions, reduction in thromboxane-induced pulmonary arterial vasoconstriction and PHT, and minimization of postadulticidal PTE.[61] Aspirin has shown success in diminishing the vascular damage caused by segments of dead worms,[61] reduced the extent and severity of myointimal proliferation caused by implanted living worms,[62] and improved pulmonary parenchymal disease and intimal proliferation in dogs receiving thiacetarsemide after previous living heartworm implantation.[59] More recent studies, however, have produced controversial results. Four dogs with implanted heartworms, receiving adulticide and administered aspirin, showed no improvement in pulmonary angiographic lesions, and treated dogs had more severe tortuousity than did controls and dogs receiving heparin.[60] Boudreau and colleagues[63] demonstrated that the aspirin dose required to decrease platelet reactivity by at least 50% was increased by nearly 70% with HWI (implantation model) and by nearly 200% with a model (dead worm implantation) of PTE. There were not significant differences in severity of pulmonary vascular lesions in aspirin-treated versus control dogs. For these reasons, the American Heartworm Society does not endorse antithrombotic therapy for routine treatment of HWD.[20] Calvert and colleagues[16] have, however, successfully used the combination of aspirin and strict cage confinement with adulticidal therapy for severe HWD.

If used, aspirin is administered daily beginning 1 to 3 weeks prior to and continued for 4 to 6 weeks after adulticide administration. With protracted aspirin therapy, packed cell volume (PCV) and serum total protein, should be monitored periodically. Aspirin is avoided or discontinued in the face of gastrointestinal (GI) bleeding (melena or falling PCV), persistent emesis, thrombocytopenia (50,000/mm³), and hemoptysis.[16]

Heparin Therapy

Low-dose calcium heparin has been studied in canine HWD and shown to reduce the adverse reactions associated with thiacetarsemide in dogs with severe clinical signs, including heart failure.[64] In this study, calcium heparin administered at 50 to 100 IU/kg subcutaneously every 8 to 12 hours for 1 to 2 weeks before and 3 to 6 weeks after adulticidal therapy, reduced thromboembolic complications and improved survival, as compared with aspirin and indobufen. Dogs in both groups also received prednisone at 1 mg/kg/day. It is emphasized that this therapy has not been studied with melarsomine adulticidal therapy. Calvert and colleagues[16] advocate sodium heparin (50 to 70 U/kg) in dogs with thrombocytopenia, DIC, or both, continuing until the platelet count is greater than 150,000/mm³, for at least 7 days, and possibly for weeks.

Microfilaricidal Therapy

Despite the fact that no agent is approved by the Food and Drug Administration for the elimination of microfilaria, microfilaricidal therapy is traditionally instituted 4 to 6 weeks after adulticide administration.[16] The macrolides offer a safe and effective alternative to levamisole and dithiazanine. Microfilariae are rapidly cleared with ivermectin at 50 µg/kg (approximately eight times preventative dose) or milbemycin at 500 mg/kg (preventative dose), although this represents an extra-label use of ivermectin. Adverse reactions, the severity of which is likely related to microfilarial numbers, were observed in 6% of 126 dogs receiving ivermectin at the microfilaricidal dose.[65] Signs included shock, depression, hypothermia, and vomiting. With fluid and corticosteroid (dexamethasone at 2 to 4 mg/kg intravenously) therapy, all dogs recovered within 12 hours. One fatality, however, was observed 4 days after microfilaricidal therapy. Similar findings and frequency have been reported with milbemycin at the preventative dose.[38] Dogs so treated should be hospitalized and carefully observed for the day. Dogs less than 16 kg, harboring more than 10,000 microfilaria per milliliter of blood, are more apt to suffer adverse reactions.[61] Benadryl (2 mg/kg intramuscularly) and dexamethasone (0.25 mg/kg intravenously) can be administered prophylactically to prevent adverse reactions to microfilaricidal doses of macrolides.

A slower microfilarial kill rate can also be achieved with ivermectin, moxidectin, and selamectin at preventative doses.[23,38,39,66] Using either the rapid or "slow kill" approach rids the patient of microfilariae and sterilizes the female heartworm.

The American Heartworm Society recommends that macrolide therapy, at preventative doses, be instituted 3 to 4 weeks after adulticidal therapy.[25] Accelerated microfilarial destruction can be achieved using recommended doses of milbemycin or by reducing the dosing interval for the other topical or oral formulations to every 2 weeks. Filter or modified Knott tests are rechecked in 5 months when using a slow kill or after 2 to 3 macrolide doses when using a accelerated dose.[25] This interval for testing can be reduced if milbemycin or high-dose ivermectin (50 µg/kg) is chosen.

This author chooses an alternative approach (see Figures 206-4 and 206-10), beginning the administration of a macrolide preventative at the time of diagnosis, often days to weeks prior to adulticidal therapy. With the slow kill microfilaricides (ivermectin, moxidectin, or selamectin at preventative doses), little chance exists of an adverse reaction; however, the owner is warned of the possibility and advised to administer the medication on a day when he or she will be at home. If milbemycin is used, it is usually administered in the hospital and may be preceded by administration of dexamethasone and Benadryl (as described previously in adulticidal therapy).

COMPLICATIONS AND SPECIFIC SYNDROMES

Asymptomatic Heartworm Infection

Most dogs with HWI are asymptomatic, even though many of these have HWD (radiographic and pathologic lesions).

Treatment is as described previously, using melarsomine in the split-dose regimen, along with a macrolide preventative.

Asymptomatic dogs may, however, become symptomatic after adulticidal therapy due to PTE and lung injury (as described elsewhere). The risk of PTE can be imperfectly predicted by semiquantitation of the worm burden, using certain antigen tests, and by the severity of radiographic lesions.[22] Clearly a dog with severe radiographic lesions will not tolerate thromboembolic complications well, but not all dogs with radiographic signs have heavy worm burdens. For example, a dog with moderate to severe radiographic lesions and high antigenemia may not be at high risk for postadulticidal PTE, because it is quite possible that the worms have died, explaining both the antigenemia (release from dead worms) and radiographic abnormalities (chronic HWD). This conclusion might also be valid in the dogs with severe radiographic lesions and negative or low antigenemia (assumes most or all worms have died, and antigen has been cleared). Alternatively, antigenic evidence of a heavy worm burden in a dog with minimal radiographic signs might still portend a severe reaction after melarsomine, because the findings suggest large worm numbers but without natural worm attrition (i.e., a relatively young infection with minimal disease). Of course, low worm burden and minimal radiographic lesions would suggest the least risk of an adverse reaction to adulticide.

It bears emphasis that with each scenario, guesswork is involved and precautions should be taken. When the risk is greatest, aspirin (5 to 7 mg/kg daily—begun 3 weeks prior to and continued until 3 weeks after adulticide) or even heparin may be used,[16] and cage confinement is most important. The owners should be educated as to the risk, the suggestive signs, and the importance of prompt veterinary assistance in case of an adverse reaction.

Glomerulonephritis
The majority of dogs suffering from chronic HWI have glomerulonephritis, which can be severe (Figure 206-12).[11] Therefore when a dog demonstrates glomerular disease, HWI should be considered as a differential diagnosis. Although it is generally felt that the glomerular lesions produced by HWI are unlikely to produce renal failure, a therapeutic dilemma results when one is found in a dog with proteinuria, azotemia, and HWI. Logic suggests that adulticidal therapy is indicated

because HWI contributes to glomerular disease, but it likewise carries risks. The approach embraced by this author is to hospitalize the patient and to administer intravenous fluids (lactated Ringer's solution at 2 to 3 mL/kg/hr) for 48 hours (beginning 12 hours prior to the first melarsomine dose). The patient is then released, and a recheck appointment for blood urea nitrogen (BUN) and creatinine determination after 48 hours is advised. The second and third injections are tentatively scheduled for 1 to 3 months, with the treatment decision based on renal function and the overall response to initial adulticidal therapy.

Allergic Pneumonitis
Allergic pneumonitis, which is reported to affect 14% of dogs with HWD, is a relatively early development in the disease course.[9,16] In fact, the pathogenesis probably involves immunologic reaction to dying microfilariae in the pulmonary capillaries. Clinical signs include cough and sometimes dyspnea and other typical signs of HWD, such as weight loss and exercise intolerance. Specific physical examination findings may be absent or may include dyspnea and audible crackles in more severe cases. Radiographic findings include those typical of HWD but with an infiltrate, usually interstitial, but occasionally with an alveolar component, often worse in the caudal lung lobes (see Figure 206-8). Eosinophils and basophils may be found in excess in peripheral blood and in airway samples.

Corticosteroid therapy (prednisone or prednisolone at 1 to 2 mg/kg per day) results in rapid attenuation of clinical signs, with radiographic clearing in less than a week. The dose can then be stopped in 3 to 5 days if clinical signs subside. Although microfilaricidal therapy is typically not indicated because infections are often occult, macrolide prophylaxis is indicated to avoid further infection. Adulticidal therapy can be used after clinical improvement.

Eosinophilic Granulomatosis
A more serious, but rare, manifestation, pulmonary eosinophilic granulomatosis, responds less favorably. This syndrome is characterized by a more organized, nodular inflammatory process, associated with bronchial lymphadenopathy and, occasionally, pleural effusion. With pulmonary granulomatosis, cough, wheezes, and pulmonary crackles are often audible; when very severe, lung sounds may be muffled and associated with dyspnea and cyanosis. Treatment with prednisone at twice the dose for allergic pneumonitis is reported to induce partial or complete remission in 1 to 2 weeks. The prognosis remains guarded because recurrence within several weeks is common. Prednisone may be combined with cyclophosphamide or azathioprine in an effort to heighten the immunosuppressive effect. The latter combination appears to be the most effective. Adulticide therapy should be delayed until remission is attained. As the prognosis for medical success is guarded; surgical excision of lobar lesions has been advocated.[67]

Pulmonary Embolization
Spontaneous thrombosis or PTE associated with dead and dying worms—the most important heartworm complication—may precipitate or worsen clinical signs, producing or aggravating PHT, right heart failure or, in rare instances, hemoptysis and pulmonary infarction. Acute fatalities may result from fulminant respiratory failure, exsanguination, DIC, or may be unexplained and sudden (arrhythmia or massive pulmonary embolism). The most common presentation, however, is a sudden onset of lethargy, anorexia, and cough 7 to 10 days after adulticidal therapy—often after failure to restrict exercise. Dyspnea, fever, mucous membrane pallor, and adventitial lung sounds (crackles) may be noted on physical examination. Thoracic radiographs (Figure 206-13) reveal significant pulmonary infiltrates, most severe in the caudal lung lobes.

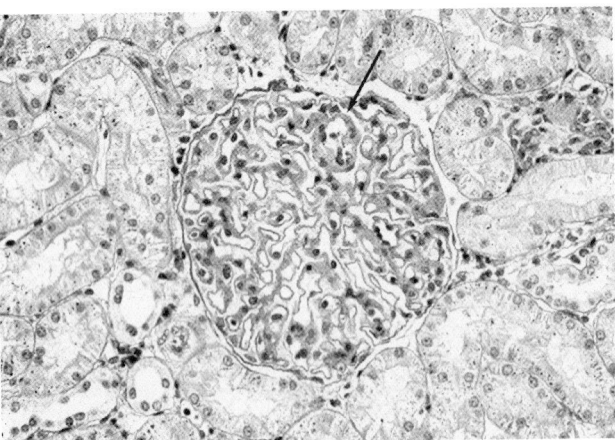

Figure 206-12 An H&E stained, 3 μm section of a glomerulus from a dog with chronic heartworm disease (HWD) and resultant membranoproliferative glomerulonephritis. The capillary walls are thickened, and an overall increase in cellularity is seen. The reader should note a thick-walled capillary containing intraluminal microfilariae. (Photograph courtesy Dr. Greg Grauer.)

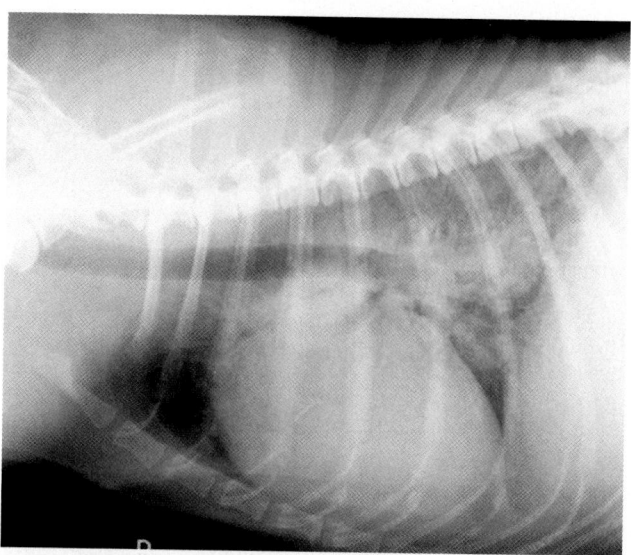

Figure 206-13 Lateral thoracic radiograph obtained from a dog with chronic heartworm disease (HWD), postadulticide. The reader should note right ventricular enlargement, enlarged apical pulmonary arteries partially obscured by pulmonary infiltrate, and an interstitial and alveolar infiltrate, most severe in the caudal lung lobes.

The degree of worsening, as compared with pretreatment radiographs, is typically dramatic. The infiltrate, typically alveolar, is most severe in the caudal lobes, and occasionally areas of consolidation are noted. Laboratory abnormalities vary with the severity of signs but may include leukocytosis, left shift, monocytosis, eosinophilia, and thrombocytopenia. The degree thrombocytopenia may provide prognostic information.

Medical management of thromboembolic lung disease is largely empiric and somewhat controversial. It is generally agreed that strict cage confinement, oxygen administration via oxygen cage or nasal insufflation (50 to 100 mL/kg), and prednisone (1 mg/kg/day for 3 to 7 days) are indicated in the most severe cases.[14,16,68] Some advocate careful fluid therapy (see recommendations for CS), measuring CVP to avoid precipitation of heart failure, to maximize tissue perfusion and

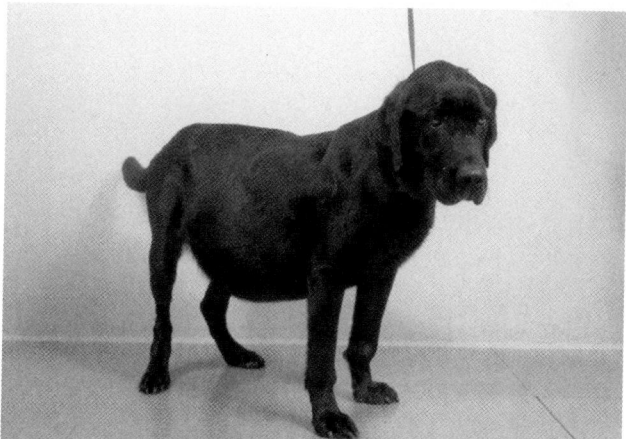

Figure 206-14 Adult male Labrador retriever with congestive heart failure (CHF) due to heartworm disease (HWD). The reader should note the distended abdomen (ascites) and cardiac cachexia.

combat dehydration.[68] The use of heparin (75 IU/kg subcutaneously three times a day until platelet count has normalized [5 to 7 days]) and aspirin (5 to 7 mg/kg/day) has been advocated by some[30] but remains controversial.[4]

Other therapeutic strategies might include cough suppressants, antibiotics (if fever is unresponsive), and, although speculative at this time, vasodilators (amlodipine, hydralazine, diltiazem; see discussion of heart failure in Chapter 197).[69,70] If vasodilatory therapy is used, one must monitor blood pressure because hypotension is a potential side effect. Clinical improvement may be rapid and release from the hospital considered after several days' treatment. For less severely affected dogs, careful confinement and prednisone at home are often adequate.

Congestive Heart Failure

Right heart failure results from increased right ventricular afterload (secondary to chronic pulmonary arterial disease and thromboemboli with resultant PHT). When severe and chronic, PHT may be complicated by secondary tricuspid regurgitation and right heart failure. Congestive signs (ascites) are worsened in the face of hypoproteinemia (see Figure 206-14). Calvert suggests that up to 50% of dogs with severe pulmonary vascular complication to HWD will develop heart failure.[16] Clinical signs (see Figure 206-13) variably include weight loss, exercise intolerance, ashen mucous membranes with prolonged capillary refill time, ascites, dyspnea, jugular venous distension and pulsation, arrhythmias with pulse deficits, and adventitial lung sounds (crackles and possibly wheezes). Dyspnea may be due to pulmonary infiltrates (PIE or PTE, but not cardiogenic pulmonary edema), abdominal distension, or pleural effusion.

Treatment aims include reduction of signs of congestion, reducing PHT, and increasing cardiac output. This involves dietary, pharmacologic, and procedural interventions. Moderate salt restriction is logical and probably useful in diminishing diuretic needs. This author chooses a diet designed for senior patients or early heart disease, because salt restriction should only be moderate. Diuretics may be useful in preventing recurrence of ascites but are typically not able to mobilize large fluid accumulations effectively. This then requires periodic abdominal or thoracic paracentesis (or both) when discomfort is apparent. Furosemide is typically used at 1 to 4 mg/kg daily, depending on severity and patient response. Additional diuretics, which provide a supplemental effect by using differing parts of the nephron, include spironolactone (1 to 2 mg/kg orally twice a day) and chlorothiazide (2 mg/kg orally daily to every other day). The ACE-inhibitors (e.g., enalapril, benazepril, lisinopril, ramipril), by their effect on the renin-angiotensin-aldosterone system, may be of use as mixed vasodilators, in blunting pathologic cardiac remodeling, and in reducing fluid retention, particularly cases of refractory ascites. Adulticide therapy is delayed until clinical improvement is noted. No evidence indicates that digoxin improves survival in HWD. Because of the risk of toxicity and pulmonary vasoconstriction associated with its use, it is not routinely used by is author in the management of HWD-induced heart failure. However, digoxin may be beneficial in the presence of supraventricular tachycardia or refractory heart failure. Aspirin, theoretically useful because of its ability to ameliorate some pulmonary vascular lesions and vasoconstriction, may be used 5 mg/kg/day orally.

The arterial vasodilator, hydralazine, has been shown by Lombard[69] to improve cardiac output in a small number of dogs with HWD and heart failure. It has also been demonstrated to reduce pulmonary artery pressure and vascular resistance, right ventricular work, and aortic pressure without changing cardiac output or heart rate in dogs with experimental HWD (but without heart failure).[70] Clinical experience has shown perceived improvement with the vasodilators diltiazem and amlodipine as well. Research and clinical experience suggest that hydralazine, amlodipine, and diltiazem might have a role in this setting, but further studies are necessary to define their role, if any. In heart failure the author uses hydralazine at 0.5 to 2 mg/kg orally twice a day, diltiazem at 0.5 to 1.5 mg/kg orally three times a day, or amlodipine at 0.1 to 0.25 mg/kg/day orally. The risk of hypotension with these therapies must be realized and blood pressure monitored.

Often heart failure follows adulticidal therapy, but if it is present prior to adulticidal therapy, the difficult question arises as when (or whether) to administer melarsomine. If clinical response to heart failure management is good, adulticidal therapy may be offered in 4 to 12 weeks, as conditions allow. Melarsomine is generally avoided if heart failure is refractory. Antiarrhythmic therapy is seldom necessary, although slowing the ventricular response to atrial fibrillation with digoxin, Diltiazem, or both (see Chapters 197 and 202) may be necessary in some cases.

Caval Syndrome

Heartworm CS is a relatively uncommon but severe variant or complication of HWD. Most studies have shown a marked sex predilection, with 75% to 90% of CS dogs being male. It is characterized by heavy worm burden (usually >60, with the majority of the worms residing in the right atrium and venae cavae) and a poor prognosis.[18]

Studies performed in the author's laboratory indicate that retrograde migration of adult heartworms to the cavae and right atrium, from 5 to 17 months after infection, produces partial inflow obstruction to the right heart and, by interfering with the valve apparatus, tricuspid insufficiency (with resultant systolic murmur, jugular pulse, and CVP increase).[71] Affected dogs also exhibit pre-existent heartworm-induced PHT, which markedly increases the adverse hemodynamic effects of tricuspid regurgitation. These combined effects substantially reduce left ventricular preload and hence cardiac output. Cardiac arrhythmias may further compromise cardiac function (Figure 206-15).

This constellation of events precipitates a sudden onset of clinical signs, including hemolytic anemia caused by trauma to red blood cells (RBCs) as they pass through a sieve of heartworms occupying the right atrium and venae cavae, as well as through fibrin strands in capillaries if DIC has developed. Intravascular hemolysis, metabolic acidosis, and diminished hepatic function with impaired removal of circulating procoagulants contribute to the development of DIC. The effect of this traumatic insult to the erythron is magnified by increased RBC fragility, due to alterations in the RBC membrane in dogs with HWD. Hemoglobinemia, hemoglobinuria, and hepatic and renal dysfunction also are observed in many dogs. The cause of hepatorenal dysfunction is not clear, but it probably results from the combined effects of passive congestion, diminished perfusion, and the deleterious effects of the products of hemolysis. Without treatment, death frequently ensues within 24 to 72 hours due to cardiogenic shock, complicated by anemia, metabolic acidosis, and DIC.

A sudden onset of anorexia, depression, weakness, and occasionally coughing are accompanied in most dogs by dyspnea and hemoglobinuria. Hemoglobinuria has been considered

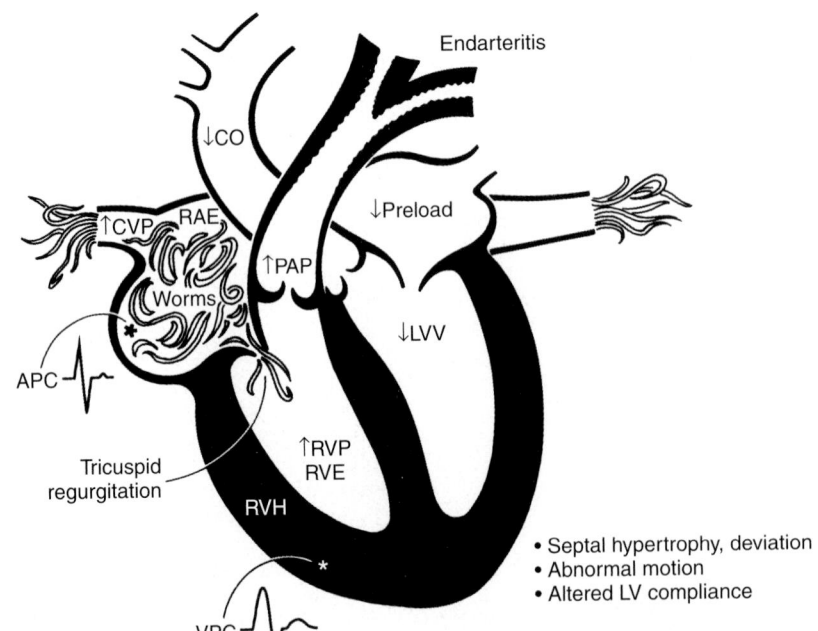

Figure 206-15 Schematic demonstrating pathogenesis of cardiac dysfunction in heartworm caval syndrome (CS). CS complicates chronic heartworm disease (HWD) when retrograde worm migration from the pulmonary arteries occurs, with the majority of worms relocating in the venae cavae and right atrium. Tricuspid valvular function is altered, resulting in incompetence. Tricuspid regurgitation is superimposed on pulmonary hypertension. Left ventricular preload is diminished. Congestive and low-output heart failure ensues. Septal deviation to the left and abnormal, rightward septal motion contributes to preload starvation of the left ventricle. Right ventricular inflow obstruction due to heartworms and cardiac arrhythmias may further contribute to cardiac dysfunction but are probably less important. CO, Cardiac output; *PAP*, pulmonary hypertension; *CVP*, central venous pressure; *RAE*, right atrial enlargement; *APC*, atrial premature complex; *VPC*, ventricular premature complex; *RVH*, right ventricular hypertrophy; *RVP*, right ventricular pressure; *RVE*, right ventricular enlargement; *LVV*, left ventricular volume; *Arrows*, increased or decreased. (From Atkins CE: Pathophysiology of heartworm caval syndrome: recent advances. *In* Otto GF: Proc Amer Heartworm Symposium '89. Batavia, Ill., American Heartworm Society, 1990, pp 27-31.)

pathognomonic for this syndrome. Physical examination reveals mucous membrane pallor, prolonged capillary refill time, weak pulses, jugular distension and pulsation, hepatosplenomegaly, and dyspnea. Thoracic auscultation may disclose adventitial lung sounds; a systolic heart murmur of tricuspid insufficiency (87% of cases); loud, split S2 (67%); and cardiac gallop (20%). Other reported findings include ascites (29%), jaundice (19%), and hemoptysis (6%). Body temperature varies from subnormal to mildly elevated.[18]

Hemoglobinemia and microfilaremia are present in 85% of dogs suffering from CS.[18] Moderate (mean PCV, 28%) regenerative anemia characterized by the presence of reticulocytes, nucleated RBC, and increased mean corpuscular volume (MCV) is seen in the majority of cases. This normochromic, macrocytic anemia has been associated with the presence of target cells, schistocytes, spur cells, and spherocytes. Leukocytosis (mean white blood cell [WBC] count, approximately 20,000 cells/cm^3) with neutrophilia, eosinophilia, and left shift has been described. Dogs affected with DIC are characterized by the presence of thrombocytopenia and hypofibrinogenemia, as well as prolonged one stage prothrombin time (PT), partial thromboplastin time (PTT), activated coagulation time (ACT), and high fibrin degradation product concentrations. Serum chemistry analysis reveals increases in liver enzymes, bilirubin, and indices of renal function. Urine analysis reveals high bilirubin and protein concentrations in 50% of cases and more frequently, hemoglobinuria.

CVP is high in 80% to 90% of cases (mean, 11.4 cm H_2O). Electrocardiographic abnormalities include sinus tachycardia in 33% of cases and atrial and ventricular premature complexes in 28% and 6%, respectively. The mean electrical axis tends to rotate rightward (mean, +129 degrees), with an S1,2,3 pattern evident in 38% of cases. The S wave depth in CV6LU (V_4) is the most reliable indicator of right ventricular enlargement (>0.8 mv) in 56% of cases. Thoracic radiography reveals signs of severe HWD with cardiomegaly, main pulmonary arterial enlargement, increased pulmonary vascularity, and pulmonary arterial tortuousity recognized in descending order of frequency (see Figures 206-5 to 206-7). Massive worm inhabitation of the right atrium with movement into the right ventricle during diastole is evident echocardiographically. This finding on M-mode and two-dimensional echocardiograms is nearly pathognomonic for CS in the appropriate clinical setting (Figure 206-16). The right ventricular lumen is enlarged and the left diminished in size, suggesting PHT accompanied by reduced left ventricular loading. Paradoxical septal motion, caused by high right ventricular pressure, is commonly observed. No echocardiographic evidence of left ventricular dysfunction exists. Cardiac catheterization documents pulmonary, right atrial, and right ventricular hypertension and reduced cardiac output.

Prognosis is poor unless the cause of the crisis—the right atrial and caval heartworms—is removed. Even with this treatment, mortality can approximate 40%.

Fluid therapy is needed to improve cardiac output and tissue perfusion, to prevent or help to reverse DIC, to prevent hemoglobin nephropathy, and to aid in the correction of metabolic acidosis. Overexuberant fluid therapy, however, may worsen or precipitate signs of CHF. In the author's clinic, a left jugular catheter is placed and intravenous fluid therapy instituted with 5% dextrose in water or one-half strength saline and 2.5% dextrose. The catheter should not enter the anterior vena cava because it will interfere with worm embolectomy. A cephalic catheter may be substituted for the

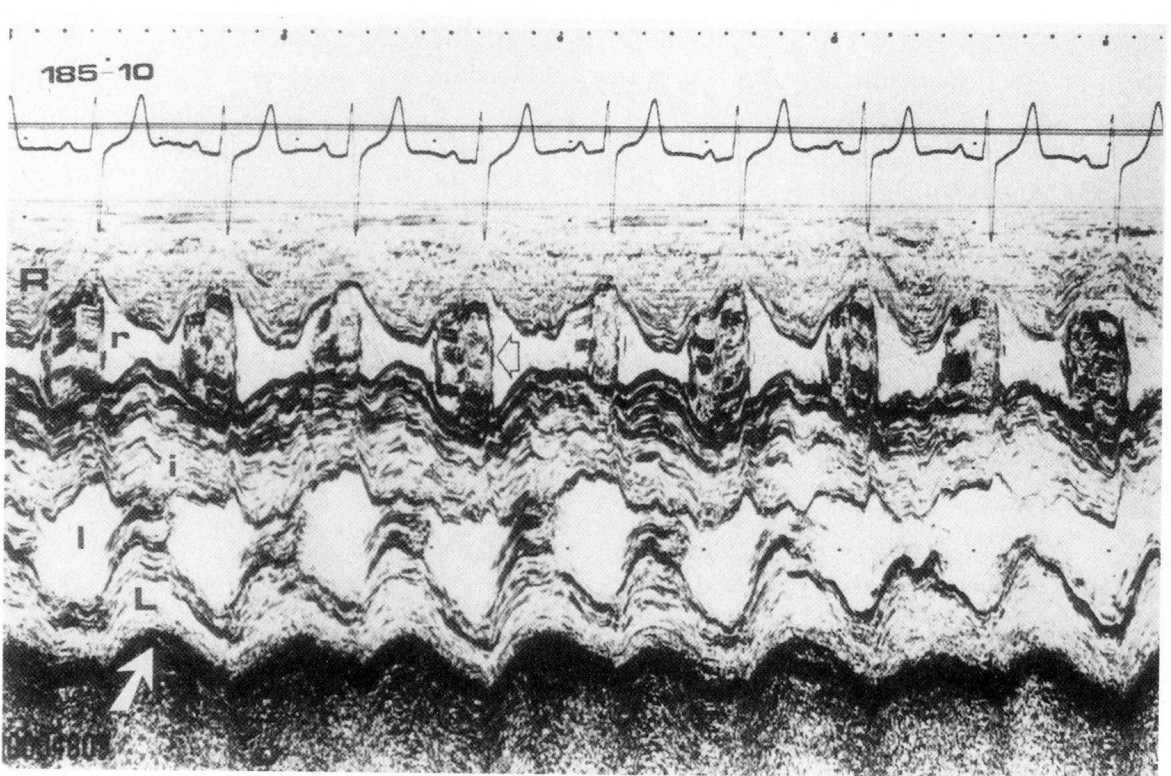

Figure 206-16 An *M*-mode echocardiogram of a dog with recent onset caval syndrome (CS), demonstrating thickening of the right ventricular and intraventricular septal walls, right ventricular eccentric hypertrophy, and a small left ventricle. An echogenic mass *(clear arrow)* of heartworms can be seen "falling" into the right ventricle with each diastole. Paradoxical septal motion is evident. The white arrow denotes the pericardium. *R*, Right ventricular wall; *r*, right ventricular lumen; *i*, intraventricular septum; *l*, left ventricular lumen; *L*, left ventricular posterior wall. (From Atkins CE: Heartworm caval syndrome. Semin Vet Med Surg 2:64-71, 1987.)

somewhat inconvenient jugular catheter, but this does not allow monitoring of CVP. The intravenous infusion rate for fluids is dependent on the condition of the animal. A useful guideline is to infuse as rapidly as possible (up to 1 cardiovascular volume during the first hour) without raising the CVP or without raising it above 10 cm H_2O if it was normal or near normal at the outset. Initial therapy should be aggressive (10 to 20 mL/kg/hr for the first hour) if shock is accompanied by a normal CVP (<5 cm H_2O), and it should be curtailed to approximately 1 to 2 mL/kg/hr if CVP is 10 to 20 cm H_2O. Whole blood transfusion is not indicated in most cases because anemia usually is not severe, and transfused coagulation factors may worsen DIC. Sodium bicarbonate is not indicated unless metabolic acidosis is severe (pH, 7.15 to 7.20). Broad-spectrum antibiotics and aspirin (5 mg/kg daily) should be administered. Treatment for DIC is described elsewhere in this text.

The technique for surgical removal of caval and atrial heartworms was developed by Jackson and colleagues.[72] This procedure should be undertaken as early in the course of therapy as is practical. Often, sedation is unnecessary, and the procedure can be accomplished with only local anesthesia. The dog is restrained in left lateral recumbency after surgical clipping and preparation. The jugular vein is isolated distally. A ligature is placed loosely around the cranial aspect of the vein until it is incised, after which the ligature is tied. Alligator forceps (20 to 40 cm, preferably of small diameter) are guided gently down the vein while being held loosely between the thumb and forefinger. The jugular vein can be temporarily occluded with umbilical tape. If difficulty is encountered in passage of the forceps, gentle manipulation of the dog by assistants to further extend the neck will assist in passage of the forceps past the thoracic inlet; medial direction of the forceps may be necessary at the base of the heart. Once the forceps have been placed, the jaws are opened, the forceps are advanced slightly, the jaws are closed, and the worms are removed. One to four worms are usually removed with each pass. This process is repeated until five to six successive attempts are unsuccessful. An effort should be made to remove 35 to 50 worms. Care should be taken not to fracture heartworm during extraction. After worm removal, the jugular vein is ligated distally, and subcutaneous and skin sutures are placed routinely. Other catheters, such as urethral stone basket catheters, horsehair brushes, snares and flexible alligator forceps have also been used.[73] Fluoroscopic guidance, when available, is useful in this procedure.

Successful worm retrieval is associated with a reduction in the intensity of the cardiac murmur and jugular pulsations, rapid clearing of hemoglobinemia and hemoglobinuria, and normalization of serum enzymatic aberrations. Immediate and latent improvement in cardiac function occurs over the next 24 hours. It is important to realize that removal of worms does nothing to reduce right ventricular afterload (PHT), and hence fluid therapy must be monitored carefully before and after surgery to avoid precipitation or worsening of right heart failure. Cage rest should be enforced for a period of time suitable for individual care.

Worm embolectomy through a jugular venotomy is frequently successful in stabilizing the animal, allowing adulticide therapy to be instituted to destroy remaining heartworms in a minimum of 1 month. Careful scrutiny of BUN and serum liver enzyme concentrations should precede the latter treatment. Aspirin therapy is continued for 3 to 4 weeks after adulticide therapy. Substantial improvement in anemia should not be expected for 2 to 4 weeks after worm embolectomy. Macrolide preventative therapy, as described previously, is administered at the time of release from the hospital.

Aberrant Migration

Although heartworms in the dog typically inhabit the pulmonary arteries of the caudal lung lobes, they may find their way to the right ventricle, and rarely (see Caval Syndrome) the right atria and venae cavae. Much less frequently, immature L5 may aberrantly migrate to other sites, including the brain, spinal cord, epidural space, anterior chamber of the eye, the vitreous, the subcutis, and the peritoneal cavity. In addition, the worms may inhabit the systemic circulation, producing systemic thromboembolic disease.[12] Treatment of aberrantly migrating heartworms requires either nothing (e.g., peritoneal cavity), surgical excision of the offending parasite, adulticidal therapy, or symptomatic treatment (e.g., seizure control with brain migration). The method for surgical removal from internal iliac and femoral arteries has been described.[12]

PROGNOSIS

The prognosis for asymptomatic HWI is generally good and, although the prognosis for severe HWD has to be guarded, a large percentage of such cases can be successfully managed.[74] Once the initial crisis is past and adulticidal therapy has been successful, resolution of underlying manifestations of chronic HWD begins. The prognosis is poorest with severe DIC, CS, massive embolization, eosinophilic granulomatosis, severe pulmonary artery disease, and heart failure. After adulticidal therapy, intimal lesions regress rapidly.[75-77] Improvement is noted as early as 4 weeks post-treatment in the main pulmonary artery, with all pulmonary arteries having undergone marked resolution within 1 year. Radiographic and arteriographic lesions of HWD begin to resolve within 3 to 4 weeks, and PHT is reduced within months and may be normal within 6 months of adulticide therapy. Pulmonary parenchymal changes are worsened during the 6 months after adulticidal therapy and then begin to lessen in severity, with marked resolution within the next 2 to 3 months. Persistence of such lesions is suggestive of persistent infection. Corticosteroid therapy hastens the resolution of these lesions. Likewise irreversible renal disease is uncommon, with glomerular lesions resolving within months of successful adulticidal therapy. Signs of heart failure are also reversible with symptomatic therapy, cage rest, and successful clearing of infection.

CONTROVERSIES IN CANINE HEARTWORM DISEASE

Yearly Testing

The remarkable efficacy of macrolide preventatives and the reduced danger of microfilaria-induced reactions with their use (see following section on preventatives), have caused some to question the need for yearly testing.[51] Many experts, however, continue to advocate this practice.[18] The issue of yearly testing is clearly important because it deals with financial and ethical, in addition to medical, issues. The veterinary profession must walk the fine line between adequate testing, by which we protect the public, and excessive testing, by which the public may feel "gouged." This is difficult because only sparse scientific detail exists to answer this question, and the answer likely differs by geographic region and even within regions, based on socioeconomic strata and client compliance.

Arguments can be put forth both for and against yearly testing.[18] Proponents might argue that this practice gets animals into the clinic yearly (vaccination may not [see Chapters 163 and 164]), thereby ensuring yearly examination and resultant health benefits and income, and provides inexpensive insurance against unrecognized infection caused by poor compliance or dogs that surreptitiously expectorate medications when orally administered. In addition, yearly antigen testing is very specific (i.e., little risk of false-positive results), prevents long-term infections from becoming established during the period between heartworm checks, and would seem to limit liability to the practicing veterinarian. They might well also point out that a recent reports have demonstrated poor compliance for heartworm prophylaxis nationwide,[32-34] and even though macrolide preventatives provide the safety net of the so-called reach-back effect (or retroactive efficacy) discussed elsewhere, that this benefit is realized only with lapses of less than 3 to 4 months, varies between products, and requires continuous administration for 1 year after the lapse.[37] Finally, yearly testing for heartworm antigen is useful to pick up latent (infections that have progressed too far to be eliminated with preventative but are not patent at the time that preventative was prescribed) or incompletely eradicated infections.

On the other hand, the opponent of yearly testing might point out that if, as a profession, we emphasize the efficacy and importance of preventive agents, we may lose credibility by also promoting yearly testing. Additionally the macrolide preventatives are very efficacious, possessing reach-back potential, in the hands of conscientious clients, and the risk of severe adverse reactions in dogs not known to be infected and receiving macrolides is small. The reason that adverse reactions are less likely is because most dogs will be rendered pharmacologically amicrofilaremic or will have small microfilarial burdens. In addition, the reactions to macrolides in microfilaremic dogs are less severe than to DEC. Furthermore, the argument can be made that the small worm burdens, most likely to result when preventative lapses are brief, will be minimally harmful and might even escape detection by immunologic tests, and that the chances of false-positive tests increase with low prevalence (as would be expected in a population of pets receiving preventative and yearly evaluation).

The American Heartworm Society addressed this question in 1995.[78] It stated "...after the initial retest, if it appears that monthly chemoprophylaxis is being given as prescribed, retesting at intervals greater than 1 year may be sufficient. However, reasonable doubt that administration has been adequate would justify retesting at shorter intervals, perhaps on an annual basis." Unfortunately little data exist on owner compliance with preventatives, and the data that have been generated are alarming. Cummings and colleagues[33] surveyed dispensing records of 50 veterinary practices in heartworm-endemic areas in the United States and found that, based on the practices' own recommendations, only enough medication was dispensed to adequately protect 41% of the canine clients. This was largely due to the fact that medication was dispensed for less than 50% of the dogs in the practices. It is important to add that this study did not identify compliance failure in which dispensed medications were not administered or in which administered medication was not swallowed. These data suggest that the majority of our canine patients should undergo yearly testing. Positive test results in this population should be carefully scrutinized, however.

YEARLONG PREVENTION

Because of the necessity of the mosquito as an intermediate host for HWI, it has been logical and accepted practice to discontinue preventatives during the winter months in the more northern climates. In warmer climates, where mosquitoes may be encountered 12 months of the year, yearlong prophylaxis has been the practice. With the advent of monthly, very effective prophylactic agents, and with improved understanding of the temperature dependence of heartworm transmission by mosquitoes, this yearlong practice has been called into question.[3] Although no supportive data exist, it might be assumed that the ease of administration of monthly preventatives may improve owner compliance and that the reach-back effect will

make up for short lapses in therapy or unexpected exposures at the beginning or end of the transmission season, thereby making the effective period of prevention longer. More importantly, recent studies have shown that transmission, even in heartworm-endemic areas, does not occur during the final quarter of the year.[2] This is because the mosquito, which is generally assumed to live 30 days, requires a minimum average daily ambient temperature to allow larval development to the infectious (L3) stage. This requirement is defined in heartworm development units (HDUs). An HDU is the degree days (in °C) that the average ambient temperature surpasses the developmental threshold of 14° C (57° F).[2] Restated, for each day that the average ambient temperature exceeds the threshold, an HDU is attained; if the average temperature is 16° C for 1 day, for example, then 2 HDUs are attained. For development of infective larvae, 130 HDUs must be attained and, to be effective, these must be attained in the lifetime of the female mosquito (~30 days). If the average temperature is 16° C, for example, it would take 65 days for L3 to develop, thereby making transmission impossible. On the other hand, a 24° C average temperature would allow the molt to L3 to occur in 13 days, well within the mosquito's life expectancy.

In a very innovative approach to this question, Knight and Lok[3] surveyed temperature extremes in 200 weather stations over a 30-year period and calculated the *worst case scenario* for transmission of heartworms. The resultant isotherm maps (Figure 206-17), constructed from this information indicate the month to begin and to cease heartworm preventative therapy by geographic region. In only Hawaii, Florida, and the southern tips of North Carolina, South Carolina, Georgia, Alabama, Mississippi, and Louisiana is yearlong preventative deemed necessary.

Therefore arguments may be drawn against this theory for yearlong prevention, or at least for a longer prevention season than indicated by the isotherm maps published by Knight and Lok.[3] First, though fascinating and backed by scientific fact, this represents only a theory, and one that can never be proven. It cannot be proven because this would require testing the hypothesis in every locale in the country in an infinite number of years and seasonal variation. Second, some aspects of the HDU model fall under question:

- Do all female mosquitoes really live only 30 days?
- Do some mosquito species live longer than others?
- Are there not other climatic factors such as humidity that play a role in larval development?
- Are there not microclimates within isotherm regions that might allow more HDUs to be attained?
- Might not mosquitoes seek microclimates (indoors perhaps) with temperatures to allow heartworm larval development?

Third, owner compliance has been shown to be less than optimal.[32-34] Fourth, the macrolide reach-back effect, which protects dogs for which compliance is imperfect, is less than 100% after a 4-month lapse in therapy, varies among preventatives, and requires 12 to 14 months of continuous therapy after the lapse.[37] Fifth, sometimes significant differences exist in adjacent isotherm regions, rendering decision making confusing and potentially hazardous. For example, in Florida, adjacent regions exist that require 10 or 12 months of preventative treatment. How does an owner or veterinarian know which protocol to use? Furthermore, in some areas, the change from current recommendations to those based on the isotherm maps is minimal. For example, in Wisconsin, current recommendations would dictate starting heartworm preventative in May and continuing through November, whereas the isotherm map suggests July through October, a difference of two doses. Sixth, animals travel, often to warmer climates during "nontransmission" seasons. Seventh, because some macrolides and macrolide combination drugs have broad spectra, their use in

Macrolide heartworm chemoprophylaxis
estimated timing of first monthly dose
1st day of month administration

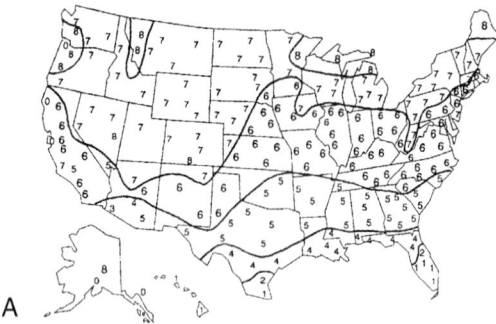

A

Macrolide heartworm chemoprophylaxis
estimated timing of last monthly dose
1st day of month administration

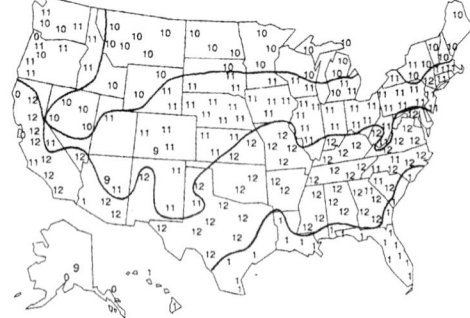

B

Figure 206-17 Isotherm maps demonstrating the month to begin **(A)** and stop **(B)** heartworm monthly preventative therapy based on data from nearly 200 weather stations (see text for detailed description). A zero (*0*) indicates no preventative necessary. (From Knight DH, Lok JB: Seasonal timing of heartworm chemoprophylaxis in the United States. In Proc Heartworm Sympos '95. Batavia, Ill., American Heartworm Society, 1996, pp 37-42.)

other parasite control might argue for their use for longer than just the projected heartworm transmission season. Lastly, the savings to clients is relatively small. If a client in North Carolina goes from yearlong prevention to the Knight-Lok recommendation (12-month administration to 7-month administration), the savings for a 25 lb dog is about $16.00 per year.

The Knight-Lok model has provided new and useful information, indicating that the risk in other than prime heartworm season is less than previously believed, and that in some instances heartworm prophylaxis is excessive. The Knight-Lok model should stand as a suggestion for the timing of prophylaxis, with practice erring to the conservative. This means extending the isotherm map suggestion 1 month in either direction and taking the earliest implementation date and the latest cessation date surrounding one's geographic region. As a profession, we are faced with the dilemma of providing the best care with fiscal responsibility. The fact that our previous assumptions have come under some reassessment should be brought to the clients' attention, using the points made previously. It then falls upon the shoulders of the client to determine if the risk of possible, but generally unlikely, infection is worth the savings.

MACROLIDES AS ADULTICIDES

It is now proven that ivermectin (and possibly selamectin) has adulticidal efficacy that can approach 100% with prolonged, continuous administration.[40,41,48] Ivermectin was demonstrated to be successful as an adulticide in experimental, young infections with 31 months' continuous administration.[41] The exact role of macrolides in the management of HWI, other than as preventatives, is unclear and likely to be a major controversy in upcoming years.

The appeal of macrolides for this use is that it takes the veterinarian out of the *complication loop*. Complications might indeed still occur but would not likely be temporally linked to the macrolide administration (as they are to arsenic use). In addition, reduced cost, patient discomfort, and inconvenience are appealing. Arguments against the use of ivermectin in this way include the following:

- Represents an off-label use of ivermectin
- Requires continuous more than 30 months' compliance from a client that often has allowed HWI to occur—often by poor compliance
- Lack of knowledge about the timing and degree of exercise restriction necessary; safe use might require 31 months of continuous exercise restriction
- Absence of a controlled kill as seen with melarsomine, reducing the ability to effectively monitor for adverse effects
- Lack of knowledge as to the effect of chronic antigen release from slowly dying adult heartworms on the kidneys and lungs
- Knowledge that macrolide "slow adulticidal therapy" does not alleviate the lung disease associated with HWI[79]
- Fact that proven efficacy is only in young (<8 months old) experimental HWIs[41]
- Concern that heartworm resistance to ivermectin might develop in dogs treated in this manner[50]

At the 2001 American Heartworm Symposium, the audience and a panel of experts were polled as to their belief as to the role of ivermectin as an adulticide in their own practices.[80] Five percent of the audience and none of the expert panelists used only ivermectin for adulticidal therapy. Approximately one third of both groups did not or would not use ivermectin as an adulticide under any circumstances. Finally, approximately 70% of the expert panel and 50% of the audience stated that they would use ivermectin for this purpose only under mitigating circumstances of financial or medical constraint.

The author recommends that melarsomine be the primary adulticidal tool and recommends or accepts the use of ivermectin in instances where a preventative is necessary in a heartworm-positive dog and the owner cannot afford arsenic therapy or in which medical conditions preclude its use; in the event of residual infection after appropriate treatment with melarsomine (assumes low worm burden); and, obviously, in unrecognized infections.

CHAPTER • 207

Feline Heartworm Disease

Clarke Atkins

LIFE CYCLE

The life cycle of *Dirofilaria immitis* is similar in the cat and the dog (see Figure 206-2). Cats differ, however, in that they are not generally the preferred target for feeding mosquitoes, that to be infected the mosquito has to have first fed on a canid, and that, as an unnatural host, cats are inherently resistant to heartworm infection (HWI). Infections in cats therefore tend to be infrequent and small. In addition, the life cycle takes longer in the cat, such that patency (noted in <20% of cats) does not occur until 7 to 8 months postinfection.

PATHOPHYSIOLOGY

The domestic cat, though an atypical host, can be parasitized by *D. immitis*, with resultant heartworm disease (HWD). The clinical manifestations of the disease are different and often more severe in this species, but the infection rate is only 5% to 20% of that of the dog.[1] Experimental infection of the cat is more difficult than in the dog; less than 25% of L3 reach adulthood. This resistance is also reflected in natural infections, in which feline heartworm burdens are usually less than 10 and typically only 2 to 4 worms.[2] Other indications of the cat's inherent resistance to this parasite are a shortened period of worm patency, high frequency of amicrofilaremia or low microfilaria counts, and shortened life span of adult heartworms (2 to 3 years).[2] Nevertheless, studies have shown a prevalence as high as 14% in shelter cats[1] and a study performed at North Carolina State University (NCSU) revealed HWD in nine of 100 cats had cardiorespiratory signs.[3] Furthermore, antibody testing showed 26% of these cats to had been exposed to HWI.[3] Similar to dogs, the male cat is at higher risk for HWI than is the female. Aberrant worm migration appears to be a greater problem in cats than in dogs.

As in the dog, immature L5 may create pulmonary and pulmonary vascular disease in cats prior to maturation. Uniquely, the disease process develops even in cats that ultimately resist a mature infection, and as in dogs, clinical signs and disease antedate clinicians' ability to diagnose the disease through conventional means. The pulmonary arterial response to adult heartworms is more severe than that of the dog, although pulmonary hypertension has infrequently been reported. Dillon demonstrated pulmonary enlargement within 1 week of transplantation of adults, suggesting an intense host-parasite interaction.[4] A severe myointimal and eosinophilic response produces pulmonary vascular narrowing and tortuosity, thrombosis, and possibly hypertension (Figure 207-1).[5] Because the feline pulmonary artery tree is smaller than that of the dog and has less collateral circulation, embolization, even with small numbers of worms, produces disastrous results with infarction and even death. Although uncommon, cor pulmonale and right heart failure can be associated with chronic feline HWD and is manifested by pleural effusion (hydro- or chylothorax), ascites, or both. The lung per se is also insulted by HWI, with eosinophilic infiltrates in the lung parenchyma (pneumonitis) and pulmonary arteries (Figure 207-2). The pulmonary vessels may leak plasma, producing pulmonary edema (possibly acute respiratory distress syndrome, ARDS), and type II cells proliferate, both potentially altering O_2 diffusion.[4] In addition, radiographic findings suggest air trapping, compatible with bronchoconstriction. The end result to this multifaceted insult is diminished pulmonary function, hypoxemia, dyspnea, cough, and even death.

CLINICAL SIGNS

Cats with HWI may be asymptomatic and, when present, clinical manifestations may be either peracute, acute, or chronic.[3,4,6-8] Acute or peracute presentation is usually due to worm embolization or aberrant migration, and signs variably include salivation, tachycardia, shock, dyspnea, hemoptysis, vomiting and diarrhea, syncope, dementia, ataxia, circling, head tilt, blindness, seizures, and death. Postmortem examination often reveals pulmonary infarction with congestion and edema. More commonly, the onset of signs is less acute (chronic form). Reported historical findings in chronic feline HWD include anorexia, weight loss, lethargy, exercise intolerance, signs of right heart failure (pleural effusion; rare), cough, dyspnea, and vomiting. The author and colleagues have found dyspnea and cough to be relatively consistent findings and, when present, should cause suspicion of HWD in endemic areas.[8] Chylo- and pneumothorax have also been recognized as unusual manifestations of feline HWD.

In a report of 50 natural cases of feline HWI in North Carolina, presenting signs were most commonly related to the

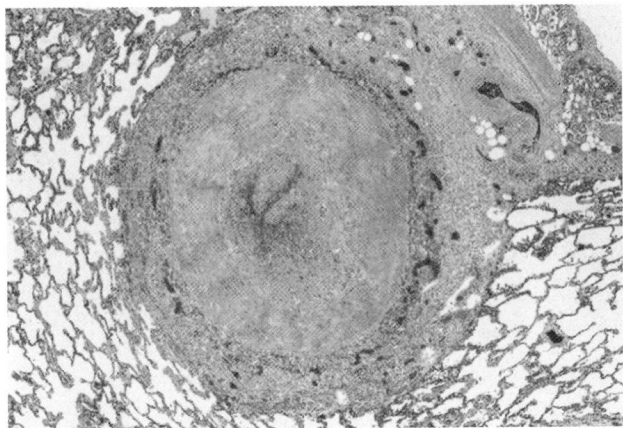

Figure 207-1 H&E stain demonstrating large pulmonary artery with obstruction of lumen due to severe medial smooth muscle hypertrophy and hyperplasia, subintimal and intimal fibrosis, endarteritis, and possibly thrombosis. The reader should also note the periarterial interstitial (probably eosinophilic) pneumonia.

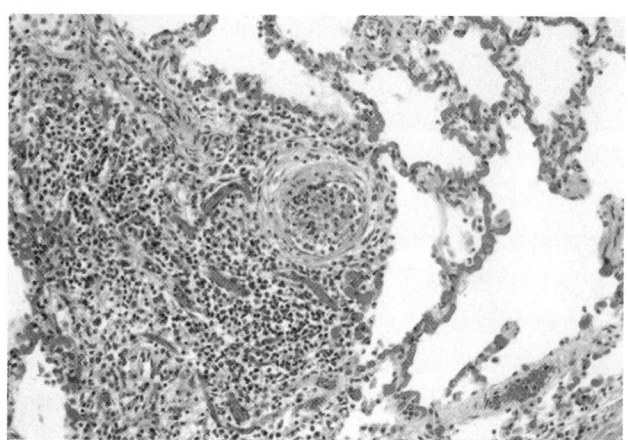

Figure 207-2 Small pulmonary artery from the cat seen in Figure 207-1 showing mild medial hypertrophy. The reader should note the extreme perivascular cuff of inflammatory cells around the vessel, representing an eosinophilic infiltrate.

respiratory system (32 cats; 64%), with dyspnea (24 cats; 48%) being most often noted, followed by cough (19 cats; 38%) and wheezing (Figure 207-3).[8] Vomiting was reported in 17 (38%) cats and was noted frequently in 8 (16%). Five (10%) heartworm-infected cats were reported to have exhibited vomiting without concurrent respiratory signs and vomiting was a presenting sign in seven (14%). Neurologic signs (including collapse or syncope [10%]) were reported in seven (14%) cats. Five (10%) of the cats were dead at the time of presentation. Murmurs were infrequently noted in cats that did not have concurrent heart disease, independent of HWI. Heart failure was present in one cat, but it had concurrent hypertrophic cardiomyopathy. HWI was considered to be an incidental finding in 14 (28%) of the cats in this study.

Physical examination is often unrewarding, although a murmur, gallop, or diminished or adventitial lung sounds (or a combination of these findings) may be noted. In addition, cats may be thin, dyspneic, or both. If heart failure is present,

jugular venous distension, dyspnea, and rarely ascites are detected.

DIAGNOSIS

The diagnosis of HWI and HWD in cats poses a unique and problematic set of issues.[4] First, the clinical signs are often quite different from those of the dog. In addition, the overall incidence in cats is low, so suspicion is lessened, eosinophilia is transient or absent, electrocardiographic findings are minimal, and most cats are amicrofilaremic.

No compelling medical reasons exist to screen cats for HWI prior to administration of macrolide preventatives because the risk of adverse reactions associated with microfilarial death is small (cats are amicrofilaremic or have small microfilarial numbers, and adverse reactions are minimized with macrolide preventatives). Nevertheless, screening allows the clinician to alert pet owners if their cats have been exposed (antibody positive) so that they might pursue confirmation of the diagnosis, if they wish. It also minimizes public relations problems if the cat develops HWD while on preventative. In addition, routine screening allows the clinician to understand the risk of heartworm exposure in the practice area. The author's approach to routine screening of cats for heartworms differs somewhat from that when suspicion of infection exists (Figure 207-4, A and B).

Immunodiagnostic methods (Table 206-2) are also imperfect in cats because of the low worm burdens (1 to 12; mean, 3) and hence, antigenic load. In a recent study, enzyme-linked immunosorbent assay (ELISA) antigen tests were positive on sera from 36% to 93% of 31 cats harboring 1 to 7 female heartworms, with sensitivity increasing as female worm burden increased.[9] Cats with male worm or worms were not detected as positive. Therefore false-negative tests occur frequently, depending on test used, maturity and gender of worms, and worm burden. All tests were, however, virtually 100% specific. It is important to realize that infection with signs may be present prior to the presence of detectable antigen (from gravid adult females). McCall and colleagues[10] report that, in natural infections, the antigen test detects less than 50% of cases. Snyder and colleagues[11] present differing data (from natural infections in which blood was obtained as

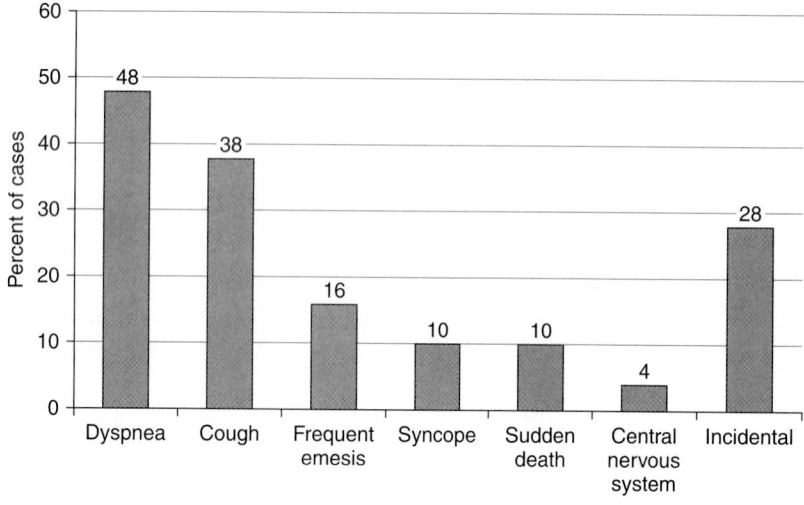

Figure 207-3 Clinical signs recorded in 50 cats with proven heartworm infection (HWI). *Freq,* Frequent; *CNS,* central nervous system signs (e.g., seizures, ataxia, circling). (From Atkins CE et al: Heartworm infection in cats: 50 cases [1985-1997]. J Vet Med Assoc 217:355-358, 2000.)

long as 2 hours posteuthanasia) that show that the antigen test is more sensitive than previous reports (74%) indicated. Recently an antigen test (IDEXX's SNAP® Feline Heartworm Antigen Test) has been marketed for cats. This is an adaptation of the canine test, with a reported increase in sensitivity of 15% over conventional antigen tests. Although less specific, heartworm antibody tests may be of use in the detection of feline HWI, even when antigen tests are negative. The antibody test may also be useful as a marker for exposure to HWI, even if the cat never develops a mature infection. Two in-clinic feline heartworm antibody tests are available (HESKA™ SOLO STEP™ FH and Synbiotics' WITNESS® FH).

Thoracic radiographs have been suggested as an excellent screening test in cats. However, Schafer and Berry[12] showed that the most sensitive radiographic criterion (left caudal pulmonary artery greater than 1.6 times the ninth rib at the ninth intercostal space on the ventrodorsal projection) was only detected 53% of cases. Furthermore, even though most cats with clinical signs have some radiographic abnormality, the findings are not specific to HWD. In addition, a study by Selcer and colleagues[13] demonstrated that radiographic findings were often transient, and radiographic abnormalities were found in cats that ultimately resisted heartworm maturation and were negative on postmortem. Radiographic findings include enlarged caudal pulmonary arteries (Figure 207-5), often with ill-defined margins, pulmonary parenchymal changes that include focal or diffuse infiltrates (interstitial, bronchointerstitial, or even alveolar), perivascular density, and occasionally, atelectasis (Figures 207-6 and 207-7). Pulmonary hyperinflation may also be evident, and the misdiagnosis of feline bronchial disease can easily be made (see Figures 207-5, *A*, and 207-6, *A*). Pulmonary angiography has also been used to demonstrate radiolucent linear intravascular foreign bodies and enlarged, tortuous, and blunted pulmonary arteries (Figure 207-8).

Echocardiography, in the author's experience, is more sensitive in cats than in dogs.[3,14] Typically, a *double-lined echodensity* is evident in the main pulmonary artery, one of its branches, the right ventricle, or occasionally at the right atrioventricular (AV) junction (Figure 207-9). The author and colleagues found heartworms by echocardiography in 78% of nine cases,[3] as did Selcer and colleagues in 16 experimental infections.[13]

TREATMENT AND PREVENTION

The question arises as to whether heartworm prophylaxis is warranted for cats because they are not the natural host and because the incidence is low. Necropsy studies of feline HWI in the Southeast have yielded a prevalence of 2.5% to 14%, with a median of 7% (Figure 207-10).[1] When considering the question of institution of prophylaxis, it is worth considering that this prevalence approximates or even exceeds that of feline leukemia virus (FeLV) and feline immunodeficiency virus (FIV) infections.[15] A 1998 nationwide antibody survey of over 2000 largely asymptomatic cats revealed an exposure prevalence of nearly 12% (Figure 207-11).[16] It is also noteworthy that, based on owners' information, nearly one third of cats diagnosed with HWD at NCSU were housed solely indoors.[8] Lastly, the consequences of feline HWD are potentially dire, with no clear therapeutic solutions. Therefore the author advocates preventative therapy in cats in endemic areas. Three drugs with FDA approval are marketed for use in cats (Table 207-1). Ivermectin is provided in a chewable

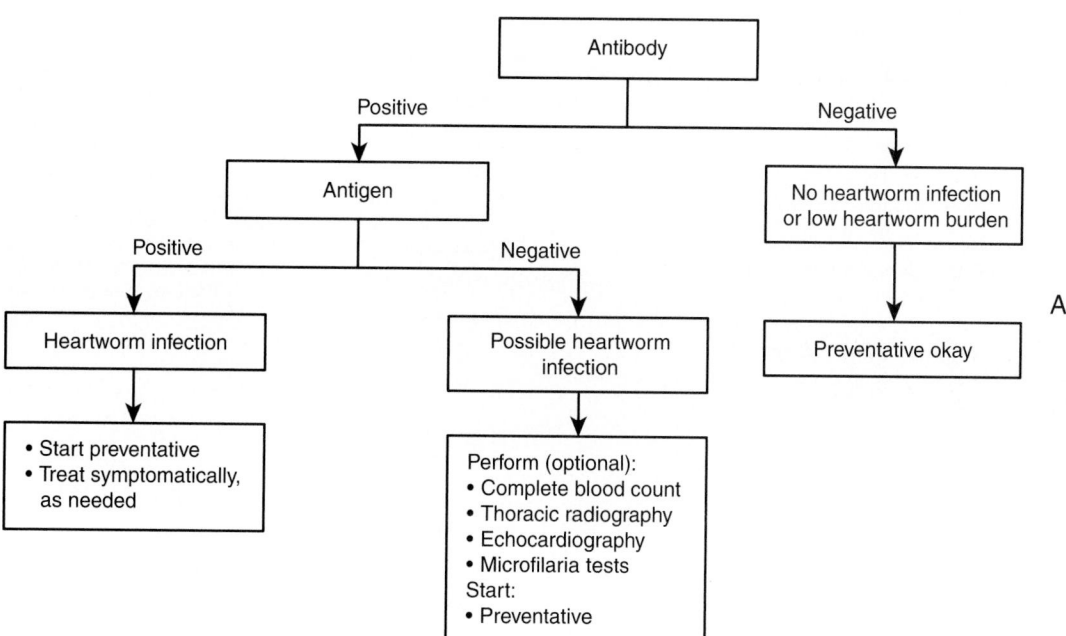

Routine Screening for Feline Heartworm Infection

Figure 207-4 **A,** Algorithm demonstrating the author's approach to screening cats for heartworm infection (HWI). **B,** Algorithm demonstrating the author's approach to the diagnosis of HWI in cats in which infection is suspected. *Continued*

Diagnosis in Cats Suspected to Have Heartworm Infection

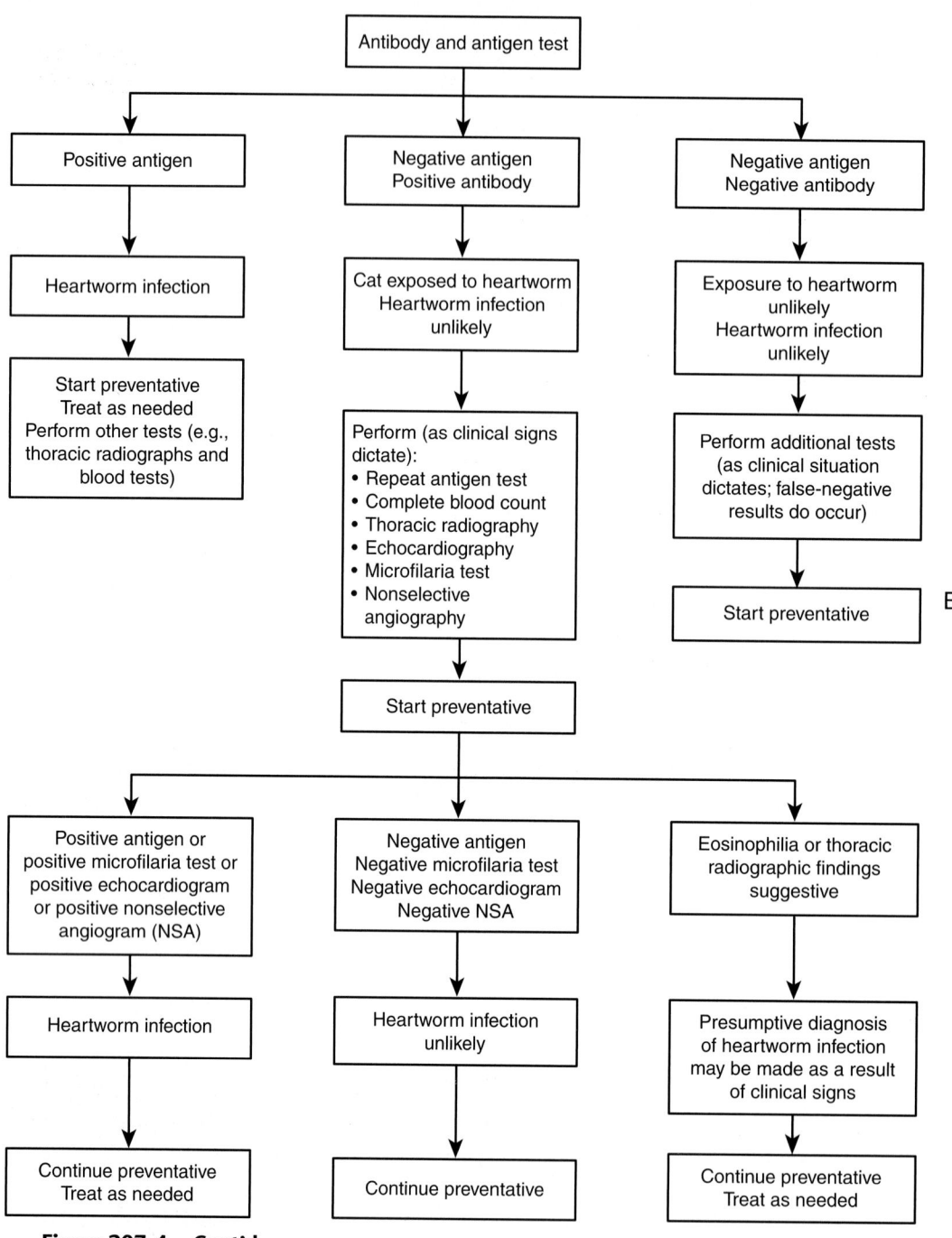

Figure 207-4   Cont'd.

formulation, milbemycin as a flavored tablet, and selamectin (a broad-spectrum parasiticide) comes in a topical formulation. The spectrum and the formulation of these products varies; hence the clients' individual needs are easily met in most cases (Table 207-1).

Because the vast majority of cats are amicrofilaremic, microfilaricidal therapy is unnecessary in this species. The use of arsenical adulticides is problematic. Thiacetarsemide

(sodium caparsolate), if available, poses risks even in normal cats. Turner, Lees, and Brown[17] reported death due to pulmonary edema and respiratory failure in 3 of 14 normal cats given thiacetarsemide (2.2 mg/kg twice over 24 hours). Dillon and colleagues[18] could not confirm this acute pulmonary reaction in 12 normal cats receiving thiacetarsemide, but one cat did die after the final injection. More importantly, a significant, though unquantified, percentage of cats with HWI develop pulmonary

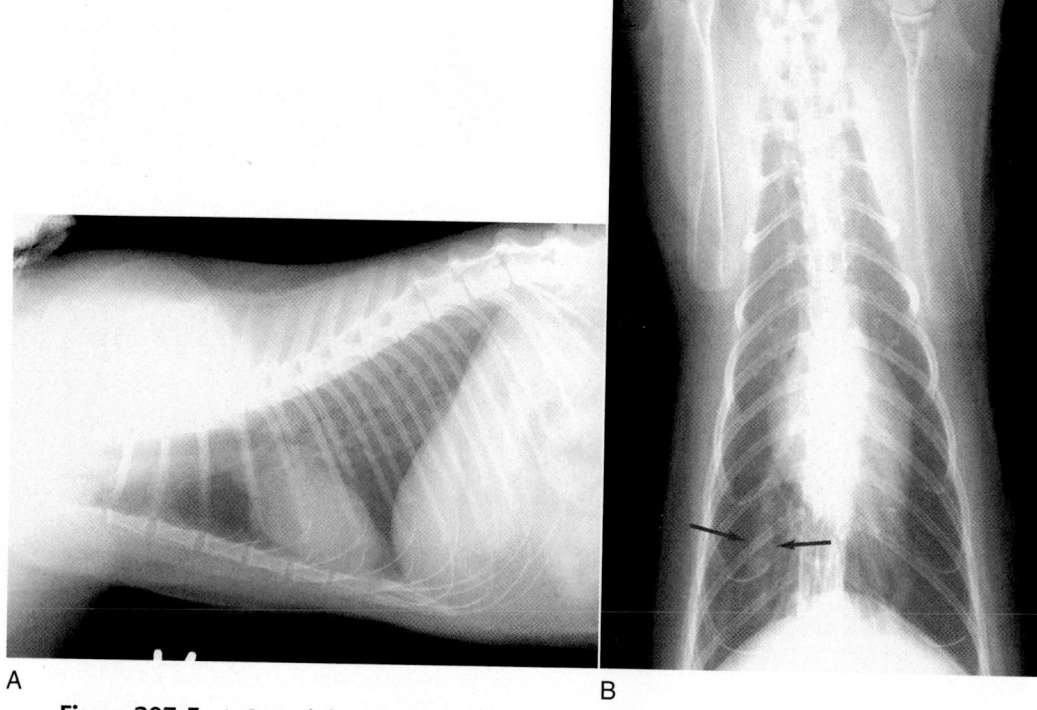

Figure 207-5 **A,** Lateral thoracic radiograph from a cat with heartworm disease (HWD). A fine interstitial pattern is seen in the caudal lung lobes, and the chest is somewhat hyperinflated. This radiographic pattern is similar to and hence confused with that of feline bronchial disease. **B,** Dorsoventral thoracic radiograph from the same cat shown in **A**. Again, the changes are not dramatic, but the right caudal lobar pulmonary artery is enlarged (>1.6 times the ninth rib at the ninth intercostals space; *arrows*). The opposite pulmonary artery can be seen to be somewhat tortuous.

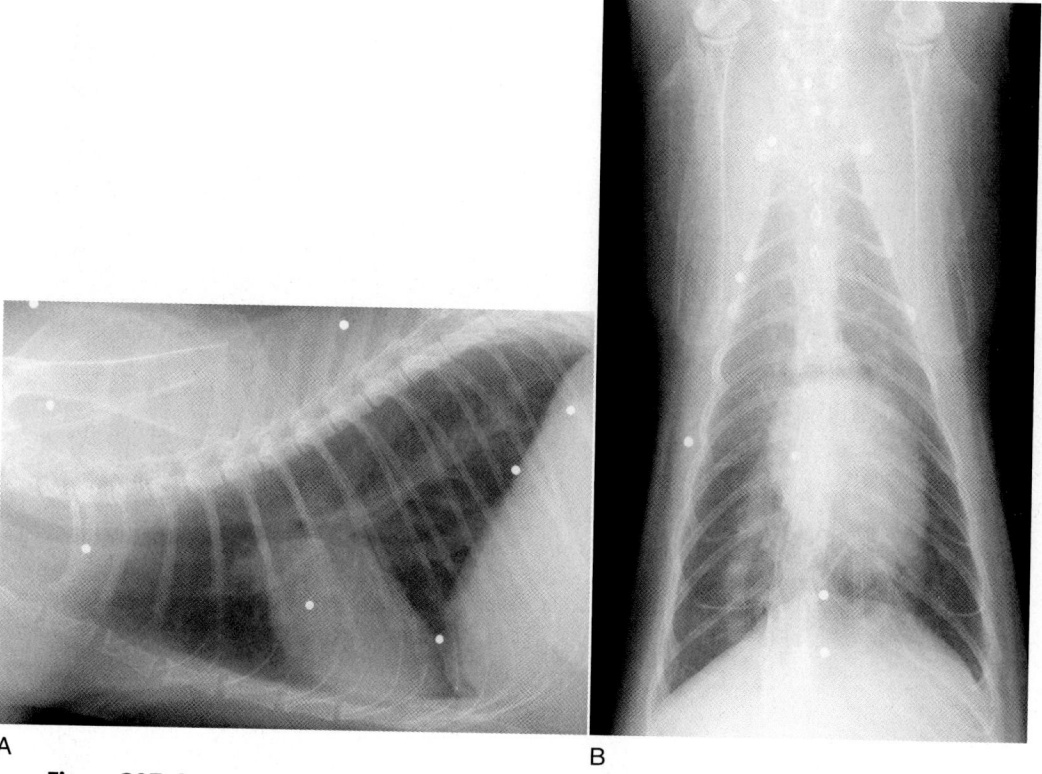

Figure 207-6 **A,** Lateral thoracic radiograph of a cat with heartworm disease (HWD) and cough. The reader should note the hyperinflated chest, flat diaphragm, and moderate interstitial pulmonary infiltrate. The right ventricle is mildly enlarged. **B,** Dorsoventral thoracic radiograph from the same cat shown in **A**. The pulmonary infiltrate is more readily appreciated in this view in the right caudal lung lobe. The reader should note the enlarged right caudal lobar pulmonary artery.

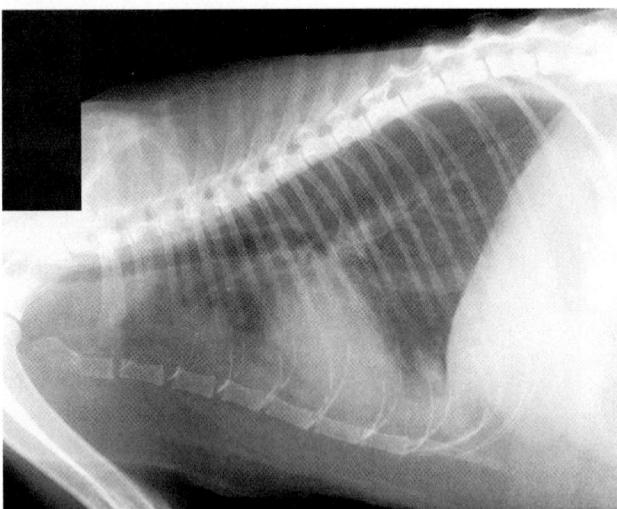

Figure 207-7 Lateral thoracic radiograph of a cat with severe respiratory distress and heartworm disease (HWD). The reader should note the alveolar infiltrate in the ventral thorax and the less severe interstitial infiltrate more dorsally in caudal lung lobes. This severe lung disease is probably due to heartworm death and may represent acute respiratory distress syndrome (ARDS).

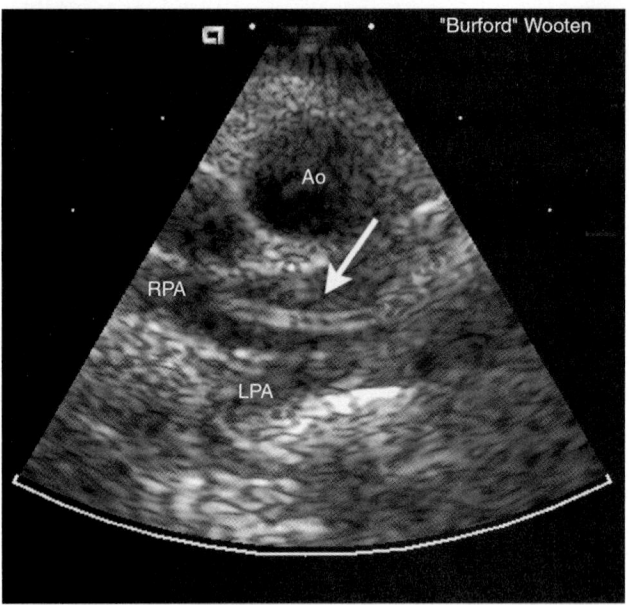

Figure 207-9 A short-axis, two-dimensional echocardiogram obtained from an 18-year-old castrate male, feline cancer patient with an asymptomatic murmur. An adult heartworm can be identified by two echo-dense parallel lines, in the right pulmonary artery *(arrow)*. *Ao*, Aorta; *RPA*, right pulmonary artery; *LPA*, left pulmonary artery.

thromboembolism (PTE) after adulticidal therapy.[4-7] This occurs several days to 1 week after therapy and is often fatal. In 50 cats with HWI, seen at NCSU, 11 received thiacetarsemide. There was no significant difference in survival between those receiving thiacetarsemide and those receiving symptomatic therapy.[8]

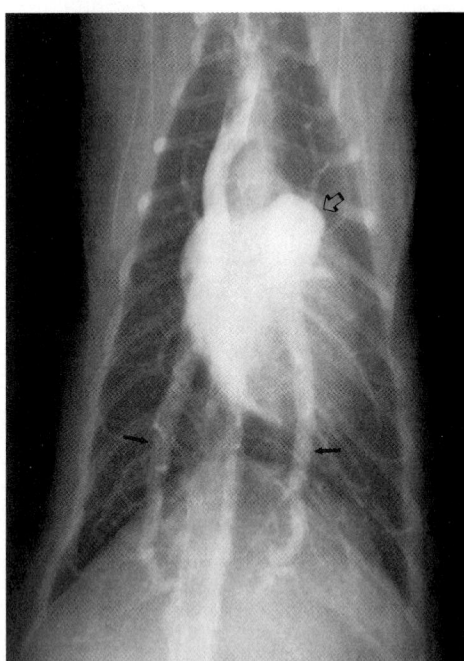

Figure 207-8 Nonselective angiogram obtained from cat with heartworm disease (HWD). The reader should note the enlarged main pulmonary artery *(open arrow)* and the enlarged, tortuous, and blunted caudal pulmonary arteries *(arrows)*. Careful scrutiny reveals linear radiolucencies in the right caudal pulmonary artery. (Photograph courtesy Dr. Kathy Spaulding. From Atkins CE: Heartworm disease. In Allen DG [ed]: Small Animal Medicine. Philadelphia, JB Lippincott Co, 1991, pp 341-363.)

Data on melarsomine in experimental (transplanted) HWI in cats are limited and contradictory. Although an abstract report exists in which one injection (2.5 mg/kg; one half the recommended canine dose) of melarsomine was used in experimentally infected cats without treatment-related mortality, the worm burdens after treatment were not significantly different from those found in untreated control cats.[19] Diarrhea and heart murmurs were frequently noted in treated cats. A second abstract report, using either the standard canine protocol (2.5 mg/kg twice over 24 hours) or the *split dose* (one injection, followed by two injections, 24 hours apart, in 1 month) described in Chapter 206, gave more favorable results.[20] The standard treatment and split-dose regimens resulted in 79% and 86% reduction in worm burdens, respectively, and there were no adverse reactions. Although promising, these unpublished data need to be interpreted with caution because the transplanted worms were young (<8 months old and more susceptible), and the control cats experienced a 53% worm mortality (average worm burden was reduced by 53% by the act of transplantation). Additionally, the clinical experience in naturally infected cats has been generally unfavorable, with an unacceptable mortality. Because of the inherent risk, lack of clear benefit, and the short life expectancy of heartworms in this species, this author does not advocate adulticidal therapy in cats. Surgical removal of heartworms has been successful and is attractive because it minimizes the risk of thromboemboli. The mortality seen in the only published case series was, unfortunately, unacceptable (two of five cats).[21] This procedure may hold promise for the future, however.

Cats with HWI should be placed on a monthly preventative and short-term corticosteroid therapy (prednisone at 1 to 2 mg/kg every 48 hours, three times a day) used to manage respiratory signs. If signs recur, alternate-day steroid therapy (at the lowest dose that controls signs) can be continued indefinitely. For embolic emergencies, oxygen, corticosteroids (dexamethasone at 1 mg/kg intravenously or intramuscularly,

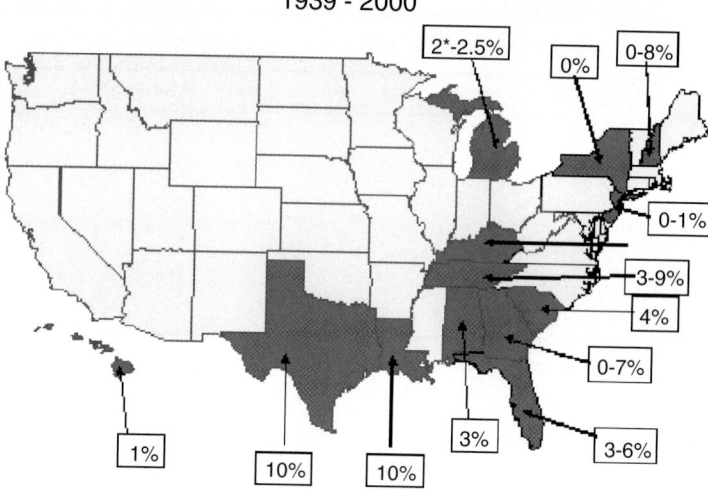

Figure 207-10 Necropsy prevalence of heartworm infection (HWI) in shelter cats. The shaded states are those in which such studies have been completed. One Michigan study, which showed a prevalence of 2%, was an antigen study. (Adapted from Ryan WG, Newcomb KM: Prevalence of feline heartworm disease—a global review. *In* Soll MD, Knight DH [eds]: Proc Heartworm Symposium '95. Batavia, Ill., American Heartworm Society, 1996.)

or prednisolone sodium succinate at 50 to 100 mg intravenously/cat), and bronchodilators (aminophylline at 6.6 mg/kg intramuscularly every 12 hours, theophylline sustained release at 25 mg/kg orally, or terbutaline at 0.01 mg/kg subcutaneously) may be used. Bronchodilators have logic, based on the ability of agents, such as the xanthines (aminophylline and theophylline), to improve function of fatigued respiratory muscles. In addition, the finding of hyperinflation of lung fields may indicate bronchoconstriction, a condition for which bronchodilation would be indicated. Nevertheless, this author does not routinely use bronchodilators in feline HWD.

The use of aspirin has been questioned because vascular changes associated with HWI consume platelets, increasing their turnover rate and effectually diminishing the antithrombotic effects of the drug. Conventional doses of aspirin did not prevent angiographically detected vascular lesions.[22] Doses of aspirin necessary to produce even limited histologic benefit approached the toxic range. Despite this, because therapeutic

options are limited, at conventional doses (80 mg orally, every 72 hours), aspirin is generally harmless, inexpensive, and convenient. Because the quoted studies were based on relatively insensitive estimates of platelet function and pulmonary arterial disease (thereby possibly missing subtle benefits), the author continues to advocate aspirin for cats with HWI. Aspirin is not prescribed with concurrent corticosteroid therapy. Management of other signs of HWD in cats is largely symptomatic.

PROGNOSIS

In the aforementioned study of 50 cats with natural HWI, at least 12 cats died of causes other than HWD. Seven of these and two living cats were considered to have survived HWD (lived ≥1000 days).[8] The median survival for all heartworm-infected cats living beyond the day of diagnosis was 1460 days (4 years; range, 2 to 4015 days), whereas the median survival of

Percent Antibody Positive by Region

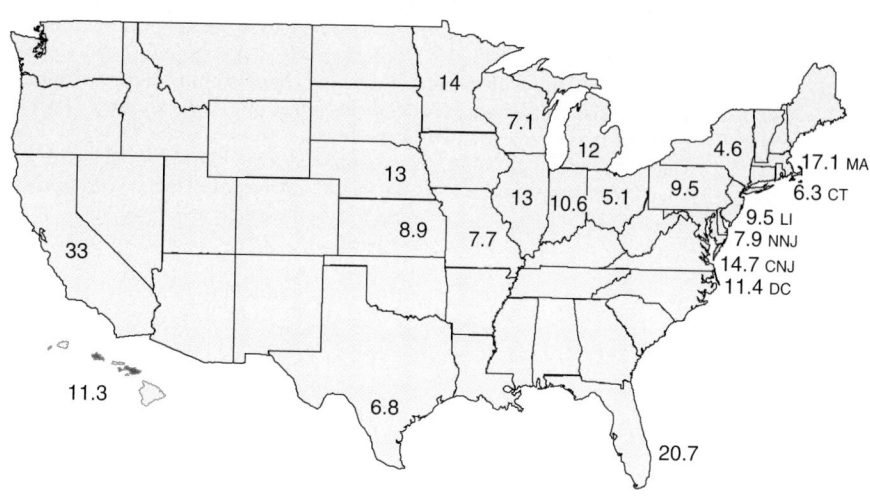

Figure 207-11 Prevalence (%) of heartworm exposure (positive antibody test) in over 2000 largely asymptomatic cats in 19 states (21 regions). *NNJ*, North New Jersey; *CNJ*, central New Jersey; *LI*, Long Island, NY. (Adapted from Miller MW et al: Prevalence of exposure to *Dirofilaria immitis* in cats from multiple areas of the United States. *In* Soll MD, Knight DH [eds]: Proc Heartworm Symposium '98. Batavia, Ill., American Heartworm Society, 1998; pp 161-166.)

Table • 207-1

Comparison of Spectra of Macrolides Currently in Use in Cats

DRUG	HW	HOOKWORMS	WHIPWORMS	ROUNDWORMS	TAPEWORMS	FLEAS & EGGS	TICKS	SARCOPTES	EAR MITES
Ivermectin (chewable)	+	+							
Milbemycin (flavored tablet)	+	+		+					
Selamectin (topical)	+	+		+		+/+	+	+	+

HW, Heartworm prevention.

all cats (n = 48 with adequate follow-up) was 540 days (1.5 years; range, zero to 4015 days). Survival of 11 cats treated with sodium caparsolate (mean, 1669 days) was not significantly different from that of the 30 managed without adulticide (mean, 1107 days). Likewise, youth (≤3 years of age), presence of dyspnea, cough, ELISA-positivity for heartworm antigen, presence of echocardiographically identifiably worms, or gender of the cat did not appear to affect survival.[8] The effect of HWI on survival has been compared with that of other cardiovascular diseases (Figure 207-12).[23]

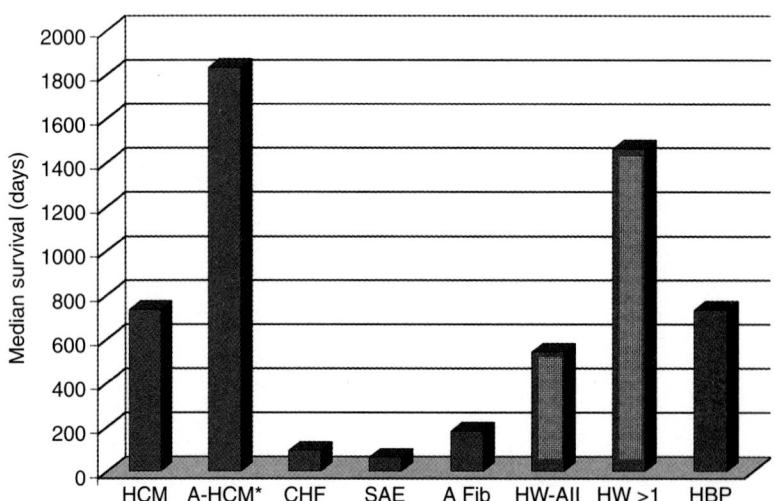

Figure 207-12 Median survival from four previous reports for cats with varying cardiovascular diseases. Median survival shown as 5 years was actually more than 5 years. *HCM*, Hypertrophic cardiomyopathy; *A-HCM*, asymptomatic hypertrophic cardiomyopathy; *CHF*, hypertrophic cardiomyopathy with heart failure; *SAE*, hypertrophic cardiomyopathy with systemic embolism; *A Fib*, atrial fibrillation; *HW-All*, heartworm infection, all cases; *HW>1*, heartworm-infection with survival beyond day 1; *HBP*, hypertension. (From Atkins CE et al: Prognosis in feline heartworm infection: comparison to other cardiovascular disease. *In* Seward LR, Knight DH [eds]: Proc Heartworm Symposium '01. Batavia, Ill., American Heartworm Society, pp 41-44.)

CHAPTER · 208

Peripheral Vascular Disease

Philip R. Fox
Jean-Paul Petrie
Ann E. Hohenhaus

Peripheral vascular disease denotes disorders of peripheral vessels including arteries, arterioles, veins, venules, and lymphatics (Box 208-1). Vascular lesions may result from primary vascular pathology or occur secondary to conditions originating in unrelated tissues or organ systems (Box 208-2). Resultant conditions may remain asymptomatic with little or no effect on morbidity and mortality, or they may progress to become life threatening. The development of newer imaging techniques, including improvements in diagnostic ultrasound, has provided accessible methods to clinically characterize these disorders. Vascular abnormalities have been classified according to the type of vessel affected and functional significance of associated lesions (see Boxes 208-1 and 208-2).

TECHNIQUES USED TO EVALUATE PERIPHERAL VASCULAR DISEASE

Angiography

Angiography is the gold standard for evaluating peripheral vascular disease owing to its superior ability to characterize and visualize normal and abnormal vascular anatomy.[1]

Diagnostic outcome requires careful attention to three important elements: (1) selection of radiopaque contrast agent, (2) technique for vascular delivery of contrast material, and (3) high-quality radiographic imaging.

Factors to be considered when selecting a contrast agent include patient safety, image quality, and cost. The features of safety and efficacy are somewhat related to the ionic composition of these materials. High osmolar ionic compounds include the diatrizoate and iothalamate salts (Conray, Mallinekrodt) (Renografin, Amersham Health). Low osmolar ionic compounds include iohexol (Omnipaque, Amersham Health), iopamidol (IsoVue), and ioversol (Optiray, Mallinekrodt). Low osmolar nonionic compounds include ioxaglate (Hexabrix, Mallinekrodt). Lower osmolar agents, both ionic and nonionic, are generally tolerated best by patients, particularly those sensitive to an increase in intravascular volume or having advanced cardiac disease (high osmolar compounds can generate a greater osmotic load).[2] Nonionic agents also have reduced risk of contrast-related anaphylactoid reactions such as urticaria, flushing, coughing, dyspnea, peripheral edema, and a sudden drop in blood pressure.[3] Contrast related nephrotoxicity is independent of the contrast agent used but can be reduced by maintaining appropriate patient hydration and minimizing the dose of contrast agent used during the imaging study.[4] Low osmolar agents are generally more expensive than high osmolar agents.

Arterial angiography, often performed using carotid or femoral arterial access, can be performed to evaluate normal or abnormal arterial vascular anatomy preoperatively; to assess vessels for occlusive disease including thromboembolism (TE); and to detect or characterize inherited or acquired lesions including peripheral aneurysms, vascular tumors, traumatic injury, and shunts. The specific catheterization technique to

be used is guided by consideration of the anatomic location of interest, anticipated lesion, status of patient health, available equipment, and operator experience. After percutaneous or surgical arterial cutdown, a catheter is directed under fluoroscopic guidance to the desired location and contrast agent is injected by hand or by the use of a mechanical injecting device. Images are acquired using mechanical rapid film changers or digitally. The advantages of digital angiography include rapid rate of acquisition, postprocessing capabilities, and reduced exposure to radiation.[1] Digital subtraction angiography may be used to

---

Box · 208-1

Peripheral Vascular Diseases

Diseases of Arteries and Arterioles
Occlusive diseases
   Arterial embolism
   Arterial thrombosis
   Angiitis, vasculitis
   Vasospasm, traumatic, toxic
   Diabetic arteriopathy
Nonocclusive diseases
   Arteriovenous (A-V) fistula
   Arterial aneurysm
   Arterial calcification
   Arteriosclerosis, hyalinosis, amyloidosis
   Atherosclerosis
   Vasculitis

Diseases of Veins
Phlebectasia
Varicosis
Phlebitis and thrombophlebitis
Venous thrombosis
Venous malformations

Diseases of Lymphatics
Lymphangitis
Lymphedema
Lymphangiectasia
Lymphatic hypoplasia, aplasia, hyperplasia
Lymphangioma, lymphocysts
Lymphangiosarcoma

Tumors of Peripheral Blood Vessels
Angioma, hemangioma, hemangiosarcoma

Box • 208-2

Causes of Peripheral Lymphatic Disorders

Lymphangitis, Lymphedema, Lymphadenitis, Lymphadenopathy
Infection
Neoplasia
Reactive hyperplasia
Granuloma

Lymphedema
Primary developmental abnormality of lymphatics
   Hypoplasia
   Aplasia
   Lymphangiectasia
   Hyperplasia
Secondary acquired abnormalities of lymphatics
   Surgical excision of lymphatics or lymph nodes
   Posttraumatic lymphangiopathy
   Neoplastic invasion
   Extrinsic compression of lymph vessels or tissue
   Acute obstructive lymphadenitis
   Chronic sclerosing lymphadenitis/lymphangitis
   Lymphatic atrophy with interstitial fibrosis
   Radiation therapy

Lymphocysts
Cystic hygroma, lymphoceles, pseudocyst

Lymphangiomas

cancel out portions of an image and thereby improve visualization of structures of interest.

Venous angiography is generally less challenging than arterial angiography, owing to easier access and lower pressures of the venous system. A small intravenous line is placed in a superficial vein distal to the site of the vascular lesion and contrast material is injected. Images are obtained similarly to arteriography. This technique is often selected to detect venous clots (appearing as vascular filling defects) or stenosis. The presence of prolific collateral vasculature can indicate chronic obstruction. Contrast venography of the cranial and caudal vena cava can be performed to assess caval patency that may be associated by a variety of neoplastic, compressive, or thrombotic disorders.

Lymphangiography helps to permit local assessment of the lymphatic system. The technique of indirect lymphangiography relies on the contrast agent, which is infused into tissue, to be selectively absorbed and transported through lymphatic channels.[5] Direct lymphangiography is more challenging (unless lymphangiectases have formed) but provides superior results when successfully performed. Selective lymphatic cannulation requires aseptic cutdown over the lymphatic region of interest. (The identification of lymphangiectases may be facilitated by subcutaneous injection of vital dyes [e.g., 3% Evans blue dye or 11% patent blue violet] into the toe web. By selective resorption of these dyes, the main lymphatic channels proximal to the metacarpus or metatarsus become grossly outlined.) The lymphatic vessel is then cannulated with a 27- or 30-gauge needle or a special lymphatic cannula.[5] An iodine-containing soluble contrast medium such as sodium

and meglumine diatrizoate (Renografin, Hypaque) is injected slowly into the vessel. Because water-soluble contrast media rapidly diffuse through lymphatic walls into surrounding tissues, the radiographic detail is blurred unless radiographs are taken shortly after dye injection. Alternatively, oily iodine-containing contrast agents (Lipiodol) are used, reducing leakage of contrast from the lymphatic vessels. The oily contrast agents are sequestered within the lymphatics and lymph nodes along the draining pathways.[1] Patency of the lymphatic channels can be appreciated in addition to the size of regional lymph nodes. Metastatic disease to the lymph nodes (or granulomas) appears as filling defects within the contrast-filled node. Lymphangiography can also be used to identify the location of lymphatic leakage.[1]

Diagnostic Ultrasound
Ultrasound imaging provides a direct, noninvasive technique for assessing anatomic abnormalities, vascular patency, and function.[6,7] Ultrasound can aid in the diagnosis of peripheral arterial occlusion, central and peripheral arteriovenous (A-V) fistulas, venous thrombosis, aneurysms, traumatic vascular disease, and compression of vascular structures from local disease processes.

Duplex ultrasonography incorporates gray-scale two-dimensional imaging, with pulsed wave (PW) and color flow Doppler techniques. Thrombi, foreign bodies, compression, and abnormal vascular anatomy can be identified with two-dimensional imaging. Color Doppler superimposed on the two-dimensional image can further help define anatomy and identify turbulence associated with vascular malformation and stenotic lesions. Normal arterial flow is laminar with the highest velocity recorded centrally, and the respective color Doppler image has a homogenous appearance. Arterial stenosis increases blood flow velocity across the narrowed lumen with corresponding change in color Doppler signal at and distal to the stenosis. PW Doppler velocity measurements are made along the length of the artery in question and at areas or interest indicated from color flow Doppler interrogation. PW Doppler imaging may help assess the degree (severity) of vascular narrowing by estimating the gradient across the stenosis by the modified Bernoulli equation: gradient (mm Hg) = (maximal velocity)^2 × 4. Moreover, arterial blood flow results in characteristic Doppler waveforms (a rapid forward flow component during systole, transient reversal of flow during early diastole, and a prolonged slow forward flow during late diastole). With mild to moderate vascular stenosis, characteristic changes in the PW Doppler waveform include acceleration of peak systolic velocities and loss of diastolic flow reversal distal to the stenosis. Of course, with complete stenosis, blood flow is interrupted.[8]

Magnetic Resonance Imaging
Magnetic resonance angiography (MRA) is a safe, noninvasive imaging technique that may be useful to evaluate the peripheral arterial system. In human medicine, both contrast and noncontrast MRA methods have been applied for planning interventional procedures (e.g., stent placements) in patients with peripheral vascular disease.[9,10] Unlike other vascular imaging techniques, noncontrast MRA displays blood flow and not the blood vessel itself. Limitations of noncontrast MRA include time of acquisition, variation of blood flow characteristics (e.g., diastolic flow reversal) in diseased vessels, and retrograde filling of arteries during complete occlusion resulting in artifacts and reduction of net forward flow on the image. Contrast-enhanced angiography using a non-nephrotoxic contrast material eliminates many of the previously mentioned limitations. Advantages of contrast-enhanced MRA include shorter acquisition times, high spatial resolution, and high signal-to-noise ratios.[10]

MECHANISMS OF THROMBOSIS

Hemostasis is a complex process that involves blood vessels, platelets, coagulation proteins, naturally occurring anticoagulants, and platelet inhibitors. Thrombosis results when one or more components of the hemostatic cascade are perturbed, tipping the balance between coagulation and fibrinolysis in favor of coagulation. Physiologic alterations leading to the formation of thrombi have frequently been classified into three main categories: (1) alterations in blood flow, (2) damage to vascular endothelium, and (3) changes in coagulation proteins and platelets, resulting in hypercoagulability.

Normal flow of blood through blood vessels is laminar, with the rapidly flowing red blood cells (RBCs) in the center of the vessel. Platelets and white blood cells (WBCs) are suspended in the blood near the vessel wall. Normal laminar flow can be disrupted by changes in the diameter of the vascular lumen and blood velocity, resulting in simultaneous regions of blood stasis and turbulence (e.g., atherosclerosis). When blood stasis occurs, increased contact occurs between platelets, coagulation factors, and the endothelium, thus promoting coagulation. Turbulent flow also causes a denuding endothelial injury that eliminates the anticoagulant function of the endothelium and promotes thrombus formation.[11]

Because under normal conditions the endothelium plays an important role for anticoagulation, factors that cause endothelial injury or dysfunction promote thrombosis. For example, the presence of atherosclerotic plaques is a well-known risk factor for thrombosis in humans and hypothyroid dogs. In addition, elevated levels of homocytseine (a sulfur-containing amino acid produced by the metabolism of methionine) act as a thrombogenic agent by promoting vascular smooth muscle cell proliferation and inhibition of endothelial cell growth. Hyperhomocysteinemia is a risk factor for thromboembolic disease in humans[12] and possibly, cats.[13,14]

Disorders that result in an imbalance of the hemostatic system toward the development of thrombosis are termed *hypercoagulable*, a physiologic alteration linked to the development of thrombosis. Either increased activity of platelets and coagulation factors or decreased activity of naturally occurring anticoagulants such as antithrombin III can result in hypercoagulability.[11]

When a thrombus becomes dislodged from the site of formation, it moves to a distal site (i.e., embolizes). Clinical consequences are generally related to local or systemic effects associated with resultant end-organ ischemia. Arterial TE can result in many organ systems. Venous thrombi may dislodge, resulting in pulmonary TE, or can result in local disruption of blood flow and venous stasis.

Arterial Thromboembolism

Vascular thrombosis is most readily identified when arteries are affected, and the clinical consequences are generally acute and severe. The aortic trifurcation is one of the most common locations for arterial TE in cats[15] and dogs (Figure 208-1). Atherosclerosis leads to the majority of human thromboembolic disease and is most commonly localized to the carotid, coronary, or cerebral arteries.[16] The differences in cholesterol metabolism in dogs and cats may partially explain the low frequency of atherosclerotic-related arterial TE in veterinary patients compared with humans. Most thrombi are formed in the left heart and embolize distally (see Figure 208-1; Figure 208-2). Thrombi formed in the arterial system where the blood flow rate is high consist primarily of platelets and have been termed *white thrombi.*

Venous Thromboembolism

Thrombi formed in the venous circulation under low blood flow conditions are composed of fibrin and erythrocytes

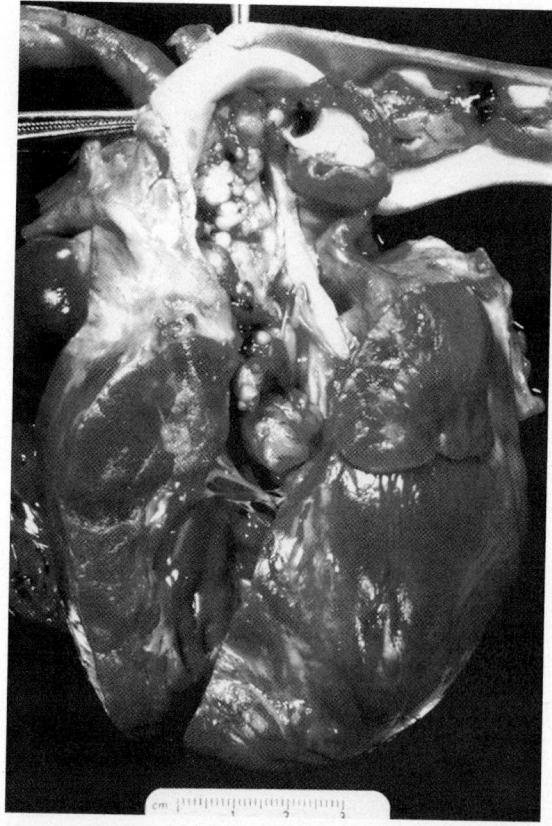

A

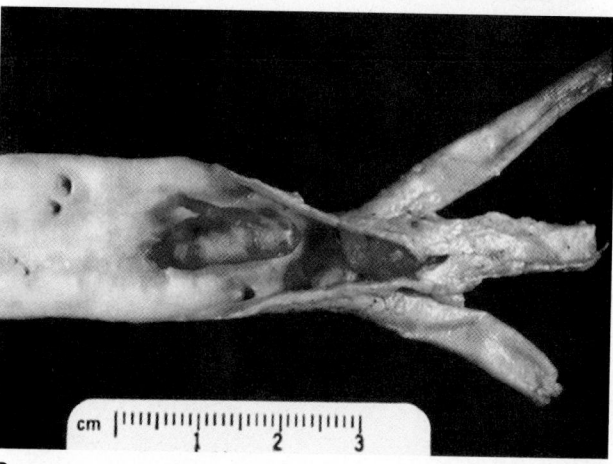

B

Figure 208-1 A, Gross heart dissected to illustrate the left ventricular outflow tract, from a dog that experienced acute posterior paresis. An extensive pedunculated mass (tumor) is present from the sinus of Valsalva and extending through the ascending aorta. B, Distal aorta from this dog containing a saddle embolus.

(Figure 208-3) and have been termed *red thrombi*. Venous thrombosis frequently causes fewer clinical abnormalities than arterial thrombosis and consequently is frequently undetected. Deep venous thrombosis, a major risk factor for pulmonary TE in over 90% of cases in humans, is not known to be a risk factor for pulmonary TE in animals. Pulmonary TE occurs in several disease states associated with hypercoagulability. These include nephrotic syndrome, hyperadrenocorticism, immune-mediated hemolytic anemia (IMHA), thrombocytosis, cardiac disease, sepsis, disseminated intravascular coagulation (DIC),

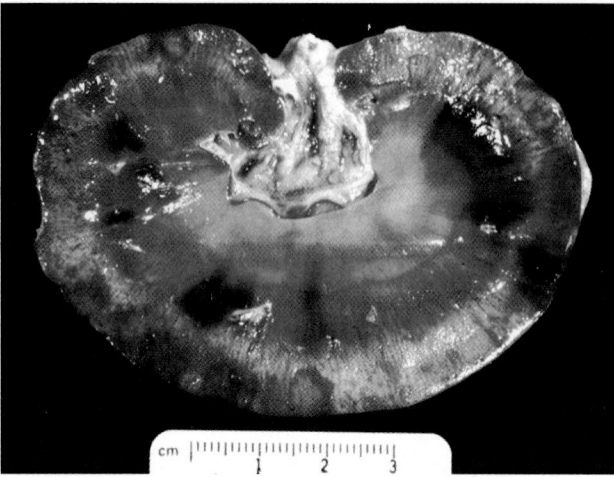

Figure 208-2 Kidney from the dog in Figure 208-1. Extensive, acute hemorrhage is seen that is associated with renal infarction.

heartworm disease, and neoplasia.[17-24] Antithrombin III deficiency may be involved in thrombogenesis as part of a number of these diseases. For example, destruction of RBCs in IMHA releases thrombogenic substances.[24] Antithrombin III inactivates thrombin and other clotting factors, and even a mild reduction in antithrombin III can result in thrombosis or TE. A deficiency of antithrombin III can be secondary to decreased synthesis (e.g., congenital), increased consumption (e.g., DIC), loss of antithrombin from the intravascular compartment (e.g., nephrotic syndrome), and increased protein catabolism (e.g., Cushing's disease). Protein C and protein S are vitamin-K dependent protein factors and major inhibitors of the procoagulant system.[11] Deficiencies of both of these proteins have been associated with clinical thrombotic disorders in humans. A single case report of protein C deficiency has been reported in a thoroughbred colt.[25] The presence of multiple concurrent disorders in patients with TE is common. For example, 47% of cats with necropsy confirmed pulmonary TE had multiple concurrent predisposing disorders.[26]

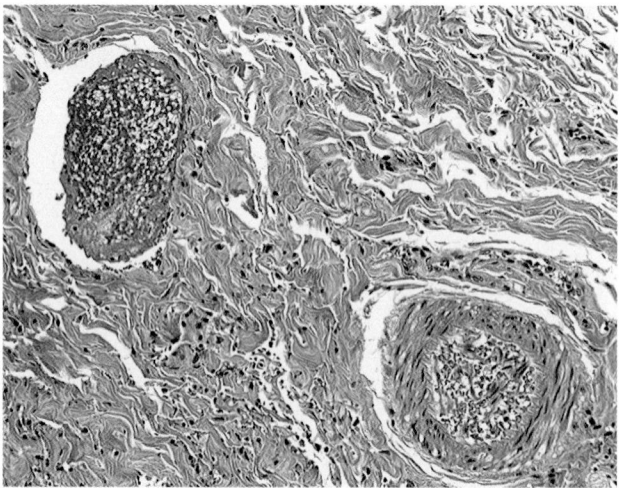

Figure 208-3 Organized thrombus fills the lumen of a vein (*upper left*) in the stomach wall from a dog with disseminated intravascular coagulation (DIC). Gastritis is also evident. A normal artery is present in the lower right.

CLINICAL DISORDERS FREQUENTLY ASSOCIATED WITH THROMBOEMBOLIC DISEASE

Hypercoagulable States
Many systemic and metabolic diseases are associated with an increased risk of arterial or venous thrombosis and TE. Primary hypercoagulable states refer to congenital abnormalities increasing the risk for thrombosis. Primary hypercoagulable states remain poorly characterized and are infrequently recognized in animals.

Secondary hypercoagulable states refer to risk factors that promote the development of thrombosis.[16] Table 208-1 lists causes and predisposing factors of thrombus and TE. Secondary hypercoagulable states resulting in TE have been described in a variety of systemic and metabolic diseases.

Disseminated Intravascular Coagulation
DIC is a specific pathologic process that involves the development of thrombi in the microvasculature and the generalized consumption of platelets and coagulation factors. This results in simultaneous hemorrhage and thrombosis, ischemia, and multiorgan failure. DIC is characterized by overwhelming thrombin and plasmin activation. Various unrelated diseases associated with DIC are unified by unregulated activation of mononuclear cell cytokines initiating simultaneous coagulation and fibrinolysis. Multiple cytokines are believed to be responsible for the initiation of DIC through induction of tissue factor expression on monocytes and endothelial cells.[16] Tumor necrosis factor (TNF)-alpha and interleukin-6 (IL-6) are two of many cytokines involved in the pathogenesis of DIC. Cytokines also inhibit natural anticoagulants including protein C and S complex, tissue factor pathway inhibitor, and antithrombin III. Cytokines affect endothelial integrity, promoting platelet adhesion and resulting in increased levels of plasminogen activator inhibitor-1 (PAI-1) and promote fibrin deposition.[11]

DIC occurs in patients with a wide variety of clinical disorders. Heatstoke, sepsis, pancreatitis, neoplasia, immune-mediated disease, trauma, and toxin exposure are common inciting causes of DIC. The trigger causing DIC in these seemingly unrelated syndromes may be systemic inflammatory response syndrome and the production of proinflammatory cytokines including but not limited to TNF, IL-1, and IL-8.[27] The most important step in treating DIC is elimination of the underlying pathologic condition or triggering mechanisms and the conditions that promote this hypercoagulable state. Anticoagulants have been advocated, although clinical data regarding efficacy are lacking.

Protein-Losing Nephropathy
Protein-losing nephropathy (PLN) results in loss of plasma proteins into the urine through injured glomeruli. The small molecular weight of antithrombin III (65,000 daltons) allows it to pass through the glomerulus similarly to albumin. The resulting hypercoagulable state is most often associated with venous thrombosis and can result in pulmonary TE.[18-22] Arterial (aortic) TE has also been reported in dogs with PLN.[7]

Hyperadrenocorticism
Both spontaneous hyperadrenocorticism and exogenous administration of glucocorticoids have been associated with the development of thromboemboli.[7] The hypercoagulable state in spontaneous hyperadrenocorticism is characterized by an increase in coagulation factors II, V, VII, IX, X, XII, and fibrinogen, coupled with a decrease in the natural anticoagulant antithrombin III.[28] Thrombin-antithrombin complexes are also increased in dogs with hyperadrenocorticism but with no clinical signs of thrombosis, suggesting subclinical thrombosis. Long-term exogenous administration of glucocorticoids is

Table • 208-1

Causes and Predisposing Factors of Thrombosis and Thromboembolism

VASCULAR ENDOTHELIAL DAMAGE	HYPERCOAGULABILITY	ABNORMAL BLOOD FLOW
Arteriosclerosis	Infection/sepsis/abscess	Neoplasia
Atherosclerosis	Neoplasia	Cardiomyopathy
Vasculitis	Hyperadrenocorticism	Congestive heart failure (CHF)
Heartworm disease	Protein losing nephropathy (PLN)	Endocarditis
Catheterization	Protein losing enteropathy (PLE)	Hypovolemia
Injection of irritating substances	Disseminated intravascular coagulation (DIC)	Shock
Neoplasia	Thrombocytosis	Anemia
Vascular incarceration/compression	Platelet hyperreactivity	Polycythemia
Hyperhomocysteinemia	Immune-mediated hemolytic anemia (IHA)	Dehydration
Feline ischemic encephalopathy (FIE)	Parvovirus infection	Hyperviscosity
Fibrocartilaginous embolism		

associated with proteinuria and glomerular changes.[29] Whether or not this ultimately results in loss of antithrombin III and hypercoagulability is unknown. Both arterial and venous TE have been diagnosed in dogs receiving exogenous glucocorticoids.[30]

Feline Cardiomyopathy

The cause of feline TE is multifactorial and principally accompanies myocardial disease with associated injury to left ventricular or left atrial endothelium. Some affected cats with aortic TE have elevated blood levels of homocysteine when compared with cardiomyopathic cats without TE,[13] and homocysteine metabolism may be abnormal in some felines.[14] Several coagulation abnormalities leading to hypercoagulability have been identified in cats with aortic TE.[31] Platelets from some cardiomyopathic cats have also been shown to be hyperaggregable in response to adenosine phosphate (ADP) in vitro.[32]

Immune-Mediated Hemolytic Anemia

Pulmonary TE is a major complicating factor to the high rate of mortality in IMHA. Because of the difficulties in antemortem diagnosis of PTE, most estimates of the number of dogs with IMHA and TE are based on necropsy results and range from 15% to 80%.[33] Use of intravenous catheters, elevated bilirubin concentration, elevated alkaline phosphatase concentration, and decreased albumin have all been associated with development of pulmonary TE.[33] Severe leukocytosis, left shift, and neutrophil toxic change may serve as laboratory markers of systemic thrombosis in some cases.[34] Derangements in routine coagulation tests, prothrombin time (PT), partial thromboplastin time (PPT), and fibrinogen concentration are common in IMHA patients.[24] Thrombocytopenia is also common and severe thrombocytopenia (platelets <50,000/μL) occurs in approximately 25% of IMHA patients. Fibrin (or fibrinogen) degradation products and D dimer are increased in greater than 50% affected of dogs. DIC is also commonly diagnosed in IMHA.[24]

THERAPY OF THROMBOEMBOLIC DISEASE

The management of primary diseases resulting in the development of TE is discussed in related chapters throughout this textbook. Therapy of TE should be directed toward the underlying disorder whenever possible. Therapeutic strategies for managing TE include short-term systemic anticoagulation and fibrinolysis followed by long-term antiplatelet or anticoagulant therapy to reduce the risk of rethrombosis.

Supportive Care

General patient care is critical for successful management of thrombosis. Analgesic agents should be considered for acute pain management. Fluid therapy should be administered when indicated to correct acid-base abnormalities and dehydration. Dextrose-containing fluids should be avoided whenever possible because they may cause endothelial damage, further promoting thrombosis. A risk of volume overload exists with heart failure or pulmonary hypertension and fluid therapy must be carefully monitored. Strict cage rest and oxygen therapy are indicated in cases of pulmonary TE or thrombosis associated with congestive heart failure (CHF).

Acute Anticoagulation

Heparin is the mainstay of acute anticoagulation. Anticoagulants prevent additional clots from forming but do not dissolve clots (see thrombolysis). Coumadin therapy for the long-term control of thrombosis is initiated after adequate heparinization has been achieved.

Heparin functions as a cofactor with antithrombin III, and together this complex exerts its effect by neutralizing factor X and thrombin. Heparin is inactivated by gastrointestinal (GI) enzymes when given orally and therefore must be administered by injection. Heparin is administered to prolong the baseline activated partial thromboplastin time (aPTT) to 1.5 to 3.0 times the baseline value. Prolongation of the aPTT or activated coagulation time (ACT) does not correlate well with heparin levels in cats and dogs, and measurement of plasma heparin levels may be more useful in monitoring heparin therapy. Although many different heparin doses have been advocated, little clinical data exist concerning efficacy. Doses of heparin required to achieve adequate heparin levels in cats with TE ranged from 175 U/kg every 6 hours to 475 U/kg every 8 hours, subcutaneously.[35] In normal dogs the dose of heparin required to achieve adequate heparin concentrations was 250 U/kg every 6 hours, subcutaneously.[36] The most common side effect of heparin therapy is hemorrhage. In the event of severe hemorrhage, heparin can be neutralized by protamine sulfate administration.[37]

Low molecular weight (LMW) heparin is being increasingly used.[38] Its anticoagulant effect is limited to blocking the activity of factor X. Because LMW heparin has a lower antithrombin effect than unfractionated heparin, LMW heparin does not markedly influence the PT or aPTT. Measurement of factor X activity has been used to assess the effect of LMW heparin. One advantage of LMW heparin is that it has a lower risk of hemorrhage than conventional heparin therapy. The optimal dose of LMW heparin in dogs and cats with thromboembolic disease remains to be determined.

Chronic Anticoagulation

Warfarin (Coumadin) is a vitamin K antagonist inhibiting the synthesis of vitamin K–dependent clotting proteins (prothrombin and factors VII, IX and X). In addition, warfarin reduces efficacy of the vitamin K–dependent regulatory proteins C and S.[11] Proteins C and S are anticoagulant factors, and their function is the first to be inhibited by warfarin administration. Therefore heparin and warfarin administration are generally overlapped for 2 to 4 days to prevent a transient hypercoagulable state. Some animals appear to do well with just warfarin. Starting doses for warfarin are 0.25 to 0.5 mg every 24 hours in the cat and 0.1 to 0.2 mg/kg every 24 hours in the dog. Due to the high individual patient variability, close monitoring of PT is essential. Early recommendations were to maintain PT 1.5 times the baseline value, and more recent recommendations suggest attaining an international normalized ratio (INR) of 2:3.[39] INR is calculated by the formula (patient PT/control PT)[ISI]. The ISI is a value specific to the tissue thromboplastin that is used in measuring the PT. Coumadin is continued on a long-term basis to prevent recurrent TE. Studies documenting the optimal dose, efficacy, and duration of Coumadin therapy for specific thromboembolic diseases in dogs and cats are unknown.

The use of Coumadin is not without risks. The major risk is fatal hemorrhage, which occurs acutely and unexpectedly. Ideally, pets maintained on Coumadin should live indoors and be well supervised to prevent trauma and to monitor for hemorrhage. Periodic measurement of the PT should be done to ensure adequate dosing. Coumadin interacts with many drugs. The addition of medications to the treatment regimen of a pet on Coumadin should be done cautiously because certain drugs will raise the activity of Coumadin and predispose patients to bleeding. Some of these drugs are phenylbutazone, metronidazole, trimethoprim sulfa, and second- and third-generation cephalosporins. Barbiturates will decrease Coumadin anticoagulant effect. If bleeding complications occur, warfarin therapy is discontinued and administration of vitamin K is recommended.[39]

Antiplatelet Therapy

Antiplatelet drugs have been advocated for long-term management to prevent rethrombosis. These drugs inhibit platelet aggregation and adhesion, preventing the formation of the hemostatic platelet plug. Aspirin inhibits cyclooxygenase, leading to decreased thromboxane A_2 synthesis. This renders platelets nonfunctional by preventing their aggregation.[40,41] Cats lack the enzyme needed to metabolize aspirin (glucuronyl transferase), making them sensitive to aspirin-induced platelet dysfunction. Doses of 0.5 mg/kg every 12 hours in the dog and 25 mg/kg twice weekly in the cat may decrease platelet aggregation.[37] However, rethrombosis generally occurs despite aspirin therapy, although it is not known whether aspirin delays recrudescence. Additional antiplatelet drugs include dipyridamole and ticlopidine. Dipyridamole is thought to inhibit platelet aggregation by inhibition of platelet phosphodiesterase, leading to increased levels of cyclic adenosine monophosphate (cAMP) within platelets. Ticlopidine impairs fibrinogen binding and inhibits platelet aggregation induced by ADP and collagen.[37] The use of these newer compounds has been limited thus far in veterinary medicine.

Thrombolysis

Thrombolytic agents such as streptokinase, urokinase, and tissue plasminogen activator (tPA) are potent activators of fibrinolysis. These agents have been used with variable and often limited success in veterinary medicine.[42-45]

Streptokinase binds plasminogen, and the complex transforms other plasminogen molecules into plasmin. Plasmin then binds to fibrin and causes thrombolysis. Streptokinase binds both free and clot-associated plasminogen. It also degrades factors V, VIII, and prothrombin, resulting in a massive systemic coagulation defect.

Streptokinase has been used to treat aortic thromboembolism (ATE) in cats with varying degrees of success. In one study of 46 cats, 15 were discharged from the hospital after streptokinase therapy with a median survival of 51 days.[45] Reperfusion injury occurred in approximately 35% after thrombolysis, with streptokinase often resulting in fatal hyperkalemia and metabolic acidosis. Eleven of the cats developed clinical hemorrhage after streptokinase therapy. In three cats, hemorrhage was significant enough to require transfusion. Others reported conservative management (treatment of heart failure plus Coumadin or aspirin) of ATE with a hospital discharge rate of 28%, which was similar to cats treated with streptokinase.[15] One recommended dose of streptokinase for dogs and cats with TE is 90,000 U, intravenously administered over 20 to 30 minutes, followed by a maintenance infusion of 45,000 U for 7 to 12 hours. Infusions may be repeated over a total of 3 days.[37]

Recombinant DNA technology produces t-PA, a serine protease. A complex forms between t-PA and fibrin, and that complex preferentially activates thrombus-associated plasminogen-resulting in rapid fibrinolysis.[47] Life-threatening hemorrhage is the number one side effect. The half-life of t-PA in dogs is 2 to 3 minutes; consequently, if bleeding occurs, stopping the infusion will result in the drug clearance from the system in 5 to 10 minutes. Because t-PA causes rapid thrombolysis, the risk of reperfusion syndrome and lethal hyperkalemia is substantial. In one report, 50% of cats with ATE died acutely during t-PA therapy, with death attributed to hyperkalemia, severe anemia, and renal hemorrhage.[46]

VASCULAR DISEASES

Diseases Of Arteries

Occlusive Arterial Diseases Arterial occlusion refers to the interruption of blood flow within an artery and most commonly results from trauma, thrombi, emboli, arteritis, degenerative lesions such as atherosclerosis, and factors associated with endothelial dysfunction or injury. Arterial thrombosis requires one or more inciting local or systemic conditions: (1) vascular endothelial damage, (2) sluggish blood flow, and (3) changes in blood constituents resulting in a hypercoagulable state.[11] Vascular endothelial injury can be induced by infectious agents (e.g., *Dirofilaria immitis*), prolonged hypotension, hypoxia, acidosis, inflammation, trauma, and immune mechanisms. Compressive lesions, such as from tumors, may promote thrombosis by a reduction in local blood flow and endothelial injury. Thromboemboli usually represent blood clots that have broken free from a site of thrombus formation. Emboli can also consist of tissue particles, fat, gas, bacterial vegetations, parasites (e.g., heartworms), tumors, or foreign bodies.[48] Entrapped emboli may themselves become thrombogenic. Arterial occlusion can be acute or chronic. Chronic gradual occlusion can occur with mural or extramural hematomas, atherosclerosis, arteriosclerosis, vasculitis, or intimal tears forming valvelike structures.

The potential clinical consequences of arterial occlusion (tissue hypoxemia, ischemia, neuropathy, tissue necrosis) are related to extent and duration of vascular obstruction, and the physiologic consequences of the affected organ or organs. Tissues supplied by the endarteries, which have no connections to collateral vascular beds, undergo greater ischemic injury than organs supplied with collateral circulation. Acute, complete arterial occlusion causes rapid ischemic injury. This is largely due to release of vasoactive substances by the clot, which induces vasoconstriction and reduces collateral circulation. In addition to the acute effects, long-term injury (days or weeks) occurs and includes fibrosis and neuromyopathy.[7]

Feline systemic thromboembolism Feline systemic TE is discussed in Chapter 204.

Canine systemic thrombosis and thromboembolism
Arterial occlusion has been reported in dogs occurring secondary to atherosclerosis, nephrotic syndrome, vegetative endocarditis, neoplastic emboli, dirofilariasis, trauma, and thrombi of left heart origin (see Figure 208-1). The distal aorta, iliac, renal, and femoral arteries are common sites of systemic TE (see Figures 208-1 and 208-2).[7]

History Acute arterial occlusion is usually indicative of systemic, metabolic, or cardiovascular disease. Clinical recognition and identification of the cause are enhanced by an insightful history, complete physical examination, and appropriate diagnostic tests. Some animals have a history of intermittent claudication, whereas in others, acute paresis or paralysis is the major presenting sign. Acute, complete arterial occlusion may cause posterior paresis, extreme hindlimb pain, and general distress.[49,50] In some cases the animal may have an unsteady gait, lameness, progression to stumbling, weakness, or collapse. Other potential signs include weight loss, exercise intolerance, hindlimb licking or chewing, and hypersensitivity over the lumbosacral region and the hindlimbs. Other signs attributable to systemic or metabolic diseases may sometimes be detected.

Clinical signs and physical examination The outcome and clinical signs of arterial occlusion depend on (1) size and number of thrombi, (2) degree and duration of vascular occlusion, (3) pathophysiologic consequences of the organ or organs supplied, (4) whether the clot is infected or sterile, (5) whether the event is solitary or repeated, (6) the adequacy of compensatory mechanisms (e.g., collateral vessel recruitment, vasodilatation, clot lysis, restoration of blood flow), (7) the effects of vasoactive chemicals elaborated by the clot on collateral vessels (i.e., vasoconstriction), and (8) related complications (e.g., tissue necrosis, local infection, hyperesthesia). A slowly progressing arteriosclerotic or atherosclerotic stenosis allows time for the development of collateral circulation and may have minimal clinical consequences. A sudden embolus, however, may not be associated with the development of collateral circulation, and presenting clinical signs may be more severe.[50] Microthrombus formation is common, and rapid clot lysis and abundant collateral circulation usually results in absence of outward clinical signs.

Classic presentation of acute arterial occlusion is described by the seven *P*s: (1) pain, (2) paleness, (3) paresthesia, (4) pulselessness, (5) polar (cold), (6) paresis or paralysis, and (7) prostration.[49] Physical examination may reveal cool distal limbs and swollen muscles. Segmental and pedal reflexes may be depressed. Hypersensitivity over the lumbar spine may exist. A slow onset and progressive peripheral neuropathy after trauma may be associated with ischemia of peripheral nerves. Arterial thrombosis of a front limb may also occur. Clinical signs are usually less severe than those described for posterior limb thrombosis.

In the central nervous system (CNS), arterial occlusion is rarely diagnosed. For signs to be recognizable, several arteries have to be occluded simultaneously, as can occur in severe atherosclerosis or with embolization after arterial catheterization. Cerebrovascular occlusions may lead to sudden disorientation, weakness, anisocoria, and hemiamaurosis. Infarction may follow TE to a localized area of the brain. *Stroke* is a generic term denoting any acute, nonconvulsive, focal neurologic deficit stemming from cerebrovascular disease. The classic presentation includes hemiparesis, but a broad spectrum of neurologic injuries may result. Neurologic signs depend on site, extent, and time course of vascular occlusion. In a series of 17 affected dogs, cerebrovascular disease was associated with coagulopathy, metastatic brain tumor, trauma, sepsis, atherosclerotic thrombus, unknown cause, and vascular malformation.[51] A cerebellar infarction caused by meningeal arterial thrombosis has also been described in a German shepherd dog with acute onset of seizure and neurologic deficits.[52] We have occasionally observed neurologic signs related to stroke in cats associated with severe systemic hypertension. Affected animals usually present acutely blind and show signs of retinal hemorrhage and detachment. Neurovascular disorders may be more common than the literature suggests. Increasing availability of advanced imaging techniques should facilitate the diagnosis of these conditions.

With endocarditis, a heart murmur of mitral or aortic insufficiency may be auscultated. Bacterial embolization from these valves may cause a systemic shower of emboli, which frequently affect abdominal organs, especially the kidneys and small intestines. Complete unilateral or bilateral renal artery occlusion invariably causes severe renal infarction. Affected dogs are depressed and may exhibit an arched back, sublumbar pain, and hematuria.

Acute occlusion of a major mesenteric artery may cause initial gastric hyperactivity, followed by ileus and intestinal infarction. Sudden anorexia, vomiting, bowel evacuation, and abdominal pain may be present. Feces may contain blood. With bowel infarction, bloody diarrhea, severe signs of an acute abdomen, and shock may develop.

Diagnosis When peripheral arterial thrombosis is suspected, a survey thoracic radiograph is indicated to evaluate cardiac size and shape and to assess for pulmonary changes including edema, thrombosis, or dirofilariasis. Chest and abdominal radiographs should be evaluated for orthopedic lesions, which could result in posterior paresis. In addition, radiographs of the pelvic and hindlimb region may be indicated to check for masses that could exert pressure on the aorta and for periosteal reactions in the sublumbar area. Doppler echocardiography may be useful for identifying vascular disturbances.[6,7]

Clinical pathology data may help characterize the underlying primary disease. Coagulation profiles are variable. Some cases of glomerulopathies and hypoproteinemia have been associated with reduced levels of antithrombin III.[22] Assessment of protein C and protein S levels should be considered when these tests are available. A clinical pathology data base is also advised to evaluate and detect renal or hepatic disease, dirofilariasis, DIC, and systemic and metabolic disorders. Blood cultures are indicated if endocarditis, bacteremia, or sepsis is suspected.

Confirmation of diagnosis may require proof of a vascular occlusion. This can be accomplished in some cases by physical examination, whereas in others, arteriography or diagnostic ultrasound are required.[1,6,8] The arteriogram can indicate the exact location of the thrombus or illustrate the extent of vascular occlusion and collateral vascular supply (Figures 208-4 and 208-5). Furthermore, radiolucent emboli such as heartworms may be outlined when present as longitudinal filling defects. Contrast angiography and other alternative imaging methods (thermography, perfusion scanning) in human medicine are being replaced by MRA and advanced ultrasound techniques such as intravascular ultrasound.[6,9]

Differential diagnoses Differential diagnoses include trauma; peripheral neuropathy; spinal, pelvic or vascular tumors; infections; toxoplasmosis; degenerative myelopathy; interventricular disc protrusion; fibrocartilaginous embolic myelopathy; and the cauda equina compression syndrome. Radiographs should be systematically evaluated for signs related to these disorders.

Prognosis The prognosis depends on the cause, extent, and severity of occlusion, presence or absence of local complications

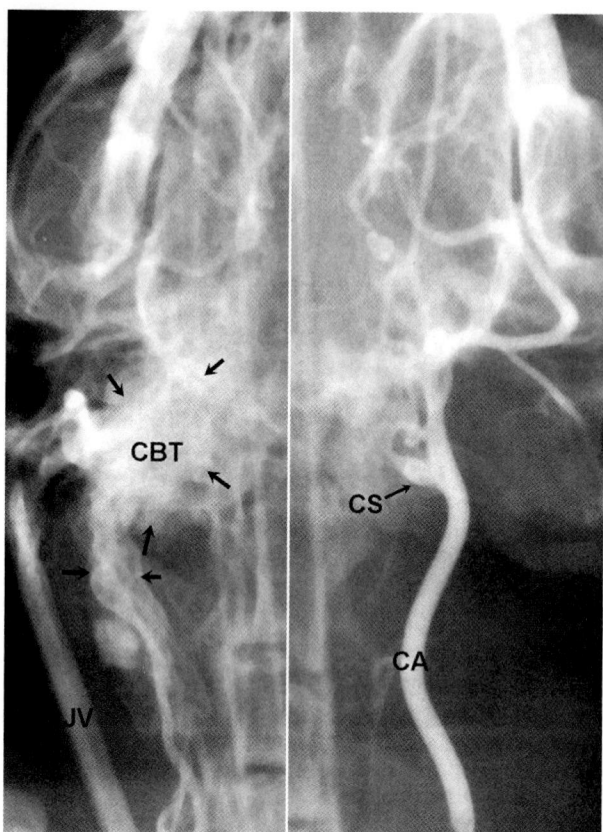

Figure 208-4 Two ventrodorsal angiograms of a dog with a carotid body tumor. The left panel demonstrates a late arterial-venous phase after injection of contrast medium into the right common carotid artery. A tumor "blush" is seen, with contrast medium opacifying vessels feeding the carotid body tumor (*CBT; arrows*). Venous return is observed via the jugular vein (*JV*). The angiogram in the right panel is a useful comparison and was taken after injection of contrast material into the left common carotid artery (*CA*). Normal flow is observed, and the carotid sinus (*CS*), an area for sensing blood pressure, is evident. (Courtesy of John Bonagura, DVM.)

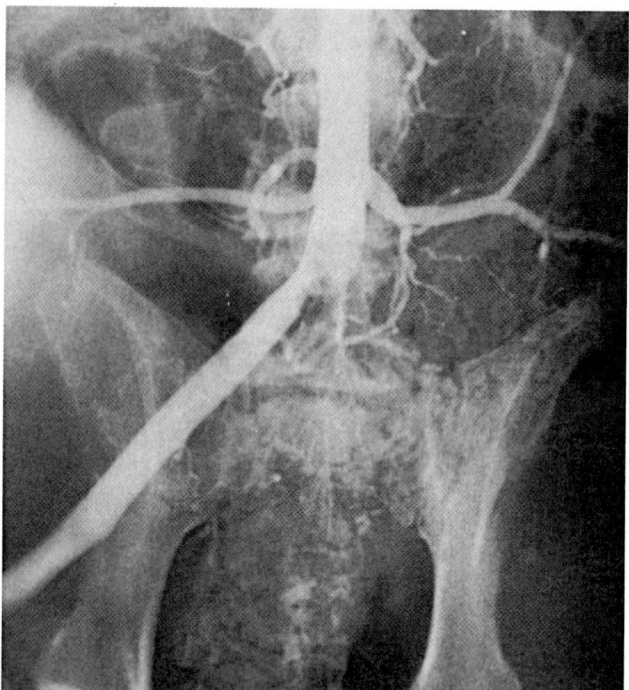

Figure 208-5 Aortogram of a 7-year-old Saint Bernard dog with a saddle thrombus at the aortic trifurcation associated with a chondrosarcoma located near the terminal aorta. The owner had observed four episodes of pain and weakness in the hindlimbs that developed gradually when the dog was taken for a walk. At the beginning of the walk, the dog was normal. If the dog was forced to continue walking after the signs of pain and lameness had appeared, it collapsed. After resting for a few moments, the dog was able to walk again. On clinical examination the femoral pulse was difficult to feel, and the periphery of the hindlimbs was cool. Pain could be elicited when the pelvic area was palpated. Aortography was performed, and a radiograph was taken 4 seconds after the beginning of the injection of contrast medium. On the aortogram the common origin of the internal iliac arteries and the left external iliac artery contain no contrast medium, suggesting that they have been occluded completely. A partial occlusion has reduced the flow of contrast medium into the right external iliac artery. Some collateral blood supply to the hindlimbs probably occurs via the seventh lumbar artery. Anticoagulation therapy was instituted, but it failed to provide relief and the dog underwent euthanasia at the request of the owner.

(ischemic neuromyopathy, ulcers), and concurrent embolization to visceral organs. Even in cases with spontaneous recovery, relapses must be expected. Rapid diagnosis and treatment are essential to avoid severe or even irreversible tissue injury.

Feline Ischemic Encephalopathy

Feline ischemic encephalopathy (FIE) results in cerebral ischemic necrosis. FIE occurs in male and female cats of all ages and is more prevalent in the summer months. The cause of FIE is uncertain. Preliminary evidence suggests *Cuterebra* infection as a potential cause in some cases.[53,54]

Clinical pathology is usually unremarkable. Cerebrospinal fluid (CSF) analysis may be normal or have mildly elevated protein levels and a mild to moderate pleocytosis. An increased proportion of large foamy macrophages have been observed in the CSF from 2 to 7 months after the onset of seizures. Suspected diagnosis can be made by T2 weighted MRI. In one study of six cats with FIE, MRI findings included mild to marked asymmetry of the cerebral hemispheres and bilateral asymmetric enlargement of the subarachnoid space.[55]

Gross lesions are usually unilateral and may involve up to 75% of one cerebral or cerebellar hemisphere (or both). Hemispheres may appear atrophic and ridged with wide sulci.

Histopathologic findings have included parenchymal atrophy and cystic degeneration, gliosis, and phagocytic macrophage infiltration. Perivascular lymphocytic cuffing of small capillaries and vascular occlusive lesions including thrombosis and vasculitis has been reported. Infarction of the middle cerebral artery represents the most common distribution.

Clinical signs are typically acute in onset, nonprogressive, and suggestive of unilateral cerebral or brainstem involvement. Seizures are the most common historical or presenting clinical sign. Other clinical signs may include depression, head tilt, anisocoria, circling, seizures, and behavior changes.

Treatment is limited to supportive care, and the prognosis is generally favorable. Clinical improvement typically occurs over several days to weeks. Multiple episodes can occur. Behavior changes and uncontrollable seizures can persist.[54,55]

Fibrocartilagenous Embolization

Fibrocartilaginous embolization (FCE) is associated with ischemic necrosis of the spinal cord parenchyma. The pathogenic

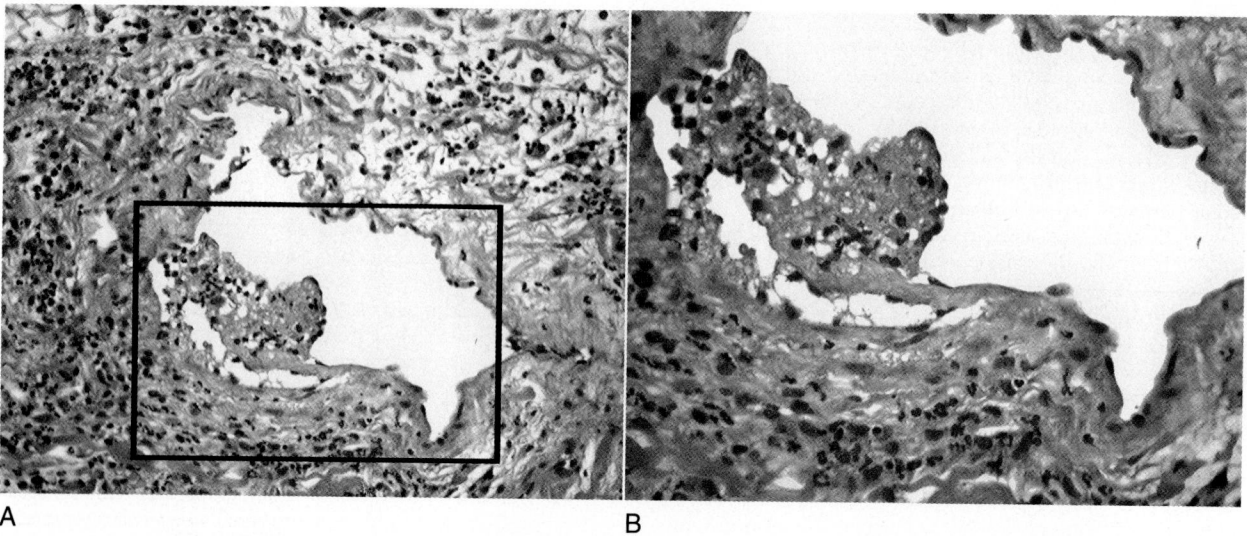

Figure 208-6 Vasculitis is indicated by inflammatory cells present within (**A**) and around (**B**) the venous vessel wall. Vascular injury associated with necrosis, degeneration of endothelial and smooth muscle cells, and fibrin deposition is evident. A small intramural thrombus is also present.

mechanism is not resolved. Spinal cord arteries and veins become occluded with fibrocartilage originating from the nucleus pulposus of the intervertebral disc. Trauma may be a predisposing factor in a large percentage of affected cases. FCE can occur at any age but is most common in adult non-chondrodystrophoid breeds. Young Irish wolfhounds and miniature schnauzers are particularly prone to the disease. FCE has been reported less commonly in cats.[55,56]

Clinical signs of myelopathy vary depending on the location and severity of the spinal cord ischemic injury. Deficits are often asymmetrical, and the clinical signs are not progressive. Affected animals do not typically show evidence of pain, although brief painful periods have been described just prior to the onset of clinical signs.

Diagnosis of FCE is based on excluding other causes of acute myelopathy. Results of plain radiographs are normal. CSF evaluation may be normal or show nonspecific abnormalities including mild protein elevations, mild pleocytosis, and xanthochromia. Myelography is typically normal, or mild spinal cord swelling is seen. MRI may reveal spinal cord edema on T2 weight images.[55]

Treatment is primarily supportive care and physical therapy. Evidence for the use of glucocorticoid therapy is lacking. If treatment is attempted, methylprednisolone succinate (MPS) should be given within the first 6 to 8 hours after the onset of neurologic signs. Prognosis for recovery is variable depending on the location and extent of the lesion. Poor prognostic indicators include lower motor neuron (LMN) signs and size of the animal because of the inherent difficulties of performing physical therapy on large breed dogs.[56]

Vasculitis and Angiitis

The terms *vasculitis* and *angiitis* refer to the pathologic syndrome that is characterized by vascular inflammation and necrosis. Although there have been many reported causes of vasculitis, only a few histologic manifestations of the disease have been diagnosed. Vasculitis can occur in toxic, immune-mediated, infectious, inflammatory, and neoplastic disorders. Blood vessels of any type in any organ can be affected, resulting in a wide variety of clinical signs. The nonspecific nature of histologic lesions, coupled with variable clinical presentations, makes the diagnosis of primary vasculitis quite challenging.

The clinical consequences of vasculitis depend on the size, number, type, and extent of blood vessels that are affected.[57]

Histologically, vasculitis is characterized by the presence of inflammatory cells within and around blood vessel walls. Vascular injury is associated with necrosis and degeneration of endothelial and smooth muscle cells and fibrin deposition (Figure 208-6). A collection of fibrin, immunoglobulins (Igs), complement, and platelets appears by light microscopy as eosinophilic material within the vessel wall and lumen and is referred to as *fibrinoid*. Eosinophilia secondary to degeneration of collagen and smooth muscle can also be present within the vessel wall.[58] These histopathologic lesions distinguish vasculitis from perivascular inflammation (Figure 208-7). Vasculitides have been classified based on specific inflammatory cell infiltrates that may include neutrophils, lymphocytes, or macrophages.[58,59] As the disease becomes chronic or begins to resolve, predominant cell populations may change. Vasculitis may develop from within a vessel as a result of infectious, immune-mediated or toxic injury or by extension from adjacent areas of inflammation. Infectious agents can injure endothelial cells directly or through the production of

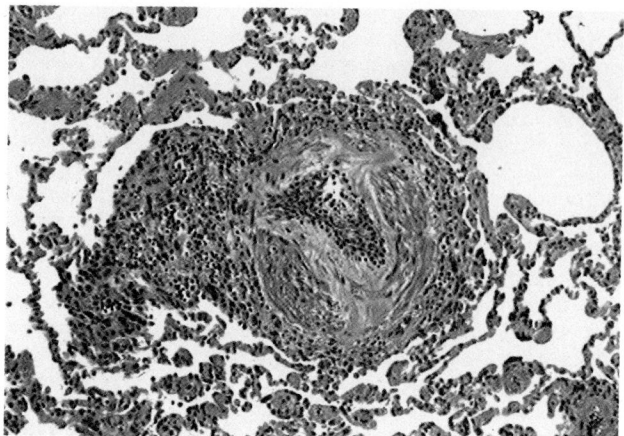

Figure 208-7 Section of lung. Perivasculitis is evident as large inflammatory infiltrate surrounding pulmonary arteriole.

endotoxins and exotoxins. The exact mechanism of endothelial injury is not known but involves the formation of oxygen free radicals, local inflammatory mediators, and the recruitment of inflammatory cells.[60] Exposure of subendothelial collagen during endothelial injury results in the activation of Hageman's factor and the subsequent activation of the complement, kinin, and plasmin systems. These lead to increased vascular permeability and inflammation.

Type III hypersensitivity reactions can cause necrotizing vasculitis from the deposition of immune complexes within the vessel walls. Activation of the complement cascade may attract neutrophils, cause immune complex phagocytosis, and result in the release of lysosomal enzymes and oxygen free radicals, thereby leading to further inflammation and necrosis. In the chronic state this reaction becomes diminished, and mononuclear cells replace the neutrophilic inflammation. Immune complex reactions of this type can occur in many disease conditions such as primary immune-mediated disease or be secondary to infectious disease. Emphasis on immune complex activity can only be misleading because immune complexes are rapidly cleared from the circulation.[59,61] In humans the discovery of antineutrophil cytoplasmic autoantibodies (specific for antigens in neutrophil granules and monocyte lysosomes) has allowed further identification of immune-mediated processes in which immune complexes were suspected but not identified. Cell-mediated immunopathogenic mechanisms are initiated in the blood vessel wall. This type of vasculitis is characterized by accumulations of lymphocytes and macrophages within vascular walls. Myocyte necrosis results in fibrinoid degeneration, endothelial hyperplasia, and occasionally thrombosis. A granulomatous type of reaction of the vessel wall can result, particularly in chronic cases. These changes may be accompanied by hemorrhage and ischemic changes in surrounding tissues.[61]

The cause of secondary vasculitides is, by definition, known, and classifications are based accordingly. These conditions usually result from infectious diseases such as feline infectious peritonitis (FIP), canine coronavirus infection, parvovirus infection (rare), Rocky Mountain spotted fever (RMSF), leishmaniasis, and dirofilariasis. They may also occur in drug reactions and in immunopathogenic connective tissue and collagen diseases, such as systemic lupus erythematosus (SLE) and rheumatoid arthritis.[62]

Microscopic Necrotizing Vasculitis

Microscopic necrotizing vasculitis (MNV) refers to a large heterogeneous group of clinical syndromes that share similar histologic properties. *Hypersensitivity vasculitis* is often referred to in dermatologic manifestations and is often clinically distinct from the multisystemic form of necrotizing vasculitis. Termed *juvenile polyarteritis syndrome* (JPS), it has been reported in young beagle dogs.[63,64] Less distinction exists between JPS and those syndromes described as *idiopathic steroid-responsive vasculitides* that can manifest as multisystemic or localized disease.[65,66] Lesions can affect mainly arterioles, capillaries, and venules.

Clinical abnormalities of MNV are often associated with phasic pyrexia, listlessness, and anorexia. In some cases, lymphadenopathy, myalgia, epistaxis, drooling, sneezing, and arthralgia may occur. In addition to the generalized signs, manifestations of specific organ lesions may occur.[67] The most common presenting clinical signs in small animals are dermatologic lesions. Hemorrhagic maculae resembling circular petechiae and ecchymoses are common. Other lesions seen include wheals, urticaria, purpura, nodules, bullae, necrosis, and ulcers. In many cases the skin lesions are associated with pain, pruritus, or both. Less frequently encountered lesions include ulcers at the mucocutaneous junctions or of the mucous membranes, especially located on the head (external ear canal and pinnae, face), bony prominences of the limbs, and the foot pads, as well as

pitting edema involving dependent areas such as limbs, ventral trunk, head, and scrotum.[62,63]

Internal organ involvement with MNV frequently goes undiagnosed. This is because clinical signs are vague, simultaneous multiorgan involvement often occurs, or organ manifestations are confused with those of infectious, degenerative, or traumatic conditions (e.g., pneumonia, glomerulonephritis, arthritis, spinal or neuromuscular conditions). The clinicopathologic findings of primary MNV vary according to severity, duration, and specific organ. Lymphopenia, eosinopenia, hypoalbuminemia, hyperglobulinemia, and hyperfibrinogenemia occur commonly. Less consistent findings include leukocytosis with a left shift and toxic neutrophils; leukopenia; neutropenia; monocytosis; a mild normocytic, normochromic anemia; and thrombocytopenia. Serum liver enzymes and triglycerides are often elevated.[57,59]

An idiopathic cutaneous and renal glomerular vasculopathy has been described in kenneled and racing greyhounds, with many characteristics similar to MNV.[68] It is characterized by fibrinoid arteritis, thrombosis, and infarction with deep, slowly healing skin ulcers and peracute renal glomerular necrosis with a predilection for afferent arterioles.

Diagnostic confirmation requires histologic examination of skin, organ, or lymph node biopsies specimen and exclusion of other immune-mediated disease. Special immunologic tests have been recommended to demonstrate a low or high concentration of complement, C3, and elevated levels of circulating immune complexes. The history may be helpful if drug hypersensitivity is suspected.

Primary periarteritis, or polyarteritis, a necrotizing vasculitis affecting small- and medium-sized muscular arteries has been identified in colonies of beagles.[69,70] This polyarteritis occurs in two forms. One form occurs mainly in young beagles, in which arteritis affects major branches of coronary arteries almost exclusively. Clinical signs are usually absent. A second form of polyarteritis is associated with vague multisystemic signs (fever, depression, anorexia, neutrophilia, decreased albumin-to-globulin ratio), a stiff gait, pain on abdominal palpation (beagle pain syndrome), or a combination of these symptoms. The signs are associated with vascular lesions including disseminated, focal, or diffuse intimal thickening and acute fibrinoid necrosis of the media resulting in occlusion and thrombosis.

The differential diagnosis includes pemphigus vulgaris and foliaceus, bullous pemphigoid, SLE; dirofilariasis, specific infectious diseases, chronic neoplasia, and cold hemagglutination disease. The prognosis is usually favorable.

Many therapies have been advocated. Administration of all unnecessary drugs should be discontinued. In many cases immunosuppressive doses of glucocorticoids with or without an antibiotic have been used successfully. Cyclophosphamide may be administered if that fails. Dogs with lesions involving only the skin can be given sulfasalazine (Azulfidine) at an initial dose of 22 mg/lb (49 mg/kg) every 8 hours.[57] Dose frequency can be decreased after lesions improve from three times to twice a day, and later, to once a day. Dogs receiving sulfasalazine should be observed for side effects such as fever, keratoconjunctivitis, and hematologic abnormalities.

Polyarteritis Nodosa

Polyarteritis nodosa (PAN) is a rare polysystemic disease associated with a necrotizing vasculitis of unknown cause. The disease affects predominantly segments and bifurcations of small and medium-sized muscular arteries. In humans, PAN is classified among immune-mediated collagen disorders and derives its name from purpural lesions that are palpable in the subcutaneous tissue. In contrast, palpable nodules are not a regular feature of PAN in animals.[71,72] The vascular lesions consist of intimal proliferation, vessel wall degeneration, necrosis, and thrombosis in all stages of development. PAN leads to a loss of vessel wall integrity, petechial and ecchymotic hemorrhages, focal areas of tissue infarction and necrosis, aneurysm formation, nodular swelling, and thickening of the major arteries. Target tissues of canine PAN include the kidneys, skin, mucous membranes, adrenals, meninges, GI tract, connective tissue, and myocardium.[72] The lungs are usually spared.

The clinical presentation includes systemic signs (pyrexia, lethargy, reluctance to walk, vague pain, or weight loss) and a wide spectrum of organ system abnormalities (linear skin ulceration, ulceration of mucous membranes, nasal discharge, spinal pain, and signs of cardiac or renal failure [or both]).[71,72] Clinicopathologic findings may include leukocytosis with a left shift and proteinuria.

The main differential diagnoses are hypersensitivity angiitis and idiopathic polyarteritis. The diagnosis is confirmed by histologic examination of a skin biopsy specimen, and the prognosis is guarded to poor. Treatment includes glucocorticoids, cyclophosphamide, or both.

Lymphomatoid Granulomatosis and Miscellaneous Vasculitides

Lymphomatoid granulomatoses and other unclassified vasculitides are characterized by a polymorpholymphocytoid, plasmacytoid, and histiocytoid granulomatous infiltration around blood vessels. Pulmonary nodular lesions of variable size due to lymphomatosis were first described in dogs.[73] Infarction, necrosis, and cavitation occur in some of the masses. The bronchial lymph nodes can be slightly to greatly enlarged, and pulmonary thrombosis is common. The cause of this rare condition is unknown. Occasionally, similar lesions are associated with eosinophilic pneumonitis in occult dirofilariasis, although they can also occur outside of endemic areas of dirofilariasis. An immune-mediated cause is likely because, in some cases, large amounts of IgG and IgM can be demonstrated in plasma cells and macrophages.[74] The differential diagnosis is primary or secondary neoplasia, with which this condition is often confused. Diagnosis is rarely made clinically and requires histologic examination of biopsy material. The prognosis is usually poor. In some patients, multicentric lymphosarcoma has developed at a later date. Surgery or treatment with glucocorticoids and cytotoxic immunosuppressive drugs is only temporarily effective.

Arterial Aneurysm

An arterial aneurysm is a circumscribed dilation of an arterial wall or a blood-containing swelling connecting directly with the lumen of an artery. Arterial aneurysms are rare in dogs and cats and only isolated cases have been reported.[75-78] Aneurysms can be categorized based on their shape (saccular or fusiform), cause (atherosclerotic, mycotic, inflammatory, arteritis, traumatic, congenital, dissecting), or their histologic appearance. Two major histologic classes of aneurysms are (1) true aneurysms (aneurysma verum) and (2) false aneurysms (aneurysma spurium).

True Aneurysm

A true aneurysm is a vascular dilatation caused by a weakened arterial or venous wall with subsequent widening of the vascular lumen. Histologically, true aneurysms involve the entire arterial wall and contain three microscopic arterial layers. Aneurysms may result from destruction of the media or the elastic fibers of large arteries (or destruction of both) by inflammatory or degenerative processes. Traumatic aneurysms can be true aneurysms or pseudoaneurysms, depending on their cause and histologic appearance. Aneurysms have been found in the aorta of dogs that were caused by migrating larvae of *Spirocerca sanguinolenta* (formerly *S. lupi*)[76] (Figure 208-8). Aneurysms can also result from turbulent blood flow with arteriovenous (AV) fistulas.

Dissecting aneurysm (aortic dissection) involves a hematoma associated with a defect in the aortic intima. Blood within the aortic lumen is forced through the intimal tear into the outer and middle layers of the aortic media, forming a second or false

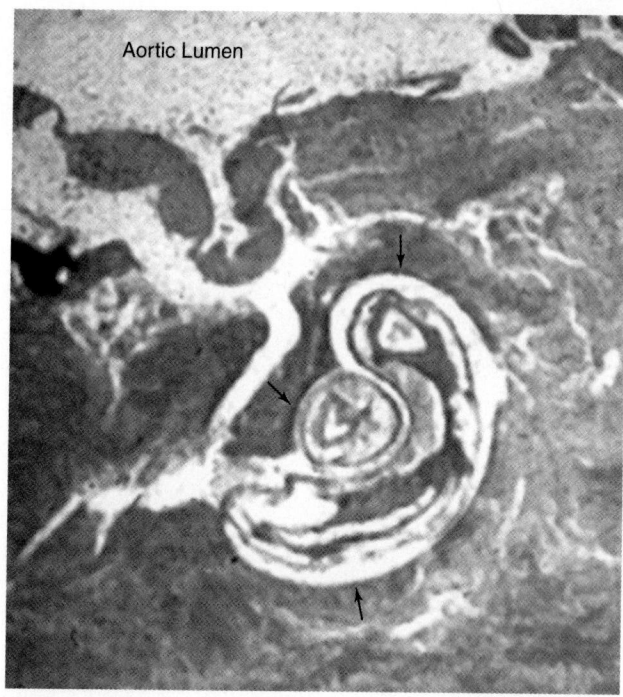

Aortic Lumen

Figure 208-8 Photomicrograph of a canine aorta. The intima and media have been disrupted by the presence of the subtropical and tropical parasite *Spirocerca sanguinolenta* (formerly *S. lupi*). The parasite is seen in cross-section (*arrows*). The aortic lumen is at the top of the figure. (Courtesy of John Bonagura, DVM.)

lumen. The dissection can then propagate proximally or distally along the aorta. A report of a dissecting aortic aneurysm was reported in a dog with clinical and histologic findings similar to that reported in humans.[75] Dissecting aortic aneurysm has also been reported in two cats: one with CHF, severe aortic insufficiency and systemic hypertension and a second cat with signs of weakness, lethargy, and cardiogenic shock.[77,78]

Peripheral aneurysms appear as soft, warm, pulsating bulges. Occasionally, a "machinery" murmur can be auscultated over these areas (see Arteriovenous Fistulas). Clinical signs are frequently absent or vague. If spontaneous vascular rupture occurs, pain, signs of anemia and shock, and pleural or mediastinal effusion may be present. Exsanguination resulting from aneurysmal rupture is possible.

Spurious (Pseudo) Aneurysm

Spurious aneurysms, also known as *pseudoaneurysms*, are caused by localized disruption of the native artery. Their histologic appearance includes arterial wall architecture that is formed by fibrous tissue. One cause of spurious aneurysms is a hematoma that communicates with an arterial lumen resulting from venipuncture.[79] Traumatic spurious aneurysms are probably more common than is usually realized. Clinical signs may include lameness, persistent pain, and deep muscular swelling unresponsive to local therapeutic measures, antibiotics, or glucocorticoids. Pitting peripheral edema may be present, and neither blood nor pus can be aspirated from the swelling. The diagnosis of spurious aneurysms may be suspected from physical examination. Survey radiographs may indicate soft tissue swelling. Diagnostic confirmation has classically relied on arteriography, which illustrates a nodular exudation of contrast medium at the arterial defect. Doppler echocardiography, especially color flow Doppler imaging, aids in identification by depicting blood flow and turbulence. Additional diagnostic tests include computed tomography (CT), radionuclide angiography, and surgical exploration. The differential diagnosis includes chronic infection, obstruction of a deep vein, or abscessation. With a spurious aneurysm, however, pyrexia and neutrophilia are not encountered. The prognosis is favorable if surgical vascular repair can be accomplished.

Arteriosclerosis

Arteriosclerosis is defined as chronic arterial wall remodeling consisting of hardening, loss of elasticity, and luminal narrowing. These changes result from proliferation of connective tissue and hyaline degeneration of media and intima. Proliferation and thickening of the intima with the deposition of ground substances leads to progressive fibrosis and vascular stenosis. Inflammation is not a feature of arteriosclerosis.[80] Arteriosclerotic lesions are commonly detected in old dogs and cats and may comprise part of the normal aging process.[80-82] These changes are typically mild and usually unimportant to health and survival. Thrombosis is rarely a complication of such microscopic lesions, and their functional significance is not known. In other instances, arteriosclerosis may be severe and associated with substantial reduction in intraluminal diameter (often referred to as *small vessel disease*) (Figure 208-9). Lesions of this nature are also common in feline myocardial diseases, particularly hypertrophic cardiomyopathy, and may be detected in canine aortic stenosis as well.[83,84] Arteriosclerotic changes may also occur in aorta and cerebral, renal, spinal, and sinoatrial node artery.[80] Intramural coronary arterial narrowing commonly occurs in association with chronic degenerative valve disease as well. Arterial lesions may have been associated with small regions of myocardial necrosis and fibrosis. Intramural coronary arteriosclerosis was found in 26.4% of old dogs undergoing necropsy.[80] Extensive nonthrombotic, nonatherogenic stenosis of extramural coronary arteries was described in two adult male Labrador retriever dogs with CHF.[85] Disease of extramural arteries is less common. Endothelial aortic plaque formation associated with arteriosclerosis was detected in 77.8% of 58 dogs brought to a small animal clinic in Helsinki for euthanasia.[86] Spontaneous arteriosclerosis, with a predilection for renal vasculature, has been demonstrated in young (<2 years old) greyhounds.[87] The severity of the lesions was correlated with increased renal vascular tortuosity and high shear stress. Clinical consequences of these lesions have not been determined.

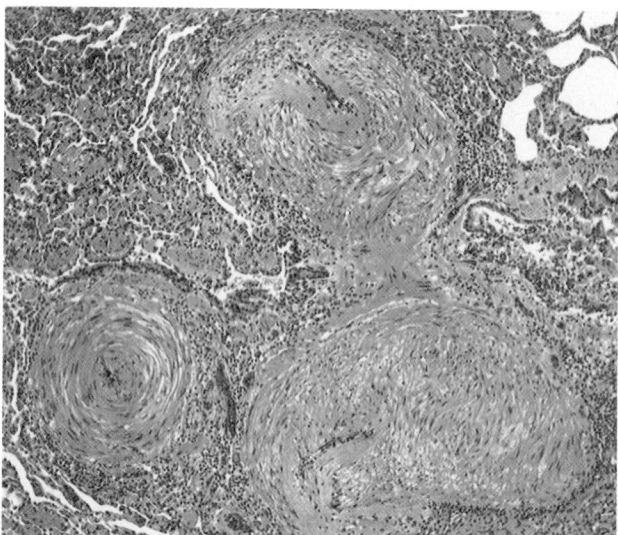

Figure 208-9 Arteriosclerosis in pulmonary arterioles. Severe thickening of the arterial intima and media and dramatic reduction of arteriolar lumen is evident. Inflammatory infiltrates are also diffusely present.

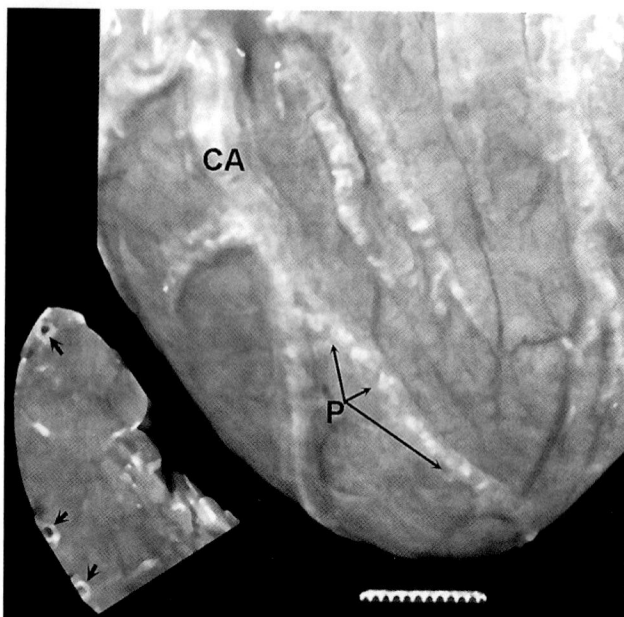

Figure 208-10 Coronary atherosclerosis of extramural coronary arteries in a dog with severe hypercholesterolemia (> 650 mg/dL) caused by hypothyroidism. Epicardial coronary arteries are evident. A larger epicardial branch is labeled *(CA)*. The reader should note numerous light plaques *(P)* within the arteries that represent deposition of lipid. The lower left portion of the figure shows a cut segment of myocardium. The lumina of the subepicardial arteries are also surrounded by a concentric layer of lipid. (Courtesy of John Bonagura, DVM.)

ATHEROSCLEROSIS

Atherosclerosis denotes inner arterial wall thickening in association with lipid deposition. Affected large coronary arteries often appear grossly thickened, yellow-white, and may have narrowed lumina (Figure 208-10). Histologically, deposits of plaque containing cholesterol, lipoid material, focal calcification, and lipophages thicken the inner sections of arterial wall (intima and inner media; Figure 208-11).[88,89] There can be widespread involvement of arteries from many organs. Unlike the disease in humans, canine atherosclerosis is uncommonly associated with extensive plaque formation, arterial calcification, or thrombosis. Atherosclerosis has not been described in cats.

Atheromas are lipoid arterial plaques and they are rare features of canine atherosclerosis. Atheromas are sometimes referred to as *xanthomatosis*. Atherothrombosis results when a localized atheroma forms on an atherosclerotic plaque, resulting in disruption of blood flow and subsequent ischemia, infarction, or both.[88] Atherothrombosis is most severe in both extramural and intramural coronary arteries, carotid arteries, and renal arteries.

Atherosclerosis has been detected in older dogs as a consequence of the hypercholesterolemia and lipidemia associated with thyroid atrophy. A predisposition for spontaneous atherosclerosis was reported in old, obese dogs with atrophied thyroid glands and hypothyroidism.[88] This observation is in accordance with experiments in which atherosclerosis could be induced in thyroidectomized dogs fed large quantities of cholesterol or cholic acids.[90,91] The spontaneous disease mainly affects male and spayed female dogs. An increased prevalence in miniature schnauzers, Doberman pinchers, and Labrador retrievers has been reported.[88] The distribution and

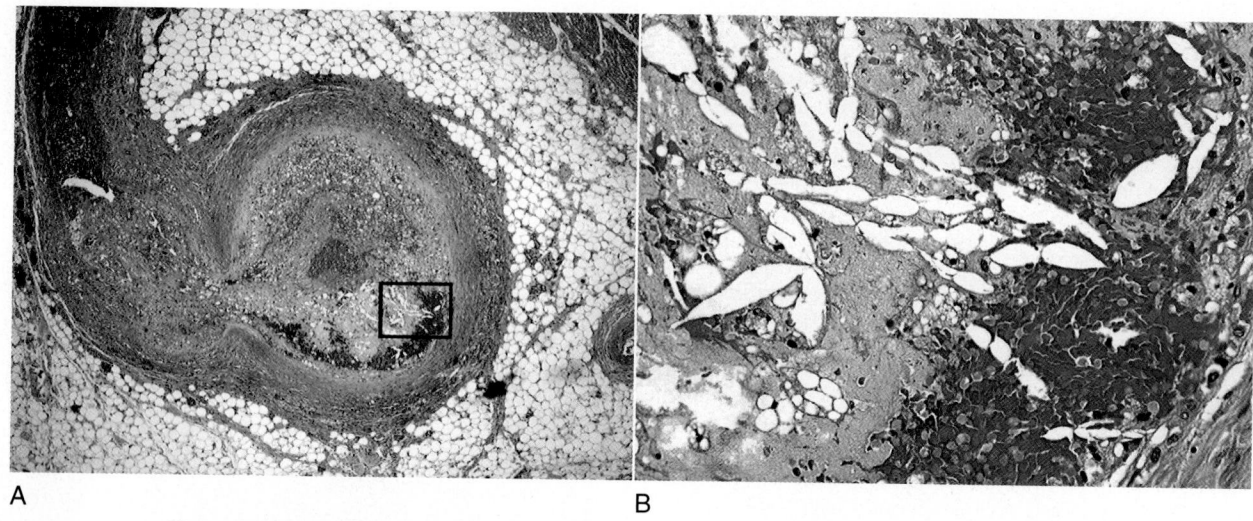

Figure 208-11 Atherosclerosis. **A,** Large coronary artery appears grossly thickened and has a narrowed lumen. The inner sections of arterial wall (intima and inner media) are thickened by deposits of plaque containing cholesterol, lipoid material, focal calcification, and lipophages. **B,** Magnified insert from **A.** Atherosclerotic plaque showing clefts of lipid material (*arrow*).

severity of arterial lesions and thyroid atrophy are typically associated with clinical signs of lethargy, anorexia, weakness, dyspnea, collapse, heart failure, vomiting, disorientation, blindness, circling, and coma.[88,92] Recorded ECG abnormalities included atrial fibrillation, notched QRS complexes, and ST segment elevation. Laboratory abnormalities included hypercholesterolemia, lipidemia, low serum triiodothyronine (T_3) and thyroxine (T_4) concentrations, elevated blood urea nitrogen (BUN) (often associated with renal infarction) and liver enzyme concentrations, and high alpha$_2$ and beta fractions in the protein electrophoresis.

Clinical diagnosis of atherosclerosis is difficult, and the prognosis for dogs with clinical signs related to stenosing atherosclerosis is poor. Potential treatments include thyroid replacement drugs, antihypertensive medication, blood cholesterol–reducing agents, or a low-cholesterol diet. Treatment strategies have not been tested in dogs, and severe lesions are essentially irreversible. Not all dogs with hypothyroidism develop atherosclerosis. Only those with increased levels of very low–density beta lipoproteins tend to be prone to develop atherosclerosis and plaques. Blood levels of low-density lipoproteins may be increased in these dogs because lipoprotein receptors are reduced and lipid removal by the tissues is decreased. The elevated lipoprotein concentrations account for arterial lipoid deposits.[91]

Atherosclerosis is strongly suspected as being an inflammatory disease developing in response to injury in the vessel wall in humans. Infiltration of the mononuclear lymphocytes into the intima, local expansion of vascular smooth muscle cells, and accumulation of extracellular matrix is believed to be the pathogenesis of the inflammation. Previously determined risk factors including hyperlipidemia and hypercholesterolemia are believed to enhance leukocyte adhesion to damaged endothelium and reduce local immune response. The role of inflammation in the development of canine atherosclerosis has yet to be determined.[93]

Arteriovenous Fistulas (Arteriovenous Malformations)

A-V fistula is an abnormal communication between an artery and vein bypassing the capillary network. The true incidence is unknown, although A-V fistulas are reported uncommonly in dogs and rarely in cats. Centrally located anomalies may occur between the cardiac chambers (e.g., ventricular septal defect) or between the great vessels (e.g., aorticopulmonary window, patent ductus arteriosus) and are reviewed in Chapter 200 In this section, only peripheral A-V malformations (A-V fistulas) are discussed.

Congenital A-V fistulas are rare and are caused by arrest or misdirection of embryologic vascular differentiation. The persistence of primitive equipotential capillaries and the subsequent failure of the existing anastomotic embryologic channels to differentiate into arteries or veins are responsible for their abnormal communications. Terminology applied to congenital A-V fistulas has been a source of confusion (e.g., hemangioma racemosum, Park-Weber syndrome, hemangioma cavernosum, strawberry birthmark, nevus angiectasis, cirsoid aneurysm, congenital A-V aneurysm).

The most common cause of an acquired A-V fistula is blunt or penetrating trauma.[94] Iatrogenic trauma is often related to venipuncture and accidental perivascular injection of irritating medicaments.[95] Additional causes include neovascularized tumors (carotid body tumor, thyroid tumor, hemangiosarcoma), ruptured aneurysm, mass ligature of arteries and veins, gunshot wounds, and erosion of contiguous vessel walls by infection or arteriosclerosis. Most A-V fistulas involve the extremities, but they can occur anywhere in the body including the neck, spinal cord, body wall, head, brain, abdomen, liver, and lung. They can also occur as a complication of mass ligation of arteries and veins during closed castration.[96-99]

Irrespective of cause and location, A-V fistulas cause similar altered blood flow dynamics. The basic principle is that blood follows the path of least resistance. The A-V malformation is an abnormal connection between a high-pressure arterial system and a low-pressure venous system with a higher capacity. Due to the difference in resistance, blood flows preferentially through the fistula rather than continuing via the artery to the capillary bed. This shunting results in a reduction of flow in the artery distal to the fistula and increased flow in the venous system. In addition to stealing blood from the distal capillary bed, these changes lead to the development of collateral circulation around the fistula. The communicating shunt increases venous pressure, venous blood oxygen saturation, and the diameter and number of anastomotic arteries and veins. Eventually an ectasia of the feeding artery and aneurysmal sacs in the venous area of the A-V communications may develop. Histologic changes occur in affected vessels so that arteries begin to look more like veins (venification) and veins like arteries (arterialization). The rapid runoff of blood through the A-V fistula into the capacitant venous circulation causes turbulence and, potentially, sound (bruit).[100]

Shunted blood flow through a large fistula can be so great that retrograde flow from a distal artery into the fistula occurs. Arterial blood supply to the tissues distal to the A-V fistula may become compromised from competition with the fistula and secondary venous hypertension, resulting in stagnation of venous blood flow in the dilated veins, or even reversal of blood flow in a distal rather than proximal direction. Local edema and ischemia followed by tissue necrosis, ulceration, or organ dysfunction may ensue. In large and mostly centrally located fistulas, the central blood dynamics also become affected. Large flow volumes across the A-V fistula compromise the blood supply to other regions of the body by shifting blood into the capacitance venous circulation. Compensatory responses to increased blood volume (cardiac preload) include elevated heart rate, cardiac contractility, and eccentric cardiac hypertrophy. Augmented cardiac output and gradual expansion of the blood volume partially restore the blood supply to deprived tissues. Eventually, however, the increased venous return and the elevated cardiac workload may induce high-output heart failure.[101]

Clinical history and signs vary according to the location, size, duration, etiopathology, and topography of the fistula. A-V fistulas of the extremities may appear as painless, easily compressible, warm bulges or varicosities (Figure 208-12). Sometimes they are detected incidentally during routine clinical examination. With medium-sized or large fistulas of the extremities, a continuous palpable thrill and pulsation, along with a machinery murmur, can be detected. The leg or region distal to the fistula may be swollen, warmer, or colder than the proximal area (sometimes with severe local ischemia), painful, and affected by pitting edema. Lameness, cyanosis, therapy-resistant toe ulcers, scab formation, or gangrene can occasionally occur distal to the fistula with severe local ischemia. In the dilated superficial veins, a faint pulsation may be felt. In the feeding arteries a *water-hammer* pulse is often present. Animals with high-output heart failure may develop a cardiac murmur of mitral regurgitation and moist lung sounds, indicating pulmonary edema.

When firm pressure is applied proximal to the A-V fistula, or if the feeding artery is compressed, the thrill and bruit disappear and the pulse, and heart rate may drop as a result of diminished venous return and reduced cardiac output. This is referred to as *Branham's bradycardia sign*, and the maneuver is called *Branham's* or *Nicoladoni-Branham's test*. Together with the local thrill or fremitus and the bruit, the Branham's sign is pathognomonic for A-V fistulas.

Other signs have been reported and vary with respect to location and hemodynamic alterations caused by the A-V fistula. An A-V fistula in the orbit was reported to cause exophthalmos.[102] Recurrent bleeding from the mouth was observed in an A-V fistula of the tongue.[98] Restless behavior and lethargy followed by progressive seizures and hemiparesis were reported in a 10-year-old mixed breed dog with a subcortical cerebral A-V malformation.[103] An A-V fistula of the spinal cord at the thoracolumbar junction in a 10-month-old female Australian shepherd dog caused a deteriorating hindlimb ataxia, difficulty in getting up and down, hypersensitivity over the lumbosacral region, and urinary incontinence.[104] Cardiomegaly and pulmonary overcirculation were detected radiographically in a dog with a postsurgical AV fistula, and these changes regressed after the fistula was surgically closed.[97] An A-V fistula was found surgically in the jejunum of an 8-month-old dog with persistent anemia and melena.[105] A-V fistulas in tumors have been recognized as a strong pulsation and fremitus detectable during palpation of the tumor mass.[94] Auscultation of the tumor mass may reveal a machinery-type murmur or bruit.

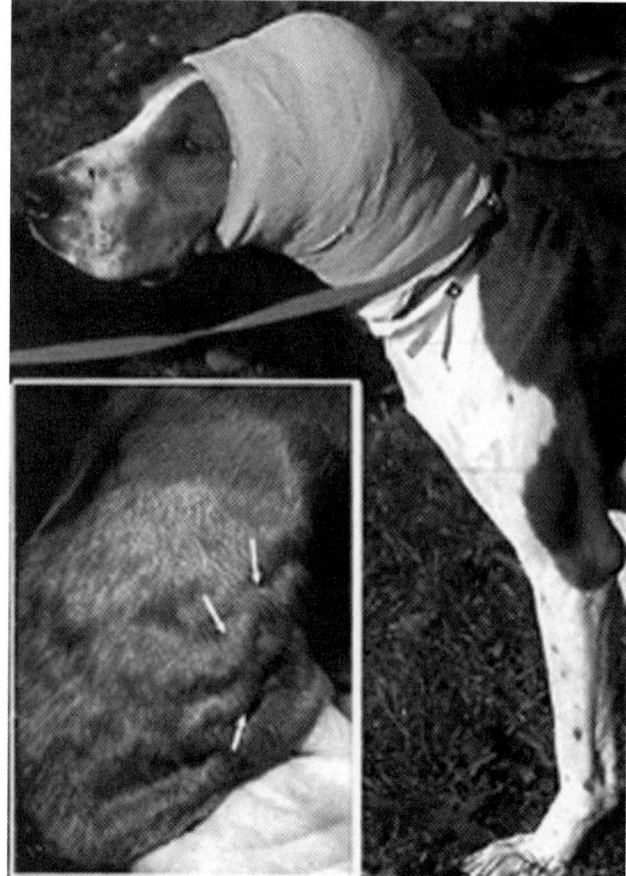

Figure 208-12 Coon dog with an arteriovenous (A-V) fistula of the ear. The dog was presented for severe bleeding caused by trauma to large distended veins *(inset, arrows)*. A continuous murmur was ausculted over the ear, and Doppler studies demonstrated continuous arterial-to-venous flow. Venous distention is secondary to direct transmission of arterial pressure and marked increases to flow. (Courtesy of S.E. Johnson, DVM, and J. Bonagura, DVM.)

Congenital hepatic A-V fistulas have been reported in young dogs. The hepatic artery connects to the portal vein and causes portal hypertension or reversal of the blood flow in the portal vein.[106,107] There can be a single fistula or multiple fistulas that can be distinctly visualized by abdominal color Doppler ultrasonography and coeliac arteriography.[108] Clinical signs include lethargy, vomiting, diarrhea, anorexia, weight loss, ascites, polyuria, and neurologic signs related to hepatic encephalopathy.[109]

Pulmonary A-V fistulas can lead to respiratory distress and cyanosis. Survey thoracic radiographs of animals with large fistulas may indicate cardiomegaly, a prominent aortic arch, a hypervascular lung field, and an increased interstitial or patchy pulmonary radiodensity, indicating pulmonary congestion or edema, respectively.

Diagnostic ultrasonography, especially color Doppler imaging, has been clinically useful for identifying and localizing A-V fistulas (Figure 208-13).[108,110,111] Findings included the presence of focal intra-arterial flow at the fistula site throughout the cardiac cycle, turbulent pulsatile venous flow at the fistula site, and nonpulsatile venous flow proximal to the fistula. Angiography may be used to define fistula anatomy and size more accurately and to plan management strategies. The absence of a normal capillary phase and premature outlining of the veins are typical arteriographic findings in shunting

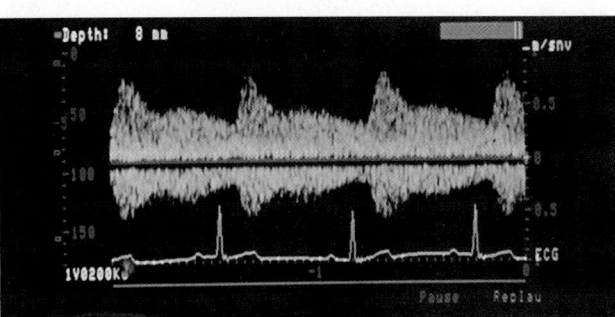

A

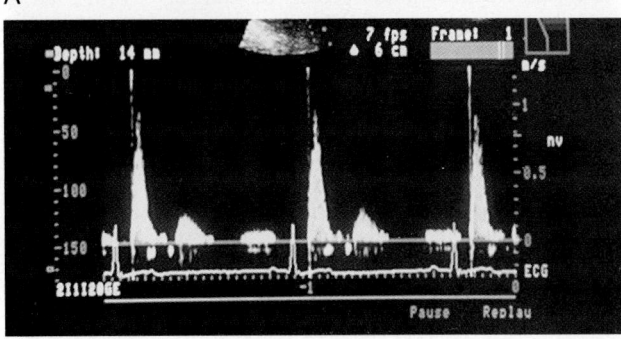

B

Figure 208-13 Pulsed wave (PW) Doppler recordings from a 5-year-old female golden retriever dog with traumatic A-V fistula. **A,** Doppler interrogation of a large, pulsatile, dilated vessel associated with the right radial artery identified by color flow Doppler at the medial right brachium. The reader should note the continuous flow best seen during diastole. **B,** Pulsed wave (PW) Doppler flows recorded from the normal left radial artery in the same dog.

lesions. The differential diagnoses of A-V fistulas include neoplasms, varices, abscesses, cystic skin lesions, aneurysms, lymphedema, and scarring.

Management of A-V fistulas has historically required surgical intervention.[112] This usually involves careful ligation of all proximal and distal arteries feeding the fistula, ligation of the draining veins, and complete excision of the A-V collaterals with the venous aneurysmal sacs (so called quadruple ligation). If relapse occurs or if multiple fistulas are present, a wide excision of the involved areas or limb amputation may be the only alternative.

Surgical approaches can often be technically difficult, mutilating, hazardous, and can have a high failure rate with residual clinical symptoms.[113] Consequently, arterial embolization techniques using special embolization wire coils have begun to be used to occlude A-V fistulas, owing to the minimally invasive nature of these procedures.[113,114] In a cat with a forelimb fistula, cyanoacrylate embolization was used to obliterate the fistula followed by en bloc surgical resection of vessels.[115] Transcatheter embolization using vaso-occlusive coils was described in three cats and two dogs with peripheral A-V fistulas.[116]

The prognosis for animals with small A-V fistulas is often good. Morbidity is highest with centrally located A-V fistulas, with fistulas that cause organ dysfunction, with large fistulas that induce a high cardiac output, and with fistulas that cannot be successfully occluded using embolization techniques.

Traumatic and Functional Arterial Disease

Trauma from direct accidental injury or iatrogenic trauma (e.g., surgery or vascular interventional procedures) is a common cause of vascular disease. Direct trauma may result in direct vascular wounds, or it can result in mural contusions leading to delayed thrombosis, necrosis, late hemorrhage, and false aneurysm formation. Vascular wounds can also occur

from fractures because adjacent vessels are relatively fixed and vulnerable. Clinical features of traumatic arterial injuries may include diminished or absent pulse, enlarging hematoma, pulsatile arterial bleeding, symptoms of ischemia distal to the wound, injury of anatomically related nerves, and hypotension with major hemorrhage. Compressive forces from local tissue trauma (compartment syndrome) and vascular stenosis may delay or inhibit return to normal function of the affected area. Accurate diagnosis and extent of traumatic vascular injuries can be accomplished by direct examination, arteriography, ultrasound, and magnetic resonance imaging (MRI).[117]

Vasospasm refers to reversible localized or diffuse vasoconstriction of arteries or small blood vessels. If short lived, the ischemia is reversible and permanent damage does not result. However, prolonged vasospasm with ischemia may lead to tissue damage and ulceration. Vasospasm is a common response to blunt and perforating vascular trauma and may also result from perivascular injection of irritating substances. When this occurs, tissue injury and vasospasm can be minimized by local infiltration with procaine hydrochloride or lidocaine. Uncommonly, vasospasm occurs in association with spontaneous arterial rupture (e.g., ruptured cerebral aneurysm, stroke). Angiography is usually required for confirmation. Vasospasm may be elicited by exotoxins. The best-known example is ergotism that produces intense vasospasm of the digits and large vessels by stimulation of the alpha-adrenoceptor. The differential diagnosis of vasospasm includes polycythemia, cold agglutinins, thrombosis, arteriosclerosis, and vasculitis.

Diseases of Veins

Diseases of the venous system frequently cause minor clinical problems, despite the fact that veins are commonly affected by or involved in trauma, TE, edema, local inflammation, and septic processes. Many conditions, however, often go unrecognized. Venous disorders include traumatic injuries, superficial and deep phlebitis and thrombosis (thrombophlebitis), catheter embolization, aneurysms, venous compression syndromes, varices, and ulcers.

Pulmonary thromboembolism (PTE) is a common and often life-threatening complication associated with a variety of systemic and metabolic diseases. A thrombus formed in the right heart or the peripheral or central venous system can embolize to the pulmonary arterial vasculature. Contributing factors include prolonged immobilization, trauma, surgery, and a range of disorders including IMHA, hyperadrenocorticism, nephrotic syndrome, DIC, sepsis, cardiac disease, amyloidosis, neoplasia, proteins C and S deficiency, and antithrombin III deficiency. PTE is covered in detail in Chapter 218.[21,26]

Varicosis and ulceration are rare in dogs and cats. When detected, they often accompany A-V fistulas. Cutaneous phlebectasia is a benign lesion sometimes erroneously called *telangiectasis*. It is reported almost exclusively in dogs with spontaneous or iatrogenic Cushing's syndrome.[118] Phlebectasia is an abnormal dilatation, extension, or reduplication of veins or capillaries or a combination of these changes.

Venous perforation or *blunt trauma* to veins is usually well tolerated because rapid clotting results in venous occlusion. If when venous occlusion or venous severance is severe, however, resultant edema and cyanosis are usually temporary because of collateral circulation. If all veins draining an area are compromised, marked edema and necrosis can ensue. Blunt trauma has been associated with caudal vena caval obstruction or kinking of the intrathoracic caudal vena cava and ascites.[119]

Venous malformations have been previously referred to as *cavernous hemangiomas*. They can be localized or extensive and appear as cystic dilation of blood vessels. They generally permit only low blood flow, and small lesions are generally asymptomatic. Expansion of the lesion may occur, however, especially after trauma. Thrombosis may occur due to sluggish blood flow,

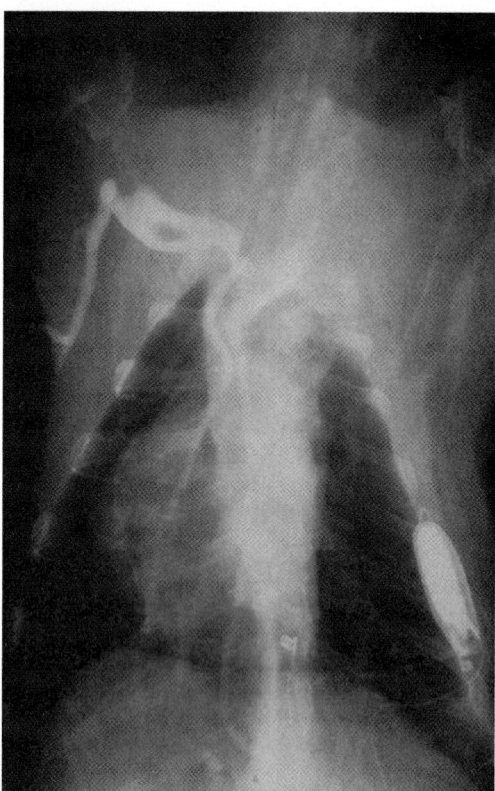

Figure 208-14 Angiogram of a dog with a cranial vena caval thrombus. The animal developed lymphedema of the neck, face, and front legs 1 week after a transvenous pacemaker lead had been inserted through the jugular vein to facilitate temporary cardiac pacing for complete heart block. Contrast medium was injected into an accessory cephalic vein with the animal positioned in sternal recumbency. Extensive collateral circulation is seen, but filling of the cranial vena cava is not identified. An epicardial electrode is visible in the cardiac apex, and the pulse generator can be seen subcutaneously in the left lateral thorax. (Courtesy of Nancy Morris, DVM.)

resulting in local swelling and tenderness. Larger lesions in dependent areas may enlarge, causing significant vascular dilation. This may result in changes in skin color, ulceration, and hemorrhage. The affected area appears as a warm, soft, compressible mass. No thrills or bruits are present due to the low flow. Pain may result from pressure exerted on deep tissues and nerves.

Diagnosis is made using history, physical examination, and ultrasound. Venography may be needed to define the lesion. Symptomatic therapy using light, compressive wraps is sometimes helpful for acute management. Surgical excision of affected vessels is occasionally required, but complete resection is difficult and local recurrence is common.[120]

Thrombosis commonly follows blunt trauma and perforating injuries, particularly with venipuncture or prolonged venous catheterization (Figure 208-14). Phlebitis is a major cause of intimal damage leading to thrombosis. The thrombosis is usually of little local consequence. However, emboli may be carried to the lung and cause PTE. In most animals, blood clots carried to the lung are rapidly lysed and cause no problems. However, when inflammatory diseases, dehydration, or circulatory failure occurs, clot formation may continue in the pulmonary vessels and lead to vascular occlusion, severe dyspnea, pain, and death.[21] In infectious thrombophlebitis, bacterial emboli may be carried to the lungs and cause thromboembolic pneumonia. Spontaneous venous thrombosis

is rare, although portal vein thrombosis has been reported. Clinical signs include ascites, peripheral pitting edema, and portosystemic shunting.[121]

Embolization of severed intravascular catheter fragments is an occasional complication of intravenous catheter placement.[122,123] In humans, reported complications of catheter embolization include perforation of cardiac walls, endocarditis, pulmonary embolism, and severe arrhythmias. Therefore it is generally considered prudent to remove catheter fragments. Nonsurgical, transvenous removal of catheter fragments using loop-snare catheters, forceps, and basket catheters have been described. Whenever possible, however, steps should be taken to avoid situations predisposing to catheter fragmentation, including inadequate restraint during catheter placement, withdrawal of catheters through their placement needles during repositioning, failure to properly secure catheter to the patient, and inadvertent severing of catheters during bandage changes.

Phlebitis can occur from a local inflammatory process extending to the veins or can originate from a venous intimal lesion. Common causes of venous intimal lesions are perivenous injection of irritating drugs, infusion of large amounts of fluid, and long-term placement of intravenous catheters. Infusion-related phlebitis occurs in three forms: (1) chemical (injury to vein by irritating drugs), (2) physical (trauma to the intima by catheters, needles, hypertonicity, or particulate matter in infused fluids), and (3) microbial (infected fluids, skin, or catheter tip). Sterile or septic thrombophlebitis may result, usually remains localized, and is characterized by pain, swelling, and exudation (Figure 208-15). Patients with serious illnesses or compromised immune systems, however, may develop sepsis, thromboembolic pneumonia, or endocarditis.

In cases of venous occlusion, clinical signs depend on the anatomic location, extent, and duration of the obstruction. Acute obstruction of centrally located and deep veins causes edema, cyanosis, discomfort, and venous dilatation distal to the obstruction site. Obstruction of the cranial vena cava causes edema in the neck, head, front limbs, and dependent portions of the chest wall (Figure 208-16). Pleural effusion commonly results from central venous obstruction. Clinical disorders of the intrathoracic caudal vena cava have been reported (Figure 208-17).[119] Obstructions of the renal or pelvic area cause edema of the hindlimbs and the scrotum. Clinical signs depend upon collateral vessel reserve and capacity of regional lymphatics. In addition to thrombosis, common causes of venous obstruction include invasive malignant processes and venous compression by abscesses, hematomas, tumors, and lymphadenopathy. A number of tumors have a tendency for venous invasion, including chemodectomas, adrenal tumors, and hemangiosarcomas. Angiography may indicate the occlusive or compressive lesion or highlight increased collateral circulation (or it may do both) (Figure 208-18). Diagnostic ultrasonography can often detect masses or flow disturbances.

The prognosis and therapy of venous obstruction depend on the primary disease. These are discussed in various chapters throughout this book.

Diseases of the Peripheral Lymphatics

The lymphatic system plays a critical role in regulating body fluid volume and immune function. Lymphatics originate within the interstitium as specialized endothelial-lined capillaries transporting fluid, solutes, and macromolecular particles back into the venous system. Fluid, protein, cells, and macromolecular particles from the interstitial space empty into the initial lymphatics composed of a series of small lymphatic capillaries that begin blindly in the tissues. The lymph then flows through a system of lymphatic vessels that progressively increase in diameter. As lymph flows centrally it passes through at least one lymph node before emptying into larger

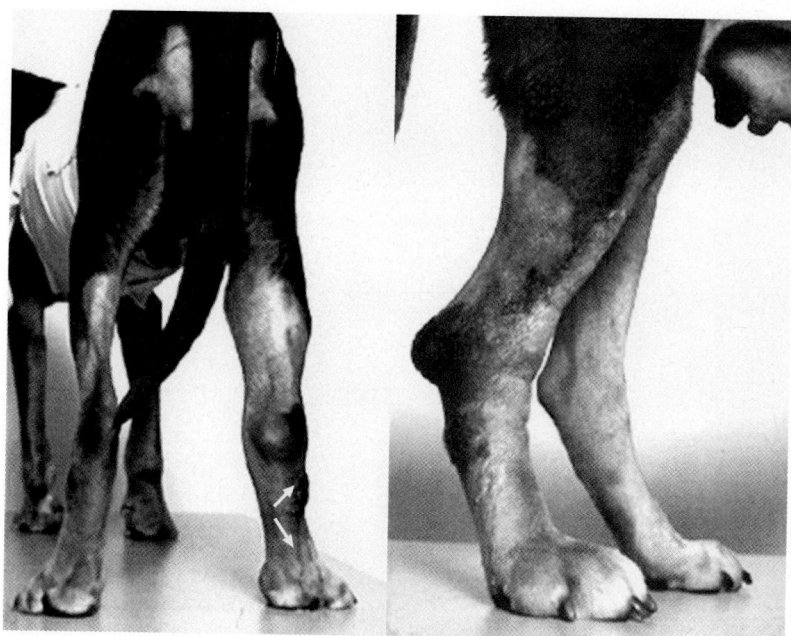

Figure 208-15 Caudal (left) and lateral (right) views of the right rear limb of a young dog with severe edema caused by thrombophlebitis. The problem developed after placement of saphenous vein catheter. The limb is markedly swollen and edema fluid *(arrows)* is leaking through a small ulcer in the skin. Thrombosis of the vein prevents venous drainage and increases lymphatic fluid formation. (Courtesy of John Bonagura, DVM.)

lymphatic trunks.[124] The deep trunks unite to form two major lymphatic vessels: (1) the thoracic and (2) right lymphatic duct. The thoracic duct drains most of the body and returns fluid into the venous system at the brachycephalic vein or the left subclavian vein. The right lymphatic duct drains the right side of the head and neck and right forelimb.

Lymphatic vessels contain many junctions between individual endothelial cells that are connected to the surrounding extracellular matrix by reticular fibres and collagen. These junctions open when tissue hydrostatic pressure becomes elevated and the anchoring filaments stretch, allowing fluid to move into the vessel. As the fluid is cleared from the interstitium, the connecting fibers contract and the junctions between the endothelial cells close. The opening and closing of these junctions allow them to act as inlet valves, preventing the backflow of lymph into the interstitium. The larger vessels of the lymphatic system have progressively fewer open junctions, increasingly muscular walls, and frequent intralymphatic valves that also prevent backflow of lymph. The action

of external muscular contraction along with intrinsic contractility of the lymphatic vessels aid in the movement of lymph through the lymphatic system. Lymph is filtered by at least one lymph node before entering the venous circulation. While in the lymph node, the lymph is in contact with the blood circulation and approximately half of the fluid is drained before leaving into the larger lymphatic ducts.[124]

In addition to its transport function, the lymph system plays a major role in the immunologic responses to infectious agents. It serves as a filtering system to impede the spread of microorganisms and neoplastic cells. The cellular components, in particular the lymphocytes, are indispensable for immunologic reactions and antibody formation.[125]

Lymphatic disorders can be subdivided into those of internal organs, such as intestinal lymphangiectasis, and peripheral lymphatic disorders. Several lymphatic diseases have been recognized in animals, including lymphedema, intestinal lymphangiectasia, chylothorax, lymphadenitis, lymphocysts, lymphoma, lymphangioma, and lymphangiosarcoma. Types and causes of peripheral lymphatic disorders are summarized in Box 208-2.

Inflammatory Lymphatic Disorders (Lymphangitis and Lymphadenitis) Lymphangitis and lymphadenitis often occur secondary to local inflammation, particularly involving the skin, mucous membranes, and subcutaneous tissues. Lymphangitis can also result from bacterial or fungal infection or adjacent neoplastic and inflammatory disease. Lymphatics may be affected and occluded as they drain inflammatory agents and their by-products from tissue spaces. In lymph nodes, microorganisms are phagocytized and inactivated or killed by humoral and cellular mechanisms. During this process, lymph nodes may become obstructed, enlarged, warm, and painful. Affected limbs may be locally swollen, and lameness can result. Pyrexia, anorexia, and depression are common, and leukocytosis may be present with acute, severe lymphangitis.

Lymphangitis may become chronic when associated with a granulomatous or static lesion, such as a foreign body, or with unsuccessfully treated acute inflammation. Persistence of inflammatory edema results in mesenchymal cell proliferation, which in turn can cause irreversible thickening of skin and subcutis.

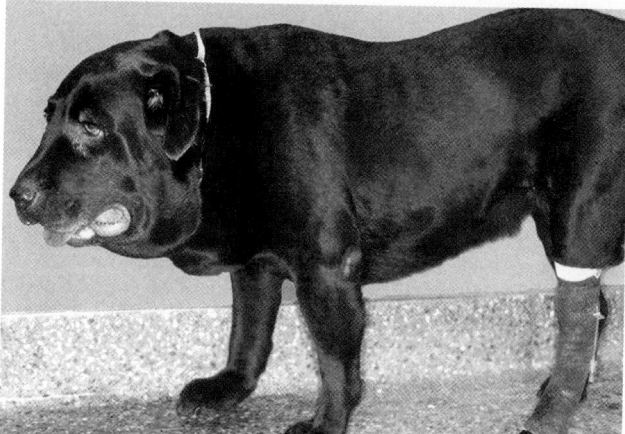

Figure 208-16 Cranial vena cava syndrome associated with a mediastinal mass and cranial vena caval occlusion. Severe peripheral edema of cranial extremities is present.

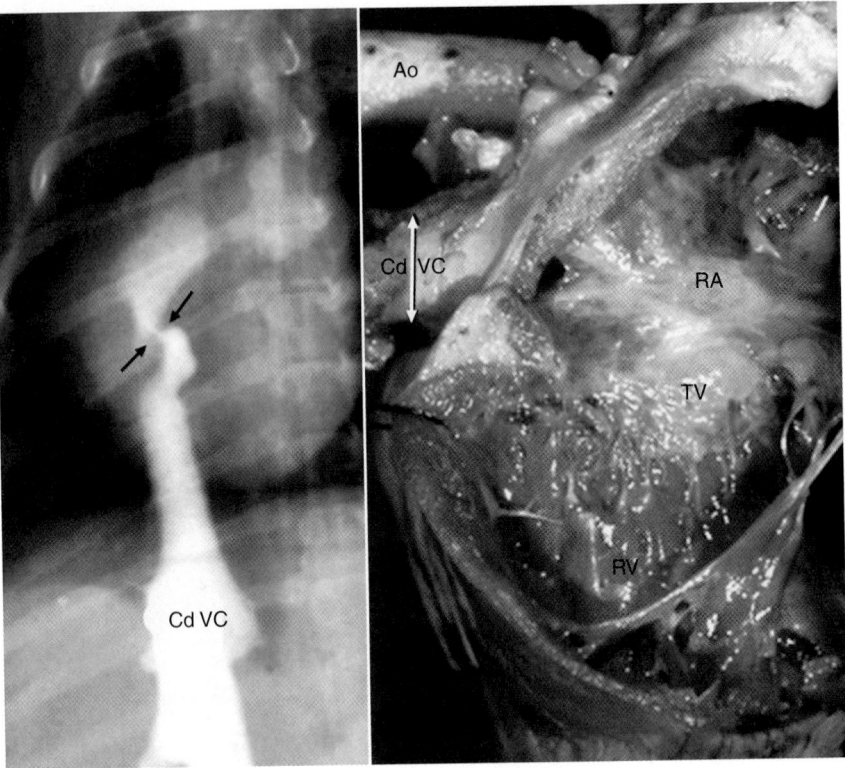

Figure 208-17 Acquired stenosis (fibrosis) of the caudal vena cava in an older dog. The left panel shows an angiogram of the caudal vena cava (*Cd VC*), which demonstrates a severe narrowing of the dye column *(arrows)* at the venous entry into the caudal right atrium. The right panel is a postmortem view of the heart taken from the right lateral perspective. The right atrial and ventricular walls have been retracted to demonstrate the stenotic, caval orifice *(small arrows)*. The reader should compare this opening with the diameter of the caudal vena cava *(to the left, large vertical arrow)*. The right ventricle (*RV*), tricuspid valve (*TV*), right atrium (*RA*), and descending aorta (*Ao*) are shown. (Courtesy of John Bonagura, DVM, and Matthew W. Miller, DVM.)

The prognosis is favorable with early treatment. Therapy consists of moist, warm, local compresses or soaks, which reduce swelling and promote drainage. Aggressive local and systemic antibiotic therapy usually promotes recovery in animals with fever and anorexia. Bacterial culture and sensitivity testing should be performed if acute lymphangitis fails to respond to treatment and in cases of chronic lymphangitis.

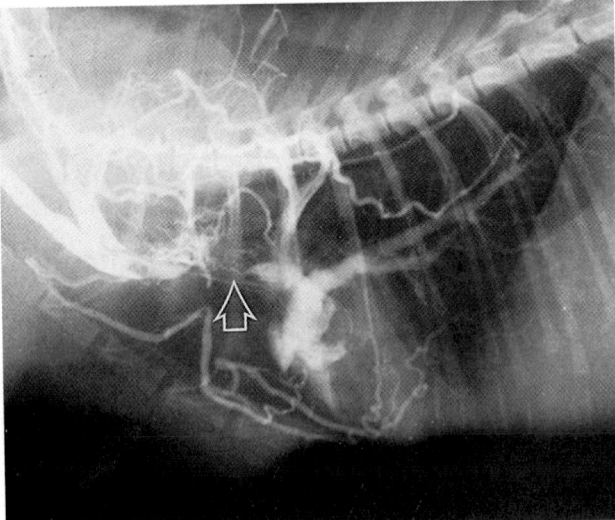

Figure 208-18 Angiogram of a 10-year-old domestic short-haired cat with pleural effusion and edema of the head and neck. Radiocontrast dye was injected into the external jugular vein. Interruption of venous return occurs in the cranial vena cava *(arrow)* caused by compression and obstruction of this vessel by a mediastinal tumor. The reader should note the prominent collateral venous network.

Contrast studies and surgical exploration may be indicated if fistulous tracts or abscesses are present or if a foreign body is suspected.

Lymphedema *Lymphedema* refers to an accumulation of fluid in the interstitial space resulting from abnormal lymphatic drainage.[124] This term should not be used for other forms of edema, such as circulatory edema related to venous obstruction or generalized edema related to hypoproteinemia. Lymphedema may result when capillary filtration exceeds the resorptive capacity of the veins and lymphatics. The protein rich fluid (2 to 5 g/dL) causes a high osmotic gradient and exacerbates fluid accumulation.[125] Numerous classification schemes have been used to categorize lymphedema. Commonly used causative categories of lymphedema include: overload, inadequate collection into lymphatic capillaries, abnormal lymphatic contractility, insufficient lymphatics, lymph node obstruction, and main lymphatic ductal defects.

Traditionally, clinical effort is undertaken to differentiate primary versus secondary lymphedema. *Primary lymphedema* refers to an abnormality of the lymphatic vessels or lymph nodes. *Secondary lymphedema* refers to disease in the lymphatic vessels or lymph nodes due to a different disease process. Secondary lymphedema can occur as a result of neoplasia, surgery, trauma, parasites, radiation therapy, or infection and is more common than primary lymphedema. Distinguishing between primary and secondary lymphedema is often difficult. A disease process involving a lymph node can result in fibrosis and obstruction with secondary lymphedema developing.

Primary lymphedema Primary lymphedema can result from three principle morphologic and functional abnormalities including (1) abnormalities of large vessels including aplasia or hypoplasia of the thoracic duct and cisterna chyli, (2) aplasia of the peripheral lymphatics or congenital valvular incompetence, and (3) lymph node fibrosis or a deficient lymph node size and number.[126]

Lymphedema caused by aplasia, hypoplasia, or dysplasia of proximal lymph channels or popliteal lymph nodes (or dysplasia of both) occurs most often in the hindlimbs of young dogs (Figures 208-19 and 208-20). The edema can be transient, observed only during the juvenile period, or permanent. Mild cases are restricted to the hindlimbs, whereas severe cases may progress to whole body edema.[127-130] Although the condition is frequently bilateral, one limb is often more swollen than the other. A number of cases of suspected congenital lymphedema have been reported.[129-132] Reported breeds include bulldogs, poodles, Old English sheepdogs, and Labrador retrievers, although it is not clear whether these breeds are at increased risk.

The history may identify chronic limb swelling since birth or edema appearing later in life. The swelling represents a pitting edema of varying magnitude that is neither too warm nor cold. The edema is not usually accompanied by lameness or pain unless massive enlargement or cellulitis occurs. Growth and activity are usually normal, but rest and limb massage do not typically reduce the severity of edema. Total plasma protein, serum protein electrophoresis, hemogram, and blood chemistry are generally unremarkable. The diagnosis of primary lymphedema is based on history (age of onset, disease progression, affected limbs, and distribution of edema), and clinical signs. Previous surgery, trauma, or infections should also be noted. Radiographic lymphography may be needed to confirm the diagnosis in subtle cases and is helpful in determining morphology of anomalous lymphatic systems (see Figure 208-20).

The prognosis for resolution of congenital lymphedema is guarded and depends on the cause. Occasionally, dogs that develop hindlimb edema during the neonatal period may improve spontaneously. More frequently, dogs with severe edema of the limbs and trunk succumb during the first few weeks after birth.[127] Chronic lymphatic vessel dilation leads

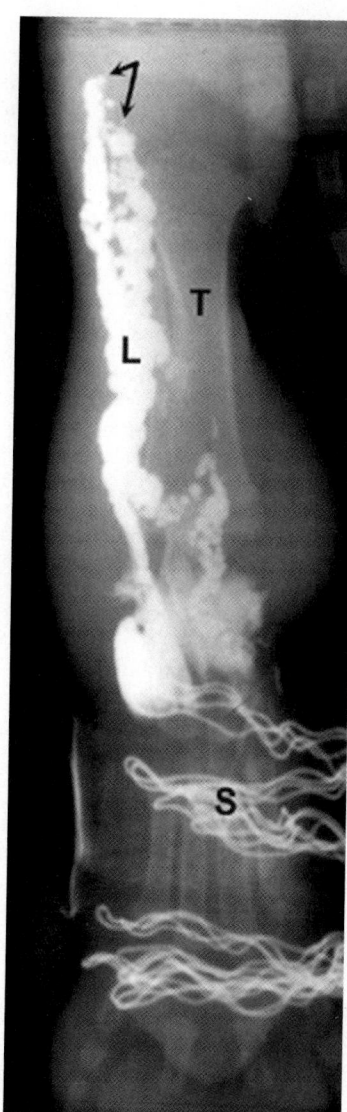

Figure 208-20 Lymphangiogram of a young dog with lymphatic dysplasia. After cannulation of a distal lymphatic vessel, contrast medium was infused into the lymphatic system. The reader should note the dilated, tortuous, lymphatic channels *(L)* that end blindly at the stifle *(arrows). T,* Ttibia; *S,* radiopaque surgical sponges. (Courtesy of C. Wendy Myer, DVM, and John Bonagura, DVM.)

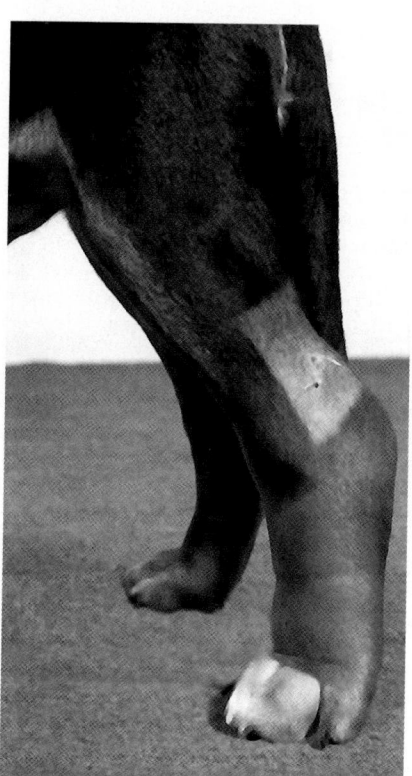

Figure 208-19 Marked, nonpainful edema of the left rear limb in a young dog with congenital lymphatic dysplasia. (Courtesy of John Bonagura, DVM.)

to loss of contractility and permanent lymphatic valvular dysfunction. Metabolic by-products accumulate and lead to collagen deposition and fibrosis. Complications such as abrasions and infection often develop. Dogs with primary lymphedema should not be used for breeding. Test matings of dogs with congenital lymphedema support the hypothesis of autosomal dominant inheritance with variable expression.

Secondary lymphedema Persistent lymphedema occurs only after destruction or blockage of a considerable number of major lymph channels (or several sequential lymph nodes with their afferent or efferent lymphatics).[125] Factors that can delay or prevent edema formation include opening of collateral vessels, rerouting of lymph flow through peripheral lymphaticovenous anastomoses and perilymphatic routes of lymph drainage, and increased venous fluid uptake. Secondary lymphedema is often related to a combination of lymphatic and venous obstruction. Inhibited venous return increases lymphatic flow by altering Starling's forces toward increased tissue fluid accumulation. This overloads the lymphatic capillaries and results in the accumulation of fluid in the interstitial space.[133] Distal lymphatics may become more distended, causing loss of valvular competency, stagnation of lymph flow, mural insufficiency, and further accumulation of proteinaceous fluid in subcutaneous tissues. Other common causes include posttraumatic or postsurgical interruption of lymphatics or lymph node excision and blockage of lymph nodes and lymph vessels by compression or invasive neoplasms. Lymphedema resulting from local neoplasia is usually a sign of a widely disseminated and highly invasive malignant process. Several causes of secondary lymphedema have been summarized in Table 208-2.

Clinical signs associated with secondary lymphedema vary depending on the underlying systemic causes. Lymphedema may be localized to the periphery of an extremity (Figure 208-21) or extend proximally to the subcutaneous tissues.[134] The location and severity of obstruction determine the extent of edema formation. For example, sublumbar or intrapelvic obstruction induces bilateral hindlimb edema and edema of the thighs and external genitalia. Mediastinal masses and thrombosis of the cranial vena cava induce bilateral edema of the front limbs and tissue of the ventral thorax, neck, and head. The clinician must palpate all lymph nodes carefully for enlargement and pain. With bilateral hindlimb edema, it is important to perform rectal or abdominal palpation to assess sublumbar lymph nodes. The prostate and anal region or mammary glands and vaginal area should be carefully inspected for neoplasms, which can lead to obstructive intrapelvic processes. Intrapelvic masses should be suspected in all dogs with hindlimb edema and vague signs of sublumbar pain, discomfort during ambulation, or difficulties with defecation or urination. Depending on the type and extent

of underlying systemic illness, limb edema may be the only detectable abnormality or may be accompanied by fever, anorexia, and weight loss. Clinicopathologic findings depend on the underlying primary disorder.[135]

Diagnosis is based largely on history and clinical examination and is facilitated by diagnostic imaging. Survey radiographs should be taken of suspicious areas, which often include the pelvis or cranial thorax. In a substantial number of cases, soft tissue masses or destructive bony lesions can be detected. Abdominal ultrasonography can provide information about soft tissue masses and readily identifies enlarged lymph nodes and other structures. Lymphography or other imaging techniques may be indicated if the diagnosis remains unclear. Lymphography is often relied upon for definitive diagnosis of lymphatic disorders. In some cases the lymphatics are hypoplastic throughout their course. When aplastic, lymphatics suitable for cannulation and injection of radiocontrast agent may not be found. Failure to outline a lymph node after lymphography is not absolute proof of its absence.[127] Lymphographic features of primary lymphedema include lymph node aplasia and small lymphatics that end blindly or anastomose into collateral vessels around (instead of into) lymph nodes where they would be normally found.

Lymphoscintigraphy is an alternative approach for imaging peripheral lymphatics. This technique requires a gamma-camera system and intradermal injection of high molecular weight–radiolabeled colloids.[136-137] Such equipment and specialized training are not widely available. When compared with conventional lymphography, lymph nodes only appear as hot spots, preventing adequate assessment of nodal structure.

Differential diagnoses for dogs with edema confined to one limb include inflammation, trauma, vascular obstruction, hemorrhage, cellulitis, phlebitis, and A-V fistula. Diagnostic considerations for dogs with edema involving both forelimbs include thrombosis or compression or invasion of the cranial cava by a mediastinal mass. With the latter, edema usually involves the head and neck regions and the limbs. Causes of only bilateral hindlimb edema include obstruction of sublumbar lymph nodes by neoplastic infiltration. If all four limbs are involved, the differential diagnoses should include hypoproteinemia, CHF, renal failure, or portal hypertension. The close association of lymphatic and venous structures can make it difficult to distinguish between lymphatic and venous obstruction, and both can occur at the same time. Ulceration, dermatitis, cyanosis, weeping varices, and fat necrosis are signs of venous obstruction rather than lymph stasis.

Therapy is usually unrewarding. In the early stages of lymphedema, medical management is directed to maintaining the patient's comfort and reducing swelling. Infectious disorders require long-term antimicrobial therapy. Some neoplastic conditions may benefit from chemotherapy or radiation therapy. Long-term heavy bandage application (e.g., Robert Jones splint) may encourage lymphatic flow and reduce subcutaneous lymph accumulation. Local topical skin care and intermittent antibiotic therapy are helpful in reducing cellulitis. With the exception of isolated instances, pharmacologic therapies are generally unrewarding. The benzopyrones (e.g., rutin) are a group of drugs that have been advocated to reduce high-protein lymphedema by stimulating macrophages, promoting proteolysis, and enhancing absorption of protein fragments.[138] Long-term diuretic administration may be contraindicated, because after reduction of interstitial fluid, proteins in the residual interstitial space proteins may promote tissue injury.[135] Surgical options may include (1) procedures to facilitate lymph drainage from affected limbs (lymphangioplasty, bridging procedures, shunts, omental transposition), and (2) procedures to excise abnormal tissue. Surgical excision of the subcutaneous edematous tissue should be staged to decrease devascularization.[135] Short-term administration of

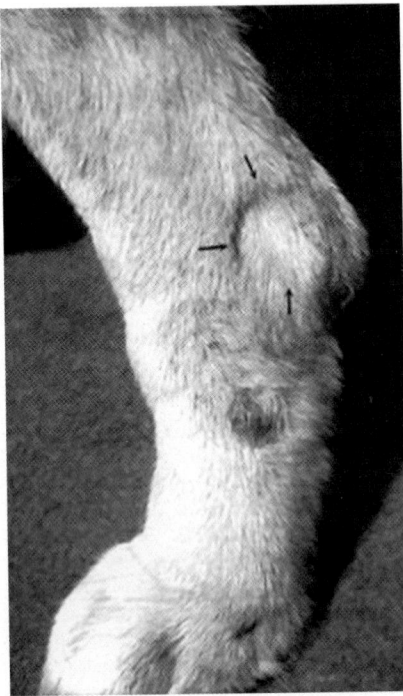

Figure 208-21 Pitting edema in a dog with a caudal lumbar mass. The edema was caused by either obstruction of venous return in the rear limbs or obstruction of lymphatic drainage. Tissue fluid was deformed by light digital pressure, resulting in a visible subcutaneous pit in the rear limb (*arrows*). (Courtesy of John Bongura, DVM.)

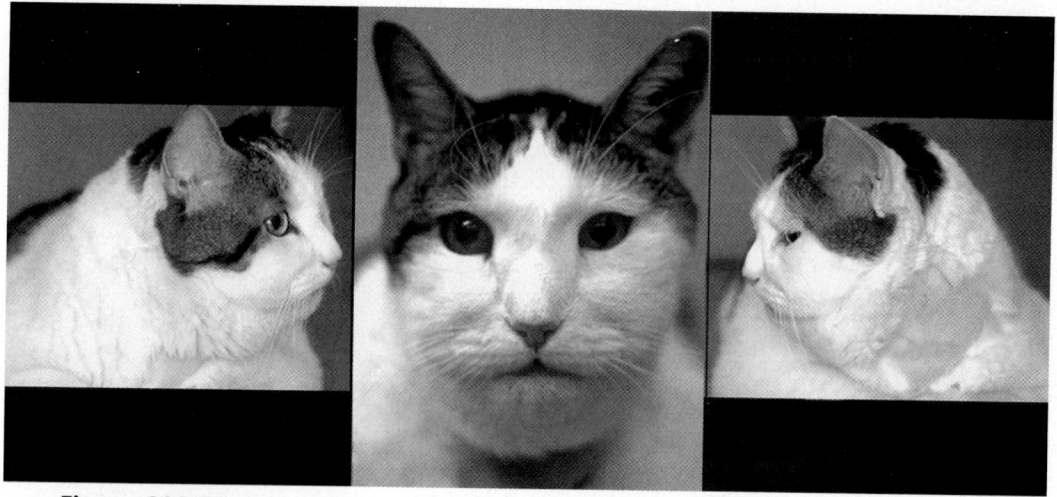

Figure 208-22 Cat with peripheral edema secondary to lymphatic obstruction by lymphangiosarcoma.

anti-inflammatory agents or diuretics, bandaging, and physical therapy may be helpful in cases of traumatic and postsurgical induced lymphedemas.

LYMPHANGIOMA, LYMPHANGIOSARCOMA

Lymphangiomas are benign tumors of lymphatic capillaries and are thought to develop when primitive lymphatic sacs fail to establish venous communication.[139] Lymphangiomas can be classified into three categories based on their histologic appearance: (1) capillary lymphangiomas comprised of a network of capillary-sized lymphatic channels, (2) cavernous lymphangiomas composed of dilated lymphatics that infiltrate the surrounding tissue, and (3) cystic hygromas (unilocular or multilocular, cystic masses lined by a single layer of endothelium supported by a connective tissue stroma and containing a straw-colored, proteinaceous [1.3 to 4.5 gm/dL] fluid).[140] The lesions present as large, fluctuant masses in the subcutaneous, fascial, mediastinal, and retroperitoneal spaces.[141] Lymphangiomas have also been diagnosed on the extremities, metacarpal pads, nasopharynx, axilla, inguinal and mammary region, retroperitoneal space, and skin of dogs.[139,142,143] Clinical signs are related to the size, location, and extent of the lymphangioma. They can exert pressure on surrounding structures and may interfere with muscle function, breathing (compression of the trachea), urination, or intestinal function. Lymph may ooze to the skin surface through single or multiple fistulous tracts. Differential diagnoses include other space-occupying masses such as abscesses, enlarged lymph nodes, neoplasms, and congenital cysts of nonlymphogenic origin. The prognosis can be good after appropriate surgical excision, marsupialization, or

radiation therapy.[144] Risk of recurrence is high due to inherent inability to identify distinct boundaries.

Lymphangiosarcoma originates from lymphatic endothelial cells (Figure 208-22).[145] It is a rare malignant tumor in dogs and cats, although it is frequently reported secondary to chronic lymphedema in humans.[146,147] A breed or sex predisposition has not been detected, but medium to large breeds may be at highest risk, and both young and older animals are affected.[145,148] Metastasis occurs commonly in dogs and cats, although an isolated case without metastasis has been reported.[145,149] Clinical signs include pitting edema of the extremities, inguinal region, axilla, and head and neck (see Figure 208-22). In a report of 12 cats with lymphangiosarcoma, nine presented with fast-growing, noncircumscribed subcutaneous masses and the others with a thoracic or abdominal mass. In all cats affected the tumor was invasive, and complete surgical resection was not possible.[149] Associated chylous effusions (pleural, abdominal, subcutaneous) have been reported.[150-153] Pulmonary lymphangiosarcoma was diagnosed in one dog with a chylous effusion.[153] Diagnosis is confirmed by obtaining a biopsy specimen. Histologically, tumors of lymphatic endothelial origin are characterized by a neoplastic proliferation of endothelial cells. Immunocytochemical stains have been used to confirm the diagnosis in dogs. The identification of the factor VIII–related antigen and vimentin indicates the cells are of endothelial origin. The intensity and distribution of the stain has been used to attempt to differentiate lymphangiosarcomas from hemangiosarcomas but is often inaccurate. Newer specific markers to identify lymphatic endothelial cells have been identified in humans and remain to be validated in the canine patient.[153] The prognosis with lymphangiosarcoma is poor, with a high rate of local recurrence and metastasis.

Diseases of the Ears, Nose, and Throat

CHAPTER 209

Diseases of the Ear

MaryAnn G. Radlinsky
Diane E. Mason

GENERAL CONCEPTS

Many different disease processes affect otic health and should be considered when evaluating a dog or cat with possible ear disease. Signalment may implicate certain diseases over others. A complete history begins with general questions about the animal's health (e.g., appetite, sneezing, coughing, vomiting, diarrhea, water consumption) and questions pertaining to primary conditions associated with ear disease. Because the ear is a specialized extension of the integumentary system, a complete dermatologic history should be obtained (i.e., appearance of lesions at the onset of the condition; duration, progression, presence of pain or pruritus; past medical therapy and response to therapy; the presence of other dermatologic problems). A complete physical examination should be performed with special attention paid to the skin to evaluate for hypersensitivities, disorders of keratinization, endocrine disorders, and other dermatologic conditions. A complete neurologic examination may reveal abnormalities associated with the middle ear (e.g., abnormalities of cranial nerves VII and VIII, Horner's syndrome, keratoconjunctivitis sicca, head tilt). Involvement of the inner ear results in other neurologic signs (e.g., head tilt, ataxia, strabismus, abnormal nystagmus), and differentiation from central vestibular disease is extremely important.

Specific examination of the ear includes evaluation of the concave and convex pinnal surfaces, palpation of the ear canals, and otoscopic examination. The ear may need to be cleaned before a thorough examination can be completed. Sedation or anesthesia is occasionally necessary to perform a complete otic exam. This is especially true with chronic conditions of the ear. Abnormalities of the otic exam include pain on palpation of the auricular cartilages, nonpliable cartilage, ossified cartilage, epithelial hyperemia, swelling, erosion, ulceration, exudate accumulation, and hyperemia or lack of transparency of the tympanic membrane. Pain upon opening the mouth is not specific to, but can occur with, ear disease. Other diagnostic tests should include cytologic examination of otic exudate and culture and susceptibility testing based on the cytology and clinical signs of the patient. Skull radiographs, computed tomography (CT), and magnetic resonance imaging (MRI) may be indicated for evaluation of the middle and inner ear. Specific diagnostic tests are available to evaluate tympanic membrane integrity, and one should not assume that the tympanic membrane is intact prior to initiation of medical therapy, including ear cleaning, which may cause immediate exposure of the middle ear to ototoxic substances.

DISEASES OF THE PINNA

Many different disease conditions can affect the pinna—some are specific to the pinna and others represent distribution of part of a systemic condition (Table 209-1). Following are specific diseases that primarily affect the pinnae (or affect the pinnae as an early manifestation of the disease).

NONPRURITIC PINNAL ALOPECIA

Canine Pinnal Alopecia

Canine pinnal alopecia is most commonly diagnosed in dachshunds but also occurs in Chihuahuas, Boston terriers, whippets, Yorkshire terriers, and Italian greyhounds.[1,2] The condition usually occurs in dogs over 1 year of age and results in slowly progressive, bilateral pinnal alopecia. Small vellus hairs remain, and complete pinnal alopecia, when it occurs, may not be present until 8 to 9 years of age. The pinnae may become chronically hyperpigmented and thickened. The remainder of the haircoat is usually normal. The condition is benign and requires no specific treatment. Differentiation from other alopecic conditions is by exclusion and histopathologic examination. Miniaturized hair follicles are typically seen on histopathology. Minoxidil, pentoxifylline, melatonin, and milbolerone have anecdotally been reported to induce hair growth in some cases.[2]

Pattern Baldness

Symmetrical alopecia or hypotrichosis of the pinnae, ventrum, and caudal or medial thigh has been recognized in the dachshund and Staffordshire bull terrier.[3] Hair loss begins with the pinnae at 6 to 9 months of age and may progress to complete pinnal alopecia. Total body alopecia with pigmentation may occur with age. Treatment with oral melatonin may cause hair regrowth with this and other pattern baldness syndromes.[2]

Periodic Alopecia of Miniature Poodles and Siamese Cats

Hair loss is usually adult-onset and acute with periodic alopecia of miniature poodles and Siamese cats. Progression of the condition may result in complete, bilateral, pinnal alopecia; however, in cats the alopecia may be patchy or complete.[1,2] The skin appears grossly normal. The pathophysiology of the condition is not known, no treatment has been described, and the hair may regrow over a period of several months.

Congenital Hypotrichosis

A lack of pelage or loss of hair within the first month after birth has been diagnosed in the Belgian shepherd, cocker spaniel, toy poodle, miniature poodle, whippet, German shepherd, Yorkshire terrier, bichon frise, Lhasa apso, Labrador retriever, rottweiler, and basset hound. The condition is seen more commonly in males and usually involves the pinna, temporal region, caudal dorsum, and ventrum. Complete hair loss may occur by 12 to 14 weeks of age. Areas of alopecia may be well delineated from normal skin, and the condition can be diagnosed by finding a marked decrease in the density of hair follicles on skin biopsy of the affected area.[2] A similar condition exists in Birman, Burmese, Devon Rex, and Siamese cats but involves the entire coat, whiskers, claws, and tongue. No treatment exists for this condition; it is heritable, and the client should be discouraged from breeding the animal.[2]

Table • 209-1

Disease Conditions Affecting the Pinna

Nonpruritic Alopecia
Canine

Periodic alopecia of miniature poodles	Color dilution alopecia	Pattern baldness
Pinnal alopecia of short-coated breeds	Alopecia areata	Demodicosis
Idiopathic follicular dysplasia	Congenital alopecia	Drug eruption
Congenital hypotrichosis	Dermatophytosis	Hypothyroidism
Estrogen-responsive dermatosis	Ectodermal defects	

Feline

Idiopathic pinnal alopecia	Dermatophytosis	Demodicosis
Iatrogenic hypothyroidism	Congenital hypotrichosis	Alopecia areata
Iatrogenic hyperadrenocorticism	Hyperthyroidism	

Crusting and Scaling Dermatoses
Canine

Fly strike dermatitis	Frostbite	Sarcoptic mange
Proliferative thrombovascular necrosis	Demodicosis	Harvest mites
Zinc-responsive dermatosis	Pemphigus complex	Vasculitis
Idiopathic hyperkeratosis of Boston terriers	Ear margin dermatosis	Sebaceous adenitis
Idiopathic lymphocytic/plasmacytic dermatitis	Lupoid dermatosis	Ear fissures
Idiopathic lichenoid keratosis	Superficial necrolytic dermatitis	Hypothyroidism
Lichenoid psoriaform dermatosis	Dermatomyositis	Pediculosis
Cold agglutinin disease	Systemic lupus erythematosus (SLE)	Leishmania

Feline

Squamous cell carcinoma	Actinic dermatitis	Notoedric mange
Insect bite hypersensitivity	Frostbite	Vasculitis
Pemphigus complex		

Papular and Nodular Dermatoses
Canine and feline

Leoproid granuloma (canine)	Neoplasia	Bacterial pyoderma
Sterile nodular histiocytic granuloma (canine)	Deep mycoses	Leishmania
Eosinophilic folliculitis, furunculosis (canine)	Foreign body	Dermatophytosis
Eosinophilic granuloma (canine)	Tick infestation	Xanthoma (feline)

Pustular, Vesicular, and Bullous Dermatoses
Canine and feline

Pemphigus foliaceus	Pemphigus erythematosus	SLE
Epidermolysis bullosa	Drug eruption	Contact or irritant dermatitis

Concave Pinnal Disorders
Canine and feline

Atopy	Allergic contact dermatitis	Hypothyroidism
Sex hormone aberrations	Seborrhea	Juvenile cellulitis
Food sensitivity	Idiopathic erythema/edema (canine)	

Auricular Cartilage Disorders
Canine and Feline

Aural hematoma	Auricular chondritis

CRUSTING AND SCALING DERMATOSES

Scabies and Mange

Erythematous, papular dermatitis of the distal pinnae associated with significant pruritus is an early manifestation of *Sarcoptes scabiei* in dogs. Crust and scale will usually first affect the tip of the pinna or ear margin. The pinnal-pedal reflex (i.e., rubbing the pinna resulting in a pelvic limb scratch reflex) is often associated with sarcoptic mange but is not pathognomonic for the condition. Concurrent lesions often involve the lateral hocks and elbows and may spread to the rest of the body. The diagnosis is usually made with skin scrapings; however, multiple scrapings may be necessary to achieve the diagnosis.[3] The presence of a single mite, egg, or fecal droppings is diagnostic for the disease. All animals in the household should be treated, and the condition is zoonotic, so owners and handlers should be made aware of the condition. Initial treatment consists of removal of crusts and debris, followed by an acaracidal dip such as lime sulfur, permethrin, organophosphate, or amitraz, which may shorten time to resolution of clinical signs and diminish zoonotic potential. Ivermectin administered subcutaneously, twice at 14-day intervals, or orally three times at 7-day intervals, results in cure. A similar dose schedule exists for milbemcyin. Topical application of selamectin or fipronil may also be curative.[1,2]

Feline mange, caused by *Notoedres cati*, results in alopecia, pruritus, excoriations, and thick crusts of the rostral pinnae and is usually restricted to the ears and head. The extremities and perineum may also be affected due to the sleeping and grooming habits of cats. The parasite may also inhabit dogs, foxes, and rabbits; transient lesions have been reported in humans.[2] The diagnosis is made with skin scrapings, and lime sulfur or amitraz dips are effective treatments. Ivermectin given two or three times subcutaneously is also effective.[2]

Fly Strike Dermatitis

Insect bite dermatitis, primarily caused by the stable fly, *Stomoxys calcitrans*, results in serosanguineous, crusting dermatitis on the ear tips in dogs with erect ears or on the folded edge of the pinna in dogs with pendulous ears. Chronic fly strike dermatitis can become granulomatous in nature. Horse flies (Tabanus species) and deer flies (Chrysops species) may also plague dogs that are housed outdoors, but their bites are usually less reactive than stable flies. The diagnosis is based on an environmental history and response to limiting outdoor exposure. Fly repellents containing permethrin, citronella, or diethyltoluamide (DEET) in petroleum jelly may be used to diminish repeated fly bites. Topical corticosteroid with an antibiotic may hasten the resolution of clinical signs.[1,2] Black flies (Simulium species) may also cause papular dermatitis and alopecia in dogs.

Cats can develop a seasonal hypersensitivity to mosquito bites. Papules, erythema, alopecia, and hypopigmentation occur on the pinnae and face. Pyrexia, lymphadenopathy, and footpad lesions may also occur.

Actinic Dermatitis and Squamous Cell Carcinoma

Damage to the skin by long-term sun exposure occurs most often in white cats, although the condition is also reported in dogs and in cats with pigmented skin. The pinna is most often affected due to its sparse hair covering; the nose, lips, and eyelids may be similarly affected. Waxing and waning ear tip erythema may progress to the development of fine scale and alopecia early in the disease. Erosive, crusted, hemorrhagic lesions and folding of the pinna occur as a precancerous condition, which may ultimately lead to carcinomatous change.[1,2,4] Squamous cell carcinoma is most often diagnosed in older cats (mean age, 12.8 years) with either skin scrapings or biopsy.[5]

Treatment of actinic dermatitis ideally consists of limiting sun exposure between the hours of 10 AM and 4 PM by housing indoors and eliminating sunbathing behavior. Application of sunscreen of SPF 15 or greater may also decrease the effects of solar radiation. β-carotene and canthaxanthin administered orally and the use of retinoic acids (i.e., isotretinoin, etretinate) have also been reported.[1,2] An initial response to therapy may be seen, but long-term effectiveness has not been thoroughly investigated.[6] Strontium plesiotherapy has been used in the treatment of actinic dermatitis. Failure to respond to medical management is an indication for pinnectomy.

Squamous cell carcinoma is usually locally invasive and slow to metastasize to either local lymph nodes or the lung. Pinnectomy is an effective mode of therapy for severe actinic dermatitis and squamous cell carcinoma. Cryosurgery, radiotherapy, brachytherapy, hyperthermic, and photodynamic therapy have also been used on focal lesions; systemic chemotherapy is not considered effective.

Frostbite

Animals affected by frostbite are usually systemically ill or have recently moved to a cold environment. The ear tips are pale, cyanotic, hypoesthetic, and cool to the touch after exposure. With warming, the tissues become hyperemic and develop scale, crust, and alopecia. The ear tips may curl, necrose, and eventually slough. Initial treatment consists of rewarming with warm water and subsequent symptomatic therapy for scaling and crusting dermatitis. Amputation of necrotic tissue results in improved cosmesis with haired skin and decreases the risk of recurrent freezing, which is more likely in previously frostbitten tissue.

Vasculitis

The underlying cause of vasculitis is often unknown, but the condition occurs subsequent to Type I and Type III hypersensitivity reactions and the deposition of antigen and antibody complex within the vascular wall.[2] The lesions are characterized by erythema, edema, and eventual necrosis and sloughing, leading to a "punched out" or ulcerated appearance to the pinnae. Other affected areas include the lips, tail, pads, and nails. A neutrophilic, eosinophilic, or lymphocytic vasculitis may be evident on histopathology. Proliferative thrombovascular necrosis of the pinnae is a form of vasculitis reported in dogs. Inflammatory vasculitis is not evident in this syndrome and cause is unknown. Conditions such as rickettsial disease, drug eruption, immune-mediated disease, and other underlying systemic conditions should be ruled out. Therapy should be directed at treating the underlying cause. Idiopathic vasculitis cases may respond to immunosuppressive doses of corticosteroids. Other reported treatments include pentoxyphylline, sulfasalazine, or dapsone.[1] Surgical excision of the affected portion of the pinna with wide surgical margins may be indicated if medical management is unsuccessful.[2]

Hyperkeratosis

Crusting and scaling of the pinnae may be caused by idiopathic defects in keratinization, primary disease conditions causing seborrhea, and secondary changes in keratinization due to parasitism. Ear margin dermatosis is common in dachshunds and other breeds with pendulous ears. Seborrheic changes begin at the ear margin and progress to confluence of scale and significant alopecia. Pruritus is variable but may be present in severe cases. The condition is not curable but controllable with keratolytic keratoplastic shampoos (e.g., sulfur-asalicylic acid, benzoyl peroxide or benzoyl peroxide-sulfur, selenium sulfide).[2] Severe cases may require topical or systemic corticosteroid treatment due to inflammation associated with removal of crusts or ear fissure formation.

Sebaceous adenitis is associated with an inflammatory process of the sebaceous glands. Follicular disruption, alopecia, and surface scale initially affect the pinna and may involve the ear canal and trunk.[7] No direct therapy exists for lost sebaceous glands, and supportive care with fatty acids, humectants, and anti-inflammatory corticosteroids can be useful. Retinoids have been used in cases with a granulomatous response to the process.[2]

Other less common disorders can cause hyperkeratosis of the pinna. Idiopathic benign lichenoid keratosis has been diagnosed in four dogs with multiple wartlike papules and hyperkeratotic plaques on the pinnae.[3] Lichenoid psoriaform dermatosis is a rare condition in which erythematous papules and lichenoid plaques appear on the concave surface of the pinna, external ear canal, and ventral head and trunk. Treatment consists of antimicrobial shampoo, systemic antibiotics, and corticosteroids.[2]

Lupoid dermatosis is a heritable condition of German short-haired pointers in which progressive, nonpruritic scale occurs on the pinnae, face, and trunk. No therapy is available for the condition.

Nutritional Dermatoses
Zinc deficiency caused by dietary insufficiency or inability to absorb dietary zinc results in crusting lesions of the pinna, and perioral, periorbital, perianal, and perivulvar sites of dogs. Food allergy can result in steroid-resistant alopecia, crust, scale, hyperpigmentation, and lichenification of the pinnae. Dietary restriction followed by feeding trials is diagnostic of the condition, which may be associated with lesions and pruritus on other parts of the body.

DERMATOSES CAUSING PAPULES AND NODULES

Tick Infestation
The following ticks may cause local irritation and secondary granuloma formation of the pinna in dogs: American dog tick (*Dermacentor variabilis*), lone star tick (*Amblyomma americanum*), brown dog tick (*Rhipicephalus sanguineus*), and Ixodes species.[3] Of these ticks, Ixodes spp. is least likely to be identified on the pinna or head. Treatment should be aimed at insect removal and prevention of reinfestation.

Neoplastic Lesions
Auricular tumors are more common and more often malignant in cats than dogs. Commonly diagnosed canine pinnal tumors include squamous cell carcinoma, cutaneous histiocytoma, mast cell tumor, sebaceous adenoma, and papilloma. Squamous cell carcinoma, mast cell tumor, basal cell tumor, and fibrosarcoma are commonly diagnosed in cats.

Granulomatous Lesions
Pinnal granulomas may be associated with bacterial infection (Staphylococcus species, *Nocardia*, *Actinomyces*, mycobacteria, atypical mycobacteria), dermatophytosis, deep mycoses, algae, *Leishmania*, and foreign bodies. Canine leproid granuloma occurs in short haired dogs primarily in cool, moist environments. Two millimeter to 5 cm nodules have been described with superficial alopecia and ulceration occurring on the dorsal pinna and head. Although acid-fast bacilli have been identified on histopathologic examination, cultures are usually negative. Lesions usually resolve spontaneously or respond to surgical excision.[8]

DERMATOSES CAUSING PUSTULES, VESICLES, AND BULLAE

Autoimmune disorders commonly affect the concave aspect of the pinnae. Lesions are usually symmetrical; vesicles, erosions, and blisters may appear on the pinna prior to the occurrence of generalized disease. Pemphigus complex, systemic lupus erythematosus (SLE), bullous pemphigoid, and epidermolysis bullosa[9] have been associated with pinnal lesions. The diagnosis may be made with cytology and skin biopsy. Differential diagnoses include bacterial infection, drug eruption, and contact hypersensitivity.[2]

CONCAVE PINNAL DERMATOSES

Atopy
Erythema and hyperplasia of the pinna and upper external ear canal are early signs of atopy. Hyperpigmentation, lichenification, and erythematous ceruminous otitis may result if the condition is allowed to progress.

Allergic Contact Dermatitis
Allergic contact dermatitis is a rare condition described in middle-aged animals due to the long period of induction required for development of delayed hypersensitivity to the offending substance. The condition is often diagnosed secondary to topical medication used to treat otitis externa and may result in pinnal alopecia.

Defects in Keratinization
Systemic conditions such as hypothyroidism, sex hormone aberrations, and seborrhea may affect the concave surface of the pinna. Grease accumulation and hyperkeratotic dermatosis may result.

Juvenile Cellulitis
Juvenile sterile granulomatous dermatitis and lymphadenitis is a rarely diagnosed condition; predisposed breeds include the golden retriever, dachshund, Labrador retriever, and Lhasa apso. Dogs are usually less than 6 months of age when they develop significant mandibular and prescapular lymphadenopathy and edema, exudate, papules, and pustules of the pinna, muzzle, and periocular skin.[1] The diagnosis is based on clinical presentation, culture and susceptibility testing, and skin biopsy. Treatment consists of immunosuppression with corticosteroids, which are tapered over 3 to 4 weeks after remission of clinical signs. Systemic antimicrobial therapy is indicated for the treatment of secondary bacterial pyoderma.

AURICULAR CARTILAGE DISORDERS

Aural Hematoma
Aural hematomas occur in both dogs and cats secondary to the self-induced trauma of head shaking or scratching. Blood accumulates within the fractured cartilage of the pinna, although swelling is most visible on the concave aspect. Any animal diagnosed with an aural hematoma should undergo a complete evaluation and treatment for otitis externa, because continued head shaking will predispose the animal to enlargement or recurrence of the hematoma. Small hematomas may resolve without therapy; however, second-intention healing may cause deformation of the pinna with a poor cosmetic result. Treatment of the hematoma may consist of corticosteroid injection, evacuation and bandaging, teat cannula drainage, Penrose drain placement, or closed suction drainage.[10] Surgical incision, drainage, curettage, and closure with mattress sutures is preferred because it provides apposition of the cartilage edges and cosmetic results. Sutures remain in place for 21 days to allow adequate cartilage healing. Treatment of the concurrent otitis externa and its underlying cause are vital to the prevention of recurrence.

Auricular Chondritis
Auricular chondritis (*relapsing polychondritis* in cats) is an inflammation and destruction of auricular cartilage usually classified as an immune-mediated disorder. The pinnae are bilaterally swollen and deformed in most cases, although unilateral involvement is possible. Diagnosis is based on biopsy findings of lymphoplasmacytic inflammation with cartilage necrosis, and treatment may be minimal if no significant systemic signs exist. Attempted treatment with immunosuppressive doses of corticosteroids was not successful in cats; dapsone therapy may induce remission.[2]

DISEASES OF THE EXTERNAL EAR CANAL: OTITIS EXTERNA

Normal Anatomy and Physiology
The external ear canal collects and delivers sound to the tympanic membrane. The ear canal is composed of auricular and

annular cartilages that roughly approximate with the vertical and horizontal portions of the canal. The normal dog has a 45-degree angle of the horizontal canal; the angle is approximately 90 degrees in cats. Stratified squamous epithelium with sebaceous glands, ceruminous or apocrine glands, and hair follicles line the canal. Sebaceous glands located in the superficial dermis secrete neutral lipids that assist in maintenance of keratinization, in capturing and removing debris, and in decreasing the humidity of the ear canal. Acid mucopolysaccharides and phospholipids are the main secretions of ceruminous glands located deeper in the dermis. The glandular secretions help to maintain proper humidity and pH in the ear canal, and a normal flora of bacteria and yeast have been identified in the external ear canal of normal dogs and cats.[11] Removal of debris from the deeper portion of the ear canal is achieved in many ways. The ratio of apocrine to sebaceous glands decreases from proximal to distal in the ear canal, resulting in more aqueous cerumen deeper in the canal, and the number of glands and hair follicles also decrease deep in the ear canal. The tympanic membrane is composed of three layers, with epithelial cells migrating away from the center of the tympanum, which aids in the removal of debris and secretions from its surface.

Diagnostic Principles

Physical Examination Complete examination of the pet with otitis includes general physical, dermatologic, otoscopic, and neurologic examinations. An otoscopic examination should be performed slowly and deliberately with dorsal and lateral traction on the pinna, keeping the otoscope centrally located in the canal to avoid placing pressure on the epithelium. Hyperemia, erosions, ulcers, exudate, foreign bodies, stenosis, and masses should be noted. The tympanum should be thin, pale, gray, and translucent, with a visible manubrium of the malleus. The tympanum is usually seen in 75% of dogs with normal ears and in 28% of dogs with otitis.[3] Otoscopy is not sensitive for rupture of the tympanic membrane but can be diagnostic of obvious ruptures.

Cytologic Examination Cytologic examination of exudate within the ear canal is a mandatory part of assessing pets with otitis. Cytology should be done at initial examination and at each re-evaluation, because gross appearance of exudate does not correlate with microscopic character. Material should be collected prior to cleaning the ear canal; specimens collected from the horizontal canal through the otoscope cone may be more representative of the disease process.[3] Mineral oil cytology is the technique most often recommended for identification of parasites. A cerumen sample is mixed with mineral oil on a glass slide prior to microscopic examination. Heat-fixed otic exudate should also be stained with modified Wright's stain (Diff Quik American Scientific McGraw, IL) and Gram stain for evaluation of bacterial pathogens and yeast under oil immersion microscopy (×100). The morphologic type of bacteria, gram-staining characteristics, and presence or absence of inflammatory cells, cerumen, and debris should be noted.

Many clinicians use a scale of 1+ to 4+ in describing numbers of yeast, bacteria, and inflammatory cells to allow evaluation of the progression of the disease process. However, low numbers of bacteria and yeast per high-powered field (hpf) (×40 dry) may be identified in normal ears.[12] Dogs and cats should have two yeast and five bacteria or less per hpf.[12] Yeast numbers 5/hpf or greater in dogs and 12/hpf or greater in cats are abnormal. Bacteria 25/hpf or greater in dogs and 15/hpf in cats are associated with otitis.[12] Persistence of the same pathogens on re-evaluation suggests lack of efficacy or inappropriate therapy, incorrect identification of the primary disease process, or lack of owner compliance with therapy. Any change in the cytologic appearance may suggest reaction to medication or a change in either the type of inflammatory process or secondary pathogens.

Culture and Susceptibility Testing Cultures need not be done if external ear canal cytology is negative for bacteria; it is unlikely that either yeast or bacteria would be present on cultures or would contribute to the disease process in those cases. Culture with susceptibility testing should be considered whenever resistant bacteria may be present or when prolonged or systemic therapy are indicated (e.g., gram-negative bacteria and inflammatory cells identified on cytology, chronic bacterial otitis, suspected otitis media, failure to respond to appropriate medical therapy).[13,14] Cultures should be collected from the tympanic bulla in all suspected cases of otitis media, because horizontal ear canal samples do not correlate with those from the middle ear in over 89% of cases, and cytologic examination of the middle ear may be negative despite the presence of otitis.[15] Because bacteria may not cross the tympanic membrane, cultures from both sites should provide the highest yield of pathogenic bacteria. Yeast cultures are not routinely performed, because cytology is more sensitive than culture for yeast organisms, which may require specific lipid supplementation of the growth media for some species.[16,17]

Radiology, Computed Tomography, and Magnetic Resonance Imaging Diagnostic imaging may be used to evaluate the patency of the external ear canal and may be necessary to evaluate the integrity of the tympanic bulla. Underlying otitis media should be identified because it perpetuates otitis externa and requires specific therapy separate from that for otitis externa. Evaluating the tympanic membrane to diagnose otitis media, however, can be difficult in cases with significant secondary changes in the external ear canal. Treating otitis externa may decrease secondary changes and allow tympanic visualization at a later date, or imaging may be pursued. Radiographs are not as sensitive as CT or MRI for detecting abnormalities of the tympanic bulla.[18-20] If obstructive external ear disease does not respond to therapy or if the ear canals are palpably fibrotic or ossified, total ear canal excision and bulla osteotomy are required. Imaging of the middle ear is not necessary in those cases, because the middle ear can be evaluated at surgery via bulla osteotomy. Radiographic changes or changes on CT or MRI are valuable in patients with otic neoplasia. Significant changes of the tympanic bulla suggest that complete surgical excision may not be possible. Advanced imaging is also valuable in cases of otitis interna and central vestibular disease.

PATHOPHYSIOLOGY

Otitis externa describes any inflammatory condition of the external ear canal. The estimated incidence of otitis in dogs and cats ranges from 4% to 20% and 2% to 6.6%, respectively.[1,13] Clinical signs associated with the condition vary, depending on the cause of the otitis. General signs consist of head shaking, scratching, otic pain, and a variable accumulation of cerumen or exudate. The external canal responds to chronic inflammation of the dermis and epidermis with epithelial hyperplasia and hyperkeratosis, sebaceous gland hyperplasia, and ceruminous gland hyperplasia and dilation. These changes are associated with increased cerumen production; however, increased humidity, increased pH, and decreased lipid content of the cerumen predispose the animal to secondary infection. Apocrine gland rupture, sebaceous gland degeneration, ear canal stenosis, and fibrosis or ossification of the canal (or both) usually occur with the end stages of otitis.[21] Because permanent changes of the ear canal can occur with any cause of otitis externa, primary, predisposing, and perpetuating factors should be investigated in all cases of otitis.

Primary Factors

Primary factors are capable of causing otitis in normal ears. Primary factors may not be cured but often are controlled with appropriate therapy.

Hypersensitivities

Atopy and food hypersensitivity   Otitis externa is a clinical sign in 50% to 80% of atopic or food-sensitive dogs and may be the sole clinical sign associated with atopy.[22,23] Erythematous ceruminous otitis is most commonly associated with allergic skin disease.[24] Early clinical signs of bilateral pruritus, concave pinnal erythema, and mild erythematous and ceruminous otitis of the proximal ear canal may progress to significant otitis externa and pinnal hyperpigmentation. The pet can develop end-stage otitis if the primary cause is not identified and treated. Aural pruritus is common to atopy and food hypersensitivity; however, steroid responsiveness is usually only seen with atopy. Atopic dogs also tend to have a slower progression of disease than food-sensitive dogs. Secondary infection with either *Malassezia pachydermatis* or bacterial cocci is common. A definitive diagnosis is based on biopsy, intradermal skin testing, serologic testing, or dietary restriction and subsequent diet trials.

Contact hypersensitivity and irritant reaction   Topical otic preparations may cause a delayed hypersensitivity or irritant reaction to the ear canal. A response to initial therapy is followed by progression of disease or change in the character of the otitis with continued therapy. Worsening of clinical signs can occur if the medication is discontinued then readministered. Neomycin, propylene glycol, and dimethyl sulfoxide have been associated with irritant otitis. Reactions are occasionally noted with alcohol, glycerin, povidone-iodine, and concentrations of acetic acid greater than 2%.[3] Contact hypersensitivity or an irritant reaction should be suspected any time otitis externa is exacerbated by therapy or upon changes in the gross or cytologic appearance of the otitis. Both contact hypersensitivity and irritant reaction act as perpetuating factors of otitis externa despite control of the primary factor.

Ectoparasites

Otodectes cynotis is the cause of otitis externa (otocariasis) in up to 50% of cats and 10% of dogs with otitis externa.[3] The infestation in cats may be classified as one of the following: (1) otitis externa, (2) ectopic infestation, or (3) asymptomatic carrier. Signs of otitis include significant pruritus, pinnal erythema and crusting, and accumulation of cerumen in the external ear canal. Gross character of the cerumen is not correlated to the microscopic findings, but is usually dark brown to black in color. Mites may be observed on otoscopic examination; however, mineral oil cytology is recommended, because few mites are required to cause clinical signs. Mites may concurrently inhabit the skin of the head and neck in animals with otitis. True ectoparasite infestation usually results in miliary dermatitis and patchy alopecia in cats. Treatment can include any of the following: carbamates, pyrethrins, rotenone, ivermectin, thiabendazole, or fipronil.[25] Selamectin has recently been proven safe and effective for treating otocariasis in both dogs and cats.[26,27] The 3-week cycle of the parasite should be considered in treatment planning.

Demodex canis has been associated with mild otitis and excessive cerumen production in dogs with the generalized form of demodicosis. The diagnosis is made with mineral oil cytology; other diagnostics (e.g., biopsy) are less often required. Other parasites such as harvest mites (*Neotrombicula autumnalis* and *Euotrombicula alfredugesi*) and ticks (*Otobius megnini*) may

cause otitis externa. Reinfestation is a common problem due to environmental exposure to these parasites.

Foreign Bodies

Younger dogs, especially hunting or working breeds, are predisposed to otic foreign bodies. The most common foreign body associated with otitis is the grass awn; however, other foreign bodies include dirt, sand, cerumen, exudate mixed with hair, and conglomerates of dried ear medication. All can incite inflammation. Dogs are usually acutely painful, bilateral foreign bodies are possible, and approximately 20% of otic foreign bodies penetrate the tympanic membrane, leading to otitis media.[3]

Keratinization Defects

Hypothyroidism, male feminizing syndrome, Sertoli cell tumor, hyperestrogenism, and idiopathic seborrhea may be associated with mild otitis externa. Idiopathic seborrhea in cocker spaniels and hereditary defects in cats leading to seborrhea may cause erythematous ceruminous otitis. Changes in the microenvironment of the ear canal lead to secondary purulent otitis.

Idiopathic Inflammatory or Hyperplastic Otitis

Cocker spaniels may be affected by severe, proliferative otitis externa at a young age. Concurrent dermatologic conditions are not necessarily present but should be ruled out for proper management. The cause of the condition is unknown but may be due to a primary glandular disorder.[2]

Other Primary Factors

Immune-mediated disorders such as pemphigus complex may be associated with both pinnal lesions and otitis externa. Pemphigus foliaceus may involve only the ears in some cases, but lesions on other parts of the body are usually present. Drug eruption from systemically administered drugs may also cause both pinnal lesions and otitis externa. Older animals with chronic or recurrent otitis should be evaluated for benign or malignant neoplasia of the skin or adenexal structures of the ear.

Predisposing Factors   Predisposing factors make otitis more likely by altering the environment of the external ear canal, thereby making the ear more susceptible to inflammation and secondary infection.

Anatomic Changes

Increased soft tissue within the ear canal, increased compound hair follicles in the canal, and stenotic canals (e.g., Shar Pei, bulldog, chow chow) or chronic changes associated with previous bouts of otitis may be predisposing factors for otitis externa. Dogs with pendulous ears are predisposed to otitis, and otitis is common in breeds of dogs exhibiting increased ceruminous compared with sebaceous gland area (e.g., cocker spaniel, Labrador retriever, springer spaniel).[28] Hair is normally present in the ear canal, and increased numbers of hairs or presence of compound hair follicles have not been correlated to the incidence of otitis in dogs. Routine hair plucking is therefore not recommended and may incite an inflammatory response within the epithelium, perpetuating otitis externa.

External Environment

Increases in temperature and humidity in the environment may be reflected in the ear canal. The incidence of otitis externa is seasonally related to temperature, humidity, and rainfall. A lag period of 1 to 2 months is associated with cases of canine otitis and may vary with geographic location. Positive cultures of the ear canal are more likely during times of increased environmental temperature and humidity.[3]

Perpetuating Factors Perpetuating factors exacerbate the inflammatory process and can maintain the disease after the primary factor has been eliminated. They can induce permanent pathologic changes to the ear canal and are the main reason for treatment failure in otitis externa.

Secondary Bacterial Colonization and Infection

Normal bacterial flora exist in the ear canal of dogs and cats. Staphylococcus species and Streptococcus species are often cultured, *Pseudomonas* is rarely cultured, and *Proteus* was not cultured from the normal canine ear canal.[13] *Malassezia* has also been identified on cytologic examination in normal dogs and cats, and its numbers are significantly increased in erythematous ceruminous otitis.[13] Bacteria and yeast are opportunistic pathogens but can cause significant secondary changes of the ear canal with chronic infection. Increased numbers of bacteria without an inflammatory response may represent colonization, which often responds to topical therapy. The presence of inflammatory cells suggests true infection, and culture and susceptibility is recommended due to resistance patterns of many bacteria. In colonization and infection, cleaning the external ear canal removes exudate, debris, toxins, free fatty acids, and bacteria that perpetuate inflammation and secondary changes of the ear canal.[29]

Staphylococcus species are common in dogs with otitis as are *Pseudomonas aeruginosa*, Proteus species, *Escherichia coli*, Corynebacterium species, and Streptococcus species.[15,30] Acute purulent otitis externa is less common than chronic, but with chronicity and repeated treatment, gram-negative bacteria, such as *Pseudomonas* and *Proteus*, predominate. The associated otitis may have surface erosions or ulcers and copious exudate. Cats may be secondarily infected with *Pasteurella multocida* and less often *Pseudomonas aeruginosa*, Proteus species, or *E. coli*.[1]

Malassezia Pachydermatis Budding yeast has been identified on ear cytology of normal dogs (up to 50%) and cats (up to 17.6%).[17] *Malassezia* are considered part of the normal flora and an opportunist in cases of otitis externa, particularly in cases of erythematous ceruminous otitis. *Malassezia* are lipid-dependent yeast that overgrow in conditions of increased moisture, increased surface lipids, and compromised barrier function of the stratum corneum.[31,32] Enzymes produced by the yeast may allow depolymerization of the interstitial matrix (e.g., hyaluronidase, chondroitin-sulphatase) and cell membranes (e.g., proteinase, phospholipase), increasing tissue invasion and penetration.[32] Cytologic examination is more valuable than culture, because some species of *Malassezia* require specific media supplemented with long-chain fatty acids.[17,31]

Chronic Anatomic Changes

Increased soft tissue volume within the ear canal associated with chronic otic inflammation leads to ear canal stenosis and alters the otic microenvironment. Chronic changes of the epidermis, adenexa, dermis, and cartilage are described in the previous pathophysiology section. The microenvironmental alterations associated with chronic ear canal stenosis and inflammation favor bacterial and yeast proliferation and the retention of exudate. The changes also hinder proper cleaning and medication of the deeper portions of the external ear canal.

Otitis Media

Untreated infection of the middle ear serves as a source for perpetuating otitis externa. Failure to identify the bacteria, yeast, or byproducts of inflammation in the middle ear may result in recurrent otitis externa and chronic pathologic changes of the middle and external ear.

Treatment Errors, Undertreatment, and Overtreatment

Incorrect treatment of otitis allows bacterial or yeast overgrowth or infection and denies treatment of the primary factor causing otitis. Overapplication of medication or use of occlusive medications increases the humidity of the ear canal, leading to epithelial maceration and inflammation, perpetuating otitis; accumulation of dried medication acts as a foreign body within the ear canal. Undertreatment allows progression of the disease and the development of resistance in the bacteria causing secondary infection.

GENERAL PRINCIPLES OF MANAGEMENT

The therapeutic plan for otitis externa requires identification of the primary disease process and perpetuating factors. Ideally management is aimed at thoroughly cleaning and drying the ear canal, removing or managing the primary factors, controlling perpetuating factors, administering appropriate topical or systemic therapy (or both), and evaluating response to therapy.

Ear Cleaning

Ear cleaning serves several functions: (1) it removes material that supports or perpetuates infection; (2) it removes bacterial toxins, white blood cells (WBCs), and free fatty acids that stimulate inflammation; (3) it allows complete evaluation of the external ear canal and tympanum; (4) it allows topical therapy to contact all portions of the ear canal; and (5) it removes material that may inactivate topical medications.[3,13] Significantly painful ears may benefit from initial anti-inflammatory therapy to decrease pain and swelling of the ear canal prior to cleaning. Severe cases of otitis externa often require general anesthesia to facilitate complete cleaning and evaluation of the external and middle ear.

Many different solutions are available for removing cerumen, exudate, and debris from the ear canal (Table 209-2). If the tympanic membrane cannot be visualized, only physiologic saline solution or water should be used, because many topical cleaning agents are ototoxic or incite inflammation of the middle ear. An operating otoscope, ear loops, and alligator forceps facilitate manual removal of large amounts of cerumen or debris. Debris is carefully removed under direct visualization, and care is taken deeper in the ear canal (close to the tympanic membrane). Aggressive hair removal is not advised, because inflammation and damage to the epithelium can result in secondary bacterial colonization and infection. Flushing may be performed after large accumulations of cerumen and debris are mechanically removed from the ear canal.

Flushing and evacuation of solution is done under direct visualization through an operating otoscope. A bulb syringe and red rubber catheter system may be used to both flush and evacuate solutions and accumulations from the ear canal. The operator, avoiding drastic pressure changes within the external ear canal that could damage the tympanum, should carefully control suction and manual evacuation of the contents of the bulb syringe from the ear canal. Other alternatives include tomcat catheters (3.5 F) or flexible, intravenous catheters (14 gauge, Teflon); stiff, narrow catheters should be used cautiously and under direct visualization deep in the external ear canal. Other reservoir systems for delivery or evacuation of solutions include a 12 mL syringe or suction tubing attached to in-house vacuum systems. In-house vacuum systems should be used cautiously and under direct visualization. Care should be taken to avoid trauma to the tympanic membrane until its integrity can be assessed. Initial flushes should be done with physiologic saline solution or water until the integrity of the tympanic membrane is established.

Table • 209-2

Otic Cleaning Solutions

TRADE NAME	ACETIC ACID	BORIC ACID	SALICYLIC ACID	ISOPROPYL ALCOHOL	PROPYLENE GLYCOL	DSS	OTHER
Ace-Otic Cleanser	2%		0.1%				Lactic acid 2.7%
Adams Pan-Otic					X	X	Parachlorometaxylenol, tris EDTA, methylparaben, diazolidinyl urea, popylparaben, octoxynol
Alocetic Ear Rinse	X			X			Nonoxynol-12, methylparaben, alovera gel
Cerulytic Ear Ceruminolytic					X		Benzyl alcohol, butylated hydroxytoluene
Cerumene							25% Isopropyl myristate
DermaPet Ear/Skin Cleanser for Pets	X	X					
Docusate Solution					X	X	
Earmed Boracetic Flush	X	X					Aloe
Earmed Cleansing Solution & Wash					X		50A 40B alcohol, cocamidopropyl phosphatidyl and PE dimonium chloride
Earoxide Ear Cleanser							Carbamide peroxide 6.5%
Epi-Otic Ear Cleanser			X		X	X	Lactic acid, chitosanide
Fresh-Ear	X	X	X	X	X		Lidocaine hydrochloride, glycerin, sodium docusate, lanolin oil
OtiCalm			X				Benzoic acid, malic acid, oil of eucalyptus
Otic Clear	X	X	X	X	X		Glycerin, lidocaine hydrochloride
Oticlean-A Ear Cleaning Lotion	X	X	X	35%	X		Lanolin oil, glycerin
Oti-Clens			X		X		Malic acid, benzoic acid
Otipan Cleansing Solution					X		Hydroxypropyl cellulose, octoxynol
Otocetic Solution	2%	2%					
Wax-O-Sol 25%							Hexamethyltetracosane

Other solutions may aid in the removal of wax in the ear canal. Ceruminolytics are emulsifiers and surfactants that break down ceruminocellular aggregates by causing lysis of squamous cells. A ceruminolytic agent in an alkaline pH may more effectively lyse squamous cells via cell surface protein disruption.[3] Oil-based products soften and loosen debris to aid in their removal but do not cause cell lysis. Water-based ceruminolytics are easier to remove and dry more quickly than oil-based solutions, which are occlusive if they remain in the ear canal. Water-based products include dioctyl sodium sulfosuccinate, calcium sulfosuccinate, and carbamate peroxide, which has a foaming action with the release of urea and oxygen. Oil-based products include squalene, triethanolamine polypeptide, hexamethyltetracosane, oleate condensate, propylene glycol, glycerin, and mineral oil. In a recent study only the combination of squalene and isopropyl myristate in a liquid petrolatum base had no adverse effects on hearing, the vestibular system, and histopathologic examination.[33] Other agents tested contained glycerin, dioctyl sodium sulfosuccinate (2% or 6.5%), parachlorometaxylenol, carbamide peroxide (6%), propylene glycol, triethanolamine polypeptide oleate condensate (10%), and chlorobutanol (0.5%).[33]

Alcohol-based drying agents added to ceruminolytics include boric acid, benzoic acid, and salicylic acid, which decrease the pH of the ear canal, cause keratolysis, and have a mild antimicrobial effect. Drying the ear canal is important to combat increased humidity, which potentiates infection.

If the tympanum is intact, the ear canal is filled with a ceruminolytic agent for at least 2 minutes and the pinna is cleaned at the same time. The solution is flushed twice with warm water, and the canal inspected. The procedure is repeated until cleaning is complete. Other solutions commonly advocated for ear flushing include dilute chlorhexidine solution (0.05%), dilute povidone-iodine, and acetic acid (2.5%). The first two agents are potentially ototoxic or induce inflammation and should not be used if the tympanum is ruptured. A combination of propylene glycol malic, benzoic, or salicylic acid; 2% acetic acid; or dilute povidone-iodine have been suggested for use in dogs with a ruptured tympanum.[3]

Owners may clean the ears at home with mild preparations of ceruminolytics and drying agents if mild otitis is present without severe accumulation of cerumen or exudate. Aqueous solutions are usually recommended because they are less occlusive and easier to clean from the ear, dog, and home environment.

The ear should be filled with the solution, then massaged for 40 to 60 seconds. The pet should be allowed to shake its head to remove the majority of the solution, and the excess should be wiped from the ear canal and pinna with a tissue. Daily flushing is usually recommended, followed by every other day, weekly, then as needed, depending on the solution. Ear swabs are not recommended for home use, because cerumen and debris may be forced into the horizontal ear canal and impact against the tympanic membrane.

Topical Therapy

Erythematous ceruminous otitis externa is diagnosed 2.7 times more often than acute suppurative otitis according to one report.[24] Yeast ± cocci were identified in those cases, with cocci or rods identified in suppurative otitis.[24] Topical therapy should be based on the cytologic examination to diminish the incidence of inappropriate treatment (Table 209-3). Many preparations combine anti-inflammatories and antimicrobials in an attempt to decrease the inflammation and combat bacterial or yeast overgrowth. All topical medications should be considered supportive, and specific treatment should be aimed at controlling the primary disease process.

Topical glucocorticoids benefit most cases of otitis externa by decreasing pruritus, exudation, swelling, and proliferative changes of the ear canal. The most potent glucocorticoids available in topical preparations are betamethasone valerate and

Table • 209-3

Topical Medications Used in the Treatment of Ear Disease

GENERIC NAME	TRADE NAME	DOSE	FREQUENCY	DESCRIPTION
Fluocinolone 0.01% DMSO 60%	Synotic	4-6 drops; total dose < 17 mL	q12h initially, q48-72h maintenance	Potent corticosteroid anti-inflammatory
Hydrocortisone 1.0%	HB101, Burrows H,	2-12 drops, depending on ear size	q12h initially, q24-48h maintenance	Mild corticosteroid anti-inflammatory
Hydrocortisone 1.0%, lactic acid	Epi-otic HC	5-10 drops	q12h for 5 days	Mild corticosteroid anti-inflammatory, drying agent
Hydrocortisone 0.5%, sulfur 2%, acetic acid 2.5%	Clear X Ear Treatment	2-12 drops, depending on ear size	q12-24h initially, q24-48h maintenance	Mild corticosteroid anti-inflammatory, astringent, germicidal
DSS 6.5%, urea (carbamide peroxide 6%)	Clear X Ear Cleansing Solution	1-2 mL per ear	Once per week to as necessary	Ceruminolytic, lubricating agent
Chlorhexidine 2%	Nolvasan	Dilute 1:40 in water	As necessary	Antibacterial & antifungal activity
Chlorhexidine 1.5%	Nolvasan	Dilute 2% in propylene glycol	q12h	Antibacterial & antifungal activity
Povidone-iodine 10%	Betadine solution	Dilute 1:10-1:50 in water	As necessary	Antibacterial activity
Polyhydroxidine iodine 0.5%	Xenodyne	Dilute 1:1-1:5 in water	As necessary, q12h, once weekly	Antibacterial activity
Acetic acid 5%	White vinegar	Dilute 1:1-1:3 in water	As necessary; q12-24h for Pseudomonas	Antibacterial activity, lowers ear canal pH
Neomycin 0.25%, triamcinolone 0.1%, thiabendazole 4%	Tresaderm	2-12 drops depending on ear size	q12h up to 7 days	Antibacterial & antifungal activity, parasiticide (mites), moderate corticosteroid anti-inflammatory
Neomycin 0.25%, triamcinolone 0.1%, nystatin 100,000 U/mL	Panalog	2-12 drops depending on ear size	q12h to once weekly	Antibacterial & antifungal activity, moderate corticosteroid anti-inflammatory
Chloramphenicol 0.42%, prednisone 0.17%, tetracaine 2%, squalene	Liquachlor, Chlora-Otic	2-12 drops depending on ear size	q12h up to 7 days	Antibacterial activity, mild corticosteroid anti-inflammatory
Neomycin 1.75 & polymyxin B 5000 IU/mL, penicillin G procaine 10,000 IU/mL	Forte Topical	2-12 drops depending on ear size	q12h	Antibacterial activity
Gentamicin 0.3%, betamethasone valerate 0.1%	Gentocin Otic Solution, Betagen Otic Solution	2-12 drops depending on ear size	q12h for 7 to 14 days	Antibacterial activity, potent corticosteroid anti-inflammatory

Continued

Table • 209-3

Topical Medications Used in the Treatment of Ear Disease—cont'd

GENERIC NAME	TRADE NAME	DOSE	FREQUENCY	DESCRIPTION
Gentamicin 0.3%, betamethasone 0.1%, clotrimazole 0.1%	Otomax, Obibiotic Ointment	2-12 drops depending on ear size	q12h for 7 days	Antibacterial & antifungal activity, potent corticosteroid anti-inflammatory
Gentamicin 0.3%, betamethasone valerate 0.1%, acetic acid 2.5%	Gentaved Otic Solution	2-12 drops, depending on ear size	q12h for 7 to 14 days	Antibacterial activity, potent corticosteroid anti-inflammatory
Polymixin B 10,000 IU/mL, hydrocortisone 0.5%	Otobiotic	2-12 drops, depending on ear size	q12h	Antibacterial activity, mild corticosteroid anti-inflammatory
Enrofloxacin 0.5%, silver sulfadiazine 1%	Baytril Otic	2-12 drops, depending on ear size	q12h for up to 14 days	Antibacterial activity
Carbaryl 0.5%, neomycin 0.5%, tetracaine	Mitox Liquid	2-12 drops, depending on ear size		Antibacterial activity, parasiticide (mites)
Pyrethrins 0.06%, piperonyl butoxide 0.6%	Ear Mite and Tick Control	5 drops	q12h	Parasiticide (mites)
Pyrethrins 0.05%, squalene 25%	Cerumite	2-12 drops, depending on ear size	q24h for 7 to 10 days	Parasiticide (mites), ceruminolytic
Isopropyl alcohol 90%, boric acid 2%	Panodry	Fill ear canal	As necessary	Drying agent
Acetic acid 2%, aluminum acetate	Otic Domeboro	Fill ear canal	q12-48h	Drying agent, antibacterial activity, lowers ear canal pH
Silver sulfadiazine	Silvadene	Dilute 1:1 with water, 1 g powder in 100 mL water	q12h for 14 days	Antibacterial & antifungal activity
Tris EDTA ± gentamicin 0.03%		2-12 drops, depending on ear size	q12h for 14 days	1 L distilled water, 1.2g Tris EDTA, 1 mL glacial acetic acid; antibacterial activity
Silver nitrate		Use sparingly	As necessary	Cauterization of ulcerative otitis externa
Miconazole 1%; ± topical glucocorticoid (7.5 mL of dexamethasone phosphate [4 mg/mL] to 10 mL of 1% miconazole)	Conofite	2-12 drops, depending on ear size	q12-24h	Antifungal activity
Ivermectin 0.01%	Acarexx	0.5 mL per ear	Once	Parasiticide (mites)
Pyrethrins 0.15%, piperonyl butoxide 1.5%	Many	2-12 drops, depending on ear size	Twice at 7-day interval	Parasiticide (mites)
Pyrethrins 0.05%, piperonyl butoxide 0.5%, squalene 25%	Cerumite	2-12 drops, depending on ear size	q24h for 7 days	Parasiticide (mites), ceruminolytic
Pyrethrins 0.04%, piperonyl butoxide 0.49%, DSS 1.952%, benzocaine 1.952%	Aurimite	10 drops	q12h	
Rotenone 0.12%, cube resins 0.16%	Many	2-12 drops, depending on ear size	Every other day	Parasiticide (mites)

fluocinolone acetonide. Less potent corticosteroids include triamcinolone acetonide and dexamethasone; the least potent is hydrocortisone. Most dogs benefit from short-term therapy with topical corticosteroids at the initiation of therapy, with concurrent therapy aimed at the primary and other perpetuating factors. Long-term therapy with topical corticosteroids can be deleterious because of systemic absorption of drug. Increased serum liver enzymes and depressed adrenal responsiveness may occur; with prolonged use iatrogenic hyperadrenocorticism is possible. Glucocorticoids alone may be of benefit for short-term therapy in cases of allergic or erythematous ceruminous otitis.

Antimicrobials are important for controlling secondary bacterial or yeast overgrowth or infection. Antimicrobials are indicated in any case with cytologic evidence of bacterial overgrowth or infection, with attention paid to the morphology and gram-staining characteristics of the bacteria. Otic preparations commonly contain aminoglycoside antibiotics. Neomycin is effective against typical otitis bacteria such as *Staphylococcus intermedium*. Gentamicin and polymyxin B are also appropriate initial topical treatments for gram-negative bacterial otitis externa. The significant risk of bone marrow toxicity in people limits the use of chloramphenicol for treating otitis in dogs and cats despite its antibacterial spectrum and availability.

Due to the frequency of resistant gram-negative bacteria such as *Pseudomonas*, other topical preparations have been developed. Enrofloxacin, ophthalmic tobramycin, and topical application of injectable ticarcillin have been used to treat otitis in dogs.[3,34] Their use should be limited to cases of resistant bacteria, and culture and susceptibility testing should be performed prior to application. Other topical agents may be used to supplement treatment of resistant *Pseudomonas*, such as silver sulfadiazine solution and tris EDTA. Tris EDTA can render *Pseudomonas* susceptible to enrofloxacin or cephalosporins by enhancing membrane permeability and altering ribosome stability. Frequent ear cleaning may also assist in the treatment of resistant bacterial otitis; ceruminolytics have antimicrobial properties, and their use in clinical cases has been evaluated.[33,35] Acetic acid in combination with boric acid is effective against both *Pseudomonas* and *Staphylococcus*, depending on concentration and duration of exposure.[36] Ear cleaning removes proinflammatory products, cells, and substances that diminish the effectiveness of topical antibiotics.

Many topical preparations control yeast organisms, which may complicate erythematous ceruminous otitis and suppurative otitis. Common active ingredients include miconazole, clotrimazole, nystatin, and thiabendazole. Preparations containing climbazole, econazole, and ketoconazole have also been evaluated.[37,38] Eighty percent of yeast were susceptible to miconazole and econazole, intermediately resistant to ketoconazole, and 90% were resistant to nystatin and amphotericin B in one in vitro study.[38] Topical ear cleaning agents have some efficacy against *Malassezia* organisms.[35] Other preparations (e.g., chlorhexidine, povidone-iodine, acetic acid) are also effective in the treatment of secondary yeast overgrowth.

Response to topical therapy should be gauged by re-evaluation of physical, cytologic, and otoscopic examinations every 10 to 14 days after the initiation of therapy. Any changes in the results of these examinations should be recorded. Most cases of otitis can be managed topically; failure to respond to therapy should prompt re-evaluation of the diagnosis and treatment.

Systemic Therapy

Systemic glucocorticoid administration may be beneficial in cases of severe, acute inflammation of the ear canal, chronic proliferative changes of the ear canal, and allergic otitis. Anti-inflammatory doses should be limited to 7 to 10 days. Cases of significant thickening or proliferative changes in the external ear canal benefit from systemic antimicrobial therapy.

Systemic therapy should be considered if concurrent dermatologic changes of the surrounding skin, pinna, or other regions of the body are present. Long-term administration of appropriate antimicrobials based on culture and susceptibility is required in all cases of otitis media. Systemic therapy for yeast is rarely recommended in animals with otitis alone. One study evaluated oral itraconazole therapy, and in ear samples evaluated on cytology and culture, no change in cytology score was found.[16]

THERAPY FOR SPECIFIC DISEASES OF THE EXTERNAL EAR CANAL

Ectoparasites

Thorough cleaning of the external ear canal, treatment of all household pets, and whole-body therapy should be considered in the treatment regimen for ear mites. Pets with no clinical signs may be asymptomatic carriers and a reservoir for reinfestation. Otic parasiticides such as pyrethrins, rotenone, amitraz, and carbaryl must be administered every 24 hours throughout the 20-day mite life cycle because they do not kill mite eggs.[13] Thiabendazole eliminates all mite stages, but it must be applied every 12 hours for 14 days. Ivermectin (0.3 to 0.5 mg/kg) may be applied topically once weekly for 5 weeks.[1] Otic administration of medication does not affect mites on adjacent or distant skin locations, and systemic or other total-body parasiticide may be indicated. Alternatively, ivermectin administered subcutaneously (0.2 to 0.3 mg/kg) 2 to 3 times at 10- to 14-day intervals or orally (0.3 mg/kg) every week for four treatments eliminates otic mites and those found elsewhere on the body.[1] Other topicals proven safe and effective for ear mite treatment include selamectin (6 mg/kg) applied to the skin between the shoulder blades and fipronil spray.[25-27] Selamectin administered once in cats and two times, 30 days apart in dogs gave results similar to topical pyrethrin therapy.[26,27]

Idiopathic Inflammatory or Hyperplastic Otitis in Cocker Spaniels

Treatment is aimed at decreasing the secondary ear canal changes associated with this condition. Anti-inflammatory doses of corticosteroids administered orally may be useful. Topical corticosteroid preparations in combination with antimicrobials decrease the soft tissue mass affecting the ear canal but may not be as effective as oral administration. Maintenance therapy may be required both topically and orally; however, low doses of corticosteroids should be used. Re-evaluation should include attention to the potential side effects of corticosteroid therapy. Intermittent treatment of secondary bacterial or yeast overgrowth and infection may be required. Surgery is often indicated due to the severe secondary changes within the ear canal.

Excessive Moisture (Swimmer's Ear)

Other primary disease conditions such as allergic otitis should be ruled out in any dog with erythematous ceruminous otitis. Dogs with frequent exposure to water, however, may require ear cleaning and drying agents to diminish the humidity of the ear canal. Many cleaning and drying agents also posses antimicrobial effects.[35] Products that combine a drying agent and corticosteroid decrease the ear canal humidity and inflammation associated with allergic otitis complicated by swimming. Care should be taken to control primary disease (i.e., allergic otitis), however, and intermittently manage the predisposing factor (i.e., excessive moisture) as necessary. The dog's ears should be cleaned and dried the day of water exposure and for 2 to 5 days after. For continued frequent exposure, maintenance cleaning may be required every other day to twice weekly.

Chronic Bacterial Otitis

Resistant bacteria play an important role in the development of chronic otitis externa. Any dog not responding to initial therapy should be re-evaluated for primary and perpetuating conditions such as allergic disease, foreign body, neoplasia, otitis media, and secondary anatomic changes of the ear canal. Primary disease processes identified in one study included hypothyroidism, atopy, food allergy, and immune-mediated disease.[34] Infection with Pseudomonas species frequently occurs with repeated treatment of otitis externa, and acquired resistance is common. Culture and susceptibility testing is imperative to guide therapy. Oral antimicrobials combined with topical therapy are used in severe cases with secondary changes of the ear canal. Identification of otitis media is vital to remove the middle ear as a source of otitis externa. Otitis media requires long-term treatment.

Ear cleaning prior to the application of topical medication may increase the efficacy of the agent by decreasing exudate in the ear canal that inactivates antimicrobial drugs such as polymyxin.[2] In cases that fail to respond to first-line drug treatments such as polymyxin or gentamicin, other topical antimicrobial agents should be tried. Ophthalmic tobramycin and injectable amikacin have been described for use as topical antimicrobials in ear disease.[2] The integrity of the tympanic membrane should be known prior to use; the clinician should avoid these medications if the tympanic membrane cannot be proven intact. Enrofloxacin or ticarcillin injectable preparations diluted in saline or water may be applied topically for resistant Pseudomonas. Parenteral ticarcillin was used in cases with a ruptured tympanic membrane until healing was observed, at which time topical therapy was instituted; clinical response occurred in 11 of 12 cases.[34] Enrofloxacin and silver sulfadiazine combination is also available in an otic preparation (Baytril Otic, Bayer Shawne Mission, KS).

Other topical therapy may assist in eliminating resistant Pseudomonas from the ear canal.

Decreasing the pH of the ear canal with 2% acetic acid is lethal to Pseudomonas; diluted vinegar in water (1:1 to 1:3) may be used to flush the ear canal. Acetic acid combined with boric acid is lethal to Pseudomonas and Staphylococcus, depending on the concentration of each agent.[36] Increasing the concentration of acetic acid may broaden its spectrum of activity but causes irritation of the external and middle ear. Silver sulfadiazine in a 1% solution exceeds the minimum inhibitory concentration of Pseudomonas and may be instilled into the ear canal. One gram of silver sulfadiazine powder mixed in 100 mL of water may be used for topical therapy and is also effective against Proteus species, enterococci, and Staphylococcus intermedium. Dilute acetic acid (2%) and silver sulfadiazine (1%) have not caused adverse effects in cases with a ruptured tympanic membrane.[1,3,13] Tris EDTA may be applied after thorough ear cleaning to increase the susceptibility of Pseudomonas to antimicrobial agents. It must be mixed, pH adjusted, and autoclaved prior to use or is available in an otic preparation (TrizEDTA, DermaPet®, Potomac, MD), which is used to clean the ears prior to instillation of topical antibiotic. Topical antiseptics such as chlorhexidine and povidone-iodine solutions may be helpful, but ototoxicity is an issue, particularly in cases in which the tympanum is ruptured or cannot be evaluated.

Re-evaluation of the pet is important for monitoring response to therapy. Evaluation of the ear canal for progressive secondary changes and cytologic examination will allow alterations in therapy as needed. Significant narrowing of the ear canal is an indication for surgical intervention. Yeast overgrowth may occur with aggressive medical management of bacterial otitis and should be identified to maintain proper medical management.

Refractory or Recurrent Yeast Infection

Malassezia infection is a common perpetuating factor with erythematous ceruminous otitis and alterations in the otic microenvironment. Primary causes of the otitis should be identified and treated. Cytologic examination, not culture, should be relied upon for the diagnosis of yeast infection.[17,31] If a case becomes refractory to therapy, reassessment of the primary condition and perpetuating factors should be done. Miconazole, clotrimazole, cuprimyxin, nystatin, and amphotericin B have all been described for treating Malassezia otitis. Climbazole had better in vitro activity against isolates of Malassezia pachydermatis in one study.[37] Yeast were more susceptible to azole antifungals than polyene antifungals; however, oral ketoconazole, itraconazole, or fluconazole have been recommended for refractory cases.[1,38] Long-term therapy may require topical antibacterial and antifungal combinations.

Ear cleaning may aid in the elimination of yeast organisms by removing cerumen, debris, or exudate and altering the microenvironment of the ear canal. Cleaning with antimicrobial agents such as chlorhexidine, povidone-iodine, and acetic acid may be beneficial; but as always the integrity of the tympanum should be established prior to use. Ear cleaning solutions may also have some efficacy against yeast organisms both in vitro and in clinical cases of otitis.[35,39]

Neoplasia

Chronic otitis externa may be the result of otic neoplasia, or otitis may be a predisposing factor in the development of neoplasia. Cocker spaniels are over-represented for benign and malignant neoplasia and otitis externa.[1,40] Tumors of the skin and adenexal structures of the ear predominate. Benign tumors in dogs include sebaceous gland adenoma, basal cell tumor, polyp, ceruminous gland adenoma, and papilloma. Cats are more frequently diagnosed with malignant neoplasms, but benign conditions include inflammatory polyps, ceruminous gland adenomas, ceruminous gland cysts, and basal cell tumors. Malignant neoplasms in both species include ceruminous gland adenocarcinoma, undifferentiated carcinoma, and squamous cell carcinoma. Ceruminous gland adenocarcinomas are the most frequently diagnosed tumors of the ear canal in dogs and cats; however, one report stated that squamous cell carcinoma occurs with equal incidence in the cat.[40,41]

The biologic behavior of otic tumors cannot be judged by their gross appearance; however, benign masses are usually nodular and pedunculated. Ulceration can be secondary to otitis associated with mass lesions, but malignant masses ulcerate more frequently than benign masses. The tympanic bulla is involved in up to 25% of aural neoplasms, and neurologic signs occur in 10% of dogs and 25% of cats with otic neoplasia.[42] The biologic behavior of malignant neoplasms tends to be local invasion with a low metastatic rate (e.g., 10% in dogs) to draining lymph nodes or lung.

Surgery is the mainstay treatment of otic neoplasia. Conservative excision may be possible for benign lesions, depending on the location of the tumor. Malignancies should be removed by total ear canal ablation and lateral bulla osteotomy. Incomplete excision results in recurrence of the mass and secondary otitis externa. Malignant neoplasia is associated with a median survival time (MST) of more than 58 months in dogs and 11.7 months in cats.[40] Extensive tumor involvement and lack of aggressive management are associated with a poor prognosis in dogs.[40,43] In cats a poor prognosis is associated with neurologic signs, squamous cell carcinoma or undifferentiated carcinoma, vascular or lymphatic invasion, and lack of aggressive therapy.[40,44] Ceruminous gland adenocarcinoma has a median disease free interval of more than 36 months and 42 months in dogs and cats, respectively.[43,44] The MST associated with squamous cell carcinoma and undifferentiated carcinoma in cats is 4 to 6 months.[40]

ROLE OF SURGERY IN THE MANAGEMENT OF OTITIS EXTERNA

The two most common surgical procedures for the treatment of otitis externa are lateral ear resection and total ear canal ablation. Total ear canal ablation is always combined with a bulla osteotomy to allow complete removal of all secretory epithelium and exudate associated with the external and middle ear. Care must be taken when choosing a surgical technique for otitis externa.

Lateral ear resection is associated with high failure rates (47% to 80%) with inappropriate patient selection.[45] The procedure should be viewed as an adjunct to medical management, not as a cure. The primary and perpetuating factors associated with otitis externa must be identified and managed or controlled even when surgery is elected. Opening the vertical ear canal improves aeration, decreases humidity, facilitates removal of cerumen or exudate, and improves the distribution of topical medication in the ear canal. Lateral ear resection may be used in cases with mild changes of the vertical ear canal but should be avoided with significant secondary changes of the vertical ear canal or horizontal canal stenosis. Owners should be educated to the continuing need for medical therapy after surgery to avoid further progression of secondary changes of the ear canal. Pets can develop end-stage otitis after lateral ear resection.

Total ear canal ablation is used to treat end-stage otitis and malignant otic neoplasia. Severe secondary changes and proliferative disease are surgically removed with the ear canal en toto. A lateral bulla osteotomy of the tympanic bulla allows complete exploration of the middle ear for the removal of secretory epithelium, exudate, and tumor. The surgery removes the site of chronic inflammation and infection to cure the vast majority of cases of otitis externa and otitis media. Complications of the procedure include facial nerve paresis or paralysis, hemorrhage, para-aural abscessation, otitis interna, Horner's syndrome, pinnal necrosis, continued pinnal dermatitis, and hearing loss. Dogs with obstruction of the ear canal from end-stage otitis or neoplasia may be partially deaf, and postoperatively only osseous conduction of sound remains.

Vertical ear canal resection may be performed in cases of tumors confined to the auricular cartilage or traumatic injury. Significant proliferative disease or changes secondary to otitis externa are rarely confined to the vertical ear canal; concurrent stenosis of the horizontal ear canal usually necessitates total ear canal ablation and lateral bulla osteotomy. The anastomosis between the horizontal ear canal and surrounding skin may undergo stenosis after surgery, necessitating reoperation. Progression of the otitis and tumor recurrence are possible after vertical ear canal resection.

DISEASES OF THE MIDDLE AND INNER EAR

Normal Anatomy and Physiology

The middle ear consists of the tympanic membrane, three cavities (epitympanic, tympanic, and ventral), and the bony ossicles (malleus, incus, and stapes). The tympanic membrane has two parts: (1) the thin pars tensa that attaches to the manubrium of the malleus and (2), above the pars tensa, the thicker, pars flaccida. The main portion of the middle ear, the ventral tympanic bulla, has two compartments in the cat (ventromedial and dorsolateral). The air-filled bulla is lined with modified respiratory epithelium, which is either squamous or cuboidal and may be ciliated. The four openings in the middle ear are the (1) tympanic opening, (2) the vestibular window, (3) the cochlear window, and (4) the ostium of the auditory tube. The auditory tube is the communication between the middle ear and caudal nasopharynx. The normal flora of the middle ear may be due to this pharyngeal communication, but the role of the auditory tube as a source of bacteria in otitis media is unknown. The tympanic opening is a common source of bacterial infection of the middle ear in dogs with otitis externa. The cochlear and vestibular windows are possible ports of entry for progression of otitis media or ototoxic substances into the inner ear.

Cranial nerve VII, or the facial nerve, the sympathetic innervation of the eye, and the parasympathetic innervation of the lacrimal gland are closely associated with the middle ear. The separation of the facial nerve from the middle ear is minimal along the rostral aspect of its course through the petrosal bone. The nerve supplies motor fibers to the superficial muscles of the head, the muscles of the external ear, the caudal belly of the digastricus, and the ossicular muscles. The nerve also supplies sensation of the vertical ear canal and concave surface of the pinna.

Postganglionic sympathetic nerve fibers course closely with those of the facial nerve to innervate the smooth muscles of the eye. Preganglionic parasympathetic fibers also pass through the middle ear to innervate the salivary and lacrimal glands.

The inner ear is located within the petrosal bone. The cochlea, vestibule (saccule and utricle), and semicircular canals form the membranous labyrinth, which is encased in bone, called the *bony labyrinth*. The vestibular system functions to maintain the position of the eyes, trunk, and limbs relative to the position of the head, responding to linear and rotational acceleration and tilting. The system consists of the saccule, utriculus, and semicircular canals and communicates with the middle ear via the vestibular window. Fluid within the semicircular canals tends to remain stationary during motion, bending the cilia of the cells in the utricle and saccule, causing depolarization. These stereocilia synapse with the dendrites of the vestibular portion of the eighth cranial nerve and the signal is conducted via cranial nerve VIII to vestibular nuclei in the myelencephalon, the spinal cord, centers in the cerebellum and cerebral cortex, and motor nuclei of cranial nerves III, IV, and VI.[46] The result is coordination of the body, head, and eye movement. Projections to the vomiting centers are responsible for nausea and vomiting associated with vestibular disorders and motion. The cochlear system, involved with the translation of sound, consists of the spiral organ, or organ of Corti, cochlear duct, scala vestibule, and scala tympani. Transmission of sound through the tympanic membrane, ossicles, and cochlear window results in undulation of the basilar membrane of the spiral organ. Cilia bend and cause depolarization and transmission of a signal to cochlear nuclei, caudal colliculi, and cerebral cortex.[46] The cochlear nuclei control reflex regulation of sound via projections to cranial nerves V and VII, which control the muscles of the ossicles. Other projections allow for conscious perception of sound.

Otitis Media

Otitis media may result from extension of otitis externa through the tympanic membrane, aspiration of pharyngeal contents up the auditory tube (e.g., a sequela to upper respiratory tract [URT] infection in cats), or from hematogenous spread. Extension from otitis externa is the most common cause of otitis media, but otitis media may serve as a perpetuating factor for otitis externa. Developmental abnormalities of the external ear canal and pharynx may also result in otitis media due to the accumulation of secretions in the middle ear.[47,48] Neoplasia, inflammatory polyps, and middle ear trauma may be associated with secondary otitis media or result in similar clinical signs.

Cholesteatoma is commonly associated with otitis media and chronic otitis externa. A cholesteatoma is a mass of keratinized squamous cells that accumulate within a structure lined with stratified squamous epithelium. The lesion is presumed to develop when a pocket of tympanic membrane becomes adhered to inflamed middle ear mucosa. Significant narrowing of the external ear canal is usually present. Radiographic signs of increased density and bony changes of the tympanic bulla predominate with loss of the air-filled lumen of the external ear canal and concurrent calcification. Treatment is usually limited to total ear canal ablation and lateral bulla osteotomy due to the changes of the external ear canal and mass or accumulation of debris in the tympanic bulla.[49]

The clinical signs associated with middle ear disease often reflect concurrent otitis externa (e.g., head shaking, lethargy, exudate, otic malodor). Significant otic pain, lethargy, inappetence, and pain upon opening the mouth are more suggestive of middle ear involvement. Neurologic signs may be present due to the course of the facial nerve and sympathetic innervation of the eye. Facial nerve paresis or paralysis result in facial asymmetry (i.e., uneven position of the lip commissures, unequal ear carriage, unilateral ptyalism) and abnormal cranial nerve reflexes on neurologic examination (e.g., menace response, palpebral and corneal reflexes, abnormal ear canal, and concave pinnal sensation). Horner's syndrome, or loss of sympathetic innervation to the eye, can also be complete or partial (i.e., ptosis, miosis, enophthalmia, prolapse of the third eyelid). Otitis interna is usually evidenced by head tilt, abnormal nystagmus, and ataxia and should be differentiated from central vestibular disease based on careful neurologic examination. Otitis interna is not usually associated with ipsilateral hemiparesis or abnormalities in level of consciousness.

Cases of para-aural abscessation usually have concurrent otitis media.[3] The primary cause may be trauma to the external ear canal, severe otitis externa, extension of otic neoplasia, or total ear canal ablation. Signs of middle or external ear disease and soft tissue swelling in the parotid area may be accompanied by draining tracts. A head tilt and pain upon palpation of the area are usually present.

The diagnosis of otitis media is based on a thorough history and physical, neurologic, and otoscopic examinations. A ruptured tympanum strongly suggests otitis media. The pharynx should also be evaluated on physical examination; identification of specific conditions may require general anesthesia due to anatomic location (e.g., inflammatory polyps) or pain associated with examination (e.g., otitis media causing temporomandibular joint (TMJ) pain, severe otitis externa). General anesthesia may also be required to perform a complete otoscopic examination in cases of severe otitis externa in which thorough cleaning of the ear is necessary for therapy and diagnosis (i.e., visualization of the tympanum). Significant otitis externa is commonly associated with otitis media; the tympanic membrane is ruptured in up to 50% of dogs with otitis externa, although 70% of dogs with otitis media had an intact tympanic membrane in one study.[15,50] The tympanic membrane in dogs with otitis externa may be difficult to examine due to secondary changes of the external ear canal, pain associated with otoscopic examination, and accumulation of exudate, cerumen, and debris. Treatment to diminish the severity of otitis externa and general anesthesia may increase the ability to evaluate the tympanum in these cases.

Any case that has significant cerumen, exudate, or debris should undergo careful cleaning of the ear canal to allow evaluation of the integrity and character of the tympanic membrane. The presence of a "false middle ear" occurs when large accumulations of debris lodge against the tympanic membrane, causing it to deviate medially into the middle ear. This makes the external ear canal appear elongated and leads to misdiagnosis of a ruptured tympanic membrane.[3]

Gentle probing of the tympanic membrane with a red rubber catheter under direct visualization may assist in the diagnosis of small tears in the membrane. If the catheter tip is consistently visible, rupture is unlikely. Alternatively, an aliquot of 1 mL of physiologic saline placed in the horizontal canal should remain stationary; disappearance suggests an opening in the tympanum, allowing the fluid to drain into the middle ear.[1] Movement of the fluid may be blocked by large amounts of debris in the middle ear, even in the presence of a tear in the tympanum.

If the tympanic membrane is visible, its character should be recorded in the medical record for comparison upon re-evaluation. Bulging, increased opacity, and hyperemia may be present with otitis media. If otitis media is suspected, radiographs of the bullae may be made. Lateral oblique and open-mouth views are most helpful for evaluating the tympanic bulla, but positioning for comparison of left and right sides is difficult and requires general anesthesia. Ventrodorsal or dorsoventral views allow evaluation of the air-filled lumen and calcification of the external ear canal. Abnormalities of the bulla include increased opacity, sclerosis, and lysis. Fluid cannot be differentiated from increased soft tissue density (e.g., neoplasia), and absence of radiographic changes does not rule out otitis media. Radiographic changes were absent in 33% of the middle ears in one study of dogs with otitis media confirmed by surgical exploration.[18] Otitis media or neoplasia and otitis interna can cause radiographic evidence of lysis of the petrosal bone.

Other diagnostic tools are available to evaluate patients with otitis media interna. Contrast introduced into the external ear canal followed by radiography, termed *canalography*, is used to diagnose tympanic membrane perforations. The method is useful for acute tympanic membrane rupture and increases the frequency of diagnosing tympanic membrane rupture with concurrent otitis externa and media beyond that of otoscope alone.[51] Advanced imaging with CT and MRI have been studied in normal dogs and dogs with otitis media (Figure 209-1).[18,52] CT is considered superior to MRI for bony changes, whereas MRI is better for detection of soft tissue abnormalities in both dogs and cats.[18,20,52,53]

If the tympanic membrane is intact in a dog with otitis media, a myringotomy is performed to obtain samples for culture and susceptibility testing and cytologic examination. Affected dogs are often more comfortable after collection of samples due to decreased pressure in the middle ear after myringotomy. The procedure must be performed with general anesthesia and is usually done after radiography or advanced imaging of the ear. The external ear canal should be thoroughly cleaned and dried prior to myringotomy to avoid contamination with external ear canal debris. Direct otoscopic visualization is used for the procedure. A 20-gauge spinal needle is used to penetrate the tympanic membrane through the caudoventral aspect of the pars tensa. Suction is applied and samples collected—culture and susceptibility takes priority over cytologic examination because cytology is frequently negative, and cultures of the external ear canal do not reflect the middle ear bacteria in the majority of cases.[15] If fluid cannot be aspirated directly from the middle ear, 0.5 to 1 mL of warm, sterile saline can be infused through the needle into the middle ear cavity and aspirated. Alternatively, an open-ended tomcat catheter or small, sterile culture swab may be passed into the middle ear cautiously under otoscopic visualization. Pseudomonas species and *Staphylococcus intermedium* are most commonly isolated, followed by yeast, β-hemolytic *Streptococcus*, Corynebacterium species, Proteus species, and Enterococcus species.[15,54] Surgical exploration is rarely required for the diagnosis of otitis media.

Medical therapy of otitis media should be guided by culture and susceptibility results. The external ear canal is flushed and dried as necessary to treat concurrent otitis externa. Flushing is usually performed under the same general anesthetic episode used for diagnostic testing. If the tympanic membrane is ruptured, the middle ear should be gently lavaged with warm saline. Cytology results, when available,

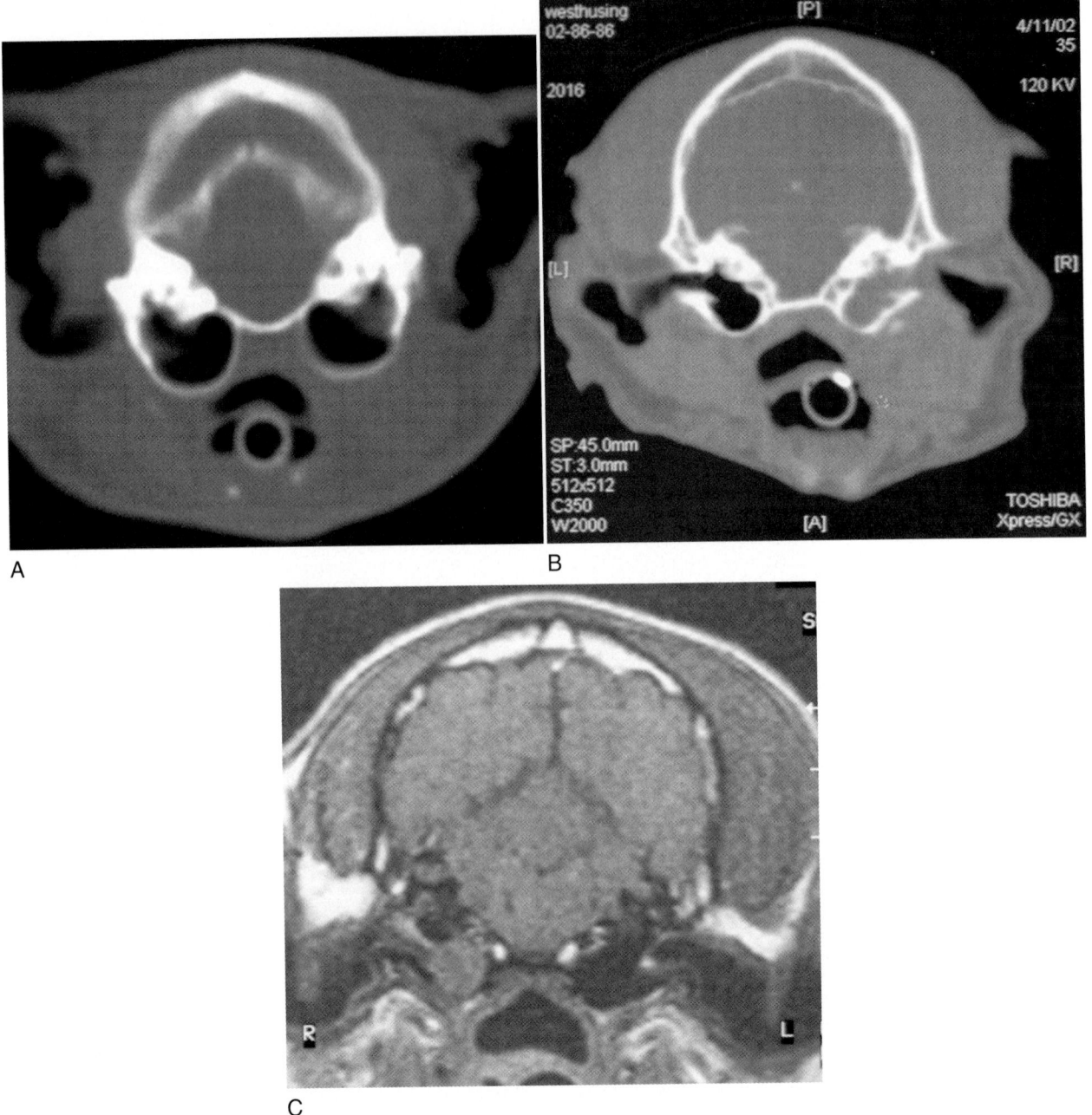

Figure 209-1 Computed tomographic (CT) image of a normal canine ear **(A)**, CT image **(B)**, and a magnetic resonance image (MRI) **(C)** of a dog with otitis media.

should be used to guide initial therapy. The integrity of the tympanic membrane must be considered when using topical agents to treat concurrent otitis externa: ototoxic medications and vehicles should be avoided if the tympanic membrane is ruptured.

Newly diagnosed cases of otitis media may be started on empiric therapy based on cytology. First-choice antimicrobials include cephalosporins, amoxicillin and clavulonic acid, and fluoroquinolones. Definitive therapy consists of administration of antibiotics based on culture and susceptibility results for a minimum of 4 to 6 weeks. Primary and perpetuating factors of otitis externa should be identified and treated or controlled. Topical medication and flushing of the external ear canal should continue until resolution of clinical signs and normalization of cytology. Gradual improvement of the otitis media is expected within 14 days. The ear canal and tympanic

membrane should be evaluated prior to and after discontinuation of therapy. Small tears in the tympanic membrane after myringotomy heal rapidly with appropriate therapy within 2 to 3 weeks.[34,55] However, re-evaluation of the tympanic membrane in dogs with otitis externa media should precede alteration of the topical agents in the therapeutic plan.

Failure to respond to therapy or chronic or recurrent otitis media warrant re-evaluation for surgical intervention. Total ear canal ablation and lateral bulla osteotomy should be considered in cases with severe secondary changes of the external ear canal and concurrent otitis media. If the external ear canal is not affected, a ventral bulla osteotomy may be performed to remove gross exudate and establish drainage from the middle ear of dogs and cats with chronic or recurrent otitis media. Caution should be taken in considering lateral ear resection and ventral bulla osteotomy in the treatment of concurrent otitis externa and media because lateral ear resection is only an adjunct to medical management of otitis externa.

Neoplasia of the Middle Ear
Neoplasia of the middle ear is rare; most cases represent extension of tumors originating in the external ear canal.

Inflammatory Polyps
Inflammatory polyps are a non-neoplastic admixture of inflammatory and epithelial cells originating in the tympanic bulla in cats. Other sites of origin include the auditory tube and nasopharynx. Macrophages, neutrophils, lymphocytes, plasma cells, and epithelial cells are usually present on histopathologic examination. The cause is unknown, but ascending infection and congenital causes have been suggested.[56] No age or sex predilection exists for the condition, but younger cats are more commonly affected (1 to 5 years of age). Signs can be unilateral or bilateral and depend on the location of the mass lesion. A single polyp can grow into the external ear canal, down the auditory tube into the nasopharynx, or both. Signs of concurrent otitis externa and media are common with polyps limited to the ear, but respiratory stridor, dyspnea, gagging, and dysphagia occur with growth into the pharynx.

Diagnosis is based on otoscopic and pharyngeal examinations. Radiographs of the bulla, nasal cavity, and pharynx may be considered, and CT or MRI can be used to diagnose the site and side of origin of inflammatory polyps.[53,57] Treatment consists of excision by traction or surgical excision via ventral bulla osteotomy.[8,58] Regrowth is a problem in half of the cats treated by traction extraction alone, and Horner's syndrome is common in cats after ventral bulla osteotomy.[8,58]

Otitis Interna
Otitis interna is usually an extension of otitis media or neoplasia of the middle ear. A careful neurologic examination is imperative to the localization of vestibular signs. Clinical signs associated with otitis interna include head tilt, ataxia, horizontal or rotary nystagmus, circling or falling toward the side of the lesion, or ipsilateral nystagmus. The fast phase of nystagmus is usually away from the side of the lesion. Occasionally, animals will become nauseated or vomit. Horner's syndrome or deficits in cranial nerve VII may accompany otitis media interna, but involvement of other cranial nerves, vertical or changing nystagmus, or the presence of conscious proprioceptive deficits or paresis indicate central rather than peripheral vestibular disease. Bilateral peripheral vestibular disease is rare, but the animal will not have a head tilt, nystagmus, or strabismus and may exhibit wide head excursions and a crouched stance or the inability to stand.

The diagnosis of otitis interna is based on history, clinical signs, and physical, neurological, and otoscopic examinations. Advanced imaging may be helpful in distinguishing the anatomic location of the disease process. Treatment with aggressive medical or surgical intervention appropriate to the localization is important in prevention of adjacent brain stem involvement.

Prognosis for Otitis Media and Interna
A fair prognosis can be given if aggressive surgical and medical therapy are possible. Cases with concurrent severe external ear canal changes require total ear canal ablation and lateral bulla osteotomy. Repeated infections after ventral bulla osteotomy or total ear canal ablation and lateral bulla osteotomy may be operated again with resolution of the condition. Resistant organisms, failure to respond to aggressive surgery, and significant osteomyelitis are associated with a poor prognosis. The neurologic signs associated with otitis media and interna may be permanent, but many animals learn to use

visual cues and can compensate for vestibular deficits. Facial nerve deficits, Horner's syndrome, and keratoconjunctivitis sicca are often permanent.

Ototoxicity
Ototoxic substances (Table 209-4) damage the cochlear or vestibular systems or both. Otic application of medication can also cause adverse effects through local inflammation of the tympanic membrane or the meatal window (or both), as well as resultant otitis media. Topical medications also cause adverse effects by systemic absorption. Ototoxic substances reach the inner ear after local application and absorption through the cochlear or vestibular windows or hematogenously. The most frequent cause of ototoxicity is the application of an ototoxic substance to the external ear canal in a pet with a ruptured tympanum, which results in distribution to the middle ear. Absorption by the inner ear is increased when inflammation of the cochlear window occurs with otitis media. Hematogenous distribution of ototoxins to the inner ear is inherent in some medications (e.g., aminoglycosides).

The development of ototoxicity also depends on the vehicle of the preparation, chemical composition, drug concentration, concurrent medications, as well as the route, frequency, and duration of administration.[3] Examples of increased risk of ototoxicity depending on the vehicle (e.g., combination of chlorhexidine and detergents) and concurrent medications (e.g., loop diuretics and aminoglycosides) have been described. Minimization of the risk of toxicity should be considered when any potentially toxic substance is administered either topically or systemically. The integrity of the tympanic membrane should be known prior to topical administration of any potentially ototoxic drug, and consequences of each drug should be considered in light of the animal's health and concurrent therapies.

Idiopathic Vestibular and Facial Nerve Diseases
A complete neurologic examination is key to differentiating peripheral from central vestibular disorders. Head tilt, ataxia, horizontal or rotary nystagmus, and cranial nerve VII deficits

Table • 209-4

Ototoxic Drugs

Aminoglycoside Antibiotics	Antiseptics
Neomycin	Chlorhexidine
Dihydrostreptomycin	Iodine & iodophores
Gentamicin	Ethanol
Streptomycin	Benzalkonium chloride
Kanamycin	Benzethonium chloride
Tobramycin	Cantrimide
Amikacin	
	Antineoplastic Agents
Other Antibiotics	Cisplatin
Polymixin B & E	Nitrogen mustard
Minocycline	
Erythromycin	**Miscellaneous**
Chloramphenicol	Quinine
Vancomycin	Salicylates
	Propylene glycol
Loop Diuretics	Detergents
Furosemide	Arsenic
Bumetanide	Lead
Ethacrynic acid	Mercury

may be seen with either condition. Central vestibular disease causes paraparesis, conscious proprioceptive deficits, other cranial nerve abnormalities, and vertical or changing nystagmus. Middle ear neoplasia, otitis media interna, idiopathic vestibular syndrome, and congenital vestibular disorders result in peripheral vestibular signs. Congenital vestibular disorders have been described in the German shepherd, Doberman pinscher, English cocker spaniel, Siamese, and Burmese breeds.[59,60] Bilateral congenital vestibular syndrome has been described in beagles and Akitas.[59,60] Clinical signs of head tilt and ataxia in these dogs and cats may be persistent or may improve; animals can be congenitally deaf.

Otitis media interna may be associated with facial paresis or paralysis if cranial nerve VII is affected by the inflammation. Otitis should be ruled out before diagnosing any animal with idiopathic facial nerve paralysis, because otitis requires aggressive management and the idiopathic condition can only be treated symptomatically or with acupuncture.[61]

Deafness

Deafness is classified as inherited or acquired, conductive or sensorineural, and congenital or late onset. Acquired deafness may be either conductive or sensorineural, depending on the etiologic agent, which also affects the time of onset. Conductive deafness results from a lack of presentation of sound to the inner ear, usually secondary to otitis externa media. Sensorineural deafness occurs with abnormalities of the cochlear system, cranial nerve VIII, or auditory pathways and higher brain centers. Inherited deafness, ototoxicity, cochlear nerve degeneration, and presbycusis (age-related deafness) are forms of sensorineural deafness.

Diagnostic Principles

Signalment can help to prioritize possible causes of deafness. Certain breeds have a high incidence of inherited deafness, and clinical signs are usually noticed at an early age if the deafness is bilateral. Most other forms of deafness occur as late-onset disorders. The history is important in establishing the nature of the deafness, because certain conditions or treatments may cause deafness (e.g., otitis externa media, ototoxic medications, head trauma, prior infectious diseases). The owner may note behavioral changes in the pet, and complete, bilateral deafness is usually easily identified. Astute owners may notice behavioral changes in puppies at an early age. Inherited deafness usually results in loss of hearing within 3 to 4 weeks of birth due to a degenerative process of the inner ear.[62] The affected pup is often more aggressive than its littermates, because it cannot hear cries of pain during play. The puppy may also be more difficult to rouse and is more vocal than its littermates, especially when they are out of view of the affected pup.

Unilateral deafness is harder to identify, but the owner may report difficulty rousing the pet when it is sleeping in lateral recumbency or difficulty in the pet's ability to orient to the origin of sounds. The physical, otoscopic, and neurologic examinations are important in differentiating peripheral from central disease and establishing whether conductive deafness is possible. The index of suspicion for conductive deafness is increased in dogs and cats with abnormalities of the external ear canal, tympanum, cranial nerve VII, or sympathetic innervation of the eye.

Abnormalities suggestive of central disease prompt more aggressive diagnostic testing such as advanced imaging and cerebrospinal fluid (CSF) analysis.

Hearing loss can be evaluated with the pet in the examination room. Different sounds can be used in an attempt to observe behavioral reactions to sound. A Preyer's reflex (i.e., movement of the pinna in response to sound) is the minimal expected response.[62] Care should be taken to avoid visual cues and air movement close to the animal's head, which cause an apparent reaction to sound in an affected dog or cat.

Unfortunately, pets may be stressed by the hospital environment and may not react to auditory cues even if hearing is normal.

Impedance audiometry and tympanometry Impedance audiometry is based on the concept that the intensity of a sound wave is dependent on the size of the cavity in which it is generated and on the compliance of the cavity's containing walls.[3] The external ear canal is occluded for the test, and a sound wave generated. Changes in the pressure within the canal are measured to evaluate the compliance of the tympanic membrane. Accumulation of fluid in the middle ear canal, rupture of the tympanic membrane, immobility of the ossicles, and other causes of conductive deafness alter the results. Normal results in a deaf animal would be supportive of sensorineural deafness.

The acoustic, or stapedial, reflex test is also known as the *acoustic decay test*. A high amplitude sound is used to cause stapedial muscle contraction that protects the structures of the inner ear. This reflex alters tympanic compliance. The afferent (cranial nerve VII) and efferent limbs (cranial nerves V and VII) must be intact for a normal reflex.[1] A normal dog will maintain this reflex for a known period of time, but decay of the reflex occurs in dogs with lesions of cranial nerve VIII.[3] Tympanometry is not commonly performed because it requires specialized equipment adapted from human kits. Ideally the generated sound affects the tympanic membrane perpendicular to its surface. This is difficult to obtain in the dog or cat due to the angle of the ear canal. The results are not sensitive or specific, but they are reliable for the diagnosis of tympanic membrane rupture.[3,63]

Brain stem auditory evoked response The brain stem auditory evoked response (BAER), or brain stem auditory evoked potential (BAEP), is an objective measure of hearing. The test identifies the presence or absence of hearing and progressive changes in hearing. Subjective determination of partial hearing loss is possible.[64] Electrodes placed on standard sites of the head record responses to an auditory stimulus generated in one ear. Sound is generated as a series of clicks, and the contralateral ear is excluded by the presentation of *white noise*. The position of electrodes, stimulus intensity, and body temperature can also alter the waves produced.[3] Electrode position is standardized and the sound generated, or stimulus intensity is presented over a range of decibels; the rate of presentation remains constant. The waves generated are subjectively and objectively evaluated. Wave I corresponds to cranial nerve VIII; wave II represents the cochlear nucleus and intracranial, extramedullary portion of cranial nerve VIII. Wave III corresponds to the dorsal nucleus of the trapezoid body, and waves IV and V originate in the rostral pons and caudal colliculi, respectively.[3]

Wave latencies and amplitudes are used to assess hearing and conduction of impulses through the brain stem, making BAER testing valuable not only in the diagnosis of hearing loss but also for evaluation of brain stem lesions. Most pets do not require sedation or anesthesia for the procedure, which is beneficial because both cause changes in wave latency. Wave latencies and amplitudes vary with the intensity and rate of delivery of the sound.[3] In general, amplitude increases and latency decreases with increasing sound intensity. Interpeak latencies are used to evaluate conduction in the brain stem, which should not change with stimulus intensity.

Conductive deafness reduces the intensity of sound reaching the inner ear. A lack of air-conducted hearing in the presence of bony-conducted hearing is diagnostic of conductive deafness during BAER. The hearing threshold is usually increased when sound is presented through air conduction, but bony-conducted hearing should remain intact. Increased hearing threshold may be accompanied by decreased wave amplitude and increased wave latency in cases of severe otitis externa.[65] Sensorineural deafness alters the appearance of the BAER, depending on the site of the lesion. Alteration of waveforms, increased hearing threshold, or complete abolition of wave-forms may be present in animals with sensorineural deafness.

Acquired Late-Onset Conductive Deafness

Conductive deafness is due to lack of transmission of sound through the tympanic membrane and ossicles to the inner ear. Conditions that block sound transmission through the external ear canal, tympanic membrane, or middle ear and ossicles, such as otitis externa, otitis media, and otic neoplasia, cause conductive deafness. Less common causes of conductive deafness include trauma-induced fluid accumulation in the middle ear, atresia of the tympanum or ossicles, fused ossicles, or incomplete development of the external ear canal, which results in fluid accumulation in the middle ear.[62,64,66,67] An increase in hearing threshold, absence of air-conducted hearing, and the presence of bone-conducted hearing on BAER suggest conductive deafness.

The application of a bone-anchored hearing aid was described in one dog with conductive deafness after total ear canal ablation.[68] It maintained bone-conducted hearing and tolerated the hearing aid anchored to the parietal bone. Use of a bone-anchored device was required, because the dog did not have an external ear canal in which to place an earpiece. The hearing aid acted as an amplifier, and the dog seemed to respond to its use.

Acquired Late-Onset Sensorineural Deafness

Presbycusis, or decline in hearing associated with aging, may be due to one of the following: loss of hair cells and degeneration in the organ of Corti, degeneration of spiral ganglion cells or neural fibers of the cochlear nerve, atrophy of the stria vascularis, or changes in the basilar membrane. Because this condition occurs in older dogs and cats from 8 to 17 years of age, animals should be evaluated for concurrent causes of conductive deafness such as chronic otitis externa or media and otic neoplasia. BAER testing may demonstrate normal waveforms in response to high-intensity sound.[69] If conduction is intact at an increased hearing threshold, use of an amplifying hearing aid may be beneficial. Pets may not tolerate occlusive types of ear pieces often used in hearing aids, and training to the ear piece should be done prior to application of the hearing aid.

Ototoxic substances, chronic exposure to loud noise, hypothyroidism, trauma, and bony neoplasia can also cause acquired late-onset deafness in dogs and cats. Ototoxicity can result in abolition of waveforms or an increase in hearing threshold on BAER.[3] BAER testing can be used to re-evaluate patients for return of function after withdrawal of medication after exposure to ototoxic medication.

Congenital Sensorineural Deafness

Inherited sensorineural deafness usually results in complete loss of hearing in the affected ear by 5 weeks of age. Many breeds can be affected with the condition (Box 209-1). The condition has been linked to coat color in many breeds of dogs and white cats. The condition is common in white cats, and mode of inheritance is thought to be autosomal dominant

---

Box • 209-1

Canine Breeds Associated with Inherited Deafness

Akita	Ibizan hound
American-Canadian shepherd	Italian greyhound
American cocker spaniel	Jack Russell terrier
American Eskimo	Kuvasz
American Staffordshire terrier	Labrador retriever
Australian cattle dog	Maltese
Australian shepherd	Miniature pincer
Beagle	Miniature poodle mongrel
Bichon frise	Norwegian dunkerhound
Border collie	Nova Scotia duck tolling retriever
Borzoi	Old English sheepdog
Boston terrier	Papillion
Boxer	Pit bull terrier
Bulldog	Pointer
Bull terrier	Poodle (toy & miniature)
Catahoula leopard dog	Puli
Chihuahua	Rhodesian ridgeback
Chow chow	Rottweiler
Collie	Saint Bernard
Dachshund	Schnauzer
Dalmatian	Scottish terrier
Doberman pincer	Sealyham terrier
Dogo Argentino	Shetland sheepdog
English cocker spaniel	Shropshire terrier
English setter	Soft-coated Wheaton terrier
Foxhound	Springer spaniel
Fox terrier	Sussex spaniel
French bulldog	Tibetan spaniel
German shepherd	Tibetan terrier
Great Dane	Walker American foxhound
Great Pyrenees	West Highland white terrier
Greyhound	Yorkshire terrier

with incomplete penetrance.[70] The condition is most common in white cats with blue irides. The correlation of white coat, blue eyes, and deafness is not perfect, but cats with two blue irides have a greater risk of deafness than cats with one blue iris, which have a greater risk of deafness than cats without blue irides.[70] Total hearing loss occurs more often in long-haired white cats.[70] The condition is common in certain breeds of dogs, such as dalmatians, which have a nearly 30% incidence of deafness (combining unilateral and bilateral deafness).

The trait is associated with the dominant merle or dapple gene in collies, Shetland sheepdogs, Great Danes, and dachshunds. The incidence of deafness tends to increase with increasing amount of white in the coat, and dogs homozygous for the merle gene are usually deaf and may be solid white, blind, or sterile.[62] The piebald or extreme piebald gene is associated with deafness in dalmatians, bull terriers, Great Pyrenees, Sealyham terriers, greyhounds, bulldogs, and beagles. Inheritance is thought to be autosomal recessive, but the trait may be polygenic.[64]

Heterochromia irides and lack of retinal pigment are associated with white color in dogs and cats. Hearing loss may be associated with absence of pigment in the cochlear stria vascularis. Diminished blood supply and disorders of endolymph production, with changes in the chemical or mechanical properties of endolymph, lead to degeneration of the organ of Corti secondary to stria vascularis atrophy. Loss of hair cells and abnormalities of the cochlear duct, Reissner membrane, tectorial membrane, and internal spiral sulcus are typical of cochleosaccular type of end-organ degeneration seen in these cases.[3,64,66,70,71]

Clinical signs of deafness may be recognized in puppies as young as 3 weeks of age by astute owners; definitive diagnosis of uni- or bilateral deafness is usually made by BAER testing at 5 to 6 weeks of age when the auditory system is completely developed and cochlear degeneration, if present, is complete.

Congenital Acquired Sensorineural Deafness   Exposure to bacteria, ototoxic drugs, low oxygen tension, and trauma in utero or during the perinatal period rarely causes deafness in young animals.

CHAPTER • 210

Diseases of the Nose and Nasal Sinuses

Anjop J. Venker-van Haagen

FUNCTIONAL CONSIDERATIONS

Functional Anatomy

The nose has four main functions: (1) to provide a portal through which air can flow to reach the alveoli, (2) to modify or regulate the flow of air, (3) to facilitate water and heat exchange (e.g., to condition the inspired air), and (4) to pass inspired air over the olfactory epithelium—the sheet of neurons and supporting cells that lines the nasal cavities. Speculation exists regarding the functions of the nasal sinuses. It seems plausible that the frontal sinuses protect the rostral portions of the brain from frontal trauma.

The apical portion of the nose, consisting of hairless integument and the nostrils, is called the *nasal plane*. It is supported by cartilage, which also supports the portion of the nose between the nasal plane and the bony portion. The levator nasolabial and levator labii superior muscles can move the cartilaginous parts. Dilation of the nostrils changes the pattern of flow of inspired air. The nostrils are dilated when increased airflow is needed, as in dyspnea, and to aid sampling of interesting odors.

The bony case of the nose is the facial portion of the respiratory passageway. The nasal cavity, comprised of bony and cartilaginous parts, extends from the nostrils to the choanae, being divided into right and left halves by the nasal septum. Each half of the nasal cavity has a respiratory and an olfactory region. The nasal conchae—slightly ossified scrolls covered by nasal mucosa—fill the nasal cavities. Together with the nasal glands, the nasal mucosa has a role in *conditioning* the inspired air. During normal inspiration, the respiratory and olfactory air currents are concurrent. When the dog or cat wants to sample environmental odors, the nostrils are dilated and forced inspiration

occurs in which a greater volume of inspired air takes a more dorsal course around the ethmoturbinates, where the olfactory receptors are most numerous.[1]

Regulation and Conditioning of the Inspiratory and Expiratory Airflow

The respiratory airflow through the nasal cavity is regulated by the ventilatory control systems. The nose represents an important part of the resistance of the airway and thereby influences gas exchange in the alveoli. The resistance has to be overcome by greater negative pressure in the thorax during inspiration, which leads to better expanding and filling of the alveoli by the inspired air and a greater venous blood flow in the lungs. In humans, a prolonged increase in nasal resistance due to severe obstruction can lead to cor pulmonale, cardiomegaly, and pulmonary edema.[2] In dogs, pulmonary edema is known to develop in laryngeal obstruction. Pulmonary edema may occur by a similar mechanism when severe obstruction of nasal airflow exists. The most common consequence of increased resistance is, however, mouth breathing.

Heating, or cooling of inspired and expired air as it passes through the nose is largely accomplished by radiation from the mucosal blood vessels. The flow of blood is from posterior to anterior, opposite to the flow of the inspired air. Humidification occurs by evaporation from the blanket of mucus covering the mucosa and the serous fluid from the nasal glands. The nasal blood flow and the activity of the nasal glands are regulated by the autonomic nervous system. The autonomic innervation of the nose consists of parasympathetic and sympathetic nerve fibers, joined together in the vidian nerve. The conditioning of the inspired air by the nose is an important function

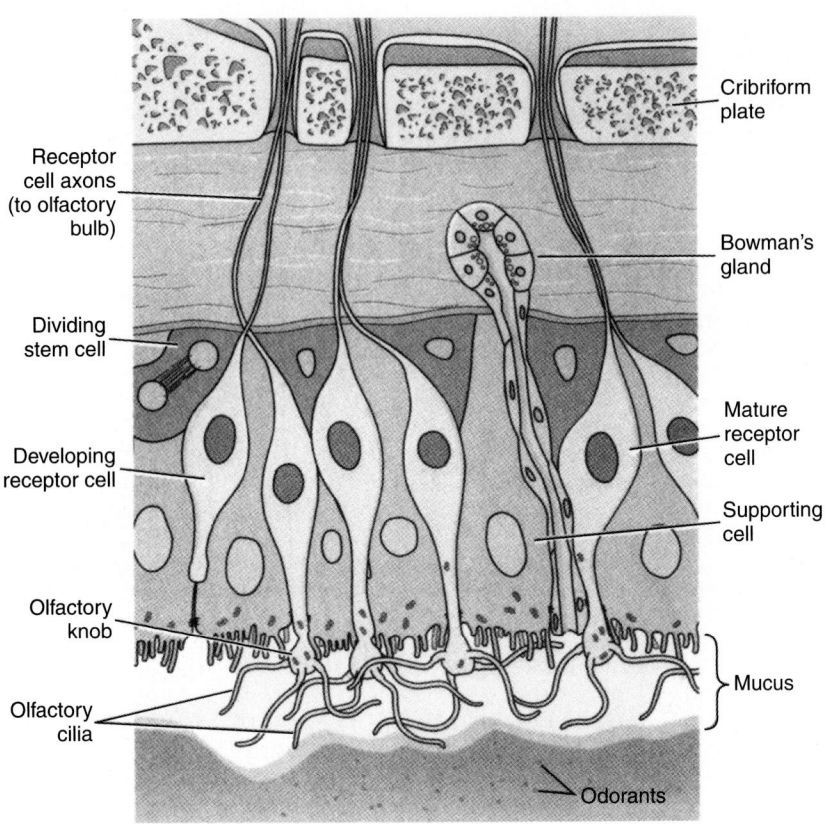

Figure 210-1 Diagram of the olfactory epithelium showing the major cell types and the projection of the olfactory receptor neurons to the bulb (see discussion of Olfaction in text). Bowman's glands produce mucus, and supporting cells help to detoxify chemicals that come in contact with the epithelium. (Courtesy Neuroscience. Sunderland, MA, Sinauer Associates, Inc., 1997, p. 267)

for protection of the alveoli. Even under extremely dry or cold conditions, the bronchi receive air warmed to body temperature with a humidity of around 98%.

Mucosal Cleaning

The pseudostratified respiratory mucosa in the nose consists of ciliated, intermediate, basal, and goblet cells. They rest on a well-defined basement membrane supported by a deep, loose lamina propria containing small blood vessels, venous plexus, and ducts of mucous and serous glands, sensory nerves, and blood cells. The tall ciliated cell is the predominant type, and it extends from the basement membrane to the luminal surface, where cilia admixed with microvilli are found. The cilia actively move the overlying blanket of mucus by a to-and-fro movement, called the *ciliary beat*. A more forceful forward movement and a less forceful recovery beat occurs. The forward movement transports the mucus blanket toward the pharyngeal end of the esophagus. The two-layer mucous blanket is sticky, tenacious, and adhesive. The outer layer is more viscid than the deeper, periciliary layer. Insoluble particles, allergens, and bacteria caught on the outer layer are thus carried to the esophagus. Soluble material reaches the periciliary layer and is absorbed.[3]

Sneezing starts with a rapid inspiration followed by an involuntary, sudden, violent, and audible expulsion of air through the nose and mouth. The reflex occurs after stimulation of sensory receptors in the nasal mucosa. It is the ultimate cleaning procedure for the nasal cavity in dogs and cats.

Olfaction

Three sensory systems are dedicated to the detection of chemicals in the environment: (1) olfaction, (2) taste, and (3) the trigeminal chemosensory system.[4] Olfactory information can influence feeding behavior, social interaction, and reproduction. A dog's sense of smell, together with its personality and intelligence, functions as a nose for humans in many circumstances.

The transduction of olfactory information occurs in the nasal olfactory epithelium, the sheet of neurons and supporting cells that lines the caudolateral wall, the ethmoidal conchae, and the dorsal part of the nasal septum.[5,6] The olfactory receptor neuron is a bipolar neuron that gives rise on its basal surface to an unmyelinated axon that carries the olfactory information to the brain. At its apex the receptor neuron has a single process that expands into a knoblike protrusion from which several microvilli, or olfactory cilia, extend into the thick layer of mucus that lines the nasal cavity and controls the ionic milieu of the olfactory cilia (Figure 210-1).

Generation of receptor potentials in response to odors takes place in the cilia of receptor neurons. The axons of the olfactory receptor cells form the olfactory nerves that pass through the cribriform plate directly to the olfactory bulb, on the anteroventral aspect of the ipsilateral forebrain. Olfactory information is passed to the amygdala and primary olfactory cortex. Further pathways for processing olfactory information include the thalamus, hypothalamus, entorhinal cortex, and hippocampus.[7]

HISTORY, CLINICAL SIGNS, AND PHYSICAL EXAMINATION

History and Clinical Signs

The medical history in nasal disease often includes clear statements of specific problems, because the signs of nasal disease—discharge, sneezing, bleeding—are obvious to the owner. Additional questions should be asked about the animal's general condition, appetite, drinking, activity, and endurance, and about changes in its habits. These questions and a general clinical examination are indicated because some systemic diseases cause nasal discharge (distemper, viral rhinotracheitis) or epistaxis (bleeding disorders), whereas some nasal diseases (such as advanced aspergillosis) can cause general malaise, and dyspnea can occur in obstructive nasal disease.

If nasal discharge is the predominant sign, the following questions should help determine whether it is from the left, the right, or both nostrils. If a nasal discharge is present, it should be characterized (watery, mucoid, pus, blood) and its frequency noted. Discharge occurring only during sneezing indicates a less productive mucosal disease than does continuous discharge. Occasional nasal bleeding is less alarming than frequent and profuse nasal bleeding, which can be fatal.

Sneezing, like coughing, is a reflex associated with protection of the mucosa. Particles, foreign bodies, inflammation of the mucosa, or abnormal turbulence in the nasal cavity associated with local drying of the mucosa can stimulate the sensory receptors in the mucosa. Continuous sneezing can cause irritation of the mucosa, leading to more sneezing and sometimes epistaxis.

Pain in the nose may only become obvious when the animal begins to react adversely to the owner's customary petting. A dog with pain in the nose may object to having a collar or the loop of a leash drawn over its head, even though this is usually associated with the pleasure of a walk. Questions to obtain information about nasal pain should be adapted to the living conditions of the dog or cat.

A nasal stridor is a soft, rustling or sniffing sound that is synchronous with inspiration, expiration, or both. Narrowing of the nasal passageway, which increases the velocity of the airflow, causes the sound.

Dyspnea may be caused by nasal obstruction in cats and dogs, both of which tend to avoid mouth breathing even in this situation, almost to the point of suffocation. Apparently, avoiding the consequent bypassing of the nasal function of air cleansing and conditioning has a high priority.

Physical Examination

After the shape of the nose as a whole is evaluated, the clinician should listen to the animal's respiration for nasal stridor. Under quiet conditions, the clinician should listen close to the dog's (and especially the cat's) nose while gently closing its mouth. If stridor is noted and the clinician suspects it is caused by nostrils that are too narrow, moving the nasal alae laterally can change the tone of the stridor. Symmetry of the airstream can be examined by watching the movement of a small fluff of cotton held in front of each nostril. At the same time, the odor of the expired air can be noted. The area around the nostrils should be inspected for nasal discharge or crusts and the nasal plane for epithelial crusts (which could be caused by pathologic dryness), epithelial lesions, and depigmentation. The ventral wall of the nasal passages, which also forms the roof of the mouth, should be inspected through the opened mouth. The teeth, especially the canine teeth, should be inspected at the same time, because dental abnormalities can cause disorders of the nose.[8] More in-depth inspections belong to special diagnostic procedures and require anesthesia.

SPECIAL DIAGNOSTIC PROCEDURES

Radiography

The standard radiographic examination of the skull consists of a lateral and a dorsoventral projection. These radiographs may provide all the information that is needed, or they may serve as a part of the *survey* examination. These standard projections are usually of limited value in examination of the nose and nasal sinuses, and special projections, such as craniocaudal radiographs, open-mouth projections, or radiographs with intraoral film, are required.

Radiography of the skull demands the most stringent and careful radiographic technique. Any unintended obliquity in positioning will hinder evaluation of the radiographs. Deep sedation or general anesthesia is mandatory. When the diameter of the skull exceeds 10 to 12 cm, a grid must be used to diminish the unfavorable effect of scattered radiation on radiographic quality. A grid is not used when part of the skull is radiographed in open-mouth projections or when radiographs are made with intraoral film. Both nonscreen film in a lightproof envelope for intraoral application and screen film in a cassette with intensifying screens should be available. Nonscreen films require a much longer exposure time but produce radiographs with greater detail.

Radiographs provide a complete overview of the anatomy, with high spatial resolution. However, superimposition of structures on the film may make it difficult and sometimes impossible to distinguish a particular detail, especially when structures differ only slightly in density.

Computed Tomography

Like conventional radiography, computed tomography (CT) is based on differences in attenuation of an x-ray beam in different parts of the body. With the x-ray beam collimated to a narrow fan shape, the x-ray tube revolves around the object during exposure and the beam is altered as it penetrates the object. An array of sensitive detectors on the opposite side of the object quantitates the x-rays passing through, thereby determining the x-ray attenuation in different parts of the object, in all projections. Computer analysis of this collection of attenuation measurements results in a cross-sectional image of the object. This product is then displayed on a monitor with high spatial resolution and higher contrast resolution than can be provided by conventional radiographs. An intravenously administered radiographic contrast agent should help to define normal from abnormal tissue and facilitate the recognition of blood vessels. Because the images represent "slices" of the object, they do not suffer from superimposition, but they also do not provide a survey view.

Positioning of the animal is just as important in CT as in conventional radiography. The position of the object within the gantry will determine the scan plane. Support is perpendicular to the opening of the gantry and perpendicular to the scan plane. Therefore CT of the body is always axial, perpendicular to the long axis of the body, with some adjustment possible through angulation of the gantry relative to the dog or cat. Other scan planes can be achieved if the object can be positioned differently relative to the gantry opening. This is important, because interfaces between organs or structures can only be imaged satisfactorily when they are perpendicular to the scan plane. The head in particular can be easily examined in different scan planes. Transverse (coronal) scans of the head are made with the animal in prone or supine position and the head extended. Dorsal (axial) scans are made with the animal in supine position and the nose pointing upward. Sagittal scans are made with the animal in lateral recumbency and the head raised on a support.

Magnetic Resonance Imaging

Magnetic resonance imaging (MRI) is based on the magnetic properties of atomic nuclei that have an odd number of protons. Because protons are in a continuous state of rotation, called the *nuclear spin*, and have an electrical charge, they may be thought of as tiny magnets. The hydrogen nucleus consists of a single proton, and hydrogen is abundant in living tissues; therefore hydrogen is eminently suitable for MRI.

In the body the magnetic forces of protons point in all directions, canceling each other out. When the body is placed in a strong, homogeneous magnetic field (in clinical imaging, usually between 0.15 and 1.5 Tesla [1 Tesla being 10,000 times the strength of the earth's magnetic field]), the protons are forced into positions parallel to the axis of this magnetic field, not only spinning around their own axes but also around the axis of the magnetic field, like a child's spinning top. The frequency of this *precession* is called the Larmour frequency, and it depends on the strength of the external magnetic field.

Using radio waves of the same frequency as the precession frequency, the protons can be made to resonate: they will precess around the axis of the external magnetic field at a larger angle, and all protons will be in phase. When the radio frequency wave is switched off, pulse relaxation occurs through two phenomena: (1) the protons realign in the magnetic field (T1 relaxation), and (2) they go out of phase (T2 relaxation). During the process of relaxation, the protons emit weak radio signals; it is these signals that are used to create the images. The images may be dominated by the concentration of protons (proton density), by T1 relaxation (T1-weighted images), or by T2 relaxation (T2-weighted images).

By using gradient coils to create small variations in the x, y, or z direction of the external magnetic field, certain scan planes and slices can be selected in which the precession of protons has exactly the right frequency to be susceptible to the radio wave pulses. Images can then be made in different scan planes without having to reposition the patient. These images are influenced by the concentration of hydrogen nuclei in the part of the body being examined, by the chemical nature of the environment the nuclei are in, and by the interactions between nuclei. MRI provides detailed anatomic images with soft tissue contrast that is superior to that of CT. The soft tissue contrast may be further enhanced by the intravenous administration of a contrast medium that is a paramagnetic substance (usually gadolinium). Its predominant effect is to shorten T1, so the regions that take it up are bright on T1-weighted images (Figure 210-2).

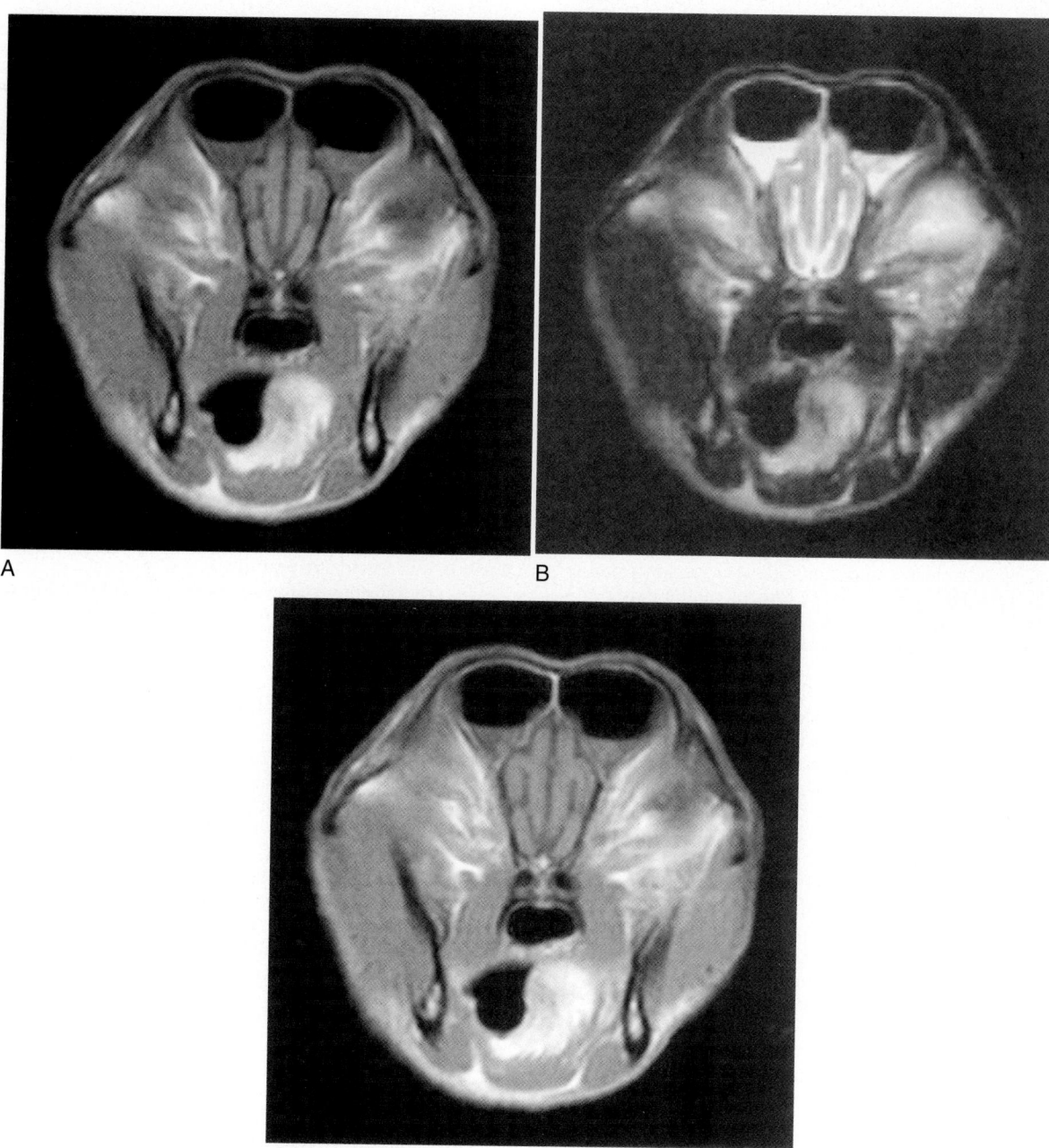

Figure 210-2 Transverse magnetic resonance image (MRI) showing fluid in the frontal sinuses of a dog. The fluid is dark on a T1-weighted image (**A**) and bright on a T2-weighted image (**B**). After the intravenous administration of contrast medium, the T1-weighted image (**C**) reveals enhancement of the well-vascularized mucosa of the frontal sinus but not of the fluid.

Rhinoscopy

Rhinoscopy is a relatively simple procedure in dogs and cats. It requires anesthesia and tracheal intubation to prevent air circulation through the nasal cavities. Most veterinarians prefer to perform the examination with the dog or cat in sternal recumbency, in a sphinxlike posture. A firm pillow is placed between the head and the front legs so that the head is stabilized but not fixed. The rhinoscopic examination is preceded by a careful inspection of the oral cavity and the pharynx.

A simple otoscope can be used for visualization. It should be of good quality, having a strong light source and dark specula, to illuminate the rostral part of the nasal cavity. The nostril is approached from the lateral side at an angle of 45 degrees to the vertical surface of the nasal plane. The tip of the speculum is placed near the lateral limit of the nostril and is then introduced by slowly turning the otoscope until its line of vision is parallel to the nasal cavity. This movement is necessary to push the nasal ala, which obstructs the opening, into a lateral position.

Once the otoscope is introduced, visibility is often poor. Nasal disease often causes discharge and the tip of the speculum can become blocked by mucus. The lens of the otoscope can be slid slightly to one side, allowing the introduction of a small suction cannula while vision through the lens is maintained. The mucus is removed under visual control, and the rostral part of the nasal cavity is then examined.

The use of an otoscope is often preferable for diagnosis and removal of foreign bodies that have entered the nasal cavity via the nostril. A forceps (called a *foreign body forceps*) developed for use through an otoscope under visual guidance can be found in catalogs for human otoscopic instruments.

An endoscope is needed for complete examination of the nasal cavity. The basic equipment includes a light source, a flexible fiber-optic cable, and a small diameter endoscope. The author and colleagues prefer the 25-degree vision rigid endoscope that is 2.7 mm in diameter and about 15 cm long. The best instruments have a wide-angle lens, which is important for orientation and facilitates the examination. This scope is adequate for most cats and dogs. For small cats, a 1.2 mm diameter rigid scope is needed. In most cats and dogs the 2.7 mm scope can be introduced, and alongside it a suction cannula (size 6) or a foreign body or biopsy forceps can be passed.

The light source for rhinoscopy can be a single-outlet model, but a combined light source and electronic flash generator is necessary to obtain photographic images. The camera should be adapted to the telescope and the timing of the flash. For teaching purposes a chip camera and a video recorder are great assets. Additional equipment for rhinoscopy includes several suction cannulas (size 6), a vacuum source, a selection of biopsy forceps, and a small dropper bottle of 0.1% adrenaline solution to stop profuse bleeding (no more than 1 or 2 drops should be used at a time).

The anatomic borders that guide the inspection of the nasal cavity are the nostril rostrally, the nasal septum medially, the roof of the nasal cavity dorsally, and the bottom of the nasal cavity ventrally. The cribriform plate is part of the caudal boundary, the other part being the ventrally positioned opening to the nasal pharynx, the choanae. The endoscopic procedure aims at bringing the greater part of the nasal cavity into view. The procedure is limited by the choanae, if not by the pathologic process. Careful maneuvering and repositioning of the endoscope should result in a reliable impression of the normal and pathologic structures in the nasal cavity.

The main indications for rhinoscopy are a history of unilateral nasal discharge, the known or probable entrance of a foreign body, obstructive disease indicating tumor with no conclusive radiographic findings, and severe rhinitis with a suspicion of aspergillosis. In all other cases of chronic nasal disease with no significant findings by radiography, rhinoscopy might be helpful but is not always conclusive.

The inspection of the nasopharynx and choanae can be accomplished with a flexible endoscope having a diameter of 4 mm and being capable of 180-degree retrospective vision, introduced via the mouth and then around the soft palate. This instrument not only provides visualization of the lesions but also affords the opportunity to biopsy.

Olfactory Tests

No simple method exists to study olfaction in dogs. The sense of smell should be tested by activation of the olfactory receptor neurons and activation of the brain. The activation of the brain is recorded by electroencephalographic olfactometry analysis. Some authors have reported results in dogs with supposed normal olfactory function and in those that have lost the sense of smell.[9-11]

CONGENITAL DISEASES

Congenital malformation of the nasal plane is a common finding in brachycephalic breeds. The cartilage supporting the nasal plane is soft; thus the alae collapse, closing the nares. Corrective surgery is a simple procedure and consists of removing a cone-shaped piece of the ala and suturing the sides of the incision together in such a way that the nasal opening is enlarged.[12]

In dogs and cats, variable congenital lesions of the nasal plane or more extensive clefts can be repaired surgically. The success of surgery is largely dependant on the available tissue around the cleft. Oronasal and oropharyngeal clefts cause rhinitis and should be considered for surgical repair. Euthanasia may be justified if repair is not possible and nasal discharge and dysphagia are causing recurrent fever and pain. Nasal dermoid sinus cysts have been reported in dogs.[13] This cyst is recognized as a fistula in the midline of the bridge of the nose, producing intermittent discharge. Exploration of the fistula may reveal skin and hair as far down as the nasal septum. This abnormally located tissue must be completely removed before the skin incision is closed. A congenital cerebrospinal fluid (CSF) fistula, causing rhinorrhea, was reported in a cat. It was closed successfully.[14]

The frontal sinuses are variable in size and sometimes even absent. Their absence is not associated with clinical signs. Congenital ciliary dysfunction has been documented in dogs of various breeds. Primary ciliary dyskinesia is a disorder in which ciliary function is ineffective and uncoordinated, resulting in rhinitis, bronchitis, bronchiectasis, and bronchopneumonia. When associated with situs inversus, the clinical syndrome is known as *Kartagener's syndrome*. The initial signs (nasal discharge and coughing) usually begin at an early age, from days to 5 weeks of age. However, some dogs have remained asymptomatic for months. Complications are caused by colonization of the mucosa and the conchae by *Pasteurella multocida* and *Bordetella bronchiseptica*, which can cause hypoplastic conchae via bone resorption.

Mucociliary clearance in the dog's nasal cavity can be measured by placing a small drop of ^{99m}Tc macroaggregated albumin deep in the cavity, via a catheter, beyond the non-ciliated rostral half. The velocity of mucus clearance ranges from 7 to 20 mm/min.[15] The test is not affected by anesthesia. However, not all normal dogs have a clearance rate within the reference range, and inflammation can change the velocity of the ciliary beat. To avoid spurious values, the test should be repeated and performed bilaterally.

Functional analysis of cilia in vitro is performed by examining transverse sections in electron micrographs after glutaraldehyde-osmium fixation. Major ultrastructural lesions in cilia of dogs with primary ciliary dyskinesia include lack of outer dynein arms, an abnormal microtubular pattern, and an electron-dense core in the basal body.[15] The prognosis is guarded.

Affected dogs that develop severe recurrent bronchopneumonia usually die of sepsis. Continuous treatment with broad-spectrum antibiotics may enable such dogs to survive longer. Therefore cultures should be repeated to maintain correct antibiotic treatment based on sensitivity testing. A worthwhile review of treatment and long-term survival in dogs is available.[15]

INFLAMMATORY DISEASES

Viral Rhinitis

Viral rhinitis is a prominent disease in cats. The initial clinical signs are paroxysmal sneezing, conjunctivitis, and serous ocular and nasal discharge. About 5 days after the onset of sneezing, the nasal discharge becomes mucopurulent and there may be ocular complications. The condition usually persists for 2 to 3 weeks. Feline herpesvirus-1 (FHV-1) and feline calicivirus (FCV) are the most prevalent and virulent respiratory pathogens of cats and account for at least 80% to 90% of their infectious upper respiratory tract (URT) infections.[16,17] The introduction of modified-live virus (MLV) vaccine against these two viruses has substantially decreased mortality and morbidity but has not eliminated the diseases. Immunization against these viruses protects the cat from development of severe disease but not from infection.[18]

Because these viruses can spread rapidly among kittens and the prevalence of chronically infected virus carriers is high, elimination of the disease is not feasible. It is estimated that 80% of cats recovering from acute infection become chronic carriers. The predominant route of infection is by direct cat-to-cat contact.[19] The chronic carrier state may develop subsequent to infection with either FHV or FCV and also occurs in vaccinated cats. Although cats carrying FHV do not necessarily shed virulent virus continuously, they should be considered infectious when they are sneezing and have nasal discharge. Calicivirus carriers shed virulent virus continuously from the oropharynx. They may have no clinical signs or mild nasal discharge, gingival ulceration, and periodontitis.

Viral rhinitis is a prominent clinical sign of canine distemper (Figure 210-3). Vaccination has reduced the occurrence of the disease to sporadic cases in countries where stray dogs are limited and veterinary care adequate. Herpes infection in newborn puppies is characterized by profuse mucopurulent nasal discharge. The diagnosis is usually made at autopsy.

Bacterial Rhinitis

Primary bacterial rhinitis is uncommon in both dogs and cats. Bacterial rhinitis develops as a sequela to viral rhinitis in cats, can be caused by foreign bodies in both dogs and cats, and occurs secondary to many other disorders due to disruption of normal mucociliary mucosal integrity.

Mycotic Rhinitis

Mycotic diseases involving the nasal cavity, the frontal sinuses, and the nasal plane occur in both dogs and cats. In dogs the most prevalent mycosis in the nasal cavity and frontal sinuses is caused by *Aspergillus* spp. The fungus is also found rarely in the nasal cavity in cats. *Cryptococcus neoformans* is a more common cause of mycotic nasal disease in cats and in certain geographic areas is quite common; nasal infections also occur in dogs. *Alternaria* spp. may infest the nasal plane in cats, causing proliferation of the skin and thereby dyspnea.

Aspergillus spp. are considered to be opportunists, producing infections in man and animals, especially when resistance to infection is reduced or when large numbers of spores are present. Spores of *Aspergillus fumigates* are present on household plants, on furniture made of plant material, around bird cages, and simply in house dust.[20]

In dogs, *Aspergillus* spp. plaques are usually found in the caudal part of the nasal cavity or in the frontal sinus. They are presumed to represent primary infections. The toxins produced by the fungus cause atrophy of the conchae in the areas of the fungus plaques and severe destruction of the mucosa and underlying structures in the entire nasal cavity and frontal sinus. There may be bone resorption and periostitis on the frontal bones, and atrophy and resorption of the internal surface of the frontal bone may open the way to the brain. The disease may spread bilaterally, destroying all internal and external bony structures, as well as the orbit, the nasal septum, and the nasal plane. *A. fumigatus* was identified in 25 of 27 of dogs (involving the sinus and related structures).[20] Disseminated aspergillosis caused by *A. terreus*, not originating from the airways, has also been reported.[21] *Aspergillus* spp. can be associated with long-standing traumatic changes in the mucosa, caused by persisting foreign bodies in the nasal cavity or oronasal fistulas. These infections are presumed to be secondary to the trauma.

Clinical signs of aspergillosis in the nose and frontal sinus are dominated by profuse mucopurulent nasal discharge and nasal pain. Depigmentation of the nasal plane below the nostril from which discharge appears is a characteristic sign (Figure 210-4). Intermittent hemorrhagic discharge occurs and

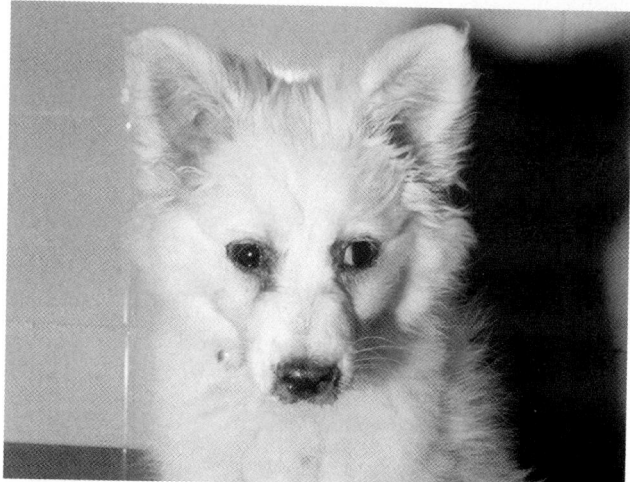

Figure 210-3 A 5-month-old Samoyed with distemper and bilateral mucopurulent discharge. Viral rhinitis is a prominent clinical sign of canine distemper.

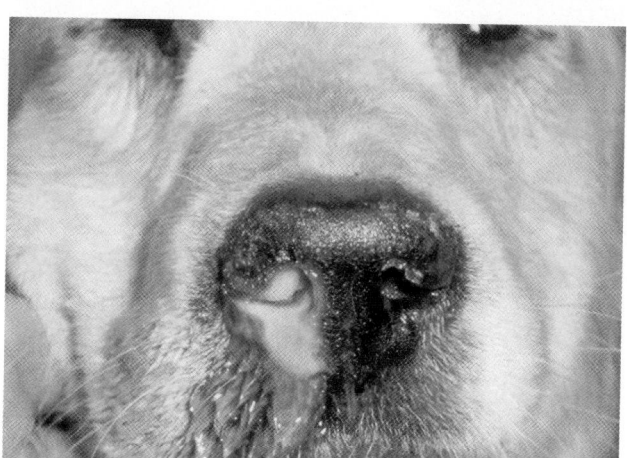

Figure 210-4 Depigmentation of the nasal plane below the nostril from which discharge appears in a dog with nasal aspergillosis in the right nasal cavity.

profuse nasal bleeding is not unusual. When only the frontal sinus is infected, hemorrhagic discharge or profuse bleeding from the nose may be the only sign. The nasal infection is often unilateral initially, becoming bilateral later. Aspergillosis is often not suspected in its initial stage, and histories of nasal discharge present for months are common. No apparent correlation exists between the duration of the initial nasal discharge and the severity or progression of signs by the time of diagnosis. Other factors, such as the number of infecting spores and the resistance of the host, may play a role. Depression is a prominent sign when the frontal sinus is infected.

The diagnosis of aspergillosis as the cause of rhinitis is made by the finding of fungal plaques or positive fungal culture results. Recognition of the fungus plaque is facilitated by the atrophy of the conchae around it, which reduces the normal obstruction to rhinoscopic vision in the caudal part of the nasal cavity (Figure 210-5). The extent of the destruction in the nasal cavities and the frontal sinuses is well demonstrated by radiography, CT, or MRI, but the diagnosis depends on finding the fungus (Figure 210-6). When the fungus is in the frontal sinus alone, radiographs usually demonstrate irregular soft tissue densities in the frontal sinus, thickening of the wall of the sinus, and sometimes reaction of the periosteum. A CT scan may reveal the severity of further bony involvement. A 3 to 4 mm diameter trephined opening in the frontal bone on the side of the affected sinus can reveal the fungus as thick, grayish-yellow material, sometimes with greenish lumps. This material should be removed and cultured. Cultures from nasal discharge are often negative because the fungus is usually located in the caudal part of the nasal cavity and is not shed in the nasal discharge. A serologic test is available for detecting antibodies to *Aspergillus* spp. in serum.

Treatment of sinonasal aspergillosis is topical or systemic. Topical treatment is usually with enilconazole or clotrimazole. The choice between these two drugs is arbitrary, because there has been no satisfactory clinical trial to compare them. The ongoing discussion is how to apply the suspensions and how long the treatment should be given. The basic idea is to flush the frontal sinus and the nasal cavity (e.g., via tubes

introduced through trephine holes). The author's clinical experience (in about 120 cases; an average of 10 per year) indicates that administration of 10 cc of a 10% suspension of enilconazole per tube twice daily for 14 days is sufficient. It is unpleasant for the dog because enilconazole has a bitter taste that most dogs dislike intensely. A retrospective study of cases treated in our clinic (unpublished data) revealed success in about 95% in over 100 cases. Hence 90% success can be expected. A less unpleasant systemic treatment would be much preferred, but the success rates and observed toxicities of other methods are not yet encouraging. Details on clotrimazole therapy have been published.[17]

Cryptococcosis is found as a cause of rhinitis in dogs and cats. The clinical signs are obstructive rhinitis and mucopurulent discharge. In cats, crusts sometimes occur on the nasal plane and the bridge of the nose. Some cats develop mucopurulent conjunctivitis. In fresh material from the nose placed on a slide and stained with India ink, *Cryptococcus* spp. organisms are recognized as thick, encapsulated, round to oval yeasts. They can be cultured on Sabouraud's agar.

Ketoconazole, itraconazole, or fluconazole can be used for therapy, which should be continued for 8 weeks. *Alternaria* spp. are found to cause granulomatous infections with crusts on the nasal plane in cats. Antimycotic treatment may be disappointing and removal of the nasal plane, as in nasal plane squamous cell carcinoma, can be a satisfactory solution.[22]

Neurogenic Rhinitis

The clinical signs of neurogenic rhinitis in dogs are dryness of the nasal plane on one or both sides, sometimes with crusts, and slight mucopurulent nasal discharge. The most frequent clinical signs are dryness of one side of the nasal plane together with ipsilateral keratoconjunctivitis sicca and mucopurulent conjunctivitis. The cause of the disorder is loss of parasympathetic innervation and when keratitis sicca is present, the dysfunction also affects the lacrimal, palatine, and nasal glands.[23] In dogs with this disorder, ipsilateral otitis media can be suspected if reddening of the tympanic membrane is noted. The lesion in the parasympathetic nerves may be caused by otitis media, because the parasympathetic nerves are carried in the chorda tympani and pass freely through the middle ear. In all cases, treatment of the otitis media with broad-spectrum antibiotics resolved all problems.

Diagnosis of neurogenic rhinitis is more difficult when it is bilateral. The Schirmer tear test should be helpful, but no values have been reported. Clinical examination and exclusion of other causes may lead to presumption of a possible neurogenic cause. Massaging nonperfumed moistening cream into the nasal plane eight times daily and administering four drops of artificial tears into the nasal cavity four times daily will resolve the clinical signs if the diagnosis is correct. This treatment will be required lifelong, because no known specific treatment for the parasympathetic nerve dysfunction exists.

Specific Rhinitis

Polyps occur in the nasal cavity in both dogs and cats. They consist of focal accumulation of edema fluid, hyperplasia of the submucosal connective tissue, and a variable inflammatory infiltrate of eosinophils, plasma cells, and lymphocytes. Hence they are not neoplastic but inflammatory polyps.[24] They are found in the nasal cavity of cats with signs of obstructive rhinitis. Bilateral obstruction may be caused by bilateral polyps or a unilateral polyp that extends into the nasopharynx.

Diagnosis is usually made by rhinoscopy. The polyp is seen as a red mass in the nasal cavity, and biopsy reveals it to be inflammatory tissue. Removal is difficult, usually requiring removal of all structures in the nasal cavity through a small opening in the nasal bone. This damages the olfactory epithelium,

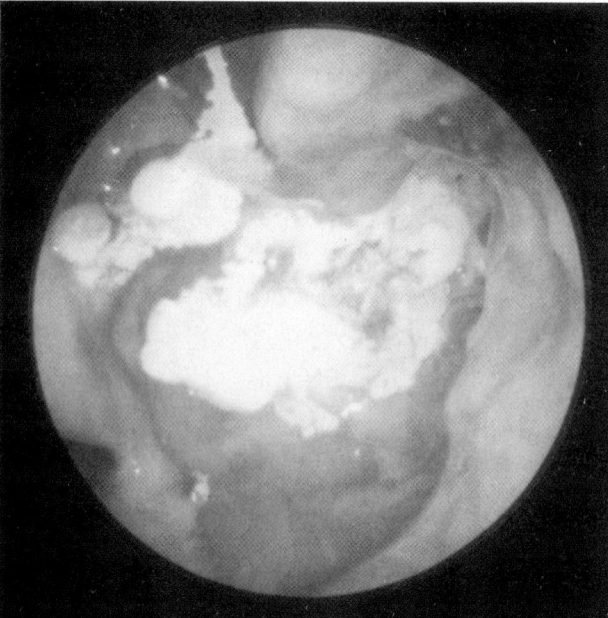

Figure 210-5 Aspergillus plaque. A rhinoscopic view in the caudal part of the nasal cavity.

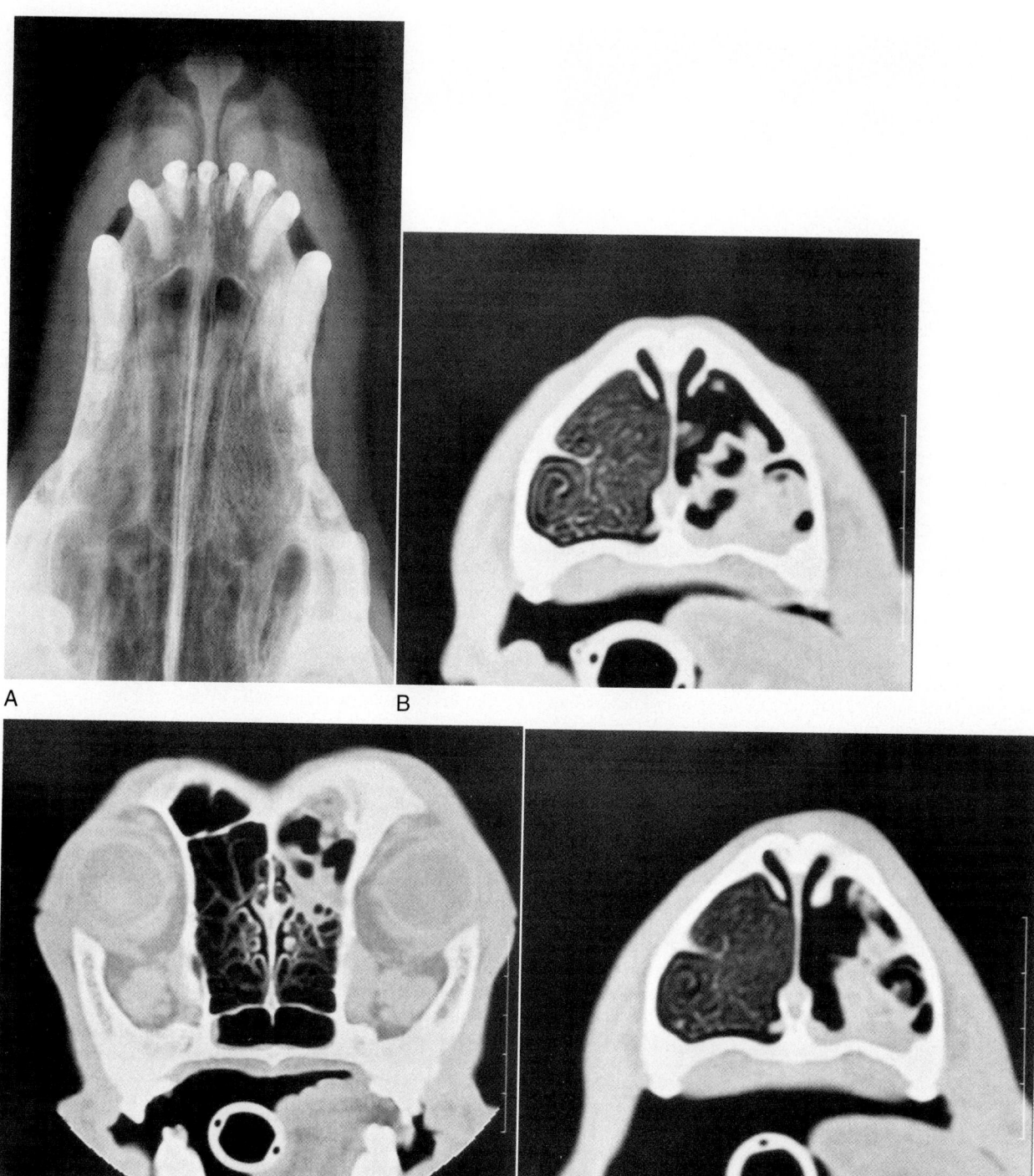

Figure 210-6 **A,** Dorsoventral radiograph (intraoral nonscreen film) of the nasal cavity of a Great Dane with aspergillosis of the left nasal cavity and frontal sinus. **B to E,** Transverse 5 mm thick computed tomography (CT) images of the nose and frontal sinuses of the same dog before (**B and C**) and 6 weeks after (**D and E**) successful treatment. The reader should note the remnants of the trephined openings in the nasal and frontal bones. No obvious differences exist between CT images before and after treatment. The extent of the destruction in the nasal cavities and the frontal sinuses is well shown by radiography and CT, but the diagnosis depends on demonstrating the fungus.

and recognition of food is disturbed. When one nasal cavity is freed of polyps, the cat regains its sense of smell with help from the intact side. Bilateral surgery should be avoided and, when necessary, only performed after the cat seems to be fully recovered from the first operation.

Polyps in the nasal cavity are rare in dogs. They are diagnosed by rhinoscopy and biopsy, which reveals inflammatory tissue. They are usually unilateral. Rhinotomy via the nasal bone and removal of all conchae and the polypous tissue relieves the obstruction. Histologic examination will reveal

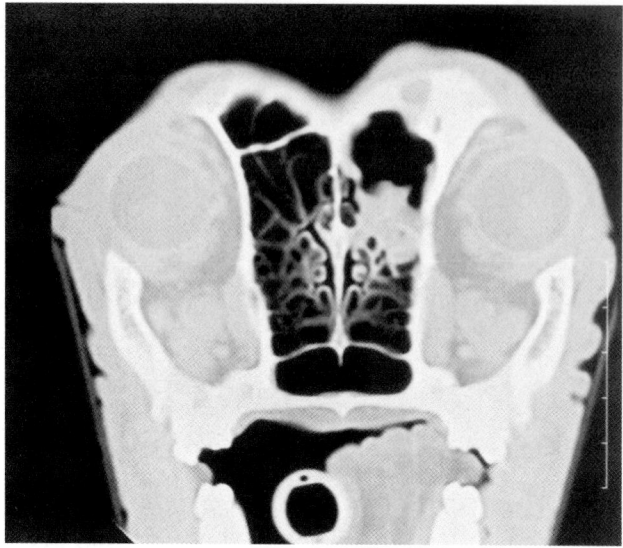

E

Figure 210-6—Cont'd

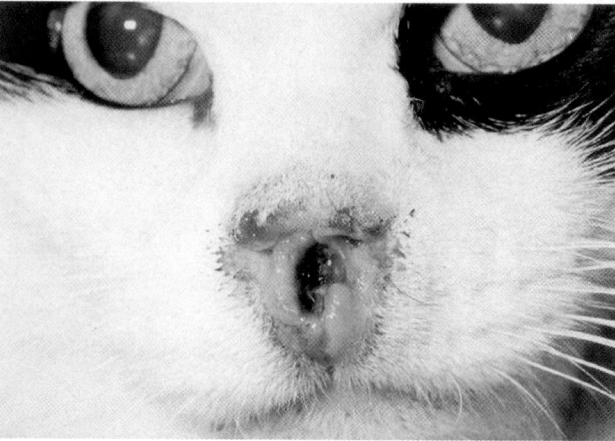

Figure 210-7 Squamous cell carcinoma of the nasal plane of a cat. Biopsy is required to differentiate tumor from inflammatory tissue.

whether the structure is a polyp or an unexpected neoplasm. In dogs, polyps usually recur after 1 or 2 years, but in cats recurrence is rare.

In young dogs and cats, foreign bodies such as grass and other plant material are common. Owners may know when the material entered the nasal cavity, usually via the nostril. Being plant material, the foreign body has the density of soft tissue and is usually not visualized on radiographs. Rhinoscopy in search of a foreign body needs patience and the use of suction, under visual control, to remove mucopurulent exudate before the foreign material is exposed and can be removed. Grass can enter the nasal cavity while a cat is chewing on it, as cats often do. Out of a ball of mucus and grass in the pharynx, a sprig of grass can enter the nasal cavity via the nasopharynx. It can be found by rhinoscopy and removed under visual control via the nostril.

Nasal allergic rhinitis is presumed to occur, but confirmation of the diagnosis has not yet been convincing, partly because IgE-based rhinitis, as occurs in human, has yet to be demonstrated.

TUMORS OF THE NASAL PLANE, NASAL CAVITY, AND FRONTAL SINUS

Tumors of the Nasal Plane

Squamous cell carcinoma of the nasal plane is found in cats in most countries of the world (Figure 210-7). The diagnosis should be made by biopsy, but the diagnosis is often delayed because initial biopsies may only reveal inflammation. When the tumor grows and destruction of tissue is in progress, total removal of the process is justified, provided that the removed tissue is submitted for histologic examination. In the differential diagnosis of processes causing proliferation of the tissue of the nasal plane, with crusts and destruction, infection by *Alternaria* spp. and eosinophilic granuloma should be included. Both are easily identified in biopsy material. Surgical removal of the neoplastic nasal plane in cats has been instructively described.[25] One firm incision will allow histologic confirmation of a tumor-free cut surface. Squamous cell carcinoma of the nasal plane sometimes occurs in dogs. The cosmetic results of removal of the nasal plane are less satisfactory in dogs than in cats. In both, the best results are obtained when

tumor growth does not yet extend around the nasal plane. Other tumors of the nasal plane are fibroma and fibrosarcoma, which grow initially beneath the epithelium and do not ulcerate primarily. Surgical removal in an early stage is possible without too much cosmetic damage.

Tumors of the Nasal Cavity

Tumors occur in the nasal cavity of dogs and cats of all ages, but most often in pets over 5 years of age. Almost all are malignant. They invade the surrounding tissue but rarely metastasize before the dog or cat is euthanized. The most frequent tumors are squamous cell carcinoma and adenocarcinoma; less frequent are chondrosarcoma, osteosarcoma, and lymphosarcoma.

The clinical signs include sneezing, hemorrhagic discharge, and mucopurulent discharge. In most cases, unilateral obstruction of the nasal cavity is recognized because of nasal stridor. No evidence of pain is observed, and the dog or cat becomes dyspneic only when the mouth is closed, which means when sleeping. As long as the tumor is unilateral, the dyspnea is moderate. When the tumor obstructs both nasal cavities, dyspnea during sleep becomes a serious hindrance, causing the animal to awaken repeatedly during the night and often be very depressed in the morning. When no therapy is offered beyond permanent tracheostomy, which is rarely accepted by the owner, recurrent nasal bleeding and dyspnea are the usual reasons for euthanasia, in both dogs and cats. Cats, however, often stop eating, which may provide a humane end point and a reason for euthanasia.

Radiographs should be obtained with the dog or cat under anesthesia. Tumor is suspected when increased density is found in one or both nasal cavities, with loss of normal maxillary and ethmoidal conchae.[26] The extension of the tumor should be considered when estimating the animal's life expectancy, but this is usually decided by the owner's interpretation of the quality of the animal's life. In all cases in which the radiographic diagnosis is uncertain, rhinoscopy is the next diagnostic procedure. Under rhinoscopic visualization the tumors vary greatly in shape and firmness, and their color ranges from gray to deep red. Biopsies are always taken for histologic confirmation of the diagnosis. If no therapy is planned, neither CT nor MRI is indicated. Radiation therapy could be considered, and details have been described.[27]

Tumors of the Frontal Sinus

Tumors in the frontal sinus develop within a bony case. The frontal sinus does not have a specific function; therefore development of the tumor will be noticed only when unilateral nasal bleeding is recurrent or when the enlarging tumor causes pressure atrophy of the frontal bone and becomes apparent as a swelling arising in the frontal sinus.

In the diagnostic investigation of recurrent nasal bleeding, radiographs will be made of the nasal cavity and the frontal sinus, and a radiographic density in the frontal sinus will be noticed. The differential diagnosis of such a density in combination with a radiographically normal ipsilateral nasal cavity includes aspergillosis, tumor, and accumulation of mucus associated with obstruction of the nasofrontal duct. Because the frontal sinus is separated from the brain by only a thin layer of bone, additional diagnostic imaging by CT or MRI is valuable. When a swelling arising in the frontal sinus is recognized by physical examination, the same procedure of taking radiographs followed by CT or MRI is indicated. With these imaging tools, extent of the lesion and differentiation of the contents of the frontal sinus may be determined. Tumor in the frontal sinus can be recognized by CT or MRI with an intravenously administered contrast medium. Vital tissue will be enhanced by the contrast medium, whereas debris will not. It must then be determined by CT or MRI whether the bony case of the frontal sinus is intact, especially whether the orbit or the brain is invaded, and whether the contralateral frontal sinus is included in the process.

When these procedures indicate that the tumor can be removed, a surgical approach via the frontal bone is indicated. At the end of the surgical procedure it is important to examine the patency of the nasofrontal duct and to relieve any obstruction. Like tumors in the nasal cavity, most tumors in the frontal sinus are malignant, and complete surgical removal is unlikely. Biopsy of the tumor through a small trephined opening in the frontal bone should be considered as an intermediate step.

TRAUMA TO THE FRONTAL SINUS AND THE NOSE

Trauma to the Frontal Sinus

Blunt or sharp objects can cause traumatic injury to the frontal sinus. The frontal bone in dogs and cats is relatively thick and provides good protection, so a fracture of it implies that a heavy blow to the head has occurred. The pet should therefore be given a thorough clinical examination for (1) signs of shock such as tachycardia, hypotension (prolonged capillary refill time, weak pulse), rapid respiration, dilation of the pupils, hypothermia, muscle weakness, restlessness, and depression or even coma[28] and (2) other fractures or wounds. Frontal bone fractures do not require immediate attention unless brain damage is suspected. In the absence of signs of brain damage, and when other traumatic injuries have been attended to, the nature and extent of the frontal bone fracture should be examined by radiography, CT, or both (Figure 210-8). Prolonged anesthesia is needed; thus these procedures are usually delayed for 24 hours or more.

When bone fragments are seen to be present in the frontal sinus they should be removed. Like any foreign body, small bone fragments are likely to become sequestered. Surgery should be performed with full attention to aseptic procedures. Before attempting reconstruction of the frontal bone, it is important to examine the patency of the nasofrontal duct and to relieve any obstruction. Airtight suturing of the subcutis, including periosteum, followed by routine skin closure prevents the development of subcutaneous emphysema. Administration of broad-spectrum antibiotics for 3 weeks and strict limitation of activity during this period (keeping a cat confined to the house) will prevent complications.

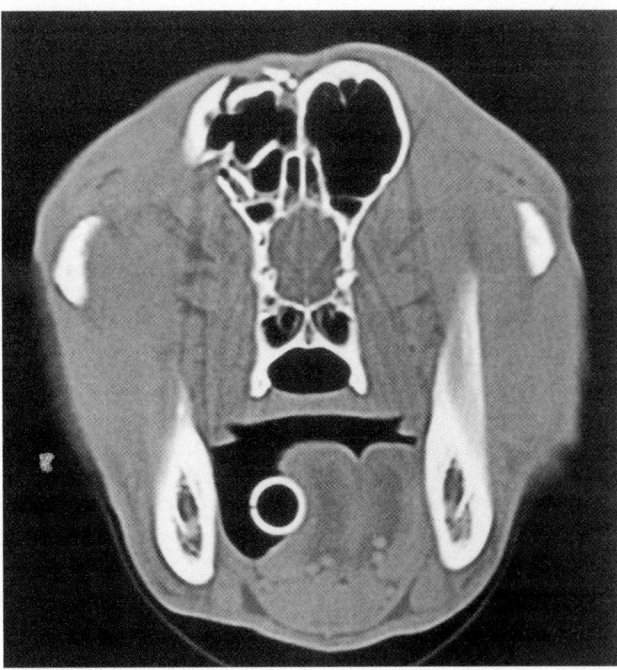

Figure 210-8 Transverse 5 mm thick computed tomography (CT) image through the frontal sinuses of a Labrador retriever with fractures of the right frontal sinus caused by being struck by a car. CT allows accurate assessment of the nature and extent of the fractures and identification of loose fragments in the frontal sinus. Bone fragments seen in the frontal sinus should be removed.

Trauma to the Nose

Trauma to the nose is characterized by massive bleeding, which adds to the other effects of the impact in promoting shock. A thorough examination for signs of this is indicated (see Trauma to the Frontal Sinus). Fractures and wounds should be noted, but priority must usually be given to the treatment of hypovolemic shock.

When the dog or cat is sufficiently stable, the larger vessels should be ligated and skin sutures should be placed as needed. Skin sutures, sometimes supported by subcutaneous sutures, may be sufficient to remodel the outer form of the nose. Fractures of the choanae are best left alone, because they are unlikely to ever result in obstruction. Severe traumatic damage to the nose almost always causes temporary obstruction, making tracheotomy necessary. Adequate oxygenation aids in avoiding general malaise and loss of appetite. Liquid or soft food facilitates eating. In dogs the tracheal cannula is often left in place for 10 days or longer. In cats that have difficulties with long-term tracheostomy, a small intranasal catheter may be placed and connected to the oxygen supply. Use of this method, however, depends on the pathway through the wounded nose. In the author's experience, the nose is functionally adequate in 2 to 3 weeks. If needed, more corrective surgery could be attempted after 6 weeks.

EPISTAXIS

Epistaxis (i.e., nasal bleeding) is often spontaneous and transient, and it is apparently due to a local cause. When it is recurrent or profuse, with considerable loss of blood, diagnostic investigation is indicated. The several causes of epistaxis should be considered in planning diagnostic procedures. Recurring epistaxis occurs in both dogs and cats, but profuse nasal bleeding occurs mostly in dogs. Recurring epistaxis in dogs and cats can be caused by ulcerative rhinitis, mycotic rhinitis, and tumor in the nasal cavity. Profuse nasal bleeding in dogs is most often caused by aspergillosis in the nasal cavity or frontal sinus, or it is caused by tumor in the nasal cavity and frontal sinus. Epistaxis can also be the sole sign of defects in primary hemostasis (platelet plug formation) or secondary hemostasis (coagulation cascade).[29] Lesions in the nasal mucosa leading to epistaxis can also occur with systemic diseases such as leishmaniasis and amyloidosis.

Epistaxis caused by local disease in the nasal cavity or frontal sinus is approached (as are all nasal diseases) by a general and specific examination for nasal disease, as described earlier in this chapter. When the bleeding has occurred recently, radiographic examination should preferably be delayed for at least 48 hours because clotted blood can be misinterpreted as a mass in the nasal cavity. Rhinoscopy should also be delayed for at least 48 hours after the bleeding has stopped, because the presence of blood clots hinders inspection and could lead to misinterpretation of findings.

In the meantime, profuse nasal bleeding should be stopped. It is best to sedate the animal (phenobarbital [2 mg/kg] is advised, because it does not affect blood pressure). After considerable blood loss, sedation that causes hypotension could lead to shock in association with hypovolemia and should therefore be avoided. Sedation will help stop bleeding.

Nasal tamponade is only acceptable for a short period and under anesthesia. For less profuse bleeding, nasal drops of 0.1% adrenaline are helpful. The use of adrenaline should, however, be restricted. Overdose could cause death due to vasoconstriction of the arteries supplying the brain. The administration of three drops in one of the nasal cavities in dogs and one drop in cats, repeated up to three times per 24 hours, is acceptable and effective when used during the bleeding. It should not be used in an attempt to prevent nasal bleeding. When examination of the nasal cavity and the frontal sinus reveals no cause for the bleeding, further investigation of primary diseases causing hemostasis is indicated.

Acknowledgement

The author acknowledges the contributions in the field of diagnostic imaging of George Voorhout, DVM, PhD, Division of Diagnostic Imaging, Faculty of Veterinary Medicine, Utrecht University.

CHAPTER • 211

Diseases of the Throat

Nolie K. Parnell

GENERAL ANATOMY AND PHYSIOLOGY

The throat is an important, but mostly ignored, communal area of both the gastrointestinal (GI) and respiratory tracts. Anatomically it is divided into the pharynx and larynx. The pharynx is further divided into the nasopharynx, the oropharynx, and the laryngopharynx. The nasopharynx is located dorsal to the soft palate, between the choanae and the intrapharyngeal opening. It is a functional space that allows the nasal cavity to communicate with the larynx. The oropharynx is ventral to the soft palate and extends from the palatoglossal arches rostrally to the base of the epiglottis caudally. The intrapharyngeal opening and the rostral border of the esophagus create the boundaries of the laryngopharynx, the most caudal part of the pharynx.[1] The laryngopharynx functions as an intersection to both the respiratory and digestive tracts. The larynx consists of three unpaired cartilages (epiglottis, cricoid, and thyroid) and one pair of arytenoid cartilages. The glottis (or cranial opening of the larynx) is composed of the corniculate and cuneiform process of the arytenoid cartilages and the epiglottis. Minor anatomic differences exist between feline and canine larynx.[2] Cats lack the interarytenoid cartilage found in dogs and instead have an interarytenoid ligament in its place. Cats also lack a vestibular ligament. Due to this deficiency the feline arytenoid cartilage is connected to the ventral aspect of the larynx by the vocal ligament. Another important anatomic difference is cats lack the laryngeal ventricles that are found between the vestibular and vocal folds in the dog. No dramatic differences exist between feline and canine innervation and muscles of the larynx.

Swallowing, or deglutition, is a complex reflex action that coordinates many structures. Cranial nerves, the swallowing center in the reticular formation of the brain stem, the muscles of mastication, tongue, soft palate, pharynx, larynx, and esophagus are all involved in what appears to be a simple act of allowing transport of material from the mouth to the stomach.[3] As a lesser recognized function, swallowing also allows saliva and debris to be removed from the pharynx. Deglutition begins as a voluntary act but during its execution becomes a reflex. Deglutition is traditionally described as having three phases: (1) oral, (2) pharyngeal, and (3) esophageal. The oral phase begins when mastication is complete. The tongue then moves the food bolus that is organized at the base of the tongue to a position that is on midline between the tongue and the hard palate. Motor fibers to the tongue are supplied by cranial nerve XII. Sensory fibers from the oral cavity and motor fibers to the masticatory muscles and soft palate originate from cranial nerve V. The oral phase is voluntary, but when the food bolus is pushed into the pharynx, receptors are stimulated that initiate the involuntary, or reflex, component of deglutition. Sensory receptors are found in the pharynx, palate, and epiglottis. Impulses from these receptors are transmitted along the glossopharyngeal nerve, recurrent laryngeal branch of the vagus nerve, and the maxillary branch of the trigeminal nerve to the swallowing center in the medulla (located in the floor of the fourth ventricle). The efferent arm of the reflex involves the motor nuclei of cranial nerves V, VII, IX, X, and XII.[4-6] These nerves supply the muscles of mastication, tongue, palate, pharynx, larynx, and esophagus. During the pharyngeal phase the goal is to pass food from the oropharynx into the esophagus and to prevent food from being aspirated into the trachea or moved into the nasopharynx. This is accomplished by elevation of the soft palate and the palatopharyngeal folds moving inward as the vocal cords are pulled together and the larynx is elevated against the epiglottis. The final act during the pharyngeal stage of swallowing occurs when the cricopharyngeal muscle relaxes, the upper esophageal sphincter opens, the bolus moves into the esophagus, the sphincter closes, and the pharyngeal muscles relax. The cricopharyngeal muscle is innervated by the pharyngoesophageal nerve, which is formed by cranial nerves IX and X.[1] The final stage of deglutition, the esophageal stage, transports the bolus from the esophagus, through the gastroesophageal sphincter, and into the stomach. The esophagus is innervated by the vagus nerve.

The larynx has three functions: (1) to act as a conduit for air, (2) to protect the lower airway from aspiration during deglutition, and (3) vocalization. The glottis remains partially open when an animal is at rest. When greater airflow is needed, the glottis is widened by abduction of the arytenoid cartilages and vocal folds (via cricoarytenoid muscles) during inspiration (and the same structures adduct during expiration). The cricoarytenoid muscles are innervated by the caudal laryngeal nerves, which are derived from the recurrent laryngeal nerves. The recurrent laryngeal nerve innervates all the muscles of the larynx except the cricothyroid muscles that are supplied by the cranial laryngeal nerves.[7] During deglutition the larynx is pulled cranially by the geniohyoideus and mylohyoideus muscles. This allows the epiglottis to close over the larynx, protecting the lower airways. The adductor muscles close the glottis concurrently. This creates an additional defense against aspiration.

HISTORY AND PHYSICAL EXAMINATION

Animals with diseases of the throat can have a variety of historical complaints. Pharyngeal diseases can be confusing because historical findings can be related to swallowing difficulties or the upper respiratory tract (URT). Historical findings secondary to laryngeal dysfunction are usually related to either inability to regulate airflow and protect the airway, or they are related to changes in vocalization. Respiratory sounds can be extremely useful in localizing the disease, whether it is pharyngeal or laryngeal, but they are not helpful if one tries to attribute a specific respiratory sound to a specific condition. Coughing, dyspnea, and nasal discharge are common clinical complaints. Stertor, a snoring sound heard on inspiration, is usually due to an intermittent obstruction such as an elongated soft palate. Stridor, an inspiratory high-pitch wheeze, is most commonly associated with laryngeal lesions. Stridor is created by air turbulence through a narrowed laryngeal opening. Any changes in vocalization would suggest a laryngeal disorder. Reverse sneezing, which is described as short periods of forceful inspiratory nasal effort with the head pulled back, indicates irritation to the dorsal nasopharyngeal mucosa.[8] Dysphagia cases can be confusing because ineffective swallowing may not be obvious to the owner and may not be the primary historical complaint. Other signs such as coughing, gagging, regurgitation, and nasal discharge may be reported in animals with either oropharyngeal dysphagia or other diseases of the throat.

A complete physical examination (including a neurologic examination) is important when evaluating animals with pharyngeal or laryngeal disease because dysfunction may be indicative of systemic disease (i.e., myopathy, neuropathy) or there may be secondary complications from the disorder (e.g., aspiration pneumonia). If laryngeal disease is suspected, the larynx should be palpated for pain or structural abnormalities. The area over the larynx should be auscultated for abnormal sounds secondary to turbulence. Part of this complete physical

examination may include exercising the patient, because occasionally manifestation of the disease only occurs after physical exertion. Many animals will have dyspnea, and a thorough physical examination may not be possible until the animal is stable. Significant airway compromise may be overlooked. It is important to assess the degree of respiratory compromise by evaluating the patient's attitude, posture, mucous membrane color, and both respiratory rate and pattern. Precluding the emergency situation, once the general examination is complete one may concentrate on examining the oral cavity. It is extremely difficult, if not impossible, to adequately evaluate the larynx and pharyngeal areas without heavy sedation or general anesthesia. In most cases it is easier for the examiner, and safer for the animal, if tracheal intubation is performed. A standard method of evaluating the oral cavity should be established so that one does not miss an important abnormality. The larynx is evaluated both for structural problems and functional abnormalities; the pharynx is evaluated for physical abnormalities. Pharyngeal function cannot be evaluated when the patient is sedated; rather, video fluoroscopy is recommended when critically assessing pharyngeal function.

DIAGNOSIS

Diagnostic Imaging
Lateral and ventrodorsal radiographic views of both the skull and cervical areas are indicated. Radiopaque foreign bodies can be identified that may be missed on laryngoscopy and pharyngoscopy (e.g., sewing needle embedded in soft tissues). Radiographs are also useful in identifying bony changes associated with chronic inflammation or neoplasia, identifying clues of unreported trauma (e.g., subcutaneous emphysema), and occasionally soft tissue masses. Suggestion of a soft tissue mass is confirmed by direct visualization and histopathology. Thoracic radiographs are also indicated. Symptoms of lower respiratory disease may be masked when a patient has concurrent, and more severe, upper respiratory symptoms. Evaluation for aspiration pneumonia, metastases, or suggestion of a motility disorder (i.e., megaesophagus) is possible.

Ultrasonography and computed tomography (CT) are noninvasive modalities to evaluate the pharynx and larynx. Ultrasonography can identify soft tissue masses, help guide fine needle aspiration, and evaluate laryngeal function.[9,10] The presence of air in these areas can limit the usefulness of this modality in establishing a definitive diagnosis. CT may be used to fully evaluate involvement of neoplasia or middle-ear disease if a nasopharyngeal polyp is suspected.[11]

Videofluoroscopy is essential for any case of dysphagia. A barium swallow allows the act of swallowing to be recorded and studied for abnormalities. The patient should be recorded attempting to swallow barium to mimic liquids and then should be given a meal (canned food mixed with barium) to be recorded. Videofluoroscopy is superior to radiography because it allows all phases of deglutition to be evaluated instead of recording one moment (intermittent moments) of the event. Unfortunately videofluoroscopy is limited to referral centers only.

Pharyngoscopy and Laryngoscopy
Laryngoscopy and pharyngoscopy allow assessment of both structural abnormalities and function of the larynx. A flexible endoscope is used for these procedures because visualization of the nasopharynx requires retroflexion. Occasionally a foreign body will be found just caudal to the larynx and may be retrieved endoscopically. The patient is placed in sternal recumbency and anesthetized with either propofol or sodium thiopental. Once anesthetized, gauze is passed under the maxilla behind the canine teeth. The gauze is used to elevate the head, so external

compression of the neck is avoided. Flexible endoscopy is ideal to evaluate the nasopharynx. If that is not possible, the caudal pharynx can be evaluated using a dental mirror and a snook hook. This will be sufficient in evaluating most nasopharyngeal polyps, masses, or caudal foreign bodies. It will not allow diagnosis of more rostral diseases such as nasopharyngeal stenosis. Laryngeal function is usually evaluated first by assessing the motion of the arytenoid cartilages. The traditional approach involves titrating anesthesia that allows both visualization of the arytenoid cartilages and deep spontaneous breaths to occur. In a normal animal the arytenoid cartilages will abduct symmetrically with each inspiration and close on expiration. The frustration with this technique is multiple. Maintaining the correct level of anesthesia is difficult (i.e., the animal is too awake to allow adequate visualization of the arytenoid cartilages or anesthetized so that the patient will not spontaneously breathe); shallow breathing can limit adequate assessment; and concerns about the effect of anesthesia on laryngeal function are legitimate concerns when performing the traditional laryngeal examination. The recently introduced technique attempts to eliminate the effects of anesthesia from the examination. Patients are premedicated with acepromazine maleate and butorphanol tartrate and induced with propofol. Doxapram hydrochloride (2.2 mg/kg intravenously) is used to increase laryngeal motion and minimize or eliminate the effects of anesthesia.[12]

Miscellaneous

Hematology and biochemical profiles should be performed on patients with pharyngeal and laryngeal dysfunction, but they will rarely confirm the definitive diagnosis. Occasionally virus isolation (feline calicivirus [FCV]) and PCR (feline herpes-1 virus [FHV-1], Chlamydia spp., and Mycoplasma spp.) are indicated in the diagnostic workup. Culture and sensitivity of tissue or secretions can provide valuable information during the diagnostic workup. Cytology and histopathology are also essential for critically evaluating infiltrative disease or mass lesions.

DISEASES OF THE PHARYNX

Nasopharyngeal Polyps

Nasopharyngeal polyps are histopathologically benign, pedunculated masses consisting mostly of fibrovascular tissue and variable severity of inflammatory cells.[13] It is the most common nasopharyngeal disease of younger cats and accounts for almost one third of all feline nasopharyngeal diseases.[14] No sex or breed predilection exists; although nasopharyngeal polyps are most commonly found in younger cats (mean range 0.4 months to 6.1 years), this disease should also be included in the differential diagnosis for older cats.[14-17] Nasopharyngeal polyps are believed to originate from the middle ear or auditory tube and then expand into the nasopharynx and external auditory canal.[18] It is unknown why nasopharyngeal polyps occur, but it does not seem likely that the polyps are a manifestation of chronic viral (FCV or FHV) infections.[17] Clinical signs are variable but include nasal discharge, sneeze, stertor, and phonation changes. Definitive diagnosis is made by direct visualization of the nasopharyngeal mass and histopathology. Quite often, nasopharyngeal polyps can be discovered with digital palpation of the soft palate. Diagnostic imaging (skull radiographs and CT) is not necessary for the diagnosis but can provide valuable information toward the extent of the mass and possible middle ear involvement. Treatment depends on clinical presentation and extent of disease. If evidence of concurrent middle ear involvement is seen, a ventral bulla osteotomy is indicated. If the disease appears to be limited to the nasopharynx, then traction avulsion to remove the polyp at its stalk is

usually attempted. The high rate of reoccurrence with this disease (33%) has led to the suggestion that ventral bulla osteotomy should be performed on all cats with nasopharyngeal polyps.[16] Nasopharyngeal polyps are considered a disease of cats, but a case of a nasopharyngeal polyp in a dog has been reported.[19]

Nasopharyngeal Stenosis

Nasopharyngeal stenosis is primarily a disease of cats but has been reported in a dog.[20,21] It is a rare disease that is characterized by scar tissue that forms a membrane or "webbing" above the soft palate and obstructs airflow through the nasopharynx. Cats are believed to develop nasopharyngeal stenosis as a consequence of healing from injuries to the area (infectious, traumatic). Cats with the nasopharyngeal stenosis have chronic histories of stertorous breathing and open-mouth breathing.[20,22] Diagnosis is made using flexible endoscopy to evaluate the nasopharynx and visualizing a pinhole-sized orifice where the caudal nares should be seen (Figures 211-1 and 211-2). Treatment of nasopharyngeal stenosis involves surgical resection of the lesion, but the prognosis should remain guarded because the webbing may reoccur.[21,23] Balloon dilation of the stenotic area has been proposed as a successful alternative to surgery.[22,24]

Pharyngeal Foreign Bodies

Foreign bodies can occur in both dogs and cats and creates both acute and chronic pharyngeal disease.[25-27] Grass awns, fish hooks, and bones are all possible, but wood sticks are the most common penetrating foreign bodies.[25,27] Medium and large breed dogs are affected more often with oropharyngeal penetrating injuries, presumptively because of their stick-chewing or retrieving behavior. Clinical signs of acute disease include pawing at the mouth or face, hypersalivation, oral pain and malodor, dysphagia, and dyspnea. Cervical or facial swellings combined with intermittently draining tracts were more commonly seen with chronic pharyngeal foreign bodies. Pharyngeal and retropharyngeal abscessation is a common complication secondary to bones, grass awns, sticks, pins, or needles. Dogs with pharyngeal or retropharyngeal abscesses will exhibit anorexia, pharyngeal pain, swelling, and will be febrile.[1] Although rare, osteomyelitis and quadriparesis are possible complications to penetrating stick foreign bodies.[28,29] In contrast, nasopharyngeal foreign bodies are more likely to create inflammation and nasal discharge. Migration of nasopharyngeal foreign bodies does not occur. Diagnosis of pharyngeal foreign bodies is difficult and frequently frustrating. Radiographs are helpful if the foreign body is radiopaque; however, if it is radiolucent the foreign body will remain elusive. Endoscopy is helpful in locating a foreign body, and if the foreign body penetrated the pharynx, endoscopy can localize the traumatized area. Aggressive search and retrieval of penetrating pharyngeal foreign bodies is important early in the course of the problem. If the foreign body is not successfully removed in its entirety during the acute stage, the prognosis decreases dramatically.[25]

Pharyngeal Mucoceles

A mucocele is a collection of saliva from a damaged salivary gland or duct. Synonyms include sialocele, ranula, or salivary cyst. Mucoceles are not true cysts because they are lined with granulation tissue and not the characteristic epithelial tissue.[30] The cause of mucoceles is unknown, although traumatic causes such as dog bites and choke collars have been purposed. Pharyngeal mucoceles are the least common type of mucocele, with sublingual and cervical being more common. Regardless, pharyngeal mucoceles are clinically important because most animals with pharyngeal mucoceles present in respiratory distress. Dogs are more affected than cats, and miniature poodles appear to be at increased risk of developing

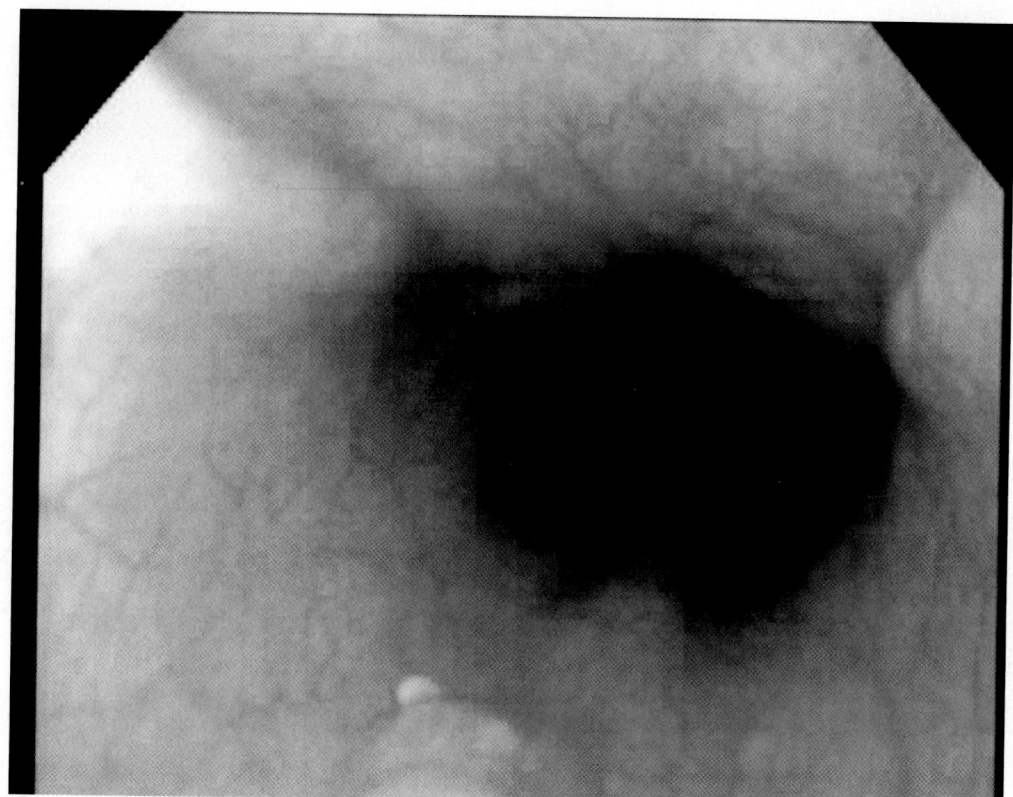

Figure 211-1 Normal nasopharynx.

pharyngeal mucoceles.[31,32] Due to the patient's respiratory compromise, it is important to establish a patent airway either via tracheal intubation or tracheostomy prior to examination. Diagnosis requires visualization of soft, nonpainful, fluctuant mass in the pharynx. Fine needle aspirate of the mass will reveal a thick, tenacious fluid that is characteristic of saliva. Drainage of fluid is important in the acute management of pharyngeal mucoceles, but surgical correction via marsupialization and resection of the associated salivary glands will need to be pursued at a later date.[31]

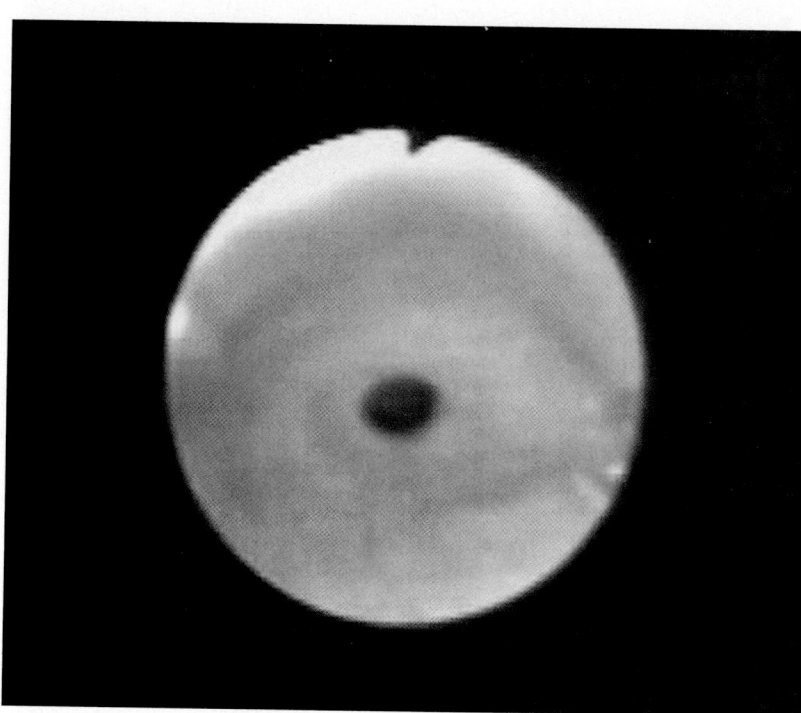

Figure 211-2 Nasopharyngeal stenosis in a young cat with a history of progressive stertor and open-mouth breathing.

SOFT PALATE ABNORMALITIES

The palate is an important anatomic structure because it divides the oral and nasal cavities. Abnormalities of the palate result from incomplete closure of the primary or secondary palate (or both) during fetal development. The primary palate develops into the lip and incisive bone.[33] The secondary palate becomes the hard and soft palate. Cleft palate and soft palate hypoplasia are two of many palatine defects that have been described. Brachycephalic breeds have a higher incidence of cleft palate. Many factors have been implicated in these abnormalities, but inherited traits seem to be found in Shih Tzus, bulldogs, pointers, Swiss sheepdogs, and Brittany spaniels.[1,34] Teratogens (e.g., vitamin A, griseofulvin) have also been shown to cause palate abnormalities.[35,36] Midline soft palate defects are most common with unilateral or bilateral defects occurring less frequently. Neonates with a cleft palate usually fail to thrive because the defect makes nursing difficult, allows milk to enter the nasal passages, or milk is aspirated into the lower airways. If the neonate is able to survive, chronic rhinitis is the most common clinical sign. Diagnosis is based on oral examination of the soft palate. A cleft palate will have a midline defect usually involving both the hard and soft palate. Soft palate hypoplasia reveals a severely shortened length, with a midline remnant of muscular tissue covered by mucosa (Figure 211-3). Animals with soft palate defects should also be evaluated for middle ear disease because concurrent middle ear disease has been identified as a potential complication.[37] Treatment of both types of soft palate defects involves surgical correction. A variety of techniques have been described to correct midline defects, with good results.[38,39] Correction of soft palate hypoplasia has a poor prognosis due to the absence of adequate tissue for repair. In animals with

this problem, it is hoped that addressing the way intake of food and water occurs (i.e., elevation) will decrease the severity of reflux into the nasal cavity.

In contrast, brachycephalic breeds can suffer from soft palate excess. Stenotic nares and everted laryngeal saccules are the other components of the upper airway obstructive syndrome known as the brachycephalic syndrome. English bulldogs, pugs, Shih Tzus, Lhasa apsos, and Himalayan cats are all breeds that suffer from brachycephalic syndrome.[40] Hypoplasia of the trachea, especially in the English bulldog, may also be present.[41] Normally the caudal edge of the soft palate should just touch the tip of the epiglottis. Because maxillae are shortened in brachycephalic breeds, the caudal edge extends beyond the tip of the epiglottis. During exercise the soft palate will be sucked into the glottis, reducing the diameter of the airway. Over time this will cause trauma and tissue edema that will further hinder airflow. Clinical signs associated with an obstructing elongated soft palate include stertorous breathing, gagging, coughing, and exercise intolerance or collapse. Diagnosis is based on oral examination and direct visualization of a soft palate that extends beyond the tip of the epiglottis. Treatment involves shortening the length of the soft palate, either with conventional techniques or carbon dioxide laser.[42-44]

Neoplasia

Oral tumors (which include pharyngeal neoplasia) are the fourth most common neoplasia in dogs. Oral neoplasms occur 2.6 times more frequently in dogs than in cats, and males are more likely to develop oropharyngeal neoplasia than females.[45] The three most common oral tumors in the dog are malignant melanoma, squamous cell carcinoma, and fibrosarcoma.[46] Squamous cell carcinoma and fibrosarcoma are the two most common oral tumors in the cat. If the feline nasopharynx is

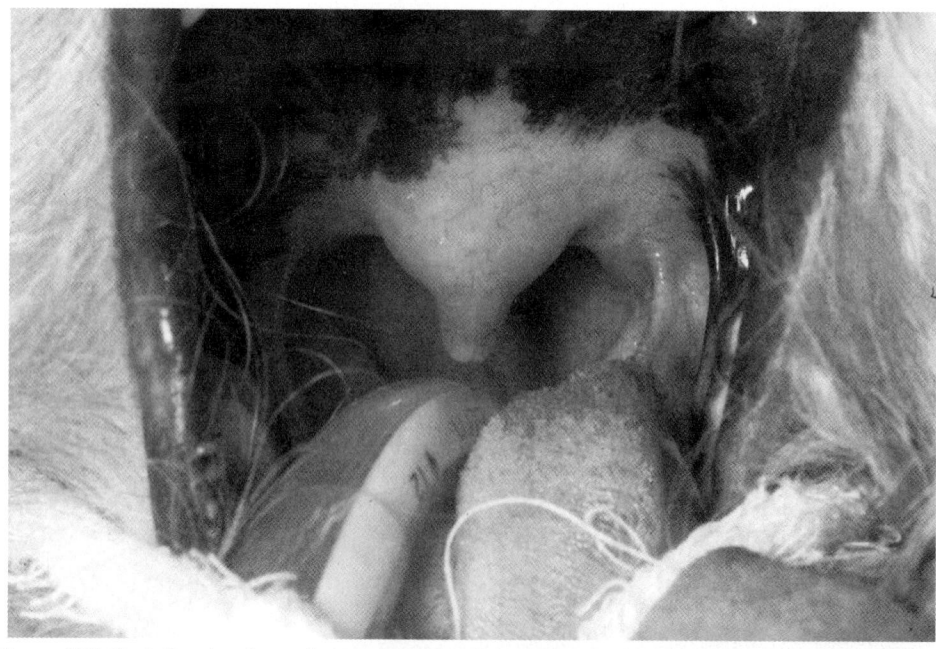

Figure 211-3 Soft palate hypoplasia in a young adult dog with a history of chronic nasal discharge.

specifically evaluated for neoplasia, lymphosarcoma is the most common tumor diagnosed.[14] Most tumors of the oral cavity are malignant, highly locally invasive, and have a variable degree of metastasis.[45,46] Clinical signs include inappetence or anorexia due to pain, dysphagia, halitosis, ptyalism, and facial deformity (swelling, exophthalmos, or bony thickening). Cats with nasopharyngeal lymphosarcoma will have nasal discharge, sneezing, stertor, or phonation changes. Diagnosis of an oropharyngeal tumor includes a histologic diagnosis and tumor staging. Direct visualization during an oral examination (and endoscopy for nasopharyngeal tumors) is performed prior to obtaining a tissue sample for cytology and histopathology. Thoracic radiographs are part of the staging, as is either skull radiographs or CT. Regional lymph nodes should be aspirated to determine metastasis. Treatment options include surgery, radiation therapy, hyperthermia, chemotherapy, and photodynamic therapy. Treatment protocol depends on tumor type and location, but local control is most effective with surgery and radiation therapy.[47] Prognosis is variable, based on a number of factors.

Tonsillitis and Pharyngitis

When discussing tonsillitis, one is referring to the palatine tonsil. The palatine tonsil is found within the palatine fossa in the lateral wall of the oropharynx. It is rare for either tonsillitis or pharyngitis to occur as a primary disease. It is much more common for the tonsils and the pharynx to be inflamed secondary to other diseases. Clinical signs are not specific for either the tonsils or pharynx but will support oropharyngeal disease. Inappetence or anorexia, ptyalism, and oral pain are all common clinical findings. Diagnosis is based on history and physical examination findings. Fever is common when infectious agents are involved. Acute tonsillitis will reveal bright-red, friable tonsils on oral examination. It is not unusual for tonsils at this stage to be enlarged and protruding from the palatine fossa. Occasionally the tonsils will have petechiae or small abscesses. The pharynx of acute pharyngitis will be visibly inflamed and can have ulcerations, petechiae, or small abscesses. Bacterial or viral isolation is usually not indicated unless clinical signs are chronic or relapsing. The most common causes of tonsillitis and pharyngitis is upper respiratory infection. FHV-1 and FCV are the two most common feline viral pathogens. FCV is more likely to cause ulcerations than FHV-1.[48,49] Canine infectious tracheobronchitis (ITB) will occasionally cause problems, although it is more likely to cause laryngitis. *Bordetella bronchiseptica* has caused URT disease in cats as well.[50] Other possibilities include chronic vomiting or regurgitation, periodontitis, and ingestion of caustic or toxic substances (e.g., cleaning detergents, liquid potpourri).[51] Rarely, bacterial infection will be incriminated as the cause. Cats can also develop a progressive, nonspecific inflammatory condition termed gingivitis-stomatitis-pharyngitis complex. Young purebred cats are predisposed to the disease, and the most severely affected cats develop ulceroproliferative lesions in the caudal oropharynx.[52] Treatment of pharyngitis or tonsillitis is directed toward eliminating the underlying cause, if possible, as well as supportive care and antibiotics, if indicated.

Oropharyngeal Dysphagia

Dysphagia refers to abnormal or difficulty swallowing. Oropharyngeal dysphagia indicates an inability to move a bolus from the oral cavity into the proximal esophagus. This symptom can be either secondary to an isolated lesion or manifestation of systemic disease. Clinical signs are variable, depending on severity and location of the problem. Signs include difficulty with prehension, dropping food from mouth, exaggerated head movements during eating, regurgitation with no correlation in time of eating, and repeated attempts to swallow food. Occasionally, respiratory signs such as nasal discharge,

coughing, and aspiration pneumonia will occur secondary to nasopharyngeal or laryngotracheal aspiration. Diagnosis of oropharyngeal dysphagia requires multiple areas to be evaluated. Accurate historical information is imperative to differentiate regurgitation from vomiting. It is rare that an owner will recognize the difference until the history and examination occurs. A standardized questionnaire has been evaluated as a sensitive tool to detect oropharyngeal dysphagia.[53] Observing the animal eating and drinking is also extremely helpful. The physical examination should include a thorough oral examination to evaluate for structural abnormalities and foreign bodies. A complete neurologic examination is also critical during the evaluation of oropharyngeal dysphagia. Radiographs of the area can identify radiopaque foreign bodies or masses. Thoracic radiographs can determine if the animal has aspiration pneumonia secondary to the dysphagia. Videofluoroscopy is an excellent diagnostic tool to localize the dysphagia.[54] Other possible diagnostics could include ANA test, evaluation for acetylcholine receptor antibodies, endocrine screening, electromyography, or biopsy for histopathology.

Causes of dysphagia include anatomic abnormalities, neoplasia, foreign bodies, or neuromuscular disorders. Brain stem tumors can also cause dysphagia, but it is usually not the only clinical or physical examination finding. The most common neuromuscular disorder is myasthenia gravis, a disease of altered neuromuscular transmission secondary to autoantibodies against acetylcholine receptors. Akitas, Scottish terriers, German shorthaired pointers, Chihuahuas, and Abyssinians are all breeds identified at increased risk for acquired myasthenia gravis.[55,56] Manifestations of myasthenia gravis may either be focal (pharyngeal or esophageal) or generalized (generalized muscular weakness or collapse). Oropharyngeal dysphagia can be one clinical sign of many that is associated with myopathies. Bouvier des Flanders have been identified with a muscular dystrophy in which oropharyngeal dysphagia is the primary clinical sign.[57] Cricopharyngeal achalasia can be acquired as a polymyopathy, or it can be congenital. Cricopharyngeal achalasia is the failure of the upper esophageal sphincter to relax and allow a food bolus into the proximal esophagus. Cocker spaniels are at increased risk for congenital cricopharyngeal achalasia, but any breed can be affected.[58] It is important to differentiate between congenital and acquired disease, because cricopharyngeal myotomy is indicated in congenital disease but should be avoided with acquired disease. Treatment of oropharyngeal dysphagia should be based on the underlying disease process. If possible, the underlying cause should be removed; if that is not possible, providing a means of adequate nutrition should be pursued.

DISEASES OF THE LARYNX

Laryngeal Paralysis

Laryngeal paralysis is a common cause of upper airway obstruction in dogs. Cats can be diagnosed as well, but it is not a common cause of upper airway obstruction for the species.[59] Laryngeal paralysis results when the arytenoid cartilage fails to abduct during inspiration, leading to narrowing of the glottic lumen. Several causes of laryngeal paralysis have been identified, but it is most often idiopathic. Most acquired idiopathic cases are older, large breed dogs. Damage to the recurrent laryngeal nerve from trauma, infiltrative disease, masses, or surgical manipulation (e.g., feline thyroidectomy) can lead to laryngeal paralysis.[59] Polyneuropathies secondary to immune-mediated disease, hypothyroidism, or other systemic disorders can be observed primarily as laryngeal paralysis.[60] Congenital laryngeal paralysis does occur but is uncommon. A hereditary form has been described in Bouvier des Flanders and is presumed in Siberian huskies and husky cross-breeds.[61,62] In Bouvier des Flanders an autosomal-dominant trait causing a loss of motor neurons in the nucleus ambiguus has been identified.[63] A laryngeal paralysis-polyneuropathy complex has been described in young dalmatians and rottweilers.[64,65]

Clinical signs are usually progressive because the ability of the arytenoid cartilage to abduct fails. Clinical signs of laryngeal paralysis include stridor, exercise intolerance, coughing, gagging, and voice change. Animals with laryngeal paralysis can present in respiratory distress, especially after an episode of excitement, exercising, and when environmental temperatures are elevated. Moderate airway obstruction is worsened by laryngeal edema and inflammation secondary to turbulent airflow in the larynx. Although ultrasound has been described as a diagnostic tool for laryngeal paralysis, most clinicians will use laryngoscopy to definitively diagnose laryngeal paralysis.[9] Laryngeal function is assessed when the animal is under a light plane of anesthesia. Paralysis may be unilateral or bilateral, although most animals with moderate to severe clinical signs have bilateral dysfunction of the arytenoid cartilages. It is important not to be fooled by paradoxic movement of the arytenoid cartilages. Paradoxic movement indicates opposite movement (i.e., medially) by the arytenoid cartilages when negative pressure occurs during inspiration. A thorough oral examination should be performed during the same anesthetic episode to identify any underlying causes. Once laryngeal paralysis has been diagnosed a complete neurologic examination that includes pharyngeal and esophageal function should occur to evaluate for concurrent or underlying problems. Thoracic radiographs are indicated to identify aspiration pneumonia or metastatic disease. When the animal presents in respiratory crisis, stabilization includes sedation and establishing an airway. This is accomplished by either tracheal intubation or tracheotomy. Short-acting corticosteroids are helpful if significant laryngeal edema exists. Once stabilized, surgery is indicated to alleviate the upper airway obstruction caused by laryngeal paralysis. Multiple surgical techniques have been described to palliate the clinical signs associated with laryngeal paralysis. The current surgical technique of choice is unilateral arytenoid lateralization, a technique that attempts to increase the area of the rima glottidis.[66] This procedure has been shown to have the most favorable outcome compared with other possible surgical techniques such as bilateral arytenoid lateralization and partial laryngectomy.[67] Postoperative complications include aspiration pneumonia, laryngeal webbing, surgical failure, and respiratory distress. Postoperative complications are common, and death can occur. In one retrospective study, 34.3% of dogs had postoperative complications and the mortality rate was 19.3%.[67] In the same study, prognosis was poor if the dog had concurrent neurologic disease. Limited information exists regarding surgical outcome in cats. The surgical technique used was unilateral arytenoid lateralization. Postoperative complications included laryngeal edema that necessitated a temporary tracheotomy tube and an altered ability to vocalize. All cats survived.[68]

Laryngeal Neoplasia

Primary neoplasms of the canine and feline larynx occur uncommonly. The most common canine laryngeal tumors reported are malignant epithelial tumors and rhabdomyoma. The most common laryngeal tumor in the cat is lymphosarcoma, with squamous cell carcinoma the second most common.[10,69,70] Most patients with laryngeal tumors are older, with 8 years as the median age.[69] Other report tumor types are adenocarcinoma, rhabdomyosarcoma, osteosarcoma, chondrosarcoma, mast cell tumor, and melanoma.[10,69-71] Clinical signs are similar regardless of tumor type and include dysphonia, coughing, gagging or choking, and respiratory distress. Occasionally an

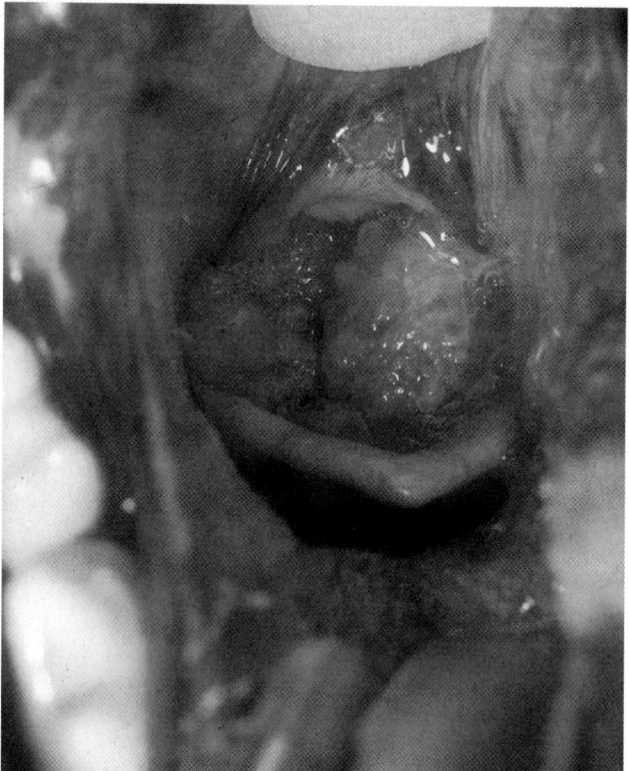

Figure 211-4 Laryngeal neoplasia in a geriatric dog, causing complete obstruction of glottis.

abnormal larynx can be palpated, but most laryngeal tumors are identified by laryngoscopy (Figure 211-4). Radiographs, CTs, and ultrasound all have diagnostic value in determination of extent of disease and potential metastasis.[10] Definitive diagnosis should be made by histopathology; caution should be used when diagnosis is based on gross appearance alone. This is especially true with feline tumors because granulomatous disease has been reported. Therapy is based on tumor type but, in general, surgical resection and creating an unobstructed airway are goals. Complete laryngectomy and permanent tracheostomy are options with variable success.[72,73] Cats with severe respiratory compromise secondary to laryngeal lymphosarcoma will respond well to radiation therapy. The prognosis of benign tumors is good if complete resection is successful; malignant laryngeal neoplasms have a poor prognosis.

Laryngeal Collapse

Brachycephalic dogs are at increased risk to develop laryngeal collapse secondary to their congenital airway malformations. Stenotic nares, elongated soft palate, and if present, a hypoplastic trachea, create an increased negative pressure during inspiration to move air through the narrowed air passages. It is believed that laryngeal cartilages become deformed from this chronic increased negative pressure and will finally weaken and collapse. Finding that older brachycephalic dogs will often have laryngeal collapse when presenting for upper airway disease support this theory. However young brachycephalic dogs are also diagnosed with laryngeal collapse, which may indicate a defect in cartilage structure.[74] Dogs with laryngeal collapse will experience stridor, episodes of respiratory distress, and a respiratory crisis due to upper airway obstruction. Determination of laryngeal collapse is possible with laryngoscopy. The corniculate and cuneiform processes of the arytenoid cartilage will be medially displaced and occasionally will touch. In severe cases these processes will overlap, and the epiglottis will appear to be rolled up or flattened.[74] No specific treatment has been effective for laryngeal collapse. Surgical treatment should be directed toward altering the underlying congenital abnormality (i.e., stenotic nares correction, soft palate resection, everted laryngeal saccule excision) to improve airflow. In cases of severe laryngeal collapse, a permanent tracheostomy is recommended.[44,75] Dogs with severe laryngeal collapse have a poor prognosis.[75]

LARYNGITIS

Inflammatory laryngeal disease is common in both the dog and the cat. The most common cause of acute inflammation of the larynx is infectious agents such as canine infectious tracheobronchitis (ITB), commonly called kennel cough, or the feline upper respiratory agents (i.e., FHV-1, FCV). ITB is a result of coinfection of *Bordetella bronchiseptica* with either canine parainfluenza virus or canine adenovirus-2 (CAV-2).[76] With most cases of ITB, the only clinical sign is paroxysmal coughing in an otherwise healthy dog. Due to inflammation of the larynx the cough is a loud, high-pitched, "goose honk" cough. Occasionally a dog may be febrile, lethargic, and inappetent. ITB is usually self-limiting, but the severity of the cough, combined with the possibility of pneumonia complicating the disease, warrants treatment. Doxycycline at 5 to 10 mg/kg orally once daily is the antimicrobial of choice for *B. bronchiseptica*. Short-term administration of an anti-inflammatory dose of glucocorticoids can be effective in decreasing laryngeal edema. Antitussives, such as butorphanol tartrate or hydrocodone bitartrate, are effective in minimizing

the severity of the cough but should not be used if pneumonia is suspected. Other causes of inflammatory laryngeal disease include endotracheal intubation, insect bites, foreign body penetration, or trauma from bite wounds, leash and choke chain injuries, or being hit by cars. Frequently no cause for acute laryngeal inflammation is found. Acute inflammatory laryngeal disease is usually self-limiting, and no specific treatment is indicated if the animal has only mild signs. However, if moderate to severe signs exist, a short course with an anti-inflammatory dose of glucocorticosteroids can be initiated to decrease laryngeal edema. Respiratory obstruction secondary to laryngeal inflammation is an uncommon clinical presentation but can occur in severe instances such as in laryngeal trauma. A tracheostomy is indicated if the patient is dyspneic, cyanotic, or extremely anxious due to laryngeal inflammation.[7]

OBSTRUCTIVE INFLAMMATORY DISEASE

An obstructive inflammatory laryngeal disease has been described in cats and dogs.[70,77-79,80] Although rare, it is a disease worth noting because the gross appearance can mimic laryngeal neoplasia. The underlying cause of inflammation is unknown. Feline immunodeficiency virus (FIV) and feline leukemia virus (FeLV) have not been found to be associated with this disease. In the feline reports, dyspnea secondary to upper airway obstruction was reported in all cats; retching, coughing, and dysphonia were also common. Stridor and dysphonia was reported in dogs. Direct visualization of the larynx reveals a laryngeal mass that cannot be distinguished from neoplasia or severe swelling and edema (Figures 211-5 and 211-6). Histopathology is imperative to distinguish between neoplasia and obstructive inflammatory disease.

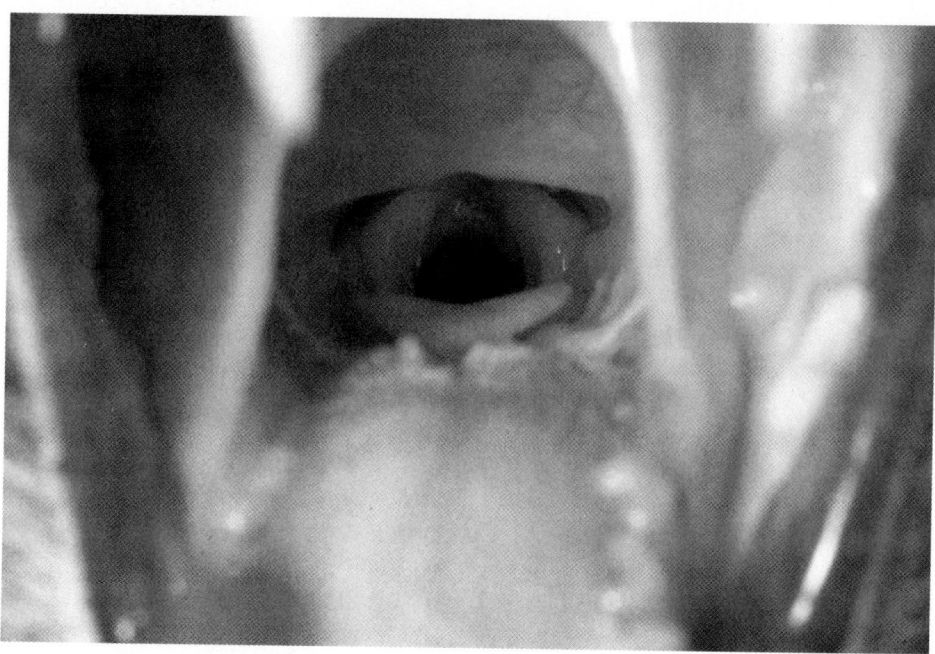

Figure 211-5 Normal feline larynx during inspiration.

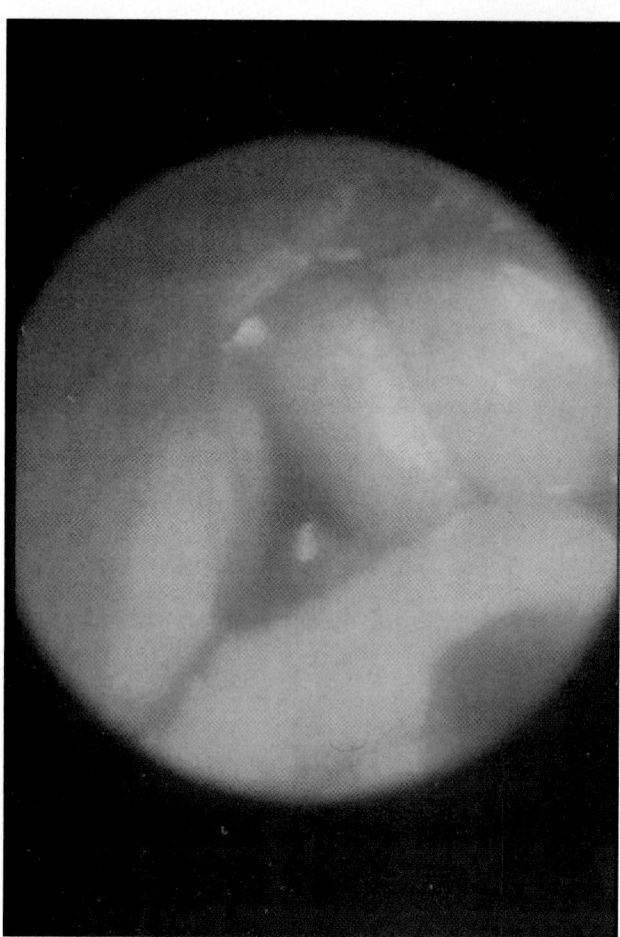

Figure 211-6 Middle-aged cat presented in respiratory distress. Laryngeal examination revealed bilateral arytenoid masses. Biopsy revealed pyogranulomatous inflammation.

Histopathology reveals either granulomatous or nongranulomatous laryngitis (neutrophilic and lymphoplasmacytic). Most patients with obstructive inflammatory laryngeal disease need to be stabilized. This is accomplished by establishing an airway through tracheostomy tube placement. Treatment with corticosteroids (dexamethasone, prednisone, or prednisolone) has variable success, and occasionally surgical resection of the proliferative tissue is indicated. The prognosis is guarded, with a high mortality rate during the initial diagnostic and treatment period.

SECTION XIII

Respiratory Disease

CHAPTER 212

Clinical Evaluation of the Respiratory Tract

Deborah Silverstein
Kenneth J. Drobatz

Respiratory diseases can be extremely challenging to manage and diagnose. The respiratory system is one of the four major body systems that require evaluation and treatment on an emergency basis. Respiratory dysfunction can result in severe physiologic compromise and imminent death if not dealt with appropriately. The respiratory workup is often dictated by the patient's condition, rather than the convenience of the clinician and the client. In patients with severe respiratory compromise, a tentative diagnosis and preliminary therapeutic plan must be guided by signalment, history, physical examination findings, and response to therapy pending stabilization for more definitive diagnostics (see Pulmonary Emergencies in Critical Care chapter). It is rare that a definitive diagnosis for the underlying cause of the respiratory problem is found using the signalment, history, physical examination, and response to therapy alone. Ancillary diagnostics are almost always required.

SIGNALMENT

The animal's signalment can provide direction for the diagnostic workup of the respiratory patient. For example, pediatric or juvenile patients are more likely to contract infectious conditions. Animals with inherited pulmonary disorders tend to manifest signs at an early age and certain breeds are predisposed to specific respiratory abnormalities. Feline asthma is noted more frequently in Siamese cats compared with other breeds. Brachycephalic breeds, particularly bulldogs, may have hypoplastic tracheas and upper airway conditions that result in respiratory difficulties. Respiratory distress due to heart failure is noted more frequently in male than female cats. Signalment provides clues to the underlying disorder but never provides a definitive diagnosis.

GENERAL MEDICAL HISTORY

A thorough history can provide important clues to the underlying respiratory problem. Questions regarding how long the owners have had the pet are important. For example, have they had the pet since it was a puppy or kitten, or did they obtain the animal when it was an adult? Obviously, owners that obtained their pet as a puppy or kitten will have a more comprehensive life history compared with owners that obtained a pet at a more advanced age. What is the travel history of the pet? This may assist in determining clinical suspicion for infectious or parasitic respiratory disease.

Establishing a clear picture of the pet's environment gives the veterinarian a sense of potential exposure to toxins or infectious diseases that might cause pulmonary problems. Animals that are allowed to run free or are unobserved can potentially be exposed to anything, such as anticoagulant rodenticide, forest fire, or house fire smoke. Was there a recent change in a living environment that is coincident with the development of the respiratory signs? Cats may develop airway hypersensitivity reactions to antigens in a new environment.

It is also important to determine the vaccination status of the animal. Similarly, is the pet in a heartworm endemic area and, if so, is the animal on an appropriate heartworm preventative plan? Are there other pets in the environment that this animal has been exposed to? Multiple animals with similar clinical signs points toward an environmental cause such as an infectious disease or a toxin. Similarly, is the owner or anyone in the family having medical problems that might suggest a zoonotic disease (e.g., trichosporonosis, rickettsial or fungal diseases, leishmania)?

Does the patient have any known hypersensitivities to dietary allergens or medications? Both are diagnostically and therapeutic important. What is the previous medical history of the patient? Has the animal had previous respiratory problems? If so, did the clinical signs improve? Has there ever been a history of trauma suggesting diaphragmatic hernia or pneumothorax?

PHYSICAL EXAMINATION

A complete physical examination is essential (see Chapter 1). In animals with severe respiratory compromise, the physical examination may point towards a tentative diagnosis from which empirical therapy can be chosen to stabilize the patient (see Approach to Respiratory Distress). Clinical signs combined with physical examination findings provide the initial steps in guiding the diagnostic workup.

Animals with nasal disorders commonly have clinical signs such as sneezing, nasal discharge, loud nasal respiratory sounds and, rarely, open mouth breathing secondary to occlusion of the nasal passages. Pure nasal disorders rarely cause severe respiratory distress, although some cats are reluctant to breathe through the mouth to relieve the obstruction. Palpation over the nasal cavities may reveal pain, asymmetry, or distortion of the nasal cavity due to destructive or proliferative diseases. Examination of the oral cavity may reveal bony abnormalities, severe dental disease, or abnormalities of the hard and soft palate that contribute to, or cause, the nasal disorder. Purulent nasal discharge may be due to primary or, more often, secondary bacterial infections. Unilateral discharge suggests tooth root abscess, cyst or hematoma, oronasal fistula, foreign body, or neoplasia. Bilateral discharge occurs secondarily to neoplasia, infectious agents, or any disease process that is caudal to the nasal septum. Epistaxis is due to any of the aforementioned causes of purulent nasal discharge, although severe bleeding is relatively rare with these conditions. Causes of epistaxis that are not due to primary respiratory abnormalities include thrombocytopenia, thrombocytopathia, coagulopathy, erosive immune-mediated diseases, or, rarely, hypertension. Definitive diagnosis of the underlying nasal disease is rarely derived from clinical signs and physical examination findings alone. Further diagnostics are typically required.

Upper and large airway disease (pharynx, larynx, and trachea) typically manifest as stridor and stertor that is audible without the stethoscope. Localization of the respiratory disease to the upper or large airways does not preclude disease in other parts of the respiratory systems but does warrant specific evaluation of the upper airways and trachea. Extrathoracic dynamic airway disease typically has louder sounds during inspiration, whereas intrathoracic dynamic lesions tend to be louder during exhalation. However, distinguishing the diseased anatomic location in the clinical patient with respiratory distress is often challenging. Auscultation over the specific location of the lesion reveals the most dramatic of sounds. Pharyngeal diseases include abscess, cyst or hematoma, cellulitis, neoplasia, foreign body, nasopharyngeal polyp, and enlarged lymph nodes. Direct visualization during physical examination or under general anesthesia usually localizes the problem. Palpation of the pharyngeal area may reveal swelling, pain, or asymmetry, indicating that the pharyngeal region is at least part of the disease process.

Laryngeal disease typically manifests as inspiratory stridor, voice change, coughing while drinking water, exercise intolerance, and an exacerbation of the clinical signs during exercise or periods of high environmental temperature. The most common laryngeal diseases include laryngeal paralysis, neoplasia, edema, and inflammation.

Tracheal disease is typically manifested as stridor and coughing, especially with exercise or excitement. A cough is easily elicited upon tracheal palpation when the trachea is inflamed. Respiratory compromise may vary from mild to severe. Distress may be more severe during inspiration, expiration, or both, depending upon whether the lesion is extrathoracic, intrathoracic, or both, respectively. The most common tracheal abnormalities include infectious tracheobronchitis (kennel cough), tracheal collapse, neoplasia, foreign body, trauma, and parasites.

Small airway and alveolar disease can be particularly challenging to diagnose. Physical manifestations of diseases in this portion of the respiratory tract include varying degrees of respiratory distress, coughing, and increased breath or adventitial sounds such as crackles or wheezes upon auscultation. Location of the increased breath or adventitial sounds may help in identifying the underlying disease process. Adventitial sounds heard loudest over the cranioventral or right middle lung lobe regions are suggestive of aspiration pneumonia. An increase in breath or adventitial sounds over the thorax in dogs with auscultable heart abnormalities is supportive of cardiogenic pulmonary edema. Auscultation abnormalities heard loudest over the caudodorsal regions of the lungs in animals with head trauma, electrocution, seizures, or upper airway obstruction may indicate neurogenic pulmonary edema. Diffuse, fine crackles throughout the thorax in a dog without significant signs of respiratory distress suggests chronic or slow onset of pulmonary parenchymal disease such as pulmonary fibrosis or metastatic neoplasia. Other lower airway and pulmonary parenchymal diseases include pulmonary thromboembolism, pulmonary contusions, pulmonary hemorrhage, acute respiratory distress syndrome (ARDS), heartworm disease, pulmonary infiltrates with eosinophilia, allergic bronchitis, feline bronchial disease, near drowning, smoke inhalation, re-expansion pulmonary edema, and inhalation of toxins.

Pleural space disease is caused by fluid, air, soft tissue, or abdominal organs in the pleural space. Patients with pleural space disorders commonly exhibit a short, shallow breathing pattern, tachypnea, and intermittent attempts at a deep respiration (especially in cats with pleural effusion). Decreased breath sounds of the thorax are auscultated. Diminished breath sounds in the ventral regions of the thorax are suggestive of fluid, whereas a dorsal distribution suggests air accumulation. Most pleural effusions and pneumothoraces are bilateral in dogs and cats, although unilateral fluid or air accumulation may occur. Diaphragmatic rupture often results in an asymmetry of auscultation findings. Diminished breath sounds are typically noted on the side where the abdominal contents are located, and loud heart and lung sounds are commonly heard on the opposite side. Rarely, a diaphragmatic hernia may result in substantial fluid accumulation on both sides of the chest, especially when the liver is present in the pleural space.

A complete, thorough physical examination should be performed even though the primary clinical signs are associated with the respiratory tract. It is rare that primary respiratory problems result in problems elsewhere in the body, but the reverse is not uncommon. Findings in other areas may provide clues as to the underlying cause of the respiratory disease or at least guide the diagnostic evaluation. Weight loss or cachexia suggests more chronic systemic disease, such as neoplasia that has metastasized to the lungs and resulted in respiratory difficulty. Additionally, the presence of masses elsewhere in the body might indicate a primary neoplastic process. Diseases that cause an acute abdomen commonly result in secondary respiratory diseases such as aspiration pneumonia or an acute respiratory distress (ARDS)-like condition subsequent to a severe inflammatory disease process. Petechiation or evidence of an abnormality of hemostasis elsewhere in the body might suggest pulmonary parenchymal hemorrhage or hemorrhagic pleural effusion as the cause of the respiratory distress.

In summary, signalment, previous medical history, clinical signs, and physical examination findings provide a solid foundation to further develop a diagnostic plan. There are numerous diagnostic modalities available to further evaluate respiratory function and identify specific disease processes in order to accurately and most effectively treat these patients.

DIAGNOSTIC TECHNIQUES

The diagnostic approach to the animal with respiratory disease largely depends on the patient's history, signalment, physical examination findings, cardiopulmonary stability, and the expected diagnostic yield versus risk of a given diagnostic test. It remains important to take into account the sensitivity and specificity of any test performed when interpreting the results. A general algorithm is displayed in Figure 212-1.

LABORATORY DIAGNOSTICS

Hematologic and biochemical profiles are important in the assessment of an animal's health status and evaluation of nonrespiratory diseases that may have a substantial effect on the respiratory system, such as acidemia, anemia, or endocrinopathies. Chronic hypoxia stimulates the release of erythropoietin from the kidneys, which results in an increased red blood cell turnover and subsequent polycythemia. Anemia leads to a decrease in total oxygen content, which increases respiratory effort and rate. Leukocytosis with a left shift with moderate to severe airway inflammation, infection, or neoplasia, and leukopenia occurs with acute bacterial bronchopneumonia or sepsis. Parasitic airway disease, asthma, bronchitis, or pulmonary infiltration with eosinophilia (PIE) commonly cause an elevated peripheral eosinophil count, and a basophilia is frequently seen in animals with Dirofilaria immitus or PIE. Hypercalcemia may be associated with a neoplastic or fungal disease process. Hypoalbuminemia may be seen in animals with pleural effusion (cause or effect), and systemic illness or multiple-organ dysfunction can lead to ARDS. Hemorrhagic infiltrates or effusions may occur secondary to severe thrombocytopenia, thrombocytopathia, or coagulopathies.

Animals with no obvious cause of respiratory distress should be examined for other systemic diseases that may predispose to pulmonary thromboembolism (PTE). Underlying diseases

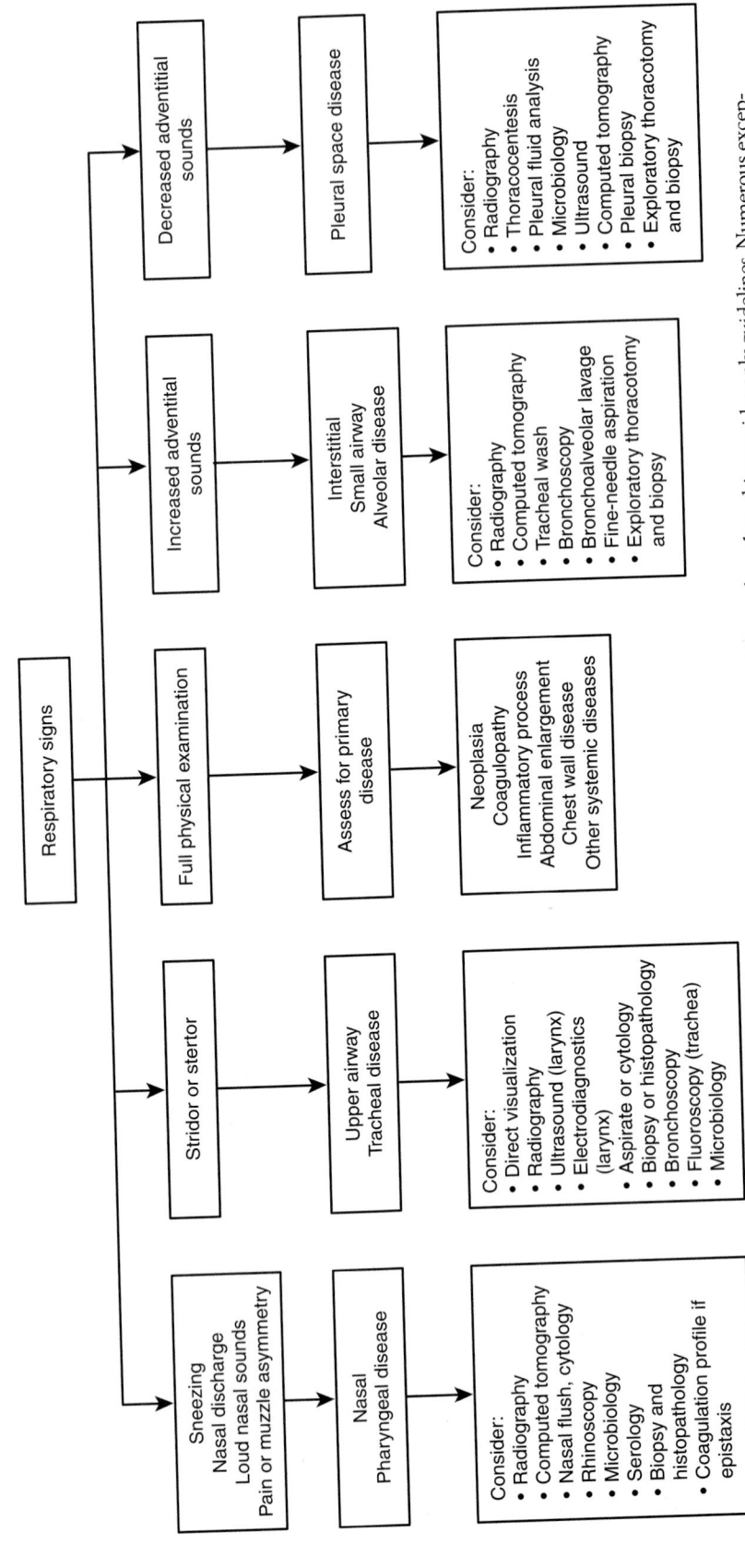

Figure 212-1 General diagnostic algorithm for evaluation of the respiratory tract. As with any algorithm, this provides only guidelines. Numerous exceptions to this algorithmic approach exist.

might include hyperadrenocorticism, diabetes mellitus, immune-mediated anemia or thrombocytopenia, protein losing nephropathy or enteropathy, or pancreatitis. Coagulation profiles, platelet counts, blood smear analysis, fibrin and fibrinogen degradation products, D-dimer assays, antithrombin III measurements, and/or thromboelastography (TEG) may be useful in the diagnosis of disseminated intravascular coagulation that might lead to PTE or pulmonary hemorrhage.

There are many serologic tests available for the identification of viral diseases, mycoses, and allergens. Specific infectious disease testing will depend on the animal's environment, travel history, and lifestyle. Feline leukemia virus and feline immunodeficiency virus infection commonly leads to secondary opportunistic infections. Additional infectious causes of respiratory disease in the dog or cat that may require further diagnostics include viral diseases (canine distemper, canine parainfluenza, canine adenovirus-2, herpevirus, feline rhinotracheitis, feline calicivirus), bacterial diseases (e.g., *Bordetella bronchiseptica*, streptococci, *Escherichia coli*, *Klebsiella*, *Pasteurella*, eugoic fermenter-4, mycobacteria, *Yersinia* spp., *Pseudomonas mallei*, *Mycoplasma* spp., *Bacteroides* spp., *Clostridium perfringens*, fusobacteria, *Peptostreptococcus* spp.), parasitic or protozoal diseases (e.g., *Dirofilria immitus*, *Paragonimus kellicotti*, *Capillaria aerophila*, *Aelurostrongylus abstrusus*, *Toxoplasma* spp., *Acanthamoeba* spp.), fungal infections (e.g., *Blastomyces*, *Histoplasma*, *Cryptococcus*, *Coccidiodes*, *Aspergillus*, and *Penicillium* spp.), or rickettsial diseases (e.g., *Rickettsia rickettsii*, *Ehrlichia canis*). Bacterial and fungal cultures, serologic testing, cytologic examination, electron microscopy, immunocytology and immunohistochemistry, immunoblotting, and/or polymerase-chain reaction amplification may be required for a definitive diagnosis of infectious diseases.[1] Heartworm disease in the cat may require echocardiography in addition to antibody and antigen testing.[2] Fecal studies should be performed in animals with suspected parasitic pneumonia. A zinc sulfate fecal flotation, including several drops of sediment, is indicated to identify *Paragonimus kellicotti* or *Capillaria aerophila* ova, and a Baermann technique should be used to identify *Aelurostrongylus abstrusus* larvae.

DIAGNOSTIC IMAGING

Radiography

Radiography remains an essential tool in the diagnostic approach to respiratory tract disease. Serial radiographic studies serve as an important method of monitoring a patient's respiratory disease and response to therapy. Proper radiographic technique is critical when viewing the nasal cavity or chest cavity owing to the nature of the fine nasal turbinates and air-tissue interface in the lungs, respectively.

Nasal radiography is typically used to evaluate animals with clinical signs of sneezing, nasal discharge, or upper airway obstruction. Morphologic changes in the air passages, turbinates, and frontal sinuses may be confirmed and the extent of the lesions defined. Nasal radiography does require anesthesia in order to obtain proper positioning and avoid motion artifact. Three views should be taken to assess the nasal cavity and frontal sinuses: a lateral, frontal, and open-mouth ventrodorsal, or intraoral dorsoventral view. It is important to look for symmetry, obliteration of air spaces between the nasal turbinates or frontal sinuses suggestive of fluid or swelling, destruction of nasal turbinates indicating a neoplastic or severe, chronic inflammatory process, or destruction/deformation of proximal facial structures which is commonly due to neoplasia or *Cryptococcus* spp.[3,4]

Radiography of the neck and extrathoracic airway is indicated in dogs or cats with inspiratory stridor or stertor, gagging, coughing, and/or recent voice change. Lateral radiographs are most useful in assessing these structures; however, tracheal displacement may be more visible on a ventrodorsal view. Both inspiratory and expiratory views are helpful in assessment of dynamic changes in airway diameter. Radiographs may assist in the identification of pharyngeal, laryngeal, or tracheal disease due to radiopaque foreign bodies or soft tissue masses (abscesses, polyps, neoplasms, granulation tissue), anatomic displacement due to mass lesions, tracheal narrowing or hypoplasia, or tracheal collapse.[5] Tracheal displacement secondary to mass lesions, soft tissue masses, hypoplasia, and invagination of the dorsal tracheal membrane are commonly seen in older symptomatic or asymptomatic dogs with chronic coughing, but rarely in cats. Cervical emphysema or pneumomediastinum following endotracheal intubation or trauma in cats is readily diagnosed with cervical radiography.[4]

Survey thoracic radiographs are commonly used in the diagnostic evaluation of dogs and cats with respiratory disease.[6] There are fewer breed-related and age-related changes seen in the feline thorax compared with the canine thorax.[4,6] A technique chart should be made to avoid over- or under-diagnosis of pulmonary disease when thoracic radiographs are viewed. In addition, a lateral and dorsoventral or ventrodorsal radiograph should comprise the minimum thoracic study. Three views (including both laterals) are commonly taken when looking for metastatic pulmonary disease or unilateral disease, although this practice has been questioned.[7] In cats, the use of high-detail x-ray intensifying screens may help in the identification of small airway disease.

The chest wall, diaphragm, pleural space, mediastinum, airways, and pulmonary parenchyma should be assessed. The thoracic wall should be evaluated for evidence of trauma (rib or sternal fractures), soft tissue masses, lytic, and/or sclerotic processes.[8]

Diaphragmatic abnormalities such as loss of the diaphragmatic silhouette or changes in the shape and position of the diaphragm are assessed in evaluation of thoracic radiographs. The diaphragmatic position and shape varies with the respiratory cycle, species and breed, conformation, coexisting diseases, and body fat content. Changes in the shape of the diaphragm are due to thoracic masses or lung disease adjacent to the diaphragm, diaphragmatic hernias, gastroesophageal intussusception, diaphragmatic masses, and chronic pleural inflammatory conditions. Cranial displacement of the diaphragm occurs secondary to abdominal disease, generalized diaphragmatic paralysis, or muscular dystrophy and caudal displacement occurs secondary to severe respiratory disease or pleural space disease. Decreased visualization of the diaphragmatic line, the presence of abdominal viscera within the thorax, displacement of abdominal or thoracic structures, pleural fluid, and divergence of the diaphragmatic crura or cranial angulation of the diaphragm might indicate a diaphragmatic hernia or diaphragmatic defect. Additional diagnostics that might be performed to confirm a diaphragmatic hernia include an upper gastrointestinal barium contrast study, horizontal beam radiographs, ultrasonography, positive contrast celiography, portography, cholecystography, angiocardiography, angiography, and nonselective cardiography, computed tomography, or magnetic resonance imaging.[9,10] Radiographs of animals with a peritoneopericardial diaphragmatic hernias also display an enlarged, round cardiac silhouette, abdominal organs within the pericardial sac, confluent silhouette between the diaphragm and heart, and an indistinguishable border of the ventral thoracic diaphragmatic surface and the caudal ventral cardiac silhouette. A dorsal mesothelial remnant between the heart and the diaphragm on the lateral view in normal cats is commonly seen.[10]

The presence of fluid, air, or soft tissue within the pleural space should be identified with thoracic radiography. As little as 100 mL of pleural fluid is detectable in a medium-sized dog using standard thoracic radiographic views. A lateral and erect ventrodorsal view enables the detection of as little as 50 mL of fluid in a 15-kg animal.[11] Removal of fluid or air prior to taking radiographs will help stabilize the animal and will improve the radiographic visualization of the lung fields, heart, and mediastinum. Radiographic changes associated with pleural effusion include blurring of the cardiac silhouette, interlobar fissure lines, rounding of the lung margins at the costophrenic angles, widening of the mediastinum, separation of the lung borders from the thoracic wall, and scalloping of the lung margins at the sternal border.[12] Hemothorax, pyothorax, chylothorax, or transudative effusions may be present. Cytology, cultures, and fluid analysis are necessary to classify the effusion (see Pleural and Extrapleural Diseases).

Radiographic changes associated with pneumothorax include dorsal displacement of the heart on the lateral view, retraction of the lung from the chest wall, and an increased density of the collapsed lung lobes. Potential causes might include chest wall trauma, an esophageal perforation leading to severe pneumomediastinum, or rupture of the trachea or lung (commonly secondary to infection, bulla, neoplasia, or positive pressure ventilation).[12]

The mediastinum should be evaluated radiographically for evidence of a mediastinal shift, masses, lymphadenopathy, fluid, or pneumomediastinum. Mediastinal shifts and mediastinal masses are most readily seen on ventrodorsal or dorsoventral radiographs. If mediastinal fluid is suspected, horizontal beam radiographs and ultrasonography may yield further diagnostic information. Pneumomediastinum is best appreciated on lateral films of the chest, and pneumomediastinum may lead to subcutaneous emphysema, pneumoretroperitoneum, and/or pneumothorax in severe cases. Potential causes of pneumomediastinum include alveolar rupture, perforation of the trachea or esophagus, extension of gas in the neck or retroperitoneal space, or a gas-producing organism within the mediastinum.[13] The cardiac silhouette and pulmonary vasculature should also be assessed since left atrial enlargement leading to compression of the left mainstem bronchus, pleural effusion, and/or pulmonary edema commonly leads to respiratory impairment. The pulmonary artery may be prominent in animals with PTE, pulmonary hypertension, or heartworm disease.[14]

Evaluation of the lungs in animals with respiratory disease may reveal an increase in opacity, hyperlucency, and/or pulmonary mass lesions. It is important to assess the distribution of pulmonary abnormalities in conjunction with clinical signs. An increase in opacity of the lung is further separated into three categories of radiographic patterns: bronchiolar, interstitial, and alveolar. Differential diagnoses for the various lung patterns can be found in Box 212-1. Cats may prove more challenging to diagnose since the pattern and distribution of lung abnormalities are often not as reliable as with dogs. For example, the distribution of pulmonary infiltrates in cats with cardiogenic pulmonary edema is often patchy and asymmetric, rather than perihilar, and cats with pneumonia often do not have cranioventral distribution and alveolar patterns, as seen in dogs (Figure 212-2).[4] Pulmonary hyperlucency might be seen secondary to overexposure, hypovolemia, hyperinflation, PTE, cavitary masses, bronchiectasis, or areas of pulmonary parenchymal dissolution (emphysema, pneumatocoele, bulla). Neoplasia is the most common cause of solitary or multifocal mass lesions in the lungs, although abscess, granuloma, or fluid-filled structures cannot be ruled out.[15]

Fluoroscopy allows for real-time imaging of the thoracic structures. The motion studies obtained are often helpful in evaluation of the animal with tracheal collapse. The animal is placed in lateral recumbency and the trachea and bronchi are examined during both quiet respiration and induced coughing. Coughing is induced by gentle digital palpation of the trachea near the thoracic inlet. A videotape of the fluoroscopic study

---

Box • 212-1

Differential Diagnoses for the Various Lung Patterns Seen on Thoracic Radiographs

Bronchial Pattern
Chronic bronchitis (irritant, allergic, parasitic)
Calcification
Peribronchial cuffing (edema, bronchopneumonia, pulmonary infiltrates with eosinophilia)

Interstitial Pattern
Nodular
    Neoplasia
    Granuloma (eosinophilic, fungal, parasitic or heartworm-associated, foreign body)
    Bulla with fluid
    Hematoma, abscess, cyst
    Mucus-filled bronchus
    Bronchiectasis
Hazy and unstructured
    Diffuse
        Artifact (underexposure, obesity, end-expiratory film)
        Degenerative changes ("old dog lung")
        Neoplasia (lymphosarcoma, metastasis)
        Pneumonitis (toxic, inhalant, metabolic, viral, parasitic)
        Acute respiratory distress syndrome
        Transitional stages of diseases such as edema, hemorrhage, bronchopneumonia
    Localized
        Hemorrhage
        PTE
        Foreign body
        Partial atelectasis
        Transitional stages of disease such as edema, bronchopneumonia, hemorrhage, or parasites

Alveolar Pattern
Diffuse
    Edema (cardiogenic or non-cardiogenic)
    Bronchopneumonia
    Hemorrhage
    Smoke inhalation
    Near-drowning
    Acute respiratory distress syndrome
Localized
    Edema
    Bronchopneumonia
    Hemorrhage
    Primary lung tumor or metastasis
    Lobar collapse or atelectasis
    Heartworm disease
    Infarct

---

is useful for reviewing the airway changes in slow motion and diagnosing subtle dynamic airway disease.

Bronchography creates an outline of the mucosal surfaces of the trachea and bronchi using radiopaque contrast material.[16,17] Since bronchoscopy is now widely available, this diagnostic test is rarely used. The current use of bronchography may be

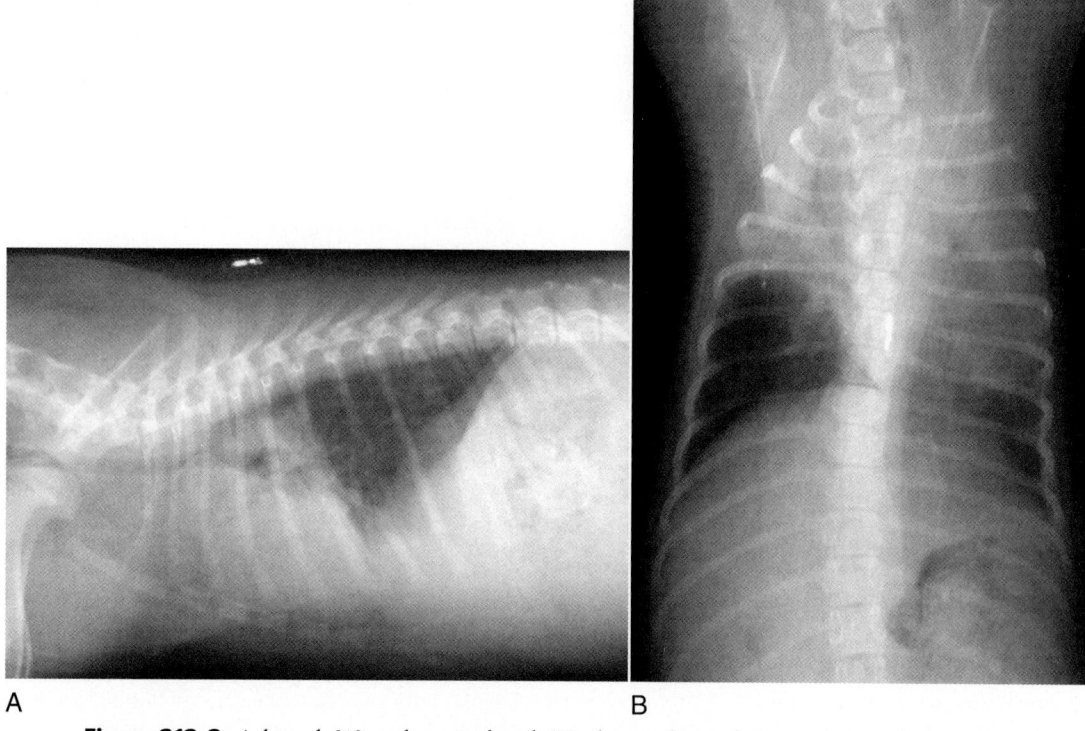

A   B

Figure 212-2 A lateral (A) and ventrodorsal (B) chest radiograph in a puppy with aspiration pneumonia. Cranioventral air bronchograms are evident.

limited to the evaluation of the severity and distribution of severe bronchiectasis prior to considering a lobectomy or pulmonectomy. Bronchography is typically performed under heavy sedation or anesthesia using fluoroscopic guidance to place a catheter through the endotracheal tube and into the pulmonary areas of interest. Contrast material such as Dionosil or sterile barium sulfate is injected and allowed to distribute during patient respiration. Fluoroscopic imaging and/or thoracic radiographs are then obtained. Potential complications (rare) include allergic reactions to the contrast, bronchospasm, retention of contrast in the small airways, or chemical pneumonitis.

Pulmonary angiography is useful for the detection of vascular anomalies (congenital or acquired) and pulmonary thromboembolism. Pulmonary angiography is performed by injecting iodinated contrast intravascularly in order to opacify the pulmonary arteries and veins. Selective pulmonary angiography is superior to nonselective angiography but does require injection of a medium-density, nonionic contrast material into a catheter in the pulmonary artery or a branch thereof. With nonselective angiography, the contrast material is injected into the jugular or cephalic vein and films are taken at a speed of 1 to 2 per second or a fluoroscopic recording is made for both procedures (up to 5 to 30 seconds with severe vascular obstruction or cardiac dysfunction).[18] Potential complications include vascular injury, thrombosis secondary to injury, embolization of air, blood clots, or catheter material, infections associated with unsterile techniques, cardiac arrythmias due to endocardial stimulation from the catheter, or immune reactions to the contrast agent (including asystole and death).[19]

Ultrasonography
Ultrasonography can be useful in animals with nasopharyngeal soft tissue or fluid-filled masses.[20] Ultrasound has also been used to assist in the diagnosis of tracheal collapse and laryngeal paralysis in dogs.[21,22] Identification of pulmonary

consolidation, masses, atelectasis, or torsion, as well as pleural or mediastinal abnormalities, may be detected using ultrasound. Ultrasound guided aspirates or biopsies are readily obtained using real-time visualization of the needle entering the tissue or fluid lesion.[23-25] Potential risks include bleeding, iatrogenic pneumothorax, or the introduction of infectious agents during the procedure. Using ultrasound, it may be easier to distinguish pleural or pulmonary opacities seen on radiographs or better visualize peripheral, pulmonary lesions that may be obscured by pleural effusion. In dyspneic patients, ultrasound is easily performed with the animal in sternal recumbency and may be better tolerated than radiographs. However, ultrasound is unable to allow visualization of lesions within an aerated lung since air impedes the transmission of sound. Ultrasound is operator-dependant and requires an experienced user for good results.

Nuclear Imaging
Nuclear scintigraphy is performed by the administration of a radioactive nuclide to the patient and detection of the energy from the radionuclides as they decay, with use of a camera that records the results to a computer monitor or photographic film.[26,27] Technetium 99m (^{99m}Tc) is the most common nuclide utilized. If pulmonary mineralization is suspected, bone-seeking radiopharmaceuticals can also be used.[28] (see Chapter 100).

Nuclear scintigraphy is most commonly utilized with lung disease in small animals to evaluate pulmonary perfusion in animals with suspected pulmonary thromboemboli or vascular anomalies.[27,29-31] It is relatively specific and sensitive for this purpose in dogs.[32] The radioactive particles are given intravenously and go through the pulmonary arteries, where they are trapped in the capillary bed. A normal animal shows uniform radioactivity throughout the lung fields. Vascular occlusion secondary to pulmonary emboli appears as deficient radioactive areas or photopenic defects on the perfusion scan.

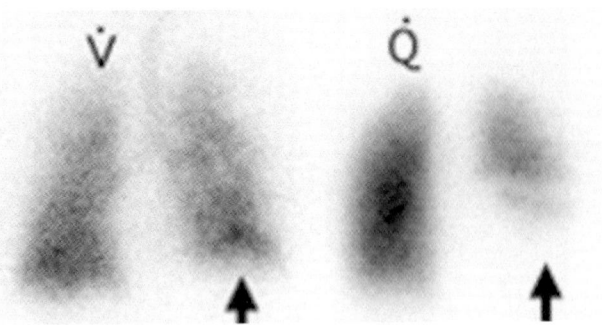

Figure 212-3 A ventilation-perfusion scan in a dog with a pulmonary thromboembolism. Normal ventilation is seen on the left (V, arrow), and a perfusion deficit is present on the right (Q, arrow).

The specificity of diagnosing ventilation/perfusion inequalities is increased if the nuclear scan is combined with a ventilation scan.[33]

The ventilation scan is performed using 99mTc-labeled diethylenetriamine pentaacetic acid, which is delivered via a nebulizer to the patient.[27,33] The radioactive aerosol is distributed in the air spaces, and areas of deficient radioactivity indicate poorly ventilated locations. A simultaneous ventilation and perfusion scan (Figure 212-3) enables the calculation of the ventilation:perfusion ratio (normal is 1:1). However, results are dependent on blood flow and ventilation differences in various parts of the lung and are difficult to interpret in the face of pulmonary interstitial lung disease.

Positron emission tomography (PET) is another noninvasive nuclear imaging technique that uses radioactive positrons to assess the chemical and physiological changes related to metabolism in a specific organ.[34] PET has been used in human medicine to diagnose and stage lung masses, monitor the size and activity of cancerous lesions, diagnose pulmonary thromboembolism, and assess changes in vascular permeability.[35,36] This technology is not often available for use in veterinary medicine but has been used experimentally in dogs to measure lung water, pulmonary vascular permeability, regional pulmonary blood flow, degree of lung injury, and regional pulmonary function.[37-45]

Alternative Imaging

Computed tomography (CT) and magnetic resonance imaging (MRI) are useful to detect or monitor nasopharyngeal, tracheal, or thoracic cavity lesions, assess the involvement of surrounding structures, and determine anatomic relationships. This imaging modality requires general anesthesia but may provide more valuable information regarding the pathogenesis, extent, and changes of many disease states.[46-55]

Computed tomography (CT) utilizes a 360-degree x-ray beam to create a three-dimensional, computer-processed cross-sectional image of body tissues or organs. The CT scanner acquires images incrementally, at a rate that varies with the type of machine and settings. The speed of the image acquisition is especially important when viewing the lung, since respiratory and cardiac motion will interfere with image quality. Most conventional CT machines have dynamic modes that acquire 8 to 12 scans per minute, although this rate is still incapable of obtaining suspended respiratory images. CT scans produce images with superior density discrimination that are free of superimposition from overlapping thoracic structures when compared with radiographs.[56] CT scanning is therefore the preferred tool for pulmonary imaging in people and is often used to differentiate pleural, extrapleural, or mediastinal tissues, or to better visualize the lungs when pleural effusion makes radiographic evaluation of the lungs difficult. A CT scan may

be indicated to evaluate the lungs when thoracic radiographs are normal, but there is clinical suspicion of pulmonary disease, in animals that have abnormalities present on radiographs that require further clarification (i.e., prior to surgical intervention), or to assist in cancer staging and monitoring changes. Metastatic nodules are more easily detected using CT than radiography, and newer technologies such as spiral CT and high-resolution CT have made CT imaging faster and more diagnostically useful.[47,50,57-60]

High-resolution CT has excellent spatial resolution and is able to demonstrate pulmonary structures that are only 300 μ, as well as monitor changes in airway and vascular diameter in vivo following various stimuli, revealing differences that may not be detectable with spirometry. It has been used in dogs to measure changes in airway diameter and assess the function of pulmonary vessels and airways.[61-63]

Helical or spiral CT utilizes a "slip-ring" technique and high-energy x-ray tubes that allow the tube and detector to continuously circle the patient, taking pictures as the patient is transported through the scanner. It takes approximately 1 second for the scanner to complete a single rotation so that 20- to 30-cm organs can be scanned in under 30 seconds, much more quickly than conventional CT methods.[64] This eliminates the motion and artifacts secondary to inconsistent lung inflation from one slice to the next, a current problem with conventional CT scanners.[65]

Spiral CT angiography enables scanning to occur simultaneously with maximum contrast medium opacification, which obviates the need for selective catheterization. This is especially beneficial in animals since catheterization requires general anesthesia, a potentially risky procedures in dyspneic animals with suspected PTE. Spiral CT angiography has been studied in humans to discover filling defects within the pulmonary arteries secondary to emboli, even in the face of underlying pulmonary disease (Figure 212-4).[66-70] Acute and chronic emboli may be differentiated by their appearance.[71] The clinical usefulness of CT angiography in small animals remains to be determined but may be preferable to nuclear scintigraphy due to its superior diagnostic accuracy and speed.[67,68] The procedure has been used experimentally to effectively diagnose pulmonary thromboembolism in dogs and clinically in dogs with metastatic pulmonary lesions.[72,73] The detection of pulmonary metastases has shown limited success.[73]

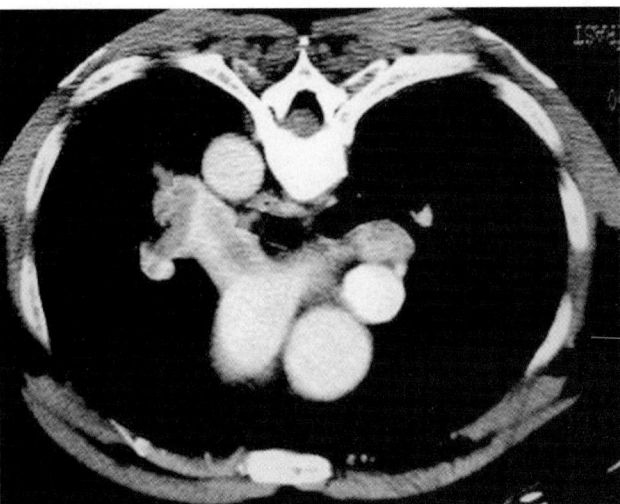

Figure 212-4 Spiral CT angiography in a dog with pulmonary thromboemboli. The arrows point to the filling defects within the pulmonary artery. (Courtesy Tobias Schwarz and Steve Cole.)

MRI is based on the principles of nuclear magnetic resonance, a spectroscopic technique that reveals chemical and physical characteristics of the examined tissues using the absorption and emission of energy in the radio frequency range of the electromagnetic spectrum. Conventional MRI is based on the spin magnetism of the hydrogen nucleus and the fact that water is abundant in biologic tissue. However, the air spaces in the lungs are challenging to image since they are porous, which causes large internal magnetic field gradients, and contain primarily air rather than water (which contains the hydrogen proton). The use of hyperpolarized (HP) noble gas (specifically ^{3}He and ^{129}Xe) has emerged over the past decade to circumvent this problem. The polarized or inert gas is inhaled by the patient and subsequently detected with the use of MRI in the airways of the lungs and dissolved in the proximal blood.[74,75] In addition, the use of novel paramagnetic aerosol ventilation and perfusion MRI imaging using gadolinium diethylenetriamine pentaacetic acid (Gd-DTPA) has been used experimentally to diagnose airway obstruction and PTE in dogs.[76] More recently, noncontrast, electrocardiography (ECG)-gated fast-spin-echo (FSE) MRI has shown promise experimentally as a means of rapidly assessing dynamically altered regional lung perfusion or airway obstruction in dogs.[77] The MRI technique has also expanded to include three-dimensional reconstruction abilities, so the user can view surface details and internal structures and dissect each layer of tissue in a mock, on-screen approach. Two-dimensional and three-dimensional techniques have been developed to perform angiographic studies without the need for contrast agents, based on the knowledge that the image intensity of flowing blood is proportional to the velocity of the flow. Although the use HP MRI, vascular MRI (VMRI) or MR angiography (MRA) is limited in veterinary medicine, future studies may prove worthwhile.

SCOPING PROCEDURES

Laryngoscopy allows visualization of the short cartilaginous lumen between the lower portion of the pharynx and the trachea. It is indicated in patients with suspected upper airway obstruction, palpable or radiographically visible mass lesions in the area of the larynx, or unexplained changes in vocalization. Clinical signs that are commonly related to laryngeal disease include coughing, choking while eating, cyanosis or syncope with exertion, inspiratory dyspnea with stertor or stridor, and changes in vocalization or sound production (meow, purr, or bark). Laryngoscopy is useful in the diagnosis of an elongated soft palate, laryngeal paralysis, laryngeal edema, acute laryngitis, laryngeal collapse, chronic granulomatous or proliferative laryngitis, traumatic lesions, everted laryngeal saccules, laryngeal or pharyngeal foreign bodies, polyps or neoplasms of the larynx, and glosso-epiglottic mucosal displacement.[78,79] In animals with severe clinical signs, stabilization with a tracheostomy or other bypassing maneuver might be necessary prior to examination.[80] The procedure can be performed with use of a standard intubating laryngoscope and mouth speculum to hold the mouth open, although a rigid or flexible bronchoscope may be required if areas distal to the vocal folds or infraglottic region require examination. The tongue is depressed to allow adequate examination of the pharynx, soft palate, lingual and glottal surfaces of the epiglottis, arytenoid cartilages, aryepiglottic folds, and vocal folds. Abnormal shape, color, and/or motility should be noted. The soft palate should be examined and palpated and the nasopharynx is examined by retracting the soft palate rostrally with a spay hook and visualizing the area with a heated dental mirror. Laryngoscopy should be performed with neuroleptanalgesia, if possible, rather than general anesthesia to prevent relaxation of the laryngeal muscles and distortion of the larynx. Propofol or thiobarbiturates are often recommended for examination of laryngeal function. The routine administration of doxapram prior to evaluation has been studied and recommended to increase intrinsic laryngeal function and aid in the diagnosis of laryngeal disease in dogs.[81] The arytenoid cartilage and vocal folds should abduct symmetrically during inspiration and relax during exhalation. The correlation of movement of these structures during the respiratory cycle should be examined.[78]

The pharynx is the crossroads of the respiratory and digestive tracts and consists of the nasopharynx, oropharynx, and laryngopharynx. If a flexible endoscope is used, retroflex nasopharyngoscopy will enable superior visualization, with or without biopsy sampling of the nasopharynx. Respiratory signs that might warrant pharyngoscopy include dyspnea, coughing after swallowing, oronasal reflux of liquid or food, open-mouth breathing, or stertorous breathing. Dysphagia, retching, gagging, and inappetance may also be present in animals with pharyngeal disorders. A standard intubating laryngoscope allows adequate visualization of the pharynx, although an endoscope may be used if further scoping is to follow. Prior to anesthesia in animals with the above clinical signs, cervical and thoracic radiographs, a thorough neurologic examination, and/or a esophagram with fluoroscopy may be indicated. Propofol or thiobarbiturates should be used and examination of the pharynx is performed prior to intubation. The soft palate, tonsils and tonsillar crypts, palatopharyngeal arches, and lateral pharyngeal wall should be carefully examined.[78]

Rhinoscopy is most commonly used in animals with chronic nasal disease, although more emergent cases may benefit as well (nasal foreign body retrieval, nasal parasite detection, and evaluation of epistaxis in animals with normal coagulation parameters).[78] Rhinoscopy has proven to be a useful tool in the animal with nasal disease, having a diagnostic success rate of 83% when performed by an experienced endoscopist and used in conjunction with rhinoscopy-assisted biopsy.[82] Rhinoscopy greatly decreases the morbidity and mortality associated with surgical rhinotomy when used to visualize the nasal passages and obtain biopsy samples. A surgical plane of anesthesia is required for rhinoscopy since the nasal mucosa is extremely sensitive (prior administration of topical anesthetic may be beneficial as well). An otoscopic speculum may be used to visualize the proximal 2 cm of the nasal passages in most animals. Since a majority of neoplastic and mycotic diseases are in the caudal half of the nasal cavity, this method has limited diagnostic usefulness. In order to perform rhinoscopy, a rigid arthroscope, flexible or rigid cystourethroscope, or flexible pediatric bronchoscope is used. Width, length, and flushing/biopsy port availability makes the various scopes more or less desirable for specific situations.

Bronchoscopy may be useful in animals with suspected lower airway disease. Clinical signs that may indicate the need for a bronchoscopic examination include chronic coughing, hemoptysis, unexplained pulmonary infiltrates on thoracic radiographs, and the suspicion of an airway mass or foreign body. Bronchoscopy allows visual inspection of the airways and the collection of samples from the respiratory tract. Bronchoscopy may be used therapeutically for the removal of foreign bodies, resolution of mucus plugs, and removal of copious secretions or blood.[83,84] Diagnostically, bronchoscopy allows the clinician to visualize, lavage, brush, and/or biopsy the airways. In animals with intraluminal tracheal tumors, bronchoscopically guided biopsies may be obtained.[85] Bronchoscopy is valuable in the diagnosis and staging of tracheal collapse in dogs (Figure 212-5).[86,87] Bronchoscopy must be performed under general anesthesia to prevent coughing and laryngospasm. Intubation may not be possible if the endotracheal tube size is equal to that of the bronchoscope. If the animal must be extubated for a bronchoscopic examination, oxygen should be supplied via a catheter placed in the trachea beside the

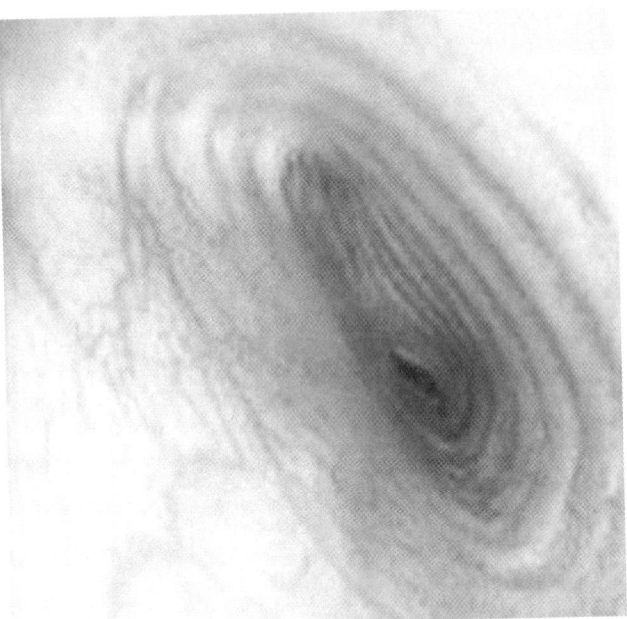

Figure 212-5 Bronchoscopic visualization of tracheal collapse in a dog. (Courtesy Candace Carter.)

bronchoscope, through the biopsy channel of the bronchoscope, or by jet ventilation through a catheter. A T-shaped adaptor can be used in larger animals so the scope can be passed through the endotracheal tube while administering inhalant anesthesia.[83,84]

RESPIRATORY SAMPLING TECHNIQUES

It is often necessary to obtain fluid, cells, and/or tissue from the respiratory tract for analysis. There are a variety of techniques that will be discussed in order to obtain specimens from the upper and lower respiratory tract.

Cytologic sampling of the upper respiratory tract can be challenging. Since there is a wide range of normal bacteria in the nasal cavity in small animals,[88] bacterial cultures of nasal swabs are not routinely performed. If a significant nonresponsive bacterial infection is suspected, a surgically obtained sample from the caudal nasal cavity may prove most useful for culture and sensitivity analysis, since cultures from this area are sterile approximately 50% of the time in dogs.[89] Most nasal disease results in inflammation of the mucosal epithelium and secondary bacterial infections, which tends to obscure the underlying disease. In addition, the disease process may be focal or multifocal, rather than diffuse. Nonsurgical techniques for the collection of diagnostic nasal samples include superficial and deep nasal swabs, nasal flushing, traumatic nasal flushing, pinch biopsy, and core biopsy. *Cryptococcus* and *Aspergillus* spp. infection can be diagnosed on examination of a superficial nasal swab; however, these agents may be encountered occasionally as normal flora or colonizers of abnormal sites. Confirmation of the disease typically requires further testing. Serologic testing, tissue biopsy, or fungal isolation should be considered in cats with a chronic nasal discharge.[90,91] Neutrophils commonly predominate in diseases such as trauma, neoplasia, infection, and foreign bodies,[92] whereas eosinophils may predominate in allergic or parasitic diseases.[93]

Biopsy collection techniques should be performed under general anesthesia. The patient should be intubated with a cuffed endotracheal tube and the caudal pharynx packed with gauze to prevent aspiration of blood or discharge.

Potential complications include hemorrhage and inadvertent puncture of the cribriform plate.

Transtracheal aspiration may be indicated in dogs with clinical or radiographic evidence of airway disease. It is contraindicated in animals with severe dyspnea or coagulopathies. The procedure is often performed on awake or lightly sedated animals in sternal recumbency or a sitting position with the neck extended. The area over the cricothyroid membrane is clipped and sterilely prepared. A local anesthetic is administered subcutaneously and a relief incision is made in the skin over the cricothyroid membrane. A shielded catheter-through-a-needle or catheter-through-a-catheter (18- to 20-gauge, 8- to 12-inch Intracath with wire stylet jugular catheter by Becton Dickinson, Sandy, UT, works well) system is used to puncture the cricothyroid membrane and the catheter is advanced into the distal trachea.[94] The needle is removed from the airway and covered. A syringe containing 1 to 10 mL of preservative-free 0.9% saline is attached to the end of the catheter. The saline is injected into the trachea and negative pressure is applied to the plunger of the syringe as the animal is gently coupaged. If possible, the catheter is moved up and down the trachea during the syringe aspiration. Fluid injection and aspiration may need to be repeated two to three times. Fluid retrieved is saved for cytologic analysis and microbiologic testing. Potential complications include catheter related trauma to the lower airways, which results in hemoptysis, coughing, and respiratory impairment or needle-related trauma to the laryngeal region that might cause bleeding, subcutaneous emphysema, pneumomediastinum, pneumothorax, or pneumopharynx and airway obstruction.[94] Airway samples from cats or very small dogs should be collected via an endotracheal tube using a long catheter inserted through the tube to infuse and aspirate fluid.[95]

Bronchoalveolar lavage (BAL) may be performed with or without bronchoscopic guidance. BAL cytology has been described in normal cats and dogs.[94,96-101] It is indicated in dogs and cats with alveolar or interstitial lung disease to help identify neoplastic, infectious, or inflammatory diseases.[102] Microbiologic, biochemical, and immunologic testing of the lavage fluid may be performed. Potential side effects are primarily related to general anesthesia, although transient hypoxemia or exacerbation of respiratory insufficiency may develop during the BAL. In order to obtain a diagnostic sample, the bronchoscope is cleaned and the biopsy port flushed with sterile saline before advancing it into the diseased airway. The scope is wedged into the smallest bronchus possible and 10 to 25 mL of warmed (37° C) nonbacteriostatic saline is instilled (alternatively, polyethylene tubing can be passed through the biopsy channel and wedged into a smaller airway). The fluid is removed by suction into a mucous suction trap or by hand using a 35 mL syringe. Between 40% and 60% of the fluid instilled is typically retrieved, depending on the wedging of the bronchoscope and patency of the airway.

At least two distant segments should be lavaged to increase the likelihood of disease identification.[102] A modified stomach technique has also been described for BAL in dogs.[103] Analysis should include a differential cell count on a cytocentrifuged sample and a culture and sensitivity if indicated. Normal cell counts in the dog and cat are approximately 200 to 400 cells per milliliter, with 65% macrophages in the cat and 83% macrophages in the dog. Neutrophils typically make up 5% of the cells in dogs and cats, lymphocytes 4% to 6%, mast cells 1% to 2%, and eosinophils up to 25% in the cat and 4% in the dog.

Bronchial brushing may be performed through the bronchoscope to obtain samples of focal lesions within the airway. This procedure should be performed after the BAL to prevent blood contamination. A sterile cytology brush with a protective polyethylene tubing is inserted through the instrument channel, placed against the bronchial wall, advanced out of the sheath, and rotated along the lesion site. A smear is made onto a glass slide or the brush is placed in sterile saline solution and swirled to release cells for cytologic analysis and culture/sensitivity testing.[104] Mild bleeding at the site is the most common complication.

Healthy dogs and cats have a certain percentage of bacteria (*Pasteurella* spp., *Mycoplasma* spp., *Streptococcus* spp., *Staphylococcus* spp., *Acinetobacter* spp., Moraxella spp., *Enterobacter* spp., *Pseudomonas* spp., *Escherichia* coli, *Klebsiella* spp., and *Bordetella bronchiseptica*) isolated from samples taken with a sterile culture swab at the level of the lower trachea or carina.[98,105,106] Therefore the culture results must be interpreted in conjunction with cytologic findings. Intracellular bacteria and suppurative inflammation are supportive of a true bacterial infection.

Biopsies may be obtained using bronchoscopic guidance for histopathologic evaluation of focal abnormalities or for electron microscopic (EM) evaluation in animals with suspected ciliary dyskinesia. Biopsy samples are acquired using the biopsy port of the bronchoscope and samples should be fixed in formalin for histopathology or glutaraldehyde for EM. The animal should be monitored for hemoptysis from biopsy-site hemorrhage following the procedure.[94,107]

Transthoracic fine-needle aspiration (FNA) or biopsy might be indicated in patients with a single or multifocal pulmonary mass lesion greater than 1 cm and easily accessible or animals with diffuse air space or interstitial disease.[108,109] Fluoroscopic or ultrasonographic guidance is useful.[110,111] Contraindications include pulmonary cysts or bullae, uncooperative patients, refractory coagulopathies, or pulmonary hypertension. Animals with respiratory distress, preexisting pneumothorax, or behavior problems are not good candidates. Animals with clinical evidence of an infectious process such as a fever, inflammatory leukogram, and lethargy may be better candidates for endotracheal, transtracheal, or bronchoalveolar lavage.

Potential complications include pneumothorax, empyema, bleeding, implantation of neoplastic cells along the needle or biopsy tract, or death. One study revealed a 12% death rate and 5% incidence of pneumothorax following transthoracic FNA procedures.[112]

THORACOTOMY AND BIOPSY

An open-chest lung biopsy may be necessary in some cases where other less invasive techniques are nondiagnostic or histopathology is required to confirm a diagnosis. Contraindications include coagulopathy or an unacceptable anesthetic candidate. It requires greater expense, invasiveness, and risk, however it does allow the opportunity to visualize the lung and obtain an adequate sample size for a diagnosis. A standard thoracotomy is typically performed, although a "keyhole" technique is often effective for obtaining a histologic diagnosis of interstitial lung disease in dogs and cats.[113] The tissue sample is cultured, an impression smear analyzed, and the remainder placed in formalin for histopathologic evaluation. Potential complications include hemorrhage, pneumothorax, or secondary infections.

PULSE OXIMETRY AND ARTERIAL BLOOD GAS ANALYSIS

Pulse oximeters are commonly used to continuously and non-invasively measure the oxygen saturation of hemoglobin. Pulse oximetry measurements can be used to determine the need for oxygen administration and to monitor patients that are receiving oxygen supplementation. A hemoglobin saturation of 95% to 100% is normal in dogs and cats. There are, however,

many limitations, especially in critically ill animals, which makes this technology less reliable than direct arterial blood gas analysis.

Arterial blood gases (ABGs) are extremely useful in the assessment of an animal's oxygenation, ventilation, and acid-base balance. ABGs are commonly used to quantitate the severity of respiratory impairment and monitor response to therapy. With the advent of fairly inexpensive, handheld blood gas analyzers, ABGs are routinely used in many private practices. Normal arterial blood gases in the dog and cat are pH=7.36−7.44, PaO_2=90−100 mmHg, $PaCO_2$=36−40 mmHg, HCO_3= 20−24 mEq/L, and BE +/− 4 mEq/L.[114]

Arterial blood gas sampling is the most accurate method of evaluating the partial pressure of oxygen in the arterial blood. In dogs, arterial puncture is commonly performed using the dorsal metatarsal or femoral arteries, although the radial artery or digital palmar arteries may also be used. In cats, the femoral artery is typically the only easily accessible artery that is large enough to readily obtain an adequate sample. Preheparinized syringes will help prevent the sample from clotting prior to analysis, and the sample should be capped with material that is not permeable to gas to prevent air contamination and equilibration. Following arterial puncture, direct pressure should be applied to the site for 3 to 5 minutes to prevent bleeding. Hypoxemia is defined as a PaO_2 less than 80 mm Hg and possible causes include a right-to-left shunt (patent ductus arteriosus, ventricular septal defects, intrapulmonary shunts due to atelectasis or consolidation), ventilation perfusion mismatch (due to various types of pulmonary disease), diffusion impairment (relatively uncommon), hypoventilation (secondary to anesthesia, neuromuscular disease, pleural space or chest wall abnormalities), or a decrease in the fraction of inspired oxygen (oxygen tank empty and hooked up to patient, high elevations).[115] The animal's ability to oxygenate is assessed by examining the PaO_2 and determining the difference between the partial pressure of oxygen in the alveolar and the arterial blood, often referred to as the "A-a gradient." This equation is based on the knowledge that there is almost complete equilibration of gases between the alveolar gas and the pulmonary capillary when alveolar ventilation and pulmonary perfusion (V/Q) are matched. The partial pressure of oxygen in the alveolus (PaO_2) is calculated as follows:

$$PaO_2=[(PB-PH_2O)FiO_2]-PaCO_2/RQ$$

where PB = barometric pressure in mm Hg, PH_2O = water vapor pressure in mm Hg, FiO_2 = fraction of inspired oxygen, RQ = respiratory quotient (normally 0.8), and $PaCO_2$ = partial pressure of carbon dioxide in the alveolus in mm Hg.

The normal alveolar to arterial difference is less than 15 mm Hg when the patient is breathing room air. The A-a gradient is increased in animals with a right-to-left shunt, low mixed venous oxygen saturation, ventilation/perfusion mismatching, and diffusion impairment. Another method of assessing the severity of oxygenation impairment is to calculate the PaO_2 : FiO_2 ratio. Healthy people and animals have a ratio of 400 to 500, but a value less than 300 is suggestive of acute lung injury and less than 200 indicates acute respiratory distress syndrome in people.[114-116]

Ventilation refers to the movement of gas into and of the alveolus and is measured by the animal's ability to maintain normal arterial CO_2 levels. The carbon dioxide tension in arterial blood represents the balance between the production of CO_2 in the tissues and CO_2 excretion in the alveolus. Carbon dioxide excretion is dependent upon the amount of CO_2 delivered to the alveolus, alveolar ventilation, and the amount of deadspace ventilation that does not contribute to gas exchange. If there is inadequate elimination of CO_2 in the lungs or excessive CO_2 production in body tissues (less common), carbonic acid and hydrogen ions accumulate, resulting in a respiratory acidosis. Potential causes of inadequate ventilation include diseases of the central respiratory center, airways, pulmonary parenchyma, pleural space, pulmonary vasculature, or chest wall. Respiratory fatigue, a primary metabolic alkalosis, or anesthetic drugs may also lead to hypoventilation. If the problem is maintained for 24 to 48 hours, the kidneys respond over hours to days by increasing the excretion of hydrogen ions and retaining bicarbonate.[114-116]

If alveolar ventilation is increased, a respiratory alkalosis will develop. Potential causes include hypoxemia, primary metabolic acidosis, and central nervous system disease. Anxiety, pain, fear, and excitement may also lead to hyperventilation. If the problem is maintained, the kidneys will again compensate slowly by retaining hydrogen ions and excreting bicarbonate.[114-116]

In order to interpret a blood gas measurement, the pH should first be assessed. Determine whether the pH is normal or if there is a primary respiratory or metabolic cause for the disorder, if there is compensation for the primary disorder, or if there are two primary abnormalities present.

PULMONARY FUNCTION TESTING

Pulmonary function testing (PFT) is used to objectively assess functional respiratory deficits. It often serves as a valuable tool to provide information regarding the severity of pulmonary dysfunction as well as response to therapy. The information acquired quantifies the degree of dysfunction and is able to localize the site of respiratory dysfunction. There are, however, a few limitations to the use of pulmonary function testing in small animal medicine. Many animals require anesthesia in order to perform the testing, the equipment utilized is expensive and requires operational expertise, and there is a large amount of individual variation that makes isolated measurements in time less valuable in an individual animal.[117]

Since veterinary patients are not able to understand instructions to perform a maximal forced exhalation, it is not possible to perform the noninvasive, rapid spirometric tests that are commonly used in human medicine. Alternatively, the tidal breathing flow-volume loop (TBFVL), which was originally developed for human infants, can be used in the unanesthetized and untrained veterinary patient to assess and quantify airflow, volume, or respiratory cycle changes.[118]

To measure TBFVL, a pneumotachograph and a differential pressure transducer are used in accordance with the size of the patient.[118-121] The Fleisch pneumotachograph is commonly used in small animals. This device measures the pressure gradient as air follows across a resistance device. The rate of airflow is proportional to the drop in pressure inside the instrument, and is plotted on the x-axis. An electronic integration of the instantaneous flow rate is used to determine flow, which is plotted on the Y-axis, generating a "flow-volume" or "F-V loop."[120] Cats or dogs are allowed to sit or stand during the testing procedure. A tight-fitting mask is placed over the muzzle, including the commisure of the lips. A 1- to 3-minute recording of the TBFVL waveforms is obtained once the animal is calm and free of extraneous movements. Computerized pulmonary mechanics analyzer systems are now available to create the F-V loops (Respiratory Loop Analysis Software, BUXCO Electronics, Sharon, CT) and provide fast, accurate data analysis.[118,122] Information acquired from the flow, volume, and time analysis may be combined to determine time ratios, inspiratory to expiratory flow ratios at indicated lung volumes, flow ratios at different lung volumes, or changes in volume during a selected period of time.[118,121] In order to improve the diagnostic sensitivity and reproducibility of the TBFVL test, application of positive pressure to the external chest wall, negative pressure to the airway, increased concentrations

of the inspired CO_2 or doxapram hydrochloride have been used.[123-126] When CO_2 is used adjunctively, an increase in the inspired oxygen concentration may be helpful to prevent hypoxic pulmonary or vascular changes.

TBFVL from normal healthy cats and dogs with differing nasal anatomy have been described.[118,121,127] TBFVL have been used clinically in veterinary medicine to diagnose and/or evaluate treatment modalities in dogs with chronic obstructive lung disease, laryngeal paralysis, tracheal collapse, brachycephalic syndrome, and cats with chronic lower airway disease.[118,121,127-134] Loops are easily obtained in most nonsedated, naïve dogs and cats. It is contraindicated in animals with severe dyspnea since placement of the mask may exacerbate the animal's condition.

The measurement of upper airway pressures can be obtained with use of a transcutaneously placed catheter into the trachea, using the same technique as described for transtracheal aspiration above. Using a pressure transducer, the pressure changes in the upper airways are readily measured. A face mask technique can be used, as described for TBFVL measurements, to obtain the flow and volume measurements and the pressure transducers matched to a defined frequency.[135] The change in pressure is divided by the change in flow to calculate resistance in the upper airway, and this is easily performed using a mechanics analyzer and designated software analysis program. Normal values for upper airway resistance have been established in dolichocephalic and mesaticephalic dogs.[136] Measurements of upper airway resistance might be beneficial in diagnosing and quantifying airway obstruction and changes in response to therapy.

Pulmonary mechanics measurements typically require general anesthesia in small animals in order to pass an esophageal balloon for the measurement of transpulmonary pressure,[137] whereas flow and volume measurements are made via an endotracheal tube. Measurements have therefore been used primarily in the research setting and it is important to recognize the potential effects of the endotracheal tube and anesthetic agents used on measurements obtained.[138-146] Clinical evaluation may be performed using a nasoesophageal canula and a tight-fitting face mask.[147-150] Dynamic pulmonary compliance is calculated as the change in lung volume divided by the change in transpulmonary pressure from the beginning to the end of inspiration. Static compliance is similarly calculated by measuring changes in volume and pressure during an incremental inflation and deflation of the lungs.

Normal values for dynamic compliance (Cdyn) and pulmonary resistance (RL) have been measured in cats and dogs.[151-154] Due to differences in body conformation, weight, age, and sex, measurements in dogs have considerable variation between studies. In medium-sized dogs, Cdyn may correlate most accurately with trunk length rather than body weight or chest circumference.[154] Measurement of pulmonary mechanics such as tidal volumes, minute ventilation, peak inspiratory pressure, resistance, and compliance may be helpful in the mechanically ventilated patient to assist in identifying pulmonary parenchymal, pleural space or chest wall disorders, deciding when to wean the patient, monitoring changes over time and in response to therapy, identifying, and detecting bronchospasm or mucous plugs during ventilation.[155-159] Clinically, the CO_2SMO (Novametrix Medical Systems Inc., Wallingford, CT) is an extremely useful pulmonary function monitoring device for the ventilated patient. However, positive pressure ventilation may interfere with esophageal pressure measurements.[160] Additional techniques that might be used to assess pulmonary function in dogs or cats include a forced oscillation measurement, forced deflation techniques, whole body plethysmography or dual-chamber plethysmography, and static thoracic compliance using a pediatric spirometer and a water manometer.[157,161-164]

ADDITIONAL DIAGNOSTICS

Nitric oxide (NO) has been shown to play a key role in the modulation of airway relaxation and responsiveness in cats.[165-168] Exhaled nitric oxide (ENO) levels might be a noninvasive means of detecting airway inflammation and its response to therapy. Preliminary data have shown that cats with a clinical diagnosis of asthma have increased ENO levels compared with control populations. (Matt Mellema, DVM, Harvard University, unpublished observations, personal communication.)

CHAPTER • 213

Diseases of the Trachea

Stephen J. Ettinger
Brett Kantrowitz

ANATOMY AND PATHOPHYSIOLOGY

The normal trachea is a semi-rigid, flexible tubular passageway connecting the larynx to the bronchi. It is made up of 35 to 45 C-shaped cartilages, each alternating with an elastic annular ligament. The cartilage-free, dorsal portion of the trachea is composed of mucosa, connective tissue, and tracheal muscle (the dorsal tracheal membrane). The trachea bifurcates into the mainstem bronchi at the level of the fourth or fifth thoracic vertebrae.

The cranial and caudal thyroid arteries are the major blood supply to most of the trachea. The recurrent laryngeal and vagus nerves supply parasympathetic innervation to the tracheal mucosa and its smooth muscle, which stimulates muscular contraction and glandular secretion. The inhibitory sympathetic fibers arise from the middle cervical ganglion and sympathetic trunk.

The tracheal mucosal layer is composed of a pseudo-stratified, ciliated columnar epithelium with goblet cells; mucus-secreting tubular glands are found in the submucosa. The ciliated cells of the epithelium act as part of the mucociliary transport system to propel mucous and inspired debris toward the pharynx.

The trachea has a limited number of ways to respond to an insult. Changes seen during examination of the trachea are usually not pathognomonic for a given disease state. The immediate response of the tracheal mucosa to irritation of any cause is increased mucus secretion. With continued insult, epithelial cells desquamate and goblet cell hyperplasia occurs. Squamous metaplasia occurs with continued insults if there is insufficient time for healing between episodes. Superficial defects in the tracheal mucosa begin to heal as early as 2 hours after cessation of an injury. Large areas of damaged epithelium devoid of functional cilia can impair the mucociliary transport system and predispose to infection and delayed healing.

The primary pathophysiologic response to stenotic disease is increased airway resistance that cannot be overcome through mouth breathing and decreased pulmonary compliance. With impaired air flow, hypoventilation and respiratory acidosis occur. Chronic obstruction can result in secondary pulmonary hypertension and right heart failure (cor pulmonale).

HISTORY AND PHYSICAL EXAMINATION

The most commonly recognized clinical signs of tracheal disease are coughing, stertorous noisy inspiratory sounds, stridulous or wheezing expiratory sounds, pulmonary edema, and occasionally cyanosis. See Chapter 53 for the clinical differentiation of coughing and its most commonly encountered causes and Chapter 54 for dyspnea and tachypnea. A thorough physical examination should follow a record of the history in evaluating patients with suspected tracheal disease. The physical examination should cover all aspects of the animal with particular attention to the entire upper and lower respiratory tracts as well as the cardiovascular system.

The neck should be palpated for evidence of surrounding disease such as subcutaneous emphysema, lymphadenopathies, abscess, cyst, neoplasia, thyroid gland enlargement, or any other mass that may involve the trachea. In most animals, except for the heavy or obese, the trachea can be palpated from the larynx to the thoracic inlet. The trachea is relatively noncollapsible, and obvious borders or angles usually cannot be felt. Often a cough can be elicited with light tracheal palpation at the thoracic inlet when laryngeal or tracheal irritation or inflammation is present.

Auscultation of the lung sounds as well as respiratory sounds directly over the trachea, larynx, and nose should be compared to help localize the site of the lesion. Sounds are usually most intense near their site of origin. Examination of the oral and pharyngeal cavities is best done with the aid of anesthesia (e.g., Propofol, Thiopental) or light sedation.

DIAGNOSTIC TESTS

Radiography
Two views of the trachea should be obtained for routine radiographic examination—lateral and ventrodorsal or dorsoventral. Radiographs to evaluate the cervical trachea should be obtained separately from those of the thoracic trachea. The lateral radiographic examination must be performed with careful positioning of the patient to avoid artifactual deviations of the trachea, especially in the caudal cervical and cranial mediastinal regions. Excessive flexion of the occipitoatlantal articulation may cause deviations of the trachea, which may artifactually suggest extra tracheal masses (Figure 213-1). Dorsal deviation of the intrathoracic trachea can be due to ventroflexion of the neck. Other causes include cardiac enlargement, pleural effusions, and cranial mediastinal masses. Ventral deviation of the thoracic trachea can be seen with a dilated esophagus or with diseases of the dorsal cranial mediastinum. Ventrodorsal (VD) or dorsoventral (DV) views are used to evaluate the course of the trachea.

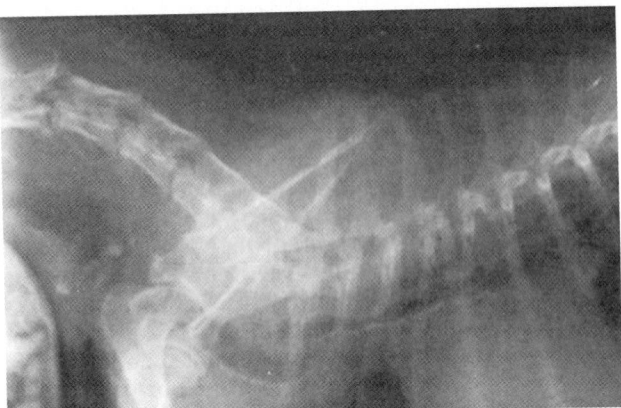

Figure 213-1 Kinking of the trachea may occur with excessive flexion of the neck in small animals and in those with tracheal malacia. These undesirable causes of narrowing of the trachea must be avoided while the dog is radiographed and, more importantly, while the dog recovers from an anesthetic.

VD oblique views are occasionally needed when the thoracic tracheal lumen is superimposed over the vertebral column and sternum to prevent sufficient radiographic detail. These views are usually not necessary since the intrathoracic trachea normally courses to the right of the vertebral column and reaches the midline only at the tracheal bifurcation (carina).

Tracheal radiographs should be surveyed for luminal filling defects, continuity of the mucosal lining, diameter, and placement within the cervical and thoracic regions. Normal aging may result in dystrophic mineralization of tracheal rings. This is not pathologic. The normal tracheal diameter generally decreases slightly from larynx to thoracic inlet but then increases.[9] The normal diameter of the trachea at the third rib should be approximately three times the width of the third rib at the level of the trachea.[1] Another method of determining tracheal diameter uses the ratio of the inner diameter of the trachea at the thoracic inlet to the distance between the ventral edge of the first thoracic vertebra and dorsal edge of the manubrium. The normal ratio is 0.16 or greater.[1] The tracheal lumen is similar to the caudal laryngeal lumen. Measurement of the degree of tracheal luminal stenosis using radiography or tracheoscopy did not correlate with necropsy measurements in one study.[2] Computed tomographic studies in 18 breed dogs determined the correlation coefficient between inner diameters the cross-sectional lumen areas and body weight and found a high correlation between the inner transverse and vertical diameters and the cross-sectional area of the lumen except at the level of the intrathoracic trachea.[48]

Motion studies (fluoroscopy) of the diseased trachea are highly desirable for evaluation of pathodynamics. Image intensification equipment is necessary to safely obtain adequate radiographic detail. These studies are extremely valuable for the evaluation of the collapsed trachea and other coughing syndromes. Patients should be placed in lateral recumbency and the entire trachea visualized. A cough usually can be induced by digital pressure applied at the thoracic inlet. Videotape recordings add to the usefulness of dynamic studies. Playback observations in slow motion can result in the detection of functional features missed during the initial examination.

Fluoroscopic equipment may not be available to the general practitioner. Motion dynamics of the trachea can often be inferred from static images obtained at different phases of respiration. Lateral inspiratory and expiratory projections are used to evaluate changes in the tracheal lumen. A forced expiration can be obtained by inducing a cough with tracheal palpation.

Mild physiologic changes in tracheal diameter during respiration are normal. The cervical trachea may narrow slightly with inspiration while the intrathoracic trachea and carina narrow slightly during expiration.

Contrast studies of the trachea and bronchi (bronchography) have been advocated in the past for further evaluation of the trachea and airways. This procedure has generally been eclipsed by bronchoscopy, a more effective and safer technique for evaluation of the lumen and lining of the major airways. Ultrasound examination of the trachea may demonstrate an alteration in the shape of the lumen on ventrodorsal projection.[49]

Tracheoscopy and Bronchoscopy

Endoscopic examination is a useful tool for evaluation of pathologic states of the trachea. It may be performed with a rigid or flexible scope to help localize the site and extent of a lesion. Endoscopy directly visualizes the tracheal mucosa and identifies inflammation, ulceration, and edema. It is used to visualize and to obtain biopsy specimens of tumors and masses; for brush cytology, fluid aspiration, and cultures; for removal of foreign bodies; for demonstration of collapsed, hypoplastic, stenotic, disrupted, or compressed areas; and for evaluation of disease progression or response to therapy.

Small animal respiratory endoscopy requires general anesthesia. The use of atropine sulfate generally is not recommended because of its detrimental effects of thickening and decreasing respiratory epithelial secretions. There are several options for sedation for tracheoscopy. Short-acting barbiturates (Propofol) permit the rapid and gentle sedation of an animal for intubation and can be given on a continuous basis if the procedure is to be relatively short. Maintenance for a longer period of time is best handled using isoflurane gaseous anesthesia since the animal may quickly awaken after the procedure with few side effects and short duration of the sedation. On occasion, ketamine-diazepam–type sedation proves useful for longer procedures, but the problems associated with waking up are enhanced, especially in difficult-to-manage pets such as those with severe lung disease, obese animals, and brachycephalic breeds. Another option is Numorphan, although its respiratory depressive effects may necessitate manual (bagged) breathing for the patient (see Chapter 104).

Tracheobronchial Culture and Cytology

Examining cytologic specimens can often be an efficient and practical means of helping to support a diagnosis while others are eliminated. There are multiple ways to obtain diagnostically significant samples from the trachea for culture and cytology. In all cases, culture specimens should be obtained before cytology specimens. If tracheal endoscopy is being performed and the equipment has a biopsy port, specimens may be obtained through this instrument with sterile endoscopic brushes. A protected sterile culture swab or cytology brush can also be introduced directly through the mouth and larynx and into the trachea for specimen retrieval.

Bronchoalveolar lavage (BAL) is the preferred method of obtaining cytologic and culture samples from the lower respiratory tract and occasionally from the upper portions of the tract. The endoscope is cleaned externally and the channels flushed with sterile saline. It is then repositioned at the sampling site and gently wedged into position. Multiple aliquots of sterile saline are passed through the channel and immediately suctioned back into the syringe. Multiple samples may be obtained in this manner from one or more positions using BAL.

Another method[1] that works well in smaller animals is to place a sterile endotracheal tube, flush a small amount of sterile saline through the tube and into the trachea, hold the animal upside down, and collect draining fluid in a sterile vial as it runs out of the endotracheal tube. Although this method is not as precise as other methods, it is practical and easy to perform with equipment found in most small animal hospital settings. An alternative technique that does not usually require general anesthesia is transtracheal aspiration. This usually requires either local anesthesia or mild sedation while a long sterile needle is used to puncture the mid-cervical trachea or cricothyroid membrane. A catheter designed to pass through the needle is threaded into the tracheal lumen and is used for aspiration.

Numerous bacterial culture studies have been made from transtracheal and bronchoscopic aspirations. These samples have principally but not exclusively been taken from the lower tracheal and respiratory tract. In a study evaluating 264 cases of lower respiratory tract specimens, 203 bacterial species were isolated in 116 of 264 dogs. Most (57%) contained a single species of bacteria. Those cultured most commonly were E. coli (45.7%), Pasteurella spp. (22.4%), obligate anaerobes (21.6%), beta-hemolytic streptococci (12.1%), Bordetella bronchiseptica (12.1%), non-hemolytic Streptococcus and Enterococcus sp. (12.1%), coagulase-positive Staphylococcus spp. (9.5%) and Pseudomonas spp. (7.8%).

Of these cultures, the most active antimicrobial agents for aerobic micro-organisms, which inhibit more than 90% of the isolates were amikacin, ceftizoxime sodium, enrofloxacin, and gentamicin sulfate.[3] In an earlier study, Mycoplasma spp. recovery in normal dogs and those with pulmonary disease was about 25%. Only young dogs under 1 year of age and those with Bordetella spp. or streptococci isolations had a significant association between their disease and Mycoplasma spp. recovery during tracheobronchial lavage.[4] Following this study, the role of Mycoplasma spp. in lower (trachea and lung) respiratory tract disease has been further elucidated. Half of 224 samples obtained from dogs and cats with lower airway disease were negative for Mycoplasma spp. but 49.5% were positive, either alone (15%) or in combination (85%) with aerobic bacteria. Mycoplasma spp. are present frequently in patients with lower respiratory tract disease. It remains to be determined whether Mycoplasma spp. play a primary or secondary role.[50] Bordetella bronchiseptica infection was reported in a series of cats mostly under 8 weeks old with dry nonproductive coughing. Transtracheal washings were positively cultured for B. bronchiseptica.[5]

Bronchoalveolar lavage cytology from 33 normal dogs identified alveolar macrophages (79.4%), lymphocytes (13.5%), eosinophils (3.6%), mast cells (2.1%), epithelial cells (0.8%), and neutrophils (0.6%).[6] These numbers vary from earlier reports of limited numbers of macrophages and lymphocytes.[7] Deviations from these numbers, although not usually diagnostic, provide valuable information on the type of response and the type of disease process present. Neutrophilic inflammation most often results from bacterial infection, which can be secondary to a number of other problems including, but not limited to, collapsed trachea, chronic bronchitis, neoplasia, allergic disease, and viral, mycotic, or parasitic infections. Such cytologic findings could include an increased number of neutrophils, degenerative changes within the neutrophils, and phagocytized bacteria.[8]

Eosinophilic inflammation is usually considered significant although it has been noted in clinically normal dogs and cats.[8,9] Eosinophils and mast cells imply an allergic or parasitic tracheobronchitis.[10] A concurrent, nonseptic neutrophilic or chronic inflammatory response is frequently present. Major differential diagnoses include allergic bronchitis, pulmonary parasites, heartworm disease, and hypersensitivity responses secondary to bacterial, protozoal, fungal, or neoplastic diseases. Chronic inflammation is indicated by a mixed inflammatory cell population with a predominant number of activated macrophages.[8] This type of response is nonspecific and has a long list of differentials.

All slides should be carefully examined for organisms or atypical cells. Tight coils of inspissated mucous can be washed out in association with small airway disease.[10] Hemorrhagic inflammation consists of chronic or chronic-active inflammatory cells with erythrophagocytosis and increased numbers of red blood cells.[8] Many diseases of the respiratory tract can cause hemorrhage including systemic clotting disorders. Large numbers of reactive lymphocytes and plasma cells are non-specific indicators of immune stimulation.[8] Primary ciliary dyskinesia may be suggested when associated with chronic bronchopneumonia, ultrastructural abnormalities, and a lack of sperm motility on testicular aspiration.[11] Neoplastic cells may be identified. Differentiation of criteria of malignancy in epithelial cells is often difficult, especially when accompanied by marked inflammation. Histologic examination may be necessary. Organisms may be found on cytology to make a definitive diagnosis but their absence does not eliminate infectious disease.

Clinicopathologic Studies

Tracheal diseases only rarely have definitive, demonstrable clinicopathologic findings. Hematologic and biochemical analysis of the blood, serology, and a urinalysis should be used as a reflection of the patient's overall health and an indication of systemic or allergic disease. Blood gas analysis is helpful to demonstrate severity of the disease and acid-base status.

SPECIFIC TRACHEAL DISEASES

Noninfectious Tracheitis
Etiology
Tracheitis refers to an inflammation of the epithelial lining of the trachea. This inflammatory response may be infectious or noninfectious; primary or secondary. The noninfectious causes of chronic tracheitis are probably more common and will be discussed as a group. Noninfectious tracheitis is usually a secondary problem to prolonged barking, collapsing trachea, chronic cardiac disease, and disease of the oropharynx. Tracheitis is unusual in cats and when it does occur in the cat it is associated with infectious feline respiratory disease. Allergic lower airway disease may also promote a secondary tracheitis.

Clinical Signs and Diagnosis
Since tracheitis may be primary (inhalation of smoke or other noxious gases) or secondary, the history varies with the etiology. Most patients with tracheitis are asymptomatic except for a cough, which is characterized as resonant, harsh, paroxysmal, and often terminated by nonproductive or slightly productive gagging. The physical examination is often normal, and no fever is present. Firm palpation of the trachea near the thoracic inlet elicits the typical tracheal cough. Examination of the oral cavity and oropharynx is unlikely to reveal abnormalities unless the tracheitis is secondary to an oropharyngeal disease process. The tonsils may be enlarged and extend further out of the crypts than normal. Auscultation of the heart is usually normal. If a cardiac murmur or arrhythmia exists, cardiac disease must be eliminated as the primary cause for the coughing (see Chapter 53) or as the cause of chronic tracheitis. A prominent snapping of the second heart sound may be present over the pulmonic valve region. Findings on auscultation of the lungs are normal unless tracheitis is secondary to pulmonary disease (see Chapters 212 and 215), in which case coarse bronchial lung sounds are expected.

Tracheitis as a primary disease often has no specific radiographic features. In acute tracheitis edema of the mucosal lining may result in a reduction of the lumen diameter. Care must be taken not to confuse this for a fixed, hypoplastic trachea. The radiographic features that occur when tracheitis is secondary to other diseases are included in the discussions of those conditions. Hematology and blood chemistries are usually within reference ranges unless a systemic disease state concurrently exists.

Table • 213-1

Drugs Used for Tracheal Diseases

GENERIC NAME (TRADE)	MECHANISM OF ACTION	DOSAGE
Theophylline/aminophylline (IV)	Bronchodilator; specific mechanism unknown	5 mg/lb q6-12h PO/IV
Terbutaline (Brethine, Bricanyl)	Beta-2 adrenergic receptor	0.625-1.25 mg BID PO-Sml
		1.25-2.5 mg BID PO-Med
		2.5-5.0 mg BID PO-Lg
		0.01 mg/kg IV, IM, SQ
Prednisone and trimprazine (Temaril-P)	Antihistamine/cortisone combination	1 tab/20 lb q12h PO
Dextromethorphan (Delsym, Silphen DM)	Antitussive-expectorant	0.5-1 mg/lb q8-12h PO
Dextromethorphan/guaifenesin (Robitussin DM)	Antitussive-expectorant	Dosage similar to dextromethorphan PO
Codeine	Narcotic antitussive	0.5-1 mg/lb q6-12h PO
Hydrocodone with homatropine (Hycodan, Tussigon)	Narcotic like antitussive	¼-1 tab (or tsp) q6-24h PO
		Approx 2 mg/kg
Tussionex syrup	Antitussive narcotic syrup-longer acting	Same dosage as hydrocodone
Butorphanol (Torbutrol)	Opioid agonist/antagonist	0.25 mg/lb q6-12h PO

Therapy

Therapy should be directed at the primary underlying disease process, and these treatments are discussed in their appropriate sections. The cough associated with secondary tracheitis may act as a continued source of irritation, which perpetuates the tracheitis, and a vicious cycle ensues. Treatment of the underlying disease process may not always be adequate to relieve the cough because of this cycle of "cough-induced tracheitis," which perpetuates the cough as well as the tracheitis. Therefore treatment aimed specifically at the tracheitis is often beneficial, if not mandatory.

Tracheal coughing is often treated with antitussive and bronchodilating preparations (Table 213-1). Many of these preparations also contain expectorants. Occasionally, short-term therapy with corticosteroids is warranted. It is important to emphasize that this provides symptomatic relief only and it could exacerbate the primary condition. With chronic coughing, nebulization four to six times daily may help to soften mucoid material collecting in the trachea. When nebulization is not possible, the dog or cat can be placed in a bathroom filled with steam from a hot shower. This should last 15 to 20 minutes, three times daily. Following either method, gentle couppage of the chest wall helps to loosen secretions and stimulate expectoration.

Infectious Tracheobronchitis

Etiology

Infectious canine tracheobronchitis, also known as *canine respiratory disease complex* and *kennel cough*, is not a single disease, but rather a clinical disease syndrome. Involved in this multi-etiology syndrome include infectious agents such as viruses, bacteria, mycoplasma, fungi, and parasites. A combination of *Bordetella bronchiseptica* with canine parainfluenza or canine adenovirus (CAV; CAD-2) is the most frequently encountered cause. Other incriminated agents are, canine herpes virus (CHV), reovirus, *Mycoplasma* spp.,[50] and occasionally canine distemper virus.[12] Most cases of infectious canine tracheobronchitis involve a primary viral infection. *B. bronchiseptica* infection in cats is unusual but has been described.[5,13] The role of *B. bronchiseptica* has recently been reviewed.[47]

Clinical Signs and Diagnosis

Infectious canine tracheobronchitis is highly contagious and most commonly occurs where groups of dogs of different ages and susceptibility are congregated. There is almost always a history of exposure to other animals, as in a kennel, hospital, or dog show. Aerosol or direct contact is considered the main source of exposure. Clinical signs usually develop 3 to 5 days after initial exposure. The clinical signs are generally mild and self-limiting. A dry, hacking, paroxysmal cough is the most consistent sign. A purulent nasal discharge may be noted. Generally, the animal is healthy in other respects.

Diagnosis is made most often on the basis of circumstantial evidence. History of exposure with a dry hacking cough is usually sufficient. Thoracic auscultation, thoracic radiographs, and hemograms are usually unremarkable. Tracheal cytology may reveal increased numbers of neutrophils and bacteria. Bacterial or *Mycoplasma* spp. isolation, as well as virus isolation and serologic evaluation, can be performed but are usually unnecessary. *B. bronchiseptica* commonly associated with this condition may require 3 months for full clearance to occur.

Therapy

Uncomplicated cases of tracheobronchitis probably do not require antimicrobials. Even though antibiotics have not been shown to reach significant concentrations in tracheobronchial secretions or to shorten the course of infection, prophylactic therapy has been recommended by some.[14] Antibiotic treatment is indicated if there is deeper respiratory involvement or if the animal is showing signs of systemic illness. Drugs chosen should be based on results of bacterial culture and sensitivity testing. In the absence of culture results, choices of oral antibiotics include chloramphenicol, fluoroquinolones, or cephalosporins. More potent injectable agents such as amikacin, gentamicin, and ceftizoxime should be chosen only after culture results indicate their effectiveness. Doxycycline (5 to 10 mg/kg once daily) is appropriate if mycoplasma are suspected.

Glucocorticoids, administered at anti-inflammatory doses can be effective in suppressing the cough of uncomplicated infectious tracheobronchitis. However, glucocorticoids do not appear to shorten the clinical course of the disease.[14] They may worsen the illness in immunocompromised individuals. If glucocorticoids are used, a bactericidal antibiotic should be chosen over a bacteriostatic one for concurrent use.

Antitussives, either alone or in combination with bronchodilators are recommended. Narcotic cough suppressants seem to be the most effective. These agents can compromise ventilation and should not be used in the presence of concurrent bacterial pneumonia. Methylxanthine bronchodilators may also be of benefit in suppressing the cough through their ability to prevent bronchospasm. Patients with tracheobronchial disease also benefit from nebulization, which can help to loosen excessive accumulations of bronchial and tracheal secretions. Nebulization with sterile saline is as acceptable as mucolytic agents.

TRACHEAL PARASITES

Lungworm (Oslerus osleri; Filaroides osleri)
Etiology
Filaroides osleri renamed *Oslerus osleri* (*O. osleri*) is a worldwide parasitic disease in dogs under 2 years of age. It can be seen in individual situations but is more often a kennel-related problem (especially in greyhounds).[1] Although most often described in young dogs, it does persist in older animals, often without significant pathophysiologic effects.

Although described as a lungworm, this parasite most commonly affects the region proximal to the tracheal carina. It may affect the lumen and lining of the larger bronchi, but only rarely does it extend deeper into the pulmonary system.

Reports of direct transmission through larvae in the stool and saliva suggest that this metastrongyle may not require an intermediate host to complete its life cycle. First-stage larvae are directly transmitted through salivary and airway secretions. These molt in the small bowel followed by migration of the larvae to the lungs and bronchi. Experimental and natural direct transmission have been demonstrated.[1] Transmission to pups has also been reported to occur through parental food regurgitation and licking and cleaning of pups by a nursing bitch.[15]

Clinical Signs and Diagnosis
Dogs usually present with chronic, mild to severe inspiratory wheezing sounds, dyspnea, coughing, and/or debilitation. Panting usually is not prominent except in advanced cases. The severity of the clinical signs may be overplayed in the literature. Most dogs experience definite but mild, often nonprogressive respiratory signs. Exercise intolerance does occasionally occur and coughing is typically characterized as a harsh tracheobronchial sound associated with attempts at terminal retching.

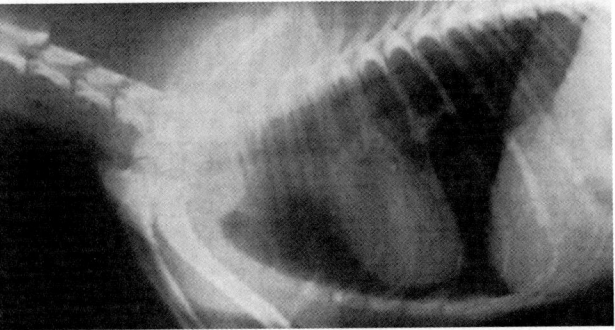

Figure 213-2 Lateral thoracic radiograph of an immature male terrier showing multiple nodules in the lumen of the caudal trachea due to *Filaroides osleri*. Note the hyperexpansion of the thoracic cavity, which is probably due to increased resistance within the trachea during expiration.

A small amount of white to blood-tinged mucus is common, but at times larger amounts of exudate are brought up.

Tracheal sensitivity occurs but physical palpation is normal. Heart sounds are normal. When obvious respiratory embarrassment occurs wheezing, ronchi, or pulmonary edema may be present.

The radiographic examination is helpful if the disease process is extensive and the nodules are large. The tracheal lining may be diffusely thickened, interrupted with indistinct solid masses, or show ill-defined, 2- to 10-mm semicircular lesions protruding into the lumen (Figure 213-2). Endoscopically, cream-colored nodules, 1 to 5 mm high and wide are usually diagnostic. The larvae are often seen peeking into the luminal edge of the growth. Brushings and biopsies of the nodules provide a definitive diagnosis (Figure 213-3).

Larvae are occasionally detected in the feces. Although some flotation methods dehydrate the larvae, zinc sulfate flotation techniques are as diagnostic as is the Baermann technique. Eggs, when seen, are 50 × 80 μm, thin shelled,

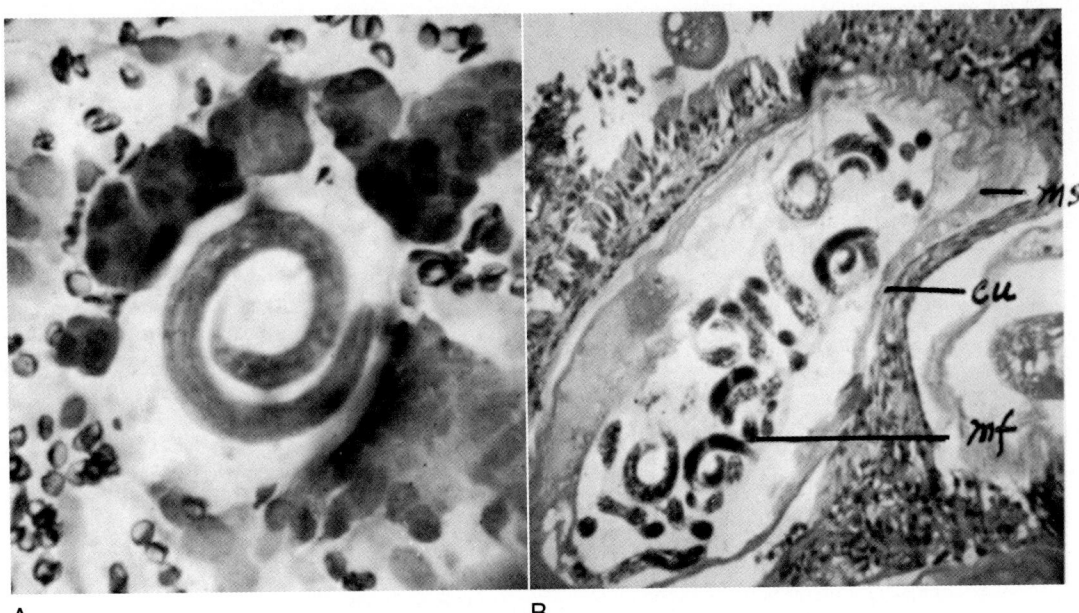

A   B

Figure 213-3 **A,** Photomicrograph of a biopsy taken from the trachea just proximal to the carina of the animal in Figure 213-2. The tracheal lining is surrounded by a larval representative of *O. osleri*. Note the kinked tail characteristic of this worm larva. **B,** Parasitic tracheitis that exhibits prominent infestation by adult filarial worms. The worms contain microfilaria (*mf*), which are within the cuticle (*cu*) and are surrounded by mucosal tissue (*ms*) from the host's pulmonary system.

colorless, and larvated. The larvae are 230 µm long with a distinct kinked tail. Both larvae and eggs may be visualized in the sputum and in washings from the trachea of an affected dog.

Therapy

Many drugs have been reported to be effective in treating lungworms, such as thiacetarsamide sodium, diethylcarbamazine, levamisole, fenbendazole, and albendazole.[1] We have treated several dogs with oral ivermectin at 1000 µg/lb once weekly for 2 months. The nodules were reduced in size but did not resolve entirely. All of these dogs became asymptomatic and continued to thrive. Thiabendazole was administered at 35 mg/kg twice daily for five days and then at 70 mg/kg twice daily for 21 days. Along with thiabendazole, prednisone at 0.5 mg/kg was given twice daily every other day.[16]

Surgical removal is not recommended owing to the large number of nodules. Removal of a large obstructing nodule may potentially be therapeutic in rare situations.

Cuterebrosis

Cuterebra spp. larvae are expected in rabbits and rodents. Several cats have been described with inspiratory dyspnea. Upon tracheoscopy, *Cuterebra* larvae were observed in the trachea, at or just cranial to its bifurcation. Successful treatment consisted of removal of the larva during tracheoscopy in one cat and by thoracotomy and removal through a tracheal incision. The cases were described by the authors as third-stage instar of the *Cuterebra* spp.[51] A fatal case of second stage instar has been reported in another cat.[37]

Tracheal Hypoplasia
Etiology

First described in 1972, the hypoplastic tracheal syndrome is a congenital defect resulting from inadequate growth of the tracheal rings.[1] The condition varies from mild to severe. This disease is recognized primarily in young, brachycephalic animals. The first complete report involved a series of dogs, most of which were English bulldogs.[1] In another report, the highest incidence was in English bulldogs (55%), with Boston terriers also being commonly affected (15% of their cases).[17] Other congenital abnormalities, including elongated soft palate, stenotic nares, cardiac defects, and megaesophagus may be associated.

Clinical Signs and Diagnosis

Since tracheal hypoplasia is a congenital disease, it can be diagnosed early in life. In one study, the median age at diagnosis was 5 months (range: 2 days to 12 years).[17] Common clinical signs include dyspnea, stridor, and coughing. Occasionally, dogs present with a moist, productive cough, moist rales on auscultation, and a fever associated with bronchopneumonia.

Physical examination may be normal (except for a palpably small trachea) or may reveal a sensitive trachea that, when palpated, evokes coughing. Excitement is likely to exacerbate the coughing episode, which is usually more severe and serious during daytime hours. Heart sounds are normal unless an associated congenital cardiac malformation is present. Clinical pathology reveals a leukocytosis with a left shift if there is a concurrent bronchopneumonia. The radiographic features are most important and usually provide a definitive diagnosis (Figure 213-4). Dorsoventral and lateral radiographs of the thorax and lateral views of the cervical region should be obtained to assess the tracheal diameter and the presence or absence of pulmonary changes. Methods for measurement and determination of normal trachea diameter have been reviewed earlier in the chapter.

The diagnosis of hypoplastic trachea is generally made when the lumen diameter is less than two times the width of the third rib where they cross. The tracheal lumen will also appear smaller than the caudal laryngeal lumen in these patients.

Care must be taken in the young patient, in which the adult proportions of the tracheal lumen may not yet be obtained. *Tracheal edema associated with tracheitis may mimic a hypoplastic trachea on the radiograph.* For this reason it is best to take radiographs when the patient is asymptomatic.

Prognosis and Therapy

The prognosis for dogs with a hypoplastic trachea depends on the degree of hypoplasia as well as the presence or absence of concurrent congenital defects. Many patients with slight to moderate hypoplastic tracheas can live normal, satisfactory lives with only an occasional need for bronchodilator therapy and antibiotics. Young dogs with this diagnosis often outgrow the condition. One report suggests that tracheal hypoplasia may be clinically insignificant in the absence of concurrent cardiac or other obstructive upper respiratory disease. Further it supports the idea that the degree of hypoplasia does not correlate with the presence or absence of clinical signs.[17]

Clinical experience has shown that many dogs present with this condition in various states of severity as puppies and young dogs. With effective empirical therapy a significant number of these dogs develop and grow into healthy mature dogs. Because the initial impression is one of a very advanced condition, the veterinarian may wish to advise the client on the potential for the dog to overcome this problem. This is particularly true if there are no associated congenital defects present. Owners who are experienced with these breeds are familiar with the problem and are often quite capable of dealing with the extensive nursing care required. One should be firm on recommending therapy for these patients. Many who have suggested euthanasia have come to regret their haste after seeing some of these dogs as mature adults. The prognosis remains guarded and it is prudent to identify the possibilities to the new pet owner who presents a pet with this condition. Similarly, the veterinarian must carefully evaluate the pet for associated congenital defects (cardiac or other upper airway).

It is important to prevent bronchopneumonia from developing by keeping the affected animal in a draft-free environment and preventing excessive exposure to moisture and cold. Prevention of excessive weight gain also helps the animal by limiting the strain placed on the respiratory system by obesity. When recurrent upper respiratory tract infections do occur, the use of antibiotics is in order, preferably as determined by culture and sensitivity testing.

It is advisable to discourage the breeding of animals affected with this congenital defect, even though at this time there is no absolute evidence indicating a hereditary basis. There are no known surgical corrective procedures.

Segmental Tracheal Stenosis
Etiology

Segmental tracheal stenosis is an unusual condition that affects small animals. It may occur as a congenital lesion or it may result from trauma to the trachea. The congenital absence of tracheal rings that causes a focal stenotic area has been described.[18] Many examples of young cats and dogs with segmental tracheal strictures of unknown cause have been recorded.[1]

Segmental tracheal stenosis can also occur secondary to a tracheotomy procedure, with necrosis and thickening of the tracheal wall from excessive endotracheal cuff pressures, as a complication of thoracic surgery, result of bite wounds to the cervical area, foreign bodies lodged in the trachea and result of massive chest trauma.

Clinical Signs and Diagnosis

This syndrome produces stridulous respiratory distress and subsequent cyanosis. Secondary upper airway tract infections may result and develop into overwhelming pulmonary disease.

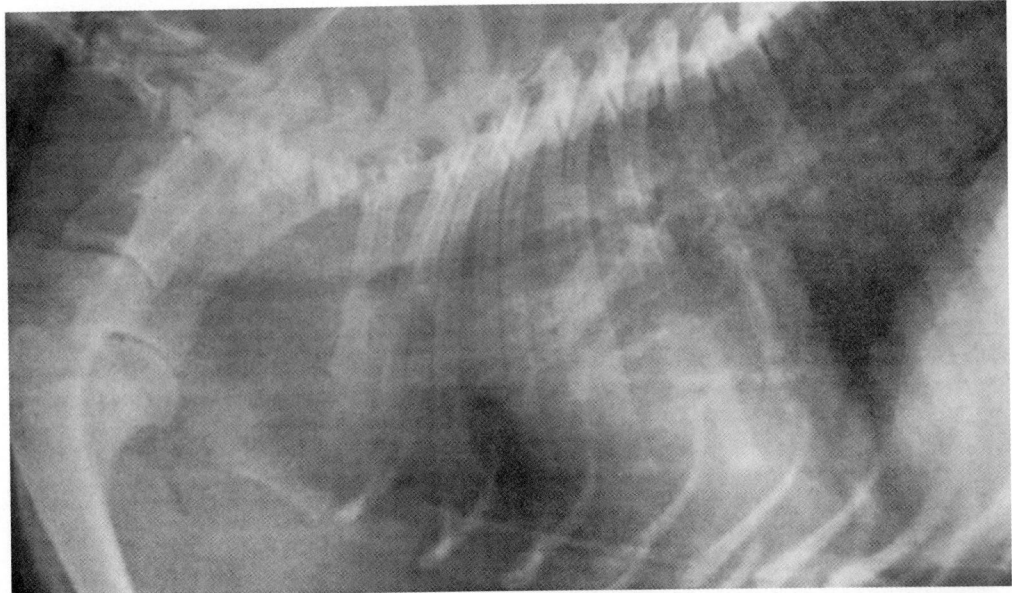

A

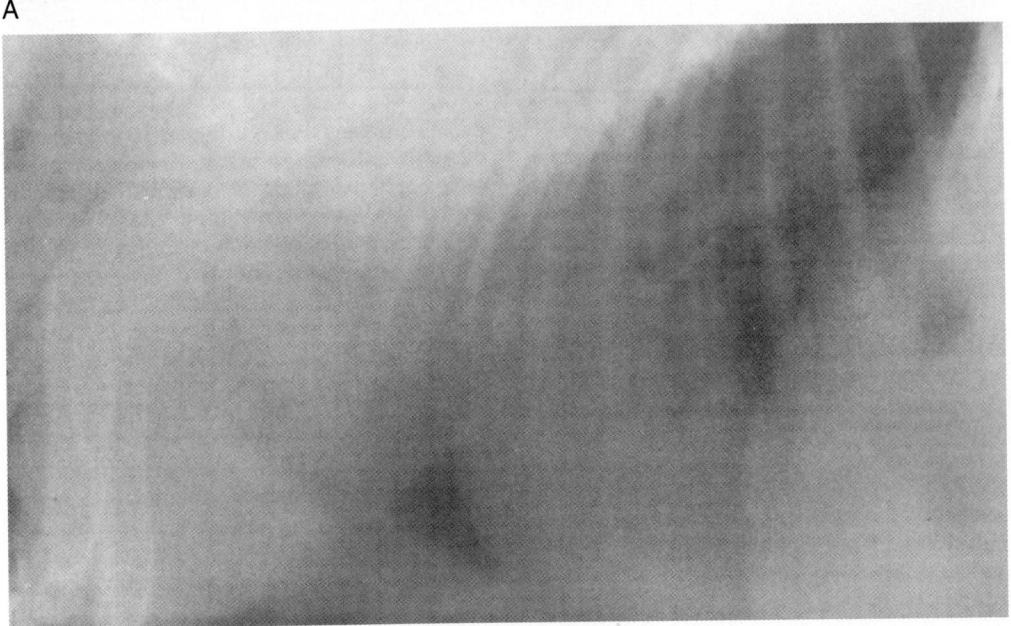

B

Figure 213-4 **A,** Lateral cervical and thoracic radiographs of a 1-year-old female bulldog. The radiograph of the thorax clearly demonstrates a markedly hypoplastic trachea in addition to pulmonary changes suggesting bronchitis. The ratio of the tracheal diameter to the height of the thoracic inlet was 0.07. The normal ratio is 0.16 or greater. The indistinct outline of the trachea is due to the accumulation of large amounts of mucous in the trachea. **B,** Hypoplasia of the trachea in a 4-month-old female boxer presented with a productive gagging cough and moderate respiratory distress. Lateral thoracic radiographs show a severely hypoplastic trachea. The ratio of the tracheal diameter to the height of the thoracic inlet was 0.05.

Radiographic studies usually establish the diagnosis. Survey tracheal radiographs often show the stenotic region as an abrupt, segmental reduction in lumen diameter. Inspiratory/expiratory projections or fluoroscopic examination demonstrate little dynamic change in the stenosis during the respiratory cycle. Bronchoscopy identifies the stenotic lesion and its severity and anatomic extent. It is possible that accurate measurement of the degree of tracheal stenosis cannot be made. Percentage of tracheal luminal stenosis as determined by antemortem methods in 15 normal dogs that underwent tracheostomy procedures were determined by radiography, tracheoscopy, and necropsy. The antemortem methods did not correlate well with control planimetric methods.[52]

Therapy

The management of segmental tracheal stenosis is similar regardless of cause. The mainstay of treatment is surgical resection of the stenotic region. Several types of procedures have been used and they are well reviewed.[1,18,19] Tracheal resection and anastamosis without excessive tension,[18,19] balloon dilatation[20], placement of polypropylene total ring prostheses applied to the external surface of the trachea and tracheal wall stent placement internally have all been used successfully.[53] The reader is referred to an appropriate surgical textbook for additional information.

Collapsing Trachea

There are two types of collapsing trachea, the dorsoventral and lateral forms. The lateral form is very unusual. It has been reported without obvious cause but it also has developed after central chondrotomy was performed to treat the dorsoventral form of tracheal collapse. Lateral collapse rarely occurs spontaneously.[21] Dorsoventral flattening (narrowing of the trachea) is a very commonly described lesion that is often associated with a pendulous, redundant dorsal tracheal membrane that prolapses into the tracheal lumen.

The collapsing trachea usually involves the cervical region, but often both the cervical and thoracic areas of the trachea are involved and the collapse may extend into the bronchi. Extension of the tracheal collapse to the bronchi is also described as collapsing of the trachea at the carina. Extension into the cartilage of the lower airways is referred to as bronchomalacia. Regardless of the focal or diffuse nature of the problem, increasing respiratory work leads to dynamic collapse of the dorsal tracheal membrane into the tracheal lumen. This further irritates and inflames the mucous membranes, disrupts the mucociliary apparatus, and increases the risk for associated small airway problems.[22] This condition has been described in cats in association with an intraluminal obstructing lesion[22] and by others but unusually.[23]

Etiology

The etiology of the collapsing trachea is unknown. The condition is an acquired disease that usually occurs in middle-aged to aged dogs, although it has been described in young dogs as a congenital lesion.[1] The clinical syndrome and findings in congenital cases are essentially similar to those described in acquired disease. In dogs with an acquired collapsing trachea, there is no loss of potential tracheal ring size, but the rings lose their ability to remain firm and thus subsequently collapse. They become hypocellular and the matrix varies from normal. Glycoprotein and glycosaminoglycan are deficient or totally lacking in dogs with collapsing tracheas.[1] The essential lesion is a deficiency in the organic matrix of the tracheal cartilage. This has led some to associate the condition with tracheal and bronchomalacia. There may be a failure of chondrogenesis or simple degeneration of hyaline cartilage, decreasing its turgidity. This in time leads to stretching of the dorsal membrane and finally collapsing of the trachea.

Biomechanical and biochemical parameters were similar when comparing cervical to thoracic tracheal rings of young and middle-aged healthy dogs.[24] Tracheal cartilages of normal adult dogs did have significantly higher proteoglycan content and lower water content than an immature group of dogs.

Chronic coughing caused by long-term airway and/or pulmonary parenchymal disease, chronic cardiac disease with tracheal and bronchial compression, tracheal trauma, denervation of the dorsal tracheal membrane, congenital defects, obesity, increased mediastinal fat, and thoracic and extrathoracic masses are likely associated problems rather than primary inciting causes of this anatomical condition. Laryngeal dysfunction and bronchial collapse significantly alter the prognosis negatively.[54]

Clinical Signs and Diagnosis

Tracheal collapse produces a "respiratory distress syndrome." The disease is usually paroxysmal in nature, often with a long history of chronic coughing. The cough may be described as chronic, harsh, or dry. If the owner is asked specifically, the cough often is described as a "goose honk" sound that occurs initially during the day and occasionally into the evening hours. With rare exception, the disease is recognized in toy and miniature breeds, most often Chihuahuas, Pomeranians, toy poodles, Shih Tzus, Lhasa apsos, and Yorkshire terriers. It may occur concurrently with chronic mitral valvular heart disease and must be differentiated from heart failure due to this condition. A slow heart rate helps to distinguish heart failure from primary collapsing trachea. Patients in a compensated cardiac state are presented with a cough due to a collapsed trachea. The pressure of the enlarged left atrium on the left mainstem bronchus may aggravate or precipitate the tracheal cough, even in the absence of heart failure. The characteristic cough is elicited by excitement, tracheal pressure (such as that caused by pulling on a leash), and drinking water or eating food. Often, the owner indicates that the dog begins to cough when it is picked up under the chest or held when excessive pressure is placed on the thoracic inlet.

Physical examination usually reveals a normal dog, which may be obese or thin. Depending on the state of anxiety and the respiratory distress of the moment, the patient's color varies form normal to cyanotic. Most dogs are afebrile but an elevated temperature develops with extreme respiratory distress and agitation. Hyperthermia may result if the distress is not relieved. Perhaps the most significant finding during the physical examination is the elicitation of a "goose honk" cough when the trachea is pressed in the region of the thoracic inlet. In thin patients, dorsoventral compression of the trachea and an angle at the lateral edges of the trachea can be palpated. This is not observed in obese dogs. The cardiac sounds vary from normal to that associated with simultaneous mitral valvular insufficiency. In the normal dog, the second heart sound is less pronounced than the snapping second heart that is often auscultated in dogs with collapsing trachea. The lung sounds vary from normal vesicular sounds to rattling, stridulous sounds associated with sibilant rales and wheezing. Stridor implies inspiratory sounds associated with upper airway obstruction, including laryngeal paresis/paralysis, everted laryngeal saccules, and cervical tracheal collapse. Varying degrees of inspiratory or expiratory dyspnea (respiratory distress), inspiratory noises, and an expiratory grunt (abdominal press) with an abdominal effort are recognized in all cases.

A significant feature of the physical examination is the frequent association of hepatomegaly. Hepatomegaly occurs in a large percentage of patients with this syndrome. It may be associated with fat deposition in the liver (see other rule outs for hepatomegaly, Chapter 225). The relationship of hepatomegaly to the clinical syndrome is unclear.

In most uncomplicated cases, there are usually no electrocardiographic abnormalities other than P-pulmonale resulting from right-sided heart strain. Examination of the oral cavity is usually normal (dental excluded). Culture of the tracheal lining using a protected brush identified aerobic growth in 24 of 29 dogs. Cytologic confirmation of inflammation or infection was not consistent.[55] Mycoplasma spp. were identified in patients cultured with lower airway disease. Some of these animals had tracheal diseases[50] and may culture commonly identified bacteria but most have no growth. Tracheoscopy reveals a decreased dorsoventral diameter of the trachea with a pendulous dorsal tracheal membrane. Dynamic changes such as intrathoracic collapse are noted as are other structural abnormalities, such as specific single or multiple flattening or collapse of tracheal rings. In most cases, the tracheal mucous membranes are hyperemic but usually show no exudate. On occasion, a copious, frothy catarrhal exudate may be present.

In a study of 20 surgically managed cases, 30% of the dogs were observed to have concurrent laryngeal paresis or paralysis.[1]

The high figure does not correlate with the authors' experience with large numbers of dogs that cough intermittently with this disease for many years. It may represent an important specific subset of patients, however, and should be looked for when a diagnosis of tracheal collapse is made. Further, laryngeal paresis results in a classic stridulous inspiratory effort in marked contrast to this expiratory wheeze, cough, and grunting syndrome. Upon completion of the visual examination, bronchoalveolar lavage, brush cytology, and/or biopsy samples are taken. The risks of bronchoscopy/tracheoscopy are relevant. Extreme caution is required. Brachycephalic dogs with diminished laryngeal motility or everted saccules are additionally at risk as may be obese patients and those with severe tracheobronchial malacia, concurrent pulmonary disease, small airway collapse, accumulated bronchial secretions, and hypoventilation. Post bronchoscopy recovery requires careful patient attention, minimized stress, occasionally long-term intubation, and on occasion intratracheal administration of 1% lidocaine spray.[25]

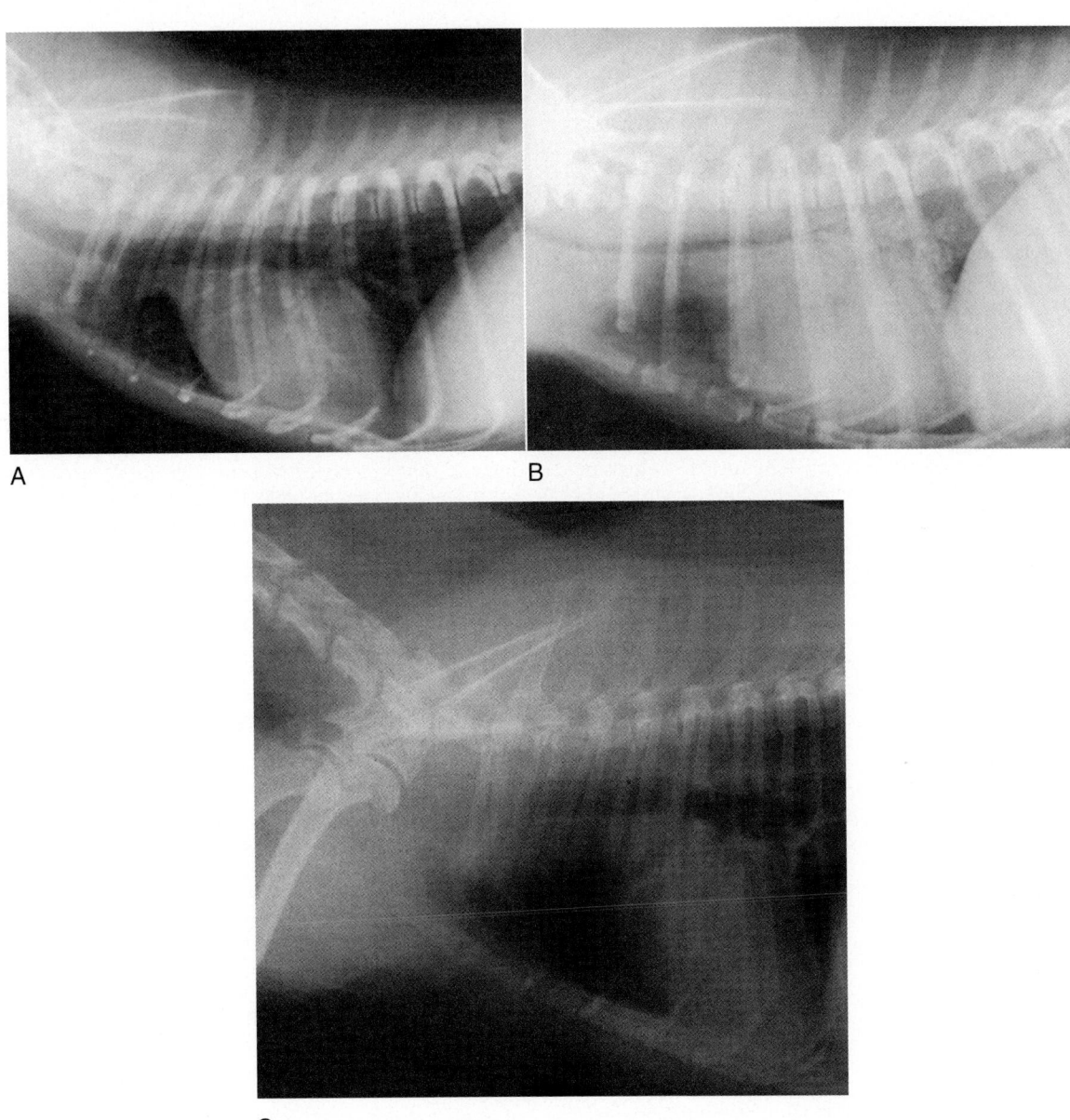

Figure 213-5 Lateral thoracic radiographs of an 8-year-old Yorkshire terrier during (**A**) peak inspiration and (**B**) peak expiration. Note the dramatic change in tracheal diameter that can occur during the respiratory cycle in animals with collapsing trachea and how important it is to obtain inspiratory as well as expiratory views. In severe cases such as this, the expiratory collapse is not limited to the thoracic segment of the trachea but extends into the cervical region as well. **C,** Collapsing trachea observed at the thoracic inlet in a dog with moderate rotation of the trachea. As a result of the rotation, the trachea appears wide rather than collapsed in the lateral view.

Continued

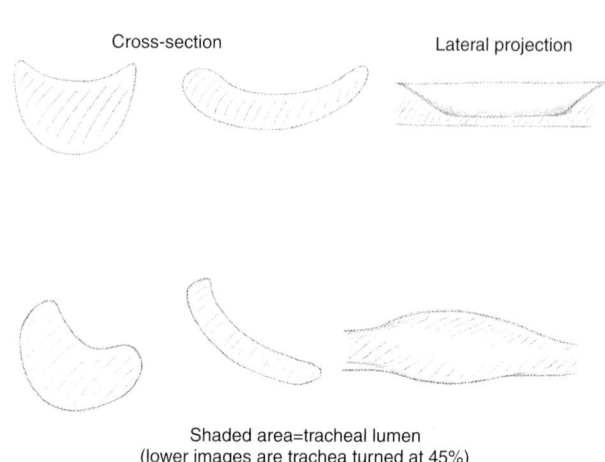

Cross-section   Lateral projection

Shaded area=tracheal lumen
(lower images are trachea turned at 45%)

D

Figure 213-5—Cont'd D, Drawing of the actual tracheal position and the line of the x-ray beam explains the appearance of the trachea on the lateral view.

Radiographic examination of patients with collapsing trachea uses both still and motion studies. The trachea should be examined on dorsoventral and lateral radiographs. Separate lateral radiographs of the cervical and cranial thoracic regions should be obtained to assess the contour of the entire trachea. Lateral radiographs made during both the maximum inspiratory phase and expiratory phase of the respiratory cycle are needed to demonstrate a dynamic collapsing trachea (Figure 213-5). Collapse of the cervical tracheal segment is usually best demonstrated during the inspiratory phase.

Conversely, the study made on expiration usually shows a collapse of the thoracic segment (and occasionally mainstem bronchi) and an unchanged or slightly dilated cervical segment. Care should be taken not to overflex or overextend the occipitoatlantal articulation when obtaining the lateral views, since this may produce pressure on the trachea that can artifactually induce narrowing of the lumen (Figure 213-6) or cause an abnormal tracheal course in the caudal cervical or thoracic region. There can be a subtle loss of radiographic detail at the dorsal luminal margin, which is produced by inversion of the dorsal tracheal membrane. The ventral margin of the tracheal lumen remains well demarcated and is unaffected by the collapsing process. The collapsed region usually involves approximately one third of the tracheal length, and the extremities of the collapse blend into normal lumen size over a distance of 2 to 3 cm. The course of the trachea is usually normal in uncomplicated cases. A redundant dorsal tracheal membrane which invaginates into the tracheal lumen can be seen as soft tissue opacity along the dorsal aspect of the caudal cervical tracheal lumen (Figure 213-5, E). This condition is seen in both small and large breed dogs, and can be distinguished from a superimposed esophagus or other structure by the sharp soft tissue-gas interface along the ventral margin. DV or VD views of the thorax do not usually demonstrate changes in the trachea. Concomitant lung disease may be seen.

Ultrasound examination of the trachea may demonstrate an alteration in the shape of the lumen on ventrodorsal projection.[49] Motion studies of normal respiratory function and cough, using fluoroscopy, can be made in order to assess the severity of the lesion. Some cases may show collapse only during the forced expiration of coughing. Slow-motion studies of videotape recordings are often helpful in delineation of the magnitude of the collapse, especially when produced by coughing.

The differential diagnosis of collapsed trachea requires consideration of such common conditions as tonsillitis, laryngeal paralysis or collapse, stenosis of the nares or trachea, eversion of the lateral saccules, elongation of the soft palate, bronchitis or primary tracheitis, foreign body tracheitis, and decompensated chronic mitral valvular disease. The list of causes of coughing that could be confused with collapsed trachea is extensive (see Chapter 53).

Therapy

The therapeutic approach to the collapsing trachea patient covers both the acute and chronic state. Although both conditions use the same common drugs, the need to deal quickly and aggressively with the acute state differs conceptually. Clients are often very anxious and the pet may be equally so, which demands immediate attention and reassurance for the owner.

In the acute state the clinician is concerned with calming the patient as quickly as possible. This may require the use of oral antitussive agents such as butorphanol or dihydrocodeinone. In the event that these products are not rapid or potent enough, injectable butorphanol may be considered. Other agents that are effective in more advanced conditions include dilute acetylpromazine, diazepam intravenously, or morphine by injection. Separating the extremely anxious pet from the client (this can often be very difficult to do) may be very useful and allows the clinician to appropriately sedate the dog and reduce the external stimuli that are continuing to occur. Not infrequently, simply removing the pet from view of the owner acts to calm the dog. In the event of cyanosis, oxygen in a humidified environment such as an oxygen-enriched cage or by nasal catheterization is suggested. The latter is made more difficult by the extreme anxiety of the patient. In such situations any physical manipulation or stress may aggravate the problem and make the cure worse than the disease. The use of short-term corticosteroids has a place in such situations since there likely is tracheal edema present. Injectable steroids initially, followed by oral dosages, tapered slowly is quite helpful during acute treatment. In some cases, pets are sent home with the owner after instructing on the administration of dilute acetylpromazine in the event of an acute exacerbation of the problem.

Throughout treatment, bronchodilators remain effective in treating this condition. The theoretical benefits accrue to reduction in spasm of the smaller airways, which reduces intrathoracic pressures and thus decreases the tendency of the larger airways to collapse. Additionally there is improved mucociliary clearance and reduced diaphragmatic fatigue. In some cases the authors even believe that the alcoholic content of an elixir compound seems to benefit the patient as much as the actual medication. Caution is required concerning the side effects of methyl xanthine drugs, which include vomiting and excitability. Similar results may be obtained by having the owner place a small dab of an alcoholic liquid in the buccal region during acute episodes of coughing at night when at home.

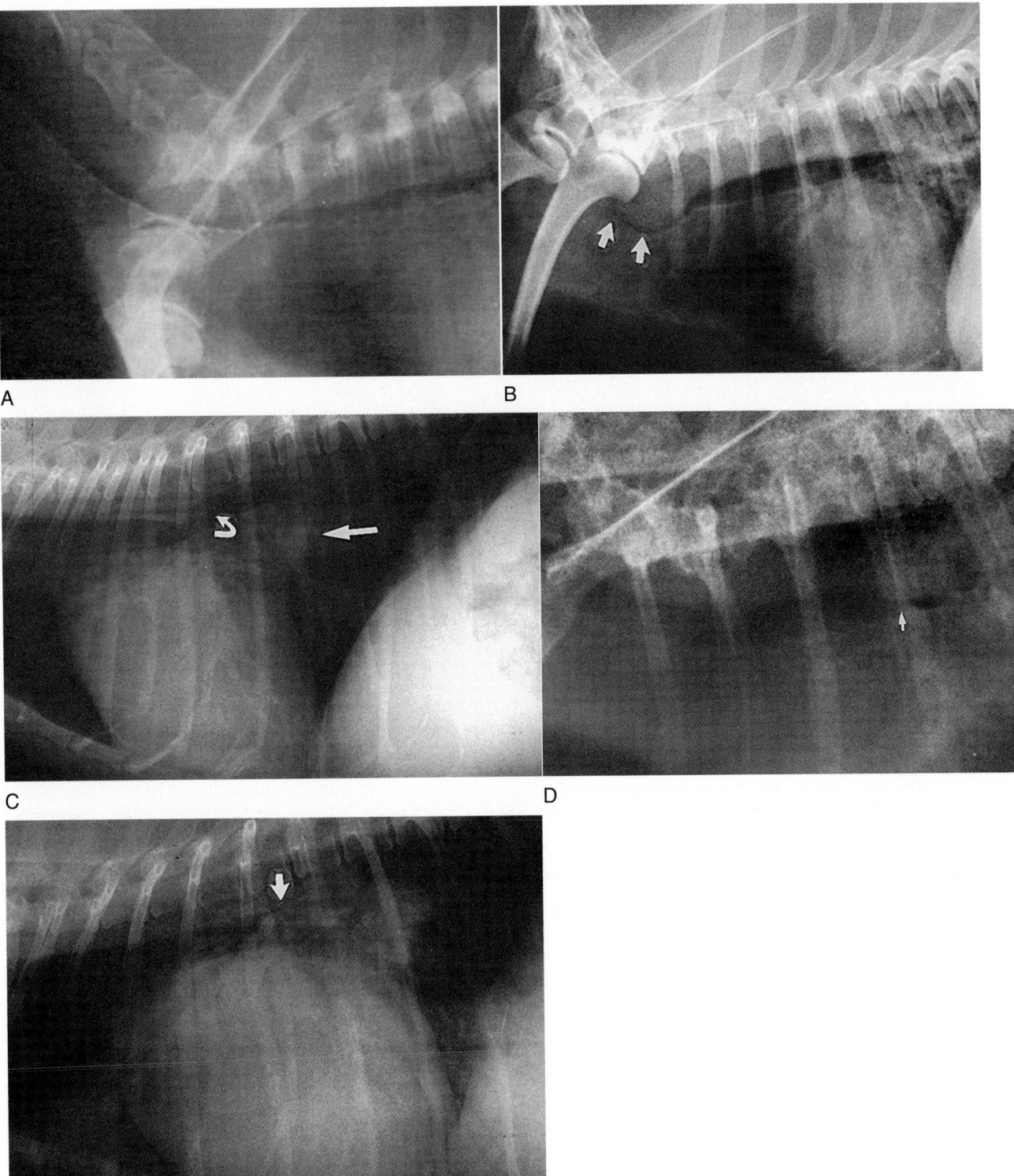

Figure 213-6 **A,** Lateral radiograph of a 13-year-old Chihuahua with a pliable, collapsible trachea showing caudal cervical tracheal collapse due to overextension of the neck. **B,** Lateral thoracic radiograph from a 14-year-old male castrate Pomeranian. Notice the reduced size of the cervical trachea as compared with the thoracic trachea on inspiration *(arrows).* **C** and **D,** 11-year-old Poodle, female spay, with severe chronic coughing. There is marked left atrial enlargement with bronchial dilatation on inspiration and on expiration there is narrowing and reduction in size of the two mainstem bronchi. Such pathology usually precludes surgical correction of the disease. **E,** Lateral radiograph from a 7-year-old Pomeranian, female spay, with severe coughing. Note the normal tracheal size until the carina at which point the mainstem bronchi shows compression and constriction *(arrow).* This patient required long-term aggressive medical therapy.

Treating the patient long term on an outpatient basis utilizes the same principles as set above except on a more relaxed level. Usually, medications can be administered on an as required basis and often may not be required throughout every day. The backbone of such therapy remains the bronchodilator agents (usually the methylxanthine derivatives such as aminophylline, theophylline elixir, or another bronchodilator, see Table 213-1). Beta-agonists (terbutaline and albuterol) are reported to be effectively used by some in place of the methylxanthine agents. No clinical studies demonstrating any proof of benefit are available. Antitussive agents butorphanol or dihydrocodeinone (hydrocodone) are quite effective in controlling symptoms. Side effects include oversedation, anorexia, and constipation. Occasionally longer use of low-dose steroids are given, often in combination with a sedative-antihistamine. Some combination products work well here (also see Table 213-1) but many have been removed from the market. Often the clinician will need to change therapies from time to time to find a newer effective agent. The neuroendocrine effect of digitalis may play a role in the effectiveness of this product, although the treatment of the cor pulmonale is considered to be another possible role.

Weight reduction in the obese patient is essential. This is accomplished principally with high-fiber, low-fat diets since exercise modification is unlikely. Weight loss alone can be curative in terms of dealing with the symptoms of this disease. Likewise removal of neck collars and utilizing only a harness when the dog is taken outside can be most effective in reducing clinical signs.

The majority of cases can be successfully treated symptomatically. Bronchodilator preparations containing expectorants and sedatives usually suffice to control this disease (see Table 213-1). Nebulization or vaporization may provide additional relief. Hospitalization with sedation for a period of several days, associated with corticosteroid therapy and nebulization, helps to reduce the degree of associated tracheitis. It is important to recognize that other disease states, specifically chronic lung disease, hepatomegaly, or chronic mitral valvular fibrosis, may be present. Antibiotics are not indicated in treating this disease unless there is concomitant bacterial infection. Removing the dog from respiratory irritants such as noxious gases, smoke, and dust is good common sense.

Several authors have reported on the surgical correction of this condition.[1,25-27] There are no evidence-based studies to link central chondrotomy with effective control of this disease. In one survey evaluating 100 dogs with tracheal collapse, 71% had long-term resolution of clinical signs with conservative care.[29] Of these 100 dogs, 4% required upper airway surgery and 11% were sent for tracheal reconstruction when no other medical conditions were recognized. Only half of this latter group had an asymptomatic recovery. These authors of this study and of this chapter suggest that surgery should be reserved only for younger dogs and those that fail to respond to aggressive medical care.[29]

Surgical methods that have been described include plication of the dorsal tracheal membrane, external tracheal ring prostheses, and intraluminal stent devices. These surgical efforts do not resolve the co-existing problem of mainstem and distal bronchial collapse and may not effectively resolve isolated thoracic inlet disease. Polypropylene C-shaped stent placement has been described with good results.[27,28,30] These authors suggest that surgery involving the thoracic portion of the trachea has been unrewarding because of high morbidity and that dogs with mainstem bronchial collapse are not good surgical candidates. In a group of dogs that did have surgery, 17 of the 90 (19%) required a follow-up tracheostomy and a high percentage of these developed complications due to occlusion with mucous or skin folds. Yet, extraluminal placement of polypropylene C-shaped stents was an effective method of controlling the clinical signs of collapsing trachea in some dogs.

Weight, severity of tracheal collapse, duration of the clinical signs, and the need for a tracheostomy did not affect the long-term outcome. Dogs over 6 years of age had more postoperative complications and a poorer long-term outcome than did dogs under 6.

Twenty-five dogs were treated surgically for tracheal collapse with use of extraluminal polypropylene ring prostheses plus a left arytenoids lateralization.[31] The authors reported a lower complication rate of 4% and a 75% success rate. They felt that this was due to reduced complications as a result of the tie back procedure.[31]

Various intraluminal stenting techniques have been considered and utilized. Varying results have been recorded using Palmaz[56] (negative), Nitinol[57] (no conclusions), Ultraflex, and Smart Stents (manufactured by Boston Scientific) with no strong positive literature to date to support unqualified recommendations. Failure to function well and migration following stent placement are problems that have been identified.

Surgical correction of a 4-year-old Poodle with a lateral collapsing trachea using ring prosthesis provided definitive relief of the symptoms. The authors evaluated the dog postoperatively and found little change anatomically. Since there was so much improvement the authors attributed the improvement to increased airway rigidity, which alleviated the effects of dynamic collapse resulting in improvement of the air flow.[21] Surgical management utilizing polypropylene spiral ring prostheses was identified in two large breed dogs with extra thoracic tracheal collapse.[32]

Obstructive Tracheal Masses
Etiology

Obstructive tracheal masses have varied etiologies. Lesions may be intraluminal, as in the case of primary tracheal neoplasia or extraluminally compressive. Tracheal tumors in dogs and cats include squamous cell carcinoma, histiocytic lymphosarcoma, lymphoblastic lymphosarcoma, osteosarcoma, adenocarcinoma, osteoma, chondroma, osteochondroma, chondrosarcoma, and leiomyoma.[1,33,34,58] Also, plasmacytoma, mast cell tumors, seromucinous carcinoma and rhabdomyosarcoma.[59] In dogs and cats, primary tumors of the trachea are uncommon. Other intraluminal masses include tracheal parasites, nodular amyloidosis, eosinophilic granulomas, abscesses, chronic granulomas,[1,35] and inflammatory polyps.[33] A single second-stage instar larval stage of *Cuterebra* spp. was identified in a 7-year-old cat's trachea.[37]

Tracheal foreign bodies can also cause an intraluminal obstruction.[1,38,39] Foreign bodies are not common, but when they do occur, they are usually small enough to pass beyond the tracheal bifurcation, causing subsequent development of inhalation pneumonia. When foreign bodies are relatively large, they are likely to come to rest at the carina.

Tracheal obstruction by external compression has been associated with thyroid and parathyroid tumors; enlargement of the mandibular, retropharyngeal, or prescapular lymph nodes due to infection, mediastinal hemorrhage and abscesses,[60,61] neoplasia, mycotic granuloma; peritracheal abscesses and cysts; extramedulary tracheal masses,[62] cranial mediastinal masses such as thymomas; esophageal tumors; and esophageal granulomas secondary to *Spirocerca lupi*.[1,40,41]

Clinical Signs and Diagnosis

Obstructive diseases are associated with a dramatic increase in airway resistance at the point of obstruction, impeding air flow, which causes hypoventilation and respiratory acidosis.[42] Clinical signs depend on the degree of obstruction. Up to one half of the airway diameter may be compromised without obvious clinical signs.[43] Even in these cases, however, close inspection of the patient will reveal an obstructive breathing pattern, which consist of a slow inspiratory phase followed by

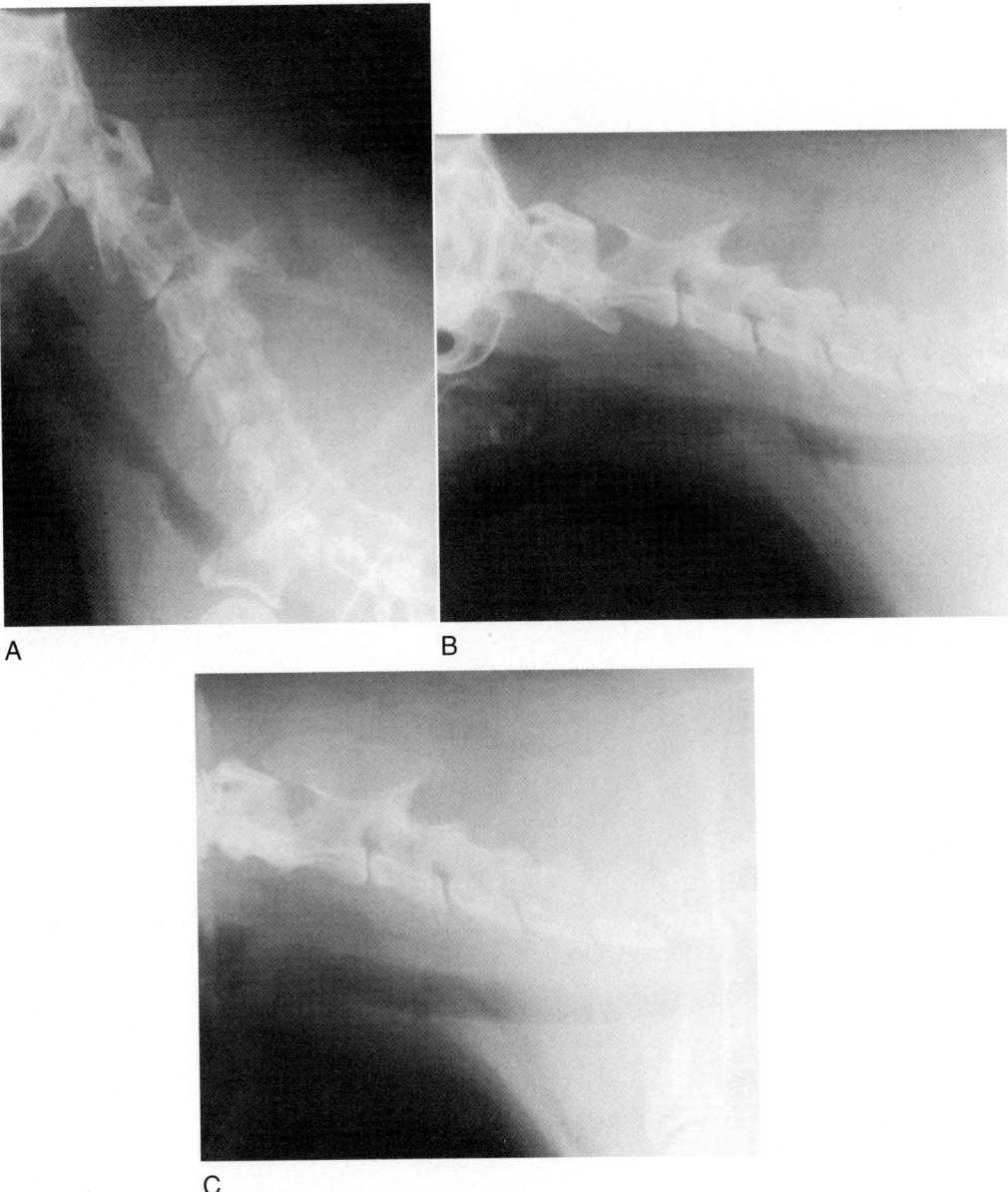

Figure 213-7 **A** and **B,** Lateral cervical radiograph of an 8-year-old cat with inspiratory dyspnea and open-mouth breathing. A tracheal mass can be seen arising from the ventral tracheal wall and growing into the lumen at the level of C4-C5. The air in the trachea provides a natural negative contrast agent. **C,** Cervical radiographs 3 months after surgical resection of the mass. The mass is no longer seen. Histopathologic diagnosis was tracheal adenocarcinoma.

a more rapid expiratory phase.[43] Most animals present with stridor, loud ronchi (rattling in the throat), and often chronic coughing. Respiratory distress and dyspnea are usually obvious.

Overzealous examination and performance of laboratory studies may disturb the patient, thereby worsening the condition. Every effort should be made to keep the animal calm, and initial diagnostic tests should be done with as little stress as possible.

The work-up for the patient with suspected tracheal obstructive disease usually begins with radiography. Lateral views should be obtained if the patient can tolerate recumbency without struggling. Ventrodorsal radiographs often put the patient in a stressful position; instead dorsoventral views should be obtained. Tracheal masses may decrease luminal size in a nonlinear manner, resulting in a mass protruding into the lumen. These masses are outlined by tracheal air, which provides a good natural negative contrast medium (Figure 213-7).

Disruption of the mucosal continuity is seen at the base of the mass. This is in contradistinction to the silhouette produced by masses that are extraluminal, in which the line produced by the luminal air-mucosa interface is seen to pass uninterrupted through the mass. Non-radiopaque foreign bodies can be rendered invisible to radiographic examination if they travel distal enough in the bronchi, which results in atelectasis of the obstructed lobe with transudation of serous fluid distal to and around the foreign body. Extraluminal masses that cause tracheal obstruction are generally recognized radiographically as linear decreases in the lumen diameter over a length determined by the size of the mass (Figure 213-8).

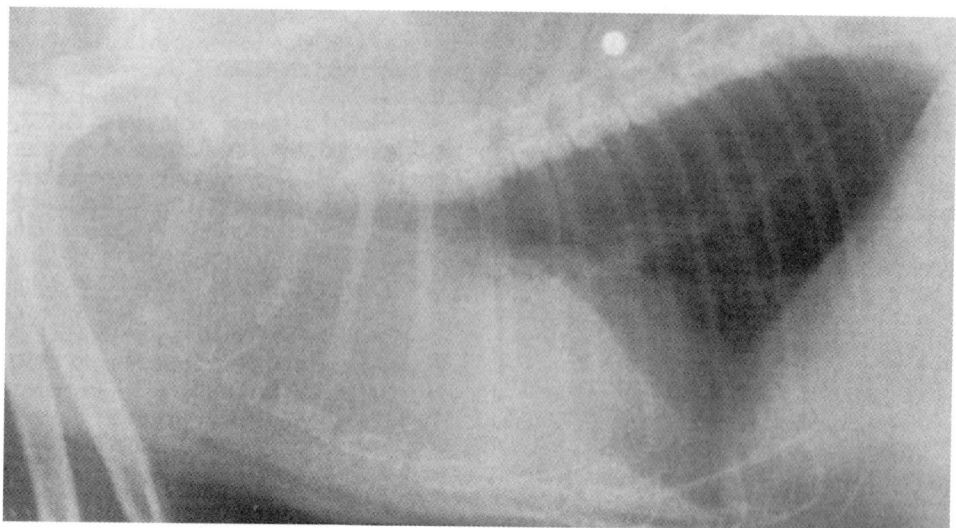

A

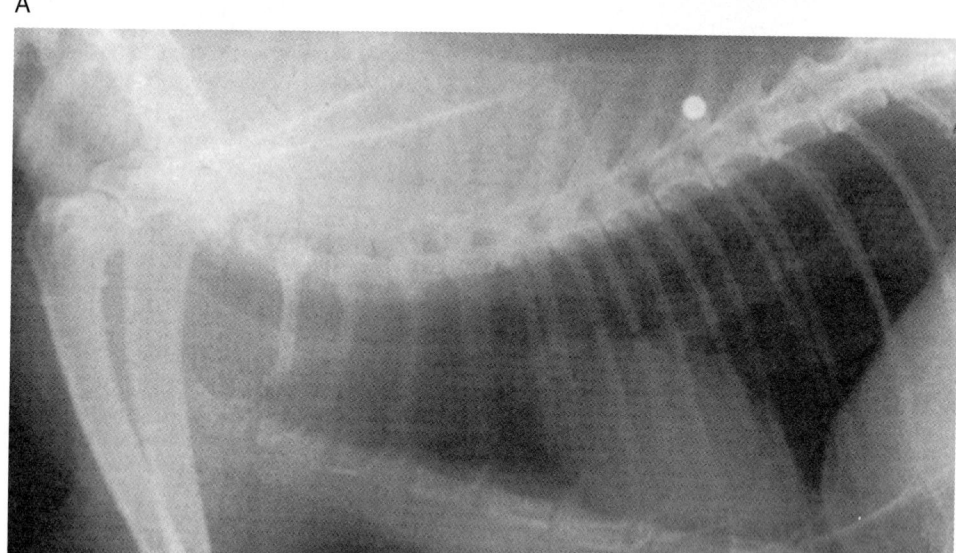

B

Figure 213-8 A, Lateral thoracic radiograph of a 5-year-old domestic short-hair cat, presented for dyspnea and emesis, shows elevation and compression of the trachea at the thoracic inlet along with pleural fluid. The cranial lung lobes are displaced caudally. These signs were secondary to lymphosarcoma of the cranial mediastinum. B, Same cat as in A, 5 weeks after chemotherapy. Notice the re-expansion of the previously compressed trachea. C, Lateral thoracic radiograph of an 8-year-old female Burmese cat with pleural fluid secondary to cardiomyopathy. Note that the tracheal elevation is not accompanied by tracheal compression as in the previous case of a mediastinal mass.

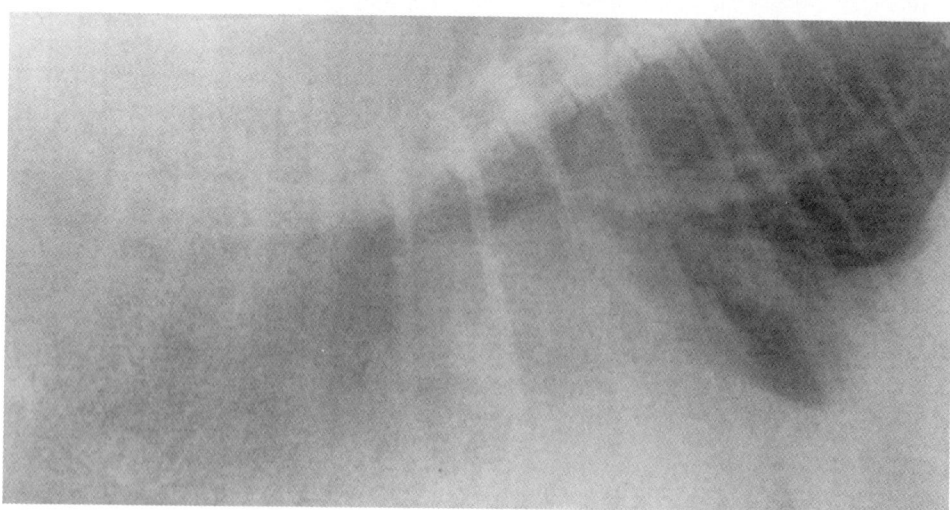

C

In the mediastinal region a mass must be quite large to result in tracheal compression. The trachea is easier to displace then to compress in this location. High-level airway obstruction is most likely to be associated with hypoinflated, small lung fields. Intrathoracic tracheal obstruction may present as a hyperinflated lung due to air trapping as a result of narrowing of the airway during expiration. This creates a ball valve effect and traps air distal to the obstructing lesion. In a cat with an inflammatory polyp partially obstructing the trachea, thoracic radiography suggested increased airway resistance during expiration (hyperinflated lungs and a caudally displaced flattened diaphragm).[36] Contrast esophageal studies are sometimes needed to differentiate the etiology of the tracheal narrowing or displacement in the cranial mediastinal region, particularly in brachycephalic breeds in which cranial mediastinal masses are often difficult to delineate. Concomitant narrowing of the trachea and esophagus in the cranial mediastinum is highly suggestive of an extraluminal mass.

Bronchoscopy allows visualizing tracheal masses and foreign bodies (especially radiolucent foreign bodies), retrieving cytologic specimens of masses, or obtaining biopsies.

Therapy

In addition to its diagnostic value, bronchoscopy can be used as part of the treatment. Some foreign bodies can be removed endoscopically, and some tracheal masses may be removed by means of a suction biopsy device attached to the bronchoscope.[34]

For foreign bodies that cannot be retrieved through the bronchoscope and for large or firm tracheal masses, the mainstay of therapy is surgical removal or resection. Surgical procedures of the trachea have been well described. Some foreign bodies may be removed in smaller patients by holding the pet upside down (head down) while under general anesthesia and gently but firmly tapping the thorax. Occasionally the foreign body is actually coughed out and other times it is moved into a more proximal position for easier bronchoscopic retrieval.

The prognosis for patients with tracheal obstruction depends on the specific primary disease as well as the present degree of respiratory embarrassment. Stressful diagnostic measures may push the patient into a state of decompensation. With tracheal tumors, the prognosis varies with the amount of trachea involved and with the specific biologic behavior of the tumor type present.

Tracheal Trauma
Etiology

Laceration of the tracheal wall causes subcutaneous and mediastinal emphysema. Traumatic injury to the trachea is unusual in small animals. Bite wounds to the neck incurred during a dog or cat fight, transtracheal wash procedure, and inadvertent laceration of the trachea during jugular venous puncture are causes. However, overinflation of endotracheal cuffs, often during dentistry in cats, is another important etiology.[63-65] An uncommon sequela to trauma is a tracheoesophageal fistula.

Clinical Signs and Diagnosis

A ventrolateral tear of the annular ligament may produce secondary subcutaneous emphysema over the entire body.[44] This latter condition develops frequently in dogs or cats involved in fights during which a tooth punctures or lacerates the tracheal wall. Air escapes from the tracheal opening and enters the subcutaneous tissue of the neck (Figure 213-9). The subcutaneous emphysema may involve only the peritracheal region or

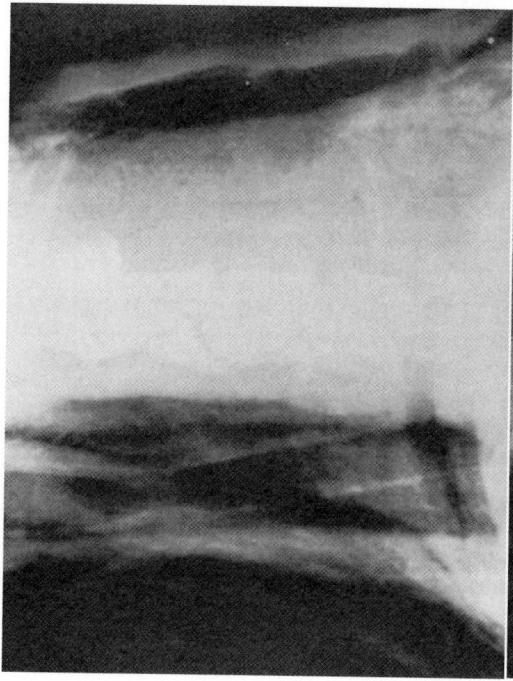
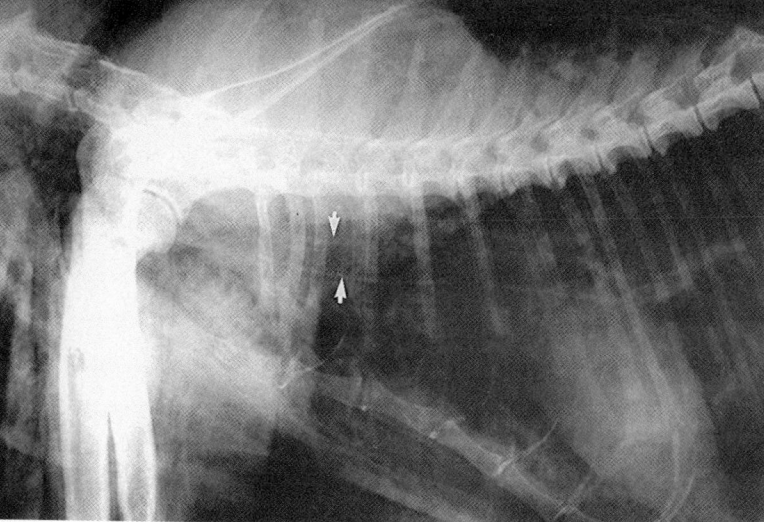

A   B

Figure 213-9 **A,** Lateral cervical radiograph of a 10-year-old male cocker spaniel with tracheal narrowing and rupture at the level of C3 resulting from a dog fight. There is extensive cervical and subcutaneous emphysema. Not that the outer tracheal wall is visible throughout its length because of the free extraluminal air that provides contrast. **B,** Pneumomediastinum in a cat associated with subcutaneous air collection. Note the prominent tracheal stripes both dorsally and ventrally as a result of the trachea being outlined by air both inside and outside of the trachea lumen.

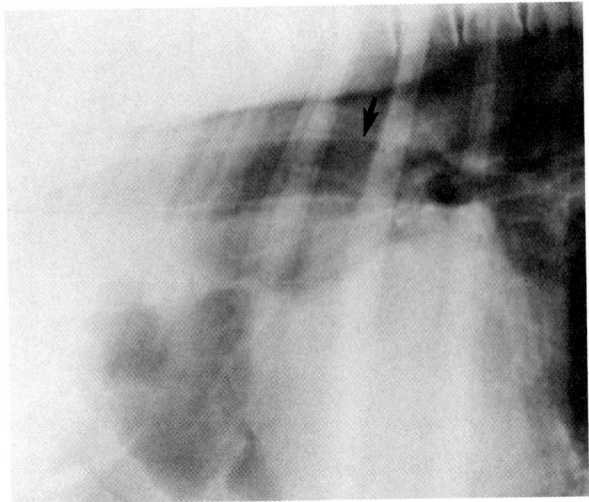

Figure 213-10 Lateral thoracic radiograph of a 10-year-old Great Dane with pneumomediastinum. Note how the free air in the mediastinum provides a negative contrast and allows detection of the dorsal tracheal wall *(arrow)*.

be more extensive and involve the entire subcutaneous area of the body. Such tears may also be responsible for the development of pneumomediastinum in both the dog and the cat (Figure 213-10). Subcutaneous emphysema is recognized by the crackling sensation of the animal's skin. The tissue beneath the skin appears swollen. The presence of such a lesion should immediately indicate the possibility of a tracheal tear.

Fractures of the trachea produce radiographic signs of peritracheal, intermuscular, and subcutaneous emphysema. Pneumomediastinum may also be present with a cervical or intrathoracic lesion. Fractures or lacerations of the trachea or tracheobronchial tree should always be considered in cases of persistent, increasing subcutaneous emphysema even when no cutaneous lacerations can be located. Bronchoscopy visualizes the point and extent of tracheal mucosal interruption. Occasionally traumatic injury of the intrathoracic trachea results in a circumferential rupture *(avulsion)*, leaving the mucosal or serosal lining intact. This prevents air from dissecting into the mediastinum. Clinical signs develop one to twenty eight days post trauma. Radiographs will reveal the separation of the tracheal rings (Figure 213-11) referred to as a "pseudo-tracheal" sign.[66-68] A focal widening of the tracheal lumen at the separation during inspiration and narrowing during expiration is often identified.

Therapy

If the subcutaneous air collection is regressing and there are no signs of pulmonary distress, it is usually recommended that the patient be cage rested, which allows the emphysema to regress by slow absorption, mild sedation, and occasionally by aspiration through a large-bore needle and wrapping the body with elastic bandages, being careful not to mechanically

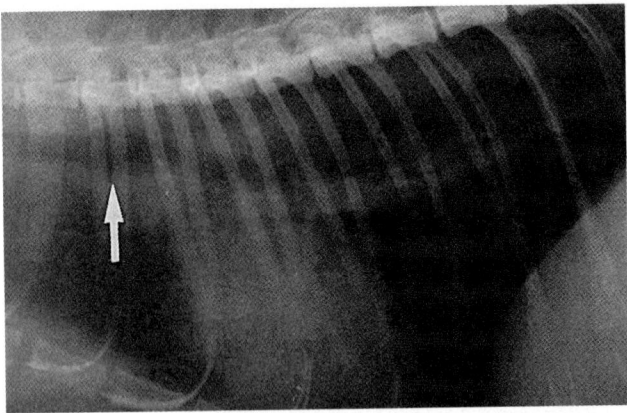

A

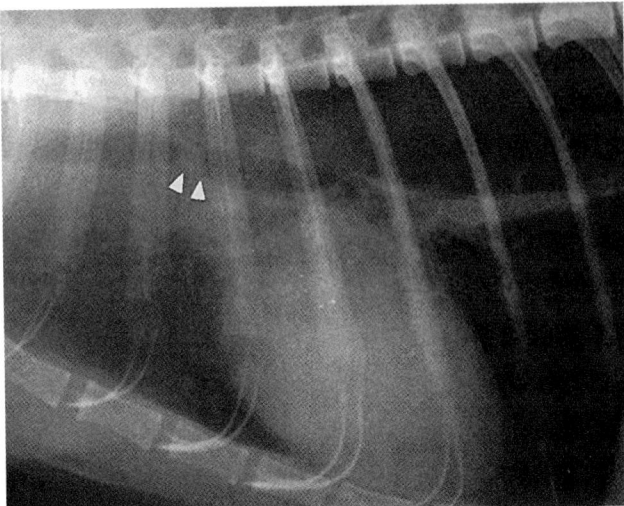

B

Figure 213-11 Lateral thoracic radiographs of a cat following thoracic trauma. **A,** Note the focal increased size of the trachea at the level of the fourth rib, which suggests trauma to the tracheal wall. In the lateral view **(B)** taken 1 week later, there is marked diminution in the size of the trachea at the fourth intercostal space due to tracheal stenosis.

restrict respiration. Medical treatment alone was effective in 15 of 20 such cases and a sixteenth case died before surgery was attempted.[63] Perhaps of greater importance is the effort to detect other pathologic conditions such as pneumothorax or hemothorax. If another such condition is present, the clinician should consider thoracocentesis.

Surgical repair of a torn tracheal ligament may be required. Most tears have been found dorsolaterally on the trachea at or near the thoracic inlet.[63] Surgical repair with good results are reported in cats with intrathoracic tracheal avulsion associated with dyspnea, exercise intolerance, and exertional cyanosis.[45]

CHAPTER 214

Diseases of the Small Airways

Lynelle R. Johnson

The primary role of the small airways is conduction of gases to and from the gas exchange region of the lung at the least energy cost to the animal. Cartilaginous support in large airways and smooth muscle tone in small airways keep airways open to facilitate gas flow. A ciliated, cuboidal epithelial layer that contains mucus-producing goblet cells and submucosal mucus glands lines smaller airways. Production of excessive airway mucus in response to inflammation or infection reduces luminal diameter, increases resistance to airflow, and augments the work of breathing. Activation of the inflammatory cascade and production of inflammatory mediators can cause bronchoconstriction in cats, which further reduces airflow.

CANINE CHRONIC BRONCHITIS

Chronic bronchitis is an inflammatory airway disease characterized by the presence of a daily cough for greater than 2 months. Neutrophilic or eosinophilic infiltration of bronchial mucosa results in production of proteases, elastases, and oxidizing products. Inflammatory cell products and oxidant injury cause increased epithelial permeability, cellular injury, and mucus hypersecretion. Histologically, chronic bronchitis is characterized by hypertrophy and hyperplasia of mucus glands and goblet cells, smooth muscle hypertrophy, fibrosis of the lamina propria, and epithelial erosion with squamous metaplasia. These changes result in obstruction to airflow and clinical signs of cough and exercise intolerance.

Presentation
Bronchitis affects middle-aged to older dogs. Although classically considered a disease of small breed dogs, bronchitis often affects larger breed dogs.[1] The primary clinical complaint is a harsh productive or nonproductive cough. Many affected dogs have a history of exercise intolerance, and some develop collapse or cough syncope.

On physical examination, dogs with chronic bronchitis appear in good health, are often overweight, and may pant excessively. Tracheal sensitivity is usually present, and auscultation reveals coarse, inspiratory crackles and expiratory wheezes. Dogs with significant bronchitis display prolonged expiration and an expiratory push. Heart rate is normal to low in dogs with respiratory disease, and an exaggerated sinus arrhythmia may be present due to increased vagal tone.

Diagnostic Evaluation
Clinicopathologic abnormalities are typically absent in dogs with bronchitis. Thoracic radiography can establish the likelihood of chronic bronchitis although normal chest radiographs do not rule out chronic airway disease. Thickening of airway walls and increased numbers of visible airway walls are found more commonly in dogs with bronchitis than in age and breed-matched controls.[2] End-on bronchi (doughnuts) and airways seen in longitudinal section (tram lines) represent airway walls thickened by inflammation (Figure 214-1). Right-sided cardiomegaly may be seen in dogs with chronic airway disease that develop pulmonary hypertension and/or cor pulmonale.

Hypoxemia and abnormal distribution of ventilation on radioaerosol scans have been reported in dogs with bronchitis.[1] Tidal breathing flow volume loops in dogs with chronic bronchitis demonstrate reduced expiratory flow and loop shapes similar to those seen in humans with chronic bronchitis.[1]

Collection of airway samples by tracheal wash or bronchoscopy characterizes the cellular infiltrate in the airways and rules out infectious causes of cough. Bronchoscopy is particularly useful in dogs that lack significant radiographic indications of bronchitis since virtually all dogs with chronic bronchitis have rough, hyperemic airway mucosa and mucoid or purulent secretions lining the airways. In animals with long-standing bronchitis, fibrous nodules can be seen protruding into the bronchial lumen. Cytologically, chronic bronchitis is characterized by a preponderance of nondegenerate neutrophils[1] (Figure 214-2), although some dogs have predominantly eosinophils in airway washings. Increased mucus and Curshman's spirals (bronchial casts of airway mucus) are sometimes noted.

Low numbers of bacteria ($<1.7 \times 10^3$ colony forming units per milliliter) can be found in airway samples from bronchitic dogs, and more than one species of bacteria may be isolated[3]; however, significant bacterial infection is not common in dogs with chronic bronchitis.[1,3] Bacteria can also be isolated from airways of healthy dogs (Box 214-1).

Treatment
Anti-inflammatories
Short-acting steroids such as prednisone or prednisolone are generally safe and effective in dogs with uncomplicated bronchitis. Remission of clinical signs can usually be achieved with initial doses of glucocorticoids that range from 0.5 to 1.0 mg/kg PO BID. The dosage should be decreased by half every 5 to 10 days, with the goal to achieve alternate day

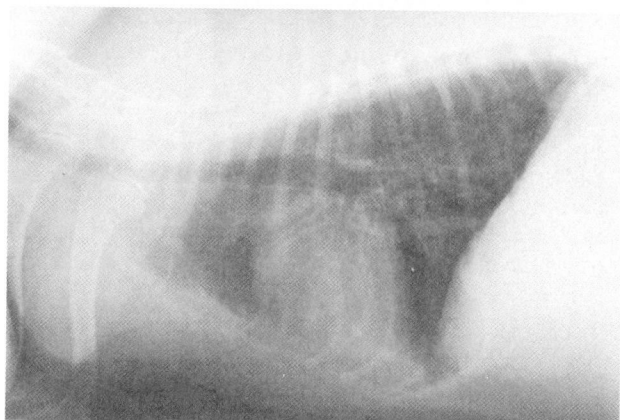

Figure 214-1 Lateral chest radiograph of a dog with chronic bronchitis. Increased bronchial markings are apparent, primarily in the caudal lung fields.

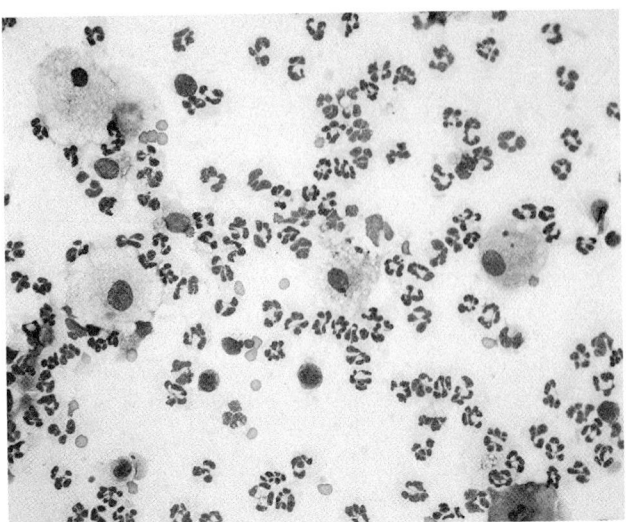

Figure 214-2 Cytology of BALF from a dog with chronic bronchitis demonstrating neutrophilic inflammation (>80% neutrophils on a differential cell count). In healthy dogs, BALF comprises predominantly macrophages (65% to 70%) and low numbers of inflammatory cells (6% to 9% each of neutrophils, eosinophils, and lymphocytes).

dosing to allow normalization of the pituitary-adrenal axis. If clinical signs recur, a return to the higher dose of glucocorticoid that controlled clinical signs is recommended. Many animals require lifelong therapy, whereas some may be successfully weaned off medication. In dogs with persistent or recurrent signs, concurrent treatment with a bronchodilator or antitussive is indicated.

Bronchodilators

Use of bronchodilators can be associated with clinical improvement due to reduced pulmonary infiltrates or improved expiratory airflow.[1] A trial on a bronchodilator is indicated when a dog exhibits marked expiratory effort and persistent cough despite anti-inflammatory therapy. Bronchodilators can improve diaphragmatic contractility, reduce respiratory muscle fatigue, stimulate mucociliary clearance, and may reduce the dosage of glucocorticoid required.

The bronchodilators used most commonly in veterinary medicine are methylxanthine derivatives and beta-2 agonists.

Box • 214-1

Bacteria Retrieved from the Airways of Healthy Animals[9,17,18]

Pasteurella spp.
Mycoplasma spp.*
Streptococcus spp.
Staphylococcus spp.
Acinetobacter spp.
Moraxella spp.
Enterobacter spp.
Pseudomonas spp.
Escherichia coli
Klebsiella spp.
Bordetella bronchiseptica

*Healthy dogs only, not cats.

Methylxanthines are believed to act through antagonism of adenosine or effects on intracellular calcium handling, since therapeutic levels do not result in accumulation of cyclic AMP. Long-acting theophylline (Theochron®, Inwood Laboratories) at 10 mg/kg PO BID achieves plasma levels in dogs that approximate the human therapeutic range of 10 to 20 µg/mL.[4] Adverse effects of methylxanthines include gastrointestinal upset, sinus tachycardia, and hyperexcitability. When toxic signs are noted, drug therapy is discontinued and then reinstituted at half the initial dose. If clinical signs improve and the dog tolerates the drug, the dosage may be increased if needed. If no response is seen, an alternate class of bronchodilator is recommended.

Beta-2 adrenergic agonists (terbutaline or albuterol) have been used successfully in management of chronic bronchitis. Dosing of terbutaline is based on animal size, and small dogs receive 0.625 to 1.25 mg PO BID, medium-sized dogs may be given 1.25 to 2.5 mg PO BID, and larger dogs receive 2.5 to 5.0 mg PO BID. Albuterol is dosed at 50 µg/kg PO TID. Beta agonists may result in excitability or tremors during initial therapy but dogs usually become accustomed to the drug.

Antitussives

Dogs with bronchitis rely on a potent cough reflex to clear secretions from the airway, and suppression of cough prior to resolution of inflammation could trap mucus in the lower airway, perpetuate airway inflammation, and worsen pulmonary function and clinical signs. When inflammation has been effectively treated but cough persists, use of cough suppressants is warranted since chronic coughing causes repeated airway injury and may lead to syncope. Potent cough suppression can be achieved with narcotic agents such as hydrocodone (0.2 mg/kg PO BID-QID) or butorphanol (0.05 to 0.12 mg/kg SQ BID-QID and 0.55 mg/kg PO BID-QID). These agents must be given at a frequent interval in order to suppress coughing without inducing excessive sedation.

Antibiotics

Airway infection is likely if greater than 3 intracellular bacteria per 50 high-power fields are seen on airway cytology,[3] and appropriate antibiotics are prescribed based on culture and susceptibility results.

Ancillary Therapy

Improvements in exercise tolerance and arterial oxygenation can be seen with weight loss alone since obesity decreases thoracic compliance, restricts expansion of the thorax, and worsens both clinical signs and gas exchange in dogs with chronic bronchitis. Exercise should be increased as tolerated. Dogs with concurrent tracheal collapse or marked tracheal sensitivity benefit from use of a harness instead of a collar. When stresses in the environment are encountered, such as cigarette smoke, pollutants, heat, or humidity, the animal should be removed to a cool, clean area.

Some animals may benefit from airway humidification to increase moisture in airway secretions and facilitate clearance. The most significant benefit can be achieved through nebulization with a pneumatic or ultrasonic nebulizer that creates small enough water particles to penetrate the airways. Standard vaporizers create larger water particles and are less effective. Nebulization can be performed two to four times daily for 10 to 30 minutes and should be followed by gentle exercise or coupage therapy to facilitate removal of secretions. Nebulization occasionally results in bronchospasm, overhydration, or distress to the animal. Some patients may benefit from administration of a bronchodilator immediately prior to therapy.

Prognosis

Bronchitis is a chronic disease that can often be controlled but never cured. The majority of patients have residual cough and exhibit clinical signs periodically throughout life. Goals of therapy are to control inflammation thus limiting clinical signs and to prevent worsening airway disease. When inadequately treated, long-standing bronchitis may lead to bronchiectasis or pulmonary hypertension due to chronic hypoxia and/or vascular remodeling.

BRONCHIECTASIS

Bronchiectasis is a focal or diffuse destructive lung condition characterized by irreversible dilatation of large cartilaginous airways, often with accumulation of pulmonary secretions. Dilatation results from destruction of muscular and elastic support structure of the airways by cytokines and proteolytic enzymes produced by inflammatory cells.[5] It can occur in association with primary ciliary dyskinesia (PCD), as a sequela to long-standing infectious or inflammatory pulmonary disease, secondary to smoke inhalation or airway obstruction, or as a complication of radiation-induced pneumonitis.[5] In cats, bronchiectasis is recognized as a histopathologic response to long-standing airway disease. Cocker spaniels seem predisposed to the disorder.[6]

Presentation

Dogs with bronchiectasis typically have a chronic history of a moist productive cough and frequent bouts of pneumonia that initially respond to antibiotics but then recur.[6,7] Hemoptysis may be present.

Physical examination is remarkable for moist crackles and expiratory wheezing. Loud bronchial sounds can sometimes be heard over dilated airways. Nasal discharge may be related to PCD or associated with pneumonia, when pulmonary secretions are expectorated into the nasal passages.

Diagnostic Evaluation

Nonspecific evidence of chronic infection includes neutrophilia, monocytosis, and hyperglobinemia due to chronic antigenic stimulation. Arterial blood gas analysis typically exhibits hypoxemia and a widened alveolar-arterial oxygen gradient.

Thoracic radiographs can demonstrate mixed bronchial, interstitial, or alveolar patterns with diffuse thickening of bronchial walls.[6] Although central or diffuse bronchial dilatation is classic for bronchiectasis, radiographs are relatively insensitive for the diagnosis. Dilated airways are more readily apparent when a severe pneumonic infiltrate is present. Computed tomography or bronchoscopy can provide evidence of bronchiectasis in dogs and cats. Classic bronchoscopic findings in bronchiectasis include dilatation of the airways with or without trapping of purulent secretions, loss of the cylindrical shape to airway lumens, and mucosal hyperemia and irregularity.

Bronchoalveolar lavage fluid (BALF) typically exhibits suppurative inflammation. Bacterial cultures for both aerobes and anaerobes are indicated since purulent secretions can favor the growth of anaerobic species. In dogs, cultures may fail to reveal bacterial growth[7] yet these cases often respond to antibiotic therapy.

Treatment

Dogs with lobar bronchiectasis or bronchial foreign bodies usually require lung lobectomy for management of disease. Dogs with pneumonia must be treated with broad-spectrum antibiotics that are efficacious against both aerobes and anaerobes. While cultures are pending, intravenous ampicillin (10 to 20 mg/kg IV q6-8h) and gentamicin (2 to 4 mg/kg q8-12h) or enrofloxacin (2.5 mg/kg IM q12h) can be used. Long-term use of antibiotics should be based on culture and susceptibility results. Animals that suffer recurrent infection due to bronchiectasis may be candidates for chronic suppressive antibiotic therapy or treatment with 1 week of antibiotics each month.

Bronchodilators can be beneficial, although animals typically have irreversible airflow limitation. Cough suppressants must be avoided since failure to remove infectious and inflammatory secretions will perpetuate disease. Maintenance of systemic and airway hydration through oral intake, intravenous fluids, and/or nebulization can be a critical factor in resolution of disease. Because dogs with bronchiectasis tend to pool secretions in lower airways, brisk coupage following nebulization is essential to assist in removal of airway secretions.

Prognosis

Owners should be aware of the likelihood of chronic recurrent infection in dogs with bronchiectasis. Resistance to antibiotic treatment may occur. Animals with significant hypoxemia and parenchymal changes may develop pulmonary hypertension or cor pulmonale. Some animals are at risk for sepsis.

Prevention

Bronchiectasis can be limited by use of appropriate antibiotic therapy in infectious lung disease, prompt recognition and removal of foreign bodies, and appropriate management of chronic bronchitis.

FELINE BRONCHIAL DISEASE

Feline bronchial disease describes a spectrum of inflammatory small airway diseases in the cat characterized by signs that range from chronic or intermittent coughing to life-threatening respiratory distress. Any age can be afflicted with bronchial disease, and Siamese cats seem to have an increased incidence of disease and may suffer from a more chronic form of bronchial disease.[8] Disease results from inflammation within the airways that induces reversible airflow obstruction through smooth muscle constriction and hypertrophy, bronchial wall edema, and hyperplasia of submucosal glands. Hyper-responsive airways and reversible airflow obstruction have been documented in some cases.[9] These conditions lead to a reduction in airway diameter and increased airway resistance, which cause clinical signs of cough and/or respiratory distress.[8,9]

Experimental models of feline bronchial disease that use antigen or allergen induction of airway hyper-reactivity describe generation of inflammatory and immunomodulatory cytokines and mediators within the airways.[10,11,12] Mast cell degranulation likely leads to recruitment and activation of T lymphocytes. Activated eosinophils release granule contents, and expose the epithelium to major basic protein (MBP), which causes ciliostasis and reduces mucociliary clearance. MBP also leads to epithelial cell lysis and desquamation.[13] Sloughing of pneumocytes exposes sensory and nerve endings to increased types and concentrations of allergens or irritants and may also result in a reduction of epithelial derived relaxant factor. Thus inflammatory damage can enhance neural responsiveness. Recent evidence suggests that inflammation can also induce oxidant stress that perpetuates airway injury.[14]

Presentation

The most frequent presenting complaints in cats with bronchial disease are coughing and abnormal respirations, such as wheezing, loud breathing, or respiratory difficulty.[9] Paroxysmal coughing is commonly reported, and the cough is often described as a dry, "hacking" cough or retch. Exercise intolerance or episodes of open-mouth breathing after exertion may be noted in some cats.

Cats with bronchial disease tend toward obesity given an inability to exercise. Bronchitic cats can appear normal at rest and exhibit normal pulmonary auscultation; however, increased tracheal sensitivity is usually present and post-tussive crackles are typically ausculted. Harsh lung sounds, crackles, or expiratory wheezes are evident in some affected cats, and the expiratory phase is prolonged.[9,15] An abdominal component to respiration may also be noted. Air trapping may occur distal to obstructed airways leading to decreased thoracic compressibility and a barrel-shaped appearance to the chest. Auscultation in this area of the lung is quiet with increased resonance on percussion.

Diagnostic Evaluation

Cats with bronchial disease have nonspecific changes on blood work, and peripheral eosinophilia was reported in only 30% of affected cats.[9] Airway parasites should be ruled out as a cause of airway inflammation and subsequent bronchoconstriction. A sedimentation technique is used to detect the single-operculated egg of *Paragonimus* spp., whereas Baermann flotation is needed to detect *Aelurostrongylus* larvae. A routine fecal flotation can be used to identify *Capillaria* eggs. Heartworm antibody/antigen tests and echocardiography could be considered in cats presenting with cough or respiratory distress.[16]

A variety of interstitial, bronchial, and alveolar infiltrative patterns may be observed in cats with bronchial disease. The severity of the radiographic pattern may not match the degree of respiratory embarrassment in cats with acute bronchoconstriction, and normal chest radiographs do not rule out the diagnosis of bronchial disease. Cats without obvious pulmonary infiltrates may show other radiographic signs compatible with bronchoconstriction, such as air trapping, flattening of the diaphragm, or hyperinflation of the lungs. The hallmark of feline bronchial disease is peribronchial cuffing caused by infiltration of inflammatory cells around the airways (Figure 214-3). Excessive mucus production and obstruction of larger airways can cause alveolar infiltrates, consolidating lesions, or atelectasis.

In the stable cat with airway disease, a transoral tracheal wash or bronchoscopy can be performed to obtain airway specimens for cytology and culture. Substantial elevation of eosinophil and/or neutrophil percentages in airway specimens correlates with the severity of clinical disease[9] and so airway cytology can be used as a guide to therapy. However, normal cats may have up to 25% eosinophils in BALF cells.[17]

Bacterial culture and susceptibility testing should be performed in all cats; however, bacteria can be isolated from a large proportion of healthy cats[9] (Box 214-1). Detection of intracellular bacteria is supportive of a true bacterial infection. *Mycoplasma* species have been isolated from tracheobronchial lavage samples in 21% to 44% of cats with respiratory disease[8,18]

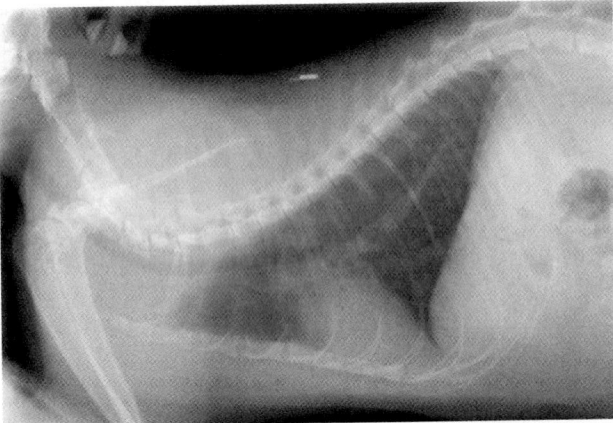

Figure 214-3 Lateral chest radiograph of a cat with chronic bronchial disease. Airway walls are thickened by peribronchial infiltrates.

but not from bronchoalveolar lavage samples from healthy cats,[17,18] and specific *Mycoplasma* culture on BALF should be considered in cats with respiratory disease.

Measurement of airway resistance and lung compliance can be performed (in anesthetized cats) at some referral institutions. Cats with bronchial disease can exhibit high lung resistance due to bronchoconstriction. Cats with bronchial disease may also exhibit airway hyper-responsiveness to a nonspecific aerosol stimulant as evidenced by a reduction in the dosage of methacholine required to increase lung resistance.[9] Whole body plethysmography can be used to study airway reactivity in awake, spontaneously breathing cats by measurement of box-pressure signals (expiratory time, peak inspiratory and expiratory flows) and calculation of enhanced pause (PENH), a variable that correlates with airway resistance.[19] Plethysmography is technically challenging, and measured variables are influenced by respiratory rate and the animal's age.

Tidal breathing flow volume loops (TBFVL) have also been evaluated in spontaneously breathing cats with bronchial disease. The cat breathes through a facemask attached to a pneumotachograph and pulmonary mechanics analyzer. Pressure measured at the pneumotachograph is proportional to flow through the mask, and signals are integrated over time to determine volume at each cycle of respiration. Significant findings in cats with bronchial disease include increased expiratory:inspiratory time, decreased peak expiratory flow rate, and decreased tidal breathing expiratory volume.[15]

Treatment
Acute Therapy

In the cat with cyanosis and open mouth breathing, diagnostic tests are kept to a minimum initially. Stabilization can be achieved by providing an oxygen enriched environment and using parenteral administration of the beta-2 agonist terbutaline at 0.01 mg/kg IV, IM, or SC.[9] Epinephrine, a sympathomimetic agent, is a potent bronchodilator but should be used only when cardiac disease has been excluded since alpha and beta-1 adrenergic stimulation can result in adverse side effects of cardiac arrhythmias, vasoconstriction, and systemic hypertension. Aminophylline is a weak bronchodilator and its use in an emergency situation may not be justified since terbutaline is more likely to be effective.

Respiratory rate and effort are monitored visually in the first hour of observation to determine therapeutic response. If the cat does not respond to terbutaline initially, use of a short-acting corticosteroid often results in rapid alleviation of airway obstruction. However, use of corticosteroids will affect further diagnostic testing by decreasing migration of inflammatory cells into the airway. Failure to respond to terbutaline and corticosteroids indicates that other causes for respiratory distress should be investigated.

Chronic Management

Anti-inflammatories Corticosteroids control airway inflammation by inhibition of phospholipase A, the enzyme responsible for initial metabolism of arachidonic acid into inflammatory agents. Corticosteroids also decrease migration of inflammatory cells into the airway, which decreases the concentration of toxic granulocyte products.

The initial dose and duration of corticosteroid therapy depends on the degree and chronicity of respiratory embarrassment, the severity of pulmonary infiltrates, and the level of inflammation detected on cytology. Initially, prednisolone is administered at 1 mg/kg PO BID for 1 to 2 weeks, and the dosage is decreased to 0.5 mg/kg BID if a good therapeutic response is seen. If the cat remains stable, the dosage can be slowly decreased to once daily and then every other day. Recurrent episodes of coughing or respiratory distress necessitate a return to a higher dosage. Cats are relatively resistant to the side effects of corticosteroids; however, an attempt should be made to achieve the lowest dose of the drug that controls signs. Approximately one half of cats require lifelong medication.

Cats that cannot be orally medicated can be treated with intramuscular injection of a repositol corticosteroid (methyl-prednisolone acetate at 10 to 20 mg IM every 2 to 8 weeks), or use of inhaled steroids (fluticasone 110 µg) can be considered. Metered dose inhalers of steroid preparations can be attached to a spacer chamber and administered to the cat via facemask. Severely affected cats usually require concurrent oral prednisolone in the initial stages of therapy. Eventually some cats can be maintained with one actuation (and 8 to 10 breaths by the cat) twice daily.

Alternative anti-inflammatory drugs might be beneficial in some cats. In an experimental model of feline asthma, cyproheptadine, a serotonin-receptor blocker, attenuated airway smooth muscle in vitro constriction.[10] Serotonin levels have not been measured in naturally occurring feline bronchial disease; however, some cats may benefit from treatment with cyproheptadine at 1 to 2 mg/cat PO BID. Cyclosporine, an inhibitor of T-lymphocyte activation, may attenuate bronchoconstriction and limit airway remodeling in cats with chronic bronchial disease[11]; however, pharmacokinetics are unpredictable and blood levels must be measured weekly until the desired trough level is achieved. Currently there are no indications for use of anti-mediator drugs such as leukotriene antagonists or 5-lipoxygenase inhibitors in the management of feline bronchial disease.[10,12]

Bronchodilators In some cases, bronchodilators may allow a reduction of the dose of steroids required to control clinical signs. Terbutaline can be administered at 0.625 mg PO BID. Inhaled preparations of beta agonists are also available. Theophylline may provide some relief of signs by prevention of acute attacks of bronchoconstriction in predisposed cats or by suppression of inflammation. Sustained-release theophylline can be administered once daily at a dosage of 10 mg/kg PO.

Antibiotics Antibiotics should be prescribed based on culture/sensitivity and cytology results if airway infection contributes to bronchial inflammation and hyperresponsiveness. If *Mycoplasma* spp. infection is suspected, a clinical trial of doxycycline can be prescribed while cultures are pending.

Prevention

Because sympathetic tone is particularly important in achieving bronchodilation in the cat, beta-blockers such as propranolol and atenolol should be avoided if bronchial disease is suspected. Cigarette smoke, dusty litters, aerosol spray, and exposure to upper respiratory viruses may trigger clinical signs in susceptible cats.

Prognosis

Therapy with anti-inflammatories and bronchodilators alleviates acute clinical signs in most cases; however, a significant proportion of cats will suffer a recurrence of signs. Continual medical management should be anticipated for many cats diagnosed with bronchial disease.

PRIMARY CILIARY DYSKINESIA

Clearance of respiratory secretions is dependent on an intact mucociliary elevator. Ciliary ultrastructure is composed of two central microtubules, nine pairs of outer microtubules, dynein arms, and connecting proteins. Primary ciliary dyskinesia (PCD) is an inherited defect in microtubule formation affecting cilia of the respiratory tract, urogenital tract, and auditory canal.[20]

Ciliary dyskinesia can also be an acquired or secondary abnormality caused by chronic respiratory disease in animals with PCD. Clinical signs result from ineffectual movement of cilia and include rhinitis, bronchiectasis, dilatation of renal tubules, infertility, loss of hearing, and hydrocephalus. Kartagener's syndrome is a specific form of PCD characterized by the triad of situs inversus (right to left transposition of thoracic and abdominal organs), chronic rhinitis/sinusitis, and bronchiectasis.

Presentation

PCD is typically diagnosed in young purebred animals. A higher incidence is reported in the bichon frise, but mix-breed dogs and cats can also be affected. Clinical signs can be observed within the first few weeks of life, but mild clinical signs might not be recognized until later in life.[20] Respiratory findings include chronic serous to mucopurulent nasal discharge, productive cough, exercise intolerance, and respiratory distress. Typically signs do not totally resolve with antibiotic treatment or are recurrent in nature. Physical examination is remarkable for nasal discharge, a moist cough, tracheal sensitivity, or adventitious lung sounds.

Diagnostic Evaluation

Standard diagnostic tests reflect the severity of underlying respiratory infection or inflammation. Radiographic findings are variable and include bronchitis, bronchiectasis, and pneumonia. Consolidating lung lesions can develop in chronic cases. Growth of one or more microorganisms is common in dogs with PCD; therefore airway samples should always be cultured for aerobes, anaerobes, and *Mycoplasma* spp. to provide appropriate antibiotic therapy.

Diagnosis of PCD requires documentation of deficient tracheal mucociliary transport and abnormal ciliary structure. Assessment of functional ciliary transport is typically performed first with nuclear scintigraphy. Because *Mycoplasma* spp. infection, acquired ciliary defects, and exposure to cigarette smoke can delay transport, the diagnosis of PCD is confirmed with transmission electron microscopy of nasal or bronchial respiratory epithelium or seminal samples. Normal animals can have structural abnormalities in 2% to 5% of cilia; therefore both the extent and the quality of ultrastructural abnormalities must be examined (Figure 214-4). Typical findings in PCD

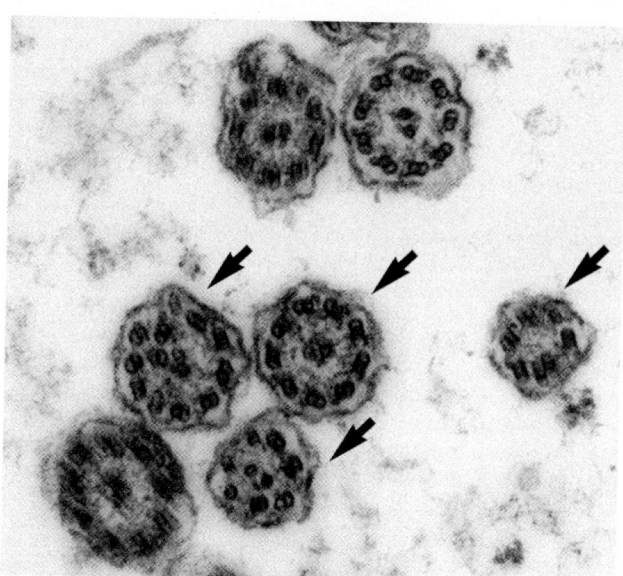

Figure 214-4 Transmission electron micrograph displaying abnormal numbers of microtubules within respiratory cilia (*arrows*).

include shortening or loss of dynein arms, atypical microtubular orientation, and duplication or deletion of central or outer microtubule doublets.[20,21]

Culture techniques can be used to differentiate primary from secondary ciliary abnormalities. In cell culture, airway epithelial cells lose cilia as a monolayer develops. With resuspension and reculture, ciliogenesis occurs. In a patient with secondary ciliary defects, the regenerated cilia are normal, however abnormalities persist in the animal with PCD.[21]

Treatment

The primary goal of therapy is to control infection with appropriate antibiotics and to facilitate clearance of respiratory secretions. Use of cough suppressants is contraindicated in PCD since these drugs can enhance trapping of secretions in the lower airway and potentiate airway inflammation.

Prognosis

Control of respiratory infection is essential to prevent debilitating sequellae in dogs with PCD. Some dogs can achieve excellent quality of life despite defective ciliary transport.

Prevention

PCD is suspected to be inherited as an autosomal recessive trait; therefore clinically normal individuals could produce an offspring with PCD. Close relatives of affected animals should not be included in a breeding program.

BRONCHIAL NARROWING

Larger airways may be compressed by external mass lesions, by an enlarged left atrium, or by loss of cartilaginous support of large intrathoracic airways. Hilar lymphadenopathy due to fungal disease, granulomatous disease, or neoplasia typically causes dorsal compression of the airway at the carina. Left atrial enlargement associated with mitral regurgitation causes dynamic collapse of the left mainstem bronchus and can be a cause of cough in the absence of heart failure. However, the most common cause of airway narrowing appears to be related to failure of the cartilage to maintain the patency of the airways.

Presentation

Bronchial compression or collapse occurs more often in dogs than in cats. This obstructive lesion leads to a chronic, nonproductive cough, respiratory difficulty, or wheezing during inspiration and expiration. An end-expiratory snap may be heard as intrathoracic airways close and open during forced expiration. In dogs with left atrial enlargement and mitral regurgitation, a systolic murmur may be present.

Diagnostic Evaluation

Hilar mass lesions can usually be seen on static thoracic radiographs; however, collapse of the mainstem bronchi or intrathoracic airways often requires fluoroscopic or bronchoscopic examination. Echocardiography assists in the diagnosis of left atrial enlargement.

Treatment

Hilar lymphadenopathy due to active fungal infection usually resolves substantially with antifungal treatment. Rare cases may require steroid therapy or surgical debulking. Collapse of the left mainstem bronchus due to left atrial enlargement may be partially alleviated by therapy directed at reduction of left atrial volume; however, many cases have persistent collapse. Chronic cough associated with deficient cartilaginous support is challenging to control. Cough suppressants are used to alleviate clinical signs when infectious and inflammatory conditions are ruled out.

AIRWAY FOREIGN BODIES

Aspiration of plant material, sticks, toys, teeth, or stones occurs when the laryngeal reflex fails to prevent access of foreign objects into the trachea. Dogs that are involved in strenuous physical activity in rural environments are especially prone to aspiration. Animals with laryngeal paralysis may be more likely to aspirate due to a combination of poor laryngeal sensation and deficient laryngeal reflexes. Animals should be intubated during dental procedures to prevent aspiration of teeth or dental tartar.

Presentation

Bronchial foreign bodies cause an acute or chronic unrelenting cough, airway obstruction, and marked tracheal sensitivity. Within a variable period of time, consolidating pneumonia develops. A bronchial foreign body should be suspected when an animal has a recurrent cough that partially responds to antibiotic therapy, or when an animal has recurrent airway infection, particularly if anaerobic bacteria are involved.

Diagnostic Evaluation

Thoracic radiography will identify a radiodense foreign object; however, foreign bodies of plant origin are not always visible. Distal atelectasis or consolidation of a lung segment can be suggestive of foreign body obstruction, although a mass lesion, mucus plug, or pneumonic condition would appear similarly. Infection secondary to a foreign body can result in diffuse interstitial or alveolar infiltrates. A pulmonary abscess may be identifiable as a discrete fluid-filled cavity encased by fibrous tissue.

Definitive diagnosis can often be made by bronchoscopic evaluation of the airways. All airway segments must be evaluated in the search for foreign bodies, and objects can often be removed if there is an edge that can be grasped by biopsy or rat tooth forceps. Stones are a challenge to remove bronchoscopically, especially when they are wedged in a bronchus. In chronic cases of plant aspiration, the foreign body is often obscured by purulent exudate, and gentle lavage and suction of the area is required to identify foreign material.

Airway samples are cultured for both aerobes and anaerobes given the high likelihood of bacterial contamination. Animals should be followed closely after removal of the foreign body since bronchiectasis may develop distal to the obstruction.

Treatment

Animals with bronchial foreign bodies are at risk for pulmonary abscess, bronchoesophageal fistula, empyema, and bronchiectasis distal to the obstruction. Lung lobectomy is often required for unretrievable foreign bodies, or when lung abscessation, bronchiectasis, or fistulation has occurred. Pleural infection requires thoracic drainage and usually thoracotomy. Long-term antibiotic therapy is based on culture and sensitivity results.

BRONCHOESOPHAGEAL FISTULA

Bronchoesophageal fistula may be congenital, or acquired due to trauma, a penetrating esophageal foreign body, or a bronchial foreign body. Affected animals present with chronic cough and recurrent pneumonia related to aspiration of esophageal contents. In some cases, difficulty eating may be the predominant sign. Respiratory signs may be relatively mild, resulting in a marked delay in the diagnosis of a congenital lesion. The diagnosis should be suspected in a young animal with recurrent aspiration pneumonia or a focal, recurrent lung density. The diagnosis is confirmed by a contrast esophagram. Endoscopic examination via the airway or esophagus can occasionally detect a fistula. Surgical resection of the abnormal connection is required, and lung lobectomy is sometimes necessary due to adhesion formation or abscessation.

BRONCHIAL MINERALIZATION

Bronchial mineralization can occur secondary to any chronic inflammatory or infectious condition and is seen with bronchitis and bronchiectasis. Prominent mineralization of airways has also been reported in hyperadrenocorticism. The contribution of bronchial mineralization to respiratory dysfunction is unclear.

BRONCHIAL NEOPLASIA

Animals with bronchial neoplasia can present with cough, an obstructive breathing pattern, or panting. Respirations are typically loud, and harsh wheezing noises are heard over large airways compressed or occluded by mass lesions. Diagnosis and treatment is described under pulmonary neoplasia (see Chapter 127).

CHAPTER • 215

Pulmonary Parenchymal Disease

O. Lynne Nelson
Rance K. Sellon

OVERVIEW OF DIAGNOSTIC CONSIDERATIONS

Dogs and cats are susceptible to a wide variety of inflammatory and noninflammatory diseases of the pulmonary parenchyma. Animals with parenchymal disease may exhibit clinical signs typical of lower respiratory tract disease such as cough and respiratory difficulty, or show no clinical signs despite sometimes extensive pulmonary disease.

When clinical information is suggestive of pulmonary parenchymal disease, a relatively finite number of diagnostic tests become available to the clinician. Thoracic radiography will be the key diagnostic tool in the majority of cases. Collection of respiratory samples by wash techniques, needle aspiration, or biopsy will be appropriate in many cases. Ancillary diagnostic tests that are often employed in patients with respiratory disease include CBC, biochemical profile and urinalysis, fecal examinations, serologic assays, and microbial culture and sensitivity. The diagnostic approach to a given patient will be influenced by the list of likely differentials, costs associated with diagnostic tests, and the patient's status. Many patients will require initial empiric therapy and supportive measures (e.g., oxygen supplementation) for alleviation of respiratory distress and stabilization before proceeding with focused diagnostic tests. A more comprehensive discussion of the diagnostic tools used in the evaluation of the patient with respiratory disease is presented in Chapter 212.

An important diagnostic tool that is underused in small animal practice is blood gas analysis. The availability of portable bedside analyzers makes blood gas measurements accessible to most small animal practitioners. Blood gas analysis provides important information regarding two important functions of the respiratory system, alveolar ventilation and oxygenation of pulmonary arterial blood. Blood gas analysis is the only means to properly assess alveolar ventilation: the capacity of a patient to properly ventilate cannot be assessed by evaluation of respiratory rate or pattern or by thoracic radiographic abnormalities. Although many parenchymal diseases are associated with hyperventilation, some can be associated with hypoventilation, particularly as respiratory fatigue develops. Knowledge of the adequacy of alveolar ventilation has important treatment ramifications. Hypoventilating animals become candidates for ventilatory support depending on the cause of the hypoventilation. Untreated, severe hypoventilation can cause respiratory acidosis, which is associated with cardiac arrhythmias and central nervous system depression.

Blood gas analysis can also help the clinician determine the mechanism that drives the development of arterial hypoxemia. The most common mechanisms that cause arterial hypoxemia in small animal practice are hypoventilation, revealed by increased P_aCO_2, and ventilation-perfusion (V/Q) mismatches. Other mechanisms, such as right-to-left shunts, and diffusion barriers, are less common. Calculation of A-a differences can reveal underlying impairments in oxygenation coexisting with hypoventilation. Hypoxemia caused by V/Q mismatches or diffusion barriers are somewhat responsive to oxygen; hypoxemia caused by right to left shunting is poorly responsive to oxygen. A more complete discussion of blood gas interpretation is presented in Chapter 212.

There are many indications for oxygen supplementation. Animals with parenchymal or other diseases associated with arterial hypoxemia through any of the mechanisms noted above, or patients with diseases that alter hemoglobin affinity for oxygen (e.g., carbon monoxide poisoning) are candidates for oxygen supplementation. Animals with clinical signs consistent with hypoxemia or tissue hypoxia, such as cyanosis, tachypnea, dyspnea, or central nervous system dysfunction are also potential candidates for oxygen supplementation. Interested readers are referred elsewhere for a more comprehensive review of the indications for oxygen supplementation.[1]

Oxygen may be administered to conscious patients via face masks, nasal oxygen catheters, intratracheal catheters, oxygen cages, or flow-by techniques.[1] The method of delivery selected will reflect availability, patient status, and patient tolerance. Increases in inspired oxygen concentration of 40% or greater can be achieved with these methods depending on flow rates. The risk of oxygen toxicity exists for patients supplemented with inspired oxygen concentrations of 50% for more than 24 hours, or 100% for more than 12 hours. If the patient's PaO_2 cannot be maintained at acceptable levels, generally 60 mm Hg or higher, on inspired oxygen concentrations less than 50% to 100%, ventilatory support may be needed. Humidification of oxygen is advised if oxygen is to be administered for more than a few hours to reduce complications associated with airway drying. Responses to oxygen supplementation can be made subjectively (changes in patient comfort, level of respiratory distress) or more objectively by repeat measurement of PaO_2 or oxygen saturation by pulse oximetry. The reader should be aware that patients monitored by pulse oximetry may still have clinically important hypoventilation and hypercarbia not detected by pulse oximetry when such patients are receiving supplemental oxygen.

As noted, ventilatory support may be needed in some patients with parenchymal disease. Hypoventilation not readily corrected, as might occur with respiratory paralysis or fatigue, CNS disease, or others, is one indication for ventilatory support. Hypoxemia refractory to supplemental oxygen administration is another. There are many different strategies for providing ventilation, which have been reviewed elsewhere.[2] Short-term ventilatory support can be provided in most practices by use of an ambu bag or the reservoir bag on an anesthetic machine.

PULMONARY EDEMA

Fluid accumulation in the interstitium and alveoli of the lung is termed *pulmonary edema*. The causes of pulmonary edema are typically divided into four major mechanisms: (1) increased vascular hydrostatic pressure, (2) decreased plasma oncotic pressure, (3) increased vascular permeability, and (4) impaired lymphatic drainage. Occasionally, a fifth miscellaneous or idiopathic category is described if edema develops without any apparent association with the other four mechanisms. When increased pulmonary venous hydrostatic pressure and left-sided congestive heart failure (CHF) are responsible for edema, the term *cardiogenic pulmonary edema* is often used. *Noncardiogenic edema* describes edema from other, non-CHF causes induced by any of the additional mechanisms listed.

The pulmonary parenchyma is somewhat resistant to the development of edema. In general, the hydrostatic pressure in the pulmonary vascular bed is relatively low compared with vascular beds in other regions of the body. Normal pulmonary wedge pressures (an estimate of capillary hydrostatic pressure) are approximately 5 mm Hg. In addition, pulmonary lymphatic drainage is relatively high due to the continual pumping action of the lungs by respiration. The capacitance of the pulmonary lymphatic system is large, and the lymphatic volume can greatly expand to further increase the removal of fluid if necessary. Alveolar surfactant surface tension helps protect against the development of pulmonary edema by decreasing the tendency for fluid to be drawn into the alveoli. Because of these protective mechanisms, acute increases in pulmonary capillary hydrostatic pressures must exceed 20 mm Hg before edema develops.[3, 4] With more slowly developing increases in hydrostatic pressure, pressures in excess of 40 mm Hg have been documented without pulmonary edema.[4,5] In these instances, time allows for stretch and greater capacitance of the pulmonary vessels, as well as an increase in lymphatic drainage to remove interstitial fluid. When fluid translocates into the interstitial space and lymphatic drainage cannot match the rate of fluid influx, interstitial edema occurs. If the pathophysiologic process driving the movement of fluid continues, the capacitance of the interstitial space is eventually overwhelmed and fluid accumulates in the alveoli. Gas exchange is impaired when airways become "flooded." Atelectasis, decreased lung compliance and airway compression, consequences of pulmonary edema, all increase pulmonary vascular resistance. The combination of impaired gas exchange and increased vascular resistance create ventilation-perfusion mismatches, which results in hypoxemia.

Left-sided CHF is the most common cause of pulmonary edema due to increased hydrostatic pressure (see Chapter 197). However, edema due to excessive fluid administration is not unusual, particularly in the setting of impaired fluid excretion as might be seen with oliguric or anuric renal failure. Pulmonary edema due to decreased plasma oncotic pressure is caused by hypoalbuminemia. Causes of hypoalbuminemia are listed on

the inside cover of this book. Pleural effusions (transudative) are more common than pulmonary edema in patients with reduced oncotic pressure as a single driving mechanism. Pulmonary edema formation is not expected from hypoalbuminemia unless serum albumin concentrations are less than 1 g/dL. Even then, subcutaneous edema, pleural effusion or other sites of edema formation typically occur prior to pulmonary edema. Pulmonary edema may be seen in patients with higher serum albumin concentrations if there is vasculitis, or if hydrostatic pressures increase because of impaired ventricular filling or excessive administration of IV fluids.

Pulmonary edema due to increased vascular permeability can occur with a wide variety of pulmonary and systemic disorders. The edema in this case is termed *noncardiogenic* and is usually relatively proteinaceous.[6,7] Capillary wedge pressures are normal. Any septic or nonseptic inflammatory condition or any cause of vasculitis may promote vascular damage and leakage. Other diseases associated with noncardiogenic edema are acute respiratory distress syndrome (ARDS, see later discussion), acute upper airway obstruction, electric shock, neurogenic edema (often secondary to seizures or head trauma), and hepatic disease.[6,8] Although the pulmonary edema that develops in association with many of these conditions is suspected to result from increased capillary permeability, the exact mechanisms driving the formation of edema are for the most part unknown. Primary pulmonary lymphatic obstruction is an uncommon cause of pulmonary edema and when it occurs, is typically the result of a neoplastic process or lymphangitis.

Presentation

Most patients will present with tachypnea and cough, or respiratory distress and hypoxia if alveolar involvement is severe. Symptoms are directly related to the cause and severity of the edema. The character of respiration is usually that of increased effort noted during inspiration and expiration due to increased lung stiffness. Severe edema may cause coughing with expectoration of blood-tinged fluid. Several abnormalities may be heard during thoracic auscultation, classically in the dorsocaudal lung fields. Crackles heard on inspiration and especially end-expiration are common; however, crackles may be absent in early or mild edema. Lungs sounds may seem exceptionally quiet with very severe edema, particularly in cats. Additional changes reflecting underlying disease processes may be noted. Abnormalities of cardiac auscultation (murmurs, transient sounds, arrhythmias) may indicate the presence of heart disease, but their presence does not always indicate an etiology of cardiogenic edema. A patient with a heart murmur and coarse crackles during inspiration without sinus tachycardia should be carefully evaluated for pulmonary diseases other than cardiogenic pulmonary edema. Patients with CHF-induced pulmonary edema would be expected to have tachycardia as a result of increased sympathetic tone. Some patients with congestive heart failure will lack abnormal heart sounds, for example those with certain forms of cardiomyopathy.

Diagnostic Evaluation

Thoracic radiographs, combined with historical and physical findings, are often diagnostic. Cardiogenic edema is characterized radiographically by "fluffy" interstitial opacities that can rapidly progress to an alveolar pattern. In the dog, the opacities are most often distributed in the hilar and caudodorsal perivascular lung regions (see Figure 215-1). In the cat, these opacities are patchy and may be diffuse or focal. Pulmonary venous enlargement suggests pulmonary venous and left atrial hypertension consistent with left-sided CHF. Enlargement of the cardiac silhouette, particularly left chambers, is commonly present in patients with cardiogenic edema. Pulmonary edema caused by increased vascular permeability is also typically most severe in the caudodorsal lung lobes.[7] The absence of cardiac

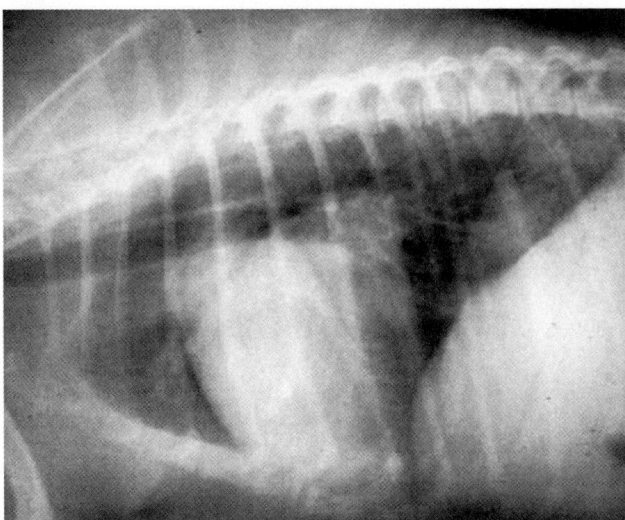

A

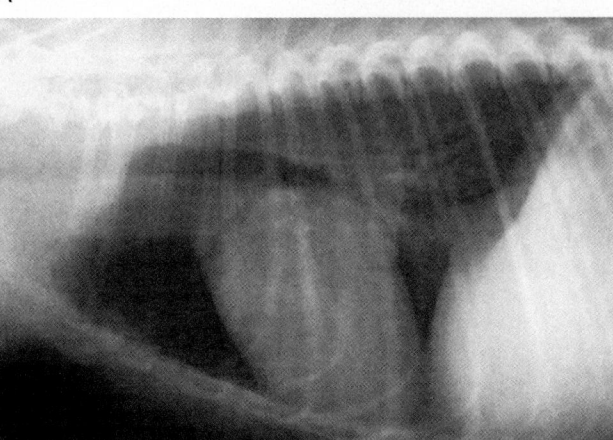

B

Figure 215-1 Lateral thoracic radiographs of a dog with cardiogenic pulmonary edema before and after treatment. Note the left atrial and ventricular enlargement and the engorged pulmonary veins, especially left cranial lobar vein. **(A)** There is an interstitial and alveolar pattern present in the pretreatment radiograph not evident in the post-treatment film **(B)**.

and pulmonary venous changes can, in most cases, distinguish such patients from those with cardiogenic edema. History and laboratory parameters are helpful in identifying underlying causes of noncardiogenic edema such as electrocution, sepsis, pancreatitis, and others. In many cases of noncardiogenic pulmonary edema, the edema is mild and not a part of the primary clinical complaint. Pulmonary edema resulting from decreased plasma oncotic pressure is typically characterized by generalized interstitial or mixed interstitial-alveolar pattern. Pleural effusion may also be present and vascular congestion is absent.

Arterial blood gas analysis typically documents hypoxemia, hypocapnia, and widened A-a gradient. Results of a CBC, serum biochemistries, and urinalysis may be helpful to determine underlying causes, particularly in noncardiogenic edema. Lung specimens obtained by respiratory washes or biopsy often do not yield a specific diagnosis unless primary pulmonary pathology is demonstrated.

Treatment

The primary therapeutic goal in the management of patients with pulmonary edema is improvement of oxygenation while stress is minimized. Minimizing stress is particularly important in severely distressed animals for which simple manipulations may lead to overt cardiopulmonary arrest. Oxygen may be administered through nasal cannula, face mask, or oxygen cage. Compromised patients may be best treated empirically based upon their initial clinical signs and presumptive diagnosis until deemed stable for additional tests, such as thoracic radiographs. Sedatives can be valuable to relieve anxiety and decrease unnecessary oxygen consumption. Morphine sulfate can be administered IV at a dosage of 0.1 to 1 mg/kg in dogs but is not suggested for use in cats. In addition to sedative benefits, mobilization of pulmonary edema has been attributed to morphine administration. Alternatively, acepromazine can be used in cats and dogs at 0.03 to 1.0 mg/kg IV, IM, or SQ. In critical cases, intubation and positive pressure ventilation may be necessary.

Narcotics and tranquilizers are likely to depress the respiratory center while severe hypoxia initiates significant anxiety. As with many medical states, an appropriate balance is sought.

Diuretic therapy is particularly effective for acute relief of pulmonary edema that develops from volume overload disorders such as CHF. Furosemide, 2 to 4 mg/kg IV every 4 to 12 hours, can be given for clinical pulmonary edema. Diuretics may be less beneficial for edema that develops secondary to increased vascular permeability disorders such as ARDS, and caution is advised when administering diuretics to patients with pre-existing hypovolemia.[9]

Bronchodilators such as the methylxanthines, aminophylline and theophylline may be beneficial to combat bronchospasm, enhance mucociliary function, and diminish diaphragmatic fatigue. Specific therapies should be also be directed at any underlying etiology such as hypoproteinemia (see Chapter 199) or cardiac disease.

Prognosis

Pulmonary function and cardiac disease, if present, are monitored often. Thoracic radiographs should be re-evaluated every 24 to 48 hours; the clinician should remember that radiographic changes often lag behind clinical response. The prognosis with treatment of pulmonary edema is variable and depends on the severity of edema and respiratory dysfunction, the nature of any underlying disorders, and aggressiveness of monitoring and therapy.

PULMONARY NEOPLASIA

Primary Pulmonary Neoplasia

Primary pulmonary tumors are not considered as common in dogs and cats as are metastatic tumors. Pulmonary neoplasia can be seen in animals of almost any age, although the majority of patients are middle-aged to older reflecting the general increase in prevalence of tumors in the pet population as it ages.

Primary lung neoplasia accounts for approximately 1% of all tumors in dogs, and fewer in cats.[10] Most primary tumors of the lung are carcinomas that arise from bronchial or alveolar epithelium, but occasionally squamous cell carcinomas can be seen.[10,11] Other less common primary lung tumors include osteosarcomas or other mesenchymal tumors.

Presentation

The clinical presentation of patients with lung tumors can be variable and may or may not reflect signs referable to the respiratory system. Chronic cough that is unresponsive to antibiotics is seen most often in dogs. Exercise intolerance, tachypnea, or overt respiratory distress can occur. Respiratory distress can result from involvement of the pleural space with development of hemothorax, pneumothorax, or pleural effusion, intraluminal obstruction or extraluminal airway compression, or pulmonary artery obstructions (inflammatory or tumor thrombus) causing ventilation-perfusion mismatches.[13] Cats with primary lung tumors may exhibit lethargy, anorexia, weight loss, dyspnea and tachypnea, wheezes, and non-productive cough. A large proportion of cats with primary pulmonary neoplasia in one study had no clinical signs referable to the presence of the lung tumor.[11] Patients with primary pulmonary neoplasia can exhibit hemoptysis.[13]

Although primary respiratory signs are expected in most patients with primary pulmonary tumors, some will have clinical signs that reflect metastasis of the lung tumor to extrathoracic organs, such as musculoskeletal structures, including the digits, abdominal organs, or brain. Clinical signs that develop from metastasis of lung tumors to other organs can thus include lameness, abdominal effusion, neurologic abnormalities, or others. Paraneoplastic syndromes that develop in conjunction with either primary or metastatic lung tumors may also be responsible for the development of clinical signs, such as lameness observed in animals with hypertrophic osteopathy (Figure 215-2).

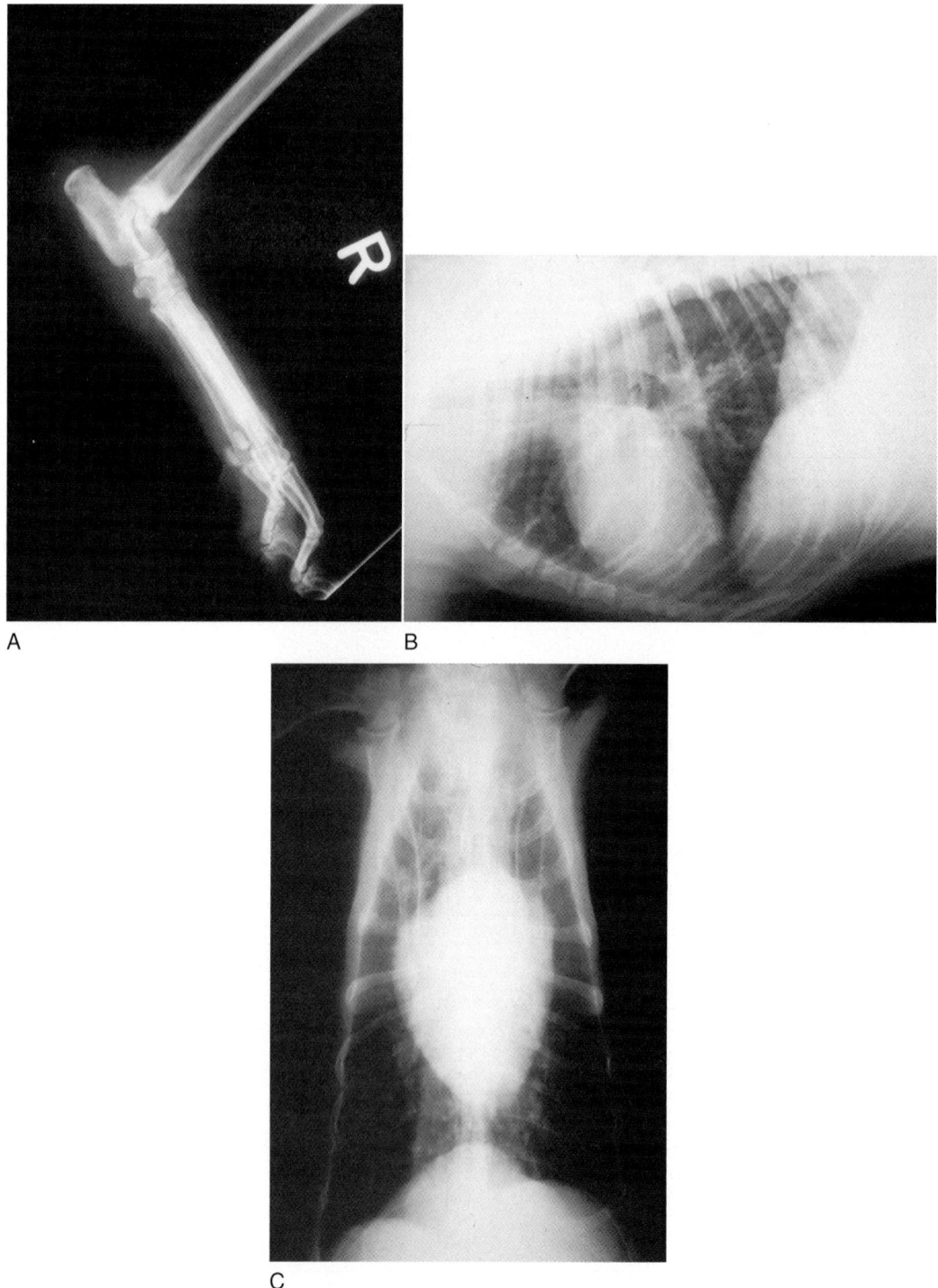

Figure 215-2   Hypertropic osteopathy in a dog with pulmonary metastatic disease. Note the extensive periosteal proliferation along the metatarsal bones.

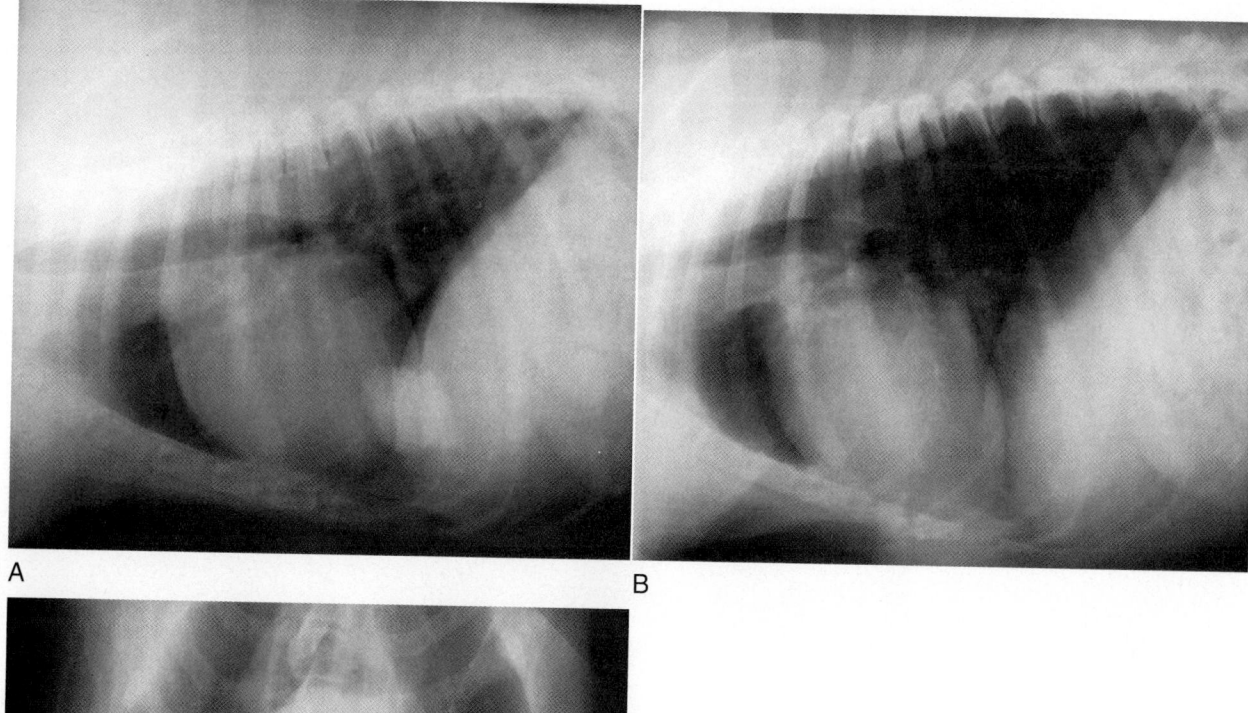

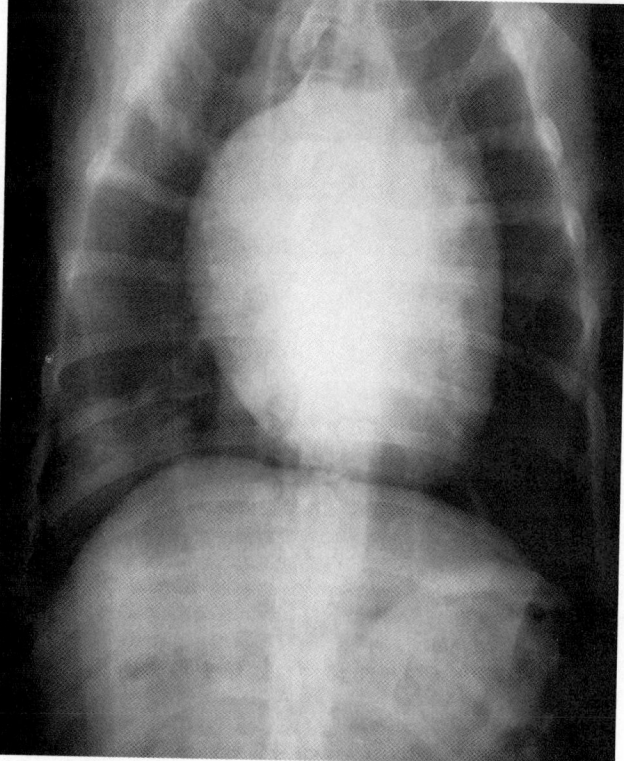

Figure 215-3 Right (**A**) and left (**B**) lateral and ventrodorsal (**C**) thoracic radiographs of a dog with a solitary lung mass best seen in only one radiographic projection.

RESPIRATORY DISEASE

Diagnostic Evaluation

Thoracic radiographs are a key tool in the diagnostic approach to patients with pulmonary neoplasia. The radiographic appearance of primary pulmonary neoplasia varies. Abnormalities observed on thoracic radiographs can range from discrete nodules of varying size and number, to ill-defined interstitial patterns, to consolidated single lung lobes. Radiographic patterns can be focal or diffuse depending on the nature of the neoplasm and whether there has been pulmonary metastasis. Enlargement of hilar lymph nodes may also be seen.

When evaluating animals radiographically for which pulmonary neoplasia or other primary pulmonary disease is suspected, it may be useful to obtain three views of the thorax, right and left laterals, and either a ventrodorsal or dorsoventral image. Three radiographic views maximize the opportunities to see lesions that might be obscured by the heart, or if in caudal lung fields, the liver (Figure 215-3). Computed tomography (CT), available at many referral centers, can provide an extra degree of sensitivity in the characterization and localization of lung lesions, including small metastatic lesions (Figure 215-4).[14-16] The size of lesions detectable with CT is influenced by several factors, including the distance between slices, amount of overlap between slices, and the location of the lesion within the parenchyma, but detection of nodules less than 5 mm in size is possible. As with other imaging modalities, false positive and false negative results are encountered with CT. CT is more expensive as compared to plain thoracic radiographs,

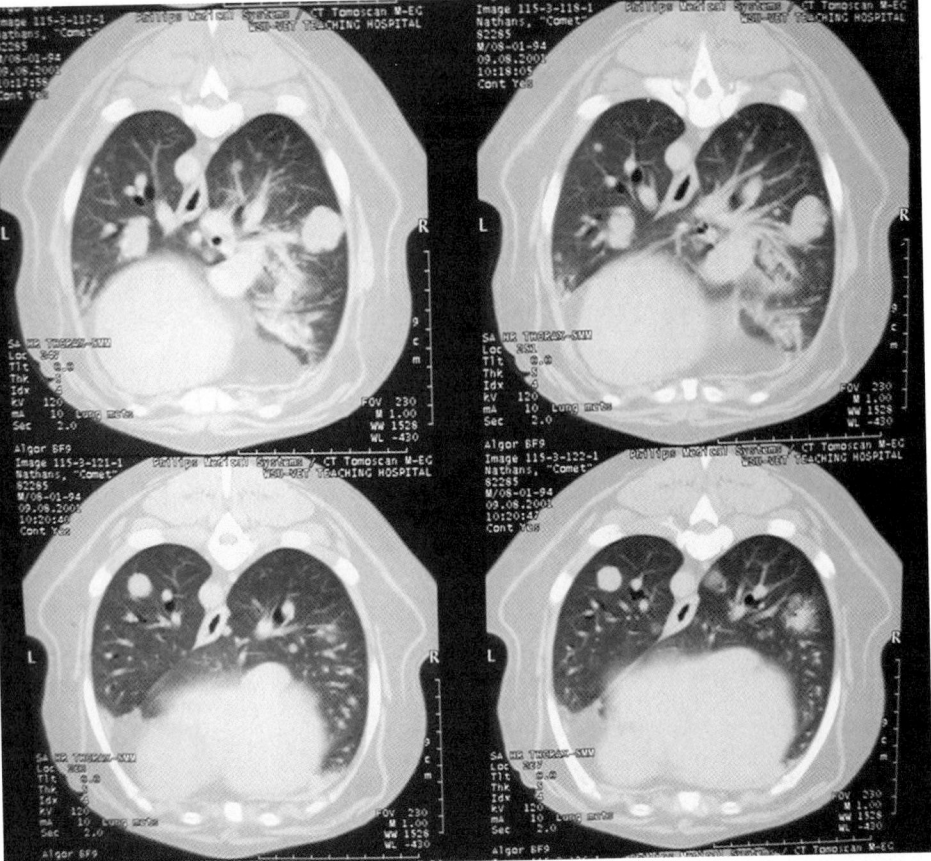

Figure 215-4 Computed tomographic scan of the thorax of a dog with pulmonary metastasis. Note the presence of numerous small densities in the lung periphery.

and general anesthesia is usually required for diagnostic CT images, which may be of concern in patients with respiratory embarrassment.

Thoracic radiographs cannot provide cytologic or histologic diagnoses, so the definitive diagnosis of primary pulmonary neoplasia hinges upon demonstration of neoplastic cells either cytologically or histopathologically. The location of lesions observed radiographically can be helpful in guiding the clinician toward appropriate sampling techniques. Some masses, particularly large masses adjacent to the thoracic wall, will be amenable to blind fine needle aspiration using anatomic landmarks observed on radiographs to guide needle placement (Figure 215-5). Smaller masses adjacent to the thoracic wall may be aspirated with ultrasound guidance; the more aerated lung around the mass, the less amenable to ultrasound-guided aspiration it will be. Techniques available at some referral centers for nonsurgical sampling of pulmonary masses include fluoroscopic and CT-guided aspiration (Figure 215-6). Respiratory wash techniques may be considered, but may have poor sensitivity for focal lesions. Bronchoscopy could be valuable to obtain brush cytology or biopsies of lesions extending into the bronchial lumen. Surgical approaches such as thoracotomy or thoracosopy can be both diagnostic and therapeutic.

The decision as to which diagnostic approach will be taken to define the origins of a pulmonary mass will be influenced by the features of the mass and by the client's willingness to tolerate expense, risk of complications, and the status of the patient. Transthoracic needle aspiration and tracheal wash are comparatively inexpensive and widely accessible because minimal equipment is needed to perform these techniques. The most common complication associated with transthoracic

aspiration is pneumothorax (see Chapter 103), so the clinician should be prepared to manage the complications of needle aspiration. A key point to be considered when attempting to establish the etiology of a pulmonary mass is that false negative, or even misleading, results with any of the techniques are common. It is possible for samples collected from pulmonary neoplasms to appear as inflammatory or even infectious processes on aspiration cytology or bronchoalveolar lavage.[17] Thus a negative result does not at all exclude neoplasia or other diseases that cause pulmonary masses. A patient may be subjected to various nonsurgical attempts at a diagnosis and still in the end need a thoracotomy or thoracoscopy to establish a definitive diagnosis.[17]

Treatment and Prognosis

The treatment for primary pulmonary neoplasia is surgical resection. Patients with small focal lesions can have a good prognosis. The prognosis for dogs is considered better in those patients that have solitary, well-differentiated lesions less then 5 cm in diameter, no metastasis to regional lymph nodes, and no malignant pleural effusion.[10] Cats have been considered in general to have a poorer prognosis in the face of primary lung tumors, with the degree of differentiation of tumors being more predictive of survival.[18] Patients with adenocarcinomas are also considered to have a better prognosis than those with squamous cell carcinomas. Because the prognosis of patients with primary lung tumors is difficult to establish without histologic information (tumor type and degree of differentiation, hilar lymph node metastasis), surgical resection can be advocated early in the course of the diagnostic process as lung lobectomy will be diagnostic, provide prognostic information, and will be the first step in providing definitive therapy.

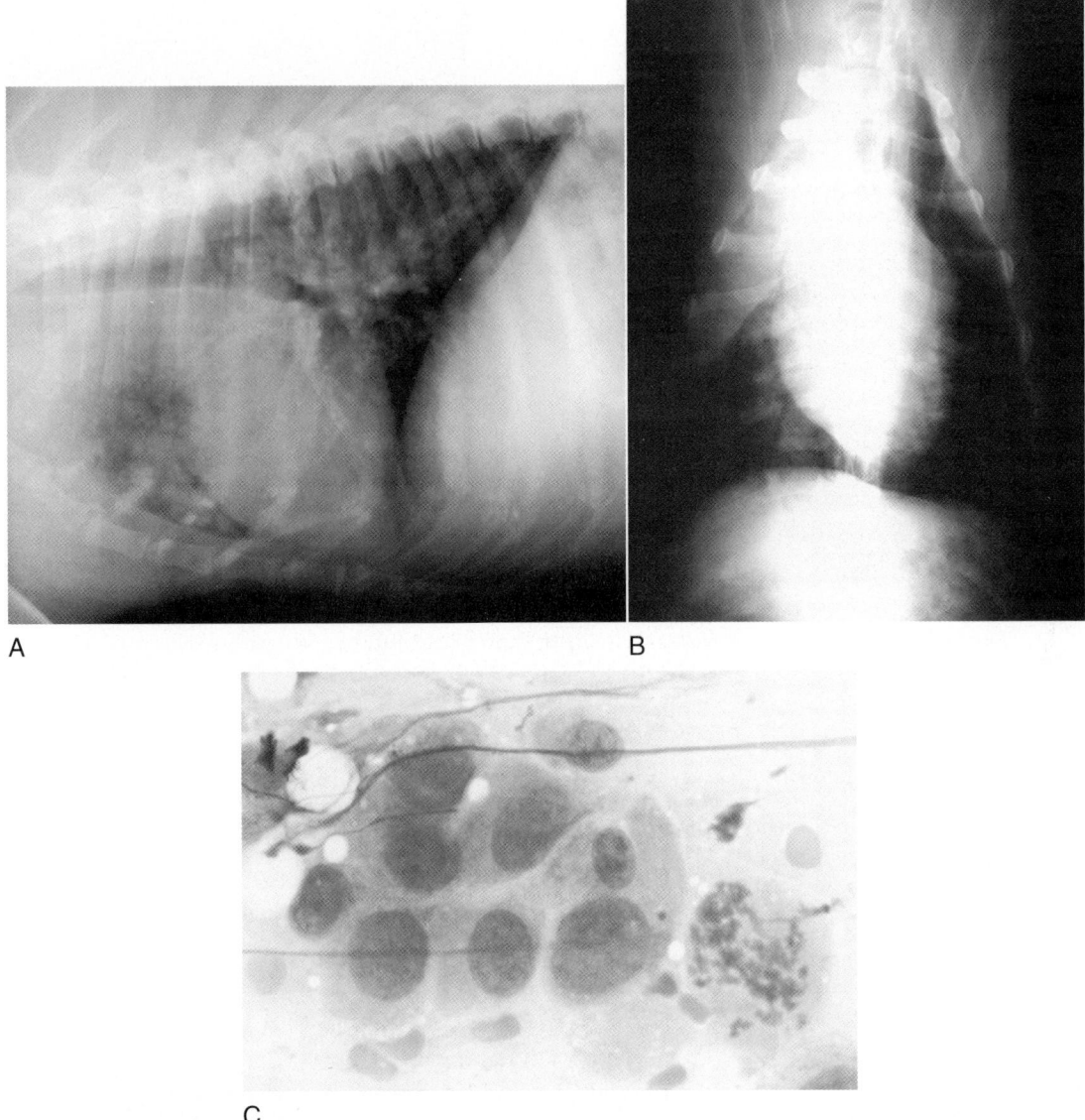

Figure 215-5 **A** and **B,** Thoracic radiographs (lateral, ventrodorsal) from a dog with primary pulmonary neoplasia. The affected lung lobe was sampled by ultrasound-guided needle aspiration. **C,** Photomicrograph of the carcinoma cells obtained by needle aspiration of the lung mass.

Metastatic Lung Disease

The respiratory system, owing to the key anatomic location of the pulmonary capillary bed, is a frequent site for the development of metastatic tumors of both carcinoma and sarcoma origin. Metastatic pulmonary neoplasia is the most common pulmonary neoplasia in dogs and cats. Although virtually any tumor can metastasize to the lungs, tumors with a high predilection for pulmonary metastasis include canine osteosarcomas, mammary carcinomas in dogs and cats, and oral and nail bed melanomas in dogs.

Presentation

Clinical signs observed in patients with pulmonary metastatic disease are widely variable and usually reflect the presence of the primary tumor. Clinical signs referable to the lower respiratory tract such as cough or exercise intolerance are frequently absent even in the face of large metastatic burdens (Figure 215-7). It is not unusual in the authors' experience to see patients with histories of lethargy, anorexia, weight loss, and unremarkable physical examinations that have radiographic lesions consistent with pulmonary metastatic disease. Because of the frequency with which vague clinical signs can be observed in dogs and cats with neoplasia that is not detectable by physical examination, a three-view thoracic radiograph is a recommended component of the initial diagnostic plan for such patients.

Diagnostic Evaluation

The diagnosis of metastatic neoplasia is often presumptive based on compatible thoracic radiographic abnormalities in a patient with a history of a histologically confirmed malignancy. Radiographically, pulmonary metastasis can be surprisingly variable in appearance and can run the gamut from multiple, well-defined interstitial nodules, to ill-defined interstitial patterns to alveolar patterns.[19] Many of these patients will not have diagnostic tests performed to confirm that observed lesions are metastatic lesions.

However, the clinician has to be careful in assuming that observed radiographic lesions are neoplastic lesions, particularly in the patient that has not had a primary tumor identified.

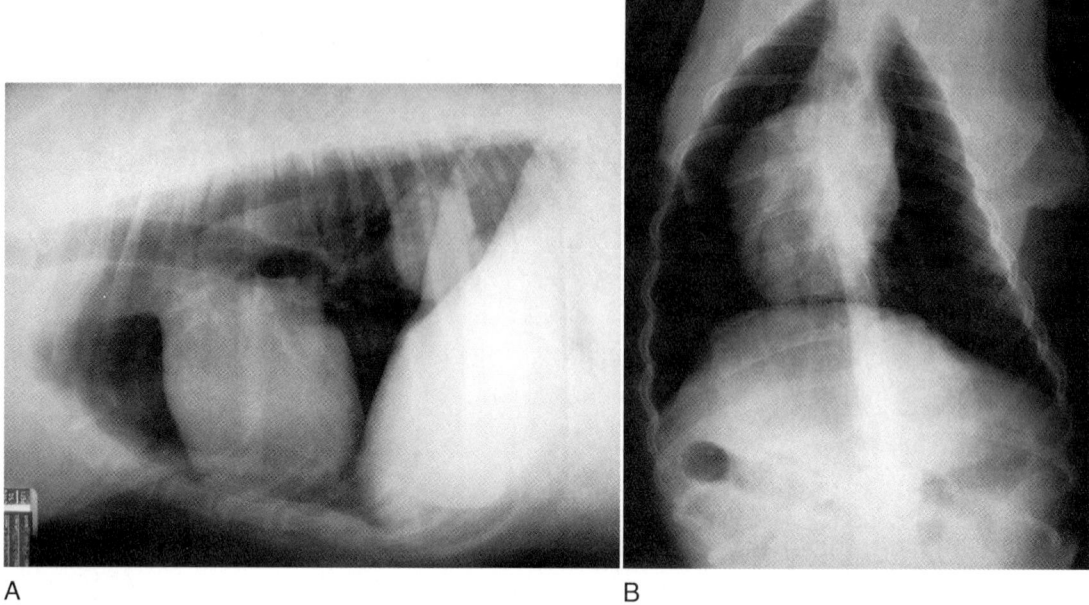

A   B

Figure 215-6 Thoracic radiographs (lateral [A], ventrodorsal [B]) of a dog with a solitary lung mass deep in the thoracic cavity. This mass was successfully aspirated with fluoroscopic guidance.

Pitfalls in such thinking include the fact that other diseases, such as the systemic fungal infections, occasional bacterial and mycobacterial infections, or hypersensitivity disorders (e.g., eosinophilic granuloma) can mimic the clinical disease and radiographic appearance of metastatic pulmonary disease. In addition, patients with one malignancy can develop other tumors that have no relationship to previously diagnosed tumors, and for which diagnostic and therapeutic intervention would be of benefit. Definitive diagnosis of metastasis can be made using the techniques described above in the diagnostic approach to primary lung tumors.

Treatment of metastatic lung disease is often unrewarding but could be of short-term benefit in patients that exhibit clinical signs referable to their pulmonary lesions. The decision to treat obviously will be weighed against other factors, such as rapidity of disease progression, quality of life concerns, owner wishes, and owner willingness to tolerate expense and

complications of treatment. Treatment of metastatic lesions could require surgical resection, best for few lesions, or chemotherapy if not already administered for the patient's primary tumor. Recently, some positive responses have been observed in dogs with metastatic pulmonary disease treated with chemotherapeutic agents or interleukin-2 via inhalation.[20,21] Such an approach offers the potential of treating pulmonary metastatic disease with fewer adverse effects as can occur with systemic administration of such agents.

Lymphosarcoma

The respiratory tract is frequently affected in dogs with lymphosarcoma, although not all dogs will have clinical signs of respiratory disease. Radiographically, lymphosarcoma can assume a variety of radiographic patters from interstitial to alveolar to mixed patterns (Figure 215-8). The diagnosis of lymphosarcoma is usually made based on assessment of other organs, but the similarities of the radiographic abnormalities to other pulmonary diseases should prompt consideration of other differentials for the respiratory component. Diagnosis of pulmonary lymphosarcoma is often readily accomplished from examination of respiratory wash specimens or needle aspiration. Treatment of lymphosarcoma is addressed in Chapter 181.

Lymphomatoid Granulomatosis

Lymphomatoid granulomatosis is characterized by infiltration around, and invasion of, pulmonary blood vessels with pleomorphic lymphoreticular and plasmacytoid cells. Eosinophils, neutrophils, and small lymphocytes are also present.[22,23] Lymphomatoid granulomatosis was once considered an immune-mediated vasculitis, but evidence in people and dogs now supports the classification of this disease as a low-grade lymphoma (see Chapter 181).[24,25] Thrombosis, necrosis, and granuloma formation are common. Intrathoracic lymph nodes are also involved.

Presentation

This disease has only been described in people and dogs. There is no obvious age or breed predilection.[23] Patients usually present with respiratory signs such as cough, tachypnea, or

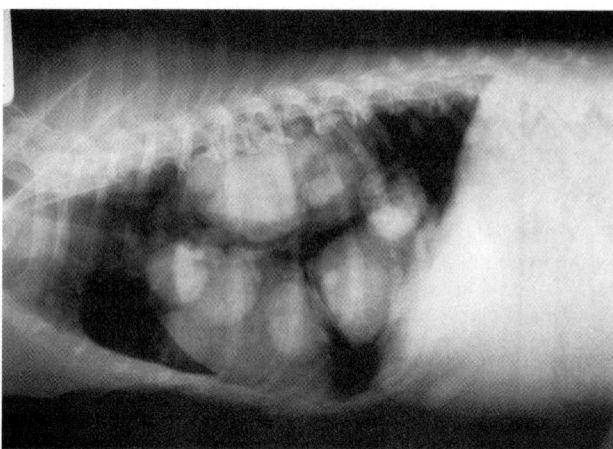

Figure 215-7 Lateral thoracic radiograph of a dog with extensive pulmonary metastasis. This dog exhibited no clinical signs of respiratory disease. (Courtesy Dan Brown, Moscow, ID.)

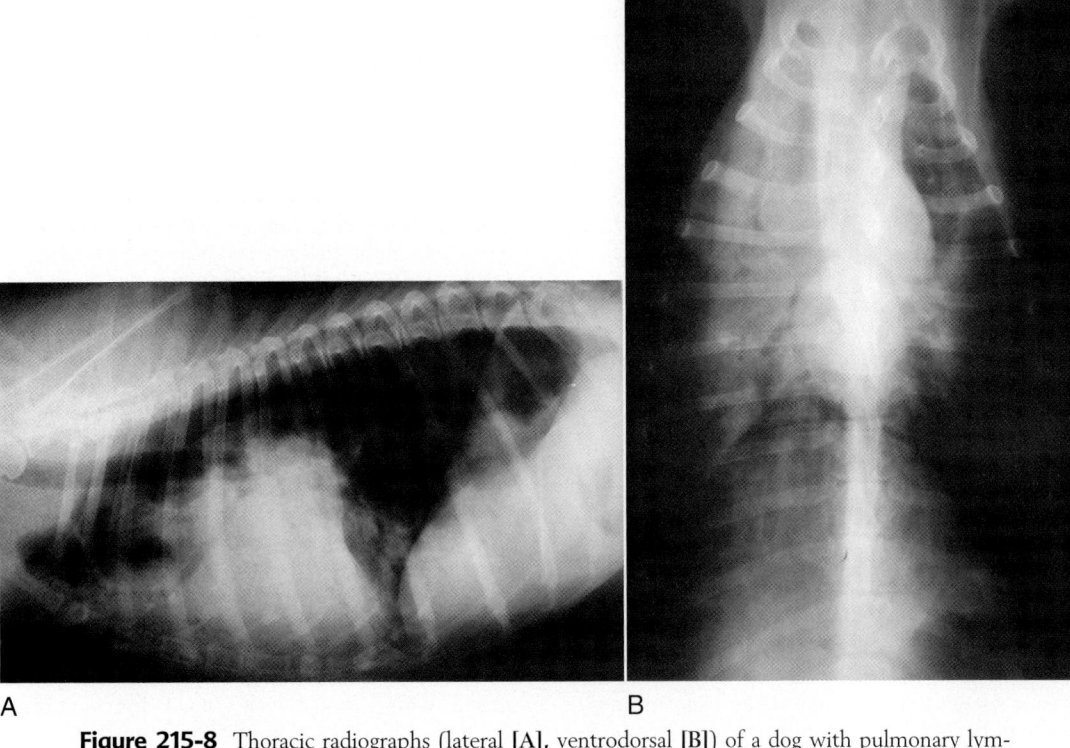

A   B

Figure 215-8 Thoracic radiographs (lateral [A], ventrodorsal [B]) of a dog with pulmonary lymphosarcoma. On the lateral view there is a marked alveolar (air bronchogram in cranial lung lobe) and interstitial pattern. On the ventrodorsal projection, note the near consolidation of the right cranial lung lobe and enlarged hilar lymph node that is compressing the mainstem bronchus to the right caudal lung lobe.

respiratory distress, although fever, anorexia, or weight loss may also be noted. Clinical signs are usually slowly progressive.

Diagnostic Evaluation
Thoracic radiographs reveal a mixed nodular interstitial pattern. The pattern is typically generalized and the nodules ill-defined. Hilar and sternal lymph node enlargement may be present.[25] Consolidation of one or more lung lobes has been reported.

Cytology preparations of bronchial wash specimens or transthoracic lung aspirates often show a nonspecific mixed inflammatory response of lymphocytes, plasma cells, eosinophils, and mast cells. The radiographic and cytologic findings can be similar to those found in animals with eosinophilic pulmonary granulomatosis, neoplasia, fungal infection, or atypical mycobacterial infection.[22,26] Heartworm tests, fungal titers, and cultures are indicated to rule out other inflammatory diseases. Definitive diagnosis usually requires surgical biopsy and histopathologic evaluation.

Treatment
Chemotherapeutic protocols described for treatment of lymphoma are utilized for lymphomatoid granulomatosis (see Chapter 181). Administration of prednisone alone is often unrewarding.[22,26] Serial thoracic radiography is used to monitor resolution of disease.

Prognosis
Prognosis is typically guarded due to the variable individual clinical responses. The small numbers of cases reported hinders comparative assessment of the efficacy of different treatment modalities used in these patients.

Malignant Histiocytosis
Malignant histiocytosis was first recognized in Bernese mountain dogs but has since been recognized in other breeds such as golden retrievers and rottweilers.[23,27,28] In Bernese mountain dogs, malignant histiocytosis has a genetic basis with a polygenic mode of inheritance suspected.[29]

Most dogs are middle-aged and exhibit respiratory signs at the time of presentation. Lethargy, anorexia, and weight loss are also common clinical complaints as most dogs have widespread systemic disease at the time of diagnosis. Thoracic radiographs commonly show multiple pulmonary nodules, lymph node enlargement, and pleural effusion. The disease is characterized by infiltration of multiple visceral organs with atypical histiocytes. The brain and spinal cord may also be affected.[30, 31] Histopathologic examination of tissue is usually necessary for a definitive diagnosis. The prognosis has generally been poor with standard chemotherapy protocols; however, one report documented successful treatment in four dogs administered a human major histocompatibility complex nonrestricted cytotoxic T-cell line.[32]

INFECTIOUS DISEASES

Bacterial Disease
Bacterial Pneumonia
The development of bacterial pneumonia in dogs and cats is often viewed as a complication of a loss of one or more pulmonary defense mechanisms. Important mechanisms that protect the pulmonary parenchyma from infection include normal laryngeal function, cough reflex, the mucociliary

RESPIRATORY DISEASE

escalator apparatus of the airways, an intact respiratory epithelial barrier with surface IgA, and in the alveoli, alveolar macrophages, and IgG.

Bacterial infection of the lung is a common complication of many diseases in dogs but is considered uncommon as a primary pulmonary disorder, which emphasizes the importance of careful assessment of patients with bacterial pneumonia for predisposing causes. Aspiration is considered the most common inciting cause, but other means of infection, such as hematogenous spread of infectious organisms, are also possible. Bacterial pneumonia may complicate viral respiratory infections following injury to the respiratory epithelium and disruption of the epithelial barrier, loss of mucociliary function, and local or systemic immune suppression.

Nosocomial infections become a concern in patients that have been in the hospital for a number of days and have risk factors such as recumbency, regurgitation or vomiting, and prolonged endotracheal tubation as would be needed for patients on ventilators.[33,34] Bacterial pneumonia is considered a less common problem in cats as compared with dogs.

Presentation Clinical signs of animals with bacterial pneumonia can be surprisingly variable. One aspect to recognize is that not all animals with pneumonia will exhibit clinical signs referable to the lower respiratory tract. Anorexia and lethargy are common but obviously nonspecific. Cough, which can be acute or chronic, tachypnea, and increased respiratory effort can be seen, with changes in respiratory character commonly reflecting the severity of underlying disease. Cough in cats with pneumonia occurs uncommonly. Some patients with bacterial pneumonia may have hemoptysis.[13] Exercise intolerance is seen in some animals. On physical examination, there may be fever, inducible cough, nasal discharge, increased lung sounds, and crackles or wheezes, but these features are not detected in every patient.

Other clinical signs in animals with pneumonia will reflect the primary diseases that put such patients at risk of

bacterial pneumonia. Such patients may exhibit neurologic abnormalities, muscular weakness, gastrointestinal signs such as vomiting or regurgitation, or other signs.

Diagnostic evaluation The diagnostic approach to a patient with bacterial pneumonia often involves some hematologic and biochemical assessment, and thoracic radiography, as first-line tests. Abnormalities of the CBC can be variable, and neutrophilia with or without a left shift and toxic changes will be expected in many but not all patients. Thrombocytopenia is associated with systemic inflammatory complications. There are no pathognomonic biochemical and urinalysis abnormalities for bacterial pneumonia, but these tests are often useful for comprehensive assessment of patient status and can give clues to diseases that are risk factors for pneumonia or other respiratory diseases. Abnormalities observed on biochemistries and urinalysis could be as much a reflection of underlying disease as of the pneumonia itself. Hypoalbuminemia reflecting increased pulmonary or systemic capillary permeability is not unusual, and animals that are clinically dehydrated may have azotemia. It is important to understand that animals with bacterial pneumonia may have normal laboratory data base results.

Although changes on arterial blood gas analysis will not be specific for bacterial pneumonia, blood gas results can be useful in the diagnostic assessment of patients with pneumonia. Arterial blood gas results will provide the clinician an indication of the adequacy of oxygenation (PaO_2) and the adequacy of ventilation ($PaCO_2$), which if severely compromised would suggest the need for ventilatory support. Evidence of ventilation-perfusion mismatches (hypoxemia, hypocarbia, widened A-a gradient) is expected in many patients.

Thoracic radiographs are useful in the assessment of patients with bacterial pneumonia. The most common radiographic appearance seen in patients with bacterial pneumonia is an alveolar pattern (Figure 215-9) that may be focal or

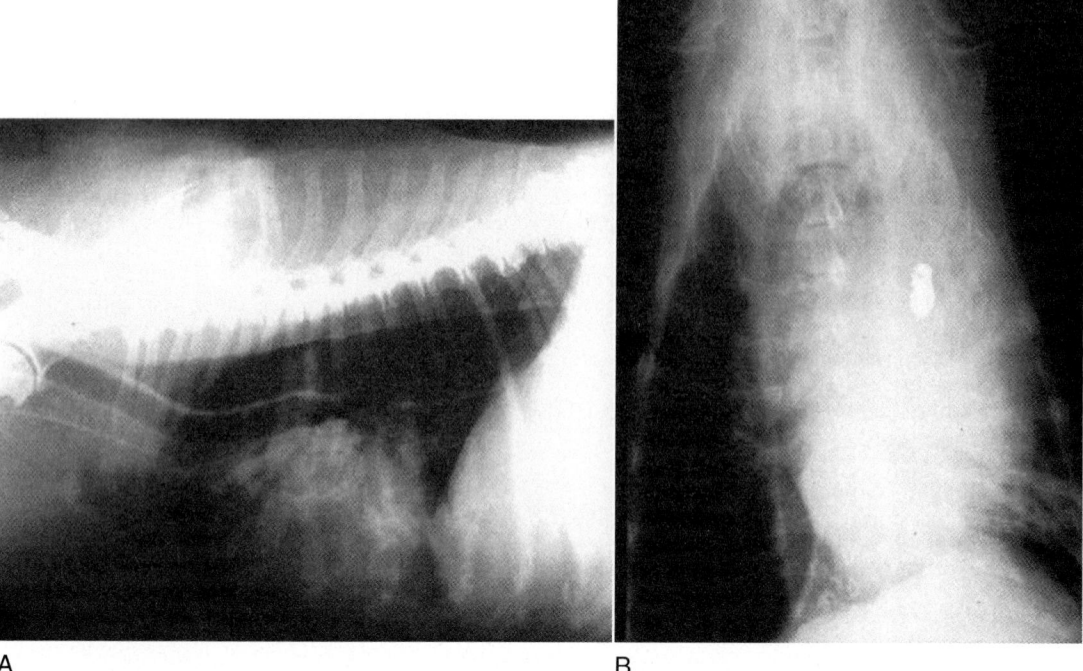

A   B

Figure 215-9 Thoracic radiographs (lateral [A], ventrodorsal [B]) of a dog with focal bacterial pneumonia secondary to aspiration. Note the prominent air bronchogram in the cranioventral lung region on the lateral projection. Note that there is also megaesophagus.

diffuse depending on the manner in which the respiratory tract was seeded with bacteria. Aspiration pneumonia (see below) is more often associated with radiographic abnormalities in the cranioventral lung regions, although not all patients will have this distribution. Depending on the causative organism, there may be pleural effusion, or soft tissue densities that reflect pulmonary abscesses. In severe cases, lobar consolidation may be apparent. Thoracic radiographs should be carefully scrutinized for other abnormalities that could suggest an underlying disorder that could predispose to bacterial pneumonia such as megaesophagus, bronchiectasis, or neoplasia.[34,35]

In some patients, extra effort may be required to demonstrate diseases that predispose to pneumonia. In a study of cats with esophageal disease, many were examined for signs of respiratory disease and required contrast esophagrams to demonstrate abnormalities in esophageal motility.[36] Since bacterial pneumonia can accompany almost any other primary respiratory disease, repeating thoracic radiographs after resolution of pneumonia is important to help uncover other underlying primary diseases. Patients with recurrence of pneumonia confined to a single lung lobe should be suspected of diseases such as endobronchial foreign bodies, airway masses, or other causes of local disruption of pulmonary defense mechanisms (Figure 215-10).

Although a presumptive diagnosis of pneumonia is possible based on history, physical examination, and radiographic findings, definitive diagnosis is established from cytology and culture of material obtained from the respiratory tract by transtracheal washes or bronchoalveolar lavage. Cytologically, suppurative inflammation is expected, with signs of septic inflammation (intracellular bacteria, degenerative neutrophils) present in some, but not all, patients. Because not all patients with bacterial pneumonia have bacteria or septic features evident on cytology, it is important to culture samples for bacteria, including *Mycoplasma* spp. If thoracic radiographs are suggestive of abscessation, anaerobic cultures would also be appropriate. Ideally, samples should be obtained by transtracheal/endotracheal washes, bronchoalveolar lavage, or less commonly, needle aspiration, before administration of antibiotics if the patient's status will allow. Collection of samples by alveolar lavage is especially useful for focal disease, particularly if performed after bronchoscopic examination, which can identify predisposing diseases such as masses or foreign bodies. Fine-needle aspiration for cytology and culture may be considered if respiratory wash techniques do not provide an etiology, if there is lobar consolidation evident radiographically, or if other procedures are cost prohibitive.

Treatment and prognosis Treatment of bacterial pneumonia requires administration of antibiotics. The specific type of antibiotic and route of administration is ideally based upon results of culture and sensitivity of lower respiratory tract secretions or exudates, and in consideration of the clinical status of the patient. Certain situations, such as a patient in severe

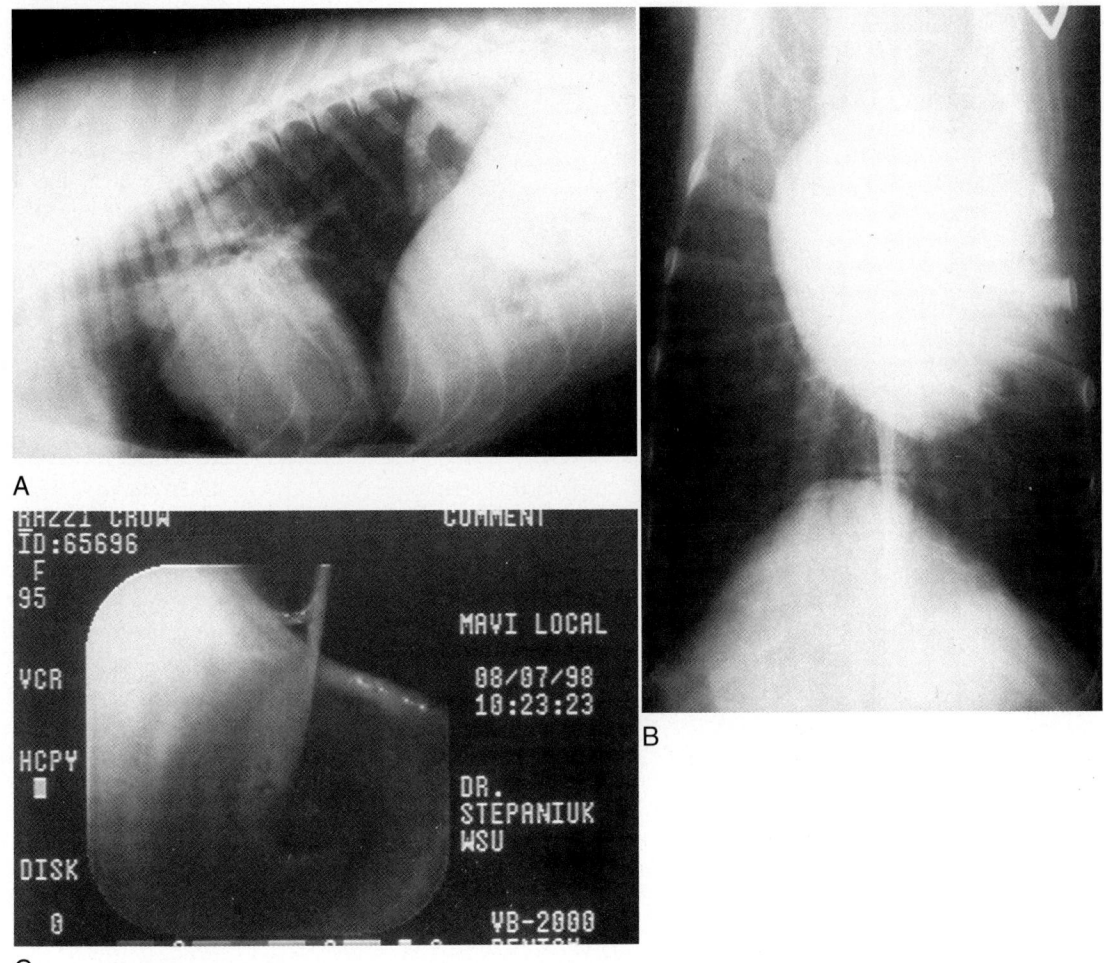

Figure 215-10 A, Thoracic radiographs (lateral [A], ventrodorsal [B]) from a dog with recurring focal pneumonia. During bronchoscopy, grass awns (C) were found in airways of this lung lobe.

respiratory distress in which collection of samples by respiratory washes may be dangerous to the patient, may preclude sample collection. Some owners may not wish to incur the financial costs of sample collection and analysis. In such cases, antimicrobial therapy may be needed on an empiric basis.

Empiric selection of antibiotics for animals suspected of having bacterial pneumonia can be facilitated by knowledge of common bacterial isolates from dogs and cats with bacterial pneumonia. Organisms often isolated from the respiratory tract of dogs with bacterial pneumonia include *Escherichia coli*, *Pasteurella multocida*, *Klebsiella* spp., *Bordetella bronchiseptica*, *Acinetobacter* spp., *Pseudomonas aeruginosa*, *Moraxella* spp., and isolates of *Staphylococcus* and *Streptococcus*.[37,38] In cats, common isolates include *P. multocida*, *Klebsiella* spp., *Proteus* spp., *Bordetella* spp., *E. coli*, and *Streptococci*.[38,39] *Mycoplasma* spp. are frequently cultured from dogs and cats with pneumonia. The role of *Mycoplasma* spp. as primary respiratory pathogens in both dogs and cats has been suggested, and recent reports are consistent with *Mycoplasma* spp. as a cause of pneumonia.[37,40,41] Less commonly, *Actinomyces* or *Nocardia* spp. can be a cause of pneumonia without pyothorax.

Initial empiric therapy can be further focused by morphologic assessment of observed organisms and gram-staining if available. Good empiric selections for canine and feline bacterial pneumonia are presented in Table 215-1. Good initial combinations would be a beta lactam such as ampicillin or first-generation cephalosporin and an aminoglycoside or fluoroquinolone. An empirically treated patient that shows no clinical improvement, or exhibits clinical deterioration, during the first 24 to 48 hours after initiation of treatment should be thoroughly re-evaluated, and another consideration given to collection of samples for analysis. A change in antimicrobial therapy could be warranted at this point, but selection becomes more difficult in the absence of sensitivity results. The patient exhibiting a positive clinical response should be treated at least 1 week beyond clinical and radiographic resolution of pneumonia as radiographic improvement may lag several days behind clinical improvement.

The route of administration of antimicrobials will, in most cases, be predicated by the patient's clinical status. Patients that are clinically stable and that have minimal clinical signs of respiratory disease are candidates for oral therapy administered at home. Patients that are clinically unstable will likely require hospitalization for administration of intravenous antimicrobials, ancillary therapy such as intravenous fluids, and oxygen supplementation. Intravenous antibiotic therapy should be continued until the patient has become stabilized and can be safely discharged on oral medications. Patients with esophageal disease may need prolonged parenteral antimicrobials or gastrostomy tubes to ensure that adequate tissue concentrations of antimicrobials are attained and to provide nutritional support.

Administration of antimicrobials via nebulization may be considered in some patients, but the clinical implementation of this route of administration has some important limitations.[42] The efficacy of nebulized medications reflects a complex set of interactions between the drug administered, the formulation of the drug, the device used to deliver the drug, and patient factors such as the characteristics of the primary disease, breathing patterns, and tolerance of delivery systems. Nebulization of antimicrobials formulated for intravenous use may prove less effective because of an inability to achieve desirable particle size, or could be harmful because of changes in pH or other properties that, when administered as an aerosol, result in respiratory mucosal irritation or injury. The best products for nebulization are those medications that have been specifically formulated for administration via nebulizer. Unfortunately, few antimicrobials, other than aminoglycosides formulated for use in people with cystic fibrosis and *Pseudomonas* infection, are available for specific use in small animal patients.

Administration of bronchodilators to patients with pneumonia has been suggested but is not universally accepted. The most appropriate use of bronchodilators would be for patients with bronchoconstriction, which may be difficult to appreciate in some patients. Bronchoconstriction is not

Table • 215-1

Antibiotic Selections for Empiric Treatment of Bacterial Pneumonia[1]

ANTIBIOTIC	ANTIMICROBIAL SPECTRUM	DOSAGE, ROUTE, FREQUENCY
Ampicillin	Gram-positive aerobes (staphylococci, streptococci), *Pasteurella multocida*, some *E. coli* Anaerobes	10-30 mg/kg IV, IM, PO q8-12h
Cefazolin (or other first-generation cephalosporin)	Gram-positive aerobes (staphylococci, streptococci), *Pasteurella multocida*, *Bordetella bronchiseptica*, some *E. coli* and *Klebsiella* spp.	10-30 mg/kg IV, IM, PO q8-12h
Gentamicin	Gram-negative aerobes (*E. coli*, *Proteus* spp., *Pasteurella multocida*, *Bordetella bronchiseptica*, some *Klebsiella* and *Pseudomonas* spp.), *Staphylococcus intermedius*	6-10 mg/kg IV q24h
Amikacin	Gram-negative aerobes (*E. coli*, *Pseudomonas* and *Klebsiella* spp., *Bordetella bronchiseptica*); *Staphylococcus intermedius*	10-15 mg/kg IV, IM, SQ q24h
Enrofloxacin	Gram-negative aerobes (*E. coli*, *Proteus* spp., *Pasteurella multocida*, *Bordetella bronchiseptica*, some *Pseudomonas* spp.); *Staphylococcus intermedius*	3-5 mg/kg PO, IV q24h (cat) 5-20 mg/kg PO, IV q24h (dog)
Doxycyline	*Mycoplasma* spp., *Bordetella bronchiseptica*	5-10 mg/kg PO, IV q12h 10-25 mg/kg PO q12h (cat)
Metronidazole	Anaerobes	15 mg/kg IV, PO q12h (dog)

[1]Selection of drugs is based ideally on culture and sensitivity. Dosages may need to be altered in the face of concurrent renal or hepatic disease.

considered an important feature in dogs with pneumonia. In cats, however, inflammation is a potent stimulus for bronchoconstriction, which may contribute to clinical signs in cats. Bronchodilators have the potential to worsen oxygenation by contributing further to ventilation-perfusion mismatchings often present in patients with pneumonia.

Coupage may help some patients with pneumonia by helping loosen mucus secretions for expectoration to clear airways. Saline nebulization to keep respiratory secretions moist can be beneficial in facilitating clearance of respiratory secretions. Limited periods of exercise in the clinically stable patient that can tolerate activity may accomplish the same purpose.

Occasionally, lung lobectomy may be necessary to treat an animal with bacterial pneumonia. There are no specific criteria that have been established for determination of which patients should receive surgery. Some candidates for lobectomy include patients that have focal disease that has not demonstrated improvement or clinical response to medical therapy, patients that have focally recurring pneumonia, or patients for which less-invasive methods have failed to establish a diagnosis and empiric therapy has failed. Retrospective studies of lobectomies for pneumonia in dogs and cats suggest that the value of surgery may lie as much in its diagnostic value as its therapeutic value. In addition to its therapeutic potential in animals with severe focal pneumonia, surgery may also help rule out other concurrent diseases such as foreign bodies, fungal infection, or neoplasms. The best prognoses reported with lobectomy for pneumonia are associated with foreign body pneumonia, and focal pneumonia, including animals with lobar consolidation, for which no etiology is discovered.[43,44] A poorer prognosis can be expected for dogs with fungal or bacterial pneumonia, or the resection of large amounts of lung tissue.

Zoonotic Respiratory Pathogens

Mycobacteria *Mycobacteria* spp. are an important cause of pneumonia in dogs and cats, not necessarily because of the frequency with which they are seen, but because mycobacterial infections can mimic other diseases such as neoplasia, systemic fungal infections, and severe bacterial pneumonia. Additionally, some *Mycobacteria* spp. are potential human health hazards. The clinical presentation of dogs and cats with mycobacterial infection is typically one of chronic cough progressing to more severe signs of respiratory disease such as tachypnea and increased respiratory effort. Radiographically, infected animals can have interstitial nodules of various numbers and sizes, or have prominent interstitial markings. Enlargement of hilar lymph nodes, lung lobe consolidation, and pleural and pericardial effusions may also be seen. As with other pulmonary parenchymal diseases, occasional animals will have hypertrophic osteopathy. Diagnosis of mycobacterial infection is made by demonstration of organisms, which are usually found in the cytoplasm of macrophages in samples collected via tracheal wash, bronchoalveolar lavage, lung aspirate, or biopsy. Mycobacterial nucleic acid can be detected in samples by the polymerase chain reaction[45] and would support a diagnosis in a patient with appropriate clinical signs and radiographic abnormalities.

Yersinia pestis and Francisella tularensis Animals in the southwestern and western United States live in areas of endemic plague (*Yersinia pestis*) and tularemia (*Francisella tularensis*). Cats are particularly susceptible to development of clinical plague, with the bubonic form most common. However, pneumonic forms of plague are seen with some regularity in endemic areas and would pose the greatest threat to people.[46] Cats infected with tularemia do not commonly show signs of

respiratory disease despite often extensive lesions in the lungs.[47] The diagnosis of these diseases can be established with fluorescent antibody assays performed on aspirates of lymph nodes or bone marrow.

Viral Diseases
Canine Distemper Virus
Canine distemper virus (CDV) infection can be associated with parenchymal disease. In CDV-infected dogs, viral infection may lead to secondary bacterial pneumonias. See Chapter 169.

Canine Adenovirus (CAV)-2, Parainfluenza (PI)
CAV-2 and canine PI are not typically a cause of parenchymal disease, although severe cases might be associated with secondary bacterial pneumonia. CAV-2 as a sole pathogen has been incriminated as a cause of pneumonia in rare instances.[48]

Feline Calicivirus
Feline calicivirus is more often a cause of upper respiratory disease in cats, but has been associated with interstitial pneumonia (see Chapter 173).[49]

Feline Infectious Peritonitis
Most cases of respiratory disease caused by feline infectious peritonitis (FIP) are associated with pleural effusion. Although pyogranulomatous pulmonary lesions are often seen in the setting of noneffusive FIP, most cats with noneffusive FIP exhibit signs referable to the eyes, CNS or liver, kidneys, or GI tract and are not commonly examined for respiratory disease.[50] Other clinical features and the diagnostic approach to cats suspected of having FIP are presented in Chapter 172.

Feline Immunodeficiency Virus and Feline Leukemia Virus
The feline retroviruses are not considered primary respiratory tract pathogens. Clinically affected cats, however, may develop parenchymal disease as a result of opportunistic infections or development of pulmonary neoplasia. Interstitial inflammation and alveolitis have been described in FIV-infected cats.[51] Diagnosis of underlying causes of respiratory disease in retroviral-infected cats will rely on the principles and techniques presented in Chapter 171, with treatment decisions based on diagnosis as well as the clinical status of the cat. FIV-positive cats may survive for long periods of time with appropriate veterinary care, so treatment decisions for such cats should not necessarily be based solely on the FIV status.

Rickettsial Disease
The primary rickettsial diseases of dogs and cats are infections caused by species in the genus *Ehrlichia* and *Rickettsia rickettsii*, the causative agent of Rocky Mountain Spotted Fever (RMSF) in dogs. RMSF causes a systemic vasculitis, and thus dysfunction of any organ system, including the respiratory tract, may cause clinical signs in affected dogs. Although not a common manifestation of infection, respiratory signs of RMSF that have been described in dogs include cough, tachypnea, and dyspnea.[52,53] Physical examination abnormalities referable to the respiratory tract can include nasal discharge and increased lung sounds. Thoracic radiographs may have an interstitial pattern, or alveolar patterns if vascular leakage secondary to pulmonary vascular inflammation is severe. Diagnosis is based on seroconversion or detection of organisms by immunohistochemical methods, and treatment involves administration of tetracycline family drugs (see Chapter 166). The canine and feline ehrlichioses are uncommon causes of respiratory tract disease despite the systemic nature of the infections.

Protozoal Disease
Toxoplasmosis and Neosporosis
Pulmonary disease in cats with *Toxoplasma gondii* infection is common. In a retrospective study of feline toxoplasmosis, fever, dyspnea, and tachypnea were common clinical signs, and pulmonary lesions were identified in approximately 25% of cats necropsied.[54] Pulmonary toxoplasmosis can be an acute, fulminant, and fatal disease. Physical examination abnormalities can reflect the multisystemic nature of the disease with increases in bronchial sounds or crackles during thoracic auscultation in cats with a respiratory component. Radiographic features of respiratory toxoplasmosis in cats may vary. Patterns reflect diffuse alveolar and interstitial disease, and areas of emphysema can create a patchy appearance to the lungs. There are no pathognomic laboratory abnormalities in affected cats.

Diagnosis is supported by serologic results (increased IgM or increases in IgG in an animal with compatible clinical disease) or established definitively with demonstration of organisms in tissues. *T. gondii* tachyzoites can be detected in bronchoalveolar washings of affected cats and should be a useful technique for cats with respiratory signs and radiographic lesions.[55] Alternatively, lung fine-needle aspiration cytology can be attempted to examine samples for tachyzoites. Toxoplasmosis in cats is discussed in further detail in Chapter 168.

Canine toxoplasmosis is not as common as feline toxoplasmosis and can involve the lungs with similar clinical signs and radiographic features as described in cats. The diagnostic approach would be similar to that for cats.

Pneumonia attributable to *Neospora caninum* infection has been described in a dog that was evaluated for persistent cough, fever, and diffuse interstitial and focal alveolar lung disease.[56] An antemortem diagnosis was established by observation of tachyzoites in a lung fine-needle aspirate and confirmed on necropsy with immunohistochemistry. There were no obvious predisposing factors (concurrent lung disease, immunosuppressive disease) apparent in this dog. Pulmonary neosporosis appears to be an uncommon manifestation of *N. caninum* infection.

FUNGAL DISEASE

Systemic Fungal Infections
The systemic fungal organisms *Blastomyces dermatitidis*, *Histoplasma capsulatum*, *Coccidiodes immitis*, and *Cryptococcus neoformans* are notorious respiratory pathogens. Clinical signs of parenchymal disease are a common reason for infected animals to be evaluated, especially dogs with blastomycosis and cats with histoplasmosis. Clinical signs of cryptococcal pulmonary parenchymal disease are less common as compared with the other systemic fungal organisms. Coccidioidmycosis is rare in cats, and blastomycosis is less common in cats than cryptococcosis or histoplasmosis. Recognition of the contributions of the systemic fungal infections to small animal respiratory disease is important because the clinical signs and radiographic features can be similar to other diseases such as metastatic neoplasia. The systemic fungal infections are easily overlooked if the clinician fails to consider recent travel history of ill patients, particularly those patients that reside in areas where the disease is not endemic. More details of the systemic fungal infections are found in Chapter 174.

Generally, infection with systemic fungi occurs primarily after inhalation of organisms present in the environment. Local infection in the respiratory tract generally precedes systemic spread, although clinical signs of respiratory disease such as tachypnea and dyspnea may not be apparent until after systemic dissemination has occurred. Most affected animals have a history that suggests slowly progressive clinical signs of multisystemic disease; poor response to antibiotic treatment is often a component of the clinical history of animals with systemic fungal infections.

Most animals with clinical signs of respiratory disease will have abnormalities evident on thoracic radiographs, although some animals can have radiographically evident pulmonary disease in the absence of clinical signs of respiratory dysfunction. Although the radiographic appearance of the systemic fungal infections can be quite variable, typical changes on thoracic radiographs include diffuse interstitial patterns that can organize into small nodules (Figure 215-11), or larger, more ill-defined interstitial nodules (Figure 215-12). Some animals will have evidence of alveolar patterns, lobar consolidation (Figure 215-13) or peribronchiolar disease. Hilar lymph node enlargement can be seen in affected animals, and may occur independent of parenchymal lesions, especially with canine histoplasmosis. Hilar lymph node enlargement is also a common feature of canine coccidioidomycosis.[57] Occasionally, calcification of pulmonary nodules can occur with histoplasmosis. Pleural effusion can be a feature of any of these infections.

For all the systemic fungi, definitive diagnosis is often accomplished by demonstration of organisms in exudates, fluid washings, and needle aspirates or tissue biopsies of affected organs. The exception is cryptococcosis, the diagnosis of which can also be made by demonstration of circulating antigen with serologic methods. The cytologic and histologic diagnosis of coccidioidomycosis can be difficult in some cases due to few numbers of organism present in material examined. Most organisms will have to be identified within a cytologic background of inflammation characterized by the presence of neutrophils, macrophages, and depending on the severity of inflammation and the method of sample collection, some evidence of hemorrhage. Samples obtained by tracheal wash, bronchoalveolar lavage, or lung needle aspiration can be negative for organisms necessitating repeating the procedures or choosing an alternative approach, including lung biopsy, to establish a definitive diagnosis. If sufficient material is obtained during sample collection, and the samples do not contain organisms cytologically, consideration can be given to submission of the material for fungal culture. Serologic detection of antibodies, particularly in suspected cases of coccidioidomycosis, can add support to the diagnosis. As with many antibody tests, positive results indicate exposure but do not necessarily confirm clinical disease. Antibody tests can remain positive in animals that have had resolution of clinical disease.

Treatment of the systemic fungal infections centers around administration of antifungal drugs in the azole category (ketoconazole, itraconazole, fluconazole) or amphotericin B. Although not proven in prospective studies, the concurrent administration of anti-inflammatory doses of glucocorticoids to animals with severe disease has been advocated to limit clinical deterioration associated with inflammation secondary to the death of large numbers of fungal organisms. Extension of antifungal therapy for an additional 2 to 4 weeks beyond typical treatment times is suggested if glucocorticoids are used.[58] The prognosis is favorable in animals diagnosed and treated early. The presence of severe respiratory signs worsens the prognosis. The reader is directed to Chapter 174 for additional details regarding the treatment of these infections.

Pneumocystosis
Pneumocystis carinii is a fungal organism that can be found in the alveoli of normal animals but can cause clinical disease in animals with immune system dysfunction. Most reported cases in dogs have been in young (<1 year) miniature dachsunds, although dogs of other breeds have also been described with the infection.[59,60] Affected dogs are evaluated for respiratory difficulty and exercise intolerance, weight loss, and skin diseases (demodicosis, bacterial pyoderma) that also reflect systemic immune system dysfunction.[61] Physical examination abnormalities include poor body condition, tachypnea, dyspnea, increased lung sounds, and skin and hair coat changes

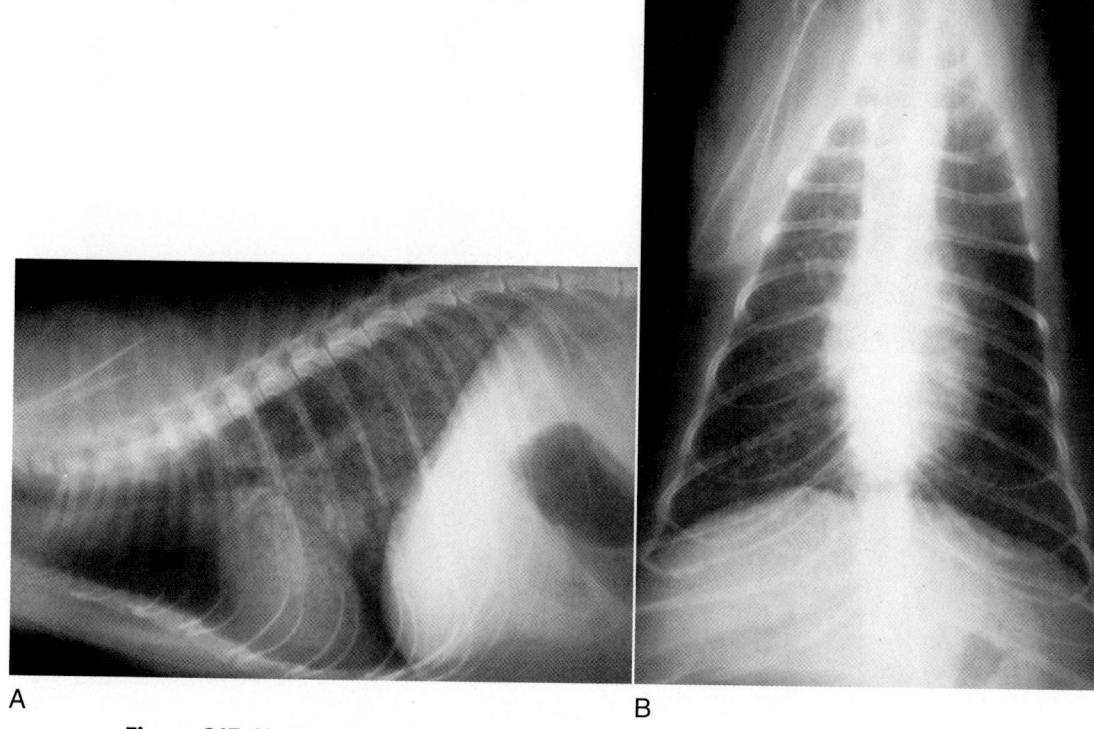

A   B

Figure 215-11 Thoracic radiographs (lateral [A], ventrodorsal [B]) of a cat with pulmonary histoplasmosis. Note the typical nodular, miliary interstitial pattern that is frequently seen with this infection. (Courtesy Dru Forrester, Blacksburg, Va.)

that reflect the secondary skin disease. Abnormalities on thoracic radiographs can vary from diffuse, mild, interstitial, or bronchial patterns to more severe interstitial and alveolar patterns. Laboratory assessment is consistent with chronic inflammation (leukocytosis, thrombocytosis, monocytosis),

except affected animals usually have low gamma globulin concentrations.

Definitive diagnosis is made by observation of organisms in respiratory washes, lung needle aspiration cytology, or histologic examination of lung tissue. Additional support for the

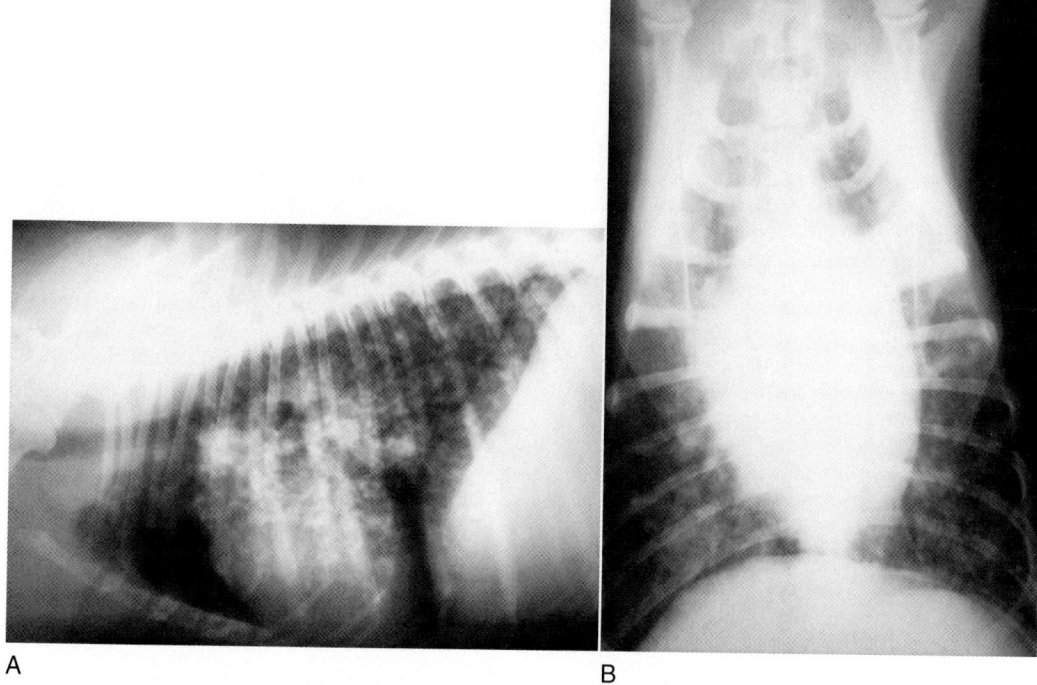

A   B

Figure 215-12 Thoracic radiographs (lateral [A], ventrodorsal [B]) of a dog with pulmonary blastomycosis. Note the larger, more ill-defined interstitial densities.

RESPIRATORY DISEASE

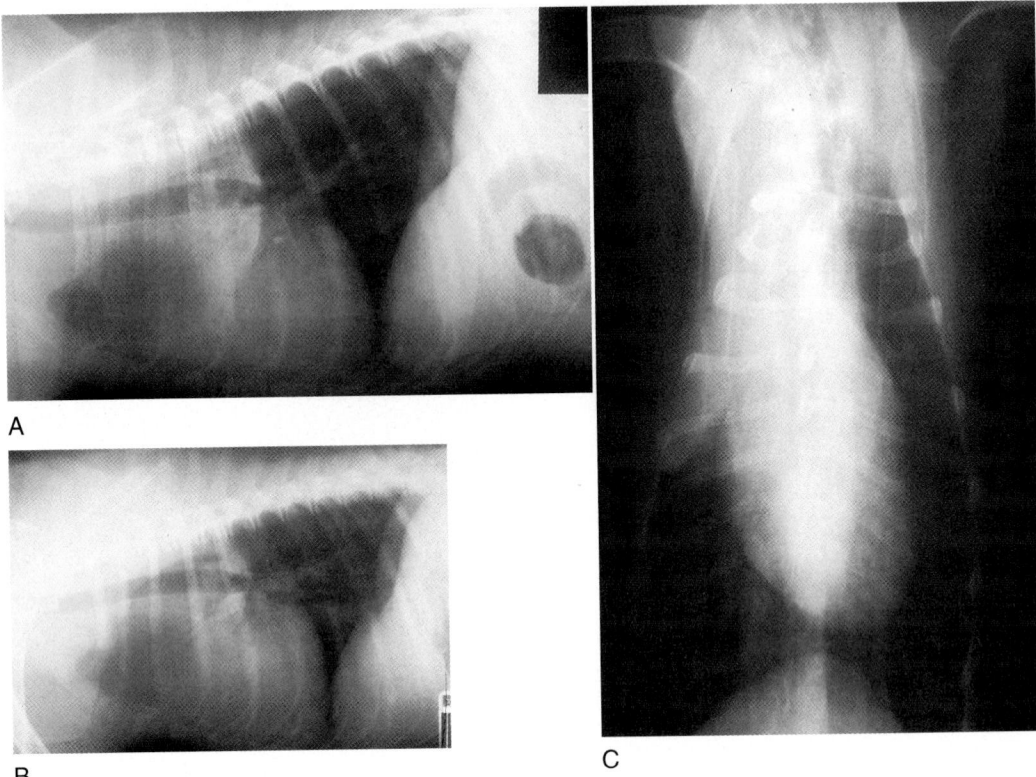

Figure 215-13 Thoracic radiographs (right [A] and left [B] lateral, ventrodorsal [C]) of a dog with *Coccidioides immitis* infection in a single lung lobe. The definitive diagnosis in this dog required lung lobectomy and histology.

diagnosis can come from immunohistochemical techniques, or polymerase chain reaction (PCR) performed on tissues from animals with compatible clinical signs. Treatment may be attempted with trimethoprim sulfa combinations (30 mg/kg PO q12h for 3 weeks) or a number of other chemotherapeutic agents including pentamidine isethionate and clindamycin/primaquine, but relapses are common. The long-term prognosis is considered guarded because relapses are common.

Aspergillosis

Aspergillus infections are most commonly a cause of nasal cavity disease in dogs. However, systemic aspergillus infection can occasionally be seen, and when it occurs, is usually caused by *Aspergillus terreus*. Rarely *Aspergillus fumigatus*, the cause of nasal aspergillosis, can cause systemic infection.[62] Systemic aspergillosis has been described most often in German shepherds, which commonly present with signs of neurologic disease from diskospondylitis. These dogs may also exhibit cough, dyspnea, and tachypnea as a consequence of pulmonary parenchymal infection. Diagnosis requires demonstration of fungal hyphae in tissues by cytologic examination of needle aspirates, biopsies, or respiratory washes. Treatment requires administration of systemic antifungals as described for the systemic fungal infections. The prognosis is considered poor.

PARASITIC DISEASES

The respiratory tract is the site of infection with a number of parasitic organisms, both flukes and helminths. As a whole, respiratory parasites are considered an uncommon cause of clinical respiratory disease in dogs and cats. The importance of the respiratory parasites is that they can cause radiographic lesions that can mimic other diseases such as metastatic neoplasia or systemic fungal infections. The eosinophilic pulmonary infiltrates caused by parasitic pneumonia require differentiation from other causes of eosinophilic pulmonary diseases.

When apparent, clinical signs from parasitic infection are usually mild, with some exceptions that can be associated with severe and life-threatening, presentations. The most common clinical sign of respiratory parasitism is cough, which can be acute or chronic. Other clinical signs that can be seen include wheezing, tachypnea, and respiratory distress in severe cases. The pathogenesis of clinical signs can reflect either the direct presence of the parasite or the immunologic response to the parasite.

As with most animals that present with clinical signs of respiratory disease, thoracic radiographs play a role in the diagnosis of respiratory parasites. Radiographic features common to most of the respiratory parasites include peribronchiolar infiltrates, interstitial patterns that can have a nodular appearance, and occasionally alveolar patterns. Other unique radiographic features of parasite infection are discussed below with the specific parasite.

The diagnosis of most of the respiratory parasites is made by detection of eggs or larvae in tracheal wash or bronchoalveolar lavage fluid, or by demonstration of larvae in stool samples, typically by the Baermann technique. Individual exceptions exist as noted below. Cytologic examination of respiratory samples typically reveals a mix of inflammatory cells, with neutrophils and eosinophils present in varying proportions but usually representing the majority of cells present. Peripheral eosinophilia is an inconsistent, although common, hematologic abnormality and its absence should not lessen the consideration of respiratory parasites as a differential diagnosis of respiratory disease if other aspects of the patient are consistent. Unique features of each of the important lower respiratory tract parasites are noted below.

Paragonimus kellicotti

Paragonimus kellicotti is the lung fluke of dogs and cats. Animals at risk of infection live primarily in the southern, midwestern, and Great Lakes regions of the United States, although infections have been seen in other parts of the world. Animals become infected following ingestion of a freshwater snail or crayfish, which serve as intermediate hosts. The fluke leaves the intestine and migrates to the lungs, where it lives in a cyst or bulla within the pulmonary parenchyma. Eggs from adult flukes are coughed, swallowed, and passed in feces to infect intermediate hosts. Animals with *P. kellicotti* may be clinically normal or be presented for coughing, which results from inflammatory reactions to adult flukes or ova in the parenchyma and airways. Of the respiratory parasites, *P. kellicotti* has potential to cause life-threatening problems to the affected patient if cysts rupture to cause pneumothorax (Figure 215-14). The physical examination can reflect crackles or wheezes, or if a pneumothorax is present, the restrictive breathing pattern and decreased lung sounds typical of pneumothorax. In cats, wheezing may be seen from inflammatory-mediator induced airway constriction.

The suspicion of paragonamiasis is raised by the observation of cystic or bullous lesions on thoracic radiographs, which may or may not be accompanied by pneumothorax. Other radiographic abnormalities that can be seen are common to other respiratory parasites. The diagnosis of paragonamiasis is made by demonstration of fluke ova in feces by sedimentation techniques, which are preferred for examination of feces. Intermittent shedding of ova dictates a need in some patients for multiple fecal examinations to establish a definitive diagnosis. Ova may also be recovered in tracheal wash or bronchoalveolar lavage fluid; the cytologic picture of such samples is characterized by mixed populations of inflammatory cells, including neutrophils, eosinophils, and macrophages.

Drugs recommended for treatment of paragonamiasis are praziquantel (25 mg/kg PO q8h for 3 days) and fenbendazole (25 to 50 mg/kg PO q12h for 14 days); treatment may need to be repeated if fecal examinations remain positive for ova. Animals with pneumothorax may require thoracocentesis, or thoracostomy tubes if repeated thoracocentesis is required.

Filaroides hirthi

Filaroides hirthi infects dogs. Adults live in the terminal bronchioles and alveolar spaces. The parasite has a direct life cycle, and larvae can develop within the primary host and contribute to cycles of autoinfection that have the potential to create large worm burdens. Most infected dogs are asymptomatic, and as with other parasitic infections, cough is a common sign. Clinically affected dogs may have conditions associated with immune system compromise. The development of widespread granulomatous inflammation and destruction of respiratory bronchioles and alveolar units is capable of inducing respiratory distress in occasional animals from loss of gas exchange regions of the lung.[63] Interstitial infiltrates, which can appear nodular, as well as alveolar infiltrates, are features of thoracic radiographs that have been described.[63] Definitive diagnosis is made by detection of larvae or larvated eggs in respiratory washes, or in fecal samples by Baermann or zinc sulfate flotation. Administration of fenbendazole (50 mg/kg PO q24h for 14 days) or albendazole (50 mg/kg PO q12h for 5 days, repeat in 3 weeks) can be given to infected dogs, but there is a risk of exacerbation of clinical signs, possibly secondary to reactions to dying worms.[63]

Capillaria aerophila

Capillaria aerophila parasitizes dogs and cats. Adults reside primarily in the trachea and bronchi. Adults deposit eggs, which are coughed, swallowed, and shed in feces. Most parasitized animals are asymptomatic; animals with clinical disease most often cough. Radiographic abnormalities are as described generally above. The diagnosis of *C. aerophila* is made by detection of ova in respiratory washes or fecal flotation. The ova have an operculum at each end and are similar, though smaller, in appearance to the ova of the whipworm *Trichuris vulpis* (Figure 215-15). As with other of the respiratory parasites, intermittent shedding of ova can cause false negative results. Administration of fendbendazole (25 to 50 mg/kg PO q12h for 14 days) is recommended.

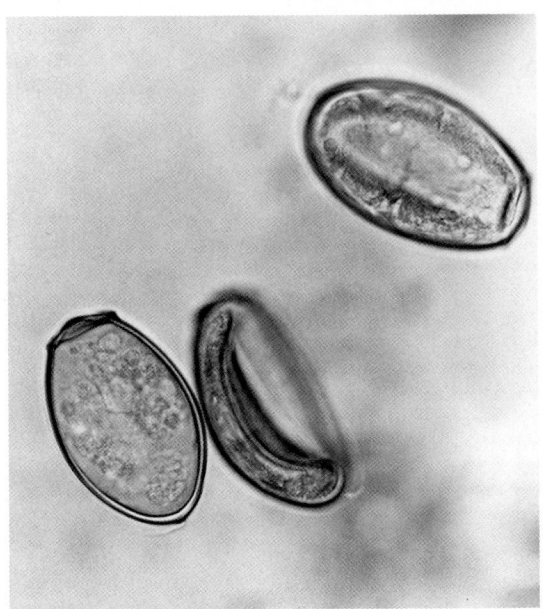

Figure 215-14 Ova of *Paragonimus kellicotti*. (Courtesy Bill Foreyt, WSU.)

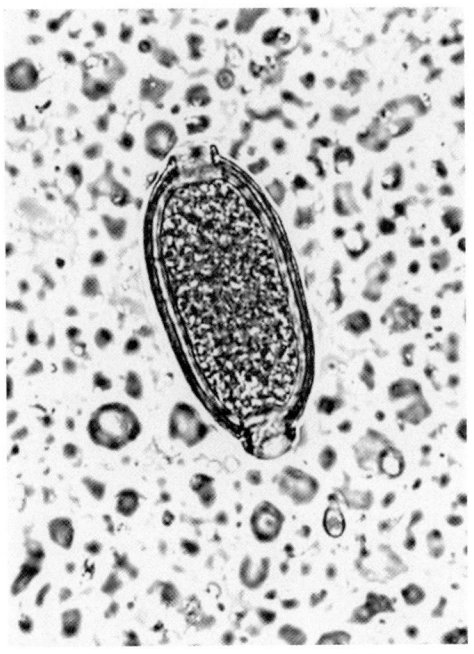

Figure 215-15 Ova of *Capillaria aerophila*. (Courtesy Bill Foreyt, WSU.)

RESPIRATORY DISEASE

Aelurostrongylus abstrusus

Cats are the principle hosts of *Aelurostrongylus abstrusus*. Adult worms live in the bronchioles, where larvae are deposited, coughed, swallowed, and shed in feces to infect a snail or slug intermediate host, which is eaten to complete the transmission cycle. Many cats are parasitized, and most are clinically normal. Clinical signs, when they occur, are attributed to inflammatory reactions to the parasites. Clinical signs can include cough, wheezing, and overt respiratory distress. Because of the overlap in clinical features, cats with a presumptive diagnosis of "asthma" should be considered candidates for *A. abstrusus* infection. Diffuse interstitial nodules are characteristic on thoracic radiographs, and peribronchiolar and alveolar patterns may also be present. Diagnosis is established by detection of larvae in respiratory washes, or in feces by Baermann technique (Figure 215-16).

Clinically symptomatic animals may be treated with fenbendazole (25 to 50 mg/kg PO q24h for 10 to 14 days) or ivermectin (400 ug/kg SC). Administration of bronchodilators and glucocorticoids has been advocated to help address the inflammation-induced bronchoconstriction that can contribute to clinical signs.[64]

Oslerus osleri

Though not a primary lower respiratory tract parasite, *Oslerus osleri* infection has been associated with secondary bacterial pneumonia, likely through disruption of normal pulmonary defenses caused by nodules in the airways. This parasite is discussed more completely in Chapter 213.

Crenosoma vulpis

C. vulpis is a lungworm that infects domestic and wild canids. Dogs acquire the parasite through ingestion of a mollusk like a slug or snail, the intermediate host that contains infective third stage larvae. Adult parasites live in the distal aspects of the bronchial tree where they produce larvated eggs that are coughed, swallowed and passed in feces. Infected dogs are seen primarily in the northeastern United States and eastern provinces of Canada.[65] Baermann techniques are the preferred method of examining feces for larvae, although centrifugal flotation techniques using zinc sulfate may also recover larvae or other parasites. Larvae and larvated eggs are usually readily recovered with airway washings. The preferred treatment is fenbendazole administered at a dosage of 50 mg/kg PO q24h for 3 days. Other anthelmintics such as ivermectin have also been suggested as effective.[65]

Angiostrongylus vasorum

Sometimes referred to as the heartworm of France,[66] *Angiostrongylus vasorum* parasitizes the pulmonary arteries of dogs primarily in Europe, Africa, and Asia. Historically *A. vasorum* has not been considered a parasite of North American dogs; however, a recent report describes the first known infection of dogs in northeastern Canada.[67] Dogs are infected following ingestion of infected intermediate hosts such as snails and slugs. Adult worms shed eggs that are transported to the pulmonary capillaries where larvae penetrate the capillary wall to migrate into the alveolar spaces. Larvae are coughed, swallowed, and passed in feces.

Adult worms cause a thrombosing pulmonary arteritis, with inflammatory responses contributing to the development of interstitial pneumonia and pulmonary hypertension. Anaphylaxis and consumptive coagulopathies can develop in some infected animals. Clinical signs reflect the pathogenesis, and signs of right-sided heart failure including cough, exercise intolerance, abdominal effusion, and hepatomegaly are possible. Animals with coagulopathies may have evidence of bleeding (anemia, hemoptysis, melena, subcutaneous hemorrhage).

Radiographic abnormalities can include those described above for other respiratory parasites; when alveolar patterns are present, they are usually more prominent in peripheral regions. In addition, dogs with *A. vasorum* may have right-sided cardiomegaly and pulmonary artery enlargement, ascites and hepatomegaly as can be seen in dogs with *Dirofilaria immitis* infection (see Chapter 206).

Detection of larvae can be accomplished by Baermann or fecal flotation. False negative results are possible as larvae are not continuously shed. Larvae may also be detected in respiratory washes. Levamisole (7.5 mg/kg PO q24h for 2 days followed by 10 mg/kg PO q24h on the next 2 days) is considered the standard treatment, but other anthelmintics, although known to stop fecal larval shedding, have not yet been adequately investigated for efficacy of killing adult worms.[66]

HYPERSENSITIVITY DISORDERS

A variety of eosinophilic disorders involving the lungs, either alone or in conjunction with infiltration of other organ systems, have been described in dogs and cats. The clinical spectrum reflects the extent of eosinophilic infiltration and ranges from disease limited to the respiratory tract to multisystemic disease involving not only the lungs, but liver, kidneys, heart, and gastrointestinal tracts. For many affected patients, the diseases are believed to be a manifestation of a hypersensitivity to an environmental or endogenous antigen. Identification of the offending antigen is infrequently accomplished.

Eosinophilic bronchopneumopathy (EB), formerly referred to as *pulmonary infiltrates with eosinophils* (PIE), is an inflammatory disease of unknown etiology that can be seen in dogs of all breeds, although a predisposition in Huskies has been reported.[68] Affected dogs can be of any age, though the majority of cases are seen in young to middle-aged dogs. The primary clinical manifestations of EB are cough, which is often accompanied by gagging, and difficulty breathing; mucopurulent or serous nasal discharge may also be seen. In the authors' experience, EB is frequently associated with coughing that results in expectoration of thick, greenish to greenish-yellow mucus.

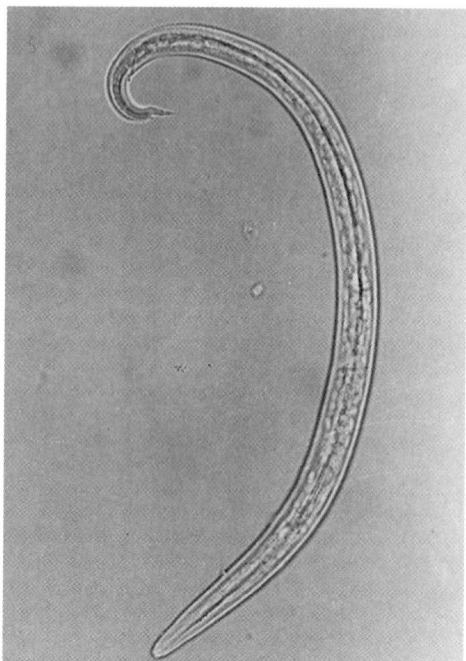

Figure 215-16 *Aleurostrongylus* larva. (Courtesy Bill Foreyt, WSU.)

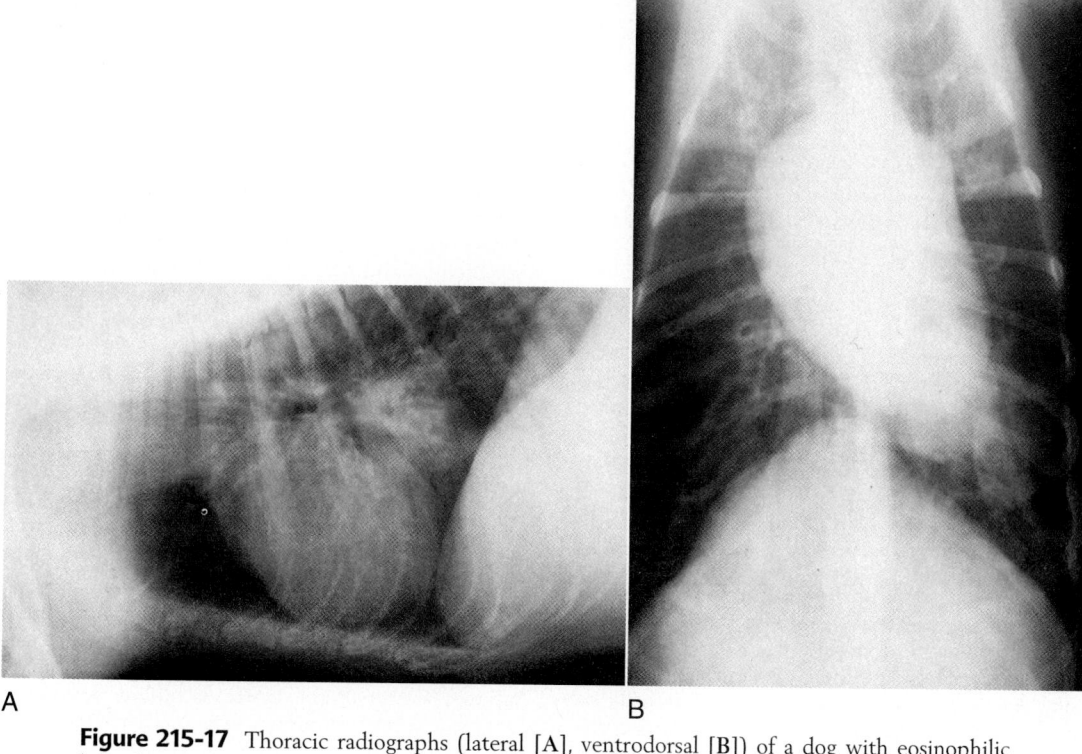

A

B

Figure 215-17 Thoracic radiographs (lateral [A], ventrodorsal [B]) of a dog with eosinophilic broncho-pneumopathy. Note the pronounced interstitial and peribronchiolar markings.

Occasionally, dogs may also exhibit lethargy and anorexia. Physical examination abnormalities are typically confined to the respiratory tract with evidence of nasal discharge, crackles, wheezes or generalized increase in lung sounds heard during thoracic auscultation. Auscultation can be normal in some dogs. Radiographically, EB is characterized by a variety of changes including diffuse bronchointerstitial, alveolar, peribronchiolar, or some combination of these patterns (Figure 215-17); bronchiectasis may be a feature of some chronically affected dogs. There are no pathognomonic laboratory abnormalities, and peripheral eosinophilia, although common, is not present in all dogs.

The diagnosis of EB is established by ruling out other causes of eosinophilic parenchymal disease such as respiratory or migrating parasites, bacterial or fungal respiratory infections, heartworm, and neoplasia. Thus fecal floats or Baermann examinations, heartworm testing, culture of respiratory washes or lavages, and bronchoscopic and cytologic examination of the respiratory tract all have a role in the diagnostic approach to EB. Bronchoscopic examination often shows evidence of green to green-yellow mucus adhered to airway walls or obstructing small airways (Figure 215-18). Airway mucosa may be thick to polypoid in appearance, and there may be airway collapse. Cytologic examination of material retrieved by transtracheal wash, bronchoalveolar lavage, or mucosal brushing typically reveals large numbers of eosinophils, but neutrophils and macrophages are also common inflammatory cells. Most dogs will have negative cultures for bacteria, but the role of bacteria in the disease in culture-positive dogs is not well defined.

Administration of glucocorticoids at immunosuppressive dosages is the mainstay of therapy for EB, with treatment

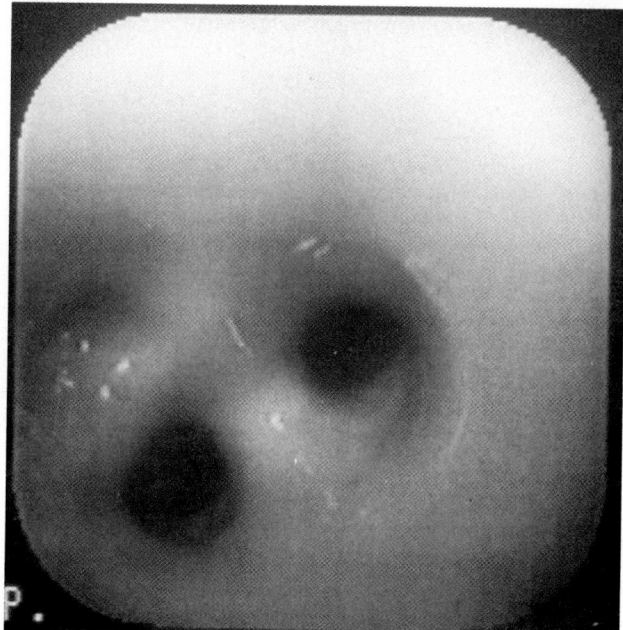

Figure 215-18 Bronchoscopic image obtained during examination of the dog in Figure 215-17 showing airways partially occluded with eosinophilic exudate.

lasting weeks to months in most dogs. Many dogs can be maintained on lower doses once the inflammation is controlled, and many can also become steroid-independent. Allergy testing and hyposensitization have been attempted with limited success in reported dogs[68] but could still be a consideration to help lower glucocorticoid doses. The prognosis is generally good with adequate therapy given for appropriate lengths of time.

Eosinophilic granulomatosus, primarily a disease of dogs, is characterized by parenchymal infiltration with eosinophils. Unlike EB, the infiltrates of eosinophilic granulomatosis have a tendency to form distinct nodules or mass-like lesions, and the radiographic appearance is thus similar to that seen in patients with systemic fungal infections or pulmonary neoplasia (see above). Clinical signs include dyspnea and cough most commonly; affected patients may also exhibit anorexia, lethargy, and weight loss. Physical examination abnormalities can include abnormal lung sounds and fever. There are no pathognomonic laboratory features, and like EB, eosinophilia is often present, but can be absent in affected dogs. Thoracic radiographic abnormalities include pulmonary nodules of various sizes and numbers, hilar lymph node enlargement, and mixes of other patterns.[69] Some, but not all dogs with EB, will have evidence of heartworm infection.[70]

Vasculitides

Inflammatory vascular diseases of the lung are uncommon in dogs and cats. Reported cases have been associated with lymphoid granulomatosis and systemic-lupus erythematosis. Some patients have presumed pulmonary vasculitis for which a cause is not discovered, but which respond clinically to administration of immunosuppressive doses of glucocorticoids.[64] Clinical features of affected animals have been coughing, interstitial patterns on thoracic radiographs, and granulomatous inflammation on respiratory washes. Other differentials for

such patients include infectious or parasitic diseases that can have a vascular component (Rocky Mountain Spotted fever, FIP, heartworm), systemic fungal infections and neoplasia. Vasculitis has also been incriminated, though not proven, as a cause of thoracic radiograph abnormalities in dogs with leptosporosis.[71] Diagnosis is made by exclusion of other causes of clinical signs and radiographic lesions and by histopathology.

Cystic-Bullous Lung Disease

Cystic-bullous lung disease is characterized by circumscribed regions of air or fluid occurring in the lung parenchyma. These lesions form as a result of cysts, bullae, or pneumatoceles. Cysts are fluid or air-filled lesions surrounded by respiratory epithelium and may be congenital or acquired.[72,73] Bullae are large areas of air accumulation formed by the loss of alveolar walls.[72,74,75] Pneumatoceles result from air entry into a necrotic lesion such as an abscess, granuloma, or tumor.

Bullae may occur as a result of emphysema (bullous emphysema), inflammation, trauma, or appear idiopathically. Emphysema results from enlargement and destruction of bronchial and alveolar walls due to obstructive pulmonary disease, such as some forms of chronic bronchitis.[76] The loss of radial traction on airway walls provided by alveoli contributes to airway collapse; alveoli may fill with air during inspiration, but negative intrathoracic pressures generated during expiration impair alveolar emptying from airway collapse. Collagen defects may predispose some animals to the formation of these lesions.[76] *Paragonimus kellicotti* (the lung fluke) can cause bullae and granuloma/pneumatocele formation in dogs and cats (see above).[77] Any of the cystic or bullous lesions may rupture creating a pneumothorax (Figure 215-19). Depending upon the number and severity of lesions, large amounts of functional lung parenchyma may be lost. Large lesions may also compress airways.

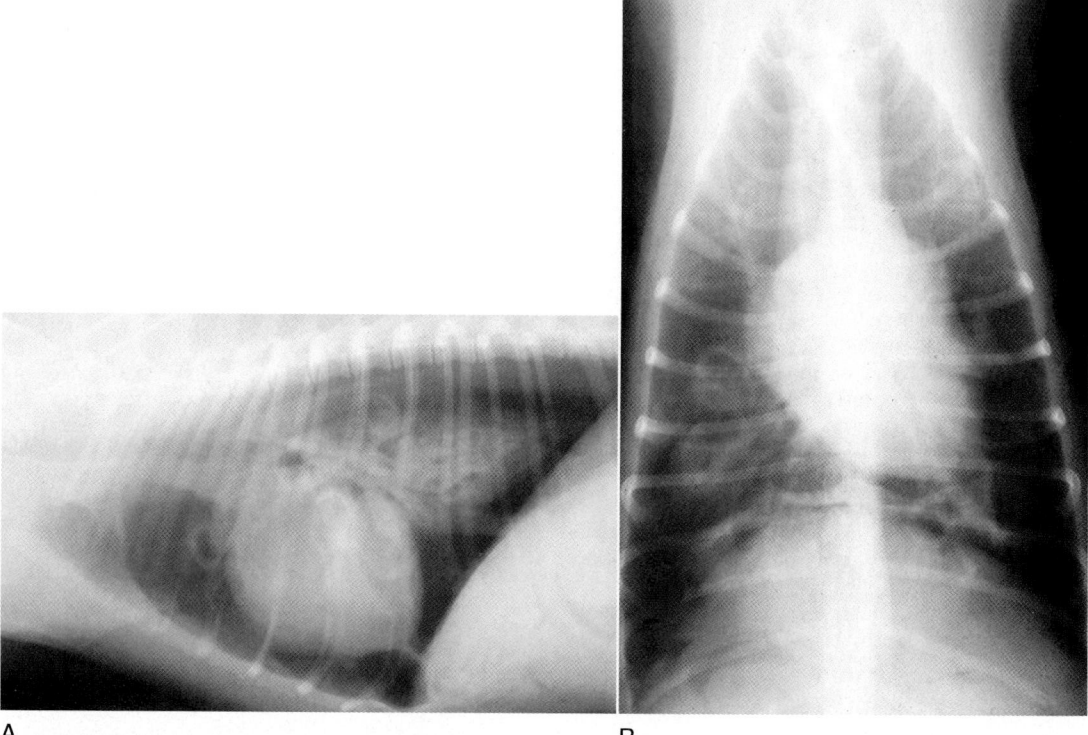

A   B

Figure 215-19 Thoracic radiographs (lateral [A], ventrodorsal [B]) of a dog with pneumothorax likely caused by rupture of a bulla. Multiple bullae remain evident in these projections. This dog had *P. kellicotti* infection.

Presentation

Symptoms and clinical complaints may relate to the primary disease processes such as chronic bronchitis or traumatic insult. Acute respiratory distress and tachypnea can occur when cysts or bullae rupture, which creates a pneumothorax. Occasionally, cystic-bullous lung disease is an incidental finding on thoracic radiographs in an animal with no clinical signs of respiratory disease.

Diagnostic Evaluation

Thoracic radiographs may reveal solitary nodules or the margins of cavitary lesions in the peripheral lung regions. Initially, these lesions may be obscured by soft tissue opacity related to primary disease processes, or by pneumothorax causing collapse of the lung tissue. Pneumothorax is commonly identified if a cavitary lesion has ruptured. Unfortunately, bullous emphysema is rarely as readily apparent per thoracic radiography as it often is during exploratory thoracotomy. Cytology from any specimens obtained via thoracocentesis (for fluid or air) may be helpful as *Paragonimus* ova might be found. Aspiration of a bullous lesion is not recommended due to the risk of inducing pneumothorax. Thoracotomy, excision, and histopathology can be required for definitive diagnosis and may also provide therapeutic benefits.

Treatment and Prognosis

Identification and treatment of acute pneumothorax is crucial (see Chapter 217). Surgical exploration and removal of cavitary lesions may be warranted in patients in which leakage of air into the pleural cavity persists in the face of conservative management (thoracocentesis or thoracostomy tubes), or for patients with recurrent episodes of pneumothorax. Removal of localized lesions carries the best long-term prognosis. Bullous emphysematous disease is difficult to correct surgically, as the bulla are numerous and the disorder is typically progressive. Pleurodesis may be considered to reduce episodes of pneumothorax.[75,76] Even though recurrence of lesions is common, survival postsurgery of greater than two years is reported.[76] When identified, successful treatment of underlying diseases, such as chronic bronchial disease or lung flukes, carries the greatest likelihood of resolution. Thoracic radiographs should be monitored frequently for the recurrence of bulla or cysts. If bullae are found radiographically, treatment is generally not advised unless the animal becomes symptomatic, for example develops pneumothorax.

TRAUMATIC LUNG DISEASE

Pulmonary Contusions

Pulmonary contusions are hemorrhages into the pulmonary parenchyma, most often caused by blunt thoracic trauma. Pulmonary contusions occur frequently in animals struck by motorized vehicles. Pulmonary hemorrhage can occur even when external thoracic damage is not detected. Hemorrhage occurs from traumatic rupture of parenchymal vessels with bleeding into the interstitium and alveoli in the region of the insult. Flooding of large regions of alveoli with blood impairs normal gas exchange and may result in clinical signs.

Presentation

Acute tachypnea and respiratory distress may be noted with severe contusions. Tachypnea may also be the result of pain, pneumothorax, or cardiovascular shock, which are common in acute trauma patients. Crackles may be ausculted over the contused area. Decreased lung sounds are suggestive of lung consolidation or pleural space disease such as effusion or diaphragmatic herniation. Some patients have minimal clinical symptoms if only mild hemorrhage has occurred.

Diagnostic Evaluation

History and physical examination abnormalities, such as fractures or abrasions, may suggest a traumatic episode. Thoracic radiographs typically reveal regional, irregular patches of mixed interstitial-alveolar densities. However, radiographic changes may be delayed for up to 24 hours following trauma. Pneumothorax, lung consolidation, or rib fractures can sometimes be identified on thoracic radiographs.[78] Contra-coup radiographic signs may occur as a result of trauma to the opposite side of thoracic wall. The lung is violently moved across the thorax, injuring the lung opposite to the stricken side. Arterial blood gas results will often show hypoxemia, which may be worsened by hypoventilation if there are injuries to the thoracic bellows (ribs, intercostal muscles, diaphragm). Traumatic myocarditis is often concurrently found in thoracic trauma cases.[79] The ECG may reveal occasional to very frequent ventricular premature contractions or sustained ventricular tachycardia.

Treatment

When indicated by clinical signs or results of arterial blood gas analysis, oxygen supplementation can be provided with nasal catheters, face mask, oxygen cage, or other strategies. Ventilatory support may be needed if hypoventilation contributes to hypoxemia. Specific treatment for the contusions is not usually necessary. Treatment for the other trauma-related problems, for example, blood loss or circulatory shock, is often more critical. Antibiotics are recommended for patients with penetrating chest wounds but not for routine prophylaxis of animals with contusions only.[80] Serial thoracic radiographs should be evaluated for the resolution of abnormalities.

Prognosis

Prognosis is excellent for recovery from pulmonary contusions, provided that other injuries sustained are stabilized and fluid therapy is monitored carefully. Improvement is usually noted within 24 to 48 hours. Secondary complications such as abscesses, lung consolidation, or the formation of cavitary lesions may occur but are unusual.

Aspiration Pneumonia

Inhalation of fluid or gastric contents, and bacteria from the oropharynx often results in profound pulmonary inflammation. Aspiration pneumonia can present as an acute fulminant illness, or a chronic and insidious process. The materials usually aspirated are acidic stomach contents and food.

Normal laryngeal and pharyngeal function typically prevent aspiration; however, certain diseases may alter normal laryngeal-pharyngeal function and predispose to aspiration events. Local or systemic neuromuscular disease, irritation and inflammation of the oropharynx secondary to chronic reflux or regurgitation (i.e., megaesophagus, esophageal obstruction, esophagitis, chronic vomiting), and anesthesia or depressed mental states resulting in prolonged recumbancy and reflux, are common causes of aspiration pneumonia.[78,81] Impaired oropharyngeal function and secondary aspiration has also been associated with brachycephalic airway conformation.[78,81] Aspiration pneumonia is a frequent complication of surgery for repair of laryngeal paralysis.[82] Accidental introduction of medications, food or contrast agents into the trachea, or lack of patient cooperation during administration of such products, can also result in aspiration pneumonia (Figure 215-20). Administration of mineral oil or similar agents by owners to prevent hair balls in cats is a particularly dangerous cause of inhalation pneumonia.

The severity of lung injury is related to various factors such as the volume of the aspirate, the pH of the aspirate (acidic stomach contents are especially damaging), and toxicity related to any particulate matter. Aspirated material may

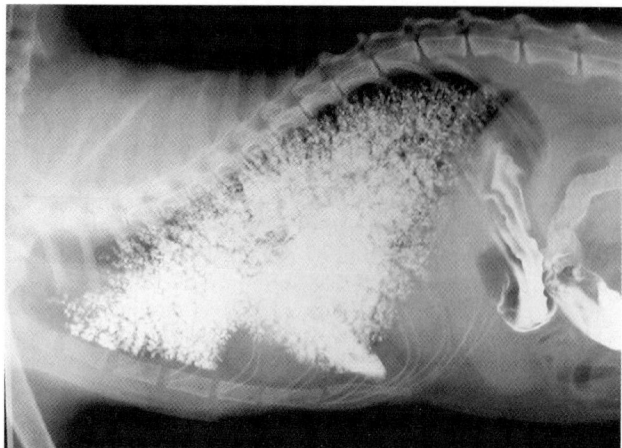

Figure 215-20 Lateral thoracic radiograph of a cat with severe barium aspiration.

cause several reactions. Obstruction and collapse of alveoli, pulmonary hemorrhage and edema, influx of inflammatory cells, necrosis of airway epithelial cells, and reactive bronchoconstriction are common sequels to aspiration. Infection frequently develops due to aspiration of oropharyngeal bacteria or impairment of pulmonary defense mechanisms from lung injury (see Bacterial Pneumonia).[78,81]

Presentation

Patients are usually evaluated for an acute onset of respiratory distress, tachypnea, and cough, although some animals will die acutely from airway obstruction. There may be a sudden onset of coughing prior to respiratory distress. Some patients are evaluated for chronic, progressive respiratory signs. Systemic signs such as fever, inappetence, lethargy, and shock are common. Inspiratory and expiratory crackles and wheezes are usually ausculted in the cranioventral lung lobes. Cats are especially prone to wheezes from bronchospasm secondary to airway inflammation.

Diagnostic Evaluation

A history of chronic vomiting, regurgitation, or medication administration that precedes the development of respiratory signs allows a presumptive diagnosis. Thoracic radiographs may support the diagnosis. Pulmonary opacities may be diffuse or focal, interstitial to alveolar. Increased alveolar opacities and consolidated regions are more common in the cranioventral and middle lung lobes (dependent areas) but can occur in any lung lobe, depending on the nature of the material aspirated and the position of the patient during the aspiration event. Nodular opacities may be noted in chronic cases or cases in which large solid particles have been aspirated. A miliary nodular pattern may be found in animals that have aspirated mineral oil mimicking neoplastic, fungal or parasitic disease. Depending on the material aspirated, evidence of aspiration may be inapparent initially on thoracic radiographs, but then pulmonary opacities develop over the ensuing 24 hours.

Respiratory secretions obtained by bronchoalveolar lavage or transtracheal wash are warranted in most patients and should be evaluated for cytology and submitted for microbial culture and sensitivity. Transthoracic aspirates may also be helpful, particularly when consolidated lesions are noted on thoracic radiographs. Cytology is typically characterized by a predominance of neutrophils and some hemorrhage. Bacteria may or may not be present. Particulate matter (e.g., food) may be found in the wash materials. Bronchoscopy may be performed to examine airways and remove large pieces of foreign material.

A complete blood count often reveals an inflammatory leukogram. Blood gas measurements and electrolytes may be helpful in emergency management. Once the patient is stabilized, investigation for an underlying cause of aspiration should be sought.

Treatment

Patients presenting in respiratory distress will need immediate measures to improve pulmonary function. Oxygen may be administered via nasal cannula, face mask, or oxygen cage.

Intubation and positive pressure ventilation may be necessary to overcome severely increased lung compliance, which increases the work of respiration. Fluid therapy is often indicated to treat a shock-like state. Vascular volume, blood pressure, and pulmonary function should be carefully monitored. Respiratory compromise, due to exacerbation of pulmonary edema from increased pulmonary capillary permeability induced by inflammation in response to aspiration, may be worsened by aggressive fluid therapy. Bronchodilators may be beneficial in the acute management of patients with bronchospasm. Methylxanthines such as theophylline may be helpful to relax bronchioles, enhance mucociliary clearance, and decrease respiratory muscle fatigue.[83]

The use of corticosteroids in the management of aspiration pneumonia is controversial. Corticosteroids may be indicated in the deteriorating patient for treatment of shock. Corticosteroids decrease the inflammatory response and stabilize cell membranes but can also inhibit normal lung protective mechanisms. If given, routine use should not be continued for longer than 24 to 48 hours. There is no evidence in people to support prophylactic use of antibiotics in patients with aspiration pneumonia as aspirated gastric contents are typically sterile.[84] Although secondary bacterial infection is common, the development of resistant infections may be encouraged if antibiotics are used initially.[84] The benefits of prophylactic antibiotics must be weighed against their potential risks. Antibiotic therapy ideally should be administered according to cytology or culture results obtained from wash or aspirate specimens. Attentive monitoring and serial radiographic, cytologic, and microbiologic analysis may be needed for some patients, particularly those with protracted illness or that exhibit clinical deterioration.

Measures should be taken to prevent further aspiration. Endotracheal intubation may be necessary to protect the airway if the patient is anesthetized or has an altered state of consciousness. Feeding tubes may need to be repositioned, or nasogastric or gastric tubes may need to be placed to facilitate removal of large volumes of gastrointestinal secretions. Institution of "upright" feeding for patients with esophageal or pharyngeal disorders may be beneficial, as may feeding through gastrostomy tubes.

Prognosis

Prognosis can vary widely depending upon the condition of the animal, the severity of lung injury, and the underlying cause of aspiration. Animals that aspirate a small amount of barium or mineral oil may have an excellent prognosis. Long-term complications may occur with aspiration pneumonia such as lung abscess, granuloma formation, or consolidation of lobes. Lung lobectomy may be indicated in these cases to eliminate sources of persistent or recurrent infections.

Near Drowning

Near drowning occurs with aspiration of water during submersion. Normal reflexes and input from higher neurologic centers cause cessation of ventilation under water; however, increased levels of carbon dioxide in the bloodstream eventually stimulate breathing efforts. Typically, only small volumes of water are typically aspirated resulting in severe pulmonary damage.

Many mechanisms contribute to lung injury.[85,86] Aspiration of water dilutes surfactant, collapses alveoli, decreases lung compliance, and severely impairs oxygenation. Near drowning from inhalation of salt water exacerbates fluid flux into alveoli due to the hypertonicity of the solution.[85,86]

Laryngospasm occurs in about 10% of cases and prevents aspiration of water and "dry drowning" results.[85,86] Aspiration of bacteria or chemicals in the water or vomitus, may contribute further to pulmonary parenchymal injury and predispose to secondary pneumonia. Severe hypoxia may cause profound neurologic disturbances from cerebral edema or herniation. ARDS (see discussion below) can occur up to 24 to 48 hours after a near drowning episode.[85-87]

Presentation

Patients are classically presented following a rescue. A loss of consciousness and severe respiratory distress or arrest is typical. Cardiovascular shock and hypothermia are commonly noted and require prompt attention. Auscultation may reveal inspiratory and expiratory crackles and wheezes, or exceptionally quiet lung sounds may be noted. Neurologic abnormalities and altered mentation may signify cerebral edema.

Diagnostic Evaluation

Diagnosis is based on the history of rescuing the patient from the water. Thoracic radiographs reveal a generalized, mixed interstitial-alveolar pulmonary pattern. Radiographic changes may not be apparent until 24 to 48 hours after the near-drowning episode. The presence of radio-opaque material in the airways (sand bronchograms) is a poor prognostic indicator.[86] Bronchial wash and cultures are indicated if there is suspicion of secondary bacterial infection.

Treatment

Ventilation is provided as soon as possible. CPR or mouth-to-muzzle resuscitation may be required during initial rescue. The Heimlich maneuver is not recommended due to the possibility of aspiration of stomach contents.[87] As soon as available, oxygen may be provided with a nasal cannula, face mask, or oxygen cage. Positive pressure ventilation is often required due to the profound decrease in lung compliance. If neurologic symptoms are present after metabolic stabilization, treatment for cerebral edema may be warranted (see Chapter 191). Animals that have been resuscitated should be observed in the hospital for up to 24 hours for the development of ARDS. Respiratory function and metabolic and neurologic status are followed closely.

Prognosis and Prevention

A poor prognosis is associated with coma, blood pH less than 7.0, the need for a CPR episode, and mechanical ventilation.[87] Educating clients as to the risks of allowing young dogs near the water is especially important; one study revealed that half the dogs presented for near drowning were 4 months old or younger.[87] Cold water and rapid currents are particularly exhausting.

Smoke Inhalation

Smoke inhalation causes direct injury to the airways and lung tissue due to heat, particulate matter, and combustion gases. Household fires are the most common cause of smoke inhalation injury in dogs and cats. A compounding factor in the pathogenesis of smoke inhalation is the secondary injury that occurs from the release of pulmonary inflammatory mediators.

In the acute phase (0 to 36 hours) of smoke inhalation, respiratory signs are caused by tissue injury, increased capillary permeability, mucosal edema, and tissue hypoxia. By 2 to 4 days post-injury, tissue edema begins to resolve. During this later phase, there is an increase in mucosal secretions, sloughing of epithelial cells, decreased mucociliary clearance, and secondary bacterial colonization leading to tracheobronchitis and pneumonia.[88] If thermal injury occurs, lesions are usually found rostral to the vocal cords because dry air has low heat carrying capacity. Carbon particulate matter can attach to airway surfaces, which results in impaired mucociliary function and contributes to bronchospasm. Numerous compounds of the gaseous by-products of combustion, when inhaled, are responsible for chemical injury, which contributes more to lung injury than does thermal injury.[88,89] Carbon monoxide inhibits oxygen binding to hemoglobin, reducing oxygen uptake in red blood cells, which results in severe tissue hypoxia. Hydrogen cyanide, hydrogen chloride, and aldehydes are irritants that cause profound airway edema and bronchospasm. In addition, hydrogen cyanide interferes with cellular aerobic metabolism compounding tissue hypoxia. Anaerobic metabolism and the generation of lactate and metabolic acidosis ensues.[90]

Presentation

Patients are classically presented following a rescue. Animals may have singed hair, and the presence of soot and smell of smoke on the fur. A loss of consciousness, and severe respiratory distress or arrest is common. Upper airway stridor may be heard in patients with laryngeal edema. Ocular and nasal discharge, and corneal edema are often present. Mucous membranes may be bright red due to carboxyhemoglobin, or cyanotic. Some patients have minimal signs on presentation but may develop severe respiratory compromise 24 to 36 hours later due to laryngeal edema, release of inflammatory mediators, decreased mucociliary function, infection or ARDS.[90]

Diagnostic Evaluation

Thoracic radiographs may be normal initially but can progress to a patchy interstitial pattern and alveolar pattern. These changes correlate with the development of pulmonary edema and pneumonia. Likewise, arterial blood gas analysis may be normal in the acute phase of injury, but PaO_2 levels will drop as pulmonary injury progresses. PaO_2 must be interpreted cautiously in animals with carbon monoxide poisoning, as PaO_2 is a measure of the amount of oxygen dissolved in plasma. In patients with carbon monoxide poisoning, PaO_2 may be normal, but the patient may still manifest severe arterial hypoxemia because carbon monoxide interferes with oxygen saturation of hemoglogin decreasing the total carrying capacity of oxygen. It is important to remember that carboxyhemoglobin is not distinguished from oxyhemoglobin with pulse oximetry, which could give a falsely high impression of the degree of hemoglobin saturation.

Assessment of carbon monoxide toxicity can be accomplished using a co-oximeter, available at most human hospitals, to measure blood carboxyhemoglobin levels.[90] In the early stages of smoke inhalation, cytology from bronchial washings, and hemograms and biochemical profiles are unremarkable. These tests may become useful in chronically managed cases to screen for secondary bacterial infections and metabolic complications. Cardiac and neurologic status should also be carefully monitored in critical patients.

Treatment

As stated earlier, animals that are rescued from fire should be observed for at least 24 to 48 hours for progressive pulmonary injury. Patients that present with severe laryngeal edema and obstruction may require tracheostomies. Oxygen supplementation should begin as soon as possible. Carbon monoxide is eliminated by the lungs and elimination is greatly facilitated by 100% oxygen administration. The half-life of carboxyhemoglobin is 4 hours in room air and 30 minutes in 100% oxygen. Oxygen should be administered until blood carboxyhemoglobin concentrations are less than 10%.[90] Positive pressure ventilation may be required in critical cases. Airway humidification and physiotherapy (chest coupage) may also be warranted.

Bronchodilators are sometimes used in the management of smoke inhalation. Ideally, antibiotic therapy should be based on documentation of infection by culture and sensitivity testing. Prophylactic therapy is generally not recommended because of predisposition to resistant infections.[90] Corticosteriods may be indicated in cases of acute cardiovascular shock; however, routine administration should be avoided due to their interference with tissue healing and protective mechanisms.

Fluid therapy is often indicated to restore lost circulatory volume and maintain tissue perfusion. Crystalloid or colloid solutions may be necessary to combat shock. If the animal has also suffered surface burns, aggressive fluid therapy will be needed. Fluids are administered with caution to smoke inhalation patients because pulmonary capillary leakage will predispose to pulmonary edema and worsening of respiratory function. Analgesics are indicated particularly if cutaneous burns coexist with smoke inhalation injury.

Prognosis

The prognosis ranges from good to grave depending upon the severity of the inhalant injury. In a study of 27 dogs with smoke exposure, 17 out of 17 dogs that had improvement or no change in respiratory signs during the first 24 to 48 hours after exposure were discharged from the hospital.[91] In this same study, dogs with deterioration in signs in the 24- to 48-hour period after hospitalization died or had prolonged stays in the hospital. The prognosis progressively worsens with severe respiratory disease requiring positive-pressure ventilation, the presence of neurologic signs, and cutaneous burns. Infection (pneumonia) and sepsis are common causes of death.

IDIOPATHIC AND MISCELLANEOUS LUNG DISORDERS

Acute Respiratory Distress Syndrome

Acute respiratory distress syndrome (ARDS) causes acute hypoxemic respiratory failure as a result of lung injury and increased pulmonary capillary permeability. ARDS is not a disease entity by itself, but rather a syndrome that develops secondary to numerous, usually critical, illnesses. Sepsis is the most common cause of ARDS in people, and has been identified as a common cause of ARDS in dogs.[8,92] Other well-described associations include aspiration of acidic substances (e.g., gastric secretions) or inhalation injury, multiple transfusions, shock, pancreatitis, microbial pneumonia, drug reaction or overdose, and major trauma or surgery.[8,92-95]

Although ARDS is a well-described syndrome, particularly in people, the pathogenesis of the syndrome is still poorly understood. Exudation of proteinaceous fluid into the interstitum in the early phase of ARDS occurs as a result of increased capillary permeability from either direct or indirect injury to the alveolar epithelium or pulmonary capillary endothelium.[96] The inflammatory response that accompanies such injuries can involve all lung parenchyma. In the later phases of ARDS (7 to 10 days post insult), increased numbers of inflammatory cells, hyaline membrane formation, and fibrosis with increased dead-space fraction are characteristic.[9,92] Severe hypoxemia that is characteristically refractory to oxygen supplementation is typical due to arteriovenous shunting and ventilation/perfusion irregularities. Pulmonary hypertension occurs as a result of hypoxic vasoconstriction and capillary obstruction from microembolization.[9]

Presentation

Most patients present with acute, severe respiratory distress and tachypnea within 24 hours of the precipitating cause, although delays of up to 3 days may occur. Tachycardia and extreme anxiety are commonly noted. Crackles and wheezes, particularly on end-inspiration and throughout expiration, are classically heard in the hilar and dorsocaudal lung fields. Sometimes lung sounds are quieter than normally expected, particularly if the patient is hypovolemic. There may be other physical examination abnormalities, such as fever or evidence of trauma, that reflect underlying causes.

Diagnostic Evaluation

ARDS is suspected when the patient demonstrates an onset of respiratory signs hours to days following a precipitating event. Thoracic radiographs usually reveal generalized interstitial or mixed patterns consistent with noncardiogenic pulmonary edema. Left cardiac and pulmonary venous silhouettes are typically normal unless another (cardiac) disorder is present (Figure 215-21).

Echocardiography is a noninvasive tool that may provide information to help differentiate ARDS from other causes of pulmonary edema. Echocardiography can rule out left atrial and ventricular abnormalities that could be associated with high-pressure (cardiogenic) pulmonary edema, which is a common differential diagnosis. Echocardiographic evidence of acute pulmonary hypertension may support a diagnosis of ARDS. Expected findings include a poorly contracting right ventricle, tricuspid regurgitation (TR), which is often present secondary to acute geometric changes of the right chambers (dilation), and elevations in right ventricular systolic pressures. Tricuspid regurgitation velocities can estimate right ventricular systolic pressure, and thus pulmonary arterial systolic pressure, which is increased in ARDS. Leftward shifting of the interventricular septum is sometimes demonstrated. The main pulmonary artery may appear dilated. Pulmonary capillary wedge pressure, if measured, is low (<18 mm Hg) with ARDS, but elevated with cardiogenic pulmonary edema.

Edema fluid analysis may provide useful information in the early stages of ARDS. Fluid may be suctioned from the airways via tubing passed through an endotracheal tube. The ratio of protein content of the edema fluid (E) to the protein content in plasma (P) in ARDS is 79% to 90%, while the E/P ratio in cardiogenic edema is less than 50%.[97]

Treatment

The mainstay of ARDS treatment is addressing the underlying condition if known. Oxygen therapy is essential. Intubation and mechanical ventilation are quite appropriate and often needed for ARDS patients so that positive end-expiratory pressure (PEEP) can be delivered. PEEP can help prevent alveolar collapse in ARDS patient and relieves the patient of the work of respiration in the face of poorly compliant lungs. It also diminishes the need for high inspired oxygen concentrations to maintain acceptable levels of oxygen saturation, thus lowering the risk of oxygen toxicity.

A low-normal circulatory volume should be maintained with cautious fluid therapy. The smallest volume of fluids that maintains cardiac output and arterial blood pressure should be administered. Overzealous fluid therapy may worsen pulmonary edema and hypoxemia. A Swan-Ganz or other hemodynamic measuring catheter may be used to monitor cardiac output, and pulmonary capillary wedge and right heart pressures. Central venous pressures can be misleading as an estimate of volume status if significant pulmonary hypertension exists. Serial measures of arterial blood pressure, packed cell volume, total protein, electrolytes, BUN, and creatinine may be useful to monitor hydration status. Nutritional support and good nursing care, especially of recumbent animals, would also be crucial to successful therapy particularly for patients surviving the initial period of ARDS. Because of the demands these patients place on clinical staff, referral of these patients to tertiary care centers would be appropriate.

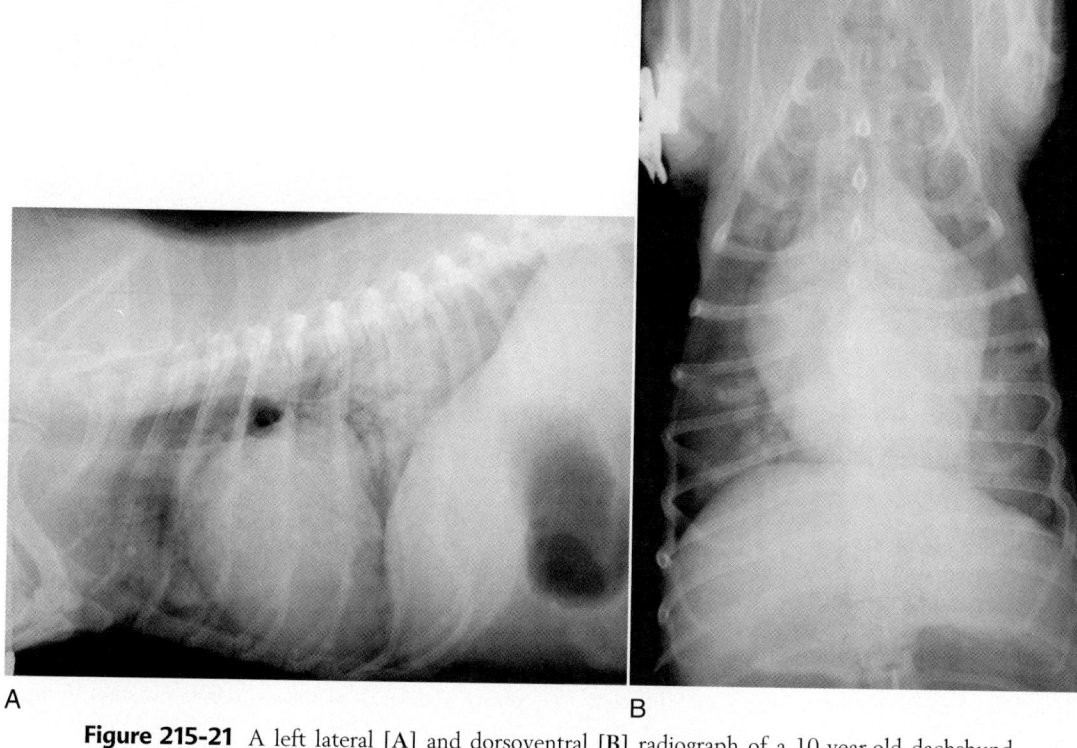

Figure 215-21 A left lateral [A] and dorsoventral [B] radiograph of a 10-year-old dachshund diagnosed with ARDS secondary to trauma. Note the severe, generalized interstitial opacities. This dog had a history of mitral valve endocardiosis, thus left-sided cardiomegaly is seen here. The pulmonary veins are not enlarged as would be expected with left-sided CHF and airway fluid aspiration revealed an E/P ratio of 86% consistent with ARDS. ARDS was confirmed on necropsy.

Corticosteriods are of unconfirmed benefit in ARDS patients. Diuretics may be helpful in the initial phase, but are of no benefit in the latter phase of ARDS (more than 5 to 7 days).[9,95] Careful attention to hydration status is required with diuretic therapy. Administration of nitric oxide as an endogenous mediator of vascular smooth muscle relaxation is under investigation.[97] Improvements in parameters of serial arterial blood gas analysis and thoracic radiographs may be helpful in the assessment of improving status.

Prognosis
ARDS patients typically progress rapidly and are notoriously fragile patients. Death can result from respiratory failure, or complications of ARDS and the underlying disease. The prognosis with severe or chronic ARDS (>3 days) is generally poor.

Lung Lobe Torsion
Lung lobe torsion is the rotation of a lung lobe around its long axis. The exact mechanism that results in increased mobility of a lung lobe is not known. Lung lobe torsion may be idiopathic, particularly in large, deep-chested breeds of dogs; however, toy breeds are sometimes affected.[44-46] Afghan hounds were overrepresented in one study.[98] Torsion can also be associated with several initiating events. Pleural effusion of various causes, thoracic surgery and manipulation of tissues, or trauma causing sudden lung lobe compression may predispose to rotation of a lung lobe.[72,99]

Rotation of the lung lobe at the hilus strangles the bronchus and vascular pedicle, which obstructs ventilation and venous drainage. Because the artery usually remains partially patent, progressive lobar engorgement with blood occurs and the lobe becomes an expansile mass. Increased hydrostatic

pressure (venous congestion) causes exudation of bloody fluid into the pleural space. Pleural effusion may further impair tidal volume and respiratory performance. Mild blood loss anemia can be observed. Necrosis, fibrosis, and shrinkage of the lung lobe may eventually occur.

Presentation
Clinical signs of pre-existing pulmonary or pleural space disease may be present in the history. Clinical signs caused by the torsion are usually acute and progressive. Respiratory distress, tachypnea and cough, with or without hemoptysis, are common presenting complaints. Other systemic signs, such as hypotension, collapse, or fever and lethargy may be present.

Diagnostic Evaluation
Signalment may provide helpful clues, as deep-chested breeds such as sight-hounds appear to have an increased incidence of idiopathic lung lobe torsion. Physical examination abnormalities are compatible with pleural effusion (see Chapters 1, 54, 57). The appearance of thoracic radiographs may vary depending upon the stage of the disease. Pleural effusion usually obscures parenchymal detail. The pleural effusion may be removed and the thorax reradiographed, at which time lobar consolidation is typically noted. Air bronchograms may occur early, but air is reabsorbed with prolonged collapse. Rounding of the lung lobe edges is noted as the lung becomes engorged. The bronchus may lie in an improper anatomic plane. Pleural fluid analysis is consistent with a hemorrhagic modified transudate (see Chapter 57). Underlying conditions may be suggested by other laboratory abnormalities, for example hypoproteinemia associated with protein-losing enteropathy resulting in pleural effusion. Bronchoscopy is sometimes

needed to verify rotation of the bronchus. Surgical exploration may be necessary to confirm the diagnosis in some cases. Histopathologic examination of the excised lung lobe should be performed to rule out underlying primary parenchymal disease such as pneumonia or neoplasia.

Treatment

Immediate improvement in tissue oxygenation is usually needed, thus supplemental oxygen is often indicated. Removal of excessive pleural fluid will enhance lung expansion and respiratory performance. Thoracostomy tubes may be warranted in some cases. Circulatory function can be supported with IV fluid therapy as needed to maintain hydration and systemic blood pressure. Surgical resection of the affected lobe is typically curative.

Prognosis

Prognosis is typically good with lobectomy, but underlying conditions may require additional therapy and monitoring. It has been suggested that the long-term prognosis may be poor in dogs that develop lung lobe torsions in association with chylothorax.[44]

Pulmonary Mineralization

Mineralization of the airways or pleura can occur in aged dogs of any breed and is often an incidental finding. Chondrodystrophic dogs may demonstrate airway mineralization at an earlier age.[47] Nodular pulmonary parenchymal mineralization of unknown etiology is occasionally misinterpreted as metastatic neoplasia. The nodules may be few or numerous and diffusely distributed (Figure 215-22). They are typically discrete and nonprogressive and are not associated with lung pathology.

Mineral opacities can also occur in areas of intense inflammation, or in necrotic lung lesions. The opacities usually occur in the center of mass lesions resulting from fungal infections, parasites, tuberculosis, or neoplastic disease.[100] Necrotic lymph nodes can also undergo mineralization and mineral-like opacities can be seen in regional lymph nodes from prior barium aspiration. Occasionally, systemic disease such as renal secondary hyperparathyroidism and hyperadrenocorticism can cause mineral deposition in lungs and other organs.

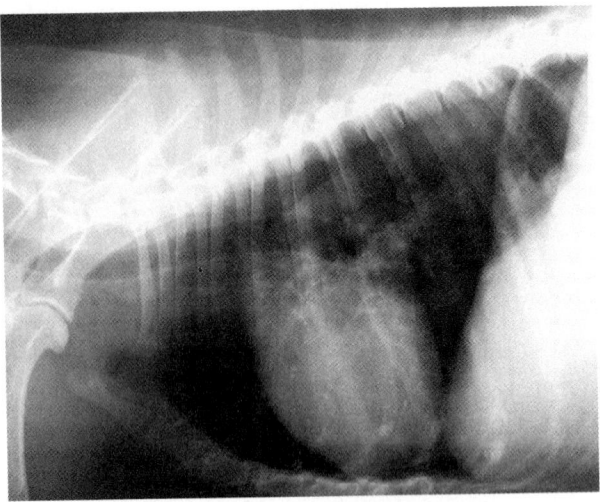

Figure 215-22 A right lateral radiograph of a dog with pulmonary mineralization. Note the multiple discrete opaque nodules, especially prominent over the cardiac silhouette.

Pulmonary Fibrosis

Interstitial lung diseases are poorly characterized in veterinary patients. Pathologically, interstitial fibrosis is characterized by alveolar septal fibrosis, interstitial fibrosis, epithelial hyperplasia, and focal calcification. Inflammation (lymphocytes and macrophages) is a variable finding.[101-103] In humans, these findings can be the result of numerous types of pulmonary injury; however, in over 50% of cases, no cause is identified.[101,102] The term *idiopathic pulmonary fibrosis* is often used to describe this disease in animals.

Idiopathic pulmonary fibrosis was first described in West Highland white terriers, but recent reports have suggested that other breeds of dogs may be affected, particularly Staffordshire bull terriers.[104-107] A form of idiopathic pulmonary fibrosis has now also been described in cats.[108] Dogs usually present with chronic and progressive pulmonary signs such as dyspnea

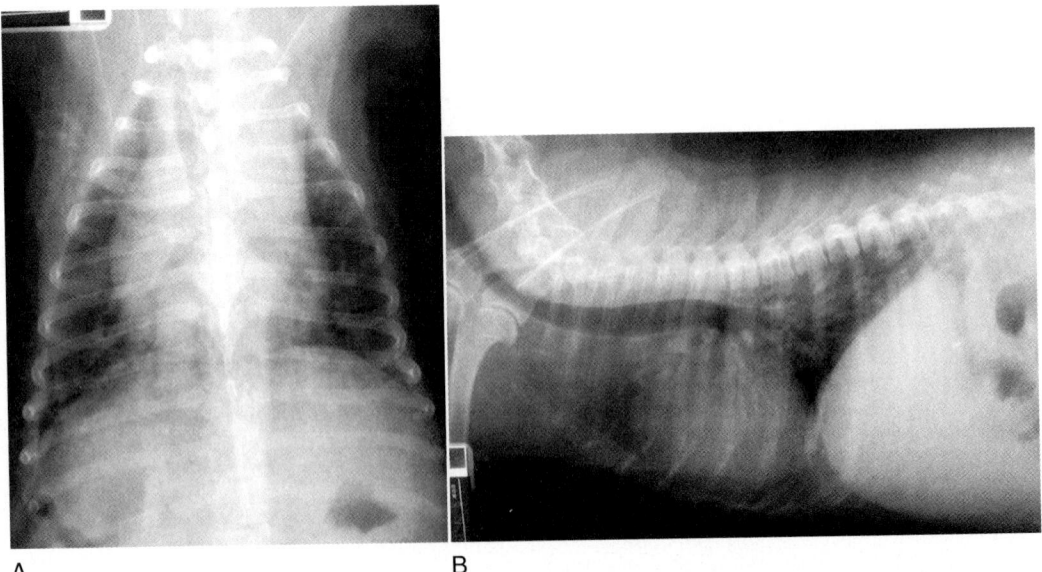

A   B

Figure 215-23 Left lateral [A] and dorsoventral [B] radiographs are shown of a 9-year-old West Highland White Terrier with idiopathic pulmonary fibrosis. Note the generalized bronchointerstitial pattern, especially prominent in the caudal lung regions. There is radiographic evidence of right heart enlargement and an enlarged caudal vena cava consistent with pulmonary hypertension.

and exercise intolerance. Cough is a variable finding.[104-107] Radiographically, there is a diffuse interstitial lung pattern with varying degrees of bronchial involvement (Figure 215-23).[104,106] Echocardiographic findings are usually indicative of moderate to severe pulmonary hypertension. A lung biopsy is generally necessary to confirm the diagnosis. The principal therapy for idiopathic pulmonary fibrosis is corticosteroids. Bronchodilators and azathioprine may be of benefit in some cases.[104,106] The prognosis for pulmonary fibrosis varies but is generally poor owing to the advanced nature of the disease at the time of diagnosis.

Obesity

Specific abnormalities of pulmonary function as a result of obesity have not been well characterized in veterinary patients. Increased oxygen consumption and myocardial work are noted in people with excess body mass with light activity. In humans, Pickwickian syndrome refers to a specific condition of obesity, lethargy, hypoventilation, and erythrocytosis. The syndrome is classically defined as elevations in $PaCO_2$ in the absence of pulmonary disease in patients who are extremely obese. A central neurological condition may be partially responsible for Pickwickian syndrome.[109] In addition, obesity is thought to worsen obstructive sleep apnea syndrome noted in humans and in English Bulldogs.[110, 111]

Excessive intrathoracic and intra-abdominal fat may interfere with lung function in numerous ways. Obese animals may have decreased thoracic wall compliance and thus have more difficulty expanding the thoracic cavity and lungs during inspiration. Hypoxia can result from decreased expansion and hypoventilation of peripheral lung regions.[109]

Increased intrathoracic fat has often been suspected to worsen airway collapse in veterinary patients with redundant dorsal tracheal membrane and associated clinical signs. Even though specific obesity-related pulmonary dysfunction has not been reported in dogs and cats, weight reduction in animals with chronic airway or pulmonary disease can dramatically affect clinical signs.

Lobar Consolidation

Lung lobe consolidation can occur as a result of many pulmonary diseases. Lobar consolidation is not a disease entity itself but may occur secondary to processes such as aspiration pneumonia, granulomatous disease, contusions, lung lobe torsion, and neoplasia.[112] Fluid, exudates, or cellular infiltrates fill the alveoli and airways, which creates a wedge-shaped, homogenous soft tissue opacity on radiographs. In the early stages, a regionally diffuse interstitial pattern or an alveolar pattern may be recognized. As the disease process spreads, lesions coalesce, and the entire lung lobe becomes involved. Radiographically, lobar consolidation appears as a soft tissue opacity with visible lung lobe margins (Figure 215-24).[112] Ventilation-perfusion abnormalities occur as blood flow persists through unventilated lung tissue. If treatment of the primary disorder does not resolve the consolidation, surgical excision of the lung lobe may be necessary.

Pulmonary Alveolar Proteinosis

Pulmonary alveolar proteinosis (PAP) is a rare disorder of dogs characterized by the accumulation of protein- and lipid-rich fluid in alveoli.[113] Clinical signs described include chronic exercise intolerance and cough. Thoracic radiographs are

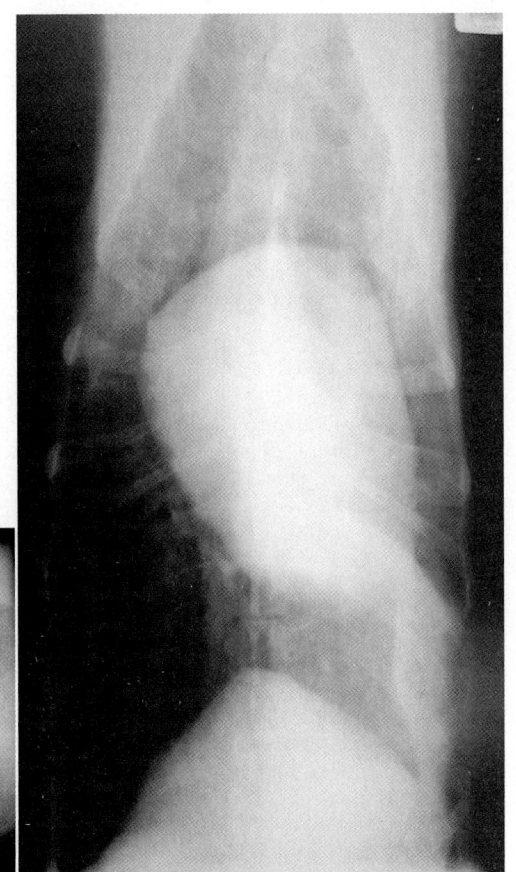

Figure 215-24 A right lateral [A] and ventrodorsal [B] radiograph of a greyhound revealing consolidation of the left caudal lung lobe. Note the wedge-shaped soft tissue opacity in the left caudal thorax on the VD view and the consolidated caudal lung opacity with air bronchograms on the lateral view. Also notice the enlarged, spherical hilar lymph node dorsal to the heart and airways on the lateral projection. This dog had coccidiomyocosis.

A   B

characterized by increased interstitial markings. Tracheal or alveolar wash samples contain few cells and moderate amounts of proteinaceous fluid. Histologic examination of lung biopsies shows distension of alveoli with PAS-positive proteinaceous material, mucus granules, and intra-alveolar cholesterol clefts with only occasional inflammatory cells. Treatment requires intermittent lavage of affected lung lobes with 0.9% saline; clinical resolution of the disease has been documented with such an approach.

Endogenous Lipid Pneumonia

Endogenous lipid pneumonia (EnLP) is an uncommon disease of dogs and cats and is usually secondary to another respiratory or systemic disease process that injures alveolar epithelial cells. In cats, the most common clinical signs are lethargy,

anorexia, and weight loss, which could reflect underlying diseases. Common signs referable to the respiratory tract include tachypnea, difficulty breathing, and cough.[114] Thoracic radiographic patterns associated with EnLP include pleural effusion, diffuse interstitial or bronchointerstitial markings, or pulmonary nodules. The cytologic features of the disease have not been well characterized. The most common underlying diseases associated with feline EnLP have been obstructive airway disease of various causes, or systemic diseases such as neoplasia, liver, kidney or heart disease, and pancreatitis. The diagnosis is not typically made antemortem, but is usually an incidental finding during necropsy, during which gross subpleural lesions are commonly found. Histologically, EnLP is characterized by alveoli filled with lipid-laden macrophages.

CHAPTER • 216

Mediastinal Disease

Lisa E. Moore
David S. Biller

ANATOMY

The mediastinum is a potential space centrally located between the right and left pleural cavities. The mediastinum is lined on each side by parietal pleura and contains and encloses the thymus, heart, aorta, trachea, esophagus, vagus nerves, lymph nodes, thoracic duct, vena cava, and other vessels and nerves that enter or leave the heart.[1] In the dog and cat, the tissue in the mediastinum is incomplete.[1,2] Therefore most unilateral pleural cavity diseases in the dog and cat ultimately become bilateral. The mediastinum is bordered dorsally by the spine, ventrally by the sternum, caudally by the diaphragm, and cranially by the thoracic inlet. The mediastinum also communicates cranially with facial planes of the neck and caudally with the retroperitoneal space through the aortic hiatus. These communications create pathways for spread of disease between the neck, thorax, and retroperitoneal areas.

Anatomic regions of the mediastinum can be subdivided to facilitate radiographic description of mediastinal disease. The mediastinum can be divided by frontal and transverse planes into five regions: craniodorsal, cranioventral, middle, caudodorsal, and caudoventral.

HISTORY AND CLINICAL SIGNS

The history and clinical signs will vary depending on the area of the mediastinum involved, the rapidity of onset, and the specific etiology of the disease process. Specific events that should prompt a clinician to consider mediastinal disease include trauma to the head, neck and/or thorax; foreign body ingestion; invasive diagnostic and/or therapeutic procedures that involve the trachea, esophagus, or cervical region. Clinical signs may include dysphagia, regurgitation, dyspnea, cough, and Horner's syndrome. Abnormal findings on physical examination that may indicate mediastinal involvement in the disease

process include poor compressibility of the cranial thorax, decreased lung sounds, dyspnea, esophageal or thoracic pain, and edema of the head and/or neck. If mediastinal disease is a component of systemic disease, extrathoracic signs of illness may also be present and include, but are not limited to, peripheral lymphadenopathy, weight loss, and polyuria/polydipsia.

DIAGNOSTIC EVALUATION

The mediastinum is not easily accessible for clinical evaluation due to its location within the thorax. Noninvasive evaluation is therefore dependent upon the utilization of appropriate imaging techniques. Invasive techniques for evaluation of the mediastinum may then be pursued if necessary.

Survey Radiography

The normal mediastinum is difficult to evaluate radiographically due to the lack of contrasting tissue densities. All mediastinal structures, with the exception of the air-filled trachea, demonstrate soft tissue opacity. This results in border effacement, which causes the structures within the mediastinum to appear confluent and prevents the structures from being visualized distinctly. The craniodorsal region is often more radiopaque than other areas of the mediastinum because of its greater thickness.

On dorsoventral (DV) and ventrodorsal (VD) projection radiographs, the craniodorsal and caudodorsal regions of the mediastinum appear as midline structures that are normally no more than two times the width of the spine. The craniodorsal region may appear wider in obese animals owing to accumulation of fat within in the mediastinum, but the boundaries remain smooth. The craniodorsal and cranioventral regions of the mediastinum are usually incompletely evaluated on DV or VD radiographs because of their superimposition on the sternum and spine. In young animals, the thymus may be visualized as a triangular, sail-shaped soft tissue dense structure in the cranioventral region along midline.

Survey radiography is the imaging modality of choice for localizing mediastinal disease. Survey radiography is used to assess the size, shape, opacity, and position of the mediastinum. Positional radiographs permit free fluid to move away from the mediastinum and may improve visualization of the mediastinum in animals with pleural effusion. Mediastinal disease can be seen radiographically as an abnormal position of the mediastinum (termed *mediastinal shift*), pneumomediastinum, or increased size and/or opacity of the mediastinum.

Abnormal positioning of the mediastinum is usually indicative of disease that originates in the lungs, bronchi, thoracic wall, or pleura. A mediastinal shift may result from the presence of an intrathoracic mass or from uneven inflation of the lungs associated with unilateral changes in lung volume. A mediastinal shift is identified by a difference in size between the right and left hemithoraces as assessed in a VD or DV view. In addition, lateral displacement of major mediastinal structures, such as the trachea or cardiac silhouette, may be apparent. Diaphragmatic asymmetry may also present with mediastinal shift.

Pneumomediastinum is characterized radiographically by visualization of mediastinal structures that are not normally seen, such as the esophagus and aorta, because the presence of air within the mediastinum provides excellent contrast to adjacent soft tissue structures (see Figure 216-1, *A*). Pneumomediastinum is usually not recognized on VD or DV radiographs. Pneumothorax, pulmonary overinflation, and deep-chested conformation in thin dogs can cause a radiographic appearance that may be mistaken for pneumomediastinum. Also, a gas-distended esophagus may drape over the trachea and rarely the great vessels, which creates a false impression of pneumomediastinum.

Increased mediastinal size is usually manifested radiographically as diffuse or focal widening of the mediastinum as assessed on a VD or DV view. Diffuse widening can be caused by mediastinal inflammation, hemorrhage, edema, or the accumulation of fluid within the mediastinum associated with pleural cavity disease. Positional radiography and ultrasonography are helpful in differentiating mediastinal fluid accumulation from other causes of diffuse mediastinal widening. Focal mediastinal widening is usually the result of a mass lesion. Pathologic widening of the mediastinum must be differentiated from diffuse widening caused by an accumulation of fat in obese animals. An accumulation of fat in the mediastinum is common in older dogs, especially brachycephalic breeds.

Contrast radiographic procedures are often helpful in further evaluation of structures within the mediastinum that cannot be adequately visualized on survey films. In the case of suspected esophageal perforation, the contrast medium of choice should be a water-soluble iodinated product.

Ultrasonography

Thoracic ultrasonography provides poor visualization of the normal mediastinum because air in adjacent lung lobes prevents transmission of the sound waves. Sonographic evaluation may provide useful information in animals with pleural effusion or cranial mediastinal disease.[3,4] Ultrasonography allows visualization of most cranial mediastinal masses. Very large masses can be imaged from almost any location in the craniolateral thoracic wall. Placing the transducer in a parasternal position or using the heart as an acoustic window may be necessary for adequate evaluation of smaller masses. Ultrasonography also helps define the internal architecture of masses as solid or cystic. In addition, ultrasonography allows localization of vascular structures relative to the mass. Although ultrasonography alone usually does not allow identification of the tissue of origin, it can be used to direct needle

placement for fine-needle aspirate (FNA) or tissue core biopsy.[3,5,6] Transesophageal ultrasonography provides excellent visualization of the heart base, major cranial mediastinal vessels, descending aorta, and part of the azygous vein.[7] Transesophageal ultrasonography eliminates imaging difficulties due to obesity, poor intercostal windows, and lung air interference.

Computed Tomography

Computed tomography (CT) provides the most detailed anatomic analysis of mediastinal structures.[8,9] It is valuable in defining the margins and size of mass lesions (see Figure 216-4, *C*) and can be used to guide placement of a needle or percutaneous biopsy instrument. Disadvantages of CT include an inability to distinguish mediastinal masses from adjacent collapsed lung lobes, limited availability in veterinary practice, and the need for anesthesia.

Further Diagnostic Evaluation

Thyroid scintigraphy using technetium 99m or iodine 131 can be used to identify ectopic or metastatic functional thyroid tissue within the mediastinum.[10,11] Technetium 99m sestamibi can be used for the detection of parathyroid secreting tissue, although the sensitivity and specificity of this method may be low.[12,13]

In humans, bronchoscopy with transbronchial needle aspiration of perihilar and other pulmonary masses has been shown to be useful in the diagnosis of various cancers.[14] Although not widely used nor reported in veterinary medicine, this technique holds promise in allowing relatively noninvasive needle aspiration of hilar and mediastinal lymph nodes. The author has performed this technique with no apparent complications.

Thoracoscopy is another technique that can be used to examine and biopsy mediastinal diseases and is a procedure that is becoming more commonly performed in veterinary medicine at referral practices and institutions.[15,16,17] Thoracoscopy allows examination of the parietal and visceral pleura, lungs, pericardium, and mediastinum. Biopsies and removal of diseased tissue can be performed with this minimally invasive technique.

DISEASES OF THE MEDIASTINUM

Pneumomediastinum

Pneumomediastinum is the presence of air within the mediastinum and can develop spontaneously, usually in animals with pre-existing respiratory disease, or as a result of damage to the esophagus, trachea, or lungs (Figure 216-1, *A*). This damage can be associated with cervical trauma, mechanical ventilation, transtracheal aspiration, tracheostomy, or central venous catheter placement.[18] Caudal extension of air from cervical fascial planes into the mediastinum and retroperitoneum may occur secondary to external trauma because of the normal communication between the mediastinum, retroperitoneum, and fascial planes of the neck (Figure 216-1, *B*). Bronchial or alveolar rupture with subsequent dissection of air along perivascular or peribronchial spaces to the pulmonary hilus and into the mediastinum is thought to be the mechanism by which pneumomediastinum occurs secondary to mechanical ventilation and pulmonary trauma.[19] A less common, iatrogenic cause of pneumomediastinum is secondary to tracheal rupture due to overdistention of the endotracheal tube cuff.[20] Severe pulmonary pathology or pre-existing respiratory disease can lead to bronchial or alveolar rupture with subsequent pneumomediastinum.

Pneumomediastinum does not occur secondary to pneumothorax. However, pneumothorax can be secondary to pneumomediastinum and is caused either by rupture of

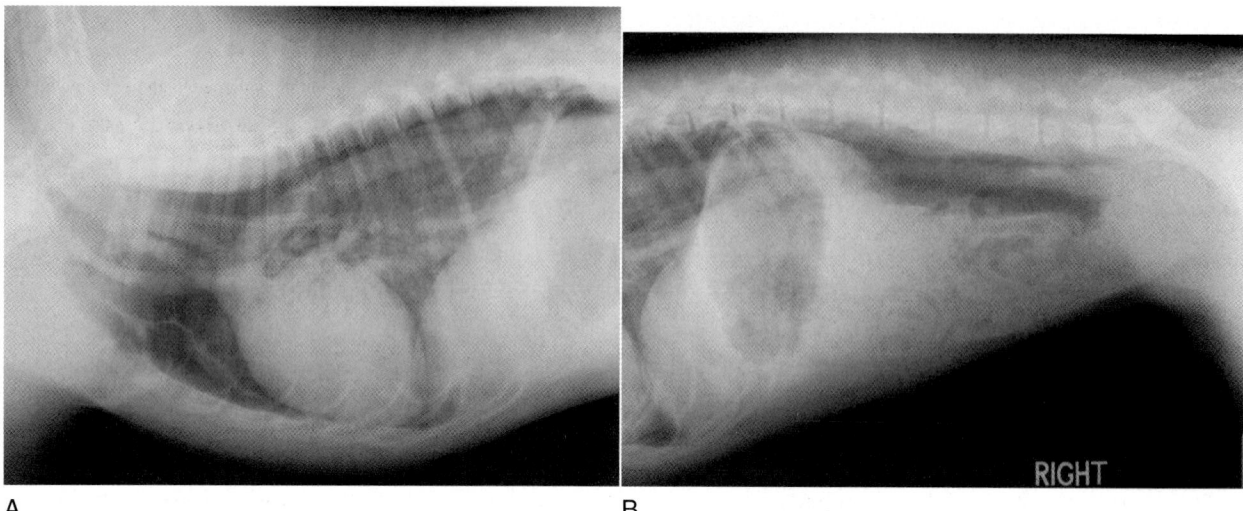

Figure 216-1 A, Lateral thoracic radiograph of a 9-month-old female Brittany Spaniel presented after being hit by a car. Numerous mediastinal structures, including the cranial vena cava, aorta, and serosal surface of the trachea, are well visualized as a result of pneumomediastinum. **B,** Lateral abdominal radiograph of the same dog. A large accumulation of air can be seen in the retroperitoneal space.

the mediastinal pleura, allowing mediastinal air to leak into the pleural space or by airway or alveolar rupture associated with underlying pulmonary disease that allows air to extend into the lung interstitium and diffuse into the mediastinum and pleural space. Subcutaneous emphysema and pneumoretroperitoneum may also occur secondary to pneumomediastinum.

Pneumomediastinum alone is usually not associated with clinical signs. If the pneumomediastinum progresses to pneumothorax, tachypnea and dyspnea are often seen. The presence of subcutaneous emphysema may be uncomfortable for the animal. Animals with pneumomediastinum associated with esophageal rupture will present with signs associated with esophageal disease, such as regurgitation, pain, and dysphagia. Acute development of severe pneumomediastinum may cause signs of circulatory collapse secondary to decreased venous return resulting from compression of the vena cava and azygous vein.

The air trapped within the mediastinum does not require treatment and will spontaneously resolve within 2 weeks if there is no ongoing source of air leakage. Concurrent subcutaneous emphysema does not usually require needle aspiration unless the volume is large enough to cause discomfort. Therapy should be aimed at resolution of any underlying disease process present.

Mediastinitis
Mediastinal inflammation is manifested radiographically as either focal or diffuse widening of the mediastinum. This may result from esophageal or tracheal perforation, deep cervical soft tissue infections extending along fascial planes into the mediastinum, or extension of infection from the pericardium, pulmonary parenchyma, or pleural space.[21,22,23,24] Chronic granulomatous mediastinitis may be caused by fungal organisms, such as *Histoplasma* or *Cryptococcus* spp., or bacterial organisms, such as *Actinomyces* or *Nocardia* spp.[24,25,26]

Mediastinitis has been documented secondary to spirocercosis in dogs.[27] Abscessation of the mediastinum may result from progression of chronic infectious or neoplastic mediastinal disorders.[23] Both mediastinal abscesses and granulomas typically appear on radiographs as mediastinal masses and thus may be mistaken for neoplasia.

Clinical signs associated with mediastinitis include tachypnea, likely related to thoracic pain, dyspnea, cough, head and/or neck edema, and regurgitation. Voice changes may occur secondary to recurrent laryngeal nerve involvement. Physical examination may reveal head and/or neck edema, tachypnea, dyspnea, fever, and decreased lung sounds if pneumothorax or pleural effusion are also present. Therapy involves resolving the underlying disorder. Esophageal perforation may require surgical repair and mediastinal masses may require surgical resection and/or drainage, along with appropriate antimicrobial therapy and supportive care.[23,26,28] Mediastinitis without a mass lesion may respond to antimicrobial therapy and supportive care alone. Thoracostomy tube placement may be necessary in animals with concurrent pyothorax or effusive mediastinitis.

Mediastinal Edema
Mediastinal edema can occur secondary to any disease that may result in edema in other areas of the body. The same pathophysiologic mechanisms apply. Although not recognized clinically very often, hypoproteinemia, lymphatic or venous obstruction, vasculitis, and heart failure may result in mediastinal edema. Edema in the mediastinum is often not clinically significant and may be overlooked due to accompanying pleural effusion.

Mediastinal Hemorrhage
Hemorrhage into the mediastinum usually results from either trauma or coagulopathy but also may be associated with neoplastic erosion of mediastinal vessels.[29,30] The clinical signs associated with mediastinal hemorrhage are related to the effects of acute blood loss. Dyspnea may occur if mediastinal hemorrhage progresses to hemothorax. Treatment is aimed at resolution of the underlying cause, such as plasma and Vitamin K_1 therapy for anticoagulant rodenticide intoxication, along with supportive care. If hemothorax due to coagulopathy or trauma is also present, auto-transfusion may be performed. Mild mediastinal hemorrhage usually does not need specific treatment.

Mediastinal Cysts
Benign cysts of pleural, branchial, lymphatic, bronchogenic, or thymic origin occur infrequently in the mediastinum.[31,32,33]

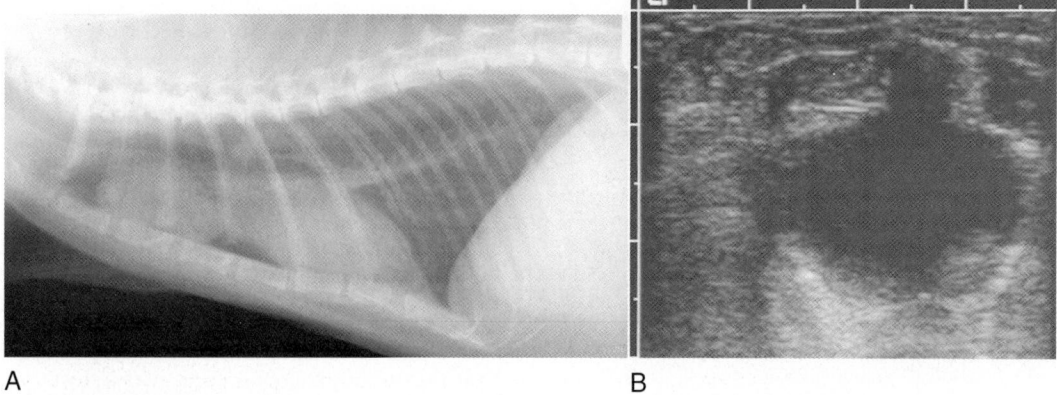

A   B

Figure 216-2 **A,** Lateral thoracic radiograph of a 19-year-old castrated male cat who presented for chronic renal failure and a heart murmur. Radiographs demonstrate a smoothly marginated soft tissue mass cranial to the heart, which causes minimal displacement of the trachea dorsally. **B,** Ultrasound of the cranial mediastinal mass. The ultrasonogram demonstrates that the mass is thin walled and cystic. Fluid obtained via ultrasound guided FNA was clear with low cellularity and protein, consistent with a mediastinal cyst.

Most animals do not have clinical signs referable to the mediastinal cyst. Radiographically, a cyst can appear as a solid mass in the cranial mediastinum due to the fluid within the cyst (Figure 216-2, *A*). A cyst can be differentiated from a solid mass ultrasonographically (Figure 216-2, *B*). Solid neoplasms, abscesses, or granulomas may have cystic components and must be differentiated from a simple cyst. Fine-needle aspiration with ultrasound guidance is the diagnostic test of choice. Cytology and culture can be performed. Mediastinal cysts typically contain a clear, colorless fluid with low cellularity and protein content.[31,32,33]

Non-Neoplastic Mediastinal Masses

Non-neoplastic mediastinal masses in dogs and cats and are usually infectious in origin. Fungal pyogranulomas, abscesses, lymphadenopathy, and hematomas have been described.[23-29] Lymphomatoid granulomatosis is a rare neoplastic/inflammatory disease of unknown etiology that causes hilar lymphadenopathy, pulmonary masses, and pleural effusion.[34] Lymphadenopathy may involve the cranial mediastinal, sternal, and tracheobronchial (hilar) lymph nodes. Cranial mediastinal lymph nodes lie along the major vascular structures and just ventral to the trachea. Sternal lymph nodes are just dorsal to the sternum, medial to the second costal cartilage, and cranioventral to the internal thoracic vessels. Sternal lymph nodes drain the abdomen, so enlargement often indicates intra-abdominal or multicentric disease.[19] The hilar lymph nodes are found at the bifurcation of the trachea and proximal bronchi. None of these lymph nodes are visible in normal animals on survey radiographs. Other lesions that may appear to be a mass include esophageal foreign bodies, diaphragmatic hernias, and gastroesophageal intussusception.

Radiographically, mediastinal masses appear as thoracic opacities on or near the midline that frequently cause displacement of adjacent mediastinal or thoracic structures, such as the heart, esophagus, and trachea. The carina is normally located at the fifth or sixth intercostal space in the dog and the sixth intercostal space in the cat. It can be displaced caudally by cranial mediastinal masses. Esophageal masses usually cause ventral displacement of the trachea. Most other mediastinal masses displace the trachea dorsally and to the right. Other radiographic changes associated with mediastinal masses include increased opacity in the cranial thorax, widening of the mediastinum, tracheal compression, and loss of

distinct, smooth, straight mediastinal borders. Masses that are in contact with a mediastinal structure may not have clearly defined borders. Enlarged sternal or hilar lymph nodes are most easily visualized on a lateral radiograph (Figure 216-3). Cranial mediastinal lymphadenopathy is better appreciated on a VD or DV view. Radiographic findings associated with enlargement of the hilar lymph nodes include separation of the main stem bronchi, elevation of the trachea cranial to the carina, and ventral deviation of the main caudal lobe bronchi caudal to the carina. Left atrial enlargement is the main differential diagnosis for this radiographic appearance. Mediastinal masses are frequently classified by location as anatomic (Box 216-1).

Pleural effusion may imitate a mediastinal mass because of the associated tracheal elevation, which is caused by the dorsal displacement of the lungs.[35] Repeat radiographs obtained after removal of the pleural fluid are often helpful in distinguishing pleural effusion from a mediastinal mass. Other lesions that may be confused with a mediastinal mass include

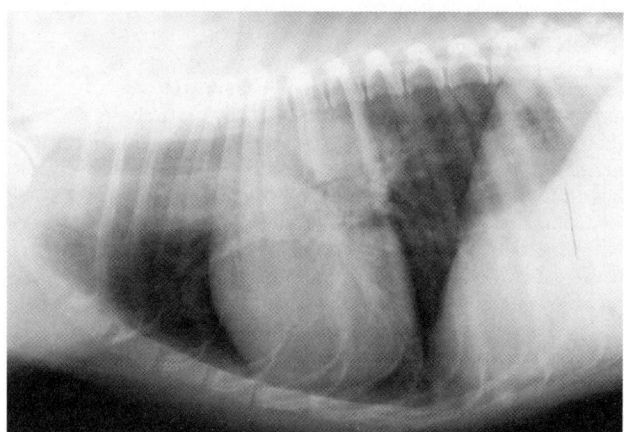

Figure 216-3 Lateral thoracic radiograph of a 3-year-old castrated male German Shorthaired Pointer presented for anorexia, weight loss, and fever. The radiographs demonstrate mass lesions and lymphadenopathy in the craniodorsal and hilar regions with displacement of the main stem bronchi ventrally. The final diagnosis was Nocardiosis.

Differential Diagnoses for Lesions Associated with Focal Mediastinal Enlargement

Region	Diseases
Cranioventral	Lymphadenopathy; abscess; thymic mass; ectopic thyroid; hematoma; granuloma; obesity; vascular mass (aorta, cranial vena cava); esophageal mass, foreign body, or dilatation; tracheal mass
Craniodorsal	Esophageal mass, foreign body, or dilatation; heart base mass; neurogenic tumor; paraspinal or spinal mass; hematoma; lymphadenopathy; aortic stenosis; patent ductus arteriosus; abscess; tracheal mass
Perihilar	Lymphadenopathy; left atrial enlargement; esophageal mass, foreign body, or dilatation; main pulmonary artery mass (post-stenotic dilatation); heart base or right atrial mass; spinal or paraspinal mass
Caudodorsal	Esophageal mass, foreign body, or dilatation; hiatal hernia; diaphragmatic hernia or mass; spirocercosis; spinal or paraspinal mass; aortic aneurysm; gastroesophageal intussusception
Caudoventral	Diaphragmatic hernia; peritoneopericardial diaphragmatic hernia; abscess; granuloma; hematoma

the normal thymus in young animals, mediastinal fat in obese animals, lung masses, especially those involving the accessory lobe or cranial tips of the left and right cranial lung lobes, very large right and left caudal pulmonary arteries, and perihilar edema. The presence of an air bronchogram within a suspected mediastinal mass indicates that it is actually a pulmonary lesion.

Mediastinal Neoplasia

Mediastinal tumors can originate from any structure within the mediastinum (lymph nodes, thymus, great vessels, trachea, esophagus, ectopic thyroid or parathyroid tissue) or from extension of neoplastic lesions in adjacent tissues.[36,37] Also, mediastinal neoplasms may be metastatic lesions or components of a multicentric neoplastic process.[38-44] Benign tumors have also been documented.[45]

Clinical signs associated with mediastinal tumors are usually caused by compression or invasion of structures such as the great vessels, thoracic duct, esophagus, and trachea. Signs include coughing, dyspnea, dysphagia, regurgitation, and edema of the head, neck, and/or forelimbs. Signs caused by peripheral nerve entrapment are less common and include laryngeal paralysis, vocalization changes, or Horner's syndrome. Signs associated with multicentric disease may reflect other sites of neoplastic involvement or may be related to paraneoplastic syndromes. These signs include anorexia, weight loss, vomiting, diarrhea, and polyuria/polydipsia.

Mediastinal lymphoma originates from either lymph node or thymic tissue in the cranial mediastinum. Mediastinal lymphoma is often associated with pleural effusion, which may initially obscure radiographic visualization of the mediastinal mass.

The diagnosis of mediastinal lymphoma can often be confirmed by cytologic identification of neoplastic lymphocytes in either a sample of pleural fluid or a sample obtained directly from the mediastinal mass via FNA. In dogs, mediastinal lymphoma may be associated with hypercalcemia. The presence of a mediastinal mass is a poor prognostic indicator in dogs with lymphoma.[46] Less common lymphatic based tumors that can cause mediastinal masses include lymphangiosarcoma and lymphangioma.[37,45]

Chemodectomas, which are usually aortic or carotid body tumors, are most often identified as heart base masses.[47] Affected animals may be presented for dysphagia, dyspnea, heart failure, or cervical swelling. Because these tumors often invade and surround roots of the great vessels at the heart base, they result in a mediastinal mass effect.

DISEASES OF THE THYMUS

The thymus extends from the thoracic inlet caudally to the fifth rib in the dog and the sixth rib in the cat. Dorsally it lies next to the phrenic nerves and cranial lung lobes. Thymic involution in small animals occurs concurrently with the onset of sexual maturity and the loss of deciduous teeth.[48] The thymus atrophies and is gradually replaced by connective tissue and fat, but remnants persist into old age.[48] Thymic branchial cysts arise from remnants of branchial pouch epithelium and may occur in the cranial mediastinum of dogs and cats (also see above).[49]

Thymic Hemorrhage

An uncommon disease of spontaneous thymic hemorrhage has been described in dogs and one cat.[49-52] Although not uniformly fatal, most animals documented with this syndrome have died. Most animals affected have been less than 2 years of age, so it appears to be associated with thymic involution. Clinical signs include lethargy, signs of thoracic pain, increased respiratory effort, and dyspnea. Physical examination findings are attributable to acute blood loss/hypovolemia and pleural effusion. Signs include pale mucous membranes, prolonged capillary refill time, tachycardia, tachypnea, and muffled lung sounds. Thoracic radiographs demonstrate a mediastinal mass (hemorrhage, hematoma) usually associated with pleural effusion. Treatment is supportive in nature and involves volume support, blood replacement, and thoracocentesis as needed.

Thymoma

Thymomas are rare tumors in the dog and cat that arise from the epithelial cells of the thymus.[53-56] They appear radiographically as large, poorly defined soft tissue masses in the cranial mediastinum (Figure 216-4, *A* and *B*). Expansion and invasion into adjacent tissues are common, but in some cases the masses are well encapsulated and fairly noninvasive. Metastasis has been reported in dogs and cats.[53,56] Pleural effusion is a variable finding and may hinder visualization of the thymic mass. Sonographically, thymomas can appear as solid, cystic, or a combination. Cytologic examination of FNA samples reveals a variable number of mature lymphocytes, which makes cytologic differentiation of thymoma from mediastinal lymphoma difficult. Mast cells are also frequently identified in cytologic samples from thymomas. Surgical or ultrasound guided percutaneous biopsy is required for definitive diagnosis. Paraneoplastic syndromes are commonly associated with thymoma in both dogs and cats.[53,55] The most well described is myasthenia gravis, which is often associated with megaesophagus in dogs with thymoma.[53] Myasthenia gravis has also been reported in cats with thymoma, but is less common. Surgical resection is the treatment of choice for thymoma, but recurrence and metastasis have been reported.

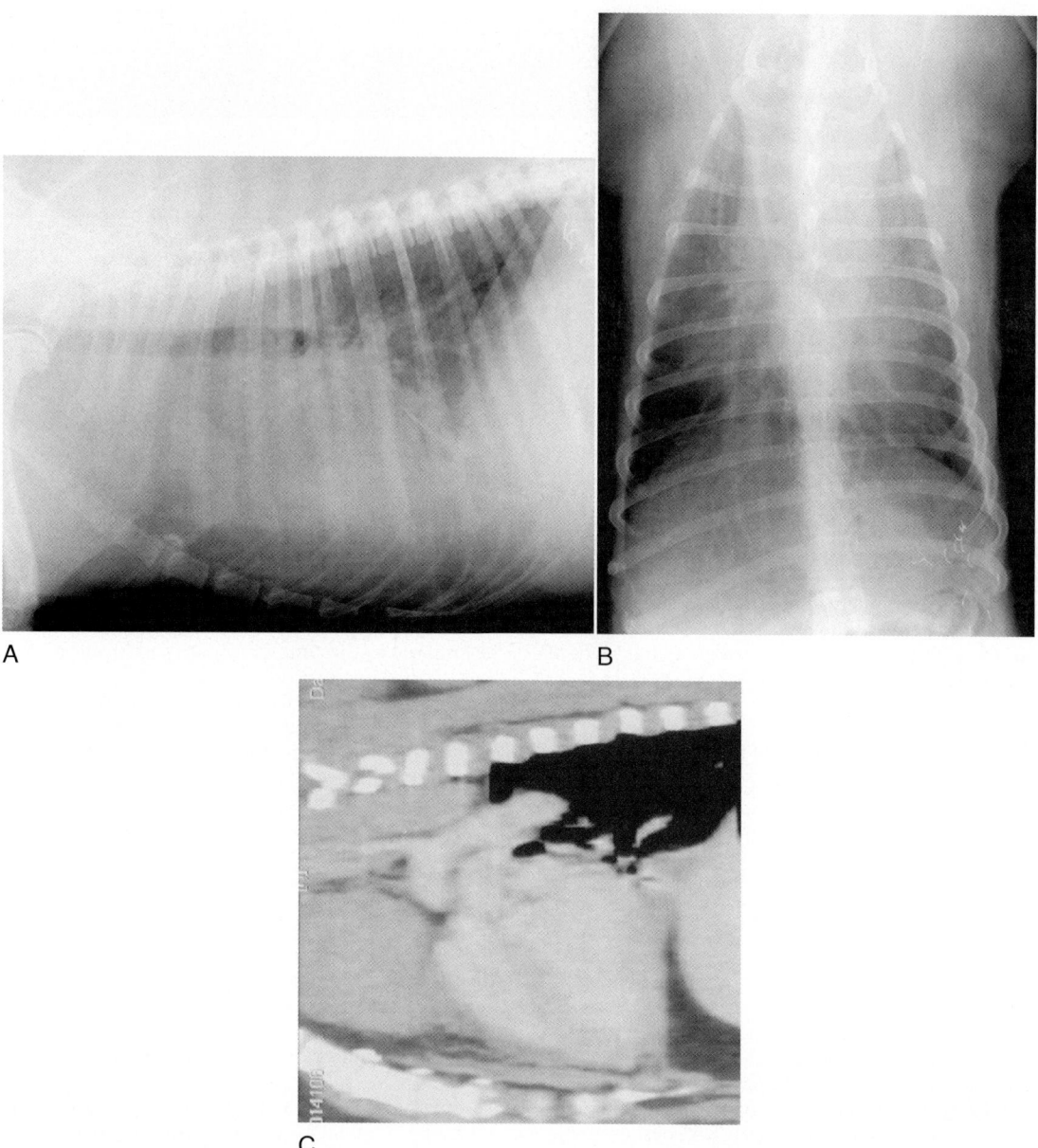

A

B

C

Figure 216-4 Lateral (**A**) and dorsoventral (**B**) radiographs of a 10-year-old castrated male Labrador Retriever presented for collapse. Radiographs demonstrate deviation of the trachea to the right. The cranial border of the cardiac silhouette is effaced by a cranial mediastinal mass. **C,** Computed tomographic 3D reconstruction of the cranial mediastinal mass in the same dog. The mass was removed surgically. Final diagnosis was thymoma with hemorrhage.

CHAPTER • 217

Pleural and Extrapleural Diseases

Michelle M. Mertens
Theresa W. Fossum

DISORDERS OF THE DIAPHRAGM

Diaphragmatic Anatomy

The diaphragm is a musculotendinous structure that separates the abdominal and thoracic cavities and is covered by pleura on its convex (thoracic) surface, adjacent to the lungs. It aids in ventilation and movement of lymphatic fluid. The phrenic nerves, which in dogs are derived from C4 to C7, provide innervation.[1] In cats, the phrenic nerves arise from C4 to C6. Prior to reaching the diaphragm, the phrenic nerves traverse the mediastinum and pericardium and are therefore subject to disruption from infiltrative masses or surgical transection (during pericardectomy or mass removal).

DIAPHRAGMATIC DISPLACEMENT AND DYSFUNCTION

Cranial or caudal displacement of the diaphragm may be associated with certain conditions and can be unilateral or bilateral. Cranial displacement results from enlargement or gas distension of abdominal contents as would be seen with late-term pregnancy or gastric dilatation-volvulus, respectively. It may contribute to respiratory compromise in such circumstances. Removal of a lung lobe or pulmonary atelectasis or consolidation results in unilateral cranial advancement of the diaphragm. Caudal diaphragmatic displacement is associated with pleural cavity disease (e.g., pneumothorax, pleural effusion) or obstructive airway disease that causes air trapping and pulmonary hyperinflation. These displacements are typically bilateral and recognition may be difficult when pleural fluid obscures the diaphragmatic silhouette. Unilateral caudal displacements are uncommon and may occur with either unilateral pneumothorax or pleural effusion, particularly chylothorax or pyothorax.

Paralysis of the diaphragm may also be uni- or bilateral. Unilateral paralysis is unlikely to be associated with clinical evidence of respiratory abnormalities; however, bilateral paralysis can result in substantial impairment of respiration. Bilateral paralysis most commonly results from cervical spinal trauma or fracture. In such cases, cranial displacement of the diaphragm may be radiographically apparent. Lack of movement of the diaphragm during fluoroscopic evaluation increases suspicion of this condition.

Diaphragmatic Hernias

Diaphragmatic hernia (DH) is a term for disorders of the diaphragm that allow abdominal contents to enter the thoracic cavity, either within the pleural space (pleuroperitoneal hernias, hiatal hernias) or pericardial sac (peritoneopericardial diaphragmatic hernias). Diaphragmatic hernias are divided by etiology into traumatic and congenital hernias.

Traumatic Diaphragmatic Hernias

Traumatic DHs are more commonly recognized in small animal veterinary patients than are congenital hernias, with studies reporting between 77% and 85% of diaphragmatic hernias being traumatic in origin.[2-4] Traumatic DHs are frequently associated with motor vehicle accidents or other forceful blows to the thorax or abdomen.[3,5] A sudden increase in intra-abdominal pressure, with an open glottis, results in rapid deflation of the lungs. The position of the glottis may be unimportant provided there is the creation of an abrupt, substantial increase in pressure with an abdominal pressure gradient.[2] The large pressure gradient causes the diaphragm to tear at its weakest points (usually in the muscular portions). The location and size of the tear(s) depend on the position of the animal at the time of impact and location of the viscera.

Signalment and History   Young male dogs between the ages of 1 and 2 years are most commonly diagnosed with traumatic DH because of their propensity to roam and sustain vehicular trauma. Affected animals may present in shock and respiratory distress, depending on the size of the hernia, which viscera have herniated, and severity of other injuries. Concurrent injuries are common. Chronic diaphragmatic hernias are reported and respiratory embarrassment may not be immediately evident. In one study, 20% of animals with traumatic DH were not diagnosed until at least 4 weeks after the injury had occurred.[2] Clinical signs associated with chronic diaphragmatic hernias are generally confined to the respiratory or gastrointestinal system and may include dyspnea, exercise intolerance, anorexia, depression, vomiting, diarrhea, weight loss, and/or pain following ingestion of food.

Physical Examination   Physical examination findings vary with the acuteness of the trauma, concurrent injuries, and organs herniated. Hypoventilation is often present and is attributable to inadequate lung expansion, voluntary decrease in chest wall motion due to pain, fractures or flail segments causing chest wall dysfunction, or pulmonary atelectasis. Signs consistent with shock include pale or cyanotic mucous membranes, tachypnea, tachycardia with variable pulse pressure, and decreased mentation. Cardiac arrhythmias, attributable to traumatic myocarditis, may be present and if severe, are associated with significant morbidity. The liver is the organ most commonly herniated and is often associated with hydrothorax as a result of venous occlusion and capsular weeping. Extrahepatic biliary obstruction has been reported.[6] Herniation and entrapment of the stomach can lead to gaseous distension, which results in a rapidly declining clinical condition and fatal respiratory impairment. Gastric dilation-volvulus has been reported with DH and should be suspected in dogs and cats presenting with abdominal enlargement and dyspnea.[7]

Diagnosis   Diagnosis of DH is made either on thoracic radiographs (Figure 217-1) or by ultrasonography of the diaphragm and cranial abdomen. The presence of gas-filled viscera in the thoracic cavity is diagnostic of a DH; however, visualization of thoracic structures and the diaphragmatic silhouette may be obscured by the presence of pleural effusion.

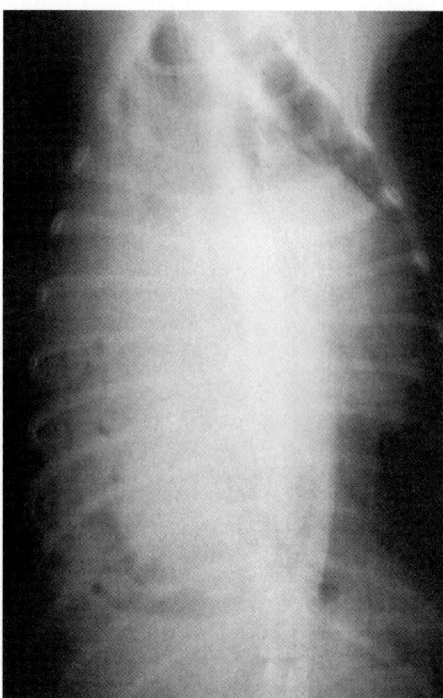

Figure 217-1 Ventrodorsal thoracic radiograph of a dog with a traumatic diaphragmatic hernia. Notice the gas-filled loops of small intestine in the right hemithorax.

In such cases, thoracocentesis may be necessary prior to obtaining diagnostic radiographs. Ultrasound examination is most helpful in cases with herniation of the liver or when large volumes of pleural fluid are present. An upper GI barium study may identify portions of the intestinal tract that have herniated into the thoracic cavity. Positive contrast celiography with a water-soluble contrast agent is occasionally used as a diagnostic aid but caution must be used when injecting radiographic contrast agents in dehydrated animals. Additionally, omental or fibrous adhesions may obscure diaphragmatic defects and result in false-negative studies.

Management Initial management should include oxygen therapy in dyspneic animals and treatment for shock, including fluids and administration of a broad-spectrum antibiotic (see Chapter 120, 124). Ventilation may be improved by positioning the animal in sternal recumbency with the front end elevated. Thoracocentesis should be performed if moderate to marked pleural fluid is present. Animals presenting with gastric distension should be considered surgical emergencies and operated on as soon as they can safely be anesthetized. Other animals with diaphragmatic hernias and associated trauma may benefit from stabilization prior to surgical intervention and definitive repair of the DH. However, these animals must be closely monitored for worsening respiratory compromise. Overall mortality rate for dogs and cats undergoing diaphragmatic herniorrhaphy is cited at approximately 20%.[8-10] Readers are referred to a surgical textbook for details of surgical correction of DH.

Congenital Diaphragmatic Hernias
Signalment and History Congenital pleuroperitoneal hernias can occur and result from improper development of the left pleuroperitoneal membrane. These hernias are infrequently recognized in dogs and cats as they generally result in death upon or shortly after birth.[11] Hernias involving the esophageal hiatus are typically congenital in nature and are known as *hiatal hernias*. (See Chapter 220.)

Peritoneopericardial diaphragmatic hernias (PPDHs) are the most common congenital pericardial and diaphragmatic anomalies in dogs and cats.[12] Herniation of abdominal viscera into the pericardial sac can result from abnormal development of the septum transversum or from failure of the lateral pleuroperitoneal folds and the ventromedial pars sternalis to unite. This defect likely occurs as a result of a teratogen, genetic defect, or prenatal injury.[13] A high incidence of right- and left-sided DH was induced when the embryotoxic herbicide nitrofen was given to rats during a critical period in gestation.[14] A teratogen was the suspected cause of PPDH and multiple cardiac defects in an entire litter of collies.[15] Unlike in humans, PPDHs are always congenital in dogs and cats because there is no direct communication between the peritoneal and pericardial cavities after birth in these species.

Cardiac abnormalities and sternal deformities often occur concomitantly with PPDHs. Reported concurrent anomalies include umbilical hernias, cranial midline abdominal wall hernias, malformed or absent sternebrae, pectus excavatum or intracardiac defects.[16,17] Polycystic kidneys have been reported in association with PPDH in a cat.[18] Although seldom noted in animals, pulmonary vascular abnormalities may occur in children with congenital DH; persistent pulmonary hypertension is thought to contribute to the morbidity and mortality associated with this condition in affected children.[19] A predisposition for PPDH has been suggested in Persian cats and Weimeraners.[17,20]

Clinical Signs and Physical Examination As with other DH, clinical signs of affected animals may vary from none to severe respiratory embarrassment, depending on the organ(s) herniated and degree of compromise of that organ(s). Vomiting and anorexia are often observed. Physical examination may reveal muffled heart sounds and lack of normally palpable organs in the abdomen.

Diagnosis Diagnosis of PPDH is usually made from thoracic radiographs and/or ultrasound and is frequently an incidental finding. Radiographic findings include apparent cardiomegaly, dorsal elevation of the trachea, and silhouetting of the heart and diaphragm; gas-filled viscera may be present. As with other diaphragmatic hernias, oral barium administration may be useful if the diagnosis is not readily apparent on radiographs or if ultrasound is unavailable.

Management Initial management of the symptomatic animal with PPDH includes oxygen therapy if dyspneic and positioning the animal in sternal recumbency with the chest elevated. Surgical repair of PPDH is recommended in most cases and should be performed at as early an age as possible. Early surgical intervention may decrease the incidence of adhesions and risk of postoperative re-expansion pulmonary edema.

DISORDERS OF THE THORACIC WALL

Chest Wall Trauma
Damage to the thoracic wall may be due to blunt (motor vehicle accidents, being kicked) or penetrating (bite wounds, gunshot wounds) injuries. Both blunt and penetrating trauma can cause extensive soft tissue damage of the thoracic wall. Although soft tissue damage is rarely the cause of major morbidity or mortality, it may be the only external evidence of severe thoracic trauma. Pain associated with thoracic wall trauma may lead to hypoventilation because the animal is unwilling to breathe; analgesics may improve ventilation. Similarly, isolated rib fractures, although unlikely to result in significant respiratory impairment, may result in decreased ventilation due to pain. Chest wall

trauma alone (without pulmonary parenchymal damage) rarely leads to significant hypoventilation resulting in hypoxia.

A flail segment (flail chest) is produced when multiple segmental rib fractures produce a free segment of thoracic wall that has lost its continuity with the remainder of the thorax. Intrapleural pressure changes during respiration result in paradoxic segment movement; the segment moves inward during inspiration and outward during expiration. Flail chest segments can initially be stabilized by positioning the animal with the flail side down. Mechanical ventilation is the preferred treatment for people with flail segments. As this may not be practical in veterinary patients, surgical stabilization of the flail segment is thought to help decrease pain, improve ventilation, and prevent further damage to thoracic structures. A recent retrospective study of the medical records from five veterinary teaching hospitals investigating the clinical management of flail chest in dogs and cats reported that the majority of cases were treated without stabilization of the flail segment.[21] The study was not able to demonstrate a difference in outcome between surgically stabilized and conservatively managed cases. It was not possible to determine from the results of the study which animals would benefit from surgery. Readers are referred to a surgical text for more details of the surgical management of flail chest.

Subcutaneous emphysema can occur with both blunt and penetrating trauma and is usually of little clinical significance. It occurs when air dissects along fascial planes under the subcutaneous tissues. Air may enter the subcutaneous tissues from direct communication with an external wound, from disruption of the pleura and intercostals muscles, or as an extension of mediastinal emphysema. The condition is usually self-limiting; treatment should be directed at the underlying cause.

Pectus Excavatum

Pectus excavatum (PE) is a deformity of the costocartilages and sternum that result in a dorsoventral narrowing of the chest. Although the causes are unknown, several theories have been proposed. It has been suggested that there may be both congenital and acquired forms of PE in people.[22] Possible etiologies include shortening of the central tendon of the diaphragm, abnormalities of intrauterine pressure, congenital deficiency of musculature in the cranial portion of the diaphragm, and abnormal respiratory gradients as may be present with upper airway obstruction.

Signalment and History

Sternal depressions are often noted early in the life of the animal and prompt owners to seek veterinary attention. The disease is progressive and the severity of the defect may increase as the animal matures. In humans, males appear to be predisposed, yet a gender predilection has not been clearly identified in animals. PE has been reported in dogs, cats, sheep, and calves. Brachycephalic dogs and Burmese cats are more commonly affected than other breeds.[23,24] PE has occurred in multiple animals of certain litters; therefore affected animals should not be used for breeding. PE can be associated with "swimmer's syndrome," a poorly characterized disease of neonatal dogs in which the legs splay to the sides.

Clinical Signs and Physical Examination

Animals with PE may be asymptomatic or may present with clinical signs associated with both respiratory and cardiovascular functional abnormalities. The sternal depression often causes malpositioning of the heart within the thoracic cavity and may result in kinking of the large veins, disturbance of venous return, restriction of ventricular filling, and decreased respiratory reserve. Direct compression of the heart may result in cardiac arrhythmias. Symptoms such as exercise intolerance, weight loss or failure to thrive, hyperpnea or dyspnea, cyanosis, recurrent respiratory infections, and vomiting may occur. A correlation between severity of clinical signs and

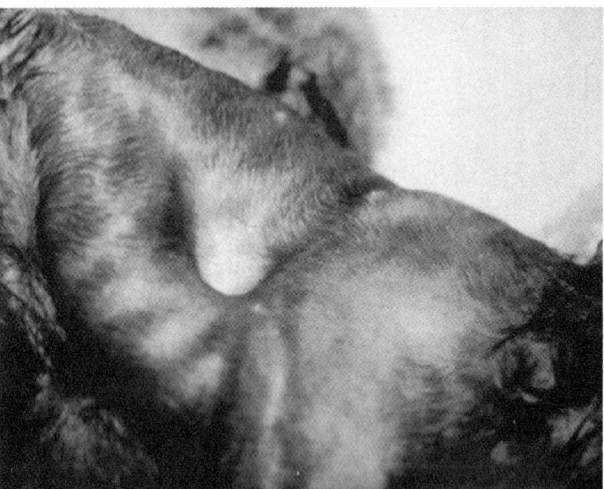

Figure 217-2 A cat with pectus excavatum. Notice the palpable depression of the caudal sternum. (From Fossum TW et al: Pectus excavatum in 8 dogs and 6 cats, J Am Anim Hosp Assoc 25:595, 1989.)

severity of the abnormality has not been identified. Other abnormalities that may be noted on physical exam include cardiac murmurs and increased or harsh lung sounds. Concurrent cardiac abnormalities such as pulmonic stenosis and atrial septal defects have been reported; care must be taken to distinguish abnormalities caused by the position of the heart from those that result from cardiac disease.

Diagnosis

Diagnosis of PE is made on physical examination by palpation of a depression in the sternum (Figure 217-2). Thoracic radiographs show an abnormal elevation of the sternum. The heart is often shifted to one of the hemi-thoraces as insufficient room exists on midline. In this abnormal position, it may appear enlarged on thoracic radiographs. Echocardiography may be necessary to distinguish cardiac disease from this apparent enlargement. Classification of the sternal deformity as mild, moderate, or severe has been described and is based on the frontosaggital and vertebral indices obtained from thoracic radiographs[24] (Figure 217-3).

Management

Animals with mild PE or those with simply a flattened ventral thorax are unlikely to require surgery. Owners should be instructed to perform medial to lateral chest compressions in such cases. In young animals with moderate to severe disease, or those with clinical signs, application of a splint to the ventral aspect of the thorax is the most commonly used treatment. Older animals with less compliant thoracic and sternal walls may require a partial sternectomy to relieve their clinical signs.

Thoracic Wall and Sternal Neoplasia

Primary tumors of the rib are uncommon in the dog; however, these tumors are usually malignant and have a high metastatic rate. Some reports cite that they generally develop in young dogs, with a mean reported age in one study of 4.5 years[25], whereas others report median ages of between 7 and 9 years.[26,27] Osteosarcomas are the most common neoplasm of the canine rib, followed by chondrosarcoma; the costochondral junction is the usual site of origin of these tumors. Fibrosarcomas and hemangiosarcomas are less frequently reported.[25,28] Most rib tumors cause a localized swelling of the thoracic wall; however, pleural effusion without evidence of a thoracic mass has been reported in two dogs with primary rib tumors and

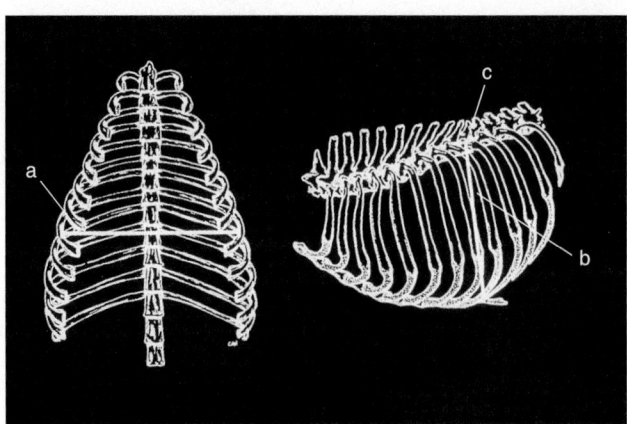

Figure 217-3 The frontosagittal index is the ratio between the width of the chest at the tenth thoracic vertebra (a) and the distance between the center of the ventral surface of the tenth thoracic vertebral body and the nearest point on the sternum (b). The vertebral index is the ratio between the distance from the center of the dorsal surface of the tenth vertebral body to the nearest point on the sternum (b and c) and the dorsalventral diameter of the vertebral body at the same level (c). (From Fossum TW et al: J Am Anim Hosp Assoc 25:595, 1989.)

metastatic pulmonary lesions.[29] Other clinical signs noted in two animals with rib tumors included weight loss and dyspnea.

Neoplasms of the ribs or sternum should be differentiated from bacterial or fungal osteomyelitis. A tentative diagnosis of the tumor cell type can usually be made by fine-needle aspiration of the mass; however, definitive diagnosis requires histologic examination of a biopsy specimen. Although pleural effusion is common in dogs with rib tumors, identification of neoplastic cells in the fluid is very uncommon. Due to the high rate of pulmonary metastasis, the prognosis for dogs with rib tumors is poor. In one study of 15 dogs with primary rib tumors, greater than 90% of the dogs died or were euthanized within 4 months of the diagnosis.[29]

Although also rare, both metastatic and primary tumors of the sternum have been reported in dogs.[30] In humans, metastatic tumors involving the sternum are more frequently recognized than primary tumors. The distant primary site is most commonly in the thyroid, kidney, breast, testicle, lung, stomach, or rectum. Primary neoplasms of the bony chest account for 7% to 8% of all bone tumors in humans, and although primary rib tumors are frequently benign, tumors of the sternum are typically malignant. Similar generalizations are difficult to make in the dog due to the infrequency with which sternal tumors have been reported. However, chondrosarcomas and osteosarcomas involving the sternebrae have been reported in dogs.[31]

When a diagnosis of sternal neoplasia is made, the diseased bone as well as normal surrounding tissue should be removed. Unlike most bones in the body, the sternebrae can be removed with little compromise of function.[32] Successful treatment of sternal osteomyelitis following resection of large portions of the sternebrae has been reported in dogs and human beings, and the procedure would likely benefit dogs with primary sternal neoplasia.

PLEURAL EFFUSION

Anatomy of the Pleural Space
The pleura consists of a single sheet of flattened mesothelial cells supported by a layer of elastic connective tissue containing vascular and lymphatic channels. The visceral pleura

covers the lung surface; the parietal pleura lines the inner surface of the ribs, diaphragm, and mediastinum. The pleural space normally contains a small amount of fluid that aids in transmission of forces and provides lubrication of the lung surfaces during respiration. Pleural fluid in the normal animal is similar to that of a plasma filtrate with a low protein concentration and a cellular composition of mesothelial cells and monocytes. Differences in electrolyte composition between pleural fluid and blood suggest modification of the plasma filtrate by an active transport or selective diffusion mechanism.[33] Filtration rate and lymphatic drainage increase with animal size and age; larger animals have small pleural fluid volumes.

Theories concerning the regulation of pleural fluid turnover have been expanded greatly over the past few decades. In 1927 Neergard described the balance of fluid formation and resorption as an equilibrium between hydraulic and colloid osmotic pressures.[34] Although these concepts are still valid, additional mechanisms must be in place to explain the stable composition of interstitial and pleural fluids. Given the differential permeability of water and solutes, pleural fluid protein concentration would increase over time if pleural fluid exchange were based solely on the difference between hydrostatic and colloid osmotic pressures. Similarly, if fluid production occurred solely at the arteriolar end of the capillary bed and resorption at the venular end as previously described, then a progressive increase in interstitial protein should occur over time.

The formation of pleural fluid is thought to be the result of filtration of fluid into the pleural space via Starling forces. It is currently thought that the absorption of pleural fluid is controlled by several mechanisms. The pressure differential across the visceral pleura favors liquid absorption; however, this is believed to contribute to only a small amount of fluid absorption.[35,36] Some believe that the pleural lymphatics provide the majority of interstitial fluid drainage[34], including particles, cells, and albumin.[37] There is evidence that stomas that help to transport albumin and water exist between the mesothelial cells of the parietal pleura and endothelial cells of the pleural lymphatics.[34] However, some albumin and liquid are also transported outside of the stomas via transcytosis.[38] A subatmospheric pressure of approximately -10 cm H_2O is generated by pleural lymphatics[39], which allows them to act as a drainage mechanism in pleural fluid accumulation. Lymphatic flow rate can increase dramatically (twentyfold) in response to increased pleural fluid filtration. Lymphatic drainage is greatest in the ventral thoracic cavity, diaphragm, and mediastinum.

More recently, the role of mesothelial cells in active transserosal transport (electrolyte coupled liquid absorption) has been investigated[40]; direct and indirect evidence of this function has been provided.[41-43] Mesothelial cell permeability to water and solutes may be equivalent to that of the capillary endothelium and these cells appear to be involved in the active transport of solutes and liquid. Thus the volume and composition of pleural fluid in the normal animal is governed by lymphatic drainage, Starling forces through the mesothelium and capillaries of the connective tissue, and activity of mesothelial cells.

Etiology of Pleural Effusions
Pleural effusions develop when there is an alteration in the balance between fluid formation and fluid resorption. This can result from changes in hydrostatic and osmotic pressures, impaired lymphatic drainage, and increased vascular or lymphatic permeability.[40] Alterations in the pleural fluid protein content and cellularity can give some evidence as to the underlying disease process. Low protein effusions are generally caused by cardiac, renal, or hepatic disease and are known as *transudates*. Effusions with a high protein count (>3.0 g/dL) suggest increased vascular permeability, decreased lymphatic removal, or both and can be caused by inflammatory or neoplastic processes or by diseases of the lymphatic system.

Alterations in osmotic pressure result in low protein effusions as disruption of Starling forces allows fluid movement out of the vascular space and decreased absorption of fluid by the capillaries of the visceral pleura. Serum albumin concentrations of less than 1.5 g/dL may result in pleural or peritoneal effusions; edema of the extremities may also occur. Hypoalbuminemia can be secondary to decreased production as seen in liver disease or increased loss as in protein-losing enteropathy or nephropathy. Hepatic hydrothorax occurs when a marked pleural effusion occurs in a patient with hepatic cirrhosis in the absence of primary pulmonary or cardiac disease.[44] These effusions often recur and may be associated with diaphragmatic peritoneopleural communications or may occur via transdiaphragmatic lymphatic drainage of the cranial abdomen.

Increased systemic venous hydrostatic pressure is most commonly seen secondarily to congestive heart failure (CHF) and may result in pleural effusion. Left-sided CHF increases visceral capillary hydrostatic pressure and decreases fluid absorption, whereas right-sided CHF increases parietal capillary pressure and tends to favor increased pleural fluid formation.[45] Increased venous pressures also decrease lymphatic drainage within the pleural cavity and can result in a transudative or chylous effusion. Venous or lymphatic obstruction, as might be seen with a lung lobe torsion or incarceration of a liver lobe through a diaphragmatic hernia, can cause transudation of fluid through the organ capsule and result in pleural effusion. Other causes of increased venous pressures include pericardial effusion and cardiac tamponade, heartworm disease, and neoplasia.

Animals with fibrosing pleuritis or severe upper airway obstruction may develop increased negative pressure in the pleural space. In fibrosing pleuritis, the lungs are unable to re-expand despite absorption or removal of pleural fluid, which result in an increase in negative pressure.[33] This negative pressure promotes rapid accumulation of pleural fluid.

Alterations in vascular or lymphatic permeability or decreased lymphatic drainage cause effusions with increasing amounts of protein and fluid accumulation. Increased vascular permeability may be induced by vasculitis, which results from release of mediators such as histamine during inflammatory processes. Diseases that commonly result in vasculitis that may cause pleural effusion include feline infectious peritonitis (FIP), pancreatitis, uremia, and immune-mediated diseases such as systemic lupus erythematosus (SLE) and rheumatoid arthritis. Lymphatic drainage may be altered by neoplastic processes such as lymphangiosarcoma, mesothelioma, or metastatic mammary carcinoma.

Clinical Signs and Physical Examination

Clinical signs associated with pleural effusion can vary according to the etiology of the increased fluid volume, rapidity with which the fluid accumulated, and the volume of fluid present. With increased pleural fluid accumulation, compensatory mechanisms are overcome and clinical evidence of decreased lung expansion and impaired gas exchange become evident. These signs are likely to have an insidious onset and substantial disease can be present before abnormalities are recognized.

Dyspnea is the most common clinical sign in animals presenting to the veterinarian with pleural effusion. Often the owner reports an acute onset. The dyspnea is usually marked by a forceful inspiration, with delayed expiration. Animals are often reluctant to lie down and may extend their heads and necks in an elevated position. Other clinical signs include tachypnea, open-mouth breathing, and cyanosis. Dogs and cats with chronic pleural effusion may present with coughing as the only clinical sign and should therefore be evaluated for pleural effusion when presenting with a persistent cough that does not respond to routine therapy. Coughing may be a result

of irritation caused by the effusion, or related to an underlying disease process (e.g., cardiomyopathy). Other physical exam findings can include muffled heart and lung sounds and dullness on thoracic percussion. Additional findings that are related to the underlying cause of the pleural effusion can include fever, weight-loss, anorexia, depression, pale mucous membranes, heart murmurs or arrhythmias, ascites, pericardial effusion, or Horner's syndrome. Animals that remain dyspneic following pleural fluid removal should be suspected of having underlying pulmonary parenchymal or pleural disease such as pneumonia or fibrosing pleuritis, respectively.

Fibrosing pleuritis is a condition that has been associated with chylothorax in both dogs and cats.[46,47] Although the cause of the fibrosis is unknown, it apparently can develop subsequent to any prolonged exudative or blood-stained effusion. Exudates are characterized by a high rate of fibrin formation.[48] Fibrin formation probably increases because chronic inflammatory exudates, such as chylothorax and pyothorax, induce changes in mesothelial cell morphologic features, resulting in increased permeability, mesothelial cell desquamation, and triggering of both pathways of the coagulation cascade.[49] Desquamated mesothelial cells have also been shown to produce type III collagen in cell culture, and promote fibrosis.[50] Additionally, the chronic presence of pleural fluid might lead to an impairment in the mechanism of fibrin degradation.[51] Fibrinolysis may decrease because direct injury to mesothelial cells may reduce inherent fibrinolytic activity of the cells, and/or the increased fluid volume may dilute local plasminogen activator. Plasminogen activator converts the precursor plasminogen to its active form, plasmin. Fibrinolytic activity in mammals is attributable primarily to this serine protease.[52]

In animals with fibrosing pleuritis, the pleura is thickened by diffuse fibrous tissue that restricts normal pulmonary expansion (Figure 217-4, A). Animals with fibrosing pleuritis may be misdiagnosed as having large amounts of pleural effusion, when in fact the pleural effusion is minimal. Diagnosis of fibrosing pleuritis is difficult. The atelectatic lobes may be confused with metastatic or primary pulmonary neoplasia, lung lobe torsion, or hilar lymphadenopathy. Radiographic evidence of pulmonary parenchyma that fails to re-expand after removal of pleural fluid should be considered possible evidence of atelectasis with associated fibrosis (Figure 217-4, B). Fibrosing pleuritis should also be considered in animals with persistent dyspnea, yet minimal pleural fluid. In human beings, computerized tomography is occasionally helpful in differentiating pleural fibrosis from other abnormalities, such as neoplasia.[53,54]

Diagnosis

Animals suspected of having pleural effusion should be thoroughly evaluated for underlying cardiac or respiratory disease. Thoracic auscultation may reveal decreased heart and lung sounds ventrally. Thoracic percussion may demonstrate a fluid line with hyporesonant sounds ventrally and normal sounds dorsally. Murmurs may be auscultated in animals with underlying cardiac disease. Animals should be evaluated for the presence of jugular pulses. In cats with cranial mediastinal masses, the cranial thorax may become less compressible. See below for radiographic and ultrasonographic findings in animals with pleural effusion.

Thoracocentesis

In addition to relieving respiratory difficulty, thoracocentesis also provides samples to aid evaluation and diagnosis. *In the dyspneic animal, thoracocentesis should be performed prior to thoracic radiographs.* Removal of even small amounts of fluid may substantially decrease the animal's ventilatory effort. The animal should be restrained in sternal recumbency with oxygen provided by mask if tolerated. Slight sedation may be required in fractious

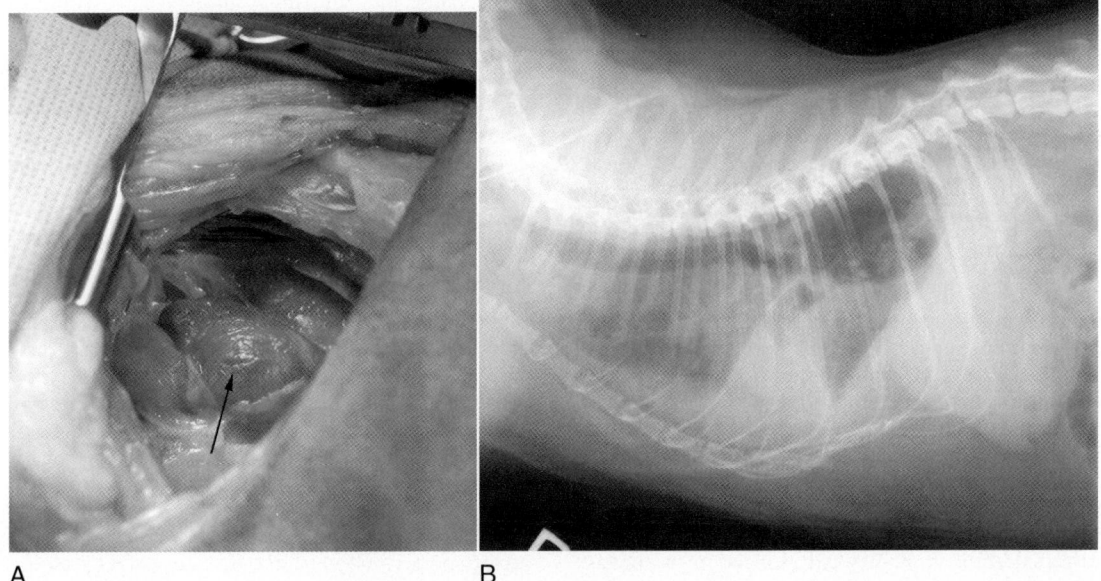

Figure 217-4 **A,** Intra-operative photo of a cat with severe fibrosing pleuritis secondary to chronic chylothorax. Notice the small, consolidated lung lobes and the thickened pleura. Decortication of the fibrous pleural was performed in this cat. **B,** Lateral radiograph of the cat from **A.** Note the rounded appearance of the caudal lung lobes. Removal of the pleural fluid did not improve the expansion of the lung lobes.

animals; general anesthetics should be avoided. Caution should be used when sedating dyspneic animals. Typically, the mediastinum in dogs and cats appears to be incomplete and fluid aspiration from either side will permit drainage of the entire thorax. However, due to chronic inflammation and thickening of the mediastinum, unilateral effusions may be noted with certain diseases such as chylothorax and pyothorax. Thoracocentesis techniques are described in Chapter 103.

Radiography and Ultrasonography

If the animal is not dyspneic, thoracic radiographs should be obtained to confirm the diagnosis of pleural effusion and allow evaluation of thoracic and intra-thoracic structures (Figure 217-5). Dorsoventral (rather than ventrodorsal) and "standing lateral" views may cause less stress to a compromised animal. Handling should be minimized and supplemental oxygen provided.

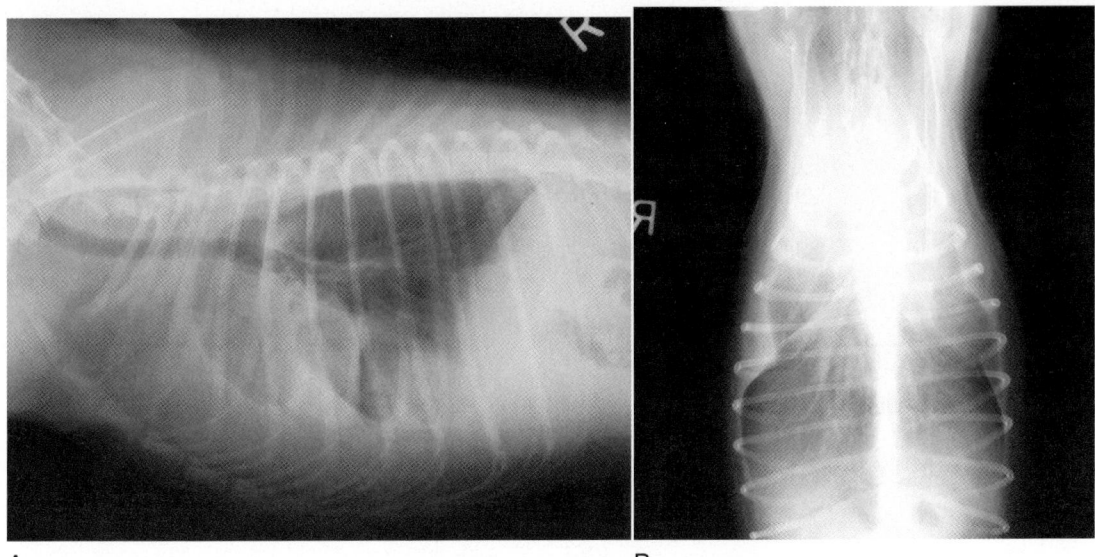

Figure 217-5 Lateral and dorsoventral radiographs of a dog with pleural effusion secondary to chylothorax. Note the loss of the cardiac and diaphragmatic silhouettes, and widened interlobar fissures.

RESPIRATORY DISEASE

Normal pleura is not generally radiographically visible. With pleural thickening, pleural lines may become visible and may be mistaken for pleural effusion. A horizontal beam radiograph will help differentiate the two. Roentgen signs associated with pleural effusion include widened interlobar fissures, retraction of the lung margins from the thoracic wall, rounding of the lung margins at the costophrenic angles, and obscuring of the diaphragmatic and cardiac silhouettes. Visualization of the cranial aspect of the cardiac silhouette in the presence of pleural effusion is occasionally possible with identification of the "pericardial fat stripe."[55] It is reported that a lucent line is occasionally evident at the cranial edge of the cardiac silhouette and represents the x-ray beam striking fat around the heart at a tangent. To permit more careful evaluation of intra-thoracic structures, radiographs should be repeated once the pleural fluid has been removed.

In the stable animal, ultrasonography should be performed prior to fluid removal as the fluid provides an "acoustic window" and may allow clearer visualization of intra-thoracic structures such as mediastinal masses. Ultrasonography can be used to diagnose cardiac functional and structural abnormalities and identify pericardial effusion. It may aid in location of encapsulated fluid and identification of the appropriate site for thoracocentesis.

Pleural Fluid Evaluation

Cytologic analysis of pleural fluid obtained via thoracocentesis is indicated. Identification of cell types and numbers, protein levels, and other physical characteristics and biochemical markers allow classification of pleural fluids into categories that aid in the identification of the underlying etiology. Fluids are generally divided into three types: transudates, modified transudates, and exudates. Additional sub-classifications include chylous, neoplastic, and hemorrhagic effusions.

Transudates and Modified Transudates

Pure transudates are clear, colorless fluids with a low total protein and low cellularity (Table 217-1). The primary cell type is mononuclear, with macrophages, and mesothelial cells most often present in small numbers; occasional lymphocytes or neutrophils can be seen. With chronicity, there is often a small increase in protein and cell numbers as a result of pleural irritation. Because of the low total nucleated cell count (TNCC), cytologic evaluation of a transudative fluid is most efficiently accomplished by concentrating cells with a cytospin preparation. Modified transudates develop from chronic transudates or they may result from increased vascular hydrostatic pressure or lymphatic leakage. In their initial stages, inflammatory processes may cause modified transudates to be produced. In addition to mesothelial cells and macrophages, neutrophils, and lymphocytes may be seen. Mast cells, eosinophils, and neoplastic cells are less commonly observed. A turbid sample may indicate a higher cell count, which allows cytologic evaluation to be performed from direct smears. A cytospin preparation may be used if there are not sufficient cells observed on direct smears. Diseases that may result in transudates and modified transudates include hypoalbuminemia, right-sided heart failure, pericardial disease, diaphragmatic hernia, and neoplasia.

Exudates

Exudates have a high protein concentration (see Table 217-1) and higher nucleated cell counts than transudates or modified transudates. They range in color from white to amber or red. The high TNCC of exudates allows accurate cytologic

Table • 217-1

Characteristics of Fluid Types

	TRANSUDATE	MODIFIED TRANSUDATE	EXUDATE	PYOTHORAX	CHYLOTHORAX	FIP
Protein content (g/dL)	<2.5	2.5-4	>3	>3.5	Variable	>5
TNCC* (cells/µL)	<1500	1000-7000	>7000	>7000	<10,000	<10,000
Color	Clear	Yellow, whitish-pink, red	White, amber, red	Amber to red or white	Usually white or pink	Straw to gold colored
Transparency	Colorless	Hazy to turbid	Opaque (usually) Turbid (rarely)	Turbid or opaque	Opaque	Hazy
Biochemical parameters			LDH >200 U/L	Glucose <10 mg/dL pH <6.9	Triglyceride > serum triglyceride	
Predominant cell types	Mesothelial cells, macrophages	Mesothelial cells, macrophages eosinophils, lymphocytes	Neutrophils (most common) Lymphocytes, macrophages, mesothelial cells, neoplastic cells	Degenerative neutrophils	Lymphocytes or neutrophils	Nondegenerative neutrophils

*TNCC, Total nucleated cell count.

evaluation to be obtained from direct smears. The predominant nucleated cell typed depends on the cause of the exudate. Neutrophils are the most common cell type seen in inflammatory processes. Other nucleated cell types found in exudates include mesothelial cells, macrophages, lymphocytes, and neoplastic cells. A predominance of lymphocytes may indicate a chylous effusion. A mixed cell population, with increased numbers of macrophages and neutrophils may be seen with more chronic chylous effusions. Fungal disease or foreign body reaction should be considered if pyogranulomatous inflammation (equally mixed population of neutrophils and macrophages) is noted.

Mesothelial cells are generally present in all effusions. Reactive mesothelial cells can exhibit characteristics of malignancy and should be interpreted with extreme caution in the presence of inflammation.[56] With the exception of lymphoma, it can be difficult or impossible to definitively identify a neoplastic process on the basis of pleural fluid evaluation. Other neoplastic cells that may exfoliate into pleural fluid include carcinoma cells, mast cells, and cells from malignant melanoma. Degenerative neutrophils indicate a septic process and the presence of bacterial toxin; careful evaluation of the smear for free or intracellular bacteria should follow.

Aerobic and anaerobic bacterial culture and sensitivity should be performed on all samples in which degenerative neutrophils are present, even if bacteria are not evident. Non-degenerative neutrophils suggest a non-septic process or low-grade sepsis. Bacterial culture and sensitivity may be indicated if alternate causes are not identified. Diseases that can result in exudative pleural effusions include neoplasia, chronic diaphragmatic hernia, feline infectious peritonitis, lung lobe torsions, lymphatic obstruction or leakage, and infectious processes.

Biochemical Parameters and Additional Fluid Evaluation

Many biochemical parameters of pleural effusions have been studied in attempts to further classify effusions and determine underlying etiologies. Most of these assays have been validated in people but have not been fully characterized in veterinary medicine. Analyses most frequently used in veterinary medicine include triglyceride, cholesterol, pH, lactate dehydrogenase (LDH), and glucose levels. Serum and fluid triglyceride concentration comparisons are used to definitively diagnose chylothorax (see below). Glucose and pH measurements can be helpful in identifying septic effusions; studies of pleural effusions in cats indicate that a glucose less than 10 mg/dL and a pH less than 6.9 are supportive of a septic effusion.[57] In people, a glucose concentration lower than normal is suggestive of tuberculosis, malignancy, rheumatoid disease, or a parapneumonic effusion. In one study of cats with pleural and peritoneal effusions, adenosine deaminase levels in effusions from cats with FIP were higher than those in unaffected cats.[58]

In humans, much work has concentrated on testing that may help differentiate neoplastic from non-neoplastic effusions. The pH of malignant effusions is typically greater than 7.2.[57] As noted above, decreased glucose concentrations can be supportive of neoplastic disease. Telomerase enzyme activity has been evaluated and was found to be equally as sensitive but less specific than cytology in differentiating fluid of malignant versus benign origin.[59] Vascular endothelial growth factor (VEGF) is expressed by some tumors and is believed to be a causative factor in the pathogenesis of both neoplastic and non-neoplastic effusions[60-62] by increasing capillary permeability.[63] Receptors for VEGF have been found in mesothelial cells.[64] In mice models, blockage of VEGF activity has led to a marked reduction in the volume of pleural effusion produced.[65] In people, high plasma or serum VEGF concentrations have been associated with a high tumor burden, presence of metastases and a poor prognosis.[66-68] However, elevations in VEGF are not specific for neoplasia and can also be found in inflammatory and infectious effusions. Very high VEGF levels have been noted in exudative effusions.[69] One study in dogs did not detect a difference in VEGF levels between neoplastic and non-neoplastic effusions.[70] In people, immunocytochemistry and chromosome analysis may also be useful in the diagnosis, classification, and prognostication of neoplastic effusions.

Eosinophilic Effusions

Pleural effusions are defined as being eosinophilic when greater than 10% of leukocytes identified are eosinophils.[71] Eosinophilic effusions have been reported in dogs in association with heartworm disease, systemic mastocytosis, interstitial pneumonia, and disseminated eosinophilic granulomatosis.[72-75] In a retrospective study of 14 cases, eosinophilic effusions were associated with diseases such as thoracic wall trauma, pneumothorax, neoplasia, congestive heart failure, and hypersensitivity states.[76] In that study, 43% of cases had neoplastic diseases. Eosinophilic pleural effusion was diagnosed 2 days after pneumothorax developed as a consequence of thoracic tube placement in one cat, and pneumothorax was diagnosed in another cat with eosinophilic peritoneal effusion. Eosinophilic pleural effusion has been associated with pneumothorax in people.[71,77] A report of a dog with pleural effusion secondary to discospondylitis cited cytology of the effusion as an exudate with Paecilomyces spp. fungal organisms present.[78] The pleural fluid contained a moderate number of eosinophils. It is believed that eosinophils may accumulate in the pleural space in response to pleural irritation.[79] Some authors suggest that leukotrienes or immune complexes may be chemotactic for eosinophils.[80] Corticosteroid responsive eosinophilic effusions have been reported[73,77]; therefore immune-mediated disease should be considered if alternate causes are not identified.

PYOTHORAX

Pyothorax is the presence of purulent material in the pleural space; bacterial pleuritis results in accumulation of hemopurulent fluid. The pleural fluid is classified as an exudate. Cytology usually reveals a very high nucleated cell count (often 50,000 to 100,000/uL) and is composed primarily of degenerative neutrophils. Nondegenerate neutrophils can be present if the animal was previously treated with antibiotics or in the presence of certain bacterial agents. Effusions caused by fungi and bacterial organisms such as Actinomyces and Nocardia spp. may contain nondegenerative neutrophils and macrophages if toxins produced affect only cells in close approximation to the organisms.[81] Multiple intra- and extracellular bacteria can be present; however, the possibility of contamination should be examined if only extracellular bacteria are noted. Macrophages are present in various numbers, depending on the causative organism and chronicity of the effusion. Leukophagocytosis is often seen in chronic infections. Reactive mesothelial cells are frequently present and should be interpreted with caution as they can exhibit criteria of malignancy. Multiple organisms are often cultured. In cats, obligate anaerobes or Pasteurella spp. are the most common isolates; in dogs obligate anaerobes or gram-positive filamentous organisms (i.e., Actinomyces and Nocardia spp.) are frequently cultured (Table 217-2).

The cause of pyothorax is often not identified. It can result from penetrating thoracic wounds, migration of foreign

RESPIRATORY DISEASE

Table • 217-2

Bacteria Commonly Associated with Pyothorax in Small Animals

BACTERIA	OXYGEN REQUIREMENTS	GRAM STAIN	MORPHOLOGY	ANTIBIOTIC SENSITIVITY*
Actinomyces spp. (most common in dogs)	Facultative anaerobe to strict anaerobe	Gram-positive	Small rods; may form filaments; often beaded and difficult to discern in clinical specimens; may form sulfur granules	**Ampicillin, amoxicillin plus clavulanic acid, penicillin,** clindamycin, chloramphenicol, erythromycin, minocycline
Bacteroides spp.	Obligate anaerobe	Gram-negative	Bacilli; pleomorphic and may be beaded or cocci, often stain poorly and are difficult to see	Most Bacteroides — **ampicillin, amoxicillin plus clavulanic acid,** clindamycin, chloramphenicol, metronidazole. *B. fragilis* — **amoxicillin + clavulanic acid, clindamycin,** chloramphenicol, **metronidazole**
Clostridium spp.	Obligate anaerobe	Gram-positive	Rods; large, frequently encapsulated, motile, spores uncommon from clinical specimens	Most Clostridium — **ampicillin, amoxicillin plus clavulanic acid,** chloramphenicol, **metronidazole**. *C. perfringens* — **ampicillin, amoxicillin plus clavulanic acid,** cefoxitin, clindamycin, chloramphenicol, metronidazole, erythromycin
Escherichia coli	Aerobe, facultative anaerobe	Gram-negative	Rods but shape can vary widely; never forms spores	**Amikacin, enrofloxacin,** ceftizoxime, potentiated sulfa drugs
Fusobacterium spp.	Obligate anaerobe	Gram-negative	Bacilli; often have a cigar-shaped appearance	**Penicillin,** clindamycin, chloramphenicol, metronidazole
Klebsiella *spp.*	Facultative anaerobe	Gram-negative	Rods; mucoid and encapsulated	**Cephalosporin,** gentamicin, tobramycin, ticarcillin
Nocardia spp. (most common in dogs)	Aerobe	Gram-positive (partly acid fast)	Long, filamentous and branching cocci or bacilli; most species produce hyphae; exudates typically have appearance of tomato soup; sulfur granules may be uncommon	**Trimethoprim-sulfa, amikacin,** imipenem, ciprofloxacin, cefotaxime, ceftriaxone
Pasteurella spp. (most common in cats)	Facultative anaerobe	Gram-negative	Coccobacilli; pleomorphic, bipolar staining	**Ampicillin, amoxicillin plus clavulanic acid, cephalosporins,** aminoglycosides
Pseudomonas spp.	Aerobe	Gram-negative	Rods; slender, motile	**Ticarcillin plus clavulanic acid, amikacin, enrofloxacin, gentamicin,** tobramycin, cefotaxime

*Boldface type denotes typical drugs of choice.
Modified from Fossum, TW: *Small animal surgery*, ed 2, St Louis, 2002, Mosby, p 813.

material (e.g., grass awns, particularly in working or hunting dogs), hematogenous spread, extension from other sites such as discospondylitis or pneumonia, pulmonary neoplasia, pulmonary or thoracic wall trauma, or from a postoperative infection. The underlying disease process should be identified and treated if possible.

These animals should be managed aggressively as treatment with antibiotics alone is not usually effective. A chest tube should be placed once the diagnosis is made. Bilateral thoracostomy tubes are sometimes necessary with chronic effusions as thickening of the pleura may create a complete mediastinum. Most animals can be successfully managed with intermittent tube aspiration. Thoracic lavage with warm saline or lactated Ringer's solution should be performed two or three times daily. Twenty mL/kg should be infused slowly into the thoracic cavity and allowed to remain for 1 hour. Animals should be closely monitored for dyspnea and the lavage fluid removed earlier if necessary.

The addition of antibiotics to the lavage fluid offers no advantage over appropriately administered systemic antibiotics.

Antibiotics should be chosen based on Gram stain and microbial culture and sensitivity results. Due to the high proportion of anaerobic infections, drugs with a spectrum against obligate anaerobic organisms should be used. Antibiotics should be continued for a minimum of 4 to 6 weeks. Surgery is mandatory in animals with underlying diseases such as foreign bodies, lung abscesses, or lung lobe torsions; and should be considered in animals that do not respond to medical treatment in the first 3 to 4 days. Readers are referred to a surgical text for additional information.

CHYLOTHORAX

Chyle is the milky fluid absorbed by the lacteals from food in the intestines. It is composed of lymph and triglyceride droplets (chylomicrons). *Chylothorax* refers to the accumulation of chyle in the pleural space. Chylothorax was once believed to be a result of trauma to the thoracic duct. Although this occasionally occurs in veterinary patients, the resulting effusion is usually self-limiting and resolves within 2 weeks. Trauma is, however, still considered a reasonable cause of chylothorax in human patients. Chylothorax may develop from increased lymphatic flow (due to increased hepatic lymph production), from decreased lymphatic drainage into the venous system, or from both. Disease processes that result in increased systemic venous pressures, such as right-sided heart failure, have been shown to cause chylothorax.[82] FeLV and FIV status should be evaluated in affected cats. Chyle is thought to exude from intact but dilated thoracic lymphatics (thoracic lymphangectasia) (Figure 217-6). Chylothorax may also occur in conjunction with diffuse lymphatic disease such as intestinal or generalized lymphangectasia. Chylothorax secondary to pulmonary lymphangiosarcoma has recently been reported in a dog.[83]

The thoracic duct (TD) arises from the cisterna chyli and is the major lymphatic vessel for the return of lymph to the venous system. Thoracic duct anatomy varies between and among species. It usually begins as a single duct, but multiple branches are often present. The convergence with the venous system occurs at the "venous angle" in the cranial vena cava where the external and internal jugular veins meet. In the dog the TD lies to the right of midline in the caudal thorax and crosses to the left side at approximately the fifth intercostal space, whereas in the cat it lies to the left side throughout its course through the diaphragm.

Animals presenting with chylous pleural effusion should be thoroughly evaluated for underlying diseases that may interfere with lymphatic flow or increase the pressure against which the thoracic duct must empty. These include heart disease (cardiomyopathy, heartworm disease, pericardial effusion, tetralogy of Fallot, tricuspid dysplasia, or cor triatriatum dexter), cranial mediastinal masses (lymphoma, thymoma), fungal granulomas, venous thrombi, or congenital abnormalities of the TD. In those cases with a defined etiology, treatment is aimed at the underlying cause. Intermittent thoracocentesis palliates the clinical signs until a definitive treatment is instituted (if possible). In the majority of animals, however, a cause is not identified (idiopathic chylothorax).

Although any breed of dog or cat may be affected, breed dispositions are suspected in Afghan hounds, Shiba Inus, and Oriental cat breeds (Siamese, Himalayan). A sex predilection has not been identified and the disease has been reported in all ages. Afghans tend to develop the disease in middle age, whereas affected Shiba Inus tend to be less than 1 year of age. In one study that showed older cats more likely to be affected than younger ones, an association with neoplasia was suspected.[84]

Coughing is usually the first and may be the only clinical sign noted in both dogs and cats. Animals with a history of a chronic cough that is unresponsive to general treatment should be evaluated for the presence of thoracic fluid. As noted earlier, coughing may be caused by irritation from the effusion or from the underlying disease process. Many animals present with acute respiratory distress as an emergent situation to the veterinarian, without overt history of previous clinical signs of respiratory disease.

Physical exam findings attributable to the presence of pleural fluid include decreased or muffled heart sounds, decreased ventral lung sounds, and increased bronchovesicular sounds dorsally. Mucous membrane color varies from normal to cyanotic, depending on the severity of respiratory compromise. Weight loss is often noted with animals with chronic disease due to the loss of fat and protein into the thoracic cavity. Other physical exam findings such as heart murmurs may be present depending on the underlying disease process.

Thoracocentesis revealing milky, opaque fluid permits a tentative diagnosis of chylothorax and should prompt the veterinarian to search for underlying causes. The fluid consistency and color will vary depending on dietary fat content and the presence of concurrent hemorrhage. Fluid samples should be placed in an EDTA tube for cytologic evaluation. Although lymph fluid is resistant to infection due to the presence of fatty acids, samples should be submitted for bacteriologic culture and sensitivity, particularly if repeated thoracocentesis has been performed. Chylous fluid may be classified as an exudate or as a modified transudate, depending on the protein levels and nucleated cell counts which can vary with chronicity and previous treatment. Lymphocytes are typical, but nondegenerate neutrophils are commonly noted with more chronic cases. Protein content is variable and may be inaccurate due to the high lipid content of the fluid. Truly chylous fluids should contain chylomicrons, should clear with the addition of ether, and be positive for the presence of lipid droplets with Sudan III stain. A definitive diagnosis of chylothorax is obtained by comparing fluid and serum triglyceride levels; in chylothorax, fluid triglyceride should be higher than that of simultaneously collected serum.

Differential diagnoses include any other causes of cough or pleural effusion. Once the diagnosis of pleural effusion is made, diseases that cause exudative effusions, such as pyothorax, are considered differentials and should be investigated. Pseudochylous effusion refers to thoracic fluid in which the fluid triglyceride level is less than that of serum and fluid

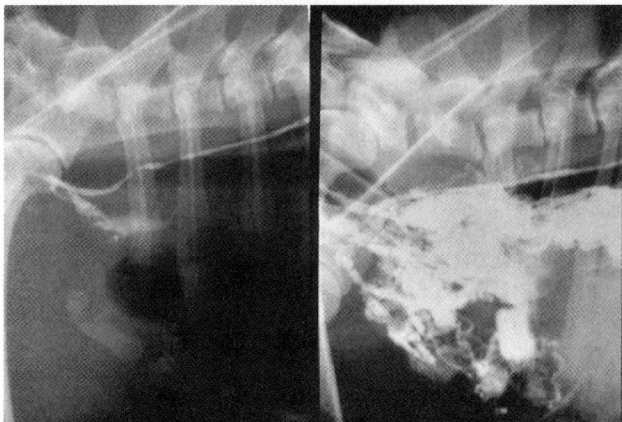

Figure 217-6 Mesenteric lymphangiogram from a normal dog (*left*) and a dog with idiopathic chylothorax (*right*). Notice the entrance of the thoracic duct into the venous system in the normal dog and the marked lymphangiectasia in the dog with chylothorax. Chylothorax is thought to occur as a result of leakage from these dilated, tortuous cranial mediastinal lymphatics.

RESPIRATORY DISEASE

cholesterol level greater. Pseudochylous effusions are rare in veterinary patients and may be associated with tuberculosis.

As noted earlier, treatment should be directed at the underlying disease process, if identified, and clinical signs palliated by intermittent thoracocentesis. Resolution of the effusion will depend on the underlying cause and may take several months. Surgical treatment should only be considered in animals with idiopathic chylothorax or those that do not respond to medical management.

Medical management of animals with chylothorax involves feeding a low-fat diet, performing needle thoracentesis as needed to relieve dyspnea (not on a regular basis), and supplementing the dog or cat with a benzopyrone such as Rutin (50 to 100 mg/kg, TID, PO). The effusion may spontaneously resolve over a period of weeks or months. If the animal cannot be managed medically, surgical intervention is typically recommended. Thoracic duct ligation is the most widely accepted method for treating animals with chylothorax, yet this intervention has not been reported to be highly successful in alleviating the chylous accumulation. Thoracic duct ligation resulted in complete resolution of pleural effusion in only approximately 50% of dogs operated; in cats, the success rate was even less (<40%).[84-86] A more recent study reported 100% efficacy in dogs and 80% in cats when TD ligation and/or pericardiotomy were performed.[88]

Advantages of thoracic duct ligation are that if it is successful it results in complete resolution of pleural fluid (as compared to palliative procedures such as pleuroperitoneal shunting) and thus it may prevent fibrosing pleuritis from developing. Disadvantages include that operative time is long, which is problematic in debilitated animals, there is a high incidence of continued or recurrent chylous or nonchylous (from pulmonary lymphatics) effusion, and mesenteric lymphangiography is often difficult to perform, particularly in cats. Without mesenteric lymphangiography, complete ligation of the thoracic duct is difficult to ensure. Ligation of the thoracic duct using thoracoscopy has been described.[87]

Thoracic duct ligation plus pericardectomy was recently reported as a treatment for chylothorax.[88] In this study, TD ligation plus pericardectomy was performed in 18 animals, and pericardectomy alone was performed in an additional two animals. Nineteen animals presented for evaluation of chylothorax (9 dogs, 10 cats), whereas one dog presented for serosanguineous pleural fluid after TD ligation that had been performed elsewhere. Echocardiography was normal in all animals with the exception of a subjectively thickened pericardium in six dogs and seven cats. Clinical signs of pleural fluid resolved in ten of ten dogs and eight of 10 cats after surgery. The overall success rate for surgical treatment of chylothorax in this study was 90%.

NEOPLASTIC PLEURAL EFFUSION

Differentiation of neoplastic and non-neoplastic effusions can be difficult. Neoplastic processes commonly resulting in pleural effusion include mesothelioma, lymphoma, multiple myeloma, carcinoma of the lung, and metastatic mammary neoplasia. Effusions caused by neoplastic processes are often hemorrhagic.

Mesotheliomas can arise from the mesothelial cells of the pleura, pericardium, or peritoneum and can be malignant or benign. Congenital mesotheliomas have been described in calves.[89] In people, mesotheliomas are frequently associated with exposure to asbestos.[90] Histologically, mesotheliomas can be fibrous or epithelial; in humans both are seen but pleural mesotheliomas in dogs are predominantly the epithelial type. Metastasis to other intrathoracic organs such as the myocardium, tracheobronchial lymph nodes, and lung is common. This tumor may also invade the diaphragm and

enter the abdomen. A diagnosis is not usually made on fluid evaluation because of the difficulty in differentiating neoplastic versus reactive mesothelial cells (see above); a surgical or thoracoscopic biopsy is generally necessary to obtain a definitive diagnosis. Readers are referred to an oncologic textbook for additional information on diagnosis and treatment of mesotheliomas.

In human medicine, pleurodesis is often used to decrease the incidence of malignant effusions. Attempts at pleurodesis in dogs have been unrewarding[91] and are not recommended by the authors. More recent research has focused on the possible etiologies of the effusions. Vascular endothelial growth factor (VEGF) is thought to play a role in the development of malignant effusions. Studies in mice have demonstrated a reduction in the formation of pleural effusion with treatment directed at VEGF receptor inhibition.[65]

PNEUMOTHORAX

Traumatic Pneumothorax

Pneumothorax in small animals is most frequently closed (no communication between the pleural space and external environment) and traumatic in origin secondary to motor vehicle accidents or other blunt trauma. Pulmonary or bronchial rupture can occur when a blow to the thorax results in a sudden increase in intrathoracic pressure, theoretically against a closed glottis. Alternatively, shearing forces on the lung may result in subpleural bleb formation, similar to that seen in spontaneous pneumothorax. Pneumothorax secondary to a bronchial tear has been reported following venipuncture in a kitten.[92]

Penetrating injuries such as bite wounds and gunshot wounds can result in an open pneumothorax, where communication exists between the pleural space and external environment. Penetrating wounds may permit influx of air into the pleural space with inspiration and rapid equilibration of intrathoracic and atmospheric pressures. The normal pressure gradient is necessary for mechanical function of the lungs and proper air exchange. Loss of negative intrathoracic pressure also decreases venous return to the heart. Abdominal wounds may result in a pneumothorax if a diaphragmatic hernia is present. A tension pneumothorax develops when the fistula between the pleura and the external environment or the pleura and the lung acts as a one-way valve, which allows air to enter on inspiration but not exit on expiration. Positive pressure develops in the pleural space causing collapse of the lungs and great veins. Fatal decreases in ventilation and cardiac output rapidly ensue. Iatrogenic tension pneumothorax has been reported secondary to lung or airway rupture in animals that receive positive pressure ventilation.[93] As with diaphragmatic hernias, young male dogs are more likely to incur vehicular or other causes of trauma and are therefore more likely to develop traumatic pneumothorax. Traumatic pneumothorax is less commonly reported in cats.

Spontaneous Pneumothorax

Pneumothorax is classified as spontaneous when no traumatic or iatrogenic cause is identified. Spontaneous pneumothorax is thought to result from rupture of pulmonary blebs or bullae and is considered primary when there is no evidence of underlying pulmonary disease. Subpleural blebs are most commonly located in the apices of the lungs. Primary spontaneous pneumothorax occurs most frequently in large, deep-chested dogs such as hounds. One recent retrospective study reported an over-representation of Siberian Huskies in their case population.[94] Middle-aged dogs are most commonly affected; there does not appear to be a sex predilection.

Secondary spontaneous pneumothorax is more common in dogs than the primary form and occurs when there is underlying pulmonary disease such as pulmonary abscesses, diffuse emphysema, neoplasia, dirofiliarisis, pneumonia or pulmonary parasites such as *Paragonimus* spp. Spontaneous pneumothorax has also been reported in cats with *Dirofilaria immitis* infection.[15] It may also be seen secondary to chronic granulomatous infections or chronic airway obstruction and subsequent overpressurization of abnormal lungs.[95,96] The majority of affected people are cigarette smokers, which suggests that the underlying pulmonary disease could be a result of interference of the normal function of alpha$_1$-antitrypsin in inhibiting elastase. It is believed that alpha$_1$-antitrypsin is inactivated in people who smoke, which allows increased elastase-induced destruction of pulmonary parenchyma.

History and Physical Examination

Animals with pneumothorax generally present with acute dyspnea and shallow, rapid respiration. A history of trauma is often vague, which makes it sometimes difficult initially to distinguish between traumatic and spontaneous pneumothorax. In animals with secondary spontaneous pneumothorax, a history attributable to underlying respiratory disease (e.g., chronic cough, fever) may be ascertained. Dogs with pneumothorax are initially able to compensate by increasing their chest wall expansion with inspiration. Animals with hypoxemia will appear cyanotic. Hypoxemia is thought to be a result of impairment of gas exchange, increased pulmonary shunting, and V/Q (ventilation-perfusion) mismatch[97] (increased alveolar-arterial PO$_2$ difference). In traumatic pneumothorax, concurrent injuries such as rib fractures and pulmonary contusions may exacerbate the clinical signs of respiratory compromise. Auscultation of the thoracic cavity may reveal decreased or muffled heart and lung sounds dorsally. Tension pneumothorax is a rapidly fatal condition. A barrel-shaped chest may be evident as pressure within the thoracic cavity increases. Cyanosis and signs attributable to markedly decreased cardiac output are evident.

Diagnosis

Thoracocentesis should be performed to stabilize the dyspneic animal prior to thoracic radiographs being taken. Pneumothorax is most commonly bilateral. Radiographic signs consistent with a pneumothorax include elevation of the heart off the sternum, collapse of the lung lobes and retraction from the chest wall, and a radiolucent area of free air in which no pulmonary vascular structures are visible, most evident in the caudal thorax (Figure 217-7). In severe cases, the diaphragm may appear flattened or caudally displaced. Apparent elevation of the heart from the sternum is a result of atelectasis of the dependent lung lobes allowing the heart to shift its position with the chest. To identify small volumes of free air, the most sensitive radiographic view is a horizontal beam taken with the animal in lateral recumbency. Although it may be difficult to identify in the presence of collapsed lung lobes, radiographs should be carefully evaluated for underlying pulmonary parenchymal or other thoracic diseases such as trauma or neoplasia. Pulmonary blebs are difficult to identify radiographically. Bullae may be an incidental finding in some cases. Removal of air with thoracocentesis is diagnostic of pneumothorax if radiographs are unclear or unavailable. Pneumomediastinum is characterized by the ability to distinguish thoracic structures (i.e., aorta and great vessels, trachea, vena cava, esophagus) within the mediastinum that are not usually apparent on thoracic radiographs.

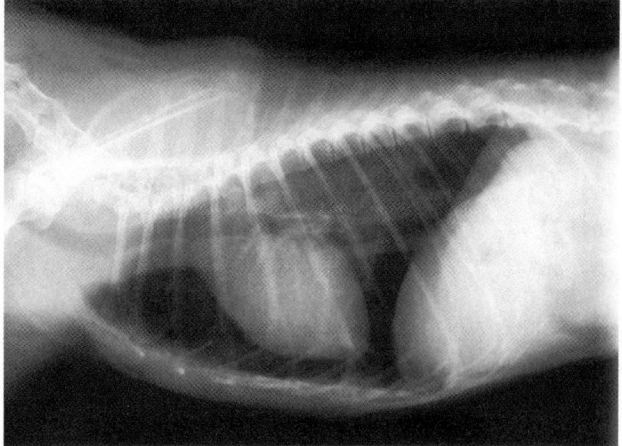

Figure 217-7 Lateral radiograph of a dog with pneumothorax. Note the apparent elevation of the heart from the sternum.

Treatment

A thoracostomy tube may be required in animals in which air rapidly accumulates. Intermittent or continuous aspiration can be used depending on the volume of air recovered from the thoracic cavity and rate at which it accumulates. Once the animal has been stabilized, the cause of the pneumothorax should be identified. Traumatic pneumothorax is most commonly managed conservatively; surgical intervention is rarely necessary. Thoracocentesis or chest tubes (see Chapter 103) can be used to manage air accumulation and dyspnea while the pulmonary lesions heal, usually within 3 to 5 days. Supplemental oxygen therapy may be beneficial in animals with pulmonary contusions or hemorrhage. Pain management is essential in animals that have experienced trauma; analgesics may help improve ventilation by decreasing the pain associated with thoracic wall movement. Recurrence of traumatic pneumothorax is uncommon. Open chest wounds should be covered immediately. Once the animal has been hospitalized, the wound can be addressed and covered with a sterile, occlusive dressing. Readers are referred to a surgical text for more detailed information on thoracic wound management.

Animals with spontaneous pneumothorax generally require thoracostomy tube placement. As opposed to animals with traumatic pneumothorax, those with spontaneous disease often require surgical intervention. A median sternotomy allows access to both sides of the lungs and permits thorough exploration of the thoracic cavity. If not immediately evident, pulmonary and airway leaks may be identified by filling the pleural space with warm physiologic saline and looking for air bubbles. Animals that undergo surgical treatment of spontaneous pneumothorax are less likely to have recurrence and have lower mortality than those that are managed conservatively.[94] Surgical exploration may permit identification of the underlying etiology that may have not been readily apparent previously. Thoracoscopic evaluation of the thorax has been reported for people and dogs with spontaneous pneumothorax and may obviate the need for surgery if a cause can be identified and treated.[98-100]

RESPIRATORY DISEASE

CHAPTER 218

Pulmonary Hypertension and Pulmonary Thromboembolism

Kristin A. MacDonald
Lynelle R. Johnson

Pulmonary Hypertension

Pulmonary hypertension (PH) is defined by a systolic pulmonary artery pressure greater than 25 mm Hg. The incidence of PH is difficult to define due to lack of clinical awareness, nonspecific clinical signs, and difficulty in confirming the diagnosis. Unfortunately, many patients with PH are diagnosed late in the course of disease when irreversible vascular pathology has developed. PH results from many diseases and pathophysiologic mechanisms and most commonly occurs secondary to chronic cardiopulmonary disease.

Relevant Pulmonary Physiology

Normal pulmonary vasculature is a low-resistance, low-pressure, high-capacitance circuit. Normal, awake dogs at sea-level have a systolic pulmonary artery (PA) pressure between 15 to 25 mm Hg, end-diastolic PA pressure of 5 to 10 mm Hg, and a mean PA pressure of 10 to 15 mm Hg.[1] When cardiac output increases, such as during exercise, there is recruitment of additional pulmonary arterioles to maintain normal PA pressure. Regional pulmonary perfusion is regulated by pulmonary arteriolar vasoconstriction. Hypoxic vasoconstriction matches pulmonary perfusion to alveolar ventilation and limits the impact of low ventilation on arterial oxygenation. However, with global alveolar hypoxia, the protective effects of hypoxic vasoconstriction are offset by widespread vasoconstriction and development of PH.

The vascular endothelium mediates vascular tone and remodeling through release of several neurohormonal factors, and endothelial injury plays a key role in development of PH. In the normal lung, there is a balance between locally acting vasodilators including prostacyclin (PGI_2) and nitric oxide (NO) versus potent vasoconstricting substances including thromboxane, endothelin-I (ET-1), and angiotensin II (AT-II). Endothelial dysfunction in PH contributes to smooth muscle cell proliferation, increased production of vasoconstrictor mediators including ET-1 and AT-II, and decreased synthesis of vasodilating substances including PGI_2 and NO.[2] Pulmonary artery thrombi are seen histologically in both primary PH (PPH) and secondary PH in people. Pro-coagulant affects may be mediated by increased TXA_2 and tissue factor, as well as reduced anti-coagulant mediators including NO, PGI_2, and thrombomodulin.[3]

Classification of Pulmonary Hypertension

Classification of PH through hemodynamic and pathophysiologic mechanisms helps to guide interventional treatment. Mean pulmonary artery pressure (MPAP) is related to pulmonary blood flow (PBF) and pulmonary vascular resistance (PVR) by the equation

$$MPAP = (PVR \times PBF) + \text{Pulmonary capillary wedge}$$
$$\text{pressure (PCWP)}$$

Abnormalities of any component of this equation can cause PH.

Pre-capillary PH occurs due to abnormalities of the pulmonary arterial vascular bed and is characterized by increased systolic, mean, and diastolic PAP, increased PVR, and normal PCWP. PVR is closely related to total cross-sectional area of the small muscular arteries and arterioles. Given the high capacitance of the pulmonary vasculature, 50% of the pulmonary vasculature must be destroyed before PH develops.[4] Diseases that cause pre-capillary PH include primary pulmonary hypertension (PPH), Eisenmenger's complex, chronic pulmonary disorders, pulmonary thromboembolism (PTE), and peripheral pulmonary artery branch stenosis. PPH has not yet been identified in veterinary medicine. Eisenmenger's syndrome is an irreversible, obliterative vascular disease that results from severe left to right shunting congenital heart disease that reverses to shunt right to left. Chronic respiratory disorders may result in PH in some individuals through hypoxic pulmonary vasoconstriction, extramural compression of the pulmonary arterioles, and destruction of pulmonary microvasculature. In the absence of pulmonary arterial pathologic changes (plexiform lesions, necrotizing arteritis, hyalinizing fibrosis), PH due to hypoxic vasoconstriction may be dynamic and respond to therapeutic intervention.

In post-capillary PH, PAP passively increases due to elevated PCWP. PA diastolic pressure is within 5 mm Hg of the PCWP, and PVR is normal. Left-sided congestive heart failure (CHF) is the most common cause of increased PCWP and may result from severe mitral valve disease, dilated cardiomyopathy, or diastolic heart disease. A mixed hemodynamic response may be seen with chronic elevations in PCWP and consists of a disproportionate elevation in PA pressures in comparison to elevated PCWP. The mechanism for increased PVR in response to elevated PCWP is not entirely clear but likely involves endothelin-1 release, endothelial dysfunction, and abnormal pulmonary vasodilatory reserve.[4] Approximately 30% of human patients with chronic pulmonary venous hypertension develop increased PVR.[4] Based on clinical experience, a low percentage of dogs with severe mitral regurgitation have a mixed hemodynamic response of PH.

Pulmonary blood flow (PBF) can be increased selectively by left to right shunting congenital heart diseases (ASD, VSD, PDA) and some patients are at risk for development of Eisenmenger's physiology. PBF is also increased by high output cardiac disease (arteriovenous fistula, chronic anemia, and hyperthyroidism); however, most patients do not develop recognizable PH. Pneumonectomy leads to selective increases in pulmonary blood flow, but PH is not recognized as a complication in dogs.

Cor pulmonale is defined as heart disease due to PH resulting from chronic pulmonary disease. The most common cause of cor pulmonale in veterinary medicine is heartworm disease in dogs. PH leads to acquired pressure overload of the right ventricle characterized by chamber dilation primarily and also concentric hypertrophy. RV myocardial failure may occur due to inadequate reduction of wall stress and may be worsened by myocardial ischemia from reduced right coronary artery perfusion pressure.[2] The extent of concentric hypertrophy and dilation of the RV ventricle depends on the age of the animal, the severity and duration of pressure overload, and the time course of progression.

Clinical Features

Clinical manifestations of PH are difficult to distinguish from those of underlying cardiopulmonary disease. Ascites may be the most obvious abnormality and is often accompanied by other signs of right heart failure including jugular vein distension or pulsation, subcutaneous edema, and cachexia. The most common clinical signs are nonspecific respiratory abnormalities such as coughing, tachypnea, and respiratory distress. Syncope is relatively common in dogs with PH. Adventitious lung sounds may be ausculted with primary respiratory disease or CHF. Cyanosis can be seen in patients with right-to-left cardiac shunts or severe respiratory disease. Cardiac auscultation may reveal a split or loud pulmonic component to the second heart sound. Right and left apical systolic murmurs are commonly heard due to tricuspid and mitral regurgitation, respectively.

A minimum database (CBC, chemistry, urinalysis) and heartworm test should be performed to identify underlying diseases that may be associated with PH. Hypoxemia and acidosis should be identified since hypoxemia can cause PH and both may worsen PH.

Thoracic radiographs are necessary to detect respiratory or cardiac diseases that may be associated with PH. Thoracic radiography is almost always abnormal, and cardiomegaly is most commonly seen. Identification of RV enlargement and dilated central pulmonary arteries with rapid tapering towards the periphery should greatly increase clinical suspicion of severe PH (Figure 218-1). Eisenmenger's complex is characterized by pulmonary undercirculation and right heart enlargement. Substantial left atrial enlargement and perihilar to caudo-dorsal pulmonary infiltrates indicate left sided CHF and possible post-capillary PH.

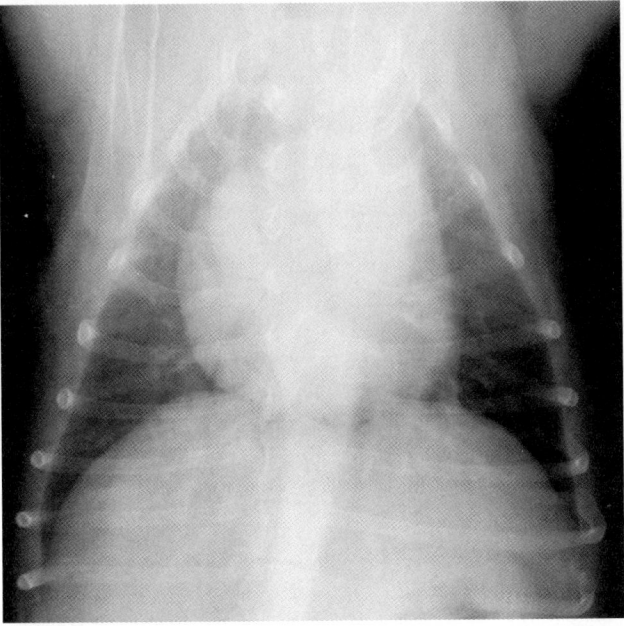

Figure 218-1 Dorsoventral thoracic radiograph of a dog with PH. There is severe right heart enlargement and dilated central portions of the pulmonary arteries.

Electrocardiographic assessment of right heart enlargement is insensitive, and abnormalities are present only with severe PH. Deep S waves and right axis deviation may be seen with severe RV hypertrophy, and tall peaked P waves may indicate right atrial enlargement. Sinus tachycardia is a common rhythm abnormality.

Echocardiography is a useful, noninvasive tool to detect PH and cor pulmonale in veterinary and human medicine.[5,6] Echocardiographic characteristics include RV concentric hypertrophy and dilation, dilation of the main pulmonary artery and main branches, systolic flattening of the interventricular septum, and paradoxical septal motion (Figure 218-2). In severe PH, the left ventricular dimensions may be reduced due to ventricular underfilling and ventricular interdependence. Pulmonic stenosis (PS) must be ruled out by a normal PA systolic blood flow velocity of less than 1.5 m/s before PH can be documented. In the absence of PS, the RV systolic pressure equals the PA systolic pressure. Using the modified Bernoulli equation (Pressure gradient = $4 \times \text{velocity}^2$), spectral Doppler allows reasonably accurate estimations of RV systolic pressure via measurement of triscuspid regurgitation velocity, and PA diastolic pressure via measurement of pulmonic insufficiency velocity (Figure 218-2). The RV:RA pressure gradient is added to the estimated RA pressure (5 mm Hg is normal, 10 to 15 mm Hg in right heart failure) for the estimated RV systolic pressure, which approximates PA systolic pressure.

Right heart catheterization is the gold standard for diagnosis of PH and determination of the hemodynamic classification. Unfortunately, catherization requires sedation anesthesia, and these patients are already at increased risk for anesthetic complications. Cardiac output and pressures can be measured, which allows calculation of PVR. Cardiac catheterization allows for pharmacologic tests of vasodilators to identify reversible lesions and evaluate potential pharmacologic treatments.

Treatment

Treatment of PH is aimed at correcting the specific hemodynamic abnormality. Left CHF is treated with diuretics, angiotensin-converting enzyme (ACE) inhibitors, and possibly careful use of afterload reducing agents (amlodipine or hydralazine). Resolution of symptomatic CHF often reduces post-capillary PH and clinical signs of syncope. Surgical or interventional techniques may be used to correct left to right shunting congenital heart diseases but should never be attempted in patients with right to left shunts since it will hasten death. Cautious use of diuretics and ACE-inhibitors are indicated for right heart failure, since patients may develop symptomatic hypotension if they become significantly volume underloaded in the face of fixed PVR. ACE-inhibitors have been shown to delay pulmonary vascular remodeling in experimental animals and have produced beneficial hemodynamic effects in people with cor pulmonale.[7] Digoxin improved cardiac output and reduced circulating norepinephrine concentration in people with primary PH and symptomatic right heart failure[2] and could be considered for treatment of severe PH and right heart failure in veterinary patients.

Treatment of precapillary PH is aimed at reducing PVR and RV pressure overload. Pulmonary vasodilator trials may be performed during cardiac catheterizations to identify responsive patients; however, most veterinary patients likely have fixed PVR at the time of diagnosis. Short-acting vasodilators (adenosine, inhaled nitric oxide, or PGI_2) may be used to identify patients that have reversible vasoconstriction, as evidenced by more than 10 mm Hg decrease in MPAP with no change or an increase in cardiac output, and/or a decrease in PVR by 25%.[4] Only about 20% of humans have a positive pressor response, and these individuals benefit from treatment with high doses of the calcium-channel blocker (diltiazem).[4]

RESPIRATORY DISEASE

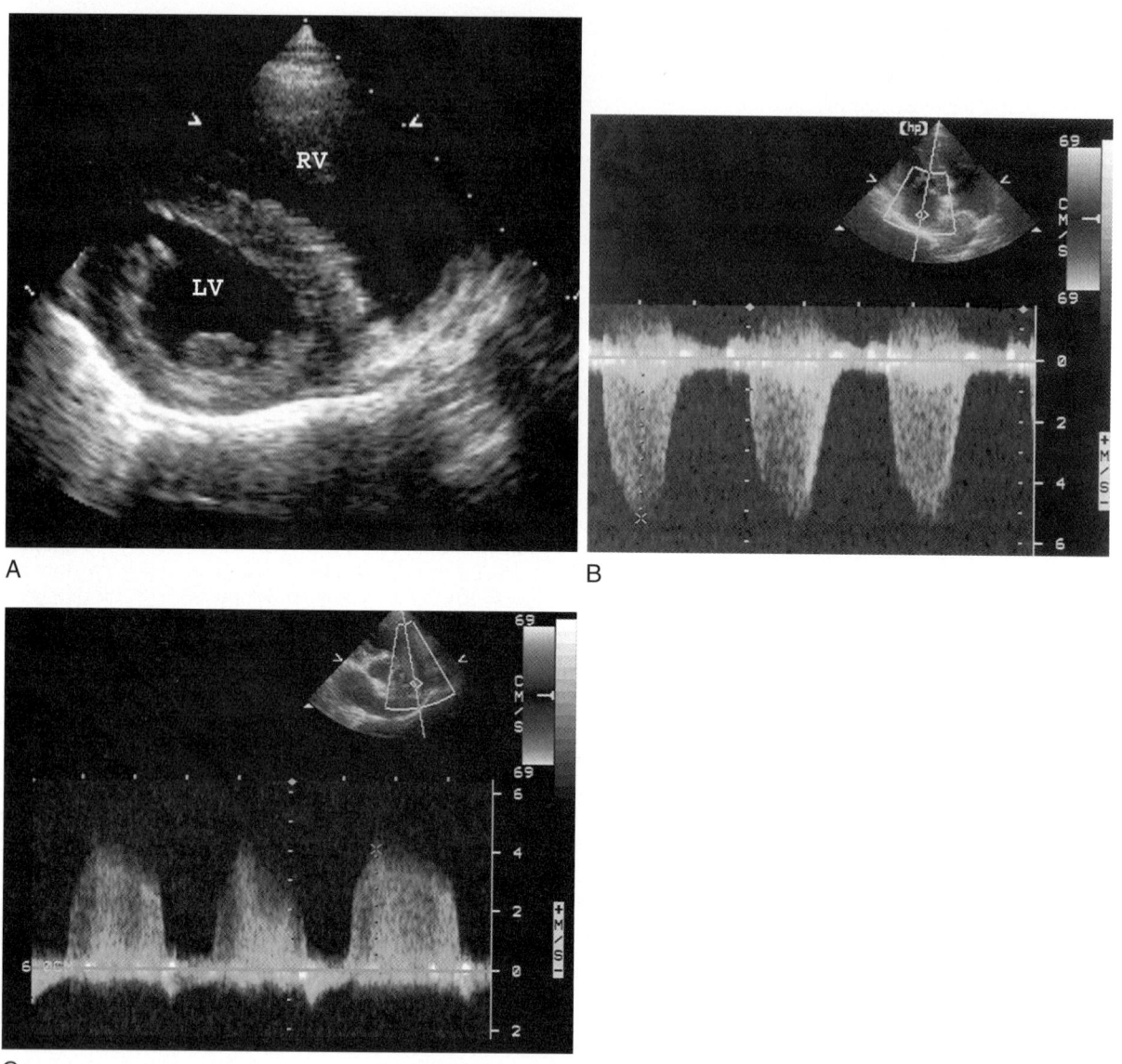

Figure 218-2 A, Two-dimensional echocardiogram of a dog with PH. The right basilar short axis view shows severe right ventricular dilation and concentric hypertrophy that is characteristic of severe acquired pressure overload. The interventricular septum is flattened, which indicates that the right ventricular pressure is greater than the left ventricular pressure. **B,** Continuous wave Doppler measurement of tricuspid regurgitation (TR) velocity in a dog with PH. The TR velocity is 5.2 m/s. Using the modified Bernoulli equation, there is a 110 mm Hg pressure gradient between the RV and RA during systole. Adding 5 mm Hg estimated RA pressure, the estimated RV and PA systolic pressure is 115 mm Hg. **C,** Continuous wave Doppler measurement of pulmonic insufficiency (PI) in a dog with PH. The PI velocity is 4 m/s, and the diastolic pressure gradient between the PA and RV is 64 mm Hg, which closely estimates the PA diastolic pressure.

No studies have evaluated short-acting pulmonary vasodilator trials and subsequent therapy with calcium channel blockers in veterinary patients with PH.

Intravenous PGI_2 has been shown to improve exercise capacity, hemodynamics, vascular remodeling, and short- and long-term survival in humans.[7] However, lifelong intravenous PGI_2 therapy is not an acceptable treatment modality in veterinary medicine. New oral (beraprost) and subcutaneous (treprostinil) synthetic prostacyclin analogs are under intense investigation in human medicine[7] and may be useful in

veterinary medicine. Other promising pulmonary vasodilators being researched for primary and secondary PH include endothelin receptor antagonists (bosentan) and phosphodiesterase inhibitors (sildenafil).[7]

Prognosis for PH is variable and depends on the type and severity of underlying etiology, degree of PH, and reversibility of vascular pathology. In humans with primary PH, mean PA pressure, RA pressure, and PVR are inversely proportional to survival.[2] Earlier identification and treatment of patients with PH may slow the progression, but prognosis remains poor to grave.

PULMONARY THROMBOEMBOLISM

Etiology and Pathophysiology

Pulmonary thromboembolism (PTE) is a life-threatening condition that occurs in more than 600,000 human patients a year.[8] Despite increased awareness and sophisticated imaging modalities in human medicine, only 30% of fatal PTE is diagnosed antemortem.[8] Similarly, PTE was suspected antemortem in only 38% of dogs and 14% of cats with postmortem evidence of major PTE.[9,10] PTE comprised 0.9% of all postmortem diagnoses in dogs, which likely underestimates the true incidence in the population.[9]

Pulmonary vascular obstruction can result from thrombus formation, or embolization of thrombi, parasites, fat, or neoplastic cells. Heartworm disease is the most common cause of PTE in dogs. It results in mechanical obstruction of pulmonary blood flow as well as enhanced reactive pulmonary vasoconstriction and reduced endothelium-dependent vasorelaxation.[11] Venous stasis, endothelial injury, and hypercoagulability contribute to thrombus formation within pulmonary arteries/arterioles (in-situ thrombosis) and to thromboembolic disease of the pulmonary capillary bed. PTE is a secondary condition, and immune-mediated hemolytic anemia (IMHA), neoplasia, cardiac disease, protein-losing nephropathy or enteropathy, hyperadrenocorticism, disseminated intravascular coagulation, sepsis, trauma, and recent surgery are associated with PTE in dogs and cats.[9,10,12] A large number of dogs and cats with PTE (47% to 64%, respectively) have multiple underlying disease processes.[9,12] Identification of risk factors and underlying diseases associated with PTE should be used to initiate early prophylactic treatment for PTE and aggressive treatment for the primary disease.

In PTE, PVR is increased due to mechanical obstruction of blood flow and reflex vasoconstriction from release of vasoactive mediators (serotonin, thromboxane) from the thrombus. Low-output cardiac failure and shock may occur with acute, major PTE. Functional status of the cardiopulmonary system plays a role in determination of the hemodynamic consequences of PTE.

Pathophysiologic consequences of PTE include abnormal gas exchange, altered ventilatory control, dysregulated pulmonary mechanics, and potentially pulmonary infarction.[2] Hypoxia results from ventilation/perfusion (V/Q) mismatch, increased alveolar dead space, and intrapulmonary or intracardiac right-to-left shunting. Hypoxia can be worsened by pulmonary edema caused by enhanced blood flow to non-thrombosed regions of the lung. Reduced surfactant function in the region of thrombosis leads to atelectasis and reduced lung compliance. Release of humoral factors causes bronchoconstriction, increased airway resistance, and tachypnea. All of these factors contribute to hypoxia, increased work of respiration, and respiratory distress.

Clinical Signs and Diagnostic Tests

PTE is seen most often in middle-aged to older animals, with no sex or breed predisposition. PTE, like PH, can mimic and often accompany other cardiopulmonary diseases. Sudden onset respiratory distress and tachypnea are common historical or physical examination abnormalities seen in 58% to 96% of dogs and 55% of cats with PTE.[11,12] The list of differential diagnoses is extensive and includes airway obstruction, pneumonia, acute CHF, ARDS or other noncardiogenic pulmonary edema, pleural space disease, or asthma in cats.

When PTE is suspected, identification of an underlying disease and definition of the degree of cardiopulmonary dysfunction are essential. Definitive documentation of PTE remains difficult in both human and veterinary medicine. CBC, chemistry, and urinalysis should be performed, and a coagulation panel can be used to support the presence of concurrent DIC.

Plasma D-dimer is used in the diagnosis of PTE in humans, with 96% sensitivity and 52% specificity.[2] Plasma D-dimer is a breakdown product of cross-linked fibrin, which is produced when fibrin is degraded by plasmin. D-dimer is produced in a number of disease conditions in both human and veterinary medicine. The utility of D-dimer in the diagnosis of PTE in veterinary medicine in unknown, but a negative test might be useful in ruling out PTE. Plasma anti-thrombin III activity should be measured if protein losing nephropathy or enteropathy is diagnosed.

Thoracic radiographic abnormalities are common but are rarely specific for PTE. In fact, 10% to 30% of dogs and 14% of cats had normal thoracic radiographs despite necropsy proven PTE[9,10], which indicates that PTE should be a top differential diagnosis in an animal with marked respiratory distress and normal thoracic radiographs. Pulmonary infiltrates may be interstitial, alveolar, or lobar in dogs and cats. Alveolar infiltrates may represent hemorrhage, edema, or infarction. Pulmonary vascular abnormalities including enlarged central pulmonary arteries, disproportionate vascular tapering, and oligemia were common in retrospective review of thoracic radiographs in cats with PTE.[10] Cardiomegaly and mild to moderate pleural effusion were common in dogs and cats.

Arterial blood gas analysis is often abnormal in dogs with PTE, and common abnormalities include hypoxemia, hypocapnea, and increased alveolar-to-arterial gradient.[9] However, normal arterial oxygenation does not exclude the diagnosis of PTE.[2] Response to supplemental oxygen administration can be variable due to the presence of additional cardiac or pulmonary pathology and pathophysiologic sequelae of embolization.

Echocardiographic abnormalities were present in 94% of people with angiographically confirmed PTE, compared with only 13% of patients with similar clinical signs.[6] Unfortunately in veterinary medicine, echocardiography is rarely utilized in the work-up of animals suspected of PTE, and in one study less than 20% of dogs with PTE were evaluated.[9] Thrombus visualization with trans-thoracic echocardiography is limited to thrombi within the heart, main pulmonary artery, or proximal left or right branches. The majority of dogs (88%) with necropsy proven PTE had thrombi located in the main PA and lobar branches.[9] Since some of these proximal thrombi might be visualized with echocardiography, cardiac ultrasound should be considered in dogs with suspected PTE.

Perfusion scanning with an intravenous injection of technetium magroaggregated albumin, is a safe, noninvasive technique for evaluation of PTE. Perfusion deficits may occur in regions of thrombosis or in nonventilated regions with reflex vasoconstriction. When combined with a ventilation scan using technetium radioaerosol, the ventilation:perfusion (V:Q) scan has enhanced sensitivity for detection of PTE. Definitive positive V:Q scans are defined as multiple segmental or lobar perfusion defects in areas of normal ventilation and no radiographic evidence of pulmonary infiltrates. Although V:Q scans are commonly used in human medicine to increase the likelihood of documenting PTE, fewer than half of patients with PTE have a high probability scan.[2] Since ventilation scans are less practical in veterinary medicine and require specialized facilities to handle radioactive materials, this imaging modality is not commonly used. However, an abnormal perfusion scan can be considered suggestive of PTE.

Pulmonary angiography is the gold standard for diagnosis of PTE in humans but is rarely used in veterinary medicine since anesthesia is usually required, and patients with severe PTE and PH are high-risk anesthetic candidates. Percutaneous right heart catheterization via a jugular sheath under deep sedation may be a safer alternative for veterinary patients. Ionic contrast agents can induce severe hypotension due to reduction in systemic vascular resistance in the face of fixed PVR, and this may worsen RV ischemia and function.[13] Selective PA angiograms and use of nonionic contrast media reduces risk of serious complications.[13] Definitive angiographic diagnosis of PTE depends on visualization of an intraluminal filling defect in the pulmonary artery, or abrupt vessel occlusion and visualization of the trailing edge of the thromboembolus.[2]

Spiral computed tomography (CT) and magnetic resonance (MR) angiography are noninvasive imaging modalities that show promise for the future diagnosis and management of PTE. However, requirement for general anesthesia in veterinary patients undergoing CT or MRI makes these modalities less attractive in unstable, high-risk patients.

Treatment

Treatment of PTE must be directed against the primary underlying condition, and efforts must be made to improve gas exchange and cardiopulmonary function. Oxygen administration is indicated to reverse hypoxemia due to V/Q mismatch or diffusion abnormalities; however, pulmonary infarction and dysregulated hypoxic vasoconstriction may result in refractory hypoxemia. Immediate stabilization is necessary for animals in low output cardiac failure. Judicious fluids and inotropic support with dobutamine can be used to improve cardiac output and restore tissue perfusion.

Early and aggressive thrombolytic treatment of PTE is reserved for hemodynamically unstable patients and is uncommonly used in veterinary medicine. The goal of thrombolysis is to reduce PA pressure rapidly, improve RV function, and improve pulmonary perfusion. Although there are reports of successful thrombolytic therapy in experimental canine PTE (in dogs with normal thrombolytic and anticoagulant systems)[14] and in animals with systemic thrombi, there are no published studies evaluating thrombolytic therapy in naturally occurring PTE in veterinary medicine. In experimental canine PTE, tissue plasminogen activator (TPA) caused a rapid, dose-limiting thrombolysis with use of 1 mg/kg intravenously over 45 minutes, and TPA appeared to cause faster and more complete thrombolysis than streptokinase and urokinase.[14] Streptokinase has been effectively used in arterial thromboembolism in dogs and cats (90,000 U IV over 30 minutes, then 45,000 U/hour IV continuous infusion for various time intervals).

Anticoagulant therapy with heparin or warfarin is used to prevent further thrombus formation. Heparin is highly protein bound and has a low bioavailability. Doses ranging from 100 to 300 IU/kg SQ q6-8h can be used to prolong partial thromboplastin time (PTT) to 1.5 to 2 times baseline for adequate anticoagulation. Fresh frozen plasma may be needed to replenish antithrombin III. Low–molecular-weight heparin (LMWH) offers an attractive alternative for anticoagulant therapy, since it is less protein bound than unfractionated heparin, has greater bioavailability, provides a more predictable dose response, and has a longer half-life than heparin. LMWH therapy does not require laboratory monitoring since it does not prolong the APTT, and it is associated with fewer bleeding episodes.[2] In normal dogs, a high dose of 150 U/kg of dalteparin produced adequate anti-Xa activity with no bleeding complications and clinically insignificant changes in APTT and thrombin time.[15] Enoxaparin has been used with anecdotal clinical success for treatment of systemic thromboembolism in veterinary medicine. Long-term anticoagulation may also be achieved with oral warfarin (0.1 to 0.2 mg/kg PO q24h). Before warfarin is given, adequate anticoagulation with heparin is needed to balance the initial hypercoagulable phase of warfarin from reduced proteins C and S.

Although rarely done, large central thrombi may be removed by surgical thrombectomy, and percutaneous removal with a specialized thrombolytic catheter has been used in an experimental canine model of PTE.

Aggressive treatment of underlying diseases that have been associated with PTE is paramount, and prophylactic anticoagulation therapy may prevent PTE in these patients. Heparin can be administered at low doses (10 to 75 units/kg SQ TID) without affecting coagulation parameters. Given its biokinetic properties and ease of monitoring, LMWH is an attractive option for preventative anticoagulant therapy.

SECTION XIV

Gastrointestinal Disease

CHAPTER 219

Oral and Salivary Gland Disorders

Mark M. Smith

ORAL NEOPLASIA

Neoplasia of the oral and pharyngeal cavities is relatively common in the dog and cat, ranking fifth and seventh most common, respectively.[1] Benign and malignant neoplastic disease may be of dental or nondental origin.[2] The annual incidence of oral and pharyngeal neoplasia in dogs is 20 per 100,000, with malignant melanoma and squamous cell carcinoma (SCC) diagnosed most commonly.[1] The annual incidence rate is lower in cats (11 per 100,000), with the predominant neoplastic types being SCC and fibrosarcoma.[1,3]

Predisposing factors in the development of oral neoplasia include the patient's age, gender, breed, and size and the pigmentation of the oral mucosa. Geriatric patients are predisposed in general, although fibrosarcoma has been reported to occur more frequently in young, large breed dogs.[2] Papillary SCC, virus-induced papillomatosis, and undifferentiated malignancies may also be included in the differential diagnosis for young dogs with oral masses.[4,5] Male dogs have been reported to be at risk for malignant melanoma and fibrosarcoma. Breeds with an increased risk for oral neoplasia irrespective of type include the German shepherd and short-haired pointer, weimaraner, golden retriever, boxer, and cocker spaniel.[6] Large breed dogs have a higher incidence of fibrosarcoma and nontonsillar SCC, whereas small breeds have a higher incidence of malignant melanoma and tonsillar SCC.[6] Dogs with heavily pigmented oral mucosa are predisposed to malignant melanoma.

Benign Neoplasms

Papilloma, fibroma, lipoma, chondroma, osteoma, hemangioma, hemangiopericytoma, histiocytoma, and epulides are reported in the oropharyngeal region in the dog.[6] Papilloma and epulis are common benign oral neoplastic conditions in the dog.

Canine oral papillomatosis (COP) are multiple lesions of viral etiology. Grossly, COPs appear on the mucosa as pale, smooth elevations that develop a rough surface early in the disease process (Figure 219-1).[7] Older lesions of 3 to 4 weeks' duration usually have deep, closely packed fronds. Lesions observed during regression appear shriveled and dark gray. Complete regression requires 1 to 2 weeks and leaves no apparent scarring.

Epulides originate from the periodontal stroma and are often located in the gingiva near incisor teeth (Figure 219-2). The epulides are separated into three types based on histologic origin: fibromatous or fibrous epulis, ossifying epulis, and squamous or acanthomatous epulis.[6] The fibromatous and ossifying epulides are pedunculated, nonulcerating, and noninvasive masses. Acanthomatous epulis, although benign, has characteristics of malignancy, including local invasiveness and bone destruction[6]; however, acanthomatous epulis does not metastasize.

Periodontal epulides may be considered odontogenic neoplasms, because they are closely associated with or may contain dental structures. Fibromatous and ossifying epulides have also been described as peripheral odontogenic fibromas, containing varying amounts of bone, osteoid, dentinoid, or cementum-like substances.[7,8] Additionally, acanthomatous epulis, sometimes referred to in the literature as an *adamantinoma*, may be more properly classified as acanthomatous ameloblastoma or peripheral ameloblastoma.[9] The more common, specific odontogenic neoplasms are ameloblastoma and odontoma. Ameloblastomas arise from vestigial layers of the dental laminae of the mandible, generally in the incisor region. The neoplasm emanates from enamel organ tissue but does not produce dental hard products. These lesions are expansile, slow-growing neoplasms.[6] Odontomas are of odontogenic origin and resemble the embryologic pattern of tooth development. The mass may comprise enamel, dentin, cementum, and sometimes small teeth. Odontomas may form on or near the crown or root of a normal tooth and may resemble displaced or extra teeth. Lesions with characteristics resembling normal teeth are considered compound, whereas complex odontomas have a more disorganized arrangement.[6]

Malignant Neoplasms

Malignant melanomas grow rapidly and are characterized by early invasion of the gingivae and bone. Metastasis to regional lymph nodes occurs early in the disease process, with lung the most common site of visceral metastasis.[6,11] Malignant melanomas are dome shaped or sessile, and they either have varying amounts of pigmentation, ranging from black and brown to mottled, or are nonpigmented (Figure 219-3). A minority of oral melanocytic neoplasms (25%) may be benign, but all suspected melanomas should be considered malignant

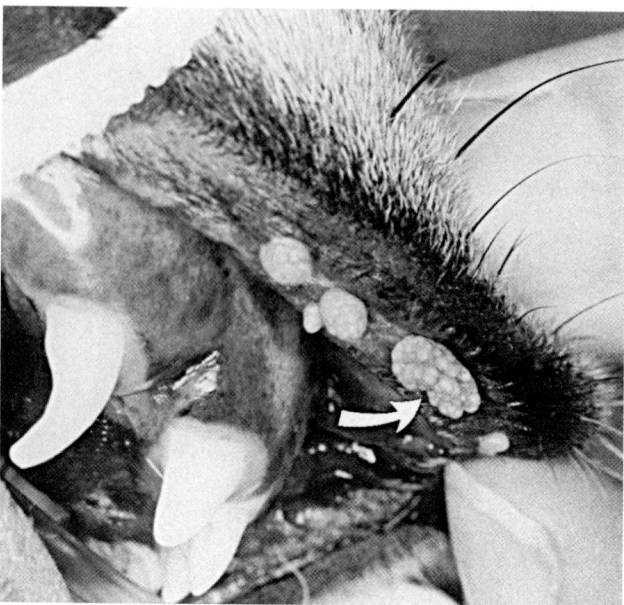

Figure 219-1 Papillomatosis (*arrow*) of the labial mucosa in a young dog.

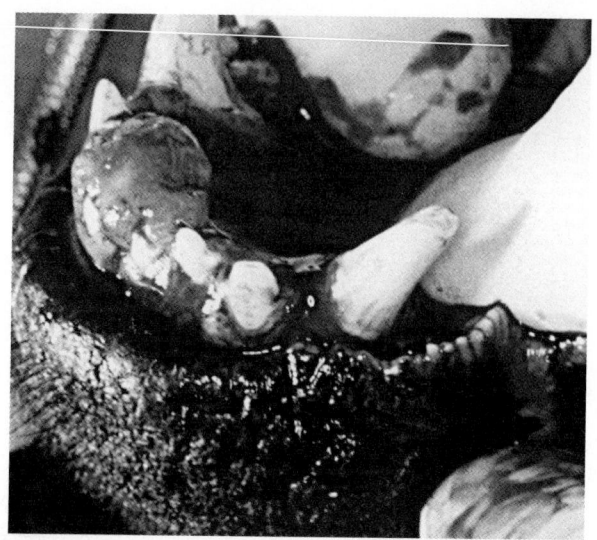

Figure 219-2 Intraoperative view of acanthomatous ameloblastoma of the mandibular incisor area in a dog.

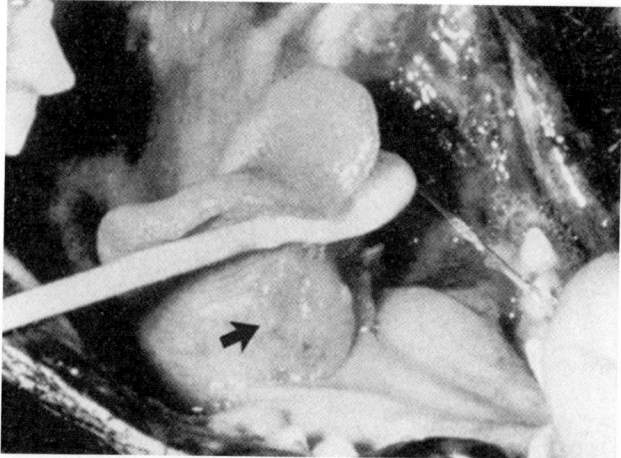

Figure 219-4 Sublingual squamous cell carcinoma (*arrow*) in a cat. (From Norris AM et al: Oropharyngeal neoplasms. In Harvey CE [ed]: Veterinary Dentistry. Philadelphia, WB Saunders, 1985.)

pending histologic evaluation. Melanomas of the mucocutaneous junction are invariably malignant.

Squamous cell carcinoma may project from the gingival mucosa but more commonly is an ulcerated, erosive lesion. It frequently involves the gingiva mesial to the canine teeth in dogs and ventral to the tongue in cats (Figure 219-4). Other common oral sites include the buccal and labial mucosa, hard palate, and tongue.[3,6,12-15] SCC destroys the mucosa and submucosa and is locally invasive in muscle and bone. Bone involvement is particularly common in dogs, showing a 77% occurrence rate. Metastasis to local and regional lymph nodes is common, whereas visceral metastasis to the lung is rare and occurs late in the disease process.

Fibrosarcoma occurs in oral locations similar to those of SCC but has a greater frequency along the lateral maxillary arcade between the canine and fourth premolar teeth.[6] The neoplasm is firm and smooth and has nodules that may become ulcerated (Figure 219-5). Fibrosarcomas are invasive,

and recurrence after local excision is common. Regional lymphatic and visceral metastasis is unusual. Conversely, low-grade fibrosarcomas appear benign clinically and rarely present with ulceration. However, these tumors are biologically malignant and require a high index of suspicion on the part of both the clinician and the pathologist.[16]

Clinical Signs, Diagnosis, and Staging

Clinical signs associated with oral neoplasms depend on the lesion's size and location. Food prehension may be abnormal and cause ulceration secondary to trauma in patients with larger neoplasms. Inability to swallow or associated pain may result in the appearance of saliva drooling from the lip commissures at inappropriate times. The saliva is blood tinged when concomitant with ulcerated lesions. Clinical signs associated with dental disease may be related to abnormal mastication. Painful dental structures or partial obstruction of functional dental areas lead to disuse. Subsequent periodontal

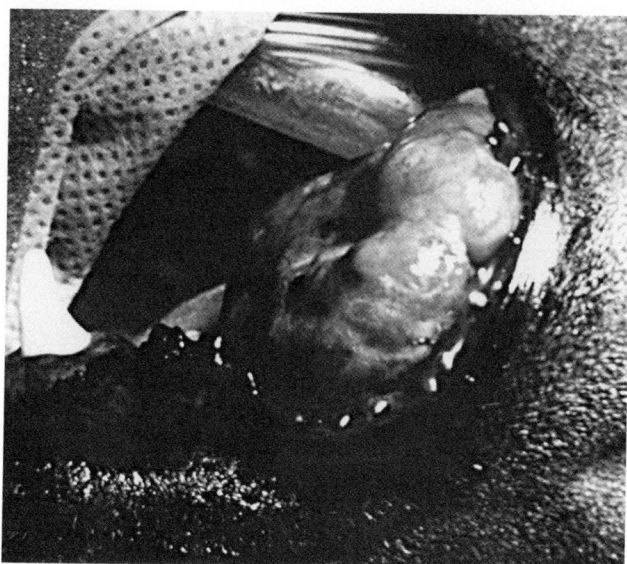

Figure 219-3 Malignant melanoma of the mandibular buccal mucosa in a dog.

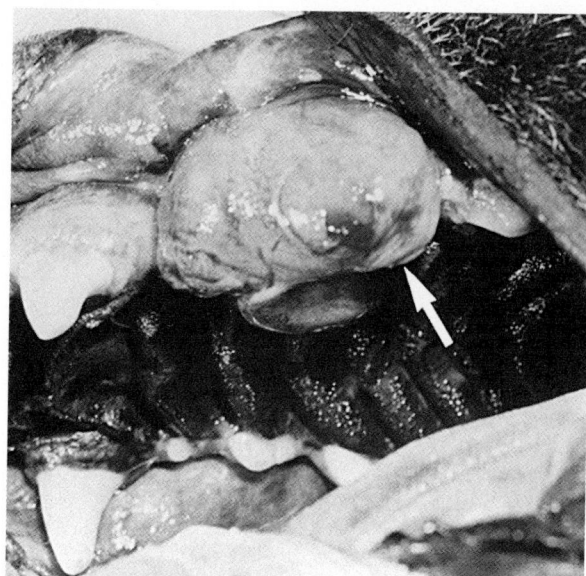

Figure 219-5 Fibrosarcoma (*arrow*) of the maxillary premolar area in a dog.

GASTROINTESTINAL DISEASE

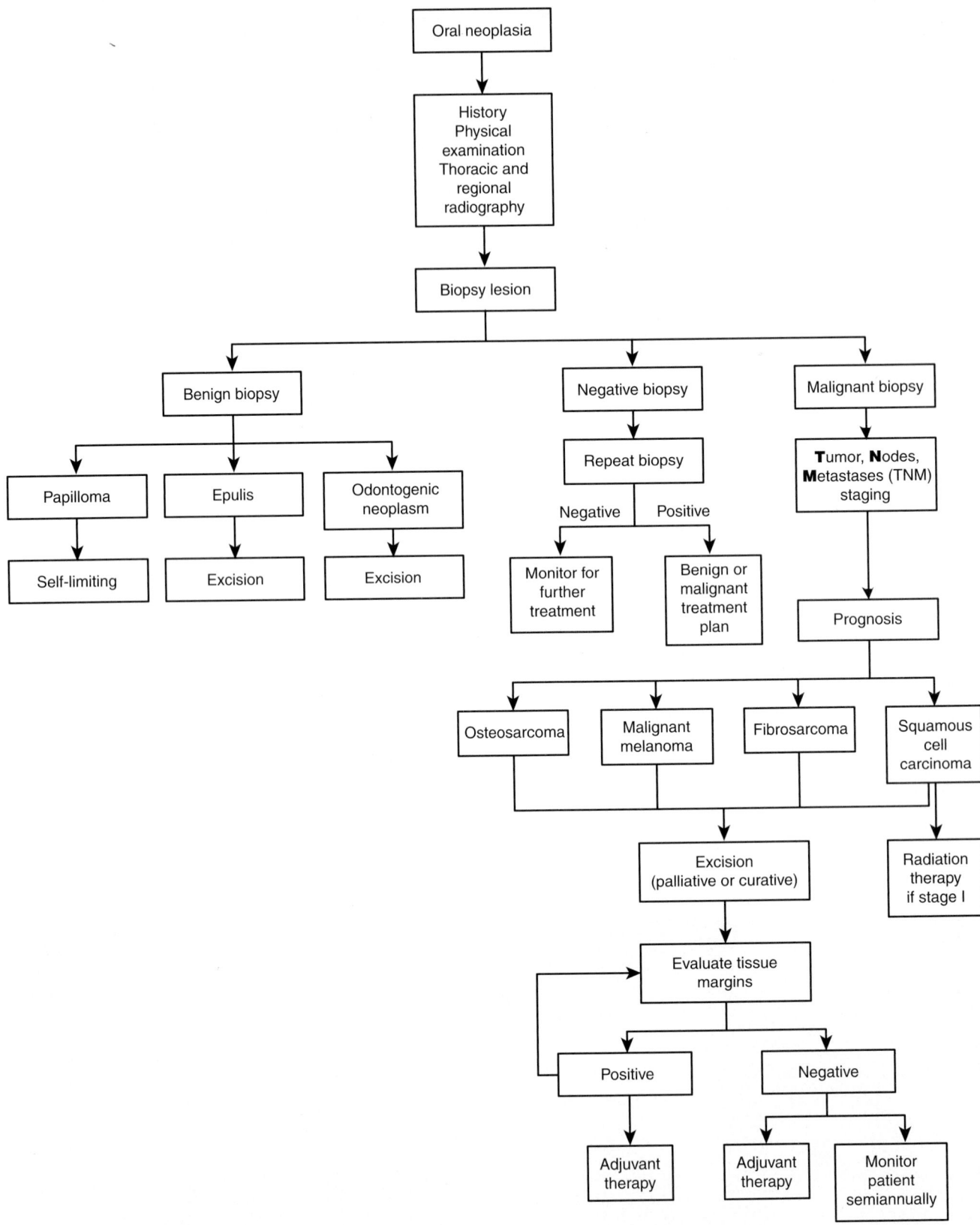

Figure 219-6 Algorithm for the diagnosis and treatment of oral neoplasms.

disease is related to excessive plaque and calculus accumulation in these areas. Severe destructive periodontal disease, halitosis, and tooth loss are potential sequelae. Although severe destructive periodontitis is not associated with a mass lesion, it is often associated with bone lysis and may resemble SCC.

Diagnosis of oral neoplastic conditions is based on histopathologic examination (Figure 219-6). The differential diagnoses include malignant and benign neoplasms. Recent advances in the development and application of immunohistochemistry techniques in veterinary medicine may provide methods for early detection of malignant neoplasms.[17-20]

Staging of the neoplastic disease should be considered as an active investigative process to be performed in concert with the diagnostic evaluation (Table 219-1).[21] The final result of this process is potentially valuable prognostic information. A complete blood count (CBC), chemistry profile, and urinalysis results should be reviewed to detect organ abnormalities related to metastatic disease or to concurrent disease that would alter the type or preclude the use of general anesthesia.

Thoracic radiographs (right and left lateral, ventrodorsal views) are taken to determine whether visceral metastasis to the lung has occurred. The size of the neoplasm is estimated in the awake patient and may be more accurately assessed after administration of general anesthesia. Skull radiographs or computed tomography (CT) performed during anesthesia can provide information on the presence of bone invasion.

The regional lymph nodes should also be evaluated. Enlargement indicates either metastasis or reactivity related to oral inflammation. Regardless of size, the regional lymph nodes should be evaluated by fine needle aspiration (false-negative results are possible) or by incisional or excisional biopsy. Minor surgery to remove a regional lymph node provides worthwhile prognostic information which may influence the owner's decision to pursue definitive treatment.[22,23] The most accessible regional lymph nodes are the submandibular and parotid nodes; the medial retropharyngeal node receives afferent lymphatics from these lymph nodes. Lymph node should be differentiated from salivary tissue, the latter having a tan color with distinct lobulations. A negative lymph node biopsy result does not preclude the possibility of regional metastasis, which may occur along perineural or vascular routes, or metastasis to other, less accessible lymph nodes, such as the medial retropharyngeal node.[23] Unfortunately, oral malignant neoplasms are often detected late in the disease process because their location may not be readily observed by the owner or veterinarian. Consequently, oral neoplasms have usually progressed to at least stage II disease at the time of diagnosis. Higher primary tumor (T)-stage tumors with bone involvement are associated with a poor prognosis.[11]

Treatment

Animals with no radiographic signs of visceral metastasis to the lung should be considered candidates for aggressive therapy. The concept of complete local excision of all visible tumor followed by, or concurrent with, chemotherapy or radiation therapy for treatment of presumed micrometastasis has achieved marked acceptance in human oncologic therapy and is being applied in veterinary medicine.[21,24-26] Surgery is integral to this multimodality treatment plan, especially for large, aggressive neoplasms.[27-30] Resective surgery plus radiation and/or chemotherapy are usually well tolerated by dogs and cats, leaving conservative management for only the more debilitated or geriatric patients.[31]

The goal of surgery for oral neoplasms in small animals is generally curative resection or palliation.[32] The ideal surgical procedure is one that offers the greatest possibility of cure, restores or maintains function, and has an acceptable cosmetic result. Benign neoplasms that do not involve bone are surgically excised. Malignant neoplasms are also excised; however, an attempt to acquire tumor-free margins is critically important.[33-35] A 2 cm margin of tumor-free tissue is recommended, often necessitating ostectomy as a component of the operative procedure.[36] Neoplasms with radiographic evidence of local bone metastasis require resective procedures, including maxillectomy and mandibulectomy. Hemimaxillectomy and hemimandibulectomy maximize the removal of the entire bony component of the neoplastic process. Segmental bone resective procedures that result in partial maxillectomy or mandibulectomy, without the opportunity for frozen section analysis of tissue margins, risk incomplete resection due to intrabony perineural and microvascular metastatic routes.[37,38] This is particularly important for mandibular lesions, for which hemimandibulectomy may be preferred to partial or segmental mandibulectomy because cosmesis and function are acceptable despite a greater degree of resection.[31,39] Extended dissection from the primary site may improve the incidence of free margins related to surgical resection of direct metastatic pathways, especially for neoplasms of the floor of the mouth. The cranial cervical area may be approached in conjunction with reconstructive surgery. Direct observation of

Table • 219-1

Clinical Staging System for Tumors of the Oral Cavity

T: Primary tumor
  T_0 No evidence of tumor
  T_1 Tumor < 2 cm maximum diameter
    T_{1a} Without bone invasion
    T_{1b} With bone invasion
  T_2 Tumor 2 to 4 cm maximum diameter
    T_{2a} Without bone invasion
    T_{2b} With bone invasion
  T_3 Tumor > 4 cm maximum diameter
    T_{3a} Without bone invasion
    T_{3b} With bone invasion

N: Regional lymph nodes (RLN)
  N_0 No evidence of RLN involvement
  N_1 Movable ipsilateral nodes
    N_{1a} Nodes histologically negative
    N_{1b} Nodes histologically positive
  N_2 Movable contralateral or bilateral nodes
    N_{2a} Nodes histologically negative
    N_{2b} Nodes histologically positive
  N_3 Fixed nodes

M: Distant metastasis
  M_0 No evidence of distant metastasis
  M_1 Distant metastasis present

STAGE GROUPINGS

STAGE	T	N	M
I	T_1	N_0, N_{1a}, or N_{2a}	M_0
II	T_2	N_0, N_{1a}, or N_{2a}	M_0
III*	T_3	N_0, N_{1a}, or N_{2a}	M_0
IV	Any T		
	Any T	Any N_{2b} or N_3	M_0
	Any T	Any N	M_1

*Any bone involvement.
From World Health Organization: *Report of the Second Consultation on the Biological Behaviour and Therapy of Tumors of Domestic Animals.* WHO, Geneva, 1978.

regional lymph nodes allows assessment of gross transcapsular spread of the tumor, which may warrant wider margins for adhered lymph nodes.[40,41]

Peripheral odontogenic fibromas are treated by aggressive, local surgical resection. Based on the common locations of this neoplasm compared with malignant neoplasms, the operative procedures would be either rostral mandibulectomy or rostral maxillectomy.[42,43]

Odontogenic tumors are treated by local excisional surgery requiring partial or segmental ostectomy.[44-46]

Radiation therapy may be particularly indicated for stage I SCC or after resective surgery for SCC with nonfree margins. This form of treatment is most effective if used in combination with surgical excision of stage II to stage IV SCC or possibly for affected regional lymph nodes.[12] Recent studies report encouraging results from radiation therapy for the treatment of canine SCC, fibrosarcoma, and malignant melanoma.[11,47] This modality should be considered for treatment of oral malignancies with or without surgery. However, as with surgery, larger, more caudally located tumors have a poorer prognosis. Severe, acute radiation reactions may occur approximately 16% of the time; the most common chronic reaction is bone necrosis and fistula formation.[11] Although the latter reaction may be difficult to treat successfully, a relatively low percentage of chronic reactions to radiation therapy may be considered an expected sequela of effective treatment.[11]

Acanthomatous ameloblastomas are sensitive to radiation therapy; however, because malignant neoplastic disease develops at the irradiated site in approximately 18% of dogs, surgical excision may be a more appropriate therapeutic option imorbidity is minimized.[48,49] The type of radiation administered (orthovoltage versus megavoltage) may influence the potential carcinogenic affect of radiation.[50] Smaller acanthomatous ameloblastomas located in the rostral portion of the oral cavity have a more favorable prognosis after radiation therapy than do larger, more caudal lesions.[50] Acute and chronic radiation reactions may occur, as in treatment for oral malignant neoplasms.

Chemotherapy or chemoradiation therapy may provide short-term palliation for oral neoplasia not amenable to surgery, for resections with non-free margins, and for recurrence after surgical excision. Cisplatin has been used in dogs for oral SCC, and doxorubicin and cyclophosphamide have been used for oral fibrosarcoma and SCC in cats.[2] The results of clinical research with radiosensitizing agents (e.g., etanidazole) may show improvement in median survival times for small animals with oral neoplasms.[51-53] Intratumoral administration of carboplatin has proved efficacious in the treatment of SCC of the nasal plane in cats[54] and may have application in the treatment of oral SCC. Systemic carboplatin may be considered as adjunctive treatment for microscopic local or metastatic malignant melanoma.[55] Chemoradiation, including hypofractionated megavoltage irradiation and cisplatin or carboplatin therapy, prolonged survival times in dogs with incompletely resected oral malignant melanoma.[56]

Prognosis

Malignant oral neoplasms have a guarded to poor prognosis regardless of their size or location in the oral cavity. The prognosis may be affected by the size of the lesion and the patient's age and species. Dogs younger than 6 years of age with SCC mesial to the second premolar have a better prognosis than older dogs with neoplasms in other locations. Cats with oral SCC have a shorter tumor-free interval than dogs regardless of the type of treatment.[57,58] The most positive prognosis for oral SCC in dogs is attained with both surgery and radiation therapy. Treatment of oral SCC in cats is strictly

palliative, with no improved survival interval.[2,57] Oral malignant melanoma may be resected locally with tumor-free margins, but regional or distant metastasis usually occurs. Tumor-free margins for oral fibrosarcoma are more difficult to achieve, which makes local recurrence likely. A 1-year survival rate of 71% has been reported for dogs with mandibular osteosarcoma treated with surgery only; another study indicated less favorable results with surgery only, reporting a median survival time of 5.5 months.[59,60]

Benign oral neoplasms and odontogenic neoplasms, including epulides, have an excellent prognosis after complete surgical excision.[43-46]

SELECTED ACQUIRED DISEASES OF THE LIPS, CHEEKS, AND PALATE

Feline eosinophilic granuloma complex (FEGC) comprises an eosinophilic ulcer, plaque, and a linear granuloma. Oral lesions are usually a linear granuloma or an eosinophilic ulcer; the latter has a predisposition for the maxillary lips (80%).[61] Intraoral lesions appear as one or more discrete, firm, raised nodules (Figure 219-7). Clinical signs include dysphagia and/or ptyalism. Although the etiology of this disease is unknown, bacterial and viral infections and immune-mediated and hypersensitivity diseases have been associated with FEGC.[61,62] Biopsy of the lesion, with the aforementioned diseases in mind, should be performed to confirm the diagnosis and to differentiate it from neoplastic disease. Ancillary tests should include a CBC, which usually shows an absolute eosinophilia. Concurrent or potentially causative hypersensitivity diseases should be considered during the diagnostic phase of treatment. The mainstay of FEGC treatment is corticosteroid therapy. Intralesional triamcinolone (3 mg weekly), oral prednisolone (1.0 to 2.0 mg/kg given twice daily), and subcutaneous methylprednisolone acetate (20 mg every 2 weeks),

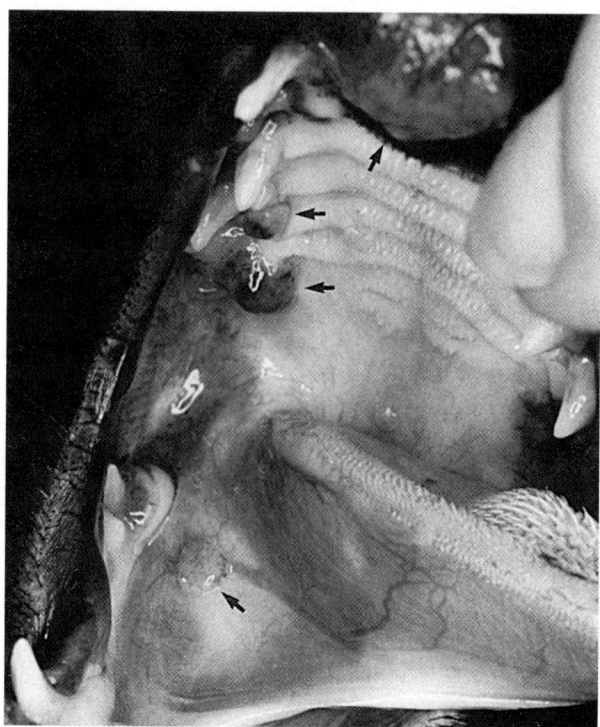

Figure 219-7 Oral lesions (*arrows*) of feline eosinophilic granuloma complex. (Courtesy Dr. M. Leib, Blacksburg, VA.)

administered until FEGC resolves, are efficacious treatments.[61] Progestational compounds (progesterone or medroxyprogesterone) are often used to treat FEGC. These compounds are not approved for use in cats and have potential side effects that make them undesirable, including adrenocortical suppression, polydipsia, polyuria, polyphagia, obesity, personality change, reproduction abnormalities, mammary hypertrophy, neoplasia, and diabetes mellitus. Cats with untreated chronic lesions, responsive previous lesions, and lesions refractory to corticosteroid therapy have a 50% recurrence rate within 5 months.[61] Failure of treatment is usually related to inadequate dosage or premature cessation of therapy. Animals that do not respond to either corticosteroids or progestational compounds have a poor prognosis and are candidates for more aggressive therapy, such as irradiation, cryosurgery, laser therapy, or immunotherapy.[62-64]

The term *stomatitis* refers to an inflammation of the oral mucosa. Oral inflammatory lesions in dogs and cats have multiple causes, necessitating a consistent and logical diagnostic approach. A complete history and thorough physical examination are essential. Dogs and cats with no evidence of debilitating systemic disease should receive a short-acting intravenous anesthetic to allow an unimpeded visual and tactile oral examination. Oral ulcerations occur in at least four different immune-mediated diseases, including systemic lupus erythematosus, bullous (pemphigus) disease, idiopathic vasculitis, and toxic epidermal necrosis. The many infectious diseases that are manifested by lesions in the oral cavity include feline leukemia virus, feline immunodeficiency virus, feline syncytium-forming virus, feline calicivirus, feline herpes virus, and feline infectious peritonitis (see Chapters 170-173).[65] Canine distemper and feline panleukopenia virus may cause stomatitis, although other organs are more severely affected. Candidiasis (infection with *Candida albicans*) may cause severe stomatitis in dogs and cats.[61,66] Many cats with stomatitis have immunosuppressive disease or systemic debilitation or have received chronic immunosuppressive therapy. Although the oral manifestation may appear as a white, pseudomembranous covering of the tongue, the lesions are usually irregular, ulcerated areas in zones of inflamed mucosa.

Feline oral inflammatory disease ranges from simple gingivitis to varying degrees of stomatitis in which inflammation extends beyond the mucogingival junction into the oral mucosa.[67] Cats with chronic gingivitis/stomatitis may have ulceration and extension of granulation tissue involving the palatoglossal folds and fauces. Clinical signs include halitosis, ptyalism, dysphagia, inappetence, and weight loss. Extensive disease is marked by root resorption and possibly bony sequestrae in edentulous areas. Unfortunately, because the causation is usually unknown, treatment is symptomatic, including professional cleaning of the teeth, therapy with antimicrobials or with systemic or local corticosteroid agents similar to those used for FEGC, and laser therapy to stimulate re-epithelialization over inflamed, ulcerated areas. It is not unusual for refractory cases to require extraction of all molars and premolars or all teeth to alleviate the symptoms of this disorder.

Stomatitis may be described as idiopathic despite a thorough diagnostic evaluation. Immunemediated ulcerative gingivitis/ stomatitis afflicts Maltese terriers, although the etiology is verified in only 20% of animals.[61] If diagnostic test results are negative in idiopathic stomatitis, it is appropriate to assume a possible immune-mediated component. A prudent treatment plan includes regular cleaning of the teeth, oral preventive medicine at home, and intermittent or chronic provocative corticosteroid therapy. Antimicrobial therapy emphasizing anaerobic pathogens (e.g., metronidazole, amoxicillin, clavulanic acid/amoxicillin) may be administered on an intermittent, chronic basis.

SELECTED ACQUIRED DISEASES OF THE SALIVARY GLANDS

Neoplasia involving the salivary glands is uncommon. There is evidence that spaniel breeds and poodles, as well as Siamese cats, are predisposed to neoplasia of the salivary glands.[68] In a report of 24 primary salivary tumors in dogs, the parotid gland was involved nearly twice as often as the other major salivary glands; the mean age of the 24 dogs studied was 10 years.[68] Another recent study indicates that the mandibular gland is most commonly affected.[69] Multiple tumor types that affect the salivary glands have been described, including mucoepidermoid tumors, SCC, malignant mixed tumors, adenoid cystic carcinoma, acinic cell carcinoma, adenocarcinoma, undifferentiated carcinoma, and sarcoma. Although primary SCC of the sublingual salivary gland occurs, it should be considered only after an invasive carcinoma involving the oral mucosa or accessory oral salivary glands has been ruled out. The prevalence of salivary gland neoplasms in cats is almost twice that in dogs, with the mandibular salivary gland most commonly affected.[68] Adenocarcinoma is the most common neoplasm affecting the salivary glands in dogs and cats.[68] Adenocarcinoma, regardless of the gland affected, is locally infiltrative, with frequent metastasis to the lung and regional lymph nodes. Cats have more advanced-stage disease at the time of diagnosis than do dogs.[68] Salivary neoplasms should be staged according to the primary tumor–regional lymph node–distant metastasis (TNM) system to allow appropriate prognostication and development of a treatment plan. Thoracic radiographs and incisional biopsy of the neoplasm and nearest regional lymph nodes provide necessary information.

Total surgical excision of salivary malignant neoplasms is difficult because of their invasive characteristics and the intricate neurologic and vascular anatomy of the salivary gland region. Therefore local treatment should include radiotherapy, with or without surgical intervention to debulk the neoplasm.

Mucocele is the most common recognized clinical disease of the salivary glands in dogs. A mucocele comprises an accumulation of saliva in the subcutaneous tissue and the consequent tissue reaction to saliva. The mucocele has a nonepithelial, nonsecretory lining consisting primarily of fibroblasts and capillaries. The incidence of salivary mucocele reportedly is fewer than 20 in 4000 dogs. Although the condition has been reported in dogs as young as 6 months of age, salivary mucocele occurs most often in dogs 2 to 4 years of age. It occurs more frequently in German shepherds and miniature poodles.

Trauma has been proposed as the cause of salivary mucocele because of the activity of young dogs and the documented damage to the salivary gland-duct complex and the formation of the mucocele. The inability to induce salivary mucocele traumatically in healthy dogs suggests the possibility of a developmental predisposition in affected dogs.

The sublingual gland is the most common salivary gland associated with salivary mucocele. Sialography has shown that the mucocele most often originates in the rostral portion (that portion of the sublingual gland superimposed on the mandible) of the sublingual gland-duct complex. Regardless of the location of origin, the mucocele usually forms near the intermandibular area (cervical mucocele). Other locations associated with the formation of a mucocele caused by a sublingual gland-duct defect are sites under the tongue, which involves the floor of the mouth (sublingual mucocele) and the pharynx (pharyngeal mucocele).

The clinical signs associated with salivary mucocele depend on the location of the mucocele. A cervical mucocele initially is an acute, painful mass resulting from an inflammatory response. Cessation of the inflammatory response results in a marked decrease in size. A decreased inflammatory response

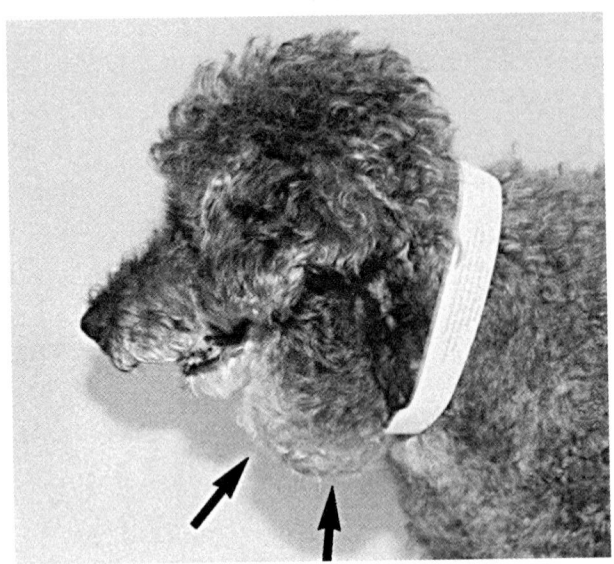

Figure 219-8 Cervical mucocele in a poodle.

of sloughed inflammatory tissue previously lining the mucocele. Sialoliths, which are concretions of calcium phosphate or calcium carbonate, may occur with chronic mucocele.

The physical examination and history usually denote the origin of the mucocele. Cervical mucoceles that appear on the midline usually shift to the originating side when the patient is placed in exact dorsal recumbency. Sialography can be used to determine the affected side if careful observation and palpation of the mucocele are unsuccessful. Sialography is also a diagnostic aid when considerations include traumatic injury to one of the salivary glands, salivary neoplasia, a mass or fistulous tract of unknown origin in the head and neck region, or a foreign body in the head or neck. The disadvantages of sialography include the need for general anesthesia and the difficulty associated with locating the duct opening or openings.

Various techniques have been used to treat cervical mucoceles. Mucocele drainage, removal of the mucocele only, and chemical cauterization of the mucocele have been reported. The basis for these therapies was the belief that a mucocele was a true cyst with a secretory lining. The fact that a mucocele is not a cyst but a reactive, encapsulating structure has prompted surgical removal of the affected gland-duct complex. The intimate anatomic association of the sublingual and mandibular glands and their ducts requires resection of both structures. Surgical removal of both the sublingual and mandibular salivary glands, combined with drainage of the mucocele, has been advocated for treatment of cervical mucoceles.

Pharyngeal and sublingual mucocele are treated by removal the mandibular and sublingual salivary glands, based on the common etiology of a sublingual gland-duct defect. Another treatment technique for these mucoceles involves marsupialization. However, resective surgery is preferred for pharyngeal mucoceles, because life-threatening upper airway compromise and morbidity from swallowing dysfunction (e.g., aspiration pneumonia) are potential complications of conservative management or recurrence.

The zygomatic salivary gland can be affected by neoplasia, inflammation, or mucocele. The clinical signs of zygomatic mucocele and neoplasia are similar. Additional signs, such as osteolytic changes of the zygomatic arch and enlargement of the submandibular lymph node, may accompany neoplasia that originate in the zygomatic gland. Surgical removal of the zygomatic gland is indicated either for neoplasia or for mucocele of zygomatic origin.

allows for the more common presenting history of a slowly enlarging or intermittently large, fluid-filled, painless mass (Figure 219-8). Blood-tinged saliva secondary to trauma caused by eating, abnormal prehension of food, or reluctance to eat are clinical signs that can be associated with sublingual mucocele. The most common clinical signs associated with a mucocele of the pharyngeal wall are respiratory distress and difficulty swallowing secondary to partial obstruction of the pharynx.

Zygomatic salivary mucoceles are infrequently reported in dogs. A visible periorbital mass is usually the presenting clinical sign of zygomatic mucocele. Ophthalmic signs secondary to the mucocele depend on the location and size of the mucocele (e.g., exophthalmos or enophthalmos).

Diagnosis of salivary mucocele is based on the clinical signs, history, and results of paracentesis (Figure 219-9). Mucocele paracentesis reveals a stringy, sometimes blood-tinged fluid with low cell numbers. Mucin and amylase analyses of the fluid are not reliable diagnostic procedures. A chronic cervical mucocele may contain palpable firm nodules that are remnants

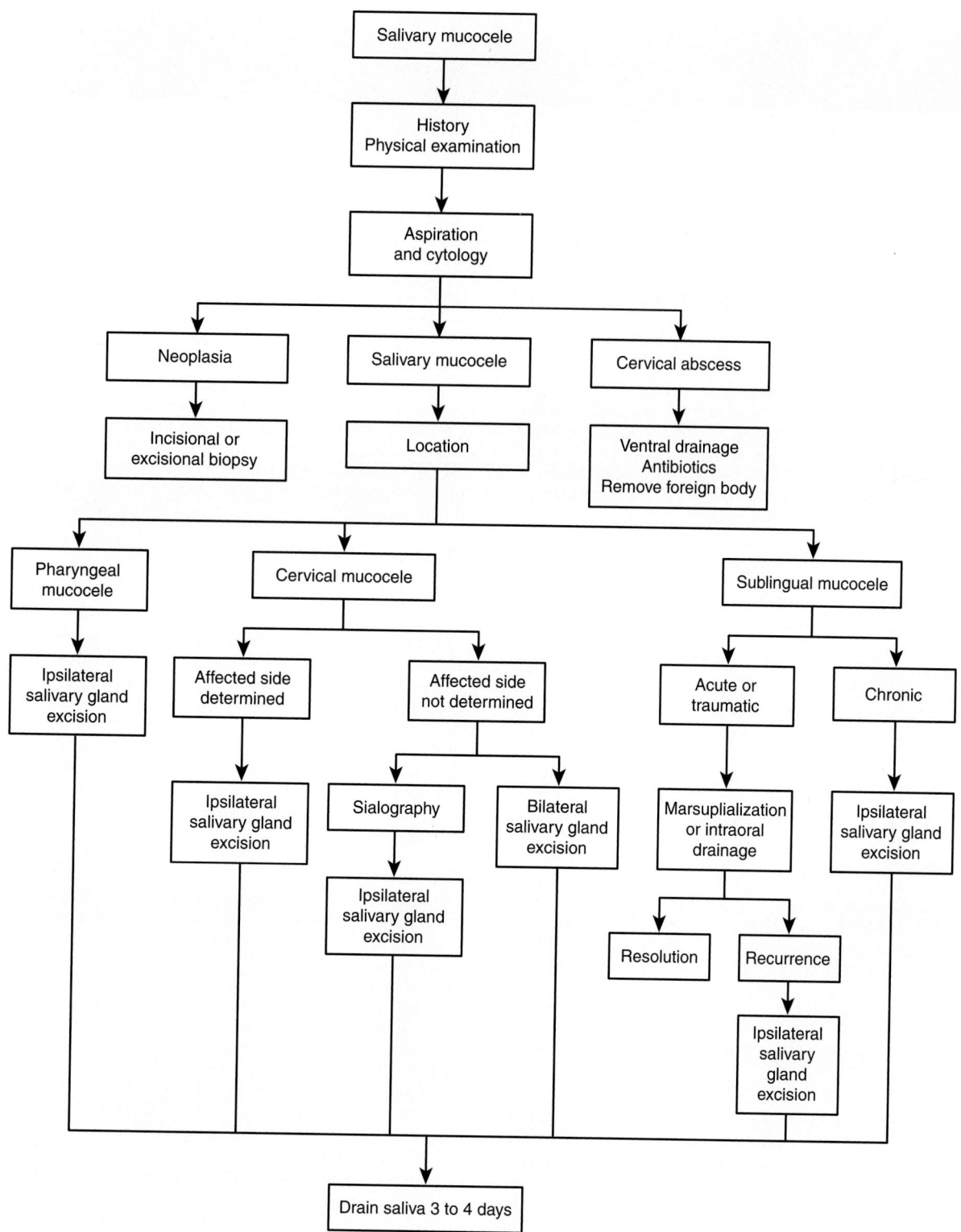

Figure 219-9 Algorithm for diagnosis and treatment of salivary mucocele in a dog.

CHAPTER 220

Diseases of the Esophagus

Albert E. Jergens

NORMAL ANATOMY AND FUNCTION

The esophagus functions to transport ingesta and liquids from the oral cavity to the stomach.[1,2] Its anatomy consists of the striated muscle (cricopharyngeus muscles) of the upper esophageal sphincter (UES), striated and smooth muscle of the body of the esophagus, and the smooth muscle of the lower esophageal sphincter (LES). The entire length of the canine esophagus is composed of striated muscle, whereas the distal one third of the feline esophagus is composed of smooth muscle. The vagus nerve and associated branches (glossopharyngeal, pharyngeal, and recurrent laryngeal nerves) innervate the esophagus. This neural network contains somatic motor nerves from the brain stem nucleus ambiguus to the esophageal striated muscle, autonomic nerves to the esophageal smooth muscle, and general visceral afferent nerves from esophageal sensory receptors.

The high pressure maintained by the UES and LES during fasting ensures unidirectional flow between the oral cavity and the stomach. The LES is also responsive to gut hormones via receptors for gastrin and secretin families. The esophageal phase of swallowing begins with relaxation of the UES, which permits movement of a bolus of food into the proximal esophagus. The peristaltic wave generated in the pharynx is further propagated through the esophagus and carries a bolus aborally to the LES (primary peristalsis). If primary peristalsis fails to propel the bolus to the stomach, then a secondary peristaltic wave is quickly generated by intraluminal distension and completes transport of the bolus to the stomach. Relaxation of the LES in advance of these propagated pressures permits food to empty into the stomach. After the bolus passes, the LES contracts to prevent reflux of gastric contents into the esophagus.

DIAGNOSIS OF ESOPHAGEAL DISEASES

History

In general, animals with overt esophageal dysfunction are not diagnostic challenges. Clients often report hallmark signs of esophageal disease including regurgitation (liquids or solids), dysphagia (difficult swallowing), odynophagia (painful swallowing), repeated swallowing attempts, and excessive salivation in affected animals. Regurgitation is the most consistent sign of esophageal disease and should be clearly differentiated from oropharyngeal dysphagia and vomiting (Table 220-1). Some animals may also have a mix of signs, such as vomiting and regurgitation, which may occur when chronic vomiting leads to esophagitis.

Other historical clues of esophageal disease may be made based on age and the character of signs. Congenital idiopathic megaesophagus shows distinct canine breed predispositions (see later), and vascular ring anomaly and cricopharyngeal dysphagia may also manifest in very young patients. Acute severe signs in either a young or older animal are suggestive of esophageal foreign body. Conversely, slowly worsening regurgitation is more commonly seen with hiatal defects (causing gastroesophageal reflux), developing stricture, or esophageal tumors. Adult animals showing esophageal dysphagia may have histories of recent anesthesia, ingestion of corrosive chemicals, or pill administration. Concurrent muscle weakness or neurologic signs may implicate extra-esophageal disorders, such as myasthenia gravis (MG) or polyneuropathy, as causes for secondary esophageal disease. Evidence of pain during swallowing is most often due to foreign body ingestion or esophagitis but is uncommonly observed with motility disturbances.

Physical Examination

The physical examination findings in animals with primary esophageal disease are variable. Most animals with acute causes for regurgitation (foreign body or mild esophagitis) show minimal abnormalities with the exception of hypersalivation and variable dysphagia. Mucopurulent nasal discharge, pulmonary crackles, and fever suggest aspiration pneumonia. Weight loss, malnutrition, and emaciation can be seen with long-standing esophageal disease, such as stricture and idiopathic megaesophagus. Observations in animals with dysautonomia may include dilated pupils and dry mucus membranes. A carefully performed physical examination serves to exclude other gastrointestinal (GI) and systemic diseases.

Diagnostic Tests

Although history provides important clues as to the likelihood of primary esophageal disease, select laboratory tests, radiography, and endoscopy are necessary for definitive diagnosis in most instances (Figure 220-1). Significant alterations in baseline laboratory tests (complete blood count [CBC], serum biochemistry, urinalysis) are uncommonly observed. Exceptions include elevations in CK (associated with myositis), nonregenerative anemia (associated with malnutrition), and proteinuria (suggestive of immune-mediated disease). Specialized serologic assays useful for the diagnosis of regurgitation include an adrenocorticotropic hormone (ACTH) stimulation test (hypoadrenocorticism) and acetylcholine receptor antibody titer (acquired MG).

Survey thoracic and soft-tissue cervical films should be performed in all animals suspected as having esophageal disease. Obvious abnormalities may include radiopaque foreign bodies, hiatal defect, esophageal dilatation (megaesophagus), alveolar opacities (aspiration pneumonia), or evidence of esophageal perforation (pneumomediastinum).

Contrast radiography is a helpful adjunct to survey imaging, being most useful in confirming luminal obstruction (stricture, mass, extraluminal compression), mucosal irregularity (mass, severe esophagitis), and significant alterations in esophageal motility. An esophagram is most often performed using liquid barium suspension followed by a barium meal. Contrast material is rapidly cleared from the normal pharynx and esophagus by a series of brisk, aborally directed peristaltic waves.[2] Persistent pooling of contrast material at any level of

Table • 220-1

Differentiation of Oropharyngeal Dysphagia, Esophageal Dysphagia, and Vomiting

PARAMETER	OROPHARYNGEAL DYSPHAGIA	ESOPHAGEAL DYSPHAGIA	VOMITING
Abdominal effort	None	None	Marked
Prodromal nausea	None	None	Present
Character of ejected food	Undigested	Undigested	Usually digested
Timing of food ejected	Immediate	Often delayed	Often delayed
Swallow attempts of a single bolus	Multiple	Usually single	Single
Ability to drink	Poor	Variable	Normal
Pain on swallowing	Possible	Possible	Absent
Associated signs	Dyspnea, cough	Dyspnea, cough	+/− Systemic signs

Modified from Guilford WG: Approach to clinical problems in gastroenterology. *In* Guilford WG, Center SA, Strombeck DR (eds): *Strombeck's Small Animal Gastroenterology*, 3rd ed. Philadelphia, WB Saunders Co, 1996, p 55.

the esophagus should be considered abnormal and confirmed on repeat films. If esophageal perforation is suspected, a water-soluble iodinated contrast agent (iohexol, gastrografin) should be used. Dynamic contrast studies (videofluoroscopy) provide more detailed quantitative information regarding esophageal motility.

Flexible endoscopy (esophagoscopy) provides the clinician the most direct means to quickly and noninvasively assess the esophagus for luminal or mucosal abnormalities. Normal esophageal mucosa is smooth, glistening, and pale pink. Abnormal findings include mass lesions (neoplastic most common), esophagitis (evidenced by mucosal erythema, hemorrhage, erosions), stricture, segmental or generalized dilatation, and perforation. Mucosal biopsy of the esophagus is uncommonly required except for intraluminal mass lesions. Exfoliative brush cytology may be superior to mucosal biopsy (due to technical constraints) for diagnosis of esophageal neoplasia. Interventional procedures allow for esophageal foreign body removal, dilatation of esophageal strictures, and feeding catheter placement via percutaneous gastrostomy or gastrojejunostomy techniques.

More specialized diagnostic procedures, such as esophageal manometry (for assessment of motility or LES competency) and distal esophageal pH monitoring (for gastroesophageal reflux), are infrequently performed in clinical practice.

CRICOPHARYNGEAL DYSPHAGIA

Cricopharyngeal dysphagia is a congenital neuromuscular disorder characterized by failure of the UES to relax (achalasia) or a lack of coordination between UES relaxation and pharyngeal contraction (asynchrony). This results in interrupted transport of a bolus through the UES into the cervical esophagus. The cause for this disorder is unknown; however, a dysfunction of the inhibitory neuron mediating UES relaxation has been incriminated.[3]

Clinical Signs

Affected animals demonstrate progressive dysphagia characterized by repeated attempts to swallow, gagging, retching, and regurgitation (often immediately after eating). Clinical signs most often appear at the time of, or shortly after, weaning. A moist, productive cough may develop as a consequence of aspiration pneumonia. Physical examination is generally unremarkable with the exception of moist crackles in animals with pneumonia.

Diagnosis

Videofluoroscopy of the pharynx and UES using liquid barium or paste is the diagnostic test of choice. Intermittent or persistent failure of UES to relax and dilate subsequent to bolus formation and pharyngeal contractions is observed. Static contrast films may demonstrate barium retention in the pharynx or aspiration into the trachea (Figure 220-2). Ancillary tests (serum CK, electromyography [EMG], muscle biopsy) should be performed in animals having more generalized signs of neuromuscular disease (muscle weakness, atrophy, neurologic deficits).

Treatment

Cricopharyngeal dysphagia is best managed by performance of cricopharyngeal myotomy. The failure rate for surgery alone may be high, especially if aspiration pneumonia or malnutrition is present.[4] In these instances, more aggressive medical management (enteral tube feeding) is warranted rather than surgery. Mature animals and those with cricopharyngeal asynchrony respond less favorably to surgical intervention. Medical therapy includes treatment of aspiration pneumonia and enteral nutritional support in emaciated patients.

ESOPHAGITIS

Esophagitis denotes acute or chronic inflammation of the esophageal mucosa which may extend to the underlying muscularis. It may be caused by chemical injury from ingested substances (corrosives, pill or capsule retention), gastroesophageal reflux (secondary to general anesthesia, hiatal defects, persistent vomiting, malpositioned nasoesophageal or pharyngostomy tubes), or esophageal foreign bodies.[5] Mucosal damage caused by reflux is attributed to prolonged contact with gastric acid, pepsin, bile salts, and trypsin. Reduced esophageal clearance by peristalsis and failure to neutralize acid by bicarbonate-rich saliva contribute to anesthesia-associated reflux esophagitis. Drug- or chemical-induced esophagitis is caused by changes in mucosal pH, hyperosmolarity, and other mechanisms. Disturbances in esophageal motility may accompany esophagitis regardless of the cause. The reported prevalence of acute esophagitis is low; however, this is likely an underestimation due the subtlety of clinical signs and radiographic findings associated with this disorder.[6]

Clinical Signs

The clinical signs vary as to the type of chemical injury, severity of inflammation, and extent of esophageal involvement.

GASTROINTESTINAL DISEASE

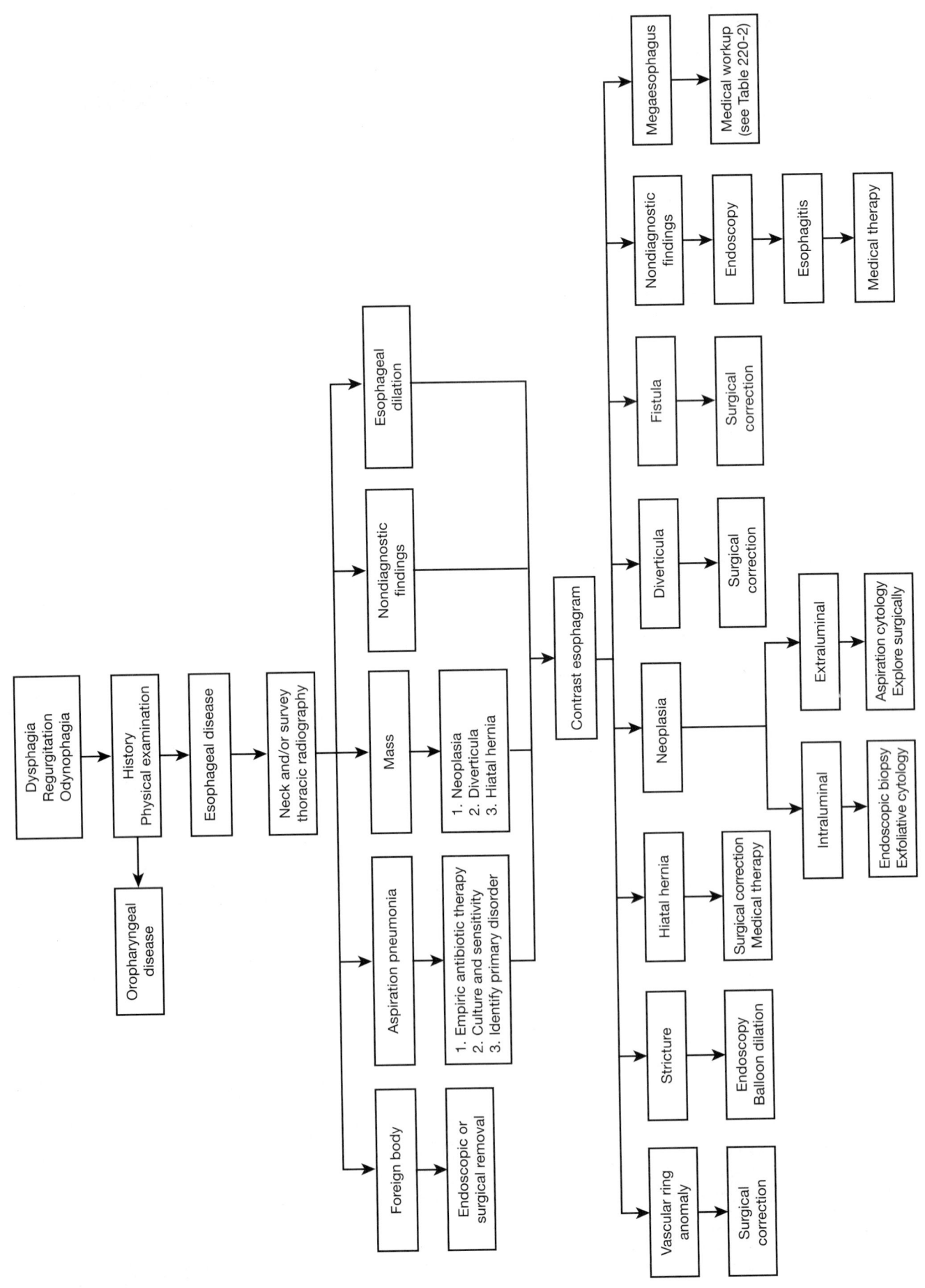

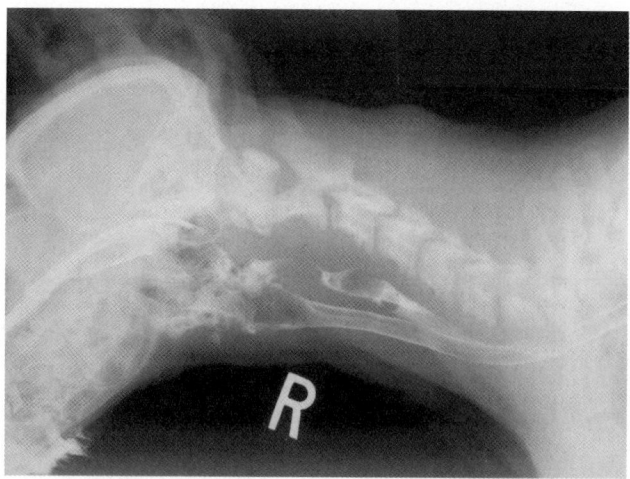

Figure 220-2 Contrast esophagram (static image) performed in a 5-month-old puppy with cricopharyngeal dysphagia. Reader should note the abnormal reflux of liquid barium into the nasopharynx.

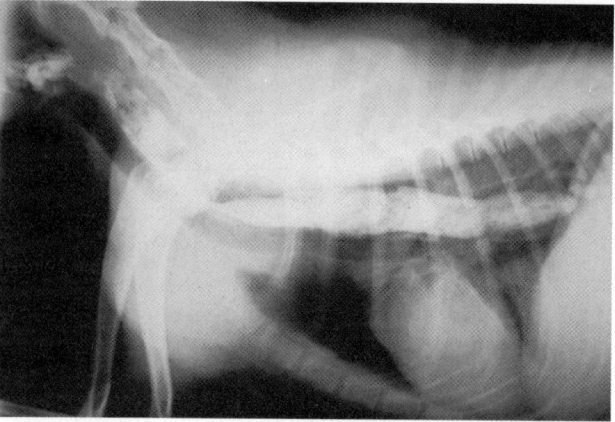

Figure 220-3 Contrast esophagram (lateral view) performed with food in a 5-year-old dog. Generalized esophageal dilatation is observed secondary to severe reflux esophagitis. Esophageal function completely normalized after medical therapy for esophagitis.

Animals with mild esophagitis may be asymptomatic. Moderate-to-severe esophagitis causes anorexia, dysphagia, odynophagia (seen as extension of the head and neck during swallowing), and hypersalivation. Regurgitation is often intermittent, but it may be persistent. Thick, ropey saliva that is blood-tinged is often expelled. The physical examination may be unremarkable in animals with mild esophagitis. Cachexia and weight loss may be seen with prolonged disease.

Diagnosis

Results of routine hematology, serum biochemistry, urinalysis, and survey thoracic radiographs are usually normal. Segmental or diffuse esophageal dilatation may be seen with severe mucosal inflammation (Figure 220-3). Barium contrast radiography is infrequently performed but may confirm esophageal dilatation, disturbances in motility, and stricture. Esophagitis is an endoscopic diagnosis that does not require mucosal biopsy. A spectrum of mucosal abnormalities may be observed during esophagoscopy including increased erythema, erosions, and alterations in mucosal texture (Figures 220-4 and 220-5). Lesions are usually most evident in the distal esophagus, adjacent to and including the LES. The presence of gastroesophageal reflux with a dilated LES is suggestive of a hiatal disorder.

Treatment

Mild esophagitis frequently resolves with minimal treatment other than dietary management. The clinician should provide frequent, smaller-sized meals of a low-fat, high-protein content to enhance LES tone and to minimize reflux. Animals having more severe esophagitis, especially those with anorexia, weight loss, or the inability to retain food, will require drug therapy and gastrostomy tube feeding. Sulcralfate suspension (0.5 to 1.0 g orally, three times a day) is the most beneficial and specific therapy for reflux esophagitis.[7] It selectively binds to eroded mucosa and provides effective barrier protection against refluxed gastric contents. Metoclopramide should

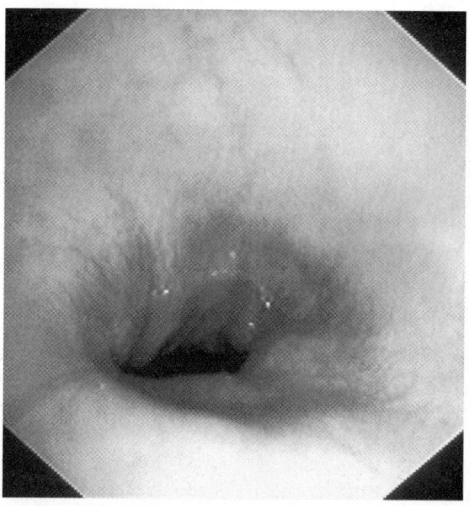

Figure 220-4 Endoscopic appearance of severe esophagitis in the distal canine esophagus. Marked mucosal erythema and dilation of the lower esophageal sphincter (LES) is evident.

be administered (0.1 to 0.2 mg/lb per os, subcutaneously, three times a day) or cisapride (0.05 to 0.25 mg/lb per os, twice a day) to decrease esophageal reflux (by increasing LES pressure) and to promote gastric emptying. Gastric acid secretory inhibitors (ranitidine 0.5 to 1.0 mg/lb orally or intravenously, twice a day; famotidine 0.25 to 0.5 mg/lb orally, once a day; omeprazole 0.35 mg/lb orally, once a day) should be given to decrease acidity of gastric juice. Broad-spectrum antibiotics are indicated in the occasional animal having concurrent aspiration pneumonia. A water bolus should be routinely administered to cats receiving tablets or capsules per os to prevent medication-associated esophagitis.[5]

The duration of drug therapy is empiric and varies with severity of signs and endoscopic lesions. Mild lesions are

Figure 220-1 Diagnostic approach to an animal with regurgitation and suspected esophageal disease. (Adapted from Washabau RJ: Diseases of the esophagus. *In* Ettinger SJ, Feldman ED [eds]: *Textbook of Veterinary Internal Medicine.* 5th ed. Philadelphia, WB Saunders Co, 2000, p 1144.)

GASTROINTESTINAL DISEASE

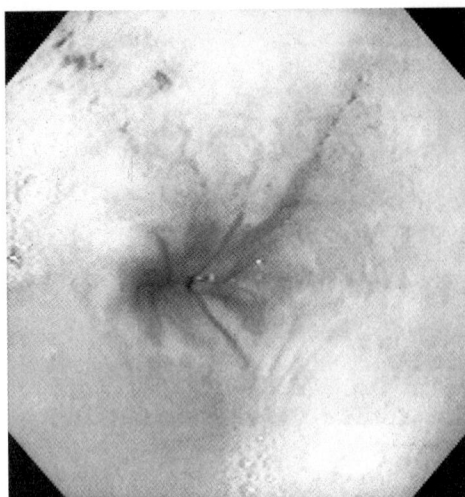

Figure 220-5 Endoscopic appearance of reflux esophagitis in the distal canine esophagus. Pooled liquid reflux and multifocal erosions are seen along the mucosa adjacent to the lower esophageal sphincter (LES).

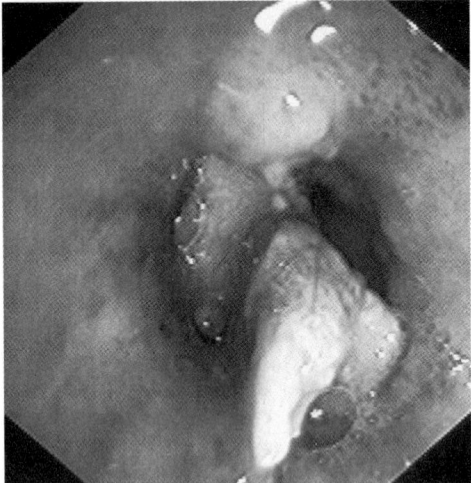

Figure 220-6 Endoscopic appearance of a large angular bone lodged in the thoracic esophagus of a 2-year-old dog. Minor erosive lesions are also present.

treated for 5 to 7 days; moderate-to-severe esophagitis is treated for 2 to 3 weeks. The prognosis in most cases of esophagitis is good with appropriate medical therapy. Animals having severe disease warrant a guarded prognosis because permanent changes in esophageal structure (stricture formation) or function (segmental or generalized hypomotility) may occur.

ESOPHAGEAL FOREIGN BODIES

The ingestion of foreign bodies is a common cause of esophageal dysphagia in the dog but is less common in cats. Foreign bodies usually lodge at points of minimal esophageal distension including the thoracic inlet, at the base of the heart, or at the diaphragmatic hiatus. The most common objects ingested are bones, fish hooks, needles, sticks, and play toys. Retained foreign bodies cause partial or complete mechanical obstruction. Muscle spasm and tissue edema occur around the foreign body, making passage of the object down the esophagus more difficult. Mucosal abrasion, laceration, and perforation may occur with sharp or angular objects that are lodged intraluminally.

Clinical Signs
The severity of clinical signs is related to the size of the foreign body and duration of esophageal obstruction.[8] Most dogs and cats with large esophageal foreign bodies are presented for evaluation of acute onset of regurgitation, dysphagia, odynophagia, gagging, and excessive salivation. Smaller foreign bodies which are undiagnosed initially may cause identical signs of several days duration.

Diagnosis
Foreign body ingestion may be reported by the owner. Physical examination is variable, ranging from unremarkable to the presence of halitosis seen with tissue necrosis. Cervical esophageal foreign bodies may be palpable. The findings of depression, anorexia, fever, and cough support aspiration pneumonia or esophageal perforation. A hemogram may reveal a leukocytosis with infection. Clinicians should evaluate thoracic radiographs for aspiration pneumonia (alveolar pulmonary opacities) or esophageal perforation (pneumomediastinum, mediastinitis). Contrast radiography is necessary to identify radiolucent objects. A water-soluble positive-contrast agent (iohexol, gastrografin) should be used rather than barium sulfate if esophageal

perforation is suspected. Esophagoscopy should be performed to confirm the diagnosis and to assess secondary mucosal damage.

Treatment
Esophageal foreign bodies are medical emergencies and should be promptly removed. Endoscopic removal of foreign bodies using a flexible instrument that accommodates a variety of retrieval (grasping) instruments is usually successful. Larger grasping forceps, normally used with rigid endoscopes, may be passed along the side of the flexible endoscope to grasp objects. Distal esophageal foreign bodies may be pushed into the stomach if they cannot be extracted orally. Gastrostomy is not required for most bone foreign bodies, but nondigestible materials retained in the stomach will require surgical removal. The clinician should thoroughly evaluate the esophageal mucosa after foreign body extraction for hemorrhage, lacerations, and perforations (Figures 220-6 and 220-7). Postprocedural thoracic radiographs should be obtained to assess for pneumomediastinum and pneumothorax.

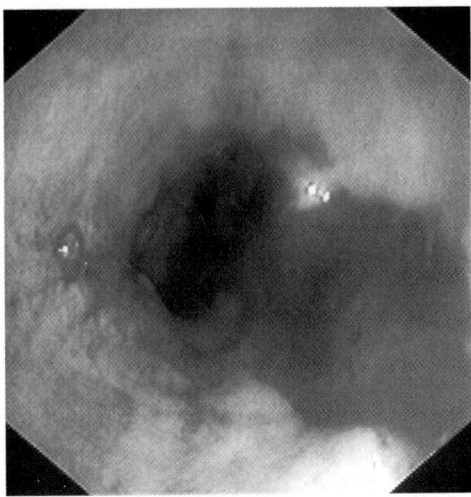

Figure 220-7 Endoscopic appearance of the thoracic esophagus after successful extraction of a bone foreign body (see Figure 220-6). Reader should note the severe trauma and hemorrhage to the esophageal mucosa as a consequence of foreign body retrieval.

Food or water should be restricted for 24 to 48 hours, depending on the extent of esophageal trauma. Animals with severe mucosal damage will require complete esophageal rest and gastrostomy tube feedings. The clinician should institute medical therapy for esophagitis (see Esophagitis earlier in this chapter). Small esophageal perforations are successfully treated with broad-spectrum antibiotics such as ampicillin (11 mg/lb subcutaneously, intramuscularly, or intravenously, three times a day).[9] Surgery (esophagotomy) is indicated if the foreign body cannot be removed endoscopically.

The prognosis after endoscopic foreign body removal is generally excellent. Significant esophageal trauma or large perforation carries a guarded prognosis. Permanent sequellae may include fistula, diverticulum, or stricture formation, as well as segmental defects in motility.

ESOPHAGEAL STRICTURE

Esophageal stricture is an abnormal circumferential narrowing of the esophageal lumen that occurs secondary to severe esophagitis. After mucosal injury, inflammation extends beyond the mucosa into the muscular layer and heals by fibrosis. Fibrotic changes (maturation with contraction) in the esophageal wall cause luminal narrowing. Strictures may occur at any point along the length of the esophagus. The time period from severe esophagitis to lumenal stenosis is approximately 1 to 3 weeks.[10] The most important causes for stricture are gastroesophageal reflux (secondary to general anesthesia) and trauma from esophageal foreign bodies.

Clinical Signs

Classical signs for esophageal dysfunction (regurgitation, dysphagia, ptyalism) are observed and tend to be progressive. Animals often are more tolerant of liquid meals rather than solid meals. A ravenous appetite with weight loss is common because of the inability to transport food past the strictured site.

Diagnosis

A diagnosis of stricture is often suggested by clinical history. The physical examination generally reveals no significant abnormalities other than weight loss. Survey thoracic radiographs are usually normal. Contrast radiography using liquid barium or barium mixed with food demonstrates esophageal lumenal stenosis (Figure 220-8). Contrast studies are useful in assessing the number, location, and length of strictures. Most animals

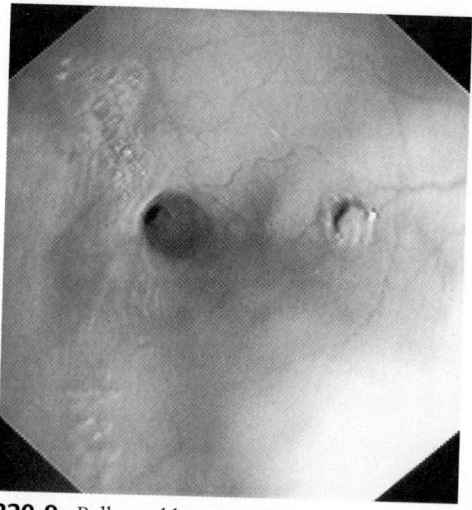

Figure 220-9 Balloon dilatation of an esophageal stricture in a cat using endoscopic guidance (see Figure 220-8). Esophagoscopy demonstrates a 4 mm diameter stricture in the thoracic esophagus.

have a single esophageal stricture. Esophagoscopy confirms stricture and permits differentiation of benign from malignant stricture via results obtained from mucosal biopsy and endoscopic exfoliative cytology.

Treatment

Benign strictures are best treated by mechanical dilatation using a balloon catheter under endoscopic guidance. Balloon catheter dilatation is superior to rigid bougienage because less likelihood of perforation exists, fewer repeated dilatations are required, and a longer clinical response occurs between dilatations.[11] A technique for balloon catheter dilatation in both dogs and cats has been previously described.[11-13] A special polyethylene catheter (Ridgiflex Dilator, Microvasive Inc., Watertown, MA) is carefully advanced adjacent to the endoscope and centered in the lumen of the stricture. The balloon is distended to a desired pressure (not to exceed the maximum pressure recommended by the manufacturer) and held for 2 to 3 minutes. The catheter is then deflated to evaluate lumenal diameter and the extent of iatrogenic trauma. The procedure is immediately repeated using a greater catheter pressure to dilate the stricture further (Figures 220-9 to 220-11).

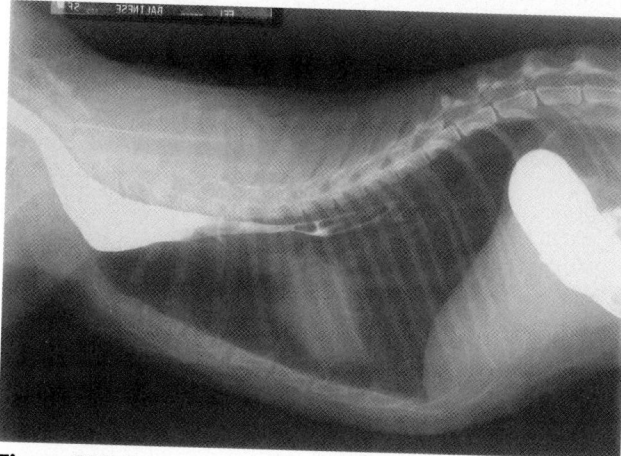

Figure 220-8 Contrast esophagram (lateral view) using liquid barium in a 4-year-old domestic shorthaired (DSH). A 1.5 cm long esophageal stricture is visualized over the base of the heart. Reader should note that the esophagus is dilated cranial to the stricture.

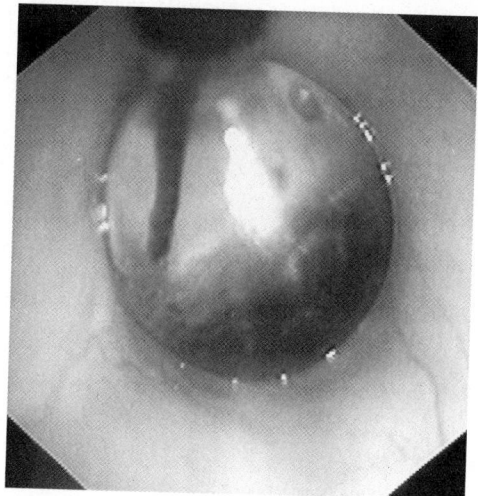

Figure 220-10 Balloon dilatation procedure using maximum balloon inflation pressure.

GASTROINTESTINAL DISEASE

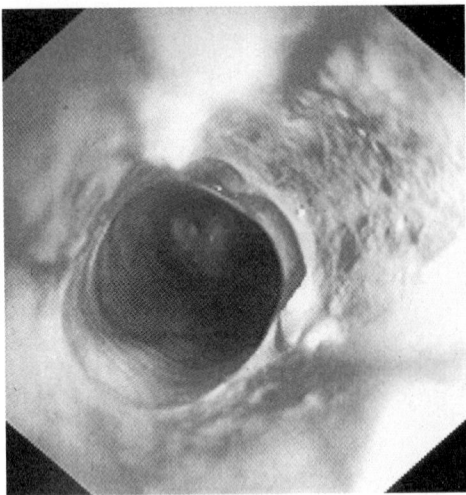

Figure 220-11 Iatrogenic esophagitis that occurs secondary to aggressive balloon dilatation. Reader should note the significant hemorrhage and fibrous tissue tears at the dilated stricture site.

Balloon dilatations are usually performed two to four times (each requiring a separate anesthetic procedures) at intervals of 2 to 3 days because restricture occurs rapidly.[14] Those strictures associated with active esophagitis will require a greater number of dilatation procedures. Complications of balloon dilatation include excessive hemorrhage (common) and esophageal perforation (rare).

Medical therapy of esophagitis is required after mechanical dilatation. The clinician should withhold feedings for 24 hours or place a gastrostomy tube for enteral feedings in animals with severe mucosal trauma. To prevent further injury to the esophageal mucosa from gastroesophageal reflux, H_2-blockers, drugs to enhance LES tone, or both should be administered. Animals with severe esophagitis are also treated with an oral sucralfate slurry (0.5 to 1.0 g dissolved into 5 ml water, orally, three times a day). The use of corticosteroids (prednisone 0.5 to 1.0 mg/lb orally, divided twice a day for 10 to 14 days) may prevent healing by fibrosis and stricture recurrence. Dietary management and medical therapy of gastroesophageal reflux should be continued for 10 to 14 days after balloon dilatation.

The prognosis for benign strictures is good with successful dilatation. Surgical resection of benign strictures is less desirable because success rates are less than with balloon dilatation procedures. Furthermore, restricture at the surgical site is a common sequellae. Malignant esophageal strictures carry a poor prognosis and are treated with a combination of surgical resection (if possible), balloon dilatation (if needed), and appropriate postsurgical irradiation, chemotherapy, or both.

MEGAESOPHAGUS AND ESOPHAGEAL HYPOMOTILITY

Megaesophagus is a disorder characterized by diffuse esophageal dilation and aperistalsis. This syndrome may occur as a congenital idiopathic disorder (uncommon), or it may manifest in adult animals as an idiopathic (common) or acquired lesion. A familial predisposition for congenital megaesophagus has been suggested for the Irish setter, Great Dane, German shepherd, Labrador retriever, Chinese Shar Pei, Newfoundland, miniature schnauzer, and fox terrier breeds.[1,3,6] Congenital megaesophagus in cats is rare, but Siamese cats may be predisposed. The pathogenesis of congenital idiopathic megaesophagus is poorly understood but may involve a defect in vagal afferent innervation of the esophagus.[15,16]

The underlying pathophysiologic mechanism for acquired idiopathic megaesophagus is unknown. Functional responses of the upper and LESs remain intact, and a defect in the afferent neural pathway responsive to esophageal distension is suspected.[17,18] Acquired secondary megaesophagus may result from many disorders, especially diseases causing diffuse neuromuscular dysfunction (Table 220-2). MG accounts for at least 25% of the acquired causes in dogs.[19,20] Dysautonomia is a generalized autonomic neuropathy in which megaesophagus and esophageal hypomotility are consistent findings.[21] This idiopathic disorder is more frequently recognized in cats and is attributed to degenerative lesions involving autonomic ganglia that affect esophageal function. Other causes of segmental or diffuse esophageal hypomotility include foreign bodies, stricture, vascular ring anomalies, and esophagitis. Esophageal dysfunction in Chinese Shar Peis may also result from segmental hypomotility and esophageal redundancy.[22]

Clinical Signs
Regurgitation is the salient clinical sign seen with megaesophagus. Considerable variability exists in the frequency and timing of regurgitation episodes after meal ingestion. Puppies with congenital megaesophagus often begin regurgitating when weaned to solid foods. Weight loss and emaciation occur secondary to malnutrition in animals having long-standing disease. Respiratory distress (moist cough, dyspnea) and fever indicate aspiration pneumonia, which is the most common complication of megaesophagus. Additional clinical signs including muscle pain and stiff gait with polymyositis, generalized weakness with neuromuscular disease, and GI signs with lead toxicity or Addison's disease may be detected in animals having megaesophagus associated with an acquired disorder.

Diagnosis
The clinician should suspect megaesophagus in any adult animal, particularly dogs, with a history of regurgitation. Survey radiographs of the cervical neck and thorax usually reveal the presence of a dilated air-, fluid-, or ingesta-filled esophagus (Figure 220-12). The presence of pulmonary alveolar opacities are indicative of aspiration pneumonia. Barium contrast radiography (esophagram) confirms dilatation and provides evidence of other structural abnormalities (mechanical obstruction). Esophageal motility is best evaluated with fluoroscopy, which assesses the presence and intensity of esophageal peristalsis. Routine hematology, serum biochemistry, and urinalysis should be performed to screen for acquired causes of megaesophagus. An acetylcholine receptor antibody titer should be performed to evaluate for acquired MG, even in the absence of generalized muscle weakness, because MG may mimic idiopathic megaesophagus. Additional laboratory tests are performed on the basis of clinical suspicion (see Table 220-2). Esophagoscopy is rarely required for diagnosis of megaesophagus, except when obstructive disease (neoplasia) or reflux esophagitis are suspected. A clinical diagnosis of dysautonomia is made in most cases based on the unique historical (depression, anorexia, constipation, regurgitation) and physical examination (dry mucous membranes, pupillary dilation, prolapsed nictitating membranes, diminished pupillary light response, bradycardia, and areflexic anus) findings.[21]

Treatment
Animals with acquired secondary megaesophagus are treated specifically for the disorder causing abnormal esophageal motor function (see Table 220-2). Treatment of idiopathic megaesophagus and those acquired forms that fail to respond to specific medical therapy is primarily supportive and symptomatic. The clinician should offer small, frequent meals from an elevated or upright position to assist passage of ingesta into the stomach. Food consistency should be varied (gruel versus

Table • 220-2

Diagnosis and Treatment of Megaesophagus

CAUSE	DIAGNOSTIC TEST	TREATMENT
Neuromuscular Disease		
Idiopathic	Diagnosis of exclusion	Small, frequent elevated feedings
Myasthenia gravis (MG)	Acetylcholine receptor antibody titer, tensilon test, +/− EMG	Pyridostigmine (0.5-1.5 mg/lb PO bid, +/− prednisone (0.5-1.0 mg/lb PO, SC bid)
Systemic lupus erythematosis (SLE)	ANA, skin biopsy	Prednisone (0.5-1.0 mg/lb PO, SC bid)
Polymyositis/polymyopathy	CK, muscle biopsy, EMG	Prednisone (0.5-1.0 mg/lb PO, SC bid)
Glycogen storage disease (type II)	Muscle/liver biopsy, urine metabolic screening	Supportive/symptomatic care
Dermatomyositis	Skin/muscle biopsy	Prednisone (0.5-1.0 mg/lb PO bid)
Dysautonomia	Clinical diagnosis	Supportive/symptomatic care
Distemper	CSF tap, distemper titer	Supportive care
Tetanus	EMG, serum toxin assay	Supportive care
Esophageal Obstruction		
Neoplasia	Contrast radiography, esophagoscopy and biopsy	Surgical resection, chemotherapy
Vascular ring anomaly	Survey/contrast radiography	Surgical correction
Stricture	Contrast radiography, esophagoscopy	Balloon dilatation
Foreign body	Survey/contrast radiography, esophagoscopy	Endoscopic retrieval
Toxicity		
Lead	Hematology, blood lead	Chelation therapy (calcium EDTA)
Organophosphate	Blood cholinesterase activity	Gastric lavage, atropine (0.1 mg/lb SC once) Pralidoxime chloride (5-7.5 mg/lb slow IV)
Miscellaneous		
Hypoad renocorticism	ACTH stimulation test	Prednisone (0.05 mg/lb PO bid), fludrocortisone (0.005 mg/lb PO bid)
Hiatal hernia	Contrast radiography, esophagoscopy	Surgical correction
Gastric dilatation-volvulus	Survey radiography	Surgical correction, supportive care
Esophagitis	Esophagoscopy	Sucralfate (0.5-1.0 g slurry PO tid), ranitidine (0.5-1.0 mg/lb PO ranitidine (0.5-1.0 mg/lb PO bid), metoclopramide (0.2 mg/lb PO tid)
Thymoma	Survey radiography, thymic aspirate	Surgical resection

Adapted from Washabau RJ: Diseases of the esophagus. *In* Ettinger SJ, Feldman ED (eds): *Textbook of Veterinary Internal Medicine,* 5th ed. Philadelphia, WB Saunders Co , 2000, p 1150.

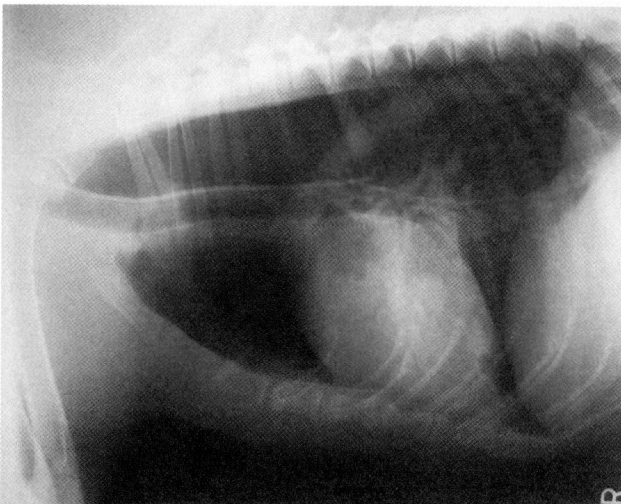

Figure 220-12 Survey thoracic radiograph (lateral view) performed in a 10-year-old dog with idiopathic megaesophagus. A diffusely dilated, air-filled esophagus is readily visualized.

bulk boluses) to determine which types of food are best tolerated. Animals that are severely malnourished or that have aspiration pneumonia should have a gastrostomy tube placed for enteral nutritional support. Broad-spectrum antibiotics should be given for treatment of aspiration pneumonia. Clients should be counseled that recurrent pneumonia is a common problem necessitating prompt detection and treatment for long-term success.

Promotility drugs are currently of unproven benefit in the management of idiopathic megaesophagus in dogs. Both metoclopramide and cisapride are smooth muscle prokinetic agents that have no effect on the striated muscle of the esophageal body.[23] Indeed, preliminary data indicate that cisapride actually decreases the esophageal transit rate of a food bolus in healthy dogs.[24] Cisapride may be a useful prokinetic agent in cats with distal esophageal motility disturbances because of the smooth muscle component in this segment of the feline esophagus.

Affected animals should be re-evaluated at 1- to 2-month intervals to monitor disease progression. Thoracic radiographs should be repeated to assess esophageal dilatation and aspiration pneumonia. Some animals with congenital idiopathic megaesophagus may improve over time (months) with diligent supportive care. The prognosis with acquired idiopathic mega-esophagus is generally poor. These animals usually succumb to repeated episodes of aspiration pneumonia or are euthanized because of their irreversible disease. Animals with acquired secondary megaesophagus may respond to specific drug therapy. The prognosis in dogs with megaesophagus caused by acquired MG is favorable, with approximately 50% of dogs responding to supportive therapy.[19]

VASCULAR RING ANOMALY

Vascular ring anomalies are congenital malformations of the major arteries of the heart that entrap the intrathoracic esoph-agus and cause esophageal obstruction. Persistent right aortic arch (PRAA) is the best-documented anomaly in both dogs and cats; it occurs when the embryonic right aortic arch (rather than the left fourth aortic arch) becomes the func-tional adult aorta. Circular entrapment of the esophagus occurs by the aorta on the right, the ligamentum arteriosum dorsolaterally on the left, the pulmonary trunk on the left, and the heart base ventrally. This anomaly is considered to have a familial tendency because German shepherds and Irish setters appear to be predisposed.[6] Other less common vascular anomalies include persistent right or left subclavian arteries, double aortic arch, persistent right dorsal aorta, left aortic arch and right ligamentum arteriosum, and aberrant intercostal arteries.

Clinical Signs

Affected puppies and kittens usually present for regurgitation of solid foods at the time of weaning. Weight loss with failure to thrive despite a good appetite is commonly observed. The presence of a moist cough, dyspnea, and fever suggest aspira-tion pneumonia. Physical examination often reveals a thin, stunted animal that is otherwise normal.

Diagnosis

Vascular ring anomalies should be differentiated from other causes of regurgitation in young animals such as congenital idiopathic megaesophagus, esophageal foreign body, and cricopharyngeal dysphagia. The signalment and a compatible history of regurgitation since weaning are very suggestive of

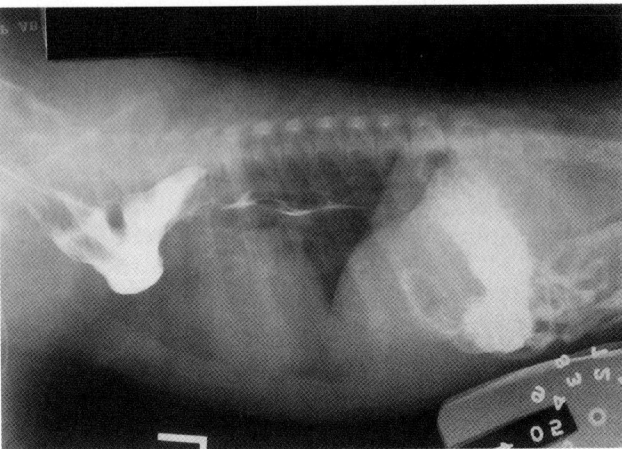

Figure 220-13 Contrast esophagram (lateral view) performed in a 7-month-old dog with a persistent right aortic arch. Abrupt attenuation of the liquid barium contrast column is observed at the base of the heart along with segmental (cranial) esophageal dilatation.

a vascular ring anomaly. Survey thoracic radiographs usually demonstrate esophageal body dilation cranial to the base of the heart. Radiographic abnormalities to the caudal esophagus are seldom seen. A barium esophagram should be performed to confirm the location of esophageal obstruction and severity of esophageal distension (Figure 220-13). Fluoroscopy is useful to evaluate for segmental or generalized esophageal motility disturbances. Angiography is occasionally performed for defini-tive confirmation of the type and location of the vascular anomaly prior to surgery. Esophagoscopy will differentiate intra-luminal stricture from extraluminal compression. Strictures appear as distinct intraluminal fibrous rings that remain static when viewed endoscopically; whereas with vascular ring anomaly, rhythmic pulsations of the great arteries compressing the esophagus externally are observed (Figure 220-14).

Treatment

Definitive therapy for PRAA is surgical ligation and transection of the ligamentum arteriosum. Animals with severe debilitation

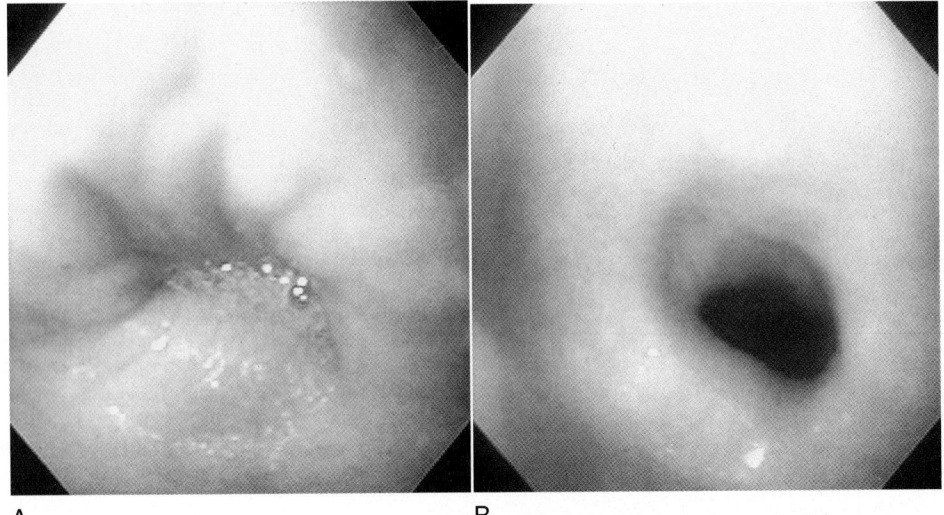

A   B

Figure 220-14 Dynamic endoscopic appearance of persistent right aortic arch in a 3-year-old dog (see Figure 220-13). Extraluminal pulsations of blood through the anomalous artery cause the stenosis to intermittently "close" **(A)** and "open" **(B)**.

from malnutrition will require enteral nutritional support via gastrostomy tube feedings. Aspiration pneumonia should be effectively treated with broad-spectrum antibiotics before surgery. Significant clinical improvement usually follows corrective surgery, although esophageal hypomotility and regurgitation may persist. In these instances, affected animals are managed with elevated feedings as described for idiopathic megaesophagus.

The best prognosis for return of normal esophageal function is obtained with early diagnosis and prompt surgical intervention. Progressive esophageal dilatation that causes irreversible myenteric nerve degeneration and esophageal hypomotility may occur if a diagnosis is not made at an early age.

ESOPHAGEAL DIVERTICULA

Esophageal diverticula are rare pouchlike sacculations of the esophageal wall that may be congenital or acquired. Congenital diverticula are due to developmental abnormalities of the esophagus that permit herniation of the mucosa through the muscularis. Acquired diverticula are classified as either *pulsion* or *traction* forms. Pulsion diverticula result from conditions of increased intraluminal pressure secondary to obstruction (stricture or foreign body) or altered motility.[25,26] Traction diverticula result from periesophageal inflammation and fibrosis. With the traction form, contraction of fibrotic adhesions leads to eversion and out-pouching of the esophageal wall. The accumulation of ingesta (impaction) within diverticula leads to esophagitis, mechanical obstruction (seen with large diverticula), and disturbed esophageal motility.

Clinical Signs
Large multilobulated diverticula are most likely to cause signs of regurgitation, odynophagia, and retching. Postprandial regurgitation results from mechanical obstruction and motility disturbances. Severe cases with mucosal ulceration may eventually perforate and cause signs of mediastinitis and respiratory distress. Clinical signs may not occur with small diverticula.

Diagnosis
Survey thoracic radiographs may reveal an air or soft-tissue opacity adjacent to the esophagus. Diverticula should not be confused with the normal esophageal redundancy seen in young brachycephalic breeds and Chinese Shar Peis. Performance of contrast radiography shows a focally dilated segment of the esophagus that fills partially or completely with contrast material. Esophagoscopy confirms a saclike out-pouching of the esophageal lumen containing impacted ingesta and having localized esophagitis.

Treatment
Diverticulectomy is the preferred therapy. Large diverticula will require greater excision and reconstruction of the esophageal wall. Small diverticula may be managed medically with smaller-sized, upright feedings of a liquid or semiliquid diet to minimize impaction of ingesta in the diverticulum. Traction diverticuli are often managed with broad-spectrum antibiotics, whereas pulsion diverticula are treated for their specific cause (see Esophagitis, Stricture, earlier in this chapter). Most cases warrant a guarded prognosis because complications, such as stricture formation and segmental hypomotility, may persist after surgery.

ESOPHAGEAL FISTULA

An esophageal fistula is an abnormal communicating tract between the esophagus and usually the respiratory system (esophagopulmonary, esophagotracheal, and esophagobronchial fistula). Both congenital and acquired fistulas have been described. Acquired fistulas are usually associated with retained esophageal foreign bodies, especially bones. Other causes include trauma, neoplasia, or periesophageal inflammation. In most cases, the lodged foreign body causes mural necrosis, esophageal perforation, and leakage of esophageal contents into adjacent tissues. Healing leads to development of a communicating tract with resultant airway contamination from esophageal contents. Esophageal fistula is relatively uncommon in the dog and cat.

Clinical Signs
Clinical signs are primarily associated with respiratory tract and include coughing and dyspnea. Coughing after drinking is a common presenting sign. Dysphagia and regurgitation are less commonly observed in association with an esophageal foreign body. Anorexia, lethargy, weight loss, and fever are seen with mediastinitis or aspiration pneumonia. The physical examination findings of cough, fever, pulmonary crackles, and weight loss reflect chronic respiratory disease.

Diagnosis
Survey thoracic radiographs usually reveal a localized alveolar, bronchial, or interstitial lung pattern (or a combination of these patterns). The right caudal lung lobe in dogs and the left caudal and accessory lobes in cats are most commonly affected.[27] Radiopaque foreign bodies may be observed in the esophagus. A barium esophagram is required for definitive diagnosis of esophageal-airway communication. Clinicians should avoid using iodinated contrast agents in these procedures because they are hyperosmolar and potentially irritating to exposed tissues. Endoscopic examination (esophagoscopy, bronchoscopy) is of limited value in confirming small fistulas. A CBC may reflect associated inflammation (periesophagitis, pneumonia) and nonregenerative anemia.

Treatment
Surgical correction of the fistulous tract is required. Esophagotomy for a retained esophageal foreign body should be performed. Lobectomy may be necessary as a result of pulmonary consolidation or foreign material contained within the airways. Postsurgical therapy includes esophageal rest and administration of appropriate antibiotics for infection (based on culture and susceptibility testing of involved tissues). A good prognosis is given to animals after successful surgery. The prognosis is guarded if severe complications, such as dehiscence, stricture, or pulmonary abscessation, are present.

ESOPHAGEAL NEOPLASIA

Tumors of the esophagus are rare, accounting for less than 0.5% of all cancers in the dog and cat.[28] Neoplasms may be of primary esophageal, periesophageal, or metastatic origin. Esophageal fibrosarcoma and osteosarcoma are the most common malignant tumors in dogs, developing from malignant transformation of esophageal granulomas associated with *Spirocerca lupi* infection.[29] Squamous cell carcinoma is the most commonly diagnosed primary esophageal tumor in cats. Other less commonly reported primary esophageal tumors in the dog and cat include leiomyo(sarco)ma and undifferentiated carcinoma. Periesophageal tumors arising from a variety of adjacent structures (lymph nodes, thyroid, thymus, and heart base) cause local esophageal invasion, direct mechanical obstruction, or both. Metastatic lesions (thyroid, pulmonary, and gastric carcinomas) commonly involve the esophagus but less frequently cause clinical signs of esophageal disease.

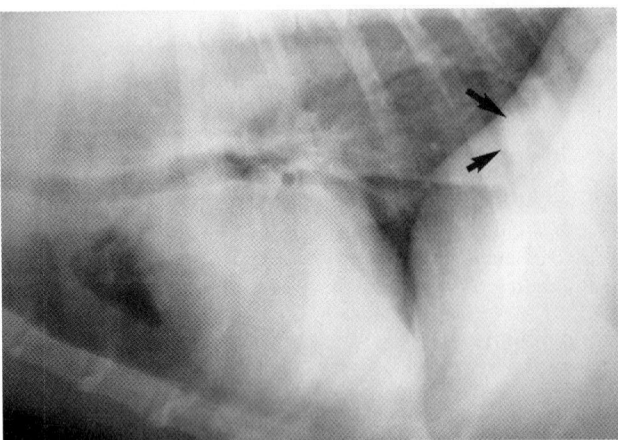

Figure 220-15 Survey thoracic radiograph (lateral view) showing generalized esophageal dilatation (megaesophagus) in a 9-year-old rottweiler. A distinct soft-tissue opacity (*arrows*) is visualized in the distal esophagus at the level of the lower esophageal sphincter (LES).

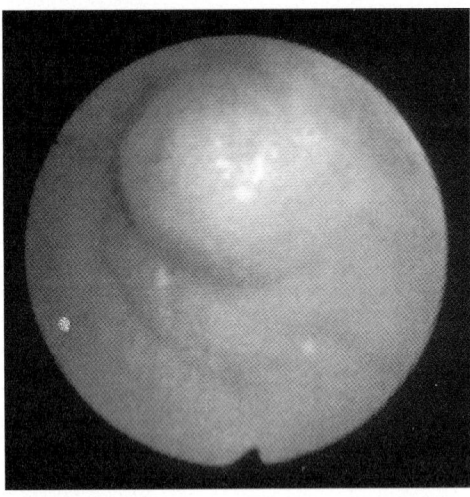

Figure 220-17 Endoscopic appearance of an esophageal mass located adjacent to the lower esophageal sphincter (LES) in a dog (see Figure 220-15). Histopathology proved the mass to be a leiomyosarcoma.

Clinical Signs

Animals with esophageal neoplasia have signs consistent with progressive esophageal obstruction, including chronic regurgitation, dysphagia, odynophagia, and ptyalism. Anorexia, weight loss, and depression are more typical of advanced disease (metastasis, systemic effects of cancer) and malnutrition resulting from the inability to retain food. The physical examination findings may reveal weight loss and emaciation, and large periesophageal masses involving the cervical esophagus might be palpable.

Diagnosis

Clinicians should consider a diagnosis of esophageal neoplasia in middle-aged and older animals having chronic progressive signs of obstructive esophageal disease. Survey thoracic radiographs may be normal or reveal variable esophageal dilatation, an intraluminal mass, or evidence of a periesophageal lesion displacing the esophagus (Figures 220-15 and 220-16). The lungs should be evaluated for aspiration pneumonia (alveolar opacities) and metastasis (nodular opacities). A barium esophagram typically confirms the presence of an intraluminal mass or obstructive lesion. Esophagoscopy with mucosal biopsy and exfoliative cytology is required for definitive diagnosis of esophageal neoplasia (Figures 220-17 and 220-18). Endoscopic biopsy of the esophagus is difficult because the

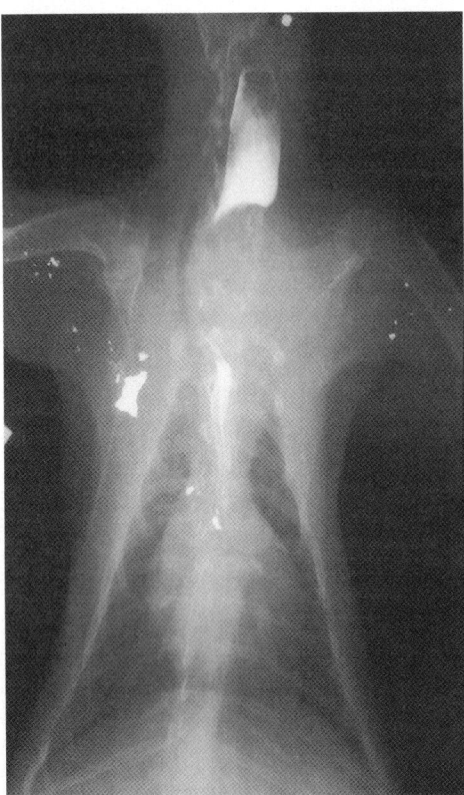

Figure 220-16 Contrast esophagram (ventrodorsal view) in a 10-year-old cat. Cervical esophageal dilation with narrowing of the barium contrast column caused by partial esophageal obstruction is observed. Reader should note the lateral displacement of the air-filled trachea suggestive of a periesophageal mass.

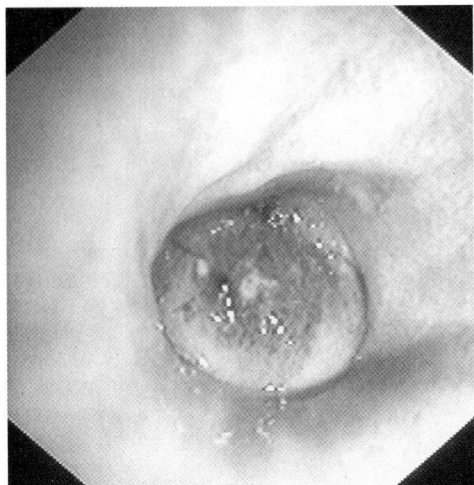

Figure 220-18 Endoscopic appearance of an invasive periesophageal mass in a cat causing near complete esophageal obstruction (see Figure 220-16). Endoscopic exfoliative cytology confirmed a diagnosis of lymphoblastic lymphosarcoma (see Figure 220-20).

mucosa is tough and it is technically demanding to position the biopsy instrument (forceps) perpendicular to the mucosa. Biopsies with small pinch forceps often provide nonrepresentative superficial epithelial specimens. Both mucosal biopsy and exfoliative cytology are most beneficial in the diagnosis of epithelial-based neoplasms, such as squamous cell carcinoma and lymphosarcoma.

Treatment

Successful treatment of malignant esophageal neoplasia is uncommon because the disease is often well advanced at the time of diagnosis. This is especially true for animals having secondary complications such as severe malnutrition, esophageal hypomotility, and aspiration pneumonia. Chemotherapy, radiation therapy, and surgery are palliative techniques for treatment of malignant tumors. In contrast, benign esophageal neoplasms (leiomyoma) carry a good prognosis with complete surgical resection.[30] Lymphosarcoma (typically diagnosed as a periesophageal mass) is generally responsive to multiple drug chemotherapy regimens.

HIATAL HERNIA

Hiatal hernia may present at two distinct entities in the dog and cat: (1) sliding hiatal hernia, which is a cranial displacement of the distal esophagus and stomach into the mediastinum through the esophageal hiatus, and (2) periesophageal hiatal hernia, which involves cranial displacement of a portion of the stomach into the mediastinum through a defect adjacent to the esophageal hiatus.[31,32] Sliding hiatal hernia is the most common form and may occur as a congenital or acquired lesion in the dog and cat.

Most hiatal hernias are probably congenital and occur as developmental defects (enlargement) of the esophageal hiatus or phrenicoesophageal ligament. Males and Chinese Shar Pei dogs appear to have an increased incidence and develop clinical signs shortly after weaning.[6] Acquired hiatal hernias occasionally occur secondary to trauma (via damage to diaphragmatic nerves and muscles resulting in hiatal laxity) and respiratory distress (caused by increased negative intrathoracic pressure seen with intermittent airway obstruction [laryngeal paralysis]). Regardless of the cause, hiatal herniation reduces LES pressure and leads to gastroesophageal reflux, esophagitis, and segmental or diffuse esophageal hypomotility.

Clinical Signs

Intermittent signs of reflux esophagitis (persistent regurgitation, vomiting, occasional hematemesis and hypersalivation) predominate. Weight loss may be observed in animals having chronic disease. Dyspnea is common due to aspiration pneumonia and compression of the lungs seen with large hernias. Affected animals may be thin on physical examination.

Diagnosis

Survey thoracic radiographs often reveal the presence of a caudodorsal, gas-filled, soft-tissue opacity. Varying degrees of esophageal dilatation and alveolar opacities (consistent with aspiration pneumonia) may also be observed. Performance of a positive contrast esophagram confirms hiatal herniation and the presence of esophageal dilatation. Fluoroscopy is useful in evaluation of the magnitude of esophageal hypomotility present. Esophagoscopy, generally not a first-choice diagnostic test, may confirm reflux esophagitis and cranial displacement of both the LES and rugal folds of the stomach into the esophageal lumen.

Treatment

Reconstructive surgery is indicated for treatment of large congenital hiatal hernias. Normal hiatal anatomy is restored by performance of diaphragmatic crural apposition, esophagopexy, and left fundic tube gastropexy techniques.[31,33] Animals having smaller, intermittent hiatal hernias should be medically managed for reflux esophagitis, using H_2 receptor antagonists (to reduce gastric acidity), sucralfate suspensions (as a mucosal cytoprotectant), and drugs (cisapride or metoclopramide) to enhance LES tone, which inhibits gastroesophageal reflux. Animals failing medical management will require surgical intervention.

A good prognosis is warranted in animals after successful surgery. A guarded prognosis is given to animals with concurrent esophageal motility disturbances.

MISCELLANEOUS ESOPHAGEAL DISORDERS

Major causes for *esophageal perforation* include esophageal foreign bodies (large or angular- shaped bones and those objects retained for a prolonged period causing pressure necrosis) and penetrating trauma to the cervical esophagus caused by bite wounds (Figure 220-19). Predominant signs of anorexia, depression, odynophagia, moist cough, fever, and a rigid stance are observed. A diagnosis is often suspected based on history and survey radiographic findings that show a pneumomediastinum, pneumothorax, and mediastinal or pleural effusion. A contrast esophagram using a water-soluble contrast agent (Omnipaque) should be performed to determine the location and extent of the esophageal tear. Esophagoscopy may detect large tears but is an insensitive tool for localizing small tears. Treatment is generally conservative, using broad-spectrum antibiotics, fluid therapy, and nutritional support by tube gastrostomy feedings. Clinicians should monitor therapeutic responses by repeating thoracic radiographs. Large perforations will require surgical correction.

Periesophageal obstruction is uncommonly associated with intrathoracic mass lesions (neoplasia, lymphadenopathy, large abscess) that cause partial extraluminal compression. Clinical signs usually indicate slowly progressive esophageal dysphagia, often accompanied by extra-esophageal signs of dyspnea, cough, and exercise intolerance. Survey thoracic radiographs usually identify an intrathoracic mass with esophageal encroachment. A contrast esophagram may or may not determine whether intraluminal versus extraluminal compression is present. Esophagoscopy is more useful in characterizing

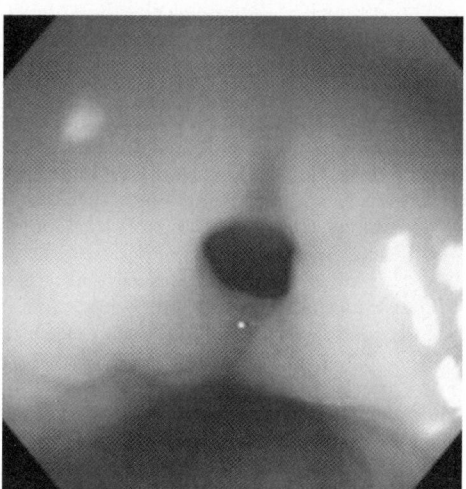

Figure 220-19 Endoscopic appearance of cervical esophageal perforation in a dog caused by penetrating bite wounds to the neck. The dog responded completely to conservative medical management.

whether or not the stenosis is extraluminal, and whether potential mucosal invasion has occurred. Definitive diagnosis depends on identification of the mass lesion with fine needle aspiration, endoscopic exfoliative cytology (Figure 220-20), or biopsy via thoracotomy.

GI intussusception is a rare disorder of young dogs caused by invagination of the stomach, and occasionally other structures such as the spleen, proximal duodenum, and pancreas, into the esophagus.[34] Prolapse of a large portion of the stomach causes abrupt clinical deterioration with mortality rates in excess of 95% reported.[35] The cause for GI intussusception is unknown; however, congenital megaesophagus possibly predisposes to this disorder due to decreased esophageal motility and reduced LES tone. Animals with GI intussusception usually have histories of acute vomiting, regurgitation, dyspnea, hematemesis, and abdominal discomfort. Survey abdominal radiographs confirm the presence of a soft tissue and gas opacity in the dorsocaudal mediastinum. A contrast esophagram usually shows gastric rugae within the esophageal lumen and the presence of esophageal obstruction. Esophagoscopy may also confirm a bulging mass (gastric rugal folds) contained within the lumen of the esophagus. Treatment of large intussusceptions necessitates manual reduction and gastropexy to prevent recurrence. Small lesions may be carefully reduced endoscopically and subsequently managed medically for reflux esophagitis.

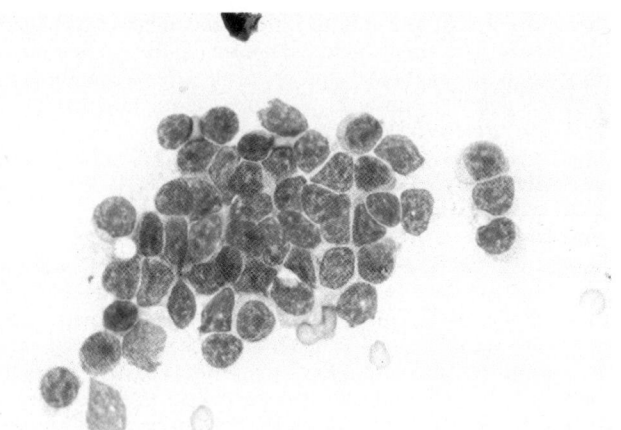

Figure 220-20 Endoscopic exfoliative cytology obtained from a cat with an invasive periesophageal mass (see Figure 220-18). A uniform population of lymphoblasts, consistent with lymphosarcoma, is present. Multidrug chemotherapy resulted in complete clinical remission for 9 months.

CHAPTER • 221

Diseases of the Stomach

Kenneth W. Simpson*

FUNCTIONAL ANATOMY

The stomach's main function is to act as a reservoir that controls the size and rate of passage of ingesta into the small intestine. The stomach also initiates the digestion of protein and fat and facilitates the absorption of vitamins and minerals.

Anatomically the stomach is composed of four regions, the cardia, fundus, body, and antrum (Figure 221-1). The fundus and body expand to accommodate ingesta. The antrum is thick and muscular and grinds food into small particles that are triturated into the duodenum. The lower esophageal sphincter prevents reflux of ingesta into the esophagus and the pyloric sphincter controls efflux into the duodenum.

The gastric wall has three layers: the mucosa, muscularis, and serosa. The mucosa has a superficial epithelium, gastric glands, and an innermost layer of smooth muscle, with fine structure and function varying depending on the gastric region (Figure 221-2). The mucosa in the cardia and pylorus is thinner and less glandular than in the fundus and body. The mucosa of the body contains mucous neck cells (pepsinogen A, gastric lipase), parietal cells (acid, pepsinogen A, intrinsic factor), and chief cells (pepsinogen A).[1-3] A variety of neuroendocrine cells involved with the secretion of gastric acid are interspersed between the glands. The predominant cells are enterochromaffin-like and somatostatin-producing cells in the fundus, and gastrin and somatostatin-producing cells in the antrum. Localized small aggregates of lymphoid tissues are observed at the base of the gastric glands. Intertwined between gastric glands is a rich network of blood vessels and lymphatics and nerves. Beneath the submucosa are two layers of smooth muscle that run perpendicuar to each other. The serosa is the outermost layer.

Regulation of Acid Secretion

Acid secretion is regulated by a variety of neurochemical and neurohumeral stimuli.[4,5] Luminal peptides, digested protein, acetylcholine, and gastrin-releasing peptide (GRP) stimulate gastrin secretion from G cells and effect histamine release from enterochromaffin-like cells (ECL cells) (Figure 221-3).

Histamine release from mast cells and binding of acetylcholine and gastrin to parietal cells also contribute to secretion. Somatostatin released in response to gastric pH levels below 3 decreases gastrin, histamine, and acid secretion.

Unstimulated acid secretion in dogs and cats is minimal (dogs <0.04 mmol/kg.75/hr)[6] and H^+/K^+-ATPase, "the acid pump," is present in tubulovesicles within the cytoplasm of parietal cells.[7] In the stimulated state H^+/K^+-ATPase and KCl transporters are incorporated into the parietal cell canalicular membrane and hydrogen ions, derived from the ionization of water within the perietal cells, are transported into the gastric lumen in exchange for K^+ by H^+/K^+-ATPase. Potassium and

*K.W. Simpson is supported by a grant from US Public Health Service DK 002938.

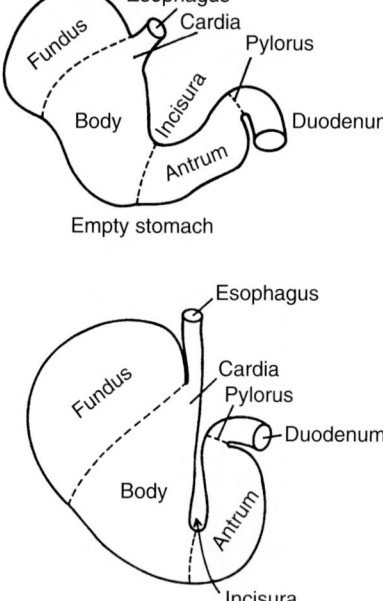

Figure 221-1 Gastric anatomy of the empty and full stomach. (From Guilford, Strombeck, 1996, p 239, Saunders.)

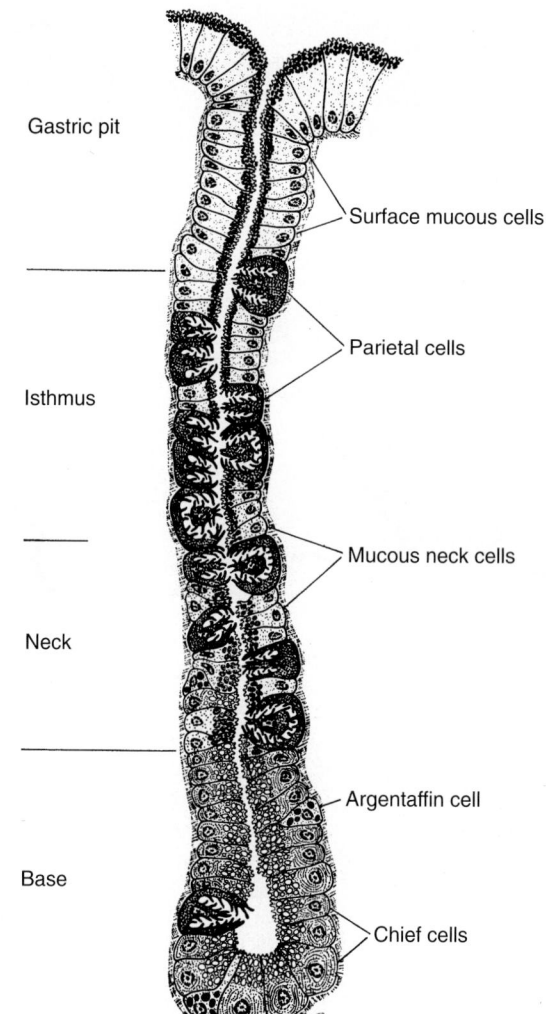

Figure 221-2 Histologic appearance of the cardiac, fundic, pyloric gastric mucosa.

chloride transporters in the canalicular membrane enable luminal transfer of potassium and chloride. OH^- combines with CO_2, catalyzed by carbonic anhydrase, to form HCO_3^-, which diffuses into the blood (the "alkaline tide"). Stimulation results in a rapid increase in fluid and hydrogen ion secretion, with pH rapidly declining to around pH 1. The concentrations of K^+ (10 to 20 mmol/L) and Cl^- (approximately 120 to 160 mmol/L) in gastric juice are higher than in plasma.

The stomach is protected from gastric acid by a functional unit known as the *gastric mucosal barrier* (GMB).[8-10] The GMB comprises tightly opposed epithelial cells coated with a layer of bicarbonate rich mucus and an abundant mucosal blood supply that delivers bicarbonate, oxygen, and nutrients. Local production of prostaglandins (PGE_2) is important in modulating blood flow, bicarbonate secretion, and epithelial cell renewal. When damage occurs, epithelial cells rapidly migrate over superficial mucosal defects aided by the local production of growth factors such as EGF (epidermal growth factor).

Gastric Motility

Normal gastric motility is the result of the organized interaction of smooth muscle with neural and hormonal stimuli. The rate of gastric emptying is determined by the difference in pressure between the stomach and the duodenum and the resistance to flow across the pylorus. Liquids are expelled more rapidly than solids and the rate of expulsion of liquids increases with volume. The rate of expulsion of solids depends on caloric density. In dogs, digestible solids smaller than 2 mm are emptied into the duodenum and gastric emptying is modulated via intestinal osmo- and chemoreceptors. Carbohydrates, amino acids, and especially fats retard gastric emptying. The release of cholecystokinin (CCK) in response to fatty and amino acids, such as tryptophan, is one factor that slows gastric emptying. Large, undigestible solids are expelled from the stomach in the fasted state by phase III of the migrating motility complex (MMC) in response to the release of motilin.

Digestion and Assimilation of Nutrients

The stomach has a limited role in the digestion of proteins, fats, and micronutrients. Pepsin, which digests proteins, is secreted as pepsinogen in response to acetylcholine and histamine in tandem with gastric acid. Dog gastric lipase, which digests fat, is secreted in response to pentagastrin, histamine, prostaglandin E_2, and secretin and parallels the secretion of gastric mucus. Although pepsin is active only at acid pH, dog gastric lipase remains active in the small intestine and constitutes up to 30% of total lipase secreted over a 3-hour period.[11] Although gastric lipase and pepsin are not essential for the assimilation of dietary fat and protein, the entry of peptides and fatty acids into the small intestine likely helps to coordinate gastric emptying and pancreatic secretion.

Intrinsic factor, which is necessary for cobalamin (vitamin B_{12}) absorption, is produced by parietal cells and cells at the base of antral glands in the dog but not the cat.[1,12] The importance of gastric intrinsic factor secretion in dogs is questionable as the pancreas is the major site of secretion in both dogs and cats. Gastric acidity may also have an effect on the availability of minerals such as iron and calcium.

Gastric Flora

The concept of the stomach as a sterile place was completely dispelled by the isolation of the gastric bacterium *Helicobacter pylori* from people in 1983.[13] The stomach of dogs and cats also harbors a diverse spectrum of large, spiral, acid-tolerant *Helicobacter* species and a variety of aerobes and anaerobes

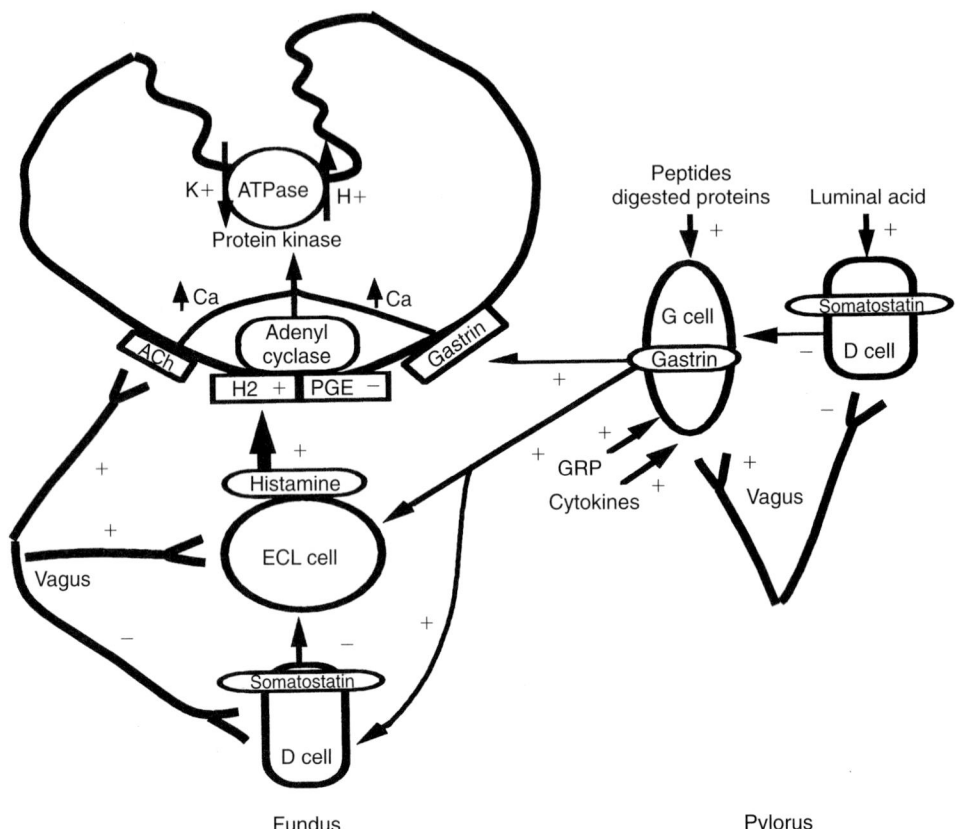

Figure 221-3 Regulation of acid secretion. *ECL*, Enterochromaffin like cell; *GRP*, gastrin releasing peptide; H_2, histamine H_2 receptor; *PGE*, prostaglandin E_2 receptor; *ACh*, acetylchline receptor. (From Simpson KW: In Dibartola, editor: *Fluid therapy in small animal practice*, ed 2, Philadelphia, Saunders, 1996.)

that may play a role in the development of gastritis or possibly cancer (see chronic gastritis). A mixed flora of aerobes and anaerobes (approximately 10^6 to 10^7 cfu/mL is rapidly established soon after birth in dogs,[14] and colonization with *Helicobacter* spp., which are likely acquired from the dam, has been documented as early as 6 weeks of age. *Helicobacter* spp. are adapted to life in an acid environment and produce urease that catalyzes the formation of ammonia from urea to buffer gastric acidity. Other bacterial species, such as *Proteus*, *Streptococcus*, and *Lactobacillus*, cultured from the canine stomach, may transiently increase after a meal or coprophagia. Acid secretion and gastric emptying likely regulate much of this transient flora and bacteria may proliferate in the event of gastric acid hyposecretion due to glandular atrophy or pharmacologic inhibition. From a diagnostic standpoint it is important to realize that bacteria such as *E. coli* and *Proteus* spp. produce urease that can lead to a false-positive test result for *Helicobacter* spp.

DISEASES OF THE STOMACH

Gastric disease is usually the result of inflammation, ulceration, neoplasia, or obstruction and manifests clinically as vomiting, hematemesis, melena, retching, burping, hypersalivation, abdominal distension, abdominal pain, or weight loss. The clinical approach is simplified by considering gastric diseases as a group of clinical syndromes based on the combination of etiology, pathology, and clinical presentation (Table 221-1). Because a large and varied group of non-gastric disorders can cause similar clinical signs, a systematic approach is essential to determine if gastric disease is the cause. The diagnostic approach

initially focuses on historical and physical findings, with clinico-pathologic testing and diagnostic imaging employed in patients with systemic involvement or chronic signs.

Signalment, History, and Physical Examination
The age and breed of the patient are helpful in diagnosis of certain gastric disorders. Young dogs are more likely to ingest foreign bodies or to suffer from outflow obstruction caused by *Pythium insidiosum*, whereas gastric cancer is typically encountered in much older dogs and cats. Gastric dilatation and volvulus are typically encountered in giant breed or dogs

Table • 221-1

Diseases of the Stomach

CLINICAL SYNDROME	PREDOMINANT FEATURES
Acute gastritis	Vomiting of sudden onset
Ulceration or erosion	Vomiting, hematemesis, melena, ± anemia
Gastric dilatation/ volvulus	Non-productive retching, abdominal distention, tachycardia
Chronic gastritis	Chronic vomiting of food or bile
Delayed gastric emptying	Acute to chronic vomiting more than 8 to 10 hr after feeding
Neoplasia	Chronic vomiting, weight loss, ± anemia

with deep chests such as Great Danes and Irish Setters. There are also breed predispositions to hypertrophic gastropathy (Drentse patrijshond, basenji, and small breed brachycephalic dogs, such as shih tzu), atrophic gastritis (Lundehund) and gastric cancer (Belgian shepherd, rough Collie, Staffordshire bull terrier, beagle, Lundehund).

Vomiting is the principal clinical sign of gastric disease (see Table 221-1), and a major objective of the history is to distinguish vomiting from regurgitation (active abdominal effort, presence of bile), and to obtain a clear picture of the vomiting episodes (duration, frequency, contents, color, progression, relation to eating). Where vomiting cannot be adequately distinguished from regurgitation it is important to observe "vomiting episodes" and the animal eating. Where regurgitation is still a possibility, thoracic radiographs help to detect esophageal dilatation or obstruction.

A thorough review of the environment (indoor, outdoor, single or multi-animal household), access to foreign bodies, toxins or medications, vaccination status, body systems (attitude, mentation, presence of polyuria, polydipsia, weight loss, diarrhea, coughing, sneezing, exercise tolerance), past medical history, and physical examination helps to discriminate many non-gastric from gastric causes of vomiting.

Physical examination is frequently normal in patients with primary gastric disease. Abdominal distension may be detected in those with GD/GDV or delayed gastric emptying. Abnormal perfusion, hydration status, temperature, respiratory rate, mucosal pallor, and abdominal pain often accompany diseases such as GD/GDV, gastric outflow obstruction, ulceration, and perforation.

Historical and physical findings are integrated to determine if the patient is systemically well or unwell, and clinical signs are acute (lasting less than 10 days), chronic, mild, or severe (Figure 221-4). Non-productive vomiting, retching, and abdominal distension in deep-chested large breed dogs are frequently associated with gastric dilatation/gastric dilatation and volvulus (GDV), which requires rapid diagnosis and treatment.

The presence of fresh or digested blood ("coffee grounds"), in vomitus, with or without melena raises the possibility of gastric ulcers or erosions.

Vomiting of food greater than 8 to 10 hours after ingestion suggests delayed gastric emptying and requires investigation to distinguish gastric outflow obstruction from defective gastric propulsion.

Weight loss is infrequently associated with gastric disease but can accompany cancer, fungal infections, outflow obstruction, and gastropathies that are part of a more generalized disease process, such as basenji and Lundehund gastroenteropathy.

If vomiting is acute and the animal is systemically well, with no historical or physical "red flags," further diagnostic testing is often postponed in favor of symptomatic therapy. If the animal is systemically unwell or has significant historical or physical abnormalities the emphasis is on efficiently identifying conditions that require surgical intervention, such as gastric dilatation and septic peritonitis, and ruling out non-gastrointestinal causes of vomiting, before proceeding to more specialized or invasive diagnostic procedures aimed at detecting primary gastric and intestinal disorders (see Figure 221-4).

Clinicopathologic Testing

Clinicopathologic testing helps to differentiate primary gastrointestinal disease form non-GI disease, and to ascertain the metabolic consequences of GI disease. Blood and urine samples should be obtained prior to treatment.

In sick patients, the rapid evaluation of microhematocrit (PCV), total solids (TS), blood glucose, blood urea nitrogen, urine specific gravity, glucose, ketones and protein, and plasma concentrations of sodium and potassium help to detect life threatening diseases such as renal failure (azotemia and

unconcentrated urine) and hypoadrenocorticism (Na:K <27:1), and guide initial management pending more definitive testing.

Abnormalities in *complete blood count* are infrequent with primary gastric disease. Hemoconcentration as a consequence of dehydration or shock frequently accompanies GDV, gastric perforation, or gastric obstruction. The combination of a hematocrit level greater than 55% and normal or decreased protein concentrations is encountered in dogs with hemorrhagic gastroenteritis (see Chapter 222). Anemia, erythrocyte microcytosis, and thrombocytosis may be present in dogs with chronic gastric bleeding. Stomatocytosis has been described in Drentse patrijshond dogs with familial stomatocytosis-hypertrophic gastritis. Basophilic stippling of red cells suggests lead toxicity.

Biochemical abnormalities in primary gastric disease are usually restricted to alterations in electrolytes and acid-base, pre-renal increases in creatinine and BUN, and occasionally hypoproteinemia.

Vomiting of gastric and intestinal contents usually involves the loss of chloride, potassium, sodium and bicarbonate containing fluid and dehydration is variably accompanied by hypochloremia, hypokalemia, and hyponatremia.[15,16] Determination of *acid-base status* by measurement of total CO_2 or venous blood gas analysis enables the presence of metabolic acidosis or alkalosis to be detected.

Metabolic acidosis is generally more common than metabolic alkalosis in dogs with GI disease.[15] Where the gastric outflow tract or proximal duodenum is obstructed, the loss of chloride may exceed that of bicarbonate, and hypochloremia, hypokalemia, and metabolic alkalosis occur.[15-17] The metabolic alkalosis is enhanced by elevated HCO_3^- conservation due to volume, and potassium and chloride depletion.[18] The net effect is a preferential conservation of volume at the expense of the extracellular pH. The renal reabsorption of almost all filtered bicarbonate and the exchange of sodium for hydrogen in the distal tubule promote an acid urine pH despite an extracellular alkalemia ("paradoxical aciduria").[18,19]

Metabolic alkalosis in patients with gastrointestinal signs is not invariably associated with outflow obstruction and has been encountered in dogs with parvovirus enteritis and acute pancreatitis.[20] Diseases characterized by acid hypersecretion, such as gastrinoma, may also be associated with metabolic alkalosis and aciduria. Basal gastric acid secretion in two dogs with gastrin-producing tumors (1.7 and 2.7 mmol/hr/kg.[75] HCl) was maximal in the unstimulated state.[21] In this situation hypochloremia, hypokalemia, metabolic alkalosis, and dehydration is likely due to the hypersecretion of gastric acid and its loss in vomitus.[21] Venous blood gases and *plasma osmolality* are often determined in animals suspected of ethylene glycol ingestion, with the findings of metabolic acidosis and a high osmolal gap (calculated by subtracting calculated from measured osmolality) supportive of ingestion.

Elevated BUN in the absence of elevated creatinine may indicate gastric bleeding. Low albumin may be detected in basenji or Lundehund dogs with protein-losing gastroenteropathy, dogs with *Pythiosis*, and dogs or cats with gastric neoplasia. Elevated globulin concentrations have been observed in basenji gastroenteropathy, *Pythium* infection, and gastric plasmacytoma. Elevations in creatinine, urea, calcium, potassium, glucose, liver enzymes, bilirubin, cholesterol, triglycerides, and globulin and decreases in sodium, calcium, urea, or albumin frequently herald non-GI causes of vomiting.

Urine should be evaluated for specific gravity, pH, glucose, casts, crystals, and bacteria. Thorough urinalysis is important; for example, white cell casts in the urine may be the only evidence that pyelonephritis is the cause of vomiting and should not be overlooked.

Coagulation testing is indicated in patients with melena or hematemesis to detect underlying coagulopathies and in those

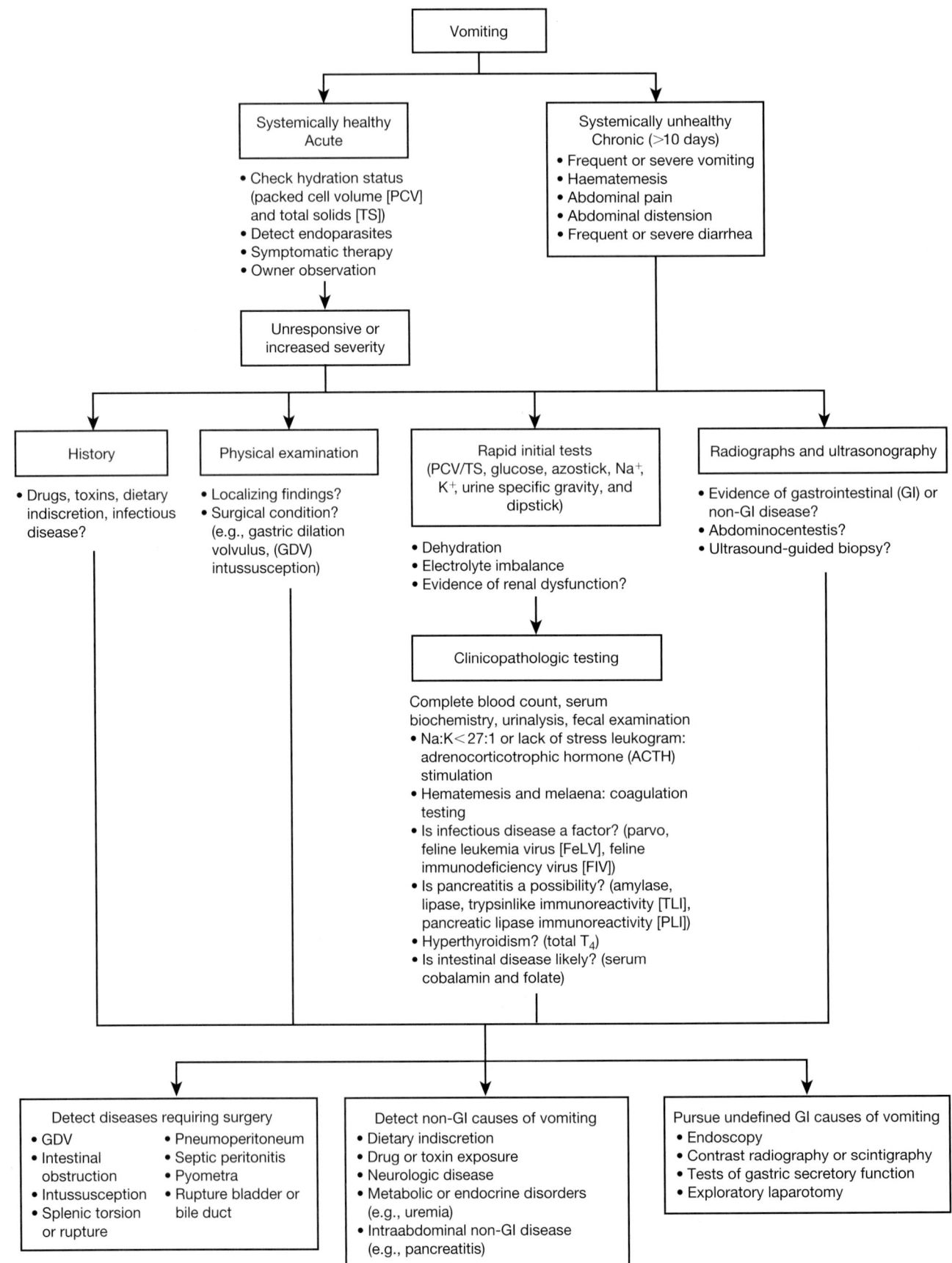

Figure 221-4 Diagnostic approach to the vomiting patient.

with acute abdomen to detect DIC. Infectious diseases associated with vomiting and diarrhea require *fecal examination* (giardia, endoparasites, *Salmonella* spp., *Campylobacter* spp., and parvovirus [ELISA] or *serologic testing* [FeIV, FIV]) for diagnosis.

Additional clinicopathologic tests are required to detect hypoadrenocorticism (ACTH stimulation), liver dysfunction (pre- and post-prandial bile acids), hyperthyroidism in cats (T_4), pancreatitis (amylase, lipase [pancreas-specific where possible], and trypsin-like immunoreactivity), and intestinal disease (serum cobalamin and folate).

IMAGING

Abdominal radiography is the test of choice for the initial evaluation of gastric disease, vomiting, and abdominal pain. Survey radiographs provide information on gastric position and contents that help to diagnose gastric distension/GDV, foreign bodies, and gastric outflow obstruction. They also enable the evaluation of the size and shape of the liver, kidneys, and spleen and detection of intussusception, peritonitis, pneumoperitoneum, and changes suggestive of pancreatitis.

Contrast radiographs may provide further information when survey radiographs are inconclusive. However, the combination of ultrasonography and endoscopy is generally more effective for detecting obstructive, inflammatory, and neoplastic GI disorders than contrast radiographic procedures, and contrast radiography is often restricted to the investigation of delayed gastric emptying associated with defective propulsion or "functional" intestinal disorders.[22] Ultrasonography can be employed to evaluate gastric wall thickness and gastric emptying, but its major value is usually the detection of non-gastric lesions in those with signs of GI disease.

When ultrasound and endoscopy are not available, distension of the stomach with air (negative contrast) may reveal gastric thickening, masses, or foreign bodies. Positive contrast with barium sulfate can provide further information and is also used to evaluate patency of the gastric outflow tract. The combination of fluoroscopy and positive contrast is helpful for evaluating pyloric patency and gastric emptying. In the absence of endoscopy and ultrasonography contrast radiographic procedures can be followed up with surgical biopsy to achieve a definitive diagnosis.

Endoscopy

Endoscopy enables direct visualization and biopsy of the stomach and duodenum and is the best way of diagnosing primary gastric inflammation, ulceration, or neoplasia; removing small foreign bodies; and evaluating patients prior to quantification of gastric emptying. It does not provide good information on submucosal lesions or functional diseases. With mural thickening or gastric masses, endoscopic biopsies are frequently too superficial and surgical biopsy is required for accurate diagnosis. Further information on equipment and techniques and photographs of a wide range of gastrointestinal lesions and can be found in endoscopic atlases.[23,24]

Evaluation of Gastric Emptying

Procedures used to evaluate delayed gastric emptying include barium contrast (liquid or mixed with food), barium-impregnated polyspheres (BIPs), nuclear scintigraphy, and the ^{13}C-octanoate breath test.[25,26] Tests of gastric emptying are often used to confirm a suspicion of delayed gastric emptying in patients with normal or equivocal survey radiographs. They are also used where gastric outflow obstruction and obvious causes of defective propulsion have been ruled out prior to and after prokinetic drugs. The limitations and benefits of these approaches are discussed under Delayed Gastric Emptying and Motility Disorders.

Gastric Secretory Testing

Gastric secretory testing is primarily performed in patients with esophagitis, gastrointestinal ulceration, mucosal hypertrophy, or copious amounts of gastric fluid that are suspected of having acid hypersecretion.

In its simplest form, fasting gastric pH and serum gastrin are measured to determine if acid hypersecretion is likely. Antisecretory therapy should be discontinued for 48 hours prior to testing, and renal and hepatic dysfunction detected, as these increase circulating gastrin. The broad range of fasting, unstimulated gastric pH in dogs and cats (pH 1 to 8) makes definitive statements regarding acid production difficult. However, the presence of a gastric pH of less than 3 in the face of a high serum gastrin rules out the possibility of achlorhydria, or mast cell tumor, and raises the possibility of gastrinoma.[21] Dogs with mast cell tumors and hyperhistaminemia induced acid hypersecretion have low serum gastrin concentrations[27], whereas dogs with achlorhydria likely have a high gastrin, but a gastric pH greater than 3.

Measurement of serum gastrin following the intravenous infusion of secretin or calcium is used to further investigate the possibility of exogenous gastrin production by pancreatic tumors, gastrinomas (Zollinger-Ellison syndrome) (see Chapter 244). Basenji dogs with gastroenteropathy and diarrhea have been reported to have elevated gastrin release in response to secretin stimulation, without evidence of gastrinoma.[28] Provocative testing of gastric acid secretion with pentagastrin or bombesin stimulation may be performed to detect achlorhydria in patients with atrophic gastritis, or elevated serum gastrin and gastric pH levels higher than 3, and in those with idiopathic small intestinal bacterial overgrowth to determine if achlorhydria is a contributing factor. Pentagastrin stimulated acid secretion in dogs reaches a peak of 28 mL/kg$^{.75}$/hr, 4.1 mmol HCl/kg$^{.75}$/hr, 0.34 mmol K$^+$/kg$^{0.75}$/hr and 0.09 Na$^+$ mmol/kg$^{0.75}$/hr.[6] Sedation with oxymorphone and acepromazine is an alternative to anaesthesia for secretion studies in dogs.[28] In cats, acid output (mean ± SD) in response to pentagastrin (8 µg/kg/hr) ranges from pH 0.9 to 1.1, with secretion rates (median values) of 1.2 mmol/15 min to 1.4 ± .5 mmol/15 min in conscious cats and 1.2 (0.6 to 2.7) mmol/kg$^{.75}$/hr in anesthetized cats.[29]

ACUTE GASTRITIS

Acute gastritis is the term applied to the syndrome of vomiting of sudden onset presumed to be due to a gastric mucosal insult or inflammation (Box 221-1). In most patients the cause is inferred from the history, such as dietary indiscretion, the diagnosis is rarely confirmed by biopsy, and treatment is symptomatic and supportive. Animals with acute gastritis

Box • 221-1
Causes of Acute Gastritis
Dietary indiscretion or intolerance (non-allergic and allergic)
Foreign bodies, e.g., bones, toys, hairballs
Drugs and toxins, e.g., NSAIDs, corticosteroids, heavy metals, antibiotics, plants, cleaners, bleach
Systemic disease, e.g., uremia, liver disease, hypoadrenocorticism
Parasitic, e.g., *Ollulanus*, *Physalloptera* spp.
Bacterial, e.g., bacterial toxins,?*Helicobacter*
Possibly viral

GASTROINTESTINAL DISEASE

associated with drug toxicity, foreign body ingestion, or metabolic disorders frequently present with hematemesis, melena, concurrent diarrhea, or other signs of systemic illness and require a more thorough diagnostic approach to determine the cause (as discussed above) and to provide optimal care. This author has found little evidence in the literature to support the role of viral infections such as parvovirus, distemper, or infectious canine hepatitis in acute gastritis.

Clinical Findings
Vomiting of sudden onset is the principal clinical sign. In some instances it is accompanied by hematemesis or melena and a variable degree of systemic abnormality. The history may reveal access or ingestion of spoiled food, garbage, toxins, medications, or foreign bodies. Signs of toxicity may be evident, such as jaundice and pallor with zinc ingestion, salivation or defecation with organophosphates toxicity or mushroom ingestion, or salivation and oral ulceration with chemical ingestion.

Diagnosis
A diagnosis of acute gastritis is usually based on clinical findings and the response to symptomatic treatment. A specific diagnosis may be sought if the patient has access to foreign objects or toxins, is systemically unwell, or has hematemesis, melena, or vomiting that fails to respond to symptomatic therapy, or other signs of more serious disease (see above). Laboratory testing in most animals with primary acute gastritis reflects mild dehydration, and is often not performed in the absence of a suspicion of more serious disease. Abdominal radiographs can be taken to detect foreign objects or gastrointestinal obstruction. Further diagnostics such as ultrasonography and endoscopy are rarely indicated as most animals with simple gastritis respond to symptomatic therapy.

Treatment
Therapy for uncomplicated acute gastritis is symptomatic and supportive and includes fluids, dietary restriction and modification, mucosal protectants or adsorbents, and possibly antacids.

Fluid Therapy
Small amounts of oral fluids, given little and often, can be given in the face of vomiting, with the volume increasing as vomiting subsides. Subcutaneous administration of an isotonic balanced electrolyte solution may be sufficient to correct mild fluid deficits (<5%) but is insufficient for patients with moderate to severe dehydration. Patients requiring intravenous fluids should undergo a more extensive diagnostic evaluation.

Dietary Restriction and Modification
Where vomiting is acute, oral intake is discontinued for at least 24 hours. Small amounts of a liquid diet can be offered in the face of vomiting to maintain GI barrier function and to determine if vomiting has resolved. A bland diet (non-spicy, fat restricted), either homemade (e.g., boiled chicken and rice, low-fat cottage cheese, and rice [1:3]) or commercial (usually fat restricted and rice based), is then introduced (fed little and often) with a gradual transition made back to a normal diet over a week or so.

Protectants/Adsorbents
Bismuth-subsalicylate, kaolin-pectin, activated charcoal and magnesium, aluminum- and barium-containing products are often administered in acute vomiting or diarrhea to bind bacteria and their toxins and to coat the gastrointestinal mucosa. These agents are probably safer and more efficacious than antibiotics or motility modifiers in acute gastroenteritis. Pepto bismol (1 mL/5 kg PO TID), bismuth subcitrate, kaolin-pectin (1 to 2 mL/kg PO TID) and sucralfate (0.25 to 1 g PO TID) are often employed. Acid-reducing drugs such as H_2-receptor antagonists can be administered but are usually reserved for patients with

Table • 221-2
Association of Gastric Ulceration and Erosion with Specific Diseases

GASTRIC PROBLEM	RELATED DISEASES
Metabolic/Endocrine	Hypoadrenocorticism, uremia, liver disease, mastocytosis, d.i.c.
	Hypergastrinemia and other APUDomas
Inflammatory	Gastritis
Neoplastic	Leiomyoma, adenocarcinoma, lymphosarcoma
Drug-induced	Nonsteroidal and steroidal anti-inflammatories
Hypotension	Shock, sepsis
Idiopathic	Stress, spinal surgery, exercise induced (sled dogs)

signs of gastric erosion or ulceration (melena/hematemesis) or persistent gastritis as described below.

The author generally avoids anti-emetics in patients with acute gastritis to enable response to therapy to be ascertained. Patients who continue to vomit require further investigation.

Prognosis
The prognosis for uncomplicated acute gastritis is usually complete recovery.

GASTRIC EROSION AND ULCERATION

Gastric erosions and ulcers are associated with a number of primary gastric and non-gastric disorders (Table 221-2). Clinical signs range in duration and severity, from acute to chronic and mild to life threatening. The pathomechanisms underlying gastric damage can be broadly attributed to impairment of the gastric mucosal barrier (defined above) through direct injury, interference with gastroprotective prostaglandins (PGE_2), mucous or bicarbonate, decreased blood flow, and hypersecretion or gastric acid.

Perhaps the most predictable recipe for gastric erosion is the combination of a non-steroidal anti-inflammatory and a glucocorticoid, either alone, or in combination with intervertebral disk disease.[30]

Nonsteroidal anti-inflammatory drugs cause direct mucosal damage and interfere with prostaglandin synthesis.[9] Flunixin meglumine, aspirin, and ibuprofen have all been associated with erosions in healthy dogs. To circumvent toxicity caused by the inhibition of "friendly prostaglandins" (PGE_2), drugs that preferentially block "inducible" cyclooxygenase (COX-2) have been developed. These COX-2 selective agents, such as carprofen, meloxicam, derccoxib, and potentially etodolac, are less ulcerogenic in normal dogs.[31,32] However, even COX-2 selective drugs such as meloxicam are ulcerogenic in combination with dexamethasone,[33] and their safety in sick animals remains to be determined.

High doses of glucocorticoids alone, such as dexamethasone and methylprednisolone, have also been associated with gastric erosions[34] but the mechanisms by which they induce damage are not clear. Unlike NSAIDs, their effects are not ameliorated by PGE_2 analogs.[35]

Hypersecretion of gastric acid in response to histamine release from mast cell tumors, and gastrin from gastrinomas has also been clearly implicated as a cause of gastroduodenal ulceration and esophagitis in dogs and cats.

Renal failure, hepatic failure, hypoadrenocorticism, and hypotension are frequently proposed as risk factors for gastric erosion or ulceration, although few details have been published on the pathogenesis, frequency, or severity of gastric damage in these conditions. In a recent study of dogs with renal failure, ulceration was present in only 1 of 28 dogs. The predominant findings in these dogs were mucosal edema, vasculopathy, and mineralization that correlated to the degree of azotemia and calcium phosphorous product.[36]

Sled dogs in the Iditarod are prone to develop gastric erosions and/or ulcers.[37] This finding is similar to exercising humans and horses in whom the pathogensis is not understood but is responsive to acid suppression.

Erosions and ulcers are also a sequela of gastric cancer and gastritis and are discussed elsewhere in this chapter.

Clinical Findings
Vomiting, hematemesis, and melena may be present in patients with gastric erosions or ulcers. Pale mucous membranes, abdominal pain, weakness, inappetance, hypersalivation (potentially associated with esophagitis as a consequence of gastric acid hypersecretion), and evidence of circulatory compromise are more variably present. Access to toxins and drugs, particularly NSAIDs, should be determined.

Clinicopathologic testing is directed at identifying diseases associated with gastric erosions and ulcers (see Table 221-2) and the consequences of erosion/ulceration. The CBC may reveal anemia that is initially regenerative but can progress to become microcytic, hypochromic, and minimally regenerative. When accompanied by thrombocytosis and decreased iron saturation or low serum ferritin, these findings are characteristic of chronic bleeding and iron deficiency. Lack of a stress leukogram and eosiniphilia in dogs is supportive of hypoadrenocorticism. Eosinophilia could also be consistent with dietary allergy, eosinophilic gastroenteritis, mastocytosis, or a hyperseosinophilic syndrome. A neutrophilic leukocytosis and a left shift may indicate inflammation or possible gastric perforation. Examination of a buffy coat smear may help to detect mastocytosis.

Biochemistry and urinalysis may reveal findings consistent with dehydration (azotemia and hypersthenuria), renal failure (e.g., azotemia and isosthenuria), hepatic disease (e.g., increased liver enzymes or bilirubin; decreased cholesterol, albumin, BUN), or hypoadrenocorticism (i.e., $Na^+:K^+$ ratio <27:1). It will also identify electrolyte and acid base abnormalities associated with vomiting and GI ulceration. The presence of a metabolic alkalosis, hypochloremia, hypokalemia, and acid urine is consistent with upper GI obstruction (physical or functional) or a hypersecretory state. Testing should be performed to detect abnormalities in primary and secondary hemostasis that may be associated with GI bleeding. Serum gastrin and potentially histamine concentrations can be evaluated where acid hypersecretion is suspected as a cause of ulceration.

Diagnosis
Diagnostic imaging
Plain radiographs are not usually helpful in diagnosing gastric erosions or ulcers but may help to rule out other causes of vomiting, such as foreign bodies, peritonitis, and gastric perforation. Contrast radiographs may reveal filling defects but do not allow detailed mucosal evaluation or sampling.

Ultrasonography can be performed to evaluate the gastric wall for thickening associated with ulcers and masses and also helps to rule out non-gastric causes of vomiting. The information provided by radiography and ultrasound is complementary to endoscopic evaluation, which is the diagnostic test of choice (Figure 221-6).

Endoscopy allows the direct evaluation of gastric damage and mucosal sampling. NSAID-associated ulcers tend to be found in the antrum and are not usually associated with marked mucosal thickening or irregular edges (Figure 221-5). This contrasts with ulcerated tumors that frequently have thickened edges and surrounding mucosa (Figure 221-17, A). Ulcers should be biopsied at the periphery to avoid perforation. Endoscopic biopsies are not ideal for diagnosing infiltrative gastric tumors and several biopsies from the same site are usually taken to enable sampling of deeper tissue. Endoscopic guided fine-needle aspirates, with use of a needle and tubing in the biopsy channel, can also be used to sample deep lesions. Even with this approach the diagnosis may be missed, and surgical biopsy required for a definitive diagnosis.

The combination of mucosal erosion or ulceration, antral mucosal hypertrophy, copious gastric juice, and esophagitis is highly suggestive of a gastric hypersecretory state (Figure 221-7). It is prudent to measure gastric pH and serum gastrin in patients with gastric erosion/ulceration that is not associated with drugs or gastric tumors. Dogs with mast cell tumors and hyperhistaminemia-induced acid hypersecretion have low serum gastrin concentrations.[38] Finding a

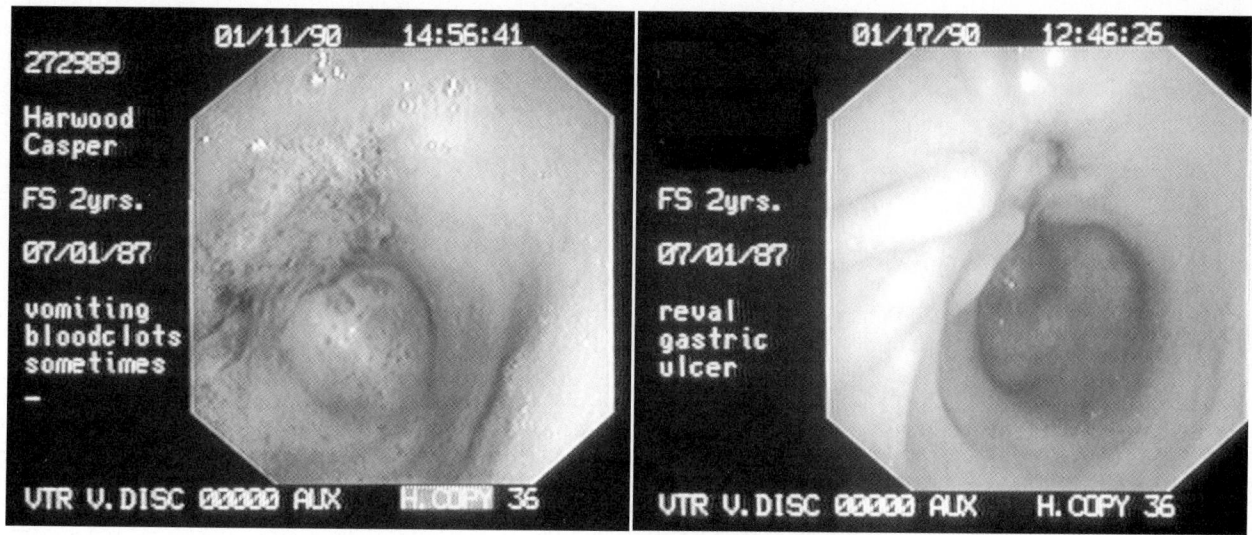

A   B

Figure 221-5 Gastric ulceration caused by ibuprofen ingestion before and after (1 week) treatment with cimetidine and sucralfate. (Images courtesy of The Ohio State University.)

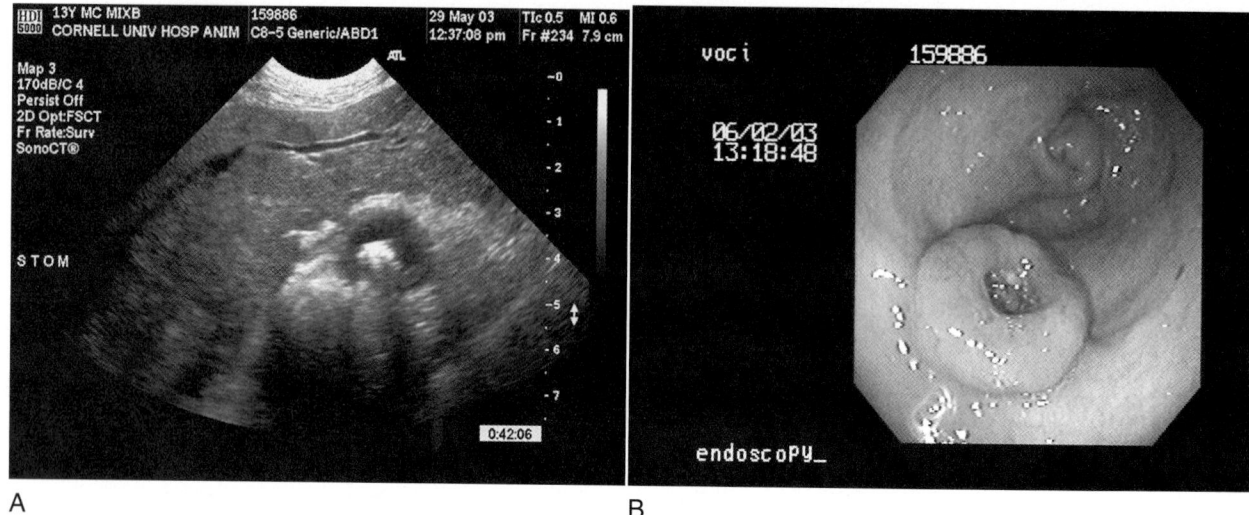

Figure 221-6 **A**, A mass projecting into the lumen of the stomach of a dog presented for vomiting and hyperglobulinemia (IgA). **B**, Presence of the mass is confirmed, enabling a biopsy diagnosis of gastric plasmacytoma.

combination of gastric pH less than 3 and a high serum gastrin concentration prompts further investigation of gastrinoma by secretin stimulation test, ultrasonography (liver and pancreas), and pentertreotide scintigraphy.[21]

Treatment

Treatment of gastric erosions and ulcers is directed at the underlying cause, which ensures adequate hydration and perfusion, including blood transfusion if needed, and restoring electrolyte and acid base disturbances. Additional support is directed at shoring up the gastric mucosal barrier by enhancing mucosal protection and cytoprotection, and decreasing gastric acid secretion. Where vomiting is persistent, antiemetics may help to reduce fluid loss, discomfort, and the risk of esophagitis.

Fluid Therapy

The rate of fluid administration depends on the presence or absence of shock, the degree of dehydration, and the presence of diseases (e.g., cardiac or renal), which predispose to volume overload. Patients with a history of vomiting who are mildly dehydrated are usually responsive to crystalloids (e.g., LRS or

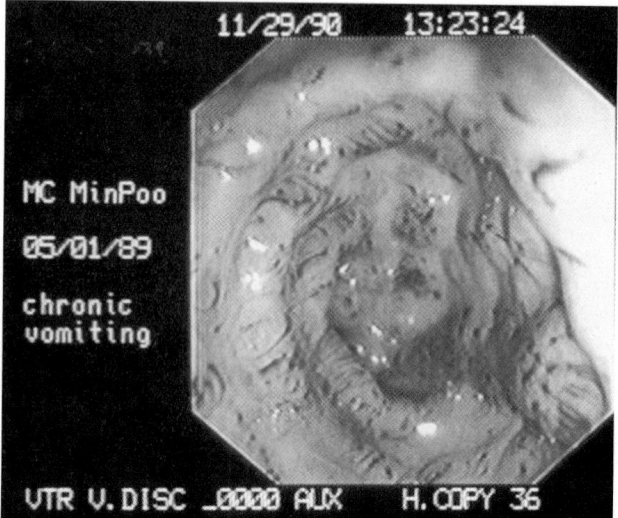

Figure 221-7 Gastric erosion and mucosal hypertophy in a dog with gastrinoma. (Courtesy of The Ohio State University.)

0.9% NaCl) at a rate that will provide maintenance and replace both deficits and ongoing losses over a 24-hour period. Potassium depletion is often a consequence of prolonged vomiting or anorexia, and most polyionic replacement fluids contain only small amounts of potassium. Therefore KCl is added to parenteral fluids on the basis of serum levels.

Patients with signs of shock require more aggressive support. The volume deficit can be replaced with crystalloids at an initial rate of 60 to 90 mL/kg/h, then tailored to maintain tissue perfusion and hydration. Colloid solutions can also be used to treat animals in shock to reduce the amount of crystalloid required (e.g., Hetastarch, hemaccel at 10 to 20 mL/kg IV over 4 to 6 hours). Plasma, colloids, packed cells, or whole blood is occasionally required to treat severe hypoproteinemia or anemia, which can develop in vomiting animals with severe ulceration or HGE.

Central venous pressure monitoring and evaluation of urine output are necessary in patients with severe GI disease, particularly those complicated by third space losses of fluid into the gut or petitoneum.

The effect of vomiting on acid-base balance is hard to predict and therapeutic intervention to correct acid-base imbalances should be based on blood gas determination. Where severe metabolic acidosis is present (pH <7.1, HCO^{3-} <10 mmol/L), sodium bicarbonate (1 mmol/kg) can be given under careful supervision for the development of worsening hypokalemia, and hypocalcemia, and CSF acidosis. Further bicarbonate supplementation is based on repeated blood gas analysis. Metabolic alkalosis usually responds to replacing volume deficit, chloride, and potassium with IV 0.9% NaCl+KCl. Diagnostic investigations should initially center on ruling out upper GI obstruction. The administration of anti-secretory drugs such as H_2 antagonists may help to limit Cl--efflux into gastric juice.

Reducing Acid Secretion and Providing Mucosal Protection

Pharmacologic inhibition of acid secretion (see Figure 221-3) can be effected by blocking H_2 (cimetidine, ranitidine, famotidine), gastrin (proglumide), and acetylcholine (atropine, pirenzipine) receptors, and by inhibiting adenyl cyclase (PGE analogs) and H^+/K^+ ATPase (e.g., omeprazole).[39] Long-acting somatostatin analogs such as octreotide directly decrease the secretion of gastrin and gastric acid.

Decreasing gastric acid secretion with an H_2 receptor antagonist has been shown to promote mucosal healing in dogs with a variety of experimentally induced ulcers and erosions (see

Figure 221-5). Famotidine is an attractive choice as it does not inhibit P450 enzymes and can be given once daily. The additional prokinetic activity of ranitidine or nizatidine (mediated by anticholinesterase activity) may make them good choices in the face of delayed gastric emptying associated with defective propulsion.[25] In patients with severe or persistent gastric ulceration that is refractory to H_2 antagonists, more complete inhibition of gastric acid secretion can be achieved with a H^+/K^+-ATPase inhibitor such as omeprazole (0.2 to 0.7 mg/kg SID PO—dogs). Omeprazole is the initial drug of choice in patients with acid hypersecretion secondary to mast cell tumors and gastrinoma (Zollinger-Ellison syndrome). Omeprazole has been shown to have few long-term side effects in dogs, but it should be used with caution in patients with liver disease and reviewed for interactions with drugs such as cisapride.

In sled dogs with exercise-associated gastric hemorrhage treatment with omeprazole significantly reduced mean gastric severity score compared to placebo but also was associated with increased frequency of diarrhea (omeprazole 54%, placebo 21%).[37] The authors recommended further investigation of diarrhea associated with omeprazole treatment before omeprazole can be recommended for routine prophylactic treatment in these athletes.[37]

The combination of omeprazole and the long acting somatostatin analog Octreotide effectively reduced vomiting in a dog with gastrinoma (Octreotide 2 to 20 µg/kg SC TID).[40] Octreotide can also be employed to rapidly decrease gastric acid secretion in patients discovered to have large ulcers at endoscopy and may also be useful for controlling gastric bleeding (see human studies).

Mucosal Protectants

The PGE_2 analog, misoprostol, protects against NSAID-induced erosions in dogs at doses that do not inhibit acid secretion (3 to 5 µg/kg PO TID in dogs) and may be given to dogs receiving chronic NSAIDs for arthritis.[41,42] The main side effect of misoprostol is diarrhea and it should not be given to pregnant animals.

The mucosal protectant polyaluminum sucrose sulfate (sucralfate) binds to areas denuded of mucosal epithelium regardless of the underlying cause and is useful for treating gastric erosions and ulcers and esophagitis. Sucralfate can be given to patients receiving injectable antacids, but it may compromise absorption of other oral medications and is probably best separated from these by 2 hours or so.

In contrast to the efficacy of misoprostol and H_2 antagonists in preventing NSAID-induced erosions, the prophylactic administration of various combinations of misoprostol, cimetidine, and omeprazole has not been shown to prevent gastric erosions in dogs with or without intervertebral disk disease receiving high-dose glucocorticoids.[34,43,44] However, these drugs may speed healing of gastric lesions in these patients. Sucralfate is probably the drug of choice for treating GI ulceration in patients receiving high doses of corticosteroids because it is not dependent on the premise that acid is causing or delaying healing.

Mast cell tumors are also worth considering separately as gastric ulceration is a frequent and severe complication. Mast cell tumors are thought to cause vomiting via the central effects of histamine on the CRTZ and the peripheral effects of histamine on gastric acid secretion (with resultant hyperacidity and ulceration). Treatment of mastocyosis with H_1 and H_2 histamine antagonists (e.g., diphenhydramine and famotidine) should reduce the central and peripheral effects of histamine. Corticosteroids are used to decrease tumor burden. Where acid hypersecretion is present, or is suspected, it is likely best managed with proton pump inhibitors (e.g., omeprazole 0.2 to 0.7 mg/kg SID). Somatostatin analogs may also be useful for controlling refractory gastric acid hypersecretion (Octreotide 2 to 20 µg/kg SC TID).[21]

Antiemetics

Antiemetics can be used where vomiting is severe or compromising fluid and electrolyte balance, or causing discomfort.[39] The initial agent used in dogs is usually metoclopramide, which antagonizes D_2-dopaminergic and $5HT_3$-serotonergic receptors and has cholinergic effects on smooth muscle (1 mg/kg/24h CRI IV). Phenothiazine derivatives such as chlorpromazine and prochlorperazine are antagons of α_1 and α_2-adrenergic, H_1- and H_2-histaminergic, and D_2-dopaminergic receptors in the vomiting center and CRTZ and are used if metoclopramide is ineffective and the patient is normotensive. Nonselective cholinergic receptor antagonists (other than the M_1 specific antagonist- pirenzipine) such as atropine, scopolamine, aminopentamide, and isopropamide are generally avoided as they may cause ileus, delayed gastric emptying, and dry mouth.

Antibiotics and Analgesia

Prophylactic antibiotic cover (e.g., cephalosporins, ampicillin) may be warranted in animals with shock and major GI barrier dysfunction. Leukopenia, neutrophilia, fever, and bloody stools are additional indications for prophylactic antibiotics in animals with vomiting or diarrhea. Initial choices in these situations include ampicillin or a cephalosporin (effective against gram-positive and some gram-negative and anaerobic bacteria), which can be combined with an aminoglycoside (effective against gram-negative aerobes) when sepsis is present and hydration status is adequate. Enrofloxacin is a suitable alternative to an aminoglycoside in skeletally mature patients at risk of nephrotoxicity from an aminoglycoside.

Analgesia can be provided using opioids like buprenorphine (0.0075 to 0.01 mg/kg IM).

Surgery may be required when the cause of ulceration is unclear or to resect large non-healing ulcers or those about to perforate.

GASTRIC DILATATION AND VOLVULUS

Gastric dilatation and gastric dilatation and volvulus are characterized by the dramatic distension of the stomach with air. With volvulus the stomach twists about its axis, moving dorsally and left of the fundus. Both dilatation and dilatation and volvulus cause caudal caval obstruction and impair venous return to the heart. This results in hypovolemic shock that can be exacerbated by devitailization of the gastric wall, splenic torsion or avulsion, congestion of the abdominal viscera, endotoxic shock, and DIC.

No single cause of gastric dilatation (GD) or dilatation and volvulus (GDV) has been identified. Large breed dogs with deep chests such as akita, bloodhound, collie, great Dane, Irish setter, Irish wolfhound, Newfoundland, Rottweiler, Saint Bernard, standard poodle, and Weimaraner are at greater risk. Cumulative incidence of GDV has been estimated at 6% for large breed and giant breed dogs. The lifetime risk is influenced by breed, ranging from of 3.9% for Rottweilers to 39% in great Danes.[45] In large breed and giant dogs, factors significantly associated with an increased risk of GDV include increasing age, having a first-degree relative with a history of GDV, having a faster speed of eating, once daily feeding, and having a raised feeding bowl and aerophagia.[46,47] The personality of the dogs may also have an impact, with happier dogs having a decreased incidence.[48]

Analysis of gastric gas supports aerophagia as the cause of distension, with dilatation explained by an inability to eructate or empty air into the intestines. Studies in dogs with GDV recovering from gastropexy suggest that abnormal electrical activity and gastric emptying may be related to the development of gastric dilatation.[49] The interrelationship of volvulus and gastric distension is unclear, although the length of the hepatogastric ligament may facilitate torsion.

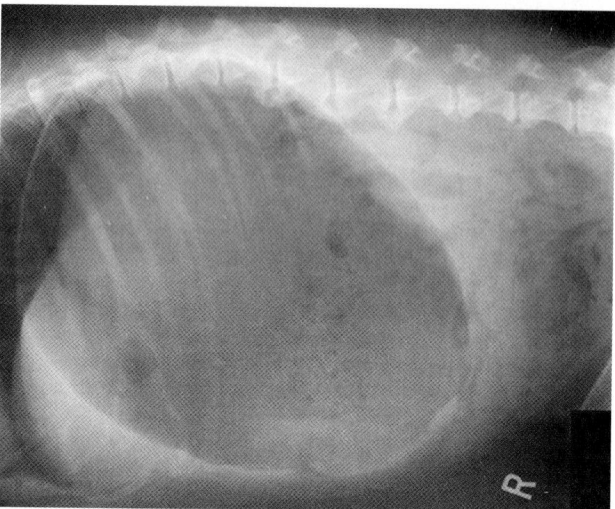

Figure 221-8 Survey radiograph of gastric dilatation (R lateral). The fundus is distended with air.

Diagnostic Features

A history of non-productive retching, salivation, abdominal distention, weakness, or collapse raises the possibility of gastric dilatation or volvulus, particularly in large breed and deep-chested dogs. Physical findings usually include abdominal distension and tympany, tachycardia, and mucosal pallor. Hypothermia, depression, and coma may be seen when shock is severe. Cardiac arrythmias such as ventricular premature beats or ventricular tachycardia may be detected on the initial examination or develop up to 72 hours after presentation.

Radiography is usually performed after fluid support and decompression and helps to distinguish simple dilatation from dilatation and volvulus. Right and left lateral recumbent views are usually acquired. Dilatation is associated with gas distension and on a right lateral position air is present in the fundus (Figure 221-8). With volvulus the pylorus moves dorally and left and the stomach is compartmentalized. On a right lateral radiograph the fundus is viewed as a large ventral compartment with the smaller, gas-filled pylorus located dorsally and separated from the fundus by a band of soft tissue, forming the "the Popeye's arm" sign (Figure 221-9). Loss of abdominal contrast may indicate gastric rupture or bleeding from avulsed splenic vessels, whereas increased contrast due to pneumo-peritoneum suggests gastric rupture.

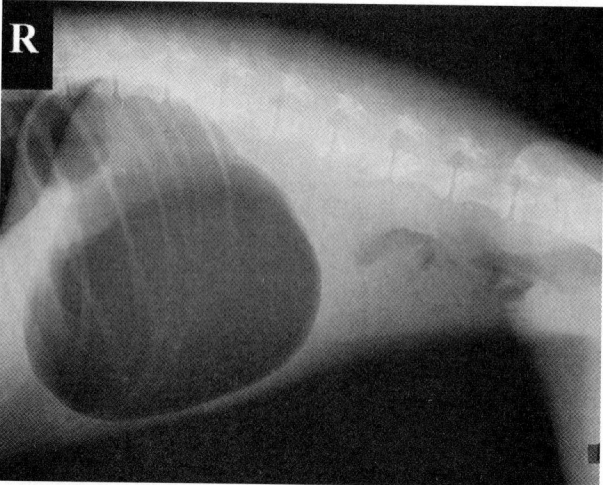

Figure 221-9 Gastric dilatation and volvulus. Right lateral radiograph showing gastric compartmentalization, with the pylorus (dorsal) separated from the fundus by a soft tissue density.

Clinicopathologic Findings

Hematologic changes are often restricted to an increase in hematocrit. A variety of acid-base and electrolyte disturbances have been observed in dogs with GDV.[50,51] Metabolic acidosis and hypokalemia were the most common abnormalities in one study and occurred in 15 out of 57 and 16 out of 57 dogs, respectively.[50] Metabolic acidosis is likely due to tissue hypo-perfusion, anaerobic metabolism, and the accumulation of lactic acid.[50] Metabolic alkalosis may also occur and may be related to the sequestration of gastric acid or vomiting.[50]

Respiratory acidosis and alkalosis have been variably observed and reflect hypoventilation or hyperventilation, respectively. The variable nature of acid-base and electrolyte abnormalities in dogs with GDV indicates that fluid therapy should be individualized on the basis of blood gas and electrolyte measurements. Monitoring and correction of acid-base abnormalities are important because they may predispose to cardiac arrythmias and muscle weakness.

Coagulation abnormalities are usually consistent with disseminated intravascular coagulopathy (thrombocytopenia, increased D-dimer or FDPs, reduced ATIII, prolongation of the APTT).

Treatment

Fluid support and gastric decompression are the most important emergency treatments.

Fluid Support

Fluid therapy has traditionally consisted of shock doses of LRS (60 to 90 mL/kg/h) given via large-bore catheters into the cephalic or jugular veins. Experimental studies that have compared crystalloids (60 mL/kg, followed by 0.9% NaCl 20 mL/kg/h) with hypertonic saline (7% NaCl in 6% dextran, 5 mL/kg, followed by 0.9% NaCl 20 mL/kg/h) in dogs with GDV-induced shock, indicate that hypertonic saline maintains better myocardial performance, higher heart rate, and lower systemic vascular resistance than crystalloid.[52] The resuscitative dose of hypertonic saline was delivered in 5 to 10 minutes versus an hour for cystalloid. Fluid therapy should be aggressively monitored by frequent measurement of blood pressure, heart rate, PCV, and total solids and urine output. Potassium and bicarbonate are best administered on the basis of blood gas and electrolyte measurements. Hypokalemia is common after fluid therapy and 30 to 40 mEq KC l/L should be added to fluids after the initial shock dose.

Gastric Decompression

Decompression can be performed by oragastric intubation with a well-lubricated stomach tube, or a 16-g catheter can be used to trocarize the stomach. Oral decompression can also be performed after trocarization. Decompression should be maintained until surgery. Sedation with butorphanol (0.5 mg/kg IV) or oxymorphone (0.1 mg/kg IV) and diazepam (0.1 mg/kg slow IV) may be necessary to pass a stomach tube.

Adjunct Therapy for Endotoxic Shock and Reperfusion Injury

Adjunct therapy frequently includes prednisolone sodium succinate (10 mg/kg IV) or dexamethasone sodium phosphate (10 mg/kg IV) for shock, and broad-spectrum antibiotics such a cephalosporin in combination with a fluroquinolone to circumvent bacterial translocation and endotoxemia. Some clinicians advocate flunixin meglumine for endotoxic shock, but the author does not.

The administration of agents to decrease lipid peroxidation (U70046F) and chelate iron (desferoxamine) has decreased mortality attributed to reperfusion injury in dogs with experimental GDV.[53,54] These agents are best given before reperfusion occurs, that is, prior to untwisting a torsion.

Cardiac Arrythmias

Cardiac arrhythmias such as ventricular premature complexes and ventricular tachycardia are relatively frequent (approximately 40% of patients) and may or may not contribute to mortality.[55,56] The arrhythmias can develop up to 72 hours after presentation and are considered a consequence of electrolyte, acid base, and hemostatic abnormalities, as well as due to reperfusion injury. Arrhythmias should be treated if they are associated with weakness or syncope, as well as if persistent ventricular tachycardia at rates greater than 150 beats per minute are demonstrated. The arrhythmias are managed by correcting underlying acid-base electrolyte and hemostatic disturbances and administering lidocaine either as a bolus (1 to 2 mg/kg IV) or continuously (up to 50 to 75 μg/kg/min) and procainamide (10 mg/kg IM q6h and then orally if effective) where persistent. It is important that plasma concentration of K^+ and Mg^{2+} are normalized to enable effective antiarrythmic therapy (see Chapter 202).

Surgery

The aims of surgery are to reposition the stomach and spleen and to perform a gastropexy to enable short-term decompression and prevent recurrence. Surgery is complicated by the presence of gastric necrosis, which requires partial gastrectomy, and avulsion or torsion of the spleen, which may require resection or removal.

Prognosis

Mortality rate for dogs with gastric dilatation and volvulus is approximately 15%.[56] Dogs with gastric necrosis, gastric resection or splenectomy have a higher mortality rate (>30%).[55-57]

The presence of gastric necrosis can be predicted by measuring plasma lactate concentration, with [lactate] greater than 6 mmol/L yielding a specificity of 88% and a sensitivity of 66% for necrosis.[57]

Prophylaxis

The recurrence rate of GD/GDV has been estimated at 11% over 3 years in one study, with median survival of 547 versus 188 days for dogs with a gastropexy versus those without.[58]

Prophylactic gastropexy in Great Danes, Irish Setters, Rottweilers, standard poodles, and Weimariners reduced mortality from as little as 2.2-fold in Rottweilers to as much as 29.6-fold in great Danes.[45]

CHRONIC GASTRITIS

Gastritis is a common finding in dogs, with 35% of dogs investigated for chronic vomiting and 26% to 48% of asymptomatic dogs affected.[59,60] The prevalence in cats has not been determined. The diagnosis of chronic gastritis is based on the histologic examination of gastric biopsies and it is usually subclassified according to histopathological changes and etiology.

Histopathologic Features of Gastritis

Gastritis in dogs and cats is usually classified according to the nature of the predominant cellular infiltrate (eosinophilic, lymphocytic, plasmacytic, granulomatous, lymphoid follicular), the presence of architectural abnormalities (atrophy, hypertrophy,

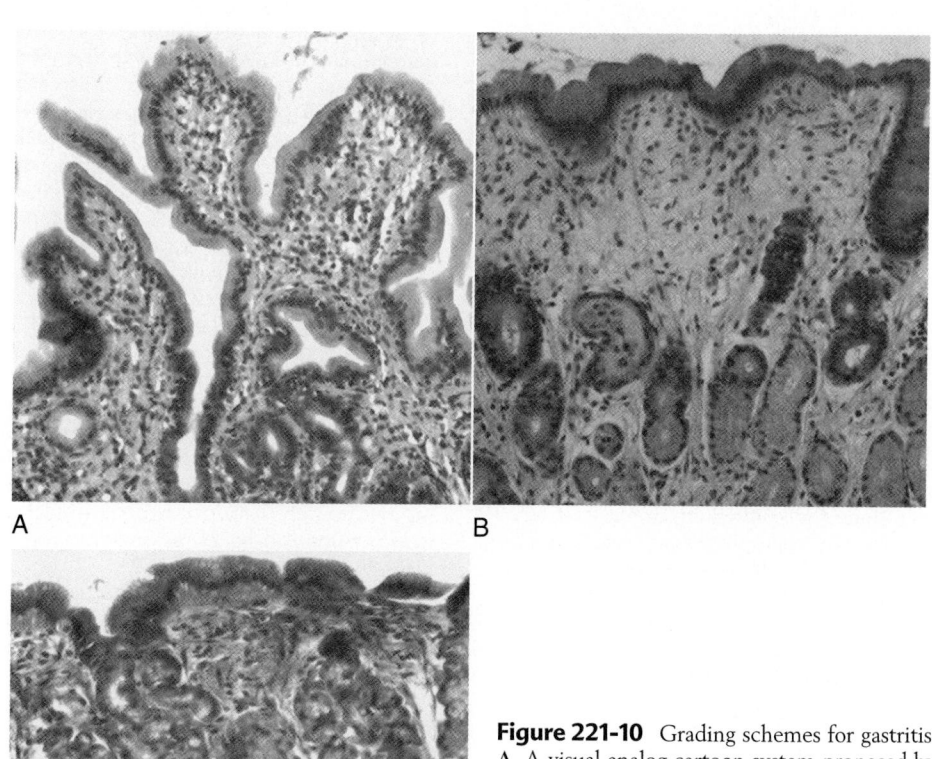

Figure 221-10 Grading schemes for gastritis. **A.** A visual analog cartoon system proposed by Happonen et al, 1998, and **B.** A standardized photograpic scale for atrophy, fibrosis and cellular infiltrate. (Courtesy Wiinberg, Simpson and MacDonough.)

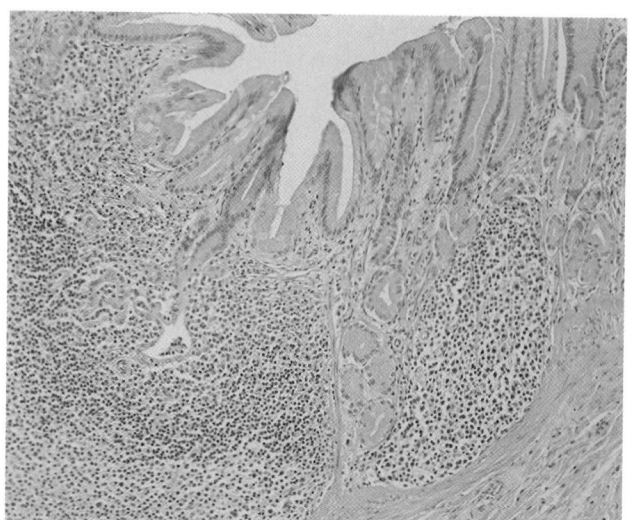

Figure 221-11 Lymphoid follicle hyperplasia and lymphoplasmacytic gastritis in a cat with *H. felis* infection.

fibrosis, edema, ulceration, metaplasia), and their subjective severity (mild, moderate, severe). A standardized visual grading scheme has been proposed by Happonen et al[60] and has been adapted for pathologists[61] (Figure 221-10).

The most common form of gastritis in dogs and cats is mild to moderate superficial lymphoplasmacytic gastritis with concomitant lymphoid follicle hyperplasia (Figure 221-11). Eosinophilic, granulomatous, atrophic, and hyperplastic gastritis are less common.

Etiology

Despite the high prevalence of gastritis an underlying cause is rarely identified, and in the absence of systemic disease, ulcerogenic or irritant drugs, gastric foreign objects, parasites (*Physalloptera* and *Ollulanus* spp.), and in rare instances fungal infections (*Pythium insidiosum, Histoplasma* spp.), it is usually attributed to dietary allergy or intolerance, occult parasitism, or a reaction to bacterial antigens, or unknown pathogens. Treatment is often empirical but can serve to define the cause of gastritis, such as diet responsive, antibiotic responsive, steroid responsive, or parasitic.

Although the basis of the immunologic response in canine and feline gastritis is unknown, recent studies in experimental animals have shed light on the immunologic environment in the gastrointestinal tract and reveal a complex interplay between the GI microflora, the epithelium, immune effector cells such as lymphocytes and macrophages, and soluble mediators such as chemokines and cytokines.[46,62] In health, this system avoids active inflammation by antigen exclusion and the induction of immune tolerance. The development of intestinal inflammation in mice lacking the cytokines IL-10, TGFβ, or IL-2 indicates the central importance of cytokines in damping down mucosal inflammation. In many of these murine models GI inflammation only develops in the presence of indigenous intestinal microflora, leading to the hypothesis that spontaneous mucosal inflammation may be the result of a loss of tolerance to the indigenous GI microflora. The role of these mechanisms in outbred species such as the dog and cat remains to be determined, but clearly loss of tolerance to bacterial of dietary antigens should be considered.

The epithelial cell is also emerging as a "general" in the inflammatory response, with gram-negative or pathogenic bacteria inducing proinflammatory cytokine (e.g., IL-8, IL1-β) secretion from epithelial cells, whereas commensal or bacteria such as *S. fecium* or *Lactobacillus* spp. induce the production of the immunomodulatory cytokines TGFB or IL-10.[62] The pro-inflammatory cytokines produced by epithelial cells are modulated by the production of IL-10 from macrophages and potentially by the epithelial cells themselves.[63] In this context, dogs with lymphoplasmacytic gastritis of undetermined etiology showed a correlation between the expression of the immunomodulatory cytokine IL-10 and proinflammatory cytokines (IFN-γ, IL-1β, IL-8).[61] Simultaneous expression of IL-10 and IFN-γ mRNA has also been observed in the intestines of beagle dogs (lamina propria cells and the intestinal epithelium) in the face of a luminal bacterial flora that was more numerous than that of control dogs.[64] Thus it is tempting to visualize a "homeostatic loop" consisting of proinflammatory stimuli and responses, countered by immunomodulation and repair, with an imbalance in either of these arms manifested as gastritis.

The importance of unknown pathogens in the development of mucosal inflammation is best demonstrated by the gastric bacterium *Helicobacter pylori*, a gram-negative bacterium, which chronically infects more than half of all people worldwide.[13] Chronic infection of human adults with *H. pylori* is characterized by the infiltration of polymorphonuclear and mononuclear cells and the up-regulation of pro-inflammatory cytokines and the chemokine IL-8. Mucosal T cells in infected individuals are polarized toward the production of gamma interferon (IFN-γ), rather than IL-4 or IL-5 indicating a strong bias toward a T_H-1 type response).[65,66] This sustained gastric inflammatory and immune response to infection appears to be pivotal for the development of peptic ulcers and gastric cancer in people.[67]

There is also a high prevalence of gastric *Helicobacter* spp. infection in dogs (67% to 100% of healthy pet dogs, 74% to 90% of vomiting dogs, 100% of laboratory beagles) and cats (40% to 100% of healthy and sick cats).[68-70] In contrast to people, in whom *Helicobacter pylori* infection predominates, dogs and cats are colonized by a variety of large spiral organisms (5 to 12 μ) (Figure 221-12). In cats from Switzerland, United States, and Germany, *Helicobacter heilmannii* is the predominant species, with *Helicobacter bizzozeronii* and *Helicobacter felis* much less frequent. In dogs from Finland, Switzerland, the United States, and Denmark *H. bizzozeronii* and *H. salomonis* are most common followed by *H. heilmanni* and *H. felis. H. bilis* and *Flexispira rappini* have also been described. Cats can also be colonized by *H. pylori* (2 to 5 μ) but infection has been limited to a closed colony of laboratory cats.

Ownership of dogs and cats has been correlated with an increased risk of infection of *H. heilmannii* in people.[71] Case reports have also suggested the transmission of *Helicobacter* spp. from pets to man. Recent studies clearly confirm that dogs and cats harbor *H. heilmannii*, but the subtypes of *H. heilmannii* present in dogs and cats (types 2 and 4) are of minor importance (approximately 15% of cases) to humans, who are predominantly colonized by *H. heilmannii* type 1 (the predominant *Helicobacter* sp. in pigs).[72]

The effect of eradicating *Helicobacter* spp. on gastritis and clinical signs, the main form of evidence supporting the pathogenic role of *H. pylori* in human gastritis, has not been thoroughly investigated to date in dogs and cats. An uncontrolled treatment trial of dogs and cats with gastritis and *Helicobacter* spp. infection showed that clinical signs in 90% of 63 dogs and cats responded to treatment with a combination of metronidazole, amoxicillin, and famotidine, and that 14 of the 19 animals re-endoscoped had resolution of gastritis and no evidence of *Helicobacter* spp. in gastric biopsies.[73]

Controlled clinical trials are required to confirm these observations but have been hampered by a much higher apparent recrudescence or re-infection rate than the 1% to 2% per year observed after treatment of *H. pylori*-infected people. With such limited information from eradication trials, most current knowledge about the pathogenicity of *Helicobacter* spp. for dogs and cats comes from the evaluation of animals with

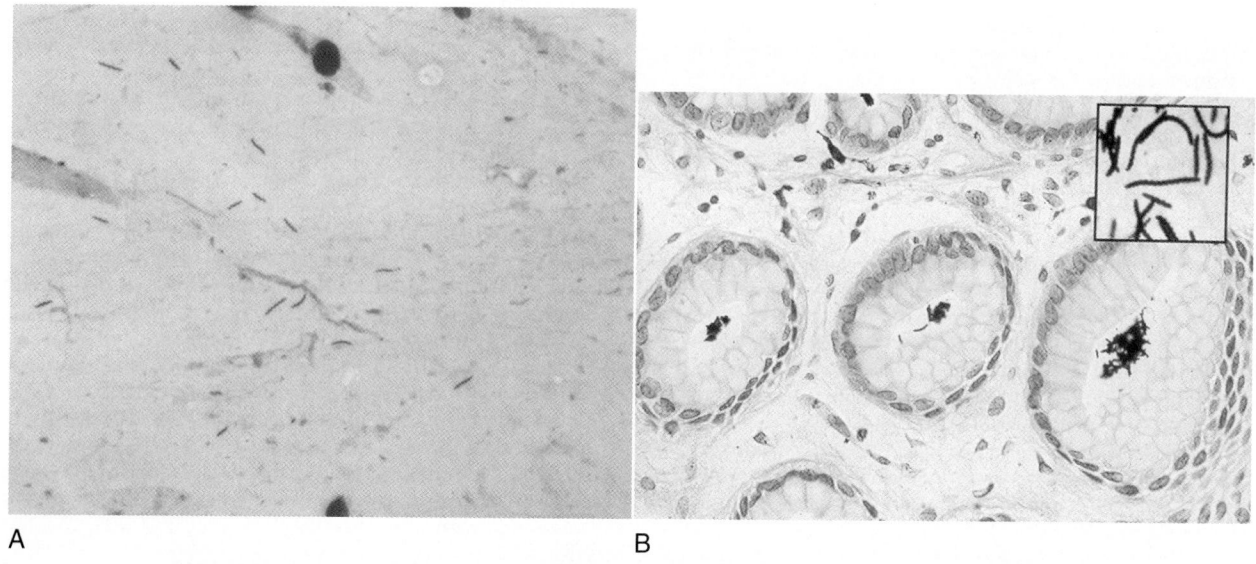

Figure 221-12 *Helicobacter* spp. visualized on **(A)** an impression smear (Diff-Quick stain) and **(B)** endoscopic biopsy (Steiner stain).

and without infections and clinical signs, and a small number of experimental infections.

The large *Helicobacter* species found in dogs an cats do not attach to the epithelium but colonize the superficial mucus and gastric glands, particularly of the fundus and cardia, and may also be observed intracellularly.[68,69] Degeneration of gastric glands, with vacuolation, pyknosis, and necrosis of parietal cells is more common in infected than uninfected animals. Inflammation is generally mononuclear in nature and ranges from mild to moderate in severity. Gastric lymphoid hyperplasia is common and can be extensive in dogs and cats infected with *Helicobacter* spp. (particularly when full thickness gastric biopsies are evaluated). In addition to this local gastric immune response, a systemic response characterized by increased circulating anti-*Helicobacter* IgG has been detected in sera from naturally infected dogs and cats. However, the gastritis observed in cats and dogs infected with large HLOs is generally less severe than that observed in *H. pylori* infected humans (where neutrophilic aggregates, and moderate to severe gastritis, are commonly encountered), and gastro-intestinal ulcers, gastric neoplasia, or changes in serum gastrin or acid secretion have not been associated with *Helicobacter* spp. infection in dogs and cats.

These differences between people, dogs, and cats may be attributed to differences in the virulence of the infecting *Helicobacter* spp., or the host response. Studies that address this issue indicate that *H. pylori* evokes a more severe proinflammatory cytokine and cellular response in dogs and cats than natural or experimental infection with large *Helicobacter* spp.[74,75] The limited mucosal inflammatory response and absence of clinical signs in the vast majority of dogs and cats infected with non-*H. pylori Helicobacter* spp., despite significant antigenic stimulation (evidenced by seroconversion and lymphoid follicle hyperplasia) suggest that large gastric *Helicobacter* spp. are more commensal than pathogenic. With this in mind, it is interesting to speculate that it is the loss of tolerance to gastric *Helicobacter* spp., rather than the innate pathogenicity of these bacteria, that explains the development of gastritis and clinical signs in some dogs and cats. However, much still remains to be learned about the role of *Helicobacter* spp. in canine and feline gastritis.

Clinical Findings

The major clinical sign of chronic gastritis is vomiting of food or bile. Decreased appetite, weight loss, melena, or hematemesis is variably encountered. The concurrent presence of dermatologic and gastrointestinal signs raises the likelihood of dietary sensitivity.[76] Access to toxins, medications, foreign bodies, and dietary practices should be thoroughly reviewed. The signalment should not be overlooked as it may increase the probability that chronic gastritis is the cause of vomiting. Hypertrophy of the fundic mucosa is frequently associated with a severe enteropathy in basenjis[77] and stomatocytosis, hemolytic anemia, icterus, and polyneuropathy in Drentse Patrijshond.[78] Hypertrophy of the pyloric mucosa is observed in small brachycephalic dogs such as Lhasa apso and is associated with gastric outflow obstruction (see Delayed Gastric Emptying and Motility Disorders). Atrophy of the gastric mucosa that may progress to adenocarcinoma has been reported in Lundehunds with protein-losing gastroenteropathy.[79]

Young, large breed, male dogs in the Gulf states of the United States may have granulomatous gastritis caused by *Pythium* spp. with infection more prevalent in fall, winter, and spring.[80] Physical examination is often unremarkable. Abdominal distension may be related to delayed gastric emptying caused by obstruction or defective propulsion. Abdominal masses, lymphadenopathy, or ocular changes may be encountered in dogs with gastric fungal infections.

Diagnosis

A biochemical profile, complete blood count, urinalysis, and T_4 (cats) should be performed as a basic screen for metabolic, endocrine, infectious, and other non-GI causes of vomiting, as well as the acid base and electrolyte changes associated with vomiting, outflow obstruction, or acid hypersecretion. Clinicopathologic tests are often normal in patients with chronic gastritis.

Eosinophilia may prompt the consideration of gastritis associated with dietary hypersensitivity, endoparasites, or mast cell tumors. Hyperglobulinemia and hypoalbuninemia may be present in basenjis with gastropathy/enteropathy, or dogs with gastric pythisosis. Panhypoproteinemia is a feature of gastroenteropathy in Lundehunds, moderate to severe generalized inflammatory bowel disease, GI lymphoma, and GI histoplasmosis. More specific testing, such as an ACTH stimulation test, or serology for *Pythium isnsidiosum*, is performed based on the results of these initial tests. Determination of food specific IgE has not been shown to be useful in the diagnosis of dietary sensitivity in dogs or cats. The utility of noninvasive tests, such as serum pepsinogen and gastric permeability to sucrose, used to diagnose gastritis in people has not been determined in dogs and cats.

Abdominal radiographs are frequently normal in dogs and cats with gastritis but may show gastric distention or delayed gastric emptying (food retained more than 12 hours after a meal). Contrast radiography may reveal ulcers or thickening of the gastric rugae or wall but has largely been supersceded by the combination of ultrasonography to detect mural abnormalities and endoscopy to observe and sample the gastric mucosa.[22]

Endoscopic examination enables the visualization of foreign bodies, erosions, ulceration, hemorrhage, rugal thickening, lymphoid follicle hyperplasia (evident as mucosal pock marks), increased mucus or fluid (clear or bile stained), and increased or decreased mucosal friability. Discrete focal or multifocal mucosal nodules may be observed with Ollulanus spp. infection.

Gastric phycomycosis can be associated with irregular masses in the pyloric outflow tract and may prompt serologic testing by ELISA, Western blotting, and culture of fresh gastric biopsies. Parasites such as Physalloptera spp. may be observed as 1- to 4-cm worms. Large amounts of bile stained fluid is suggestive of duodenogastric reflux-associated gastritis, whereas lots of clear fluid my indicate hypersecretion of gastric acid. Gastric fluid can be aspirated for cytology (Helicobacter spp., parasite ova or larvae) and pH measurement. Impression smears of gastric biopsies are an effective way of looking for Helicobacter spp. (5 to 12 μ spirals) and are more sensitive than the biopsy urease test (Helicobacter spp. produce urease). Serum gastrin should be measured in the face of unexplained gastric erosions, ulcers, fluid accumulation, or mucosal hypertrophy.

The endoscopic procedure of dribbling dietary antigens onto the gastric mucosa to ascertain the presence of food allergy has not been useful in dogs or cats: it is highly subjective, detects only immediate hypersensitivity, and does not correlate with the results of dietary elimination trials.[76] The stomach should be biopsied even when it looks grossly normal (usually three biopsies from each region- pylorus, fundus, and cardia). Thickened rugae may require multiple biopsies, and a full-thickness biopsy is often required to differentiate gastritis from neoplasia or fungal infection and to diagnose submucosal or muscular hypertrophy. The results of gastric ultrasonography can help to forewarn the clinician of these possibilities and are complement to the endoscopic findings.

Gastric sections should be stained with H&E for evaluation of cellularity and architecture, and modified Steiner stain for gastric spiral bacteria (Figure 221-12, B). Further special stains, such as Gomori's methenamine silver, are indicated if pyogranulomatous inflammation is present to detect fungi. Masson's trichrome can be used to highlight gastric fibrosis, whereas sirius red and alcian blue help to reveal eosinophils and mast cells, respectively. Immunocytochemistry can be employed to help distinguish lymphoma from severe lymphocytic gastritis. Mucin staining has been performed in Lundehunds with gastric atrophy and showed an abnormal presence of mucus neck cells and pseudo-pyloric metaplasia.[81]

The interpretation of gastric biopsies has important implications for patient care because biopsy findings are often used to guide treatment. For example, moderate lymphoplasmacytic gastritis without Helicobacter spp. infection is often treated with corticosteroids, whereas mild lymphoplasmacytic gastritis may be treated with a change in diet. As the histopathologic evaluation of gastric biopsies has not been standardized, the prudent clinician should carefully review histologic sections to get a feel for the pathologist's interpretation. Even with optimum evaluation similar histologic changes can be observed in patients with different underlying etiologies, so well-structured treatment trials often form the basis of an etiologic diagnosis.

Treatment

Treatment of gastritis initially centers on the detection and treatment of underlying metabolic disorders and the removal of drugs, toxins, foreign bodies, parasites, and fungal infections.

Parasitic Gastritis

Ollulanus tricuspis is a microscopic worm (0.7 to 1 mm long, 0.04 mm wide) that infects the feline stomach.[82] Its predominant cat-to-cat transmisison is through ingestion of vomitus. It can also undergo internal autoinfection with worm burdens reaching up to 11,000 per stomach. Mucosal abnormalities range from none, to rugal hyperplasia, and nodular (2 to 3 mm) gastritis.

Histologic findings include lymphoplasmacytic infiltrates, lymphoid follicular hyperplasia, fibrosis, and up to 100/hpf globular leukocytes. Ollulanus spp. are not detected by fecal examination and require evaluation of gastric juice, vomitus, or histologic sections for larvae or worms. Gastric lavage and xylazine-induced emesis have been described to aid diagnosis. Treatment with fenbendazole 10 mg/kg PO SID 2d may be effective.

Physalloptera spp. are about 2 to 6 cm long worms that are sporadically detected in the stomachs of dogs and cats. Physalloptera rara are most commonly described and appear to be primarily a parasite of coyotes. Diagnosis is difficult as worm burden is often low and the eggs are transparent and difficult to see in sugar floatation. Treatment with pyrantel pamoate (5 mg/kg PO:dogs single dose; cats two doses 14 days apart) may be effective. Control of infection may be difficult due to the ingestion of intermediate hosts, such as cockroaches and beetles, and paratenic hosts, such as lizards and hedgehogs.

Given the difficult diagnosis of Ollulanus and Physalloptera spp., empirical therapy with an anthelminthic such as fenbendazole may be warranted in dogs and cats with unexplained gastritis.

Gastric infection with Gnathostoma spp. (cats), Spirocerca spp. (dogs), and Aonchotheca spp. (cats) has been associated with gastric nodules that have been treated by surgical resection of affected gastric tissue.[83]

Gastric Pythiosis

The presence of transmural thickening of the gastric outflow tract (Figure 221-13, D) and histology that indicates pyogranulomatous inflammation raise the possibility of infection with fungi such as Pythium insidiosum.[80] Special staining (Gomoris methenamine silver), culture, serology, and PCR of infected tissues can be used to help confirm the diagnosis. Treatment consists of aggressive surgical resection combined with itraconazole (10 mg/kg PO SID) and terbinafine (5 to 10 mg/kg PO SID) for 2 to 3 months post-surgery. ELISA titers of pre- and post-treatment samples may show a marked drop during successful treatment and drugs can be stopped. Medical therapy is continued for another 2 to 3 months if titers remain elevated. The prognosis is poor and fewer than 25% of afflicted animals are cured with medical therapy alone.[80]

Helicobacter-Associated Gastritis

The general lack of knowledge of the pathogenicity of gastric Helicobacter spp. has meant that veterinarians are faced with the dilemma of either treating or ignoring spiral bacteria observed in biopsies from patients with chronic vomiting and gastritis. In light of their pathogenicity in man, ferrets, cheetahs, and mice, it would seem prudent that eradication of gastric Helicobacter spp. is attempted prior to initiating treatment with immunosuppressive agents to control gastritis. However, this must be decided on an individual basis. For example, in the patient with a lymphoplasmacytic infiltrate of the stomach and small intestine with a concomitant gastric Helicobacter spp.

infection, should one treat for inflammatory bowel disease, *Helicobacter*, or both?

The author recommends treating only symptomatic patients that have biopsy-confirmed *Helicobacter* spp. infection and gastritis. Current treatment protocols are based on those found to be effective in humans infected with *H. pylori*. An uncontrolled treatment trial of dogs and cats with gastritis and *Helicobacter* spp. infection showed that clinical signs in 90% of 63 dogs and cats responded to treatment with a combination of metronidazole, amoxicillin, and famotidine, and that 74% of 19 animals re-endoscoped had no evidence of *Helicobacter* spp. in gastric biopsies.[73]

Unfortunately these promising results regarding the eradication of *Helicobacter* spp. have not been borne out by more controlled studies in asymptomatic *Helicobacter*-infected dogs and cats. Treatment combinations that have been critically evaluated are (1) amoxicillin (20 mg/kg PO BID 14d), metronidazole (20 mg/kg PO BID 14d), and famotidine (0.5 mg/kg PO BID 14d) in dogs[84]; (2) clarithromycin (30 mg PO BID 4d), metronidazole (30 mg PO BID 4d), ranitidine (10 mg PO BID 4d), and bismuth (20 mg PO BID 4d) (CMRB) in *H. heilmannii* infected cats[85] and (3) azithromycin (30 mg PO SID 4d), tinidazole (100 mg PO SID 4d), ranitidine (20 mg PO SID 4d) and bismuth (40 mg PO SID 4d)(ATRB) in *H. heilmannii*-infected cats.[85] Re-evaluation of infection status at 3 days (dogs) or 10 days (cats) after treatment revealed six of eight dogs and 11 of 11 CMRB and four of six ATRB-treated cats to be *Helicobacter* spp. free on the basis of histology and urease testing (dogs) or ^{13}C-urea breath test (dogs and cats).[85,86] However, at 28 days (dogs) or 42 days (cats) after completing antimicrobial therapy, eight of eight dogs and four of eleven cats that received CMRB, five of six cats that received ATRB were found to be re-infected. A transient effect of combination therapy (amoxicillin 20 mg/kg PO TID 21d, metronidazole 20 mg/kg PO TID 21d, and omeprazole 0.7 mg PO SID 21d) on bacterial colonization has also been observed in six cats with *H. pylori* infection.

Further analysis of gastric biopsies from infected dogs and *H. pylori* infected cats using PCR and *Helicobacter*-specific primers revealed persistence of *Helicobacter* DNA in gastric biopsies that appeared negative on histology and urease testing. These studies suggest that antibiotic regimens that are effective against *H. pylori* in people may only cause transient suppression, rather than eradication, of gastric *Helicobacter* spp. in dogs and cats.

The author has recently employed the combination of amoxicillin (20 mg/kg PO BID), clarithromycin (7.5 mg/kg PO BID) and metronidazole (10 mg/kg PO BID) for 14 days to eradicate *Helicobacter pylori* infection in cats. Further controlled trials of antibiotic therapy in infected dogs and cats, particularly symptomatic patients with gastritis and *Helicobacter* spp. infection, are clearly required before guidelines regarding the treatment of gastric *Helicobacter* spp. in dogs and cats can be made.

Chronic Gastritis of Unknown Cause
Lymphocytic plasmacytic gastritis of unknown cause is common in dogs and cats. It may be associated with similar infiltrates in the intestines, particularly in cats (who should also be evaluated for the presence of pancreatic and biliary disease). The cellular infiltrate varies widely in severity and it may be accompanied by mucosal atrophy or fibrosis, and less commonly hyperplasia.

Patients with mild lymphoplasmacytic gastritis are initially treated with diet. The diet is usually restricted in antigens to which the patient has been previously exposed, such as a lamb-based diet if the patient has previously been fed chicken and beef, or contains hydrolyzed proteins (usually chicken or soy) that may be less allergenic than intact proteins. Many of these diets are also high in carbohydrate and restricted in fat,

which facilitates gastric emptying, and may contain other substances such as menhaden fish oil or antioxidants that may alter inflammation.

The test diet is fed exclusively for a period of about 2 weeks while vomiting episodes are recorded.[76] If vomiting is improved a challenge with the original diet is required to confirm a diagnosis of food intolerance. The introduction of a specific dietary component to the test diet, such as beef, is required to confirm dietary sensitivity. If vomiting is unresponsive the patient may be placed on a different diet for another 2 weeks, usually the limit of client tolerance, or started on prednisolone (1 to 2 mg/kg/day PO, tapered to every other day at the lowest dose that maintains remission over 8 to 12 weeks).

Patients with moderate to severe lymphoplasmacytic gastritis are usually started on a combination of a test diet and prednisolone. If the patient goes into remission they are maintained on the test diet while prednisolone is tapered and potentially discontinued. Antacids and mucosal protectants are added to the therapeutic regimen if ulcers or erosion are detected at endoscopy or if hematemesis or melena is noted.

If gastritis is unresponsive to diet, prednisolone, and antacids, additional immunosuppression may be indicated. Gastric biopsies should be carefully re-evaluated for evidence of lymphoma. In dogs immunosuppression is usually increased with azathioprine (PO 2 mg/kg SID for 5d then EOD, on alternating days with prednisolone). Chlorambucil may be a safer alternative to azathioprine in cats (PO) and has been successfully employed in the management of inflammatory bowel disease and small cell lymphoma (see below). Prokinetic agents such as metoclopramide, cisapride, and erythromycin can be used as an adjunct where delayed gastric emptying is present. These are discussed below.

Diffuse eosinophillic gastritis of undefined etiology is usually approached in a similar fashion to lymphoplasmacytic gastritis. The presence of eosinphilia, dermatologic changes, and eosinophilic infiltrates may be even more suggestive of dietary sensitivity. In cats it should be determined if it is part of a hypereosinophilic syndrome. Treatment for occult parasites, dietary trials, and immunosuppression can be carried out as described above. Focal eosinophilic granulomas can be associated with parasites or fungal infection that should be excluded prior to immunosuppression with corticosteroids.

Atrophic Gastritis
Atrophic gastritis in dogs and cats is often associated with a marked cellular infiltrate (see Figure 221-10). In people atrophy is associated with *Helicobacter* spp. infection and inflammation, and immune-mediated destruction.[87] Gastric disease is often not discovered until the patient presents with pernicious anemia secondary to cobalamin deficiency caused by a lack of gastric intrinsic factor. In people, atrophic gastritis, intestinal metaplasia of the gastric mucosa, and hypochlorhydia are thought to precede the development of gastric cancer.[88] The host inflammatory response is also thought to contribute to the development of atrophy and pro-inflammatory IL-1β and IL-10 gene polymorphisms in people are associated with increased inflammation, gastric atrophy, hypochlorhydria, and gastric cancer.[89,90]

Atrophic gastritis has been infrequently described in dogs and cats but does share some similarities with people. Atrophy has been associated with gastric adenocarcinoma in Lundehunds[81] and in dogs with lymphoplasmacytic gastritis of undetermined cause atrophy correlates with the expression of mRNA for IL-1β and IL-10 and the presence of neutrophils. However, there is no clear evidence that lymphoplasmacytic gastritis progresses to atrophy and gastric cancer in dogs or cats,[91] and the role of *Helicobacter* spp. or antigastric antibodies in the development of atrophy in dogs and cats remains to be determined.

In contrast to humans, dogs and cats with atrophic gastritis have not been reported to develop cobalamin deficiency. This is probably because the pancreas, rather than the stomach, is the main source of intrinsic factor in these species. Achlorhydria has been described in dogs and may enable the proliferation of bacteria in the stomach and upper small intestine, although this has not been proven. The treatment of atrophic gastritis has received limited attention, but *Helicobacter* spp. eradication and immunosuppression have been effective in people.

Hypertrophic Gastritis

Hypertrophy in the fundic mucosa is uncommon and is often part of the breed-specific gastropathies or gastroenteropathies mentioned above (Figure 221-13). Concurrent hypergastrinemia should prompt consideration of underlying hepatic or renal disease, achlorhydria, or gastrin-producing tumors, which should be pursued appropriately. Basenji gastoenteropathy is variably associated with fasting hypergastrinemia and exaggerated secretin stimulated gastrin, and anecdotal reports suggest that affected basenjis may respond to antimicrobial therapy. Antral hypertrophy of brachycephalic dogs causes outflow obstruction and is treated with surgery (see below).

DELAYED GASTRIC EMPTYING AND MOTILITY DISORDERS

Disorders of gastric motility can disrupt the storage and mixing of food and its expulsion into the duodenum.[25] Normal gastric motility is the result of the organized interaction of smooth muscle with neural and hormonal stimuli. Delayed gastric emptying is the most commonly recognized manifestation of gastric motility disorders. Rapid gastric emptying and motility disorders associated with retrograde transit of bile or ingesta are less well defined.

Delayed gastric emptying is caused by outflow obstruction or defective propulsion (Table 221-3) and is usually suspected by the vomiting of food at least 8 and often 10 to16 hours after a meal.

Diagnosis

Vomiting of food some time after ingestion (more than 8 hours) is the most common sign. Vomiting may be projectile with pyloric stenosis. Abdominal distension, weight loss, melena, abdominal discomfort, distention, bloating, and anorexia are more variably present.

The signalment and history may be helpful narrowing down the cause. Development of vomiting at weaning raises the possibility of pyloric stenosis. Access to foreign bodies, bones, and medications is of obvious relevance to outflow obstruction. Brachycephalic, middle-aged, small breed dogs, such as shih tzus, seem predisposed to the syndrome of hypertrophic pylorogastropathy, where vomiting is secondary to pyloric outflow obstruction caused by hypertrophy of the pyloric mucosa and/or muscularis.[92,93] Gastric neoplasia is usually detected in older animals, and weight loss, hematemesis, and pallor may be present. Gastric pythiosis is more prevalent in young large breed dogs in the Gulf states of the United States. Large breed, deep-chested dogs are more prone to GDV that may have an underlying problem with gastric emptying (see GD/GDV above).

A thorough physical examination is performed to detect causes of vomiting such as string foreign bodies, or intestinal masses or thickenings, non-gastrointestinal (GI) causes, including thyroid (nodules-cats), liver (jaundice, hepatomegaly) or kidney disease (renomegaly, lumpy or small), and the systemic effects of vomiting, such as dehydration and weakness.

Table • 221-3

Causes of Delayed Gastric Emptying

Outflow Obstruction
Congenital stenosis
Foreign bodies
Hypertrophy of pyloric mucosa
Granuloma
Polyps
Neoplasia
Extragastric masses

Defective Propulsion
Gastric disorders
Gastritis
Ulcers
Neoplasia
Gastroenteritis
Peritonitis
Pancreatitis
Metabolic (hypokalemia, hypocalcemia, hypoadrenocorticism)
Nervous inhibition (trauma, pain, stress?)
Dysautonomia
GDV
Surgery
Drugs (e.g., anticholinergics, narcotics)
Idiopathic

The diagnostic approach is to confirm delayed gastric emptying and to detect causes of gastric outflow obstruction that may require surgery, and non-gastric disorders associated with defective propulsion. Historical and physical findings are combined with clinicopathologic testing, plain radiographs, and ultrasonography.

Hematology, serum biochemistry, urinalysis, fecal analysis (e.g., parasites, parvo), and serology (e.g., FelV) are employed to detect non-GI causes of vomiting or delayed gastric emptying and to determine the consequences of vomiting. Laboratory findings vary depending on the severity of vomiting and completeness of pyloric obstruction and the presence of disorders associated with blood loss or inflammation. The CBC is often normal, but anemia may accompany gastric ulcers or neoplasia. Hyperglobulinemia may be present where outflow obstruction is secondary to fugal granuloma. The presence of hypochloremia, hypokalemia, and metabolic alkalosis, with or without aciduria, should increase suspicion of an upper GI obstruction or potential hypersecretion of gastric acid.

Radiographs are essential to confirm the retention of food or fluid in the stomach longer than 8 hours, and often 12 to 16 hours, after a meal, and to detect extra gastric disorders such as peritonitis. Ultrasound may detect mural thickening or irregularity of the stomach suggestive of neoplasia, granuloma, or hypertrophy. Ultrasound may also reveal radiolucent foreign objects and detect non-gastric causes of delayed emptying, such as pancreatitis. Contrast radiography can be used to detect mural abnormalities and to confirm a suspicion of gastric obstruction where plain radiographs are inconclusive (Figure 221-14). However, endoscopy is usually favored over radiographic procedures for confirming gastric outflow obstruction and gastric and duodenal causes of decreased propulsion (e.g., ulcers, gastritis) (see Figure 221-13). Measurement of gastric pH and serum gastrin can help to differentiate idiopathic

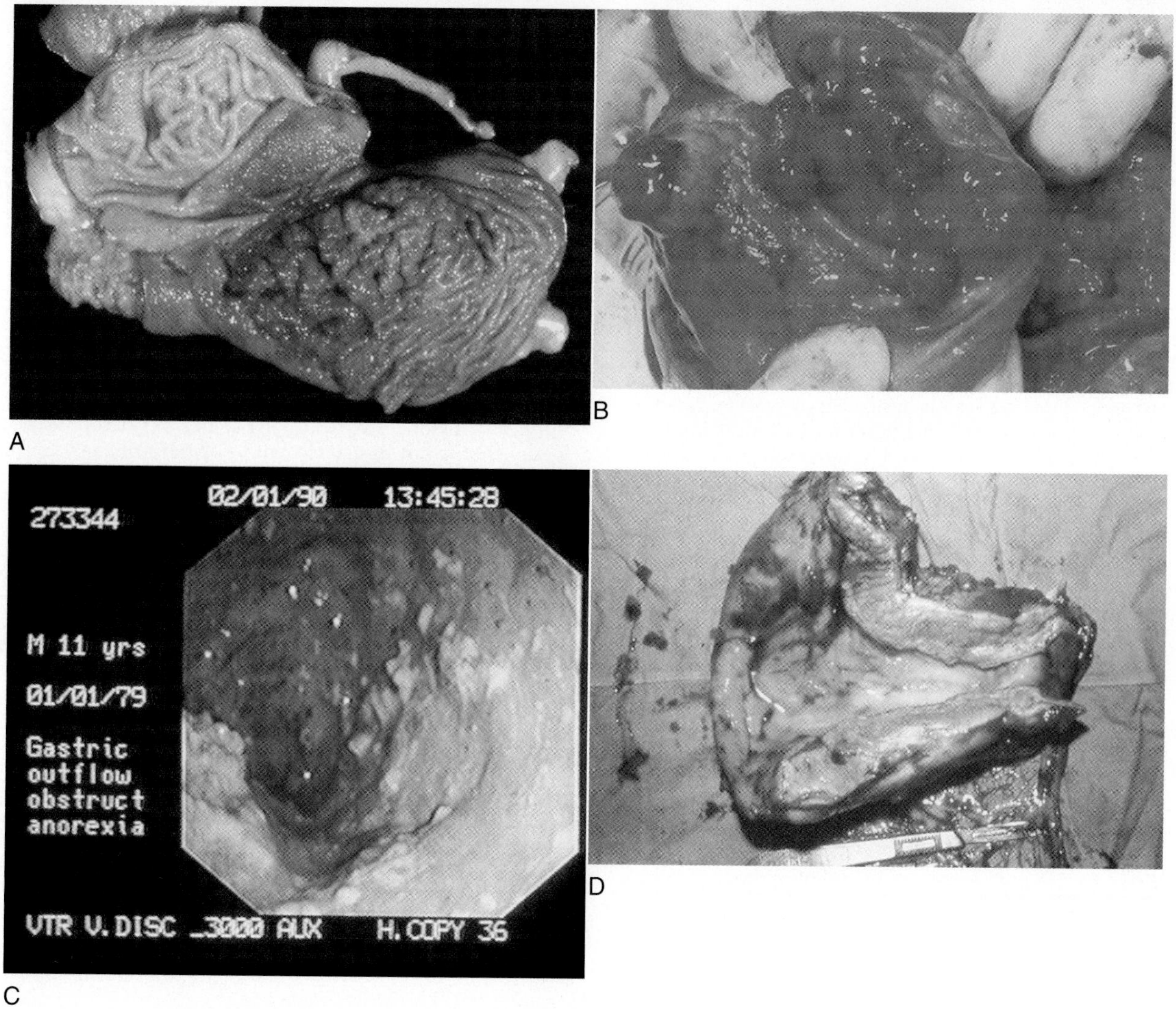

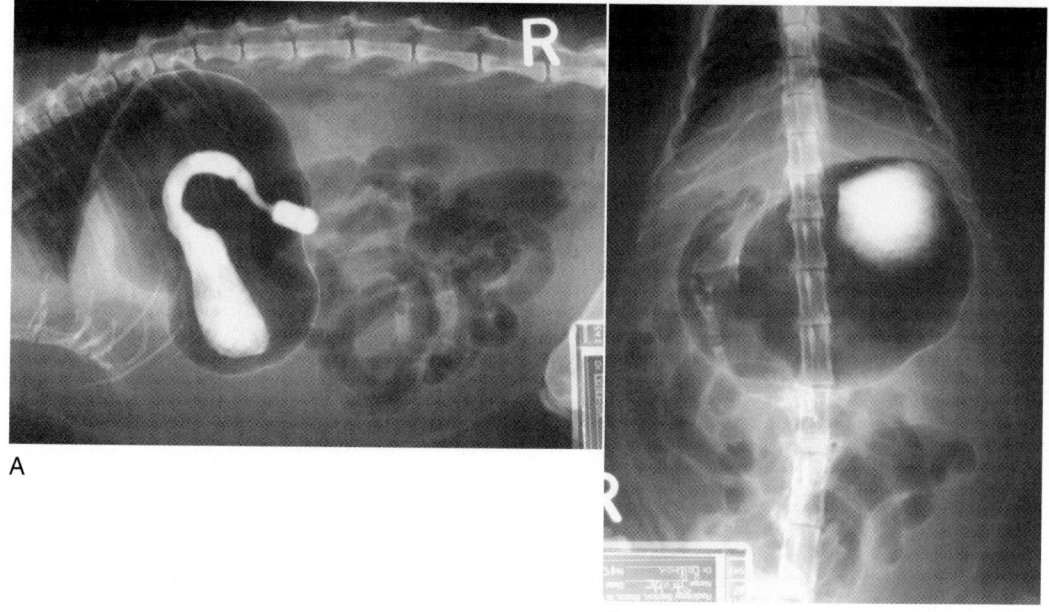

Figure 221-13 Gross appearance of hypertrophic gastropathies. **A,** Diffuse fundic hypertrophy; **B,** multifocal fundic hypertrophy; **C,** antral mucosal hypertrophy (idiopathic hyperplastic pyloro-gastropathy in a brachycephalic dog); **D,** thickening of the pyloric outflow tract due to *Pythium* spp. (*A, B,* and *D,* Courtesy of Cornell University; *C,* courtesy of The Ohio State University.)

Figure 221-14 Marked gastric dilation and retention of liquid barium in a 12-year-old domestic short hair cat. Full thickness gastric biopsies showed submucosal infiltration with neutrophils and lymphocytes. (Courtesy of Cornell University.)

hypertrophic pylorogastropathy from hypertrophy associated with hypergastrinemia. Pancreatic polypeptide-producing tumors may also be associated with mucosal hypertrophy. Endoscopy is hampered by the recent administration of barium so it is often performed first. Endoscopic biopsy is limited to the superficial mucosa and surgical biopsy is frequently required to achieve a definitive diagnosis of granulomatous, neoplastic, or hypertrophic conditions.

More sophisticated procedures to directly evaluate gastric emptying and motility are usually employed to determine if vomiting is due to an undefined gastric motility disorder and to optimize prokinetic therapy (Table 221-4).[25,26] Radiographic contrast procedures are readily available but are hampered by the wide variability in emptying times for barium in liquid or meal form. The administration of barium impregnated polyspheres (BIPS) is a simplified contrast procedure suited to routine clinical practice as it requires many fewer radiographs than traditional barium series and is standardized in terms of test performance and interpretation but its utility in clinical patients remains to be determined. Scintigraphic techniques are generally considered the most accurate way to evaluate emptying but are restricted to referral institutions. Ultrasound can be useful for detecting gastric wall abnormalities and measuring contractile activity. A test employing the labeled ^{13}C-octanoic acid has been evaluated in people and dogs and found to reflect gastric emptying (the values are longer than scintigraphy as ^{13}C-octanoate has to be absorbed and metabolized before $^{13}CO_2$ is liberated).

Treatment

Treatment of gastric emptying disorders is directed at the underlying cause. Gastric ulcers, erosions, and inflammation should be investigated and managed medically as described above. Foreign bodies are removed either endoscopically or surgically. Pyloric stenosis, polyps, and hypertrophic gastropathy that is not associated with hypergastrinemia are managed surgically. When hypertrophic gastropathy, ulcers or erosions, or excessive gastric juice is encountered at endoscopy, intravenous H_2-antagonists can be given during the endoscopic procedure to try to prevent postoperative perforation or esophagitis. Neoplasia, polyps, and granulomas may require extensive gastric resection and Billroth procedures.

Table • 221-4

A Review of Methods for Assessment of the Rate of Gastric Emptying in the Dog and Cat[26]

METHOD	SPECIES	TEST MEAL	n	GASTRIC HALF EMPTYING TIME ($t\frac{1}{2}$)*
Radioscintigraphy	Dog	Eggs, starch + glucose	27	66 min (median), 45—227 min (95% CI)
		Beef baby food + kibble	6	4.9 ± 1.96 hours (mean ± sd)
		Liver	4	About 2 hours
		Canned dog food + egg	6 (18 tests)	172 ± 17 min (mean ± se)
		Canned dog food + egg	7 (14 tests)	285 ± 34 min (mean ± sd); 294 ± 39 min (mean ± sd)
		Canned dog food	6	77 min (mean)
	Cat	Dry cat food	10	2.47 ± 0.71 hours (mean ± sd)
		Liver + cream	6 (15 tests)	163 ± 11 min (mean ± se)
		Canned cat food	20	2.69 ± 0.25 hours (mean ± sd)
		Dry cat food	20	3.86 ± 0.24 hours (mean ± sd)
		Eggs	10	330 min (median), 210—769 min (range)
Radiography		Dry dog food + radio-opaque solids	10	3.5 hours (median), 1—6 hours (range)
		Canned dog food + egg + BIPS	6 (18 tests)	Small BIPS 416 ± 81 min (mean ± se)
	Dog	Canned dog food + BIPS	20	Small BIPS 6.05 ± 2.99 hr (mean ± sd) Large BIPS 7.11 ± 3.60 hr (mean ± sd)
		Kibble + BIPS	8	Small BIPS = 8.29 ± 1.62 hr (70% of dogs ± se) Large BIPS = 29.21 ± 18.31 hr (70% of dogs ± se)
		Kibble + liquid barium	9 (27 tests)	Total gastric emptying time = 7—15 hr (range)
		Kibble + liquid barium	4	Total gastric emptying time = 7.6 ± 1.98 hr (mean ± se)
	Cat	Canned cat food + BIPS	10	Small BIPS 6.43 ± 2.59 hr (mean ± sd) Large BIPS 7.49 ± 4.09 hr (mean ± sd)
		Canned cat food + BIPS	6	Small BIPS - 7.7 hr (median), 3.5—10.9 hr (range) Large BIPS - 8.1 hr (median), 5—19.6 hr (range)
		Canned cat food + BIPS	10	Small BIPS - 5.36 hr (median) Large BIPS - 6.31 hr (median)
		Cat food + liquid barium	8	Gastric emptying time = 11.6 ± 0.9 hr (mean ± sd)
Gastric Emptying Breath Test	Cat	Canned cat food	6	Peak ^{13}C-excretion = 56.7 ± 9.8 min (mean ± sd)
	Dog	Bread, egg + margarine	6 (18 tests)	3.43 ± 0.50 hr (mean ± sd)

*Gastric emptying rate is expressed as gastric half emptying time, unless otherwise stated. (Reproduced with permission of Wyse et al, *JVIM* 2003, 17:604-621.)

Dietary modification to facilitate gastric emptying may be beneficial irrespective of cause.

Small amounts of semi-liquid, protein- and fat-restricted diets fed at frequent intervals may facilitate emptying, such as an "intestinal disease diet" blended with water and mixed with an equal volume of boiled rice.

In nonobstructive situations gastric emptying can be enhanced and duodenogastric reflux inhibited by prokinetic agents such as metoclopramide, cisapride, erythromycin, or ranitidine.[25,39,94] The choice of prokinetic depends if a central antiemetic effect is required (e.g., metoclopramide), if a combined antacid prokinetic is indicated (e.g., ranitidine), or if treatment with one agent has been ineffective or caused adverse effects (e.g., behavioral changes with metoclopramide). Metoclopramide (0.2 to 0.5 mg/kg PO SC TID) has central antiemetic properties in addition to its prokinetic activity in the stomach and upper GI tract and is frequently an initial choice in patients with underlying metabolic diseases associated with vomiting and delayed gastric emptying.

However, metoclopramide may only facilitate the emptying of liquids and is less effective in promoting organized gastroduodenal and intestinal motility than cisapride. Cisapride (0.1 to 0.5 mg/kg PO TID) has no central antiemetic effects but is generally more potent in promotion of the gastric emptying of solids than metoclopramide, but it does have more drug interactions and its availability is limited. Erythromycin (dog: 0.5 to 1.0 mg/kg PO TID, between meals) releases motilin and acts at motilin receptors and mimics phase III of the interdigestive migrating myoelectric complex (MMC) promoting the emptying of solids. Niaztidine and ranitidine (0.25 to 0.5 mg/lb PO TID) have prokinetic activity attributed to an organophosphate-like effect.

No controlled trials in dogs and cats have evaluated the efficacy of different prokinetics in different disease states, and treatment is usually based on a best guess/least harmful basis. Where true prokinetic activity is required, cisapride and erythromycin appear to be the most efficacious.[25] Treatment trials with prokinetics should probably be structured to last between 5 and 10 days to determine benefit. A diary of clinical signs and the objective assessment of gastric emptying using the tests described above, before and after therapy helps to optimize treatment. Combination therapy, such as erythromycin and cisapride, is not recommended due to the potential for adverse drug interactions. The prognosis for patients with delayed gastric emptying depends on the cause.

A suspected motility disorder characterized by duodenogastric reflux is thought to account for a syndrome known as the bilious vomiting syndrome. Affected dogs usually vomit early in the morning. Remission may be achieved by feeding the animal late at night. Prokinetic agents may also be employed.

GASTRIC NEOPLASIA

Gastric neoplasia represents less than 1.0% of all reported canine and feline neoplasms.[95] Malignant tumors are more common than benign tumors and most types of gastric neoplasms have been reported to occur more frequently in males, except adenomas, which occur more frequently in females.[95] Other gastric malignancies reported are leiomyosarcoma, lymphosarcoma, fibrosarcoma, rare anaplastic sarcomas, and gastric extramedullary plasmacytoma. Table 221-5 summarizes the prevalence, breed predisposition, and distribution of gastric tumors in dogs.

Benign Tumors
Benign tumors of the stomach include leiomyomas and less frequently, adenomatous polyps. Canine gastric leiomyoma is a tumor of old dogs, median age 16 years, and many are

Table • 221-5

Characteristics of Gastric Neoplasia in Dogs

TUMOR	MOST COMMON LOCATION	MEDIAN AGE (YEARS)	REPORTED BREED PREDISPOSITION
Adenocarcinoma	Pyloric antrum, lesser curvature	10	Belgian shepherd Rough Collie Staffordshire Bull terrier Lundehund
Leiomyoma	Cardia	16	Beagle
Leiomyosarcoma		7	none
Lymphosarcoma	Diffuse	10	none

discovered incidentally at necropsy or when they are presented for GI bleeding and microcytic anemia (Figure 221-15).

Adenomatous polyps are rare in dogs but have been reported as either raised, sessile or pedunculated, single or multiple growths in the stomach. The most common site is the terminal pyloric antrum and although most are discovered incidentally, they may also cause signs of gastrointestinal upset with vomiting (Figure 221-16). In humans, adenomatous polyps are generally regarded as possible premalignant lesions and changes considered focally malignant have been found in dogs. Benign GI neoplasia in the cat occurs at a much lower frequency than in the dog, where up to 36% of all GI neoplasia is reported to be benign.

Malignant Tumors
Adenocarcinoma
Malignant adenocarcinoma is the most common gastric neoplasm in dogs and accounts for 47% to 72% of all canine

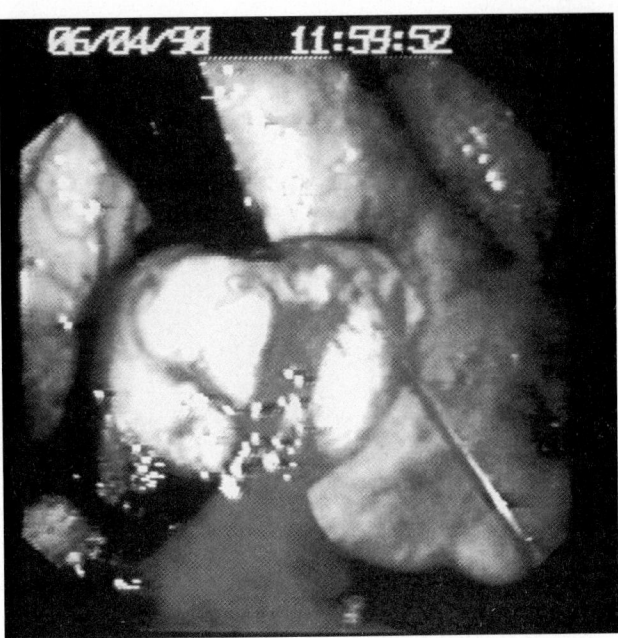

Figure 221-15 An ulcerated gastric leiomyoma in the cardia of a dog. (Courtesy of The Ohio State University.)

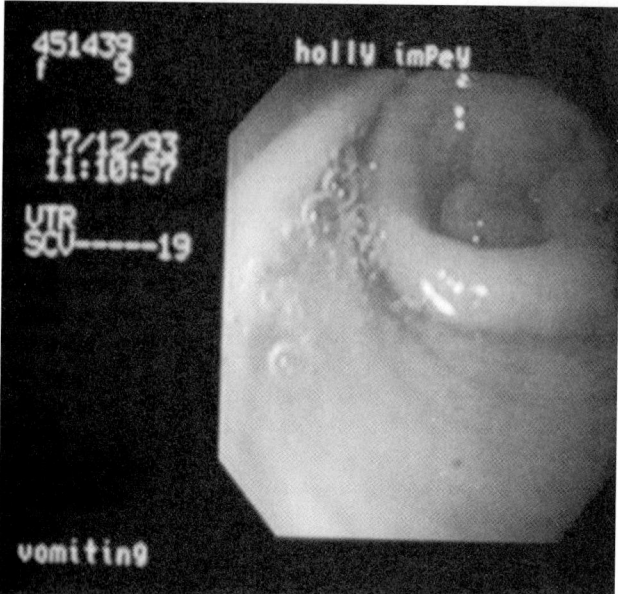

Figure 221-16 Adenomatous polyp in the pyloric outflow tract of a dog. (Courtesy of University of London.)

gastric malignancies.[96-99] Gastric adenocarcinoma is extremely rare in cats. The peak age of dogs with gastric carcinomas has been reported to be from 11 to 12 years with a range of 3 to 13 years and an average age of 9.1 to 10 years. A breed predilection for gastric carcinoma in related Belgian shepherd dogs and rough collie and Staffordshire bull terrier has been suggested, although the majority of studies show no significant breed predilections. Lundehunds with atrophic gastritis seem overrepresented, and gastric atrophy and inflammation may precede tumorigenesis as it does in humans.[79,88]

Gastric carcinomas of dogs occur most commonly in the lesser curvature and pyloric region as annular or stenosing lesions and metastasis is frequent with involvement of lymph nodes, lung, and liver (Figure 221-17). Carcinomas can be further divided into three morphologic patterns of distribution: (1) Diffusely infiltrating non-ulcerating lesions that involve most of the stomach and are consistent with the "leather bottle" appearance described in man, (2) Localized, raised thickened plaque usually containing a raised, excavating central ulcer, and (3) Raised, polypoid, sessile lesion projecting into the lumen of the stomach.

Two histologic types of gastric carcinoma exist in man: the diffuse and intestinal or tubular type. The diffuse type consists of widespread random infiltrates of neoplastic cells dispersed between stromal elements of the gastric wall. The intestinal type is characterized by a tubular, glandular structure. These same two classifications have been shown to exist in dogs with the diffuse type being more common.

Lymphosarcoma

The most common gastrointestinal neoplasm in both cats and dogs is lymphosarcoma, although it most often involves several segments of the intestinal tract. In canine lymphosarcoma (LSA) or lymphoma originating in the gastric submucosa the tumor type can be described as diffuse or nodular with the diffuse infiltrate being more common (Figure 221-18). Involvement of the liver, regional lymph nodes, small intestine, and bone marrow is common. Feline gastric lymphoma is not associated with FeLV infection and has been recently categorized as large cell or small cell, with small cell lymphoma being more localized to the GI tract and carrying a much better prognosis than large cell lymphoma.[100]

In both dogs and cats, lymphocytic-plasmacytic inflammation has been found to precede or coexist with gastric LSA, and it has been suggested that lymphocytic-plasmacytic enteritis (LPE) is a prelymphomatous change in the GI tract. The development of gastric lymphoma in response to chronic antigenic stimulation and inflammation is exemplified by gastric MALT lymphoma in people with *H. pylori*-associated gastritis. Whether a similar situation is present in dogs and cats remains to be determined.

Leiomyosarcoma

Leiomyosarcomas are slow growing tumors of smooth muscle origin. The median age for of affected dogs is greater than

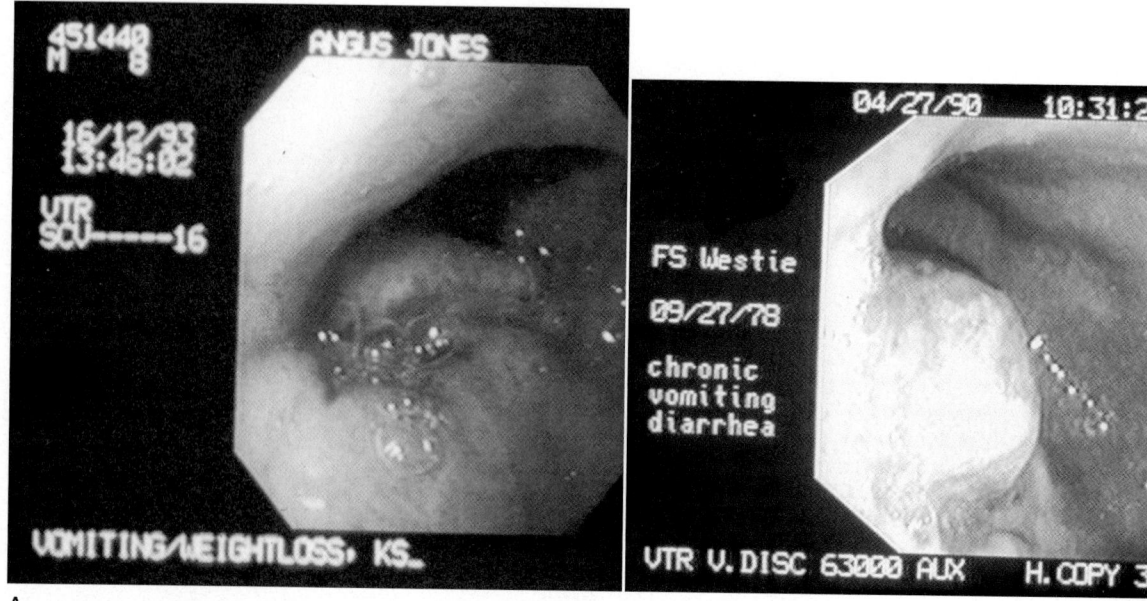

A   B

Figure 221-17 Endoscopic appearance of diffuse (**A**) and focal (**B**) gastric adenocarcinoma in a dog. (Courtesy of The Ohio State University.)

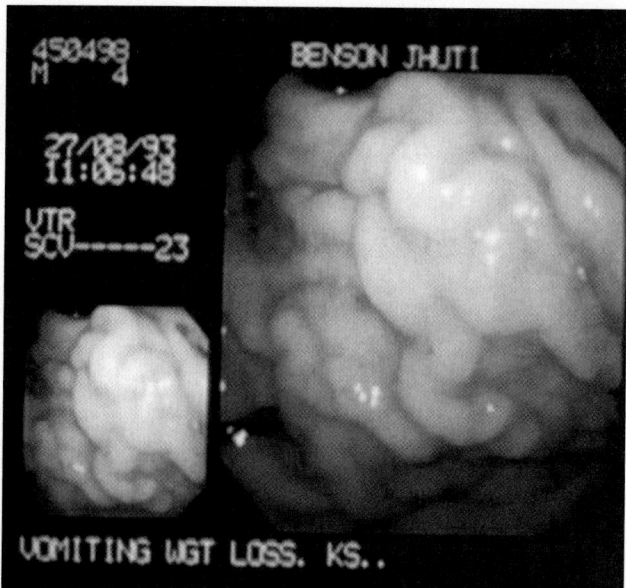

Figure 221-18 Gastric rugal thickening due to lymphoma. (Courtesy of University of London.)

10 years. Intestinal leiomyosarcoma has been found to be more common in female dogs and a predilection was reported in the German shepherd breed. However, neither breed nor sex predilection has been reported for gastric leiomyosarcoma.[101] In one study, dogs with leiomyosarcoma of the spleen, stomach, small intestine, and cecum were grouped together with 79% showing no evidence of metastases at surgery and 64% survived longer than 2 weeks.[101] Invasion of the gastric wall by leiomyosarcomas and lymphosarcomas is often diffuse. These tumors may cause ulceration, grossly resembling adenocarcinomas or appear as discrete masses. The median survival of these dogs was 10 months (range 1 month to 7 years). Of the stomach/small intestine group, 29% died of leiomyosarcoma eventually. Leiomyosarcoma and leiomyoma have been associated with paraneoplastic hypoglycemia and seizures presumed due to the production of insulin-like growth factors.[102]

Clinical Findings

The most common clinical signs associated with gastric neoplasia are chronic vomiting, weight loss, anorexia, diarrhea, and hematemesis, melena, or pallor if ulceration is present. Some dogs will also show abdominal pain or a distended abdomen. With GI lymphoma, the onset of clinical signs is often insidious and gradually increases in severity, becoming refractory to symptomatic treatment.

Diagnosis

Survey radiographs may be completely normal or suggest focal gastric wall thickening, an abdominal mass, or evidence of peritonitis, rupture of a viscus, splenomegaly, hepatomegaly, or lymphadenopathy.

Ultrasonography may reveal mural thickening or irregularities that forewarn the endoscopist the lesion may be more submucosal or muscular than superficial. Lympadenopathy or regional metasasis may be evident.

Gastroscopy is able to efficiently detect most gastric tumors and has largely replaced contrast radiography. Lymphosarcoma is seen as a diffuse, smooth, or cobblestone-like thickening of the rugae with a mucosa that is pink or white and may have scattered petechial or ecchymotic hemorrhages. Gastric carcinomas tend to be focal dark pink to red masses that may appear slightly pedunculated. Discolored purple to black areas indicate hemorrhage, whereas yellow to brown foci often represent necrotic ulcers. In some cases, lesions may be submucosal and the endoscopist gets the impression that something is indenting the stomach or the wall seems less distensible or thick.

Several biopsy samples should be taken from suspicious areas and masses should be biopsied multiple times in the same place to get deeper into tissue as gastric tumors may have superficial necrosis, inflammation, and ulceration. These centers of ulcers and craters should be avoided, taking biopsies at the periphery to avoid perforation. Surgical biopsies should be taken where the gross endoscopic appearance does not match the histologic diagnosis, such as a large focal gastric mass with an endoscopic biopsy result of lymphoplasmacytic gastritis.

When endoscopy is not available contrast radiography may be useful with features of gastric neoplasia including thickening of the gastric wall, filling defects and derangement of normal rugal pattern, and delayed gastric emptying with retention and irregular pooling of barium. Surgery is then performed to sample the affected area.

Treatment

Except for lymphosarcoma, surgery is the most common form of treatment for gastric cancer. Resection may be curative if the affected area is localized or if the tumor is benign. If a widespread area is involved, a partial gastrectomy or antrectomy followed by gastroduodenostomy (Billroth I) may be attempted. However, many patients are presented at a late stage of disease and the lesions are often too extensive to resect. Gastric adeoncarcinoma often metastasizes and regional lymph nodes and liver should be inspected and biopsied. Even with surgery the prognosis for malignant gastric neoplasia is poor, with most patients dying within 6 months from recurrent or metastatic disease. Leiomyosarcoma is an exception and carries a good to excellent prognosis if the mass is surgically resectable. Even if gross metastasis is evident at surgery, a favorable outcome may be achieved because the tumor is slow growing. Survival in dogs with stomach, small intestinal, splenic, and cecal leiomyosarcoma ranges from 0 to 47 months after surgery and the median survival is 12.5 months.[101]

Gastrointestinal lymphosarcoma has a poor prognosis in dogs.[103] In cats the prognosis depends if the tumor is small or large cell. Small cell lymphomas achieve substantial remission when treated with chlorambucil and prednisolone.[100] Large cell lymphoma is treated with combination cyclical chemotherapy and carries a much poorer prognosis.

CHAPTER 222

Diseases of the Small Intestine

Edward J. Hall
Alexander J. German

The small intestine (SI) must be capable of performing digestive and absorptive functions while simultaneously protecting the body from a multitude of environmental threats. Thus it is the largest and most complex immunologic organ in the body, and armed with an understanding of its immunologic role, the clinician will be better able to understand and treat many intestinal diseases.

Considering the complex, paradoxical roles of the small intestine, minor daily variations in stool quality must be considered normal. *Diarrhea*, a significant increase in the frequency, fluidity, or volume of feces, is the cardinal sign of SI malfunction. However, diarrhea may also be a manifestation of disease elsewhere in the gastrointestinal (GI) tract or even in other organ systems (Box 222-1). Furthermore, diarrhea is not present in all cases of SI disease, and many other signs of SI disorder are nonspecific and may be overlooked (Box 222-2). Nevertheless, an understanding of normal SI function, in particular the small intestine's role as an immunologic organ, allows a logical approach to diagnosis and treatment.

STRUCTURE AND FUNCTION OF THE SMALL INTESTINE

Normal Structure

Gross Structure
The small intestine runs from the pylorus of the stomach to the ileocolic valve (Figure 222-1, *A*). It is divided anatomically into three arbitrary segments: the proximal duodenum (Figure 222-2), the jejunum, and the distal ileum.[1]

Microstructure
The small intestine is in essence a tube connected to the external environment (Figure 222-1, *B*). Its basic cross-sectional structure of serosa, muscularis, submucosa, and mucosa is present throughout (Figure 222-1, *C*) but varies in proportions, reflecting the varying functions of each region.

The *mucosa* is the most clinically important layer of the intestine. It is responsible for secretion and absorption and serves as a barrier. It comprises the epithelium and the lamina propria and is modified by gross folds and fingerlike processes, the *villi* (see Figure 222-1, *C*). Mucosal capillaries are fenestrated; in conjunction with a central villus lymphatic (*lacteal*), they carry away protein-rich tissue fluid. Loss of epithelial integrity permits leakage of the protein-rich fluid and the development of a protein-losing enteropathy (PLE). The lamina propria contains aggregates of lymphoid tissue and nonaggregated immunocytes (see Gastrointestinal Immune System).

Functional Anatomy

Surface Area of the Small Intestine
The surface area of the small intestine is increased almost 600-fold, compared with that of a simple tube, by folds in the mucosal wall (~3 fold), cylindrical projections into the intestinal lumen called villi (~10 fold), and microscopic microvilli on the surface of each epithelial cell (~20 fold) (see Figure 222-1). Villus atrophy or even just microvillar damage is likely to produce profound malabsorption and diarrhea.

Box • 222-1

Causes of Diarrhea

Gastrointestinal Disease
Primary small intestinal disease
Primary large intestinal disease
Dietary-induced causes (food poisoning, gluttony, sudden change of diet)
Gastric disease
  Achlorhydria*
  Dumping syndromes*
Pancreatic disease
  Exocrine pancreatic insufficiency
  Pancreatitis
  Pancreatic neoplasia
Liver disease
  Hepatocellular failure
  Intrahepatic and extrahepatic cholestasis

Nongastrointestinal Disease
Polysystemic infection (e.g., distemper, leptospirosis, infectious canine hepatitis in dogs; FIP, FeLV, FIV in cats)
Endocrine disease
  Hypoadrenocorticism
  Hyperthyroidism†
  Hypothyroidism
  APUDomas (gastrinoma or Zollinger-Ellison syndrome)*
Renal disease
  Uremia
  Nephrotic syndrome
Miscellaneous
  Toxemias (pyometra, peritonitis)
  Congestive heart failure
  Autoimmune disease
  Metastatic neoplasia
  Various toxins and drugs

*Rare conditions.
†Rare in dogs only.
APUD, amine precursor uptake and decarboxylation tumor
FeLV, feline leukemia virus
FIP, feline infectious peritonitis
FIV, feline immunodeficiency virus

Box • 222-2

Clinical Signs of Small Intestinal Disease

Primary Sign
Diarrhea (increase in frequency, volume, and consistency of bowel movements)

Secondary Signs
Vomiting
Weight loss and/or failure to thrive
Hematemesis
Melena
Altered appetite (inappetence/anorexia)
Polyphagia, coprophagia, pica
Abdominal discomfort, pain
Abdominal distension
Borborygmi and flatus
Halitosis
Dehydration
Polydipsia
Ascites and edema
Shock

Crypt-Villus Unit

A villus and its associated crypts comprise the functional unit of the small intestine (see Figure 222-1, D). Crypts continually produce undifferentiated epithelial cells, mainly enterocytes. After further division of daughter cells as they pass up the crypt, cells undergo a final division before differentiating into immature enterocytes.

Mucosal Epithelial Cells

The intestinal surface is covered by an epithelial cell monolayer. Enterocytes predominate, interspersed mainly with mucus-secreting goblet cells. The epithelial basement membrane is permeable to nutrients, and by expressing glycoproteins, called *laminins*, it promotes enterocyte adhesion, growth, polarization, and differentiation through interaction with integrins expressed by enterocytes.[2]

Crypt cells have a potent secretory capacity. However, as enterocytes migrate to the villus tip, maturation involves loss of secretory activity and the development of digestive and absorptive properties. The duration of migration from crypt to villus tip is 3 to 5 days in dogs and cats. The majority of enterocytes are exfoliated at the tips of the villi.

Goblet cell density in the mucosa varies, being highest in the ileum. The cells secrete protective mucus and novel trefoil peptides, which act as growth factors. Endocrine- and paracrine-secreting epithelial cells, as well as transforming growth factors α and β (TGFα) and epidermal growth factor (EGF), have important trophic activities. Receptors for EGF on the luminal and basolateral surfaces of enterocytes suggest they respond both to blood-borne EGF and to luminal EGF secreted from salivary and pancreatic tissue or delivered in milk.

Enterocytes

The *mucosal barrier* is formed by the intestinal epithelium; tight junctions encircle the lateral aspects of enterocytes, excluding antigens and bacteria. Effete enterocytes are shed from the villus tip (see Figure 222-1, D), but the integrity of the tight junctions is probably loosest in the crypts, where fluid secretion occurs.

Enterocyte function dictates normal digestion and nutrient absorption. Function depends on the polarity of the enterocyte, involving a specialized portion of the cell membrane on the luminal surface, the *microvillar membrane (MVM)*. The MVM, also called the *brush border* because of its microscopic appearance (see Fig. 222-1, E and F), consists of thousands of parallel cylindrical processes, the microvilli, bearing digestive enzymes and specific carrier proteins (see Figure 222-1, F). Maximum enzyme and transport activities are expressed in the midvillus region. As enterocytes migrate to the villus tip, enzymes are cleaved from the brush border by bacterial and pancreatic proteases and released into the lumen to form the succus entericus, which is thus not a true secretion.

Enterocyte metabolism is geared toward the production of brush border proteins and the transfer of nutrients from the lumen to the blood. Basolateral cell membranes export sodium from the cell via energy-dependent sodium-potassium adenosine triphosphatase (Na/K ATPase). Water can follow osmotically, or compensatory sodium influx at the luminal surface can drive carrier-mediated nutrient absorption. Natural inhibition of glycolysis in enterocytes facilitates the transfer of glucose from the lumen to the blood. Enterocytes can utilize ketone bodies, but their major energy source is glutamine. Both are derived from the lumen, which explains the decline in villus structure, epithelial integrity, and absorptive function in starvation and anorexia and therefore the clinical importance of attempting to maintain enteral nutrition.[3]

Brush border enzyme activities are variable, tending to be highest in the proximal SI and declining in an aboral gradient. Digestive enzymes, especially disaccharidases and transport proteins, may be inducible in response to the composition of the diet. This has been shown in dogs[4] but not in cats,[5] perhaps reflecting the carnivorous nature of cats. A sudden change in diet in dogs may cause diarrhea through transient intolerance until either existing enterocytes upregulate expression of specific enzymes and carriers or new enterocytes expressing induced proteins differentiate, thus rendering the diarrhea self-limiting.

Digestion

Major dietary constituents must be hydrolyzed from their initial polymeric structure to monomers to be transported across the MVM. This is largely achieved in the SI by bile salts and luminal enzymes. The intestine provides the optimum environment in terms of solute, temperature, and pH. Most enzymes are secreted by the pancreas, and exocrine pancreatic insufficiency (EPI) is a major cause of malabsorption. Normally only terminal digestion is performed by MVM enzymes; the reserve capacity called into function after significant intestinal resection probably represents both increases in brush border protein expression and compensatory hypertrophy of the remaining tissue (see Short Bowel Syndrome).

Lactose is found almost exclusively in dairy products, and its hydrolysis by brush border lactase is most important in the nursing animal. At weaning, activities of lactase decline, especially in cats,[5] and animals may become lactose intolerant, although congenital lactase deficiency has not been demonstrated in dogs or cats.

Absorption

Digested nutrients are delivered to the body across the mucosal barrier and then via the lymphatics or bloodstream. Uptake can occur by passive diffusion or by active or facilitated carrier-mediated transport. Receptor-mediated endocytosis enables the uptake of small amounts of a specific intact nutrient, such as cobalamin. Endocytosis of small, antigenic peptides is of no nutritional significance but is crucial to the mucosal immune response.

GASTROINTESTINAL DISEASE

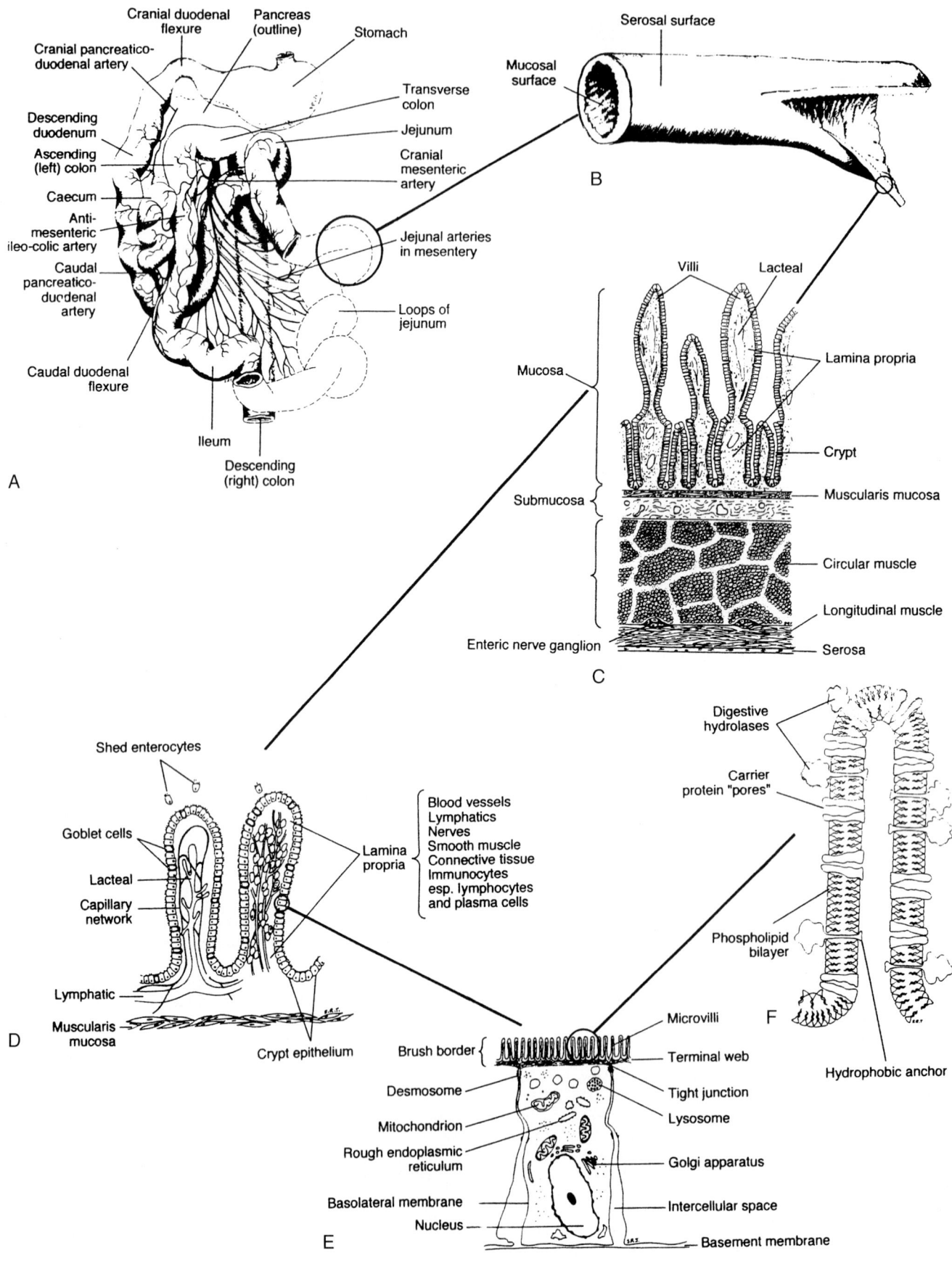

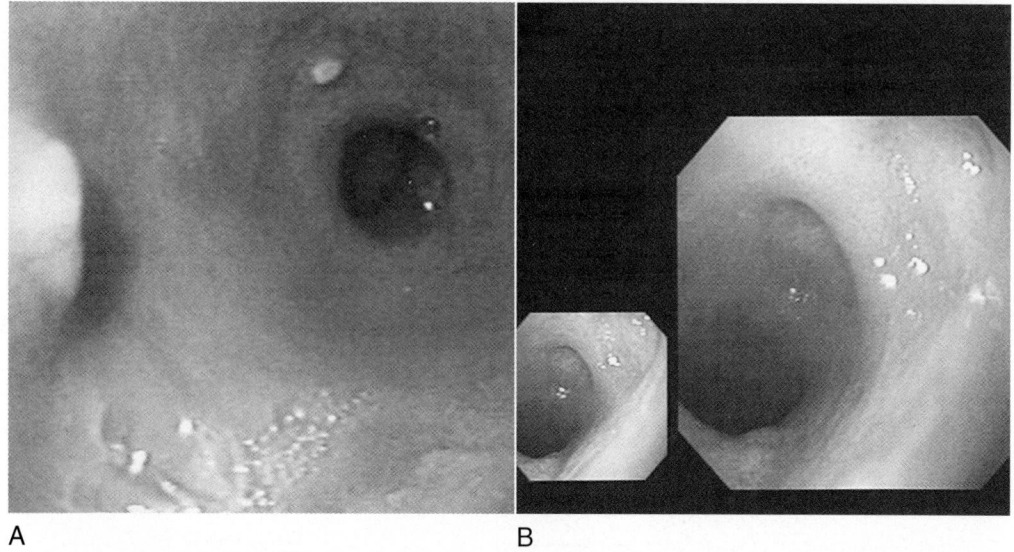

A   B

Figure 222-2 Video-endoscopic appearance of the upper small intestine. **A,** Major and minor duodenal papillae in a normal canine duodenum. **B,** Peyer's patches on the antimesenteric side of the duodenum, appearing as a line of mucosal depressions.

Carbohydrate Absorption

Glucose is transported across the MVM with energy expenditure by the basolateral Na/K ATPase on the sodium-glucose cotransporter protein SGLT 1. The glucose transporter GLUT 5 on the MVM allows facilitated diffusion of fructose and D-xylose. Fructose uptake in cats is low, which perhaps explains why the xylose absorption test is unhelpful in cats. GLUT 2 on the basolateral membrane of enterocytes shuttles glucose, galactose, and fructose out of the enterocyte by facilitated diffusion.

Protein Absorption

L-amino acids are absorbed on stereo-specific carriers by sodium-linked active transport.

Lipid Absorption

The products of fat digestion are absorbed by passive diffusion from mixed micelles. The limiting factor, assuming normal pancreatic function, is the intestinal surface area, and villus atrophy is likely to cause fat malabsorption.

Fat-Soluble Vitamins

Vitamins A, D, E, and K are solubilized in mixed micelles before passive diffusion across the brush border. Fat malabsorption associated with inadequate amounts of bile salts (i.e., biliary obstruction), lymphangiectasia, or severe villus atrophy may result in vitamin deficiency.

Water-Soluble Vitamins

Water-soluble B vitamins are absorbed by a variety of passive, facilitated, and active mechanisms. The absorptive mechanisms for folic acid and vitamin B_{12} are complex (Figure 222-3, *A*) and important clinically because they may be helpful in determining the site and nature of the intestinal disease (Figure 222-3, *B*).

Folic acid is absorbed in the proximal SI through a carrier-mediated process at low luminal concentrations. *Cobalamin*

Figure 222-1 Functional anatomy of the small intestine. **A,** Anatomic arrangement of the small intestine. **B,** The small intestine is basically a tube with a serosal surface covered by visceral peritoneum and an inner absorptive and digestive surface, the mucosa. **C,** Beneath the outer serosa, longitudinal and circular muscle layers produce peristaltic and segmental contractions for propelling and mixing the luminal contents. The submucosa is rich in blood and lymphatic vessels. The mucosa comprises the thin muscularis mucosa, the lamina propria, and the columnar epithelium; it is thrown into folds and is covered by fingerlike villi to increase the digestive and absorptive surface area. **D,** Enterocytes, which are shed from the villus tip but are continually replaced through division of crypt cells, are the site of nutrient digestion and absorption. Goblet cells secrete protective mucus. Water-soluble nutrients pass into the rich capillary network of the lamina propria, and fat is passed as chylomicrons into the lacteals. Immunocytes in the lamina propria are involved in maintaining tolerance to luminal antigens. **E,** The luminal membrane of the enterocyte is thrown into processes called *microvilli*, which increase the luminal surface area. Tight junctions between enterocytes maintain epithelial integrity. Absorbed nutrients are passed from the enterocyte into the intercellular space for distribution to the body. **F,** A schematic representation of a microvillus showing digestive hydrolases anchored in the phospholipid cell membrane and protruding into the intestinal lumen. Carrier proteins in the membrane are believed to act as "pores," shuttling nutrients across the membrane by means of conformational changes in their structure often induced by sodium influx at the expense of energy utilization through Na/K ATPase on the basolateral membrane. (From Hall EJ: Small intestinal disease. In Gorman NT (ed): *Canine Medicine and Therapeutics,* 4th ed. Blackwell Science, Oxford, 1998, p 488.)

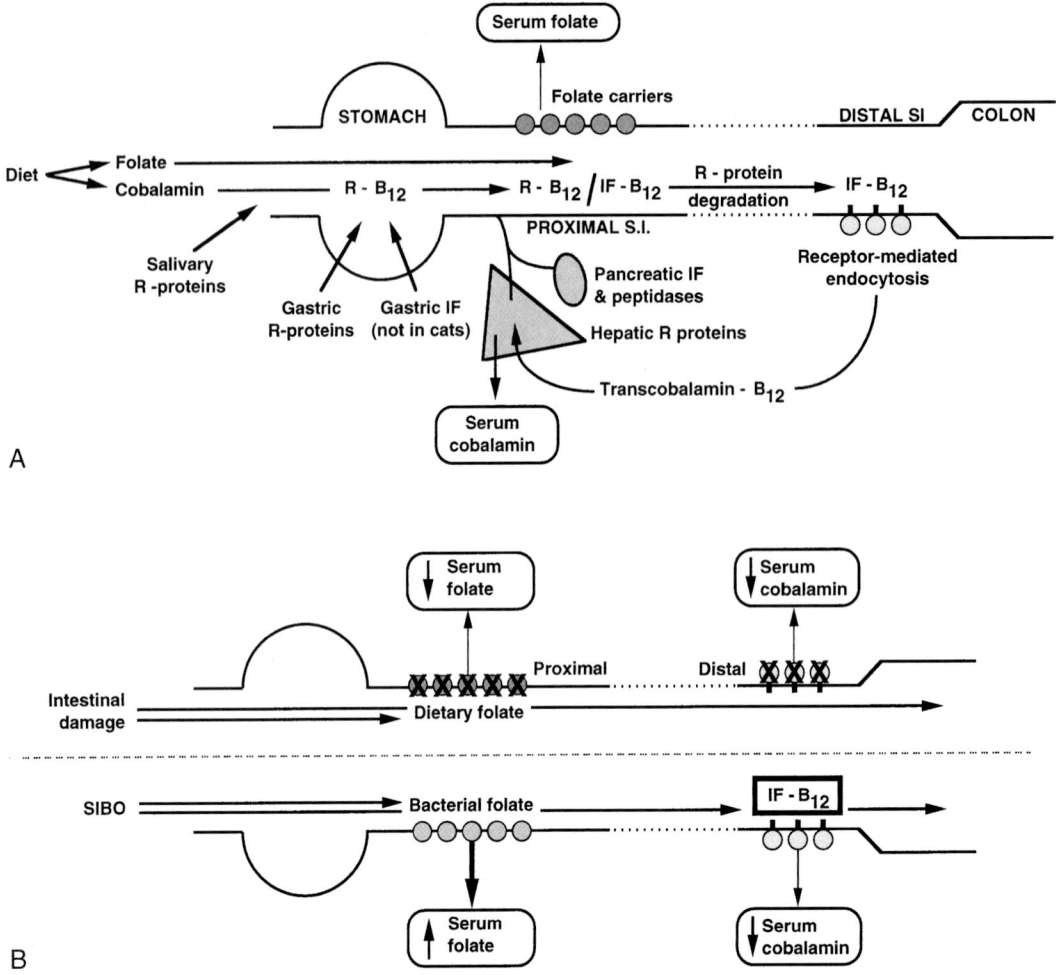

Figure 222-3 Diagrammatic representation of the absorption of folate and cobalamin. **A,** In normal intestine, folate is absorbed in the proximal SI by means of carrier-mediated diffusion, and cobalamin is absorbed in the ileum through receptor-mediated endocytosis. **B,** In diseased intestine, proximal and distal mucosal damage causes folate and cobalamin malabsorption, respectively; bacterial overgrowth may cause an increase in folate uptake because of bacterial folate synthesis and a decrease in cobalamin uptake because of bacterial binding.

(vitamin B_{12}) is absorbed by means of receptor-mediated endocytosis in the ileum, in a complex process that permits intact cobalamin absorption and exclusion of potentially harmful analogs. Intrinsic factor (IF) promotes cobalamin absorption in the ileum; IF-bound cobalamin passes to the ileum, where the complex binds specific receptors and undergoes endocytosis. The source of IF is the stomach and pancreas in dogs and solely the pancreas in cats.[6,7] Cats and dogs have less capacity to store cobalamin than do humans, and severe cobalamin malabsorption can deplete the vitamin's stores in cats and dogs within a month.

Intestinal Motility

Slow wave motion and segmental and peristaltic contractions of the SI are generated by the co-ordinated contraction of smooth muscle in response to spontaneous electrical activity modulated by co-ordinated neurohumoral and neurochemical molecules.[8] Many of these neurohumoral and neurochemical molecules are also involved in the regulation of intestinal secretion and absorption and the mucosal immune response.[9]

Intestinal motility in the fasted state in dogs is characterized by three phases. A cycle comprising a quiescent phase (lasting about 1 hour), minor contractile activity (15 to

40 minutes), and migrating myoelectric complexes (MMCs) (4 to 8 minutes) is repeated approximately every 3 hours.[10] The short MMC phase is a period of intense contractile activity that sweeps undigested food, secretions, desquamated cells, and bacteria down the intestine. This process is known as the "intestinal housekeeper" wave and is induced by motilin secretion. The pattern of intestinal motility in cats is different, but a migrating spike complex correlates with the MMC.

In the fed state, the pattern of motility is most similar to phase two fasting motility. Its duration is determined by the nature of the diet, with fats and fiber prolonging it. Segmental contractions slow intestinal transit and ensure mixing and digestion of nutrients, and peristalsis propels ingesta. Reduced segmental motility may lead to rapid transit, and decreased peristalsis delays transit, conditions manifesting clinically as diarrhea and ileus, respectively.

Fluid Balance

The ability of the intestine to absorb fluid and electrolytes varies according to the site, with water absorption becoming increasingly efficient distally. The net amount of fluid and electrolytes in the GI tract reflects a balance between absorption and secretion, with net absorption in health.

Intestinal Secretion

Intestinal secretion, a function of villus crypt cells, is believed to occur by electrogenic transport of chloride across the basolateral membrane into the enterocyte and by chloride efflux through chloride channels in the MVM. Passive flux of water follows chloride secretion into the intestinal lumen.

Absorption

In a 20-kg dog, approximately 2.7 L of fluid (oral intake, stomach juice, saliva, pancreatic juice, bile, and SI secretion) is presented to the SI each day. The jejunum absorbs 50%, the ileum, 75%, and the colon, 90% of the fluid volume presented to it, leaving 0.05 L in feces.[11] This gradient in absorptive ability is a function of enterocyte pore size, membrane potential difference, and the type of transport processes associated with each intestinal segment.[12] The site of the enterocyte on the villus is also important; villus enterocytes absorb, whereas crypt cells secrete.

The absorption of water is passive and follows transport of solutes across the GI epithelium by one of three processes: passive absorption, active absorption, or solvent drag.

Jejunum Because the jejunum is highly permeable, passive transport provides the major contribution to sodium (Na) and chloride (Cl) movement in this segment.

Ileum In the ileum, sodium is absorbed predominantly through neutral NaCl absorption.

Colon Colonic absorption is important in SI disease, because it compensates for fluid losses. Furthermore, patients with SI disease may present with signs of large intestinal (LI) dysfunction, because the colonic reserve capacity may be overwhelmed. In addition, products from the SI, such as hydroxylated fatty acids and deconjugated bile acids, stimulate colonic secretion.

Control of the Absorption and Secretion of Water and Electrolytes

Fluid balance is largely an autonomous process regulated by the neurocrine systems in the submucosal plexus.[12] Vasoactive intestinal polypeptide (VIP) and acetylcholine are major mediators of secretion; at the cellular level they increase intracellular calcium and cyclic adenosine monophosphate (cAMP), inhibit neutral sodium and chloride absorption, and facilitate transcellular chloride efflux. Many bacterial agents exert diarrheogenic effects by increasing intraenterocytic cAMP. The principal regulators of absorption—noradrenaline, somatostatin, and opioids—lower intracellular cAMP and calcium concentrations and stimulate neutral NaCl absorption and thereby can have therapeutic antidiarrheal effects.

Bacterial Flora

The normal SI bacterial flora is a diverse mixture of aerobic, anaerobic, and facultatively anaerobic bacteria. Common aerobes include *Staphylococcus* spp., *Streptococcus* spp., Enterobacteriaceae, *Escherichia coli*, *Bacillus* spp., *Proteus* spp., *Pasteurella* spp., *Corynebacterium* spp., *Lactobacillus* spp., and *Enterococcus* spp. Frequent anaerobes are *Clostridium* spp. and *Bacteroides* spp.

The flora increases in number from duodenum to colon. Factors maintaining this aboral gradient are luminal patency, motility, substrate availability, bacteriostatic and bacteriocidal secretions (e.g., gastric acid, bile, and pancreatic secretions), and an intact ileocolic valve. Abnormalities or dysfunction of any of these factors may lead to quantitative or qualitative abnormalities in the flora.

Quantitative bacteriology performed on samples of undiluted intestinal juice has revealed bacterial counts in healthy cats range from 10^2 to 10^8 colony-forming units (CFU) per milliliter of total bacteria in the proximal small intestine.[13,14] These numbers are considerably higher than the less than 10^5 CFU/mL reported in healthy humans and subsequently extrapolated to dogs. However, no consensus exists as to what constitutes a normal SI flora count in healthy dogs; some studies suggest that the proximal SI of healthy dogs can harbor up to 10^9 CFU/mL total bacteria.[15] Therefore the cutoff for normal flora in dogs and cats cannot be extrapolated from humans, and descriptions of small intestinal bacterial overgrowth (SIBO) in dogs using the cutoff value of 10^5 may be spurious.[15]

The resident bacterial flora is an integral part of the healthy SI and influences a wide variety of parameters, such as villus size, enterocyte turnover, brush border enzyme turnover, and intestinal motility. The digestion and assimilation of fats, carbohydrates, proteins, amino acids (e.g., taurine), and vitamins (e.g., cobalamin and folate) are also affected by bacteria.

The presence of a stable enteric flora is important for preventing colonization by pathogens; it also stimulates the development of the enteric immune system. The host response to a bacterium is likely to be as important as the intrinsic pathogenicity of the organism. Loss of tolerance to the normal bacterial flora may precipitate intestinal inflammation, abnormal intestinal function, and perhaps even neoplasia. Inability to tolerate a normal bacterial flora may explain antibiotic-responsive enteropathy in German shepherd dogs (see Small Intestinal Bacterial Overgrowth).

The SI flora is relatively resistant to dietary changes. Studies using different diets or the addition of fructo-oligosaccharides to the diet have failed to demonstrate significant effects on the number or type of bacteria in the proximal SI of dogs,[16,17] but some effects have been seen on the colonic flora in cats.[18] Given the intimate inter-relationship of a healthy intestine with its flora, indiscriminate use of anti-biotics in dogs and cats with diarrhea or gastroenteritis is ill-advised and may enhance antibiotic resistance. Although the consequences of inappropriate antibiotic therapy are often mild and self-limiting, postantibiotic salmonellosis has had fatal consequences in cats.[19]

Gastrointestinal Immune System

The SI mucosa has a general barrier function (Box 222-3); however, it must also generate a protective immune response against pathogens while remaining "tolerant" of harmless environmental antigens such as commensal bacteria and food. Despite recent advances in our understanding of the structure of and interactions in the immune system, it is still unclear what prompts the SI to respond to or to become tolerant of a particular antigen.

Box • 222-3

Components of the Intestinal Mucosal Barrier

Protein denaturation by gastric acid
Protein degradation by proteolytic enzymes
   and bacteria
Clearance of waste by peristalsis
Unstirred water layer
Surface mucous layer
Secretory IgA
Enterocyte microvillus membrane
Epithelial tight junctions
Mucosal-associated lymphoid tissue

Structure of the Mucosal Immune System

The gut-associated lymphoid tissue (GALT) consists of inductive and effector sites.[20] Inductive sites comprise Peyer's patches (PPs), isolated lymphoid follicles, and the mesenteric lymph nodes (MLNs); effector sites comprise the intestinal lamina propria (LP) and epithelium. Such a distinction is not absolute, however, and the functions of these different sites overlap.

The PPs are the main sites of induction of the immune response and may also function as sites of B-lymphocyte development. The PP consists of an overlying follicle-associated epithelium (FAE), a subepithelial dome (SED), multiple B-cell follicles, and interfollicular regions. Within the FAE is a specialized population of antigen transport cells (microfold cells or M cells), which act as portals through which the underlying immune cells receive antigen. The MLNs receive afferent lymph from the intestine and are also important in the generation of immune responses.

The LP consists of a matrix of connective tissue with a prominent immune cell component. A large leukocyte population, composed principally of lymphocytes (intraepithelial lymphocytes [IELs]), also exists between enterocytes. Accumulating evidence indicates that *cross-talk* (two-way immunoregulatory signals mediated by cytokines and adhesion molecules) occurs between IELs and enterocytes.[21]

Cells and Molecules of the Mucosal Immune System

Lymphocytes   *B lymphocytes* are present in the Peyer's patches and the lamina propria. In the PPs they are found predominantly in follicular regions. In the LP, B cells are largely represented by plasma cells, mostly of the IgA isotype. Most plasma cells are present around the intestinal crypts, and the numbers vary along the length of the small intestine.[22]

In the SI, most *T lymphocytes* are of the conventional alpha/beta type.[23] An evolutionarily older (gamma/delta) T-cell population also exists and is considered a primitive first-line defense.[23] T lymphocytes can be further subdivided on the basis of expression of cell surface markers, in particular CD4 and CD8 molecules. CD4+ T cells (classical "helper" T cells) recognize antigenic peptide presented by major histocompatibility complex class II (MHC II) molecules, whereas CD8+ T cells (usually cytotoxic cells) are MHC class I restricted.

In the canine LP, T cells are most numerous in the upper villus regions and are mostly the alpha/beta, CD4+ phenotype.[22-24] However, in the feline LP, CD8+ T cells outnumber the CD4+ population.[25] Most LP lymphocytes are highly differentiated, which implies that they receive continuous antigenic and mitogenic stimulation, probably from the endogenous microbial flora.

The T cells in the intestinal epithelium (i.e., IELs) are a heterogeneous population; most are CD8+ cells, which may be of either the alpha/beta or the gamma/delta phenotype, depending on the species. Known functions of IELs include cytolytic activity and cytokine production, which suggests that these cells play roles in epithelial surveillance and the maintenance of mucosal immune homeostasis.

Dendritic cells   Dendritic cells (DCs) function predominantly as antigen-presenting cells and can be found in both inductive (PP) and effector (LP) tissues. In effector tissues their main function is antigen sampling, whereas in inductive sites they are responsible for generating acquired immune responses. Follicular dendritic cells (FDCs) are a unique population of cells[26] that take up and store antigen to provide continued stimulation to memory B cells. Immature DCs can efficiently acquire and process antigen but cannot present it or initiate immune responses.[27] Conversely, mature DCs cannot take up or process antigen but are efficient at antigen presentation and lymphocyte stimulation.[27]

Other immune cells   Macrophages are present in the PP and LP. Their functions include phagocytosis, antigen presentation, and immunoregulatory roles. They secrete cytokines, chemokines, and inflammatory mediators, including tumor necrosis factor-α (TNF-α), eicosanoids, and leukotrienes. Neutrophils are present in small numbers, although their numbers increase with mucosal inflammation. Both mast cells (MCs) and eosinophils can be found in the LP; they also actively produce chemical mediators (e.g., histamine, heparin, eicosanoids, and cytokines). Mast cells express the high-affinity IgE receptor (FcεRI), which can bind IgE, causing MC degranulation and release of inflammatory mediators.[28] In dogs, eosinophils are a prominent population in the LP, especially in the crypts. Eosinophils[22] may have proinflammatory roles, especially in allergic processes, because they are a rich source of proinflammatory mediators, cytokines, and chemokines.[28] Triangular cross-talk may occur among eosinophils, MCs, and T cells.

Enterocytes   In addition to absorptive functions, enterocytes have important immune functions. First, they are an important component of the mucosal barrier, controlling uptake of antigens. Second, they may be capable of antigen presentation, through expression of MHC II and nonclassical antigen-presenting molecules. In dogs, MHC II is expressed by enterocytes, most abundantly in crypt epithelium.[29] In contrast, MHC II is largely absent from the intestinal epithelium of cats, except in regions adjacent to Peyer's patches.[25] Third, enterocytes can produce inflammatory mediators, chemokines, and cytokines and may regulate immune responses in both epithelial and LP compartments. Cross-talk between enterocytes and IELs may also occur through cell to cell interactions (e.g., between E-cadherin expressed on the enterocyte and the integrin alpha$_e$/beta$_7$, expressed by IEL).[30]

Enteric neurons   The SI also contains a well-developed nervous system with extensive ramification in both inductive and effector sites.[31] These neurons can release immunoactive neuropeptides (including substance P and VIP), which can cause *neurogenic* inflammation. Bidirectional communication may also exist, in which release of mediators by immune cells (e.g., mast cells) can generate axon reflexes and thereby perhaps modulate intestinal motility, secretion, and absorption.

Cytokines   A large array of cytokines is present in the SI, and these cells can be grouped into proinflammatory, immunoregulatory, and chemokinetic types.[32] CD4+ T cells are a major cytokine-producing cell population. Different CD4+ T-cell populations have different patterns of cytokine secretion and can differentially regulate distinct arms of the immune system (e.g., humoral and cell mediated). *In vitro*, two principal populations of CD4+ T cells exist: a T helper 1 (Th1) population (which produces interleukin-2 [IL-2], interferon-γ [IFN-γ], and TNF-β), and a T helper 2 (Th2) population (which produces IL-4, IL-5, IL-6 and IL-10).[33] Other populations with downregulatory functions also have been identified, which predominantly secrete TGF-β or IL-10.[34] Many other cell types also may produce cytokines (see above) and, consequently, an overall cytokine "milieu," which determines the predominant type of immune response that develops, is created.

Homing of Lymphocytes in Gut-Associated Lymphoid Tissue

To mount an effective immune response, lymphocytes must traffic between the inductive and the effector sites. Such homing pathways are mediated by complex leukocyte-endothelial interactions. Those governing recirculation to mucosal tissues are distinct from systemic tissues,[35] because differential expression

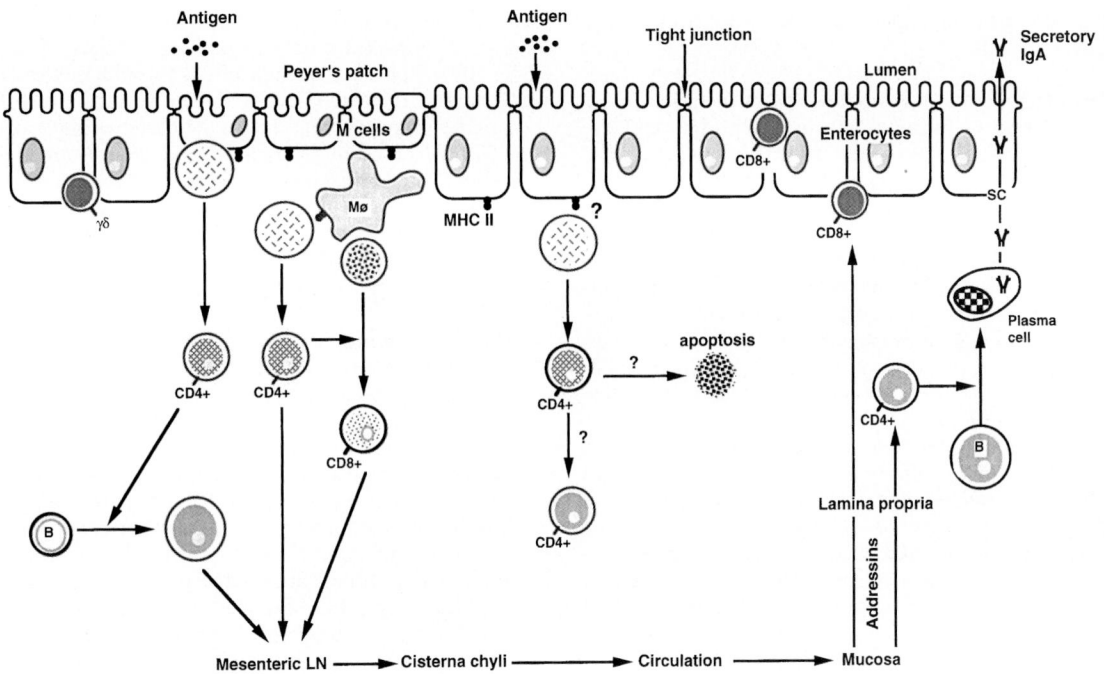

Figure 222-4 Diagrammatic representation of the mucosal-associated lymphoid tissue, showing M cells in a Peyer's patch sampling luminal antigen, presentation of the antigen to the associated lymphoid tissue, priming of B and T cells, and their circulation to the lamina propria, with subsequent IgA secretion.

of homing receptors (addressins) determines the specificity of homing. Virtually all naïve mucosal lymphocytes can home to the PPs, MLNs, and other nodes in the body. In contrast, mucosal memory lymphocytes home preferentially to effector sites in the GALT.

Tissue migration of cells from the blood vessel is a multi-stage process involving a number of molecular interactions. The most important interaction for mucosal lymphocytes occurs between alpha$_4$/beta$_7$ on the lymphocyte and mucosal addressin cell adhesion molecule-1 (MAdCAM-1) on the endothelial cell.[23]

Inflammation causes increased activation of both lymphocytes and endothelial cells, which alters the expression of both homing receptors and vascular addressins. Enhanced expression of MAdCAM-1 leads to increased recruitment of specific mucosal lymphocytes, whereas expression of other vascular addressins (e.g., E-selectin, P-selectin and peripheral node addressin) can lead to recruitment of a broader range of lymphocyte specificities.[36]

A final factor important to the homing of lymphocytes is the chemokines and their receptors.[37] Because chemokine receptors can be selectively expressed on different CD4+ T cell subsets (Th1 versus Th2), the chemokine milieu of a particular tissue determines which T-helper cell types (and which other immune cell subsets) are recruited.

Acquired Immune Responses of Gut-Associated Lymphoid Tissue

Acquired immune responses develop after a series of steps involving antigen uptake, presentation to naïve lymphocytes, costimulation by helper cells, clonal expansion, homing to effector sites, and performance of effector functions. The specific mechanisms involved are described in detail elsewhere.[38]

Antigen uptake and presentation Most antigen uptake occurs through the M cells of the Peyer's patches; the antigen

then is transported to macrophages and dendritic cells in the subepithelial dome (Figure 222-4). Macrophages and DCs act as antigen-presenting cells (APCs), presenting antigen, in the context of MHC II molecules, to lymphocytes (Figure 222-5).

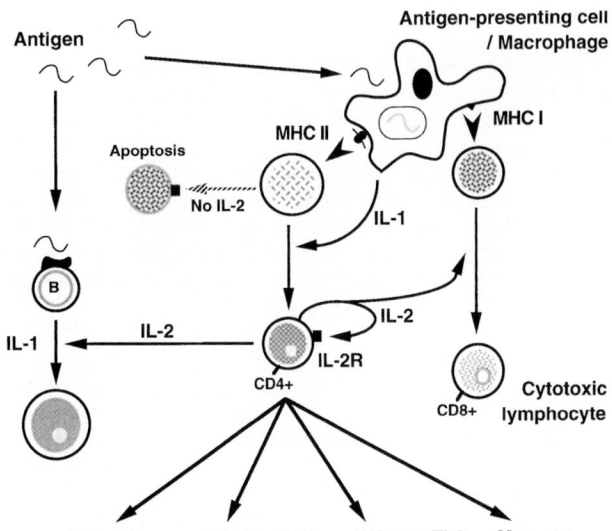

Figure 222-5 Activation of mucosal CD4+ T cells by antigen presentation in association with major histocompatibility complex (MHC) class II molecules; the result is either clonal expansion into memory and effector cells or apoptosis, depending on the synthesis of interleukin-2 receptor (IL-2R) and IL-2. CD8+ T cells are activated by antigen presentation in association with MHC class I molecules and, under the influence of CD4+ T cell–derived cytokines, develop into intraepithelial lymphocytes. γδT cells also form a part of the intraepithelial cell compartment.

Enterocytes may also be capable of taking up antigen and presenting it to T cells.

B-cell responses   The primary function of the B lymphoid lineage is generation of humoral immune responses, and the synthesis of IgA predominates in the intestinal mucosa. In the PP follicles, antigen on the surface of DCs stimulates B cells through the B-cell receptors (secretory immunoglobulin M [sIgM] and immunoglobulin D [IgD]). Costimulation to B cells is provided by CD4+ T cells, which enables the B cells to undergo clonal expansion. During the process of B-cell development, a switch occurs such that the effector cells are capable of producing a single immunoglobulin class (e.g., IgG, IgE, and IgA). The switching process is assisted by CD4 T-helper cells, which produce cytokines such as TGF-β, IL-4, and IFN-γ (for IgA, IgE, and IgG switching, respectively).

After class switching, B cells undergo further expansion and then traffic to effector sites to differentiate terminally into plasma cells. After synthesis, IgA (and to a lesser extent IgM) is released and then transported into the intestinal lumen by the polymeric immunoglobulin receptor (pIgR) on the enterocytes.[39] This complex passes through the enterocyte and is delivered across the microvillar membrane. On the luminal surface, the extracellular fragment of the pIgR is cleaved, forming *secretory component* (SC), which associates with pIgA and protects it from degradation in the intestinal lumen. The main function of sIgA is immune exclusion; that is, to bind its respective antigen and neutralize it. Immune exclusion limits the amount of antigen absorbed into the intestinal mucosa and thus the amount available to stimulate active immune responses. This helps maintain tolerance (see below) and protects the mucosa from antigen invasion.

Responses to parasites also occur through generation of antigen-specific plasma cells. These cells, found in the mesenteric lymph nodes, produce IgE that binds to the FcεRI on mucosal mast cells. When subsequently exposed to antigen, MC degranulation occurs and the associated parasite is expelled. Inappropriate IgE responses to food antigens also can be generated, providing a potential mechanism for food allergy.

Cytotoxic lymphocyte responses   Cytotoxic lymphocyte (CTL) responses are present in the SI mucosa, and their main function is to remove tumor cells or cells infected with intracellular bacteria, viruses, or parasites. CD8+ alpha/beta T cells, the main cytotoxic cells, are generated in a manner similar to B cells except that the former are found in interfollicular regions. Again, help is provided by CD4+ T cells, under the influence of cytokines such as IFN-γ. CD4+ cells themselves can participate in cytotoxicity, and γ/δ IELs may also be cytotoxic.

Mucosal Tolerance
The above descriptions relate to specific immune responses to pathogens, but such responses are the exception rather than the rule, and the default mucosal response to antigens is tolerance. This is not surprising, given that the majority of luminal antigens are derived from innocent dietary components or endogenous microflora. Generation of active immune responses to such ubiquitous molecules is both wasteful and potentially harmful, because it could lead to uncontrolled inflammation. Although the mechanisms by which mucosal tolerance actually occurs have been well characterized, the fundamental question of what prompts GALT tolerance or an immune response remains unresolved.

Mucosal tolerance can result either from anergy/deletion (apoptosis) of antigen-specific T cells or from active suppression by antigen-specific suppressor cells (secreting downregulatory cytokines, including IL-10 and TGF-β).[40]

The CD4+ α/β T-cell subsets that mediate active suppression either produce downregulatory cytokines (e.g., TGF-β or IL-10)[34,40] or achieve their effect through cell to cell interactions (e.g., through CD25+, IL-2 receptor). However, any cell capable of producing similar cytokine profiles could play a role and therefore tolerance could arise from the effects of CD8+ T cells, macrophages, stromal cells, and enterocytes. Furthermore, because TGF-β and IL-10 are also important in IgA production, generation of mucosal tolerance potentially could occur in parallel to specific IgA responses, which help to maintain tolerance through immune exclusion.

Mucosal Immune System Response or Tolerance
As mentioned previously, the mucosal immune system is prompted either to generate specific immune responses (e.g., toward a pathogen) or to remain tolerant (e.g., to commensal bacteria or food components). The best current hypothesis for the determination of which effect occurs is the "danger theory,"[41] which is based on the supposition that the type of response depends on the context in which the antigen is presented.

The normal intestinal mucosa has an intact mucosal barrier and an environment dominated by downregulatory cytokines (e.g., IL-10 and TGF-β). Therefore most immune responses that develop are tolerance responses. Furthermore, the same cytokine milieu encourages IgA responses, which limit mucosal antigen exposure through immune exclusion.

However, when the mucosa is invaded by a pathogen or toxin, cell damage leads to the release of "danger signals," such as inflammatory mediators (e.g., prostaglandins, leukotrienes), proinflammatory cytokines (e.g., IL-1, IL-6, and TNF-α), and chemokines (e.g., IL-8). In this altered environment, the nature of the immune response generated changes from tolerance to an active immune response. This active response can be either Th1 dominated (e.g., cytotoxicity and IgG responses) or Th2 dominated (i.e., IGE responses). The powerful responses that develop aim to eliminate the pathogen completely, but the potential for bystander damage to host cells is great.

If the antigenic challenge is contained, the danger signals diminish, the mucosa enters a repair phase, and the normal "tolerogenic" environment returns. However, if the danger persists, either because the mucosal barrier remains breached and the pathogenic insult continues unabated or because of an inherent abnormality in the GALT, a state of chronic inflammation ensues. This may also lead to a breakdown in tolerance to harmless environmental antigens (food components and commensal bacteria) and inflammation. Chronic inflammation ultimately leads to histopathologic changes, which are similar regardless of the inciting cause.

PATHOPHYSIOLOGIC MECHANISMS IN INTESTINAL DISEASE

Motility Disorders
Alterations of intestinal motility as a primary cause of diarrhea have not yet been well characterized.[42] Irritable bowel syndrome may be associated with altered intestinal motility (see below). Secondary alterations in motility often occur, such as with intestinal obstruction, pseudo-obstruction, adynamic ileus, or inflammatory or infectious enteropathies. In malabsorption conditions, unabsorbed solutes decrease transit time because osmotically retained fluid causes intestinal distension and hypermotility. Hyperthyroidism decreases transit time in cats and causes diarrhea. Rapid waves of contractions have been demonstrated in enterotoxigenic diarrhea.

However, in most instances diarrhea is actually associated with intestinal hypomotility. Abnormal dilatation of the intestine caused by hypomotility or obstruction is known as *ileus*. *Adynamic ileus* is a transient and reversible functional obstruction

Box • 222-4

Causes of Ileus

Physical
Intestinal obstruction
Overdistention by aerophagia

Neuromuscular
Anticholinergic drugs
Dysautonomia
Spinal cord injury
Visceral myopathies

Metabolic
Hypokalemia
Uremia
Endotoxemia

Functional
Abdominal surgery
Ischemia
Inflammatory causes
Peritonitis
Pancreatitis
Parvovirus

of the intestine with a number of causes (Box 222-4). In enteric viral infections, for example, ileus is common, promoting diarrhea by stasis, which allows bacterial fermentation. Hypomotility and constipation are expected with hypothyroidism, but occasionally antibiotic-responsive diarrhea is found.[43]

Luminal Disturbances

Lack of pancreatic enzymes in EPI or increased destruction of enzymes by acid hypersecretion (e.g., Zollinger-Ellison syndrome) or SIBO results in failure of digestion. Bacteria may also compete for nutrients (e.g., binding of cobalamin in SIBO).

Interruption of enterohepatic circulation and lack of bile salt micelles result in fat malabsorption and can be caused by portosystemic shunting, intrahepatic or extrahepatic cholestasis, bacterial deconjugation of bile salts in the gut lumen, or ileal disease. Surgical resection of the ileum (e.g., with ileocolic intussusception) and inflammatory bowel disease (IBD) affecting the distal SI cause both bile salt and cobalamin malabsorption.

Villus Atrophy

Villus atrophy causes loss of intestinal surface area and results in malabsorption of fat. Also, carrier-mediated uptake is rate limited, because there is a finite number of nutrient transporters. Villus atrophy results in a loss of carriers critical to carbohydrate and protein digestion.

Atrophy is caused either by a decrease in the production of enterocytes or an increase in the rate of enterocyte loss. Infectious agents that damage enterocytes may infect the villus tip (e.g., rotavirus) or midvillus (e.g., coronavirus), causing cell loss and a mild to moderate diarrhea. Destruction of crypt cells (e.g., parvovirus infection) causes loss of enterocyte production, complete villus collapse, and severe diarrhea.

A persistently increased rate of enterocyte loss through immune-mediated mechanisms results in a compensatory increase in the crypt cell proliferation rate, and if the cell loss is matched by the increased proliferation, villus height does

not decrease. However, a significant effect still is exerted on the digestive and absorptive ability of the SI, because prematurely lost mature enterocytes are replaced by immature, suboptimally functioning enterocytes. If enterocyte loss outpaces increased proliferation, villus atrophy results. If the initiating cause can be removed, villus atrophy is completely reversible. Cytotoxic drugs (e.g., vincristine) and parvovirus infection (which cause crypt arrest and destruction, respectively) can be devastating, causing complete villus and crypt collapse. However, assuming some stem cells survive the insult, regeneration is possible, although it is likely to take several days.

Enteroctye Dysfunction

Even if enterocytes are only damaged, the loss of brush border proteins still is often clinically important. Interference with enterocyte function can occur without histologic damage through the action of various bacterial secretions. Malnutrition and ischemia also impair function and increase epithelial permeability.

Microvillar Membrane Damage

The MVM is clearly damaged when overt histologic villus damage can be seen, but even without light microscopic changes, massive impairment of mucosal function can occur if the microvilli are damaged. Such damage is seen with enteropathogenic *Escherichia coli* infection or lectins, which cause a loss of surface area and brush border enzymes and carriers. Bacterial overgrowth is associated with subtle but specific damage to the membrane. Obligate anaerobes are very effective at degrading membrane glycoproteins or releasing brush border enzymes.[44]

Brush Border Membrane Disease

Primary brush border membrane diseases are biochemical abnormalities that occur in the absence of histologic damage. They are well characterized in humans, but equivalent defects in dogs and cats have rarely been demonstrated. Relative lactase deficiency does occur in dogs and particularly in cats.[5] Defects in ileal cobalamin–intrinsic factor complex uptake have been documented in giant schnauzers, collies, and beagles, resulting in cobalamin deficiency with consequent methylmalonic aciduria.[45] Clinical signs include inappetence, failure to thrive, neutropenia, and anemia.

Mucosal Barrier Disruption

The mucosal barrier is crucial in maintaining oral tolerance and excluding pathogens. In animal models, malnutrition results in villus atrophy with increased transepithelial macromolecular absorption, abnormal mucin, and reduced IgA secretion.[46]

In the N-cadherin dominant negative chimaeric mouse, intestinal inflammation is restricted to regions of the gut where the mutant gene is expressed and consequently where epithelial integrity is disrupted because of a lack of expression of E-cadherin.[47]

Natural causes of decreased barrier function include luminal aggressive factors and endogenous inflammatory mediators such as IFN-γ (Box 222-5). Barrier damage may lead to entry of antigens, subsequent allergic and/or inflammatory reactions, and even translocation of bacteria into the circulation. Leakage of protein-rich tissue fluid in the opposite direction is also of clinical significance, causing a protein-losing enteropathy (PLE).

Hypersensitivity

Sensitization of a patient to a dietary antigen may provoke an IgE-mediated allergic reaction when the animal is next exposed. The release of numerous mast cell mediators (e.g., histamine, serotonin, heparin, interleukins) may have remote effects (e.g., pruritus, urticaria) and even generalized systemic effects (anaphylaxis). Mast cell mediators also have local effects

Box • 222-5

Examples of Agents that Can Damage the Mucosal Barrier

Luminal Aggressive Factors
Enteric infections
Endotoxin
Drugs
Ethanol
Nonsteroidal anti-inflammatory drugs (NSAIDs)
Cytotoxic drugs
Bile salts

Endogenous Factors
Malnutrition (starvation, malabsorption)
Ischemia
Reperfusion injury
Nitric oxide
Remote inflammatory disease and burns
Intestinal inflammation
Interferon-γ
Neutrophil migration
Mast cell mediators (e.g., histamine, bradykinin)

Table • 222-1

Experimental Rodent Models of Chronic Intestinal Inflammation

TYPE OF INFLAMMATION	MODEL
Spontaneous	Ulcerative colitis in Cotton-top tamarin
	C3H/HeJBir mouse
Induced	Chemical
	Acetic acid enema
	Immune complex/formalin enema
	TNBS/ethanol enema
	Indomethacin
	Microbial products
	Dextran sulphate sodium
	Carrageenan
	Lymphogranuloma venereum
	Peptidoglycan-polysaccharide
Genetically manipulated	Cytokine perturbations
	IL-2 deficiency
	IL-2R deficiency
	IL-10 deficiency
	TGF-β deficiency
	IL-7 transgenic
	T-cell or MHC perturbations
	TCR-α chain deficiency
	HLA-B27/β2m transgenic
	Cyclosporin A colitis
	Epithelial perturbations
	Gαi2 deficiency
	N-cadherin—dominant negative transgenic chimera
	Mdr-1 deficiency
Leukocyte transfer to immunodeficient mice	CD45RBhiCD4 T cell into SCID mouse
	CD45RBhiCD4 T cell into RAG-deficient rats
	T-cell transfer into SCID mouse
	Bone marrow transfer into Tgε26 mice
	Transfer of cells from mice infected with murine retrovirus

From German AJ et al: Chronic intestinal inflammation and intestinal disease in dogs. J Vet Intern Med 17:8, 2003.
CD, cluster of differentiation; IL, interleukin; HLA, human leukocyte antigen; MHC, major histocompatibility complex; SCID, severe combined immunodeficiency; TCR, T cell receptor; TGF, transforming growth factor.

on the intestine, acting directly on epithelium, muscle, and endothelium and indirectly through fibroblast and nerve activity.[48] They induce rapid changes in absorption and secretion, mucus secretion, epithelial and endothelial permeability, and gut motility, causing vomiting and diarrhea.

Mucosal Inflammation

Inflammation is a cellular and vascular response to a number of inciting causes, including infection, ischemia, trauma, toxins, neoplasia, and immune-mediated reactions. The normal mucosa is continually bombarded by a vast array of antigens derived from endogenous bacteria and food components and can be considered to be in a state of "controlled inflammation." Anything that overloads this system is likely to trigger uncontrolled inflammation.

Experimental models of gastrointestinal inflammation have allowed researchers to understand better the pathogenesis of mucosal inflammation and the mechanisms that trigger it (Table 222-1). These genetically engineered rodents have a variety of spontaneously arising or induced disruptions of the mucosal immune system that lead to chronic inflammation, the end results of which are histologically similar. The disruptions usually are induced in one of three ways: through disruption of the mucosal barrier (e.g., the N-cadherin dominant negative chimaeric mouse)[47]; through dysregulation of the mucosal immune system; or through disruption of the endogenous microflora. Disruption of the mucosal immune system, either through targeted deletion of cytokines (e.g., IL-2, IL-10, or TGF-β knockout mice) or through abnormalities in the CD4+ T-cell compartment, results in dysregulated immune responses and, consequently, uncontrolled mucosal inflammation.[49] Extracellular proteolysis by matrix metalloproteinases is critical in the pathogenesis of IBD in humans.[50]

Either mucosal barrier disruption or immune system dysregulation (or both) is required for the development of uncontrolled inflammation; however, the presence of an enteric flora is essential for expression of disease. In this regard, chronic intestinal inflammation generally does not develop when the rodent in these model systems is reared in a germ-free environment.[49]

This demonstrates the importance of the endogenous flora in the pathogenesis of uncontrolled mucosal inflammation, as confirmed by studies showing that normal humans are tolerant to their own intestinal microflora but that this tolerance is broken in patients with IBD.[51]

Neoplasia

Solitary tumors can cause diarrhea, probably through the effects of partial obstruction, stasis of ingesta, and secondary bacterial overgrowth. More typically the tumor is associated with such signs as intestinal obstruction (i.e., vomiting, abdominal pain, absence of feces), bleeding, and cancer-associated anorexia. Mast cell tumors may cause duodenal perforation and peritonitis through histamine-mediated gastric acid hypersecretion.

Diffuse tumors, such as lymphoma, that infiltrate the mucosa cause diarrhea. Malignant cells may simply obstruct blood and lymphatic flow, but enterocyte function is likely to be impaired or the mucosa may be ulcerated.

Nutrient Delivery Failure

After absorption nutrients are delivered to the body via blood and lymph; only lymphatic diseases are described in animals. Primary lymphatic obstruction (lymphangiectasia) that causes malabsorption may be idiopathic or may be associated with lymphangitis. Secondary lymphangiectasia is seen with lymphatic obstruction.

SMALL INTESTINAL DISEASE

Signs

Diarrhea

Diarrhea is an increase in fecal mass caused by an increase in fecal water and/or solid content. It is accompanied by an increase in frequency and/or fluidity and/or volume of feces. Yet it must be remembered that the absence of recognizable diarrhea does not preclude the possibility of significant SI disease.

Diarrhea can be classified in several ways (Box 222-6). These categories are not mutually exclusive, and they allow the problem to be viewed from different perspectives, facilitating diagnosis and the choice of appropriate treatment. A mechanistic approach is simple, and many SI diseases have a component of osmotic diarrhea, but even in a situation as simple as lactase deficiency, other mechanisms become involved (Figure 222-6). Osmotic diarrhea in lactose malabsorption causes intestinal distension, which induces peristalsis and rapid transit, and bacterial fermentation products in the colon cause secretion. Bacterial fermentation of unabsorbed solutes is often a complicating factor in malabsorption. The fecal pH is often low because of the production of volatile fatty acids, and some products of fermentation (e.g., hydroxylated fatty acids, unconjugated bile acids) can cause colonic inflammation and secretion, and therefore signs of LI diarrhea frequently accompany prolonged SI disease.

Osmotic diarrhea   Excess water-soluble molecules in the intestinal lumen retain water osmotically and overwhelm the absorptive capacity of the SI and colon (e.g., sudden diet change, overeating, and malabsorption). The diarrhea typically resolves when food or laxatives are withheld.

Secretory diarrhea   Stimulation of SI secretion such that the reserve absorptive capacity is overwhelmed results in diarrhea even though the absorptive ability of the SI and colon may not actually be impaired. Treatment with oral rehydration

---

Box • 222-6

Classifications of Diarrhea

Mechanistic
Osmotic
Secretory
Permeability (exudative)
Dysmotility
Mixed

Temporal
Acute
Chronic

Anatomic
Extraintestinal
Small intestinal
Large intestinal
Diffuse

Pathophysiologic
Biochemical
Allergic
Inflammatory
Neoplastic

Etiologic
Diet; bacterial, viral, parasitic causes; other

Causal
Exocrine pancreatic insufficiency, salmonellosis, lymphoma, other

Clinical
Acute, nonfatal, self-limiting
Acute potentially fatal
Acute systemic disease
Chronic

---

fluids containing glucose and amino acids (e.g., glycine) to increase water absorption is appropriate.

Typically secretory diarrhea does not resolve with fasting but does not cause weight loss unless anorexia, vomiting, or additional SI damage is a factor. Morbidity and even

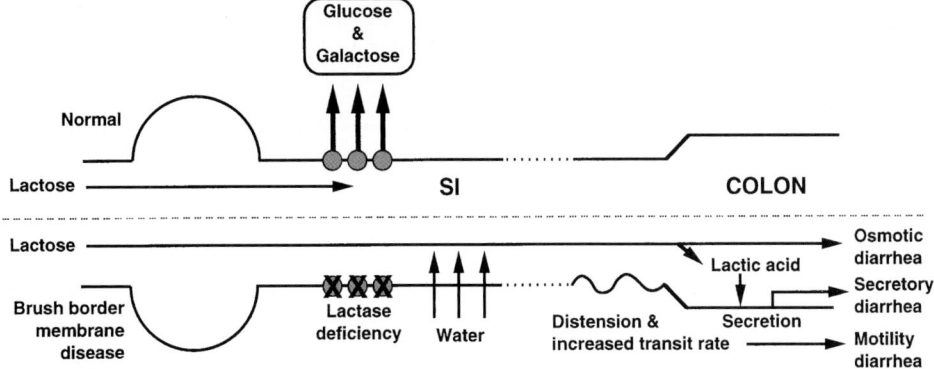

Figure 222-6 Diagrammatic representation of the mechanisms of diarrhea caused by lactase deficiency.

Box • 222-7

Causes of Secretory Diarrhea

Bacterial enterotoxins and endotoxins (e.g., *Clostridium perfringens*, *Escherichia coli*, *Salmonella* spp., *Shigella* spp., *Yersinia enterocolitica*)
Unconjugated bile acids from bacterial fermentation
Hydroxylated fatty acids from bacterial fermentation
Giardia infection
Possibly hyperthyroidism
Laxatives (castor oil, dioctyl sodium sulfosuccinate, bisacodyl)
Cardiac glycosides
Amine precursor uptake and decarboxylation (APUD) neoplasms (excess vasoactive intestinal polypeptide, serotonin, prostaglandins, substance P)
Intestinal inflammation

Table • 222-2

Pathophysiologic Mechanisms of Malabsorption

MECHANISM	EXAMPLE
Luminal Phase	
Dysmotility	
Rapid intestinal transit	Hyperthyroidism
Defective substrate hydrolysis	
Enzyme inactivation	Gastric hypersecretion
Lack of pancreatic enzymes	Exocrine pancreatic insufficiency
Fat maldigestion	
Decreased bile salt delivery	Cholestatic liver disease, biliary obstruction
Increased bile salt loss	Ileal disease
Bile salt deconjugation	Bacterial overgrowth
Fatty acid hydroxylation	Bacterial overgrowth
Impaired release of CCK, secretin	Impairment of pancreatic secretion due to severe small intestine disease
Cobalamin malabsorption	
Intrinsic factor deficiency	Exocrine pancreatic insufficiency Giant schnauzer defect
Competition for cobalamin	Bacterial overgrowth
Mucosal Phase	
Brush border enzyme deficiency	
Congenital	Trehalase (cats)
Acquired	Relative lactose deficiency
Brush border transport protein deficiency	
Congenital	Intrinsic factor receptor
Acquired	Secondary to diffuse SI disease
Enterocyte defects	
Enterocyte processing defects	Abetalipoproteinemia
Reduction in surface area	Villus atrophy
Immature enterocytes	Increased enterocyte turnover
Mucosal inflammation	Inflammatory bowel disease
Transport Phase	
Lymphatic obstruction	
Primary	Lymphangiectasia
Secondary	Obstruction caused by neoplasia, infection, or inflammation
Vascular compromise	
Vasculitis	Infection, immune mediated
Portal hypertension	Hepatopathy, right heart failure, cardiac tamponade

mortality are associated with the dehydration that results from excessive fluid loss. Secretory diarrhea typically is caused by chemical toxins and toxins elaborated by enteric bacteria (Box 222-7).

Permeability (exudative) diarrhea Intestinal inflammation can stimulate increased fluid and electrolyte secretion and impair absorption. Leakage of tissue fluid, serum proteins, blood, and mucus may occur from sites of inflammation, ulceration, or infiltration or if portal hypertension or lymphatic obstruction is present. Increased permeability severe enough to cause loss of plasma proteins in excess of their rate of synthesis results in a PLE.

Malabsorption
Failure of food assimilation is sometimes classified as primary failure to digest (maldigestion) or primary failure to absorb (malabsorption). However, such a classification is misleading, because failure of absorption is an inevitable consequence of failure to digest. The preferred use of the term *malabsorption* is to describe defective absorption of dietary constituent resulting from interference with the digestive and/or absorptive phases in the processing of that molecule.

Within this broad definition, the site of the primary abnormality may be found in the luminal, mucosal, or transport phase (Table 222-2). Also, the reserve capacity of the distal SI and colon may prevent overt diarrhea despite significant malabsorption and weight loss. The clinical manifestations of malabsorption, namely diarrhea, weight loss, and altered appetite (polyphagia, coprophagia, pica), are largely a result of the lack of nutrient uptake and the losses in feces. Animals are often systemically healthy and have an increased appetite unless an underlying neoplastic or a severe inflammatory condition is present. Only when the patient is quite malnourished or develops hypoproteinemia does it become ill.

Melena
The presence of dark, tarry, oxidized blood in feces, a condition called *melena*, reflects either swallowed blood or generalized or localized GI bleeding, which usually occurs proximal to the large intestine (Table 222-3). Medication with ferrous sulfate or bismuth subsalicylate (Pepto-Bismol) also can impart a black color to the feces. It has been estimated that the loss of 350 to 500 mg/kg of hemoglobin into the GI tract is required for melena to be visible.[52] The presence of microcytosis with or without thrombocytosis is suggestive of iron deficiency secondary to chronic blood loss. An increased blood urea nitrogen (BUN) to creatinine ratio (from bacterial digestion of

blood) provides supporting evidence. Hypoproteinemia may indicate significant blood loss or the presence of a PLE.

The general approach to melena is to rule out bleeding diatheses, ingestion of blood, and underlying metabolic disorders before pursuing primary GI causes. Ultrasonography is particularly useful for detecting gastrointestinal masses and thickening. The next step for investigating upper GI blood loss is endoscopy. If the source of GI bleeding is still undetermined, tagged red cell scintigraphy, exploratory laparotomy, angiography, and enteroscopy may be used to localize the site.[53]

Table • 222-3

Causes of Melena

MECHANISM	SOURCE
Ingestion of blood	Oral, nasal, pharyngeal, or pulmonary bleeding
Coagulopathies	Thrombocytopenia, factor deficiencies, DIC
Gastrointestinal erosion/ulceration	
Metabolic	Uremia, liver disease
Inflammatory	Gastritis, enteritis, HGE
Neoplastic	Leiomyoma, adenocarcinoma, lymphosarcoma
Paraneoplastic	Mastocytosis, hypergastrinemia and other APUDomas
Vascular	A-V fistula, aneurysms, angiodysplasia
Ischemia	Hypovolemic shock, hypoadrenocorticism, thrombosis/infarction, reperfusion
Drug induced	Nonsteroidal and steroidal anti-inflammatory agents
Foreign objects	

APUD, amine precursor uptake and decarboxylation tumor; A-V, arteriovenous; DIC, disseminated intravascular coagulation

Table • 222-4

Protein-Losing Enteropathies

CAUSES	EXAMPLES
Lymphangiectasia	Primary lymphatic disorder, venous hypertension (e.g., right heart failure, hepatic cirrhosis)
Infectious	Parvovirus, salmonellosis, histoplasmosis, phycomycosis
Structural	Intussusception
Neoplasia	Lymphosarcoma
Inflammation	Lymphocytic-plasmacytic, eosinophilic, granulomatous
Endoparasites	Giardia, Ancylostoma spp.
Gastrointestinal hemorrhage	HGE, neoplasia, ulceration

HGE, hemorrhagic gastroenteritis

Borborygmi and Flatulence

Borborygmus is a rumbling noise caused by the propulsion of gas through the intestines. Swallowed air and bacterial fermentation of ingesta are the main causes of borborygmi and flatulence. Feeding a diet that is highly digestible, with a low fiber content (e.g., cottage cheese and rice in a 1:2 ratio) leaves little material present in the intestine for bacterial fermentation and can effect a cure in some cases. If borborygmi or flatulence continues despite dietary modification, the animal may be excessively aerophagic or may have malabsorption, especially if diarrhea or weight loss are also present.

Weight Loss or Failure to Thrive

General causes of weight loss are reduced nutrient intake, increased nutrient loss, and increased catabolism or ineffective metabolism. The history should reveal whether the type and amount of diet fed is adequate and whether anorexia, dysphagia, or vomiting is a potential cause. Weight loss or failure to thrive accompanied by diarrhea often is a feature of malabsorption, and the diagnostic approach is the same as for chronic diarrhea. However, diarrhea does not invariably accompany malabsorption that causes weight loss.

Protein-Losing Enteropathy

When SI disease is severe enough for protein leakage into the gut lumen to exceed protein synthesis, hypoproteinemia develops.[54] Chronic diarrhea associated with hypoproteinemia usually requires intestinal biopsy to define the cause of the PLE (Table 222-4). Nonintestinal diseases, which may potentially be associated with intestinal protein loss (e.g., portal hypertension), usually present with ascites before diarrhea. Hypoproteinemia associated with GI disease is much less common in cats than in dogs and most often accompanies GI lymphoma.

Clinical presentation Breeds that appear to be predisposed to PLE are the basenji, lundehund, soft-coated wheaten terrier, Yorkshire terrier, and Shar Pei (see below). Clinical signs associated with PLE include weight loss, diarrhea, vomiting, edema, ascites, and pleural effusion. Weight loss frequently is the predominant feature, and diarrhea is not invariably present, particularly with lymphangiectasia and focal intestinal neoplasia. Physical findings may include edema, ascites, emaciation, thickened intestines, and melena. Thromboembolism is a feature of some cases of PLE.

Diagnosis The serum concentrations of both albumin and globulin are reduced in most patients with PLE. Exceptions are raised hyperglobulinemia with hypoalbuminemia found in histoplasmosis and immunoproliferative SI disease in the basenji (see below). Hepatic and renal causes of hypoalbuminemia are eliminated by assay of serum bile acids and urinary protein loss respectively. Hypocholesterolemia and lymphopenia are common in PLE. Hypocalcemia and hypomagnesemia are also reported.[55] Measurement of fecal loss of alpha$_1$-protease inhibitor may be a sensitive test for PLE.[56]

Survey abdominal radiographs often are normal in patients with PLE, but ultrasound scans may reveal intestinal thickening, mesenteric lymphadenopathy, or abdominal effusion. Thoracic radiographs may show pleural effusion, metastatic neoplasia, or evidence of histoplasmosis. Although intestinal function tests may confirm the presence of malabsorption, they rarely provide a definitive diagnosis, and intestinal biopsy is more appropriate. Because many intestinal causes of PLE are diffuse, endoscopy is the safer way to obtain biopsies, but surgical biopsy may be required to obtain a definitive diagnosis for lymphoma and for diseases that cause secondary lymphangiectasia (Box 222-8).

Treatment Plasma transfusion may be indicated during the perioperative period when collecting biopsy specimens, and diuretics may reduce ascites. Spironolactone (1 to 2 mg/kg given orally twice daily) may be more effective than furosemide for treating ascites. Thromboembolism is a feature of some cases of PLE. Specific treatments are discussed later.

Diagnosis of Small Intestinal Disease

Most cases of diarrhea are acute, nonfatal, and self-limiting and require only symptomatic support without a definitive diagnosis. However, some cases are life-threatening, may have an infective potential for other animals, or may present a potential zoonotic risk to humans. If significant hypovolemia or dehydration is present, fluid and electrolyte deficits must be addressed simultaneously with the diagnostic effort. The extent of diagnostic investigations required for acute diarrhea

Box • 222-8

Relative Advantages of Endoscopic and Surgical Intestinal Biopsy

Endoscopy
Advantages
Minimally invasive
Allows visualization and biopsy of focal lesions
Permits multiple biopsies
Minimal adverse reactions
Allows steroids to be started early

Disadvantages
Requires general anesthesia
Permits access only to duodenum (and distal ileum?)
Allows only small, superficial (and crushed) biopsies
Requires expensive equipment
Technically demanding

Laparotomy
Advantages
Allows biopsy of multiple sites
Permits large, full-thickness biopsies
Allows inspection of other organs
Offers potential for corrective surgery

Disadvantages
Requires general anesthesia
Poses a surgical risk
Requires convalescence
Requires delay before steroids can be started

Table • 222-5

Clinical Signs Associated with Small and Large Bowel Disease

SIGNS	SMALL INTESTINAL DISEASE	LARGE INTESTINAL DISEASE
Feces		
Stool volume	Large	Small
Mucus	Rare	Common
Blood (if present)	Melena	Fresh blood
Fat	Sometimes	Absent
Color	Variable	Normal
Defecation		
Tenesmus	Rare	Common
Undigested food	Occasionally	Absent
Frequency	Normal: Two to three times a day	Normal: More than three times a day
Urgency	Uncommon	Common
Other signs		
Vomiting	Sometimes	Uncommon
Gas	Sometimes	Absent
Weight loss	Common	Rare

Box • 222-9

Historical Information Useful in the Diagnosis of Small Intestinal Disease

Patient Information
Age
Gender
Breed (see Table 222-6)

Environmental History
Indoor versus outdoor
Free roaming
Scavenging
Exposure to parasites
Contact with infected animals
Recent change of environment
Endemic disease area

Past Medical History
Vaccination status
Worming status
Previous abdominal surgery
Previous excision of cutaneous mast cell tumor
Drug history

Progression of Clinical Signs
Severity
Duration
Frequency
Continuous or intermittent in nature
Length of sign-free intervals
Factors that improve or worsen signs (e.g., treatments, diets)
Order of appearance of signs

varies; investigations are appropriate if diarrhea is hemorrhagic, accompanied by systemic signs, or unresponsive to symptomatic treatment. By definition, chronic diarrhea is not self-limiting, and an etiologic diagnosis usually is required to allow specific treatment. Diagnostic approaches to acute and chronic diarrhea are discussed in detail elsewhere.

The aim of the diagnostic approach is to eliminate extraintestinal diseases and to differentiate SI from LI disease (Table 222-5). The history (Boxes 222-2 and 222-9 and Table 222-6) and physical examination (Table 222-7) are crucial steps toward reaching a diagnosis and in some cases may be all that is required. Preliminary investigations may also include collection of baseline data (i.e., hematology, serum biochemistry, urinalysis, and fecal examination). Diagnostic imaging may be indicated, especially if a disease requiring surgical intervention is likely. Further investigations include exclusion of EPI, indirect tests of intestinal function and damage and, ultimately, direct examination of the SI by endoscopy or surgery with histologic examination of biopsies.

Fecal Examination

Fecal examinations are an important part of the investigation of SI disease. Tests such as quantification of fecal fat excretion are unsuitable for practice, and bacteriologic culture is sometimes of questionable value, but identification of parasites is important.

Direct smear Staining of smears for undigested starch granules (Lugol's iodine), fat globules (Sudan stain), and muscle fibers (Wright's or Diff Quik stain) may indicate malabsorption but is unreliable. Fungal elements and sporulating clostridia may be seen, but rectal cytology is more useful.

Table • 222-6

Some Suspected and Confirmed Breed Susceptibilities to Small Intestinal Disease in Dogs and Cats

BREED	CONDITION
Basenji	Lymphocytic-plasmacytic enteritis (also called immunoproliferative disease)
Beagle	Cobalamin deficiency
Border collie	Cobalamin deficiency
German shepherd	Idiopathic antibiotic-responsive; inflammatory bowel disease (lymphoplasmacytic, eosinophilic)
Giant schnauzer	Defective cobalamin absorption
Irish setter	Gluten-sensitive enteropathy
Lundehund	Lymphangiectasia
Retrievers	Dietary allergy
Rottweiler	Susceptibility to parvovirus
Soft-coated wheaten terrier	Protein-losing enteropathy/nephropathy
Shar Pei	Lymphocytic-plasmacytic enteritis, cobalamin deficiency
Toy breeds	Hemorrhagic gastroenteritis
Yorkshire terrier	Lymphangiectasia

Table • 222-7

Significant Physical Findings in Animals with Signs of a Small Intestinal Disorder

FINDINGS	INTERPRETATION
General	Rule out other systemic disease
Oropharynx	
Mucous membranes	Hydration status, cardiovascular status, anemia, icterus
Tongue	Linear foreign body
Cervical Region	
Thyroid gland	Thyroid nodule (hyperthyroidism)
Abdominal Palpation and Auscultation	
Palpation	Effusions, masses, bunching of intestinal loops, foreign bodies, abnormal accumulations of ingesta, associated pain, feces, lymphadenopathy, other systemic disease
Auscultation	Ileus, borborygmi
Rectal Examination	
Digital examination	Masses, foreign bodies, hemostatic disorders, dehydration
Collection of stool sample	Laboratory analysis, melena
Rectal mucosal scrape	Cytology
Cutaneous Examination	
Poor coat condition, scale	Malnutrition
Pruritus	Food hypersensitivity
Pedal pruritus	*Uncinaria stenocephala* infection (larval migration)

Unstained wet mounts may be used to identify protozoal trophozoites.

Enterotoxin production by *Clostridium perfringens* is a potential cause of diarrhea. The presence of a large number of clostridial endospores (more than 5 per oil field) on Diff Quik–stained smears may be suggestive, but a positive fecal enterotoxin assay (enzyme-linked immunosorbent assay [ELISA] or reverse passive latex agglutination) is more significant.

Fecal concentration methods   For detection of most parasites, fecal concentration methods are more rewarding (Figure 222-7). Examination of three fecal samples by zinc sulfate flotation is recommended to detect *Giardia* oocysts. A direct smear, sedimentation, or the Baermann technique can identify larvae of *Strongyloides* spp.

Bacteriologic examination   Routine culture of all bacteria from a fecal sample is of little value, but targeted evaluation for potential pathogens may be helpful. Culture of feces is indicated in animals with hemorrhagic diarrhea or pyrexia or with an inflammatory leukogram or neutrophils on rectal cytology. Identification of *Salmonella* spp., *Campylobacter jejuni*, and *Clostridium difficile* may be helpful, although the significance of a positive isolate should be interpreted in the light of the clinical history, because these organisms can be present in clinically healthy animals. Furthermore, although fecal flora might be representative of colonic bacterial populations, they do not necessarily reflect the SI flora and cannot be used to diagnose SIBO. *E. coli* can be cultured from most fecal samples, but only certain strains are pathogenic, and molecular probes have recently been used to detect pathogenicity markers of *E. coli* in small animal medicine.[57] However, the significance of a positive result needs further assessment, because these organisms can be isolated from both healthy and ill dogs. Feces can be cultured for fungi, such as *Histoplasma capsulatum*, but isolation is difficult and slow.

Virologic examination   Viral diarrhea is usually acute and self-limiting and does not require a positive diagnosis.

Electron microscopy can be used to identify the characteristic viral particles of rotavirus, coronavirus, and parvovirus. A fecal ELISA for parvovirus is also available (see below).

Giardia antigen   A commercially available ELISA can be used to detect *Giardia* antigen in feces.

Occult blood

These tests are used to search for intestinal bleeding from ulcerated mucosa and benign or malignant tumors. Unfortunately, all versions nonspecifically test for hemoglobin and are very sensitive, reacting with any meat diet and not just patient blood. Therefore the patient must be fed a meat-free diet for at last 72 hours for a positive result to have any reliability.[52,58]

Alpha₁-protease inhibitor   This test assays the presence in feces of a naturally occurring endogenous serum protein that is resistant to bacterial degradation if it is lost into the intestinal lumen. To improve diagnostic accuracy, three fresh fecal samples should be sampled. The assay is valid only if used on fecal samples collected after voluntary evacuation, because abrasion of the colonic wall during manual evacuation is enough to elevate alpha₁-protease inhibitor (alpha₁-PI) concentrations. It appears to be of value for the diagnosis of PLE[59] and may prove to be more a sensitive marker than measurement of serum albumin for the detection of early disease.[60]

EGG SIZES

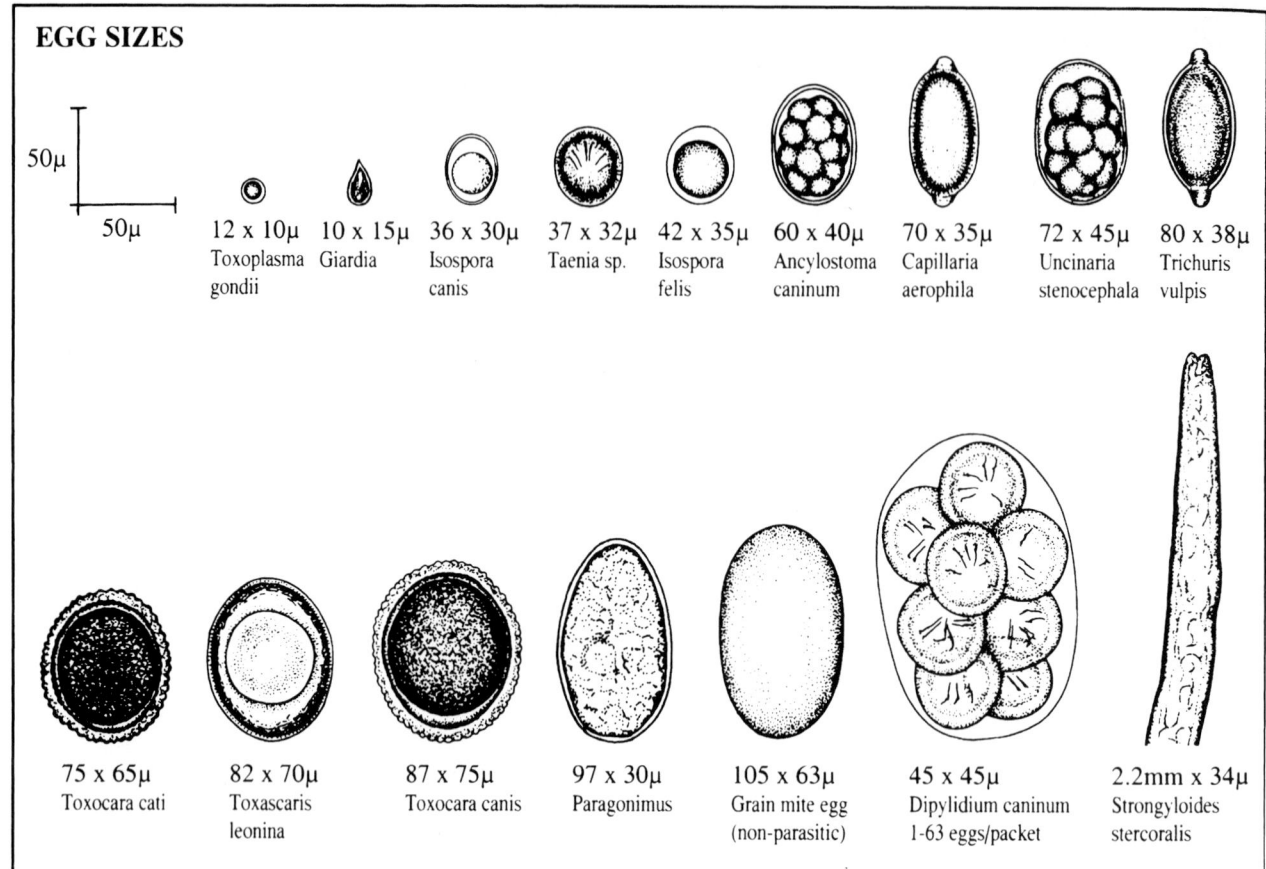

Figure 222-7 Identification of protozoan cysts and worm eggs that may be found in the feces of dogs and cats. (Hoechst-Roussel-Agri Vet Company, USA.)

Rectal cytology At the end of the rectal examination, the rectal wall is mildly abraded, the gloved finger rolled on a microscope slide, and the smear stained. Although the result is often negative and, when positive, probably more representative of LI disease, an increased number of neutrophils may be suggestive of a bacterial problem, indicating the need for fecal culture. Clostridial endospore elements (*Histoplasma*, *Aspergillus*, *Pythium*, and *Candida* spp.) may be identified. The test is fast and simple but in all cases confirmatory tests are indicated.

Imaging
Until recently, imaging of the intestinal tract was limited to plain and contrast radiographs. This has been dramatically altered by the use of ultrasound and endoscopy. Scintigraphy, computed tomography (CT), and magnetic resonance imaging (MRI) scanning are rapidly being adopted, and "virtual endoscopy" by helical CT is becoming available.

Radiography
Survey radiographs Plain radiographs are most useful in the investigation of primary vomiting, diarrhea associated with vomiting, abdominal pain, and palpable abnormalities. Diagnostic yield is improved if both lateral views are taken,[61] although a single lateral radiograph is all that is required if radiography is combined with ultrasonography. Generally the aim is the detection of (acute) surgical disease; these radiographs allow detection of foreign bodies, masses, obstructions, decreased serosal detail, free peritoneal gas, and ileus (Table 222-8).

Ileus is an abnormal dilatation of an immotile segment of intestine, and the differential diagnosis depends on whether it

is localized or generalized and whether an accumulation of gas or fluid is present (Box 222-10). The usefulness of plain radiographs in malabsorption is minimal.

Contrast radiography Since the introduction of abdominal ultrasonography and endoscopy, contrast radiographic studies have had limited value in the assessment of SI disease.

Barium follow-through examinations. Studies using microfine barium suspensions can identify ulcers and irregular mucosal detail and may confirm the presence of radiolucent foreign bodies. Such studies are of limited use in identifying mural masses and partial obstructions, and they rarely provide more information than a good-quality survey film (Figure 222-8). Furthermore, although contrast studies allow assessment of the intestinal transit rate, they provide limited etiologic information, and dysmotility may occur secondary to other causes. Also, administration of barium may delay endoscopy for at least 24 hours.

Barium-impregnated polyethylene spheres (BIPS). BIPS are solid-phase radiopaque markers that provide information on gastric emptying, intestinal transit, and obstructive disorders (Figure 222-8, *D*). Given that the transit time of BIPS is highly variable,[62] their use for transit studies is limited. However, they may be more helpful in the detection of obstructive disorders.

Ultrasonography
Transabdominal ultrasound examination of the SI is now a routine part of the investigation of intestinal disease. In the future, endoscopic ultrasound will allow the mucosal wall and

Table • 222-8

Helpful Survey Abdominal Radiograph Findings in Patients with Intestinal Disease

FINDINGS	INTERPRETATION
Radiopaque foreign bodies	Visible on survey films
Ileus	Either adynamic/paralytic or obstructive (see Box 222-4)
Abnormal soft tissue shadow	Abdominal mass
Displacement of viscera	Abdominal mass, enlargement of intraperitoneal or retroperitoneal organ, rupture or hernia
Bunching of intestines	Excess intra-abdominal fat, large mass, adhesions, linear foreign body
Bowel wall thickness	Edema, infiltrative (inflammatory, neoplastic disease)
Bowel wall irregularity	Enteritis, neoplasia, ulcers
Loss of serosal detail	Emaciation and immaturity, peritoneal effusion (ascites in hypoproteinemia and/or portal hypertension, peritonitis, carcinomatosis)

adjacent viscera (e.g., pancreas) to be examined in more detail. A conventional ultrasound examination can detect layering of the wall, peristalsis, and luminal contents and can measure intestinal wall thickness.[63] It has excellent sensitivity for the detection of lesions such as intussusceptions,[64] masses,[65]

Box • 222-10

Differential Diagnosis of Ileus

Gas Ileus
Generalized
Aerophagia
Smooth muscle paralyzing drugs
Generalized peritonitis
Enteritis

Localized
Localized peritonitis (e.g., pancreatitis)
Early-stage bowel obstruction
Disruption of mesenteric arterial supply

Fluid Ileus
Generalized
Enteritis
Diffuse intestinal neoplasia

Localized
Foreign body
Tumor causing obstruction
Intussusception

radiolucent foreign bodies, intestinal wall thickening, and lymphadenopathy in chronic inflammatory and neoplastic enteropathies (Figure 222-9). Values for normal SI wall thickness have been reported for dogs and cats,[63] and thickness decreases from proximal to distal. Ultrasound-guided fine needle aspiration for cytologic examination is possible. Disruption of the normal five-layered sonographic appearance (mucosal surface, mucosa, submucosa, muscularis, serosa) is typical of neoplasia, although loss of layering can also result from other infiltrative disorders and bowel wall edema. Intussusceptions are usually recognized in the transverse plane as multiple concentric rings[65] and longitudinally as a thick, multilayered segment.

Special Tests

In cases of malabsorption, intestinal biopsy is usually necessary to obtain a definitive diagnosis. However, EPI should be ruled out before biopsy, because signs of malabsorption are nonspecific. It is also well recognized that biopsies from up to 50% of patients are considered normal by light microscopy. Therefore, usually before biopsy, a number of indirect tests are performed to assess for intestinal damage, altered permeability, and dysfunction.

Diagnosis of Exocrine Pancreatic Insufficiency

Because the signs of EPI cannot be distinguished from primary causes of SI, serum trypsin-like immunoreactivity (TLI) measurement must be performed in all cases.

Serum Folate and Cobalamin Concentrations

The assay of serum folate and cobalamin concentrations can be performed on the same serum sample taken for the TLI test. This assay has limited value in the diagnosis of SI diseases, but subnormal folate and cobalamin concentrations secondary to GI disease may be detected. Cobalamin deficiency is more common, and the response to treatment of the underlying GI disease may be suboptimal if this vitamin deficiency is not corrected. In dogs, the severe cobalamin deficiency recognized in several breeds has been linked to an IF-cobalamin receptor deficiency.[45,66] Cobalamin deficiency is a common sequel to small intestinal disease in cats,[67] and systemic metabolic consequences have been recognized. Determination of the serum folate and cobalamin concentrations is not recommended for the diagnosis of canine SIBO (see below).

Indirect Assessment of Intestinal Absorption

Attempts to assess intestinal function by measuring the mediated absorption of numerous substrates (e.g., lactose, glucose, vitamin A, D-xylose, triglyceride, and starch tolerance tests) are no longer performed because of a similar lack of sensitivity and specificity.

Xylose/3-O-methyl-D-glucose test The differential absorption of these two sugars eliminates the nonmucosal effects that blight the xylose test, and initial results suggest that the test may be of value in dogs and cats.[68]

Intestinal Permeability

Intestinal permeability is an index of mucosal integrity and is assessed by measuring unmediated uptake of nondigestible probe markers. Tests use a nonmetabolizable probe marker that is excreted in the urine. The permeability probe chromium-51-labeled ethylenediamine tetra-acetic acid (^{51}Cr-EDTA) was used in original studies,[69] but the need for a γ-emitter limited its safe use.

Errors related to nonmucosal factors (including the gastric emptying rate, intestinal transit time, and completeness of urine collection) can be eliminated by concurrently measuring the absorption of two probes with different pathways of

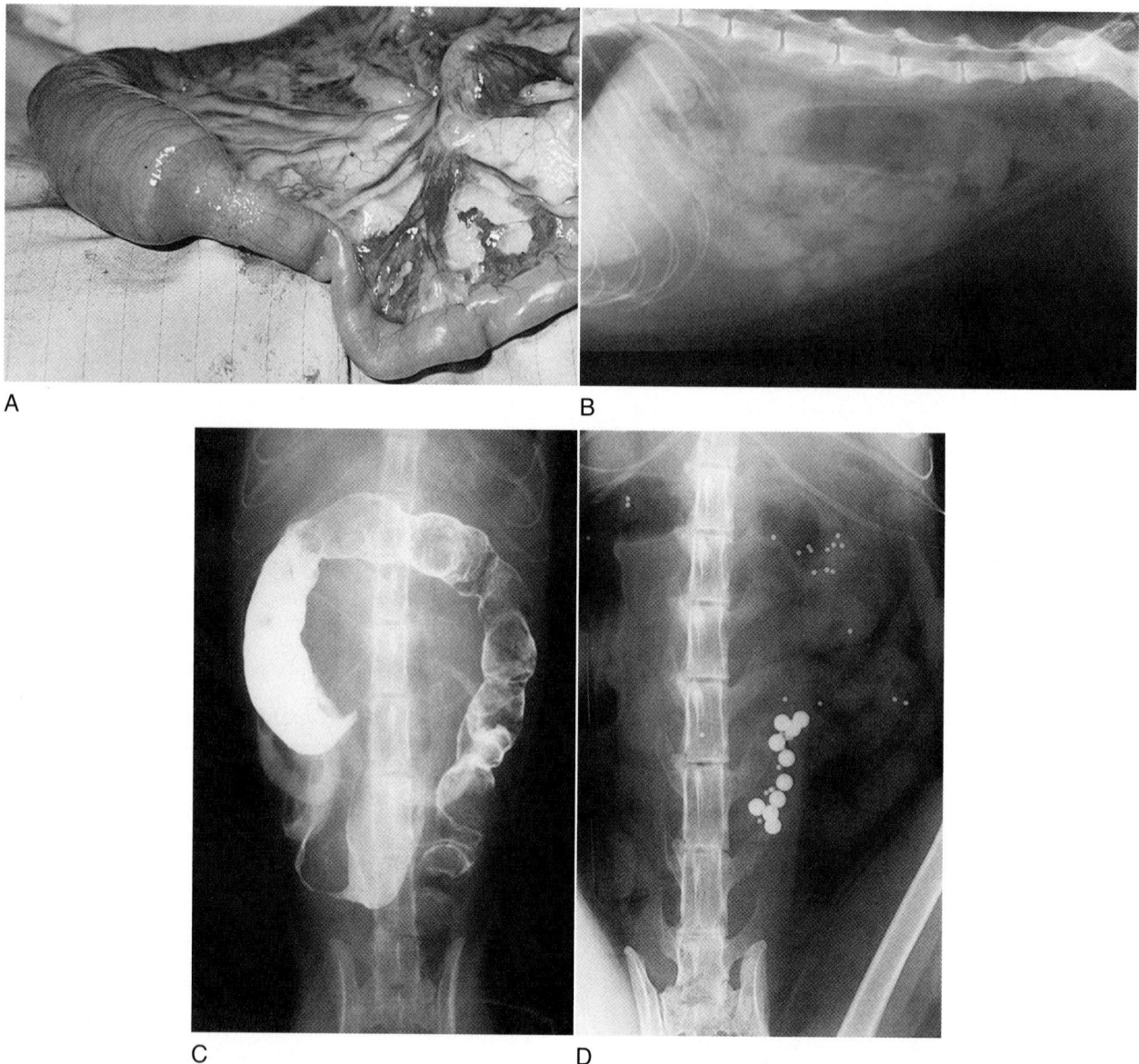

A

B

C

D

Figure 222-8 Identification of an intestinal mass in a Siamese cat. **A,** Annular adenocarcinoma in the ileum demonstrated at laparotomy. **B,** Prior plain lateral radiograph showing a dilated loop of bowel associated with this caudal abdominal mass. **C,** Ventrodorsal radiograph after oral administration of barium suspension showing a dilated loop of SI in the midline, colonic filling, and narrowing of the intestinal lumen at the site of the mass. **D,** Ventrodorsal radiograph after oral administration of BIPS showing accumulation of the larger markers at the site of the partial obstruction caused by the mass. (Courtesy A.H. Sparkes.)

absorption (Figure 222-10). Calculation of their excretion ratio eliminates errors from extramucosal factors because both probes should be affected equally. The ratio, which is altered by villus atrophy or epithelial damage or both, offers a simple, sensitive diagnostic test.

A 5-hour urine collection is performed after oral administration of two sugars. A number of candidates can be used for the probe molecules, and a mixture of one large simple sugar (e.g., lactulose, cellobiose, raffinose) and one small one (e.g., rhamnose, arabinose, mannitol) can be chosen. The cellobiose/mannitol excretion ratio and lactulose/mannitol ratio have been used in companion animals,[70] but with advances in the high-performance liquid chromatography (HPLC) assay of these sugars, the lactulose/rhamnose test has become the standard test of SI permeability.

Tests for Protein-Losing Enteropathy
Historically, intestinal protein loss has been detected by measuring the fecal loss of ^{51}Cr-labeled albumin.[71] The test is unpleasant to perform and potentially hazardous and has largely been discarded, although it remains the standard by which other tests, such as the assay of fecal alpha1-PI (see above), are judged.

Breath Tests
Breath tests are used to assess bacterial metabolism in the GI tract. Bacteria synthesize a gas, which is absorbed and excreted in breath. Breath hydrogen tests have been used most extensively because mammalian cells cannot produce hydrogen, and therefore any that is measured must be bacterial in origin. Such tests can assess carbohydrate malabsorption, bacterial colonization of the SI, and oro-cecal transit time.

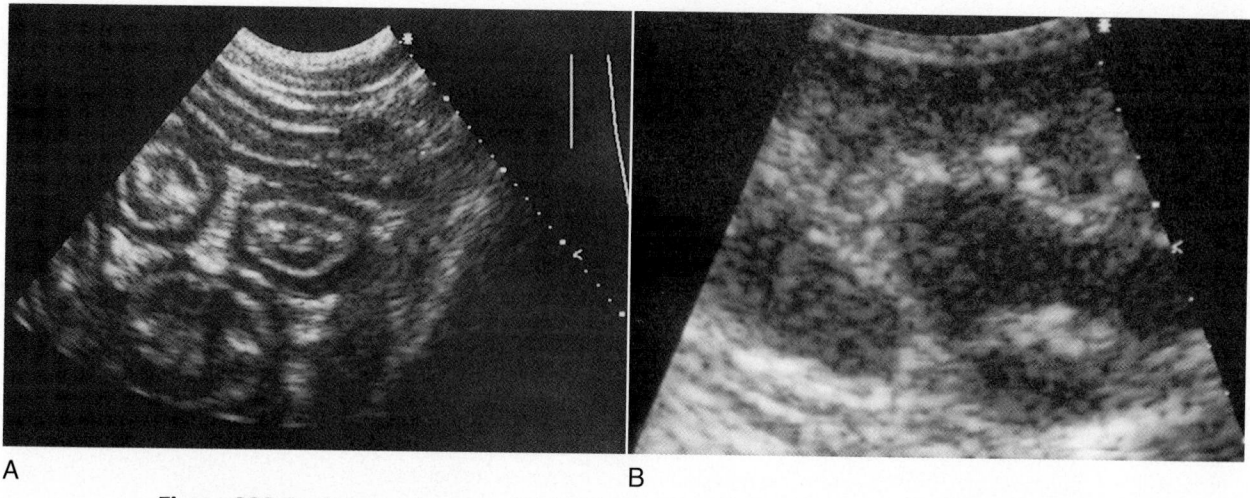

A   B

Figure 222-9 Ultrasound images of the abdomen showing **(A)** transverse image of three loops of bowel with normal layering of the small intestinal wall in a dog and **(B)** mesenteric lymphadenopathy in a cat with alimentary lymphoma. (**A,** Courtesy F.J. Barr. **B,** Courtesy H. Rudorf.)

A variety of protocols has been used, including xylose to assess malabsorption, lactulose to assess oro-cecal transit, and a test meal to assess SI bacterial fermentation. Also, a number of recent studies have attempted to standardize the techniques for companion animals.[72-75] However, these techniques are not widely used even in referral centers.

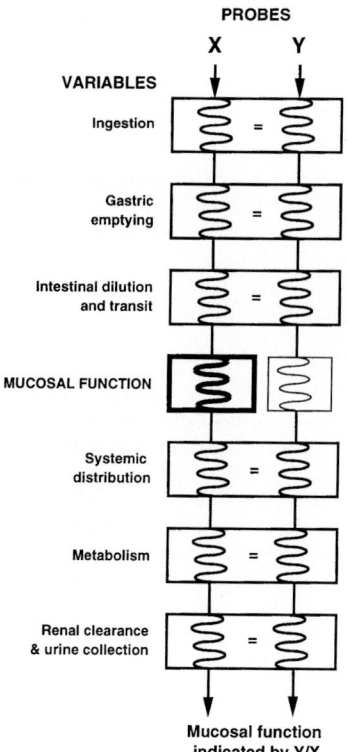

Figure 222-10 Principle of differential permeability testing. Simultaneous administration of two probes selected to respond identically to each variable except mucosal permeability. The Y/X ratio provides a specific index of mucosal permeability. (Hall EJ: Small intestinal disease: Is endoscopic biopsy the answer? J Small Anim Pract 35:408, 1994.)

Labels in Figure 222-10:
PROBES
X   Y
VARIABLES
Ingestion
Gastric emptying
Intestinal dilution and transit
MUCOSAL FUNCTION
Systemic distribution
Metabolism
Renal clearance & urine collection
Mucosal function indicated by Y/X

Unconjugated Bile Salts

The principle of the serum conjugated bile acids test is that conjugated bile salts secreted into the intestine in bile are deconjugated by certain bacterial species and absorbed by the SI. Therefore, in theory, increases in SI bacterial numbers might result in an increase in serum unconjugated bile acids (SUBA). Preliminary work suggested that the test was sensitive and specific for canine SIBO,[76] although a recent study has questioned its utility.[77]

Miscellaneous Tests

A number of tests for intestinal bacterial metabolites have been devised to detect SIBO. These include the nitrosonaphthol test, urinary indican excretion, bacterial release of sulfapyridine from sulfasalazine, and bacterial release of p-amino benzoic acid (PABA) from a bile salt conjugate (PABA-UDCA). However, none of these tests are widely used in companion animals.

Endoscopy

Flexible endoscopy allows gross examination of the SI mucosa and collection of tissue samples without the need for invasive surgery. The proximal small intestine can be viewed during gastroduodenoscopy (see Figure 222-2), and the distal SI often can be visualized by passing the endoscope retrograde through the ileocolic valve. Therefore only the midjejunum cannot be satisfactorily examined by routine endoscopy. However, given that most cases of malabsorption involve diffuse disease, this limitation may not be significant. Enteroscopy, which was developed in humans and which uses a much narrower, thinner endoscope, may allow examination of most of the jejunum.

Abnormal findings on gross endoscopic examination include mucosal granularity and friability, erosions/ulcers, retained food, mass lesions, and hyperemia/erythema. However, none of these characteristics is pathognomonic for particular disease conditions, and gross findings frequently do not correlate with those of the histopathologic examination. A milky white appearance or a milky exudate is suggestive of lymphangiectasia, and the presence of intraluminal parasites may be diagnostic in some cases.

Intestinal Biopsy

In most cases of acute diarrhea, a tissue diagnosis is not needed, and intestinal biopsy is never performed. However, in chronic diarrhea a definitive diagnosis often depends ultimately on histologic examination of intestinal tissue, although this procedure has major limitations (see below). Biopsy specimens are collected, either endoscopically or surgically. The clear advantages of endoscopy to the patient and client are balanced by a number of drawbacks (see Box 222-8), and the client should always be warned that surgical biopsy might ultimately be required for definitive diagnosis. A surgical option is also preferred if there is any possibility of extraintestinal disease or focal intestinal pathology. Biopsies should always be taken, even in the absence of gross abnormalities, because microscopic changes may be present. Multiple endoscopic biopsies (eight or more) should be taken, because the size of the specimens, crush artifacts, and fragmentation can make interpretation difficult.[78]

The duodenum and proximal jejunum (if possible) are biopsied routinely by endoscopy, whereas ileal biopsies may be obtained via colonoscopy. Full-thickness, longitudinal, elliptical surgical biopsies usually are taken from at least three sites, the duodenum, the jejunum, and the ileum.

Examination of Biopsies

Although histopathologic assessment of intestinal biopsies remains the gold standard for diagnosis of intestinal disease, it has marked limitations. Biopsy specimens can be normal by light microscopy, which suggests that many diseases have a functional rather than a morphologic abnormality (Box 222-11) or that sampling problems have occurred.[78] Agreement between histopathologists often is poor. In a recent study, some histopathologists made a diagnosis of lymphoma after assessing tissues from healthy dogs.[79] Histopathologic scoring schemes and standardized criteria have been suggested as a means of improving agreement (Box 222-12), but marked variability still exists. Therefore the primary clinician should always interpret results cautiously and in light of the clinical presentation, and results should be questioned if the tissue diagnosis does not fit the clinical picture or if the response to apparently appropriate therapy is poor. In some cases, repeat biopsy (e.g., by exploratory laparotomy) may be required. Cytologic examination of endoscopic biopsy squash preparations or mucosal brushings may be a useful adjunct to

histopathologic examination.[80] Alternate examinations are largely research tools, but they can provide significant information. Examinations available include electron microscopy; biochemical assay of brush border enzymes; immunocytochemical characterization of B cells, T cells, and their subsets (e.g., CD4 and CD8 cells)[22-24] and MHC expression[24,29]; cytokine expression[81]; and assessment of T-cell clonality.[82]

Duodenal Juice

Duodenal juice can be collected during duodenoscopy through a sterile polyethylene tube passed down the biopsy channel or by needle aspiration through the intestinal wall at laparotomy. However, collection of sufficient sample without blood and tissue contamination can be difficult. The sample can be examined for *Giardia* trophozoites, although this has not proved reliable in diagnosis.[83] Alternatively, quantitative and qualitative aerobic and anaerobic cultures can be performed. This is the gold standard for diagnosis of SIBO, although there are major problems in interpretation. First, problems may arise from differences in the methods of collection (e.g., endoscopic aspiration versus needle aspiration) and from insufflation with air during endoscopy or dilution with endoscopic wash fluid, gastric juice, bile, or blood. Second, laboratory protocols for bacteriology may vary among laboratories, especially for obligate anaerobes. Third, large intraindividual variation exists in duodenal juice culture results,[16] with one report documenting a 7 log-unit difference between bacterial counts obtained on two separate occasions from an individual animal.[84] Fourth, because bacterial overgrowth may occur in pockets, a single upper SI culture may

---

Box • 222-12

Criteria for Histologic Assessment of Intestinal Biopsies

Crypt-Villus Unit
Villus height and width
Villus clubbing/fusion
Crypt depth
Mitotic index
Crypt abscessation
Crypt to villus ratio

Epithelium
Erosions
Enterocyte height
Intraepithelial lymphocyte density
Goblet cell number/size

Lamina Propria
Immune cell density
Predominant cell type
Lymphangiectasia

Miscellaneous
Hyperemia or congestion
Edema
Fibrosis
Infective agents
Neoplasia

Box • 222-11

Causes of Chronic Diarrhea for which Small Intestinal Biopsy May Be Normal*

SIBO, ARD
Dietary indiscretion
Food intolerance
Type I hypersensitivity to food (if dog is starved before biopsy)
Toxigenic/secretory diarrheas
Motility disorders/irritable bowel syndrome
Brush border membrane disease (e.g., hypolactasia)
Patchy mucosal disease not sampled
Intestinal sclerosis (if biopsies are not full thickness)
Undiagnosed EPI or colonic or systemic disease

*Detection of histologic abnormalities depends on the size and quality of the biopsy, the quality of processing, and the expertise of the pathologist.
ARD, antibiotic-responsive diarrhea; EPI, exocrine pancreatic insufficiency; SIBO, small intestinal bacterial overgrowth.

not be entirely representative. Despite these problems, a strict cutoff for the upper limit of normal bacterial counts is often applied; this is inappropriate, because healthy dogs can have numbers in excess of this limit without showing clinical signs. Finally, a recent study has suggested that it does not aid in decision making for cases of GI disease.[77] Therefore, given all these limitations, routine diagnostic use of duodenal juice bacterial culture is not recommended.

Acute Small Intestinal Disease

Potential causes of acute diarrhea are listed in Table 222-9, but whether a complete diagnosis is pursued and when therapy is instituted are clinical judgments. The diagnostic approach to acute diarrhea is discussed elsewhere.

Patients that are bright, alert, and not dehydrated may require no further investigation, because signs are often self-limiting. Further investigation of acute diarrhea is indicated under the following circumstances:

- The patient is dull or depressed, febrile, dehydrated, tachycardic or bradycardic or is having abdominal discomfort, melena, bloody mucoid stools, or frequent vomiting.
- Obvious physical abnormalities (e.g., intestinal masses, thickening, or plication) localize the problem to the SI, and diagnostic imaging, noninvasive biopsy, or surgery can define the cause.
- Systemic abnormalities are present, as defined by a minimum database and other clinicopathologic tests.

It is important that the patient be regularly re-evaluated to monitor the response to therapy and to detect any new abnormalities that may arise.

Treatment of Acute Diarrhea

The initial management of acute diarrhea associated with systemic illness is symptomatic and supportive, and is commenced on the basis of clinical findings, in particular the presence of dehydration, while the results of the initial data base and further tests are pending.

Fluid therapy   Oral fluid and electrolyte replacement therapy may be sufficient if acute diarrhea is associated with only mild or insignificant dehydration, and if vomiting is infrequent or absent,[85] although its efficacy should still be monitored. However, when diarrhea is accompanied by significant vomiting or dehydration, parenteral fluids should be administered at a rate that replaces deficits, supplies maintenance needs and compensates for ongoing losses. Patients with marked hypovolemia require more aggressive support.

The type of fluid and requirement for potassium supplementation is best judged by performing a minimum data base and blood gas analysis. Parenteral fluids are usually best given intravenously. The intraosseous route can be used if venous access is unavailable, but subcutaneous administration of fluids is likely to be inadequate.

Diet   Studies examining the role of diet in the treatment of acute diarrhea in dogs and cats are scarce.[86] Current recommendations are based on common sense and anecdotal evidence. Best practice generally is considered to be withholding food for 24 to 48 hours and then feeding a bland diet, given little and often, for 3 to 5 days. Thereafter the original diet is gradually reintroduced. In animals with no other significant clinical findings, this may be the only therapy required. Common choices of a bland, fat-restricted diet for dogs are boiled chicken or white fish or low-fat cottage cheese with boiled rice. Cats seem to have a lower tolerance to dietary starch and may benefit from a diet with a higher fat content. Little attention is paid to the overall nutritional adequacy of home-prepared bland diets when fed in the short term.

This dogma of *intestinal rest* has been challenged by studies that demonstrate that feeding human infants during diarrhea promotes recovery. The success of such *feeding through diarrhea* varies depending on the cause, with most benefit seen in secretory diarrhea. However, in dogs and cats, secretory diarrhea is less common, the increased volumes of diarrhea may be cosmetically unacceptable, and the frequently contemporaneous vomiting may preclude this approach. The inclusion of glutamine, a nutrient utilized preferentially by enterocytes, may also promote recovery and decrease bacterial translocation,[87,88] although experimental proof of improved intestinal integrity in animals is lacking.[89]

Theoretically, any intestinal disease may predispose the animal to the development of a food sensitivity, therefore feeding of a novel protein source during these periods may preclude the development of sensitivity to the staple diet. However, this concept of feeding of a *sacrificial protein* is supported only by circumstantial evidence.

Protectants and adsorbents   Bismuth-subsalicylate, kaolin-pectin, montmorillonite, activated charcoal and magnesium, and aluminum and barium-containing products are often administered in acute diarrhea to bind bacteria and their toxins and to coat and protect the intestinal mucosa, but they may also have an antisecretory effect. Therapy for acute diarrhea with protectants, adsorbents or motility modifying agents (see below) should not exceed 5 days.

Motility- and secretion-modifying agents   Anticholinergics and opiates or opioids (loperamide, diphenoxylate) are frequently used for the symptomatic management of acute diarrhea, but anticholinergic agents can potentiate ileus and are not recommended. Opiate analgesics were thought to exert their effects by stimulating segmental motility, but they actually act mainly by decreasing intestinal secretion and promoting absorption and can be used in the short-term symptomatic management of acute diarrhea in dogs. They are contraindicated in cases involving obstruction or an infectious etiology.

Antimicrobial therapy   Antimicrobials are indicated only in animals with a confirmed bacterial or protozoal infection,

Table • 222-9

Causes of Acute Diarrhea

CAUSES	EXAMPLES
Dietary	Hypersensitivity (allergy), intolerance, sudden diet change, food poisoning (poor quality, spoiled foods/bacterial)
Toxic	Food or other sources
Infectious	Parvovirus, coronavirus, paramyxovirus, adenovirus, may or may not be FeLV/FIV related; also *Salmonella, Campylobacter, Clostridium* spp. (?) and *Escherichia coli* (?) Helminths; *Coccidia, Giardia* spp.
Parasites	
Acute pancreatitis	
Anatomic	Intussusception
Metabolic	Hypoadrenocorticism

FeLV, feline leukemia virus; FIV, feline immunodeficiency virus.

GASTROINTESTINAL DISEASE

those in which a breach of intestinal barrier integrity is suspected from evidence of GI bleeding, and hence in those at risk of sepsis. Leukopenia, neutrophilia, pyrexia, the presence of blood in the feces, and shock all are indications for prophylactic antibiotics in animals with diarrhea. Initial choices in these situations include ampicillin or a cephalosporin (effective against gram-positive and some gram-negative and anaerobic bacteria). If systemic translocation of enteric bacteria is suspected, antimicrobials effective against anaerobic organisms (e.g., metronidazole or clindamycin) and "difficult" gram-negative aerobes (e.g., an aminoglycoside or a fluoroquinolone) are indicated. Intravenous quinolones have been shown to reach therapeutic concentrations in the canine gut lumen and can be effective against enterococci, *E. coli*, and anaerobes.[90] Oxytetracycline, tylosin, and metronidazole are suitable for the treatment of SIBO.

A four-quadrant, intravenous antibacterial regimen may be required if septicemia is likely, and suitable combinations would be a cephalosporin (or amoxicillin) or a fluoroquinolone (or amikacin) with metronidazole or clindamycin. However, aminoglycosides should not be given until the patient is volume-expanded.

Probiotics Traditionally, many practitioners have recommended feeding live yogurt as a way of repopulating the intestine with beneficial lactobacilli after an acute GI upset. There is evidence in other species that probiotics do exert a positive effect on intestinal permeability and mucosal immune responses, although the effects may be species specific and present only while the probiotic is continuously administered.[91] Probiotics are now available for use in dogs and cats, and emerging data exist to support their use.[92]

Acute Diarrhea Induced by Diet, Drugs, or Toxins

Altered food intake, probably the most common cause of acute, self-limiting diarrhea in dogs, includes rapid diet change, dietary indiscretion, dietary intolerance, hypersensitivity, and food poisoning. Dietary hypersensitivity (food allergy) is probably rare. Ingestion of drugs (e.g., nonsteroidal anti-inflammatory drugs [NSAIDs] or antibacterials) or toxins (e.g., insecticides) also may cause vomiting and diarrhea. The history may allow an educated, presumptive diagnosis to be made. However, the exact cause often is never determined because the patient is not systemically unwell and responds to symptomatic therapy. The prognosis usually is excellent, and only if the diarrhea does not respond or the patient deteriorates is further investigation necessary.

Hemorrhagic Gastroenteritis

There are numerous potential causes of bloody vomiting and diarrhea, but *hemorrhagic gastroenteritis* (HGE) is the name given to a syndrome characterized by acute hemorrhagic diarrhea accompanied by marked hemoconcentration. The cause of the syndrome is unknown. It may represent an intestinal type 1 hypersensitivity reaction or could be a consequence of *C. perfringens* enterotoxin production.[93]

Clinical findings Dogs present with acute hemorrhagic diarrhea, with small breed dogs most frequently affected. Pyrexia is unusual, but vomiting, depression, and abdominal discomfort are common. The onset may be peracute and can be associated with marked fluid shifts into the SI, leading to severe hypovolemic shock even before signs of dehydration (e.g., decreased skin turgor) appear.

Diagnosis A presumptive diagnosis of HGE can be made on the basis of appropriate clinical findings associated with a packed cell volume (PCV) of 55% to 60% or more. Total protein is often normal or not as high relative to the PCV, probably because of intestinal plasma loss. Radiographs may demonstrate ileus.

The absence of leukopenia and the presence of marked hemoconcentration help distinguish HGE from parvovirus. Positive fecal tests may support a diagnosis of clostridiosis, but direct evidence of SI infection is rarely obtained.[93]

Treatment Intravenous fluids are essential in treating patients with HGE. Some patients become hypoproteinemic, and plasma or colloid support may be required. Parenteral antibiotics are often administered because of potential clostridial infection and the high risk of sepsis. Clinical improvement is usually noted within a few hours, though the diarrhea may take several days to resolve. Close patient monitoring is essential; patients that have not responded within 24 hours should be re-evaluated for parvovirus, intussusception, or foreign objects. Once the patient is in the recovery phase, standard dietary therapy for acute diarrhea can be instigated. The prognosis for most animals with HGE is good, but if HGE is complicated by severe hypoproteinemia or sepsis, the prognosis is more guarded.

Infectious and Parasitic Causes of Acute Diarrhea

Diarrhea caused by infectious and parasitic agents is considered common in animals that are young, immunologically naïve or immunocompromised, housed in large numbers, or housed in unsanitary conditions. Parvovirus, *Giardia*, *Salmonella*, and *Campylobacter* spp., and some helminths can be significant causes of diarrhea. The importance of coronavirus, *C. perfringens*, and *E. coli* as causes of diarrhea has yet to be defined. The zoonotic potential of many of these infections has not been clearly elucidated, but basic hygienic precautions should always be adopted. Specific SI infections are discussed below, but the reader is referred elsewhere for detailed information on other viruses such as paramyxoviruses, adenoviruses, feline leukemia, and immunodeficiency viruses, which also cause diarrhea but affect many other organ systems apart from the GI tract.

VIRAL ENTERITIDES

Most viral enteritides of dogs and cats, especially the parvovirus infections, cause an acute and usually self-limiting diarrhea, although severe cases in young or immunocompromised patients may be fatal. Canine parvovirus infection is described here as the index case for viral enteritides.

Canine Parvovirus

Canine parvovirus type 2 (CPV-2) is a highly contagious cause of acute enteritis.[94] It emerged as a pathogen in the late 1970s, perhaps from a mutation of a feline vaccine as it is related to feline panleukopenia and mink enteritis viruses. CPV-2b has emerged as the most prevalent antigenic variant. There have been reports of cats being infected with CPV-2, but the severity of signs is much reduced.

Infected dogs shed massive quantities of virus particles in feces during the acute illness and then for about 8 to 10 days afterward. Parvovirus is extremely stable and can remain infectious in the environment for many months. Infection is acquired via the fecal-oral route and is more common in the summer months. The virus has an affinity for rapidly dividing cells and localizes to the intestine (crypt cells), bone marrow, and lymphoid tissues. It causes apoptotic cell death, leading to intestinal crypt necrosis and severe diarrhea, leukopenia, and lymphoid depletion.[95]

Clinical Findings

Clinical signs of diarrhea typically occur 4 to 7 days after infection. Anorexia, depression, fever, vomiting, diarrhea (often profuse and hemorrhagic), and dehydration are common.

Hypothermia and disseminated intravascular coagulation (DIC) are associated with terminal bacterial sepsis or endotoxemia. Dogs of any age can be affected, but the incidence of clinical disease is highest in puppies between weaning and 6 months. Puppies younger than 6 weeks usually are protected by maternal antibody. In dogs older than 6 months, males are more likely to become infected than females. Overcrowding, intestinal parasitism, concurrent infection with distemper virus, coronavirus, *Giardia*, *Salmonella*, or *Campylobacter* spp. can increase the severity of illness.

Puppies infected *in utero* or shortly after birth may develop myocarditis and either die suddenly or develop cardiomyopathy if maternal antibody is absent. This situation rarely arises nowadays because widespread vaccination and infection have left few seronegative dams. Yet death still occurs, especially in young puppies, and particularly in susceptible breeds such as rottweilers, Dobermans, English springer spaniels, and American pit bull terriers.[96] Death is usually attributed to dehydration, electrolyte imbalances, hypercoagulability, endotoxic shock, or overwhelming bacterial sepsis related to mucosal barrier disruption and leukopenia. Infected dogs are immunosuppressed and susceptible to catheter infections.[97] Endotoxemia, TNF activity, coliform septicemia, and proliferation of enteric *C. perfringens* determine morbidity and mortality.[98]

Diagnosis

Parvovirus should be suspected in young dogs with sudden onset of vomiting and diarrhea, especially if they are also depressed, febrile, or leukopenic or if they have been in contact with infected dogs. Leukopenia (often 500 to 2000 white blood cells per microliter) may be detected in up to 85% of field cases and is very suggestive of parvovirus infection. It reflects neutropenia and lymphopenia. Neutropenia results from impaired bone marrow production with concurrent neutrophil loss through the damaged GI tract, and severe neutropenia crudely correlates with a poor prognosis.

In the absence of leukopenia, clinical signs are indistinguishable from those of other bacterial or viral enteritides, GI foreign bodies with peritonitis, or intussusception. Abdominal radiographs may reveal non-specific gas and fluid accumulation, and ileus. Biochemical abnormalities often include hypokalemia, hypoglycemia, prerenal azotemia, and increased bilirubin or liver enzymes.

Definitive diagnosis requires demonstration of CPV-2 virus (or viral antigens) in the feces. Fecal ELISA is regarded as an accurate and specific diagnostic test but is most sensitive in the first 7 to 10 days when virus excretion is greatest. Single anti-CPV antibody determination in serum (by hemagglutination inhibition) is not useful for diagnosis except in the presence of typical clinical signs in an unvaccinated animal. A rising IgG titer by paired serology provides only a retrospective diagnosis. Serum IgM analysis may provide evidence of recent infection.

Treatment

Treatment is supportive and is similar to regimens used in most animals with severe gastroenteritis. Intravenous fluid therapy usually is indicated and is continued until vomiting stops and oral intake resumes. A balanced electrolyte solution (e.g., lactated Ringer's solution) supplemented with potassium and 2.5% glucose is often used. Plasma or whole blood infusions are given to treat severe hypoproteinemia or anemia. Antibiotics are used to control potentially fatal sepsis (see above).

Traditionally, oral intake is withheld until vomiting has stopped for at least 24 hours; this may take 3 to 5 days in severe cases. Rather than avoid the oral route completely, it may be better to trickle feed small amounts of glutamine-containing solutions to reduce bacterial translocation.[87,88] Once vomiting has been controlled, small amounts of a bland diet are fed initially. Frequent or persistent vomiting can be managed with intermittent injections or constant-rate infusion of metoclopramide, once intestinal obstruction has been ruled out. Phenothiazines (e.g., chlorpromazine) can be used if metoclopramide is ineffective and the animal has been rehydrated.

Administration of corticosteroids is of unproven benefit and is probably best limited to dogs with severe endotoxic shock. Flunixin meglumine is best avoided because of its adverse effects on the GI tract and kidneys. Antiendotoxin therapy has been useful in some patients,[99] but the timing of antiendotoxins in relation to antibiotic therapy may be important. Because antibiotics may increase endotoxin liberation, it may be preferable to administer antiendotoxin serum before antibiotics. However, one study showed that the use of the antiendotoxin rBPI$_{21}$ had no beneficial effect on survival,[100] and in another study, use of antiendotoxin was correlated with decreased suvival.[101] Administration of recombinant human granulocyte colony-stimulating factor (G-CSF) to neutropenic parvoviral enteritis patients may raise neutrophil counts but is of no clinical benefit,[102] because the endogenous G-CSF concentration is already elevated.[103] In contrast, administration of feline interferon-omega was found to improve clinical signs and reduce mortality.[104]

Prognosis

Severe infection and leukopenia are associated with a high mortality rate, but most dogs with parvovirus recover if dehydration and sepsis are treated appropriately. Complications include hypoglycemia, hypoproteinemia, anemia, intussusception, and secondary bacterial or viral infections.

Prevention

Prevention is achieved by limiting exposure to the virus, adequate disinfection (1:32 dilution of sodium hypochlorite bleach), and vaccination.[94] Vaccination is an effective means of preventing and controlling CPV-2, but maternal antibody interference is a problem. Maternally derived antibodies (MDAs) can persist for up to 18 weeks and can interfere with vaccination, although most modern vaccines can overcome MDAs by 10 to 12 weeks of age. Modified live CPV-2 vaccines are most commonly used; killed vaccines provide less duration of immunity but may be recommended in pregnant dogs and puppies younger than 5 weeks. Vaccines may differ in efficacy; low-passage, high-titer vaccines are considered most effective, and only one injection at or after 12 weeks may be needed.[105] In susceptible breeds and dogs in high-risk areas, vaccination may begin at 6 to 8 weeks of age and be repeated every 3 to 4 weeks until 18 weeks of age. There is good correlation between the antibody titer and resistance to infection with canine parvovirus. Annual revaccination is currently recommended.

Feline Parvovirus (Feline Panleukopenia)

Feline panleukopenia is a highly contagious infection of cats that causes severe acute diarrhea and death, similar to canine parvovirus. Mortality in young kittens is high (50% to 90%), therefore the prognosis is guarded until the vomiting and diarrhea stop and the leukopenia resolves.

Canine Coronavirus

Canine coronavirus (CCV) can cause diarrhea of variable severity in dogs.[94] Transmission is by the fecal-oral route. The incubation period is 1 to 4 days, and infected dogs may shed virus intermittently for months after clinical recovery. However, the significance of coronavirus as a primary pathogen is unclear. Experimental inoculation is associated with only mild disease and CCV infection, and antibodies against CCV are present in many healthy and diarrheic dogs. Infection is very prevalent, particularly in animal shelter and laboratory dogs. Most CCV infections are probably subclinical, although severe enteritis may occur in dense populations

GASTROINTESTINAL DISEASE

or with concurrent infections. In such situations, vaccination may be helpful.

Feline Enteric Coronavirus

Feline enteric coronavirus (FECV) is ubiquitous in the cat population. Mild to moderately severe diarrhea, which may be associated with weight loss, is seen in kittens infected with FECV. Inapparent infection is common in normal cats, many of which shed FECV in feces and are seropositive. FECV infection is important, because enteric coronaviruses may mutate to feline infectious peritonitis virus (FIPV).

Intestinal Feline Infectious Peritonitis

An unusual manifestation of feline infectious peritonitis (FIP) of isolated mural intestinal lesions has been reported.[106] Predominant clinical signs were diarrhea and vomiting, and all cats had a palpable mass in the colon or ileocecocolic junction. Affected intestine was markedly thickened and nodular, with multifocal pyogranulomas extending through the intestinal wall.

Feline Immunodeficiency Virus

Infection with feline immunodeficiency virus (FIV) is associated with a 10% to 20% incidence of chronic enteritis. Although secondary and opportunistic infections may be responsible for signs, sometimes no other etiologic agent can be identified.[107] Anorexia, chronic diarrhea, and emaciation are typical. Palpably thickened bowel loops reflect chronic enteritis with transmural granulomatous inflammation.

Feline Leukemia Virus

Among its many manifestations, feline leukemia virus (FeLV) infection can be associated with fatal peracute enterocolitis and lymphocytic ileitis.

Torovirus

A torovirus-like agent has been isolated from the feces of cats afflicted with a characteristic syndrome of chronic diarrhea and protruding nictitating membrane.[108] However, a clear association with clinical signs was not demonstrated.

BACTERIAL ENTERITIDES

Most GI infections by pathogenic bacteria are associated with acute diarrhea; however, because these bacteria sometimes can be isolated from healthy animals and from those with chronic diarrhea, confusion exists about the significance of these organisms. Enteroinvasive bacteria such as *Campylobacter* spp., *Salmonella* spp., *Shigella* spp., and *Yersinia enterocolitica* all can be pathogenic and yet may be isolated from healthy animals. The incidence of infection is greatest in young, kenneled animals and immunocompromised patients. Although these organisms may present a zoonotic risk, attempting to eradicate them with antibiotics may be unhelpful and unnecessary and may even induce a carrier state.

Campylobacter spp.

Campylobacter jejuni and *C. upsaliensis* have been associated with intestinal disease in dogs and cats, although experimental infection of dogs causes only transient signs.[109] Most infections are asymptomatic, with carriage rates in healthy dogs and cats of up to 50%; kenneled and young animals have the highest isolation rates. Clinically significant disease is usually restricted to young, parasitized, or immunocompromised animals. Clinical signs are watery, mucoid, or hemorrhagic diarrhea accompanied by vomiting, tenesmus, pyrexia, and anorexia. Concurrent infection with *Giardia* or *Salmonella* spp., parvovirus, or coronavirus causes more severe disease.

Diagnosis

Because the bacteria are fragile, the diagnosis is best made by isolating them from fresh feces. The presence of slender, seagull-shaped bacteria on a stained fecal smear yields a presumptive diagnosis.

Treatment

Animals with severe hemorrhagic mucoid diarrhea should be treated with erythromycin, or quinolone antibiotics such as enrofloxacin. Fluoroquinolones may be preferred, because erythromycin may cause vomiting, but the efficacy of the former has not been critically evaluated. Resistance to antibiotics has been reported, and post-treatment cultures should be performed to document eradication. It is important that the owner be instructed in hygienic precautions to prevent zoonotic infection.

Prognosis

The prognosis for recovery usually is good.

Salmonella spp

Salmonella organisms are gram-negative motile rods that can cause significant clinical signs in dogs and cats and that have a zoonotic potential. Asymptomatic carriage is common, and *Salmonella* bacteria have been isolated from the feces of up to 30% of healthy dogs and 18% of healthy cats. Clinically significant disease is unusual and occurs most frequently in young, parasitized, kenneled, or immunocompromised animals.

Clinical Findings

Three scenarios may follow infection: asymptomatic carriage, gastroenteritis, or bacteremia and endotoxemia. Significant infection causes acute diarrhea that ranges from mild to severe and bloody, as well as anorexia, pyrexia, abdominal pain, and vomiting. Bacterial translocation from the gut lumen may result in septicemia, endotoxemia, DIC, and death in susceptible animals.

Cats with *Salmonella* infection may show only vague signs (e.g., pyrexia, leukocytosis, and conjunctivitis) and no gastrointestinal signs. An acute febrile illness and diarrhea, known as songbird fever, has been reported in cats after ingestion of dead songbirds infected with *Salmonella typhimurium*.

Diagnosis

Diagnosis is based on the isolation of *Salmonella* organisms from feces or from blood in septicemic patients. Clinicopathologic features are nonspecific. Hyperkalemia and hyponatremia, suggestive of hypoadrenocorticism, may occur.

Treatment

Antibiotic treatment may promote bacterial resistance and a carrier state and is not recommended when *Salmonella* bacteria are isolated from healthy infected animals or stable animals with acute diarrhea. In animals with severe hemorrhagic diarrhea, marked depression, shock, persistent pyrexia, or sepsis, parenteral antibiotics should be given. The choice of antibiotic should be governed by sensitivity testing when possible, but fluoroquinolones appear to be effective against many *Salmonella* spp.[110] Therapy initially should be given for 10 days, but prolonged therapy may be required. The feces should be recultured on several occasions to ensure that the infection has been eliminated.

Prognosis

The prognosis for diarrhea associated with *Salmonella* infection in most cases is good. A guarded prognosis should be given in patients with septicemia. Negative prognostic indicators include peracute onset, marked pyrexia (temperature over 40° C), hypothermia, severe hemorrhagic diarrhea, degenerative left shift, and hypoglycemia.

Clostridium spp.

C. perfringens, C. difficile, and other clostridial species are part of the normal resident microflora of dogs and cats but may cause diarrhea as a consequence of enterotoxin production.[111,112]

C. difficile can produce two toxins (A and B) and is responsible for antibiotic-associated pseudomembranous colitis in humans. It has been incriminated as a cause of chronic diarrhea in dogs.

Enterotoxin-producing C. perfringens has been associated with diarrhea in hospital kennels and with acute and chronic GI signs. Examination of a Diff Quik–stained fecal smear for safety pin–shaped, C. perfringens–containing spores has been suggested as a simple screening test, because enterotoxin elaboration was believed to coincide with sporulation. However, this supposition has been disproved by the measurement of C. perfringens enterotoxin in feces in the absence of spore formation.[113] Furthermore, enterotoxin can be detected in the feces of healthy dogs, Although SI diarrhea may occur, most dogs show signs of LI diarrhea, and a causal relationship to diarrhea remains to be proven.

Escherichia coli

The role of enteropathogenic (EPEC) and enterotoxigenic (ETEC) E. coli as a cause of diarrhea in dogs and cats is unresolved. Although many strains are normal commensals, some are a significant cause of acute diarrhea, and other isolates may cause chronic diarrhea.[57] The attachment of ETEC organisms and subsequent release of heat-labile, heat-stable and Shiga-like toxins may cause acute diarrhea. EPEC bacteria attach to the mucosa, cause effacement of microvilli, and produce profound malabsorption and diarrhea without causing marked changes on light microscopy (Figure 222-11).[114] Identification of pathogenic strains requires specialized assays, such as bioassays for toxins and genome probes for identification of pathogenicity markers, and isolation does not prove causation.[57]

Enteroadherent Organisms

Enteroadherent E. coli and other adherent organisms, including Streptococcus spp., have been reported to cause chronic diarrhea in dogs.

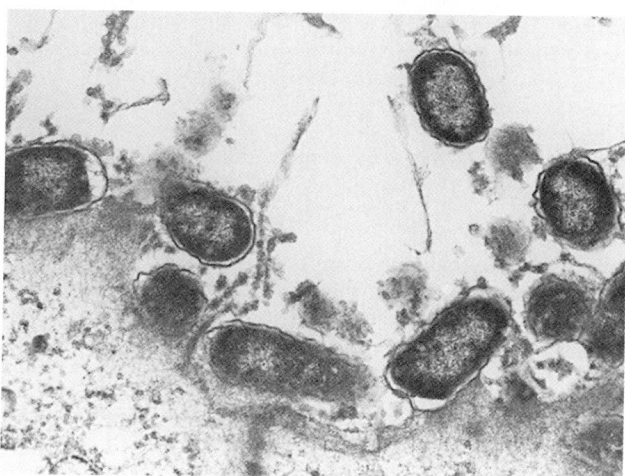

Figure 222-11 Electron micrograph showing attaching and effacing Escherichia coli organisms on the luminal surface of an enterocyte, causing widespread microvillus damage. (Courtesy R.J. Higgins and G.R. Pearson.)

Yersinia pseudotuberculosis

Yersinia pseudotuberculosis can be ingested when cats eat infected rodents or birds. The bacteria infect the GI tract, liver, and lymph nodes, causing marked weight loss, diarrhea, anorexia, lethargy, jaundice, and mesenteric lymphadenopathy. Treatment may be attempted with oxytetracycline or trimethoprim-sulfa, but the disease usually is progressive and fatal.

Tuberculosis

In dogs and cats, Mycobacterium spp. cause multisystemic, granulomatous infections that occasionally involve the GI tract. Cats may develop SI infection with Mycobacterium bovis from drinking infected cow's milk; the infection is associated with vomiting, diarrhea, weight loss, mesenteric lymphadenopathy, and peritonitis.

Miscellaneous Bacteria

Many GI bacteria may be opportunistic pathogens, and occasionally clinical signs are related directly to a specific organism. Bacillus piliformis is a rare disease that causes acute, fatal diarrhea in puppies and kittens (Tyzzer's disease). No effective treatment has been described. Providencia alcalifaciens was reported to cause primary bacterial enteritis in three dogs.[115]

RICKETTSIAL DIARRHEA (SALMON POISONING)

Neorickettsia helminthoeca and Neorickettsia elokominica are found in the metacercariae of the fluke Nanophyetus salmonicola, which is present in salmon in the western regions of the Cascade Mountains from northern California to central Washington. About a week after ingestion of infected salmon by dogs, the rickettsiae emerge from the mature fluke and cause a disease characterized by high fever, hemorrhagic gastroenteritis, vomiting, lethargy, anorexia, polydipsia, nasal-ocular discharge, and peripheral lymphadenopathy. Mortality is extremely high in untreated patients.

The diagnosis is based on a history of ingestion of raw fish in an endemic area, the detection of operculated fluke eggs in feces, and the presence of intracytoplasmic inclusion bodies in macrophages from lymph node aspirates. Oxytetracycline (7 mg/kg given intravenously three times a day) is the treatment of choice and should be continued for at least 5 days. The trematode vector is eradicated with praziquantel.

ALGAL INFECTIONS

Toxic algal blooms can lead to acute gastroenteritis and death in animals that drink contaminated water. Blue-green algae can synthesize an anticholinesterase that induces vomiting, diarrhea, ataxia, and rapid death in dogs. Prototheca spp. are achlorophyllous algae that cause protothecosis. Typically a cutaneous infection in cats, in dogs it can involve the intestine. LI disease is more common, but fatal disseminated disease affecting the SI has been reported.

FUNGAL INFECTIONS

Low numbers of fungi are found in the normal intestinal microflora and are generally not pathogenic. However, under the right circumstances, such as immunosuppression, they may invade the intestinal mucosa and even disseminate throughout the body. The incidence of these diseases varies worldwide; some are ubiquitous, some are localized to tropical and subtropical areas, and some are endemic in restricted areas. Intestinal infection with a variety of poorly septate molds and fungi is called phycomycosis. Of all cases, infection with

Pythium spp. (pythiosis) is by far the most common. *Pythium insidiosum* may cause a primary intestinal infection.

Pythiosis

Pythiosis occurs sporadically throughout the world in tropical and subtropical climates. In the United States, pythiosis is most common in the states bordering the Gulf of Mexico. Animals may develop intestinal infection by ingestion of zoospore-contaminated water. Intestinal disease is seen most commonly from fall to spring after infection in late summer, when environmental conditions of warm, swampy water favor fungal growth.

History and Clinical Signs

Infection is more common in dogs than cats and typically occurs in young, large breed dogs under 3 years of age. Hunting dogs working in swamplike environments are the most likely to be exposed to infection. The organism can infect any part of the GI tract, but SI infection causes chronic, intractable, and sometimes bloody diarrhea. Vomiting, anorexia, depression, and progressive weight loss are usually noted. Infection is characterized by regions of transmural pyogranulomatous inflammation and ulceration. The bowel wall becomes greatly thickened, which may eventually result in partial or complete obstruction.

Diagnosis

On physical examination the most consistent findings in dogs with intestinal pythiosis are emaciation, with either one or more palpable abdominal masses or a thickened, irregular segment of bowel. Mild to moderate nonregenerative anemia and a mild neutrophilia with or without a left shift are typical. Definitive diagnosis can be made only by demonstration of branching, poorly septate or nonseptate hyphae in the tissues, because grossly, the mass or masses can resemble neoplasia at laparotomy. The organisms stain poorly with hematoxylin and eosin or periodic acid–Schiff (PAS) but are evident with Gomori methenamine silver stain. Recently an ELISA and a polymerase chain reaction (PCR) test have been developed.[116,117]

Treatment and Prognosis

The prognosis for phycomycosis is grave. Conventional treatment involves surgical excision followed by antifungal treatment. However, lack of ergosterol in the cell membrane makes azole derivatives largely ineffective. Euthanasia is often necessary, either because surgical excision is impossible or because of recurrence and wound dehiscence.

Zygomycosis

Other organisms have been isolated sporadically from cases of phycomycosis and are opportunistic pathogens in immunosuppressed patients. They are from the Zygomycetes class (zygomycosis), and include members of the Entomophthoraceae (e.g., *Basidiobolus* spp., *Conidiobolus* spp.) and Mucoraceae (e.g., *Absidia* spp., *Rhizopus* spp., *Mucor* spp., *Mortierella* spp.).

Histoplasmosis

H. capsulatum sometimes disseminates throughout the body, including the GI tract.

HELMINTHS

Helminthic infestation is common in dogs and cats. Some species are pathogenic in large numbers, and others are nonpathogenic.

Roundworm Ascarids

Toxocara canis and *Toxascaris leonina* are found in dogs, and *Toxocara cati* and *Toxascaris leonina* are found in cats. *T. canis* can be transmitted across the placenta and *T. canis* and *T. cati*

through the milk. Infection is also caused by ingestion of the ova or of other hosts, such as rodents. The adult nematodes live in the SI. Migrating juvenile *T. canis* can cause hepatic, pulmonary, and occasionally ocular damage. *T. canis* presents a public health problem (i.e., visceral and ocular *larva migrans*).

Clinical Findings

Roundworms most often cause disease in young animals, and common signs are diarrhea, weight loss, or failure to thrive. A poor haircoat and a potbelly may be evident in puppies or kittens. Intestinal obstruction and perforation have been described in severe cases.

Diagnosis

Almost all puppies can be presumed to have *T. canis* infection. The diagnosis is made by fecal flotation (see Figure 222-7).

Treatment

A wide range of anthelmintics is effective against roundworms (Table 222-10). Treatment should be repeated at 2- to 3-week intervals in affected animals. Young animals should be routinely wormed at 2, 4, 6, 8, 12, and 16 weeks of age and then at least at 6-month intervals. It is important to ensure proper hygiene to stop reinfection or spread. *T. canis* can be controlled by administering fenbendazole to pregnant bitches at an oral dosage of 50 mg/kg given daily from day 40 to 2 days after whelping.

Hookworms

Ancylostoma caninum is the most important hookworm of dogs and is associated with blood loss and hemorrhagic enteritis. *Ancylostoma tubeforme* is the most common hookworm in cats but is less pathogenic. *Ancylostoma braziliense* occurs in dogs in the southern United States.

Uncinaria stenocephala is the hookworm of dogs in western Europe, although it also occurs in the northern United States and in Canada. Infection is most commonly reported in kenneled dogs, particularly greyhounds, and can be acquired prenatally, during lactation, by ingesting larvae, by migration of larvae through the skin, and by ingestion of a paratenic host.

Clinical Findings

Diarrhea, weakness, pallor, vomiting, dehydration, poor growth, and anemia are common in puppies with *A. caninum* infection. The infection can cause a rapid and fatal anemia or a more chronic iron deficiency anemia. *U. stenocephala* does not suck large quantities of blood and cause anemia, although severe infestations may be associated with diarrhea. Larval migration of *U. stenocephala* causes pedal pruritus.

Diagnosis

The diagnosis is made by demonstrating ova in feces (see Figure 222-7).

Treatment

Appropriate anthelmintics are detailed in Table 222-10. For *Ancylostoma* infection in anemic puppies, pyrantel pamoate has been suggested as the treatment of choice because it acts very rapidly and is comparatively safe. Anemic puppies may require blood transfusion and supportive care. Monthly administration of milbemycin or ivermectin plus pyrantel pamoate has been approved for the prevention or control of hookworm in dogs.

Tapeworms

Dipylidium caninum is the most common tapeworm infecting dogs and cats in the United States and Europe. Fleas are the intermediate host. *Echinococcus granulosus* is a tapeworm that uses dogs as definitive hosts, but humans and sheep are

Table • 222-10

Common Anthelmintic Medications for Dogs

| DRUG | DOSAGE | USUAL FORMULATION | SPECTRUM OF ACTIVITY | |
			NEMATODE	CESTODE
Piperazine	83.2—300 mg/kg	Tablet	Yes	No
Pyrantel	5 mg/kg	Paste	Yes	No
Selamectin	6 mg/kg monthly	Topical Spot-on	Yes	No
Fenbendazole	20—100 mg/kg for 1—3 days	Granules, paste, suspension	Yes	*Taenia* sp.
Mebendazole	50 mg/kg for 2 days	Tablet	Yes	*Taenia, Echinococcus* spp.
Nitroscanate	50 mg/kg	Tablet	Yes (not *Trichuris* sp.)	*Taenia, Dipylidium caninum, (Echinococcus)* spp.
Pyrantel, febantel, praziquantel (combination)	1 tablet/10 kg	Tablet	Yes	*Taenia, Echinococcus* spp., *D. caninum*
Pyrantel, febantel (combination)	1 mL/kg	Suspension	Yes	*Taenia* sp., *D.caninum*
Dichlorophen	200 mg/kg	Tablet	No	*Taenia* sp., *D.caninum*
Praziquantel	5 mg/kg	Injection, tablet	No	*Taenia, Echinococcus* spp., *D. caninum*

intermediate hosts. *E. granulosus* infection is not associated with clinical signs in dogs but is an important zoonosis. Various other *Taenia* spp. are also common in dogs and cats.

Clinical Findings

Heavy infestations of *D. caninum* are only rarely associated with diarrhea, weight loss, and failure to thrive. There are usually no clinical signs except "rice grains" (proglottids) in the perineal area or feces.

Diagnosis

A diagnosis of *D. caninum* infection is made by demonstrating characteristic egg capsules, contained in proglottids, obtained from the perineal area or feces (see Figure 222-7).

Treatment

Treatment of *D. caninum* infection involves adequate flea control (the animal and the environment) and administration of an appropriate anthelmintic (see Table 222-10). *E. granulosus* and other *Taenia* spp. are best controlled by routine administration of praziquantel (see Table 222-10).

Strongyloides sp.

Strongyloides stercoralis is a small nematode that may cause hemorrhagic enteritis in young puppies. Infective larvae are ingested, transmitted transmammary or through penetration of the skin, and after migration through the lung develop in the SI.

Clinical Findings

Signs of hemorrhagic enteritis occur in young puppies.

Diagnosis

Fecal evaluation using the Baermann technique or demonstration of motile first-stage larvae in smears of fresh feces (see Figure 222-7) helps differentiate larvae from Filaroides and mature hookworms.

Treatment

Infection is treated with thiabendazole or possibly fenbendazole or ivermectin (see Table 222-10).

PROTOZOA

Coccidia

Isospora spp.

Isospora spp. are the most common coccidial parasites of dogs (*Isospora canis, Isospora ohioensis*) and cats (*Isospora felis, Isospora rivolta*). Transmission occurs by ingestion of ova or paratenic hosts. Sporozoites are liberated in the SI and enter cells to begin development. The prepatent period ranges from 4 to 11 days, depending on the species. *Isospora* organisms are rarely associated with clinical signs. Puppies and kittens kept in unhygienic conditions or immunosuppressed animals may develop heavy infestations, which occasionally are associated with diarrhea that is often mucoid but sometimes bloody.

Isospora oocysts are found on direct examination of a fecal smear or by flotation. The infection is often self-limiting, but sulfadimethoxine (50 mg/kg given orally once daily for 10 days) or trimethoprim-sulfa (15 to 30 mg/kg given orally once daily for 5 days) can be used when clinical signs warrant treatment. The prognosis for recovery is good.

Cryptosporidium sp.

Cryptosporidium parvum, a significant pathogen in humans, is not a single species but is composed of genetically distinct genotypes. Transmission occurs by the fecal-oral route. Molecular studies have shown that dogs may transmit the cattle genotype to humans but that specific cat and dog genotypes also exist.[118] *C. parvum* has been associated with self-limiting diarrhea in dogs and cats and severe hemorrhagic diarrhea in immunocompromised animals.

Cryptosporidial oocysts are extremely small (approximately 1/10 the size of *Isospora* oocysts) and require identification by fecal flotation and oil immersion microscopy or by intestinal biopsy.

Paromomycin was reported to be effective against *Cryptosporidium* organisms in a cat. However, more recent studies have demonstrated that the drug's efficacy is poor and that it may cause acute renal failure. No other drugs are consistently efficacious, although nitazoxanide may prove to be effective. Fortunately, the disease is usually self-limiting in immunocompetent animals.

Giardia sp.
Giardia sp. can affect both dogs and cats. The prevalence of infection in canine studies ranges from less than 2% to 100% in kennels. Cats are less commonly infected than dogs. The parasite is usually transmitted via the fecal-oral route. Ingested oocysts excyst in the upper SI, and trophozoites attach to the intestinal mucosa from the duodenum to the ileum. After multiplication of trophozoites, oocysts are passed in the feces at 1 to 2 weeks after infection. Molecular epidemiologic studies indicate that giardiasis may be a zoonosis.[119]

Clinical Findings
Most infections are not associated with clinical signs. Clinical signs range from mild, self-limiting, acute diarrhea to severe or chronic small bowel diarrhea associated with intestinal protein loss and weight loss.

Diagnosis
Giardia infection can be diagnosed by demonstration of motile trophozoites in duodenal juice or on a fresh fecal smear or by demonstration of cysts by zinc sulfate fecal flotation. Shedding of cysts occurs intermittently, and three fecal analyses are 95% sensitive. *Giardia* antigen can also be detected by means of a fecal ELISA, and this is the preferred method of diagnosis compared to zinc sulfate flotation performed by inexperienced technicians.

Treatment
Metronidazole is the drug most commonly used to treat *Giardia* infection in small animals. The standard dosage recommended for dogs is 25 mg/kg given orally twice daily for 5 days; the standard dosage for cats is 10 to 25 mg/kg given orally twice daily for 5 days. The drug is effective in eliminating *Giardia* infection in two thirds of infected dogs but may cause side effects at these high doses.

Albendazole (25 mg/kg given orally twice daily for 2 days) and fenbendazole (50 mg/kg given orally twice daily for 3 days) also eliminate *Giardia* infection.[120] Fenbendazole is preferred, because albendazole has been associated with bone marrow toxicosis.[121] Febantel (in a combination product with praziquantel and pyrantel pamoate) is also effective in dogs.

Decontamination of the patient's coat by bathing and the patient's habitat by steam cleaning or cleaning with quaternary ammonium compounds is advised to prevent reinfection. A *Giardia* vaccine is available for use in high-risk areas, and it has been shown to be effective in clearing infection from dogs that failed to respond to standard drug therapy.[123]

Prognosis
The prognosis is usually good. Some patients may require several treatments to eliminate infection, because reinfection is a significant problem.

CHRONIC IDIOPATHIC ENTEROPATHIES

Chronic enteropathies have historically been defined by histologic description of the tissue, which provides little information as to the nature of the intestinal dysfunction or its etiology.

Furthermore, tissue samples collected from many cases have no obvious morphologic changes. In the future, new methods of investigation may better characterize functional and immunologic abnormalities.

Management of Chronic Enteropathies
The management of idiopathic enteropathies is essentially symptomatic. If a specific diagnosis is made (e.g., lymphangiectasia, severe IBD, lymphoma), specific treatment modalities can be used (see below). However, in many circumstances the diagnosis is not obvious, often because of a lack of specific or marked histopathologic changes, and it usually is most appropriate to perform treatments sequentially. It is safest to commence with antiparasiticides, then a dietary trial, followed by an antibacterial trial, before finally attempting immunosuppression. Such an approach may identify occult parasitism, antibiotic-responsive diarrhea (ARD) and diet-responsive conditions. However, because different treatments also lack specific activities, caution should be exercised in using treatment trials for diagnosis without prior investigation.

Antiparasiticides An appropriate trial of an antiparasiticide should eliminate the possibility of parasitic diseases, such as chronic giardiasis, that are difficult to diagnose. Fenbendazole (50 mg/kg given orally every 24 hours for 3 days) is the most appropriate drug for these circumstances, although alternatives exist (e.g., metronidazole or a febantel/pyrantel/praziquantel combination). Given the highly infectious nature of *Giardia* organisms, all in-contact animals may need to be treated concurrently or reinfection may occur, which might suggest apparent treatment failure.

Dietary management Dietary management is a very important treatment modality in most chronic enteropathies and can be used in different ways. For diagnosis and treatment of adverse food reactions, an antigen-limited exclusion diet is most appropriate (see below). Dietary management also can be important in the symptomatic management of many idiopathic enteropathies. The ideal diet is highly digestible, moderately fat restricted, lactose free, gluten free, not markedly hypertonic, nutritionally balanced, and palatable.

Inclusion of moderately fermentable fiber (e.g., psyllium, ispaghula) is known to promote colonic health, and soluble fiber also promotes small intestinal health.[124] However, because dietary fiber can delay intestinal transit, its inclusion may be contraindicated for some intestinal diseases. Feeding the daily requirement in divided meals (usually between two and four) reduces the load on a compromised intestine. Feeding more frequently is unnecessary, because the rate of gastric emptying imposes natural trickle feeding of the intestine.

Additional supplements include prebiotics such as fructooligosaccharides (FOS) and mannanoligosaccharides.[16,17,125,126] FOS has been shown to alter the constituents of the fecal flora, but the effect on the SI flora is limited.

Antibacterials Antibacterials are indicated for specific conditions in which a bacterial pathogen has been documented (see above), in the treatment of ARD or secondary SIBO, and in other chronic enteropathies, such as IBD, in which modulation of the flora may be required. The drugs most commonly used in these circumstances are oxytetracycline, metronidazole, and tylosin. The beneficial effects of such drugs may go beyond their antibacterial activity, with potential effects on the mucosal immune system.

Immunosuppressive medication Immunosuppressive or anti-inflammatory drugs are indicated when evidence of mucosal inflammation is present and no underlying cause is found. However, given that immunosuppression may lead to clinical deterioration in some cases, the diagnosis should be reviewed before institution of such therapy, especially if the diagnosis was made on the basis of endoscopic biopsy alone.

ADVERSE REACTIONS TO FOOD

An adverse reaction to food is a repeatable, unpleasant response to a dietary component that is a manifestation of an immunologic reaction to a dietary antigen (i.e., a true food allergy) or a nonimmunologic reaction (i.e., an intolerance). Although different pathogenetic mechanisms are responsible for the two groups, the clinical signs are similar, and the approach to treatment is the same, usually involving exclusion of the offending food component.

Food intolerance may be associated with a single ingredient of a prepared food (e.g., lactose, preservative) that may be present in immunologically unrelated foods. Conversely, confirmed allergy to a specific food may impart allergy to related foods. In humans, food intolerance is diagnosed more frequently than hypersensitivity, but its true prevalence in small animals is unknown. A recent study in cats demonstrated that 29% of cats had adverse food reactions, and a further 20% responded completely to diet and did not relapse.[127] However, the number of these reactions that were immunologically mediated was not documented.

Food Allergy (Hypersensitivity)

The prevalence of true food allergy is unknown because no reliable diagnostic tests are available. Furthermore, food allergy with GI signs may be more difficult to prove than cases in which dermatologic signs prevail. This is partly because other GI diseases may also respond (for nonallergenic reasons) to dietary manipulation (Box 222-13). The management of food allergy is simple: feed any food that does not contain the allergen, and the animal will be healthy. The difficulty for the clinician lies in the recognition of food allergy and the identification of foods that must be excluded.

Mechanisms

Currrent hypotheses of food allergy propose one or a combination of mechanisms that lead to breakdown of oral tolerance: an inadequate mucosal barrier, abnormal presentation of dietary antigens to the mucosal immune system, or immune system dysregulation (see earlier discussion). Such hypotheses could explain both genetic susceptibility to the development of allergy and the development of allergies after a primary GI insult that damages the mucosal barrier. For example, viral or parasitic enteritis can both damage the mucosal barrier and provide danger signals in the intestinal mucosa. Active immune responses, rather than tolerance, can then occur to bystander antigens (i.e., sensitization to dietary antigen). Dietary hypersensitivity may involve a variety of mechanisms, including type I (IgE mediated, immediate), type II (immune complex mediated), and type IV (delayed hypersensitivity) reactions.

Clinical Signs

A contemporaneous association between ingestion of a particular food and the onset of signs is suggestive of an immediate (type I) IgE-mediated hypersensitivity, but mixed or delayed reactions are also possible. In such cases the inevitable delay between food ingestion and onset of signs obscures any causative link, particularly if repeated ingestion causes chronic disease.

Clinical signs of food allergy generally involve the skin and GI tract (Box 222-14). Most case studies have focused on dermatologic signs, with few reports of food-allergic GI disease.[128] Systemic signs (anorexia, lethargy) are rarely recorded, and urticaria-angioedema and even anaphylaxis seem rare. Concurrent skin and GI signs can occur but have been reported only rarely.[129] However, only 5% of human patients with gluten-sensitive skin lesions (dermatitis herpetiformis) have GI signs, yet intestinal histologic examination shows a subclinical enteropathy in 95% of these individuals.

Food-allergic skin disease The major sign of food-allergic skin disease is pruritus, which is nonseasonal and has no

---

Box • 222-13

Conditions that May Improve Clinically in Response to Dietary Modification

Food allergy
Food intolerance
Small intestinal bacterial overgrowth
Inflammatory bowel disease
Lymphangiectasia
Exocrine pancreatic insufficiency
Pancreatitis
Chronic gastritis
Gastroesophageal reflux
Gastric emptying disorders
Portosystemic shunt

Box • 222-14

Clinical Signs Recognized as Manifestations of Food Allergy

Systemic Signs
Anorexia
Lethargy
Peripheral lymphadenopathy (cats)
Urticaria-angioedema
Anaphylaxis

Cutaneous Signs
Primary papules
Erythroderma
Pruritus and self-trauma
Secondary pyoderma
Scaling
Otitis externa
Miliary dermatitis (cats)
Eosinophilic granuloma complex (cats)

Gastrointestinal Signs
Vomiting
Hematemesis
Diarrhea
Small intestinal—like signs
Colitis-like signs
Abdominal pain, "colic"
Weight loss and/or stunting
Altered appetite

pursued; immunosuppressive medication is used only as a last resort. However, in some cases, clinical signs or mucosal inflammation is so severe that early intervention with immunosuppressive medication is essential. If clinical signs are intermittent, the owners should keep a diary to provide objective information as to whether treatments produce genuine improvement.

Dietary modification   The diets recommended for patients with IBD are antigen limited, based on a highly digestible, single-source protein preparation. An exclusion diet trial should be undertaken to eliminate the possibility of an adverse food reaction, and most clients are happy to try this, given concerns over the side effects of immunosuppressive drugs. An easily digestible diet decreases the intestinal antigenic load and thus reduces mucosal inflammation. Such diets may also help resolve any secondary sensitivities to dietary components that may have arisen from disruption of the mucosal barrier. After the inflammation has resolved, the usual diet often can be reintroduced without fear of an acquired sensitivity.

Well-cooked rice is the preferred carbohydrate source because of its high digestibility, but potato, corn starch, and tapioca are also gluten free. Fat restriction reduces clinical signs associated with fat malabsorption. Modification of the n3 to n6 fatty acid ratio may also modulate the inflammatory response and may have some benefit both in treatment and in maintenance of remission, as in human IBD.[165,166] However, no direct studies have been done to prove a benefit in canine IBD. Supplementation with oral folate and parenteral cobalamin is indicated if serum concentrations are subnormal.

Antibacterial therapy   Treatment with antimicrobials can be justified in IBD, partly to treat secondary SIBO and partly because of the importance of bacterial antigens in the pathogenesis of IBD.[50] Ciprofloxacin and metronidazole are often used in human IBD,[167] and metronidazole is the preferred drug for small animals. The efficacy of metronidazole may not be related just to its antibacterial activity, because it may exert immunomodulatory effects on cell-mediated immunity. Furthermore, other antibacterials (e.g., tylosin) may also have immunomodulatory effects and have efficacy in canine IBD.

Immunosuppressive drugs   The most important treatment modality in idiopathic IBD is immunosuppression, although this should be used only as a last resort. In human IBD, glucocorticoids and thiopurines (e.g., azathioprine, 6-mercaptopurine) are used most widely.[168] In dogs, glucocorticoids are used most frequently, and prednisone and prednisolone are the drugs of choice. Dexamethasone should be avoided, because it may have deleterious effects on enterocytes. In severe IBD, prednisolone can be administered parenterally, because oral absorption may be poor. The initial dosage of 1 to 2 mg/kg given orally every 12 hours is given for 2 to 4 weeks and then tapered slowly over the subsequent weeks to months. In some cases therapy can be either completely withdrawn or at least reduced to a low maintenance dose given every 48 hours.

Signs of iatrogenic hyperadrenocorticism are common when the highest glucocorticoid dose is administered. However, signs are transient and resolve as the dosage is reduced. If clinical signs of IBD consistently recur when the dosage is reduced, other drugs can be added to provide a steroid-sparing effect (see below). Budesonide, an enteric-coated, locally active steroid that is destroyed 90% first-pass through the liver, has been successful in maintaining remission in human IBD with minimal hypothalamic-pituitary-adrenal suppression. A preliminary study showed apparent efficacy in dogs and cats,[169] but limited information is available on the use of this drug.[170]

In dogs, azathioprine (2 mg/kg given orally every 24 hours) is commonly used in combination with prednisone/prednisolone when the initial response to therapy is poor or when glucocorticoid side effects are marked. However, azathioprine may have a delayed onset of activity (up to 3 weeks) and, given its myelosuppressive potential, regular monitoring of the hemogram is necessary. Azathioprine is not recommended for cats; chlorambucil (2 to 6 mg/m² given orally every 24 hours until remission, followed by drug tapering) is a suitable alternative. Other immunosuppressive drugs are methotrexate, cyclophosphamide, and cyclosporine. Methotrexate is effective in the treatment of human Crohn's disease,[171] but it is not widely used in companion animals; it often causes diarrhea in dogs. Cyclophosphamide has few advantages over azathioprine and is rarely used. However, cyclosporine may show promise for the future, given its T lymphocyte–specific effects and efficacy in canine anal furunculosis. Unfortunately, it is expensive, and studies in human IBD have shown variable efficacy and toxicity.[172,173]

Novel therapies for IBD   Novel therapies are increasingly used for human IBD in an attempt to target more accurately the underlying pathogenetic mechanisms. These therapies include new immunosuppressive drugs, monoclonal antibody therapy, cytokines and transcription factors, and dietary manipulation (Table 222-11).[174] In the future, such therapies may be adopted for small animal IBD.

Mycophenolate mofetil recently has been used to treat human IBD, although its efficacy is variable.[175] Drugs that target TNF-α (e.g., thalidomide and oxpentifylline) may be suitable for the treatment of canine IBD because of the importance of this cytokine in disease pathogenesis. Human open-label trials have demonstrated a beneficial effect for thalidomide in refractory Crohn's disease.[176] Oxpentifylline has shown efficacy in studies *in vitro*, but clinical results have been less rewarding.[177] Anti–TNF-α monoclonal antibody therapy, which has also undergone trials in human IBD, has the additional beneficial effect of inducing apoptosis in inflammatory cells.[178] Species-specific monoclonal antibodies will be needed for canine and feline IBD.

Finally, modulation of the enteric flora with probiotics or prebiotics may have benefits in targeting the pathogenesis of IBD. A *probiotic* is an orally administered living organism that exerts health benefits beyond those of basic nutrition. In addition to having direct antagonistic properties against pathogenic bacteria,[91] they modulate mucosal immune responses by stimulating either innate (e.g., phagocytic activity) or specific (e.g., secretory IgA) immune responses.[179] However, care should be taken to select the most appropriate organisms, which are likely to vary between host species.

Prebiotics are selective substrates used by a limited number of "beneficial" species, which therefore cause alterations in the luminal microflora. The most frequently used prebiotics are nondigestible carbohydrates, such as lactulose, inulin, and FOS. Both probiotics and prebiotics can reduce intestinal inflammation in mouse models of IBD.[180] Preliminary placebo-controlled trials with probiotics and prebiotics in human IBD patients have shown promising results,[181] although similar trials in canine and feline IBD are still awaited.

Lymphocytic-Plasmacytic Enteritis

Lymphocytic-plasmacytic enteritis (LPE) is the most common form of idiopathic IBD. It is characterized by a mucosal infiltrate of lymphocytes and plasma cells (see Figure 222-12). However, there are numerous other causes of lymphocytic-plasmacytic infiltration of the SI (see Box 222-17 and Figure 222-12), including enteric pathogens, bacteria, and *Toxoplasma* organisms. All such underlying causes must be excluded before a diagnosis of idiopathic LPE is confirmed.

Table • 222-11

Novel Therapies for Human Inflammatory Bowel Disease

THERAPY	MECHANISM OF ACTION
Drug Therapy	
Tacrolimus	Immunosuppressant macrolide
Mycophenolate	Inhibits lymphocyte proliferation; reduces IFN-gamma production
Leukotriene antagonists (zileuton, verapamil)	Inhibit arachidonic acid cascade
Prostaglandin (PG) targeting agents	Mucosal protection from PG analogs; anti-inflammatory effects from PG antagonists
Thromboxane synthesis inhibitors	Anti-inflammatory effects
Ridogrel	
Picotamide	
Oxpentifylline	Inhibits TNF-alpha expression
Thalidomide	Inhibits TNF-alpha and IL-12 expression; reduces leukocyte migration; impairs angiogenesis
Bone Marrow and Stem Cell Transplantation	
Bone marrow grafts	Unknown; immunomodulation (?)
Dietary Manipulation	
Protein hydrolysate diets	"Hypoallergenic"
Fish oil therapy	Diverts eicosanoid metabolism to LTB_5 and PGE_3
Short chain fatty acid therapy	
Butyrate	Provides nutrition for enterocytes
Probiotics and prebiotics	Antagonize pathogenic bacteria; immunomodulatory effects
Cytokine Manipulation	
Systemic IL-10	Down-modulatory cytokine
Anti—IL-2 monoclonal antibody (MAb)	Counteracts proinflammatory effects
Anti—IL-2R (CD25) MAb	Inhibits IL-2 effects
Anti—IL-12 MAb	Counteracts proinflammatory effects
Anti—IL-11 MAb	Downregulates TNF-alpha and IL-1beta
Recombinant IFN-alpha	Anti-inflammatory; antiviral (?)
Anti—IFN-gamma MAb	Immunomodulatory effect on Th1 cells
Anti—TNF-alpha MAb	Counteracts proinflammatory effects; induces inflammatory cell apoptosis
Endothelial Cell Adhesion Molecules and Their Manipulation	
ICAM-1 (antisense oligonucleotide)	Reduces immune cell trafficking
Anti-alpha$_4$/beta$_7$ MAb	Reduces immune cell trafficking
Other Immune System Modulations	
Intravenous immunoglobulin	Saturates Fc receptors; other (?)
T-cell apheresis	Immunomodulation
Anti-CD4 antibodies	Immunomodulation
Transcription Factors	
NF-κB antisense oligonucleotide	Inhibits proinflammatory cytokine expression
ICAM-1 antisense oligonucleotide	Reduces immune cell trafficking

Modified from Forbes 2003, German and others 2003.
IFN, interferon; IL, interleukin; ICAM, intercellular adhesion molecule; LTB, leukotriene B; MAb, monoclonal antibody; PG, prostaglandin; PGE, prostaglandin E; Th1, T helper 1; TNF, tumor necrosis factor

Pathogenesis

Idiopathic LPE is believed to reflect immune dysregulation, and the spectrum of severity ranges from mild to severe infiltration. Alterations in immune cell populations in canine LPE have been documented, including increases in lamina propria T cells (especially CD4+ cells), IgG+ plasma cells, macrophages, and granulocytes.[154]

Increased concentrations of acute-phase proteins (e.g., C-reactive protein), which normalize after treatment, have been documented in canine LPE.[164] Marked alterations in cytokine patterns also were recently documented in canine LPE, with increased expression of Th1 (IL-2, IL-12, and IFN-gamma), Th2 (IL-5), proinflammatory (TNF-alpha), and immunoregulatory (TGF-beta) cytokines.[81] These studies

GASTROINTESTINAL DISEASE

confirm that the mucosal immune response is upregulated in canine IBD.

Clinical Signs

Clinical signs of LPE include diarrhea and weight loss, but these are not pathognomonic. Chronic vomiting may be the predominant sign, especially in cats. LPE is prevalent in German shepherds, Shar Peis, and purebred cats, and in dogs it often causes a PLE. Severe LPE (immunoproliferative disease) is recognized in basenjis. Protein-losing enteropathy with or without concurrent protein-losing nephropathy has also been described in soft-coated wheaten terriers.[144] LPE typically affects older animals; it is uncommon (but not impossible) in individuals less than 2 years of age.

Diagnosis

The approach to diagnosis of LPE is the same as for any chronic enteropathy, although definitive diagnosis ultimately depends on documentation of characteristic histopathologic changes in the absence of an underlying cause. Such changes include the presence of increased numbers of lymphocytes and plasma cells in association with architectural disturbances. Complete or partial villus atrophy may be present, and villus fusion and crypt abscessation may be noted in severe cases. The distinction between severe LPE and alimentary lymphoma is sometimes difficult, and discrepancies may arise between endoscopic biopsies and postmortem examination of the same patient. It is hypothesized that such discrepancies arise because the two conditions may be present concurrently in the SI, because prolonged intestinal inflammation may ultimately result in transformation to lymphoma, or because low-grade lymphoma is initially misdiagnosed.

Another major concern is the criteria by which a diagnosis of LPE is made. In this regard, major discrepancies exist in interpretation of intestinal biopsies by different histopathologists.[79] Interpretation of the degree of inflammation is subjective; inflammation may be patchy, and the presence of edema (due to hypoproteinemia) may make cell density difficult to assess. Furthermore, discrepancies exist between gross endoscopic and histologic findings, and proximal endoscopic biopsies may not be representative. Attempts have been made to standardize interpretation by using grading schemes; those that assess morphologic abnormalities in conjunction with changes in cellularity are most appropriate.[158]

Treatment and Prognosis

The treatment of LPE is that outlined for idiopathic IBD above. First-line treatment usually involves dietary manipulation and metronidazole. The prognosis for severe LPE is guarded. Some patients respond dramatically and can ultimately be weaned off all medication; other cases, however, require persistent, low-dose maintenance immunosuppressive therapy.

Basenji Enteropathy

A severe, hereditary form of LPE has been well characterized in basenjis,[182] although the mode of inheritance is unclear.[183] It has been likened to immunoproliferative small intestinal disease (IPSID) in humans, because both conditions involve intense intestinal inflammation. However, IPSID is characterized by an associated gammopathy (alpha heavy chain disease) and a predisposition to lymphoma. Affected basenjis often have hyperglobulinemia but not alpha heavy chain disease and may be predisposed to lymphoma. The intestinal lesions in basenjis are characterized by increases in CD4+ and CD8+ T cells.[182]

Clinical Signs

Signs of chronic intractable diarrhea and emaciation are most common. Lymphocytic-plasmacytic gastritis, with hypergastrinemia and mucosal hyperplasia, may be seen in addition to the enteropathy. PLE often occurs, with consequent hypoalbuminemia, although edema and ascites are not common. Clinical signs are usually progressive, and spontaneous intestinal perforation may occur.

Diagnosis

The approach to diagnosis is the same as before, and ultimately depends on histopathological examination of biopsy specimens.

Treatment

Treatment generally is unsuccessful, with dogs dying within months of diagnosis. However, early, aggressive combination treatment with prednisolone, antibiotics, and dietary modification may achieve remission in some cases.

Familial Protein-Losing Enteropathy and Protein-Losing Nephropathy in Soft-Coated Wheaten Terriers

Recently a clinical syndrome unique to soft-coated wheaten terriers was characterized.[144,184] Affected dogs present with signs of PLE or PLN or both. A genetic basis is likely, and although the mode of inheritance is not yet clear, pedigree analysis of 188 dogs has demonstrated a common male ancestor.[185] The disease is probably immune mediated, given the presence of inflammatory cell infiltration. A potential role for food hypersensitivity has been suggested, because affected dogs have demonstrated adverse reactions during provocative food trials and alterations in antigen-specific fecal IgE concentrations.[145,184,186]

Clinical Signs

Signs of PLE tend to develop at a younger age than PLN. Clinical signs of the PLE include vomiting, diarrhea, weight loss, and pleural and peritoneal effusions. Occasionally, thromboembolic disease may occur.[187]

Diagnosis

Preliminary laboratory investigations, as in most dogs with PLE, demonstrate panhypoproteinemia and hypocholesterolemia. In contrast, hypoalbuminemia, hypercholesterolemia, proteinuria, and ultimately azotemia are seen with PLN.[185] Histopathologic examination of intestinal biopsy material reveals evidence of intestinal inflammation, villus blunting, and epithelial erosions, as well as dilated lymphatics and lipogranulomatous lymphangitis.

Treatment and Prognosis

The treatment for PLE is similar to that described for general IBD, but the prognosis is usually poor.

Eosinophilic Enteritis

Eosinophilic enteritis (EE) is reported to be the second most common form of IBD. It frequently also involves the stomach and/or colon in eosinophilic gastroenteritis (EGE) and/or colitis. Segmental EE has also been reported.[188] Histologically, variable mucosal architectural disturbances (e.g., villus atrophy) are present in conjunction with a mixed infiltrate of inflammatory cells in which eosinophils predominate (see Figure 222-12). However, as with LPE, diagnostic criteria vary among pathologists; some define EE based purely on subjective increases in mucosal eosinophil numbers, whereas others apply stricter criteria, requiring that eosinophils predominate in the lamina propria. Another criterion is the presence of eosinophils between epithelial cells of the villus and crypt, which suggests transepithelial migration. Nevertheless, the number of mucosal eosinophils can vary markedly in normal dogs,[22] and therefore this condition may be overdiagnosed. As with other forms of IBD, a diagnosis of EE should be made only after other causes of eosinophilic infiltration have been eliminated.

Clinical Signs

EE may be seen in dogs and cats of any breed and age, although it is most common in younger adult animals. Boxers and Dobermans may be predisposed, and an increased incidence in German shepherds has been suggested. EGE may also be associated with systemic eosinophilic disorders in both cats and dogs. The clinical signs reported, which depend on the area of GI tract involved, include vomiting, SI diarrhea, and LI diarrhea. Mucosal erosion/ulceration may occur more frequently in EE than in other forms of IBD, therefore hematemesis, melena, or hematochezia may be seen. Severe EGE has been associated with PLE and hypoproteinemia and, rarely, spontaneous perforation of the GI tract.[189]

Pathogenesis

An eosinophilic mucosal infiltrate may be related to dietary sensitivity, endoparasitism, or idiopathic EGE. The eosinophil infiltration is likely to be the result of local and systemic production of cytokines and chemokines, such as IL-5, and members of the eotaxin family.[190] These mediators may be produced by the Th2 subset of CD4+ T cells.

Diagnosis

The diagnosis of EGE is made by histopathologic assessment of intestinal biopsies after exclusion of parasites and food allergy. Peripheral eosinophilia is neither invariably present nor pathognomonic for EGE, because it may also be seen in parasitism, hypoadrenocorticism, allergic cutaneous or respiratory disease, and mast cell neoplasia.

Treatment

Given that eosinophilic mucosal infiltrates may also be related to endoparasitic diseases, empirical treatment with fenbendazole is always advisable. Subsequent to this, an exclusion diet trial should be instigated to eliminate the possibility of dietary sensitivity before immunosuppressive therapy is considered. The prognosis in idiopathic EGE is guarded, even with a good initial response to treatment, because recurrence is common.

Other Forms of Inflammatory Bowel Disease
Granulomatous Enteritis

Granulomatous enteritis is a rare form of IBD characterized by mucosal infiltration with macrophages, resulting in the formation of granulomas. The distribution of inflammation can be patchy. This condition is probably the same as "regional enteritis," in which ileal granulomas have been reported. Granulomatous enteritis has some histologic features in common with human Crohn's disease, but obstruction, abscessation, and fistula formation are not noted. Conventional therapy is not usually effective, and the prognosis is guarded, although a combination of surgical resection and anti-inflammatory treatment was reported to be successful in one case.[191] In cats, a pyogranulomatous transmural inflammation has been associated with FIPV infection.

Proliferative Enteritis

Proliferative enteritis is characterized by segmental mucosal hypertrophy of the intestine. Although many species can be affected, the condition is most common in pigs. A similar but rare condition has been reported in dogs.[192] There have been suggestions of an underlying infectious etiology, and Lawsonia intracellularis has been implicated, although this has not yet been proved. Other infectious agents with a proposed link are Campylobacter spp. and Chlamydia organisms.

LYMPHANGIECTASIA

Definition and Cause

Intestinal lymphangiectasia is characterized by marked dilatation and dysfunction of intestinal lymphatics. Abnormal lymphatics leak protein-rich lymph into the intestinal lumen, ultimately causing PLE and hypoproteinemia. Lymphangiectasia may be a primary disorder or can develop secondary to lymphatic obstruction.

Primary lymphangiectasia usually is limited to the intestine, although it may be part of a more widespread lymphatic abnormality involving, for example, chylothorax.[193] It is considered congenital, although clinical signs are not usually present from birth. The development of associated lipogranulomatous lymphangitis, superimposed on the congenital abnormalities, is one reason for a progressive disorder. The disease is most commonly seen in small terrier breeds (e.g., Yorkshire, Maltese) and the Norwegian lundehund (Figure 222-13), suggesting a genetic predisposition.

Secondary lymphangiectasia is caused by intestinal lymphatic obstruction. Underlying causes include (1) infiltration or obstruction of lymphatics by an inflammatory, fibrosing, or neoplastic process; (2) possibly obstruction of the thoracic duct; and (3) right heart failure due to congestive heart failure or cardiac tamponade. Lipogranulomatous lymphangitis is sometimes reported in association with lymphangiectasia, but it is not clear which is the primary event; lymphangitis could cause lymphatic obstruction, or leakage of lymph could cause granuloma formation.

History and Clinical Signs

The clinical manifestations of lymphangiectasia are largely attributable to the effects of the enteric loss of lymph. Other intestinal functions remain intact, and hypoproteinemia may be present without diarrhea.[194] Diarrhea, steatorrhea, profound weight loss, and polyphagia are more typical, and vomiting, lethargy, and anorexia are reported occasionally. Signs may have an insidious onset and an intermittent pattern. Ascites or subcutaneous edema may develop if hypoproteinemia is marked. The ascitic fluid usually is a pure transudate, but if right heart failure causes secondary lymphangiectasia, a modified transudate develops through portal hypertension. Lymphangiectasia has been associated with granulomatous hepatopathy[195] and in lundehunds with chronic gastritis and gastric carcinoma.[196]

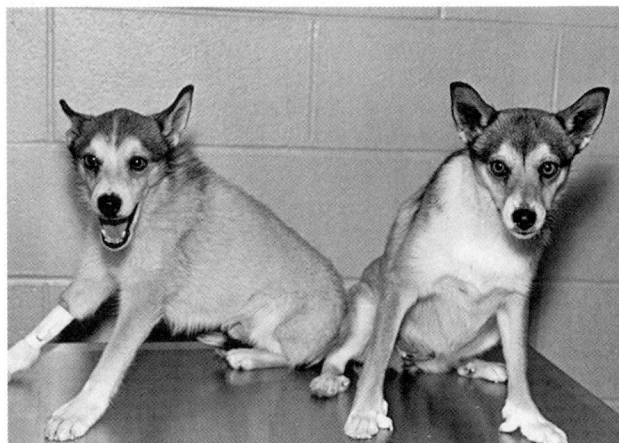

Figure 222-13 Normal lundehund (*left*) and one affected with lymphangiectasia, showing abdominal distension caused by hypoproteinemic ascites. (Courtesy D.A. Williams.)

Diagnosis

Given that lymph is rich in lipoproteins and lymphocytes, laboratory analysis often shows panhypoproteinemia, hypocholesterolemia, and lymphopenia. Hypocalcemia and hypomagnesemia have been reported.[55,197] The hypocalcemia is the result not only of hypoalbuminemia, but also of the development of ionized hypocalcemia. Therefore other mechanisms, including vitamin D and calcium malabsorption, may be involved. PLE can be documented by measuring[51] Cr-albumin leakage or fecal concentrations of alpha$_1$-PI. In affected lundehunds, increased permeability has been documented by both methods, and the increases in the fecal alpha$_1$-PI concentration were seen before changes in serum proteins.[198]

Gross findings at endoscopy include the presence of white lipid droplets or prominent mucosal blebs, which are likely the result of villus tip distension with chyle. Endoscopic biopsies may be supportive of the diagnosis, but full-thickness biopsies may be required to make a definitive diagnosis. At exploratory laparotomy, most dogs show gross abnormalities, including thickened small intestine, dilated lymphatics (in the mesentery and intestinal serosa), and occasionally adhesions.[199] Mesenteric lymph nodes may also be enlarged, and yellow-white nodular masses (1 to 3 mm in diameter) are often observed in and around the mesenteric and serosal lymphatics. The nodules are lipogranulomas, consisting of accumulations of lipid-laden macrophages, and result from perilymphatic extravasation of chyle or are associated with a lymphangitis.

Characteristic histopathologic changes include "ballooning dilatation" of lymphatics, not only in the mucosa but also in the submucosa. This true lymphangiectasia must be distinguished both from normal postprandial dilatation of lacteals and from the secondary lacteal dilatation occasionally noted in other enteropathies (e.g., IBD) (Figure 222-14). Genuine cases are less common than currently believed, and failure to recognize an underlying inflammatory cause may explain the success of steroid treatment in some cases. Assessment of the degree of inflammatory cell infiltrate in the lamina propria is subjective, and if edema is present, the LP cell density may be underestimated.

Treatment

Secondary lymphangiectasia is managed by specific treatment of underlying disease, such as pericardiocentesis or pericardectomy for cardiac tamponade. The aim of treatment of primary lymphangiectasia is to decrease the enteric loss of plasma protein, resolve associated intestinal or lymphatic inflammation, and control any edema or effusions. Dietary manipulation and glucocorticoids are the most important treatment modalities.

The ideal diet for cases of lymphangiectasia is markedly fat restricted, calorie dense, and highly digestible. Weight reduction diets, although low in fat, are inappropriate, because patients require a high level of nutrition. Previously, administration of medium chain triglycerides (MCT) was recommended, because these lipids were thought to be absorbed directly into the portal blood. However, this theory was recently contradicted.[200] Supplementation with fat-soluble vitamins is advised, and there are anecdotal reports of improvement with glutamine supplementation.

Glucocorticoid therapy (prednisolone, 1 to 2 mg/kg given orally divided daily and then tapered) may be beneficial in some cases, especially if associated lymphangitis, lipogranulomas, and a lymphocytic-plasmacytic infiltrate are present in the lamina propria. Unfortunately, not all cases respond to

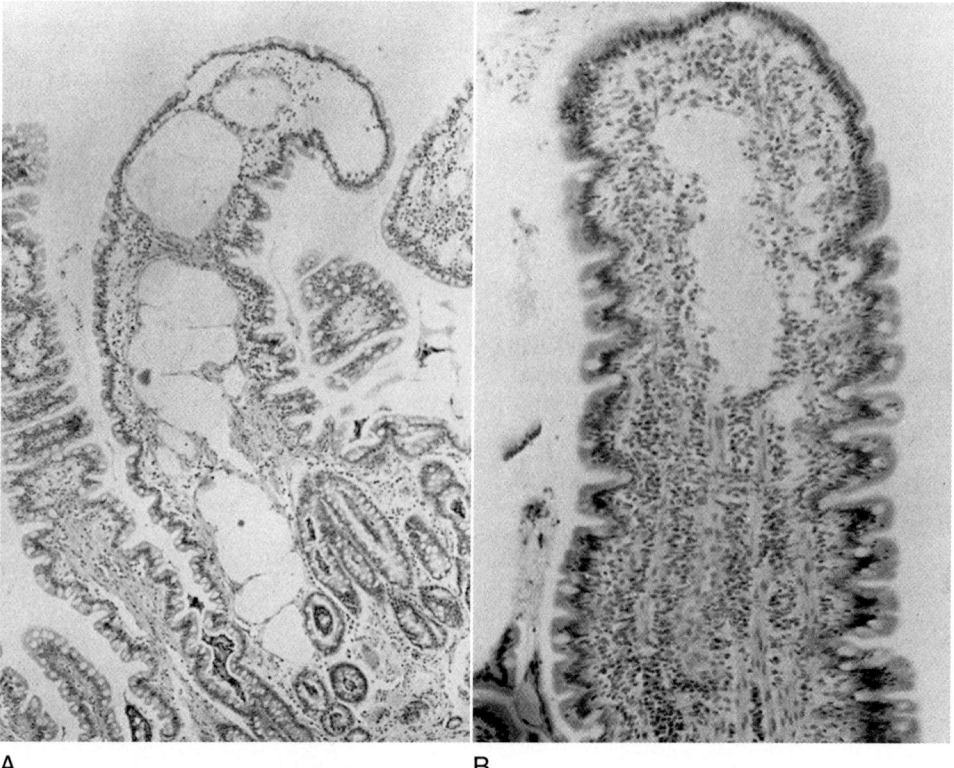

A   B

Figure 222-14 Histologic appearance of a jejunal biopsy from **(A)** a Jack Russell terrier with a protein-losing enteropathy, in which markedly dilated lacteals consistent with a diagnosis of lymphangiectasia are present, and **(B)** a retriever with moderate lymphoplasmacytic enteritis and mild secondary ectasia of the lacteals.

such therapy. The use of antimicrobials such as tylosin or metronidazole has not shown any obvious success. Diuretics are indicated in the management of effusions, and combinations of diuretics are preferred (e.g., furosemide and spironolactone); administration of plasma or colloid may also help if hypoproteinemia is marked. The response to treatment is unpredictable, but cessation of clinical signs may be achieved temporarily, with remissions of months to several years. However, the overall long-term prognosis is poor, and patients eventually succumb to severe malnutrition, incapacitating effusions, and intractable diarrhea.

MISCELLANEOUS CAUSES OF PROTEIN-LOSING ENTEROPATHY

Common causes of PLE include lymphoma and IBD. However, there have also been recent reports of PLE associated with intestinal crypt lesions[201,202] without evidence of lymphangiectasia or inflammation in most cases. The underlying etiology of such lesions is not known. Response to therapy with antibacterials and immunosuppressive medication is variable; some dogs deteriorate suddenly and can die from thromboembolic disease.

INTESTINAL NEOPLASIA

Lymphomas, adenocarcinomas, and mast cell tumors are the most common GI tumors in cats, whereas adenocarcinomas and leiomyomas are more common in dogs. Intestinal fibrosarcomas, hemangiosarcomas, carcinoids, and plasma cell tumors are rare. Clinical signs usually include weight loss, although a spectrum of signs may be seen, including diarrhea, anorexia, melena, vomiting, abdominal discomfort, abdominal effusion, and anemia. Other consequences of intestinal neoplasia include intussusception, intestinal perforation, and a variety of paraneoplastic effects.

Intestinal Lymphoma

Lymphoma is characterized by mucosal, submucosal, and/or epithelial infiltration of neoplastic lymphocytes,[203,204] which can invade the intestine in either a diffuse or a focal manner (Figure 222-15). Focal forms may cause obstruction; diffuse infiltration is more common and usually results in malabsorption. Most affected cats test negative for the feline leukemia virus (FeLV) at the time of diagnosis. Progression from LPE to lymphoma has been reported.

Clinical findings Middle-aged or older dogs and cats are most commonly affected. Weight loss, chronic diarrhea, and progressive inappetence are common features, although vomiting and melena may also be noted. Diffusely thickened intestines, intestinal mass lesions, mesenteric lymphadenopathy (see Figure 222-15), or abdominal pain may be noted on abdominal palpation. Concurrent hepatosplenomegaly and generalized lymphadenopathy are suggestive of multicentric lymphoma or an alimentary form involving the liver. Clinical signs of hypoproteinemia may develop if diffuse lymphoma results in severe PLE.

Diagnosis Hematologic examination may demonstrate anemia, characterized as either normocytic-normochromic nonregenerative or microcytic and hypochromic. Neutrophilia may also be evident. Routine biochemistry tests may reveal panhypoproteinemia in dogs and cats with diffuse lymphoma, although B-cell neoplasms may present with hyperglobulinemia as a result of monoclonal gammopathy. Alterations in serum folate or cobalamin concentrations may be the result of

malabsorption or of SIBO secondary to intestinal obstruction. Ultrasonography may demonstrate diffuse or focal intestinal wall thickening, loss of intestinal wall layering, and mesenteric lymphadenopathy; it also facilitates fine needle aspiration of focal lesions. Samples for cytologic evaluation can be collected at endoscopy by cytology brush or squash preparation, but in many cases intestinal biopsy is required. Full-thickness biopsy material is preferable to endoscopic pinch biopsies, which may miss the lesion or simply demonstrate adjacent LPE. However, exploratory laparotomy is a risky procedure, because many patients are severely debilitated and hypoproteinemic.

Although histopathologic assessment of biopsy material is the gold standard for diagnosis of alimentary lymphoma, differentiation from LPE can be difficult. Immunohistochemistry may aid in the diagnosis if all lymphocytes are of a single lineage. In the future, immunohistochemistry,[204] flow cytometry,[205] and assessment of T-cell clonality by PCR may prove to be more accurate methods of diagnosis.[82]

Treatment and prognosis Dogs with diffuse alimentary lymphosarcoma (LSA) usually respond poorly to therapy, and there is a risk of intestinal perforation. In contrast, the prognosis in cats is more favorable; some attain prolonged remission.[206,207] Response to combination chemotherapy has been reported, either with standard multidrug protocols or with an "oral only" regimen (e.g., prednisolone and chlorambucil).[206] The latter treatment is well tolerated and may be particularly applicable to cases in which the differentiation between lymphoma and LPE is uncertain.

Intestinal Adenocarcinoma

Intestinal adenocarcinoma is most common in middle-aged to older dogs and cats, and Siamese cats may be over-represented. In dogs these tumors have a predilection for the duodenum, whereas the jejunum and ileum are more commonly affected in cats (see Figure 222-8).

Clinical findings and diagnosis Adenocarcinomas are locally infiltrative, and clinical signs usually relate to partial obstruction or peritonitis when perforation has occurred. Abdominal palpation may reveal focal thickening of the intestine. Melena and signs of anemia may be present if significant ulceration has occurred. Hematologic examination may demonstrate anemia, which usually is strongly regenerative and either normocytic-normochromic or hypochromic and microcytic. Occasionally the anemia is Coombs' positive. Diagnostic imaging may delineate a mass lesion, although definitive diagnosis requires percutaneous aspiration or surgical biopsy.

Treatment and prognosis Surgical resection is the treatment of choice. However, the prognosis is usually grave, because tumors almost invariably have spread at the time of diagnosis. Metastatic spread commonly involves local lymph nodes and the liver, and metastasis to the testes was recently reported.[208] Remission times from surgery of up to 2 years have been reported, but survival time is usually less than 6 months. Chemotherapy has not been demonstrated to be effective.

Smooth Muscle Tumors of the Small Intestine

Smooth muscle tumors of the intestine (including leiomyoma and leiomyosarcoma) are uncommon in dogs and rare in cats.[209] Differentiation of smooth muscle tumors from other types of stromal neoplasia can be difficult and may require immunohistochemical procedures.[210] Presenting clinical signs can vary but may include vomiting, diarrhea, anorexia, polyuria, polydipsia, melena, acute collapse, and weight loss. Although some of these signs are the result of local tumor effects (i.e., obstruction, hemorrhage), paraneoplastic effects are reported, especially hypoglycemia,[211,212] which is thought

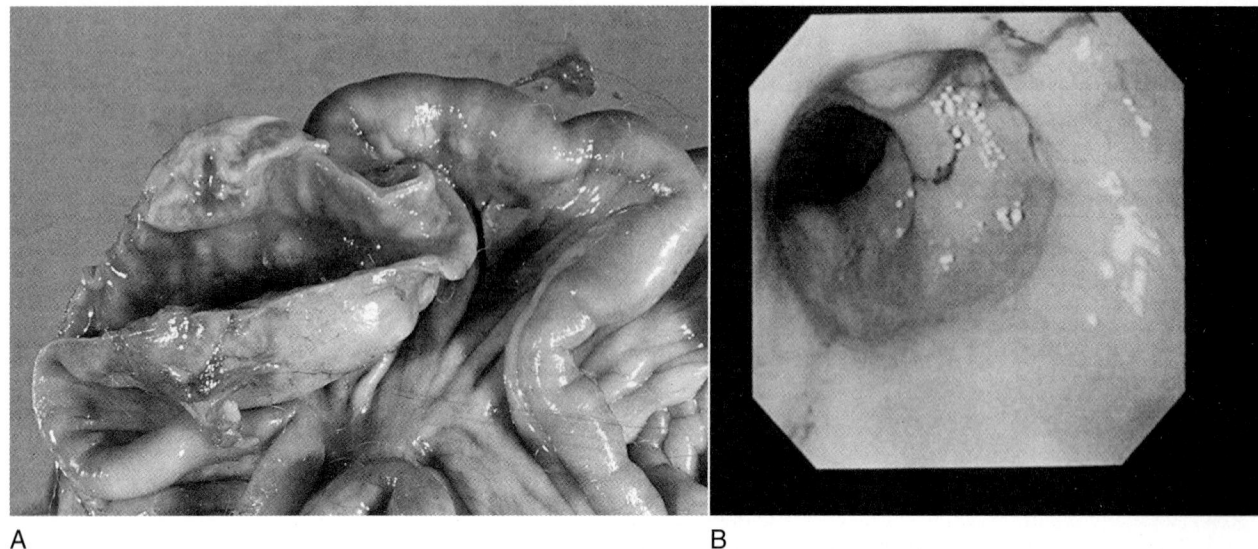

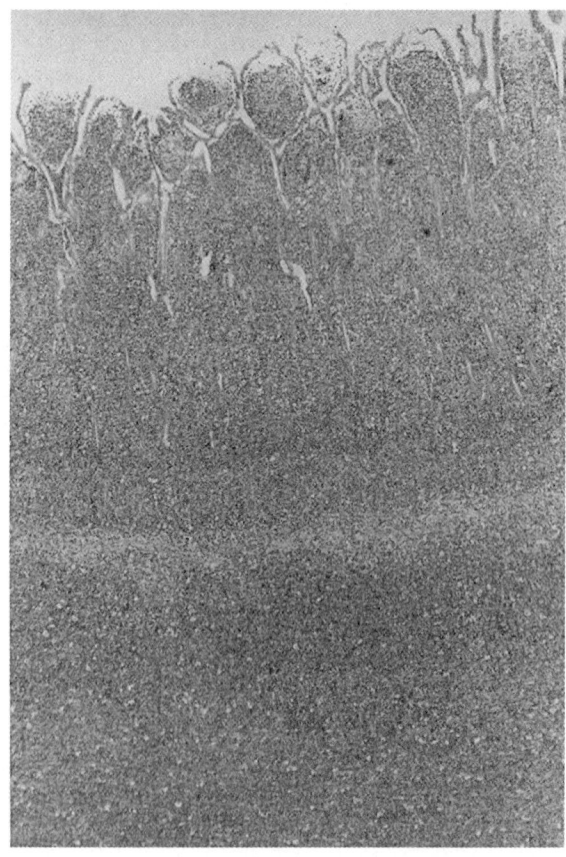

Figure 222-15 Intestinal lymphosarcoma. **A,** Nodular mass in the jejunum of a 10-year-old Pekinese cut open to demonstrate the mucosal wall thickening caused by focal lymphoma. **B,** Endoscopic image of the duodenum of a 6-year-old retriever, showing bulging of the mucosa caused by diffuse infiltration of lymphoma. **C,** Histologic appearance of lymphoma, showing loss of the normal epithelium and infiltration of all layers with malignant lymphocytes. (Courtesy G.R. Pearson.)

to be the result of production of an insulin-like growth factor II–like peptide.[213] Other paraneoplastic syndromes associated with leiomyosarcomas include nephrogenic diabetes insipidus[214] and erythrocytosis.[215]

Laboratory findings may reflect the consequences of direct or paraneoplastic effects, but they also may be unremarkable. Diagnostic imaging may aid the identification of a mass lesion, and upper GI endoscopy may confirm the presence of a lesion if it is within reach and disrupting the mucosa. However, pinch biopsies are too superficial, and exploratory laparotomy is the technique of choice both for diagnosis and for treatment. Leiomyosarcomas are slow to grow and metastasize. If surgical resection is complete and if the dog survives the

initial postoperative period, the prognosis is good, with median survival times of 21 months reported.[209] Even if metastasis is evident at the time of surgery, the prognosis is reasonable, with prolonged survival reported in some cases. The prognosis for leiomyomas is excellent after surgical excision.

Amine Precursor Uptake and Decarboxylation Tumors
Other functional amine precursor uptake and decarboxylation tumors (APUDomas), such as vasoactive intestinal peptide tumors (VIPomas), pancreatic polypeptide tumors (PPomas), and functional carcinoids, have yet to be adequately described in dogs and cats.

Other Neoplasms

Fibrosarcomas, mast cell tumors, and nonfunctional carcinoid tumors tend to be focally invasive and usually present with clinical signs similar to those of intestinal adenocarcinomas. The diagnosis is based on histologic and occasionally immunohistochemical confirmation of the tumor type. Hemangiosarcoma rarely arises in the SI, and signs relate to hemorrhage. Adenomatous polyps affecting the SI have been reported in middle-aged cats,[216] with clinical signs that include vomiting, hematemesis, or diarrhea. However, in some cases chronic, low-grade blood loss may occur, and animals instead present with microcytic anemia.

ADYNAMIC ILEUS AND INTESTINAL PSEUDO-OBSTRUCTION

Adynamic ileus is a common sequel to parvoviral enteritis, abdominal surgery, pancreatitis, peritonitis, endotoxemia, hypokalemia, and dysautonomia (see Box 222-10).[217] The term *intestinal pseudo-obstruction* describes a condition in which patients show clinical evidence consistent with an obstruction, but no mechanical cause can be found.[218-220] The condition has been associated with both visceral neuropathies and myopathies in humans, and such causes may occur in small animals. Most canine cases are associated with idiopathic sclerosing enteropathy, with fibrosis and a mononuclear cell infiltrate of the tunica muscularis. A case of feline intestinal pseudo-obstruction occurred secondary to intestinal lymphoma.

After the possibility of a mechanical obstruction has been eliminated, management of both adynamic ileus and intestinal pseudo-obstruction is aimed at identifying any underlying cause and providing specific treatment. Symptomatic therapy to stimulate intestinal motility is also indicated.[221] Suitable prokinetic agents include the 5-HT$_4$ receptor agonist cisapride, the D$_2$ dopaminergic antagonist metoclopramide, and motilin-like drugs such as erythromycin. In dogs and cats cisapride appears to be the most effective agent, but it is no longer marketed in many countries. Antibacterials may also be appropriate, given the probability of secondary SIBO, and immunosuppressive medication may be appropriate if an underlying IBD is suspected. Feeding is beneficial in humans, and nutritional support can be continued indefinitely, although vomiting, constipation, and diarrhea usually continue. Unfortunately, most cases reported in the veterinary literature responded poorly to therapy, and the prognosis is grave.

INTESTINAL OBSTRUCTION

Intestinal obstruction can be classified as acute or chronic, partial or complete, and simple or strangulated. Obstruction can be the result of extraluminal, intramural, or intraluminal mass lesions.[222] The most common extraluminal cause of obstruction is intussusception. Younger animals are more likely to develop intussusception after a case of gastroenteritis or after having intestinal surgery, although an increased risk in postparturient queens has also been reported.[223] Intestinal neoplasia is the more frequent cause of intussusception in middle-aged and older animals. Intramural causes include intestinal neoplasia (most common), hematomas, granulomas (e.g., focal FIP), IBD, stricture, and phycomycosis. Most intraluminal obstructions are caused by foreign objects, such as stones, fruit pits, and toys in dogs and linear foreign objects in cats.[224] *Intestinal volvulus* describes a condition in which the intestines rotate around the mesenteric axis, compromising the cranial mesenteric artery, and complete vascular obstruction may lead to strangulation. Reports are sporadic, but a predisposition in German shepherds has been reported.[225]

The prognosis depends on the cause of the obstruction and the severity of associated abnormalities. The outcome is likely to be favorable with simple foreign bodies, but it is grave for animals with volvulus or metastatic intestinal neoplasia. The patient may be at risk of developing short bowel syndrome if a significant length of intestine must be removed (see below).

SHORT BOWEL SYNDROME

Short bowel syndrome refers to a syndrome that occurs when large lengths of the SI (more than two thirds) are absent because of resection or, rarely, a congenital anomaly.[226,227] Clinical signs (e.g., diarrhea) result because the animal has an insufficient functional mass of SI for assimilation of nutrients and electrolytes. The degree of malabsorption depends on the length of intestine resected; in dogs, experimental studies suggest that removal of up to 85% of the intestine can be tolerated. The site of resection is also important; resection of the jejunum causes malabsorption of food, water, and electrolytes; resection of the ileum causes malabsorption of cobalamin and bile acids. Massive resection of the SI also precipitates changes in GI hormonal regulation, leading to hypergastrinemia and subsequently increased acid secretion. In some cases, the syndrome may occur only transiently after resection, because adaptive hyperplasia in the remaining intestine may lead to subsequent improvement.

Clinical Signs
The signs of intestinal malabsorption, i.e., intractable diarrhea and weight loss.

Diagnosis
The diagnosis usually is based on a history of intestinal resection with consequent diarrhea and weight loss. If a congenital lesion is suspected, contrast radiography can demonstrate the shortened SI length.

Treatment
After massive resection, aggressive parenteral fluid therapy and total parenteral nutrition should be instigated. Oral feeding is restricted but not withheld completely, because the presence of food, bile, and pancreatic secretions in the gut are important stimuli for intestinal adaptation. An isotonic, oligomeric, fat-restricted liquid diet can be fed initially, with a gradual transition first to a polymeric liquid diet and then to an easily assimilable, fat- and fiber-restricted diet. Malabsorption of fat- and water-soluble vitamins and of minerals (zinc, copper, and calcium) may also occur, and dietary or parenteral supplementation may be required. Parenteral cobalamin supplementation is essential if the ileum has been resected. Acid blockers (e.g., H$_2$-receptor antagonists) may be used in the postoperative period to counteract possible hypergastrinemia. Antimicrobial agents may be necessary if the ileocecocolic valve has been resected or if secondary SIBO is suspected. If the response to diet and antibiotics is poor, antisecretory agents (loperamide, diphenoxylate, or octreotide) may be required. Bile salt–binding resin (e.g., cholestyramine) may help reduce colonic secretion caused by bile salts malabsorbed after ileal resection.

Complications of short bowel syndrome in humans include gallstones, oxalate uroliths, and lactic acidosis. In refractory cases, experimental surgical modifications of the gut to try to slow intestinal transit and increase absorptive surface area have been described. Intestinal transplantation may be feasible in the future.

Prognosis
The prognosis depends on the amount of intestine left and the response to therapy. Some animals undergo remarkable

GASTROINTESTINAL DISEASE

adaptive hyperplasia and may return to a normal diet, whereas others never respond adequately.

IRRITABLE BOWEL SYNDROME

Irritable bowel syndrome (IBS) is characterized by recurrent, usually acute, episodes of abdominal pain, borborygmi, and diarrhea. In the absence of morphologic changes, a functional disorder is considered the cause of this enigmatic problem. Disordered intestinal motility may be of primary importance, and a number of mechanisms have been proposed for IBS in humans (Box 222-19).[228] However, it is not known whether any are responsible in dogs and cats. A variety of treatments, including antispasmodics (anticholinergics and also smooth muscle relaxants, such as mebeverine), anxiolytics (e.g., diazepam, chlordiazepoxide) and dietary modification

Box • 222-19
Causes of Irritable Bowel Syndrome
Primary motility disorders Visceral hyperalgesia Psychosomatic disorders Food intolerance Undiagnosed inflammatory disease

(low-fat diet, increased fiber) have been tried with no consistent results. IBS probably will remain a frustrating condition to diagnose and treat successfully until its etiology is better understood.

CHAPTER • 223

Diseases of the Large Intestine

Robert J. Washabau
David E. Holt

The large intestine of the dog and cat has evolved to serve two major functions: (1) extraction of water and electrolytes from the fluid contents of the lumen and (2) control of defecation. The large intestine accomplishes these functions by regulating fluid transport, bacterial fermentation, motility, immune surveillance, and blood flow. Sodium and water absorption serve to dehydrate the feces prior to defecation; mucus glycoproteins serve to trap bacterial pathogens and prevent bacterial translocation; epithelial cells, lymphocytes, plasma cells, macrophages, and dendritic cells serve to regulate the bacterial flora and the immune response to microbes; and motility serves to facilitate storage or defecation of feces. Perturbations in any of these functions may result in the problems of diarrhea, constipation, or the systemic inflammatory response syndrome (SIRS).

STRUCTURE

Macroscopic Anatomy

The large intestine consists of the cecum, colon, rectum, and anal canal (Figure 223-1). In dogs and cats, the ileum communicates directly with the colon, and what is referred to as the *cecum* in the dog and cat is actually a diverticulum of the proximal colon. The colon is further compartmentalized into ascending, transverse, and descending portions, each segment having slightly different functions and properties. The right colic or hepatic flexure separates the ascending and transverse colon, and the left colic or splenic flexure separates the transverse and descending colon. In dogs and cats, the large intestine contributes 20% to 25% of the total (small and large) intestinal length.[1,2]

The cranial and caudal mesenteric arteries provide the arterial blood supply to the colon, and venous return from the colon is transmitted to the main portal vein via the cranial and caudal mesenteric veins. Lymph is circulated from the colon to the right, middle, and left colic lymph nodes, and eventually into the cisterna chyli and thoracic duct. Parasympathetic innervation arises from the vagus nerve in the proximal colon, and from the pelvic nerves in the distal colon. Sympathetic innervation arises from the paravertebral ganglia and follows the lumbar splanchnic nerves and mesenteric arteries to the colonic mucosa and muscularis. Parasympathetic preganglionic fibers and sympathetic postganglionic fibers synapse on cell bodies and neurons of the enteric nervous system, respectively.

Microscopic Anatomy

As with the small intestine, the cross-sectional structure of the large intestine consists of four distinct layers (i.e., mucosa, submucosa, muscularis, serosa) (Figure 223-2). The large intestine differs from the SI in the following important ways: villi are absent in the large intestine, the microvilli of the large intestine epithelial cells are much less abundant, goblet cells are more prominent in the large intestine, endocrine cells are less prominent in the large intestine, and crypt-to-epithelial migration is a much slower process in the large intestine.

The mucosa of the large intestine is a flat absorptive surface area differing from the small intestine in that villi are not present. However, numerous straight tubular glands (400 to 600 μm) are present in parallel cylinders, and they extend from the muscularis mucosa to the mucosal surface.[3] The glands are lined by a continuous sheet of columnar epithelial cells, which are separated from the mesenchymal tissue of the lamina propria by a well-defined basement membrane. The epithelium in the lower half of the crypts is composed of proliferating undifferentiated columnar cells, mucus-secreting

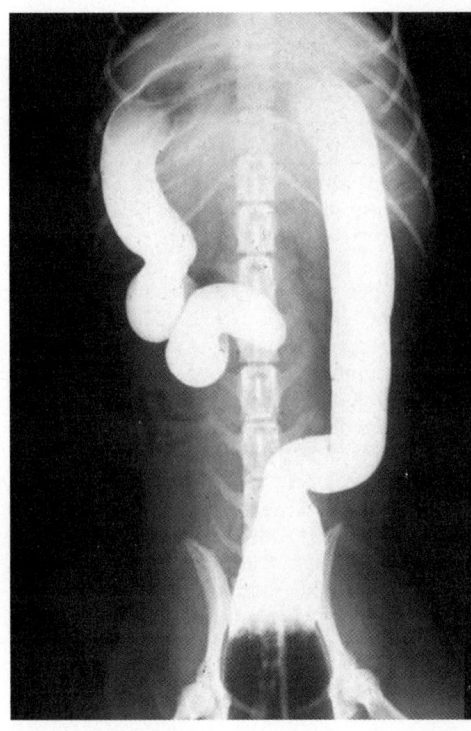

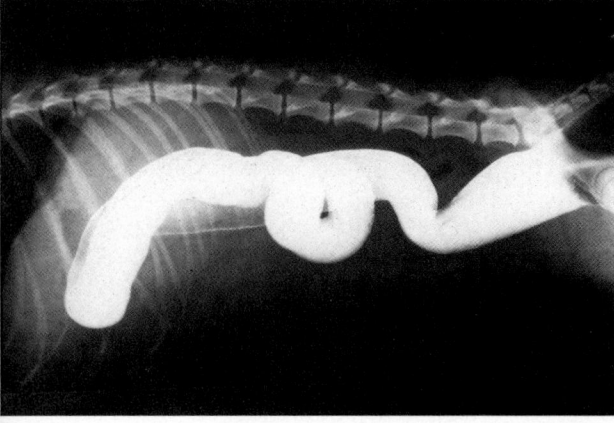

A

B

Figure 223-1 **A,** Radiographic anatomy of the feline colon—lateral projection, barium enema. **B,** Radiographic anatomy of the feline colon—ventrodorsal projection, barium enema.

goblet cells, and at least three types of endocrine cells.[4] Cellular proliferation is predominantly in the lower part of the crypts in both dogs and cats. The epithelium of the upper half of the crypts consists of differentiating columnar cells, goblet cells, and a few endocrine cells. The flat absorptive surface is lined by many columnar cells and a moderate number of goblet cells (10 to 25 goblet cells per 100 epithelial cells),[3,5] most of which are largely depleted of their mucous granules. Intraepithelial lymphocytes (IELs) are relatively sparsely distributed throughout the epithelium (one to seven lymphocytes per 100 epithelial cells),[3,5] and as in the small intestine, the predominant T cell subset is the cytotoxic-suppressor (CD8+) type.[6,7] The cellular elements of the lamina propria of the large intestine resemble closely those found in the small intestine and include lymphocytes, many plasma cells, mast cells, macrophages, eosinophils, enteric neurons, and fibroblasts.

The innermost layer of the mucosa is separated from the submucosa by the muscularis mucosae, a layer of smooth muscle cells roughly 8 to 10 cells (or 70 to 80 μm) thick. The submucosa of the colon resembles the submucosa of the other tubular digestive organs. It contains many blood and lymph vessels, dense connective tissue sparsely infiltrated by cells (fibroblasts, lymphocytes, plasma cells, mast cells, macrophages, and eosinophils), and the unmyelinated nerve fibers and ganglion cells that form the submucosal plexus.

The muscularis is composed of an inner circular muscular layer forming a tight spiral circumferentially along the course of the colon and an incomplete outer longitudinal muscle layer. The ganglion cells of the myenteric plexus of Auerbach are found between the circular and longitudinal muscle layers. Unmyelinated postganglionic fibers are also found in the circular muscle layer and communicate with the submucosal (Meissner's) plexus. The interstitial cells of Cajal, which are located on the submucosal surface of the circular smooth muscle, play a dual role as pacemaker cells and as mediators of neuromuscular transmission in the colon.[8-10]

The serosa is composed of mesothelial cells and covers only the portions of the large bowel found within the peritoneal cavity (cecum and colon). Several classification systems for colonic mucosal architecture and cellularity have been proposed. One such classification system[11] is outlined in Table 223-1. It should be emphasized that important *age*,[12] *site*,[1,3] *diet*,[13-16] and *procedure*-related[3] differences exist in the cellularity and architecture of the colonic mucosa, and these differences must be taken into account when interpreting colonic histology. For example, the protein and fiber content of the diet have significant effects on colonic mucosal morphology (e.g., crypt depth, cellularity).[14-16] The pathologist

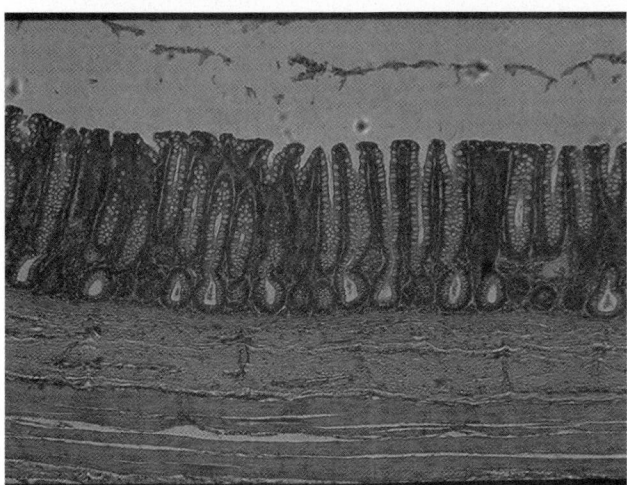

Figure 223-2 Microscopic anatomy of the canine colon.

Table • 223-1

Guidelines for Histologic Interpretation of the Canine and Feline Colonic Mucosa

PARAMETER	NORMAL	FREQUENT ABNORMAL FINDINGS
Overall mucosal appearance	Crypts straight, dominated by goblet cells throughout, separated from muscularis mucosae by no more than four layers of leukocytes (or 15 to 20 μm)	Crypts irregularly distributed, tortuous, lifted from muscularis mucosae by more than four-cell thicknesses
	Lamina propria sparse so that crypts are closely applied to adjacent crypts	Crypts obviously separated from adjacent crypts by edema, fibrosis, or leukocytes
	Proprial cell population is sparse and leukocytes almost all lymphocytes and plasma cells; neutrophils absent and eosinophils sparse except at base of crypts	Increase in lymphocyte and/or plasma cell numbers; presence of eosinophils in superficial half of lamina propria. Neutrophils anywhere are abnormal
	Mitotic figures are found in basilar 50% to 60% of each crypt, averaging 2 to 3 per crypt	Basal third of crypts excessively basophilic, mitotic figures in superficial third of crypt
	Overall crypt length 10 or 20 cm proximal to the anus averages 384 to 406 μm	Overall mucosal thickness substantially < or > 400 μm (only valid if section is well oriented and includes muscularis mucosae)
Epithelium	Columnar epithelium, basal oval nucleus; a few surface enterocytes may be cuboidal and more basophilic than the neighboring cells	Surface epithelium focally missing with pyknosis or flattening of adjacent enterocytes (versus artifactual loss in which adjacent cells are normal); surface or cryptal epithelium cuboidal or squamous, abnormally basophilic, with suprabasilar nucleus
	Intraepithelial lymphocytes are few (1 to 2 per 100 enterocytes)	Obvious increase in intraepithelial lymphocytes
	Goblet cells diffusely distributed, least numerous at crypt base and on luminal surface; mucin expulsion easily induced by pre-biopsy manipulations (so clinician should evaluate mucin loss into dilated crypt lumens with caution)	Loss of mucin from goblet cells, thus crypts seem depleted of goblet cells and may be dilated with intraluminal mucin
Lamina propria	Inconspicuous except in zone between base of crypt and muscularis mucosae that normally contains mixture of lymphocytes, plasma cells, and eosinophils	Increase in distance between crypts and between crypt base and muscularis mucosae; increases in lymphocytes, plasma cells, eosinophils, and collagen are frequent but not mutually exclusive
	Edema is a frequent biopsy artifact, impossible to distinguish from serious inflammation; similarly, physiologic congestion or hyperemia cannot be distinguished from inflammatory hyperemia	Edema must be regarded with skepticism unless accompanied by other evidence of inflammation or other changes in vascular permeability (e.g., hemorrhage, thrombosis)
Submucosa	Few lymphocytes or plasma cells; no neutrophils or eosinophils	Any type of leukocyte around dilated submucosal vessels (rarely observed except in eosinophilic colitis or invasive bacterial infection); if lymphocytes cross muscularis mucosae into submucosa, clinician should consider lymphoma
	Loosely interwoven collagen	Fibrosis

Adapted from Wilcock B: Endoscopic interpretation in canine or feline enterocolitis, *Semin Vet Med Surg (Small Anim)* 7:162, 1992. Used with permission.

should always take these factors into account when interpreting colonic biopsy specimens. The method of biopsy also influences the architecture and cellularity of the mucosa. Compared with full-thickness biopsies, gland length is 25% to 30% shorter and goblet cell numbers are 70% to 75% less in endoscopic biopsies from the same animals. The shallow depth of the endoscopic biopsy apparently causes glandular collapse, and enema or cathartic preparative solutions are believed to cause discharge of mucous goblets.[3,11]

FUNCTION

Electrolyte Transport

The large intestine regulates the electrolyte and water composition of the feces. Distinct differences exist in the mechanisms of electrolyte transport between the ascending and descending colon,[17,18] but in general the canine and feline colon absorbs water, sodium, and chloride while secreting potassium and bicarbonate.

Table • 223-2

Anatomic and Physiologic Differences—Large versus Small Intestine

	LARGE INTESTINE	SMALL INTESTINE
Villous projections (villi)	Absent	Present
Brush border microvilli	Sparse	Prominent
Goblet cells	Abundant	Sparse
Endocrine cells	Three cell types	> 20 cell types
Crypt-to-epithelial migration	Slow	Rapid
Amino acid + glucose absorption	Absent	Present
Lipid absorption	Absent	Present
Vitamin absorption	Absent	Present
Glucose-stimulated Na absorption	Absent	Present
Electrogenic Na absorption	Present	Absent
Mineralocorticoid-stimulated Na absorption	Significant	Negligible
SCFA production and absorption	Prominent	Minimal

The mechanisms of absorption and secretion in the large intestine are in many ways similar to those of the small intestine (Chapter 222), but several important differences exist (Table 223-2). Active nutrient (glucose, amino acid, monoglyceride) transport is prominent in the small intestine, but no evidence indicates active glucose or amino acid absorption in the colon except during the early neonatal period. Sodium transport also differs in the colon. Glucose- and amino acid–stimulated sodium transport is a well-established property of the small intestine, so much so that oral glucose-electrolyte solutions have been used to reduce the morbidity of cholera and other infectious diarrheal diseases of the small intestine. In contrast, glucose-coupled sodium transport does not take place in the colon and glucose-electrolyte solutions are of no benefit in diarrheal diseases of the large intestine. Sodium transport in the colon instead relies upon electrogenic transport.[18,19] The large intestine also differs in its response to mineralocorticoids. Aldosterone markedly increases sodium transport in the colon, but it has only a modest effect in the small intestine. Net sodium absorption ceases in the colon only when the luminal sodium concentration is reduced below 30 to 50 mEq/L, whereas net sodium absorption in the jejunum occurs only at luminal sodium concentrations above 130 mEq/L.[19]

Chloride absorption in the colon has both passive and active properties. Passive chloride absorption primarily represents a potential-dependent process secondary to the electrical potential generated by electrogenic sodium absorption.

Bicarbonate secretion is an important feature of colonic electrolyte function and helps to neutralize acids produced by bacterial fermentation. Chloride-bicarbonate ($Cl-HCO_3$) exchange is the primary cellular mechanism responsible for bicarbonate secretion.

The descending colon possesses both potassium absorptive and potassium secretory processes that are regulated by luminally and hormonally mediated mechanisms, and the overall net potassium movement represents the balance of these oppositely directed transport mechanisms.[18,19] Therefore the colon

has the potential to serve as an important regulatory system for the maintenance of overall potassium balance. Although renal potassium transport is critical in the overall control of potassium balance, the colon also contributes to the maintenance of potassium balance by modifying both potassium secretion and absorption, especially when kidney function is impaired.

Water Absorption

In health, approximately 2.7 L of fluid (oral intake, saliva, gastric fluid, bile, pancreatic fluid, and intestinal secretions) is presented each day to the small intestine of a 20 kg dog. About 1.35 L is absorbed in the jejunum, 1.0 L in the ileum, and 315 mL in the colon, leaving 35 mL in feces.[20] Thus the jejunum absorbs 50%, the ileum 75%, and the colon 90% of fluid volume presented to it (Figure 223-3). This fluid absorptive capacity of the colon is largely determined by basal electrolyte (primarily sodium) transport and by the ability of several agonists (aldosterone and glucocorticoids) to augment electrogenic and electroneutral sodium absorption. As long as ileocecal flow is less than the colonic absorptive capacity, significant alterations in small intestinal fluid movement may be present, but colonic absorption will prevent the development of diarrhea. On the other hand, when small intestinal absorption and ileocecal flow are normal, a relatively small decrease in colonic absorption (inflammatory bowel disease [IBD]) will produce significant increases in fecal water output.

Mucus Secretion

A lubricant layer of mucus forms a crucial physiologic barrier between the colonic mucosa and the luminal environment. Mucus is a constantly changing mix of secretions and exfoliated epithelial cells, the chief determinants of which are high molecular weight glycoproteins or mucins.[21] Gastrointestinal (GI) mucins are secreted from goblet cells as they ascend from their origin in the crypts up to the colonic epithelium. Mucin secretion is dependent upon the close integration of the cystic fibrosis transmembrane regulator (CFTR), chloride secretion, and granule exocytosis. In addition to their physiologic role as a mucosal barrier, mucins may also have a pathologic role in the metastases of epithelial tumors and enhanced susceptibility to infection.[21]

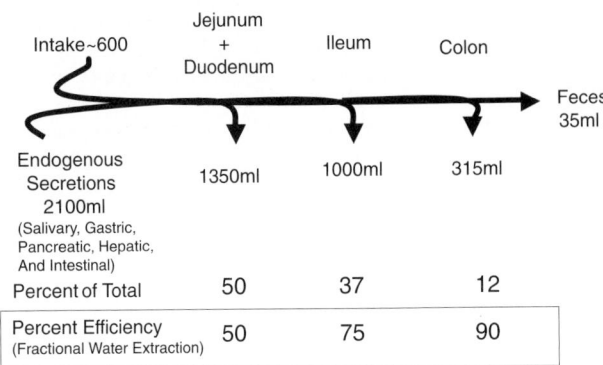

Regional Daily Net Water Turnover in the Canine Gastrointestinal Tract
(Approximate Figures 20 Kg Dog, ml/24 hr)

Figure 223-3 Regional daily water turnover in the canine gastrointestinal (GI) tract. (Adapted from Burrows CF: Chronic diarrhea in the dog. Vet Clin North Am Small Anim Pract 13:521, 1983, with permission.)

Bacterial Fermentation

The colon contains the largest concentration of bacteria in the GI tract, up to 10^{11} organisms per gram of feces. The colonic microflora play an important role in the nutrition of the animal primarily via the production of short chain fatty acids (SCFAs).[22] Major fiber fermentation substrates include cellulose, hemicellulose, and pectin, substrates that typically are not digested by pancreatic or intestinal amylases. Acetate, propionate, and butyrate account for more than 85% of formed SCFAs, and they accumulate in concentrations up to 150 mmol/L in the colon of dogs.[23] SCFAs are rapidly absorbed by the colonic mucosa, are readily metabolized by colonic epithelial cells, and have various physiologic effects. Among their physiologic effects, SCFAs promote differentiation and proliferation of colonocytes,[24] stimulate absorption of water and electrolytes,[25] provide 7% to 10% of an animal's overall energy requirements,[23] and influence or modify motility of the GI tract.[26]

The colonic flora is influenced by many factors, including host species, breed, developmental stage, dietary history, environmental conditions, geographic locale, colonic motility patterns, disease, and medication history.

In general, anaerobic bacteria (*Bacteroides* spp., *Bifidobacterium* spp., *Clostridium* spp., and *Lactobacillus* spp.) predominate in the canine colon, accounting for up to 90% of the colonic microflora. Most are facultative or aerotolerant anaerobes, not true obligate anaerobes.[27] Enterobacteria and streptococci are the predominant aerobic bacteria found in the canine colon. In the cat, approximately equal numbers of anaerobic and aerobic bacteria are found in the colonic lumen.[28]

The colonic flora changes significantly with developmental stages. The aging canine colon becomes more readily populated by *Clostridium perfringens* and other obligate anaerobes, and less populated by aerobes and aerotolerant anaerobes.[27,29] This change takes place in the ascending and descending colon, but it is most significant in the descending colon where anaerobic conditions tend to predominate. Senescent changes in bacterial populations of the colon conform to the principles of successional ecology.[30] Over time, changes in pH, redox potential, bacterial competition, and nutrient availability facilitate the proliferation of anaerobic bacteria permitting them to eventually displace the aerotolerant forms.

An animal's breeding and genetic background may also influence the colonic flora. For example, far fewer *Bifidobacterium* spp. are recovered from the feces of beagle dogs than are recovered from other dog breeds.[29,31] This represents a problem for studies of colonic bacteriology because many of the reference studies have been generated from beagle dogs.

Diet has a major impact on numbers and types of bacteria recovered from the colon. *Bacteroides* spp. appear to be particularly susceptible to changes in the diet.[31-33] The protein, carbohydrate, and fiber content of the diet all appear to influence the ability of bacteria to grow within the colon. Thus dietary history should always be considered when interpreting results of fecal or colonic bacterial cultures.

Geographic locale and environmental conditions can also influence colonic bacteriology in the dog. *Bifidobacterium* spp. are readily isolated from dogs from Japan, but they are inconsistently found in American dogs.[29,31] Housing conditions appear to be another confounding factor. Open housing environments[27] appear to facilitate colonization of a greater proportion of facultative anaerobic bacteria compared with closed facility conditions.[34]

Motility patterns of the colon influence the bacterial ecology of the colon. The antiperistaltic activity of the ascending and transverse colon particularly facilitates the mixing of fecal material with endogenous bacteria. Abnormalities in the motility patterns of this part of the colon lead to changes and proliferation of obligate anaerobes similar to that found in the descending colon.[35]

Disease and medical therapies, particularly antibiotics, alter the microbial characteristics of the colon. These changes are poorly understood in dogs and cats, but they very likely contribute to clinical symptomatology.

Immune Surveillance

The colon contains a diverse array of immune cells, including T and B lymphocytes, plasma cells, macrophages, dendritic cells, antigen-presenting cells, mast cells, eosinophils, and neutrophils.[3,5-7,36-39] Immune cells are found in the epithelium, lamina propria, and submucosa of the colon. As in the small intestine, appropriate interactions between these different cell types are essential in generating either immune responsiveness or tolerance to the large array of luminal antigens.[40,41] Much less is known about colonic immunity, but some generalizations may be made. In the colon, CD8+ T cells are found primarily in the epithelium; very few CD8+ T cells are found in the lamina propria or submucosa. Most IELs are CD3+ and CD8+, a phenotype consistent with suppressor-cytotoxic functions. Lamina propria T cells, on the other hand, are predominantly of the CD4+ helper phenotype. Immunoglobin A (IgA)-containing plasma cells are more prominent than IgG- or IgM-containing plasma cells in the lamina propria. Thus in the normal colonic mucosa, a balance would appear to be maintained between helper and suppressor T cell populations, which allows specific antigen responsiveness while avoiding hyper-reactivity.[5,6,42] A more detailed discussion of GI immunity may be found in Chapter 222, Diseases of the Small Intestine. Many similarities exist in the immune systems at both sites, but important differences exist in the immune response of the small and large intestine (discussed in Inflammation).

Motility

The colon has evolved to serve two important functions: (1) extraction of water and electrolytes from the luminal contents in the ascending and transverse colon and (2) control of defecation in the descending colon. This specialization of function has been attributed to regional differences in colonic motility patterns.[35,43-46] Electrical slow wave frequency and rhythmic phasic contractions (RPCs) are slower in the proximal portion of the colon, thus facilitating extraction of water from the fecal mass by diffusion and active transport. Retrograde giant contractions (RGCs) and antiperistalsis further facilitate the mixing of contents in the proximal colon. In contrast to that of the proximal colon, motility of the distal colon is characterized primarily by migrating spike bursts and powerful giant migrating contractions (GMCs) that propagate the fecal mass toward the rectum.[46]

Colonic smooth muscle generates at least four different types of contractions to perform the complex motility functions of mixing and propulsion: (1) tone, (2) RPCs, (3) RGCs, and (4) GMCs. The time course, frequency, and force generated by each of these contractions are significantly different from each other.[43-46] The precise role of tone in circular muscle cells is not known, but the resulting decrease in the diameter of the colon may enhance the efficiency of the phasic contractions in mixing and propulsion. Tone is normally of small to moderate force and can last for prolonged periods of time (several minutes to hours). RPCs produce mixing and net slow distal propulsion of luminal contents in the postprandial and fasting state. Phasic contractions occur rhythmically at a few cycles per minute, last for about 3 to 5 seconds, and generate a moderate force (75 to 100 g). RGCs occur infrequently, last for about 20 seconds, generate a very strong force (> 150 g), and are propagated from their point of origin into the ascending colon. RGCs facilitate mixing in the ascending colon. The GMCs are of a similar magnitude and frequency to the RGCs, but they generate mass movements from their point of origin to the anorectal junction. It has been suggested that different signal transduction pathways are used by smooth muscle cells to trigger different contractions.[47,48] It is remarkable that the same smooth muscle cells can generate so many different types of contractions using a limited number of second messengers.

DIAGNOSTIC EVALUATION

History and Physical Examination

Inflammation is the most important pathophysiologic condition of the colon. Colitis is responsible for the major clinical signs of hematochezia, mucus in the feces, dyschezia, abdominal discomfort, tenesmus, urgency, and increased frequency of defecation. The colon is an important target organ for IBD in the dog, whereas the upper GI tract (stomach and small intestine) is more frequently involved in feline IBD. Clinical signs are useful in localizing the anatomic site of the diarrhea to the small or large bowel (Table 223-3), although some animals will have diffuse involvement of the small and large intestines.

The history should include specific questions about diet, parasite control, environment, travel history, concurrent medical disease, and drug history. Dietary sensitivity reactions[49] and parasitism are major causes of colitis in many pet populations. Dietary history should include information regarding type of diet, incidence of dietary indiscretion, supplements, snacks, and treats. Information concerning previous fecal examinations and anthelmintic use may provide useful clues to the cause of the diarrhea. Environmental history should identify other pets in the household, the composition of their diets, and any behavioral interactions or hierarchies that might influence the development of clinical signs. The travel history may yield important information about exposure to histoplasmosis, pythiosis, and heterobilharziasis, all of which have regional distributions. Concurrent medical disease (e.g., Addison's disease, IBD, pancreatitis) will also help place the current episode of colitis in context. The drug history should include information about the use of alternative and complementary medicines that could contribute to clinical symptomatology.

The physical examination may be normal in many cases of colitis. The most consistent physical examination findings are pain and irregularities of the colonic mucosa on digital rectal examination. The perineum should be examined carefully to exclude perineal diseases such as perineal hernia and perianal fistula. Physical examination may reveal other important findings, including *fever* (IBD, cecal or colonic perforation, fungal infection), *abdominal pain* (IBD, colonic neoplasia, cecal or colonic perforation), *abdominal mass* (colonic neoplasia, granulomatous colitis, intussusception), *small intestinal thickening* (concurrent SI IBD, SI lymphoma), *mesenteric lymphadenopathy* (SI IBD, SI lymphoma), *hepatosplenomegaly* (lymphoma, disseminated fungal infection), and *uveitis* (prototothecosis, lymphoma). A scoring system has been developed to relate clinical signs with histologic findings in canine IBD.[50]

Constipation is the second most important pathophysiologic condition of the colon. Clinical signs include reduced, absent, or painful defecation for a period of time ranging from days to weeks or months. Physical examination findings will depend on the severity and pathogenesis of constipation. Dehydration, weight loss, abdominal pain, and mild to moderate mesenteric lymphadenopathy are common findings in cats with idiopathic constipation. Physical examination might also reveal *abdominal mass* (cecal or colonic neoplasia, granulomatous colitis), *abdominal pain* (foreign bodies, colonic perforation), *autonomic neuropathy* (dysautonomia), *hindlimb paresis* (lumbar spinal cord pathology), *pelvic fracture* (pelvic outflow obstruction), and *perineal hernia* (cause or complication of constipation).

Laboratory Data

For both inflammation and constipation, the scope of the medical investigation will be shaped by prior history, suspected cause, chronicity, and signs of systemic illness[51,52] (Figure 223-4).

Complete blood count (CBC), serum chemistry, and urinalysis should be considered in animals with signs of colonic disease, particularly those with signs of systemic disease. These tests may provide evidence of *anemia* (chronic disease, GI blood loss), *leukocytosis* (IBD, neoplasia, cecal or colonic perforation), *eosinophilia* (parasitism, Addison's disease, mast cell disease, hypereosinophilic syndrome), *thrombocytopenia* (concurrent immune thrombocytopenia), *hypoproteinemia* (protein-losing enteropathy [PLE]), *hyperglobulinemia* (FIP, IBD, infection, neoplasia), *hypercalcemia* (neoplasia, fungal disease), *hypoglycemia* (leiomyosarcoma), and *hyponatremia* and *hyperkalemia* (Addison's or pseudo-Addison's disease). This minimum data base is also useful to screen animals prior to anesthesia and colonoscopy. If fungal, *Oomycetes*, or algal infections are possible causes in the pet's geographic area, special serologic tests are available for the diagnosis of some of these diseases (Table 223-4). Feline leukemia virus (FeLV) and Feline immunodeficiency virus (FIV) testing are warranted in cats with unexplained, chronic diarrhea.

Fecal Parasitic Evaluation

Direct fecal smears and fecal flotation studies should be performed to evaluate for helminth, protozoa, and some bacterial infections (see Table 223-4). Direct fecal smears may be useful in detecting *Giardia*, *Tritrichomonas*, and *Campylobacter* organisms. Zinc sulfate flotation is the most accurate and practical fecal flotation test available, and it may be more sensitive for the detection of *Giardia* and *Tritrichomonas* infections. Some animals may have intermittent shedding of helminth ova, *Giardia* trophozoites and cysts, or both; therefore suspected infections should always be treated with anthelmintics or antiprotozoal agents before animals are subjected to colonoscopy.

Fecal Bacterial Culture

Fecal cultures should be considered in animals with suspected bacterial infections of the intestine and colon. Risk factors for bacterial colitis include young age, crowded or poor hygienic environmental conditions, co-infection with helminth or protozoal parasites, viral immunosuppression,[53] boarding or kenneling conditions, and multiple-pet households. Bacterial pathogens associated with colitis or enterocolitis lesions in dogs

Table • 223-3

Clinical Signs Associated with Diarrhea—Large Bowel versus Small Bowel

SIGNS	SMALL BOWEL	LARGE BOWEL
Weight loss	May be present	Uncommon
Vomiting	May be present	Uncommon
Flatulence	Present with malassimilation	Unusual
Defecation frequency	Normal to mild increase	Marked increased frequency
Fecal volume	Increased	Normal to mild increase
Urgency	Absent	Usually present
Tenesmus	Absent	Usually present
Mucous in feces	Usually absent	Frequently present
Hematochezia	Absent	Often present
Melena	Sometimes present	Absent
Steatorrhea	Present with malassimilation	Absent

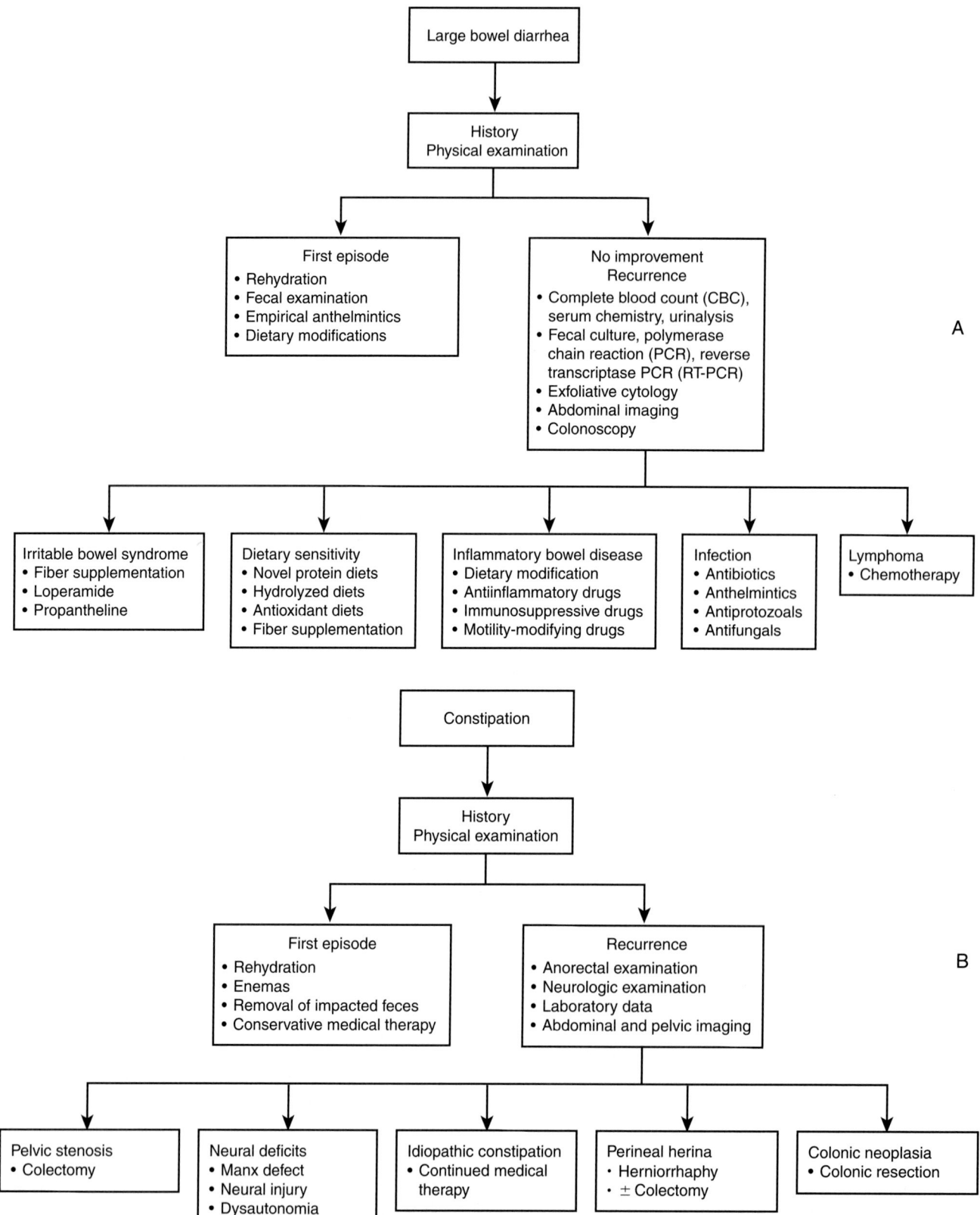

Figure 223-4 A, Diagnostic approach to large intestinal diarrhea. **B,** Diagnostic approach to constipation. *PCR,* Polymerase chain reaction; *RT-PCR,* reverse transcriptase polymerase chain reaction.

Table • 223-4

Definitive, Suspected, and Unproved Pathogens of the Large Intestine of Dogs and Cats

CLASSIFICATION/ ORGANISM	TISSUE TROPHISM	EVIDENCE OF PATHOGENICITY	DIAGNOSIS	REFERENCES
Helminths				
Trichuris vulpis	Cecum, colon	Good evidence	Fecal flotation	63,64
Trichuris serrata, T. campanula	Cecum, colon	Moderate evidence	Fecal flotation	63,64
Ancylostoma caninum	Intestine, colon	Good evidence	Fecal flotation	63,71,116,117
Heterobilharzia americana	Colon	Good evidence	Fecal flotation, histology	66,67,68
Protozoa				
Balantidium coli	Colon	Poor evidence	Fecal flotation	69,70
Entamoeba histolytica	Colon	Weak evidence	Fecal flotation	71,72,73
Giardia spp.	Intestine, colon	Moderate to good evidence	Fecal flotation, ELISA, IFA, duodenal/colonic aspiration	74-87
Isospora ohioenesis—dogs	Intestine, cecum, colon	Weak evidence	Fecal flotation	88,89
Tritrichomonas foetus—cats	Ileum, cecum, colon	Moderate to good evidence	Fecal flotation, culture, PCR	90-95
Fungi				
Histoplasma capsulatum	Intestine, colon	Good evidence	Exfoliative cytology, histology	96-100
Oomycetes				
Pythium insidiosum	Stomach, intestine, colon	Good evidence	Histology, immunohistochemistry, ELISA, PCR	101-107
Algae				
Prototheca zopfii/wickerhamii	Eyes, skin, colon, CNS	Good evidence	Exfoliative cytology, histology	108,109
Bacteria				
Brachyspira pilosicoli	Ileum, colon	Moderate evidence	Culture, PCR, histology	110-114
Campylobacter coli, C. jejuni, C. upsaliensis, C. helveticus	Intestine, colon	Moderate to good evidence	Culture, PCR	115-124
Clostridium perfringens	Colon	Moderate to good evidence	Gram staining, culture, ELISA, PCR	126-133
Clostridium difficile	Colon	Weak to moderate evidence	Culture, Toxin A ELISA, genotyping	131-136
E. coli (ET, EI, EP, EH, EA)	Intestine, colon	Good evidence	Culture, serotyping, PCR	137-144
Salmonella spp.	Intestine, colon	Good evidence	Culture, serotyping, PCR	145-147
Yersinia enterocolitica	Colon	Poor evidence	Culture	148,149

ELISA, Enzyme-linked immunosorbent assay; IFA, indirect fluorescent antibody; PCR, polymerase chain reaction.

and cats have included *Brachyspira pilosicoli, Campylobacter* spp., *Clostridium perfringens* and *C. difficile*, certain *Escherichia coli* (enterotoxigenic, enteroinvasive, enteropathogenic, enterohemorrhagic, enteroadherent), *Salmonella* spp., and perhaps *Yersinia enterocolitica* (see Table 223-4). Culture results should always be interpreted in light of clinical signs, other findings such as coinfections, and substantiating laboratory data such as serologies or polymerase chain reaction (PCR) results. Fecal cultures should not be performed for the purpose of diagnosing small intestinal bacterial overgrowth (Chapter 222).

Molecular Diagnosis

A number of PCR and reverse transcriptase (RT)-PCR assays have been developed for gene amplification products and messenger RNAs of infectious organisms. Assays are now available for the molecular diagnosis of *Tritrichomonas foetus, Pythium insidiosum, Campylobacter jejuni, Clostridium perfringens,*

C. difficile, E. coli, Salmonella spp., and *Brachyspira pilosicoli*, and many more are likely forthcoming. Molecular detection has become the standard for infectious disease diagnosis in many instances.[54]

Exfoliative Cytology

Exfoliative rectal or endoscopic cytology may be useful in identifying causative agents (e.g., fungal elements, neoplastic cells) and inflammatory cells (e.g., lymphocytes, eosinophils). Rectal smears may be obtained with cotton-tipped applicator or conjunctival spatula during anorectal examination or with a cytology brush at the time of endoscopy. A good correlation (specificity: 97%; sensitivity: 93%) has been shown between exfoliative cytology and subsequent endoscopic or surgical biopsy in one study.[55] Additional studies will be needed to verify the diagnostic value of this test.

Imaging

Survey abdominal radiographs may occasionally document colonic foreign objects, mesenteric or sublumbar lymphadenopathy, intussusception, and extraluminal compression; however, survey radiographs are generally nonspecific in the diagnosis of colonic disease. Contrast studies (i.e., barium enema) are performed infrequently because of their poor sensitivity and requirement for general anesthesia. Ultrasonographic imaging has proved more useful in documenting mass lesions, lymphadenopathy, intussusceptions, and bowel thickening. Abdominal ultrasound may also be used to facilitate percutaneous aspiration of luminal masses, mucosal thickenings, and lymph nodes.[56,57] Computed tomography (CT) colonography, also known as *virtual colonoscopy*, has been successfully implemented in human medicine and has been studied experimentally in the dog.[58]

Colonoscopy

Colonoscopy is indicated for the diagnosis of colitis-type diarrhea unresponsive to dietary modification and medical therapy, suspected colorectal neoplasia, chronic constipation, unexplained stricture, and evaluation of prior surgical or medical treatment.[59] Colonoscopy is performed after other noninvasive diagnostic tests (e.g., fecal parasitologic examination, fecal bacteriologic examination, exfoliative cytology, abdominal ultrasonography, survey ± barium contrast radiography) have failed to diagnose the disease.

Rigid or flexible endoscopy may be performed, but flexible endoscopy provides better visualization and examination of the entire colon. The normal colonic mucosa is pink in color, smooth in texture, and glistening in appearance (Figure 223-5). Unlike the esophageal, gastric, and duodenal mucosa, submucosal blood vessels are readily apparent. The mucosa should not hemorrhage when abraded by the endoscope; active hemorrhage usually implies an underlying disorder such as inflammation or infection. The colonoscopic procedure should include examination of the more proximal structures (e.g., ascending colon, cecum, ileocecal sphincter, distal ileum) whenever possible. The proximal colon is an important site of inflammation, parasitism, ileocolic intussusception, cecal inversion, and neoplasia.

Fecal materials must be completely evacuated before the colonic mucosa can be properly examined. Incomplete bowel preparation is the major reason for an unsuccessful colonoscopic examination. Patient permitting, food should be withheld for 36 to 48 hours so that fecal material does not accumulate in the colon. The patient should also be given warm-water enemas, GI lavage solutions, or both. Lavage solutions are preferable to warm-water enemas,[60-62] but both may be given to facilitate successful colonoscopy. Polyethylene glycol solutions are isosmotic, administered orally, and induce a diarrhea that rapidly removes fecal material from the bowel.

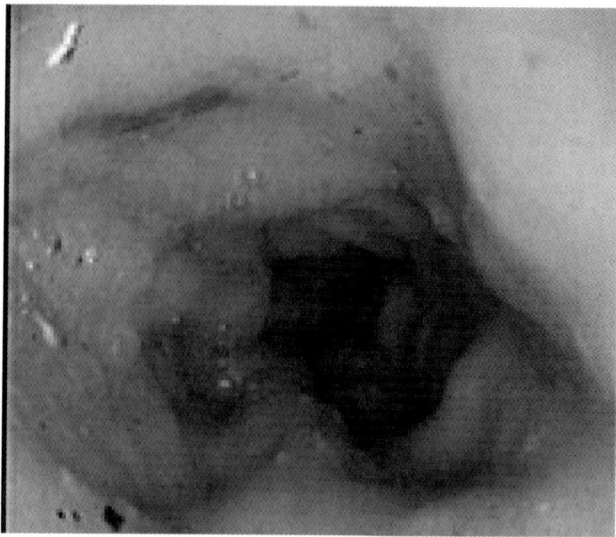

Figure 223-5 Normal endoscopic appearance of the canine large intestine.

Large volumes may be administered without inducing significant changes in water or electrolyte balance.[60] Electrolyte solutions should be given at a dose of 25 mL/kg at 24 and 12 hours prior to colonoscopy. Warm-water enemas should be performed gently, without irritating substances, at 24, 6, and 2 hours before colonoscopy. The combination of a 36 to 48 hour food-fast, GI lavage solution, and enemas will usually result in a colon that is free of fecal fluids and solids. Endoscopic examination of the colon is described in detail (see Chapter 101).[59]

Diseased tissue, nondiseased tissue, and the transition zone between diseased and nondiseased tissue should be biopsied during colonoscopic procedures. This standard helps to verify the extent of the disease, ensures that disease in the submucosa has not been missed, and provides representative tissue samples to the pathologist to diagnose the disease. In some cases of severe IBD or colonic neoplasia, advanced tissue necrosis may prevent the diagnosis of the disease process in the central part of the lesion. In the absence of gross mucosal abnormalities, three to five biopsy specimens should be obtained from each of the midascending, midtransverse, and mid-descending colonic regions.

INFECTION

The colon may be colonized by several types of infectious organisms. The most important of these are the helminths (*Trichuris* spp., *Ancylostoma* spp., *Heterobilharzia* spp.), protozoa (*Giardia* spp., *Tritrichomonas* spp.), fungi (*Histoplasma* spp.), Oomycetes (*Pythium* spp.), algae (*Prototheca* spp.), and bacteria (*Brachyspira* spp., *Campylobacter* spp., *Clostridium* spp., enteropathogeneic and enterotoxigenic *E. coli*, and *Salmonella* spp.). The routine medical investigation of any dog or cat affected with chronic large bowel diarrhea should include direct and indirect fecal examinations for helminth and protozoa, bacterial culture of feces, and serologies (see Table 223-4). Some organisms appear to be of low pathogenicity, but it should be emphasized that even commensal organisms may become pathogens given the appropriate circumstance.

Helminths
Trichuris

Cause *Trichuris vulpis* is perhaps one of the most common causes of chronic large bowel diarrhea in dogs.[63]

Cats are occasionally infected with *T. serrata* and *T. campanula*. Clinical signs in *Trichuris*-infected dogs and cats may vary from asymptomatic infections to mild intermittent episodes of mucousy feces to acute-onset bloody diarrhea with tenesmus and dyschezia.

Pathophysiology The fecal-oral route of transmission is the canonical route of infection. After ingestion of infective *Trichuris* ova, eggs hatch in the small intestine and larvae migrate to the cecum and colon where they attach to the mucosa. The pathogenicity of any infection is generally related to the magnitude of the host immune response. Factors contributing to the pathogenicity and clinical signs include the number of mature worms present, the location of the worms, the degree of inflammation, the severity of anemia or hypoproteinemia, nutritional status of the host, and the presence of other GI parasites and micro-organisms.[64]

Clinical examination Affected animals generally have mild clinical signs of typhlitis and colitis, although some dogs develop a clinical scenario of signs and laboratory findings (e.g., hyponatremia, hypochloremia, hyperkalemia) consistent with hypoadrenocorticism. When tested, *Trichuris*-infected dogs are normoreactive to ACTH stimulation and are instead referred to as *pseudo-Addisonian*.[65] Eosinophilia, anemia, and hypoalbuminemia are possible, but these are more common laboratory findings with other GI helminth infections (e.g., hookworms).

Diagnosis *Trichuris* ova can be identified on routine fecal flotation procedures; however, they may be missed because of intermittent shedding. Empiric treatment for occult *Trichuris* infection should always be performed before moving on to a more detailed, costly, and unnecessary medical investigation.

Treatment Many safe and effective therapeutic agents are available for *Trichuris* spp. Fenbendazole, febantel with praziquantel, milbemycin, and ivermectin with pyrantel pamoate all have established efficacy against whipworms. Treatment should be repeated in 3 weeks and again in 3 months, and pet owners should be advised to decontaminate the environment.

Prognosis The prognosis for recovery and cure is excellent.

Ancylostoma caninum. Hookworms are primary pathogens of the small intestine (Chapter 222), but they occasionally infect the cecum and colon with overwhelming infestations. Diagnosis is achieved by demonstrating hookworm ova in the feces, and treatments are similar to those used for whipworm infections (Chapter 222).

Heterobilharzia americana
Cause *H. americana* is considered the primary agent of schistosomiasis in dogs. It is an uncommon infection in dogs and is encountered almost exclusively in the southern Atlantic and Gulf Coast states in the United States. In addition to the dog, nutria, raccoons, rabbits, and mice serve as important reservoir hosts. Although uncommon, heterobilharziasis is an important consideration in the differential diagnosis of acute and chronic large bowel diarrhea in endemic areas.[66,67]

Pathophysiology The life cycle of *H. americana* is complex and involves an intermediate (snail) and definitive (dog) host and various life stages. Dogs are infected when motile cercaria from snails penetrate their skin. The schistosomulae migrate from the skin to the liver of the definitive host, where they develop into mature male and female worms. Adult schistsomes lay eggs in the terminal mesenteric venules, and

egg migration through the bowel wall elicits an intense granulomatous response. It is usually the host response that gives rise to the clinical symptomatology.

Clinical examination Clinical signs vary from none to acute signs of vomiting, weight loss, bloody diarrhea, and progressive emaciation. Affected animals may have biochemical evidence of hypoalbuminemia, hyperglobulinemia, hypercalcemia, and liver enzyme elevation.[68]

Diagnosis Diagnosis is confirmed by demonstration of ova on direct fecal examination or tissue biopsy. Serologic tests have not yet been successfully implemented in companion animals.

Treatment Fenbendazole in combination with praziquantel appears to be effective in the treatment of *H. americana*.

Prognosis The prognosis for acute infections is generally favorable, although severe liver involvement may portend chronic liver disease and cirrhosis.

Protozoa
Balantidium coli *B. coli* is primarily a pathogen of sheep. Only one case report of natural infection in the dog has ever been published.[69] In another report, a total of 375 fecal samples of 56 mammalian species belonging to 17 families of 4 orders were examined for the detection of *Balantidium coli*. *B. coli* organisms were detected in several animal species, but not in dogs or cats.[70]

Entamoeba histolytica Two isolated case reports of colitis in dogs[71] and one in cats[72] are associated with recovery of *E. histolytica* from the feces. *E. histolytica* can be recovered from the feces of healthy dogs and cats, but it appears to be of low pathogenicity in dogs and cats.[73]

Giardia
Cause *Giardia* spp. are protozoal parasites that primarily infect the small intestine of dogs and cats. The cecum and colon are only occasionally colonized by *Giardia*. All mammalian isolates are currently classified as *Giardia lamblia*, although some nomenclature systems use the name *G. duodenalis* or *G. intestinalis*.[74] Recent DNA sequence technology suggests that one or two distinct *Giardia* genotypes can be isolated exclusively from dogs,[75,76] and a distinct genetic group can be isolated from cats.[77] It is not clear whether differences in pathogenicity exist between these genotypes. *Giardia* species have a worldwide distribution. Because *Giardia* is maintained in nature primarily by fecal-oral transmission, more cases are associated with crowded and unsanitary conditions. A recent study showed a prevalence in the dog of 7.2%.[78]

Pathophysiology *Giardia* spp. are found on the surface of enterocytes, where the trophozoites attach to the brush border of the epithelium. Specific histologic changes have not been reported, but persistence of infection may promote apoptosis and inhibition of re-epithelialization.

Clinical examination Although infected animals may remain asymptomatic, clinical signs such as acute or chronic diarrhea, weight loss, or even acute or chronic vomiting may develop. Although *Giardia* cysts and trophozoites have been found in the feces of dogs with both small bowel and large bowel diarrhea, *Giardia* infection is primarily a problem of the small intestine (Chapter 222).

Diagnosis *Giardia* infections can be diagnosed by demonstrating motile trophozoites on fresh fecal smears or cysts by zinc sulfate sedimentation.[79,80] Commercial enzyme-linked immunosorbent assay (ELISA) kits have also been used to detect *Giardia* antigen in fresh fecal samples. ELISA assays may be slightly more sensitive and specific than a single zinc sulfate concentrating technique in diagnosing *Giardia* infections in dogs.[78,80] A direct immunofluorescent antibody test has been used in the diagnosis of *Giardia* infections in humans, but it has not yet been validated in the dog. Duodenal aspirates during GI endoscopy appear to be ineffective in diagnosing *Giardia* infection.[81]

Treatment   Metronidazole, ipronidazole, fenbendazole, albendazole, and a praziquantel, pyrantel pamoate, febantel combination have all been used in the treatment of *Giardia* infections with varying levels of success.[82-85] A *Giardia* vaccine has been shown to be effective in prevention and therapy in dogs,[86,87] but efficacy has not yet been established in cats.[74]

Prognosis   The prognosis for long-term health and recovery is generally very favorable.

Isospora canis, I. ohioensis, I. felis, I. neorivolta.

The *Isospora* species are the most common coccidial parasites of dogs (*I. canis* and *I. ohioensis*) and cats (*I. felis* and *I. neorivolta*). The coccidia are primarily parasites of the small intestine (Chapter 222), but *I. ohioensis* may induce cecal and colonic pathology in puppies and young dogs.[88,89] Sulfadimethoxine (50 mg/kg orally, once a day for 10 days) or sulfatrimethoprim (15 to 30 mg/kg orally, once a day for 5 days) may be used where clinical signs warrant treatment.

Tritrichomonas foetus

Cause   *Tritrichomonas foetus* is a flagellated protozoan parasite that is an important venereal pathogen in cattle. *T. foetus* has also been identified as an intestinal pathogen in domestic cats from which intraluminal infection of the colon leads to chronic large bowel diarrhea.[90] Infected cats are usually young and frequently reside in densely populated housing such as catteries or animal shelters. Cats often have a history of infection with *Giardia* spp.; these infections are subsequently identified as *trichomoniasis* after failure to eradicate the organisms with standard antiprotozoal treatment (e.g., metronidazole or fenbendazole).

Pathophysiology   After experimental inoculation in cats, *T. foetus* organisms have been shown to colonize the ileum, cecum, and colon, reside in close contact with the epithelium, and are associated with transient diarrhea that is exacerbated by coexisting cryptosporidiosis.[91]

Clinical examination   Infected animals have clinical signs that are consistent with chronic colitis-type diarrhea.

Diagnosis   Diagnosis of trichomonosis in cats is made by direct observation of trichomonads in samples of freshly voided feces that are suspended in physiologic saline (0.9% NaCl) solution and examined microscopically at ×200 to ×400 magnification.[92] *T. foetus* can also be grown from feces via incubation at 37° C in Diamond's medium.[93] The sensitivity of direct examination of a fecal smear for diagnosis of *T. foetus* in naturally infected cats is unknown but is suspected to be poor. A commercially available culture system that is sensitive and specific for culture of *T. foetus* will improve the diagnostic outcome. These kits are most useful when inoculated with less than or equal to 0.1 g of fresh feces at 25° C. More recently, a single-nested tube PCR technique has been developed that is ideally suited for diagnostic testing of feline fecal samples that are found negative by direct microscopy

and by definitive identification of microscopically observable or cultivated organisms.[94]

Treatment   At this time the origin of the infection in most cats is unknown, and no effective antimicrobial treatment exists for *T. foetus* infection. Metronidazole and fenbendazole may improve clinical signs but generally do not resolve infection. Nitazoxanide eliminates shedding of *T. foetus* and *Cryptosporidium* oocysts, but diarrhea and oocyst shedding recur with discontinuation of treatment. A series of cats that were treated with paromomycin for *T. foetus* infection subsequently developed kidney failure.[95] Consequently, paromomycin should probably not be used in cats.

Prognosis   The prognosis for eradication of the organism is not encouraging at this time.

Fungi

Histoplasma capsulatum

Cause   Histoplasmosis is a systemic fungal disease of dogs and cats caused by *H. capsulatum*. In the environment, *H. histoplasma* organisms are mycelial, saprophytic soil fungi. In infected tissue or when cultured at 30 to 37° C, the organism is a yeast. The fungus is endemic throughout most of the temperate and subtropic regions of the world. Most cases of histoplasmosis in the United States occur in the central states, with the geographic distribution following the Mississippi, Ohio, and Missouri Rivers.[96,97]

Pathophysiology   Infection is probably via inhalation or ingestion of infective conidia from the environment. The respiratory system is thought to be the primary route of infection in cats and dogs, although the GI tract may also be an important route in the dog. After inhalation or ingestion, conidia transform from the mycelial phase and are phagocytized by macrophages, where they grow as facultative intracellular organisms. Hematogenous and lymphatic dissemination results in multisystemic disease. Organisms can be disseminated to any organ system, but the lungs, GI tract, lymph nodes, liver, spleen, bone marrow, eyes, and adrenal glands are the most common organs of dissemination in the dogs; lungs, liver, lymph nodes, eyes, and bone marrow are most commonly affected in cats. Cell-mediated immunity induces a granulomatous inflammatory response in most infections.[98]

Clinical examination   Dogs with GI histoplasmosis typically have mild fever, anorexia, lethargy, weight loss, vomiting, diarrhea, hematochezia, and tenesmus. Cachexia is a common physical examination finding. Other historical and physical examination findings (dyspnea, cough, ascites, lameness, oropharyngeal ulcerations, chorioretinitis, neuropathy) will depend upon organ and tissue involvement. The full clinical spectrum of histoplasmosis infection is outlined in Chapter 174.

Diagnosis   Endoscopic examination usually reveals severe granulomatous inflammation of the large intestine (Figure 223-6, *A*). Organism identification is required for definitive diagnosis. The most common means of organism identification is cytology. Cytology from affected tissue reveals pyogranulomatous inflammation, often with numerous small, round to oval intracellular yeast cells (2 to 4 μm in diameter) characterized by a basophilic center and a light halo (Figure 223-6, *B*). Exfoliative cytology during colonoscopy is particularly useful in diagnosing the disease.[55] Histopathology is helpful if cytology is nondiagnostic or inconclusive. Multiple endoscopic colonic biopsies are usually sufficient to diagnose the disease. The yeast form does not stain well with routine hematoxylin-eosin (H&E) stains, so special stains such as PAS and Gomori's

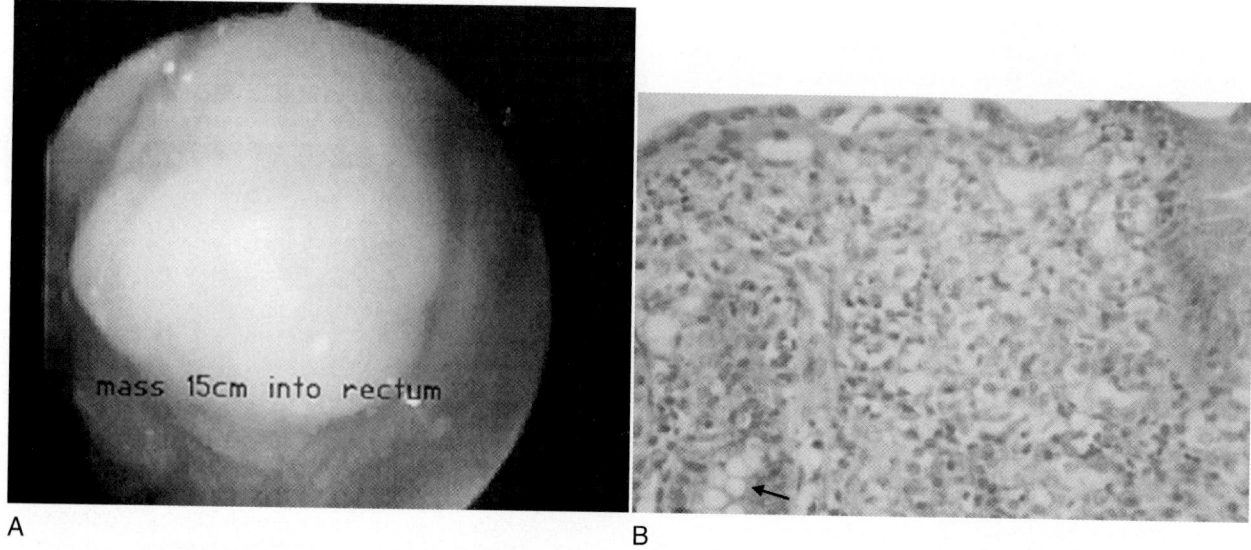

Figure 223-6 A, Endoscopic appearance of granulomatous colitis in a dog infected with *Histoplasma* spp. B, Histologic appearance of granulomatous colitis in a dog infected with *Histoplasma* spp. Arrow indicates numerous small, round to oval intracellular yeast cells (2 to 4 μm in diameter) (Hematoxylin-eosin [H&E] stain).

methenamine silver stain are often used to demonstrate organisms. Fungal culture from affected tissue can be used for diagnosis but is rarely needed in clinical cases. Currently available serologies have poor specificity and sensitivity.[98]

Treatment Itraconazole (5 mg/kg orally, twice a day for 2 to 4 months) is considered the treatment of choice for feline histoplasmosis. In one study, itraconazole therapy cured histoplasmosis infections in all eight study cats.[99] Ketoconazole and amphotericin B have been described as the treatments of choice for canine histoplasmosis. With colonic involvement, additional GI therapy may be useful in affected dogs (e.g., dietary modification, treatment for small intestinal bacterial overgrowth, direct antidiarrheal therapy). Corticosteroids may have been used successfully in the treatment of airway obstruction secondary to hilar lymphadenopathy in chronically infected dogs.[100]

Prognosis There may be important species differences in prognosis, although the paucity of reports, especially of prospective clinical trials, makes it difficult to generalize. It would seem that the prognosis is guarded in dogs but fair to good in cats.

Oomycetes
Pythium insidiosum
Cause *P. insidiosum* is an aquatic oomycete that causes severe GI pathology in a range of hosts in the tropic and subtropic climates.[101] Based on ribosomal RNA gene sequence data, members of the Class Oomycetes are phylogenetically distinct from the Kingdom Fungi and are more closely related to algae than to fungi.[102] The Oomycetes differ from fungi in two important properties (i.e., cell wall and cell membrane composition). Chitin is an essential component of the fungal cell wall, but it is generally lacking in the oomycete cell wall. Oomycetes also differ from fungi in that ergosterol is not a principal sterol in the oomycete cell membrane. This difference may explain why ergosterol-targeting drugs like itraconazole are less effective in the medical treatment of pythiosis.[102]

Pathophysiology The infective state of *P. insidiosum* is thought to be the motile zoospore, which is released into stagnant water in warm environments and likely causes infection either by encysting in the skin or by being ingested into the GI tract. Ingested zoospores encyst and adhere to the gastric, jejunal, and colonic epithelium with a polarity oriented toward the submucosa for rapid tissue penetration after germ tube eruption. *Pythium* induces a chronic pyogranulomatous response in the GI tract and mesenteric lymph nodes. The gastric outflow tract and ileocolonic junction are the most frequently affected portions of the GI tract, and it is not uncommon to find two or more segmental lesions in the same patient.[103] Inflammation in affected regions is typically centered on the submucosa, with variable mucosal ulceration and occasional extension of disease through serosal surfaces, resulting in adhesion formation and peritonitis.

Clinical examination Weight loss, vomiting, diarrhea, and hematochezia are the most important clinical signs. Physical examination often reveals emaciated body condition and a palpable abdominal mass. Signs of systemic illness such as lethargy and depression are not typically present unless intestinal obstruction, infarction, or perforation occurs.

Diagnosis Ileocolonic wall thickening, obliteration of the normal layered appearance, and regional lymphadenopathy are common ultrasonographic features of canine intestinal pythiosis.[104] Of course, these findings cannot be readily differentiated from those associated with intestinal malignancy. Definitive diagnosis requires histologic demonstration or immunohistochemical staining of the organism, positive ELISA or PCR assays, or a combination of these techniques. The histologic findings associated with pythiosis generally are characterized by eosinophilic granulomatous to pyogranulomatous inflammation with fibrosis. Affected tissue typically contains multiple foci of necrosis surrounded and infiltrated by neutrophils, eosinophils, and macrophages. Discrete granulomas composed of epithelioid macrophages, plasma cells, multinucleate giant cells, and neutrophils and eosinophils may

GASTROINTESTINAL DISEASE

also be observed. *Pythium* zoospores may be cultured directly from affected tissue in antibiotic-containing (e.g., strepto-mycin, ampicillin) media. More recently, sensitive and specific ELISA and PCR assays have been developed for the accurate diagnosis of pythiosis in dogs.[105-107]

Treatment Aggressive surgical resection remains the treatment of choice for pythiosis in dogs. Because it provides the best opportunity for long-term cure, complete resection of infected tissue should be pursued whenever possible. Segmental lesions of the GI tract should be resected with 3 to 4 cm margins whenever possible. Medical therapy for the oomycetes has not been very promising. This may relate to the absence of ergosterol (cell membrane target of most currently available antifungal drugs) in the oomycete cell membrane. Clinical and serologic cures have been obtained in a small number of dogs after therapy with amphotericin B lipid com-plex (2 to 3 mg/kg every other day, administered to a cumu-lative dose of 24 to 27 mg/kg) or itraconazole (5 mg/kg every 12 hours for 6 to 9 months).

Prognosis Unfortunately, most dogs with GI pythiosis are not presented to the veterinarian until late in the course of the disease, when complete excision is not possible. The anatomic site of the lesion (e.g., pylorus, ileocolic sphincter) may also prevent complete excision. Consequently, the prog-nosis is usually grave in most animals.[102]

Algae
Prototheca zopfii and P. wickerhamii
Cause Three species have been recognized within the genus *Prototheca*: *P. stagnosa*, *P. wickerhamii*, and *P. zopfii*; a fourth species, *P. salmonis*, has been proposed. Of these three species, *P. wickerhamii* and *P. zopfii* have demonstrated pathogenicity. *Prototheca* spp. are ubiquitous in nature and are found in sewage systems, soil, lakes, rivers, ponds, and in feces. The organism has been documented to cause disease in dogs and cats and a variety of other species. *P. wickerhamii* is the causative organism in virtually all instances of cutaneous pro-tothecosis, and *P. zopfii* is the causative organism in most instances of disseminated disease.[108]

Pathophysiology Cutaneous infection with granuloma formation is the most common manifestation of prototothecosis in most species, including cats and humans. Dissemination does not readily occur in cats or humans, but the infection readily disseminates to distant sites in dogs.

Clinical examination Of the 26 canine cases reported in the veterinary literature, 20 either had ocular signs on presen-tation or developed them later.[108] Sixteen cases had GI signs, usually colitis-type diarrhea, vomiting, and weight loss. Six cases had neurologic signs in the form of paresis, head tilt, cer-vical pain, circling, and ataxia. *P. zopfii* accounts for most of the cases of canine disseminated prototothecosis.

Diagnosis Contrast radiography or abdominal ultra-sonography may reveal diffuse colonic wall thickening or obstruction, but these are nonspecific findings. Fecal parasito-logic examination is generally of little use in demonstrating the organism, but exfoliative cytology, histology, or both read-ily identifies the organism.[109] Aqueous or vitreous centesis can also be performed in dogs with ocular pathology and is gener-ally useful in documenting organisms in the ocular fluid.

Treatment The management of systemic prototothecosis has been challenging in all animal species. Amphotericin B and itraconazole (5 mg/kg orally, twice a day for 1 month and then 5 mg/kg orally, once a day thereafter) have been used in

several patients. Short-term improvement was reported in only two dogs.

Prognosis Like pythiosis, the prognosis for prototothecosis is grave. The course of the disease is so insidious that, by the time a definitive diagnosis has been reached, the organism has often disseminated throughout the body.

Bacteria
Brachyspira pilosicoli
Cause *Brachyspira* spp., formerly *Serpulina* spp. or *Treponema* spp., are intestinal spirochetes of dogs, pigs, guinea pigs, rodents, nonhuman primates, and humans.[110] In pigs, they cause two important diarrheal syndromes: (1) *B. hyo-dysenteriae* causes swine dysentery and (2) *B. pilosicoli* causes porcine intestinal spirochetosis. The consequences of colo-nization by intestinal spirochetes in animals other than pigs and in humans is controversial. Some investigators believe the bacteria may be responsible for various GI disturbances, whereas others have questioned their clinical importance and claimed that shedding of large numbers of spirochetes in con-nection with diarrhea may be blamed on dislodgment from the crypts by diarrhea induced by other causative agents.

Intestinal spirochetes have been found in both healthy and diarrheal dogs. In a recent study it was suggested that canine intestinal spirochetes consist of *B. pilosicoli* and a group of nonpathogenic spirochetes, provisionally designated *Brachyspira (Serpulina) canis*.[111] Infection with *B. pilosicoli* in the colon of dogs might be subclinical, but massive infection, which may occur in environments with poor hygiene or in dogs with a compromised intestinal function because of concurrent causative factors, may cause diarrhea.[111] *B. pilosicoli* may be associated with diarrhea in colony[112] and pet shop dogs.[113]

Pathophysiology Severity of clinical signs appears to be associated with attachment of spirochetes to the epithelial surface of the colon, persistence of *B. pilosicoli* in the cecal and colonic crypt lumina, chronic inflammation caused by sprio-chetal invasion into the lamina propria, and translocation to extraintestinal sites.[114]

Clinical examination Infected animals have clinical signs consistent with large bowel-type diarrhea.

Diagnosis *Brachyspira* infections can be diagnosed by fecal culture, colonic histopathology, and PCR of fresh fecal samples. *Brachyspira* spp. are most effectively grown on either trypticase soy agar with 5% sheep blood or selective BJ agar at 42° C under anaerobic conditions. PCR amplification of the 16S rRNA gene has been used to further clarify natural infections.[111]

Treatment The best treatments for *Brachyspira* spp. infection have not yet been identified.

Prognosis The prognosis for health and recovery appears to be quite favorable.

Campylobacter
Cause *Campylobacter jejuni*, *C. coli*, *C. upsaliensis*, and *C. helveticus* are commensal organisms found in the GI tract of healthy dogs and cats throughout the world.[115-117] The high prevalence of these organisms in healthy nondiarrheic dogs (*C. jejuni*, 49%; *C. coli*, 5%; *C. upsaliensis*, 19%) and cats (*C. jejuni*, 46%; *C. coli*, 1%; *C. upsaliensis*, 5%; *C. helveticus*, 22%) complicates diagnosis.[118-121] Under certain conditions, however, *Campylobacter* can induce significant GI tract pathol-ogy. Young age, immunoincompetence, concurrent GI infec-tions, prior therapeutic interventions (e.g., antibiotics), and

poor hygienic conditions appear to be the greatest risk factors for the development of infection.[122]

Pathophysiology At some point, *Campylobacter* organisms become enteroinvasive and induce the host inflammatory response. *C. jejuni* localizes in mucus-filled crypts of the intestine and colon where it induces a superficial erosive enterocolitis.[122,123] Colonic epithelial glands undergo hyperplasia and thickening with exfoliation of the brush border and goblet cells. The colonic epithelium becomes cuboidal, crypt height is reduced, and crypt abscess is present. Shallow crypts and blunt irregular villi are features of the ileum response to infection.

Clinical examination Clinical signs are watery diarrhea, often containing mucous and blood pigments, tenesmus, anorexia, fever, and vomiting.[123,124] Concurrent infections with *Salmonella*, *Giardia*, or parvovirus cause more severe disease.

Diagnosis Direct examination of a fresh fecal sample is the method of diagnosis in many instances. Large numbers of curved, highly motile bacteria along with increased numbers of leukocytes is presumptive evidence of *Campylobacter* infection. With Gram staining, large numbers of faintly staining gram-negative, slender, curved (gull wing shaped) rods are evident. Fecal cultures or PCR are the most conclusive ways to determine the presence of *Campylobacter*.[118,120] *C. jejuni* is best cultured microaerophilically at 42 °C for 48 hours on special *Campylobacter* blood agar plates.

Treatment Erythromycin is the treatment of choice, although tetracyclines, aminoglycosides, clindamycin, and quinolones are also effective. Post-treatment cultures should be performed to confirm eradication. Pet owners should be advised on the importance of proper hygiene.

Prognosis The prognosis for recovery and cure are generally excellent unless an underlying immunosuppressive condition has increased the susceptibility to infection.

Clostridium perfringens

Cause *C. perfringens* is a gram-positive, spore-forming, obligate anaerobic rod-shaped bacterium that contributes to the microbial ecology and nutrition of the colon in healthy dogs and cats.[27] Under certain conditions, proliferation and sporulation of *C. perfringens* permits enterotoxin A (or CPE) production which may then induce mucosal damage, fluid secretion and large bowel-type diarrhea. Evidence for and against a role for *C. perfringens* in the pathogenesis of large bowel diarrhea has been put forward. Enterotoxigenic *C. perfringens* has been associated with canine nosocomial diarrhea,[125] hemorrhagic enteritis,[115] and acute and chronic large bowel diarrhea.[126,127] On the other hand, many dogs harbor *C. perfringens* and CPE in the GI tract without developing clinical signs.[116,117,122] Until more definitive evidence is obtained, including the fulfillment of Koch's postulates, *C. perfringens* should probably be considered as a suspected pathogen in large bowel diarrhea.

Pathophysiology The presumed pathogenicity of *C. perfringens* requires an anaerobic environment, sporulation, and enterotoxin production. However, problems exist with this hypothesis: enterotoxin may be demonstrated in the feces without sporulation, and enterotoxin may be found in the feces of healthy dogs. *C. perfringens* isolates are classified as one of five toxigenic types (A to E) based on the production of one or more of four major (α, β, ϵ, ζ) and seven minor (δ, θ, κ, λ, μ, ν, and sialidase) toxins.[128] Although all five types of

C. perfringens are capable of producing CPE, the majority is produced by type A strains. As with enterotoxigenic *E. coli* (ETEC) strains, CPE is believed to induce crypt epithelial cell secretion.

Clinical examination *Clostridium perfringens*-associated colitis is believed to be a major cause of acute, nosocomial, chronic large bowel diarrhea. Acute nosocomial diarrhea often begins within 1 to 5 days of boarding or kenneling. Affected dogs develop diarrhea, often with blood pigments, mucous, and tenesmus. These diarrheas are usually self-limiting and may resolve with supportive care alone. Chronic large bowel diarrheas associated with *C. perfringens* are similar to other large bowel-type diarrheas (i.e., chronic, intermittent, and recurring signs of colitis).

Diagnosis No gold standard exists for the diagnosis of *C. perfringens*–associated diarrhea. Ideally, the diagnosis would be made on the basis of positive test results with Gram staining, fecal culture, ELISA enterotoxin (CPE) assay, PCR enterotoxin (*cpe*) genotyping, and rule-out of other colonic diseases on colonoscopy and biopsy.[129-132] Compared with normal dogs (without diarrhea), diarrheic dogs are more often CPE ELISA and *cpe* PCR positive, but many normal dogs are positive on both assays.

Treatment Recent *in vitro* antimicrobial susceptibility testing suggests that *C. perfringens* should be susceptible to ampicillin, erythromycin, metronidazole, and tylosin.[133] These antibiotics have also been used in vivo with good success. It should be emphasized that many of the same patients respond to supportive care, including intravenous fluids, intestinal protectants, and bland or fiber-supplemented diets.

Prognosis Affected animals usually respond to appropriate therapy within a matter of days. The prognosis for recovery is excellent.

Clostridium difficile

Clostridium difficile is believed to share many ecological factors with *Clostridium perfringens*,[134,135] but the role of this organism as a pathogen in dogs and cats has not been firmly established. Compared with normal dogs (without diarrhea), diarrheic dogs are more often toxin A ELISA positive, even though they may be *toxin A* PCR negative.[132] As with *C. perfringens*, many healthy dogs and cats carry *C. difficile* without developing clinical signs. In one recent study, it was difficult to experimentally infect dogs with this organism, and those that were infected did not develop clinical signs.[136] Antibiotic-associated diarrheas develop in dogs and cats, but they may have a pathogenesis other than *C. difficile*.

Escherichia coli

Cause Most strains of *E. coli* are true commensal organisms that are not associated with clinical signs. Strains of *E. coli* that cause diarrhea in animals can be grouped into five main categories: (1) enterotoxigenic (ETEC), (2) enteroinvasive (EIEC), (3) enteropathogenic (EPEC), (4) enterohemorrhagic (EHEC), and (5) enteroadherent (EAEC) organisms.[137] Identification of pathogenic strains requires modern molecular technology such as bioassays, DNA hybridization, and PCR amplification.

Pathophysiology Infection may result in enteritis, colitis, or both.[138] Enterotoxigenic (ETEC) strains adhere to the surface of epithelial cells and produce toxins that are heat labile, heat stable, or both, and that induce crypt epithelial cell secretion. EIEC strains of *E. coli* invade, replicate in, and destroy epithelial cells. EPEC strains are neither enterotoxigenic nor enteroinvasive, but they do attach to and efface the brush border of the enterocytes. EHEC strains produce verocytotoxins that induce hemorrhagic ileitis and colitis. EAEC strains of *E. coli* also induce enterocyte pathology, but their mechanism of action is poorly understood. Enterotoxigenic, enteropathogenic, and enterohemorrhagic *E. coli* have all been isolated from dogs and cats with diarrhea. *E. coli* endotoxin colonic absorption of water and sodium and contributes to the diarrhea seen during and after episodes of sepsis.[139]

Clinical examination Affected animals typically have diarrhea and hematochezia with clinical signs relevant to the small intestine, colon, or both.

Diagnosis *E. coli* can be grown from the feces of healthy dogs and cats, so a positive culture does not necessarily reveal the identity of an underlying pathogen. In addition to positive culture, diagnosis may require enterotoxin assays and DNA hybridization and PCR amplification.[140-144]

Treatment Antibiotics should be used only in those cases in which firm evidence of bacterial infection exists. Fluoroquinolones appear to be a very effective classification for the treatment of enteric *E. coli* infections.

Prognosis The prognosis is generally good for recovery and cure if infection is recognized early in the clinical course.

Salmonella

Cause *Salmonella* spp. are predominantly motile, gram-negative facultative anaerobic rod-shaped bacteria found in the feces of normal and diarrheic animals.[116-117] As with many other commensal organisms of the GI tract, the high prevalence of these organisms complicates diagnosis. From 1% to 30% of the fecal samples or rectal swabs taken from healthy domestic pet dogs, 16.7% of dogs boarded in kennels, and 21.5% of hospitalized dogs were found to be positive on bacteriologic culture for *Salmonella*. From 1% to 18% of healthy cats and 10.6% of random source research colony cats are also culture-positive for *Salmonella* (summarized in reference 122). Despite these findings, several species of *Salmonella* have been impugned in the pathogenesis of acute enterocolitis in dogs and cats. *S. typhimurium* is the species most commonly isolated from diarrheic feces of dogs and cats, although other species have been identified.[145-147]

Pathophysiology Those most at risk for *Salmonella* infection are young and immunoincompetent animals, those with concurrent GI infections (e.g., parvoviral or parasitic infections), and those animals who have had prior therapeutic interventions (e.g., antibiotics or glucocorticoids).[122] *Salmonella* is an enteroinvasive organism that induces an acute inflammatory response resulting in enterocolitis, mucosal sloughing, and secretory diarrhea. Most *Salmonella* infections are resolved via the local immune response, but bacterial translocation and septicemia may evolve into SIRS and multiple organ dysfunction syndromes (MODS) in some patients. Early recognition is important in preventing this sequela.

Clinical examination The main clinical signs of *Salmonella* enterocolitis are anorexia, lethargy, fever, vomiting, diarrhea with mucous and blood pigments, dehydration, abdominal pain, and tenesmus. With bacterial translocation and septicemia, affected animals may have evidence of pale mucous membranes, weakness, tachycardia, tachypnea, and vascular collapse.

Diagnosis Culture, serotyping, and PCR are the best methods of diagnosing *Salmonella* infections.[145]

Treatment Treatment varies according to the severity of the clinical signs. Mild, self-limiting forms of enterocolitis may in fact resolve with little more than supportive therapy. Antibiotic therapy in such cases may prolong fecal shedding and encourage development of the carrier state. In animals with severe hemorrhagic diarrhea, history of immunosuppression, suspected or documented septicemia, evidence of SIRS, or a combination of these symptoms, parenteral antibiotics should definitely be used. If culture results are unavailable, therapy should include enrofloxacin, amoxicillin, or trimethoprim-sulfa, all of which are effective against *Salmonella*. Posttreatment cultures should be performed to confirm eradication, and pet owners should be advised of the public health importance of the disease.

Prognosis The prognosis for recovery in nonsepticemic patients is generally good, although some animals may remain chronic carriers with recrudescence during periods of stress or unrelated disease. The prognosis for the septicemic patient is more guarded.

Yersinia enterocolitica *Y. enterocolitica* is a commensal organism of the GI tract of some dogs and cats that may be a rare cause of acute colitis.[148] It is a motile, gram-negative facultative anaerobic coccobacillus bacterium that may be transmitted to animals via ingestion of raw pork[149] or contaminated water. If suspected, animals should be treated with cephalosporins or trimethoprim-sulfa. The prognosis is unknown because of the paucity of case reports.

INFLAMMATION

Inflammatory Bowel Disease

Cause IBD may be defined using clinical, histologic, immunologic, pathophysiologic, and genetic criteria.

Clinical criteria IBD has been defined clinically as a spectrum of GI disorders of an unknown cause that is associated with chronic inflammation of the stomach, intestine, or colon.[40] A clinical diagnosis of IBD is considered only if affected animals have: (1) persistent (> 3 weeks in duration) GI signs (anorexia, vomiting, weight loss, diarrhea, hematochezia, mucosy feces), (2) failure to respond to symptomatic therapies (parasiticides, antibiotics, GI protectants) alone, (3) failure to document other causes of gastroenterocolitis by thorough diagnostic evaluation, and (4) histologic diagnosis of benign intestinal inflammation.[50] Small bowel and large bowel forms of IBD have been reported in both dogs and cats, although large bowel IBD appears to be more prevalent in the dog.

Histologic criteria IBD has been defined histologically by the type of inflammatory infiltrate (neutrophilic, eosinophilic, lymphocytic, plasmacytic, granulomatous), associated mucosal pathology (villus atrophy, fusion, crypt collapse), distribution of the lesion (focal or generalized, superficial or deep), severity (mild, moderate, severe), mucosal thickness (mild, moderate, severe), and topography (gastric fundus, gastric antrum, duodenum, jejunum, ileum, cecum, ascending colon, descending colon).[11] Typical histologic changes associated with IBD are shown in Figure 223-7. As with small intestinal IBD, subjective interpretation of large intestinal IBD lesions has made it difficult to compare tissue findings between pathologists. Subjectivity in histologic assessments has led to the development of several IBD grading systems.*

---

*References 3, 11, 13, 36, 37, 38, 150, 151.

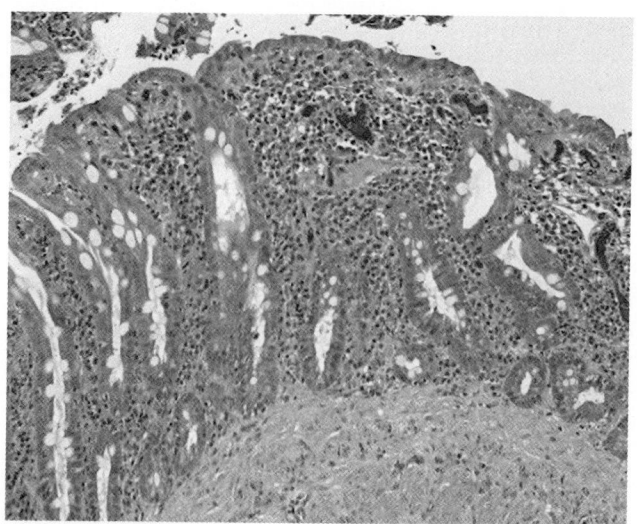

Figure 223—7 Histologic appearance of inflammatory bowel disease (IBD) of the canine colon. Crypts are separated from adjacent crypts by edema, fibrosis, and inflammatory cells. Increased numbers of lymphocytes are present in the lamina propria, and reduced goblet cells are present in the epithelium. (Photomicrograph courtesy of Dr. Mattie Hendrick, University of Pennsylvania.)

Immunologic criteria IBD has been defined immunologically by the innate and adaptive response of the mucosa to GI antigens. Although the precise immunologic events of canine and feline IBD remain to be determined, a prevailing hypothesis for the development of IBD is the loss of immunologic tolerance to the normal bacterial flora or food antigens, leading to abnormal T cell immune reactivity in the gut microenvironment.[152] Genetically engineered animal models (e.g., IL-2, IL-10, T cell receptor knockouts) that develop IBD involve alterations in T cell development, function, or both, suggesting that T cell populations are responsible for the homeostatic regulation of mucosal immune responses.[153] Immunohistochemical studies of canine IBD have demonstrated an increase in the T cell population of the lamina propria, including CD3+ cells and CD4+ cells, macrophages, neutrophils, and IgA-containing plasma cells. Many of the immunologic features of canine IBD can be explained as an indirect consequence of mucosal T cell activation. Enterocytes are also likely involved in the immunopathogenesis of IBD. Enterocytes are capable of behaving as antigen-presenting cells, and interleukins (e.g., IL-7, IL-15) produced by enterocytes during acute inflammation activate mucosal lymphocytes. Up-regulation of Toll-like receptor 4 (TLR4) and Toll-like receptor 2 (TLR2) expression contribute to the innate immune response of the colon.[154] Thus the pathogenesis and pathophysiology of IBD appears to involve the activation of a subset of CD4+ T cells within the intestinal epithelium that overproduce inflammatory cytokines with concomitant loss of a subset of CD4+ T cells and their associated cytokines, which normally regulate the inflammatory response and protect the gut from injury. Enterocytes, behaving as antigen-presenting cells, contribute to the pathogenesis of this disease.[155]

Pathophysiologic criteria IBD may be defined pathophysiologically in terms of changes in transport, blood flow, and motility. The clinical signs of IBD, whether small or large bowel, have long been attributed to the pathophysiology of malabsorption and hypersecretion, but experimental models of canine IBD have instead related clinical signs to the emergence of abnormality motility patterns.

Genetic criteria IBD may be defined by genetic criteria in several animal species. Crohn's disease and ulcerative colitis are more common in certain human genotypes, and a mutation in the NOD2 gene (nucleotide-binding oligomerization domain2) has been found in a subgroup of patients with Crohn's disease.[155] Genetic influences have not yet been identified in canine or feline IBD, but certain breeds (e.g., German shepherds, boxers) appear to be at increased risk for the disease.

Pathophysiology The pathophysiology of large intestinal IBD is explained by at least two interdependent mechanisms: (1) the mucosal immune response and (2) accompanying changes in motility.

Immune responses A generic inflammatory response involving cellular elements (B and T lymphocytes, plasma cells, macrophages, and dendritic cells), secretomotor neurons (e.g., vasoactive intestinal polypeptide, substance P, cholinergic neurons), cytokines and interleukins, and inflammatory mediators (e.g., leukotrienes, prostanoids, reactive oxygen metabolites, nitric oxide [NO], 5-HT, IFN-γ, TNF-α, platelet-activating factor) is typical of canine and feline IBD.[156,157] Many similarities exist between the inflammatory response of the small and large intestine, but recent immunologic studies suggest that IBD of the canine small intestine is a mixed Th1 and Th2 response,[40,158,159] whereas IBD of the canine colon may be more of a Th1 type response with elaboration of IL-2, IL-12, INF-γ, and TNF-α[160] (Figure 223-8). Other studies of canine colonic IBD have demonstrated increased numbers of mucosal IgA- and IgG-containing cells,[36,161-163] nitrate,[162] CD3+ T cells, NO,[164] and inducible nitric oxide synthase (iNOS)[164] in the inflamed colonic mucosa (Table 223-5). Increases in the CD3+ positive T cell population of the inflamed colon are consistent with changes reported in the inflamed canine intestine. Thus important similarities exist, as do differences between small (Chapter 222) and large bowel IBD.

Motility changes Experimental studies of canine large intestinal IBD have shown that many of the clinical signs (diarrhea, passage of mucus and blood, abdominal pain, tenesmus, and urgency of defecation) are related to motor abnormalities

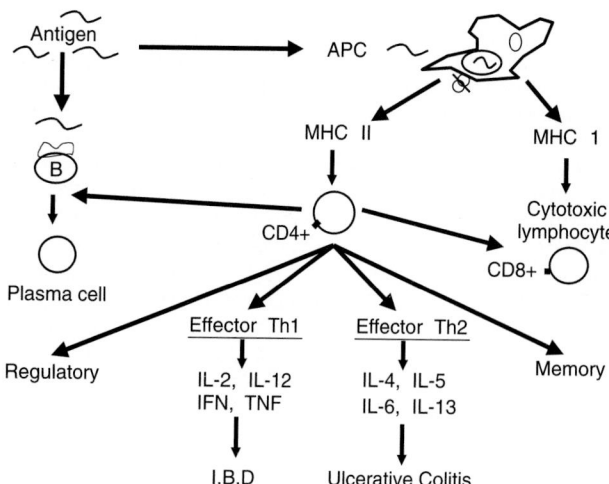

Figure 223-8 Immunopathology of canine large bowel inflammatory bowel disease (IBD) and canine ulcerative colitis. IBD of the canine colon may be more of a Th1-type response, whereas ulcerative colitis is more a Th2-type response. *MHC,* Major histocompatibility complex; *APC,* antigen-presenting cell; *IL,* interleukin; *IFN,* interferon; *TNF,* tumor necrosis factor.

Table • 223-5

Immunologic and Motility Abnormalities in Canine Large Bowel Inflammatory Bowel Disease

HISTOLOGIC FINDINGS	IMMUNOLOGIC ABNORMALITIES	REFERENCE
Lymphocytic-plasmacytic colitis	Increased nitric oxide and IgG in colonic lavage fluid	162
Lymphocytic-plasmacytic colitis	Increased expression of inducible nitric oxide synthase mRNA	164
Lymphocytic-plasmacytic colitis	Increases in T cells and B cells in lamina propria	36
Lymphocytic-plasmacytic colitis	Increases in CD3+ T cells and in IgA+ and IgG+ plasma cells	163
Lymphocytic-plasmacytic colitis	Increased IL-2 and TNF-α mRNA expression	160

TISSUE/CELL TYPE	MOTILITY ABNORMALITIES	REFERENCE
Colon	Loss of spontaneous phasic contractions	165,166
	Decreased frequency of migrating motor complexes (MMCs)	165,166
	Increased frequency of giant migrating contractions (GMCs)	165,166
Colonic circular smooth muscle cells	Decreased amplitude and duration of the slow wave plateau potential	167
	Shift from the M_3 to M_2 muscarinic receptor subtype	169
	Reduced calcium influx through L-type calcium channel	170
	Reduced L-type calcium channel expression	171
	Decreased open probability of K_{Ca} channels	172
	Down-regulation of PKC α, β, ε, expression and activation	174
	Reduced phospholipase A_2 expression	173
	Increased NF-κB expression and activation	175
Colonic enteric neurons	Sensitization to substance P during colonic inflammation	168
Colonic interstitial cells of Cajal	Reduced density of interstitial cells	167
	Cytoplasmic vacuolation and damage to cellular processes	167

IgG, Immunoglobulin G; *IgA*, immunoglobulin A; *IL-2*, interleukin-2; *TNF-α*, tumor necrosis factor alpha; *PKC*, protein kinase C; *M*, muscarinic; *NF-κB*, nuclear factor-κB; K_{Ca}, calcium-activated potassium channel.

of the colon. Ethanol and acetic acid perfusion of the canine colon induces a large bowel form of IBD syndrome indistinguishable from the natural condition.[165,166] Inflammation in this model suppresses the normal phasic contractions of the colon, including the migrating motility complex, and triggers the emergence of GMCs. The appearance of these GMCs in association with inflammation is a major factor in producing diarrhea, abdominal cramping, and urgency of defecation. GMCs are powerful lumen-occluding contractions that rapidly propel pancreatic, biliary, and intestinal secretions in the fasting state (and undigested food in the fed state) to the colon to increase its osmotic load.[43,45,46] Malabsorption results from direct injury to the epithelial cells and from ultrarapid propulsion of intestinal contents by GMCs so that sufficient mucosal contact time is not allowed for digestion and absorption to take place.

Inflammation impairs the regulation of the colonic motility patterns at several levels (i.e., enteric neurons, interstitial cells of Cajal, circular smooth muscle cells; summarized in Table 223-5). Inflammation-induced changes in the amplitude and duration of the smooth muscle slow wave plateau potentials contribute to the suppression of RPCs.[165] These alterations likely have their origin in structural and functional damage to the interstitial cells of Cajal.[167] At the same time that inflammation suppresses the RPCs, inflammation sensitizes the colon to the stimulation of GMCs by the neurotransmitter substance P.[168] These findings suggest that SP increases the frequency of GMCs during inflammation and that selective inhibition of GMCs during inflammation may minimize the symptoms of diarrhea, abdominal discomfort, and urgency of defecation associated with these contractions.[168]

Inflammation suppresses the generation of tone and phasic contractions in the circular smooth muscle cells through multiple molecular mechanisms (see Table 223-5; Figure 223-9). Inflammation shifts muscarinic receptor expression in circular smooth muscles from the M_3 to the M_2 subtype.[169] This shift has the effect of reducing the overall contractility of the smooth muscle cell. Inflammation also impairs calcium influx[170] and down-regulates the expression of the L-type calcium channel,[171] which may be important in suppressing phasic contractions and tone while concurrently stimulating GMCs in the inflamed colon. Changes in the open-state probability of the large conductance calcium-activated potassium channels (K_{Ca}) partially attenuate this effect.[172] Inflammation also modifies the signal transduction pathways of circular smooth muscle cells. Phospholipase A_2 and protein kinase C (PKC) expression and activation are significantly altered by colonic inflammation,[173,174] and this may partially account for the suppression of tone and phasic contractions. PKC α, β, and ε isoenzyme expression is down-regulated, PKC ι and λ isoenzyme expression is up-regulated, and the cytosol-to-membrane translocation of PKC is impaired.[174] The L-type calcium channel, already reduced in its expression, is one of the molecular targets of PKC. Inflammation also activates the transcription factor NF-κB that further suppresses cell contractility.[175]

Clinical Examination The clinical signs of large intestinal IBD are those of a large bowel-type diarrhea (i.e., marked increased frequency, reduced fecal volume per defecation, blood pigments and mucous in feces, and tenesmus). Anorexia, weight loss, and vomiting are occasionally reported in animals with severe IBD of the colon or concurrent IBD of the stomach, small intestine, or both. Clinical signs usually wax and wane in their severity. A transient response to symptomatic therapy may occur during the initial stages of IBD. As the condition progresses, diarrhea gradually increases in its frequency and intensity and may become continuous. In some cases the first bowel movement of the day may be normal or nearly normal, whereas successive bowel movements are reduced in volume and progressively more urgent and painful.

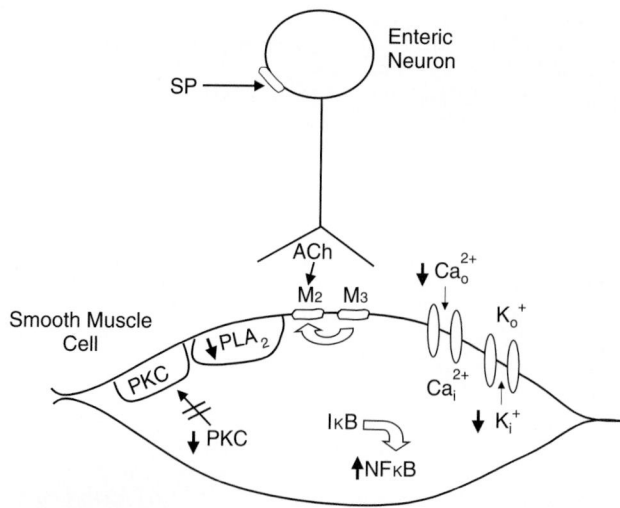

Figure 223-9 Motility abnormalities in canine large bowel inflammatory bowel disease (IBD). Inflammation impairs motility by inducing changes in receptor, signal transduction, and ion channel activity in smooth muscle cells and enteric neurons. Changes include but not are limited to a shift in muscarinic receptor expression from M_3 to M_2 receptor subtype; impaired calcium mobilization; down-regulation of L-type calcium channel expression; changes in the open-state probability of the large conductance calcium-activated potassium channels (K_{Ca}), down-regulation of phospholipase A_2 and protein kinase C (PKC) α, β, and ε isoenzymes; and activation of the transcription factor NF-κB in smooth muscle cells. Inflammation also sensitizes the colon to the stimulation of GMCs by the neurotransmitter substance P. *PKC*, Protein kinase C; *PLA₂*, phospholipase A_2; *M*, muscarinic; *NF-κB*, nuclear factor-κB; K_{Ca}, calcium-activated potassium channel; *SP*, substance P; *Ach*, acetylcholine.

During severe episodes, mild fever, depression, and anorexia may occur.

There does not appear to be any sex predilection, but age may be a risk factor, with IBD appearing more frequently in middle-aged animals (mean age approximately 6 years with a range of 6 months to 20 years).[50,51] German shepherd and boxer dogs are at increased risk for IBD, and pure-breed cats appear to be at greater risk. Cats more often have an upper GI form of IBD, whereas dogs are at risk for both small and large bowel IBD.

Physical examination is unremarkable in most cases. Thickened bowel loops may be detected during abdominal palpation if the small bowel is concurrently involved. Digital examination of the anorectum may evoke pain or reveal irregular mucosa, and blood pigments and mucous may be evident on the examination glove.

Diagnosis CBCs, serum chemistries, and urinalyses are often normal in mild cases of large bowel IBD. Chronic cases may have one or more subtle abnormalities. One review of canine and feline IBD reported several hematologic abnormalities including mild anemia, leukocytosis, neutrophilia with and without a left shift, eosinophilia, eosinopenia, lymphocytopenia, monocytosis, and basophilia.[51] The same study reported several biochemical abnormalities including increased activities of serum alanine aminotransferase and alkaline phosphatase, hypoalbuminemia, hypoproteinemia, hyperamylasemia, hyperglobulinemia, hypokalemia, hypocholesterolemia, and hyperglycemia. No consistent abnormality in the CBC or serum chemistry has been identified.

A scoring index for disease activity in canine IBD was recently developed that relates severity of clinical signs to serum acute-phase protein (C-reactive protein [CRP], serum amyloid A) concentrations.[50] The canine IBD activity index (CIBDAI) assigns levels of severity to each of several gastroenterologic signs (e.g., anorexia, vomiting, weight loss, diarrhea), and it appears to be a reliable index of mucosal inflammation in canine IBD. Interestingly, both the activity index and serum concentrations of CRP improve with successful treatment, suggesting that serum CRP is suitable for the laboratory evaluation of therapy in canine IBD.[50] Other acute-phase proteins were less specific than CRP. One important caveat that should be emphasized is that altered CRP is not *prima facie* evidence of GI inflammation. Concurrent infections or other inflammatory conditions could cause an acute-phase response, including CRP, in affected patients.

Treatment

Dietary therapy The precise immunologic mechanisms of canine and feline IBD have not yet been determined, but a prevailing hypothesis for the development of IBD is the loss of immunologic tolerance to the normal bacterial flora or food antigens. Accordingly, dietary modification may prove useful in the management of canine and feline IBD.[176,177] Several nutritional strategies have been proposed including novel proteins, hydrolyzed diets, antioxidant diets, medium chain triglyceride supplementation, low-fat diets, modifications in the omega-6 (ω-6) and omega-3 (ω-3) fatty acid ratio, and fiber supplementation. Of these strategies, some evidence-based medicine has emerged for the use of novel protein, hydrolyzed, and fiber-supplemented diets.

Food sensitivity reactions were suspected or documented in 49% of cats presented because of gastroenterologic problems (with or without concurrent dermatologic problems) in a prospective study of adverse food reactions in cats.[178] Beef, wheat, and corn gluten were the primary ingredients responsible for food sensitivity reactions in that study, and most of the cats responded to the feeding of a chicken- or venison-based selected protein diet for a minimum of 4 weeks. The authors concluded that adverse reactions to dietary staples are common in cats with chronic GI problems and that they can be successfully managed by feeding selected protein diets. Further support for this concept comes from studies in which gastroenterologic[179-181] or dermatologic[182] clinical signs were significantly improved by the feeding of novel proteins.

Evidence is accruing that hydrolyzed diets may be useful in the nutritional management of canine IBD. The conceptual basis of the hydrolyzed diet is that oligopeptides are of insufficient size and structure to induce antigen recognition or presentation.[183,184] In one preliminary study, dogs with IBD showed significant improvement after the feeding of a hydrolyzed diet, although they had failed to respond to the feeding of a novel protein.[183] Clinical improvement could not be solely attributed to the hydrolyzed nature of the protein source because the test diet had other modified features (i.e., high digestibility, cornstarch rather than intact grains, medium-chain triglycerides, an altered ratio of ω-6 to ω-3 polyunsaturated fatty acids). Additional studies will be required to ascertain the efficacy of this nutritional strategy in the management of IBD.

Fiber-supplemented diets may be useful in the management of irritable bowel syndrome (IBS) in the dog. IBS is a poorly defined syndrome in the dog that may or may not bear resemblance to IBS in humans. Canine IBS has been defined as a chronic large bowel-type diarrhea without known cause and without evidence of colonic inflammation on colonoscopy or biopsy.[185] Dogs fulfilling these criteria were successfully managed with soluble fiber (psyllium hydrophilic mucilloid) supplementation of a highly digestible diet.[185]

Exercise   Experimental IBD in the dog is accompanied by significant abnormalities in the normal colonic motility patterns. Physical exercise has been shown to disrupt the colonic MMCs and to increase the total duration of contractions that are organized as nonmigrating motor complexes during the fed state.[186] Exercise also induces GMCs, defecation, and mass movement in both the fasted and fed states. The increased motor activity of the colon and extra GMCs that result from physical exercise may aid in normal colonic motor function.[186]

Pharmacologic therapy   Animals with mild to moderate forms of large bowel IBD generally respond favorably to dietary modification alone, but pharmacologic therapy will be required with more severe forms of large bowel IBD. Medical therapy includes *anti-inflammatory* (sulfasalazine and other 5-aminosalicylates, metronidazole, prednisone, budesonide), *immunosuppressive* (azathioprine, cyclosporine, chlorambucil), and *motility-modifying* (loperamide) drugs (Table 223-6).

Sulfasalazine   Sulfasalazine is a highly effective prostaglandin synthetase inhibitor that has proven efficacy in the therapy of large bowel IBD in the dog. Sulfasalazine is a compound molecule of 5-aminosalicylate (meselamine) and sulfapyridine linked in an azochemical bond. After oral dosing, most of the sulfasalazine is transported to the distal GI tract where cecal and colonic bacteria metabolize the drug to its component parts. Sulfapyridine is largely absorbed by the colonic mucosa but much of the 5-aminosalicylate remains in the colonic lumen where it inhibits mucosal cyclooxygenase and the inflammatory cascade. Sulfasalazine has been recommended for the treatment of canine large bowel IBD at doses of 10 to 25 mg/kg orally, three times a day for 4 to 6 weeks. With resolution of clinical signs, sulfasalazine doses are gradually decreased by 25% at 2-week intervals and eventually discontinued while maintaining dietary management.[187] Salicylates are readily absorbed[188] and induce toxicity in cats; therefore this drug classification should be used with great caution in cats. If used in cats, some authors have recommended using half of the recommended dog dose (i.e., 5 to 12.5 mg/kg orally, three times a day).[187] Sulfasalazine use has been associated with the development of keratoconjunctivitis sicca in the dog,[189,190] so tear production should be assessed subjectively (by the pet owner) and objectively (by the veterinarian) during use.

Other 5-aminosalicylates   This drug classification was developed to reduce the toxicity of the sulfapyridine portion of the parent molecule (sulfasalazine) and to enhance the efficacy of the 5-aminosalicylate portion. Meselamine (Dipentum, Asachol) and dimeselamine (olsalazine) are available for use in the treatment of canine large bowel IBD. Olsalazine has been used at a dose of 5 to 10 mg/kg orally, three times a day in the dog. Despite the formulation of sulfa-free 5-aminosalicylate preparations, instances of keratoconjunctivitis sicca have still been reported in the dog.[189,190]

Metronidazole   Metronidazole (10 to 20 mg/kg orally, twice a day to three times a day) has been used in the treatment of mild to moderate cases of large bowel IBD in both dogs and cats. Metronidazole has been used either as a single agent or in conjunction with 5-aminosalicylates or glucocorticoids. Metronidazole is believed to have several beneficial properties, including antibacterial, antiprotozoal, and immunomodulatory effects.[191] Side effects include anorexia, hypersalivation, and vomiting at recommended doses and neurotoxicity (ataxia, nystagmus, head title, and seizures) at higher doses.[192] Side effects usually resolve with discontinuation of therapy, but diazepam may accelerate recovery of individual patients.[193]

Glucocorticoids   Anti-inflammatory doses of prednisone or prednisolone (1 to 2 mg/kg orally, once a day) may be used to treat IBD in dogs that have failed to respond to dietary management, sulfasalazine, or metronidazole, and as adjunctive therapy to dietary modification in feline IBD. Prednisone or prednisolone are used most frequently, because both have short durations of action, are cost-effective, and are widely available. Equipotent doses of dexamethasone are equally effective but may have more deleterious effects on brush border enzyme activity. Prednisone should be used for 2 to 4 weeks depending upon the severity of the clinical signs. Higher doses of prednisone (e.g., 2 to 4 mg/kg orally, once a day) may be needed to control severe forms of eosinophilic colitis or hypereosinophilic syndrome in cats.

Combination therapy with sulfasalazine, metronidazole, or azathioprine may reduce the overall dose of prednisone needed to achieve remission of clinical signs. As with sulfasalazine, the dose of glucocorticoid may be reduced by 25% at 1- to 2-week intervals while (it is hoped) maintaining remission with dietary modification.

Because of steroid side effects and suppression of the hypothalamic-pituitary-adrenal axis, several alternative glucocorticoids have been developed that have excellent topical (i.e., mucosal) anti-inflammatory activity but are significantly metabolized during first pass hepatic metabolism. Budesonide has been used for many years as an inhaled medication for asthma, and an enteric-coated form of the drug is now available for treatment of IBD in humans (and animals). Little clinical evidence supports of the use of this medication in canine or feline IBD, but doses of 1 mg/cat or 1 mg/dog per day have been used with some success in anecdotal cases.

Azathioprine   Azathioprine is a purine analog that, after DNA incorporation, inhibits lymphocyte activation and proliferation. It is rarely effective as a single agent and should instead be used as adjunctive therapy with glucocorticoids. Azathioprine may have a significant steroid-sparing effect in IBD. Doses of 2 mg/kg orally, every 24 hours in dogs and 0.3 mg/kg orally every 48 hours in cats have been used with some success in IBD. It may take several weeks or months of therapy for azathioprine to become maximally effective. Cats particularly should be monitored for side effects, including myelosuppression, hepatic disease, and acute pancreatic necrosis.

Cyclosporine   Cyclosporine has been used in the renal transplantation patient for its inhibitory effect on T cell function. In more recent times, cyclosporine has been used in a number of immune-mediated disorders, including keratoconjunctivitis sicca, perianal fistula (anal furunculosis), and IMHA. Evidence-based medicine studies will be needed to establish efficacy, but anecdotal experience would suggest that cyclosporine (3 to 7 mg/kg orally, twice a day) may be useful in some of the more difficult or refractory cases of IBD.

Chlorambucil   Chlorambucil (2 mg/m² orally, every other day) has been used in place of azathioprine in some difficult or refractory cases of feline IBD.

Motility-modifying drugs   The mixed μ,δ-opioid agonist, loperamide, stimulates colonic fluid and electrolyte absorption while inhibiting colonic propulsive motility.[194-197] Loperamide (0.08 mg/kg orally, three times a day to four times a day) may be beneficial in the treatment of difficult or refractory cases of large bowel-type IBD.

Probiotic therapy   Probiotics (see Table 223-6) are living organisms with low or no pathogenicity that exert beneficial effects (e.g., stimulation of innate and acquired immunity) on

Table • 223-6

Drug Index—Large Bowel Diarrhea

DRUG CLASSIFICATION AND EXAMPLES	DOSE	INDICATION
Anthelmintic Drugs		
Albendazole	25 mg/kg PO SID x 2 days	Giardia infection
Febantel	10 mg/kg PO SID x 3 days—adult dogs	Trichuris infection
	15 mg/kg PO SID x 3 days—puppies	Trichuris infection
Fenbendazole	50 mg/kg PO SID x 3 days	Trichuris, Ancylostoma, Giardia infection
Ivermectin	200 µg/kg SQ once	Larvicidal for T. canis
Mebendazole	22 mg/kg PO SID x 3 days	Trichuris infection
Metronidazole	25 mg/kg PO BID x 5 days	Giardia infection
Milbemycin oxime	0.5 mg/kg PO once per month	Trichuris preventive
Praziquantel	44 mg/kg PO once	Heterobilharzia
Pyrantel pamoate	5 mg/kg PO dog, 20 mg/kg cat	Ancylostoma, Toxocara
Antibiotics		
Ampicillin	22 mg/kg PO IV TID	Salmonella, E. coli, Clostridium perfringens
Cefadroxil	22 mg/kg PO BID	Salmonella, E. coli
Chloramphenicol	44 mg/kg PO TID—dogs	Campylobacter
	11 mg/kg PO BID—cats	Campylobacter
Enrofloxacin	5 mg/kg PO IM SQ BID	Salmonella, E. coli
Erythromycin	15-20 mg/kg PO TID	Campylobacter, C. perfringens
Metronidazole	10-20 mg/kg PO BID-TID	C. perfringens
Orbifloxacin	2.5-7.5 mg/kg PO SID	Salmonella, E. coli
Trimethoprim sulfonamide	30 mg/kg PO IM SQ BID	Salmonella
Tylosin	40-80 mg/kg PO SID	IBD, C. perfringens
Antifungal Drugs		
Amphotericin B	2-3 mg/kg IV QOD administered to a cumulative dose of 24-27 mg/kg	Histoplasmosis, pythiosis, protothecosis
Itraconazole	5 mg/kg PO BID for several months	Histoplasmosis, pythiosis, protothecosis
Ketoconazole	10-15 mg/kg PO BID several months	Histoplasmosis, pythiosis, protothecosis
Anti-Inflammatory Drugs		
Budesonide	1 mg/cat or 1 mg/dog PO SID	IBD
Meselamine	10 mg/kg PO TID	IBD
Metronidazole	10-20 mg/kg PO BID-TID for 4-6 weeks	IBD
Olsalazine	5-10 mg/kg PO TID for 4-6 weeks	IBD
Prednisolone	4.0-6.0 mg/kg PO SID for 4-6 weeks	Feline eosinophilic colitis
Prednisone	1.0-2.0 mg/kg PO SID for 4-6 weeks	IBD
Sulfasalazine	10-25 mg/kg PO TID for 4-6 weeks—dogs	IBD, ulcerative colitis
	5-12.5 mg/kg PO TID for 2-4 weeks—cats	Refractory IBD
Immunosuppressive Drugs		
Azathioprine	2 mg/kg PO SID for 4-6 weeks—dogs	IBD
Chlorambucil	2 mg/m² PO every other day for 4-6 weeks	IBD
Cyclosporine	3-7 mg/kg PO BID for 4-6 weeks	IBD
Motility-Modifying Drugs		
Loperamide	0.08 mg/kg PO TID-QID	IBD, IBS
Propantheline	0.25 mg/kg PO BID-TID	IBS
Aminopentamide	0.01-0.03 mg/kg PO BID-TID	IBS
Probiotics		
Enterococcus faecium (SF68)	5×10^8 colony-forming units/day	IBD
Lactobacillus rhamnosus GG	1×10^9 to 5×10^{11} colony-forming units/day	IBD

PO, per os; SID, once per day; IV, intravenous; TID, three times per day; BID, twice per day; QOD, every other day.

the health of the host. The gram-positive commensal lactic acid bacteria (e.g., Lactobacilli) have many beneficial health effects, including enhanced lymphocyte proliferation, innate and acquired immunity, and anti-inflammatory cytokine production.

Lactobacillus rhamnosus GG, a bacterium used in the production of yogurt, is effective in preventing and treating diarrhea, recurrent Clostridia difficile infection, primary rotavirus infection, and atopic dermatitis in humans.[198]

Lactobacillus rhamnosus GG and *Lactobacillus acidophilus* (strain DSM13241) have been safely colonized in the canine GI tract, although probiotic effects in the canine intestine have not been firmly established.[199a,199b] The probiotic organism, *Enterococcus faecium* (SF68), has been safely colonized in the canine GI tract, and it has been shown to increase fecal IgA content and circulating mature B (CD21+/MHC class II+) cells in young puppies. It has been suggested that this probiotic may be useful in the prevention or treatment of canine GI disease.[200] This organism may, however, enhance *Campylobacter jejuni* adhesion and colonization of the dog intestine, perhaps conferring carrier status on colonized dogs.[201]

Two recent studies have shown that many commercial veterinary probiotic preparations are not accurately represented by label claims. Quality control appears to be deficient for many of these formulations.[202,203] Until these products are more tightly regulated, veterinarians should probably view product claims with some skepticism.

Behavioral modification IBD and IBS very likely have underlying behavioral components. Abnormal personality traits and potential environmental stress factors were identified in 38% of dogs in one study.[185] Multiple factors were present in affected households, including travel, relocation, house construction, separation anxiety, submissive urination, noise sensitivity, and aggression.[185] The role of behavior in the pathogenesis and therapy of canine and feline GI disorders remains largely unexplored.

Prognosis Most reports indicate that the short-term prognosis for control of IBD is good to excellent. After completion of drug therapy, many animals are able to maintain remission of signs with dietary management alone. Treatment failures are uncommon and are usually due to (1) incorrect diagnosis (it is especially important to rule out alimentary lymphosarcoma), (2) presence of severe disease such as histiocytic ulcerative colitis and PLE or irreversible mucosa lesions such as fibrosis, (3) poor client compliance with appropriate drug and dietary recommendations, (4) use of inappropriate drugs or nutritional therapy, and (5) presence of concurrent disease such as small intestinal bacterial overgrowth or hepatobiliary disease.[187] The prognosis for cure of IBD is poor, and relapses should be anticipated.

Histiocytic Ulcerative Colitis

Cause Histiocytic ulcerative colitis is a rare disorder of the dog that has been reported sporadically since 1965.[204-209] Most cases have been reported in the boxer breed, although recent reports have included the French bulldog, mastiff, Alaskan Malamute, and Doberman pinscher breeds. The disease typically affects the young boxer, with the majority (78%) developing clinical signs before 2 years of age. Males and females appear to be equally affected. The pathogenesis of this disorder is incompletely understood, but a bacterial pathogenesis has recently been proposed.[209a] As with Whipple's disease in humans and Johne's disease in cattle, the presence of periodic acid-Schiff (PAS)-positive macrophages and intralesional bacteria have suggested a number of infectious agents such as mycobacteria, rickettsiae, chlamydiae, and mycoplasmae.[208] Vascular abnormalities of the colonic mucosa and intrinsic abnormalities of the PAS+ histiocytes have also been implicated in the pathogenesis of this syndrome.

Pathophysiology Histiocytic ulcerative colitis lesions are characterized by increased numbers of IgG+, IgG3+, and IgG4+ plasma cells, CD3+ T cells, MHC class II+ cells, L1+ cells, and PAS+ cells in the lamina propria, and decreased goblet cell numbers in the epithelium (see Figure 223-8).[208] Canine histiocytic ulcerative colitis appears to be more typical of a Th2-type response (similar to human ulcerative colitis), whereas canine large intestinal IBD appears to be more of a Th1-type response.[160]

Clinical Examination Affected animals have classic signs of large bowel disease (e.g., mucoid bloody diarrhea, frequent episodes of urgency and straining to defecate). As the disease progresses, continuing intestinal blood and protein loss causes some animals to lose significant amounts of body weight. The most remarkable findings on physical examination are pain during digital palpation of the anorectum and thickened rectal mucosa along with blood pigments. Moderate to severe cachexia may be a clinical feature of more chronically affected animals.

Diagnosis Colonoscopy and biopsy are the diagnostic methods of choice.[206] Endoscopic findings are variable and include diffusely hyperemic and irregular colonic mucosa with multifocal, petechial hemorrhages; nodular and corrugated mucosa; edema and fibrosis; and, multifocal, scattered ulcers throughout the mucosa.[206,207] Histopathologically, a marked expansion of the lamina propria occurs with a diffuse infiltration of PAS-positive histiocytes. Histiocytic infiltration is often accompanied by multifocal, superficial mucosal ulcers with neutrophil, lymphocyte, and plasma cell infiltration.

Treatment. Sulfasalazine has been the drug of choice for this disorder, and affected animals showed some initial clinical improvement only to experience relapses during the course of the disease. The disease was thought to be progressive and requiring lifelong therapy. More recently, therapeutic cures have been reported with enrofloxacin therapy, again implying an underlying bacterial pathogenesis.[209a]

Prognosis If histiocytic ulcerative colitis is at an advanced stage at the time of diagnosis, treatment often does not improve clinical signs and a poor prognosis is warranted.

Typhlitis

Cause Primary inflammation or infection of the cecum is a rare clinical problem in the dog and cat. Typhlitis more often develops secondarily as part of a typhlocolitis or ileotyphlocolitis syndrome.[210] Eosinophilic typhlitis, for example, has been reported in association with eosinophilic coloproctitis and ileitis in one dog,[210] and neutrophilic typhlocolitis was observed in a group of gnotobiotic dogs experimentally infected with *Campylobacter* spp.[124] Typhlitis usually responds to the same medical therapies that are used to treat ileocolitis. In rare cases, surgical resection may be required due to obstruction and abscessation.[211]

Pathophysiology The cecum responds pathophysiologically in much the same way that the colon responds to inflammation, except that size and orientation predispose the cecum to obstruction, abscessation, and rupture.

Clinical Examination Dogs affected with typhlocolitis may have mild discomfort on abdominal palpation, or there may be severe abdominal pain with cecal obstruction and abscessation.

Diagnosis Abdominal ultrasonography may be useful in documenting thickening of the cecal mucosa in some cases of typhlocolitis, but definitive diagnosis usually requires direct endoscopic examination. Ultrasonography is more useful in the diagnosis of obstructive lesions of the cecum (e.g., abscessation, neoplasia). Survey radiography is not that useful unless sequelae to infection are noted (e.g., abscessation, inversion, rupture).

Treatment Infectious typhlitis is best treated with antimicrobial and other therapy as outlined for treatment of inflammatory and infectious colitis.

Prognosis The prognosis for typhlocolitis lesions is generally favorable, particularly if they are diagnosed prior to the onset of smooth muscle hypertrophy and obstruction.

Colitis Associated with Perianal Fistula

Perianal fistula or anal furunculosis is a chronic and painful perianal disease of dogs, characterized by inflammation, ulceration, and sinus tracts involving the tissues surrounding the anus.[212,213] Clinical signs include tenesmus, hematochezia, and an ulcerated malodorous perianal region, resulting in pain, anorexia, and weight loss. Inflammation and sinus tracts may involve the rectum and descending colon in some animals, and it may be difficult, if not impossible, to attribute clinical signs to the colitis or the perianal fistula. Because of the high incidence of colitis in dogs affected with perianal fistula, it has been suggested that colonic biopsies should be obtained in all animals affected with perianal fistula.[213] It has also been suggested that affected animals should be managed with a novel protein diet as part of the overall medical therapy.[212] A more detailed discussion of perianal fistula may be found in Chapter 224.

OBSTRUCTION

Neoplasia

Cause In dogs, tumors of the large intestine are more common than tumors of the stomach and small intestine. The mean age of dogs affected with colonic neoplasia is variably reported between 7 and 11 years of age.[214] Most colonic tumors of dogs are malignant and include the adenocarcinomas, lymphosarcomas, and GI stromal tumors (leiomyosarcoma, neurofibrosarcoma, fibrosarcoma, and ganglioneuroma).[215-224] Leiomyosarcomas are the most common (91%) of the GI stromal tumors.[217-220] Most colonic neoplasia develop in the descending colon and rectum, although leiomyosarcomas more frequently develop in the cecum.[217,219] Local tumor invasion apparently occurs at a slower rate with canine colonic neoplasia, and metastasis to distant sites is relatively uncommon. Benign colonic neoplasia (e.g., adenomas, adenomatous polyps, leiomyomas) also occur, although they are less common than malignant tumors. Malignant transformation of adenomatous polyps to carcinoma *in situ* and invasive adenocarcinoma has been demonstrated in the dog just as it has in humans.[214,225,226,226b] Extramedullary plasmacytomas are an uncommon tumor of the GI tract but occur in the large intestine and rectum.[227,228] All of the aforementioned tumors are associated with signs of inflammation and obstruction (i.e., hematochezia, tenesmus, dyschezia). Carcinoids (rare 5-hydroxytryptamine [5-HT]-secreting tumors) are occasionally associated with diarrhea because of the effects of 5-HT on secretion and motility.

In cats, adenocarcinoma (46%) is the most common tumor of the large intestine, followed by lymphosarcoma (41%) and mast cell tumors (9%).[229-231] The mean age of cats affected with colonic neoplasia is 12.5 years. The descending colon (39%) and the ileocolic sphincter (28%) are the most common sites of colonic neoplasia in the cat. Unlike colonic tumors in the dog, feline colonic tumors have a high rate (63%) of metastasis and, of course, metastasis is associated with decreased survival time. Metastatic sites include colonic lymph nodes, mesenteric lymph nodes, liver, spleen, bladder, urethra, omentum, mesocolon, lungs, duodenum, and peritoneum.

Pathophysiology Mechanical obstruction is the most common pathophysiologic consequence of locally invasive colonic tumors. Other non-neoplastic processes such as intussusception, FIP granuloma, fibrosing stricture, linear and non-linear foreign bodies, hematoma, and phycomycosis lesions also cause intraluminal obstruction. Prolonged obstruction induces smooth muscle hypertrophy proximal to the site of the obstruction.[232] Other pathophysiologic consequences of intestinal obstruction are pronounced fluid secretion and malabsorption of water and solutes; fluid, electrolyte, and acid-base disturbances; proliferation and translocation of luminal bacteria; and inflammation, devitalization, and perhaps even perforation of the colon. Secretory diarrheas have been reported with carcinoids of the rectum, colon, and intestine.

Clinical Examination Most affected dogs have signs of hematochezia, mucoid feces, tenesmus, and dyschezia of varying severity. Importantly, the clinical signs observed with colorectal neoplasia are often indistinguishable from other causes of obstruction or chronic colitis. Hematochezia is infrequently reported with leiomyosarcomas or leiomyomas, presumably because these tumors do not typically involve the mucosa. Other clinical signs depend on the tumor type and location. Vomiting, malabsorption, and cachexia may be observed, for example, when multifocal or diffuse tumors (e.g., lymphosarcoma) involve the proximal portions of the GI tract. GI stromal tumors, particularly the leiomyomas, have been associated with hypoglycemia and the resulting clinical signs of muscular weakness and seizure activity.[233] Functional plasmacytomas secrete a single class of immunoglobulin and affected animals may go on to develop hyperviscosity syndrome (e.g., retinal bleeding, epistaxis). If colonic perforation has occurred, animals may be presented moribund with fever, lethargy, anorexia, vomiting, abdominal pain, and collapse.

Vomiting (65%), diarrhea (52%), and weight loss (46%) are common clinical signs in cats with colonic neoplasia.[229] Most cats with colonic (and alimentary) lymphosarcoma are FeLV-negative. These lymphomas are thought to be caused by FeLV, with integrated virus causing neoplastic transformation in the absence of viral replication. Although most lymphomas in cats appear to be comprised of malignant T lymphocytes, most colonic (and alimentary) lymphomas are of B cell origin. Alimentary and colonic lymphomas originate primarily from submucosal lymphocytes, mucosal lymphoid follicles, or both, although one recent study reported an epitheliotropic form of T cell intestinal lymphomas.[234] Epitheliotropic T cell lymphomas have not yet been reported in the feline colon.

Diagnosis Canine rectal adenocarcinomas are palpable in 60% to 80% of clinical cases, but colonic and cecal lesions are not as readily apparent on physical examination.[214,226,232,235,236] More than 50% of cats with colonic masses have a palpable abdominal mass.[229]

Survey and contrast radiographic and ultrasonographic studies have been used with varying levels of success in the diagnosis of canine and feline colonic neoplasia. Annular stenotic lesions associated with adenocarcinoma of the colon may manifest as proximal colonic dilation on survey radiographs.

Radiographic contrast material more precisely outlines the narrowing of the lumen at the site of the tumor. Although still of some clinical utility, contrast studies have been largely superceded by ultrasonography and other imaging modalities. Ultrasonography is presently considered to be the most effective means of diagnosing colonic tumors in dogs and cats and appears to be useful in evaluating mural lesions and associated abdominal changes such as lymphadenopathy.[236] Ultrasonography was reported to be useful 84% of the time in localizing feline colonic neoplasia in one study.[229] Ultrasonographic features of colonic tumors include transmural wall thickening with complete loss of the normal wall layering, fluid accumulation proximal to the lesion, and reduced regional motility.[236]

Transabdominal fine needle aspiration, peritoneal fluid cytology, and endoscopic exfoliative cytology may be useful in the diagnosis of lymphoma, but histopathology is generally required for a definitive diagnosis of other colonic neoplasia. CT and magnetic resonance imaging (MRI) scanning have not been sufficiently evaluated at this time for reasonable comparisons to be made with ultrasonography.

Flexible colonoscopy with mucosal biopsy is the preferred method of diagnosis for colonic neoplasia. Endoscopic abnormalities may include mass effect, mucosal bleeding, increased mucosal friability, erosions and ulcers, and circumferential luminal narrowing with submucosal infiltrative lesions. Multiple biopsy specimens should always be taken from diseased tissue, adjacent healthy tissue, and the transition zone between healthy and diseased tissue. With tumor necrosis, the pathologist will have a much better chance of diagnosing and staging the disease by evaluating non-necrotic tissue.

Treatment The treatment of colonic neoplasia will depend upon tumor type, anatomic location, and presence and extent of metastases. Complete surgical excision is the recommended therapy for focal adenocarcinomas, cecal leiomyosarcomas, and obstructive lymphomas. Multiagent chemotherapy (prednisone, vincristine, cyclophosphamide) has been used to treat colonic lymphoma, but it does not appear to alter survival time in affected cats.[229] Cyclo-oxygenase II (COX II) up-regulation may contribute to the growth characteristics of some canine colonic neoplasia.[237-239] Selective COX II inhibitors (e.g., piroxicam, meloxicam) may therefore be useful in the treatment of some canine colonic neoplasia. Plasmacytomas may be managed with adjuvant chemotherapy (e.g., prednisone, melphalan) after surgical excision. Radiation therapy has been used to palliate recurrent adenocarcinomas with varying results and complications; however, postradiation peritonitis and perforation have been reported in some cases.[240]

Prognosis The prognosis for adenomatous polyps, leiomyomas, and fibromas is generally favorable. Adenocarcinomas, lymphosarcomas, and plasmacytomas tend to recur, metastasize, or both to distant sites. Dogs with annular colorectal adenocarcinomas have a particularly poor prognosis with a median survival time (MST) of only 1.6 months.[214,235] The prognosis for most malignant tumors is generally guarded. Surgical resection alone results in 22 month (dogs) and 15 month (cats) average survival times in dogs and cats.[214,229] It should be noted that cats undergoing subtotal colectomy for colonic adenocarcinoma had a longer survival time than those receiving mass resection only (MST of 138 days versus 68 days).[229] Not surprisingly, cats with metastatic lesions had much shorter survival times, 49 days versus 259 days.[229]

Intussusception

Cause Intussusception is an invagination of one segment of the GI tract into the lumen of an adjoining segment. The *intussusceptum* is the invaginated segment of the alimentary tract, whereas the *intussuscipiens* is the enveloping segment. Invagination may occur in an antegrade (aborad) or retrograde (orad) direction, but is most commonly in the antegrade direction. Any portion of the alimentary tract may be involved, but enterocolic intussusceptions account for almost two thirds of the published cases in dogs and cats. Enterocolic intussusceptions can be further divided into three types: (1) cecocolic (or cecal inversion), with the inverted cecum forming the apex[241]; (2) ileocolic, with the ileum forming the apex; and (3) ileocecal, with the ileum forming the apex.[242] Of these three forms of enterocolic intussusception, the ileocolic intussusception is the one most frequently encountered in clinical practice. A number of conditions are reported to predispose to intussusception, including intestinal parasitism, viral enteritis, foreign bodies, and masses, but in dogs and cats most intussusceptions are idiopathic.[243-245]

Pathophysiology The initiating events in an intussusception are often difficult to identify retrospectively, but all intussusceptions appear to share three important features: (1) inhomogeneity in a bowel segment—a region in which the GI tract undergoes a sudden anatomic change in diameter (e.g., ileocolic junction) or a bowel segment that is either flaccid or indurated; (2) mechanical linkage of nonadjacent segments—which can be intraluminal (e.g., linear foreign bodies, parasites) or extramural (e.g., fibrous adhesions or bands); and (3) peristaltic activity of the gut.[242]

Invagination begins as a result of peristaltic contraction. Once the invagination has begun, its progress may be rapid, involving as much as several centimeters of intestinal tract within just a few hours. Invagination and intussusception result in luminal obstruction, which may be partial or complete. Obstruction usually results in distension of the bowel segment proximal to the intussusception. The degree of distension is dependent upon the completeness and duration of the obstruction, volume of fluid secretion, degree of vascular compromise, and volume of gas production from bacterial fermentation. Because the mesentery and blood supply are included in the invaginating segment, vascular compromise can occur, which initially leads to intramural hemorrhage and edema and eventually to ischemia and necrosis of the bowel. Full-thickness necrosis may ensue, but perforations are rare.

Clinical Examination The most important clinical signs with ileocolic intussusceptions are intermittent vomiting, progressive loss of appetite, mucoid bloody diarrhea, and a palpable cylinder-shaped mass in the cranial abdomen. Abdominal pain is not a consistent finding in affected animals. Clinical signs may persist for several weeks, and affected animals eventually succumb to the effects of starvation rather than dehydration, electrolyte imbalances, or acid-base disturbances.

Diagnosis With some ileocolic intussusceptions, the intussuscepted bowel may protrude through the anus and must be differentiated from a rectal prolapse. This is accomplished by passing a blunt probe between the protruding segment and the anal sphincter. If the probe can be passed cranial to the pubis without reaching a fornix, then the protruding bowel is the apex of an intussusception rather than rectal prolapse.

Survey abdominal radiographic findings may be suspicious for intussusception (Figure 223-10, *A*). Barium contrast studies (barium enema or upper GI series) are often diagnostic, but abdominal ultrasonography is the preferred method of diagnosis. The appearance of a targetlike mass (consisting of two or more hyperechoic and hypoechoic concentric rings in transverse section) or the appearance of multiple hyperechoic and hypoechoic parallel lines in longitudinal section is virtually diagnostic of an intussusception (Figure 223-10, *B*).[246] The ultrasound scan might also identify a mass associated with the intussusception. Endoscopy may be performed in suspected cases of suspected neoplasia, otherwise endoscopy does not confer any additional benefits over abdominal ultrasound or CT scanning.

Treatment The surgical management of ileocolic intussusception involves either reduction or resection, and anastomosis, or both.[247,248] Secretory diarrhea may persist after relief of the obstruction, and affected animals may need continuous crystalloid and colloidal therapy. If possible, the ileocecal sphincter should be preserved to reduce reflux and contamination of the distal small bowel. Cecocolic intussusceptions or inversions should also be treated with surgical resection. Surgical resection of the cecocolic intussusceptions

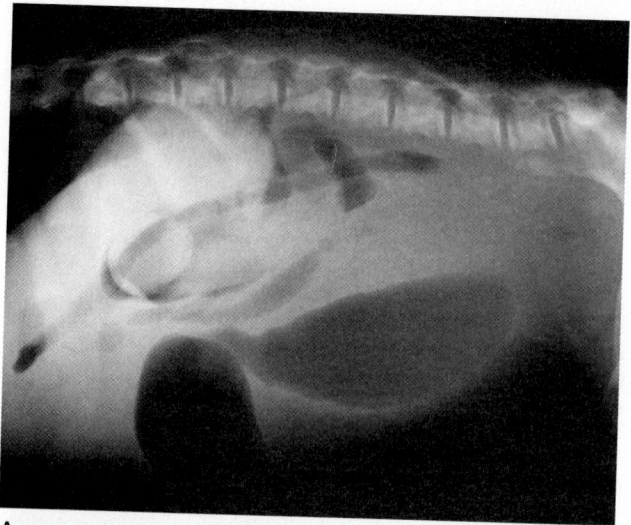

A

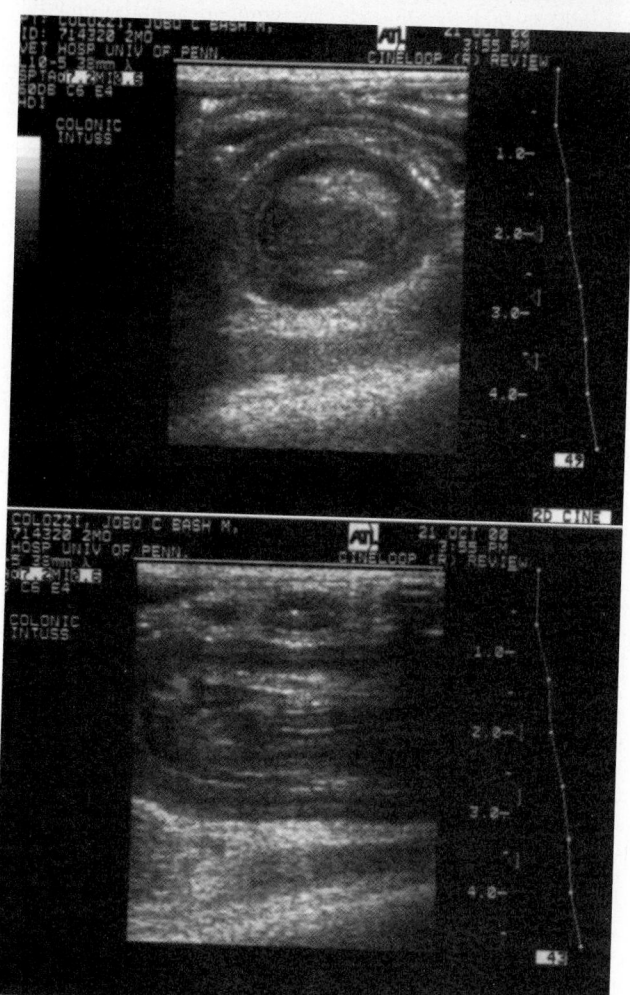

B

Figure 223-10 A, Survey lateral radiographic appearance of ileocolic intussusception in a 6-month-old puppy. B, Ultrasonographic appearance of ileocolic intussusception in a 10-year-old cat. (Digital image courtesy of Dr. Rafe Van Knox, University of Pennsylvania.)

is generally curative. Enteroplication procedures have been recommended,[249] but they do not appear to reduce recurrence rates.[247,248]

Prognosis The most common complications after treatment of intussusception are recurrence, dehiscence of the anastomosis, ileus, intestinal obstruction, peritonitis, and short bowel syndrome. The recurrence rate in dogs is reported to be between 11% and 20%. In dogs in which no surgical procedure was performed to prevent recurrence, intussusception recurred in 25% of dogs that underwent manual reduction alone and in 19% of dogs that underwent resection and anastomosis. Enteroplication does not appear to reduce recurrence rates any further.[247,248] Indeed, 19% of dogs undergoing enteroplication in one study experienced severe complications that required a second surgery. Intestinal obstruction was a complication of the enteroplication in those patients.[248]

HYPOMOTILITY AND DYSMOTILITY

Constipation
Cause The etiopathogenesis of idiopathic megacolon is still incompletely understood. Several reviews have emphasized the importance of considering an extensive list of differential diagnoses (e.g., neuromuscular, mechanical, inflammatory, metabolic and endocrine, pharmacologic, environmental, and behavioral causes) for the obstipated cat (Box 223-1; reviewed in reference 250). A review of published cases suggests that 96% of cases of obstipation are accounted for by idiopathic megacolon (62%), pelvic canal stenosis (23%), nerve injury (6%), or Manx sacral spinal cord deformity (5%).[52] A smaller number of cases are accounted for by complications of colopexy (1%) and colonic neoplasia (1%); colonic hypo- or aganglionosis was suspected, but not proved, in another 2% of cases. Inflammatory, pharmacologic, and environmental and behavioral causes were not cited as predisposing factors in any of the original case reports. Endocrine factors (e.g., obesity, hypothyroidism) were cited in several cases, but were not necessarily impugned as part of the pathogenesis of megacolon. It is important to consider an extensive list of differential diagnoses in an individual animal, but it should be kept in mind that most cases are idiopathic, orthopedic, or neurologic in origin. Behavioral (e.g., stress) or environmental (e.g., competition for the litter box) factors, or both, may play an important role in the development of this lesion, but they have not been very well characterized in retrospective or prospective studies.

Pathophysiology Megacolon develops through two pathologic mechanisms: (1) *dilation* and (2) *hypertrophy*. *Dilated megacolon* is the end stage of colonic dysfunction in idiopathic cases. Cats affected with idiopathic dilated megacolon have permanent loss of colonic structure and function. Medical therapy may be attempted in such cases, but most affected cats eventually require colectomy. *Hypertrophic megacolon*, on the other hand, develops as a consequence of obstructive lesions (e.g., malunion of pelvic fractures, tumors, foreign bodies). Hypertrophic megacolon may be reversible with early pelvic osteotomy, or it may progress to irreversible dilated megacolon if appropriate therapy is not instituted.[251]

Constipation and *obstipation* are earlier manifestations of the same problem. Constipation is defined as infrequent or difficult evacuation of feces but does not necessarily imply a permanent loss of function. Many cats suffer from one or two episodes of constipation without further progression. Intractible constipation that has become refractory to cure or control is referred to as *obstipation*. The term *obstipation* implies a permanent loss of function. A cat is assumed to be obstipated only after several consecutive treatment failures. Recurring episodes

GASTROINTESTINAL DISEASE

(70% male, 30% female) of domestic shorthair (DSH) (46%), domestic longhair (15%), or Siamese (12%) breeding.[52] Affected cats are usually presented for reduced, absent, or painful defecation for a period of time ranging from days to weeks or months. Some cats are observed making multiple, unproductive attempts to defecate in the litter box, whereas other cats may sit in the litter box for prolonged periods of time without assuming a defecation posture. Dry, hardened feces are observed inside and outside of the litter box. Occasionally, chronically constipated cats have intermittent episodes of hematochezia or diarrhea due to the mucosal irritant effect of fecal concretions. This may give the pet owner the erroneous impression that diarrhea is the primary problem. Prolonged inability to defecate may result in other systemic signs, including anorexia, lethargy, weight loss, and vomiting.

Physical examination Colonic impaction is a consistent physical examination finding in affected cats. Other findings will depend upon the severity and pathogenesis of constipation. Dehydration, weight loss, debilitation, abdominal pain, and mild to moderate mesenteric lymphadenopathy may be observed in cats with severe idiopathic megacolon. Colonic impaction may be so severe in such cases as to render it difficult to differentiate impaction from colonic, mesenteric, or other abdominal neoplasia. Cats with constipation due to dysautonomia may have other signs of autonomic nervous system failure, such as urinary and fecal incontinence, regurgitation due to megaesophagus, mydriasis, decreased lacrimation, prolapse of the nictitating membrane, and bradycardia. Digital rectal examination should be carefully performed with sedation or anesthesia in all cats. Pelvic fracture malunion may be detected on rectal examination in cats with pelvic trauma. Rectal examination might also identify other unusual causes of constipation, such as foreign bodies, rectal diverticula, stricture, inflammation, or neoplasia. Chronic tenesmus may be associated with perineal herniation in some cases.[250] A complete neurologic examination, with special emphasis on caudal spinal cord function, should be performed to identify neurologic causes of constipation (e.g., spinal cord injury, pelvic nerve trauma, Manx sacral spinal cord deformity).

Diagnosis Although most cases of obstipation and megacolon are unlikely to have significant changes in laboratory data (e.g., CBC, serum chemistry, urinalysis), these tests should nonetheless be performed in all cats presented for constipation. Metabolic causes of constipation, such as dehydration, hypokalemia, and hypercalcemia may be detected in some cases. Basal serum T_4 concentration and other thyroid function tests should also be considered in cats with recurrent constipation and other signs consistent with hypothyroidism. Although hypothyroidism was documented in only one case of obstipation and megacolon, obstipation is a frequent clinical sign in kittens affected with congenital or juvenile-onset hypothyroidism.[52] Constipation could also theoretically develop after successful treatment of feline hyperthyroidism.

Abdominal radiography should be performed in all constipated cats to characterize the severity of colonic impaction and to identify predisposing factors such as intraluminal radiopaque foreign material (e.g., bone chips), intraluminal or extraluminal mass lesions, pelvic fractures, and spinal cord abnormalities (Figure 223-11). The radiographic findings of colonic impaction cannot be used to distinguish between constipation, obstipation, and megacolon in idiopathic cases. First or second episodes of constipation in some cats may be severe and generalized but may still resolve with appropriate treatment.

Ancillary studies may be indicated in some cases. Extraluminal mass lesions may be further evaluated by abdominal ultrasonography and guided biopsy, whereas intraluminal mass lesions are best evaluated by endoscopy. Colonoscopy may also be used to evaluate the colon and anorectum for

of constipation or obstipation may culminate in the syndrome of *megacolon*.

The pathogenesis of idiopathic dilated megacolon appears to involve functional disturbances in colonic smooth muscle. *In vitro* isometric stress measurements have been performed on colonic smooth muscle obtained from cats suffering from idiopathic dilated megacolon.[252,253] Megacolonic smooth muscle develops less isometric stress in response to neurotransmitter (acetylcholine, substance P, cholecystokinin), membrane depolarization (potassium chloride), or electrical field stimulation, when compared with healthy controls.[252,253] Differences have been observed in longitudinal and circular smooth muscle from the descending and ascending colon. No significant abnormalities of smooth muscle cells or of myenteric neurons were observed on histologic evaluation. These studies initially suggested that the disorder of feline idiopathic megacolon is a generalized dysfunction of colonic smooth muscle and that treatments aimed at stimulating colonic smooth muscle contraction might improve colonic motility. More recent studies suggest that the lesion may begin in the descending colon and progress to involve the ascending colon over time.[254]

Clinical Examination

History Constipation, obstipation, and megacolon may be observed in cats of any age, sex, or breed; however, most cases are observed in middle-aged (mean: 5.8 years) male cats

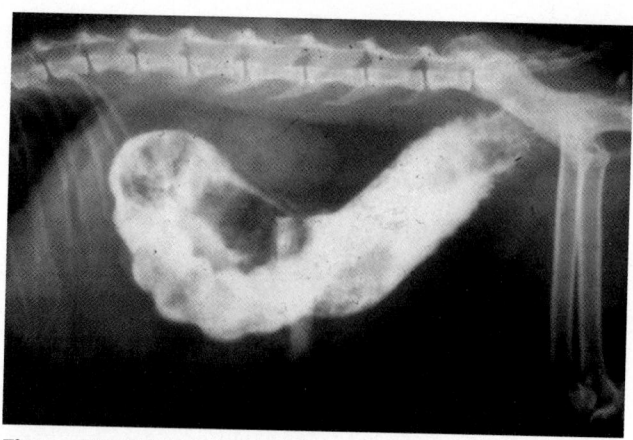

Figure 223-11 Barium enema in a 12-year-old cat with idiopathic constipation and megacolon.

Treatment The specific therapeutic plan will depend upon the severity of constipation and the underlying cause (Figure 223-12; Table 223-7).[250] Medical therapy may not be necessary with first episodes of constipation. First episodes are often transient and resolve without therapy. Mild to moderate or recurrent episodes of constipation, on the other hand, usually require some medical intervention. These cases may be managed, often on an outpatient basis, with dietary modification, water enemas, oral or suppository laxatives, colonic prokinetic agents, or a combination of these therapies. Severe cases of constipation usually require brief periods of hospitalization to correct metabolic abnormalities and to evacuate impacted feces using water enemas, manual extraction of retained feces, or both. Follow-up therapy in such cases is directed at correcting predisposing factors and preventing recurrence. Subtotal colectomy will become necessary in cats suffering from obstipation or idiopathic dilated megacolon. These cats, by definition, are unresponsive to medical therapy. Although pelvic osteotomy is described for cats with pelvic canal stenosis,[225] subtotal colectomy is an effective treatment and is considered the standard of surgical care.[280] An algorithm for the therapeutic approach to the constipated, obstipated, and megacolonic cat is outlined in Figure 223-12.

Removal of Impacted Feces Removal of impacted feces may be accomplished through the use of rectal suppositories, enemas, or manual extraction.

Rectal suppositories A number of pediatric rectal suppositories are available for the management of mild constipation.

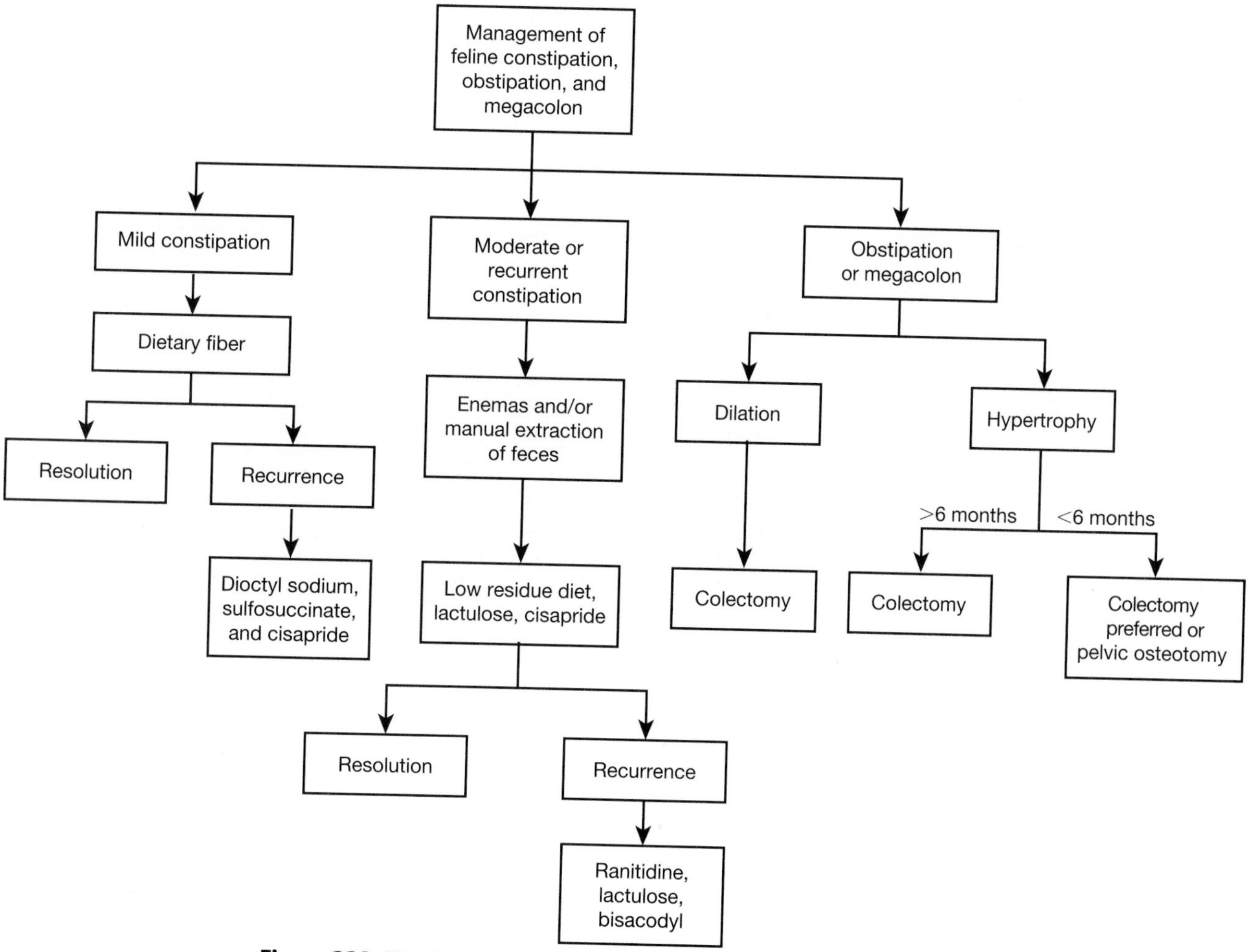

suspected inflammatory lesions, strictures, sacculations, and diverticula. Barium enema contrast radiography may be used if colonoscopy is not possible. Both colonoscopy and barium enema contrast radiography will require general anesthesia and evacuation of impacted feces. Cerebrospinal fluid analysis, CT or MRI, and electrophysiologic studies should be considered in animals with evidence of neurologic impairment. Finally, colonic biopsy or anorectal manometry will be necessary to diagnose suspected cases of aganglionic megacolon.

Management of feline constipation, obstipation, and megacolon

- Mild constipation
  - Dietary fiber
    - Resolution
    - Recurrence
      - Dioctyl sodium, sulfosuccinate, and cisapride
- Moderate or recurrent constipation
  - Enemas and/or manual extraction of feces
    - Low residue diet, lactulose, cisapride
      - Resolution
      - Recurrence
        - Ranitidine, lactulose, bisacodyl
- Obstipation or megacolon
  - Dilation
    - Colectomy
  - Hypertrophy
    - >6 months
      - Colectomy
    - <6 months
      - Colectomy preferred or pelvic osteotomy

Figure 223-12 Therapeutic approach to feline constipation and megacolon.

GASTROINTESTINAL DISEASE

Table • 223-7

Drug Index—Constipation

DRUG CLASSIFICATION AND EXAMPLE	DOSE
Rectal Suppositories	
Dioctyl sodium sulfosuccinate (Colace, Mead Johnson)	1-2 pediatric suppositories
Glycerin	1-2 pediatric suppositories
Bisacodyl (Dulcolax; Boehringer Ingelheim)	1-2 pediatric suppositories
Enemas	
Warm tap water	5-10 mL/kg
Warm isotonic saline	5-10 mL/kg
Dioctyl sodium sulfosuccinate (Colace, Mead Johnson)	5-10 mL/cat
Dioctyl sodium sulfosuccinate (Disposaject, PittmanMoore)	250 mg (12 ml) given pre rectum
Mineral oil	5-10 mL/cat
Lactulose (Cephulac, Merrell Dow; Duphalac, Reid Rowell)	5-10 mL/cat
Oral Laxatives	
Bulk laxatives	
Psyllium (Metamucil, Searle)	1-4 tsp mixed with food, every 24 or 12 hours
Canned pumpkin	1-4 tsp mixed with food, every 24 hours
Coarse wheat bran	1-4 tblsp mixed with food, every 24 hours
Emollient laxatives	
Dioctyl sodium sulfosuccinate (Colace, Mead Johnson)	50 mg orally, every 24 hours
Dioctyl calcium sulfosuccinate (Surfax, Hoechst)	50 mg orally, every 24 or 12 hours as needed
Lubricant laxatives	
Mineral oil	10-25 ml orally, every 24 hours
Petrolatum (Laxatone, Evsco)	1-5 ml orally, every 24 hours
Hyperosmotic laxatives	
Lactulose (Cephulac, Merrell Dow; Duphalac, Reid Rowell)	0.5 ml/kg orally, every 12 to 8 hours as needed
Stimulant laxatives	
Bisacodyl (Dulcolax, Boehringer Ingelheim)	5 mg orally, every 24 hours
Prokinetic Agents	
Cisapride (compounding pharmacies)	0.1-1.0 mg/kg orally every 12 to 8 hours
Tegaserod (Zelnorm, Novartis)[257] - dogs	0.05-0.10 mg/kg orally, twice a day
Ranitidine (Zantac, Glaxo SmithKline)	1.0-2.0 mg/kg orally, every 12 to 8 hours
Nizatidine (Axid, Eli Lilly)	2.5-5.0 mg/kg orally, every 24 hours

These include dioctyl sodium sulfosuccinate (emollient laxative), glycerin (lubricant laxative), and bisacodyl (stimulant laxative). The use of rectal suppositories requires a compliant pet and pet owner. Suppositories can be used alone or in conjunction with oral laxative therapy.

Enemas Mild to moderate or recurrent episodes of constipation may require administration of enemas, manual extraction of impacted feces, or both. Several types of enema solutions may be administered, such as warm tap water (5 to 10 mL/kg), warm isotonic saline (5 to 10 mL/kg), dioctyl sodium sulfosuccinate (5 to 10 mL/cat), mineral oil (5 to 10 mL/cat), or lactulose (5 to 10 mL/cat). Enema solutions should be administered slowly with a well-lubricated 10 to 12F rubber catheter or feeding tube. Enemas containing sodium phosphate are contraindicated in cats because of their propensity for inducing severe hypernatremia, hyperphosphatemia, and hypocalcemia in this species.[256]

Manual extraction Cases unresponsive to enemas may require manual extraction of impacted feces. Cats should be adequately rehydrated and then anesthetized with an endotracheal tube in place to prevent aspiration should colonic manipulation induce vomiting. Water or saline is infused into the colon while the fecal mass is manually reduced by abdominal palpation. Sponge forceps may also be introduced rectally (with caution) to break down the fecal mass. It may be advisable to evacuate the fecal mass over a period of several days to reduce the risks of prolonged anesthesia and perforation of a devitalized colon. If this approach fails, colotomy may be necessary to remove the fecal mass. Laxative or prokinetic therapy (or both) may then be instituted once the fecal mass has been removed.

Laxative Therapy Laxatives promote evacuation of the bowel through stimulation of fluid and electrolyte transport or increases in propulsive motility. They are classified as bulk-forming, emollient, lubricant, hyperosmotic, or stimulant laxatives according to their mechanism of action. Hundreds of products are available for the treatment of constipation. Table 223-7 summarizes those products that have been used with some success in cats.

Bulk-forming laxatives Most of the available bulk-forming laxatives are dietary fiber supplements of poorly digestible polysaccharides and celluloses derived principally from cereal grains, wheat bran, and psyllium. Some constipated cats will respond to supplementation of the diet with one of these products, but many require adjunctive therapy (e.g., other types of laxatives or colonic prokinetic agents). Dietary fiber is preferable because it is well tolerated, more effective, and more physiologic than other laxatives. Fiber is classified as a bulk-forming laxative, although it has many other properties. The beneficial effects of fiber in constipation include increased fecal water content, decreased intestinal transit time, and increased frequency of defecation.[26,257] Fiber supplemented diets are available commercially, or the pet owner may wish to add psyllium (1 to 4 teaspoon per meal), wheat bran (1 to 2 tablespoon per meal), or pumpkin (1 to 4 tablespoon per meal) to canned cat food. Cats should be well hydrated before commencing fiber supplementation to maximize the therapeutic effect. Fiber supplementation is most beneficial in mildly constipated cats, prior to the development of obstipation and megacolon. In obstipated and megacolon cats, fiber may in fact be detrimental. Low-residue diets may be more beneficial in obstipated and megacolonic cats.

Emollient laxatives   Emollient laxatives are anionic detergents that increase the miscibility of water and lipid in digesta, thereby enhancing lipid absorption and impairing water absorption. Dioctyl sodium sulfosuccinate and dioctyl calcium sulfosuccinate are examples of emollient laxatives available in oral and enema form. Anecdotal experience suggests that dioctyl sodium sulfosuccinate therapy may be most useful in animals with acute but not chronic constipation. As with bulk-forming laxatives, animals should be well hydrated before emollient laxatives are administered. It should be noted that clincial efficacy has not been definitively established for the emollient laxatives. Dioctyl sodium sulfosuccinate, for example, inhibits water absorption in isolated colonic segments *in vitro*, but it may be impossible to achieve tissue concentrations great enough to inhibit colonic water absorption *in vivo*. Dioctyl sodium sulfosuccinate at a dose of 30 mg/kg/day had no effect on fecal consistency in beagle dogs.[258] Further studies are required to determine the clinical efficacy and therapeutic role of dioctyl sodium sulfosuccinate in the management of the constipated cat.

Lubricant laxatives   Mineral oil and white petrolatum are the two major lubricant laxatives available for the treatment of constipation. The lubricating properties of these agents impede colonic water absorption and permit greater ease of fecal passage. These effects are usually moderate, however, and, in general, lubricants are beneficial only in mild cases of constipation. Mineral oil use should probably be limited to rectal administration because of the risk of aspiration pneumonia with oral administration, especially in depressed or debilitated cats.

Hyperosmotic laxatives   This group of laxatives consists of the poorly absorbed polysaccharides (e.g., lactose, lactulose), the magnesium salts (e.g., magnesium citrate, magnesium hydroxide, magnesium sulfate), and the polyethylene glycols. Lactose is not effective as a laxative agent in all cats.[259] Lactulose is the most effective agent in this group. The organic acids produced from lactulose fermentation stimulate colonic fluid secretion and propulsive motility. Lactulose administered at a dose of 0.5 mL/kg body weight every 8 to 12 hours fairly consistently produces soft feces in the cat. Many cats with recurrent or chronic constipation have been well managed with this regimen of lactulose. The dose may have to be tapered in individual cases if flatulence and diarrhea become excessive. Magnesium salts are not currently recommended in the treatment of feline constipation and idiopathic megacolon. Some veterinarians have reported anecdotal successes with the polyethylene glycols.

Stimulant laxatives   The stimulant laxatives (bisacodyl, phenolphthalein, castor oil, cascara, senna) are a diverse group of agents that have been classified according to their ability to stimulate propulsive motility. Bisacodyl, for example, stimulates NO-mediated epithelial cell secretion and myenteric neuronal depolarization.[260] Diarrhea results from the combined effect of increased mucosal secretion and colonic propulsion. Bisacodyl (at a dose of 5 mg orally, every 24 hours) is the most effective stimulant laxative in the cat. It may be given individually or in combination with fiber supplementation for long-term management of constipation. Daily administration of bisacodyl should probably be avoided, however, because of injury to myenteric neurons with chronic use.[250]

Colonic Prokinetic Agents   Previous studies of feline colonic smooth muscle function have suggested that stimulation of colonic smooth muscle contraction might improve colonic motility in cats affected with idiopathic dilated megacolon.[252,253,261] Unfortunately, many of the currently available GI prokinetic agents have not proved useful in the therapy of feline constipation, either because of significant side effects (e.g., bethanechol) or because the prokinetic effect is limited to the proximal GI tract (e.g., metoclopramide, domperidone, erythromycin). The $5-HT_4$ serotonergic agonists (e.g., cisapride, prucalopride, tegaserod, mosapride) appear to have the advantage of stimulating motility from the gastroesophageal sphincter to the descending colon with relatively few side effects. Cisapride, for example, increases gastroesophageal sphincter pressure, promotes gastric emptying, and enhances small intestinal and colonic propulsive motility.[262] Cisapride enhances colonic propulsive motility through activation of colonic neuronal or smooth muscle 5-HT receptors in a number of animal species.[263,264] *In vitro* studies have shown that cisapride stimulates feline colonic smooth muscle contraction,[253,264] although it has not yet been conclusively shown that cisapride stimulates feline colonic propulsive motility *in vivo*. A large body of anecdotal experience suggests that cisapride is effective in stimulating colonic propulsive motility in cats affected with mild to moderate idiopathic constipation; cats with long-standing obstipation and megacolon are not likely to show much improvement with cisapride therapy. Cisapride was widely used in the management of canine and feline gastric emptying, intestinal transit, and colonic motility disorders throughout most of the 1990s.[262,265,266] Cisapride was withdrawn from the American, Canadian, and certain Western European countries in July 2000 after reports of untoward cardiac side effects in human patients. Cisapride causes QT interval prolongation and slowing of cardiac repolarization via blockade of the rapid component of the delayed rectifier potassium channel (I_{Kr}).[267] This effect may result in a fatal ventricular arrhythmia referred to as *torsades de pointes*. Similar effects have been characterized in canine cardiac Purkinje fibers,[267] but *in vivo* effects have not yet been reported in dogs or cats. The withdrawal of cisapride has created a clear need for new GI prokinetic agents, although cisapride continues to be available from compounding pharmacies throughout the United States. Two new prokinetic agents, tegaserod and prucalopride, are in differing stages of drug development and may prove useful in the therapy of GI motility disorders of several animal species.[261]

Tegaserod is a potent partial nonbenzamide agonist at $5-HT_4$ receptors and a weak agonist at $5-HT_{1D}$ receptors.[269,270] Tegaserod has definite prokinetic effects in the canine colon, but it has not yet been studied in the feline colon. Intravenous doses of tegaserod (0.03 to 0.3 mg/kg) accelerate colonic transit in dogs during the first hour after intravenous administration.[269] Tegaserod at doses of 3 to 6 mg/kg orally has also been shown to normalize intestinal transit in opioid-induced bowel dysfunction in dogs,[271] and it may prove useful in other disorders of intestinal ileus or pseudo-obstruction. Gastric effects of tegaserod have not been reported in the dog, so this drug may not prove as useful as cisapride in the treatment of delayed gastric emptying disorders. *In vitro* studies suggest that tegaserod does not prolong the QT interval or delay cardiac repolarization as has been occasionally reported with cisapride. Tegaserod was marketed under the trade name of Zelnorm in the United States in September 2002 for the treatment of constipation-predominant IBS in women. As with many other drugs in companion animal medicine, tegaserod has not been licensed for the treatment of canine or feline GI motility disorders.

Prucalopride is a potent 5-HT$_4$ receptor agonist that stimulates GMCs and defecation in the dog and cat.[272,273] Prucalopride also appears to stimulate gastric emptying in the dog.[274] In lidamidine-induced delayed gastric emptying in dogs, prucalopride (0.01 to 0.16 mg/kg) dose-dependently accelerates gastric emptying of dextrose solutions. Prucalopride has not yet been marketed in the United States or elsewhere.

Misoprostol is a prostaglandin E$_1$ analogue that reduces the incidence of nonsteroidal anti-inflammatory drug (NSAID)-induced gastric injury. The main side effects of misoprostol therapy are abdominal discomfort, cramping, and diarrhea. Studies in dogs suggest that prostaglandins may initiate a giant migrating complex pattern and increase colonic propulsive activity.[275] *In vitro* studies of misoprostol show that it stimulates feline and canine colonic smooth muscle contraction.[276] Given its limited toxicity, misoprostol may be useful in cats (and dogs) with severe refractory constipation.

Ranitidine and nizatidine, classic histamine H$_2$ receptor antagonists, may also stimulate canine and feline colonic motility. These drugs stimulate contraction apparently through inhibition of tissue acetylcholinesterase and accumulation of acetylcholine at the motor endplate. It is not yet clear how effective these drugs are *in vivo*, although both drugs stimulate feline colonic smooth muscle contraction *in vitro*.[277] Cimetidine and famotidine, members of the same classification of drug, are without this effect.

Surgery   Colectomy should be considered in cats that are refractory to medical therapy (Figure 223-13; see Surgery). Cats have a generally favorable prognosis for recovery after colectomy, although mild to moderate diarrhea may persist

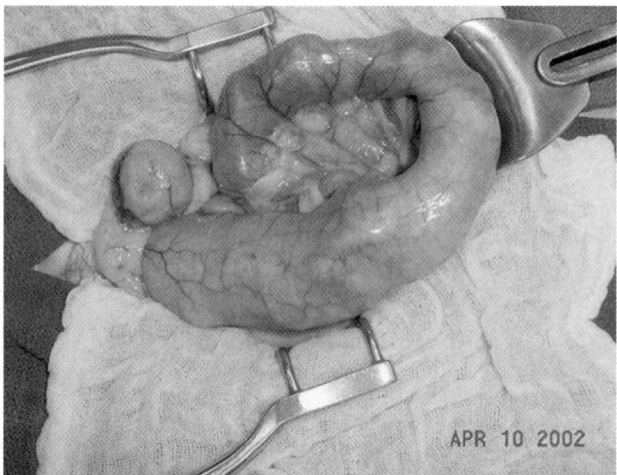

Figure 223-13 Surgical appearance of feline idiopathic megacolon.

for weeks to months postoperatively in some cases.[278,279] Although pathologic hypertrophy may be reversible with early pelvic osteotomy in some cases,[255] subtotal colectomy is an effective treatment for this condition regardless of duration, and pelvic osteotomy is not required.[280]

Prognosis   Many cats have one or two episodes of constipation without further recurrence, although others may progress to complete colonic failure. Cats with mild to moderate constipation generally respond to conservative medical management (e.g., dietary modification, emollient or hyperosmotic laxatives, colonic prokinetic agents). Early use of colonic prokinetic agents (in addition to one or more laxative agents) is likely to prevent the progression of constipation to obstipation and dilated megacolon in these cats. Some cats may become refractory to these therapies, however, as they progress through moderate or recurrent constipation to obstipation and dilated megacolon. These cats eventually require colectomy. Cats have a generally favorable prognosis for recovery after colectomy, although mild to moderate diarrhea may persist for 4 to 6 weeks postoperatively in some cases.

Irritable Bowel Syndrome

A fiber-responsive large bowel diarrheal syndrome similar to IBS in humans has been characterized in dogs.[185] Affected animals have a chronic idiopathic large bowel-type diarrhea characterized by excessive fecal mucous, hematochezia, and tenesmus. Pet owners occasionally report abdominal pain and weight loss. Multiple diet changes and empiric medications fail to relieve clinical signs. Medical investigation is negative for bacterial and other pathogens, colitis, and colonic neoplasia, and the term *chronic idiopathic large bowel diarrhea* is applied to the patient's disorder. Dogs affected with this syndrome may respond to the feeding of a highly digestible diet that is supplemented with soluble fiber.[185] Dogs that have failed to respond to fiber supplementation may respond to medical treatment with loperamide or anticholinergic agents.[187]

ULCER

Cause

Colonic ulcers may develop after glucocorticoid therapy and neurosurgery in dogs with spinal cord injury.[281,282] Gastric ulcers are of greater prevalence in this circumstance, but colonic ulcers may be equally devastating. Several factors are likely to contribute to colonic ulcerogenesis, including glucocorticoid-induced inhibition of immune function, epithelial renewal, prostaglandin production, mucus secretion, and collagen production; neurosurgery-induced increases in sympathetic tone; and the inhibitory effects of spinal injury on colonic motility and blood flow. The risk of colonic ulcer formation is greatly increased by concurrent NSAID administration. Why this lesion develops in some dogs but not others is not readily explained.

Pathophysiology

The left colic flexure or proximal portion of the descending colon appears to be at greatest risk for colonic ulceration and perforation; two thirds of the published cases were reported at this site.[282] Nonambulatory neurosurgical patients treated with dexamethasone are at greatest risk for development of colonic perforation. Colonic perforation is often preceded by variable nonspecific signs, most frequently depression, anorexia, and emesis. Perforation appears to be associated with 100% mortality, emphasizing the importance of prevention and early clinical recognition.

Clinical Examination

Middle-aged, male dogs are most often affected, usually within 5 to 7 days of surgery. Depression, anorexia, emesis, abdominal pain, constipation, melena, and fever are the most important clinical signs. Many of these signs are subtle and easily missed by some pet owners. The immunosuppressive properties of glucocorticoids may mask the initial signs of peritonitis associated with colonic perforation.

Diagnosis

If suspected, patients at risk should be carefully evaluated for perforation and peritonitis. Imaging studies (radiography and ultrasonography), abdominocentesis, peritoneal lavage, and exploratory surgery, if indicated, should be considered in patients at risk.

Treatment

Patients with colonic ulcer, perforation, and peritonitis should be explored immediately. Therapy should be aimed at excision of the ulcer, anastomosis of healthy bowel segments, lavage of the peritoneal cavity, open peritoneal drainage (if indicated), and postoperative antibiotics.

Prognosis

Colonic ulcer and perforation is generally associated with a poor prognosis. A preventive approach to this complication appears to be warranted in high-risk patients: (1) use of less-potent glucocorticoids (e.g., prednisone, prednisolone) instead of dexamethasone, (2) limited or no use of glucocorticoids.

SURGERY

Indications

In dogs the most frequent indication for colonic and rectal surgery is either neoplastic disease or rectal prolapse. Other conditions, including cecal neoplasia, cecocolic volvulus, colonic entrapment, congenital anomalies, traumatic perforation, and perforation associated with intervertebral disc disease and corticosteroid treatment are less common indications for large intestinal surgery.[283] The most frequent indications for colonic surgery in cats is intractable megacolon.

Preoperative Considerations

In dogs with rectal or colonic tumors, appropriate staging is vital to determine the extent of local and systemic disease. In many cases, a careful digital rectal examination can delineate the extent of local disease in the rectum and provide subjective information on the enlargement of regional lymph nodes. Thoracic radiographs are made to rule out pulmonary metastatic disease. Abdominal ultrasonography is used to rule out abdominal metastatic disease and to guide aspiration and biopsy of enlarged iliac lymph nodes. Proctoscopy and colonoscopy show the local extent of neoplastic disease. It is vital that the entire colon be assessed with colonoscopy even after a rectal tumor has been identified, because additional neoplasms are reported in the colon in a percentage of these cases.[235,284] Preparation for evaluation and biopsy of the rectum and colon is performed using an orally administered GI lavage solution.[60,61]

Animals with anal or rectal prolapse are carefully examined to determine the underlying cause of tenesmus. In younger animals, parasitism is the most frequent predisposing cause identified. In older animals, tumors, colitis, urolithiasis, dystocia, and perineal herniation have all been associated with rectal prolapse.[284,285]

Mechanical cleansing is recommended before surgery of the large intestine in humans.[286] However, in cats undergoing surgery for megacolon, preoperative enemas are probably unwarranted because they create a liquid slurry that oozes through noncrushing clamps and contaminates the surgical field. Instead, the dry, hard feces associated with chronic constipation can easily be manipulated into the segment of colon to be resected and then removed. Preoperative enemas are contraindicated in cases of suspected large intestinal perforation.

Perioperative antibiotics are administered to minimize the chance of surgical infection. Randomized, controlled clinical trials of antimicrobial prophylaxis in canine and feline colonic surgery have not been conducted. However, based on human trials,[287] antibiotics effective against aerobes and especially the anaerobes that predominate in the large intestine are administered intravenously once at the beginning of surgery. Antibiotics are not administered again unless either contamination occurs at surgery or the procedure takes longer than 2 hours. In the latter case a second intravenous dose of antibiotics is administered. Antibiotics are continued postoperatively in cases with preoperative or surgical contamination based on the results of operative culture and sensitivity testing.

Surgical Considerations

In animals requiring surgery for cecal or colonic disease, a ventral midline laparotomy is performed. After conducting a thorough abdominal exploration for concurrent or metastatic disease, the affected area of the large intestine is packed off with moistened laparotomy sponges. Resection of the cecum can be performed with or without preservation of the ileocolic junction, depending on the extent of the local disease. In most cases of cecal neoplasia a complete resection and jejuno- or ileocolonic anastomosis is performed to ensure adequate tumor removal.

Subtotal colectomy is an effective treatment for feline idopathic megacolon or megacolon secondary to the mechanical obstruction created by old, healed pelvic fractures. Recommendations for removal of the ileocolic valve and ileum vary in cats with megacolon. The ileocolic blood vessels tether the distal ileum and proximal ascending colon, preventing anastomosis to the distal colon; therefore if a complete colectomy is performed, these vessels must be sacrificed. This necessitates removing the ileum, which has important normal functions in water, vitamin B_{12}, and bile salt resorption, and performing a jejunocolonic anastomosis. In spite of this concern, postoperative intestinal function was normal in four cats evaluated after subtotal colectomy and jejunocolonic anastomosis.[279] The ileocolic valve also minimizes colonic bacterial access to the small intestine,[288] so preservation of the valve would be ideal to minimize small intestinal bacterial overgrowth and deconjugation of bile salts. However, preservation of the ileocolic junction necessitates leaving several centimeters of the ascending colon to ensure a tension-free anastomosis, possibly predisposing these cats to recurrent constipation. To evaluate these concerns, cats with megacolon treated with colectomy were studied retrospectively. Cats with excision of the ileocolic junction had significantly looser stool on long-term follow-up.[289] However, there was no difference in the incidence of constipation between cats with preservation versus excision of the ileocolic junction.[289] This is perhaps explained by in vitro experiments with ascending and descending colonic smooth muscle from cats with clinical megacolon showing that smooth muscle dysfunction is less severe in the ascending colon.[254]

When the ileocolic junction is preserved, the ascending colon is transected approximately 3 cm distal to the ileocolic junction to ensure a tension-free anastomosis. An end-to-end colocolostomy is performed using single interrupted sutures of 4/0 polydioxanone.[283] The omentum is wrapped around the anastomotic site and the abdomen is thoroughly lavaged with a warm, balanced electrolyte solution. All lavage fluid is aspirated from the peritoneal cavity before the incision is closed.

Prior to surgery, rectal prolapse must be differentiated from a prolapsed intussusception of intestine or colon. A well-lubricated, blunt instrument is passed between the anus and the prolapsed tissue. In animals with a prolapsed intussusception, the probe passes easily. Conversely, in animals with a simple rectal prolapse, the probe cannot pass because the prolapsed tissue joins the mucocutaneous junction of the anus.[284] The viability of the prolapsed tissue is assessed based on gross appearance, color, and bleeding. In cases of simple prolapse where the tissue is healthy, the prolapse is digitally reduced and a purse string suture is inserted in the mucocutaneous junction of the anus, avoiding the anal sacs and the anal sac ducts. The suture is tightened sufficiently to prevent prolapse while leaving a small orifice for the passage of soft feces. The suture is removed after several days and the animals carefully observed for recurrence of the prolapse. In cases of recurrent or substantial prolapse where the rectal tissue is still healthy, a colopexy is performed. Rectal resection is performed in animals with traumatized, necrotic, or irreducible rectal prolapse. The reader is referred elsewhere for the details of these procedures.[284]

Various techniques and surgical approaches have been described for removal of rectal tumors.[284] The approach and technique vary with the extent and location of the mass or masses. Tumors in the proximal rectum may be accessed by a ventral midline laparotomy combined with a pelvic osteotomy. Healing of the distal colon, the proximal rectum, or both is complicated by the poor blood supply to this area of the large intestine.[290] A dorsal approach has been described for tumors involving the middle third of the rectum,[284,291] however, many tumors in this area are also amenable to resection via a rectal pull-through.[284,292] The plexus of pelvic nerves at the peritoneal reflection is vital to postoperative fecal continence. In an experimental study on healthy dogs, transection alone or resection of 4 cm of rectum via a dorsal approach resulted in fecally continent dogs. Resection of 6 cm of the rectum, including the peritoneal reflection, caused fecal incontinence.[291] This limitation on resection is problematic in animals with larger rectal tumors, as a 2 cm gross margin is recommended on both sides of the tumor.[284]

Postoperative Considerations

Postoperative treatment depends largely on the underlying reason for cecal, colonic, or rectal surgery. Pre- or postoperative epidural anesthesia using a combination of local anesthetic and narcotic provides effective pain relief. Animals receiving epidural anesthesia may not be able to urinate normally for 12 to 24 hours; hence bladder size must be evaluated frequently and the bladder gently expressed or catheterized if needed. Narcotics, mixed narcotic agonists and antagonists, partial mu opioid agonists, and COX-II inhibitory class NSAIDS are alternatives for pain management in dogs. Mixed narcotic agonists and antagonists are effective in cats.

Cats recovering from colectomy are maintained on intravenous fluids until they commence eating and drinking. Electrolytes are supplemented if necessary. Bowel movements may be soft or loose and more frequent than normal. A highly digestible, low residue diet is fed. In cats with profuse postoperative diarrhea in which small intestinal bacterial overgrowth is suspected, a short course of antibiotics is administered.

Adequate nutrition is vital for dogs and cats recovering from large intestinal surgery. Early feeding increases anastomosis strength and promotes enteric epithelial proliferation and function.[293,294] Ideally, the diet should provide a source of soluble fiber which, when hydrolyzed to SCFAs, stimulates colonic mucosal proliferation.[293] In animals with fecal continence difficulties after extensive rectal resection, a low-residue diet is fed twice daily. The animal is then walked for 20 to 30 minutes after eating. In many cases the gastrocolic reflex will result in defecation and near complete emptying of the colon during this time, minimizing subsequent fecal soiling in the house.

CHAPTER • 224

Rectoanal Disease

Debra L. Zoran

The storage and voluntary evacuation of feces are under the control of the muscles and nerves serving the pelvic canal, rectum, and anus. These elimination functions are controlled by complex interactions involving smooth muscles, striated muscles, and the intrinsic and extrinsic neurons that innervate them. The ability to retain fecal content, to perceive that the rectum is full, and to determine appropriate defecation is called *fecal continence*. Abnormal function of these muscles or nerves results in loss of fecal continence or constipation but rarely leads to hematochezia or mucoid diarrhea. Alternatively, inflammatory disorders of the rectal mucosa result in tenesmus, increased fecal mucus, hematochezia, or frequent defecation. In dogs with severe rectal inflammatory disease, fecal incontinence may occur secondary to reservoir function failure. Even though many of these conditions are not as serious as other diseases of the gastrointestinal (GI) tract, their social impact makes them a significant influence on the human-animal bond and on the owners' willingness to manage their pet's condition.

ANATOMY

The rectum, anal canal, internal and external anal sphincters, muscles of the pelvic canal, and the skin and subcutaneous structures of the perianal region make up the anorectum (Figure 224-1).[1] The rectum originates at the pelvic inlet, a continuation of the distal colon, and ends at the anal canal.[1] The rectal muscularis layer includes the longitudinal muscles, which are continuous with the muscularis layers of the colon, and the inner circular muscle layer. The two layers, which provide tone and structural support for the rectal mucosa and

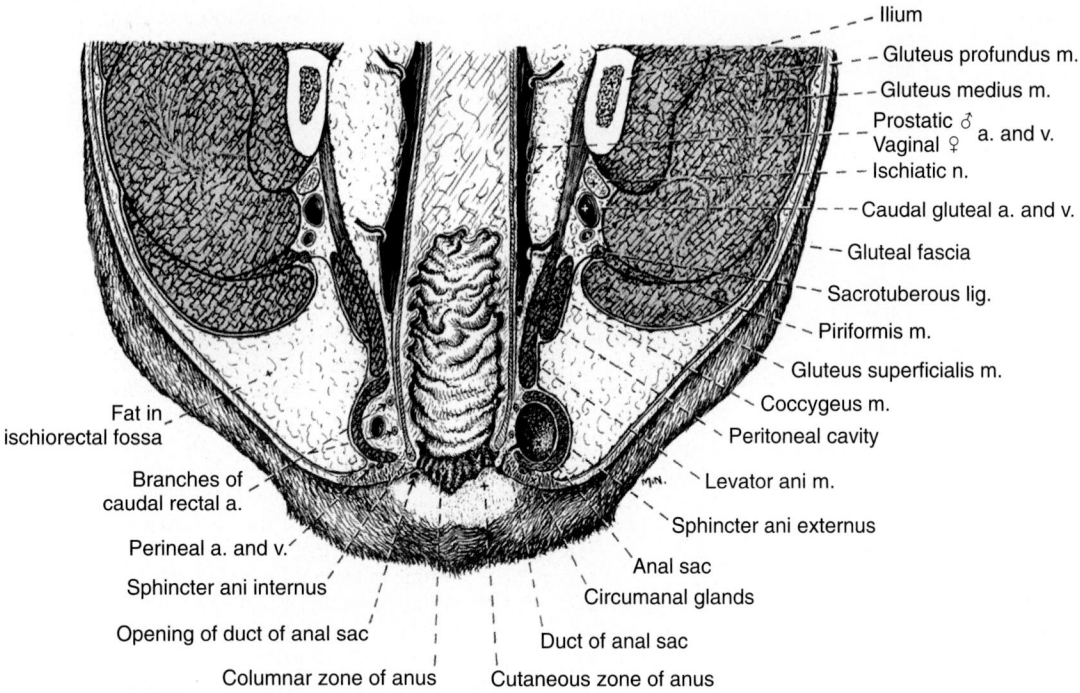

Ilium
Gluteus profundus m.
Gluteus medius m.
Prostatic ♂
Vaginal ♀ a. and v.
Ischiatic n.
Caudal gluteal a. and v.
Gluteal fascia
Sacrotuberous lig.
Piriformis m.
Gluteus superficialis m.
Coccygeus m.
Peritoneal cavity
Levator ani m.
Sphincter ani externus
Anal sac
Circumanal glands
Duct of anal sac
Cutaneous zone of anus

Fat in ischiorectal fossa
Branches of caudal rectal a.
Perineal a. and v.
Sphincter ani internus
Opening of duct of anal sac
Columnar zone of anus

Figure 224-1 Cross section through the anorectum of a dog. (From Evans HE: Miller's Anatomy of the Dog, 3rd ed. Philadelphia, WB Saunders, 1993.)

submucosa, are controlled and supported by the myenteric plexus neurons and the caudal rectal arteries, respectively.[2] The rectal mucosa contains columnar epithelium rich in goblet cells and numerous solitary lymph follicles. The secretion of mucus from goblet cells is regulated by a submucosal neuronal plexus in the rectal mucosa.[2] Inflammation of the mucosa causes stimulation of this neuronal plexus, resulting in the clinical signs of anorectal disease (e.g., mucoid feces, hematochezia, tenesmus, and dyschezia). As with Peyer's patches in the small intestine, these lymph follicles can be visualized endoscopically as either raised or punctuate depressions in the rectal mucosa. At the junction of the rectum and anus, the mucosal epithelium transitions to squamous epithelium. This transition point defines the junction of the rectum and the internal and external anal sphincters.

The short anal canal extends from the rectum to the anal opening and forms the terminal opening of the alimentary canal. The involuntary smooth muscle of the internal anal sphincter and striated skeletal muscle of the voluntary external anal sphincter surround the anal canal and determine its function. The mucosa of the anal canal is divided into three zones, the columnar, intermediate, and cutaneous zones.[2] The columnar zone connects the rectum to the anus and is composed of longitudinal ridges of columnar mucosa. The intermediate zone is the transition area between the columnar mucosa and the stratified squamous epithelium that makes up the cutaneous zone. The cutaneous zone is the most caudal portion of the anus and is subdivided into two regions. The innermost region contains the paired anal sacs, which lie ventrolateral to the anus, and the termination of the anal sac ducts.[2] The outermost region is keratinized and hairless and peripheral to the anus itself. The anal opening is formed by the plane that separates the two cutaneous zones. The anal sacs contain coiled, apocrine, sudoriparous glands and a few sebaceous glands.[2,3] The secretions from these glands, which are serous to pasty in composition, accumulate in the anal

sacs, along with desquamated epithelium and bacteria. Anal sacs are of clinical importance because they may become impacted with secretions, which often causes discomfort and sometimes leads to infection or abscessation.

Two other types of glands present in the anal area. *Circumanal (hepatoid) glands* are nonsecretory, subcutaneous sebaceous glands in the anal subcutaneous zone.[2,3] These glands may become clinically important in intact male dogs, because they grow throughout life and form adenomas late in life as a result of constant androgen exposure. The *anal glands* are tubuloalveolar sweat glands located craniolateral to the circumanal glands.[2,3] The anal glands produce a fatty secretion, the function of which is unknown. The ducts from these glands open in the intermediate zone of the anus.

The innervation of the anorectum is similar to that of the colon in that it comprises a well-defined enteric nervous system consisting of a myenteric and a submucosal plexus.[2] This segment of the autonomic nervous system controls the many sensory, integrative, and motor neurons that characterize the functions of the rectum and anus (Figure 224-2).[1] In particular, these neurons control the secretions of goblet cells and integrate movements of the colon and rectum to ensure appropriate storage and transport of feces. The innervation of the anus is more complex. The pelvic plexus, specifically the sacral nerve branches of the pelvic nerve, provides parasympathetic fibers that are excitatory to the rectum and inhibitory to the internal anal sphincter.[2,4] Conversely, the sympathetic fibers that arise from the hypogastric nerves of the caudal mesenteric ganglion are inhibitory to the rectum (i.e., cause relaxation) and excitatory to the internal anal sphincter (i.e., cause contraction), thus allowing appropriate storage of feces.[2,4]

Relaxation of the internal and external anal sphincters in conjunction with rectal contraction permits defecation. The external anal sphincter is a striated muscle with several muscle bundles that surround the internal sphincter. These muscles are reflexively able to increase anal sphincter pressure, mediated

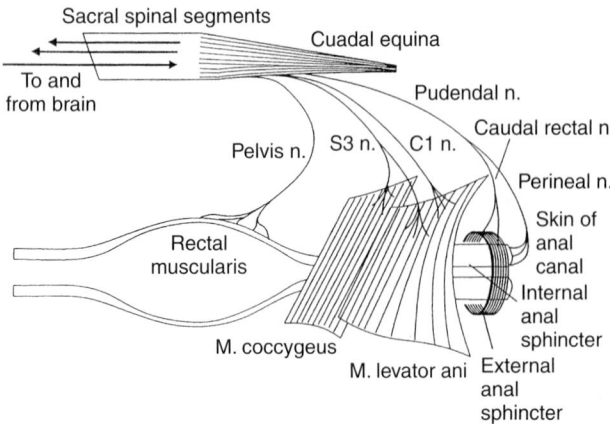

Figure 224-2 Neural control of defecation. (From Strombeck DR, Guilford WG: Small Animal Gastroenterology, 2nd ed. Davis, California, Stonegate Publishing, 1990.)

via somatic nerve fibers in the anal branch of the pudendal nerve, while still allowing accommodation of feces in the rectum.[2,4] A properly functioning external anal sphincter allows maximal distention (e.g., storage of feces in the rectum) while maintaining anal control. When the pudendal nerve is damaged, the external anal sphincter is incompetent, and clinically apparent fecal incontinence develops.

The pelvic diaphragm constitutes the final aspect of anatomic control of anorectal function. These muscles support the rectal and anal canal and participate in the maintenance of fecal continence and appropriate defecation by providing structural support and additional muscular control. The muscles that participate in this activity include the right and left ventral sacrococcygeal muscles and the levator ani.[2] The sacrococcygeal muscles originate on either side of the rectum and attach dorsally to the base of the tail (see Figure 224-1).[1] These smooth muscles, which are innervated by the pelvic plexus, shorten the rectum during defecation, assisting in the evacuation of feces. The levator ani muscles are striated muscles (innervated by the sacral and caudal nerves) that surround the rectum and assist in compression of the rectum during defecation.[2]

PHYSIOLOGY OF DEFECATION

Normal anorectal function and the act of defecation are primarily pressure-based functions that rely heavily on complex interactions between peripheral pressure receptors, myenteric neurons, somatic and autonomic afferent nerve fibers, spinal cord, brain stem, somatic and autonomic efferent nerve fibers, and smooth and striated muscle of the rectum and anal sphincters[1,5-7] (see Figure 224-2). When the rectum is empty, intraluminal rectal pressure is low. Increased intraluminal pressure is the primary component of maintenance of fecal continence; it is generated by contraction of the internal anal sphincter, either in response to a sudden increase in intra-abdominal pressure (e.g., coughing or sneezing) or by an increase in rectal filling.[1,5] The main stimulus for defecation is increased pressure in the rectum caused by distention. The rectoanal inhibition reflex allows relaxation of the internal anal sphincter, along with contractions of the external anal sphincter, to allow slow but continuous filling of the rectum.[1,5,8] As the fecal volume increases in the rectum, conscious awareness of rectal filling is perceived by means of sensory signaling of information transmitted via sacral afferent fibers to the cerebral cortex.[4,6,9] The rectoanal inhibition reflex allows

continued filling of the rectum until defecation is appropriate. If the volume of feces remains small (and stretch is minimal) or if defecation is not appropriate, the internal anal sphincter returns to a state of contraction, resulting in propulsion of feces back into the colon. This activity is also stimulated by descending inputs from motoneurons in the sacral spinal cord and pudendal nerve that mediate voluntary contraction of the external anal sphincter and levator ani.[4,6,9,10] This back-and-forth process is repeated until the volume of feces is sufficient both to initiate rectal distention and to come into contact with the anal mucosa, resulting in a stronger urge to defecate.

When defecation is initiated, distention of the rectum activates parasympathetic efferents that control contraction of colonic smooth muscle (resulting in mass movement of the distal colon) and inhibition of the external anal sphincter and pelvic muscles (resulting in relaxation of the sphincters).[11-13] The rectum itself produces only small contractions that are not propulsive, therefore the main propulsive force for expelling feces from the body is the contraction of colonic smooth muscles. Thus the rectum serves primarily as a conduit during the process of defecation and as a storage depot in the periods between. Defecation is facilitated by proper posture and generation of increased abdominal pressure (closure of the glottis, fixation of the diaphragm, and contraction of the abdominal wall muscles).[2,5,12,13] Conscious suppression of defecation is facilitated by descending impulses to sacral nerves and the pudendal nerve, which mediate contraction of the levator ani and external anal sphincter, resulting in maintenance of fecal continence.[9,12,13]

HISTORY AND PHYSICAL EXAMINATION

The close association of the anorectum and colon results in similar clinical signs of disease for these two components and creates difficulty in localizing signs to a specific region of the lower GI tract. A careful history and complete physical examination are required to determine whether tenesmus and dyschezia are the result of colonic disease or of anorectal disease alone. In general, diseases of the anorectum are either inflammatory (with signs of hematochezia, tenesmus, mucoid feces, or dyschezia predominating) or they result in altered motility (e.g., constipation or fecal incontinence). It is unusual for systemic signs, such as anorexia, weight loss, vomiting, or diarrhea, to occur in animals with rectoanal disease; their occurrence suggests concurrent systemic disease or disorders in other segments of the GI tract.

The physical examination of the perineum should always include careful visual inspection for evidence of inflammation, swelling, tumor masses, herniation, rectoanal prolapse, or fistulas. After the visual inspection a digital examination should be performed, including palpation of the anal sphincter tone, the pelvic diaphragmatic musculature, and the size and expressibility of the anal sacs; determination of the diameter of the rectal lumen; and tactile examination of the texture, regularity, and surface of the mucosa. Other structures that should be palpated are the prostate in males, the vaginal vault in females, and the pelvic urethra. In pets with severe inflammation of the anorectum, digital palpation may be impossible without sedation or complete anesthesia. In general, cats should be sedated prior to rectoanal palpation to prevent patient or operator injury.

Hematochezia, blood dripping from the anus, or excess mucus with normally formed feces is often a good indicator of rectoanal disease, especially inflammatory diseases such as proctitis, perianal fistulas, anal sacculitis, polyps, or neoplasia. Tenesmus is a hallmark of both anorectal and colonic disease and must be differentiated from *dyschezia* (painful defecation), which is much more typical of diseases of the anorectum.

Box • 224-1

Causes of Tenesmus and Dyschezia

Colorectal Disease
Constipation
Colitis-proctitis
 Inflammatory bowel disease
 Histoplasma capsulatum (histoplasmosis)
 Clostridium perfringens (enterotoxicosis)
 Prototheca zopfii (prototothecosis)
Rectal stricture
Neoplasia—polyps
Foreign material
Irritable bowel syndrome

Perineal-Perianal Disease
Anal sacculitis, impaction, or abscess
Anal sac neoplasia
Perianal fistula
Perineal hernia

Urogenital Disease
Cystitis-urethritis-vaginitis
Cystitis—urethral calculi
Prostatitis—prostatic abscess
Parturition
Neoplasia of the urethra, bladder, prostate, or vagina

Miscellaneous Causes
Caudal abdominal cavity mass
Pelvic fracture—neoplasia

Both conditions are typically associated with inflammatory diseases of the colon or anorectum; they result in increased frequency and urgency of defecation and straining during defecation (Box 224-1).[14] Because many owners may confuse the signs of dyschezia and tenesmus, it is often necessary to observe the animal during the act of defecation. Furthermore, owners often are unable to determine whether straining is associated with defecation or urination, therefore urogenital disease must be considered until the clinical signs can be localized.

In most cases of anorectal disease, routine hematology and biochemical tests are seldom helpful for identifying a specific diagnosis. However, they are important in the identification of concurrent or complicating conditions that may influence further diagnostic tests or therapy, especially in older animals. In any animal with an abnormal fecal stream, multiple fecal flotations, cytologic examination of feces, and specific tests for infectious causes of GI disease (e.g., enzyme-linked immunosorbent assay [ELISA] for clostridial toxin, *Giardia* spp., cryptosporidia, and viruses) are strongly recommended. The most common parasitic cause of tenesmus and hematochezia in dogs is *Trichuris vulpis* (whipworm) infection, and because of the pattern of intermittent shedding, empirical anthelmintic therapy is recommended even in the absence of identification of ova in feces.

In dogs and cats with acute onset of hematochezia and tenesmus, dietary therapy using high-fiber diets is a reasonable initial therapeutic approach. If further diagnostic evaluation is deemed necessary, specific imaging techniques directed toward assessment of the anorectum are indicated. Imaging of the anorectum by conventional means (e.g., abdominal radiography and ultrasonography) is generally unrewarding for most cases of anorectal disease. However, these modalities can be helpful for identifying some causes of colonic disease (e.g., neoplasia, infiltrative disease, constipation, or foreign bodies) that may have a similar clinical presentation. Intrarectal ultrasonography can help the examiner to determine the extent of intraluminal or intramural tumor involvement and to evaluate pararectal structures. However, ultrasound units with these probes are not universally available. Contrast radiography is rarely helpful in the diagnosis of anorectal disease, because most rectal strictures, polyps, or hernias can be either palpated or observed during proctoscopic examination. However, in dogs with severe rectal strictures or tumors that obstruct passage of a colonoscope or proctoscope, this technique may provide the examiner with additional information.

In general, rigid proctoscopy, with or without colonoscopy, is the diagnostic tool of choice for examination, biopsy and, in some cases, treatment of rectoanal disease. Proctoscopy is technically less difficult, and the instrumentation is less expensive, than that required for flexible colonoscopy. With either a proctoscope or colonoscope, the rectal mucosa can be visualized for color, texture, friability, masses, and bleeding, and biopsies of the colonic or rectal mucosa can be readily obtained. Furthermore, any lesions of the terminal rectum (e.g., polyps) that are identified can often be directly visualized by gently prolapsing the rectum and anus using tissue forceps. This technique also allows surgical removal of small polyps or masses.

DISEASES OF THE RECTUM

Perineal Hernia

Perineal hernias have been clinically recognized in the dog for more than 100 years and are most common in older, intact male dogs.[15,16] They are rarely seen in cats or female dogs.[17] Four types of perineal hernias have been described, but the most common type is the caudoventral perineal hernia, which occurs between the levator ani, external anal sphincter, and internal obturator muscles.[18,19] Sciatic hernias occur between the sacrotuberous ligament and the coccygeus muscle, dorsal hernias occur between the levator ani and coccygeus muscles, and ventral hernias occur between the levator ani and ischiourethralis or ischiocavernosus muscles.[19] Most perineal hernias are unilateral, although bilateral herniation can occur, with the right side being predisposed.[15,16] Herniation may involve only rectal tissues, but eventually prolapse of pelvic organs, such as the urinary bladder, prostate, or other abdominal tissues (e.g., fat, intestine), into the weakened area can occur. In dogs, neurogenic atrophy of the levator ani muscles, gender-based variations in pelvic muscle anatomy, and gonadal hormonal influence are all thought to be factors in the development of perineal hernias.[19] The degree of stretching and deviation of the rectal wall and the presence or absence of abdominal organs in the hernia are all factors that determine clinical signs.

History and Physical Examination

In more than 90% of affected dogs, perineal swelling and tenesmus are the most common clinical signs[15,18,19]; however, constipation, dyschezia, and hematochezia are also reported. Dysuria and stranguria accompany the signs of rectoanal disease if the bladder is retroflexed and trapped in the ischiorectal fossa. With longstanding bladder entrapment, azotemia and signs of renal failure (e.g., anorexia, vomiting) also occur. Less commonly, persistent dribbling of urine or other signs of urinary incontinence may be present instead of signs of urinary obstruction. In cats with perineal herniation, concurrent

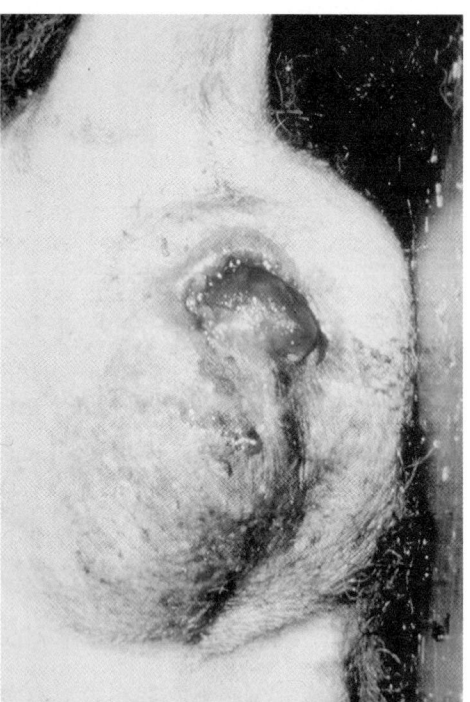

Figure 224-3 Perineal swelling in an 8-year-old dog with a perineal hernia.

severe obstipation or megacolon is the most common predisposing factor.[17] The physical examination often reveals a visible perineal swelling or a reducible perineal swelling (Figure 224-3). External palpation of a defect in the musculature just lateral to the external anal sphincter is often sufficient for confirmation of the hernia. However, in some pets the hernia is palpated rectally only as a defect in the pelvic diaphragm. A digital examination can also be performed to detect any other rectal wall abnormalities (e.g., deviation, sacculation, or diverticulum). In general, the combination of historical and physical examination findings is sufficient to confirm the diagnosis of perineal hernia. Further evaluation, either with ultrasonography or contrast studies, may be necessary to determine the extent of hernia contents (e.g., the presence of intestine, bladder, or prostate) prior to repair. The major differential diagnoses are rectal diverticulum, neoplasia, prostatic or paraprostatic cyst, and seroma/hematoma.

Pathogenesis
The pathogenesis of perineal hernias is not completely understood. Because most patients are older male dogs, gonadal hormonal influences have been strongly suggested. The evidence supporting this idea derives from the fact that castrated dogs are rarely affected with perineal hernia; however, no difference in the levels of testosterone and estrogen 17-beta have been found between normal dogs and dogs with perineal hernia.[20] Some have suggested that, rather than hormone concentrations, the number or affinity of hormone receptors may be the important factor in the development of perianal muscle weakness.[21] Another potential factor is that in male dogs, the levator ani muscles are weaker and thinner and have a weaker attachment to the external anal sphincter.[18,22,23] The fact that brachycephalic breeds (e.g., Boston terrier, boxer, Welsh corgi, and Pekinese) appear to be predisposed to the development of perineal hernias suggests that an anatomic or breed-specific defect is important.[19] Evidence against a strictly hormonal cause for hernia development is the fact that in cats,

the benefits of castration have not been demonstrated, a finding illustrated by a retrospective study in which 19 of 20 cats with perineal hernias had been either castrated or spayed.[17]

Aside from anatomic and hormonal theories, another factor considered important in disease development is damage to the pudendal nerve or to the first, second, or third sacral nerves, which results in neurogenic atrophy of the levator ani muscles.[23] However, it is not known whether damage precedes development or occurs as a result of the hernia.

In addition to primary predisposing factors, perineal hernias in dogs may occur secondary to persistent tenesmus and constipation, which results in muscular weakness in the pelvic floor[15,16] or may occur as a result of severe prostatic disease or paraprostatic cysts.[24] In cats, perineal hernias most commonly occur secondary to constipation resulting from megacolon.[17] Other factors associated with perineal hernias in cats are perianal masses, chronic fibrosing colitis, and previous perineal urethrostomy.[17]

Therapy
Definitive surgical repair (perineal herniorrhaphy) is the treatment of choice in most instances. The primary aim of the surgical repair is to replace muscular support of the pelvic diaphragm. Preoperative preparations may include preanesthetic blood work, electrocardiography, abdominal ultrasound, and chest radiographs if indicated to rule out complicating factors for anesthesia or secondary causes of hernia formation. Stool softeners (e.g., lactulose) and a highly digestible diet (i.e., to reduce fecal volume) should be initiated several days before surgery.[19] If the bladder is retroflexed and trapped within the hernia, catheterization should be attempted immediately. If this is unsuccessful, the bladder should be emptied by cystocentesis; then, with the bladder decompressed, the hernia is reduced and the bladder is pushed back into the abdominal cavity if possible.

Regardless of whether the bladder is properly repositioned, a transurethral Foley urinary catheter should be placed and a closed collection system should be attached until surgery can be performed. Urine cultures should be obtained and appropriate antibiotics administered for all animals with perineal hernia involving bladder entrapment. Preoperative antibiotics (e.g., cefoxitin used as a single agent) are recommended for protection against contamination by enteric coliforms.

Several techniques for perineal hernia repair have been reported, including standard herniorrhaphy, transposition of the superficial gluteal muscle, an internal obturator transposition technique, a combination of the gluteal and obturator muscle transpositions, and a special technique in which small intestinal submucosa is used to repair the defect.[19,25-28] The reader is referred to a surgical text for a detailed description of the specific surgical techniques used in herniorrhaphy. Traditional hernia repair involves closure of the triangular area formed by the external anal sphincter, levator ani, coccygeus, and obturator muscles. However, with this method of repair, the rate of hernia recurrence is high (10% to 45%), and postoperative complications are common.[27]

The current standard for repair is the obturator transposition technique because of its much lower rate of recurrence and lower complication rate. The use of porcine small intestinal submucosa as a biomaterial for perineal herniorrhaphy is relatively new and has shown promise both as a primary means of repair and as an augmentation technique when the internal obturator muscle is weak or when a salvage procedure is required.[19,28] Other surgical procedures that may be required in the repair of this disorder include repair of diverticuli or rectal deviations, removal of prostatic cysts and, in cats with megacolon, a subtotal colectomy. Castration is recommended but is not an essential aspect of treatment, especially if the length of the procedure increases the risk for an older dog.

After surgery, a highly digestible (low residue) diet and stool softeners should be provided indefinitely to prevent straining and recurrence. Local perineal swelling is common and resolves with application of hot compresses. In dogs for which surgical repair is not possible, the treatment approach is to reduce fecal volume, impaction, and straining by feeding a low-residue diet and administering stool softeners, laxatives (e.g., lactulose), and enemas as needed. In most cases, dietary and conservative management of hernias is not rewarding in the long term.

Prognosis

In general, the prognosis for long-term repair of perineal hernias is guarded. The rates of recurrence are related to the type of surgical repair done and the skill of the surgeon. Most surgeons agree that the obturator transposition technique, combined with one of the other approaches, is the best surgical option currently available.[19,26,28] However, the more severe the preoperative clinical signs, the longer the signs have been present, and the existence of bilateral involvement all increase the likelihood of a higher recurrence rate, regardless of the technique used. Other postoperative complications include infection, seroma or hematoma formation, fecal incontinence, rectal prolapse (especially if a bilateral repair is required), sciatic nerve paralysis or sciatic pain, and urinary complications, including incontinence or obstruction (caused by sutures in or scarring of the urethra).[18,19]

Rectal Tumors

Tumors of the intestine, which are uncommon in dogs and cats, represent fewer than 1% of all malignancies reported.[29] In dogs, rectal or colonic adenocarcinoma is the most common malignant intestinal tumor, whereas adenomatous polyps of the rectum are the most common benign tumor.[29] Lymphoma is the most common intestinal tumor of cats, and although it occurs more frequently in the small intestine, colorectal lymphoma is the most common large bowel tumor of cats.[29] Lymphosarcoma of the rectum is less common in dogs than in cats, but it is more prevalent than colonic lymphosarcoma. Siamese cats are reported to have a higher incidence of intestinal (including colonic) adenocarcinoma, but in one study, domestic shorthair cats had a higher frequency of rectal adenocarcinoma than Siamese cats.[29,30] Other rectal tumor types that have been reported include leiomyoma, leiomyosarcoma, plasmacytoma, and fibrosarcoma.[29-33] Polyps that occur in the rectum are generally focal, pedunculated, or sessile and rarely metastasize, although they can in some instances invade locally into the lamina propria and submucosa.[1,29,34] In dogs, locally invasive polyps, although histologically benign, are referred to as *carcinoma in situ*.[29]

History and Physical Examination

The signalment of dogs and cats affected with rectal tumors is typical in that older dogs (mean, 9 years of age) and cats (mean, 10 years of age) are more likely to be affected.[29] In dogs the incidence is higher in males, whereas in cats the opposite is true.[29,35] Breeds predisposed to the development of intestinal cancers include boxers, collies, and German shepherds, and this appears to be true for rectal tumors as well.[29] The clinical signs seen in animals with rectal tumors include hematochezia, mucoid feces, tenesmus, and dyschezia of varying severity. Other clinical signs may be observed (e.g., weight loss, inappetence), depending on the tumor type, location, and behavior.

A digital rectal examination may reveal a prominent mucosal mass, narrowing of the rectal lumen, pain during the examination, or blood on the gloved finger. Rectal adenocarcinomas may have either a prominent mass or a stenotic annular ring lesion that encircles the rectum. If significant obstruction is present, colonic distention may be detected on abdominal palpation due to persistent constipation or incomplete evacuation of the bowel. Conversely, in animals with persistent straining, rectal prolapse may occur.

Diagnosis

Palpation of a rectal mass or annular ring stricture in a dog or cat with a typical signalment and clinical signs is often suggestive; however, biopsy of the affected tissue, either using proctoscopy or by direct visualization, is necessary to make the definitive diagnosis. In most cases a mucosal tissue biopsy is adequate for analysis; however, in some submucosal tumors (e.g., lymphosarcoma, leiomyosarcoma), an excisional biopsy or collection of deeper tissues is required. Radiography and ultrasound examination of the region and drainage of lymph nodes are very helpful for defining the depth of the lesion and staging the extent of metastasis.

Therapy

For all tumors of the rectum except lymphosarcoma, surgical excision of the cancer is the recommended initial course of action, because this provides patient relief and debulks the tumor mass.[29,35] For dogs with rectal lymphosarcoma, treatment with standard chemotherapy protocols is initiated unless a mass is obstructing the rectum and debulking is necessary.[29]

Radiation therapy, cryosurgery, and laser therapy have all been used to treat colorectal tumors after surgical excision, with variable success.[36-39] Electrosurgery or cryosurgery is recommended for dogs with nonannular masses or polyps that can be easily prolapsed. Full-thickness resection of annular rectal cancers can be attempted, but wound dehiscence, infection, rectal stricture, and fecal incontinence are common complications.

More recently, local excision combined with cryosurgery has been used to extend the life of affected dogs significantly; however, the complication rate (e.g., for strictures, prolapse, and perineal hernia) is still high (82%).[36] As an alternative, high-dose radiotherapy has been reported to be an effective form of treatment for distal rectal adenocarcinomas that can be completely prolapsed through the anal opening. Polyps and carcinoma in situ are generally easily excised or treated with cryosurgery or electrocautery, with good to excellent postsurgical results and few recurrences.[29,34] Preliminary work suggests that treatment of dogs with rectal tubulopapillary polyps using piroxicam is also effective.[40]

Prognosis

The prognosis for rectal polyps, carcinoma in situ, leiomyoma, and fibroma is generally good; postoperative complications are few, and the recurrence rate is low. Adenocarcinoma, lymphosarcoma, and plasmacytomas all tend to recur, and because of their aggressive nature, treatment with surgery or other means may lead to secondary complications.[29] Annular colorectal adenocarcinoma is a particularly aggressive tumor and is often associated with a very poor prognosis (e.g., mean survival of 1 to 2 months) because of the complications of treatment, secondary effects (e.g., constipation), and recurrence (e.g., due to difficulty in removing all of the tumor).[29,39]

Rectal Prolapse

Rectal prolapse is defined as eversion or prolapse of the rectum through the anal opening. A prolapse can be partial or complete; a *partial prolapse* involves a protrusion of the rectal mucosa, whereas a *complete prolapse* involves the entire rectum and may include part of the anus as well.

History and Physical Examination

Rectal prolapse shows no breed, age, or gender predisposition in dogs or cats. However, it is more prevalent in young animals with typhilitis or proctitis secondary to endoparasites.[1] Manx cats with neurologic dysfunction of the anorectum also appear to have a higher predilection for the condition.[19] Other factors that increase tenesmus and are associated with an increased risk of rectal prolapse include rectal polyps or neoplasia, rectal deviation, dystocia, urolithiasis, prostatic disease, and colonic or rectal foreign bodies.[1,19,41] Rectal prolapse has also been reported as a sequela of perineal urethrostomy in the cat.[42] The diagnosis is made by finding the everted, edematous, and hyperemic prolapsed rectal tissue. In longstanding cases of rectal prolapse, the tissues may be ulcerated and necrotic. A complete rectal prolapse typically appears as a cylindrical mass with a depression at the end, which represents the bowel lumen. The mass usually is sensitive or painful to the touch (Figure 224-4).

Diagnosis

Although a diagnosis of rectal prolapse is made by finding the everted rectal tissue on physical examination, the condition must be distinguished from a small or large intestinal intussusception, which can cause similar presenting signs and can have a similar physical appearance. The easiest way to differentiate the two is to pass a well-lubricated, blunt probe between the rectal wall and the prolapsed tissue. With a rectal prolapse, the probe cannot pass between the tissues because the everted rectal tissue converges with the mucocutaneous junction of the anus.[1,14] Intussusception is also typically associated with signs of intestinal obstruction (e.g., vomiting, anorexia),

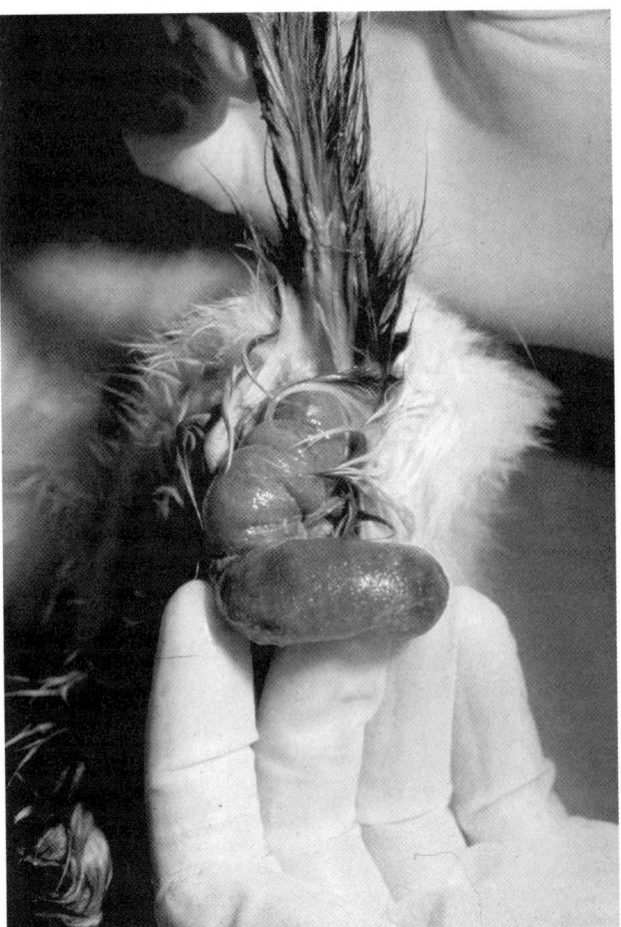

Figure 224-4 Complete rectal prolapse in a cat with colorectal adenocarcinoma and severe tenesmus.

whereas a rectal prolapse is not associated with systemic signs. Anal prolapse must also be distinguished from rectal prolapse; however, in most cases anal prolapse is not associated with a large amount of protruding mucosa and may appear to worsen after defecation. Most cases of anal prolapse are self-limiting and temporary, and the condition frequently occurs secondary to repair of a perianal hernia.

Pathogenesis

Dyschezia and tenesmus are common signs of rectoanal disease, yet concurrent development of rectal prolapse is uncommon. This suggests that an individual predisposition probably contributes to the development of a prolapse; such predispositions may include weakness of the perirectal and perianal connective tissues or musculature or uncoordinated peristaltic contractions of the rectum in association with rectal or anal inflammation.[1,43] However, no carefully conducted studies have been done that further evaluate these possible connections.

Therapy

The first goal of treatment is to identify and eliminate, if possible, any underlying causes of the prolapse. If the prolapsed tissue is healthy and the amount of exposed mucosa is minimal, a conservative treatment approach can be used. This technique involves rehydrating the tissue with a warm isotonic saline solution, followed by application of a water-soluble gel lubricant, gentle massage and manipulation to reduce edema, and gentle but immediate attempts to reduce the prolapsed tissue. If this regimen is successful, a loose purse-string perianal suture (enough to allow passage of soft feces) is placed to prevent recurrence. Postoperative straining can be prevented by administration of a narcotic epidural or topical anesthetic drops. Adjunctive therapy includes feeding a highly digestible diet and administration of a stool softener or laxative for 2 to 3 weeks. The purse-string suture can be removed in 2 to 3 weeks, once the underlying problem has been corrected.

If conservative therapy fails, a colopexy procedure, to fix the rectum and colon in place, is indicated.[43,44] This procedure places a slight amount of cranial traction on the descending colon, because four to six nonabsorbable mattress sutures are placed in the descending colon, which is attached to the left abdominal wall. If the rectal or colonic tissue is devitalized, lacerated, or irreducible, it must be amputated in conjunction with a full-thickness anastomosis of the remaining rectal segments.[43,44] Postoperative management of these animals is the same as the conservative management of rectal prolapse: a purse-string suture is placed to reduce the possibility of recurrence, a low-residue diet is fed to reduce stool volume, and stool softeners are given for 2 to 3 weeks to keep feces soft and able to pass through the purse-string opening.

Prognosis

The prognosis for the first rectal prolapse episode or for animals with a partial prolapse is generally good. Animals with a complete prolapse or recurrence after conservative therapy often require a colopexy and have a guarded to good long-term prognosis. The prognosis for patients that require amputation of the prolapsed tissue is more guarded because of the technical demands of the surgery, the great potential for leakage and infection during the postoperative period, and the increased risk of development of a rectal stricture.[14,43]

Rectal or Anal Stricture

Rectal or anal strictures cause narrowing of the lumen due to scar tissue that forms as a result of rectal inflammation, rectal trauma (from injury or surgery), or proliferative neoplastic disease in the rectum. The clinical picture (e.g., constipation, dyschezia, and, ultimately, vomiting or anorexia) is indistinguishable from that presented by extraluminal narrowing of the colon due to neoplasia, prostatic disease, or pelvic fracture.

History and Physical Examination

The typical history is an older dog that has chronic constipation or progressively more difficulty defecating. Affected dogs have persistent tenesmus, prolonged posturing to defecate, and frequent attempts to defecate, with only a narrow ribbon of feces or no feces produced.[14] If concurrent colorectal inflammatory or neoplastic disease is present, hematochezia, mucoid feces, or diarrhea may be observed. As the duration and severity of the obstruction worsen, other systemic signs may be observed (e.g., lethargy, anorexia, vomiting, weight loss). Several conditions can predispose dogs to the development of a rectal stricture, including recent rectal or anal surgery, chronic rectal or anal inflammation, rectal neoplasia, and ingestion of foreign material that causes rectal trauma as it is passed.

Digital rectal examination is sufficient to identify a narrow and often very tight rectal or anal opening (Figure 224-5). Benign strictures are firm, thick, annular fibrotic bands that must be differentiated from neoplastic strictures, which tend to be asymmetric, masslike formations. However, annular rectal adenocarcinoma cannot be distinguished from a benign fibrotic stricture by palpation alone. The only other physical abnormality found in dogs with rectal stricture is an enlarged colon with hard or impacted feces.

Diagnosis

In most dogs, the history and physical examination are sufficient to identify a stricture. The key aspect of diagnosis is determining whether the stricture is malignant or benign. Radiographs and ultrasound scans of the abdomen and pelvis are important, because they rule out other causes of constipation/obstipation, such as pelvic fractures, prostatomegaly, and abdominal masses that affect the colon or sublumbar lymphadenopathy. Contrast radiography is not usually necessary to make a diagnosis of stricture, but it may be helpful for determining the extent of the stricture if the opening is too narrow for physical analysis. Rectal probe ultrasonography can be used to determine the extent of rectal involvement or to detect other lesions. Ultimately, however, biopsy is necessary to determine whether the lesion is benign or malignant. Biopsy of tissue can be obtained through rigid proctoscopy, flexible endoscopy, or direct visualization by prolapse of the affected rectal tissues. A major limitation on the use of either

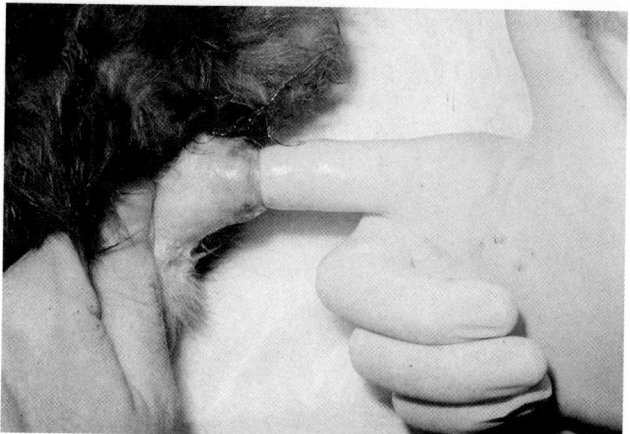

Figure 224-5 Severe rectal stricture identified on digital rectal examination.

a rigid or a flexible scope to obtain biopsy specimens is that passage of the scope and distention of the rectum (for visualization) often is impossible. In such cases, direct prolapse or surgical biopsies must be obtained.

Therapy

Previously, rectal strictures were managed by surgical techniques, such as rectal pull-through or rectal myotomy procedures.[14] More recently, bougienage and balloon dilatation techniques have gained favor, because when performed properly, they are often successful in dilating the stricture site without incurring the severe complications that frequently accompany surgical correction (e.g., fecal incontinence, infection, dehiscence, or restricture).[14] To facilitate appropriate visualization and comfort for these procedures, the dog or cat should be anesthetized, and if possible the procedure should be done with endoscopic or fluoroscopic assistance.

For bougienage of rectal strictures, a metal bougie of increasing size (over several separate but successive procedures) is passed into the stricture site and advanced slowly, stretching the fibrous tissue without causing significant tearing, which tends to increase inflammation and the likelihood of restricture.

Like esophageal strictures, rectal strictures also can be successfully dilated using balloon dilatation techniques, and this approach is frequently preferred over bougienage. The diameter of the balloon and the number of dilatations required to achieve a sustained opening in the rectal lumen are quite variable, but chronic strictures in larger animals may require several procedures to achieve functional success. In general, for small dogs (less than 7 kg) and cats, balloons with a diameter of 10 to 15 mm are used; for medium-sized dogs, the balloon diameter is 20 to 30 mm; and for large dogs (greater than 16 kg), it is 30 to 40 mm.[14] These numbers are guidelines, because animals with severe rectal strictures may require much smaller balloons for the initial procedure to prevent excessive tissue tearing. In dogs with recent strictures or those without excessive fibrosis, one or two dilatation procedures 4 to 5 days apart may be all that is required to dilate the affected tissue successfully. However, when rectal wall thickening is present or the reduction in the lumen is greater than 75%, four to six dilatation procedures may be required to achieve functional success.[14] The purpose of performing multiple procedures several days apart (but no more than 7 days) is to increase the diameter of the stricture waist gradually, without excessive tearing or inflammation; this gradual approach reduces the likelihood of restricture (which tends to occur in 7 to 10 days).[14] Careful visualization of the procedure ensures that tearing and hemorrhage are kept to a minimum and reduces the risk of deep tears or significant hemorrhage, which increase the likelihood of restricture or rectal perforation. Adjunct therapy should include administration of broad-spectrum antibiotics, a highly digestible (low-residue) diet, and use of lactulose or stool softeners to maintain a soft fecal consistency. The use of corticosteroids to reduce the occurrence of restricture has not been studied, and such therapy should be undertaken cautiously if rectal tears or bacterial contamination is suspected.

Prognosis

For most benign rectal strictures, the prognosis is guarded to fair, because balloon procedures may allow return to near normal functionality; however, unless the predisposing cause of the stricture is corrected, it is likely to recur. The risk of severe complications after balloon procedures is lower than for surgical repair techniques, primarily because the risk of inducing fecal incontinence is greatly diminished. The prognosis for all neoplastic strictures is poor, owing both to the difficulty in managing the primary problem and to the poor response to balloon or other management techniques.

DISEASES OF THE ANUS

Atresia Ani

Atresia ani, a congenital condition that affects the anal opening and rectum, may occur in both puppies and kittens. The several anatomic variations of atresia ani have been classified as types I through IV, but all generally result in an abnormal anal outlet and/or rerouting of feces from the rectum to another outlet.[14,45] Pets with type I, or imperforate anus, have a membrane over the anal opening, but the rectum ends as a blind pouch just cranial to the anal opening. Type II is similar to type I, but the rectal pouch ends much more cranial to the anal opening. In type III, or rectal atresia, the rectum ends in a blind pouch in the abdomen (cranial to the pelvis), and the remaining rectum and anus are normal. Type IV, which occurs only in females and may occur with or without imperforate anus, is characterized by a persistent communication between the rectum and vagina (rectovaginal fistula) or urethra (rectourethral fistula).[45]

History and Physical Examination

The clinical signs are often noticed at weaning (4 to 6 weeks) or earlier in affected puppies and kittens. In general, types I, II, and III create similar problems: straining to defecate, bulging of the perineum, absence of feces, no visible anal opening, abdominal distention with palpable fecal material, and abdominal or perineal discomfort.[14] Initially, the puppy or kitten eats and appears to grow, but with increasing fecal distention of the colon, lethargy or restlessness, loss of appetite, and vomiting are noted. Type IV often is associated with tenesmus but is characterized by the passage of small amounts of watery feces via the vagina or urethra, with associated perivulvar erythema and infection.

Diagnosis

The diagnosis is based on finding the typical physical abnormalities in a puppy or kitten of appropriate age that has a concurrent history of tenesmus or lack of ability to defecate normally. For type I or II atresia ani, absence of an anal opening is diagnostic. In type III, radiography or ultrasonography may be helpful for defining the end of the rectal pouch. In type IV, the presence of fecal material exiting through the vaginal opening is suggestive.

Another congenital anomaly that may occur in dogs and cats and that can be confused with atresia ani is anogenital cleft. This condition occurs in females and is characterized by continuity of the mucosa of the anus, rectum, and vagina along the perineal midline.[45] A similar anomaly can occur in male cats resulting from a rectourethral cleft, which is a communication that allows a common opening for the rectum and urethra.

Therapy

The only treatment available is surgical correction, which may require staged procedures, depending on the type of anomaly present. Type I atresia ani is the simplest to correct, because opening of the anus and ballooning of the stricture may be all that is required in some animals. In animals for which this procedure is unsuccessful, the stenotic segment often must be surgically removed. Types II and III require significant and technically demanding surgical procedures to return functionality. In all three circumstances, fecal incontinence is a major and often life-threatening complication. Type IV lesions require technically demanding surgery to close the rectal, vaginal, and urethral defects.

Prognosis

Regardless of the anomaly, young and weak puppies or kittens often do not survive the procedure. In addition, the prognosis is guarded to poor for complete return of normal anal or rectal function for any type of atresia ani. This is primarily because of the likelihood of injury to the external anal sphincter or its innervation during surgical repair. Another common surgical complication of this procedure is the development of rectal or anal strictures. Also, many affected puppies and kittens have concurrent megacolon, which develops as a result of persistent fecal impaction and which may be irreversible, requiring indefinite aggressive medical management or a subtotal colectomy.

Perianal Fistula

Perianal fistula is a chronic, often debilitating disease of the perianal tissues in dogs characterized by one or, more often, multiple draining tracts surrounding the anus. Anal furunculosis, an alternate descriptor, is typically a progressive disease characterized by ulcerative, painful, malodorous lesions resulting from the associated tissue destruction and infection. In severe cases, the entire anus is surrounded with ulcerative, draining tracts that often lead to fecal incontinence or rectal stricture formation (Figure 224-6). The fistulas usually do not involve the anorectal canal directly; however, typical signs include self-mutilation, dyschezia, and rectal stenosis, resulting in fecal incontinence or constipation.

History and Physical Examination

Perianal fistulas occur primarily in older, large breed dogs with a broad-based tail and lower tail carriage, which may create an environment that predisposes these breeds to perianal problems. The two breeds with the highest incidence of perianal fistula are German shepherds and Irish setters, but sheepdogs, retrievers, and spaniels also may develop the disorder.[46-49] No distinct gender or age predilection appears to exist, but the condition is more prevalent in male dogs over 5 years of age.[46,49] Because of the animal's low tail carriage, the disease may not be noticed by the owners until obvious lesions are present or the discharge or odor becomes overpowering. The only abnormality reported by some owners, especially early in the course of the disease, is persistent licking of the anus. Other clinical signs that may be reported include hematochezia, dyschezia, perianal discharge, constipation, and tenesmus. In severely affected dogs, anorexia, weight loss, and behavioral changes may occur as a result of the discomfort.

Physical examination may be difficult, if not impossible, without sedation because the simple act of having the tail lifted is painful to the animal. The examiner may also need to clip the hair and cleanse the area to fully assess the extent of

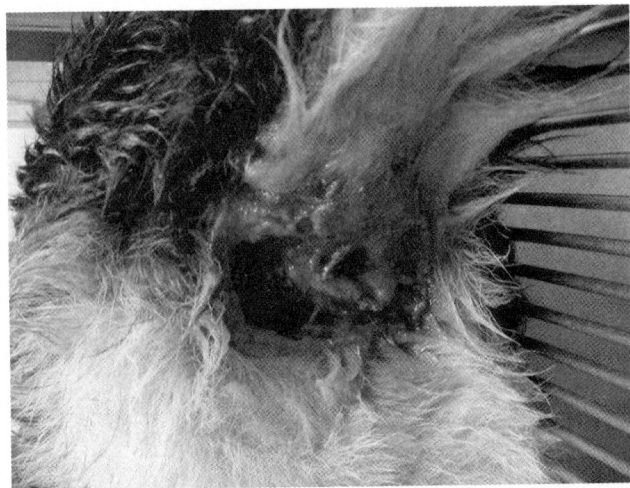

Figure 224-6 Severe fistulating and ulcerative perianal fistula in a German shepherd.

the perianal involvement. Visual inspection reveals multiple, ulcerated, draining tracts that extend into the tissues surrounding the anus. The lesions are often extremely malodorous and, in outdoor dogs, may contain fly maggots. Rectal strictures, abnormal anal tone, or granulomatous rectal mucosa may be found during a digital rectal examination. In addition, in some dogs with perianal fistulas, the anal sacs are involved in the fistulation, which may result in anal sac obstruction or abscessation.

Diagnosis

A diagnosis of perianal fistula is usually made based on the combination of typical signalment and history and physical examination findings. Important differentials for this condition include chronic anal sac abscessation with secondary fistulas, aggressive perianal tumors (e.g., adenocarcinoma), caustic injury, and untreated dog bite wounds.[14] A digital rectal examination and probing of the extent of the lesions while the dog is under general anesthesia confirms the diagnosis. Because German shepherds are predisposed to this condition and often have other concurrent colonic or rectal abnormalities, a proctoscopic or colonoscopic examination is also recommended.[48]

Pathogenesis

The factor long considered to be the most important contributor to formation of perianal fistulas is anatomic predisposition,[47] including (1) a broad-based tail (e.g., German shepherds), (2) low tail carriage (e.g., Irish setters), and (3) increased density of apocrine sweat glands in the zona cutanea.[47,49] More recently, an immune-mediated basis for the disease has been suggested by clinical trials, which have demonstrated a positive response to prednisone therapy in affected German shepherds.[48] This proposed etiology is further supported by the positive response to treatment seen in clinical trials using azathioprine, cyclosporine, and tacrolimus.[50-54] In humans, food allergy is believed to be a component of the development of perianal fistulas; although this has not been proved in dogs, it may also be a contributing factor in this species. The development and pathogenesis of perianal fistulas likely constitute a multistage process, in which an inflammatory condition sets the stage (e.g., immune-mediated, allergic, or anatomic causes) and is followed by the development of a secondary bacterial infection that results in severe epidermal ulceration and necrosis.

Therapy

The two basic approaches that have been used in the management of perianal fistulas are medical management and surgical excision. In many cases, medical management alone is sufficient for control; however, in severe cases, a combination of medical and surgical treatment often is necessary. Recently, laser surgical excision has met with some success in a limited number of cases; however, as with surgical approaches, fecal incontinence is a potential complication.[19,37,55]

Medical management of perineal fistulas has four components: (1) removal of perineal hair and tissue cleansing, (2) immunosuppressive therapy, (3) antibacterial therapy, and (4) dietary therapy.[19] In one study, a combination of high-dose prednisone (2.2 mg/kg PO2) and dietary therapy using novel antigen diets resulted in complete resolution of signs in one third of the dogs, improvement in another third, and no change in the remaining one third.[48] More recently, immunosuppressive therapy with azathioprine (50 mg/kg every 24 hours PO) or cyclosporine (1 mg/kg every 12 hours PO) has proved effective in controlling (90% had complete resolution within 2 weeks, 50% had no recurrence in 12 months) or reducing disease, whether used alone or in combination with surgical therapy.[50,51,53,54] In another study, the addition of

ketoconazole to cyclosporine therapy proved helpful by allowing a dramatic reduction in the cyclosporine dose (by 80% to 90% in all dogs).[50,54] In most dogs, antibacterial therapy with a first-generation cephalosporin is used to control bacteria typically associated with infections of the skin (e.g., staphylococci). The use of novel antigen diets in the management of perianal fistulas in dogs has not been evaluated in a controlled setting, therefore the effectiveness of this aspect of therapy is unknown; however, in one study the use of these diets was helpful.[48]

For dogs with severe perianal fistulas or those who do not respond to medical management alone, surgical or laser surgical excision of the affected tissue is recommended. A variety of surgical procedures may be necessary, including deroofing (removing the skin covering the fistulous tract) followed by electrofulguration (or electrocoagulation), anal sacculectomy, excision or debridement of diseased tissue, rectal pull-through procedures when rectal strictures are involved and, in some cases, tail amputation.[46,49,55] Carbon dioxide (CO_2) laser therapy may be a very effective means of debridement for dogs requiring surgical therapy, because the laser reduces bleeding, pain and postsurgical swelling.[37]

Prognosis

The overall prognosis is guarded in dogs with a perianal fistula, even though most methods, whether medical or surgical, have met with some degree of success. The most common complications of surgical approaches are fecal incontinence, rectal stricture, and recurrence. Therefore medical therapy with prednisone and cyclosporine should be used as the first-line approach in the majority of dogs, with surgical palliation kept a last resort.

DISEASES OF THE ANAL SACS

Impaction, Anal Sacculitis, and Abscessation

Several common infectious or inflammatory diseases affect the anal sacs, including anal sac impaction, anal sacculitis, and abscessation of the anal sacs. These diseases are more common in dogs than cats, affecting up to 12% of the canine population.[56]

History and Physical Examination

The most common clinical signs of anal sac disease are anal pruritus or pain, which elicits licking or biting at the tail or anal region, "tail chasing" behavior, scooting or rubbing of the anus on the ground, and reluctance to sit or discomfort when sitting.[14,57] In more severely affected dogs, pain may cause dyschezia, tenesmus, or reluctance to defecate. Dogs with longstanding anal sac disease may develop large swellings in the area over the anal sac, and if the abscessed sac ruptures, a draining fistula will extend from the affected anal sac.

External or internal digital palpation of the anal sacs may be required in some cases to detect diseased or impacted anal sacs. Normal anal sac secretions are liquid, brown, and foul smelling but easily expressed from the sac through the ducts to their openings on the anus.[57,58] In dogs with anal sac impaction, the material often becomes pasty or even dried and may be difficult to express without causing the animal pain. The material present in infected or abscessed anal sacs is often thicker, may be purulent or bloody, and frequently is very malodorous.

Diagnosis

In most pets the history of anal pruritus, along with visual inspection of a perianal swelling at either the 4 to 5 o'clock or the 7 to 8 o'clock position lateral to the anus, is highly suggestive. In the absence of significant visible external swelling, a digital rectal examination is sufficient to confirm anal sac involvement. Some dogs and all cats require sedation for safe performance of a rectal examination because of the accompanying discomfort. Impaction of the anal sacs is confirmed by removal of thick, pasty anal sac material or by inability to empty the sacs easily with appropriate technique. If the anal sacs are painful when gently palpated or if the material expressed is purulent or a color other than light tan to brown, anal sacculitis should be suspected. If doubt exists, a sample of the material can be cytologically examined for large numbers of neutrophils, bacteria, or yeast (e.g., *Malassezia* sp.).[58] If the anal sac is infected or abscessed, fever may also be present. The major differentials in dogs and cats with these clinical signs are perianal fistulas, perianal or anal tumors, and bite wounds (cats) or other trauma.

Pathogenesis

The most common cause of inflammation or infection of the anal sac is obstruction of the ducts, which prevents normal (frequent) expulsion of the material and allows bacteria normally present (e.g., *Escherichia coli*, *Streptococcus faecalis*, and *Clostridium* spp.) to set up a secondary infection.[58] Anatomic conformation also may play an important role in the tendency to develop anal sacculitis or abscessation; for example, smaller than normal ducts or aberrant duct placement on the anus decreases effective emptying. Other contributing factors may be dogs that produce thicker secretions, the development of abnormal anal tone, the production of soft feces, and recent estrus in females.[57,59]

Therapy

Treatment of simple anal sac impaction is straightforward, requiring that the anal sacs be emptied by gentle digital manipulation. If the sacs cannot be easily or completely emptied, they should be gently flushed with warm saline or mineral oil to loosen the concretions and pasty material. Once the sacs are empty, an antibiotic and steroid ointment or solution can be instilled to reduce local infection and inflammation. The sacs should be kept empty for several weeks to prevent recurrence or possible abscessation. In dogs with chronic impaction, the owners can be taught to express the anal sacs at home or, as an alternative, the anal sacs can be surgically removed.

Dogs with anal sacculitis or abscessed anal sacs must also have the sacs emptied, but because of the associated discomfort, sedation or anesthesia is usually required. In dogs with anal sacculitis alone, the sacs should be gently flushed with an antiseptic solution (e.g., dilute [0.5%] chlorhexidine) and antibiotic solution instilled into the sacs. Broad-spectrum oral antibiotic therapy is recommended for 10 to 14 days, along with application of hot compresses to reduce swelling and pain and frequent anal sac expression. In most cases managed this way, the infection resolves completely, and further therapy is not necessary. However, for dogs that have frequent recurrence of anal sacculitis, anal sac removal should be considered.[60-62]

Abscessation of the anal sacs is managed as is other abscessed tissue: the abscess must be surgically opened, flushed, and debrided. This procedure should be repeated daily for 2 to 4 days to help keep the area open and draining and to help remove any additional material that forms in the sacs. A broad-spectrum antibiotic should be administered for 10 to 14 days. Application of hot compresses several times daily for 3 to 5 days also helps reduce the swelling and pain. Surgical removal of the abscessed anal sac is not recommended unless there is recurrence after appropriate treatment. In addition, the surgery should not be performed until antibiotic therapy has been administered long enough to ensure tissue healing. Anal sac removal is recommended when all other options fail, primarily because of the risk of complications, especially

fecal incontinence. A recent retrospective report revealed that closed anal sacculectomy procedures were 13 times less likely to have postoperative complications compared with open techniques,[60] which makes the closed approach considerably more viable.

Prognosis

The prognosis for anal sac impactions and anal sacculitis is generally good, because these cases typically respond completely to conservative medical management. Most dogs and cats with anal sac abscesses also respond well to aggressive medical management of the infection; however, because these conditions may be more difficult to treat or may recur, surgical anal sac removal may be required. The prognosis for animals requiring anal sacculectomy is guarded to good, depending on the technique used and the surgeon's skill. The primary risk postoperatively is the development of fecal incontinence, especially in older dogs that have reduced anal sphincter tone or function.

Anal Sac, Anal, and Perianal Tumors

Tumors of the anus and perianal integument are relatively uncommon in dogs, and their clinical importance can vary widely. These tumors can range from the benign perianal gland adenoma of older intact male dogs to the malignant perianal gland adenocarcinoma that is most common in older intact or spayed female dogs.[63,64] Anal sac adenocarcinomas and perianal gland tumors are reported primarily in dogs, although a Siamese cat with an anal sac adenocarcinoma recently was reported.[65] Other anal and perianal tumors can occur in cats and dogs but are extremely uncommon. These tumors include perianal adenocarcinoma, squamous cell carcinoma, and melanoma.[64] Large breed dogs, especially German shepherds and Alaskan huskies, appear to be predisposed to the development of perianal adenocarcinomas.[64]

History and Physical Examination

The typical history of a dog with an anal sac adenocarcinoma is an older (greater than 10 years) female dog with dyschezia or perineal swelling. However, male dogs are occasionally affected, and the tumor can occur in younger dogs without an identifiable external swelling. This aspect of the disease illustrates the importance of a digital rectal examination as part of a complete physical examination, even in female dogs without clinical signs of tenesmus, dyschezia, or hematochezia. In dogs with paraneoplastic hypercalcemia of malignancy, a common complication of this tumor, the owner may also note polyuria, polydipsia, muscle weakness, or vomiting. Tumors of the anal sac are detected by careful palpation of the anal sac and its associated structures. Most of these tumors are unilateral, and they may be quite small (0.2 to 1 cm), which is why the examination must be performed carefully.[64] With few exceptions, these tumors, regardless of their size, have metastasized to the external iliac (sublumbar) lymph nodes by the time of the examination.[66] Other sites of metastasis include the liver, spleen, abdominal lymph nodes, and lungs. Most hypercalcemic animals become systemically ill, which suggests the need for a complete hematologic and biochemical evaluation; however, all hypercalcemic animals should have a thorough digital rectal examination initially to rule out anal sac adenocarcinoma.

The benign perianal gland tumors (circumanal gland, or hepatoid, adenomas) affect all breeds of dogs, but cocker spaniels, bulldogs, beagles, and Samoyeds appear to be overrepresented.[64] Because these tumors develop and grow under the influence of plasma androgens, more than 85% of them are found in older intact male dogs. In most dogs, the tumor is visible in the perianal integument, but it can be found in a variety of sites, including the prepuce, inguinal region, or ventral tail skin.[64] The tumors are usually firm, single, nodular masses of variable size. They can ulcerate, bleed, necrose, or cause intense pruritus of the anal region that may lead to difficulty in defecation, scooting, and other signs of anal disease.

Diagnosis and Pathophysiology

Diagnosis of benign perianal tumors is based on the finding of a mass in an intact male dog with the typical signalment and history and physical examination findings. The diagnosis is confirmed by fine needle aspiration cytology or excisional biopsy. The main differences between malignant perianal tumors and their benign counterparts are that the malignant tumors are not influenced by androgens, they behave more like anal sac adenocarcinomas (e.g., have metastasized by the time of diagnosis), and they are difficult to excise completely because of their location, rapid spread, and local infiltration.[64]

A presumptive diagnosis of an anal sac adenocarcinoma, based on the history and physical examination findings and with or without concurrent hypercalcemia, should be followed by histopathologic confirmation. In addition to diagnosis of the tumor, the evaluation should include a thorough systemic examination, including a complete blood count, serum biochemistry profile, urinalysis, and survey radiographs of the chest and abdomen to assess for tumor metastasis and paraneoplastic effects. Abdominal ultrasonography is also frequently used to assess the size and involvement of abdominal lymph nodes or the liver, because metastasis has occurred in greater than 50% of affected dogs by the time of diagnosis.[66] Humoral hypercalcemia of malignancy is present in 50% to 90% of dogs with anal sac adenocarcinoma. The molecular basis for the development of these anomalies is not completely understood, but the tumor results in expression of a gene for parathyroid hormone–related peptide (PTH–rP), which has functions similar to that of naturally occurring parathyroid hormone.[63,64] In some cases, the hypercalcemia may be severe enough to lead to multiple organ dysfunction. After complete removal of the tumor, hypercalcemia may resolve; however, hypercalcemia persists in dogs with metastatic disease or incomplete removal of the anal sac tumor.

Therapy and Prognosis

Castration and removal of the primary tumor by surgical excision or cryotherapy constitute the treatment of choice for perianal gland adenomas.[64] It is a more difficult procedure for large tumors and in those cases is more frequently associated with postoperative side effects (e.g., wound dehiscence, fecal incontinence, and hernia). In general, benign perianal gland tumors are slow growing; consequently, they are effectively treated with surgical excision, cryosurgery, electrocautery, and laser surgery, and they rarely recur (rate is less than 10%). The long-term prognosis is excellent except in cases of large tumors that cannot be completely excised.

Malignant perianal tumors are rapid growing, do not regress after castration, and because of their rapid metastasis are often not completely removed by surgical excision. For both perianal and anal sac adenocarcinomas, aggressive surgical removal with adequate margins, along with excision of regional lymph nodes, is recommended.[64] Despite aggressive surgical approaches, a local recurrence rate of 50% is reported for female dogs with adenocarcinoma.[64] Some oncologists suggest combination therapy, comprising surgical removal followed by platinum or doxorubicin chemotherapy to further control metastasis and local recurrence. Intraoperative irradiation of regional lymph nodes has proved successful at stopping metastasis in a limited number of cases.[64]

Nevertheless, the average survival of dogs with anal sac adenocarcinoma is reported to be 8 months (range, 2 to 39 weeks).[60,64] If the tumor is discovered early, before metastasis, and is completely excised, the prognosis is good. The prognosis

for smaller tumors is slightly better (e.g., fair) than for those greater than 5 cm, because the surgery is more effective and is associated with fewer complications. With large tumors, tumors with obvious metastasis, or concurrent hypercalcemia, the long-term prognosis is poor (survival rate of less than 40% at 1 year).

Fecal Incontinence

Fecal incontinence is defined as the inability to control defecation and retain feces until voluntary, conscious defecation is initiated.[14] Animals with fecal incontinence pass feces involuntarily and are often euthanized because of the difficult social issues that result. Fecal incontinence can be caused by neurologic disorders that affect function of the anal sphincter, primary disorders of the external anal sphincter (e.g., non-neurogenic sphincter disorders), or diseases that affect the normal reservoir function of the colon or rectum (e.g., reservoir incontinence) (Box 224-2).[14] In general, animals with sphincter incontinence have more severe signs (e.g., lack of

---

Box • 224-2

Causes of Fecal Incontinence

Neurologic Disease
Sacral spinal cord
Congenital vertebral malformation
Meningomyelocele
Sacrococcygeal hypoplasia of Manx cats
Sacral fracture
Sacrococcygeal subluxation
Lumbosacral instability
Viral meningomyelitis
Discospondylitis
Degenerative myelopathy
Neoplasia

Peripheral neuropathy
Trauma
Repair of perineal hernia
Perianal urethrostomy
Penetrating wounds
Dysautonomia
Hypothyroidism
Diabetes mellitus

Non-Neurologic Disease
Colorectal causes
Inflammatory bowel disease
Neoplasia
Constipation

Anorectal causes
Trauma
Surgery (anal sac, perineal hernia, rectal resection)
Perianal fistula
Neoplasia

Miscellaneous causes
Severe diarrhea
Irritable bowel syndrome
Decreased mentation
Old age

conscious posture to defecate, uncontrolled passage of feces) and are likely to be irreversibly affected. Animals with severe inflammatory disease may also have loss of voluntary control of defecation as a result of urgency to defecate, tenesmus, or hematochezia, but the problem may resolve with appropriate treatment of the disease.

History and Physical Examination

Determination of the cause of fecal incontinence requires a careful, complete history. In particular, it is important to distinguish fecal incontinence from urgency to defecate. Furthermore, the mere presence of fecal material accumulating around the anus must be distinguished from lack of ability to control the anal sphincter and fecal dribbling. Examples of diseases or circumstances that may damage nerves or muscles and lead to fecal incontinence include previous spinal cord disease, pelvic trauma, dystocia, chronic constipation, and anorectal surgery.[14] Animals with frequent, conscious defecation associated with normal posturing usually have normal anal sphincter and nerve function but may have incontinence as a result of loss of reservoir function. The most common causes of reservoir dysfunction are inflammatory, infectious, and neoplastic diseases of the colon, rectum, or anus that cause decreased compliance and abnormal motility. Severe large bowel diarrhea secondary to colonic inflammation can cause fecal incontinence for the same reason. In most animals with neurogenic or non-neurogenic sphincter incontinence, the fecal stream is normal. Furthermore, in animals with neurogenic sphincter incontinence, abnormal micturition often occurs concurrently because of the common neural pathways.[4] The urinary abnormalities may include dribbling urine, incomplete voiding, or inability to void, and when these occur in conjunction with fecal incontinence, neurologic dysfunction should be strongly considered.

The physical examination should include careful inspection of the perineum for evidence of abscesses, fistulas, hernias, masses, or other abnormalities. After the visual inspection, a digital rectal examination is performed to assess for normal anal sphincter tone, fecal impaction, strictures, or masses. Abdominal palpation is necessary to determine the presence of colonic impaction, as well as bladder size and expressibility. A distended, flaccid bladder from which urine is easily expressed is consistent with a lesion of the sacral spinal cord, the sacral nerves, or the pudendal nerve.[4] A complete neurologic examination, including observation of gait and posture, evaluation of myotactic and postural responses, and assessment of lumbosacral pain, is required in any animal suspected of having fecal incontinence. The neurologic deficits that may be present in dogs with neurogenic sphincter incontinence are abnormal posture, hindlimb gait abnormalities, decreased myotactic reflexes, or an abnormal pudendal (anal) reflex.[67] The anal reflex, which is a measure of perianal sensation and sacral spinal cord function (via the pudendal nerve), is tested by pinching the perianal skin, which results in an immediate contraction of the anal sphincter. This reflex should be present on both the right and left sides of the anus. The pudendal-anal reflex (bulbocavernosus reflex) is tested by squeezing the penis or vulva while observing for normal anal contraction. Lesions of the perineal afferent nerves, the sacral spinal cord, or the pudendal efferent nerves can decrease or abolish these

reflexes and cause a dilated anus, loss of perineal sensation, and a loss of micturition control.[67]

Diagnosis

When loss of colorectal reservoir function is suspected, the diagnostic plan should include an examination of the fecal stream (e.g., fecal floatation, cytology) and proctoscopy or colonoscopy with biopsy to identify the primary disease. If signs of systemic disease are also detected, further evaluation (e.g., hematology, serum chemistries, radiographs, ultrasonography) is warranted as indicated. Sphincter incontinence (either neurogenic or non-neurogenic) is usually apparent from the history and physical examination. Neurogenic and non-neurogenic dysfunction are differentiated by neurologic examination. If further confirmation is necessary, anal sphincter electromyography or monometry is used to prove sphincter incompetence; however, this is rarely necessary and not universally available. When lesions of the lumbar spinal cord or the cauda equina are suspected, vertebral radiographs, myelography, computed tomography, magnetic resonance imaging, or cerebral spinal fluid analysis may be indicated.[67] The causes of fecal incontinence are listed in Box 224-2.

Pathophysiology

Control of fecal continence is maintained by the muscles of internal and external anal sphincters, the rectum, and the coccygeus and levator ani muscles of the pelvis, which are innervated by the pelvic, hypogastric, pudendal, and sacral nerves.[4,67] Both motor and sensory impulses are integrated into the sacral spinal cord to coordinate normal fecal continence. The non-neurogenic causes of sphincter incontinence are usually due to reservoir incontinence (e.g., colitis, neoplasia) or to trauma to the anorectal muscles (e.g., surgery, hernia, fistula, neoplasia) (see Box 224-2).[14]

Therapy and Prognosis

The treatment of fecal incontinence depends entirely on the primary cause; for example, loss of reservoir function due to colitis often resolves completely with appropriate treatment, whereas loss of neurologic function is permanent and rarely treatable. Some forms of non-neurogenic incontinence are transient (e.g., postoperative complication, trauma), and some forms of neurogenic incontinence may improve after specific treatment (e.g., spinal surgery to reduce compression or subluxation). However, in these cases no specific drugs or diets are particularly effective. Highly digestible diets may be beneficial, because they reduce the volume of fecal material. Enemas and exercise may stimulate defecation at desired times and can be used to help control the social unacceptability of the problem.[68] A surgical technique using an implanted Silastic sling, and placement of an autogenous muscle graft to augment the muscles of continence, have been described, but the success rates for these procedures are not satisfactory.[69] Recently, a technique to create a new sphincter using muscle transplants has shown promise for providing a functional stomal sphincter in dogs with chronic fecal incontinence.[70] Nevertheless, in many pets euthanasia is chosen because in most cases the prognosis is poor for return to normal or acceptable sphincter function.

SECTION XV

Liver and Pancreatic Diseases

CHAPTER 225

History, Clinical Signs, and Physical Findings in Hepatobiliary Disease

Cynthia R. L. Webster

The liver plays a central role in a diverse array of processes including carbohydrate, lipid, and protein metabolism; detoxification of metabolites and xenobiotics; storage of vitamins, trace metals, fat and glycogen; fat digestion; and immunoregulation. The clinical signs, physical findings, and clinicopathologic abnormalities that accompany hepatic disease reflect deficiencies in these varied functions. The liver, however, has a tremendous reserve capacity to perform these functions. Thus the appearance of relatively specific signs of hepatobiliary disease such as icterus, hypoglycemia, bleeding tendencies, hepatic encephalopathy (HE), or ascites, which reflect exhaustion of the liver's functional reserves, occur only late in disease progression. Early clinical signs of hepatic disease, such as intermittent anorexia, polyuria/polydipsia (PU/PD), vomiting, and lethargy, mimic those seen with disease in other organ systems. In most cases, early detection of hepatobiliary disease relies on clinicopathologic evaluation and histopathologic examination of hepatic tissue.[1]

Although most early signs of liver disease are nonspecific, several clues should raise one's awareness as to the presence of hepatobiliary disease; these include strong breed predispositions and the occurrence of several clinical recognizable syndromes that accompany hepatobiliary disease, including gastrointestinal (GI) ulceration, HE, tissue jaundice, coagulopathies, and ascites.

Several breed predispositions occur in hepatobiliary disease. Congenital portosystemic vascular anomalies (PSVASs) are most frequent in purebred dogs particularly Irish wolfhounds, Australian cattle dogs, Maltese terriers, Cairn terriers, miniature schnauzers, Yorkshire terriers, dachshunds, Labrador retrievers, and golden retrievers. Feline PSVASs occur most often in mixed breed cats, but Persians and Himalayans are over-represented. Bedlington terriers have a congenital abnormality in hepatic copper metabolism that results in hepatic copper overload and subsequent development of chronic inflammatory hepatobiliary disease. Less well-defined copper-associated hepatopathies occur in West Highland white terriers, dalmatians, Skye terriers, and Siamese cats. Several breeds have a predisposition to develop idiopathic chronic inflammatory hepatobiliary disease, including Doberman pinschers, American and English cocker spaniels, standard poodles, and Labrador retrievers. Hepatic amyloidosis occurs in Chinese Shar Pei dogs and in Abyssinian, Oriental, and Siamese cats.

Historical findings that suggest the presence of hepatobiliary disease include recent ingestion of a known hepatotoxic substance or treatment with a potentially hepatotoxic drug.[2] Stunted growth or anesthesia or drug intolerance (or a combination of these factors) in a young animal, particularly in a predisposed breed, suggests the presence of PSVASs. A recently stressed obese cat that becomes anorexic is a classic historical example of a cat with idiopathic hepatic lipidosis.

The clinical signs associated with hepatobiliary disease are typically referable to the GI, renal, neurologic, or hematopoietic systems (Table 225-1). In addition, a rare dermatologic syndrome called *superficial necrolytic dermatitis* marked by ulcerative crusting dermatitis of the face and distal extremities, accompanies a unique form of chronic liver disease in the dog (hepatocutaneous syndrome).

Intermittent GI signs such as diarrhea, anorexia, and vomiting, are common signs of hepatobiliary disease. Chronic hepatic disease predisposes dogs to gastroduodenal ulceration, so a myriad of clinical signs referable to ulcer disease, such as hematemesis, abdominal pain, and melena, should prompt consideration of an underlying hepatopathy.

HE is neurologic condition associated with failure of the liver to detoxify inhibitory neurotoxins generated in the intestinal tract. The clinical signs are those of diffuse cerebral disease. HE is most often seen with PSVASs or with hepatopathies associated with acquired portosystemic shunts, but may also accompany acute fulminant hepatic failure. In acute failure the neurologic signs of HE can be confused with those associated with hypoglycemia. Either or both problems commonly accompany severe acute hepatic failure. Cerebral edema, an ominous consequence of fulminant hepatic failure, can also cause neurologic signs mimicking HE. These signs include disorientation, stupor, and coma.

An important differential for the presence of abdominal fluid accumulation is hepatobiliary disease. Chronic liver disease, particularly in the dog, can be associated with the development of ascites secondary to the presence of portal hypertension. Portal hypertension develops either due to capillarization of the hepatic sinusoidal endothelium from fibrosis, increased hepatic blood flow such as occurs with arteriovenous fistula, or is secondary to disease or obstruction of the portal vein or its tributaries. Ascites may accompany primary or metastatic hepatobiliary disease or can signal the presence of bile peritonitis from rupture of the biliary tract.

A highly variable, but often predominant, early clinical sign in many dogs and cats with chronic hepatobiliary disease or PSVASs is the presence of polyuria, polydipsia, or both. The mechanism for the polyuria and polydipsia is unknown, but the following six have been hypothesized[3]: (1) psychogenic polydipsia, (2) alterations in portal vein osmoreceptors, (3) decreased hepatic urea production resulting in disruption of the renal medullary concentration gradient, (4) potassium depletion, (5) stimulation of thirst centers due to HE, and (6) increased endogenous cortisol levels associated with increased adrenal production or decreased hepatic degradation.

Animals with hepatobiliary disease may also have signs referable to ammonium biurate urolithiasis such as stranguria, pollakiuria, or hematuria. Ammonia biurate stones form secondary due to chronic hyperammonemia and decreased hepatic processing of uric acid.

The most significant physical finding that should prompt a consideration of hepatobiliary disease is icterus, a yellow discoloration of the mucous membrane associated with accumulation of bilirubin. Pale mucous membranes, abdominal enlargement due to ascites or hepatomegaly, and poor body

Table • 225-1

Pathophysiology of Common Clinical Signs and Physical Examination Findings in Hepatobiliary Disease

CLINICAL SIGNS	PATHOPHYSIOLOGY	PHYSICAL FINDINGS	PATHOPHYSIOLOGY
Gastrointestinal (GI)		Icterus	Decreased uptake, conjugation or export of bilirubin into bile
Vomiting	Direct stimulation of CRTZ Gastroduodenal ulceration Concurrent intestinal inflammatory disease	Hepatomegaly	Hepatic infiltration with inflammatory cells, neoplasia, amyloid, fat, glycogen
Diarrhea	Concurrent intestinal inflammatory disease Steatorrhea Portal hypertensive enteropathy	Abdominal fluid	Ascites: Portal hypertension Avid renal sodium and water retention Hypoalbuminemia Bile: rupture gallbladder/biliary tract Neoplastic effusion
Acholic feces	Extrahepatic bile duct obstruction	Poor body condition score	Poor appetite Increased metabolic rate GI malabsorption
Melena	Gastroduodenal ulceration Coagulopathy	Abdominal pain	Cholecystitis GI ulceration Bile peritonitis Pancreatitis
Neurologic		Fever	Leptospirosis Rickettsial disease Protozoal disease: *Toxoplasma, Neospora* Feline Infectious Peritonitis (FIP) *Salmonella* Bacterial cholecystitis Supporative hepatitis
Personality change Weakness Anorexia, lethargy Ptyalism (cats) Head pressing Disorientation → stupor → coma Irritability/aggression Seizures	Hepatic encephalopathy (HE) Hypoglycemia Cerebral edema Vitamin B$_1$ deficiency		
Renal			
Polyuria/polydipsia (PU/PD)	Primary polydipsia Decreased hepatic urea production with subsequent disruption renal medullary interstitial gradient Increased circulating cortisol Manifestation of HE		
Pollakiuria, stranguria, dysuria	Ammonium biurate urolithiasis		
Bilirubinuria	Hyperbilirubinemia		
Hematologic	Anemia		
Pale mucous membranes	Blood loss from coagulopathy or GI bleeding Anemia chronic disease		

condition score might be other findings on physical examination of dogs or cats with hepatobiliary disease.

LABORATORY EVALUATION OF HEPATOBILIARY DISEASE

Clinical Enzymology

Evaluation of serum values of hepatobiliary enzymes such as alanine aminotransferase (ALT), aspartate aminotransferase (AST), alkaline phosphatase (ALP), and γ-glutamyl transpeptidase (GGT), are commonly used to screen for the presence of hepatobiliary disease, because consistent increases in the serum concentration of these enzyme activities occur after hepatobiliary injury.[4] Although these serum enzymes have a high sensitivity for the detection of hepatobiliary disease, interpretation of abnormalities is hampered by their lack of specificity for hepatobiliary disease. The central role of the liver in metabolism and its high blood flow make it uniquely sensitive to secondary injury. Thus several clinical conditions exist in which liver enzymes may be elevated but in which clinically significant hepatobiliary disease may not be present (Table 225-2). Although the magnitude of serum enzyme elevation is usually proportional to the severity of active hepatobiliary damage, the degree of elevation is not predictive of hepatobiliary functional capacity. Marked increases in serum enzymes may indicate substantial hepatobiliary injury but, due to tremendous hepatic regenerative capacity, are not necessarily indicative of a poor prognosis. Alternatively, in severe end-stage chronic liver disease, serum enzymes may be normal or only mildly increased, because replacement of hepatocytes by fibrosis, prolonged enzyme leakage, or both has resulted in depletion of total liver enzyme content. A single serum enzyme determination should never be used to establish a prognosis. The prognostic value of serum enzymology is improved by following sequential serum enzyme determinations, especially in conjunction with a hepatic function test or hepatic biopsy.

Alanine aminotransferase (ALT) is a liver-specific cytosolic enzyme. The largest increases in serum ALT, a leakage enzyme, are seen with acute hepatocellular necrosis and inflammation. The magnitude of ALT elevation is roughly proportional to the number of injured hepatocytes. The serum $t_{1/2}$ in dogs is around 2.5 days. No published values exist for feline serum ALT $t_{1/2}$. In acute liver disease in the dog, the finding of a 50% decrease in sequential serum ALT determinations over 2 to 3 days is considered a good prognostic sign. In dogs, serum ALT may also increase with severe muscle necrosis.

In dogs, phenobarbital and corticosteroids increase serum ALT.[4-7] In most dogs, drug induction results in mild increases in ALT (two- to fourfold), but in some individuals increases approach those seen with acute hepatocellular injury. Whether these larger elevations in serum ALT activity represent enzyme induction or are reflective of possible corticosteroid or phenobarbital hepatotoxicity is still unclear. Serum ALT may increase with primary or metastatic hepatic neoplasia.[8] Mild to moderate increases are seen in 70% to 80% of dogs with hepatocellular or bile duct carcinoma. Occasionally hepatic nodular hyperplasia results in increased serum ALT.

Serum AST is more sensitive than serum ALT in the detection of hepatobiliary disease, although considerably less specific because significant amounts of AST are also contained in muscle. The $t_{1/2}$ of serum AST is 5 to 12 hours in the dog and 77 minutes in the cat. In general, increases in serum AST parallel increases in serum ALT and, like ALT, are associated with leakage after altered membrane permeability. In instances where serum AST is much higher than serum ALT, a muscle source for the elevations should be explored. Alternatively, because AST is

Table • 225-2

Conditions in which Increases in Serum Hepatobiliary Enzyme Concentrations May Occur in the Absence of Primary Liver Disease

Drug Induction:
Corticosteroids (dogs):
(↑↑↑ ALP, ↑↑ GGT, ↑ ALT, ↑ AST)
Anticonvulsants:
(phenobarbital, phenytoin, primidone)
(↑ ALT, ↑ ALP, ↑ AST, ↑ GGT)

Endocrinopathies:
Hyperthyroidism (cats):
(↑ ALP, ↑ ALT)
Hypothyroidism (dogs):
(↑ ALP)
Diabetes mellitus:
(↑ ALP)
Hyperadrenocorticism (dogs):
(↑↑↑ ALP, ↑ ALT, ↑ GGT, ↑ AST)

Neoplasia:
Adenocarcinomas:
pancreatic, intestinal, adrenocortical, mammary
Sarcomas:
hemangiosarcoma, leiomyosarcoma
Hepatic metastasis:
(↑ AST, ↑ ALT, ↑ ALP)
Unique enzyme induction:
(↑↑ ALP, ↑↑ GGT)

Miscellaneous:
Systemic infections
Pregnancy (cats):
(↑ placental ALP)
Colostrum fed neonates (dogs):
(↑ GGT)

Hypoxia/Hypotension:
(↑↑ ALT, ↑ ALP, ↑ GGT, ↑ AST)
Congestive heart failure (CHF)
Septic shock
Hypoadrenocorticism
Circulatory shock
Severe acute blood loss
Status epilepticus
Hypotensive crisis
Surgery

Muscle Injury:
(↑ ALT, ↑↑ AST)
Acute muscle necrosis/trauma
Malignant hyperthermia
Myopathies

Bone Disorders: (↑ ALP)
Young animals (up to 7 months)
Osteosarcoma
Osteomyelitis

present within the mitochondria and the cytosol, an elevated AST to ALT ratio may be indicative of acute severe irreversible injury. In dogs, serum AST is mildly increased by corticosteroids and phenobarbital. Increases in serum AST may be more sensitive than ALP or ALT in the detection of hepatic metastasis.[8]

Although serum ALP elevation is a sensitive indicator of hepatobiliary disease, its low specificity for liver disease confuses interpretation. ALP's low specificity is associated with the presence of several isoenzymes and a unique sensitivity to drug induction. Isoenzymes of ALP are present in the liver, kidney, intestine, bone, and placenta. The intestinal, kidney, and placental isoenzymes do not contribute to serum ALP due to their short $t_{1/2}$. An exception is in late-term feline pregnancy, where the placental ALP isoenzyme represents a significant source of the serum enzyme. The bone isoenzyme, B-ALP, contributes about one third of total serum ALP.[9] Increased osteoblastic activity associated with growing bones in young animals or with pathologic conditions such as osteomyelitis or osteosarcoma can increase serum B-ALP. These conditions typically cause mild increases in the total serum ALP.

Two liver isoenzymes contribute to the serum ALP in dogs; a liver (L-ALP) and corticosteroid-induced isoenzyme (C-ALP). Cats have only one liver isoenzyme. In the dog and cat, L-ALP is a membrane-bound enzyme found on the hepatocyte canalicular membrane and the luminal surface of biliary epithelial cells.[10] Canine C-ALP is a hyperglycosylated form of the isoenzyme produced by hepatocytes and is also located on the hepatocyte canalicular membrane. The serum $t_{1/2}$ of both L-ALP and C-ALP in the dog is about 70 hours. The $t_{1/2}$ of the cat liver isoenzyme is only 6 hours. Increases in serum ALP in the dog and cat are the result of increased de novo synthesis, elution of the enzyme from cellular membranes, or both.

In a series of 270 dogs with histologically confirmed hepatic disease, the highest serum ALP activities were seen with cholestasis (median: tenfold increase) followed by chronic hepatitis, corticosteroid-induced hepatopathy, and hepatic necrosis (approximately sixfold).[4] Although the specificity of serum ALP determination for hepatobiliary disease was only 51%, the sensitivity was quite high (approximately 80%). Canine bile duct carcinoma and hepatocellular carcinoma can be accompanied by moderate to marked increases in serum ALP (see Table 225-2). Hepatic nodular regeneration, a common hepatic lesion in old dogs is frequently accompanied by mild to moderate increases in ALP.

Exposure of dogs to excess endogenous or exogenous corticosteroids increases serum ALP.[5,6,11] In experimental studies, dogs given immune-modulating doses of prednisone had increases in serum ALP by the third day that continued to rise throughout the period of corticosteroid administration. Serum ALP elevation in corticosteroid-treated dogs is accompanied by changes in hepatic morphology. Morphologic changes include ballooning enlargement of hepatocytes and development of intracytoplasmic hepatic vacuolation due to glycogen accumulation.[6] In some studies, focal areas of hepatocyte necrosis have been described. In dogs treated with prednisone, these morphologic changes begin by the second day and gradually progress in severity as corticosteroid treatment continues.

One of the challenges in the interpretation of canine serum ALP elevations is distinguishing between increases associated with cholestatic hepatic disease and those secondary to exposure to corticosteroids. In theory, serum ALP isoenzyme analysis should separate these two groups, because hepatobiliary disease should increase L-ALP and corticosteroid exposure should increase C-ALP. In reality, considerable overlap exists between isoenzyme distributions in these two conditions. The most widely used technique for serum ALP isoenzyme analysis is levamisole inhibition.[9] This technique is based on the fact that levamisole inhibits L-ALP and B-ALP but not C-ALP. In dogs with normal total serum ALP, C-ALP represents from 5% to 20% of total serum ALP. In experimental dogs treated with corticosteroids, the initial rise in serum ALP is associated with induction of L-ALP, and only after several days of treatment does C-ALP become the prominent isoenzyme. Chronic corticosteroid exposure due to hyperadrenocorticism or iatrogenic hypercortisolism from parenteral, oral, or topical corticosteroid administration, is consistently associated with increases in C-ALP. Serum C-ALP also increases in chronically ill animals, apparently from long-term endogenous cortisol excess. Although highly sensitive for the detection of exposure to corticosteroids, the specificity of isoenzyme analysis is low. Further, many dogs with hepatobiliary disease also have increases in serum C-ALP.[12]

Phenobarbital induces mild (two- to sixfold) increases in serum ALP.[2,7] Phenobarbital may induce either L-ALP, C-ALP, or both.[10] Interpretation of increased serum ALP activity in phenobarbital-treated dogs is complicated by the fact that this drug is a hepatotoxin. Because ALT, AST, and GGT are also mildly induced by anticonvulsants, they may be of no value in differentiating serum ALP increases due to microsomal induction from those associated with morphologic injury. If the serum abnormalities in these enzymes are greater than two to three times the upper limit of normal, the possibility of phenobarbital-induced hepatotoxicity should be explored. Dogs on chronic anticonvulsant therapy with enzyme induction should have determination of serum albumin, bilirubin, and bile acids to monitor hepatobiliary function.

Because feline ALP is not susceptible to drug induction, elevations in serum ALP are more specific for feline hepatobiliary disease. The magnitude of serum ALP elevations in feline hepatobiliary disease, however, are not as great as those in the dog due to the short $t_{1/2}$ of feline ALP and the fact that hepatic stores of feline ALP are less than in the dog. Thus feline serum ALP is a less sensitive indicator of hepatic disease than in the dog. Clinically, the largest increases in feline ALP are seen in hepatobiliary conditions associated with intrahepatic or extrahepatic cholestasis.

GGT is present in many tissues, although serum GGT concentrations are primarily derived from the liver. Hepatic GGT is located on the hepatocyte canalicular membrane. Serum elevations in GGT are most common with cholestatic disorders and are associated with increased de novo synthesis and membrane elution.

In dogs, moderate to marked increases in GGT are seen with intrahepatic and extrahepatic cholestasis, whereas mild elevations are seen with acute hepatocellular injury. In a series of dogs with histologically confirmed hepatic disease, serum GGT was more specific (87%) than serum ALP (51%) in the detection of hepatobiliary disease, but it was less sensitive (50%) than SAP (80%).[4]

When serum GGT and ALP were used in series, their specificity for the detection of hepatobiliary disease increased to 94%. In a series of 36 dogs with primary or metastatic hepatic neoplasia, 39% had high serum GGT values. Phenobarbital and corticosteroids cause mild (two to threefold) increases in serum GGT in the dog.

In a series of 69 cats with hepatobiliary disease, the largest increases in serum GGT were associated with extrahepatic bile duct obstruction (EHBDO) and cholangiohepatitis. Serum GGT had a higher sensitivity than serum ALP (86% versus 50%, respectively), but lower specificity (67% versus 93%, respectively) for the detection of hepatobiliary disease.[4] In some cats with cirrhosis, EHBDO, or cholangitis, serum GGT may be considerably greater than serum ALP values. In idiopathic hepatic lipidosis, however, serum GGT values may be normal or mildly increased (two- to sixfold), whereas serum ALP values are markedly increased (tenfold).

PLASMA PROTEINS IN HEPATIC DISEASE

The liver synthesizes many plasma proteins and detoxifies ammonia, the major breakdown product of protein metabolism. The clinical consequences of disruptions in hepatic protein metabolism are decreases in plasma oncotic pressure due to hypoalbuminemia, bleeding tendencies associated with coagulation protein deficiencies, and the development of HE due to ammonia retention.

Albumin

The liver is the exclusive site of albumin synthesis. Because synthesis occurs at 33% of maximum capacity and the serum $t_{1/2}$ of albumin is 8 to 9 days, serum hypoalbuminemia is most often seen in chronic hepatic disorders such as cirrhosis and PSVASs. In cirrhotic dogs, serum hypoalbuminemia, portal hypertension, and avid sodium and water retention lead to the development of ascites. In ascitic animals, serum hypoalbuminemia may reflect both third-party sequestration of albumin in the abdominal fluid and hepatic synthetic failure. Hypoalbuminemia is not specific for hepatic disease and may occur with protein-losing enteropathies, protein-losing nephropathies, exudative cutaneous lesions, vasculitis, or acute blood loss. Inadequate nutrition can curtail hepatic albumin synthesis. Because albumin is a negative acute phase reactant, systemic inflammatory disease may shut down hepatic albumin synthesis.

Globulins

The serum globulin fraction is composed of immunoglobulins and nonimmunoglobulins. Because the liver synthesizes many of the nonimmunoglobulins including α-globulins and β-globulins, hepatic synthetic failure can be accompanied by serum hypoglobulinemia. However, because many nonimmunoglobins are acute-phase reactants whose production that is increased in response to systemic inflammatory disease, early chronic inflammatory liver disease may be accompanied by hyperglobulinemia.[4,13,14]

Immunoglobulins are not synthesized in the liver but may be increased in chronic inflammatory hepatic disease. A polyclonal increase in γ-globulins has been documented in chronic canine hepatic disease and is seen in 50% of feline cases of chronic cholangiohepatitis. Hypergammaglobulinemia in chronic liver disease may be associated with enhanced systemic immunoreactivity due to abnormal Kupffer cell processing of portal antigens or secondary to autoantibody production. Low titers of antinuclear antibodies have been detected in 50% of dogs with chronic inflammatory hepatic disease.[15] In a series of dogs with chronic inflammatory hepatic disease, 48% had antibodies that reacted with canine liver membrane preparations.[16] Although dogs with positive titers tended to have higher serum ALT and bilirubin values and more severe histopathologic lesions than dogs without antibody responses, it remains to be determined whether these autoantibodies have any role in disease progression.

Coagulation Proteins

The liver plays an important role in hemostasis. Hepatocytes synthesize all of the coagulation factors, except factor VIII, as well as critical inhibitors of coagulation and fibrinolysis (antithrombin III, antiplasmin) and fibrinolytic proteins (plasminogen). In addition, the liver is responsible for clearance and catabolism of activated coagulation factors, plasminogen activators, and breakdown products of fibrinolysis such as fibrin degradation products (FDP). The liver is also the site of vitamin K–dependent activation of factors II, VII, IX, and X and protein C.

Assessment of coagulation status is important in animals with liver disease because altered hemostasis can contribute to clinical manifestations of hepatic disease and complicate invasive diagnostic procedures. The complexity and overlap of the liver's synthetic and clearance functions, however, makes the interpretation of hemostatic testing difficult. The commonly used tests to assess coagulation include determination of prothrombin time (PT), activated partial thromboplastin time (APTT), fibrinogen, and FDPs. Abnormalities in these coagulation tests in hepatobiliary disease may be indicative of hepatic synthetic failure, vitamin K deficiency, or the presence of a consumption coagulopathy such as disseminated intravascular coagulation (DIC).

Coagulation abnormalities are quite common in dogs and cats with hepatobiliary disease.[4] In dogs with naturally occurring hepatic disease, 50% and 75% had an abnormal PT and APTT, respectively. Specific factor analysis revealed that greater than 90% of the dogs had at least one abnormality. Because factor depletion must be greater than 70% to show prolongation of coagulation times, it is not surprising that many more dogs had abnormalities in the concentration of coagulation factors than had prolongation of PT or APTT. In cats with naturally occurring hepatobiliary disease, 82% had at least one coagulation abnormality.[17] The most common abnormalities were an increase in PT (16 of 22) and low factor VII activity (15 of 22).

Despite the presence of abnormalities in coagulation tests, spontaneous hemorrhage in animals with hepatic disease is rare. Hemorrhage is more likely to occur after a challenge to hemostasis such as venipuncture, hepatic biopsy, or gastric ulceration. Because coagulation tests are relatively poor predictors of an individual's tendency to bleed, one should assume that animals with hepatobiliary disease have a higher than normal risk of bleeding after provocative procedures regardless of the results of coagulation testing.

Assessment of coagulation has prognostic significance in hepatic disease. In dogs with chronic inflammatory liver disease, prolongation of PT and PTT to 1.3 to 1.4 times normal was associated with survival less than 1 week.[18] Although prognostic and useful in managing and predicting the complications of hepatic disease, PT and APPT are not sensitive or specific indicators of hepatic disease and should not be used as screening or diagnostic tests.

Vitamin K deficiency may develop during hepatobiliary disease for several reasons. Prolonged bile duct obstruction interrupts the enterohepatic circulation of bile acids resulting in intestinal bile acid deficiency and resultant fat-soluble vitamin K malabsorption. Oral antibiotics may alter the normal intestinal bacterial flora, resulting in the destruction of vitamin K–generating bacteria. Inadequate dietary consumption of vitamin K, although rarely a primary cause of vitamin K deficiency, may be contributory. This is especially true in disorders such as feline idiopathic hepatic lipidosis, which is marked by prolonged anorexia. Vitamin K is a cofactor in the carboxylation and resultant activation of factor II, VII, XI, and X and protein C. Prolongation of PT is the first coagulation abnormality seen with vitamin K deficiency, because factor VII has the shortest plasma $t_{1/2}$. In vitamin K deficiency, vitamin K–dependent factors circulate in an inactive form. The concentration of these inactive factors can be measured and is referred to as *proteins induced by vitamin K absence or antagonists* (PIVKAs). The presence of increased PIVKAs is more sensitive than changes in PT to detect vitamin K deficiency.[19] When either PIVKAs or prolongation of PT were used to detect vitamin K deficiency, 50% to 75% of cats with naturally occurring hepatobiliary disease had vitamin K deficiency.[19,17] Failure to activate vitamin K–dependent factors also may occur as the result of hepatic synthetic failure. Parenteral administration of vitamin K readily (within 24 to 48 hours) corrects coagulation abnormalities due to vitamin K deficiency, but has little to no effect on coagulation abnormalities due to hepatic synthetic failure.

Due to the liver's central role in coagulation and fibrinolysis, it can be quite challenging to differentiate whether coagulation abnormalities are associated with DIC or are due to severe liver disease. Typically DIC is recognized by prolongation of PT, APTT, decreased fibrinogen, thrombocytopenia, and increased FDPs, all of which may accompany hepatic failure. Increases in PT and APTT may accompany hepatic synthetic failure or vitamin K deficiency. In early liver disease, fibrinogen concentrations may be normal to increased (fibrinogen is an acute-phase reactant), but as hepatic function deteriorates, fibrinogen concentrations typically decrease due to reduced hepatic synthesis. Increases in FDPs have been detected in 14% of dogs with chronic hepatic disease and in 30% of cats with idiopathic hepatic lipidosis.[4,11] These increases may represent impaired hepatic clearance of FDPs.

Both quantitative and qualitative platelet defects accompany hepatobiliary disease. Although quantitative platelet abnormalities have been poorly documented in small animals with hepatic disease, many dogs with chronic hepatic disease have mild thrombocytopenia (120,000 to 180,000). The reason for this thrombocytopenia is unknown. Thrombocytopenia is rare in cats with hepatobiliary disease unless DIC is present. Studies in dogs with hepatobiliary disease have demonstrated the presence of qualitative defects in platelet aggregation.

BLOOD AMMONIA

The liver is responsible for the majority of ammonia detoxification. Ammonia is generated primarily in the GI tract by bacterial degradation of amines, amino acids, and purines; by the action of bacterial urease on urea; and by intestinal catabolism of glutamine. Ammonia readily diffuses through the intestinal mucosa and into the portal circulation where it travels to the liver. After uptake by hepatocytes, ammonia is detoxified either by enzymatic conversion to urea in the mitochondrial urea cycle or by consumption in the synthesis of glutamine. Urea then undergoes renal excretion. Ammonia, which escapes hepatic metabolism, enters the systemic circulation where other tissues, including the kidney, muscle, brain, and intestines, detoxify it by the formation of glutamine.

Failure of the liver to detoxify ammonia or shunting of portal blood away from the liver results in hyperammonemia. Because the urea cycle operates at only 60% capacity, hepatic failure must be fairly advanced for blood ammonia concentrations to rise. Because intrahepatic or extrahepatic shunting of portal blood directly deposits ammonia in the systemic circulation, blood ammonia concentrations are more sensitive in the detection of hepatobiliary disorders associated with shunting.[4,20] Hyperammonemia also occurs in animals with urea cycle enzyme deficiencies and with pathologic conditions that result in decreased availability of urea cycle substrates. Hyperammonemia has been described in dogs with a deficiency of the urea cycle enzyme, argininosuccinate synthetase, and in cats fed a diet deficient in arginine, an essential substrate in the urea cycle.[21,22]

The biggest obstacle in the clinical use of blood ammonia determinations is the difficulty in sample handling. Samples must be drawn directly into cold heparinized tubes, immediately transferred to the laboratory on ice for refrigerated centrifugation, and preferably assayed within 1 hour. Feline, but not canine, plasma samples may be frozen at $-20°$ C for 48 hours without sacrificing accuracy. Because erythrocytes contain two to three times the amount of ammonia as does plasma, if they are not separated from the plasma immediately or if hemolysis is found in the sample, spurious increases in blood ammonia will result.

Technical limitations aside, blood ammonia determination is important for evaluating dogs and cats suspected of having hepatobiliary disease. Hyperammonemia is an important, although not exclusive, cause of HE and is the only toxin implicated in this condition that can be measured clinically. The presence of hyperammonemia can therefore be used to verify the presence of HE. Not all animals with HE, however, will have abnormal blood ammonia levels. Hyperammonemia also reliably occurs in pathologic conditions associated with significant shunting of portal blood away from the liver. Thus 80% of dogs and 90% of cats with PSVASs demonstrate fasting hyperammonemia. Fasting hyperammonemia occurs less often with chronic parenchymal disease, being abnormal in approximately 50% of dogs with chronic hepatitis.[13] Elevations in blood ammonia are unusual with acute hepatic disease, unless it is fulminant.

The diagnostic value of blood ammonia can be improved by performing an ammonia tolerance test (ATT).[4] In an ATT,

a baseline blood ammonia value is determined after a 12-hour fast. The animal is then given an exogenous load of ammonium orally or per rectum and blood ammonia determined postchallenge. In the classic oral ATT, NH_4Cl_2 is given at a dose of 100 mg/kg in a dilute solution (not to exceed a concentration of 20 mg/mL and a total dose of 3 g) and blood ammonia determined 30 minutes later. In the rectal ATT, a warm-water enema is given 12 hours prior to the administration of 2 mL/kg of 5% NH_4Cl_2 via a catheter inserted into the rectum. Samples for blood ammonia are taken at 20 and 40 minutes postchallenge. In normal animals after oral or rectal challenge, blood ammonia should not increase any more than twofold. In animals with hepatic insufficiency or PSVASs, ammonia values generally increase three to tenfold. Virtually all dogs and cats with PSVASs and 90% of dogs with chronic hepatitis have abnormal ATT.[9,11] Rarely an ATT will precipitate HE.

A recent study evaluated a modified oral ATT in which dogs were fed a small test meal supplying 33 kcal/kg (25% of daily metabolizable energy requirement) with a protein concentration of 30.3% dry matter.[20] When blood ammonia concentrations were determined at zero time and 6 hours later, a sensitivity of 81% and 91% was found for the detection of PSVASs. The test had poor sensitivity in detecting dogs with parenchymal hepatocellular disease. Unlike classic ammonia tolerance tests, this provocative test was not associated with adverse side effects such as the induction of vomiting or HE.

SERUM UREA NITROGEN

Approximately 65% of dogs and cats with PSVASs have a decreased serum urea nitrogen (SUN).[3] Decreases in SUN are thought to arise secondary to decreased urea production in the atrophied liver. Decreased SUN is not specific for liver disease because it can be influenced by hydration status and dietary protein content, GI hemorrhage, glomerular filtration rate, and fluid or solute diuresis.

BILIRUBIN

Bilirubin is a yellow pigment formed in the reticuloendothelial cell system (RES) by the enzymatic processing of heme. Bilirubin released from RES cells is not water soluble and is transported in plasma reversibly bound to albumin. This unconjugated bilirubin is extracted by the liver and conjugated by esterification with glucuronic acid. Water-soluble conjugated bilirubin is actively secreted against a concentration gradient into the bile. The bilirubin in bile enters the intestinal tract via the bile duct, where it is either excreted unchanged in the feces or is converted to urobilinogen by the action of enteric bacteria. Most of the urobilinogen is further degraded into the brown-pigmented stercobilins. The absence of stercobilins in the feces results in pale-colored acholic stools. Small amounts of urobilinogen enter the portal venous system and undergo enterohepatic circulation. The majority is re-excreted into the bile, but a small amount undergoes urinary excretion.

Icterus is the clinical manifestation of bilirubin retention within tissues (see Figure 225-1). Although less sensitive than serum liver enzymes for the detection of hepatobiliary disease, serum hyperbilirubinemia is more specific. Hyperbilirubinemia occurs when an abnormality in the processing of bilirubin exists and can be divided into three categories: (1) prehepatic, (2) hepatic, and (3) posthepatic. Prehepatic hyperbilirubinemia is associated with increased production of bilirubin due to the need to process large amounts of heme such as occurs during severe hemolytic anemia. It is readily differentiated from hepatic and posthepatic causes by determining hematocrit. Hepatic hyperbilirubinemia is associated with impaired hepatic uptake, conjugation, or excretion of bilirubin. It is seen in hepatic disorders in which severe intrahepatic cholestasis develops. Hepatic hyperbilirubinemia may also accompany severe extrahepatic infections.[23,24] In this condition, referred to as the *cholestasis of sepsis*, circulating cytokines directly inhibit hepatocyte bilirubin transport. In a series of 29 septic cats, 63% had hyperbilirubinemia.[23] Posthepatic hyperbilirubinemia is associated with interruption of flow within the extrahepatic bile ducts.

The differentiation of hepatic and posthepatic icterus can be quite challenging clinically and yet is extremely important because these conditions demand different interventional strategies. Posthepatic hyperbilirubinemia usually requires surgical decompression of the biliary tract, whereas hepatic hyperbilirubinemia is typically treated medically. The clinical differentiation between hepatic and posthepatic hyperbilirubinemia is best made by ultrasound evaluation of the biliary system combined with careful consideration of clinical history, physical examination, and ancillary laboratory testing.

During prolonged cholestasis, excess conjugated bilirubin may become irreversibly bound to albumin. These so-called biliproteins are clinically significant in that they are measured as direct reacting bilirubin, but their $t_{1/2}$ approximates that of albumin.[4] Their presence can result in persistently elevated serum bilirubin weeks after the resolution of the underlying cholestatic liver disorder.

BILE ACIDS

Bile acids are synthesized exclusively in the liver from cholesterol. After conjugation to either taurine or glycine, bile acids are excreted into bile and collected, stored, and concentrated in the gallbladder. After ingestion of a meal, cholecystokinin release stimulates gallbladder contraction and the transport of bile acids into the intestine. In the intestinal lumen, bile acids aid in the solubilization and absorption of fats. When the bile acids reach the ileum, they are efficiently transported back into the portal circulation from which they are re-extracted by the hepatocyte sinusoidal bile acid transporter. This enterohepatic circulation of bile acids operates at 98% efficacy.

Disruption of the enterohepatic circulation of bile acids results in increases in the concentration of total serum bile acids (TSBAs). In normal animals, TSBA concentrations are determined by the spillover of bile acids that escape from the enterohepatic circulation. During fasting, when the enterohepatic circulation of bile acids is low, TSBAs are low. After a meal, bile acids are released into the intestines and subsequently absorbed into the portal circulation. Increased portal vein bile acid concentrations are reflected in a transient elevation in TSBAs. This endogenous challenge to the enterohepatic circulation of bile acids is used clinically. In a typical bile acid test, TSBAs are determined after a 12-hour fast, a test meal is fed and then postprandial TSBAs determined 2 hours later.

The most commonly used method for the determination of TSBAs is an enzymatic method that relies on the reaction of 3-α-hydroxy bile acids with bacterial 3-α-hydroxysteroid dehydrogenase. Normal values for fasting TSBA concentrations using this method are 1.7 ± 0.3 μM and 2.3 ± 0.4 μM in cats and dogs, respectively. Two-hour postprandial values are 8.3 ± 2.2 μM in the dog and 8.3 ± 0.3 μM in the cat.[4] Sample collection for this assay is easy because serum bile acids are stable even at room temperature. Hemolysis and lipemia should be avoided because they interfere with the assays spectrophotometric endpoint.

Numerous studies have demonstrated the efficacy of fasting and postprandial TSBAs in the diagnosis of feline and canine hepatobiliary disease and PSVASs.[3,4] In a series of 108 cats with hepatobiliary disease, when cutoff values of greater than 15 μM were used as abnormal, fasting TSBAs were more specific (96%) than increases in serum ALP, ALT or GGT in predicting the presence of hepatobiliary disease. The sensitivity at this cutoff value (54%) was about the same as for serum enzyme determination. The determination of postprandial TSBAs using a cutoff of greater than 20 μM as abnormal improved both the sensitivity (100%) and the specificity (80%) of bile acid testing in the detection of feline hepatobiliary disease. Postprandial TSBAs had a greater sensitivity than fasting TSBAs for the detection of all categories of feline hepatobiliary disease except hepatic necrosis.

In a series of 107 dogs with histologically confirmed hepatic disease, the specificity of fasting TSBAs using a cutoff of greater than 5 μM as abnormal was 83%.[4] Using a cutoff of greater than 15 μM as abnormal, postprandial TSBAs had a specificity of 89% and a sensitivity of 82%. When cutoff values for abnormal fasting and postprandial TSBAs were increased to greater than 20 μM and greater than 25 μM respectively, the specificity of both tests was 100%. Sensitivity at these cutoff values was 59% and 74% for fasting and postprandial samples, respectively. At the higher cutoff values, neither fasting nor postprandial TSBAs outperformed the other. A notable exception was improved performance of postprandial TSBAs in the detection of inactive cirrhosis or PSVASs.

Maltese dogs may have increased postprandial TSBAs in the absence of hepatobiliary disease.[25] In a screening of 200 Maltese dogs, 79% had postprandial TSBAs above the reference range using the enzymatic method. Nine dogs with abnormal postprandial TSBAs had normal rectal ATT and no evidence of hepatobiliary disease on hepatic biopsy. Two dogs with abnormal postprandial TSBAs had abnormal ATT and PSVASs. The cause of increased postprandial TSBA values in Maltese dogs with normal liver biopsies remains undetermined.

A number of factors that influence the enterohepatic circulation of bile acids in normal animals can affect TSBA values.[4] These include the completeness of gallbladder emptying, the rate of gastric emptying, intestinal transit rate, the efficiency of ileal bile acid reabsorption, and the frequency of enterohepatic cycling. Inadequate fat or amino acid content in the test meal or consumption of an insufficient amount of food can result in failure of cholecystokinin release and gallbladder contraction. In general it is recommended that the animal eat a meal of regular dog or cat food, although 2 teaspoons of food for pets less than 10 lbs and 2 tablespoons for larger animals has been reported to be adequate. Visual confirmation of meal consumption is mandatory. The presence of concurrent disease that delays gastric emptying may result in failure to stimulate gallbladder contraction. Alterations in intestinal transit time so that the movement of conjugated bile acids to the ileum is delayed can result in less than optimum timing for determination of the postprandial values. Severe ileal disease can result in decreased bile acid reabsorption and inadequate challenge to the enterohepatic circulation. The presence of small bowel overgrowth leads to bacterial deconjugation of bile acids and decreased ileal absorption of bile acids.

Occasionally, fasting TSBA concentrations are higher than postprandial values. This happens when interdigestive gallbladder contraction occurs during the course of the fast preceding the test. It may also be associated with individual variations in gastric emptying, response to cholecystokinin release, and intestinal transit time.

The interpretation of abnormal TSBA is subject to a number of limitations. First, TSBAs are not capable of discriminating one hepatobiliary disease from another. A second limitation of TSBA determination is that little, if any, correlation exists between the severity of histologic changes or the degree of portosystemic shunting and the extent of TSBA elevation. A TSBA value is either normal or abnormal. When evaluating serial determinations of TSBAs to monitor disease progression or response to therapy, only a return to normal can be used as a reliable indicator of clinical remission.

CARBOHYDRATE METABOLISM

The major function of the liver in carbohydrate metabolism is to maintain normoglycemia during the fasting state. The liver has a large reserve for maintaining glucose homeostasis so that greater than 70% of hepatic function must be lost before hypoglycemia occurs. Hypoglycemia occurs most often in acute fulminant hepatic failure and in small breed dogs with PSVAs.[3] In acute hepatocellular injury, hypoglycemia may be a relatively early indicator of severe hepatic failure. Up to 35% of dogs with congenital PSVAs are periodically hypoglycemic. In these dogs, hypoglycemia may be due to impaired hepatic glucose production, decreased hepatic glycogen stores, reduced responsiveness to glucagons, or a combination of these factors. Inadequate glycogen stores may reflect immaturity of the carbohydrate metabolizing enzyme systems or be a consequence of chronic stimulation of glycogenolysis. Hypoglycemia is a rare complication of end-stage chronic inflammatory liver disease and is a negative predictor of survival.[18]

Hypoglycemia may occur as a paraneoplastic syndrome in dogs with hepatic neoplasia.[8] Proposed mechanisms for the hypoglycemia include increased glucose use by the tumor or secretion of an insulin-like substance that inhibits gluconeogenesis and promotes glycogenolysis. Insulin levels, when measured, have been normal.

Glycogen storage diseases may cause hypoglycemia.[11] In dogs, a congenital deficiency in amylo-1,6-glucosidase has been associated with fasting hypoglycemia and the development of hepatomegaly due to glycogen accumulation.

CHOLESTEROL AND LIPID METABOLISM

The liver has several functions in lipid metabolism. Plasma fatty acids released from adipose tissue are extracted by the hepatocytes, after which they are either converted to triglycerides or undergo mitochondrial β-oxidation. Triglycerides are either stored or packaged as very low–density lipoproteins and released into the vasculature. The liver also extracts chylomicron remnants and low-density lipoproteins from plasma. This is the major route by which cholesterol enters into the liver, although the liver is also capable of cholesterol synthesis. Hepatic cholesterol can be esterified and then packaged and secreted in lipoproteins or stored in the liver. The majority of unesterified (free) cholesterol in the liver undergoes biliary excretion.

Hypercholesterolemia is associated with increased hepatic synthesis, decreased biliary excretion of cholesterol, or both. In the dog and cat, EHBDO is accompanied by increases in serum cholesterol. Hypocholesterolemia occurs in approximately 62% of dogs and 67% of cats with PSVAs and may be due to decreased cholesterol synthesis or increased incorporation of cholesterol into bile acids.[3] Hypocholesterolemia also occurs with late-stage chronic liver disease in dogs.[13]

URINALYSIS

Between 40% to 74% of dogs and 15% of cats with PSVAs have ammonia biurate crystalluria.[3] Repeated examination of fresh urine specimens may be necessary to document the presence of these crystals. Uric acid, a by-product of purine nucleotide catabolism, is normally converted to allantoin by hepatic urate oxidase. In hepatic disease, a deficiency of this enzyme may lead to hyperuricemia. In the presence of concurrent hyperammonemia, increased concentrations of both ions appear in the urine, resulting in the precipitation of ammonia biurate crystals.

Bilirubinuria is the presence of conjugated bilirubin in the urine. Bilirubinuria in the dog is not abnormal, because dogs have a low renal threshold for bilirubin and their renal tubular epithelium is capable of bilirubin production. Because cats have a high renal threshold for bilirubin and feline kidneys do not make bilirubin, feline bilirubinuria is always abnormal and suggests the presence of a hepatobiliary or hemolytic disorder.

HEMATOLOGIC ABNORMALITIES

Anemia may be present in dogs or cats with hepatobiliary disease. Regenerative anemia is most often associated with blood loss. Although spontaneous bleeding associated with coagulopathies is rare in animals with hepatic disease, blood loss may occur after provocative procedures or secondary to GI ulceration. Nonregenerative anemia, a more common finding in hepatic disease, is usually normocytic and normochromic and often associated with inefficient use of systemic iron stores (anemia of chronic disease). A microcytic, hypochromic, nonregenerative anemia should prompt consideration of chronic GI blood loss. Erythrocyte microcytosis occurs in dogs and cats with congenital PSVAs,[3] in dogs with acquired shunting secondary to cirrhosis and in some cats with idiopathic hepatic lipidosis. Studies investigating the cause of this microcytosis in dogs with PSVAs have documented a relative iron deficiency that may be associated with impaired iron transport.[26] Target cells and poikilocytes may be seen in dogs and cats with hepatic disease. These morphologic changes may be associated with alterations in the erythrocyte plasma membrane lipoprotein content resulting in altered cell deformability.

HEPATIC BIOPSY ACQUISITION AND INTERPRETATION

Because patterns of clinicopathologic abnormalities do not reliably differentiate one form of hepatic disease from another, it is often necessary to obtain hepatic tissue for histopathologic or cytologic evaluation. The indications for examination of hepatic tissue include persistent increases in serum liver enzymes, increased serum bile acids or bilirubin, unexplained abdominal effusion or ascites, unexplained hepatomegaly, to assess response to therapy or disease progression, and to evaluate for breed-specific hepatopathies. Because the most common complication encountered in the procurement of hepatic tissue is hemorrhage, before undergoing hepatic tissue acquisition, all dogs and cats should have a PT, APTT, and platelet count assessed. Determination of PIVKAs and buccal mucosal bleeding time may improve the sensitivity of detecting bleeding tendencies. Due to the high frequency of vitamin K deficiency in hepatic disease and the ease with which it is treated, many clinicians routinely pretreat all patients with parenteral vitamin K_1 24 hours prior to hepatic biopsy. Acquisition of hepatic tissue is contraindicated in the presence of a severe coagulopathy, although some animals may be biopsied safely after the administration of fresh frozen plasma to supply deficient coagulation factors.

In general, hepatic biopsy is preferred over fine needle aspirate (FNA) to characterize liver disorders. However, in animals with bleeding disorders or those with large cavitary lesions or suspected abscesses, ultrasound guided fine needle aspiration (22 gauge needle) can safely be performed with minimal danger of hemorrhage or spread of infection. In studies done comparing FNA to hepatic biopsy, complete agreement is typically seen in around 30% of cases. While FNAs may be helpful in identifying vacuolar or neoplastic disease such as lymphoma, they frequently miss the presence of necroinflammatory or vascular disease.

Hepatic biopsy can be obtained by ultrasound-guided needle biopsy, laparoscopic biopsy, or wedge biopsy by laparotomy. The advantages of the latter two methods are the ability to grossly evaluate the liver at the time of biopsy, the acquisition of relatively large tissue samples, and the identification and control of postbiopsy hemorrhage. An obvious disadvantage of these techniques is their invasive nature and, in the case of laparoscopy, the need for special equipment and technical expertise. Ultrasound-guided needle biopsy using automated spring-triggered biopsy needles has proven to be a safe, effective, minimally invasive means of obtaining biopsy material in most animals. Ultrasound guidance allows accurate sampling of focal lesions and permits visualization of the needle tract to minimize complications. When obtaining ultrasound-guided needle biopsy, particular care should be taken to obtain adequate samples (two to three specimens that fill at least three fourths of the 18- (in cats) or 16- (in dogs) gauge biopsy needle chamber should be obtained). Complications of ultrasound-guided needle biopsy (other than hemorrhage) are rare but include perforation of biliary structures, pneumothorax, and bacterial peritonitis. When an intrahepatic abscess is suspected or a highly vascular lesion is present, hepatic needle biopsy is contraindicated due to the high probability of infection and bleeding, respectively. Postbiopsy, animals should be monitored with ultrasound for the presence of postbiopsy bleeding and have PCV checks for up to 6 hours after the procedure.

Because the tissue obtained by wedge or needle biopsy represents only a tiny fraction (maybe 1/10,000) of the entire liver, one of the major limitations of hepatic biopsy is sampling error. Sampling error arises due to uneven distribution of lesions in what appears by diagnostic imaging to be diffuse disease. A recent study demonstrated significant discordant between the morphologic diagnoses obtained when needle and wedge biopsies from the same animal were evaluated by the same pathologist.[28] This discordance most likely reflects sampling error. This same study also demonstrated that individual pathologists disagree on the morphologic diagnosis 44% and 65% of the time when the same wedge or needle biopsies, respectively, were evaluated. This emphasizes the need for a constant stream of communication between clinician and hepatic histopathologists. Clinicians should always be the final judges as to whether the histopathologic morphologic diagnosis fits with the clinical picture. Opinions from more than one pathologist on hepatic biopsy material may be necessary to arrive at an accurate morphologic diagnosis. In addition, internist and pathologist should both be willing to accept the limitations of hepatic biopsy and be prepared to rebiopsy, if warranted.

To fully appreciate the value of histopathologic evaluation of the liver, one must understand what information to reasonably expect from tissue samples.[29] One should expect the sample to determine the category of disease (necroinflammatory, neoplastic, vacuolar, or vascular), to define the extent of disease (mild, moderate, or severe) and to access the chronicity of the lesion (presence of fibrosis, type of cellular infiltrate). One should not expect every hepatic biopsy to provide a etiologic diagnosis. The biopsy, however, may provide clues as to cause. Special stains can help to identify infectious agents or determine if copper overload exists. Samples for anaerobic and aerobic culture may confirm suspicion of primary or secondary bacterial infection. Certain infectious diseases or toxins may cause lesions with characteristic anatomic distributions

(e.g., passive congestion and acetaminophen toxicity cause centrilobular lesions), whereas infections such as salmonellosis or toxoplasmosis cause focal or multifocal lesions. Vacuolar change indicates cytoplasmic accumulation of lipid, water (hydropic degeneration), or glycogen (steroid hepatopathy). The liver can have a similar histologic reaction pattern to different insults. Macroscopic or microscopic PSVAs, primary hypophasia of the portal vein and arteriovenous fistula cause a characteristic histologic pattern (hepatic cord atrophy, portal vein attenuation, and portal arteriolar proliferation). Chronic inflammatory lesions provide the biggest challenge in interpretation, because the liver responds to many chronic insults (whether caused by toxins, infection, or immune stimulation) with the same reaction pattern. The important points to remember in evaluating inflammatory biopsies is to pay attention to the type of inflammatory cell present (neutrophilic: acute, active, or both; eosinophilic: allergic or parasitic; lymphoplasmacytic: subacute to chronic), whether inflammation breaks through the limiting plate (the disease is more severe if it does), and to note the extent of fibrosis (confined to portal regions, bridging portal tracts). Bridging fibrosis is consistent with severe disease and is a negative prognostic factor.[18]

DIAGNOSTIC IMAGING

Radiography

Radiography can be used to assess changes in the size and opacity of the liver.[30] Diffuse hepatomegaly is indicated by rounding of the liver edges, extension of the hepatic shadow beyond the costal arch, and caudal displacement of the stomach axis. Hepatomegaly may occur due to congestion, infiltrative disease (neoplasia, lipidosis, glycogen accumulation, amyloidosis), inflammatory disease, RES cell hyperplasia, or extramedullary hematopoiesis. Focal hepatomegaly can be discerned by observing displacement of the structures bordering the liver, and it may occur with cysts, granulomas, neoplasia, regenerative nodules, hematomas, or abscesses. Microhepatica is visualized radiographically by a decreased size of the hepatic shadow and a shift of the gastric axis to a more upright orientation with cranial displacement. Microhepatica is observed with hepatic atrophy and fibrosis.

Normally the liver is visualized as a homogenous soft tissue opacity. Cholelithiasis or choledocholithiasis may be visualized as mineralization in the liver. The former is recognized as a discrete round opacity in the cranial right ventral liver shadow, and the latter is seen as diffuse mineralization. Focal mineralization may also be seen with chronic gallbladder infection or neoplasia, granulomatous lesions, abscesses, resolving hematomas, and within regenerative nodules.

Gas opacities in the liver may be associated with hepatic abscesses, emphysematous cholecystitis, or after long-term bile duct obstruction. The finding of gas within the portal vessel indicates the entry of GI gas or infection with gas-producing organisms and is a grave sign seen with gastric torsions and severe necrotizing gastroenteritis.

Radiographic contrast imaging of the portal venous system is used to localize PSVAs. It can be accomplished via three methods. The first, cranial mesenteric arteriography, involves cannulation of the cranial mesenteric artery via the femoral artery and injection of iodinated contrast followed by rapid fluoroscopic imaging. These studies are fraught with technical difficulties and are seldom performed. The second method, splenoportography, involves injection of contrast agent directly into the spleen, either percutaneously or at the time of laparotomy. Complications include splenic infarction and hemorrhage. The best method to demonstrate PSVAs is operative mesenteric portography. This involves intraoperative jejunal vein catherization and injection of iodinated contrast.

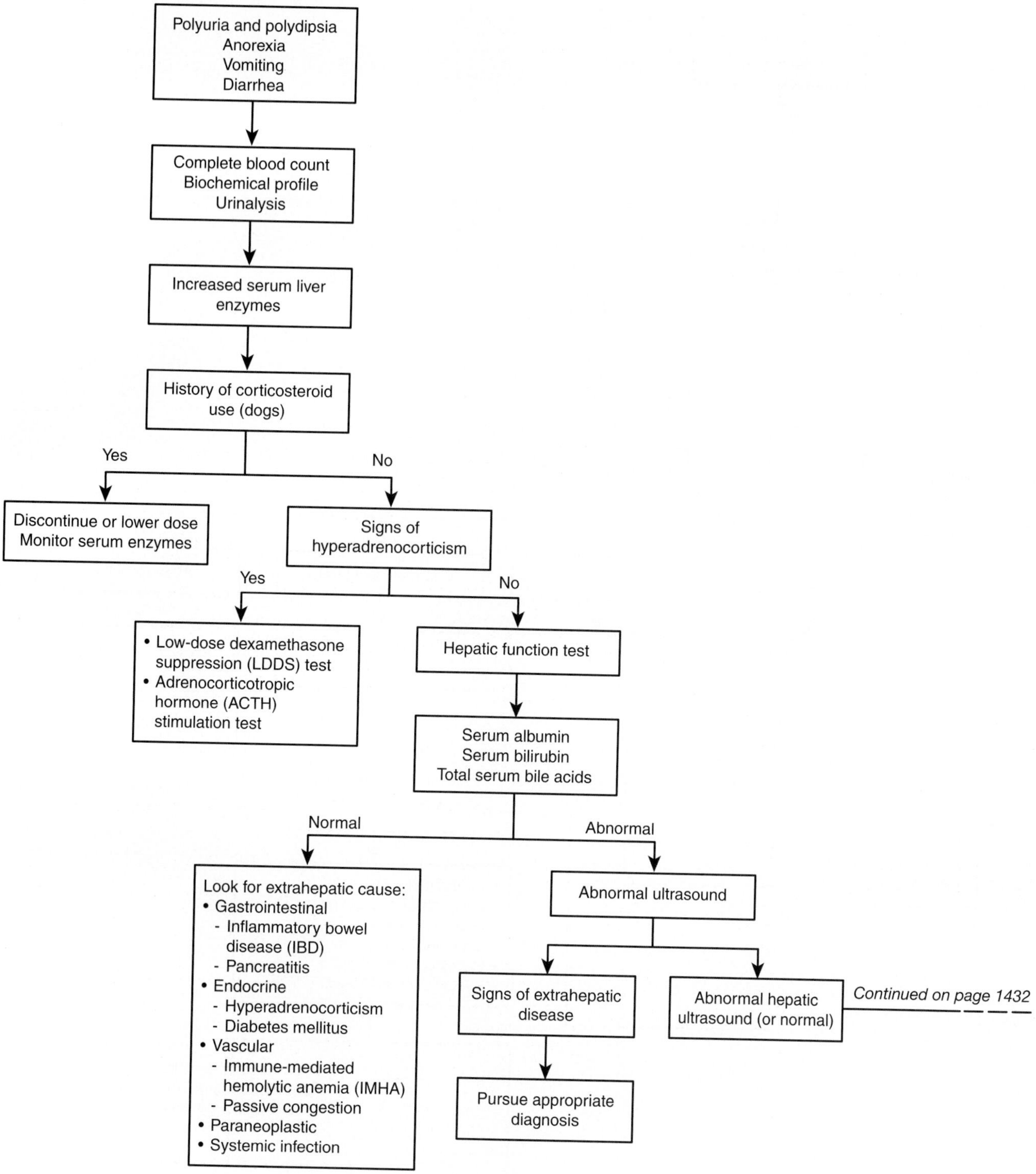

Polyuria and polydipsia
Anorexia
Vomiting
Diarrhea

↓

Complete blood count
Biochemical profile
Urinalysis

↓

Increased serum liver
enzymes

↓

History of corticosteroid
use (dogs)

Yes →

Discontinue or lower dose
Monitor serum enzymes

No →

Signs of
hyperadrenocorticism

Yes →

- Low-dose dexamethasone
  suppression (LDDS) test
- Adrenocorticotropic
  hormone (ACTH)
  stimulation test

No →

Hepatic function test

↓

Serum albumin
Serum bilirubin
Total serum bile acids

Normal →

Look for extrahepatic cause:
- Gastrointestinal
  - Inflammatory bowel
    disease (IBD)
  - Pancreatitis
- Endocrine
  - Hyperadrenocorticism
  - Diabetes mellitus
- Vascular
  - Immune-mediated
    hemolytic anemia (IMHA)
  - Passive congestion
- Paraneoplastic
- Systemic infection

Abnormal →

Abnormal ultrasound

Signs of extrahepatic
disease

↓

Pursue appropriate
diagnosis

Abnormal hepatic
ultrasound (or normal)

Continued on page 1432

Figure 225-1 Laboratory diagnosis of hepatobiliary disease.

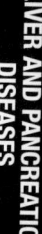

LIVER AND PANCREATIC
DISEASES

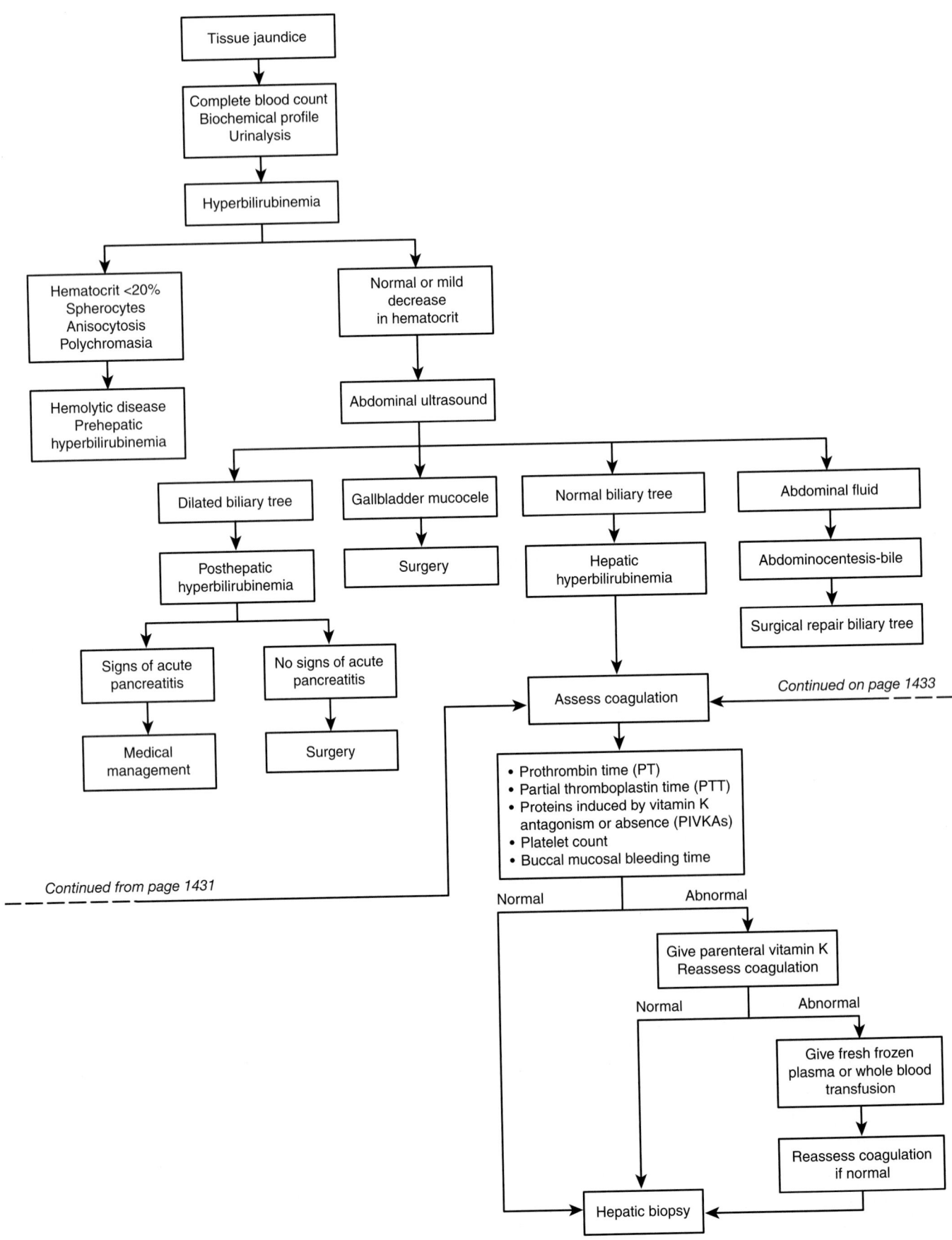

Figure 225-1 Cont'd

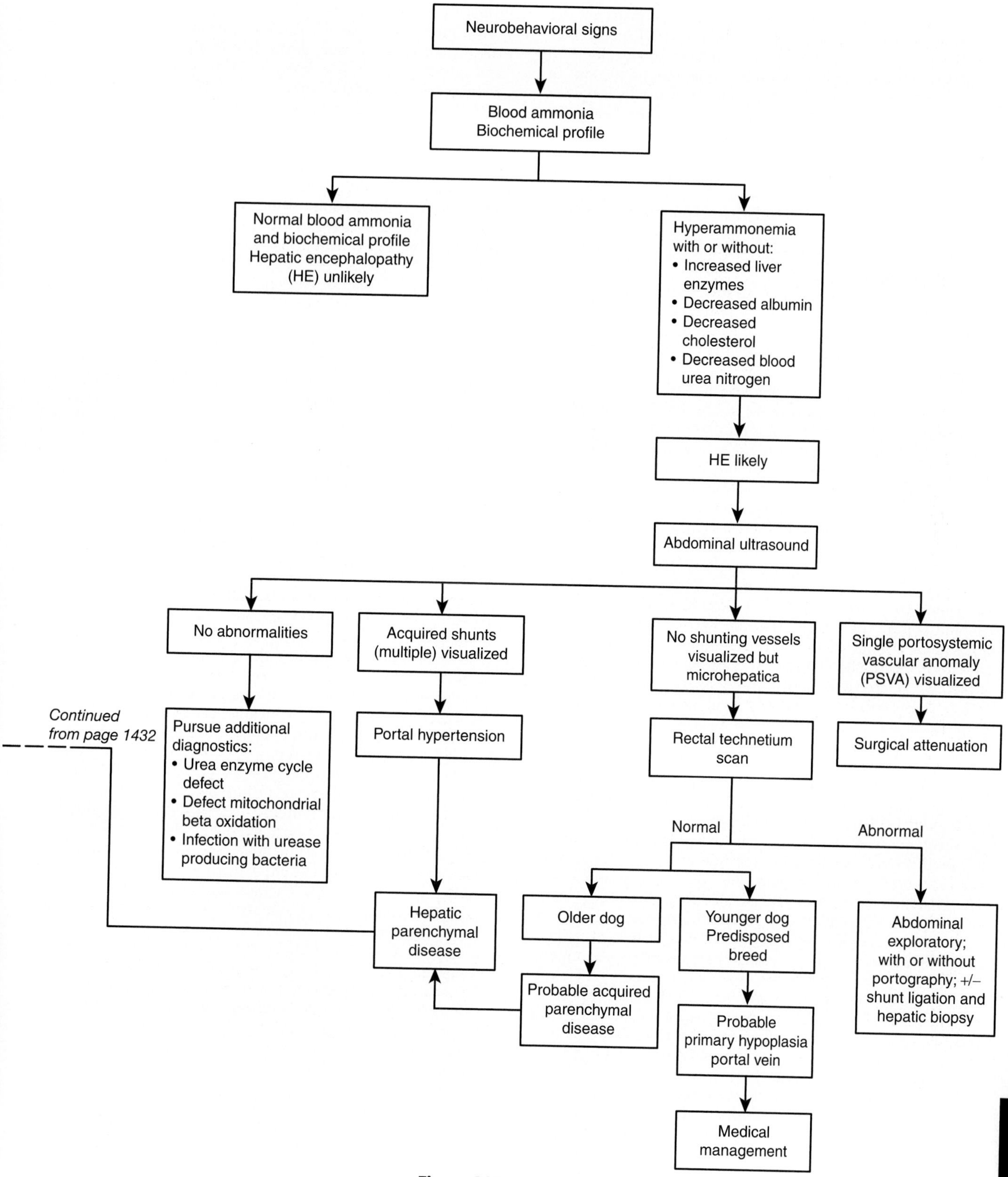

Neurobehavioral signs

→

Blood ammonia
Biochemical profile

Normal blood ammonia
and biochemical profile
Hepatic encephalopathy
(HE) unlikely

Hyperammonemia
with or without:
• Increased liver
  enzymes
• Decreased albumin
• Decreased
  cholesterol
• Decreased blood
  urea nitrogen

HE likely

Abdominal ultrasound

No abnormalities

Acquired shunts
(multiple) visualized

No shunting vessels
visualized but
microhepatica

Single portosystemic
vascular anomaly
(PSVA) visualized

Pursue additional
diagnostics:
• Urea enzyme cycle
  defect
• Defect mitochondrial
  beta oxidation
• Infection with urease
  producing bacteria

Portal hypertension

Rectal technetium
scan

Surgical attenuation

*Continued
from page 1432*

Normal

Abnormal

Hepatic
parenchymal
disease

Older dog

Younger dog
Predisposed
breed

Abdominal
exploratory;
with or without
portography; +/–
shunt ligation and
hepatic biopsy

Probable acquired
parenchymal
disease

Probable
primary hypoplasia
portal vein

Medical
management

Figure 225-1 Cont'd

Colorectal scintigraphy is used in small animals for the detection of PSVAs.[31] In these studies, a small amount of [99m]technetium pertechnetate is administered rectally and absorbed across the colon into the portal venous system. In the normal dog, radioactivity is visualized in the liver within 10 to 22 seconds and subsequently moves to the heart and lungs. In animals with PSVAs, radioactivity reaches the heart and lungs first or at the same time as the liver. Rectal technetium scans are abnormal in dogs with macroscopic PSVAs or acquired shunts from chronic parenchymal disease and normal in dogs with microvascular dysplasia or parenchymal disease without acquired shunts.

Ultrasonography

Ultrasonography enables differentiation between focal and diffuse disease, evaluation of alterations in hepatic parenchyma in diffuse disease, evaluation of the biliary system and portal vasculature, and procurement of tissue for hepatic histopathology.[32,30]

The normal liver has a homogenous echogenicity that is isoechoic to slightly hyperechoic to the renal cortex. It has sharp, smooth edges and contains numerous variably sized circular and tubular anechoic structures that represent hepatic and portal veins. Hepatic arteries and intrahepatic bile ducts are not routinely visualized. The gallbladder is seen as an anechoic structure with thin walls varying from oval to pear shaped. It may be bilobed in the cat. The common bile duct can be visualized as a tubular anechoic structure just ventral to the portal vein. During hepatobiliary disease, changes in hepatic size, vascularity, and echogenicity may occur. It must be emphasized that few hepatic lesions have diagnostic sonographic features and that a normal hepatic ultrasound does not rule out the possibility of diffuse hepatic disease.

The determination of liver size by sonography is, at best, subjective. A large liver may be easily imaged and has rounded edges. There will be a relatively large distance between the diaphragm and stomach. A small liver may be difficult to image, with a narrow distance identified between the diaphragm and stomach.

In diffuse hepatic disease the liver may appear hyperechoic or hypoechoic. The hyperechoic liver is brighter than the renal cortices. Portal vein margins become indistinct in the hyperechoic liver. Increased echogenicity may accompany fibrotic liver disease, lipidosis, corticosteroid hepatopathy, or hepatic neoplasia (lymphoma, bile duct adenocarcinoma). The fibrotic liver can be distinguished from the other causes of increased echogenicity by its small size, the presence of regenerative nodules, and its association with ascites. In a series of cats with various hepatobiliary disorders, the finding of a hyperechoic liver that was isoechoic to falciform fat was highly suggestive of the presence of hepatic lipidosis. A hypoechoic liver is less echogenic than the renal cortices and has enhanced visualization of portal vasculature. It may accompany moderate to severe suppurative hepatic disease, passive congestion, or hepatic lymphoma.

The sonographic appearance of hepatic lymphoma can be quite variable. The liver may be diffusely hyper- or hypoechoic. There may be focal or multifocal poorly circumscribed hypoechoic masses or well-circumscribed hyperechoic nodules surrounded by areas of hypoechogenicity (so called target lesions).

A variety of focal hepatic lesions can be recognized with ultrasonography. Hepatic cysts appear as round, smoothwalled, anechoic structures with acoustic enhancement.

Biliary cysts appear as thin-walled, circular, anechoic structures. Hematomas have a variable appearance, depending on their state of resolution. Early hematomas are hyperechoic and progress to hypoechoic; once they mature, they are anechoic. They may have areas of mineralization. Regenerative nodules also have a variable appearance. They may be hypoechoic, isoechoic, hyperechoic, or have mixed echogenicity. Variably sized multiple hypoechoic areas often exist; some areas may appear anechoic if necrosis occurs within them. Abscesses or granulomas have a variable appearance, depending on their cellular composition and duration. Early abscesses are hyperechoic with poorly defined margins. As they mature they become more hypo- to anechoic and may have mixed echogenicity. The presence of gravity-dependent hyperechoic cellular material may be demonstrated. Occasionally they may contain gas or mineralization. Some posterior acoustic enhancement may occur.

Primary hepatic neoplasia may have a variable appearance.[8] It usually is a large, solitary, moderately circumscribed mass that bulges beyond the normal liver margins with an echo texture similar to normal liver. Metastatic neoplasia appears as one or more spherical lesions that may be hypoechoic, hyperechoic or isoechoic. It may also appear as a target lesion.

Ultrasonography is important in determining the presence of EHBDO.[32] The first indication of EHBDO is distention of the gallbladder with loss of tapering of the neck into the cystic duct. This occurs 24 hours after experimental bile duct ligation in the dog. The common bile duct distends by 48 hours postligation. Extrahepatic bile ducts dilate by 72 hours and are visible as many tortuous anechoic structures at the portal hepatis between the gallbladder and the pancreas. Intrahepatic bile ducts distend by 1 week and are seen as tortuous, irregularly branching anechoic structures with echogenic walls throughout the liver. In cats, distention of the common bile duct to greater than 5 mm is consistent with EHBDO.[33] Ultrasound also enables visualization of the cause of the obstruction that may be associated with intraluminal (neoplasia, strictures, choleliths) or extraluminal (pancreatitis, neoplasia) disorders.

Abdominal ultrasonography has an accuracy rate of about 90% for the diagnosis of PSVAs.[31] Animals with PSVAs have small livers with a decrease in portal vascular structures and may have bilateral renomegaly and uroliths. The abnormal connection between the portal vein and the systemic vasculature may be visualized. In general, intrahepatic shunts are easier to visualize than extrahepatic shunts. Portoazygous shunts are the most difficult extrahepatic shunts to identify. Doppler capabilities can enhance the ability to detect extrahepatic shunts. Dogs with extrahepatic shunts have high-velocity turbulent flow in the portal vein, and preliminary studies show a decreased portal vein size as assessed by comparison of the portal vein with the aorta or caudal vena cava. Acquired portosystemic shunts are more difficult to visualize by ultrasound but can be seen in the retroperitoneum near the kidneys or medial to the spleen. Other signs of portal hypertension such as ascites, decreased or reversed portal blood flow, and microhepatica are seen when acquired shunts are present.

Hepatic arteriovenous fistulas can be seen with as tortuous, tubular, anechoic structures within or adjacent to the liver. Doppler-assisted ultrasonography demonstrates areas of turbulent blood flow. The hepatic artery and portal vein branches may be dilated and tortuous. Celiac arteriography is used to identify arteriovenous fistulas and to define the limits of surgical resection.

CHAPTER 226

General Principles in the Treatment of Liver Disease

Jan Rothuizen

INTRODUCTION

Many generally accepted and clinically used medications for liver disease lack critical evaluation of their effectiveness. A scientific basis for proof of effect of a medication may be obtained in different ways.

First, there may be a well understood and direct connection with the pathophysiologic basis of the disease. An example is the use of thyroid hormone to treat hypothyroidism caused by decreased production in the thyroid glands. A firm and direct relationship should be present between cause of disease and medication to accept such as a basis. A proven pathophysiology-based therapy in human medicine supports the use for comparable lesions in veterinary medicine. An example is ursodeoxycholic acid (UDCA) therapy in non-obstructive cholestatic diseases. Proof in humans, however, is not proof for dogs or cats and does not eliminate the need for veterinary studies.

The second way a therapy can be accepted as scientifically based is when an effect has been proven in clinical trials. The best method is a randomized, double-blind, placebo-controlled study. No reports exist in the literature of any randomized, placebo-controlled, double-blind studies on the effect of a treatment of liver disease of dogs or cats. Because few, if any, clinics have a sufficient case load to perform a number of such studies within a reasonable time, the only way to test therapies for liver diseases is to perform multicenter studies. Bearing in mind that sound studies on the effectiveness of a drug can only be performed by evaluating one (additional) drug per trial, it is clear that a lot of work must be done. Accepting the need for multicenter studies identifies the need for standardization of the nomenclature and diagnostic criteria for diseases. The diagnosis of the majority of canine and feline liver diseases depends largely on the histologic evaluation of liver tissue, obtained by one of several possible biopsy techniques. It is well known that evaluation of one liver specimen by different histopathologic produces different interpretations, often even a range of different diagnoses. Moreover, in different countries or continents, the same disease may be known under different names without clinicians realizing that it is one disease. The need for standardization of diagnostic criteria of diseases and stages of disease, as well as the unification of nomenclature, has recently been recognized by the World Small Animal Veterinary Association (WSAVA), in cooperation with the American and European Colleges of Veterinary Internal Medicine, ACVIM and ECVIM. This group has agreed on the standardization of nomenclature and histopathologic interpretation of liver tissues of known liver diseases of dogs and cats. The results are being published in a book (see www.wsava.org), providing descriptions and color slides of histologic features. These standards will be updated every 3 years. The availability of standardized criteria and nomenclature will aid multicenter studies on liver diseases.

DRUGS USED FOR TREATMENT OF LIVER DISEASES

Glucocorticoids (Prednisone and Prednisolone)

The use of corticosteroids has been common practice in human medicine for 30 to 40 years. Mononuclear inflammatory cells, lymphocytes, and plasma cells in chronic hepatitis leads to the assumption that (auto-) immune reactions were the main cause of ongoing, chronic hepatitis leading to the development of cirrhosis. The recognition of hepatitis viruses A and B limited this category to nonA-nonB hepatitis and later nonA-nonB-nonC hepatitis after discovery of hepatitis C virus. These terms have been abandoned in human medicine. Many different viruses cause many different forms of hepatitis. Only a small and well-defined group remains classified as autoimmune hepatitis that is treated with corticosteroids. The different forms of viral hepatitis require specific antiviral treatment or only supportive treatment. Recognition of new canine viral and metabolic causes may lead to development of specific treatments for different forms of hepatitis that are now taken together as idiopathic hepatitis. Presently, steroid therapy is the best-documented and most generally used therapy for chronic hepatitis. Many anecdotal reports exist. Only one publication[1] reports the evaluation of the effect of glucocorticoids on the survival in a large series of dogs with chronic hepatitis in which there was a highly significant increased survival found in treated compared with untreated dogs. Complete remission was described, and no relapse occurred when recovery from hepatitis was reached. This report was a retrospective, uncontrolled study. The general experience of veterinary hepatologists is that glucocorticoids are often effective in treating chronic hepatitis in dogs. Prednisone needs to be metabolized into prednisolone by the liver. It is logical to use prednisolone in case of liver disease. Prednisolone can be regarded as a treatment of first choice for idiopathic chronic hepatitis. For cases in which a defect in copper metabolism is known, leading to copper storage and oxidative damage of the liver, specific chelating therapy instead of steroids is indicated. Corticosteroids have anti-inflammatory effects but also anti-fibrotic and choleretic effects. Their principle indication remains immunomodulation. For stimulation of choleresis, UDCA is much more effective, and the weak effect on formation of fibrosis does not justify the use of corticosteroids for treatment of fibrosis without mononuclear inflammation.

Glucocorticoids are contraindicated for infectious diseases of the liver and biliary system. They should be reserved for chronic hepatitis with mononuclear inflammation of which no infectious cause is known. Toxins, viruses, and so on may cause acute hepatitis, but the specific cause remains unknown in most cases. Most acute hepatitis cases recover spontaneously without treatment or with only symptomatic support (antiemetics, fluid therapy). Given the similarities between hepatitis in dogs and other species in which hepatitis is nearly always caused by viral infections, at least some dogs with acute hepatitis may have an active viral infection. This may be overcome by the immune response so that the dog recovers or in some cases develops a chronic inadequate (auto-) immune response. In the chronic stage of disease, immunosuppression may help to reduce the inflammatory effects without treating the underlying cause. In acute cases such medication is contraindicated. The author has seen a number of dogs with acute hepatitis develop a sudden fatal deterioration when corticosteroids were given. Side effects of glucocorticoids are detailed in Chapter 242.

Azathioprine

If immunosuppression is the desired action of therapy and glucocorticoids yield unacceptable adverse effects, azathioprine is an alternative drug. By combining azathioprine and glucocorticoids, the steroid dose can be reduced so that side effects can be avoided or made acceptable. A disadvantage of azathioprine is bone marrow suppression. It is more expensive than glucocorticoids and is also potentially toxic to humans. The owner should use gloves during administration, and tablets should be chosen so that they do not need to be broken, thereby exposing the owner to inhalation of small particles. No studies have reported the effects of azathioprine in liver diseases. Azathioprine is not a preferred drug to treat liver diseases other than in rare cases that do not tolerate glucocorticoids. Azathioprine should be avoided in cats because severe side effects are common.[2]

Ursodeoxycholic Acid

UDCA is one of the natural bile acids in the enterohepatic circulation.[3] It is synthesized and manufactured as tablets or capsules (e.g., Actigall, Ursochol) that are used in both human and veterinary medicine. Bile acids are produced and conjugated in the liver, and they are kept very efficiently in the enterohepatic cycle. The primary bile acids (those primarily formed in the liver) are transformed by intestinal bacteria into secondary and tertiary bile acids so that a mixture of bile acids circulates. Some bile acids are highly toxic, especially in the liver where they are concentrated. The less hydrophilic the more toxic the specific bile acid tends to be[4]; the most toxic bile acid is lithocholic acid. The hydrophilic UDCA is nontoxic in concentrations encountered in normal or diseased liver. Toxic bile acids have a number of negative effects. They induce apoptosis[5] of hepatocytes by activation of the Fas receptor, which activates intracellular signaling of the apoptosis pathway. Liver cell necrosis is also induced by altered permeability of the mitochondrial membrane due to high concentrations of bile acids. Disruption of the mitochondrial electron transport chain leads to formation of free radicals and oxidative damage to the cells.

The proposed positive actions of the nontoxic bile acid UDCA are fourfold. UDCA has been shown to prevent cells from entering the apoptosis pathway and to prevent mitochondrial damage. The exact mode by which these actions occur is not known. One explanation is that toxic bile acids, such as lithocholic acid, circulate in the enterohepatic circulation and accumulate in the liver cholestasis. They are displaced from the bile acid pool by constant enrichment of the pool with UDCA. Another explanation is induction of an increased bile flow by UDCA. Active bile acid excretion into the bile canaliculi by hepatocytes is one of the main mechanisms in which bile is formed because excretion of bile acids against a huge concentration gradient is followed by water, building the flow of bile.[6] Addition of external bile acids to the pool induces the need for hepatocytes to excrete more bile acids, thereby enhancing the bile flow and efflux of toxic bile acids. The enhanced bile flow explains also why UDCA is contraindicated in cases of extrahepatic bile duct obstruction.

The third action of UCDA is modulating the immune system, resulting in reduction of the immune response, which may be favorable in cases where autoimmunity is part of the trigger for ongoing disease.

Finally, UDCA has recently been shown to increase the production of glutathione (GSH)[4] and metallothionein in hepatocytes, which could help to prevent oxidative damage.

Both dogs and cats are given 15 mg/kg/day, divided over two doses. UDCA has virtually no side effects in therapeutic doses. It is therefore a safe drug that at least does no harm to the patient. However, no published studies are available on the clinical effect of UDCA in dogs or cats. Although in theory UDCA may be used in a wide spectrum of diseases, it has only been proven effective in human chronic cholestatic disease such as primary biliary cirrhosis.[7-9] At present, the main indication in analogy to use in human medicine seems to be chronic severe cholestatic diseases such as destructive cholangiolitis in dogs and lymphocytic cholangitis in cats.

Antioxidants

Oxidative stress and damage of cells by free oxygen radicals is a mechanism extensively studied in recent years. Factors such as reduced blood perfusion, inflammatory reactions, and accumulation of copper or iron in the liver may be incriminated in the development of hepatocyte necrosis and hepatitis. Copper toxicosis results in chronic hepatitis or hemolysis, specifically by oxidative damage caused by free copper in the cell. Oxidation is also the principle mechanism by which phalloidin,[9-11] produced by the mushroom *Amanita phalloides* and acetaminophen[12-14] may cause severe, sometimes fulminant liver failure. Oxidative stress is also a key step in the pathogenesis of ethanol-associated liver injury in man. The main sources of free radicals are hepatocyte mitochondria, cytochrome P450 enzymes, and endotoxin-activated macrophages (Kupffer cells).[15] Free radicals take up electrons from neighboring molecules, causing oxidative damage to lipids, proteins, and DNA. The normal cellular defense mechanisms against oxidative stress are superoxide dismutase (SOD), catalase, and GSH peroxidase. Depletion of GSH may cause exhaustion of part of the cellular defense and oxidative damage. Nutritional vitamins C and E act also as free-radical scavengers.

It is logical to separate the liver diseases in which oxidation is the principle event leading to tissue damage and inflammation (such as amanita and acetaminophen intoxication and copper storage diseases) and liver diseases (such as viral or idiopathic hepatitis) where oxidative stress may be one factor in a series of events but not the key factor. The beneficial effect of antioxidant therapies has been well-proven in amanita- and acetaminophen-induced damage, both in experimental animal models[9,11-13] and in human[10] and veterinary medicine.[14] For copper storage diseases in which free intracellular copper is the trigger for free-radical formation, the best therapy remains direct elimination of free copper by copper-chelating drugs such as penicillamine. No reports exist on the effect of antioxidant therapy in copper storage diseases of dogs; therefore clinicians have no reason to consider such therapies in addition to chelating drugs. The only event in copper storage diseases in which use of antioxidants is logical is hemolytic crisis that has at least been described in Bedlington terriers, similar to humans with Wilson's disease. Such an acute and severe oxidative stress requires all possible medications available to save the animal, and chelating therapy together with antioxidants may be life saving. The use of antioxidant therapy in other liver diseases is much more speculative, because oxidative damage is only one factor in a complex pathogenesis. Several antioxidants may be used as therapy; however, no scientific reports exist on efficacy and use is speculative. The main antioxidants are vitamin C, vitamin E, silymarin, and S-adenosyl-L-methionine (SAMe). In addition, zinc and UDCA have antioxidant function.

Vitamins C and E

These vitamins are normally synthesized by dogs and cats, whereas humans cannot make vitamin C (ascorbate). Vitamin C is one of the physiologically soluble intracellular antioxidants. It is not known whether deficiency can occur in disease, and no reports exist regarding the clinical effect of supplementation. In LEG rats with hepatic copper storage due to Wilson's disease, addition of vitamin C to the diet prolonged their lives and retarded hepatitis and jaundice.[16] Vitamin E (alpha tocopherol) is also a nutritional antioxidant that protects against different routes of membrane peroxidation. It is not known if vitamin E is deficient in liver diseases, and no systematic evaluations of the effect of supplementation in such diseases exist. It is a lipid-soluble vitamin so, theoretically, it is expected to be helpful in cholestatic diseases. Excess of vitamin E has no side effects.

S-Adenosyl-L-methionine

SAMe is a natural metabolite in the hepatocytes. It is a precursor for cysteine, which is one of the amino acids of GSH. GSH forms one of the main defense mechanisms of the cell against intoxications, and depletion causes oxidative stress. Depletion might occur by exhaustion due to exposure to toxic substances. SAMe is important in the defense against free oxygen radicals.[12-14] The precursor of SAMe is methionine, which is activated by SAMe-synthetase. Theoretically, deficient capacity of this liver enzyme as a consequence of liver disease could cause inadequate production of SAMe and GSH. SAMe is nontoxic, and administration of exogenous SAMe could restore deficient GSH in the hepatocytes. One report[17] exists of GSH levels in the liver of naturally occurring liver diseases of dogs and cats. This report showed greater variation (both decreased and increased) of GSH levels in disease than in health, which makes it difficult to conclude that low levels are a critical factor in the pathogenesis of such liver diseases. No evidence-based reports are available of clinical trials on the effect of SAMe treatment.

Silymarin

Silymarin or silibilin is the active component extracted from the fruit of *Silybum marianum*, milk thistle. Silymarin has been used for centuries in human medicine as treatment for liver diseases. It appears to be a strong free-radical scavenger by increasing cellular SOD. Many reports exist concerning its protective and even life-saving actions on the liver after intoxications with the mushroom toxin phalloidine[9-18] or acetaminophen, both of which exert their toxic effects by oxidation. Both experimentally and in human clinical medicine it appears very effective against these toxins. The typical oxidative changes of the mitochondria can be prevented in experimental intoxications with mushroom toxins, and this leaves no doubt about the therapeutic potential of silymarin. Treated dogs had lower liver enzymes, reduced prolongation of prothrombin times, and survived in one trial, whereas one third of the placebo-treated dogs died.[9] It is not known how long after intoxication silymarin has beneficial effects; reports vary from 10 minutes[9] to 5 hours.[18] This may also depend on the amount of toxin and the effective dose of the milk thistle extract. No studies have compared the protective effect of silymarin with other antioxidants such as vitamin E, SAMe, or N-acetyl-cysteine.[10]

No evidence proves that antioxidants have a beneficial effect in liver diseases not primarily caused by oxidative damage. For intoxications with phalloidine or acetaminophen, both silymarin and SAMe proved to be protective in experimental rodent studies and dogs; however, no comparison exists that is most effective. For liver diseases caused by congenital copper storage diseases, antioxidant therapy may be additional to chelating drugs. A beneficial effect has only been proven in LEG rats with Wilson's disease,[16] and no studies have shown that combining chelating drugs with vitamin yields better results than chelation alone.

Antifibrotic Drugs

Fibrosis is the unavoidable sequel of chronic liver disease, and untreated or untreatable chronic liver diseases end in fibrosis, cirrhosis, and incapacity of the liver to regenerate. Increased lipid peroxidation in hepatocytes activates the mesenchymal hepatic stellate cells (HSCs). Transforming growth factor beta-1 (TGF-β) is the principle and most potent fibrogenic cytokine and is produced by Kupffer cells and HSCs.[19,20] HSCs are also the primary target cells that produce extracellular collagen matrix.[21] Specific drugs to inhibit TGF-β[20] are not clinically available. Hepatocyte growth factor (HGF) is the principle hepatotrophic factor for liver regeneration, and it suppresses hepatic fibrogenesis in animal experiments. Inhibitors of HSC also exist.[19,20] These three most promising routes (inhibition of TGF-β, inhibition of HSC, and stimulation of HGF) to actively reduce liver fibrosis and stimulate liver regeneration are not beyond the experimental stage. Presently the reduction of lipid peroxidation (which reduces HSC activation) is the only clinically available method. Silymarin, SAMe, and vitamin E are most promising in this respect, but no clinical studies exist. One certain way to stop fibrogenesis of the liver to prevent cirrhosis is to treat the underlying disease and thereby stop progression of fibrosis. This is certainly an explanation of why drugs such as prednisolone, azathioprine, penicillamine, zinc, and vitamin E have been mentioned as having antifibrotic effects.

Colchicine is the only drug used specifically to stop and reduce fibrosis. It is thought to act via stimulation of collagenase activity. The disadvantage is that side effects have been reported, such as vomiting, diarrhea, and neurologic signs but side effects are rare. Neither in human medicine nor in veterinary medicine has the clinical effect been proven. In large clinical studies in humans, no effect was shown[22,23]; in veterinary medicine only several anecdotal reports exist in which colchicine was always part of multidrug therapy. No reports exist concerning the use of colchicine to treat liver diseases in cats. The use of colchicine in veterinary medicine should be postponed until it has been firmly proven effective.

Anticopper Medications

One cause for chronic hepatitis which is rare in humans but may be much more important in dogs is storage of copper in the liver, which can induce oxidative damage due to free intracellular copper. Copper toxicosis in Bedlington terriers has been the historical example of this form of chronic hepatitis that is caused by a deletion in the Murr1 gene.[24] A number of forms of chronic hepatitis exist in different breeds that have been attributed to copper storage as the causative factor. These breeds are Bedlington terriers,[24] Skye terriers,[25] Dalmatians,[26] West Highland white terriers,[27] and Turkish shepherds.[28] Copper may also accumulate as a result of impaired biliary excretion secondary to cholestatic diseases. Thus hepatitis in Dobermans and Labrador retrievers may be a primary copper metabolic disease or secondary copper accumulation due to intrahepatic cholestasis in the course of hepatitis.[29] The increasing list of diseases in which hepatic copper accumulation may be the primary cause, indicates that specific therapies aimed at reducing free copper in the liver may become more important. Excessive copper is generally stored and encapsulated in the hepatocyte lysosomes, and cannot be reached by chelating drugs. Because it is the free cytoplasmatic (and not the lysosomal copper) that causes oxidative damage, quantitative copper measurement does not necessarily reflect the success of chelating or other therapy. Only diseases in which copper accumulation is the primary defect need specific anticopper medication. If copper accumulates as the consequence of a cholestatic disease, specific treatment of the underlying disease will reduce the amount of free cellular copper. The rationale for additional chelating medication has never been proven for such diseases. Chelating drugs should be used with some care because dogs treated for long periods with chelators can develop copper deficiency.

Three forms of anticopper medications are available for treatment of primary copper storage diseases. First, chelating drugs can actively bind free extracellular copper, upon which the complex is excreted into the urine by the kidneys. Extracellular copper exchanges with free intracellular copper so that by constant exhaustion of the extracellular copper pool, the toxic intracellular excess is also removed. At present two copper chelators are available. D-penicillamine has been the first drug successfully used to treat humans with Wilson's disease, and it has also been widely used to treat Bedlington terriers with copper toxicosis.[30,31] The author's experience in about 100 Bedlington terriers diagnosed at 1 year of age is that medication with penicillamine from young age on prevents the development of hepatitis and clinical signs. This was, however, not tested in a double-blind, placebo-controlled, and randomized study. The alternative copper chelating drugs are 2,2,2- and 2-3-2-tetramine tetrahydrochloride.[32] The 2-3-2-tetramine form gives higher cupriuresis in healthy dogs, and it has been used in one clinical study. However, only the 2,2,2-tetramine form (Trientene) is commercially available. Trientene may be more efficient in copper chelation than penicillamine, because copper deficiency as a result of chronic use has only been reported for Trientene.[31] The advised dose for both chelators is identical: 10 to 15 mg/kg twice daily. The effect of Trientene in copper storage diseases has only been mentioned anecdotally. It is therefore difficult to advise that it is the most appropriate copper chelating drug for dogs. Based on the facts that much more experience exists with D-penicillamine in dogs, and that it remains the preferred drug for humans with Wilson's disease, the author's preference is to use D-penicillamine. Penicillamine may have infrequent side effects, mainly nausea and vomiting. It is therefore preferred to give it twice daily together with meals. This is also the best time of administration because the blood levels will be highest at the time alimentary copper is absorbed. A second anticopper medication is zinc[33] gluconate or acetate in capsules for oral use (10 mg elemental zinc/kg twice a day). In the intestinal tract, zinc induces metallothionein in the enterocytes. This protein binds copper, and the complex is sequestered with the senescent enterocyte into the intestinal lumen. Unlike chelating drugs, zinc salts should be given 1 hour before each meal, so induction of metallothionein has taken place when alimentary copper is absorbed. Combinations of chelators and zinc salts should be avoided, because when the chelator binds zinc the removal of copper becomes less effective. The positive effect of zinc therapy has been evaluated critically in humans and has been reported anecdotally in dogs with copper storage disease. The indications for zinc therapy and chelating drugs are different. Chelators bind free copper actively and thus are an effective way to quickly remove the free intracellular copper that causes the hepatic damage. Copper chelators should be used as a routine for about 3 months to achieve complete inactivity of the hepatitis. Zinc should be used as a preventive drug to avoid accumulation of free copper in the liver. It is therefore especially effective when given to young dogs in which copper storage has been diagnosed but in which no hepatitis is present yet. This was usually done by copper measurement in liver biopsies of Bedlington terriers when they were 1 year old. At that age copper accumulation is sufficient to be diagnostic but not yet enough to produce hepatitis. The author's clinic has treated about 70 young Bedlington terriers with

subclinical copper toxicosis life-long with zinc gluconate (clinical disease has been prevented in all cases). Presently, DNA tests can be performed at young age so that liver biopsies can be avoided. It is also possible to treat dogs with clinical disease due to copper excess for several months with D-penicillamine; when liver biopsies prove recovery from hepatitis, renewed accumulation can be prevented with life-long zinc medication. Zinc gluconate has side effects other than transient inappetence in rare cases. Very long treatment can induce copper deficiency.[32] It is cheap and therefore the preferred form of treatment to prevent copper-associated hepatitis. When higher than the recommended doses are given very long, zinc intoxication can cause hemolytic anemia. The third potential form of medication for copper storage diseases is through antioxidants. It is more logical to treat the cause by removing copper by chelation rather than to fight the effects. However, in rare cases in which excessive copper causes hemolytic crisis,[34] it may be advisable to combine chelating drugs and antioxidants such as SAMe, silymarin, or vitamin E.

Treatment of Ascites in Chronic Liver Disease

Ascites typically is a late sign of decompensation in the course of chronic liver diseases, such as chronic hepatitis, cirrhosis, and portal vein hypoplasia in dogs. Cats very rarely have ascites due to chronic liver disease. The portal blood pressure is only high enough to cause ascites without hypoalbuminemia in cases of acute complete obstruction of the portal vein by thrombosis and congenital arteriovenous fistulas. Whatever the cause, in all liver diseases associated with ascites the high portal pressure may also lead to formation of portosystemic collateral vessels and various grades of hepatic encephalopathy (HE). The potential risk for HE brings the need to use diuretics with caution.[35] The main complicating factors by which HE may induce coma that may be lethal are alkalosis and hypokalemia. Only the nonionized NH_3 form of ammonia penetrates cellular (neuronal) membranes. In any form of alkalosis the reaction equilibrium: $NH_3 + H^+ \leftrightarrow NH_4^+$ shifts to the left. Therefore ammonia is much more toxic in alkalosis. In case of hypokalemia the plasma potassium is replenished by shift of potassium from the cells, in exchange with sodium and hydrogen ions. The resulting hydrogen shift causes alkalosis in the extracellular fluid and acidosis in the cells so that ammonia can easily penetrate cells. Intracellularly it becomes ionized in which form it cannot leave the cell. Blood ammonia, which is the best parameter to monitor HE, may then be surprisingly low in relation to the severity HE because most of it is trapped inside the cells. This cellular ammonia trap is easily activated with the use of most diuretics. It is therefore better to use potassium-sparing aldosterone receptor antagonizing diuretics, such as spironolactone (2 to 4 mg/kg twice a day). Only if the dog eats well enough to have adequate supply of alimentary potassium to substitute the renal loss can loop diuretics be used. Combinations of furosemide and spironolactone may be very effective to treat ascites. It is important to monitor blood pH and potassium and to correct potassium deficiency.

In a relatively short period of several days or weeks, the abdominal accumulation of free fluid can account for more fluid than the entire circulating volume. In this period the renin-angiotensin-aldosterone system is highly activated, resulting in sodium and water retention and potassium loss. Intravenous fluid therapy and potassium compensation is necessary when the dog does not eat or drink sufficiently. Complete paracentesis of ascetic fluid may complicate HE and should be avoided in liver patients.

Chronic hepatitis and even cirrhosis with active inflammation may improve so much upon treatment with corticosteroids that the disappearance of the inflammatory infiltrates provides enough reduction of portal pressures to induce remission of ascites. A low-sodium diet may help to keep the ascites controlled.

Treatment of Hepatic Encephalopathy

The source of the known toxins causing brain neurotransmitter changes known as *HE* is protein digestion in the intestinal tract. Ammonia and aromatic amino acids are the two main factors.[35] Both require portosystemic collateral circulation, either congenital or acquired due to chronic portal hypertension, to reach the systemic circulation and the blood-brain barrier. The reserve capacity of the liver in dogs is enough to prevent HE in liver disease without collateral circulation. Cats do not make the essential amino acid arginine, and HE may occur without shunting as a result of fasting. Arginine is an essential intermediate of the hepatic urea cycle, and deficiency causes inadequate detoxification of ammonia. These cats often develop hepatic lipidosis simultaneously. Lipidosis and HE are a manifestation of their inability to synthesize several essential amino acids. Large variations in susceptibility to these effects exist between cats.

Management of HE is different for dogs and cats with congenital or acquired portosystemic shunting and cats with HE due to fasting hyperammonemia resulting from arginine deficiency. Portosystemic encephalopathy, which is by far the most common form, should be treated with an appropriate diet of reduced protein content with specific reduction of sources of aromatic amino acids. Very strict reduction of proteins may be counterproductive; dog studies have shown that prevention of catabolism (i.e., negative energy balance) is more important than strict maintenance of low-protein intake. Another important factor is that lactulose and soluble fiber in the diet helps to reduce ammonia uptake from the large intestines. Lactulose and soluble fibers have many effects on ammonia metabolism; the most important effect is that it is metabolized by the colonic bacterial flora to produce acids that reduce the pH of colonic content. Ammonia is then present in the ionic form that is not absorbed and thus lost with the feces. Well-balanced commercial liver-support diets are available that meet these requirements of adequate energy content, sufficient reduction of protein with special emphasis on aromatic amino acids, and presence of soluble fiber. These diets are also low in copper and sodium. Sodium reduction may be important if portal hypertension is present, because in these cases not only HE but also ascites may form with interrelated metabolic complications as described previously. Low copper is not necessary in relation with HE or ascites, but is important in the management of those forms of canine hepatitis that are thought to be caused by copper metabolic diseases.

If diet alone is not sufficient to manage cases with portosystemic encephalopathy, clinicians can improve the HE status by giving oral lactulose. Lactulose was developed to treat constipation, because the disaccharide molecule is metabolized in the colon into multiple smaller molecules that increase the osmotic content of the colon and attracts water into the feces. The best guideline for use of lactulose for management of HE is to give just enough (twice daily) to reach slightly softer stool. The combination of diet and lactulose is often sufficient to manage chronic HE for many years in cases in which the underlying cause cannot be treated (inoperable portosystemic shunts, arteriovenous fistula, portal vein hypoplasia, inactive cirrhosis).

Deterioration of HE may occur due to several instances (see Ascites), the most important being catabolism, dehydration, alkalosis, hypokalemia, and formation of ascites. Sudden high intestinal ammonia production in the face of portosystemic collateral circulation may also cause sudden aggravation of HE. This may be caused by intestinal bleeding from gastroduodenal ulcers, which may be associated with chronic liver diseases. Blood is the most ammoniagenic protein, and in sudden deterioration it may be important to examine and treat possible gastrointestinal (GI) bleeding. Furthermore, key rules to control HE are measurement of blood pH, potassium, and ammonia, correction of hypokalemia, correction of hypovolemia, and intravenous feeding to correct catabolism. It should be understood (see Ascites) that the blood level of ammonia and potassium are reflections but not exact representations of what is going on in the neurons.

One factor in the pathogenesis of HE is an increased activity of the neuronal GABA/benzodiazepine receptor system, which suppresses neuronal activity. For this reason, one should be extremely careful in using any sedation or anesthesia exploiting this receptor system. If necessary, inhalation anesthesia is safest, because it exploits different receptors and does not depend on liver function.

Finally, additional measures exist with beneficial effects that have never been proven in veterinary cases. One of them is the use of antibiotics such as neomycin to eradicate or change the intestinal flora. In humans, lactulose and neomycin can have synergistic effects. Neomycin may be an option to use as an enema in combination with lactulose in rare cases of HE crisis.

Hepatic Encephalopathy and Liver Lipidosis in Cats

Cats can have portosystemic encephalopathy just like dogs and humans. However, the cats, which are susceptible to develop liver lipidosis when fasting, are also prone to develop HE due to deranged metabolism. Having a shared metabolic basis, feline hepatic lipidosis and nonportosystemic HE require essentially the same therapy. With this understanding, the general rules concerning the influence of hypokalemia and alkalosis also apply to HE in cats.

Hepatic lipidosis in cats is essentially a consequence of catabolism from anorexia due to any cause. Lipidosis can develop within a few days but may also take 2 weeks to occur. Some cats can withstand prolonged fasting without developing clinically significant lipidosis at all. The precise pathogenesis of lipidosis is not known in detail, but catabolism leads to decreased insulin-to-glucagon ratio in the circulation, which stimulates hormone-sensitive lipase to release fatty acids. The liver is the main place for their metabolism. One of the principle routes by which the liver can make fat stores suitable for use in other tissues is by the formation of very low–density lipoproteins (VLDL). One of the essences of this complex metabolic disorder is the unavailability of essential amino acids. These are necessary for different liver functions, such as formation of apoproteins for composition of VLDL in which form accumulating triglycerides can be exported from the liver cells, and the urea cycle in which arginine is essential. For treatment of both HE and lipidosis it is therefore essential to restore the energy balance especially by giving proteins. High-energy diets containing predominantly fats or sugars do not help these cats. Feeding liquefied baby food or commercial high-energy and high-protein veterinary formulations are equally good. The goal is to restore the energy balance and supplement amino acid deficiencies, especially arginine and taurine. L-carnitine may be an important factor because it may help the hepatocytes to exploit fatty acids in beta oxidation.[36] This is the only form of HE requiring high- instead of low-protein feeding. A daily caloric intake around 75 kcal/kg is adequate. The supplementation of vitamins by multivitamins may be beneficial in cats with long-term anorexia. When the cat is not yet too ill, a dedicated owner can often force-feed with a syringe. Otherwise a gastrotomy tube is most appropriate for long-term force-feeding without stress for the cat.[37] Force-feeding is often required for several weeks until the cat starts eating spontaneously. It is dangerous to stimulate appetite by diazepam administration. The risk for HE is a contraindication for drugs activating the GABA/benzodiazepine receptor system, over stimulation of which is part of the pathogenesis of HE. Cats with hepatic lipidosis can easily develop insulin resistance with hyperglycemia, which may gradually increase to glucose levels as seen in diabetes mellitus. The insulin resistance implies that very large doses of insulin would be needed, with the inherent risk for sudden hypoglycemia. A benefit of treatment with insulin has never been demonstrated, and it is advised to restrict therapy to forced feeding.

Glucocorticoids are contraindicated because they stimulate lipolysis and fatty acid accumulation in the liver, induce catabolism, and increase the risk for hyperglycemia. Some authors advocate the use of antibiotics for cats with hepatic lipidosis, but a positive effect has never been proven. In the author's clinic, antibiotics are not given as a routine.

It is essential to try to identify the primary cause of anorexia. Not eating is very nonspecific and occurs for multiple reasons. It is often impossible to find an underlying disease. The reader should note that this may also be a primary liver disease[38] that may remain undiscovered when the diagnosis of lipidosis is based on thin needle aspirates of the liver. Neutrophilic or lymphocytic cholangitis and hepatic lymphosarcoma are the most frequent hepatobiliary diseases causing lipidosis. Finally, it is important to realize that some cats are metabolically predisposed to develop lipidosis and nonportosystemic HE, whereas other cats can withstand negative energy balance reasonably well. The predisposed cats will easily develop the same syndrome later in their lives, and it is important that owners understand this risk. Successful management is primarily dependent on early recognition of these metabolic disorders.

Dietary Therapies for Liver Disease
The most important requirements for dietary management of liver diseases have already been mentioned under ascites, HE, and feline hepatic lipidosis. Only the copper content of dog food requires an additional remark. Several copper-associated forms of chronic hepatitis exist in dogs. With careful evaluation of the causes of hepatitis in different breeds, clinicians may discover more forms of hepatitis in which abnormal copper metabolism is the primary problem. The goal is not only to treat these cases successfully with chelating and other drugs but also to prevent disease. This may at least in part be achieved by feeding a low-copper diet. It is very difficult to formulate a home-cooked diet containing very low copper. A realistic alternative is to use one of the commercial liver diets that contain much lower copper than regular diets.

PARENCHYMAL LIVER DISEASES

Parenchymal liver diseases may be divided into metabolic diseases affecting the liver (such as steroid hepatopathy, lipidosis of the liver in case of diabetes, or induced by catabolism in fasting cats), systemic diseases secondarily involving the liver (hypoxic necrosis of the liver, nonspecific reactive hepatitis due to endotoxemia), primary hepatitis (chronic or acute) of toxic, viral or unknown cause, copper storage diseases with secondary hepatitis, and the end-stage of each form of chronic hepatitis: cirrhosis. Many of the metabolic diseases and the diseases in which the liver is secondarily involved do not require specific treatment. The regenerative capacity of the liver will result in spontaneous recovery upon successful treatment of the underlying disease. Parenchymal liver diseases that need specific treatment are acute and chronic hepatitis (including lobular dissecting hepatitis) and copper-associated hepatitis in dogs, cirrhosis in dogs, hepatic abscesses in dogs, and hepatic lipidosis in cats.

HEPATITIS IN DOGS

Acute Idiopathic Hepatitis
The cause of hepatitis is not known in most cases. Viruses may be the cause of acute idiopathic hepatitis in dogs in analogy to many other species. This implies that treatments with immunosuppressive drugs (prednisolone, azathioprine) that are being used for chronic hepatitis are contraindicated for acute hepatitis in which there may be florid viral infection. Most cases of acute hepatitis recover spontaneously and need only supportive care with antiemetics and fluid therapy. Oxidative intracellular damage may in theory be part of the pathogenesis of many liver diseases, including acute and chronic hepatitis. However, a positive effect of antioxidants has never been shown in acute idiopathic hepatitis. Acute hepatitis in dogs is almost never caused by bacterial infection. Therefore treating with antibiotics is not needed. In acute hepatitis the liver reserve capacity is almost never exhausted, so prevention of sepsis resulting from insufficient liver function by antibiotic medication is also not necessary. As a routine, idiopathic acute hepatitis, which is a histopathologic diagnosis, does not need specific treatment. Supportive care may be indicated: antiemetics in case of severe vomiting and fluid therapy in case of dehydration. The most important point in making the diagnosis of acute idiopathic hepatitis is that the disease may progress into chronic hepatitis. Usually recovery takes place in about 3 weeks. In a small number of cases, the author has seen acute hepatitis become chronic. This usually begins as a subclinical chronic hepatitis without clinical signs and is often unnoticeable with blood examination. It is therefore recommended to take a control biopsy 4 to 5 weeks after the diagnosis of acute idiopathic hepatitis so that the onset of chronic hepatitis can be discovered in an early phase. Beginning forms of chronic hepatitis can be treated very successfully with prednisolone (5 to 6 weeks 1 mg/kg/day, divided over two doses), preventing advanced fibrosis or cirrhosis. Untreated cases will become clinical in the very chronic stage, which is about 4 to 8 months later. In that stage it is usually not possible to achieve complete recovery of fibrotic damage.

Hepatitis and Necrosis Due to Phalloidine or Acetaminophen Intoxication
It is important to ask the owner if acetaminophen or mushroom toxins (phalloidine) may have been ingested recently. These toxic forms of hepatitis are caused by oxidative damage and require specific treatment. Phalloidine intoxication should be treated with silymarin (50 mg/kg/day) for 3 to 5 days. The success depends on early recognition and immediate therapy. Silymarin has been reported to lose its effect when given a few hours after intoxication. Any other antioxidant therapy such as SAMe should also be useful, but reports have focused on silymarin.[9] Supportive care, induction of vomiting in very acute intoxication, and measures to prevent or reduce HE are also indicated. Many dogs die within 1 week due to liver and kidney failure. Acetaminophen intoxication should be treated similar to phalloidine intoxication. Several reports exist concerning the favorable effect of SAMe treatment[12-14] for acetaminophen intoxication (800 mg/kg/day), but the classical treatment is with the combination of N-acetylcysteine[10] (140 mg/kg orally, every 6 hours during 3 days), vitamin C (25 to 35 mg/kg orally, every 6 hours for 2 days), and cimetidine 5 mg/kg twice a day for 4 days. Historically, acetaminophen and phalloidine intoxication have different treatments, but it is logical to expect good effect of both silymarin and SAMe, in conjunction with symptomatic therapy. Dogs with acetaminophen intoxication may have hemolysis and blood transfusion may be required.

Leptospirosis

Leptospirosis is an acute disease, primarily of the kidneys, but it also causes a nonspecific reactive hepatitis with intrahepatic cholestasis. Icterus is therefore common, although the symptoms arise mainly from acute nephritis.[39-40] Each dog with acute disease displaying icterus and acute renal failure should be treated immediately with ampicillin or amoxicillin and clavulanate.[40,41] Early institution of antibiotic therapy may be life saving. If the diagnosis is confirmed by high immunoglobulin M (IgM) titers, antibiotics are continued until kidney function is restored. Then latent bacteria in tubular epithelial cells that may cause leptospiruria should be eradicated with streptomycin given for 2 consecutive days. The acute renal failure should also be treated with fluid therapy.

Liver Abscess

Liver abscesses are rare in dogs and cats. Treatment is by surgical removal after pretreatment with antibiotics. The choice for specific antibiotics should be based on culture of an ultrasound-guided thin needle aspirate. *Staphylococcus* and *Clostridium* are most common. Antibiotics should be administered long-term, (6 to 8 weeks). Hepatic abscesses occur predominantly in older dogs, and in the author's experience many cases have a liver cell carcinoma with central necrosis that became secondarily infected. This can easily be missed; therefore clinicians should also take histologic biopsies from the margins of the abscess.

Chronic Idiopathic Hepatitis

Chronic hepatitis is one of the most frequent liver diseases in dogs. In most cases it is not possible to indicate a cause (idiopathic hepatitis). The inflammatory cells are lymphocytes and plasma cells, indicating that at least part of the pathogenesis may be immune-mediated. The only well-documented therapy is with glucocorticoids. Prednisolone should be given until the inflammation (liver cell necrosis and infiltration with inflammatory cells) has recovered completely.[1] This cannot be concluded based on clinical signs or blood examination because both will be influenced by the glucocorticoid treatment. Therefore the only reliable way to evaluate the result is with repeated liver biopsies. It is usually possible to predict approximately how long the medication should be continued. High activity (necrosis of hepatocytes and presence of inflammatory cells) of the inflammation and high degree of fibrosis indicate the need for longer treatment than in cases of low active inflammation with little fibrosis. As a rule, chronic hepatitis should be treated for at least 6 weeks; severe cases require longer treatment up to 10 to 12 weeks. Dose regimens vary. Our routine is to use a continuous dose of 1 mg/kg/day, divided over two daily doses. In the author's experience, lower doses (0.5 mg/kg/day), medication on alternating days, or both is often less effective to achieve complete remission of the disease. If unacceptable side effects indicate the need to decrease the prednisolone, combination therapy with azathioprine can be given (both drugs 0.5 mg/kg/day).

Complete remission of the disease occurs in most of the cases. Fibrotic changes are usually permanent. When inflammation disappears the dogs are usually symptomless. Severe fibrosis or cirrhosis may require life-long support by dietary measures and lactulose.

Copper-Associated Hepatitis

Copper-associated forms of hepatitis occur in Bedlington terriers, West Highland white terriers, Skye terriers, Dalmatian dogs, and Turkish shepherds. If active hepatitis is found, treatment should be with copper chelating drugs such as penicillamine. Prevention of clinical disease in cases diagnosed early or maintenance therapy with chelation when the inflammation has stopped can be achieved with zinc salts. Details are given in the general section of this chapter. Dobermans, especially 5 to 7 years old females, may display a specific form of hepatitis, called *Doberman hepatitis*. The prognosis of this disease has generally been reported to be bad, and in the author's clinic almost all Dobermans with this disease die on the usual medications. In the author's clinic, Doberman hepatitis has been treated with penicillamine alone, and this has resulted in complete remission of the disease. This may be regarded as support for the hypothesis that copper storage plays a causative role in this disease. Double blind, placebo-controlled, randomized studies are needed.

Lobular Dissecting Hepatitis

This is a very severe form of hepatitis that develops rapidly and is usually lethal within 2 to 4 weeks. Extremely pronounced fibrosis occurs, which is the reason that despite the acute course, this disease is classified under the chronic forms of hepatitis. The disease occurs more in younger dogs and affects all breeds and both sexes. Medication with immunosuppressive drugs is usually without success. No reports exist on successful medical treatment for this disease. Treatment with colchicine[22,23] is appropriate for this disease.

DISEASES OF THE BILIARY SYSTEM

Destructive Cholangiolitis in Dogs

This is strictly not a form of hepatitis but an idiosyncratic reaction in dogs, nearly always to drugs containing sulfonamides. Necrosis of the smaller intrahepatic bile ductules is the result, and these dogs display extremely severe intrahepatic cholestasis. The first action is immediate withdrawal of the sulfonamide medication. The necrosis of the intrahepatic bile ductules is irreversible, and the only hope is that it is possible to save and exploit the remaining biliary system. In the author's experience, it is essential to start treatment with UDCA immediately. As a rule, life-long medication is needed to exploit the remaining biliary system optimally. When the dog shows enough response to justify hope for a long-term survival, the clinician should evaluate the long-term reaction in the liver. Chronic cholestasis may induce a chronic damage to the liver with continuous loss of functional hepatocytes and activation of the deposition of fibrous tissue. This may finally produce portoportal bridging fibrosis in the liver (biliary fibrosis) that, although the architecture of the liver lobules remains in tact, can give rise to portal hypertension. Ascites and formation of acquired portosystemic shunting may result. Long-term progress can often be predicted by evaluating liver biopsies 2 to 3 months after the start of treatment. If enough capacity of the intrahepatic biliary system remains, some dogs may be maintained with continuous ursodeoxycholic acid medication. In decompensating cases, supportive treatment or prevention of HE or ascites is indicated.

Neutrophilic Cholangitis in Cats

This disease is characterized by a neutrophilic inflammation of the biliary tract. The synonym is suppurative or acute cholangitis. This is essentially a septic disease, and it is therefore required to sample bile from the gall bladder by ultrasound-guided puncture with a thin needle for cytologic evaluation and both aerobic and anaerobic culture with sensitivity testing. In the vast majority of cases *E. coli* is cultured, but *Staphylococci* or other bacteria may also be identified. It may in some cases be an infection superimposed on pre-existing bile duct obstruction associated with cholelithiasis, pancreatic, or intestinal disease.[42] Bile duct obstruction requires surgical decompression and antibiotic medication guided by culture of bile. The true uncomplicated neutrophilic cholangitis is an acute disease characterized only by bacterial infection of the bile ducts, as evaluated with the combination of bile culture, liver histology, and ultrasonography. Uncomplicated neutrophilic cholangitis responds quickly to antibiotic therapy. Amoxicillin-clavulanate, amoxicillin, or ampicillin may be the first choice treatment until the results of culture become available. Treatment for at least 4 weeks is necessary. If pre-existing bile duct disease is present, the treatment should be adjusted accordingly. The additional use of UDCA is often advised, but in the author's experience single antibiotic therapy is adequate in nearly all uncomplicated cases.

Lymphocytic Cholangitis in Cats

This is a very chronic disease of the bile ducts (both intra- and extrahepatic). Secondary inflammation with fibrosis may also affect the portal tracts. Both in the bile system and in the portal tracts, lymphocytes are the predominant inflammatory cell type. Because the principle site of the disease is the bile system and not the liver, the standardized name is *lymphocytic cholangitis* (synonyms cholangiohepatitis, chronic or lympho-plasmacytic or nonsuppurative cholangitis, sclerosing cholangitis). The cause is unknown, but a similar form of chronic cholangitis may be due to liver fluke infestation, which occurs on all continents. The very chronic bile duct inflammation of lymphocytic cholangitis causes irregularly distended, fibrotic bile ducts that are prone to secondary bacterial infection. The wide, irregular, but still more or less patent bile ducts that are visible on ultrasonography, should be distinguished from distension due to extrahepatic bile duct obstruction. In case of obstruction, treatment with UDCA is contraindicated,[4] whereas it is one of the most useful medications for lymphocytic cholangitis. In most cases the difference can only be made with histologic examination of a liver biopsy. The two diseases have different histological characteristics. Liver fluke eggs may also be visible histologically in the bile ducts, but they should also be evaluated with fecal examination.

Agreement on treatment of lymphocytic cholangitis is not yet settled. Similarities exist (with human primary sclerosing cholangitis and primary biliary cirrhosis) for which the pathogenesis is equally unknown but has been proposed to be autoimmune. This has prompted treatment of these cats with glucocorticoids (2 to 4 mg/kg/day). However, this has been found to be ineffective in most cases.[42] As confirmed by the author's experience, any response to even very long-term high-dose glucocorticoid medication is rare. Alternatively, methotrexate in addition to glucocorticoids has been proposed,[42] because this is used for human autoimmune disorders. However, this treatment is not without risk, and a positive effect has not yet been reported. Similarly, metronidazole may have an effect on cell-mediated immunity, and it has been advocated in combination with glucocorticoids. However, no reports are available on the evaluation of this combination.

UDCA may be the only generally advised drug for which at least a theoretic basis exists. It has beneficial effects on cholestatic diseases in different ways. Positive effects on non-obstructive cholestatic disease have been proven in human cholestatic diseases. UDCA (15 mg/kg/day, divided over two doses) is advised as the main therapy for this disease. Treatment should be given until the disease has resolved, which in many cats implies life-long medication. No adverse effects of this therapy have been reported in dogs or cats. It is imperative to exclude extrahepatic bile duct obstruction before starting UDCA medication.

Antibiotics may have a place in the treatment of cats with lymphocytic cholangitis, but no reports exist concerning the effect of chronic antibiotic medication. It is not logical to treat all cats with antibiotics. The bile culture (aerobic and anaerobic) is positive in some cats, presumably due to secondary infection of the abnormal biliary system. It is advised to perform gall bladder puncture to obtain bile for culture and cytologic examination in all cats with cholangitis. Cats with a positive culture require antibiotics, based on the sensitivity tests. Long-term treatment is needed (6 to 8 weeks). At present, one should accept that the cause and pathogenesis of lymphocytic cholangitis is unknown, and that therapy is in most cases does not induce remission. Clinical improvement and slackening of the progression may occur.

If liver fluke infestation is present or suspected based on liver histology, the preferred treatment is with praziquantel (Droncit). Medication for 3 days (20 mg/kg/day) is most commonly given, but reinfections may occur. It is important to evaluate feces for fluke eggs after medication.

CHAPTER • 227

Inflammatory Canine Hepatic Disease

Michael D. Willard

CHRONIC HEPATITIS

Chronic hepatitis (CH) refers to a syndrome that has previously been identified by several names (e.g., chronic active hepatitis, chronic persistent hepatitis, chronic lobar hepatitis). In this chapter, *CH* will refer to chronic (i.e., ≥6 months) canine hepatic disease in which a hepatocellular necrosis exists that is associated with a predominately lympho-plasmacytic inflammation that typically progresses to fibrosis and cirrhosis. The cause, if known, should be included as an adjective (e.g., drug-induced CH, copper-associated CH); otherwise the CH is termed *idiopathic*. Additional descriptors (i.e., mild, moderate, severe) of the severity of the inflammation and of the chronicity as indicated by fibrosis are desirable.[1-3]

CH may have various causes (e.g., copper, drugs, infectious agents), and familial tendencies exist. Breeds that have been reported to have an increased frequency of CH include Doberman pinschers, Bedlington terriers, West Highland white terriers, Cocker spaniels, dalmatians, Skye terriers, standard poodles, Labrador retrievers, German shepherd dogs, Scottish terriers, and beagles.[1,2,4,5] Dogs 4 to 7 years old seem more commonly affected. Some papers suggest that females are more commonly affected, whereas others suggest that both sexes are at risk. However, particular breeds have definite sex predilections (e.g., female Doberman pinschers, male cocker spaniels).[1-3]

Most dogs with CH have idiopathic disease, and immune mechanisms may play an important role in some animals.[2,3] In one recent study, CD3+ lymphocytes were the most common lymphoid cells in the liver of 16 dogs with CH. The number of CD3+ cells was positively correlated with necrosis, and these lymphoid cells occasionally surrounded degenerating hepatocytes. Inflammation was worse in the earlier stages but then decreased as the livers became cirrhotic.[6] Whether this immune response was the cause of or an effect of the hepatitis remains to be elucidated. This is in keeping with another report that found that 54% of the hepatic lymphocytes in normal dogs were CD3+ cells.[7] Antinuclear antibodies and antibodies to liver membrane proteins have also been found in some dogs with CH, but again, cause and effect has not been clarified.[1,2]

Copper accumulation has been associated with CH in several breeds (Box 227-1). In Bedlington terriers, hepatic copper accumulation is the cause of the hepatitis; however, copper may accumulate secondary to cholestasis. In most other breeds the relationship between copper and CH is either uncertain or the copper accumulation is thought to be an epiphenomenon. Excessive hepatic copper accumulation secondary to hepatitis may be clinically insignificant, but hypothetically it might be able to further aggravate hepatic injury. Normal dogs generally have less than or equal to 400 µg copper/gm hepatic tissue, dry weight (i.e., parts per million [ppm]).[8] Dogs with greater than 2000 ppm usually have hepatic disease caused by copper, although one author stated that dogs may have 3500 ppm before hepatic disease occurs.[9] In dogs with hepatic disease, hepatic copper levels less than 1000 ppm are probably secondary to hepatic disease, concentrations greater than 2000 ppm are probably primary causes of hepatic disease, and concentrations greater than 1000 ppm are possibly primary causes.[8,10]

Iron also accumulates in the livers of dogs with hepatic disease. In one study, 54 of 95 dogs (56 of which had histologic evidence of hepatic disease) had excessive hepatic iron,[11] whereas in another study, 32 of 34 dogs with CH had increased hepatic iron.[12] Normal hepatic iron is 400 to 1200 ppm, but some dogs had up to 7680 ppm with a mean of 1354 ppm.[11] The presence of iron was correlated with the presence of hepatic injury, but there was not a linear relationship between the amount of iron and the degree of hepatic pathology. The iron accumulated in Kupffer cells and macrophages but not hepatocytes; therefore it was not hemochromatosis as reported in people. Rather, iron accumulation seems secondary to inflammation, necrosis, or copper accumulation (or a combination of these conditions). Some have hypothesized that such secondary iron accumulation in the hepatic parenchyma may aggravate existing hepatic damage.[11]

Alpha-1 antitrypsin (α1-AT), also known as alpha-1 protease inhibitor, has been hypothesized to be a cause of canine CH.[1] Accumulation of a genetically defective α1-AT in hepatocytes in people causes hepatocyte death and low circulating concentrations of α1-AT. As hepatocytes accumulate α1-AT, they die and attract mononuclear cells with cytokines that cause production of more α1-AT. In a study of 57 dogs with hepatic disease, 37 had α1-AT in their livers.[13] The authors noted that α1-AT accumulation was more frequently seen in dogs with chronic progressive hepatitis or cirrhosis. However, it was uncertain whether the α1-AT was the cause or effect of hepatic disease.

Clinical signs of dogs with CH vary with the stage at which they are diagnosed. Because CH is a slow, insidious disease, clinical signs are seldom apparent until the disease is relatively advanced. A patient with a sudden onset of clinical signs may have advanced disease. Dogs presenting in severe hepatic failure (e.g., with cirrhosis) typically are lethargic, depressed, anorexic, vomiting, weak, and have weight loss, polyuria/polydipsia (PU/PD), and/or ascites (or a combination of these problems).[1,2] Diarrhea is relatively common, but is typically not as prominent as is seen in patients with intestinal disease. Icterus is relatively uncommon, and seizures (e.g., hepatic encephalopathy), bleeding, and fever tend to be relatively rare. Dogs that have somewhat advanced disease but are not in severe failure often show lethargy, poor appetite, weight loss, and vomiting as prominent findings. Some animals are fortuitously diagnosed when routine health screening or blood testing for other diseases reveals occult hepatic disease. These patients may be clinically normal and yet have reasonably advanced disease (even hepatic fibrosis) for which the patient is still compensating. This has major ramifications when considering anesthetic procedures. Hepatocutaneous syndrome is not typically associated with CH, although West Highland white terriers and Cocker spaniels seem to be at increased risk for both.[14]

Clinical laboratory findings in dogs with CH are primarily characterized by increased alanine aminotransferase (ALT),[1-3,12] and approximately 90% have ALTs five to 18 times the upper

---

Box • 227-1

Breeds That Have Been Associated with Increased Hepatic Copper Concentrations

Bedlington terrier
Airedale terrier
Bull terrier
Bulldog
Cocker spaniel
Collie
Dachshund
Dalmatian
Doberman pinscher
German shepherd dog
Golden retriever
Keeshond
Kerry blue terrier
Labrador retriever
Norwich terrier
Old English sheepdog
Pekingese
Poodle
Samoyed
Schnauzer
Skye terrier
West Highland white terrier
Wire fox terrier

From Rolfe DS, Twedt DC: Copper-associated hepatopathies in dogs. Vet Clin North Am Small Anim Pract 25:399, 1995.

LIVER AND PANCREATIC DISEASES

limit of normal.[2] Serum alkaline phosphatase (SAP) is often increased, but the pattern is often not that of the common steroid hepatopathies in which the SAP is typically many times higher than the ALT. However, if CH progresses to cirrhosis, hepatic enzymes may decrease to the reference range. Hypoalbuminemia, hypocholesterolemia, or both are often present when hepatic insufficiency occurs, and finding these two changes simultaneously strongly suggests either hepatic insufficiency (e.g., cirrhosis) or protein-losing enteropathy. Hyperglobulinemia occurs less commonly (25%) than hypoalbuminemia (40%).[2] Decreased blood urea nitrogen (BUN) may be due to hepatic insufficiency, decreased protein intake, or excessive loss due to polyuria; all of which may occur in patients with CH. Serum bile acids and ammonia tolerance testing are usually abnormal in dogs with CH.

Hypoalbuminemia was reported to be prognostic in one study[2] but not in another.[15] Approximately 75% of cirrhotic patients are hypoalbuminemic[2]; however, not all dogs with hypoalbuminemia have progressed to cirrhosis. Hypoalbuminemia coupled with normal or increased alpha-1 antitrypsin and haptoglobin has been reported in patients with severe hepatic disease that have the potential to recover.[16] Hypoglycemia is rare and has been suggested to have ominous prognostic implications.[2]

Expected hematologic abnormalities include minor anemia (e.g., anemia of chronic disease), sometimes with microcytosis, leukocytosis, and thrombocytopenia (if consumption of platelets occurs). Approximately 10% to 60% of cases have prolonged prothrombin time (PT) and partial thromboplastin time (PTT),[2,3] and a prolonged PT may be prognostic.[2] If ascites is present, it is usually either a modified transudate or a low-protein transudate associated with fibrosis or cirrhosis.

Physical examination is often relatively unremarkable unless ascites is present. Icterus is uncommon, but poor body condition is reasonably typical. Abdominal radiographs are usually unrevealing unless ascites or microhepatia is present. Ultrasonographic changes are typically nonspecific unless obvious microhepatia, ascites, or nodularity of the liver is found. Sometimes multiple acquired portosystemic shunting is detected. Rarely, ultrasound will reveal target lesions.

Definitive diagnosis of CH requires histology. Tru-Cut® needle biopsies can be diagnostic, but they can also miss important histologic changes that surgical or laparoscopic samples are more likely to find. Laparoscopy and surgery allow biopsy of multiple hepatic lobes and can detect gross changes not revealed with ultrasound, thus allowing one to direct biopsy to specific areas of the liver.

Diagnosing CH requires finding inflammation and piecemeal necrosis (i.e., necrosis of the hepatocytes adjacent to the portal tract—the "limiting plate").[1,3] The inflammation consists primarily of lymphocytes and plasma cells. Small numbers of neutrophils and macrophages may be present; however, granulomatous reactions are not expected in CH. Necrosis first involves destruction of hepatocytes adjacent to the limiting plate, but with time the necrosis extends from the portal area to the central veins (i.e., bridging necrosis). Copper is often present and can be detected by special stains (e.g., rubeanic acid and rhodanine) when it exceeds 400 ppm or by quantitative analysis.[1] Atomic absorption analysis requires approximately 1 g of tissue. The tissue sample should be shipped frozen or refrigerated to the lab in a copper-free serum blood tube. Formalin may contain copper and can confuse the analysis.[8] Increased Kupffer cell iron stores have been reported in some affected dogs.

Hydropic change (i.e., vacuolar change typical of steroid hepatopathy) is common and may reflect excessive endogenous steroid release due to disease. Nodular regeneration is also commonly seen.[2] Fibrosis is expected in dogs with advanced CH, and cirrhotic change (i.e., regenerative nodules plus severe bridging fibrosis) may be seen. Rarely, portal vein thrombosis occurs, although this is more commonly seen in other inflammatory disorders.

Therapy for CH involves reducing inflammation, alleviating the cause when possible (e.g., reducing hepatic copper levels when they pose a risk to the patient), antioxidant therapy, reducing or preventing fibrosis, treating hepatic encephalopathy, and supportive therapy. (See elsewhere in this text for a detailed discussion of therapeutic principals.)

Reducing inflammation typically involves glucocorticoid therapy.[1,2] Steroids are thought to benefit the patient by their anti-inflammatory effects and by their ability to inhibit fibrosis and stimulate appetite. Glucocorticoids purportedly also decrease intestinal copper absorption. Glucocorticoids typically make the patient feel better and seem to prolong life in patients diagnosed before end-stage hepatic disease occurs.[5] However, if the patient shows signs of advanced hepatic failure, steroids seldom help much. Dexamethasone tends to cause more side effects (e.g., hemorrhagic gastroenteritis) than prednisolone. Iatrogenic hyperadrenocorticism should be avoided. Prednisolone (2.2 mg/kg orally, once a day) is administered, and the dose is tapered as soon as clinical signs and hepatic enzymes evidence substantial improvement. Repeated pulses of high-dose therapy may be needed. Steroids typically cause a further rise in the SAP, although the ALT should decrease if the CH is being controlled. If steroid therapy is ineffective or if excessive side effects occur, azathioprine (Imuran) given at 2.2 mg/kg orally, every other day may be beneficial. Concurrent use of allopurinol increases the likelihood of toxicity from azathioprine.[2]

Oxidation is a significant mechanism of hepatic damage, as seen when excessive copper is accumulated[2]; therefore antioxidants are typically administered. Although no critical studies are available that demonstrate efficacy in dogs with CH, water-soluble Vitamin E is typically administered (400 to 600 IU orally, once a day) because of its safety, minimal cost, and potential benefit. S-adenosyl-L-methionine (SAMe), a precursor of glutathione and a methyl donor for methylation reactions, has benefited animals and people exposed to excessive alcohol.[17] Milk thistle, a herbal compound used for hepatic disease in people, has silymarin as the active complex. Silymarin increases superoxide dismutase in cells and serum concentrations of glutathione and glutathione peroxidase.[18] A meta-analysis showed that milk thistle was safe and well tolerated in people with chronic hepatic disease. It did not have a demonstrable effect on outcome in most cases, but one study showed that people with alcoholic cirrhosis were benefited.[18]

Ursodeoxycholic acid has a hepatoprotective effect, probably due to displacing hydrophobic bile acids (e.g., lithocholic acid) from hepatocyte membranes, and has also been touted as having immunomodulatory properties.[2] Its use at 15 mg/kg orally, once a day in a dog with CH was associated with improvement of hepatic enzymes.[1] It rarely causes diarrhea, but does have a hypercholeretic effect and should not be administered to dogs with biliary tract obstruction.

Patients with excessive hepatic copper accumulation (2000 ppm) should be treated with copper chelation therapy, oral zinc therapy, or both to prevent absorption of copper. Copper chelation typically involves administering penicillamine (10 to 15 mg/kg orally, twice a day). Affected Belingtons treated with penicillamine can lose 900 ppm copper per year,[8] whereas other breeds (e.g., Doberman pinschers) may respond faster.[1] Some patients experience clinical improvement despite persistence of hepatic copper concentrations. Penicillamine seems to have anti-inflammatory effects and inhibits fibrosis. Penicillamine therapy causes vomiting in approximately 30% of treated animals, and administering it with food may decrease such side effects. Trientine (10 to 15 mg/kg orally, twice a day) may be substituted if penicillamine cannot be tolerated. Trientine causes fewer side effects, may affect a different body pool of copper than penicillamine, and is effective in patients with hemolytic anemia due to copper release from necrotic hepatocytes.[8] One dog developed clinical copper deficiency (i.e., microcytic anemia and hepatic dysfunction) due to trientine chelation therapy coupled with a controlled copper diet.[19] 2,3', 2-tetramine is more effective at chelating copper than trientine, but it is not commercially available.[8]

Chelation therapy can be combined with oral administration of zinc to decrease intestinal copper absorption. It has been suggested that zinc therapy only prevents further accumulation of copper; however, in one study of three Bedlingtons and three West Highland white terriers administration of zinc significantly decreased hepatic copper concentrations after 2 years of therapy.[8] Administering zinc salts (e.g., zinc acetate or zinc gluconate initially given at 5 to 10 mg elemental zinc/kg twice a day) 1 hour before meals induces metallothionein (a copper-binding protein) in enterocytes. Dietary copper binds to this protein, is not absorbed, and is eventually evacuated from the body when the enterocyte is sloughed. Excessive zinc can cause hemolytic anemia, and blood zinc concentrations need to be checked periodically. Diets lower in copper can augment other therapy, but such diets are inadequate by themselves if the patient is already symptomatic for excessive hepatic copper concentrations.[8]

H-2 receptor antagonists, Carafate, or both are sometimes administered because hepatic disease has been suggested to cause gastroduodenal ulceration.

FIBROSIS AND CIRRHOSIS

Fibrosis and cirrhosis may result from any severe or chronic hepatic insult. Inflammatory cells cause hepatocellular necrosis, which creates space (i.e., hepatocyte dropout) that is filled by more inflammatory cells. The liver's response to necrosis is to produce hepatocytes and bile duct epithelium. However, lysosomal proteases and radicals released by inflammatory cells disrupt normal hepatic extracellular matrix (ECM) and cellular membranes causing release of substances (e.g., transforming growth factor-beta [TGF-β]) that attract collagen-producing cells. Fibrosis causes ECM modification, and hepatocytes growing on it may have functional alterations.[2,20]

Dogs with acute massive necrosis or CH often develop hepatic fibrosis. Because fibrosis follows the course of inflammation and necrosis, a disease that produces inflammation in the portal areas that reaches out to lobules and other portal areas causes bridging fibrosis (i.e., there is a "bridge" of fibrous connective tissue from one portal area to another). In some cases, fibrosis extends from the portal triad to the hepatic veins. When bridging fibrosis causes permanent distortion of the liver associated with regenerative nodules, it is termed *cirrhosis*. Fibrosis that cuts across acinar zones causes micronodular cirrhosis. Fibrosis that divides the liver into groups of acini with more than one portal tract within each nodule causes macronodular cirrhosis. Fibrosis that only surrounds bile ducts causes biliary cirrhosis. If fibrosis is severe, collagen limits the ability of vessels and sinusoids to distend, thereby increasing resistance to blood flow. Collagen around hepatocytes impairs sinusoidal blood flow and the sinusoidal endothelium's selective permeability, decreasing hepatocyte function. As cirrhosis persists, the type of collagen laid down may be less susceptible to collagenase activity, making it harder to remove.[2] Cirrhotic patients are at increased risk for anesthetic-related complications.

Preventing fibrosis is an important long-term goal in patients with any chronic inflammatory disease. Prednisolone,

azathioprine, penicillamine, zinc, and vitamin E appear to have antifibrotic effects.[1,20] Once severe fibrosis has occurred, colchicine therapy may be considered. Colchicine is a microtubule assembly inhibitor that increases collagenase activity. Colchicine (0.03 mg/kg orally, once a day) was associated with improved histology (i.e., decreased fibrosis) in one dog. It has been used in other dogs, but it is difficult to confidently ascribe beneficial results to colchicine because of limited experience.[2] Although frequently prescribed, no controlled drug trials have proven its value.

Chronic Hepatitis in the Doberman Pinscher

Middle-aged, female Doberman pinschers are at increased risk for severe CH with subsequent cirrhosis.[1,2,21] Clinical presentation and clinical pathology findings are as described under CH, but PU/PD, splenomegaly, neutrophilic leukocytosis, normal to increased PCV,[2] and bleeding may be more common than in affected patients of other breeds. Because these dogs are particularly prone to severe CH and cirrhosis, they are noticeably fragile; even minimal anesthesia can cause severe, acute decompensation. Many patients with clinical illness die within weeks of first signs of disease. Some affected Dobermans are referred for suspected diabetes insipidus due to severe PU/PD. If CH is diagnosed fortuitously in an asymptomatic dog, the life expectancy after diagnosis is presumably longer; however, early therapy in asymptomatic patients has not been proven to substantially increase life span.

Approximately 8% of Dobermans in Finland had an increased ALT; however, not all Dobermans with an increased ALT had CH.[1] Some Dobermans with increased ALT values lived for months and in some cases years without clinical signs of CH.[22] In a more recent study, 18 Dobermans with subclinical CH were biopsied, and all had excessive hepatic copper concentrations. Initially there was parenchymal and portal inflammation, but the parenchymal inflammation diminished and the portal inflammation increased as the disease progressed. There was expansion of portal areas with necrosis, fibrosis, and bile duct proliferation.[21] Five dogs lived for 3 years; as a group they were asymptomatic for an average of 19 months.

Even though female Doberman pinschers are clearly at risk for severe CH, not all Doberman pinschers with hepatic disease have CH. Doberman pinschers also appear to be at risk for drug- induced hepatic disease (e.g., diethylcarbamazine, oxibendazole, amiodarone). Therefore hepatic biopsy is recommended for Dobermans with an increased ALT if the patient is not an undue anesthetic and biopsy risk. Periportal copper accumulation, hepatonecrosis, and inflammation are expected in early cases,[1,2] although one report suggested that the earliest inflammatory and fibrotic lesions are around hepatic veins.[23] Eventually a substantial hepatic necrosis occurs, with neutrophilic and macrophage infiltrates. Excessive hepatic copper levels are common, and Doberman pinschers as a breed have been suggested to have higher hepatic copper levels than some other breeds. However, five of 35 Dobermans with CH had normal hepatic copper levels,[23] and even Dobermans with substantial copper accumulation generally do not attain the concentrations often seen in severely affected Bedlington terriers.[2] Therefore although it is not clear if the copper accumulation is innocuous or pathogenic, it is not an initiating cause of CH as in Bedlington terriers. Hepatic iron concentrations tend to be increased. Because of their increased risk for CH, it is reasonable to routinely screen Doberman pinschers for biochemical evidence of hepatic disease. Therapy depends upon the stage of the disease, but usually consists of antioxidants and glucocorticoids ± azathioprine. Copper chelation and antifibrotic therapy are used as indicated by histopathology.

Chronic Hepatitis Associated with Copper Accumulation in the Bedlington Terrier

Bedlington terriers in the United States have historically had a high incidence of an autosomal-recessive metabolic defect in biliary copper excretion (approximately 60% of tested dogs).[8] The gene responsible for this defect is different from that causing Wilson's disease in people. Bedlingtons homozygous for the trait progressively accumulate copper in their livers, which typically causes oxidative mitochondrial damage after reaching approximately 2000 ppm. Bedlingtons may begin accumulating copper in utero.[24] Their hepatic copper content continually increases throughout their lives (see following) and may reach 12,000 ppm.[2] Once sufficient copper has accumulated in the liver, otherwise insignificant stress may trigger acute hepatic necrosis, possibly with acute hemolysis and renal failure due to release of large amounts of copper from dying hepatocytes.[1,2]

An increased ALT is usually the first clinicopathologic evidence of disease; however, this increase does not occur until excessive hepatic copper accumulation is associated with hepatocyte damage and inflammation. Younger dogs with excessive hepatic copper but no inflammation often have normal ALTs.[2] As hepatic damage occurs, increased ALTs may be found in clinically normal animals. Clinical signs may be those of acute hepatic disease (e.g., vomiting, anorexia, lethargy) from which they may recover; chronic hepatic failure (e.g., anorexia, vomiting, depression, loss of body condition) that ultimately progresses to obvious hepatic failure with jaundice, ascites, and hepatic encephalopathy; or acute hepatic failure coupled with hemolytic anemia and jaundice.[2]

Measuring serum or plasma copper or ceruloplasmin concentrations is not helpful; definitive diagnosis requires hepatic histopathology. Accumulation of copper in lysosomal granules is the first histologic abnormality. As hepatic copper levels increase, random areas of focal inflammation occur. Inflammatory infiltrates extend out from the portal triads as the disease progresses, with occasional bridging necrosis and some fibrosis. Finally cirrhosis occurs.[8] Hepatic copper levels increase until about 6 years of age, and then they begin to decrease, probably because copper-laden hepatocytes are replaced with scar tissue or regenerative nodules.[1,2] Hepatic iron concentrations are also increased.

Identifying and removing affected dogs from the breeding pool is the desired approach. Selective breeding in the Netherlands has decreased the prevalence from 46% (1976 to 1986) to 11% (1990 to 1997).[25] When screening asymptomatic animals, one may biopsy at 6 and 15 months of age. Unaffected dogs will have normal amounts of hepatic copper both times, heterozygotes will initially have a high copper concentration that lessens by the second biopsy, and homozygotes will initially have excessive copper that is increased at the second biopsy.[8] The Orthopedic Foundation for Animals (www.offa.org/index.html) has a registry for unaffected Bedlington terriers that uses a DNA marker tightly linked to the expression of copper toxicity.[26] However, a study of 154 hepatic biopsies from Bedlingtons found that the DNA marker did not reliably identify copper intoxication in individual dogs.[27] This discrepancy may have been due to studying different subpopulations of Bedlingtons. Fecal excretion of [64]copper discriminates between affected and nonaffected West Highland white terriers and Bedlingtons.[28] However, the test requires special facilities and is not as specific as desired.

Feeding a relatively low copper diet and administering oral zinc is usually beneficial in affected, asymptomatic dogs. Chelator therapy may also be used, and penicillamine therapy has apparently prevented disease progression in some dogs that continue to have excessive copper. Affected animals may live a normal life if therapy starts when they are young.[8]

West Highland White Terriers

West Highland white terriers have a genetic tendency toward higher hepatic copper concentrations than most other breeds, and CH is more common in West Highland white terriers. However, not all West Highland white terriers with CH have inflammation that is clearly associated with excessive hepatic copper accumulation.[1,2] Furthermore, many West Highland white terriers with modest copper accumulation do not develop CH. In distinction to what occurs in Bedlington terriers, West Highland white terriers that accumulate copper in their livers do not do so for their entire lives, and the values tend to decrease over time.[9] Finally, West Highland white terriers usually do not achieve hepatic copper levels greater than 3500 ppm, in distinction to Bedlington terriers, which often achieve levels greater than or equal to 5000 ppm.

Histopathology of West Highland white terriers livers may show normal liver with excessive copper; multifocal hepatitis with excessive copper, and cirrhosis with excessive copper.[2] Dogs with CH are treated as previously described.

Dalmatians

Dalmatians have recently been recognized to develop necroinflammatory hepatitis associated with increased hepatic copper concentrations.[4] Too few animals have been diagnosed to delineate whether or not an age or sex predilection exists. Affected animals have typical signs of hepatic disease (e.g., anorexia, vomiting, lethargy). Increased ALT was the predominant clinicopathologic finding, whereas lesser increases in SAP were common. Hypoalbuminemia and hyperbilirubinemia were seen in some dogs. Ultrasound findings were typically normal. Piecemeal necrosis and bridging fibrosis were the most common histologic findings, and inflammatory infiltrates were either lymphocytic or neutrophilic. Hepatic copper concentrations ranged from 754 to 8390 ppm, with an average of 3197 ppm. Average life span after diagnosis was 80 days, with some animals living to 240 days postdiagnosis.

Skye Terriers

At least some bloodlines of Skye terriers seem to have a tendency to have CH. Although not well characterized, it appears that the CH occurs first and that hepatic copper accumulation is an inconsistent secondary effect of the inflammatory lesion. Hepatic copper concentrations up to 2257 ppm have been reported. The first histologic lesion is intracanalicular cholestasis.[1,2]

Cocker Spaniels

Young male cocker spaniels are at increased risk for early onset CH that quickly becomes cirrhotic. The mean age at presentation of 16 affected dogs was 5.6 years, and males were preferentially affected.[29] Most had ascites (11 of 16) of less than 2 weeks' duration. A mature neutrophilic leukocytosis and ascites (either a transudate or a modified transudate) were typical. ALT was usually increased, but hyperbilirubinemia was a mild, inconsistent finding. Biopsy typically reveals a periportal hepatitis consisting primarily of plasma cells and lymphocytes with limiting plate destruction. Severe bile duct duplication was common. Copper accumulation was inconsistent. One study looking at α1-AT and its relationship to CH in cocker spaniels concluded that the two were not related.[13] Because the disease is typically advanced at the time of diagnosis, prognosis is grim. Most clinically affected dogs die within a month of diagnosis, although occasional patients may live for up to a year with supportive therapy.[2]

Infectious Canine Hepatitis and its Possible Association with Chronic Hepatitis

Canine adenovirus was found in the liver of five out of 53 dogs with CH; however, another study failed to find it in any of 45 dogs with hepatic disease.[1,2] Whether a cause-and-effect relationship exists is unknown. Some people have hypothesized that the viral infection initiates a self-perpetuating inflammatory hepatic disease. Experimental exposure of partially immunized dogs has produced CH.[2]

CHOLANGIOHEPATITIS

Cholangiohepatitis is diagnosed by finding mixed inflammatory infiltrates in the periportal (i.e., zone I) area, usually with inflammation extending through and into the bile ducts.[12,15] Icterus is common, and ALTs, SAPs, and serum bile acids tend to be higher than is seen with CH. However, one cannot discriminate between dogs with CH and those with cholangiohepatitis based upon laboratory values. In one study, median survival time (MST) was 25 months.[2,15]

DRUG-ASSOCIATED HEPATITIS

Although almost any drug will eventually be associated with hepatotoxiciy in some individual, some drugs are frequently associated with hepatic damage. Most hepatotoxic drugs cause hepatocellular degeneration, necrosis, or fibrosis with minimal inflammation. Inflammatory infiltrates have been associated with trimethoprim-sulfadiazine, phenobarbital, diethylcarbamazine and oxibendazole, and amiodarone, although they are usually relatively mild and do not closely resemble CH. However, the degree of inflammation associated with apparent drug toxicity is variable, and some animals have substantial inflammation. Whether the inflammation is due to the drug or some other, concurrent problem is unknown.[1,30,31]

ACIDOPHIL CELL HEPATITIS

This is a transmissible disease (apparently viral) that has been reported affecting dogs in the United Kingdom. In the acute phases, it is associated with relatively little hepatic inflammation. However, it is believed that CH and cirrhosis may result. Increased hepatic enzymes are expected, and diagnosis requires hepatic biopsy. The characteristic lesion is finding acidophil cells throughout the parenchyma with an angular shape and acidophilic cytoplasm.[1,2]

LEPTOSPIROSIS

The most common clinical presentation of dogs with leptospirosis is acute renal failure. Depending upon the serovar involved, dogs may or may not have concurrent hepatic disease (i.e., increased SAP and hyperbilirubinemia). In one recent study, 20 of 36 dogs with leptospirosis had hepatic involvement[32]; however, the lesion characteristic of acutely affected dogs is edema and sinusoidal congestion, with perhaps a mild neutrophilic and eosinophilic infiltrate. Serovar grippotyphosa has been suggested to be able to cause CH. In one kennel, five American foxhounds were diagnosed with CH. Four had leptospires in their canaliculi. In another report, beagles vaccinated against leptospirosis developed CH, and leptospires were found in their bile canaliculi.[1,2]

LOBULAR DISSECTING HEPATITIS

This is characterized by finding inflammatory cells diffusely throughout the hepatic lobule as opposed to primarily in the periportal regions, and collagen and reticulin fibers dissecting around small groups of hepatocytes and sometimes single hepatocytes.[1,2] Copper may be found in the liver, but it appears to be a secondary event. This syndrome appears most commonly in neonatal and juvenile dogs (e.g., mean of 11 months old in one series). Hepatic enzymes are typically increased, and ascites associated with portal hypertension is probably the most common presenting clinical sign. Standard poodles may be at increased risk for hepatitis, but it is not certain that it is lobular dissecting hepatitis. One paper reported three standard poodles with a disease that resembled lobular dissecting hepatitis but which did not cause ascites.[33] Regardless of whether or not these dogs had lobular dissecting hepatitis, a breed predisposition seemed likely.

GRANULOMATOUS HEPATITIS

Granulomatous hepatitis is an uncommon hepatopathy differing from CH in that macrophages are a predominate finding. The lesion tends to be multifocal and can be caused by numerous bacteria (e.g., *Nocardia*, *Mycobacterium*, *Rhodococcus*, *Borrelia*, *Bartonella*), fungi (e.g., histoplasmosis, coccidioidomycosis), and parasites (e.g., *Hepatozoonosis*, *Heterobilharzia*). In people, occult lymphoma has been implicated. However, many cases of canine granulomatous hepatitis are idiopathic.[2] One report of nine dogs with granulomatous hepatitis found intestinal lymphangiectasia in two, lymphosarcoma in one, and histiocytosis in one.[34] In three cases, the cause was uncertain. Clinical signs vary widely, and no breed or age predisposition is recognized for idiopathic disease. Special stains for bacteria and fungi are warranted, as is serology for selected agents. Culture for bacteria including atypical mycobacteria (which can be hard to find, even with special stains) is desirable. If one cannot find a cause, it is usually prudent to first treat for a possible undiscovered agent (e.g., atypical mycobacteria, *Bartonella* spp.) and only resort to immunosuppressive therapy after diagnostic efforts and therapeutic trials have failed.

CHAPTER 228

Feline Inflammatory Liver Disease

Sarah M. A. Caney
Timothy J. Gruffydd-Jones

The most important and common hepatic disorders of cats in which inflammation is the predominant pathologic change are the different forms of the cholangitis and cholangiohepatitis complex. Inflammatory lesions are a feature of some other feline disorders that affect the liver, but other pathologic features dominate. These include infectious diseases such as feline infectious peritonitis (FIP), protozoal infections (most notably toxoplasmosis), bartonellosis, and hepatotoxicities particularly associated with drugs including diazepam and tetracyclines.

CHOLANGITIS AND CHOLANGIOHEPATITIS COMPLEX

The cholangitis and cholangiohepatitis complex is regarded as the second most common hepatic disorder in cats in the USA after idiopathic hepatic lipidosis.[1] In countries in which hepatic lipidosis is less common, such as the United Kingdom, the cholangitis and cholangiohepatitis complex may constitute the most common primary hepatic disorder of cats.

Considerable confusion exists over the classification and terminology used to describe different forms of the cholangitis and cholangiohepatitis complex, and this is the most contentious issue relating to feline inflammatory liver disease.

Pathology and Classification

Different variants of the complex have been described based on histopathologic features of the lesions including the predominant nature of the inflammatory cellular infiltrate (i.e., neutrophilic, lymphocytic) and bile duct proliferation and presence of fibrosis.[2]

It is currently difficult to devise a classification of feline inflammatory liver diseases incorporating cholangitis and cholangiohepatitis that will reconcile all the previously reported cases and forms of the classification used. The most striking feature of the lesions is generally whether they are suppurative with a prominent neutrophilic infiltration or whether the inflammatory infiltrate is predominantly lymphocytic in nature. This is the basis for the classification of cholangitis and cholangiohepatitis. It correlates with distinctly different clinical presentations and has practical relevance to the management of affected cats.

Suppurative Cholangitis and Cholangiohepatitis

The dominant feature in suppurative cholangitis and cholangiohepatitis is evidence of a suppurative process within the bile ducts. The infiltrate is primarily of neutrophils, although there may be a range of inflammatory cells including lymphocytes and plasma cells. Disruption of the limiting plate occurs with infiltrate extending into the portal areas.[2] Periportal necrosis is common. The bile ducts themselves show necrosis and degeneration with pyknosis, variation in nuclear appearance, and cytoplasmic vacuolation. The extent of fibrosis is variable and probably reflects the duration or stage of the disease process (Figure 228-1B).

Other specific disease entities frequently accompany suppurative cholangitis. The most commonly reported of these is pancreatitis, characterized histologically by periductal infiltration, acinar degeneration, fibrosis, and nodular hyperplasia. The extent of the pancreatitis is generally mild. Coexisting pancreatitis has been described in the majority of reported cases of cholangiohepatitis and was identified in 50% of 18 cases of cholangiohepatitis in a retrospective pathologic study.[3]

Inflammatory bowel disease (IBD) has been recognized more recently as a coexisting feature in cholangiohepatitis. It was diagnosed in 83% of cats with cholangiohepatitis in a retrospective pathologic study.[3] Although the intestinal inflammatory infiltrate was predominantly lymphocytic and plasmacytic in nature, in some cases a neutrophilic element was present.

The term *triaditis* has been used to describe a syndrome of concurrent cholangiohepatitis, pancreatitis, and IBD. The association of these entities may indicate a common underlying disease process in some cases. Suppurative cholangitis is believed to result from ascending infection of the biliary tract. Bacteria can generally be cultured from the bile of affected cats, and a mixed growth of bacteria is often recovered (comprised of common inhabitants of the intestinal gut flora). Ascending infection from the intestine is also believed to be an important factor in the development of pancreatitis.[4] The pancreatic and bile ducts are joined before entering the duodenum and this may predispose to concurrent development of pancreatitis and suppurative cholangitis. It is possible that the presence of IBD may predispose to ascending infection. In triaditis the predominant clinical features are most often associated with the cholangitis, with the pancreatitis and IBD being identified as complications.

Lymphocytic Cholangitis

In some cases of feline inflammatory liver disease the inflammatory infiltrate is predominantly lymphocytic.[5,6] (Figure 228-2B) In a proportion of these cases the inflammatory infiltrate consists purely of lymphocytes and is restricted to the portal areas. It has been suggested that this is a specific form of feline inflammatory liver disease that has been termed *lymphocytic portal hepatitis*.[7] It is reported to occur in older cats.[7] Assessment of the significance of this pathologic change is complicated by the recognition that lymphocytic portal infiltrates are common in older cats not showing any clinical evidence of liver disease. Over 90% (29 of 30) of cats more than 15 years of age were described as having portal lymphocyte infiltrates in one survey.[8]

In other cases, although lymphocytes predominate, the inflammatory infiltrate is mixed with variable numbers of other inflammatory cells, particularly neutrophils. The infiltrate may be more extensive, appearing as marked aggregates of lymphocytes in the form of lymphoid follicles sometimes surrounding bile ducts or as a more diffuse infiltrate within portal areas. Changes are evident in the biliary tree, with bile

Table • 228-1

Comparison of Suppurative and Lymphocytic Cholangitis

	LYMPHOCYTIC CHOLANGITIS	SUPPURATIVE CHOLANGITIS
Predispositions	Younger cats Persians	Middle aged/older cats
Clinical Features	Often bright	Usually depressed, ill
Appetite	May show polyphagia	Usually anorexic
Jaundice	±	+
Ascites	±	−
Lymphadenopathy	±	−
Hepatomegaly	±	−
Laboratory Changes		
Neutrophilia	±	+
Lymphopenia	±	−
↑ ALT	+	+
↑ ALP	+	+
± Bilirubin	+	+
+ Bile acids	±	+
↑ Globulins	+	−
Ultrasound	± Hyperechoic liver	± Hyperechoic liver biliary stasis
Pathology		
Cellular infiltrate	Primarily lymphocytes	Primarily neutrophils
Distribution of lesions	Mainly portal	Mainly bile ducts
Fibrosis	Variable/can be extensive	−
Association with other disorder	? Pancreatitis	Pancreatitis/IBD
Treatment	Immunosuppressive corticosteroids	Antibiotics Choleretics

duct proliferation and sometimes inflammatory changes within the walls of the bile ducts. However, usually no epithelial degeneration or inflammatory infiltrate exists within the lumen of the bile ducts. Fibrosis is present to a variable extent, and this may be severe in chronic cases. This initially has a distinctive septal or monolobular pattern, with bridging fibrosis between the portal areas. The fibrosis is not associated with venules and does not lead to pseudolobule formation but frequently results in prominent nodular hyperplasia. There may be disruption of the vasculature with increased prominence of small blood vessels on the surface of the liver.

Parallels have been drawn between lymphocytic cholangitis and some forms of inflammatory liver disease in man that are characterized by lymphocytic infiltration such as sclerosing cholangitis, biliary cirrhosis, and pericholangitis; however, important differences in the histopathologic features exist. In occasional cats the fibrosis may be prominent around the bile ducts as a concentric distribution, and this has been termed *sclerosing cholangitis*.[9] However, differences exist compared with sclerosing cholangitis in man, and it may simply represent a variant form in the distribution of fibrosis of lymphocytic cholangitis.

It is not clear whether what has been termed as *lymphocytic portal hepatitis* is a distinct separate entity or a variant of lymphocytic cholangitis. The similarities in terms of the lymphocytic predominance, biliary involvement, and pattern of fibrosis, are more striking than the differences; therefore the latter appears more likely. IBD and pancreatitis have been reported to be common in cases described as lymphocytic portal hepatitis.[3] Pancreatitis has been recognized in combination with lymphocytic cholangitis but previous reports do not reveal any evidence of a striking association.[5]

There has been some preliminary characterization of the immune-cell infiltration in lymphocytic cholangitis.[10] The infiltrative lymphocytes are predominantly CD3-positive T cells with smaller numbers of associated B cells. Occasional IgA-positive plasma cells are present, and increased MHC II expression by a variety of immune cells occurs. The nature of this infiltrate suggests, not unexpectedly, that an immune-mediated mechanism may play a role in the pathogenesis of the liver pathology. In the liver diseases of man that bear some similarity, sclerosing cholangitis and biliary cirrhosis, autoantibodies against liver cell components are identified. However in the limited studies that have been reported, no evidence of such antibodies have been found in affected cats.[5]

There may be some initiating factor that triggers the development of lymphocytic cholangitis leading to immune-mediated mechanisms that perpetuate liver pathology. Clinical signs may not arise until this stage has been reached.

It has been postulated that lymphocytic cholangitis and suppurative cholangitis may be essentially part of the same disease syndrome, with lymphocytic cholangitis representing a chronic stage of an earlier suppurative process.[1] A mixed inflammatory cell infiltrate in some cats is identified that probably represents progression of suppurative cholangitis to a more chronic form (see following), but the authors believe that this is distinct from lymphocytic cholangitis. Key features suggest lymphocytic cholangitis is a separate, distinct disease syndrome:

- No evidence suggests that cats diagnosed with lymphocytic cholangitis have had earlier episodes of liver disease or that cats with suppurative cholangitis are at greater risk of developing lymphocytic cholangitis.
- Lymphocytic cholangitis occurs most frequently in younger cats, but suppurative cholangitis tends to occur in middle-aged to older cats.
- An inflammatory infiltrate is found in the bile ducts of cats with suppurative cholangitis but not in lymphocytic cholangitis.
- Concurrent pancreatitis is common in cats with suppurative cholangitis but is unusual in lymphocytic cholangitis.

These two latter findings implicate ascending infection in the pathogenesis of suppurative cholangitis, but no evidence suggests it plays a role in the development of lymphocytic cholangitis.

Mixed Inflammatory Infiltrates

A small proportion of cats with inflammatory liver disease show a mixed cell infiltrate consisting of both neutrophils and lymphocytes. They show bile duct proliferation with epithelial degeneration and necrosis but also have inflammatory infiltrates within the lumen of the bile ducts that differentiate them from the cases of lymphocytic cholangitis with a mixed cell infiltration. It is plausible that these cases represent a chronic stage of earlier episodes of suppurative cholangitis.

SUPPURATIVE CHOLANGITIS AND CHOLANGIOHEPATITIS

Clinical Features

Suppurative cholangitis occurs more frequently in middle-aged and older cats. In one series of reported cases, all affected cats were over 10 years of age.[7] No apparent sex or breed predisposition exists. Most cats in which a diagnosis of suppurative cholangitis is made are presented as sick cats with acute illness.[1] They are usually anorexic and may be pyrexic. Jaundice is the most consistent specific clinical sign and is caused by intrahepatic cholestasis, sometimes with extrahepatic biliary obstruction. There may be evidence of abdominal pain and resentment on abdominal palpation. Some cats with suppurative cholangitis may have milder or more chronic disease that may be overlooked.

Diagnosis

The most consistent changes on routine laboratory evaluation are increases in ALT and bilirubin. Cholestatic enzymes, ALP, and γGT are usually increased, and usually raised fasting or postprandial (or both) serum bile acid concentrations are found. It is reported that some cats with cholangitis have normal liver enzymes, although in the authors' experience this is rare. The most common finding on hematology is a leukocytosis with neutrophilia and left shift. There may be suppression of hepatic production of clotting factors in the form of prolonged clotting times and increased PIVKA levels,[11] although spontaneous clinical complications of impaired hemostatic function are rare.

The principal abnormalities on imaging are related to the extrahepatic biliary tract. Evidence of gallbladder distension usually exists, and the bile duct may appear prominent.

Cholelithiasis is occasionally seen in cases of suppurative cholangitis, and the majority of reported cases of cholelithiasis have been associated with suppurative cholangitis. It is not clear whether cholelithiasis is the primary problem leading to suppurative cholangitis as a complication, or, as seems more plausible, suppurative cholangitis predisposes to cholelithiasis. Gallstones can be radiolucent, although calcification is a common feature (Figure 228-1A). On ultrasonography, choleliths cause acoustic shadowing. This can aid diagnosis of translucent stones, although inspissated bile, inflammatory, and neoplastic masses may have a similar appearance. Other ultrasonographic features that may be seen with suppurative disease include thickening of the gallbladder (wall thickness >1 mm), distension of the bile duct (>5 mm), and the presence of sludging or inspissation of bile.[12] There may be general patchy echogenicity of the liver.[13]

Histopathology is necessary for confirmation of diagnosis of suppurative cholangitis. A number of techniques can be used to obtain suitable biopsies for histopathologic examination. Fine needle aspirates offer the most noninvasive method of collecting samples. These may confirm the presence of a suppurative process but do not allow assessment of liver architecture and can be misleading.[14,15] Fine needle aspirates can be submitted for bacteriologic isolation and should be maintained in an anaerobic environment until culture is performed. Wedge biopsy at exploratory laparotomy enables direct visualization of the liver and biliary tree and provides the ideal specimen for pathologic assessment. The patency of the bile duct can be established by applying gentle pressure to the gallbladder. Bile should be aspirated for gross assessment and to provide a sample for culture. Immediate cytologic evaluation of a smear of bile will confirm neutrophilic infiltration in suppurative cases. The bile frequently becomes extremely inspissated in suppurative cholangitis, and aspiration may necessitate use of a wide bore needle. Exploratory laparotomy provides the opportunity to examine the pancreas for evidence of pancreatitis and to obtain biopsies where appropriate. It also enables collection of full-thickness intestinal biopsies to investigate the possibility of concurrent IBD. Biopsies suitable for assessment of hepatic architecture can be obtained percutaneously using a suitable liver biopsy needle such as a Tru-Cut® biopsy needle. Ultrasound guidance allows more accurate placement of the biopsy needle. If the required equipment and expertise is available, laparoscopy offers the best compromise between minimizing invasiveness while allowing visualization and biopsy. Hepatic biopsies should be submitted for bacteriologic culture in addition to histopathology.

Treatment

Antibiotic treatment is the priority for suppurative cholangitis. The choice of antibiotic should ideally be based on the results of culture of bile and sensitivity tests. However initial selection of antibiotic must be made before results of bacteriologic culture are available. E. coli is the most frequently isolated organism but a mixed growth (including anaerobes such as Bacteroides spp. and other organisms that constitute the normal small intestinal bacterial flora), is frequently found, reflecting ascending infection from the gut. The ideal feature of an antibiotic selected for empiric use is that it should be broad spectrum, bactericidal, achieve therapeutic levels in bile, and not require hepatic metabolism for activation or excretion. The authors' initial choice is therefore generally a potentiated synthetic penicillin (e.g., amoxicillin-clavulanate), cephalosporin (e.g., cephalexin), or fluoroquinolone combined with metronidazole for additional activity against anaerobes. Chloramphenicol has sometimes been recommended[1]; however, high levels can accumulate in the presence of biliary stasis, and toxic effects may result. Antibiotic treatment is maintained for at least 4 to 6 weeks to minimize the risk of recurrence.

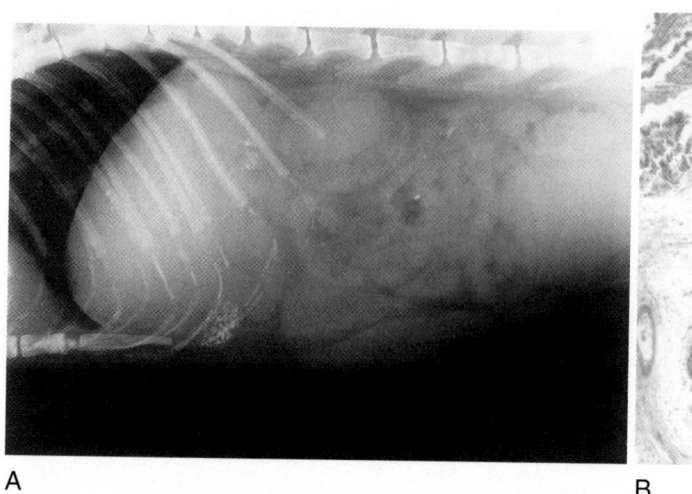
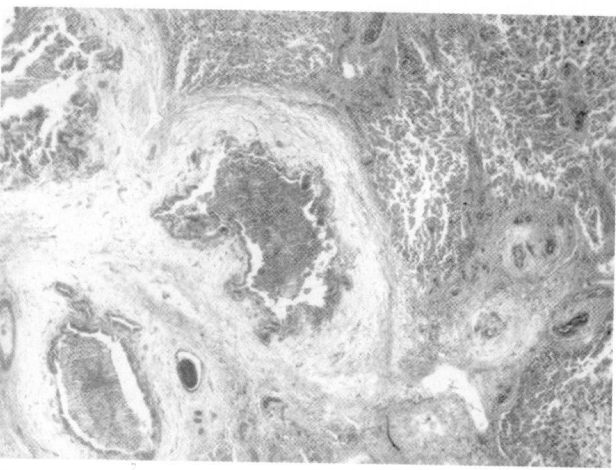

A   B

Figure 228-1 **A** and **B**, Lateral radiograph of a cat with suppurative cholangitis showing a calcified choleliths. Hepatic histology from the same case.

The benefits of corticosteroid therapy are widely accepted for lymphocytic cholangitis (see following) and probably also for chronic nonsuppurative cholangitis associated with mixed inflammatory infiltrates. The use of corticosteroids for acute suppurative cholangitis may have benefits in some cases when used judiciously at anti-inflammatory doses for short periods (e.g., prednisolone at 1 mg/kg daily) based on facilitating bile flow through reducing biliary tract inflammation.

Cholecystectomy may be necessary in some cases to remove inspissated bile. This should be followed by lavage and flushing to ensure patency. This may require cannulation of the duodenal papilla. If complete obstruction of biliary flow is identified at laparotomy, cholecystoduodenostomy is indicated to re-establish biliary flow. The peri- and postoperative mortality rate for cats requiring surgical intervention is high.[16]

Supportive measures aid in the management of suppurative cholangitis. Fluid therapy is likely to be required initially, and in most cases nutritional support is also needed. In the longer term modified diets formulated for liver support are indicated, but in the early stages maintenance of calorific intake is the priority. Suitable diets should be easily digested with reduced protein and supplemented with arginine and carnitine.

Choleretics are of value in promoting bile flow, and this is indicated if extraheptic biliary obstruction is not present. The beneficial effects of ursodeoxycholic acid include changing the composition of the bile acid pool by reducing the proportion of hydrophobic bile acids that have toxic effects on hepatocellular membranes. A dose of 10 to 15 mg orally, once a day is used. No controlled clinical trials have been reported to demonstrate a beneficial effect of UDCA, but it is widely used and appears to be safe.[17] Vitamin K supplementation is indicated if defects in clotting function are identified, particularly prior to any biopsy or surgical procedure. A dose of 5 mg of Vitamin K is given orally or subcutaneously. The response to treatment can be assessed by monitoring PIVKA concentrations and clotting function, which are usually restored to normal in a few days.[11]

More recently S-adenosyl-L-methionine (SAMe) has been used as a nutraceutical agent in the support of cats with liver disease. One beneficial effect is believed to be the restoration of glutathione levels that are reduced in liver disease, leading to increased oxidative damage and exacerbation of liver disease. Other beneficial effects may be to increase levels of cysteine and taurine, which are required for bile acid conjugation and a cytoprotective effect. Although theoretic potential benefits to SAMe exist, no trials have been reported that confirm this.

Prognosis

Information on the prognosis for suppurative cholangitis is limited. In one study just over half (8 of 15) of cats survived for more than 1 year after the diagnosis was made with a median survival time (MST) of 29 months.[18] This concurs with the authors' limited experience that suppurative cholangitis has a reasonable prognosis. Some cases do appear to recur shortly after initial treatment and this risk may be reduced by ensuring prolonged antibiotic treatment, preferably selected on the basis of culture and sensitivity testing. Suggestions that suppurative cholangitis may progress to lymphocytic cholangitis is not supported by evidence, and the authors have not observed any cases of such progression. The prognosis for cats that require surgical intervention to restore bile flow is much more guarded.[16] Concurrent presence of pancreatitis and IBD complicates the prognosis for suppurative cholangitis and the choice of treatment. Management of pancreatitis in cats is challenging. It is not known whether the high doses of corticosteroids usually used for cats with IBD have any deleterious effects on cholangitis and pancreatitis in cats with triaditis. The authors' clinical impression, based on limited experience, is that while this may produce short-term clinical improvements, the longer-term benefits are more questionable.

LYMPHOCYTIC CHOLANGITIS

Clinical Features

In contrast to suppurative cholangitis, lymphocytic cholangitis occurs more often in young cats, with more than 50% of cases in cats under 4 years of age.[5] A predisposition exists in Persian cats, but no sex bias is seen.[5] This form of inflammatory liver disease is seen much more frequently than suppurative cholangitis in the authors' clinic.

The etiology of this disease is unknown, although an immune-mediated mechanism is believed to contribute to the pathogenesis.

The two main presenting signs in lymphocytic cholangitis are (1) jaundice and (2) progressive ascites. Occasionally both clinical signs are present. In contrast to suppurative cholangitis,

LIVER AND PANCREATIC DISEASES

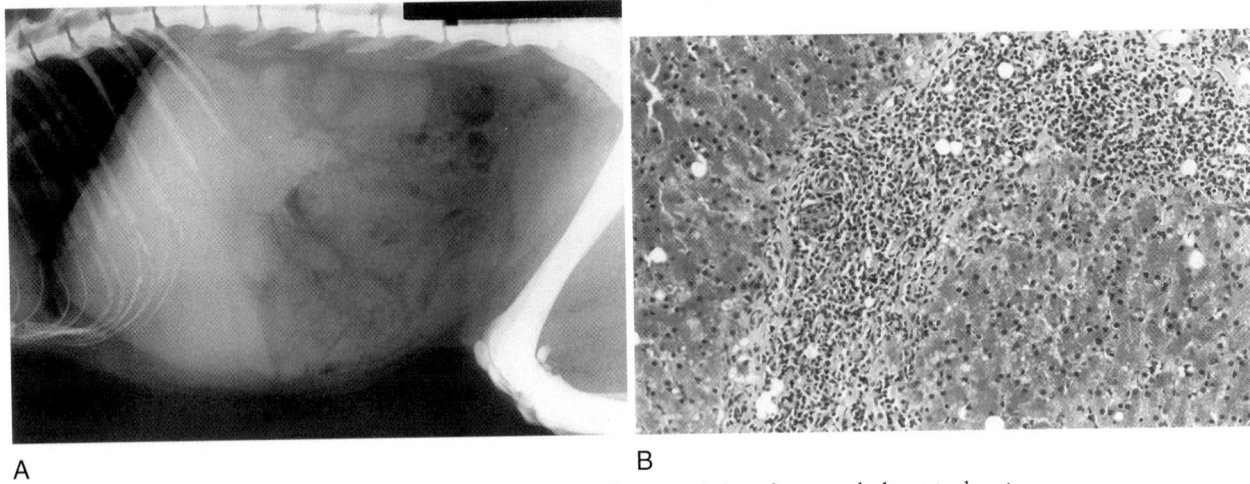

A   B

Figure 228-2 **A** and **B,** Lateral radiograph of a cat with lymphocytic cholangitis showing severe hepatomegaly. Hepatic histology from the same case.

cats with lymphocytic cholangitis often do not appear ill. Appetite is often maintained and some cases show a noticeable polyphagia. There may be severe weight loss, but other cases retain reasonable bodily condition. It is unusual for pyrexia to be present. Hepatomegaly may be detectable on abdominal palpation, and in some cases this can be striking. Mild generalized lymph node enlargement is a common finding. This is most apparent on palpation of the superficial lymph nodes but may also involve the mesenteric lymph nodes. In the later stages of the disease with extensive cirrhosis and portal hypertension, hepatic encephalopathy may develop.

Diagnosis
An increase in liver enzymes (ALT, ALP, and GGT) and bile acids is usually seen that can be severe. Bilirubin levels may be increased, frequently corresponding with jaundice. Serum globulin levels are often raised, and this may reflect an increase in γ globulins detectable on serum protein electrophoresis. The most consistent change on hematology is lymphopenia. There may be some neutrophilia and mild anemia. If ascitic fluid is present, abdominal paracentesis will show this to be clear to yellow tinged. It is generally thick with a high protein content, the majority of which is globulin. The cellular content is generally low, with a nonspecific mixture of inflammatory cells.

Radiography may be complicated by the presence of ascites but may reveal hepatomegaly (Figure 228-2A). The liver may have a heterogeneous appearance on ultrasonography with irregular margins. If extensive cirrhosis occurs, the liver may have a hyperechoic appearance.

Histopathology is required to make a definitive diagnosis. Fine needle liver aspirates may reveal a lymphocytic infiltrate but will not show the characteristic changes in liver architecture, the location of the infiltration, or the pattern of fibrosis. Percutaneous core biopsy techniques generally provide diagnostic samples. However, the prominent presence of blood vessels on the surface of the liver, together with possible compromise of liver-dependent clotting factors, leads to a significant risk of postbiopsy hemorrhage; therefore biopsy at laparotomy provides the advantage of enabling better hemostatic control. Laparotomy also enables larger biopsies to be obtained, as well as selection of biopsy sites, including assessment and biopsy (if appropriate) of other abdominal organs.

The most important differential diagnoses for lymphocytic cholangitis are other causes of jaundice and ascites but

particularly FIP and other liver diseases. The lymphadenopathy and preponderance of lymphocytes infiltrating the liver can potentially lead to confusion with lymphosarcoma, especially if needle aspirates are used, but can be differentiated on histopathology. Many similarities exist in the clinical and laboratory features of FIP and lymphocytic cholangitis—jaundice, ascites, raised liver enzymes, hyperglobulinemia, neutrophilia, lymphopenia, and ascitic fluid with high globulin content. There may be pointers in the clinical presentation that may help to differentiate these two diseases, but this is complicated by the very variable clinical presentation of cats with FIP. Other features suggestive of FIP may be identified such as uveitis, neurologic signs, and pleural effusion. Reliable differentiation may depend on histopathologic investigations.

Treatment
Corticosteroids are the mainstay of treatment used based on countering immune-mediated damage to the liver. Considerable clinical experience supports their beneficial effect. Prednisolone is frequently used at an initial immunosuppressive oral dose of 1 to 2 mg/kg twice a day, which is gradually reduced over an extended period of 6 to 12 weeks

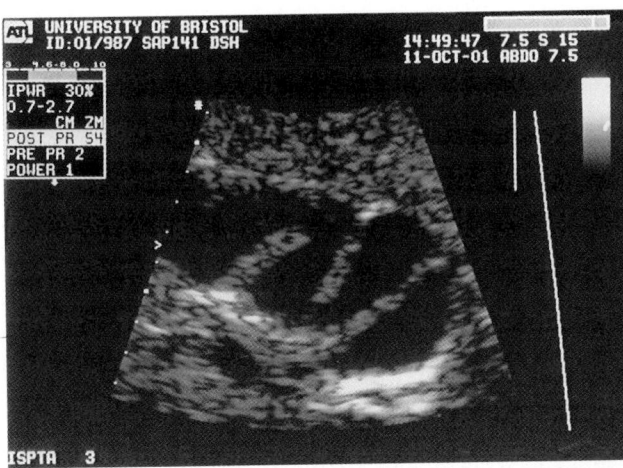

Figure 228-3 Ultrasound of abdomen of a cat with suppurative cholangitis showing a dilated, tortuous bile duct.

according to the progress of the case. Other immunosuppressive agents are occasionally used (e.g., cyclosporine, chlorambucil, methotrexate, cyclophosphamide), but experience of their use and value is limited. Colchicine may be used at a dose of 0.03 mg/kg once a day in an attempt to combat fibrosis, although there have been no controlled trials to confirm any beneficial effect. Choleretics, SAMe, and nutritional support (see Suppurative Cholangitis) may be helpful. If ascites is severe, particularly if this is causing dyspnea due to pressure on the diaphragm, drainage by abdominal paracentesis may be indicated. Loop diuretics such as furosemide (1 to 2 mg/kg twice a day) combined with restriction of dietary salt may be helpful in mild ascites. Potassium-sparing diuretics (e.g., spironolactone) and angiotensin-converting enzymes (e.g., enalapril) are alternative agents for treating ascites.

Prognosis

Limited information is available about the prognosis for cats with lymphocytic cholangitis, but the majority of cats respond well to treatment. The mean survival in 25 cats in which portal hepatitis was described was 37 months, with 16 cats surviving for more than 1 year.[18] The authors' experience is that the prognosis is better in cats with jaundice compared to those with ascites. Lymphocytic cholangitis has been seen to resolve spontaneously in occasional cases. Some cats will need repeated courses of prednisolone or may need to be maintained on long-term lower doses. Response to treatment is based initially on resolution of clinical signs. Monitoring of liver biopsies can be used to assess response to treatment but is usually declined by owners, and subsequent progress has to be based on monitoring laboratory features (particularly liver enzymes and bile acids).

MIXED INFLAMMATORY CHOLANGITIS

This form of cholangitis is seen less frequently and is less well characterized. It usually appears as a chronic disease with gradual loss of condition, although in some cases an initial episode of acute illness occurs with depression that may reflect acute suppurative cholangitis, leading to subsequent chronic liver disease. Jaundice is frequently present. The laboratory changes are similar to those seen in the other forms of cholangitis but are less consistent and frequently milder. The major dilemma in treatment of cats with cholangitis-involved mixed inflammatory infiltrates is whether antibiotics or corticosteroids are most appropriate for treatment. Limited experience suggests that the best response is achieved with prolonged corticosteroid treatment, but antibiotics are frequently administered in combination initially.

CHAPTER • 229

Vascular Liver Diseases

Kyle G. Mathews
Susan K. Bunch

EMBRYOLOGY AND ANATOMY

The portal vein is formed within the mesentery dorsal to the right limb of the pancreas by the confluence of the cranial and caudal mesenteric portal branches. It receives blood from the gastrointestinal (GI) tract and spleen via numerous mesenteric veins, the gastroduodenal, splenic, and gastric veins.[1] As the portal vein approaches the liver, it sweeps from right to left and divides into right and left branches, which further divide into branches supplying the individual liver lobes. The main right branch supplies the right lateral and caudate process of the caudate lobe, whereas the main left branch supplies all other lobes.[2] Within the hepatic parenchyma, the portal blood exits the portal triads, traverses the sinusoids, and ultimately enters the systemic circulation via the hepatic veins. The left hepatic vein is the only hepatic vein not hidden by hepatic parenchyma as it enters the caudal vena cava just caudal to the diaphragm.

Congenital extrahepatic portosystemic shunts (PSSs) are usually single vessels that connect the portal venous system to the systemic circulation, and as such may arise from any portal vessel. Most empty into the abdominal vena cava, but many will traverse the diaphragm prior to emptying into the thoracic vena cava or azygos vein. Intraoperatively, clinicians can easily locate most shunts by retracting the descending duodenum and examining the vena cava cranial to the left renal vein. If the shunt vessel is not located in this area, the surgeon retracts the liver to the right so that the esophageal hiatus may be examined for evidence of a portoazygous shunt. Occasionally, the omental bursa must be opened to gain access to shunt vessels dorsal to the stomach. This is done by tearing the ventral leaf of the greater omentum followed by cranioventral retraction of the stomach. Intraoperative imaging may be required in some cases to locate the shunt or to help make or exclude a diagnosis of microvascular dysplasia (MVD).

Many intrahepatic venous PSSs result from failure of the ductus venosus to close in infancy. Oxygenated blood from the placenta is carried from the left umbilical vein and umbilical sinus to the systemic circulation via the ductus venosus. It is not known why the ductus fails to close in some individuals. Pathology of the ductus wall or portal hypertension due to inadequate development of the portal venous tree has been speculated.[2] The cause of right-sided congenital intrahepatic and extrahepatic PSSs is unknown. Congenital extrahepatic PSSs are abnormal communications between the cardinal and vitelline venous systems.[3] Intrahepatic PSSs connect portal vein branches after their divergence from the portal vein proper to the hepatic veins or abdominal vena cava, thereby bypassing the hepatic sinusoids. They are usually hidden from view by the hepatic parenchyma. Left-sided shunts (patent ductus venosus [PVD]) arise from the left portal vein branch, pass through the left liver lobes or papillary process of the caudate lobe, and then empty into a venous ampulla cranial to the liver at its confluence with the left hepatic vein.[4,5] Central shunts pass through the right medial or quadrate lobes, and right-sided shunts pass through the caudate process of the caudate lobe or the right lateral liver lobe before emptying into the vena cava.[5,6]

Arterioportal fistulae (APF) are congenital vascular malformations that allow communication between the hepatic arterial blood supply and the portal venous system. The location of APF can vary; one or more lobes may be involved.[7-11]

Diagnostic Evaluation
History and Clinical Findings For vascular anomalies that connect the portal venous system to the systemic venous system as the primary defect (i.e., single PSS, congenital mild diffuse or multifocal intrahepatic portovascular dysplasia), the signs, physical examination abnormalities, clinicopathologic changes, and certain histopathologic findings in liver biopsy specimens are directly related to diversion of portal blood flow around the liver. Intrahepatic portal pressure is normally higher than caudal vena cava pressure; therefore in the presence of a single patent anomalous conduit, portal blood flows preferentially around the liver. Exposure of the central nervous system (CNS) to shunted gut-derived toxins (e.g., ammonia and other encephalotoxins, absorbed bacteria, endotoxins) that would otherwise be removed by the liver results in signs of hepatic encephalopathy (HE), whereas lack of trophic factor-rich portal blood and oxygen (50% of that delivered) leads to poor hepatocyte growth and function.

In conditions that are characterized by high portal pressure (i.e., severe chronic hepatitis such as idiopathic noncirrhotic portal hypertension [NCPH] or single or multiple APF), previously rudimentary multiple extrahepatic shunt vessels connecting the portal vein with the caudal vena cava open to modulate portal pressure. These vessels are commonly found clustered around the left kidney, and occasionally in the submucosa of the esophagus, primarily in dogs and rarely in cats. Additional pathophysiologic consequences and signs of this acquired shunting are directly related to the underlying cause (e.g., high alanine transaminase activity in dogs with chronic hepatitis) and the existence of high portal pressure (e.g., ascites, GI bleeding).

Portosystemic shunt Most cats and dogs with PSSs are examined because of signs of illness at less than 2 years of age,[12-28] but some animals have been 10 years of age or older at presentation.[14,15,27] Diagnosis may be missed in some individuals because the signs are subtle, or because owners believe that certain long-standing behaviors are "normal." A gender bias has not been convincingly identified, although one study from Britain describing 45 dogs with intrahepatic PSSs reported that twice as many affected dogs were male as were female.[23] Male cats often outnumber females in the literature. A familial predisposition for single extrahepatic PSS is suspected in several small purebred dogs.* The inheritance pattern of PSS in Yorkshire terriers has been investigated through pedigree analysis and trial breeding, but it remains unclear.[25]

A recent study that evaluated breed association in over 2000 dogs with vein-to-vein PSS in North America identified six breeds as having odds ratios near 20 or greater for having PSS: Havanese, Yorkshire terrier, Maltese, Dandie Dinmont terrier, Pug, and miniature schnauzer.[15]

Large purebred dogs, such as retrievers, Australian cattle dogs, Old English sheepdogs, and Irish wolfhounds, are more likely to have intrahepatic PSS.* PSSs are much less common in cats than in dogs.[20] As with small breed dogs, the majority of feline PSSs are congenital, single, and extrahepatic. Most cats with PSS are domestic shorthairs, but among purebred cats, the Himalayan and Persian are predisposed.[20,22,26] The history most commonly includes failure to thrive, neurologic signs that could include bizarre behavior such as yelping, staring, aggression, head pressing, and wall hugging, seizures, and intermittent blindness. These signs are usually present in cats by 6 months of age. Intermittent ptyalism, which is a consistent finding in approximately 75% of cats, may be a subtle manifestation of GI disturbance or HE.[18,20,26,28] GI signs, including intermittent anorexia, vomiting, or diarrhea, are observed in about 30% of affected dogs[13] but less frequently in cats.[20,22,26] Anesthetic or sedative intolerance has also been recorded infrequently. Dogs that are older at the time of diagnosis can be presented because of polyuria-polydipsia (PU/PD), which has been reported to be associated with increased ACTH secretion and hypercortisolism,[29,30] or urate stone formation.[15,31]

Owners of affected dogs may remark that their pets have a dietary preference for fruits and vegetables. Onset of signs correlates with meal ingestion approximately 30% to 50% of the time. Some cats have a history of improved behavioral arid neurologic signs after antibiotic therapy.[12]

High portal pressure is not a feature of vein-to-vein vascular anomalies, so abdominal effusion does not form in animals with PSS unless they have profound hypoalbuminemia. Many cats are of small stature, poor body condition, and have an unkempt haircoat[12,14,20,22]; neurologic signs (e.g., amaurosis, dementia) and ptyalism may also be evident on examination. There may be evidence of other congenital defects; cryptorchidism was noted in about 30% of male cats in one study[20] and 50% of the male dogs in another study. Coexistent heart murmur has also been reported.[16,20,26] Bilateral renomegaly is seen in both species, and copper-colored irises inappropriate for the breed in cats may also be noted in dogs (Yorkshire terrier, Maltese, Dandie Dinmont terrier, pug, and miniature schnauzer).[15]

Mild diffuse or multifocal intrahepatic portovascular dysplasia A disorder first described in 82 dogs and 23 in cats in which the signalment and signs resemble those of animals with PSS but a macroscopic vascular anomaly cannot be identified[32] has been termed microvascular dysplasia (MVD).[32,39] This condition can occur as the sole anomaly or jointly with PSS. Based on histopathologic changes in liver specimens and detailed portography, the anatomic site of vascular abnormality is believed to be the terminal portal veins. In Cairn terriers, MVD is believed to be an autosomal inherited trait; the specific mode of inheritance has not been established.[35]

The same dog breeds that are predisposed to PSS are those that have been described with MVD,[33,34,38,39] and cats are typically domestic shorthairs.[32] Common presenting signs include vomiting, diarrhea, and signs of HE, especially in dogs with both defects. Dogs with only MVD are somewhat older,[34,36] and many have mild to no signs of illness.

Idiopathic noncirrhotic portal hypertension A category of hepatopathies in human patients characterized by

*References 13,16,18,19,21,25,27.

*References 13,16,18,19,21,23.

intra-abdominal portal hypertension, a patent portal vein, and relatively unremarkable liver biopsy findings has been described and termed noncirrhotic portal hypertension (NCPH).[40-44] Two unusual previously reported diseases of primarily young dogs (≤2.5 years) might be able to be grouped under this same name: *hepatoportal fibrosis* in 3 dogs[45,46] and *primary hypoplasia of the portal vein* in 42 dogs).[47] Two more recent reports describe a syndrome resembling idiopathic NCPH in four Doberman pinscher dogs,[48] three of which were related, and a similar condition in 33 dogs of various breeds.[49] NCPH has also been reported as an incidental finding in a colony of dogs with mucopolysaccharidosis Type I.[50] This condition is seen most often in purebred dogs 4 years of age or younger, of either gender, weighing over 10 kg. Individual cases had been described earlier but were buried in reports of PSS. Presenting signs include abdominal enlargement associated with effusion, GI abnormalities, polydipsia, weight loss, and less consistently, signs of HE. The cause for this group of conditions has not been identified, but the unifying thread amongst the theories is severe, diffuse intrahepatic vascular malformation. Dogs with NCPH have similar signs, clinicopathologic test results, and diagnostic imaging findings as dogs with cirrhosis, but they differ substantially in histopathologic changes in liver biopsy specimens and prognosis. This condition may represent severe diffuse or multifocal intrahepatic portovascular dysplasia.

Arterioportal fistulae Clinical signs associated with APF are usually acute in onset during the first year of life and are primarily associated with the portal hypertension that results from conference of high-pressure arterial blood to the normally low-pressure portal venous system. Young medium to large breed dogs are most commonly reported, although small breeds may also be affected.[10] This appears to be a rare condition in cats.[51] Nearly all animals with APF have ascites[9,11,51,52] (Figure 229-1). Vomiting, diarrhea, lethargy, and weight-loss are also commonly reported.[8] Signs consistent with HE have been reported less frequently. In some animals with APF, the sound of turbulent blood flow through macroscopic fistula or fistulae, resembling the heart murmur in animals with patent ductus arteriosus, can be auscultated across the body wall over the affected lobe or lobes.

Clinicopathologic Test Results Clinicopathologic findings in over 50% of affected dogs, regardless of the type of vascular anomaly, are typical of global hepatic dysfunction: hypoalbuminemia, euglycemia, hypoglycemia, hypocreatinemia,

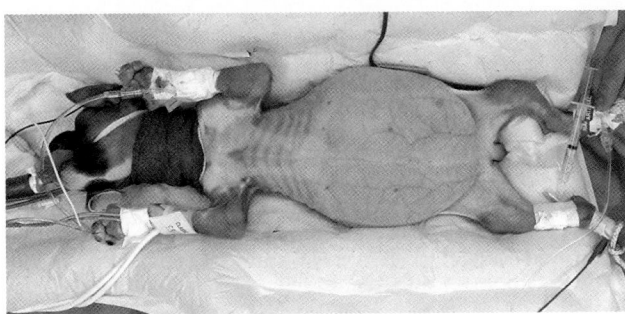

Figure 229-1 Preoperative photograph of a typical puppy with an hepatic arterioportal fistula. Ascites has resulted in a pot-bellied appearance. Numerous catheters and monitors have been placed, including a cephalic venous catheter for fluid and plasma administration, arterial catheter to monitor blood pressure, and a jugular catheter to monitor central venous pressure (CVP). The patient is placed on a warm-air blanket to help prevent hypothermia. (Courtesy of Dr. Chick Weisse.)

hypocholesterolemia, normal to low blood urea nitrogen (BUN) concentration, postchallenge hyperammonemia, and normal or high fasting with high postprandial serum bile acid (SBA) concentrations.[13,16,18,28] Clinicopathologic evidence of hepatic dysfunction eliminates the possibility of certain inborn errors of metabolism that cause hyperammonemia in young animals (e.g., urea cycle enzyme deficiency,[53] methylmalonic academia[54]) or hyperammonemia associated with urethral obstruction.[55] Target cells can be seen in some dogs, but microcytosis is the most common hematologic change in dogs; iron sequestration or ineffective iron transport have been proposed as causes for iron-deficient erythropoiesis.[56,57] Two to threefold increases in serum alkaline phosphatase (AP) and alanine aminotransferase (ALT) activities are commonly recorded; the origin of high serum AP activity is unknown. The AP isoenzyme of bone origin could be part of the high serum total AP activity in growing dogs, but subcellular hepatic organelle injury and increased release or decreased elimination of canalicular AP has also been proposed.[58] A study comparing dogs with intrahepatic PSS versus dogs with extrahepatic PSS made no particularly surprising discoveries; dogs with intrahepatic PSS weighed more and had higher blood glucose concentration and serum AP values than did dogs with extrahepatic PSS.[19]

Dogs with MVD may have similar but less dramatic changes as dogs with other vascular anomalies, but never have microcytic red blood cells (RBCs).[35-37,39] In fact, high SBA concentrations may be the only clinicopathologic finding in young purebred dogs with MVD that have been screened for PSS before sale or that are ill for nonhepatic reasons. The authors of one study attempted to distinguish dogs with MVD from dogs with MVD and PSS by use of a regression equation developed from four variables that were the most discriminating values in multiple regression analyses:

$$diagnosis = 2.851 - (0.00135 \times cholesterol\ concentration)$$
$$- (0.234 \times albumin\ concentration)$$
$$(0.0209 \times MCV) + (0.000517$$
$$\times postprandial\ SBA\ concentration).$$

Values approaching one were most consistent with a diagnosis of MVD and PSS, where values closer to 0 were likely associated with MVD alone.[36] Essentially, the lower the values for serum cholesterol and albumin concentrations, and MCV, and the higher the SBA concentration, the more likely the diagnosis of PSS.

In cats, poikilocytosis is common, and about 30% have erythrocytic microcytosis. Serum albumin, urea, and cholesterol concentrations can be strikingly normal or in the low-normal range. Serum glucose concentration is usually normal as are liver enzyme activities. The most consistent clinicopathologic abnormality in cats with PSS is high SBA, hyperammonemia, or both.*

As many as 50% or more of affected animals of both species may have dilute or hyposthenuric urine, but fewer numbers inconsistently have ammonium biurate crystalluria in a freshly voided and analyzed urine specimen. Persistent hyperammonemia and decreased ability to convert uric acid to allantoin favor formation of ammonium urate uroliths independent of urinary pH,[63,64] which, in some cats and dogs with PSS, may be the only presenting complaint.[20,31] Rarely, bilirubinuria can be seen in the absence of other chemical or sediment abnormalities. Other than concentrating defects and urinary sediment findings typical of animals with hepatic vascular anomalies, little information is available concerning characteristic renal consequences. Arising from preliminary observations that a small group of dogs with PSS had

---

*References 12,14,20,24,25,59-62.

glomerular sclerosis, renal tissue from 12 dogs with PSS that had died or were euthanatized was examined retrospectively.[66] In six of nine dogs in which urinalysis was done, trace to 1± protein by dipstick analysis was found. All 12 dogs however, had light microscopic evidence of glomerulopathy, with severity scores assigned as moderate to severe in nine of 10 dogs in which paraffin-embedded tissue was available. The renal changes were believed to be associated with shunted antigens from the GI tract; direct immunoperoxidase staining failed to consistently identify immunoglobulin deposition. Renal volume and glomerular filtration rate were compared with reference values in 21 dogs with confirmed PSS, with renal volume compared pre- and postsurgical correction in five dogs. Values for both decreased after surgery, perhaps explaining in part why many dogs with PSS are polydipsic before surgery and that this directly relates to the presence of shunting.[67] Primary polydipsia was also documented in three dogs with PSS and theorized to be another reason for increased water consumption.[68] In animals with abdominal effusion associated with NCPH or APF, fluid analysis is consistent with a pure transudate.

Hepatic Histopathologic Findings   Microscopic findings in liver specimens from dogs and cats with naturally occurring PSS mimic those of dogs with surgically created PSS, which was first described by Nicholas Eck in 1877.[69] Mild to moderate lobular hepatocellular atrophy with close approximation of portal venules, inconspicuous portal vein tributaries of small caliber, arteriolar duplication, lipidosis and vacuolar change, smooth muscle hypertrophy and increased lymphatics around central veins, and Ito cell hypertrophy are the findings in both species. Some animals have mild fibrosis around central veins. Minimal, if any, evidence of necrosis or inflammation is seen.[12,18,23,70-72] Random intralobular thin-walled blood vessels can also be seen and may represent a compensatory response to decreased portal blood flow. The histopathologic changes in the liver are considered identical in dogs with PSS, MVD, and NCPH,[32,35,37,39,47-50] and can be over- or misinterpreted among boarded pathologists (Table 229-1).

Histologic changes in liver tissue at some distance from the vascular malformation or malformations in animals with APF are similar to those of other vascular anomalies, presumably associated with portal blood deprivation.[9,11,52] Findings in liver tissue in close proximity to the fistula include dilated portal venules, marked arteriolar hyperplasia, and sinusoidal capillarization. Some portal veins in resected lobes manifest evidence of previous thrombus formation and recanalization.[9]

Diagnostic Imaging   Microhepatia is found on survey radiographs in about 50% of cats,[12,14,20] and 60% to 100% of dogs[15,17,18,36] with PSS. Bilateral renomegaly may also be documented. In dogs with MVD, the liver and kidneys are usually of normal size radiographically,[35,37] but the liver can be small in some cases.[36] Ammonium biurate uroliths are discovered in the bladder most commonly, but they can develop in the kidney, urethra, or both. They can be radiolucent, but usually contain enough calcium salts and magnesium ammonium phosphate to make them moderately radiopaque.

Confirmation of vascular communication or communications between the portal system and the systemic circulation may be achieved by using a variety of imaging modalities including ultrasonography, nuclear scintigraphy, portography, computed tomography (CT), and magnetic resonance imaging (MRI).

Ultrasonographic evaluation of potential PSS is both sensitive (80% sensitivity for canine extrahepatic shunts, 95% overall for canine shunts) and specific (67% specificity for extrahepatic shunts, 98% overall).[6,73] It is less invasive than portography, doesn't require the licensure and handling precautions needed for administration of radioisotopes, and

Table • 229-1

Histopathologic Diagnoses of Two Pathologists Compared with the Medical Record Diagnosis in 33 dogs with Hepatic Vascular Anomalies and in Two Normal Dogs

CASE NUMBER	MEDICAL RECORD DIAGNOSIS	PATHOLOGIST 1 (BLIND EVALUATION)	PATHOLOGIST 2 (BLIND EVALUATION)
1	CPS	MVD	CPS
2	CPS	NCPH	CPS
3	CPS	CPS	N/CPS
4	CPS	MVD	N
5	CPS	CPS	CPS
6	CPS	MVD	CPS
7	NCPH	MVD	CPS/NCPH/MVD
8	NCPH	CPS	CPS/NCPH/MVD
9	CPS	CPS	CPS
10	NCPH	NCPH	NCPH
11	NCPH	MVD	CPS
12	NCPH	CPS	N
13	MVD	MVD	CPS/NCPH/MVD
14	NCPH	NCPH	NCPH
15	CPS	NCPH	CPS
16	CPS	CPS	CPS
17	MVD	N	N
18	CPS	MVD	CPS
19	NCPH	NCPH	NCPH
20	NCPH	MVD	N
21	NCPH	NCPH	CPS
22	MVD	MVD	N
23	MVD	CPS	N
24	NCPH	MVD	CPS/NCPH/MVD
25	NCPH	NCPH	Unclear
26	CPS	MVD	CPS/NCPH/MVD
27	CPS	CPS	CPS
28	NCPH	CPS	CPS/NCPH/MVD
29	CPS	MVD	Lobular dissecting hepatitis
30	N	N	N
31	N	N	N
32	MVD	N	N
33	MVD	CPS	N
34	MVD	N	N
35	MVD	NCPH	N

CPS, Portosystemic venous shunt; *MVD*, microvascular dysplasia; *NCPH*, noncirrhotic portal hypertension; *N*, normal.

unlike CT does not require general anesthesia. Abdominal ultrasonography should therefore be strongly considered for all patients with possible PSS. Sensitivity improves with intrahepatic PSS (100%) as the shunt vessel is surrounded by hepatic parenchyma (Figure 229-2), whereas extrahepatic PSSs are generally smaller and may be obscured by sound wave attenuation "shadowing" secondary to the presence of gastric or intestinal gas.[6,73] The authors' experience with ultrasonographic evaluation of canine extrahepatic PSS suggests that results are highly operator dependent. The experience level of the operator must be taken into account when evaluating results. Origin and termination of the shunt vessel or vessels may be

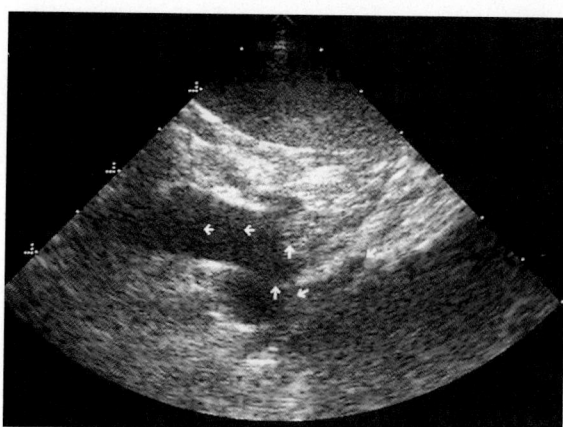

Figure 229-2 Sonogram of an intrahepatic portosystemic shunt surrounded by hepatic parenchyma. The arrows indicate direction of blood flow determined by color flow Doppler ultrasonography. (Courtesy of Dr. Kathy Spaulding.)

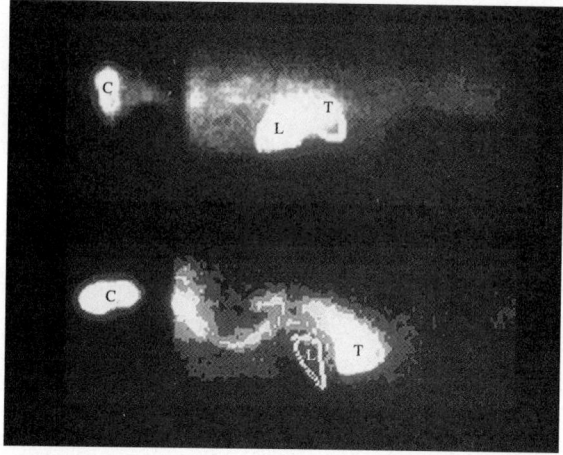

Figure 229-3 Lateral per rectal technetium scintigrams. The head is to the right. Colonic technetium deposition site (C), liver (L), and thoracic (T) regions of interest. Technetium reaches the liver prior to the thorax in a normal dog (top). The situation is reversed in a dog with a portosystemic shunt (bottom).

identified in many cases, but an understanding of the geometry and location of complex, tortuous shunts may be difficult to appreciate using two-dimensional ultrasonography. In patients with complex intrahepatic shunts, intraoperative ultrasonography may improve the surgeon's ability to locate and define the morphology of the shunt, although this has not been well described. Color flow and pulse wave Doppler ultrasonography offers the added advantage of visualization of blood flow direction, turbulence, and measurement of portal blood flow velocity. Portal flow velocity was decreased in dogs with experimentally induced cirrhosis with secondary portal hypertension and multiple extrahepatic shunts[74]; therefore it may also be decreased in dogs that develop multiple shunts secondary to naturally occurring liver disease or after surgical attenuation of shunt vessels. The normal portal flow velocity for dogs is around 15 cm/sec, and flow velocity and direction is relatively uniform. Portal flow velocity was increased or variable in 9/17 (53%) dogs with a congenital extrahepatic shunt, and in 12 of 13 (92%) dogs with an intrahepatic shunt. Increased flow velocity may be due to decreased resistance to cranial flow because of the presence of the shunt.

A variety of rectally administered radiopharmaceuticals have been used to identify the presence of PSSs.[76-79] 99mTechnetium pertechnetate is most commonly used because it is rapidly absorbed, relatively inexpensive, and has a short half-life.[76,79,80] After absorption by the colonic mucosa, 99mtechnetium enters the colonic venous (portal) circulation and is transported cranially to the liver. The patient is placed in right lateral recumbency on the surface of a gamma camera, which detects the location of the isotope. This information is displayed on a computer monitor. In dogs with normal portal circulation, the liver is visualized as a bright area on the monitor as the isotope is initially delivered to the hepatic microcirculation (Figure 229-3). With time, the isotope enters the hepatic veins, caudal vena cava, and cardiopulmonary vasculature at which time the heart can be visualized on the monitor.

Although special handling of the isotope and patient are required, the study may be performed in less than 5 minutes and requires only light sedation. Morphology, number, and location of PSSs, if present, often cannot be ascertained using scintigraphy. By drawing regions of interest (ROI) around the liver and thorax using computer software, an estimate of shunt fraction is calculated based on the counts per pixel within each ROI (Figure 229-4). Normal dogs have a shunt fraction less than 15% (i.e., the image of the liver is significantly more intense than that of the thorax at the time of image acquisition).[81] In contrast, in animals with PSS the

image of the heart is initially more apparent as the isotope bypasses the liver via the shunt (see Figure 229-3). Shunt fractions in dogs with macrovascular intra- and extrahepatic shunts often exceed 80%, whereas the reported mean shunt index for five cats was only 52% in one study.[82] The range of

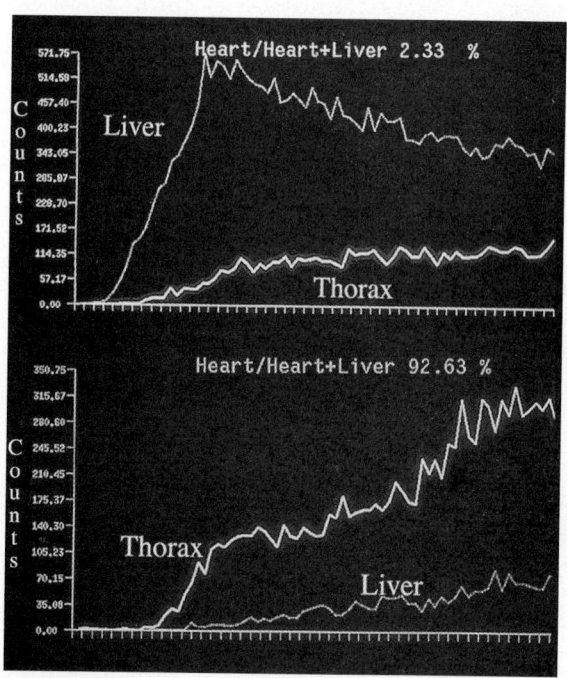

Figure 229-4 Time (seconds)/radioactivity (counts) curves of the normal (top) and shunt dog (bottom) depicted in Figure 229-3. Radioactivity in the liver is greater than that in the thorax in the normal dog (top). The situation is reversed in the dog with a portosystemic shunt (bottom). Shunt fraction is calculated by using data collected over 12 seconds starting at the separation of the curves using the formula:

[Σ total heart counts over time]/[Σ(total heart counts) + (total liver counts) over time].

Shunt fraction was 2.3% in the normal dog and 92% in the dog with a shunt.

shunt fractions for dogs with MVD is thought to be lower than those with macrovascular shunts, although this has not been reported. Shunt fraction estimation is inexact and prone to inter- and intraoperator variability.[83] As such, changes in shunt fraction over time should be cautiously interpreted. Despite its limitations, per rectal scintigraphy is quite useful in determining if significant shunting is present. If ultrasonography has failed to identify the presence of a shunt, yet clinical signs or laboratory test results are consistent with shunting, then scintigraphy should be considered.

Portography, although less commonly performed because it is more invasive than ultrasonography and scintigraphy, has the advantage of offering a "global snapshot" of the patient's portal circulation. By injecting contrast medium into the portal circulation, the relative location and number of PSSs may be identified with fluoroscopy, plain radiography, or CT (Figure 229-5).[84] Percutaneous splenoportography may be performed preoperatively by injecting contrast into the splenic parenchyma with or without ultrasound guidance. Caudally located shunts may be missed with this technique. Injection of contrast medium into the mesenteric artery via a femoral artery catheter is now rarely performed because of less invasive options and because it results in a poorer quality study due to dilution as the contrast medium passes from the intestinal arterial to the portal circulation. Alternatively, a fluoroscopically guided catheter may be inserted in the right jugular vein and advanced into the caudal vena cava, shunt, and portal system in dogs with large intrahepatic shunts prior to insertion of thrombotic coils (see discussion of treatment of intrahepatic shunts), or it may be used in the minority of dogs in which the results of ultrasonography and scintigraphy are inconclusive or discordant.[85,86] Portographic imaging may be used intraoperatively by catheterization of a mesenteric or splenic vein to evaluate the morphology of the portal vasculature, to confirm the location of hard to find macrovascular shunts, or to rule out their presence in dogs suspected of suffering from MVD.[34,35,38,87,88] The same catheter is used to measure portal pressures during shunt manipulation. Intraoperative portography can be cumbersome, because it requires either a portable radiographic unit or temporary closure of the abdominal incision and transport of the patient. Sensitivity of intraoperative portography has been reported to be between 85% and 100% and is dependent on patient positioning.[89]

Computed tomography (CT) is primarily performed in dogs with complex intrahepatic shunts. Contrast medium injected into a peripheral vein highlights both the systemic and portal venous circulation. Alternatively in large dogs, the contrast medium may be injected into a splenic vein using ultrasound guidance.[90] Because the radiopacity of the vasculature changes rapidly, helical CT is preferred because it allows rapid acquisition of data over a large anatomic area.[91,92] Transverse images of the liver and its vasculature are then reconstructed after data acquisition. Three-dimensional images of the shunt created with specialized computer software are especially useful to surgical planning. Disadvantages to CT are the need for general anesthesia and the cost. A second anesthetic event may be eliminated if the CT scan is performed immediately prior to surgery; however, this allows the surgeon little time for evaluation of the images, especially if three-dimensional reconstruction is contemplated.

Two- and three-dimensional magnetic resonance angiography (MRA) have been reported as reliable techniques for evaluating shunt vessels in human patients.[93] Two-dimensional MRA, without contrast enhancement, has been evaluated in dogs with shunts and found to have the following sensitivities and specificities: multiple extrahepatic shunts (63% to 97%)[94] and single congenital shunts (79% to 97%). The use of gadolinium-enhanced and three-dimensional MRA as preoperative planning tools for animals with complex shunt anatomy has not been reported to date.

APF are seen as numerous tortuous vascular communications with ultrasound or celiac arteriography (Figure 229-6).[11] Microscopic hepatic arteriovenous fistulae were suspected in one young dog.[52] Ultrasonographic evidence of reversed portal blood flow (hepatofugal flow) and diminished forward (hepatopetal) flow are present in all cases. The portal venous system is often markedly distended. Multiple acquired PSSs may develop as a compensatory mechanism to diminish portal blood pressure and protect against splanchnic congestion (Figure 229-7).[9,11] Multiple shunts are most easily imaged in the region of the left kidney.

Differential diagnoses If an animal suspected of having PSS is older than average at presentation, or if a young dog has signs of portal hypertension, other primary hepatopathies must be considered, such as chronic hepatitis; liver biopsy is needed. If a PSS cannot be identified by ultrasonography, transcolonic scintigraphy, surgery, or portography in a dog (or

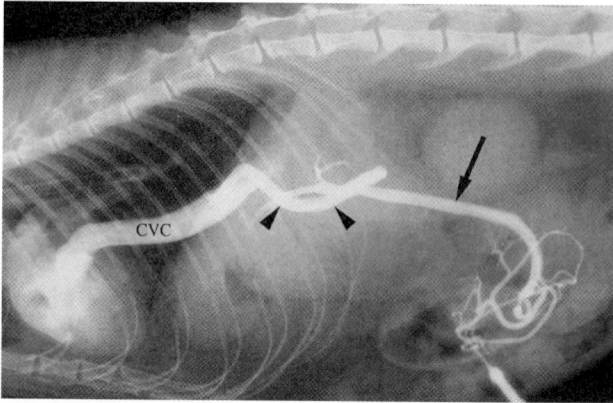

Figure 229-5 Lateral intraoperative mesenteric portogram of a cat. A large extrahepatic shunt vessel (*arrowheads*) originates from a branch of the portal vein (*arrow*) and terminates at the caudal vena cava (*cvc*). (Courtesy of Dr. Daniel Brockman.)

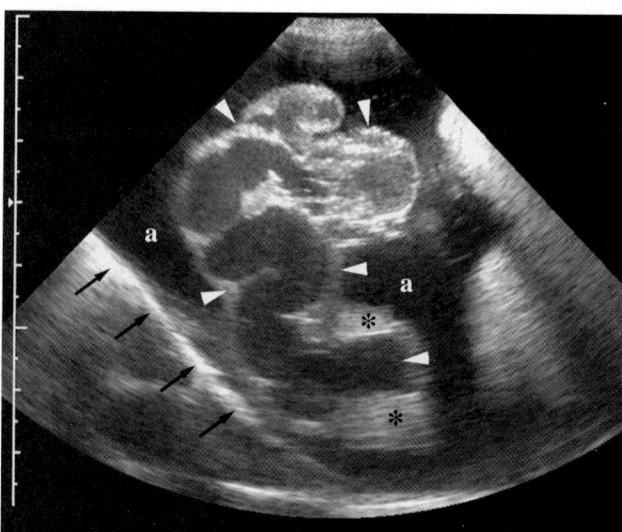

Figure 229-6 Sonogram of a left-sided arterioportal fistula. The patient's head is to the left, and ventral is toward the top of the image. Diaphragm (*arrows*), ascites (*a*), atrophied hepatic parenchyma (*). The APF (*arrowheads*) is seen as numerous thin-walled tortuous vessels. (Courtesy of Dr. Kathy Spaulding.)

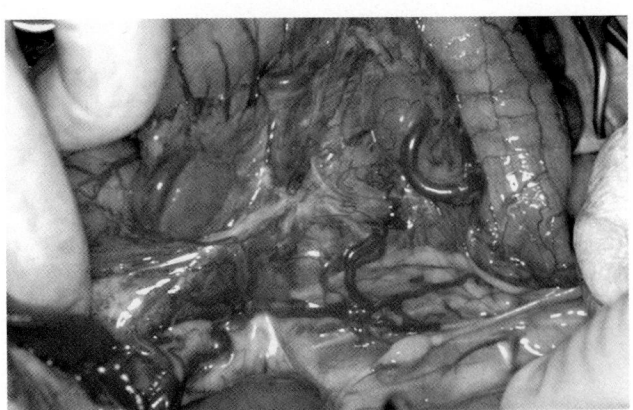

Figure 229-7 Intraoperative photograph of multiple acquired extrahepatic shunt vessels, which resulted from portal hypertension in a dog with an APF. (Courtesy of Dr. Chick Weisse.)

less commonly, a cat) suspected of having PSS, MVD is likely. Liver biopsy in such cases would provide evidence to exclude a more serious hepatopathy.

If APF are not found in a young dog with ascites, a normalized to small liver and clinicopathologic evidence of hepatic dysfunction, lobular dissecting hepatitis (or other form of chronic hepatitis), and NCPH are possibilities. Histopathologic examination of liver tissue will distinguish these disorders. An algorithm to facilitate diagnosis of vascular disorders in dogs and cats is provided in Figure 229-8.

Surgical Management
Preoperative and Operative Considerations Clinicians have good reason to believe that signs of HE should be controlled before surgical correction is attempted. In one study, asymptomatic dogs had a better prognosis for complete recovery after surgery. To start, a diet moderately restricted in protein (minimum 20% on a dry matter basis [2 g protein/kg/day] for dogs; 30% on a dry matter basis [3 g crude protein/kg/day] with adequate amounts of taurine and arginine for cats) is recommended.[95-98] If signs are not controlled with dietary modification alone, an oral disaccharide (e.g., lactulose, lactitol), antibiotics, and soluble fiber may be added. For animals with ascites secondary to portal hypertension, a diet that is moderately restricted in sodium (0.20% to 0.25% on a dry-matter basis) is beneficial.

After a diagnosis of PSS has been made, many clinicians prefer to preload patients with PSS on anticonvulsant medications to diminish the risk of postoperative seizure activity. Potassium bromide (dogs: 100 mg/kg, orally every 24 hours; cats: 30 mg/kg, orally every 24 hours) may be started 2 weeks prior to surgery, and the dose adjusted (30 to 100 mg/kg, orally every 24 hours) to obtain a serum concentration of 100 to 200 mg/dL.[99] The lower end of the dose should be used in cats, because many develop coughing as an adverse effect.[100] Similarly, phenobarbital may be started (2.2 mg/kg, orally every 12 hours) and the serum concentration evaluated prior to surgery. Oral lactulose, antibiotics, and a low-protein diet are generally started at the same time.

Given that most animals undergoing surgical correction of a PSS are hypoalbuminemic, and because current methods used to detect diminished hepatic production of clotting factors are insensitive (e.g., prolonged PTT), fresh frozen plasma is commonly administered pre- and intraoperatively (6 to 10 ml/kg, intravenously).[101] Dextrose-containing fluids should also be considered in the perioperative period. Anemia combined with intraoperative fluid loading and blood loss may result in the need for cross-matching and blood transfusions.

Intraoperative portography may be needed if the macrovascular shunt is difficult to locate, or if MVD is suspected and macrovascular shunting needs to be ruled out.

Placement of a jugular catheter preoperatively is recommended so that central venous pressure (CVP) can be monitored during shunt attenuation and postoperatively.[102] An arterial catheter is also helpful in many cases for monitoring blood pressure.

Without intraoperative warming, PSS shunt patients are at risk for developing profound hypothermia. Fluid-line warmers, warm-air devices, heating blankets, or a combination of these devices should be used in all cases.

Patients undergoing surgical correction of an intrahepatic shunt may require additional surgical exposure cranial to the liver. A partial median sternotomy and diaphragmatic incision may need to be performed. In these cases, placement of a chest tube will be required prior to surgical closure.

Correction of Extrahepatic Portosystemic Shunts
Many extrahepatic PSSs (48% to 68%) cannot be completely occluded with a single surgery without causing life-threatening portal hypertension.[102-104] Once the shunt has been surgically identified, surrounding tissues are dissected away as close to the vena cava or diaphragm as possible (Figure 229-9). A suture is passed around the shunt so that temporary occlusion may be performed while measuring portal pressures. A variety of parameters are then evaluated during temporary occlusion to determine if complete ligation of the vessel is prudent. Significant increases in portal pressure as measured by a manometer attached to a catheter placed within a jejunal vein, increased intestinal peristalsis, intestinal and pancreatic venous congestion, and decreases in CVP are all indications that complete occlusion should not be attempted.[102,105] Perioperative mortality rates after partial or complete ligation are generally between 10% to 20%.[13,28,103,105] Most dogs with a partially ligated shunt vessel improve clinically and often can be taken off of symptomatic treatment for some time. However, up to 41% to 50% of animals with partially ligated extrahepatic shunts redevelop clinical signs months to years postoperatively (mean: 3 years).[28,103,106] Because of this, repeat laparotomy to attempt complete ligation, before clinical signs recur, has been recommended. Parameters to determine appropriate timing for reoperation have not been documented. Of 24 dogs that underwent partial occlusion of their extrahepatic shunt, complete shunt occlusion occurred spontaneously in 15 (63%) 1 to 6 months postoperatively.[107] This would argue against repeat surgery within this time period.

Staged or gradual occlusion of the shunt vessel can result in complete resolution of shunting in many animals. By placing materials around the shunt that result in its gradual closure, acute portal hypertension associated with complete ligation may be avoided and perioperative mortality diminished. In addition, multiple surgeries are not required. Two implantable materials (ameroid rings and cellophane bands) have been evaluated for this purpose. Ameroid rings are composed of hydrophilic casein that swells over time (Figure 229-10). They are surrounded by a stainless steel collar, which limits outward expansion. They were originally designed as a cardiovascular research tool to create gradual occlusion of coronary and other vessels and have been adopted as a treatment tool by veterinary surgeons. Placement around a shunt vessel results in occlusion in 30 days in most animals, although delayed closure of up to 90 days has been reported.[72] Shunt occlusion has been thought to be due partly to ring swelling, and partly due to an inflammatory reaction with fibrosis around the ring. The mechanisms by which the portal circulation accommodates increased flow have not been reported, but it is clear that acute increases result in life-threatening

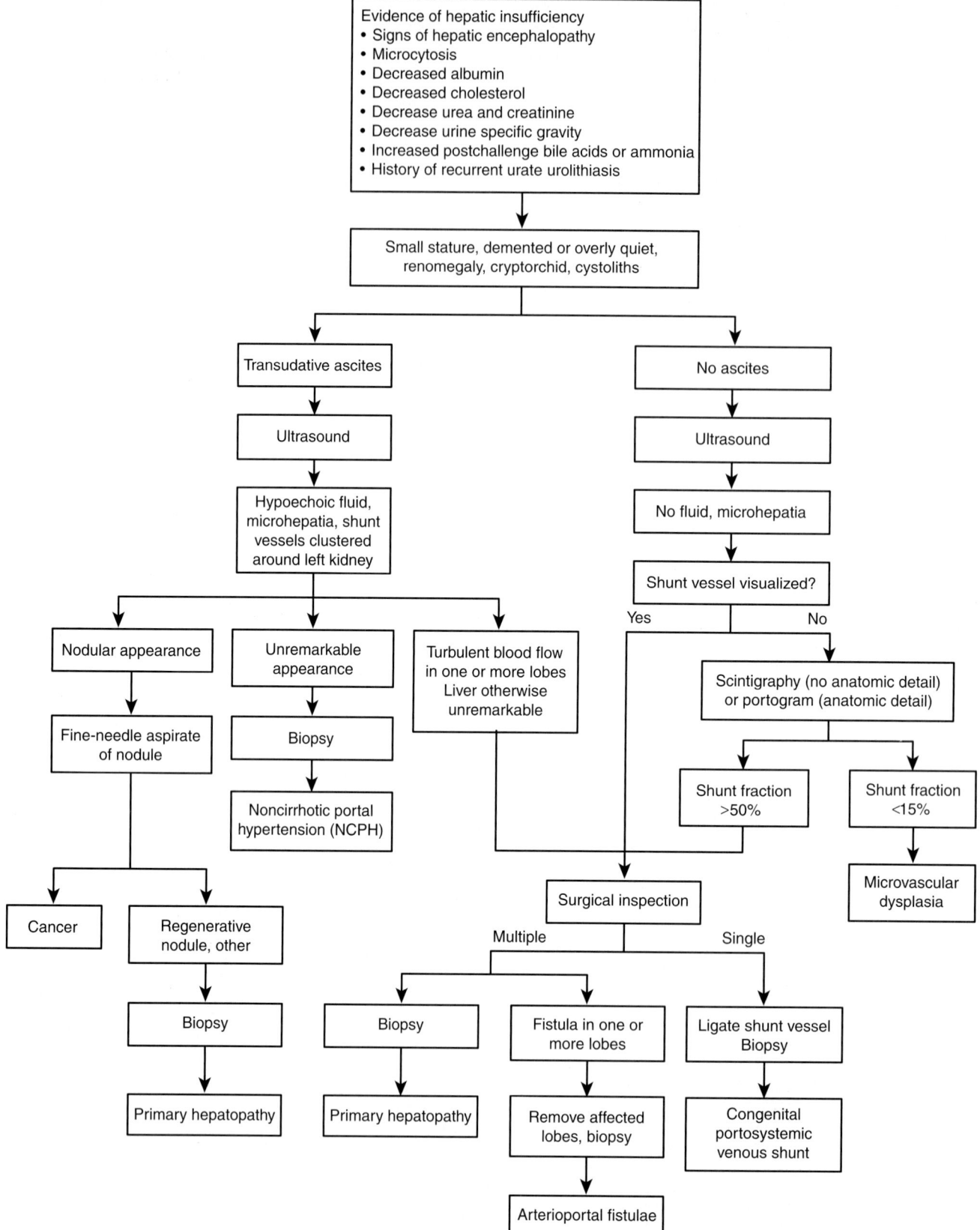

Figure 229-8 Suggested diagnostic path for animals suspected of having a portovascular anomaly.

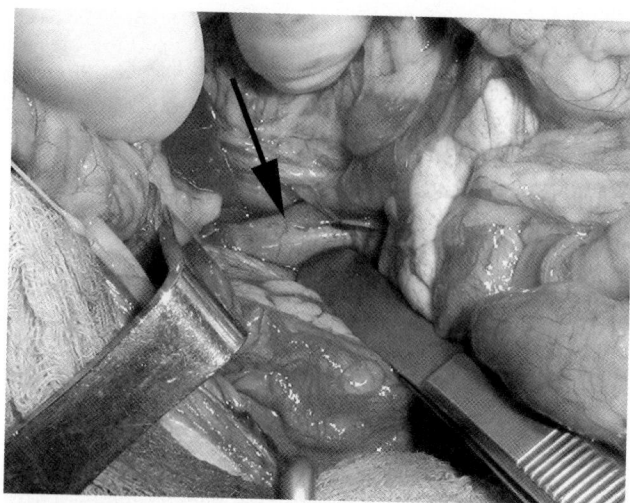

Figure 229-9 Intraoperative photograph of a large splenic vein to abdominal vena cava portosystemic shunt vessel (*arrow*). (Courtesy of Dr. Chick Weisse.)

portal hypertension, whereas gradual increases in portal flow lead to increased liver size. Portal hypertension associated with sudden complete shunt occlusion is generally not a problem after ameroid ring placement unless the weight of the ring kinks the vessel postoperatively, or excessive manipulation of the shunt vessel during ameroid placement results in thrombotic shunt occlusion.[72] A recent study investigating ameroid ring placement on external iliac veins in six dogs showed that the luminal area of the ring only decreased by 23%. All dogs had evidence of venous thrombosis at the site, with complete occlusion occurring by the sixth day in half of the dogs.[108] This rate of PSS occlusion after ameroid placement may be too rapid, and could theoretically result in subclinical portal hypertension and subsequent development of multiple extrahepatic PSSs. Multiple acquired shunts have been reported in approximately 10% to 20% of dogs, and are even more common in cats, after ameroid placement (see Feline Portosystemic Shunts: Unique Considerations).[72,109] In these patients, symptomatic treatment may need to be continued indefinitely. It is interesting to note that four of 24 dogs (17%) < in one study that had an extrahepatic PSS partially ligated) also

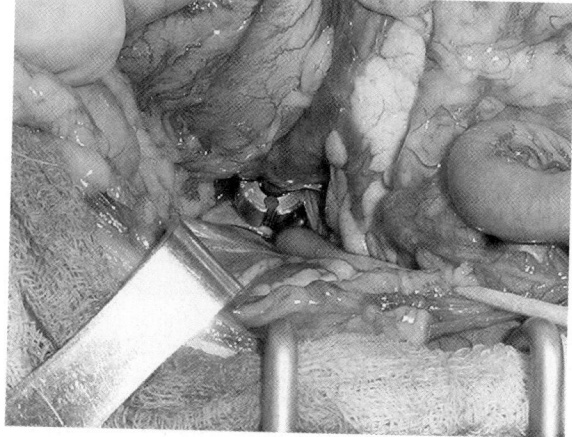

Figure 229-10 Intraoperative photograph of the same PSS seen in Figure 229-5 after placement of an ameroid ring around the vessel. (Courtesy of Dr. Chick Weisse.)

went on to develop multiple acquired shunts despite continued flow through the original shunt.[107]

An alternative to the ameroid ring is cellophane tape or film, which is derived from plant cellulose. Cellophane incites an inflammatory reaction that results in gradual attenuation of the shunt vessel. Progressive occlusion is slower and potentially less complete than with ameroid constrictors; however, potentially diminished risks are associated with placement, including less risk of tearing the shunt, less shunt manipulation required, and less risk of kinking the shunt postoperatively. Additionally, because occlusion is slower, there may be a diminished risk of developing multiple acquired shunts. When placed around the femoral vein in six dogs occlusion was progressive over a 6-week period in four of six dogs, and was incomplete in all.[110] Of eleven dogs with extrahepatic PSSs treated with cellophane banding, 10 had resolution of shunting. In eight dogs, shunt occlusion occurred by 8 weeks, whereas occlusion did not occur until 7 and 11 months in the remaining two dogs.[111]

Correction of Intrahepatic Portosystemic Shunts

Intrahepatic shunt vessels are hidden from the surgeon by hepatic parenchyma in most cases. Because of their large diameter, complete ligation is rarely accomplished with one surgery. The location of the shunt may be confirmed intraoperatively by a variety of means. Palpation of the liver will often reveal a soft spot with accompanying fremitus in the affected liver lobe. Intraoperative mesenteric portography or ultrasonography may also be performed.[112] The portal vein branch that feeds the shunt vessel, as well as the exit point of the shunt, can be identified by passing a catheter through a purse-string suture and small incision in the portal vein. The catheter is passed cranially through the shunt and into a prehepatic venous ampulla or thoracic caudal vena cava. A left-sided shunt (PDV or patent ductus venosus) empties into a venous ampulla, which also receives the LHV prior to emptying into the vena cava at the level of the diaphragm.[113] The shunt vessel , LHV-ampulla, or both are bluntly dissected free from the surrounding tissues between the liver and the diaphragm. The shunt vessel, LHV-ampulla, or both are then either partially ligated while monitoring portal venous pressures, or a large ameroid constrictor or strip of cellophane is placed.[114] Experimental occlusion of the LHV in normal dogs resulted in transient congestion of the left and central hepatic lobes, but it had no clinical effect.[115] New information indicates that dissection and partial ligation of the LHV or ampulla is not needed because left-sided shunts may be dissected prior to their entry into the ampulla in most cases.[5] If the shunt vessel empties directly into the vena cava (most right-sided and central shunts), a determination is made as to whether the portal vein branch that feeds the shunt can be dissected free from the surrounding tissues.[116,117] If possible, partial ligation, ameroid ring or cellophane band placement on this vessel is performed.[118] Shunt vessels that empty directly into the vena cava, and for which the feeding portal branch cannot be isolated, are either partially ligated after inflow vascular occlusion of the liver, or an extrahepatic shunt may be created by placing a jugular vein graft or grafts between the portal vein and abdominal vena cava. After graft placement, complete resection of the shunt and its surrounding liver lobe has been reported. Inflow vascular occlusion of the liver requires that the patient or liver be hypothermic at the time of surgery to limit ischemic damage to the liver. Whole body hypothermia has been reported in dogs with good results, despite complications that include severe hypotension, arrhythmias, acidemia, and cardiac arrest secondary to increased myocardial irritability.[119] Topical cooling of the liver with cold saline may protect it from ischemia and reperfusion injury without the systemic side effects seen with whole-body hypothermia; however, this has not been evaluated in dogs with PSS.[120] To perform inflow occlusion, the aorta (or celiac and cranial mesenteric arteries), portal vein, and abdominal and thoracic vena cava are temporarily occluded. This allows the surgeon to make an incision into the thoracic vena cava or the portal vein, identify the shunt, and place a circumferential suture around it.[116,121] Once the venotomy has been closed and blood flow to the liver has been reestablished, the circumferential ligature is slowly tightened while monitoring portal pressures as for extrahepatic shunts. The significant blood flow through large intrahepatic shunts cannot be suddenly obstructed by the surgeon without the development of life-threatening portal hypertension. Intraoperative shock (hemorrhagic and septic), cardiac arrest, and portal hyper- and hypotension have been listed as causes of intraoperative death. Postoperative survival rates vary from 75% to 89%, with peritonitis, portal vein thrombosis, and portal hypertension listed as the most common causes of death in the postoperative period.[17,19,23,28,116] Predictors for the development of postoperative complications were low body weight (<10 kg) and hypoproteinemia or hypoalbuminemia in one study.[122] Shunt location had no effect on short or long-term outcome. One- and 2-year survival rates were 60% and 55%, respectively, for partially attenuated shunts. After 4 months, euthanasia because of failure to show clinical improvement, was the most common cause of death. Another study followed 37 dogs that survived initial intrahepatic PSS attenuation. Twenty-eight (76%) became clinically normal and required no medical management (mean follow-up: 16 months).[23] Nine dogs had persistent or recurrent encephalopathy of which three were euthanized without surgery. Six dogs were reoperated, three successfully ligated, and three euthanatized at surgery.

Complete occlusion requires multiple-staged procedures, unless a vein graft is placed between the portal vein and the vena cava. By placing the graft, portal hypertension may not develop after complete occlusion of the intrahepatic shunt. Splenectomy followed by anastomosis of the splenic vein to the abdominal vena cava has been used to alleviate portal hypertension in one dog as an emergency procedure.[123] Intraoperative hemorrhage from an intrahepatic PSS in this dog necessitated resection of the involved liver lobe and created life-threatening portal hypertension. As a planned procedure, a jugular vein may be harvested and used to create a bridge between the portal vein and the abdominal vena cava. With this technique, the surgeon essentially moves the shunt to an extrahepatic location, which allows for ligation or resection of the intrahepatic shunt. This new extrahepatic shunt can then be treated by placing an ameroid constrictor around the graft in an attempt to achieve complete resolution of all portosystemic shunting. This technique has been reported in a limited number of cases.[124,125] Eight of 10 dogs could have their intrahepatic PSS completely ligated using this technique in one study.[124] Nine of these dogs had an excellent clinical outcome, despite the development of multiple PSS in four of eight dogs reevaluated 8 to 10 weeks postoperatively.

Given the invasiveness and complexity of surgical correction, interventional radiologic techniques may become more routinely performed in the future. Transjugular coil embolization of canine intrahepatic PSS has been reported, and the short-term results are promising.[86,126] A fluoroscopically guided catheter is advanced from the right jugular vein to the caudal vena cava and shunt vessel. Contrast studies and measurement of portal pressures before and after coil placement are performed. A cylindric wire mesh stent is placed in the caudal vena cava at the level of the shunt to prevent coil migration. Catheter-delivered thrombogenic coils are then placed in the shunt (Figure 229-11). Complete or near complete occlusion of the shunt requires multiple-staged coiling sessions to prevent the development of acute portal hypertension.

Feline Portosystemic Shunts: Unique Considerations

Complete ligation of feline PSS is only possible in one of three cases. Most importantly, the prognosis after partial surgical ligation is less favorable than that reported for dogs. Although clinical improvement is usually seen after surgery, only 57% of 22 cats had a good to excellent long-term outcome.[60] Persistence or recurrence of clinical signs has been reported in the majority of partially ligated cases.[12,20,59-61] For this reason, staged attempts to completely ligate the shunt vessel are advocated,[20,24] with resolution of clinical signs possible if complete ligation is eventually achieved.

Given the poorer prognosis associated with partial ligation when compared with dogs, gradual occlusion of feline PSSs with ameroid constrictors has also been investigated.[25,62] After ameroid placement, many cats (33% to 77%) experience postoperative complications, including central blindness (zero to 45%), hyperthermia (zero to 27%), seizures (8% to 14%), and frenzied behavioral changes (zero to 23%). Most of these complications are temporary. It should be noted that postoperative hypothermia and hypoglycemia are commonly reported in studies evaluating feline response to PSS ligation. Despite the high frequency of complications, the postoperative mortality rate is low (zero to 4%) and compares favorably

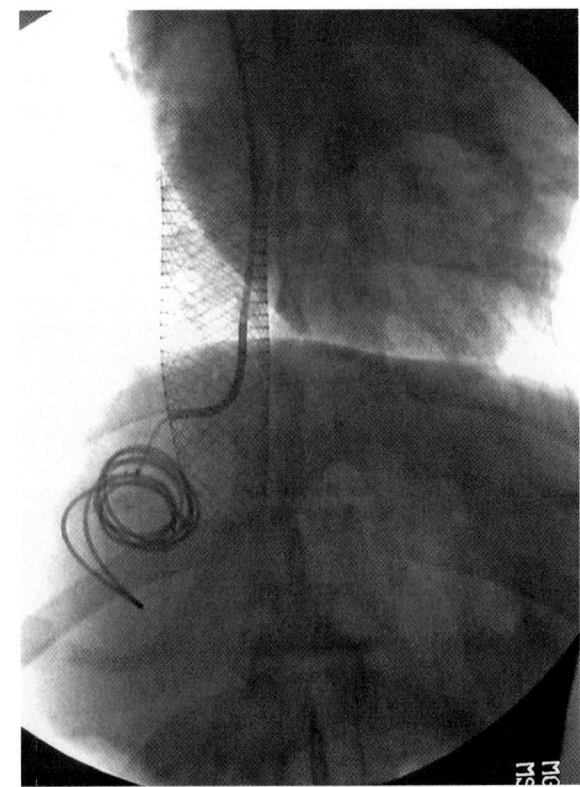

Figure 229-11 Ventrodorsal fluoroscopic image of a catheter-delivered thrombogenic coil being placed into a large right-sided intrahepatic portosystemic shunt (PSS). The dog's head is toward the top of the image. A cylindric braided wire stent has been placed in the caudal vena cava at the level of the diaphragm to prevent cranial migration of the coil. (Courtesy of Dr. Chick Weisse.)

to surgical attenuation (complete or partial ligation) of feline PSS (11%).[20] However, at recheck evaluation 8 to 10 weeks postoperatively, persistent shunting is common (57%). This is most likely due to the development of subclinical portal hypertension resulting in multiple acquired extrahepatic shunts, although this has been documented in only a few cases. As with dogs, too rapid closure of the shunt vessel or an underdeveloped portal system (or both) may contribute to portal hypertension. Long-term results vary between studies with 33% to 75% of cats reported as having a good to excellent clinical outcome[25,62] and 18% to 66% having a poor outcome. Owners contemplating surgical treatment for their cats' extrahepatic PSSs should be made aware of the discordant results reported in the current literature.

Fewer than 10% of feline shunts are intrahepatic, and acquired shunts are rarely reported, therefore less can be said regarding their long-term prognosis.[20,127] A left-sided intrahepatic shunt consistent with a PDV is most common, although shunts involving the right and central liver lobes have been reported. As in dogs, feline PDVs empty into a venous dilatation or ampulla that receives contributions from the PDV, left hepatic veins, and phrenic veins prior to emptying into the caudal vena cava at the level of the diaphragm.[128,129] Partial ligation of the intrahepatic shunt cranial to the hepatic parenchyma has been reported in 10 cats.[129] Most cats survived these procedures.[70,128,129] Complete occlusion of the shunt by ligation of the portal vein branch feeding the shunt and transjugular coil embolization has been reported in one cat each.[70,130] Both cats survived and were clinically normal at long-term follow-up. This is in contrast to canine intrahepatic shunts, which can rarely be completely occluded with a single procedure.

Correction of Arterioportal Fistulae

Surgical treatment by resection of the affected liver lobe is successful in the majority of cases that have not gone on to develop multiple shunts. Partial hepatectomy has been successfully performed with and without temporary occlusion of the hepatic vasculature.[7,8,10] Portal hypertension resolves immediately after liver lobectomy, although this resolution is incomplete in many cases.[7,8,10] After surgery, animals that have formed multiple shunts may need to be treated medically with low-protein diets and medications as previously discussed for other forms of portosystemic communications. Upon review of 11 dogs with APF from four reports, eight of the dogs had developed multiple shunts by the time of surgery.[7,10,131,132] Two dogs died or were euthanatized at surgery; one died 15 hours postoperatively (hypovolemic shock); one dog each was euthanatized at 1 month (esophageal stricture), 14 months (recurrent hepatoencephalopathy), 26 months (hemorrhagic diarrhea), and 31 months (recurrent vomiting). Four of the 11 dogs (36%) were still alive at 5, 24, 26, and 36 months postoperatively. One dog still suffered from episodic HE 24 months postoperatively; the others were reportedly normal and off all medications and dietary management.

Multiple Acquired Portosystemic Shunts

Multiple acquired shunts form in response to increase portal blood pressure. Cirrhosis, APF, and NCPH are some conditions that may result in formation of multiple shunts (see Figure 229-11). Treatment is aimed at controlling the underlying problem if possible, and the prognosis is guarded unless the underlying problem can be ameliorated (see discussion of symptomatic treatment of PSS). Surgical treatment has been performed in the past by partially occluding the abdominal vena cava in an attempt to raise caval pressures above portal pressures and thus eliminate portosystemic shunting. Long-term survival and quality of life were no different between medically managed and surgically managed groups after hospital discharge in one study.[133] There

appears to be no place for vena cava banding in animals with conditions causing portal hypertension.

Postoperative Complications

Despite preloading with anticonvulsants, postoperative seizure activity can still occur in PSS in some patients regardless of the shunt type or the surgical procedure performed.[104,134-138] Other residual neurologic deficits, such as transient blindness in cats, have also been reported.[62] In some cases, life-threatening status epilepticus may develop up to 3 days postoperatively. Some reports suggest that older animals are more prone to developing this complication,[135,137] but this complication may occur regardless of age.[139] A few of the causes that have been suggested include alterations in brain amino acid and neurotransmitter profiles, and withdrawal of gut-derived benzodiazepine agonists.[140-142] Postoperative seizures in these patients appear to be most responsive to intravenous barbitutate[134] or a continuous rate infusion (CRI) of propofol (0.01 to 0.25 mg/kg/mm),[136] and management may require ventilatory and parenteral nutritional therapy.

Life-threatening portal hypertension is uncommon, but it may develop in the early postoperative period.[36,72,102,103] Clinical signs may include abdominal pain, hypotension, ascites, and vomiting. Reoperation to remove the suture or ameroid ring that is obstructing blood flow through the shunt vessel must be performed immediately. Successful outcome after reestablishment of shunt patency is uncommon.

Portal vein thrombosis may occur after shunt manipulation regardless of the surgical procedure.[105,143,144] Potential contributing factors to this condition include portal venous stasis or turbulent flow, endothelial damage, and hypercoagulability.[144] The authors have seen this occur in both dogs and cats with both intra- and extrahepatic shunts. Increases in portal venous pressures may result in the development of multiple shunts and continuation of clinical signs, or they may be severe enough to result in life-threatening GI venous stasis. The optimal method and duration of treatment is not clear. Treatment with anticoagulants, thrombolytic compounds such as tissue-plasminogen activator,[145] or both should be considered.

Treatment for Animals with Nonsurgical Conditions

For dogs with partially occluded PSS, inoperable PSS, NCPH, or for animals with owners who decline definitive treatment, symptomatic management is recommended for life. Quality of life is improved temporarily, but fluctuating neurologic signs and occurrence of urate urolithiasis can be expected. The current ability to manage clinical signs in dogs with congenital PSS primarily with diet is limited unless a purified diet is used, but it is no substitute for surgical correction. In a study of the long-term effects of surgically created end-to-side portocaval shunts in adult dogs, the diet used was a purified, carbohydrate-based diet formulated with a specific ratio of branched chain amino acid to aromatic amino acid composition. Both dogs with created portocaval shunt and sham-operated dogs lived comfortably for nearly 1 year, free of signs of HE and weight loss. These diets are not made commercially, so they are inaccessible to owners. Another study evaluated 23 dogs with congenital PSS that did not have corrective surgery but had symptomatic treatment for at least 3 years.[147] About half of the dogs had been euthanatized within 1 year of diagnosis, mostly because of uncontrollable HE, but nine dogs lived a reasonable quality of life for 3 to 8 years. Similar studies have not been performed in cats. Despite these encouraging findings in dogs, hepatic deterioration associated with poor portal blood flow progresses as long as the abnormal vascular pattern persists. The same regimen is used for cats with inoperable PSS or for cats whose owners decline surgery.

No surgical remedy for MVD exists, so symptomatic management for HE (if present) is the only treatment recommended. Affected dogs seem to live comfortably in good to excellent condition for at least 5 years without serious consequences.[25]

For dogs with NCPH, one study concluded that affected dogs might live as long as 9 years after diagnosis with minimal

symptomatic treatment for ascites, and for some, HE. Four dogs were euthanized because of problems related to persistent portal hypertension (e.g., duodenal ulceration, urate urolithiasis).[49]

For treatment of animals that have acquired portosystemic shunting associated with primary hepatobiliary disease, see elsewhere in this text.

CHAPTER • 230

Toxic, Metabolic, Infectious, and Neoplastic Liver Diseases

Margie A. Scherk
Sharon A. Center

INTRINSIC AND IDIOSYNCRATIC XENOBIOTIC HEPATOTOXICITY

Deriving 75% of its circulation directly from splanchnic venous drainage, the liver receives direct and concentrated delivery of xenobiotics (drugs and environmental chemicals) absorbed from the gut. Consequently, because of this central position in drug metabolism and disposition, the liver is a preferential target for adverse xenobiotic reactions. Many xenobiotics are capable of causing some degree of liver injury; these are broadly classified as intrinsic or idiosyncratic, although a combination of reactions also may occur.[1] Intrinsic hepatotoxicity is a result of the direct action of a xenobiotic or its metabolite on vital cell targets; a prototype of this form of injury is acetaminophen. Biochemical and morphologic features of intrinsic hepatotoxins reflect either extrinsic mechanisms or

intracellular events and many damage zone 3 (Figure 230-1). The most common hepatic reaction with intrinsic drug toxicity is necrosis without an inflammatory infiltrate. Although drug-metabolizing enzymes detoxify many xenobiotics and toxins, they also enhance the toxicity of some.

Unlike intrinsic toxicity, idiosyncratic injury is thought to commonly involve immune-mediated mechanisms that either invoke specific cell surface death receptors, signaling apoptosis or necrosis, or involve hapten and neoepitope expression on the hepatocyte surface. Idiosyncratic hepatotoxicity can exhibit either a regional or mixed zonal pattern.

Because the liver has an enormous regenerative capacity, replacement of lost hepatocytes may mask detection of drug-induced injury. The outcome of intrinsic and idiosyncratic xenobiotic hepatotoxicity varies widely, ranging from cell survival to apoptosis or complete cytolytic necrosis. Nutritional status affects

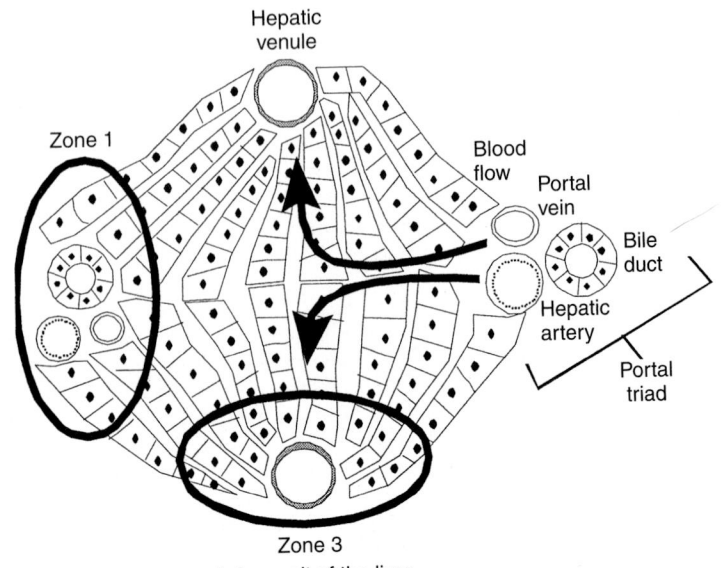

Figure 230-1 Microscopic liver architecture: acinar unit of the liver.

xenobiotic toxicity, with obesity favoring the accumulation of lipid-soluble toxic metabolites and anorexia or protein: calorie restriction resulting in reduced hepatic glutathione (GSH) concentrations that can increase the hepatotoxicity of certain agents.

Xenobiotic Hepatotoxicity: Morphologic Lesions

Drug-induced liver injury can mimic all forms of spontaneous liver disease. Lesions that may be linked with xenobiotic hepatotoxicity, include hepatocellular necrosis, toxic hepatitis, steatosis, and cholestasis (canalicular stasis with periportal inflammation). A summary of xenobiotics-related hepatotoxic reactions is provided in Table 230-1. The most common effects are described below.

Hepatocellular necrosis associated with xenobiotic toxicity may be zonal (often zone 3) or panlobular. Clinically, illnesses may range from an asymptomatic increase in transaminase activity to jaundice and overt hepatic failure. Intrinsic hepatotoxins can produce vague gastrointestinal (GI) signs, abdominal discomfort within a few hours to days of exposure (e.g., diazepam (cats) and carprofen (dogs)). In some cases, clinical signs resolve within days of xenobiotic withdrawal, however, in others, overt liver failure develops within 1 week and is associated with sequentially increasing liver enzymes, jaundice, coagulopathies, evidence of proximal renal tubular injury (i.e., granular casts, renal glucosuria), acute renal failure, and neurobehavioral changes indicative of hepatic encephalopathy.

Toxic hepatitis is characterized by diffuse or multifocal hepatic necrosis and degeneration with or without canalicular cholestasis. Hepatic acinar structure is maintained, but areas of necrosis and degeneration are surrounded by viable hepatocytes (+/− degenerative features) and an inflammatory infiltrate (mononuclear, macrophages, or eosinophils). Illness can range in spectrum from asymptomatic increases in transaminases to signs of overt liver failure and jaundice.

Steatosis (cytosolic fatty vacuolation) reflects the abnormal accumulation of triglycerides in hepatocytes in either a macrovesicular or microvesicular pattern. With the exception of hepatic lipidosis in cats, mild to moderate fatty vacuolation of hepatocytes may accompany "toxic" hepatitis. Microvesicular steatosis is thought to reflect severe metabolic disruptions associated with abnormal mitochondrial function. When diffuse, this lesion often accompanies inflammation and hepatocellular necrosis.

Cholestasis induced by xenobiotic toxicity results from the disruption of bile production or flow and may present as a periportal inflammatory lesion causing hepatocanalicular cholestasis or a less obtrusive, canalicular dysfunction without inflammation or necrosis. The major evidence for this form of injury involves

---

Box • 230-1

Known Hepatotoxins

Azathioprine
Carprofen (dogs)
Clonazepam (cats)
Diazepam (cats)
Danazol (dogs)
Acetaminophen (dogs and cats)
Diethylcarbamazine (*Dirofilaria immitis* microfilaria-positive dogs)
Diethylcarbamazine
Galactosamine
Glucocorticoids (dogs)
Halothane (dogs)
Ketoconazole
Mebendazole (dogs)
Methimazole (cats)
Methoxyflurane (dogs)
Mitotane (dogs)
Oxibendazole (dogs)
Phenytoin (dogs)
Primidone (dogs)
Phenobarbital (dogs)
Stanozolol (cats)
Thiacetarsemide (dogs)

Commonly Reported Toxins

Amanita mushrooms
Aflatoxins/mycotoxins
Blue-green algae: cyanobacteria
Cycad (Sago palm nuts)
Chlorinated compounds
Dimethylnitrosamine
Dinitrophenol
Heavy metals (Pb, Zn, Mn, Ar, Fe, Cu)
Phenols (especially cats)

Endotoxins and Enterotoxins

Enteric organisms: *Clostridium perfringens*, *C. difficile*
Food poisoning: Staphylococcal, *Escherichia coli*, *Salmonella*, *Bacillus cereus*

Table • 230-1

Histologic Patterns of Xenobiotic Associated Hepatic Injury

PATTERN OF INJURY	MECHANISMS	PROTOTYPE XENOBIOTICS
Zonal necrosis	Xenobiotic adducts, free radicals, neoantigens	Acetaminophen, halothane
Toxic hepatitis	Hapten formation → neoantigen	Phenytoin, sulfonamide, isoniazid
Microvesicular steatosis	Impaired hepatic B-oxidation of fatty acids	Tetracycline, valporic acid, tamoxifen
Macrovesicular steatosis	Increased triglyceride synthesis, reduced egress	Anabolic steroids in inappetent cats
Phospholipidosis	Formation of lysosomal inclusions	Amiodarone
Canalicular Cholestasis	Decreased membrane fluidity, Na/K ATPase	Anabolic hormones, estrogens, androgens
Hepatic cholestasis	Inflammation, Damage to bile canaliculi	Chlorpromazine
Veno-occlusive disease	Occlusion of terminal hepatic venules	Azathioprine, 6-thioguanine
Peliosis hepatica	Damage to sinusoidal membranes	Anabolic androgenic hormones
Hepatic xeoplasia	Unclarified	Sex hormones
Mixed inflammatory patterns	Immune-mediated to product/adduct	Many drugs

sequential increase in alkaline phosphatase (ALP) and GGT activity, and the development of hyperbilirubinemia.

Specific Hepatic Xenobiotic Toxicities

A list of known hepatoxins follows.

Antimicrobial Hepatotoxicity   Antimicrobial hepatotoxicity, Table 230-2, has been widely recognized in humans and less commonly reported in veterinary patients. Trimethoprim-sulfa reactions are the best recognized example in dogs. Tetracycline therapy can result in fulminant hepatic failure in both dogs and cats as well as hepatic lipidosis.

Anticonvulsants: Phenobarbital, Phenytoin, and Primidone
Phenobarbital hepatotoxicity is the best-characterized "idiosyncratic" reaction in the dog, and has been well studied

in this species as an enzyme inducer. It is clinically recognized as a hepatotoxin in some epileptic dogs. Clinical signs may include sedation and ataxia due to impaired drug metabolism. Anorexia, ascites, jaundice, and coagulopathy develop when liver damage is severe. A direct dose-related hepatotoxicity is not consistent. Clinical signs can develop within several months or years of phenobarbital initiation. Most dogs have been treated for over 1 year before showing clinical signs. Despite substantial hepatic injury, dogs may appear to be physically healthy despite abnormal serum chemistry values. Remission of clinicopathologic features and improvement in hepatic injury may occur after drug discontinuation. Dose reduction may produce improvement, but this is not well documented. Necropsies in dogs succumbing to hepatic insufficiency usually confirm chronic liver injury or cirrhosis. Lesions are identical to those described in dogs with primidone hepatotoxicity

Table • 230-2

Antimicrobial Hepatotoxicity

ANTIBIOTICS	TYPE OF LIVER INJURY
Penicillins	
Amoxicillin	Hepatocellular
Ampicillin	Hepatocellular
Amoxicillin/clavulanic acid	Cholestatic*, mixed vanishing bile duct lesions, granulomatous
Carbenicillin	Mixed
Nafcillin	Cholestatic
Oxacillin	Cholestatic, granulomatous
Penicillin G, V	Hepatocellular
Timentin	Cholestatic
Cephalosporins	Mixed, cholestatic
Ceftriaxone	Biliary sludge/stones
Cephalexin	Granulomatous
Tetracyclines	Hepatic lipidosis*, fulminant hepatic failure* (dogs, cats)
Macrolides	
Erythromycin	Cholestatic*, vanishing bile duct lesions
Azithromycin	Cholestatic
Clarithromycin	Cholestatic
Clindamycin	Acute hepatocellular injury
Sulfonamides	Cholestatic*, hepatocellular*, mixed, granulomatous, fulminant liver failure*
Trimethoprim-Sulfa	Cholestatic, hepatocellular, mixed, granulomatous, fulminant liver failure* (dogs)
Antifungal	
Ketoconazole	Hepatocellular*, mixed, fulminant liver failure
Fluconazole	Hepatocellular*, cholestatic
Itraconazole	Hepatocellular
Flucytosine	Hepatocellular
Griseofulvin	Hepatocellular, cholestasis (cats)*
Antiparasitic Agents	
Albendazole	Hepatocellular, mixed
Mebendazole	Hepatocellular*, mixed, fulminant hepatic failure*
Thiabendazole	Mixed*, vanishing bile duct syndrome with diethylcarbamazine, necrosis (dogs)
Oxibendazole	

*Antimicrobial drug hepatotoxicity reported in humans but pertinent to veterinary patients.
From Brown SJ, Desmond PV, Hepatotoxicity of antimicrobial agents. *Seminar Liver Dis* 2002; 22:157-67

as 25% of primidone is metabolized to phenobarbital, and cannot be differentiated from dogs with other forms of chronic parenchymal liver injury.[2] Combination therapy of phenobarbitol and primidone increase the risk of hepatotoxicity.

Phenytoin, a potent enzyme inducer can cause hepatitis, jaundice, and death in dogs when used as an anticonvulsant, especially when administered in combination with either phenobarbital or primidone. A dose-independent chronic hepatitis may progress to cirrhosis and appears to be reversible if the drug is discontinued promptly after initial signs of illness. Rarely, acute hepatotoxicosis has been observed.

Diazepam Diazepam-associated hepatotoxicity in cats appears to be an idiosyncratic reaction. It causes severe panlobular hepatocellular necrosis sparing the biliary epithelium. Affected cats received these agents for behavior modification (e.g. inappropriate urination). Hepatotoxicity is recognized within the first week (several days) of oral drug administration. Initial clinical signs include inappetence, vomiting, and severe lethargy associated with transaminases progressively rising levels. After several days, ALP GGT and bilirubin levels progressively increase activities progressively and cats become overtly jaundiced. Clinicopathologic abnormalities may progress to reflect fulminant hepatic failure, including hypoglycemia, profound coagulopathies, high creatinine kinase activity (muscle and myocardial necrosis), granular casts, and acute renal failure. Cats who have survived fulminant hepatic failure have received blood transfusions, plasma, vitamin K_1, water-soluble vitamins, parenteral feeding, and aggressive fluid and electrolyte support. Administration of N-acetylcysteine (NAC) is recommended. Surviving animals have persistently high ALP and GGT activity for several weeks to months after recovery due to regeneration, and hyperplastic biliary epithelium. Similar toxicity has been observed in cats receiving oral clonazepam.

Oxibendazole and Mebendazole Administration of a combination heartworm-hookworm preventative containing diethylcarbamazine and oxibendazole has been associated with lethal hepatotoxicity in dogs. Clinical signs developed 2 to 4 weeks after the initiation of treatment and included lethargy, anorexia, vomiting, diarrhea, polydipsia, polyuria, and weight loss. Biochemical profiles reflected hepatocellular injury and cholestasis.

Methimazole Methimazole used to treat hyperthyroid cats may be associated with cholestatic hepatotoxicity. This usually occurs within the first month of therapy and is indicated by increased liver enzyme activity (transaminases, ALP) and jaundice. Liver injury appears to be reversible with early drug discontinuation. Because metabolism of toxic intermediates involves GSH, it is postulated that patients with subnormal hepatic GSH concentrations may beat an increased risk for hepatotoxicity.[3] Although not yet studied in the cat, hyperthyroidism in other species reduces hepatic GSH concentrations, possibly from to increased oxidative stress associated with the enhanced metabolic rate. Because catabolism and protein deficiency states can enhance hepatic GSH depletion, certain symptomatic hyperthyroid cats may be at increased risk for methimazole toxicity. Cats with pre-existent liver disease associated with GSH depletion (e.g., cholangitis, cholangiohepatitis) may also be at increased risk.[4] This coincides with the observation that cats with cholangitis/cholangiohepatitis may become increasingly symptomatic when hyperthyroid.

Nonsteroidal Anti-inflammatory Drugs Because NSAIDs are being used more often in the treatment of inflammatory and painful conditions, it is important to be observant for not only gastric and renal effects of prostaglandin inhibition but also for potential hepatotoxic effects. The mechanism by which hepatic toxicity occurs with most NSAIDs is not known, but it is not related to prostaglandin inhibition. NSAID-associated hepatopathy is believed to be idiosyncratic. Thus it is reasonable to obtain baseline biochemistry values (alanine aminotransferase [ALT], alkaline phosphatase [ALP], blood urea nitrogen [BUN], creatinine, total protein, packed cell volume [PCV]) because these agents can be associated not only with idiosyncratic hepatotoxicity but also with dose-dependent GI bleeding and exacerbation of renal insufficiency.

Nearly all nonsteroidal anti-inflammatory drugs (NSAIDs) can cause an asymptomatic increase in transaminase activity in humans. Usually enzyme activity normalizes rapidly upon treatment of cessation. Virtually all NSAIDs can cause some form of liver injury. There is no clear correlation between chemical class of NSAID and risk of hepatotoxicity. The histologic type of injury varies within and between classes. Although hepatocellular injury is most common, cholestatic injury, mixed injury, steatosis, and granulomatous reactions also are described in humans. Since many toxic metabolites are normally detoxified by GSH, some metabolites may become more injurious when hepatic GSH stores are depleted (e.g. in patients with chronic necroinflammatory and cholestatic liver disease).[5]

Two NSAIDs are directly hepatotoxic: aspirin and phenylbutazone. In humans, the effects of aspirin are predominantly dose-dependent, anicteric, rarely fatal, and are reversible when treatment is discontinued. Carprofen (see below), a propionic acid derivative is recognized to cause severe and sometimes lethal idiopathic hepatotoxicity in dogs. Reye's syndrome, an unusual adverse response to aspirin, occurs in children with viral infections and results from mitochondrial toxicity.

Acetaminophen Acetaminophen is widely recognized to provoke hepatotoxicity through induction of the p450 enzyme and impairment of hepatic GSH concentrations. Treatment with thiol donors to restore circulating and liver GSH status, or that directly conjugate toxic adducts can attenuate acetaminophen hepatotoxicity. Both NAC and S-adenosyl-L-methionine (SAMe) have been proven to do this. Dogs have an apparent predisposition to acetaminophen-induced liver damage due to their intrinsically low hepatic GSH concentrations relative to that of other species.[5] Cats have higher hepatic GSH concentrations and do not succumb to hepatotoxicity. Rather, they develop oxidative damage to their rbcs (red blood cells) (Heinz body anemia, methenoglobinemia) because of labile sulfhydry bonds in their hemoglobin, and endothelial toxicity.

Carprofen Carprofen is a lipophilic, propionic acid class NSAID useful for the amelioration of pain associated with osteoarthritis. It can provoke idiosyncratic cytotoxic hepatotoxicity in some dogs.[6] Severity of cytotoxic injury varies among dogs and appears unrelated to dose or duration of treatment. Most dogs have received treatment for at least 2 weeks before showing vague signs of toxicity: anorexia, vomiting, lethargy, and polyuria/polydipsia (PU/PD). Some dogs with occult hepatic injury lack clinical illness. Common clinicopathologic abnormalities include modest to markedly increased transaminases (exceeding increases in ALP). Renal toxicity (granular casts, glucosuria in the absence of hyperglycemia, and proteinuria) may also occur. Some dogs succumb to fulminant hepatic failure, although most recover after drug withdrawal and 1-2 weeks of hospitalized supportive care. It is unclear whether chronic inflammatory liver disease precedes or follows acute toxicity.

Natural or Herbal Remedies Awareness of the potential hepatotoxicity of herbal preparations and other botanicals Many herbal remedies are believed to be harmless and are

Table • 230-3

Herbal Remedies Associated with Hepatotoxicity

AGENT/PRODUCT NAME	TOXIC INGREDIENT	EVIDENCE/TYPE HEPATOBILIARY INJURY
African remedy (Mediterranean/African regions)	Atractylis gummifera	Diffuse hepatic necrosis; acute onset within hours
	Callilepsis laureola	Mitochondrial toxins
Bajiaolian	Podophyllotoxin	Abnormal liver tests
Chaparral leaf	Larrea tridentata, nordihydroguaiaretic acid	Fulminant hepatic necrosis, zone 3 necrosis, chronic hepatitis, cholestasis, cirrhosis
Chinese Herbal Medicine	Glycyrrhizin	Vanishing bile duct syndrome
Chinese Herbal Tea	T'u san-chi'l (Compositae)	Veno-occlusive disease
Comfrey (Symphytum officinale) (gordolobo yerba, tea, maté)	Pyrrolizidine alkaloid	Veno-occlusive disease
Dai-saiko-to (differs from Sho-saiko-to in proportion of components)		Acute and chronic hepatitis
European remedy	Chelidonium majus, other Neoclerodane diterpenes, Teucrium chamaedrys	Hepatitis, fibrosis, eosinophilic inflammation
Germander		Zone 3 hepatitis, necrosis, fibrosis, cirrhosistoxicity enhanced by p450 cytochrome induction and glutathione (GSH) depletion
Herbal teas comfrey, Heliotroprium, Senecio, Crotalaria, Symphytum, T'u-san-chi'l [Compositae]	Pyrrolizidine alkaloid	Veno-occlusive disease
Jin Bu Huan	Lycopodium serratum	Acute/chronic hepatitis, fibrosis, steatosis
Kombucha "mushroom"	Yeast-bacterial aggregate	Abnormal liver tests
Ma-huang	Ephedrine many other ingredients	Acute hepatitis
Margosa oil	Azadirachta indica	Hepatic lipidosis associated with diffuse mitochondrial failure (Reye's syndrome)
Mediterranean traditional remedy	Teucrium polium	Zone 3 necrosis, fibrosis, acute liver failure
Mixed preparations: mistletoe, valerian, skullcap	Unknown	Hepatic injury, laboratory abnormalities
Natural laxatives	Senna, podophyllin, aloin	Abnormal liver tests
Oil of cloves	Eugenol	Direct-dose hepatotoxin
Pennyroyal oil (home-made tea)	Labitae (mint) Mentha pulegium; pulegone → menthofuran pulegone	Zone 3 necrosis, liver test abnormalities, pulegone depletes glutathione
Prostata	Saw palmetto Serenoa serrulata, Pygeum africanum, other ingredients	Hepatitis, fibrosis, cholestasis
Sassafras	Sassafras albidum	Hepatic carcinogen (animals)
Sho-saiko-to (TJ-9)	Scutellaria, others	Zonal, bridging necrosis, fibrosis, microvesicular steatosis, cholestasis
Chinese name: Xiano-Chai-Hu-Tang	Many components	Acute hepatitis, focal steatosis
	Venencapsan (horse chestnut leaf, sweet clover, celandine, milk thistle, dandelion root, milfoil)	
Zulu remedy	Callilepsis laureola	Hepatic necrosis

commonly used without adequate medical supervision. The true frequency with which botanicals cause hepatic damage is unclear but it is important to remain alert for a causal relationship when liver injury is identified. A list of hepatotoxic associations with different herbal remedies is provided in Table 230-3.[5]

General Treatment Recommendations

If acute ingestion of a hepatotoxin within the preceding 8 hours, prompt is suspected emesis, gastric lavage, high enema cleansing, and administration of activated charcoal (orally and by enema) is recommended. Animals with reduced consciousness or active enteric bleeding should not be made to vomit or have vigorous enema manipulations performed for fear of causing aspiration pneumonia or exacerbating hemorrhage. Activated charcoal may importantly reduce enterohepatic circulation of certain toxins and should be administered. Antioxidant supplementation is warranted. Although not clearly a direct antidote for every form of xenobiotic hepatotoxicity, administration of NAC is safe, and may guard against hepatocellular thiol depletion. It is important that NAC be injected as a slow bolus rather than as a constant rate infusion. Using a nonpyrogenic 0.2 μm filter, give 140 mg/kg; subsequently give 70 mg/kg up to 4-6 times daily slow IV. Once oral medications can safely be administered, initiate SAMe 20 mg/kg PO. SAMe is best administered on an empty stomach to ensure availability of this pivotal metabolic substrate. Supplementation with alpha-tocophetol (vitamin E, 101 u/kg orally per day) is also suggested. In fulminant hepatic failure, provision of clotting factors by administration of fresh frozen plasma is advised (2 to 5 mL/kg intravenously), along with vitamin K_1 (0.5 to 1.5 mg/kg subcutaneously, every at 12-hour intervals for three doses). For certain xenobiotics, particularly early after acetaminophen ingestion, cimetidine is administered with the intent of impairing cytochrome p450 activity responsible for generation of toxic adducts. Fluid therapy is provided to ensure adequate hydration, not only for normal circulatory support, but also for maximal biliary and renal excretion of toxic adducts. Fluids should be supplemented with B complex vitamins (1 to 2 mL/liter of fluid), along with KCl (judiciously using conventional sliding scale doses), phosphate, and magnesium according to needs. Glucose supplementation is important for patients in fulminant hepatic failure or demonstrating proximal renal tubule injury with glucosuria when hypoglycemia is recognized. For toxins that are highly protein bound and difficult to eliminate, administration of medications with competitive protein binding may exacerbate toxicity. For animals with declining oncotic pressure, administration of synthetic colloids (hetastarch, Dextran-70) is advised. Because colloids may result in platelet-associated bleeding tendencies, fresh frozen plasma is preferred in animals in fulminant hepatic failure prior to colloid administration.

Clinical use of Milk Thistle (silibinin) remains controversial, except for intervention of amanitin-associated mushroom toxicity.[5] The active constituents, flavonolignans including silibinin, isosilibinin, silidianin, and silicristin, are collectively known as *silymarin*; silibinin is the principle active ingredient. This herbal product is thought to be a hepatoprotective, antioxidive, antiinflammatory, antifibrotic, and to promote hepatic regeneration. No evidence indicates that silymarin poses a toxic effect, although standardization of products and purity is unregulated. Doses of 20 to 50 mg/kg of 60% to 80% potency silymarin extract may be appropriate for dogs; studies of *Amanita phalloides* hepatotoxicosis used 50 to 150 mg/kg successfully.[5]

Nutritional support is critical for animals recovering from acute xenobiotic toxicity. Protein restriction should not be imposed unless signs of hepatic encephalopathy are recognized; undue restriction may impair a positive nitrogen balance needed for tissue regeneration.

Sequential evaluation of liver enzymes (transaminases in particular), total bilirubin (where elevated), and serum bile acids (SBA) (in those with normal bilirubin) can be used to monitor resolution of hepatocellular toxicity and improving liver functions. For lesions associated with reactive biliary epithelial hyperplasia, the serum ALP and GGT activities may increase for days after clinical improvement is firmly established.

Discontinuation of the suspected hepatotoxin is the most important interventional treatment for chronic xenobiotic hepatotoxicity. Intervention with glucocorticoids or other immunomodulating medications should only be based on liver biopsy findings. Common involvement of *oxidative stress* argues for intervention with antioxidants, especially thiol donors (SAMe), and vitamin E until clinicopathologic findings indicate recovery. Ursodeoxychol acid is specifically indicated when high bile acid concentrations are a part of the disease process, but it has limited value in acute xenobiotic toxicity.

If cholestasis is a component of chronic disease, accumulation of membranocytolytic hydrophobic bile acids justifies its use.[3]

METALS AND LIVER DISEASE

Because the liver is the first organ perfused by portal blood containing absorbed minerals, it can serve as a "sink" or "reservoir" for excessive quantities of absorbed materials or toxic metals. Copper and iron play a critical role in formation of reactive oxygen species (ROS); selenium and zinc contribute to ROS detoxification. Excess copper is primarily eliminated through the biliary system, thereafter undergoing an enterohepatic circulation. The transition metals copper and iron have been proven to accumulate in the liver tissue of dogs and cats with necroinflammatory liver disorders where they may enhance hepatic vulnerability to oxidant injury.[8]

Copper

Because copper is a transition metal, it has both pro-and antioxidant effects. Pathologic hepatocellular copper overload has been well described in Bedlington terriers as a genetic defect and has been observed randomly in other pure and mixed breed dogs and in a few cats. Serum ALT activity has been shown to correlate with mitochondrial copper concentrations, hepatocellular oxidant damage, and cytolysis in patients with inherited copper storage hepatopathy. The familial tendency for hepatic copper accumulation described in the West Highland white terrier does not consistently lead to liver injury. Copper retention is more commonly observed as a complicating feature of chronic cholestatic liver disease.

Iron

In approximately 80% of dogs with chronic necroinflammatory liver disease, tissue iron concentrations exceed the normal range.[9] Recent work suggests that although this iron appears morphologically isolated in hepatic Kupffer cells, other macrophages or lipogranulomatous inflammatory foci in liver tissue, it remains biologically active and may contribute to ROS formation and hepatic fibrosis.[7,9]

It is clear that iron is a profibrogenic factor based on extensive study of humans with hemochromatosis, a genetic defect resulting in hepatocyte iron loading. A central role in liver fibrogenesis associated with iron overload is the Kupffer cell, which in turn, activates nearby stellate cells, directly mediating collagen gene activation.

Therapeutic intervention in iron-related liver injury has been studied. High hepatic iron concentrations are associated with subnormal concentrations of vitamin E and a reduced GSH/GSSG balance in liver tissue. Hepatocytes depleted of GSH are more susceptible to iron-induced lipid peroxidation. In hemochromatosis, phlebotomy is the treatment of choice along with administration of antioxidant and hepatoprotective agents. Both vitamin E and silibinin attenuate iron-associated oxidative liver injury in this disorder.[10,11] One of the authors has rarely diagnosed apparent hemochromatosis-like hepatic disease in dogs and cats. These have been managed with phlebotomy (i.e., biweekly removal of no greater than 15% of blood volume), repeated based on circulating ferritin concentrations and serum iron indices (as well as chronic supplementation with antioxidants).

METABOLIC DISORDERS

Amyloidosis

Amyloidosis involving the liver is uncommon but may occur as a component of systemic amyloidosis, a syndrome resulting from multiorgan extracellular amyloid deposition. Amyloid is made up of a number of different amyloidogenic proteins reflecting a diversity of disease processes. All amyloid proteins share a pleated structure, resulting in a characteristic green birefringence when stained with Congo red and viewed with polarized light. In systemic amyloidosis of dogs and cats, the precursor protein is typically amyloid A (AA), an amino terminal fragment of the acute-phase protein, serum amyloid A (SAA). This protein may occur secondary to sustained acute-phase reactions associated with chronic inflammatory, infectious, or neoplastic diseases or as a familial trait as it does in man.

In systemic amyloidosis, the clinical signs vary corresponding to the pattern and extent of tissue involvement. In familial AA amyloidosis in Chinese Shar Pei dogs and in Abyssinian cats, the most common presentation involves renal involvement. Systemic familial amyloidosis involving the liver has been described in a small number of dogs, and in Siamese, Oriental shorthair, Devon Rex, Burmese, and DSH cats.[12-15] Investigation of amyloid protein in Siamese and Abyssinian cats suggests a unique isotype in the Siamese. Diffuse hepatic involvement predisposes to spontaneous hepatic rupture, owing to increased organ fragility and the presence of a coexistent coagulopathy (inhibition or deficiency of factors, binding of ionized calcium, or deficiency of vitamin K). Cats present suddenly dead or hypothermic with acute signs of hemorrhage from ruptured liver lobes (anemia, hemorrhagic abdominal effusion). A regenerative anemia, presence of Howell Jolly bodies due to splenic dysfunction from amyloid deposition, a "stress" leukocytosis, and poikilocytes are observed. Thrombocytopenia and abnormally prolonged clotting times are common in cats with hepatic rupture; some cats respond to vitamin K_1. Increased ALT is common, but some cases lack biochemical features indicating hepatic involvement. A familial cluster of cases is common. Hepatic ultrasonography initially may reveal a diffusely hypoechoic liver.

Definitive diagnosis requires tissue biopsy and histopathologic demonstration of amyloid. Cytologic evaluation of an hepatic aspirate may suggest (but not definitively confirm) the presence of amyloid, based on the identification of pink amorphous material adjacent to hepatocytes (with a modified Wright's-Giemsa stain). Caution is warranted before collecting liver samples because either aspiration or biopsy may initiate uncontrollable hemorrhage. On gross inspection, affected liver or spleen appear pale and enlarged, with rounded edges. The intestines may be dilated reflecting dysmotility secondary to amyloid deposition.

Colchicine is used in the treatment of familial Mediterranean Fever in man (similar to the periodic fever syndrome in Shar Pei dogs). It attenuates inflammation by interfering with release of inflammatory mediators, neutrophil participation, and deposition of amyloid fibrils. Clinical signs (several dogs) and histologic severity of hepatic amyloid deposition (as reported in one dog) have been blunted in Shar Pei dogs treated with colchicine (0.03 mg/kg orally per day). No experience exists with colchicine in cats with systemic amyloidosis and liver involvement. Colchicine has been used in a few cats with hepatic fibrosis (0.03 mg/kg orally, once a day to every other day). Acute treatment of liver hemorrhage requires generous provision of fresh whole blood and plasma transfusions. A grave prognosis is warranted for cats with hepatic amyloid; survivors eventually succumb to renal failure or acute hypovolemic shock from liver lobe fracture.

Feline Lipoprotein Lipase Deficiency

Lipoprotein lipase (LPL) regulates the dispersal of fatty acids to muscle and adipose. Deficiency disturbs fat metabolism leading to hypertriglyceridemia, hyperchylomicronemia, and systemic sequela of these aberrations. Several kindreds of cats with familial LPL deficiency have been studied; this defect is an autosomal recessive trait.[16,17] Compared with normal cats,

affected cats have more than tenfold increase in circulating triglycerides yet normal total cholesterol. Kittens do not exhibit clinical signs other than fasting lipemia; they grow normally and show clinical signs at 8 to 9 months of age, including fasting hyperlipemia, lipemia retinalis, cutaneous xanthogranulomas (lipogranulomas), and peripheral neuropathies due to the compression of lipogranulomas in areas of minor trauma. Treatment involves feeding a diet restricted in fats and triglycerides. Peripheral neuropathies may resolve or improve after several months on a fat-restricted diet.

Canine Hyperlipidemia

Abnormalities in canine lipid metabolism have received limited attention. Affected breeds include Miniature Schnauzers, Shetland Sheepdogs, Briards, Beagles, certain terrier breeds (especially Scottish terriers, West Highland white terriers, Cairn terriers), and some mixed breed dogs. Hyperlipidemia in the dog predisposes to development of a diffuse vacuolar hepatopathy or biliary mucocele. Vacuolar hepatopathy may be associated with excess hepatocyte glycogen and/or lipid inclusions. Biliary mucocele formation may reflect the influence of hypercholesterolemia on biliary cholesterol concentrations and appears to be augmented by age-related cystic hyperplasia and possible dysmotility of the gallbladder wall.

In the developmental stage, biliary mucoceles are asymptomatic and are serendipitously discovered during abdominal ultrasound performed for unrelated reasons. Dogs with large biliary mucoceles may present for associated necrotizing cholecystitis or they may be found ultrasound investigation for high liver enzyme activity (especially ALP). Many cases have a coexistent diffuse vacuolar hepatopathy causing a diffuse or multifocal hepatic parenchymal hyperechogenicity, hypoechoic nodules, nongravitational gallbladder "sludge," and a thickened, bi- or trilaminar appearance of the gallbladder wall. The appearance of a "kiwi" fruit echoimage within the gallbladder lumen is diagnostic for a firm, well-established mucocele. These must be surgically removed, the urgency depending on clinical evidence of necrotizing cholecystitis (hyperbilirubinemia, high liver enzymes, cranial abdominal pain, leukocytosis). Dogs with severe hypothyroidism can also develop pathologically significant hypercholesterolemia, hepatic vacuolation, high liver enzyme activity associated with abnormally increased SBA concentrations, hyperbilirubinemia, and biliary mucoceles. Initiating thyroxin therapy for 1 to 2 weeks before elective surgical removal of a biliary mucocele is advised in these dogs if clinical signs of the mucocele are minimal. Although liver lesions resolve with institution of thyroxine, mucoceles usually require surgical removal. At surgery, the gallbladder should be excised because mucoceles have been observed to reform. Chronic life-long treatment with a fat-restricted diet (in hyperlipidemic patients) and chronic administration of ursodeoxycholic acid (15 mg/kg orally per day) is recommended for dogs with biliary mucoceles, even after their removal.

Canine "Steroid or Glycogen" Vacuolar Hepatopathy

The hepatic response to glucocorticoids varies remarkably among species. In the dog, rapid change in hepatic morphology and induction of liver enzymes is well recognized. High dose glucocorticoid administration usually causes significantly increased ALP and ALT activity within 2 to 3 days if given by injection and within 1 to 2 weeks if given orally.[18] Individual variation in response, different potencies of glucocorticoid agents, and route of exposure (endogenous, parenteral, oral, cutaneous, ocular) influence changes in hepatic morphology, clinicopathologic features, and clinical signs. Typically, increased ALP and GGT activity develop in parallel as these enzymes undergo induction and subsequent release from sinusoidal and canalicular membranes. Initially, (during the first week of glucocorticoid exposure) a liver-ALP isoenzyme predominates. This is rapidly replaced (within 1 week) with a glucocorticoid-ALP isoenzyme.[19] Because most canine patients with increased ALP activity produce the glucocorticoid-ALP isoenzyme, clinical utility of isoenzyme fractionation is low.

In the seminal study of glucocorticoid hepatopathy in the dog (injectable prednisone daily for 14 days), hepatocellular glycogen gradually increased, achieving maximal values on the fifteenth day. Glycogen accumulated first in zone 1 but thereafter predominated in zone 3 resulting in typical *ballooning degeneration*. After discontinuation of glucocorticoids exposure, hepatocellular glycogen slowly diminished over a period of weeks. Ultrasonographic features of vacuolar hepatopathy include diffuse or multifocal parenchymal hyperechogenicity with variable appearance of hypoechoic nodules. Distinction from other chronic necroinflammatory or fibrosing liver disorders is impossible without tissue sampling.

A similar clinical scenario as that described for exogenous glucocorticoids occurs in dogs with adrenal hyperplasia syndromes, where high steroid sex hormone production or high cortisol production occurs. A confusing aspect of the vacuolar hepatopathy syndrome in dogs is its association with a variety of chronic health problems. These may reflect an aspect of patient stress response correlating with acute phase responses, resulting in enhanced production of endogenous corticosteroid or nonglucocorticoid steroid hormones (Box 230-2). If clinical scrutiny fails to disclose an underlying health problem or cortisol values consistent with classic hyperadrenocorticism in a dog with a prominent vacuolar hepatopathy associated with high ALP activity (often with modestly increased SBA concentrations), a sex hormone profile conducted before and after ACTH administration should be pursued. Samples may be sent to the University of Tennessee Endocrinology laboratory (UTCVM Clinical Endocrinology Laboratory Tests, Department of Comparative Medicine, Room A105, 2407 River Drive, Knoxville, TN 37996-4500; (865) 974-5638). Because severe vacuolar hepatopathy has been observed to progress to the severe lesions associated with the hepatocutaneous syndrome, one of the authors (SAC) has recently taken a more aggressive approach. Treatment is undertaken in patients with abnormally high sex steroids (single or multiple abnormalities involving androgen, progesterone, or estrogen hormones, without cortisol abnormalities) in the following circumstances: marked vacuolar remodeling with formation of reticulin-bound nodules, or clinical signs such as PU/PD, polyphagia, or evidence of compromised liver function (e.g., high bilirubin, high bile acids). Treatment with mitotane (op' DDD) has been successful; experience with trilostane is limited at present. L-deprenyl and melatonin treatment has been discouraging, and no experience exists with estrogen aromatase inhibitors in this syndrome.

Hepatic Lipidosis Syndrome in the Cat

Cats have a propensity for accumulating triglycerides (TG) in their hepatocytes. Systemically ill cats usually develop some degree of hepatocellular fatty vacuolation. The development of lipid vacuoles within hepatocytes is not directly noxious but rather reflects an underlying metabolic disorder. Hepatic TG accumulation is not problematic until the degree of vacuolation is morphologically severe. In a normal feline liver, the fat content comprises less than 5% of total organ weight. The liver of a cat with the HL syndrome may double or triple in weight from accumulated fat.

TGs accumulate when the rate of hepatic synthesis exceeds their dispersal. Hepatic TGs are produced from fatty acids derived from the systemic circulation (dietary lipids, adipose stores) and from *de novo* hepatic synthesis. Overnutrition, especially with carbohydrates, augments hepatic fat accumulation

---

Box • 230-2

Differential Diagnoses for Canine Vacuolar Hepatopathy

Hyperadrenocorticism
Spontaneous disease
Pituitary or adrenal origin
Iatrogenic: glucocorticoids therapy:
    PO, IM, SQ, topical: skin, eye, ear

Adrenal Hyperplasia Syndrome
Abnormal sex hormone production

Hepatocutaneous Syndrome

Chronic Stress
Illness > 4 weeks

Severe Dental Disease:
Infection

Chronic Infections or Inflammation
(e.g., Pyelonephritis, chronic dermatitis)

Inflammatory Bowel Disease (IBD)
Chronic
Lymphoplasmacytic
Eosinophilic

Neoplasia
Lymphoma, other

Disorders Influencing Lipid Metabolism
Diabetes mellitus
Idiopathic hyperlipidemia
    (e.g., schnauzer, sheltie, other)

Pancreatitis
Chronic

Hypothyroidism: Severe

Congestive Heart Failure (CHF)

---

as a result of a positive energy balance and an inhibitory metabolic influence on mitochondrial fat oxidation. Many cats developing HL are obese; unrestricted release of fatty acids from excessive adipose stores promotes HL, because up to one third of mobilized fat resides in the liver at any time. HL reflects the liver's inability to match fat dispersal with delivery from systemic sources. The balance of TG lipolysis and accumulation is modulated by blood glucose concentration, hormonal, neural, and pharmacologic mechanisms. The activity of hormone sensitive lipase (HSL, promoting lipolysis) and LPL (promoting fat uptake) directly regulate adipocyte fat metabolism. Norepinephrine, epinephrine, growth hormone, glucagon, corticosteroids, and thyroxin increase HSL activity, whereas insulin inhibits HSL. Because cats release catecholamines readily, stress may exacerbate HSL activity. This effect is augmented in the absence of insulin resulting in occult or overt HL in unregulated diabetic cats. The LPL activity promotes fat uptake into adipocytes in the well-fed individual. In starvation however, although LPL activity declines, HSL increases, this balance favoring hepatocellular fat accumulation. An obese individual undergoing self-imposed starvation (anorexia) consequently has increased risk for peripheral fat mobilization and hepatocellular uptake.

The fate of fatty acids is diverse, including their consumption by beta-oxidation, conversion to phospholipids, use in formation of TG, cholesterol esters, to be packaged with apoproteins for dispersal as lipoproteins. An important mechanism of hepatic TG egress or dispersal is through formation of very low–density lipoproteins (VLDL). A variety of subcellular activities regulate VLDL dispersal from the hepatocyte, including lipid transport through subcellular compartments, combination with apoprotein, formation of secretory particle and vesicle, and expulsion into the perisinusoidal space. Impairment at any step or imbalance between essential lipoprotein components may compromise hepatic fat mobilization. The essential interaction of fatty acids and L-carnitine at the mitochondrial membrane for intraorganelle delivery and formation of activated fatty acid necessary for beta-oxidation may also play a role in development of the HL syndrome. The recently demonstrated deficiency of GSH in hepatocytes of these cats could represent dysfunction of the transsulfuration pathway. This, collectively considered with the common finding of B_{12} deficiency in the HL cat (especially those with substantial intestinal disease), supports defective availability or use of SAMe necessary for methylation reactions and de novo synthesis of L-carnitine. Studies of the influence of L-carnitine on fatty acid oxidation in the cat, and in modeled HL, support this association.[20,21]

Ultrastructural study of hepatocytes in HL cats documents reduced number of peroxisomes—organelles needed for oxidation of long chain fatty acids prior to mitochondrial delivery. This may further interfere with normal fat oxidation. Given the complexity of lipid metabolism, a multitude of factors likely predisposes any given cat to HL. Possible scenarios include an increased presentation of fat to the liver as a result of obesity, catabolism, chronic over-nutrition, enhanced *de novo* hepatic fatty acid synthesis, or impaired fatty acid oxidation or VLDL dispersal.

Cats of any age may be affected by HL; most commonly cats are between 4 to 15 years of age. Domestic shorthair cats are more commonly affected, which may reflect breed popularity. Initial clinical features include inappetence and anorexia, weight loss, vomiting, lethargy, and weakness.[22] Physical findings include dehydration, variable icterus, an unkempt appearance, and palpable liver margins. Although fat may become depleted on the limbs and dorsal trunk, abdominal fat stores are spared.

Hematologic tests may disclose a nonregenerative anemia and a stress leukogram reflecting the disease causing anorexia. Poikilocytosis is common and may reflect altered red blood cell (RBC) membrane lipids, metabolism and oxidative stress altering cell membrane flexibility.

Biochemical changes reflect cholestasis, and to a lesser degree, altered hepatocellular membrane permeability and viability. Because the feline HL syndrome lacks necroinflammatory lesions, release of transaminase and ALP usually coexist. Rarely, a cat with HL will have high transaminases with only modest ALP activity. In HL without pancreatitis or inflammatory disease involving biliary structures, the GGT activity usually remains quiet. Hyperbilirubinemia and high SBA concentrations are common. Hypokalemia reflects inappetence and is significantly associated with failure to survive if uncorrected.[22] Hypochloremia may reflect vomiting. Hypophosphatemia reflects a multitude of effects on the intercompartmental homeostasis of phosphate, but most importantly it may occur as a consequence of a refeeding syndrome. A urinalysis reveals urobilinogen, bilirubin crystals, and bilirubin pigmenturia.

Ultrasound evaluation characteristically shows a hyperechoic hepatic parenchyma. Liver aspirates demonstrate hepatocellular lipid vacuolation. Aspiration cytology is good for identifying HL, hepatic lymphoma, and overt hepatic sepsis, but it is unreliable for detection of necroinflammatory disorders, especially cholangitis and cholangiohepatitis. Ultrasound examination is also important for inspection of disorders involving the pancreas, stomach, intestines, and biliary structures, which may have initiated the inappetence resulting in HL. Surgical or laparoscopic biopsy of the liver reveals a yellow-tan hepatic color and friable tissue. Histopathology of hepatic biopsies reveals profound vacuolation of hepatocytes. Presence of lipid within vacuoles is verified using Oil Red-O stain on frozen sections not paraffin embedded. It is important to look for other findings in the liver biopsy and in other sampled tissues for an underlying primary disease process.

Appropriate treatment requires client education regarding the likelihood of an underlying primary disease, the importance of critical supportive care, without which the condition has a poor prognosis and the infrequency of recurrence of lipidosis in survivors. Treatment may require weeks to months of assisted alimentation and metabolic support. Concurrent medical conditions must be managed. A recovery rate exceeding 85% can be achieved if a primary disease is identified and ameliorated or cured and the patient survives the initial 72 hours of critical supportive care.

The most important treatment is provision of a balanced feline diet delivering adequate energy intake (60 kcal/kg/day). Feeding is usually achieved using a feeding tube (esophagostomy tube being least invasive and easiest to manage with fewest complications). The number of feedings per day is determined based on the volume of food tolerated per meal. The diet is balanced to prevent protein-to-calorie malnutrition. Fat supplementation is contraindicated. Carbohydrate supplementation is ill advised (e.g., dextrose infusion) because of its inhibitory influence on fatty acid oxidation. Dietary protein restriction is reserved only for patients with irrefutable signs of hepatic encephalopathy. Placement of a large bore feeding tube is recommended after the patient is stable enough to tolerate anesthesia and bleeding tendencies have been circumvented by administration of vitamin K_1. Nasoesophagostomy tubes are used only short term to start patient nutritional support. Gastrostomy tubes may be placed at the time of surgery; esophagostomy tubes may be placed under a shorter anesthetic or at the time of surgery. The inappetent cat has increased risk for food aversion when confronted with forced oral alimentation. Tube placement is discussed in Chapter 92.

Vomiting must be controlled. Although this can be achieved medically (see Chapter 38), it may also be alleviated by reducing the feeding volume, increasing the number of meals per day, or by use of a *trickle feeding approach* with a syringe or fluid pump. Trickle feeding is accomplished by placing liquefied food into an empty fluid bag and administering it gravitationally or by pump assistance via an intravenous line attached to the large bore feeding tube or by use of a large syringe filled with food and syringe pump. Care must be taken to renew food and delivery tubing and syringe at 6- to 8-hour intervals to avoid bacterial contamination.

Fluid support is best provided intravenously with a nonlactate and nonglucose containing fluid. Lactate intolerance is suspected in the severe HL cat, and steady glucose infusion is thought to potentiate hepatic TG accumulation. Hydration is critical in any animal with severe hepatic insufficiency as is thought to exist in the HL cat. Dehydration impairs hepatic circulation, which can compromise normal detoxification processes. Azotemia increases diffusion of urea into the gut and subsequently, enteric ammonia production. Constipation may be augmented by dehydration and prolongs contact with and absorption of endotoxic enteric material. Cats demonstrating signs consistent with hepatic encephalopathy may benefit from lactulose administration. Aggressive attention to correction of hypokalemia is essential; this is accomplished using the customary sliding scale for fluid potassium supplementation.

Hypophosphatemia may precede initiation of nutritional support but more commonly reflects a refeeding phenomenon. Treatment of hypophosphatemia accomplished using potassium phosphate (delivered at 0.01 to 0.03 nmol/kg/hr) monitoring serum phosphate every 6 hours. Phosphate supplementation is discontinued when serum phosphorus greater than 2 mg/dL. Iatrogenic hyperkalemia is possible if the clinician fails to appropriately reduce KCl infusion rate given concurrently. Parenteral phosphate requirements resolve once alimentation is established.

Water-soluble vitamins should be added to intravenous fluids (1 to 2 mL vitamin B complex per liter). Cobalamin (vitamin B_{12}) deficiency should be suspected in HL cats with thickened intestines on palpation; treat by giving 1 mg B_{12} subcutaneously. Administration of B_{12} in a deficient cat with HL is critical because this imposes a significant metabolic deficit, limiting methylation reactions and endogenous SAMe production. Thiamine (vitamin B_1) deficiency also has been observed in cats presented for HL based on dramatic response to vitamin supplementation. Affected cats usually show severe neck ventroflexion; this also may occur with substantial hypophosphatemia, hypokalemia, hepatic encephalopathy, and a variety of disorders influencing neuromuscular or cervical vertebral function. Anaphylaxis may occur as a result of injected thiamine; oral rather than parenteral thiamine administration (50 to 100 mg per cat per day for 1 week in those demonstrating consistent clinical signs) may be preferable.

Cats with HL are often deficient in vitamin K as proven by the PIVKA (proteins induced in vitamin K absence or antagonism) or prothrombin time (PT) tests. Lack of dietary intake, altered intestinal bacterial flora as a consequence of antimicrobial treatment, impaired vitamin K epoxidase cycle associated with hepatic dysfunction are considered underlying causes. Subcutaneous treatment with vitamin K is recommended for three doses (0.5 to 1.5 mg/kg at 12-hour intervals). Further treatment may induce RBC oxidation and hemolysis. Correction of PIVKA clotting abnormalities typically occurs within this time. Vitamin K treatment must precede insertion of feeding appliances, jugular venipuncture, cystocentesis, hepatic aspiration, or hepatic biopsy.

Supplementation with 250 to 500 mg L-carnitine per day is warranted based on experimental data and on observed clinical response. L-carnitine is an essential cofactor of fatty acid oxidation. Although it may be derived from the diet, it also is normally synthesized endogenously from lysine and methionine. Methionine metabolism may be compromised in the HL cat, limiting transformation of methionine to SAMe. Because SAMe generates GSH through the transsulfuration pathway and L-carnitine via methylation reactions, both depletion of GSH and L-carnitine may result. L-carnitine prevents accumulation of free fatty acids in the hepatocyte cytoplasm, as well as acetyl groups in the mitochondria where they inhibit beta-oxidation. It is surmised that the HL cat maintains a "relative" local hepatocellular carnitine deficiency regardless of adequate plasma or muscle carnitine concentrations. Taurine may also be supplemented (250 to 500 mg/day); this essential amino acid in the cat is necessary for normal bile acid conjugation. Owing to the compromised hepatic GSH shown in a small number of HL cats tested, antioxidant supplementation using vitamin E (10 IU/kg per day in food) and the thiol donor NAC intravenously during initial crisis (Heinz body hemolysis, recumbency) followed by SAMe there, (20 to

---

Box • 230-3

Treatment of Hepatic Lipidosis in Cats

1. Supply 60 kcal/kg/day of balanced diet: protein restriction is contraindicated unless encephalopathy is present.
2. Correct dehydration and maintain hydration using non-lactate, non-glucose—containing fluids.
3. Supplement with vitamin K1 (0.5-1.0 mg/kg/day SC for 3 treatments at 12-hr intervals).
4. Place a large bore-feeding tube as soon as possible.
5. Correct hypokalemia.
6. Correct hypophosphatemia.
7. Supplement with 250-500 mg L-carnitine/day.
8. Supplement with water-soluble vitamins.
9. Supplement with 250-500 mg tawire/day.
10. Supplement with vitamin E (10 IU/kg/d PO), NAC for crisis intervention, SAMe (20-40 mg/kg/d via feeding tube).

---

40 mg/kg through feeding tube is suggested. A higher dose SAMe than is normally used may be necessary because removal of the enteric coating for administration through the feeding appliance theoretically limits SAMe availability. Alternately administer 90 mg/day in an uncrushed tablet orally. Treatment of HL is summarized in Box 230-3.

STORAGE DISORDERS INVOLVING THE LIVER

Lysosomal Storage Disorders

Lysosomal storage disorders comprise a group of inherited juvenile or adult-onset disorders that show different clinical features depending on the particular metabolic aberration. Most of these are autosomal recessive traits and express as a consequence of line breeding.[24,25] Normal lysosomes degrade cellular and extracellular macromolecules, providing amino acids, fatty acids, nucleic acids, and carbohydrate residues for reuse. Primary lysosomes, derived from the Golgi apparatus, may fuse with other membrane-bound vesicles forming secondary lysosomes. Secondary lysosomes contain material derived from outside the cell through endocytosis or from within the cell by autophagy. Storage diseases are defined by the nature of the lysosomal hydrolase deficiency and resultant accumulating metabolic substrates or products. Disorders are suspected based on clinical signs, including progressive neurologic dysfunction, ocular abnormalities, visceromegaly (including hepatomegaly), and skeletal abnormalities; signs may overlap clinically with nonlysosomal storage disorders.[24]

The different disorders that may be associated with hepatocellular or Kupffer cell storage product accumulation are described in Table 230-4. The mucopolysaccharidoses (MPSs) and disorders associated with interrupted catabolism of oligosaccharides can be crudely determined by specific urine tests (e.g., toluidine blue for detection of glycosaminoglycans reflecting MPS). Evaluation of peripheral leukocytes (looking for unusual lysosomal granules in granulocytes, lymphocytes, and monocytes) and staining blood smears with acid phosphatase (to confirm lysosomal vacuolation) can be helpful. Juvenile forms of certain storage diseases may be suspected from the appearance of vacuolated lymphocytes or monocytes in peripheral blood (e.g., mannosidosis, GM1-GM2-gangliosides, mucolipidoses). Ultrastructural examination of skin also can demonstrate lysosomal storage disorders, however it is not specific. Genetic testing for many disorders is available. Where this isn't possible, plasma, leukocyte, and tissue sampling with verification of storage products and enzyme deficiencies is necessary. For reliable assessments, samples from an age- and sex-matched peer group should be evaluated concurrently.

Treatment is limited for these disorders. Bone marrow transplantation and enzyme replacement studies have been conducted on canine MPS type I and VII, feline MPS type VI, canine fucosidosis, and feline α-mannosidosis. Although variable improvements have been documented, this is not a practical recommendation and without neutering permits perpetuation of the genetic defect. Bone marrow transplant failed to improve advanced ceroid-lipofuscinosis in English setters.

HEPATOBILIARY INFECTIONS

The central position of the liver between the enteric and systemic circulation makes it an important interventional mechanism guarding against infectious agents. Normally, enteric flora entering the portal venous circulation by enteric transmural migration are killed or extracted by the hepatic macrophages (Kupffer cells), migrating macrophages, with neutrophils, and some being eliminated in bile. Locally produced immunoglobulins, primarily IgA, cooperate in providing innate immune defense. A number of conditions are known to predispose to hepatobiliary infections (Box 230-4).[23] Ischemic and hypovolemic injury decrease hepatic perfusion and impair macrophage function. The interruption of normal choleresis as occurs in cholestasis of any cause may result in infections derived from normal enteric organisms as rapid elimination of bacteria becomes compromised.

Infection, sepsis, and endotoxemia may each cause hepatic injury and cholestasis. Clinical signs variably include hepatosplenomegaly, fever, lethargy, and jaundice. Hematologic abnormalities may include a nonregenerative anemia (chronic inflammation), leukopenia, or leukocytosis with a left shift, and toxic changes in neutrophils. Biochemical abnormalities include increased transaminase and ALP activities and variable hyperbilirubinemia. Sepsis-related hypoglycemia might be recognized. Successful therapy requires judicious provision

Table • 230-4

Storage Disorders Involving the Liver

CLASS	STORED PRODUCT/ DEFICIENT ENZYME	TISSUES IMPACTED	REPORTED IN
Sphingolipidoses	Sphingolipids	Nervous tissues, liver, macrophages, granulocytes	Dogs and cats
Glycoproteinosis Mannosidosis Fucosidosis	Sugars	Hepatocytes, renal and neural cells	Cats: Persians, DSH Springer spaniels, other dogs
Mucopolysaccharidoses (MPSs) MPS I MPS II MPS IIIA MPS VI MPS VII	Glycosaminoglycans (GAGs) (sulfates of dermatan, heparan, keratan, & chondroitin)	Wide tissue involvement, growth deformities, may observe storage produce in: Hepatocytes, Kupffer cells, neural cells, MPS VI skeletal tissues	Dogs and cats Dogs Dogs Cats (Siamese, DSH) Dogs
Mucolipidoses	Features of sphingolipidosis & MPS, deficiency of acetylgucosamine-1-phosphotransferases	Growth deformities; involves many tissues including: cartilage, skin, connective tissue, Kupffer cells, no hepatomegaly	Cats
Ceroid-lipofucinoses	Lipopigments (lipofuscin, ceroid) protein products	Neural cells, Kupffer cells	Dogs and cats
Niemann-Pick types A & C (Sphingomyelinosis)	Cholesterol (defective esterification)	Hepatocytes, fibroblasts	Dogs and cats
Glycogen storage diseases	Storage: glycogen	Liver, heart, skeletal muscle, kidney, CNS, RBCs: varies with defect	Dogs and cats, depending on form
GSD IA	Deficiency: Glucose-6-phosphate dehydrogenase	Fail to thrive, obtunded, hepatomegaly causing abdominal distention	Maltese dog, toy breed puppies
GSD II	α-glucosidase	Muscle, megaesophagus, neurons	Swedish Lapland dog
GSD III	Amylo-1,6-glucosidase	Like GSD IA, but mild hypoglycemia	German shepherd dog, Akita
GSD IV	α-1,4-D-glucan (glycogen branching enzyme)	Lethal perinatally, cardiac signs, skeletal muscle atrophy	Norwegian Forest cat
GSD VII	Phosphofructose kinase deficiency	RBC hemolysis (with alkalosis), skeletal muscle weakness, lacks hepatic involvement	English springer spaniel American cocker spaniels, cross breed dogs

Box • 230-4

Conditions Predisposing to Hepatobiliary Infections
Disorders in Dogs and Cats with Culture Positive Hepatobiliary Infections

Obstructed Bile Flow
Extrahepatic bile duct occlusion
Disease of the gall bladder:
   Dysmotility
   Cholelithiasis
   Cystic duct occlusion
   Cholecystic neoplasia
Parenchymal cholestasis
   Destruction of intrahepatic bile ducts: ductopenia (e.g., certain cats with chronic cholangitis/cholangiohepatitis)
   Microcholelithiasis (intrahepatic bile ducts)
Pancreatitis

Impaired Hepatic Perfusion ± Oxidant Injury:
Chronic necroinflammatory liver disease: chronic hepatitis, chronic cholangiohepatitis
Cirrhosis
Copper storage hepatopathy
Acquired portosystemic shunting
Congenital portosystemic shunting
Liver lobe torsion
Hepatic neoplasia
   Primary: development of a necrotic center
      Hepatocellular carcinoma, Hepatoma
   Metastatic:
      Lymphosarcoma, adenocarcinoma, malignant histiocytosis
   Portal venous thrombosis
Pancreatitis
Trauma: automobile accident, bite wounds, penetrating wounds

Compromised Immunocompetence
Hyperadrenocorticism
Diabetes mellitus
Severe hypothyroidism
FIV/FeLV
Treatment with immunomodulatory drugs: glucocorticoids, azathioprine, methotrexate, chemotherapy
Amyloidosis

Increased Translocation of Enteric Organisms
Inflammatory bowel disease
Enteric neoplasia: lymphosarcoma, adenocarcinoma
Chronic liver disease
Extrahepatic bile duct occlusion
Reduced bowel motility
Pancreatitis

Neonatal
Omphalitis

Visceral larval migrans
Toxocara

Iatrogenic
Extension from a feeding device
Surgical infection

From Center SA[23]; in press.

---

of fluid and electrolyte support, supplemental glucose for sepsis-related hypoglycemia, and appropriate antimicrobial coverage. Importantly, the underlying causal factor must be identified and either eliminated or controlled. Nutrition should focus on avoiding a negative nitrogen balance. Antioxidant support with thiol donors (NAC in crisis that can be used as an intravenous treatment; SAMe for more chronic oral administration) and vitamin E may be helpful.[23]

In general, hepatobiliary infections, and especially focal abscesses, are uncommon. Focal abscesses may result from trauma, ascending biliary tree infection, or ischemic lesions within the liver (e.g., necrotic liver tumor, thromboembolic lesions).[23,26,29] Immunocompromised patients are at greatest risk especially for hepatic abscessation.[23] Multifocal abscess formation and microabscessation may involve a variety of organisms derived from systemic infections by hematogenous or lymphatic distribution, or by infection ascending the biliary tree.[23,27,28] Early signs of hepatic abscessation are often vague (lethargy, fever, dehydration, trembling, anorexia, vomiting, diarrhea, and weight loss). Localization of disease to the abdomen may be indicated by abdominal tenderness and hepatomegaly. Hematologic features usually include a leukocytosis with or without a left shift and toxic neutrophils, as well as monocytosis; if chronic, a nonregenerative anemia may develop. Biochemical features include increased transaminase and ALP activities, hyperglobulinemia, and sometimes, sepsis-induced hypoglycemia. Should an abscess rupture, septic peritonitis and abdominal effusion develop. Diagnosis is greatly facilitated by abdominal ultrasound, which may disclose discrete focal lesions in the hepatic parenchyma and abdominal effusion. Cytologic evaluations of abdominal effusion or aspiration from discrete parenchymal lesions usually disclose neutrophils in various conditions (necrotic, degenerative, toxic) and bacterial organisms. Culture of blood or urine may identify occult infectious agents. Submission of both aerobic and anaerobic microbial cultures from sampled lesions or effusion is critical for optimized therapy. Polymicrobial infections nearly always involve an anaerobic organism; approximately 50% of solitary hepatic abscesses in dogs appear to be polymicrobial.[23] Because anaerobes are difficult to culture, they should be suspected and treated when cytologic evaluation discloses a polymicrobial population. Further, therapy should continue even if no organisms are cultured or only a few aerobic organisms are grown. Anaerobes may potentiate infection with other organisms and alter the course of disease.[28,30,31] When causal factors remain illusive, hepatic biopsy may be indicated looking for underlying neoplasia or other primary hepatic processes predisposing to infection.

Good initial therapy for hepatic abscessation is achieved with combination of penicillin and a fluoroquinolone or an aminoglycoside. Metronidazole or clindamycin can be substituted for penicillin to provide an anaerobic spectrum.[23] Dose reduction of metronidazole by 50% is indicated in patients with jaundice or reduced hepatic function (adjusted dose for dogs and cats is 7.5 mg/kg orally, twice a day to three times a day).[23] Fluoroquinolones provide broader gram-positive coverage compared with aminoglycosides and are thought to have better penetration across an abscess wall. First-generation cephalosporins, potentiated sulfonamides, and aminoglycosides, are uniformly ineffective against anaerobes. Animals with cholestasis also should receive ursodeoxycholic acid (10 to 15 mg/kg per day) to facilitate brisk choleresis. Hydration must be maintained to achieve this objective.

Ultrasound-guided abscess aspiration as a primary mode of abscess treatment has been successfully applied to veterinary patients.[23] This approach is recommended for several reasons: (1) as a method of confirming the diagnosis, (2) to provide time for patient stabilization before surgical exploration for liver lobe resection, and (3) because it is successful as a solitary means of therapy in a subset of patients. Major factors arguing against this technique are unsafe access, contamination or lesion depth exceeding aspiration needle length. It is always essential to anticipate a need for immediate surgical intervention when aspirating a suspected hepatic abscess in the event of abscess rupture into the peritoneal cavity.

Successful management of multifocal microabscessation can be accomplished with intravenous antibiotics if the involved organisms are identified and sensitivity defined. Treatment requires extensive supportive care and long-term administration (months) of a tailored antibiotic regimen targeting involved pathogens along with identification and management of the underlying predisposing cause. Disseminated sepsis should initiate a search for an underlying condition compromising immune defense.[23]

Hepatic Involvement in Systemic Infectious Disease

A number of systemic infectious diseases can involve the liver (see Box 230-4).[23,32] Agents with tropism for endothelium, parenchymal hepatic cells or macrophages are particularly prone to secondarily involve the liver. Infectious canine hepatitis caused by adenovirus type 1 is a unique pathogen because it is the only recognized virus with primary tropism for the liver. Along with severe hepatic necrosis and initiation of chronic hepatitis, glomerulonephritis, corneal edema, and uveitis may develop. This is currently a rare condition in North America due to high efficacy of vaccination programs.[33,34]

Granulomatous Hepatic Inflammation Granulomatous hepatic inflammation is an uncommon diagnosis characterized by multiple discrete, sharply defined nodular infiltrates consisting of macrophage aggregates (and with or without epithelioid cells), surrounded by or intermixed with lymphocytes and plasma cells. Lesions may be focal, multifocal, or diffuse. Underlying causes include many infectious agents.

Differential diagnoses that should be considered include metazoal (e.g., schistosomiasis, dirofilariasis), fungal (e.g., histoplasmosis, paecilomycosis), protozoal (e.g., visceral leishmaniasis, toxoplasmosis), bacterial (e.g., mycobacteria, *Nocardia*, *Bartonella*, *Brucella*, *Borrelia*, *Propionibacterium acnes*), and viral (e.g., feline coronavirus infectious peritonitis [FIP]) infections, and visceral larval migrans (*Toxocara* migration). Noninfectious disorders may be caused (drug reactions, lymphangiectasia, histiocytosis or histiocytic neoplasia, lymphosarcoma, and immune-mediated inflammation. The last may be associated with a positive antinuclear antibody test.[1] Until recently, causative factors have remained elusive in at least 50% of cases. However, with increased molecular surveillance for infectious causes, more definitive diagnoses are anticipated.

HEPATOBILIARY NEOPLASIA

The most common primary and secondary types of hepatic neoplasia in the dog and cat are shown in Table 230-5. Retrospective studies show an incidence of primary hepatobiliary neoplasia in less than 1.5% of all canine and less than 2.9% of all feline neoplasms.[35-41] Hemolymphatic neoplasia in the liver is more common. The peak incidence of hepatobiliary cancer occurs at 10 to 12 years of age in both species. In cats, malignant tumors develop at a younger age than benign tumors do.[38-41,48] It remains unclear whether previously eliminated feline leukemia virus (FeLV) may induce oncogenic transformation resulting in feline hemolymphatic neoplasia in the liver. In dogs, hepatic carcinoids occur at a mean age of 8 years.[37,43] No significant breed predilections exist for primary liver cancer; however, female dogs may be predisposed to biliary carcinoma (BC), while male dogs and cats to hepatocellular carcinoma (HCC).[37,43-46] Although no evidence indicates that chronic

Table • 230-5

Hepatic Neoplasia

DOGS	CATS
*Primary Hepatic Tumors (26%)	***Primary Hepatic Tumors (20%)**
Hepatocellular carcinoma	Biliary carcinoma
Hepatocellular adenoma	Hepatocellular carcinoma
Hepatic hemangiosarcoma	Hepatic hemangiosarcoma
Biliary carcinoma	
Other	**Other**
Leiomyosarcoma	Biliary cystadenoma
Liposarcoma	Myelolipoma
Myxosarcoma	Hepatic carcinoid
Fibrosarcoma	
Biliary adenoma	
Hepatic carcinoid	
Hemolymphatic Neoplasia (28%)	**Hemolymphatic Neoplasia (60%)**
Lymphosarcoma	Lymphosarcoma
Mast cell tumor (MCT)	MCT
Plasma cell tumor	Plasma cell tumor
Metastatic Neoplasia (46%)	**Metastatic Neoplasia (20%)**

*Primary tumors: in order of prevalence.

inflammatory liver disease predisposes to HCC in dogs, cats with chronic cholangitis may have an increased predisposition to BC.

Primary liver tumors may be classified as hepatocellular, biliary, neuroendocrine or as sarcomas. Secondary metastasis of neoplasia to the liver is common in both species, and represents the largest proportion of hepatic cancers in dogs.[47-49] Lymphoreticular neoplasia involving the liver occurs in both species and represents the largest proportion of cancer in feline liver.[50]

Hepatic nodular hyperplasia is common in geriatric dogs, but unlike in humans, does not appear to represent a preneoplastic change. Biliary cystadenomas are considered benign tumors in older cats, and may be focal or multifocal.[51-53] Some of these may have a malignant behavior due to location in the porta hepatis. In younger cats, multiple hepatic cysts may express as a manifestation of polycystic disease, with or without renal lesions. Confusion in histologic diagnosis of these lesions with biliary cystadenomas may occur in some patients.

Clinical signs of hepatic neoplasia are often vague and nonspecific including chronic lethargy, inappetence, dehydration, PU/PD, and fever. Less commonly, vomiting, diarrhea, jaundice, and ascites may develop. PU/PD is more commonly linked to primary liver tumors (up to 50% of dogs). Rarely, neurologic signs may occur in dogs and these reflect hypoglycemia or hepatic encephalopathy.[37,54,55] Weakness due to myasthenia gravis associated with carcinoma was described in a dog.[56] Many animals (25% dogs, 50% cats) will be asymptomatic. Finding a cranial abdominal mass or hepatomegaly is the most common physical abnormality.

Clinicopathologic features are usually vague and nonspecific. Hematologic tests may reveal a nonregenerative anemia and a neutrophilic leukocytosis reflecting neoplasia-associated inflammation. Hepatic hemangiosarcoma may produce a regenerative anemia, acanthocytosis, and schistocytosis. Mast cell tumors (MCTs) may produce eosinophilia and signs associated with release of biogenic amines.[54,55] Lymphoma may be accompanied by circulating lymphoblasts, eosinophilia, thrombocytopenia, thrombocytosis, and hematologic effects attributable to bone marrow involvement.

Biochemical changes reflect hepatocellular or biliary epithelial damage or biliary stasis (increased transaminase and ALP activities, hyperbilirubinemia, high SBA concentrations). Hepatic enzyme activity does not reflect the degree of hepatic neoplastic involvement. High SBA concentrations develop in 50% to 75% of dogs and in 33% of cats with hepatic cancer. Despite the more common prevalence of biliary neoplasia in the cat, only 33% have hyperbilirubinemic. In dogs, hypercalcemia (implying lymphoma), hyperglobulinemia, and hypoglycemia are more common. Hypoglycemia may be a dominant marker of large tumor mass (metabolic consumption) or reflect paraneoplastic phenomena due to production of an insulin-like protein.[54,55] Hypoalbuminemia, more common in dogs, may reflect a negative acute phase response, catabolism and poor nutritional intake, or hepatic insufficiency. Increased serum pancreatic lipase (PL) activity was reported in dogs (n = 6) with either pancreatic or hepatic neoplasia.[57] It was proposed that some hepatic tumors produce PL. Alpha-fetoprotein (AFP), a glycoprotein produced by fetal, neoplastic, and regenerating hepatocytes, may increase in dogs with hepatocellular carcinoma, chronic hepatitis, or rapidly regenerating liver tissue.[50,58,59]

If ascites is present, fluid should be evaluated for protein, cell typers, #'s, and morphology. Imaging remains the most valuable, noninvasive method for localizing hepatic mass lesions and for detecting of overt metastasis. Abdominal radiography may show caudal and lateral displacement of the stomach. Occasionally, dystrophic mineralization of mass lesions or involved biliary tissues may be recognized. Pulmonary metastases occur late in the disease process.

Abdominal ultrasound is a better imaging modality for the detection of mass lesions, with a sensitivity (true positive, all patients with neoplastic lesions) ranging between 20% to 84% depending on operator, equipment and tumor type.[60,61] Although echogenicity and distribution can suggest a tumor type, broad overlap of patterns occur and findings do not closely correlate with histologic type.[62] Lesions may be localized or diffuse, hypo-, hyper-, or of mixed echogenicity; target lesions (hypoechoic margin surrounding a hyperechoic core) may be observed with carcinomas and other tumor types. Most variable in appearance are lymphomas as these may assume nearly any echogenic appearance or remain indiscernible despite diffuse hepatic involvement. Ultrasound may fail to detect neoplasia, and mass lesions from other causes may be erroneously assumed to be neoplasia.[63] Hematomas acquired from needle aspiration or Tru-Cut® biopsy sampling may subsequently be observed as mass lesions. Doppler (color flow) assessment of the mass may show vascularization more consistent with a tumor versus a benign process.[50,64] Computed tomography (CT) or magnetic resonance imaging (MRI) can provide information valuable in tumor staging and planning for attempted surgical resection.

Collection of cells by fine needle aspiration or tissue (via Tru-Cut® needle, laparoscopic, or surgical biopsy) for histopathology is required for definitive diagnosis.[65,66] Cytologic diagnoses of lymphoma, MCT, and carcinomas may be accomplished in some cases. Bleeding tendencies must be considered before invasive tissue sampling. Usually, fine needle aspiration poses little threat.

Treatment and prognosis of different forms of hepatic neoplasia depends on its distribution, localization, and tumor type. Removal of focal mass lesions or liver lobe resections are recommended for neoplasia restricted to the liver. Tumors involving the porta hepatis cannot be resected. The considerable regenerative capability of the liver can permit successful resection of up to 80% of the liver if the remaining tissue is normal functionally and critical supportive care provides fluid, electrolyte, glucose, water-soluble vitamin, and coagulation factor support.[67] Caution is warranted in diagnosing apparent metastatic disease on the basis of gross appearance of the liver at the time of surgery, because hyperplastic nodules may be mistaken for cancer. Mass resection may offer palliation in the circumstance of a bleeding mass, despite irrefutable evidence of metastasis. Biliary tree diversion (biliary enteric anastomoses) should be considered for obstructive lesions involving the extrahepatic biliary structures because long-term palliation is possible. Chronic biliary tree occlusion results in cirrhosis within 6 to 8 weeks.

A fair to good prognosis may follow excision of focal canine HCC and benign feline tumors. However, dogs with BC and cats with malignant tumors have a poorer prognosis. HCC can be confusing because it may present as diffuse, multifocal, or solitary lesions. Histopathologic subtype and anaplastic characteristics also influence whether a HCC will metastasize. Metastasis is highest (100%) with diffuse HCC and lowest (37%) with solitary mass HCC. After surgical resection of HCC, a median survival time (MST) of 377 days was reported (n = 18).[42] Adjunctive, postoperative chemotherapy (5-fluorouracil, cisplatin, actinomycin D) has not been shown to provide significant benefit in dogs. However, one of four dogs treated with mitoxantrone had a complete response.[68] No comparable information is available for cats.

Biliary carcinoma shows a high metastatic rate in both dogs and cats (56% to 88% and 67% to 78%, respectively).[48,69] Surgical resection is more difficult than for HCC due to multifocal or diffuse extension and involvement of the porta hepatis. Little information exists regarding adjunctive chemotherapy. In cats, surgical resection of biliary adenomas or myelolipomas may provide several years of tumor-free survival or cure. Despite the benign character of these tumors, removal is recommended because malignant transformation has been suggested.[49]

Postoperative adjunctive chemotherapy has been beneficial in inducing remission and prolonging survival in dogs with hepatic hemangiosarcoma. Surgery is indicated for removal of bleeding or large resectable masses. Chemotherapeutic protocols include a combination of vincristine, doxorubicin, and cyclophosphamide.[50]

Hepatic carcinoids and lymphosarcomas in dogs have a high metastatic rate (86% to 93%). Carcinoids are a rare and aggressive neuroendocrine tumor.[35,37,43]

Hepatic tumors metastasize first to regional lymph nodes then lung, and peritoneum in the dog and peritoneum in the cat. Biliary tumors in the cat may extend into the pancreas. Metastatic extension to brain, spinal cord, bone, kidney, adrenal gland, and spleen is less common in each species.

Canine MCT involving the liver can be controlled with cyclophosphamide, vinblastine, and prednisone.[50,70] Many protocols are recommended for control of lymphoma in dogs and cats; most include vincristine, cyclophosphamide, and prednisone, with variable combinations of L-asparaginase, methotrexate, and doxorubicin.

Radiation therapy is not a feasible option for hepatic cancers, owing to the exquisite sensitivity of this organ to even low amounts of radiation.[71] Although liver transplantation, directed delivery of chemotherapeutic agents (intra-arterial chemotherapy), transarterial chemoembolization, and immunotherapeutic regimes using a-FP as a tumor-specific antigen have been used in humans with HCC, these have not been explored in animals.[72,73]

CHAPTER • 231

Diseases of the Gallbladder and Extrahepatic Biliary System

Michael D. Willard
Theresa W. Fossum

ANATOMY

Bile is formed by hepatocytes and discharged into the canaliculi lying between the hepatocytes. Canaliculi unite to form interlobular ducts, which ultimately merge to form lobar or bile ducts. The gallbladder plus the hepatic, cystic, and common bile ducts constitute the extrahepatic biliary system. Bile drains from the bile ducts into the cystic and common bile ducts and is stored and concentrated in the gallbladder (Figure 231-1). The gallbladder lies between the quadrate lobe of the liver medially and the right medial lobe laterally.[1] It is a pear-shaped organ that, in a medium-sized dog, normally holds approximately 15 mL of bile. The rounded end of the gallbladder is the fundus. Between the neck of the gallbladder (i.e., the tapering end leading into the cystic duct) and the fundus is the body.

The cystic duct extends from the neck of the gallbladder to the junction with the first tributary from the liver.[1] From this point to the opening of the biliary system into the duodenum, the duct is termed the *common bile duct*. The common bile duct runs through the lesser omentum for approximately 5 cm and enters the mesenteric wall of the duodenum. The canine common bile duct terminates in the duodenum near the opening of the minor pancreatic duct. This combined opening of the minor pancreatic duct and common bile duct is the major duodenal papilla. The feline common bile duct usually joins the major pancreatic duct before entering the duodenum.[1]

PHYSIOLOGY

Bile primarily contains water, conjugated bile acids, bile pigments, cholesterol, and inorganic salts. Over 90% of bile salts are reabsorbed from the intestinal tract, transported back to the liver via the portal vein, and re-excreted (i.e., enterohepatic circulation). Bilirubin and biliverdin produce the typical yellow color of bile. Bile is continually secreted into the gallbladder, where it is stored and modified. Gallbladder emptying is normally induced by neural (vagal parasympathetics) and humoral (cholecystokinin) stimuli. Parasympathomimetic drugs and magnesium sulfate[2] cause gallbladder contraction, whereas anticholinergic drugs and somatostatin inhibit contraction.[1]

DIAGNOSTIC TOOLS FOR EVALUATING THE GALLBLADDER AND BILE DUCTS

Icterus, vomiting, abdominal pain, and ascites are all consistent with biliary tract dysfunction. Complete blood count (CBC), serum biochemistry profile, and urinalysis are indicated if biliary tract dysfunction is suspected. The CBC inconsistently reflects cholecystic inflammation. Increased alanine aminotransferase (ALT) is common if inflammation ascends into the hepatic parenchyma. Increased serum alkaline phosphatase (SAP), with or without hyperbilirubinemia, is typical

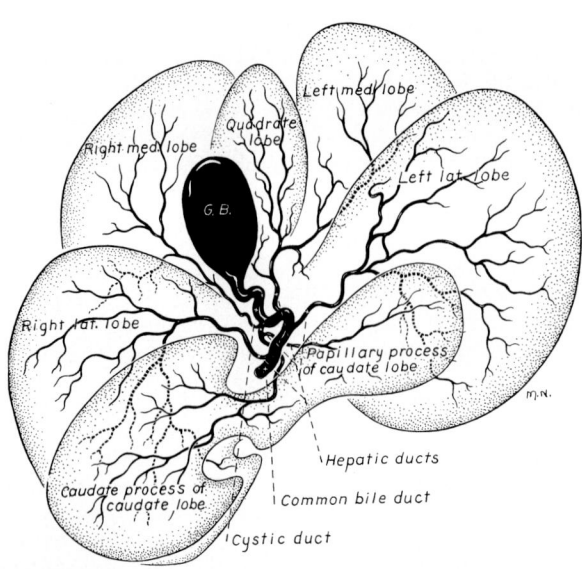

Figure 231-1 Anatomy of the canine gallbladder. (From Evans HE, Christensen GC: Miller's Anatomy of the Dog, 3rd ed. Philadelphia, WB Saunders Co, 1993, p 750.)

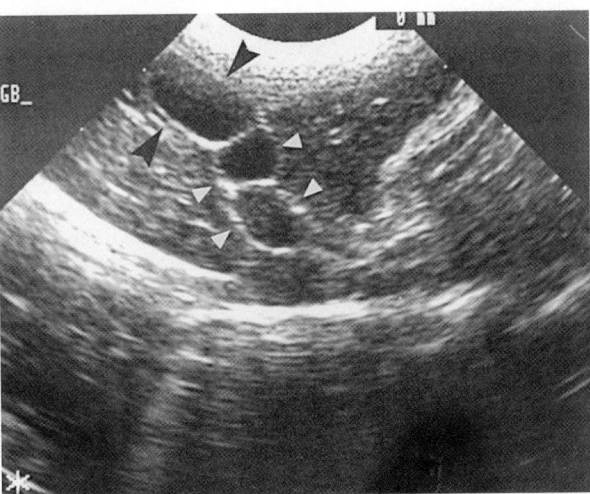

Figure 231-2 Distention and convolution of the gallbladder body *(black arrowheads)* and neck *(white arrowheads)* in a cat with common bile duct obstruction. (Courtesy of Dr. L. Homco, Texas A&M University.)

in extrahepatic biliary tract obstruction (EHBO)[3] and inflammatory disease ascending from the biliary tract. Cats tend to have lesser elevations of SAP than dogs.

Hypercholesterolemia may occur secondary to EHBO. Bilirubinuria occurs before hyperbilirubinemia. Imaging, surgery, or both are usually required to differentiate icterus due to hepatic disease versus biliary tract disease.

Abdominal radiographs may reveal radiodense objects (e.g., gallstones) or air in the gallbladder. Animals with EHBO due to pancreatitis may have a soft tissue mass or poor serosal detail in the region of the pancreas. Contrast radiographs of the biliary tree are rarely useful, and endoscopic retrograde pancreatography is rarely performed in icteric animals.

Ultrasonography is the most useful nonsurgical technique to distinguish hepatic parenchymal from biliary tract disease. It can identify abnormalities within the lumen of the gallbladder (e.g., stones, tumors, flocculent material) and most biliary tract obstructions (Figure 231-2).[3] Finding "sludge" is not informative because many normal dogs have this finding.[4] Anorexic animals often have marked cholecystic enlargement, which can be misdiagnosed as obstruction. Dilatation of the gallbladder neck plus loss of the tapering of the gallbladder neck typically occur within 24 hours of ligation of the bile duct. This is followed by dilatation of the common duct at 48 hours and of the extrahepatic ducts at 72 hours. Similar changes occur in the intrahepatic bile ducts within 1 week.[5] The common bile duct is typically less than 3 mm in diameter in medium-sized dogs[6] and less than 2.5 mm in cats.[3] One study found that 28 cats without EHBO had a common bile duct 4 mm or less in diameter, whereas a common bile duct greater than 5 mm in diameter meant EHBO in six of seven cats.[7] Distension of the gallbladder plus the common bile duct was the most common finding in 22 cats.[8] If the clinician is unsure whether EHBO is present after performing ultrasonography, repeating the examination in 2 to 4 days or after inducing gallbladder contraction (e.g., feeding a high-fat meal) is often definitive. However, loss of elasticity of the bile ducts may occur as a result of aging, inflammation, or chronic obstruction (especially in cats), and some ducts never return to their original diameter after obstruction.[5,6] Rarely, EHBO will not be diagnosed until laparoscopy or laparotomy.

Gallstones are typically identified ultrasonographically as hyperechoic foci or by the observation of acoustic shadowing originating from the gallbladder.[5] Sediment (sometimes referred to as *sludge*) is occasionally noted in the gallbladder, but its significance is uncertain. Supposedly, bile becomes progressively thicker as water is absorbed during biliary stasis.

Soft tissue changes of the gallbladder (e.g., tumors, granulation tissue, congenital defects) may be seen ultrasonographically. Cholecystitis may cause gallbladder wall thickening, edema, or both, which can produce a layered or "double-wall" ultrasonographic appearance[5]; however, one cannot reliably diagnose cholecystitis ultrasonographically. Finding a stellate or striated pattern within the gallbladder with immobile contents is suggestive of mucocele.[9]

Bile (for culture or cytologic examination) can be aspirated from the gallbladder by ultrasound-guided fine-needle aspiration using a 22- to 25-gauge needle.[10] As much bile as possible is withdrawn to lessen the likelihood of subsequent bile leakage into the abdomen. This procedure appears to be relatively safe, although vagal-induced severe bradycardia and other problems have occurred in people.[1] Aerobic and anaerobic cultures of bile (and hepatic parenchyma) are recommended if bacterial cholecystitis is suspected.

Laparoscopy or exploratory laparotomy should be performed in animals with suspected leakage of bile into the abdomen, as well as those with EHBO, neoplasia, parasites, stones, infiltrates, and other mass lesions of or within the biliary tract. Laparoscopy can be particularly valuable in helping the clinician decide if exploratory surgery is warranted. During exploration, patency of the common bile duct must be ensured by compressing the gallbladder or catheterizing the duct. Readers are referred to surgery texts for detailed information regarding extrahepatic biliary tract surgery.[11] Nuclear scintigraphy is rarely used to define canine or feline biliary disease, owing to the need for specialized equipment and facilities.

SPECIFIC PROBLEMS SEEN WITH GALLBLADDER AND BILIARY TRACT DISEASE

Vomiting, icterus, and anorexia are common in animals with inflammatory or obstructive biliary tract disease.[12,13] Fever and abdominal discomfort also occur, but not as consistently. Icterus is often helpful for localizing the problem to the biliary tract. After hemolytic disease is eliminated, ultrasonography helps distinguish hepatic parenchymal from biliary tract disease. Ascites may occur owing to leakage of bile into the peritoneal cavity. Bilious effusions are obvious because the fluid looks like bile. If one is unsure whether abdominal fluid is bilious or bile stained, bilirubin concentrations in serum and in effusion should be compared. Bilious effusions have fluid bilirubin concentrations greater than serum concentrations.

Acute abdomen (i.e., shock, sepsis, pain due to abdominal disease) may be caused by leakage of bile into the peritoneal cavity, particularly if the bile is septic. Hematemesis is uncommon in animals with cholecystic disease, but intracystic bleeding may allow blood to exit into the duodenum, where it is refluxed into the stomach and vomited.

SPECIFIC DISEASES OF THE GALLBLADDER

Obstructive Disease

Pancreatic disease is the most common cause of canine EHBO,[3] whereas tumors and inflammatory disease of the biliary tract, pancreas, or both are the most common causes in cats.[8] Stones can cause EHBO, but they do so uncommonly.[14] Therefore the prognosis for dogs with EHBO is generally much better than it is for cats.

Pancreatitis may cause scar formation in or around the duct or compress the duct by inflamed tissue, abscesses, or cysts. Treatment of EHBO secondary to benign pancreatitis initially consists of medical management of the pancreatitis. If this is unsuccessful or if ascending bacterial infection is suspected, cholecystoduodenostomy or cholecystojejunostomy may be considered but should generally be avoided unless absolutely necessary. In extremely ill animals with EHBO that cannot undergo surgical exploration, temporary decompression of the gallbladder with a Foley catheter or a self-retaining accordion catheter may be warranted.

Neoplasia (especially biliary tract or pancreatic adenocarcinomas) may cause EHBO. Surgery for pancreatic neoplasia is generally unrewarding, because most such tumors are malignant. Cholecystojejunostomy may be palliative if the intestinal lumen is patent. Pancreatic-duodenal resection (i.e., Billroth II) is possible; surgical cures are unlikely, whereas morbidity may be substantial. Biliary, intestinal, hepatic, or lymph node malignancy may also obstruct the bile ducts; biopsy is imperative to obtain a diagnosis. The prognosis is typically poor; however, chemotherapy benefits some animals with lymphosarcoma.

Choleliths (see Nonobstructive Disease) that obstruct the common bile duct should be removed. Cholecystectomy is the treatment of choice when clinical signs are secondary to cholelithiasis.[13] If stones are present in the common bile duct, the duct can be catheterized via the duodenum and the stones flushed into the gallbladder. Alternatively, enlarged bile ducts can be incised (choledochotomy) and the stones removed; however, care is needed when closing the common bile duct to avoid iatrogenic stricture formation. Much greater mortality occurs in people with cholelithiasis when a choledochotomy is performed versus cholecystectomy.

A gallbladder mucocele is an abnormal accumulation of inspissated mucus that distends the gallbladder and often causes some degree of EHBO.[9] Affected dogs will usually be icteric and have abdominal pain plus increased ALT, SAP, or bilirubin. Mucoceles typically cause a striated or stellate appearance on ultrasound with immobile bile. Cocker spaniels might be over-represented. Infection sometimes occurs. Left untreated, necrosis of the gallbladder with subsequent rupture may occur. Cholecystectomy seems the preferred therapy. Miscellaneous causes of EHBO include diaphragmatic hernia[15] and biliary pseudocysts.[16]

Nonobstructive Disease

Cholecystitis (i.e., inflammation of the gallbladder) usually involves the associated bile ducts. It is typically due to a bacterial infection caused by bacteria ascending from the intestine via the common bile duct or by hematogenous seeding, and it can often be cured with antibiotics. However, if cholecystitis recurs repeatedly despite appropriate use of antibiotics, cholecystectomy is usually curative. Cholecystitis may take one of several courses.

Bacterial cholangitis and cholangiohepatitis occur if the infection ascends the biliary tree into the liver. This appears to be more common in cats than in dogs, but Shetland sheepdogs may have a higher than expected incidence. Any bacteria may be responsible; *Escherichia coli* seems especially common. These animals often present to veterinarians because of icterus, anorexia, vomiting, or a combination of these symptoms. Fever is uncommon. Increased serum ALT, SAP, and bilirubin are typical, but neutrophilia is inconsistent. Imaging is seldom diagnostic but helps eliminate other diseases. Cats with a gallbladder wall greater than 1.0 mm thick typically have histologic abnormalities of the gallbladder, but cats with a less thick gallbladder wall may also have disease.[17] Fine needle aspirate of the gallbladder with subsequent cytology of bile may reveal bacteria (Figure 231-3). Hepatic biopsy with aerobic and anaerobic culture of bile and hepatic parenchyma is indicated. The prognosis is variable, but good results are expected when the correct antibiotics are promptly administered. Enrofloxacin plus amoxicillin is reasonable until culture results are available. Vitamin K_1 should be administered if coagulopathy is suspected.

Necrotizing cholecystitis occurs when a bacterial infection severely damages the gallbladder wall, sometimes rupturing it (Figure 231-4) and spilling bile into the abdomen.[18] This usually causes generalized septic peritonitis. If the bile is inspissated, rupture causes spillage of a relatively thick, gelatinous mass into the cranial abdomen, producing a localized peritonitis. These animals tend not to become as sick as quickly as those with diffuse peritonitis. Sometimes pain can be localized to the anterior abdomen. If diagnosed before the gallbladder ruptures, signs are similar to those of localized peritonitis. Adhesions or fistulous tracts around the gallbladder occasionally occur. Diagnosis is usually made by ultrasonography or exploratory laparotomy. Surgical exploration should be performed once the animal is stable. Treatment consists of cholecystectomy, antibiotics, and appropriate therapy for peritonitis. Salvaging the gallbladder by closing the defect is inappropriate because the wall is typically necrotic and will dehisce. The common bile duct must not be ligated when the

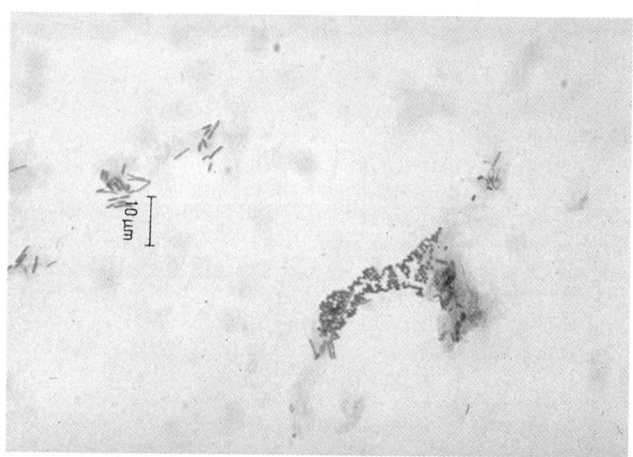

Figure 231-3 Photomicrograph of bile obtained by cholecystocentesis showing bacteria.

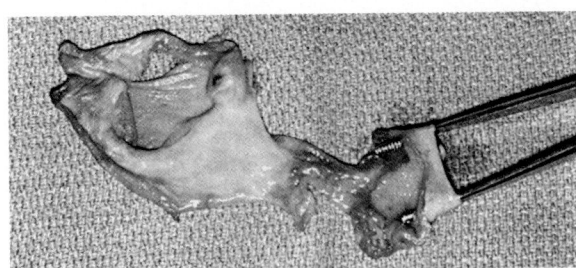

Figure 231-4 Photograph of a ruptured gallbladder that has been resected from a dog. Rupture was spontaneous and was due to necrotizing cholecystitis. Forceps are in the cystic duct.

gallbladder is removed. The mortality rate was 39% in a study of 19 dogs with necrotizing cholecystitis; delayed diagnosis probably contributed to this high mortality.[18]

Emphysematous cholecystitis occurs when gas-forming bacteria infect the gallbladder and gas fills the lumen or invades the wall (tympanic and emphysematous cholecystitis, respectively).[19] Once considered pathognomonic of diabetes mellitus, emphysematous cholecystitis can develop in any animal. Signs may be similar to those described for bacterial and necrotizing cholecystitis. Plain radiographs are diagnostic (Figure 231-5), and treatment consists of antibiotics. Knowing that gas-forming bacteria (e.g., *E. coli*, *Clostridium perfringens*) must be responsible helps guide antibiotic selection (e.g., enrofloxacin plus amoxicillin).

Choleliths are often fortuitous findings at necropsy or during imaging.[1] They often cause no problems (Figure 231-6); however, they may be associated with cholecystitis or rupture.[13] If found in an animal with biliary tract disease, they should be removed. Although people commonly develop dietary-induced cholesterol gallstones, canine gallstones usually contain bilirubin, calcium, and mucin.

Parasites of the gallbladder, bile ducts, or both are seldom diagnosed. *Platynosomum fastosum* (previously *P. concinnum*) is a fluke principally found in animals from Florida, Hawaii, and the Caribbean. It typically infects cats that eat lizards or toads (i.e., a second intermediate host). The fluke may

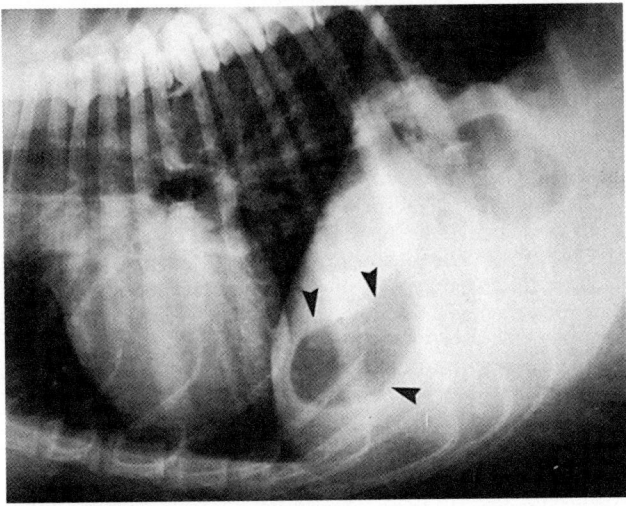

Figure 231-5 Lateral radiograph of a dog showing a pear-shaped, air-filled structure (*arrows*). This is the gallbladder of a dog with emphysematous, tympanic cholecystitis. (Courtesy of Dr. Robert Toal, College of Veterinary Medicine, University of Tennessee.)

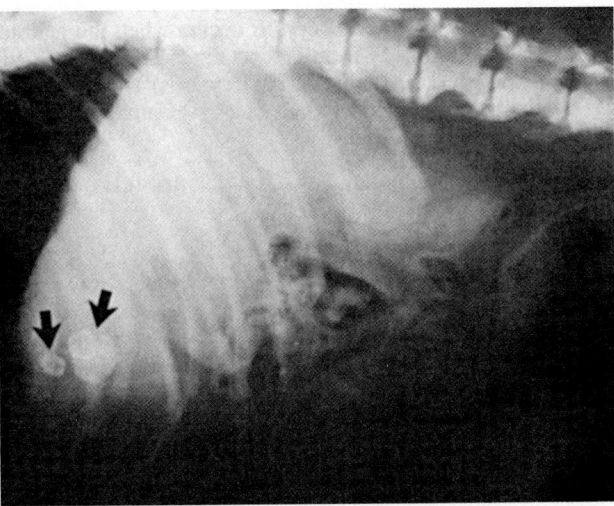

Figure 231-6 Lateral radiograph of a dog showing mineral densities in the region of the gallbladder (*arrows*). These were gallstones that were not causing clinical disease in this dog.

ultimately be found in the gallbladder, bile ducts, or both, where it may be asymptomatic or cause fibrosis, obstruction, or both. Signs of infection can be similar to those of cholecystitis. Diagnosis is by ultrasonography or by finding ova by fecal sedimentation examination (not fecal flotation), assuming that complete biliary tract obstruction does not occur. Therapy may be attempted with praziquantel (20 mg/kg subcutaneously, once a day for 3 days). Prognosis is uncertain, but severe hepatic disease warrants a guarded prognosis.[1] *Amphimerus pseudofelineus* has also been associated with cholangitis, cholangiohepatitis, and distention of the feline common bile duct.[20] High-dose (40 mg/kg) praziquantel therapy administered orally once a day for 3 days reportedly eradicated the infection. *Metorchis conjunctus* and *Eurytrema procyonis* may also be found in the feline biliary tract.

Neoplasia of the gallbladder or extrahepatic biliary tract is rare. Bile duct carcinomas have been reported in cats and dogs.[19] Metastasis of bile duct carcinomas commonly occurs before clinical signs manifest; therefore surgery is rarely curative. Surgical therapy of cholecystic tumors may be curative if no metastasis exists.

Congenital dilatation of intrahepatic and extrahepatic bile ducts may occur without obstruction in dogs with Caroli's disease. Affected animals are generally less than 3.5 years old and usually experience vomiting, polyuria, anorexia, ascites, and increased hepatic enzymes. The gallbladder and common bile duct are generally normal in size. Renal fibrosis and cystic changes are common in affected animals.[21]

Rupture of the Gallbladder or Extrahepatic Biliary Ducts

Extrahepatic biliary duct or gallbladder rupture may be iatrogenic or associated with blunt abdominal trauma, cholecystitis, or obstruction secondary to stones, neoplasia, or parasites. Trauma usually causes rupture of the bile duct rather than the gallbladder. Ductal rupture probably occurs when a force is applied adjacent to the gallbladder sufficient to cause a shearing force on the duct. The most common site of ductal rupture appears to be the common bile duct just distal to the entrance of the last hepatic duct; however, rupture may occur in the distal common bile duct, cystic duct (rare), or hepatic ducts. Gallbladder rupture is more commonly associated with necrotizing cholecystitis or cholelithiasis, with or without obstruction of the common bile duct.[18]

Early diagnosis of biliary tract rupture is imperative. Leakage of infected bile causes clinical signs of bile peritonitis to develop quickly. In a study of 24 dogs and two cats with biliary tract rupture, there was 54% mortality, which was limited to animals with infected bile. *E. coli* was the bacterium most commonly cultured from infected animals.[12] Ascites and icterus may be the only signs in dogs with sterile bile in the peritoneal cavity due to traumatic rupture; however, necrosis and changes in mucosal permeability secondary to the bile can allow secondary bacterial infection.[19] Delayed diagnosis of a ruptured biliary tract results in necrotic tissues and adhesions, which complicate surgical repair. Diagnostic peritoneal lavage may assist in the early diagnosis of sterile bile peritonitis.

Surgical treatment for a ruptured common bile duct involves repair of the duct or biliary diversion. Repair is often possible if the rupture is diagnosed early, but it becomes difficult once adhesions develop. In such cases, cholecystojejunostomy is generally easier and safer. Ruptured hepatic ducts are usually ligated. Gallbladder rupture should be treated by cholecystectomy.

Miscellaneous Findings

Cystic mucinous hypertrophy is occasionally found in older animals, either at necropsy or during ultrasonography. It is not clearly associated with disease, although progestational drugs may produce it.[1] Unless evidence of significant gallbladder dysfunction exists, this lesion does not warrant further evaluation. Congenital defects of the gallbladder are occasionally observed. Bifid gallbladders have been reported in cats, although their significance is unknown. Nonbiliary tract disorders may also produce cholecystic lesions. Gallbladder edema is reportedly common in infectious canine hepatitis. In other diseases, however, gallbladder lesions are seldom significant. Even in canine salmonellosis, the gallbladder is rarely important as a reservoir of infection.

CHAPTER • 232

Canine Exocrine Pancreatic Disease

David A. Williams
Jörg M. Steiner

Exocrine pancreatic disease occurs commonly in dogs. Pancreatitis is by far the most common disorder, followed by pancreatic adenocarcinoma, exocrine pancreatic insufficiency (see Chapter 234), and other less commonly observed conditions.

PANCREATITIS

Classification of inflammatory disease of the pancreas in human beings has been standardized and simplified during the last two decades; however, the same is not true in veterinary medicine, and different authors classify pancreatitis differently. The following classification is based on the system currently used in humans.[1] *Acute pancreatitis* refers to pancreatic inflammation that, after removal of the inciting cause, is completely reversible.[1] Chronic pancreatitis, on the other hand, is a long-standing inflammation of pancreatic tissue associated with irreversible histopathologic changes, most importantly fibrosis and atrophy.[1] Acute and chronic pancreatitis cannot be differentiated clinically and can be mild or severe; however, chronic cases are more commonly mild and acute cases more commonly severe. Although mild pancreatitis is associated with few systemic effects, minimal pancreatic necrosis, and a low mortality, severe pancreatitis is characterized by extensive pancreatic necrosis, multiple organ involvement, and a poor prognosis.[1] Another classification parameter is the presence or absence of pancreatic complications, such as acute fluid accumulations around the inflamed pancreas (previously also known as *pancreatic phlegmon*), infected necrosis, pancreatic pseudocyst, and pancreatic abscess.[1] Classification based on cause is desirable but unfortunately cannot be achieved in most cases.

Numerous experimental procedures including hyperstimulation by administration of caerulein, carbamylcholine, or scorpion venom; obstruction of the pancreatic duct; intraductal injection of bile, fatty acids, or enzymes; pancreatic ischemia; and certain dietary manipulations all induce pancreatitis in dogs.[2] Some of these factors may also play a role in the development of spontaneous pancreatitis.[2,3] Ultimately, pancreatitis develops as a consequence of autodigestion of the pancreas resulting from premature zymogen activation within acinar cells. An early event in many experimental models of pancreatitis is abnormal fusion of lysosomes and zymogen granules (Figure 232-1). Lysosomal proteases, such as cathepsin B, are capable of activating trypsinogen, and the low pH in the fusion vacuoles also favors trypsinogen activation.

Several mechanisms are in place that prevent autodigestion of the pancreas by the enzymes it secretes. First, proteolytic and phospholipolytic enzymes are synthesized, stored, and secreted in the form of catalytically inactive zymogens. These zymogens are activated by enzymatic cleavage of a small peptide—the activation peptide—from the amino-terminal of the polypeptide chain.[2] Enzymes from several sources, including some lysosomal proteases, are capable of activating pancreatic zymogens, but ordinarily activation of zymogens does not occur until they are secreted into the small intestine. The enzyme enteropeptidase, which is synthesized by duodenal enterocytes, is particularly effective at cleaving the activation peptide from trypsinogen and plays a crucial role in the

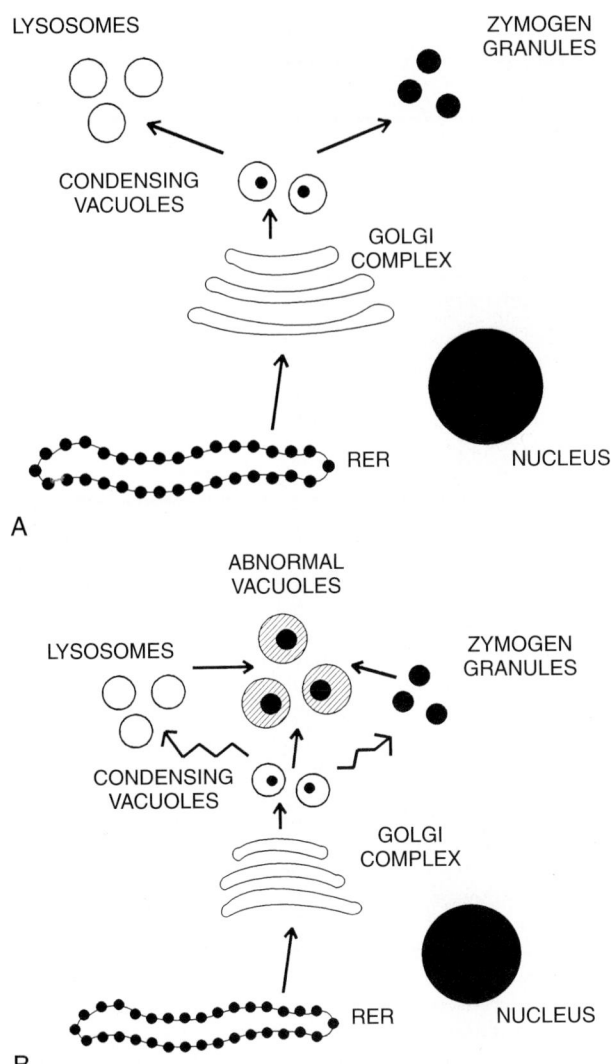

Figure 232-1 Normal **(A)** and abnormal **(B)** intracellular routing of digestive and lysosomal enzymes by the pancreatic acinar cell. The abnormal intracellular routing of digestive enzymes during pancreatitis results in mixing of zymogens and lysosomal proteases in intracellular vacuoles. Subsequent activation of zymogens by lysosomal proteases is considered to initiate the development of pancreatitis.

activation of digestive enzymes.[2] Active trypsin subsequently cleaves the activation peptide from other digestive zymogens. During synthesis, processing, storage, and secretion, digestive enzymes are strictly segregated from other, potentially damaging, cellular enzymes, such as lysosomal enzymes.[2] Should spontaneous intrapancreatic activation of trypsinogen occur, at least two mechanisms help to limit activation of other zymogens. Trypsin is quite effective at hydrolysing itself, so that activation of small amounts of trypsin tends not to be catastrophic. However, should significant activation occur, acinar cells contain a specific trypsin inhibitor—pancreatic secretory trypsin inhibitor (PSTI)—that is synthesized, segregated, stored, and secreted along with the digestive enzymes (Table 232-1).[2] PSTI is believed to inhibit trypsin activity should there be significant activation of trypsinogen within the acinar cell or duct system.[2] However, this mechanism fails at the low pH in the fusion vacuoles.

Once intracellular and intraductal activation of trypsinogen to trypsin takes place, further activation of all zymogens (particularly proelastase and prophospholipase) will amplify pancreatic damage. Activation of progressively larger amounts of protease and phospholipase within the gland is associated with progression of mild edematous pancreatitis to hemorrhagic or necrotic pancreatitis with multisystem involvement and consumption of plasma protease inhibitors.[2,4]

Plasma protease inhibitors (see Table 232-1), particularly α-macroglobulins, are vital in protecting against the otherwise fatal effects of proteolytic enzymes in the vascular space.[2,4] Dogs die rapidly from acute disseminated intravascular coagulation (DIC) and shock once α-macroglobulin is depleted, because free proteases concurrently activate the kinin, coagulation, fibrinolytic, and complement systems.[2,4] Binding of proteases by α-macroglobulin results in a conformational change that allows the complex to be rapidly cleared from the plasma by the reticuloendothelial system (RES). This removal of α-macroglobulin–bound proteases by the RES is important because proteases bound to α-macroglobulin retain catalytic activity, particularly against low molecular weight substrates.

The primary function of α_1-proteinase inhibitor (α_1-PI) is to inhibit neutrophil elastase during inflammation (see Table 232-1). Although pancreatic proteases do bind to α_1-PI and are effectively inhibited, the binding is reversible and the availability of α_1-PI during pancreatitis is not life saving.[2] Alpha$_1$-PI probably serves as a transient inhibitor and intermediary in the transport of proteases to α-macroglobulin, particularly in the extravascular space, into which the large α-macroglobulin molecules cannot permeate.

Once enzyme activation is initiated, numerous inflammatory mediators and free radicals are important in the progression of pancreatitis.[4,5] These mediators are mostly released from neutrophils and macrophages and include tumor necrosis factor-α (TNF-α), interleukin-1 (IL-1), IL-2, IL-6, IL-8, IL-10, interferon-α (INF-α), INF-γ, nitric oxide (NO), and platelet activating factor (PAF).[5]

Cause

The inciting cause of pancreatitis in the dog is usually unknown, but the following potential causes and risk factors should be considered.[2] It has been suggested that pancreatitis is more prevalent in obese animals,[2] and it has been shown that the disease is less severe when induced in lean dogs.[2] Evidence also shows that a low-protein high-fat diet induces pancreatitis, and that pancreatitis is more severe when induced in dogs being fed a high-fat diet.[2]

Hyperlipidemia, often grossly apparent, is common in dogs with acute pancreatitis, and may develop as a result of abdominal fat necrosis or may be a cause of the disease in some cases. Some familial hyperlipidemias in human beings are associated with frequent episodes of pancreatitis that respond to control of serum triglyceride concentrations. It is widely believed that the high prevalence of pancreatitis observed in Miniature Schnauzers may be related to idiopathic hyperlipidemia.[2]

Hereditary pancreatitis is well-documented in human beings. Several mutations of the cationic trypsinogen gene (and some other genes) have been identified, the most prevalent being replacement of the arginine in position 117 with a histidine (R117H) or replacement of the asparagine in position 21 with isoleucine (N21I).[6] The two mutations mentioned lead to conformational changes that protect trypsin from autodigestion. As a consequence, prematurely activated trypsin persists and can trigger activation of other zymogens.[6] The high prevalence of pancreatitis in the Miniature Schnauzer suggests a possible hereditary component; however a recent study failed to identify any mutations in the cationic trypsinogen gene in this breed.

Table • 232-1

Major Protease Inhibitors in Canine Pancreas and Plasma

INHIBITOR	PANCREATIC SECRETORY TRYPSIN INHIBITOR (PSTI)	α_1-PROTEINASE INHIBITOR (α_1-ANTITRYPSIN) (α_1-PI)	MACROGLOBULINS (α-M$_1$ AND α-M$_2$)
Principal locations	Pancreas, pancreatic juice	Plasma, intercellular space	Plasma
Approximate molecular weight	6000	55,000	750,000
Specificity	Trypsin only	Broad spectrum (serine proteases)	Broad spectrum (serine and other proteases)
Inhibition	Temporary (slowly degraded by trypsin)	Transient (transfers enzyme to α-M)	Irreversible (permanent trap for captured enzyme)
Function	Inhibits intrapancreatic autoactivation of trypsin	Readily diffusible inhibitor present in the intercellular space	Traps proteases prior to removal by reticuloendothelial system (RES)

More than 50 drugs and drug classes have been implicated as a cause of pancreatitis in human beings, although absolute proof of a causal relationship is often lacking.[7] Suspect drugs that are also commonly used in veterinary medicine include L-asparaginase, azathioprine, estrogen, furosemide, potassium bromide, salicylates, sulfonamides, tetracyclines, thiazide diuretics, and vinca alkaloids.[2,8] Corticosteroids have recently been removed from the list of drugs that may induce pancreatitis in human beings. There is little credible evidence that glucocorticoid administration causes pancreatitis in dogs with the possible exception of the use of high doses in association with spinal trauma (e.g., surgical intervention for intervertebral disc disease). Nonetheless, it is probably wise to discontinue the use of any drug in patients with pancreatitis of undetermined cause unless a specific indication for continued use exists and no alternatives are available.

Administration of cholinesterase inhibitor insecticides and cholinergic agonists has been associated with the development of pancreatitis, probably by causing hyperstimulation.[2] Scorpion stings cause pancreatitis in human beings in Trinidad, and experimental administration of scorpion venom to dogs also elicits pancreatitis. Zinc toxicosis has also been reported to cause pancreatitis in the dog. Also, both spontaneous or iatrogenic hypercalcemia may cause pancreatitis in dogs.[2]

Experimental obstruction of the pancreatic ducts produces atrophy and fibrosis, although inflammation and edema may also develop when pancreatic secretion is stimulated.[9] Clinical conditions that may lead to partial or complete obstruction of the pancreatic ducts include biliary calculi, sphincter spasm, edema of the duct or duodenal wall, neoplastic conditions, parasites, trauma, and surgical interference. Biliary calculi are a major cause of pancreatitis in man, but this has not been reported in dogs, presumably because of the low prevalence of biliary stones in this species and because dogs have an accessory pancreatic duct that does not communicate with the common bile duct and serves as the main pancreatic duct.[10] Congenital anomalies of the pancreatic duct system may predispose to pancreatitis in man, and similar mechanisms may occur in the dog but have not been documented.

Reflux of duodenal juice into the pancreatic ducts secondary to surgical creation of a closed duodenal loop causes severe acute pancreatitis. Under normal circumstances such reflux is unlikely to occur because the duct opening is surrounded by a specialized compact smooth mucosa over the duodenal papilla and is equipped with an independent sphincter muscle; however, this antireflux mechanism may sometimes fail owing to an abnormally high duodenal pressure, such as may occur during vomiting or after blunt trauma to the abdominal cavity.

Surgical manipulation and blunt abdominal trauma are also potential causes of pancreatitis, but reports of pancreatitis after such insults are rare.[2] Pancreatitis after pancreatic biopsy is extremely rare, and is also uncommon after resection of pancreatic neoplasms.[2]

Experimental and clinical reports have indicated that ischemia is important in the pathogenesis of acute pancreatitis, either as a primary cause or as an exacerbating influence. Pancreatic ischemia may develop during shock, secondary to hypotension during general anesthesia, or during temporary occlusion of venous outflow during surgical manipulation in the anterior abdomen. In some cases this may explain some instances of postoperative pancreatitis when areas remote from the pancreas have undergone surgery.

Viral, mycoplasmal, and parasitic infections may be associated with pancreatitis, although this is usually recognized as part of a more generalized disease process.[2] Recently, pancreatitis has been recognized as a potential complication of babesiosis.[11] It is unknown whether bacterial infection plays a role in the development of pancreatitis in some cases, but concomitant bacterial infection does increase the severity of experimental pancreatitis.[2] Pancreatitis may occur in association with end-stage renal failure, but this is rare. It is likely that renal failure secondary to acute pancreatitis is encountered more frequently.[2] Finally, autoimmune mechanisms have been incriminated in a small subset of human patients with pancreatic inflammation that responds to glucocorticoid therapy.[12]

DIAGNOSIS

History and Clinical Signs

Although dogs of any age and body condition may develop pancreatitis, affected animals are usually middle aged or older and are often overweight. Dogs with acute pancreatitis are usually presented because of vomiting, weakness, abdominal pain, depression, or diarrhea.[13] Severe acute disease may be associated with shock and collapse. Some dogs demonstrate abdominal pain by assuming a "prayer" position, with the forelimbs stretched out, the sternum on the ground, and the hindlimbs raised. Signs of pain may also be elicited by abdominal palpation, although some animals do not react even though they have severe acute pancreatitis. Abdominal pain is the most consistent clinical sign in human patients, being reported in more than 90% of cases. By comparison a study in dogs reported abdominal pain in only 59% of cases.[13] This probably reflects failure to detect abdominal pain rather than its absence. An anterior abdominal mass is palpable in some cases, and occasionally mild ascites occur. Dogs with severe disease are often dehydrated and may be febrile. Uncommon systemic complications of pancreatitis that may be apparent on physical examination include jaundice, respiratory distress, bleeding disorders, and cardiac arrhythmias.[2] In some patients the onset of signs may have followed ingestion of a large amount of fatty food.[13]

The clinical signs of mild, acute, and chronic pancreatitis in dogs are poorly documented but are probably extremely variable and nonspecific. The disease may not be clinically apparent at all. As a consequence, mild disease remains undiagnosed in the vast majority of cases.

Diagnostic Imaging

Radiographic findings in dogs with pancreatitis include an increased density, diminished contrast (*ground glass* appearance), and granularity in the right cranial abdomen, displacement of the stomach to the left, widening of the angle between the pyloric antrum and the proximal duodenum, displacement of the descending duodenum to the right, presence of a mass medial to the descending duodenum, static gas pattern in or thickened walls of the descending duodenum, static gas pattern in or caudal displacement of the transverse colon, gastric distension suggestive of gastric outlet obstruction, and delayed passage of barium through the stomach and duodenum with corrugation of the duodenal wall. Unfortunately these findings are subjective, and definitive radiographic evidence of pancreatitis is usually not present. However, abdominal radiographs may provide evidence to rule in or rule out alternative diagnoses.

Abdominal ultrasonography is highly specific for pancreatitis when stringent criteria are applied, with a sensitivity of up to approximately 70% in dogs and 30% in cats.[13] Enlargement of the gland, localized peritoneal effusion, or both are not sufficient for a diagnosis. Changes in echogenicity are quite useful. A decrease in echogenicity indicates pancreatic necrosis, which is often associated with hyperechogenicity in the peripancreatic region (Figure 232-2). Hyperechogenicity of the pancreatic parenchyma itself indicates pancreatic fibrosis and can be seen in cases of chronic pancreatitis. Pancreatic duct dilation also has been reported in cats.[2,3] Serial examinations are particularly useful for identification and management of pancreatic complications such as pancreatic pseudocyst or abscess.

Computed tomography (CT) is the most useful modality for visualizing the pancreas and for identifying pancreatic necrosis in human patients, but financial considerations and the much smaller size of the pancreas will likely limit its usefulness in the dog.

Clinical Pathology

Leukocytosis, often associated with a left shift, is a common hematologic finding in acute pancreatitis. The packed cell volume (PCV) may be increased as a result of dehydration, but anemia is also frequently observed.[2,3,13] Azotemia is often present, usually reflecting dehydration, but it may also reflect secondary acute renal failure.[14] Activities of hepatic enzymes are often increased, reflecting either hepatic ischemia or exposure of the liver to high concentrations of toxic products from the pancreas.[2,15] Hyperbilirubinemia and clinically apparent icterus may occur, possibly indicating severe hepatocellular damage, intrahepatic and extrahepatic obstruction of bile

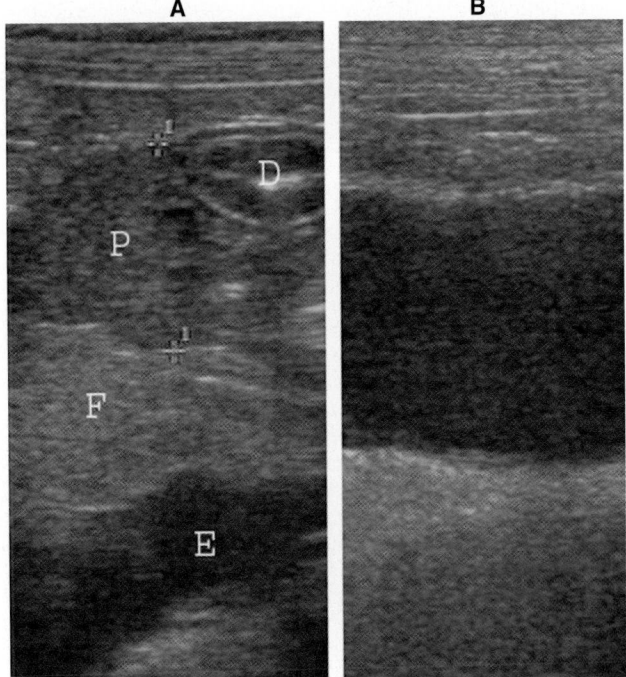

Figure 232-2 Ultrasonographic scans of the cranial abdomen in two dogs. The dog in panel **A** had severe pancreatitis. The duodenum can be seen in the upper right hand corner (*D*). The pancreas can be seen as an irregular mixed echoic structure (*P*). The dark areas within the pancreas represent areas of pancreatic necrosis. The hyperechoic area right below the mixed echoic structure represents peripancreatic fat necrosis (*F*). The hypoechoic area below the peripancreatic fat suggests peritoneal effusion (*E*). The changes seen here are highly specific for acute pancreatitis. The dog shown in panel **B** had a pancreatic abscess. A large uniformly hypoechoic structure exists that suggests a fluid-filled mass. Such a fluid-filled mass could represent a pancreatic pseudocyst or a pancreatic abscess and was diagnosed as a pancreatic abscess in this patient. (Images courtesy of Dr. Sharon Shull.)

flow, or both. Hyperglycemia is common as a result of hyperglucagonemia, stress-related increases in the concentrations of catecholamines and cortisol, or destruction of islet cells by pancreatic inflammation. Some dogs remain diabetic after recovery from acute episodes of pancreatitis.[2] Hypocalcemia has often been reported, usually secondary to hypoalbuminemia but is usually mild to moderate and rarely associated with clinical signs of tetany.[2,3] Hypocalcemia can also be due to deposition of calcium as soaps after excessive generation of fatty acids by the breakdown of fat. Hypercholesterolemia and hypertriglyceridemia are common, and hyperlipemia is often grossly apparent even though food has not been ingested recently. Hyperlipidemia may prevent accurate determination of some serum biochemical values.[2]

Assays for several pancreatic enzymes and zymogens in serum have been evaluated for the diagnosis of canine pancreatitis, including amylase and lipase activities, serum trypsin-like immunoreactivity (cTLI), pancreatic lipase immunoreactivity (cPLI), trypsin-α_1-proteinase inhibitor complexes, and serum and urinary trypsinogen activation peptide (TAP).[2,3,16]

Serum amylase and lipase activities have been used to diagnose canine pancreatitis for several decades, but both have been repeatedly shown to lack sensitivity and specificity.[10] In general, approximately 50% of patients with an elevated serum amylase activity, lipase activity, or both do not have pancreatitis. Trypsin complexed with plasma α_1-proteinase inhibitor and TAP in plasma or urine should act as specific markers for pancreatitis.[16] However, a recent study found urinary TAP concentration to be very insensitive even though it was highly specific.[16] Plasma TAP concentration was slightly more sensitive but also had a lower specificity of 77%.[16] Taking into consideration the cost of the assay, the limited availability of laboratories providing the assay, and the lack of stability of TAP, this assay is of little clinical usefulness for the diagnosis of canine pancreatitis. A recently developed assay for serum trypsin-α_1-proteinase inhibitor complex concentrations did not prove to be useful for the diagnosis of spontaneous pancreatitis in the dog. Serum cTLI concentration is specific for exocrine pancreatic function and is the test of choice for EPI, but its short half life renders it fairly insensitive for the diagnosis of canine pancreatitis.

Serum cPLI concentration is highly specific for exocrine pancreatic function and appears to be a useful marker for pancreatic inflammation. In a recent study of 11 dogs with biopsy-confirmed pancreatitis, all 11 dogs had serum cPLI concentrations above the upper limit of the reference range, and nine of 11 dogs (82%) had concentrations above a cutoff value of 200 µg/L.[18] Serum cPLI is not elevated in dogs with gastritis and experimentally induced chronic renal failure; it is also not affected by administration of prednisone. Thus serum cPLI is the most sensitive (Figure 232-3) and specific diagnostic test for canine pancreatitis currently available.

Pancreatic biopsy obtained by exploratory laparotomy or laparoscopy is often considered the gold standard for diagnosing canine pancreatitis, but it has limitations. In a recent study, less than 10% of dogs with pancreatitis showed gross anatomic evidence of pancreatitis. In addition, histologic examination often reveals the distribution of pancreatitis to be patchy and highly localized. Thus although the presence of pancreatic inflammation, necrosis, or both can be considered definitive evidence for pancreatitis, a lack of such findings (even if multiple biopsies are evaluated) does not definitively exclude pancreatitis. Moreover, the risk of anesthesia may be elevated in patients with pancreatitis, making the collection of a biopsy potentially detrimental in such cases.

TREATMENT

The classic therapy for acute pancreatitis is maintenance of fluid and electrolyte balance while the pancreas is "rested" by withholding food.[2] Recent reports have challenged the logic and wisdom of withholding food, however, and both parenteral and enteral nutrition have been well tolerated by patients with pancreatitis.[19] Evidence also indicates that enteral nutrition may be superior to parenteral nutrition. Oral intake should probably be restricted only in those patients with incessant vomiting, and then for as short a period as possible.

If drug-induced pancreatitis is suspected, any incriminated agents should be withdrawn and replaced by an unrelated alternative drug, if necessary. Other potential causative factors (see previous discussion) should similarly be investigated and, if possible, eliminated. Balanced electrolyte solution should be given intravenously to replace fluid deficits and provide maintenance requirements. Mild cases of pancreatitis are probably self-limiting and may improve without therapy. Other patients require aggressive fluid therapy over several days to treat severe dehydration and ongoing fluid and electrolyte loss due to vomiting. Many animals become hypokalemic during such therapy, and serum potassium should be monitored and supplemented parenterally if required. Serum creatinine and blood urea nitrogen (BUN) should also be monitored to document resolution of azotemia, thereby ruling out associated renal failure. Although metabolic acidosis is probably common in acute pancreatitis, this may not always be the case, and vomiting patients may be alkalotic. Therefore blind correction of suspected acid-base abnormalities should not be attempted.[2] It is common practice to administer antibiotics to dogs with pancreatitis, particularly when toxic changes are evident on the hemogram or when the patient is febrile. Antibiotic therapy appears to be beneficial in human patients and in some experimental models of pancreatitis; in contrast to humans, dogs with pancreatitis rarely have infectious complications, and antibiotic therapy would appear to be of minimal benefit. However, for cases where good evidence for pancreatic infection exists, it should be noted that trimethoprim sulfa and enrofloxacin penetrate well into the exocrine pancreas in dogs.

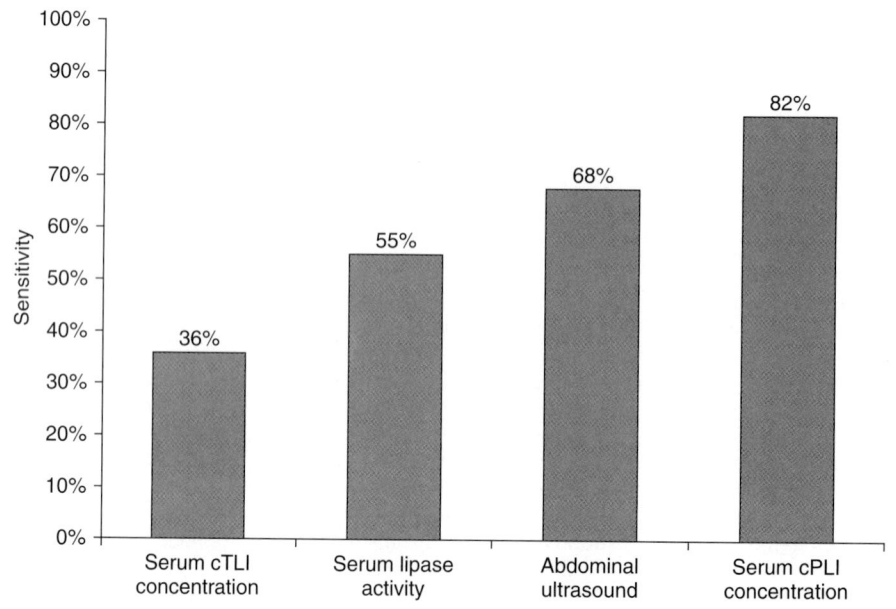

Figure 232-3 This figure shows a comparison of the sensitivity for different diagnostic modalities for a diagnosis of canine pancreatitis. The reader should note that serum cTLI concentration, abdominal ultrasound, and serum cPLI concentration have a high specificity for canine pancreatitis, whereas only approximately 50% of dogs with an elevated serum lipase activity have pancreatitis.[13,18]

Analgesic therapy (subcutaneous meperidine hydrochloride, transdermal fentanyl, morphine by constant rate intravenous infusion, or intraperitoneal lidocaine) should be given to provide relief of pain, even if obvious signs of pain are not apparent.[20] Hyperglycemia is often mild and transient, but in some cases diabetes mellitus may develop, requiring treatment with insulin. Respiratory distress, neurologic problems, cardiovascular abnormalities, bleeding disorders, and acute renal failure are all poor prognostic indicators. Attempts should be made to manage these complications by appropriate supportive measures.

Some affected animals do not improve or continue to deteriorate in spite of intensive supportive care. Evidence indicates that, in severe pancreatitis, marked consumption of plasma protease inhibitors occurs and that saturation of available α-macroglobulins is rapidly followed by acute DIC, shock, and death.[21] Transfusion of plasma or whole blood to replace α-macroglobulins may be life saving in these circumstances, and it has the additional benefit of maintaining plasma albumin concentrations.[22] Low-molecular-weight dextrans have also been used to expand plasma volume, but they may aggravate bleeding tendencies, contain no protease inhibitor, and provide no major advantages over plasma administration. The use of corticosteroids in pancreatitis has been recommended by some because they stabilize lysosomal membranes, reduce inflammation, and alleviate shock, but they have not been shown to be of value in experimental studies.[2] Unless autoimmune pancreatitis is suspected, they should be given only on a short-term basis to animals in shock. Attempts to rest the pancreas by use of direct inhibitors of secretion such as atropine, acetazolamide, glucagon, calcitonin, and somatostatin or its analogues have not proved effective. Recent data have suggested that somatostatin may even have detrimental effects in experimental pancreatitis, and its use cannot be recommended. Administration of a variety of naturally occurring and synthetic enzyme inhibitors with selective actions against individual pancreatic digestive enzymes has shown promise in experimental studies, but these agents have not been shown to be beneficial in human patients with pancreatitis. Inhibition of gastric secretion by use of antacids or cimetidine and suctioning off gastric secretions have been used in an attempt to inhibit pancreatic secretion, however, none of these methods has been consistently shown to be effective. In one study the use of sodium selenite as an antioxidant was reported to lead to a significant decrease in mortality in dogs with pancreatitis. This study was not controlled, and controlled studies in human patients with pancreatitis failed to show any clinical benefit. The use of peritoneal dialysis to remove toxic material accumulated in the peritoneal cavity is believed by some to be useful in human patients with pancreatitis, but it has not been shown reproductivity to be useful and is rather impractical in canine patients with pancreatitis. In some cases pancreatitis may be localized to one lobe of the gland, and surgical resection of the affected area may be followed by complete recovery. Future clinical and experimental trials will probably be directed at the use of agents to modify events currently believed to be important in the pathogenesis of pancreatitis, including inhibitors of inflammatory mediators, free-radical scavengers, enzyme synthesis and transport inhibitors, and factors that may stabilize lysosomal and other cell compartment membranes.[5]

After vomiting has subsided, small amounts of water should be offered; if no exacerbation of clinical signs occurs, food may be gradually reintroduced. The diet should preferably have a high carbohydrate content (rice, pasta, potatoes) because protein and fat are more potent stimulants of pancreatic secretion and are perhaps more likely to promote a relapse. If improvement continues, gradual introduction of a low-fat maintenance diet should be attempted.[19]

In many patients with a single episode of pancreatitis, the only long-term therapy recommended is to avoid feeding high-fat meals. In patients with repeated bouts of pancreatitis occur, and it may be beneficial to feed a fat-restricted diet permanently. In some patients, hypertriglyceridemia may need to be controlled pharmacologically. Despite all efforts, some animals experience recurrent disease.[23]

Some reports have indicated that oral pancreatic enzyme supplements decrease abdominal pain and discomfort that accompanies chronic pancreatitis in humans. It is unknown whether they are of similar value in dogs, but a trial period of enzyme therapy may be warranted in dogs with chronic signs of abdominal pain or anorexia.

PROGNOSIS

Pancreatitis is an unpredictable disease of widely varying severity, and it is difficult to give a prognosis. Life-threatening signs accompanying acute fulminating pancreatitis are usually followed by death in spite of supportive measures, but some dogs recover fully after an isolated severe episode. In other cases relatively mild or moderate chronic or recurrent pancreatitis persists despite all therapy, and the patient either dies during an acute severe exacerbation of the disease or undergoes euthanasia because of failure to recover and the expense of long-term supportive care. Most patients with uncomplicated pancreatitis probably recover spontaneously and do well as long as high-fat diets are avoided.

PANCREATIC PSEUDOCYST

A pancreatic pseudocyst is a collection of sterile pancreatic juice, enclosed by a wall of fibrous or granulation tissue and occurs as a complication of pancreatitis.[1] Recently, several cases of pancreatic pseudocysts in dogs have been described.[24] Clinical signs are usually nonspecific and mimic those of pancreatitis. On abdominal ultrasound a cystic structure in close proximity to the pancreas can be identified. Aspiration of the pseudocyst is relatively safe and should be attempted for diagnostic and therapeutic purposes.[24] In contrast to fluid from a pancreatic abscess, the drained fluid from a pancreatic pseudocyst should be of low cellularity and should not contain any evidence of inflammation. Pancreatic pseudocysts can be treated medically or surgically. Surgical correction can involve extirpation of the pseudocyst, external drainage, or internal drainage, but internal drainage is the preferred treatment in human patients. Medical management of pancreatic pseudocysts involves ultrasound-guided percutaneous aspiration and close monitoring of the size of the pseudocyst. This approach was successful in several cases described in the human medical literature.[24] However, surgical intervention should be considered in cases in which clinical signs persist or when the size of the pseudocyst does not decrease significantly over time.

PANCREATIC ABSCESS

A pancreatic abscess is another possible complication of pancreatitis.[1] A pancreatic abscess is a circumscribed collection of pus, usually in proximity to the pancreas, containing little or no pancreatic necrosis.[1] In dogs, bacterial infection is only rarely present.[25,26] Clinical signs are nonspecific, but may include vomiting, depression, abdominal pain, anorexia, fever, diarrhea, and dehydration. In some patients a mass in the cranial abdomen can be identified upon abdominal palpation.[25] Common clinicopathologic findings are neutrophilia with a left shift, elevation of serum amylase and lipase activities, elevations of hepatic enzyme activities, and hyperbiliru-binemia.[25,26] Surgical drainage and aggressive antimicrobial therapy are the treatment of choice in human patients with pancreatic abscess. Dogs may also respond favorably to surgical drainage.[25] However, in one report only five of nine patients survived the immediate postsurgical period.[26] Thus given the mixed results, risks, difficulties, and expenses associated with anesthesia, surgery, and postoperative care, one may want to avoid surgical intervention unless clear evidence exists of an enlarging mass, sepsis, or both in a patient that is not responding well to medical therapy. Antimicrobial therapy in dogs is of questionable value unless an organism is identified upon bacterial culture.

EXOCRINE PANCREATIC NEOPLASIA

Pancreatic adenomas are benign tumors that are usually singular and can be differentiated from pancreatic nodular hyperplasia by the presence of a capsule. Pancreatic adeno-carcinoma is the most common neoplastic condition of the exocrine pancreas in the dog; however, in contrast to humans, where pancreatic adenocarcinoma is the fifth most common malignancy, it occurs rather infrequently in dogs. Adenocarcinomas usually originate from the duct system but can also originate from acinar tissue. A few cases of pancreatic sarcomas (i.e., spindle cell sarcoma, lymphosarcoma) have been reported. Whether these tumors are primary neoplastic lesions of the exocrine pancreas, metastatic lesions of tumors of other organs, or a localized lesion of a multicentric neoplasia is open to question.

Cause and Pathogenesis

The cause of neoplastic conditions of the exocrine pancreas is unknown. Benign neoplastic lesions can lead to transposition of cranial abdominal organs. However, these changes are subclinical in most cases, and the diagnosis is often made as an incidental finding at necropsy examination. In very few cases a benign growth can obstruct the pancreatic duct and cause secondary atrophy of the remaining exocrine pancreas leading to EPI. Adenocarcinomas can also cause transposition of cranial abdominal organs and obstruction of the pancreatic duct. In addition, adenocarcinomas can be associated with tumor necrosis and resulting pancreatic inflammation when the tumor outgrows its vascular supply. Pancreatic adenocarcinomas can also spread to neighboring or distant organs.

Clinical Signs and Diagnosis

The presentation of canine patients with exocrine pancreatic neoplasia is nonspecific, and clinical signs observed are often those of chronic pancreatitis such as vomiting, anorexia, diarrhea, or chronic weight loss. Multifocal necrotizing steatitis has been described in a few dogs that were ultimately diagnosed with pancreatic adenocarcinoma. Clinical signs related to metastatic lesions, such as lameness, bone pain, or dyspnea, have also been reported in some cases of pancreatic adenocarcinoma.

Neutrophilia, anemia, hypokalemia, bilirubinemia, azotemia, hyperglycemia, and elevations of hepatic enzymes have all been reported in affected patients, but results of routine blood tests may be unremarkable. Elevations of hepatic enzymes and serum bilirubin concentration are identified most commonly.[27] Hyperglycemia, when present, is related to concurrent destruction of pancreatic beta cells. Some dogs with pancreatic adenocarcinoma have extremely high serum lipase activities that reach values that are as high as 25 times the upper limit of the reference range. A single dog with a pancreatic adenocarcinoma and pseudohyperparathyroidism, leading to hypercalcemia, has been described in the literature.

Radiographic findings are also nonspecific in most cases. Abnormal findings include decreased contrast in the cranial abdomen, suggesting peritoneal effusion into this area, transposition of the spleen caudally, and shadowing in the pyloric region. In some cases abdominal radiographs can suggest the presence of a mass in the cranial abdomen.[27] In most cases a soft tissue mass can be identified by abdominal ultrasonography in the region of the pancreas.[27,28] However, in many if not most cases, the pancreatic origin of the mass cannot be conclusively established.[27] Similarly, neoplastic lesions of neighboring organs may be falsely presumed to be of pancreatic origin. In addition, patients with severe pancreatitis may show an ultrasonographic mass effect in the area of the pancreas that must not be confused with a pancreatic adenocarcinoma. If peritoneal effusion is identified on abdominal ultrasound, a sample should be aspirated and evaluated cytologically, but in most cases carcinoma cells do not readily exfoliate into the peritoneal effusion, and neoplastic cells are not routinely identified on cytology. Fine needle aspiration or transcutaneous biopsy under ultrasound guidance can be attempted when suspicious masses are identified and has been reported to be successful in approximately 25% of all cases.[27] The low success rate of fine needle aspiration is probably due to the lack of exfoliation of pancreatic adenocarcinoma cells. In other cases carcinoma cells can be identified, but the origin of the cells cannot be determined conclusively.[27] Ultrasound-guided biopsy with histopathologic evaluation of biopsies has been reported infrequently; however, in one study ultrasound-guided biopsy of a pancreatic mass resulted in a diagnosis of pancreatic adenocarcinoma in two of two cases.[27] In two of three more cases, biopsy of the liver revealed metastatic carcinoma.[27] In many cases the diagnosis is made at exploratory laparotomy or even on necropsy examination.

Therapy and Prognosis

Pancreatic adenomas are benign and theoretically do not need to be treated unless they cause clinical signs. However, because the definitive diagnosis of pancreatic adenocarcinoma is often made by histopathology, a partial pancreatectomy should be performed even in cases of suspected pancreatic adenoma. The prognosis in these cases is excellent. Pancreatic adenocarcinomas often present at a late stage of the disease. In human patients with pancreatic adenocarcinoma, metastatic disease is usually present at the time of diagnosis; this is also common in dogs with this disease. The most common sites of metastatic disease are the liver, abdominal and thoracic lymph nodes, mesentery, intestines, and the lungs, but various other metastatic sites have also been reported.[27] In those few cases when gross metastatic lesions are not identified at the time of diagnosis, surgical resection of the tumor may be attempted, but owners should be forewarned that clean surgical margins are only rarely achieved. Total pancreatectomy and pancreatico-duodenectomy, though theoretically possible, have not been described in dogs with spontaneous disease. Extrapolation from human patients suggest high morbidity and mortality for these procedures.[29] To this point, chemotherapy or radiation therapy have shown little success in human or veterinary patients with pancreatic adenocarcinomas. Overall, the prognosis for dogs and cats with pancreatic adenocarcinoma is grave.

NODULAR HYPERPLASIA

Nodular pancreatic hyperplasia occurs quite frequently in older dogs.[10] Disseminated small nodules can be found throughout the pancreas and can be differentiated from pancreatic adenomas by the absence of a capsule.[10] Nodular hyperplasia does not lead to functional changes or clinical signs and is thus most frequently diagnosed incidentally during necropsy of older dogs.

CHAPTER 233

Feline Exocrine Pancreatic Disease

Jörg M. Steiner
David A. Williams

Diseases of the exocrine pancreas, once believed to be rare in cats, are now known to occur frequently in this species. Pancreatitis is the most common disorder, followed by exocrine pancreatic neoplasia, exocrine pancreatic insufficiency (see Chapter 234), and other miscellaneous conditions.

PANCREATITIS

The overall prevalence of feline pancreatitis is unknown but as the diagnostic accuracy for this disease is improving, this disease is being diagnosed with increasing frequency. The classification of feline pancreatitis is analogous to the dog (see Chapter 232), but in contrast to dogs, cats are more likely to have chronic disease.

Pancreatitis is ultimately due to autodigestion of the exocrine pancreas by prematurely activated digestive enzymes, most importantly proteases and phospholipases. Pathogenetic mechanisms that initiate clinical disease are the same as in the dog, as are the protective mechanisms that normally protect the pancreas from autodigestion (see Chapter 232).

Etiology

The majority of feline pancreatitis cases are idiopathic; however, a number of causes and risk factors have been identified. A cause-and-effect relationship has been established for *Toxoplasma gondii* and the hepatic fluke *Amphimerus pseudofelineus* (see below), but other infectious organisms, such as panleukopenia and feline infectious peritonitis, have also been implicated. Blunt trauma to the abdominal cavity such as seen in cats that have been hit by car or fallen from great heights ("high-rise syndrome") can cause pancreatitis, as can surgical manipulation and ischemia secondary to hypotension during anesthesia.

Drugs are an important cause of pancreatitis in human patients and a variety of drugs have been implicated in causing pancreatitis in human beings. However, a cause-and-effect relationship, although likely, has yet to be confirmed in cats. Pancreatitis due to organophosphate intoxication has been documented in cats.[1] The role of inflammatory diseases of the liver and the intestines in the pathogenesis of feline pancreatitis is unknown, but many cats with chronic pancreatitis also have inflammatory infiltrates of these organs. Indeed, diagnosis of chronic pancreatitis in cats should prompt diagnostic evaluation for potential concurrent inflammatory bowel disease (IBD), and vice versa.

Diagnosis
History and Clinical Signs
The history of cats with pancreatitis is extremely variable. Most cats with severe disease present with a history of lethargy and anorexia.[1] Key clinical signs of acute pancreatitis

in dogs and human beings, vomiting and abdominal pain, have been reported in only 35% and 25%, respectively, of cats with severe pancreatitis.[1] Hypothermia, dyspnea, diarrhea, and ataxia have also been reported.[1] Mild chronic pancreatitis may be subclinical or may cause anorexia and weight loss.

Diagnostic Imaging
Abdominal radiographs are only of limited usefulness for the diagnosis of pancreatitis. Possible findings are the same as in dogs and are also nonspecific in cats (see previous chapter). Thoracic radiographs may show pleural effusion in severe cases. Abdominal ultrasound is highly specific for feline pancreatitis if stringent criteria are applied. Again, findings are the same as in the dog (see Figure 232-2), but additionally pancreatic duct dilation has been reported during abdominal ultrasound examination.[2,3] Although highly specific for feline pancreatitis the sensitivity of abdominal ultrasound for pancreatitis has been reported to be only 10% to 35% when performed by a board-certified ultrasonographer.[4] A recent report assessing the clinical usefulness of contrast-enhanced computed tomography in cats with pancreatitis found this diagnostic modality to be even less sensitive than abdominal ultrasonography.[4]

Clinical Pathology
Changes in the complete blood count and serum chemistry profile are often mild and nonspecific.[1] Elevations of liver enzymes are common in severe cases and indicate secondary hepatic lipidosis or concurrent cholangitis or cholangiohepatitis.[5,6]

Serum lipase activity increases and serum amylase activity decreases in feline experimental pancreatitis.[7] However, the only study that evaluates the clinical utility of these serum enzyme activities in cats with spontaneous disease found no difference in the mean or the ranges of serum lipase or amylase activities between 12 cats with severe pancreatitis, 43 normal cats, and 31 cats with other diseases. These results suggest that these tests are of no value in the diagnosis of feline pancreatitis.[8] Serum feline trypsin-like immunoreactivity (fTLI) concentration is specific for exocrine pancreatic function in the absence of azotemia, but depending on the study the sensitivity of this diagnostic test for feline pancreatitis ranges between 30% and 60%.

An assay for serum feline pancreatic lipase immunoreactivity (fPLI) has recently been developed and initial clinical studies have been promising. In a group of cats with experimentally induced pancreatitis, both serum fTLI and fPLI concentrations increased initially, but serum fPLI concentration stayed elevated much longer than did serum fTLI concentration (Figure 233-1).[9] Another study of cats with spontaneous pancreatitis showed serum fPLI concentration to be both more sensitive and more specific for diagnosing pancreatitis than serum fTLI concentration or abdominal ultrasonography.[10]

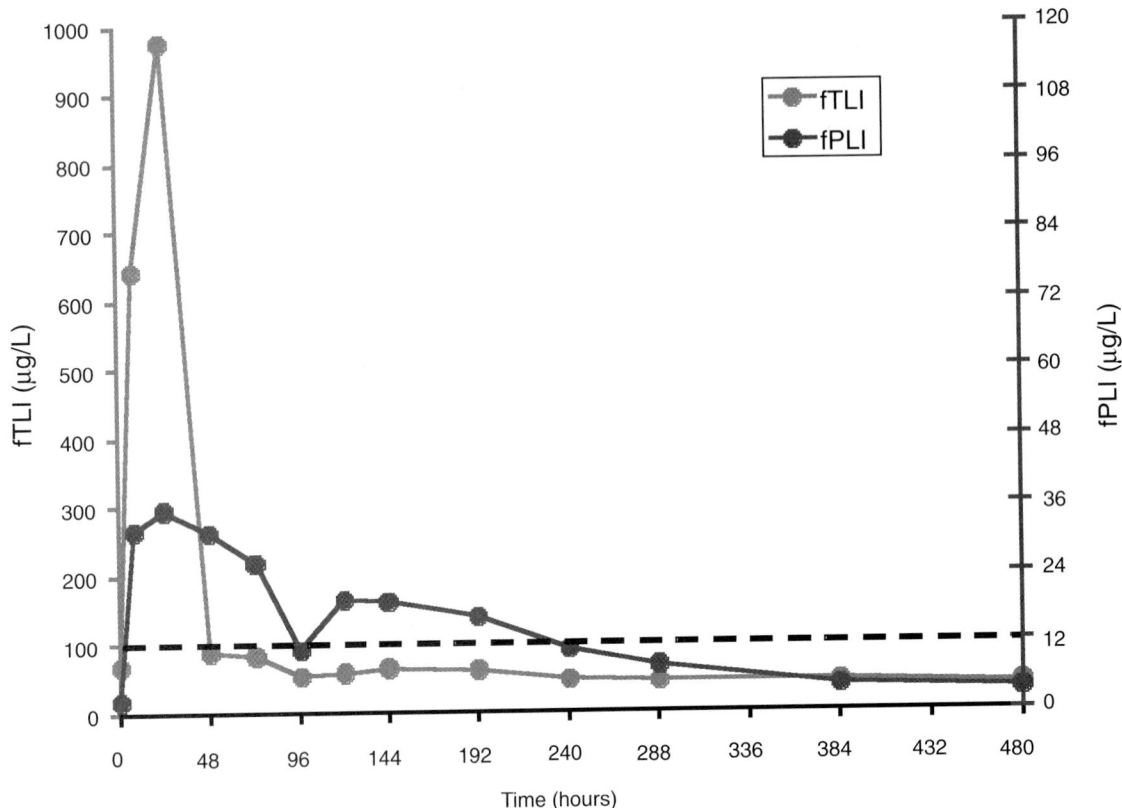

Figure 233-1 Mean serum fTLI and fPLI concentrations over time in six cats with experimentally induced pancreatitis. The gray line shows the mean serum fTLI concentrations over time and the black line shows the mean serum fPLI concentrations. The broken line displays the currently recommended cut-off value for the diagnosis of pancreatitis for serum fTLI concentration of 100 μg/L and that for serum fPLI concentration of 12 μg/L. The elevation of mean serum fPLI concentration is of far greater duration than that of mean serum fTLI concentration. These data indicate that serum fPLI concentration is more sensitive than serum fTLI concentration for the diagnosis of feline pancreatitis.[9]

At the time of writing both the fTLI and the fPLI assay are performed only at the authors' laboratory.*

Traditionally, histopathology of a pancreatic biopsy has been considered the gold standard for diagnosis of feline pancreatitis. However, gross anatomic lesions are not consistently seen and pancreatic inflammation is often localized to a small area of the gland in both acute and chronic pancreatitis. Furthermore, although pancreatic biopsy per se is safe, it is expensive and may be contraindicated in patients at risk for anesthetic complications.

Treatment

Treatment of Severe Pancreatitis

For the most part treatment of severe pancreatitis mirrors that of dogs (see previous chapter). However, special consideration must be given to nutritional support as most cats with pancreatitis present with a history of anorexia and hepatic lipidosis is common in these patients.[6] Cats that do not vomit should be offered a low-fat diet orally. If the cat is anorectic, as most cats will be, a nasogastric, esophageal, or gastrostomy

tube is the most practical route of alimentation. If these routes are contraindicated a jejunostomy tube should be placed. Partial or total parenteral nutrition are other alternatives but a jejunostomy tube is preferable.

Abdominal pain is infrequently recognized in cats with pancreatitis but probably occurs in most patients. In many patients previous abdominal pain becomes apparent after analgesia has been instituted and thus analgesic therapy is indicated in all patients.

Mild Pancreatitis

As stated earlier, cats with mild pancreatitis often have evidence of concurrent inflammatory bowel disease and or cholangiohepatitis. Although corticosteroids are believed to be of no benefit in most patients with acute pancreatitis, the authors' experience indicates that corticosteroids can be safely used in cats with concurrent chronic pancreatitis and inflammatory bowel disease. Indeed, successful treatment of IBD with prednisolone appears to lessen the severity of pancreatitis in some of these cats. Cats with concurrent IBD often have subnormal serum cobalamin concentrations, and cobalamin supplementation is essential for optimal therapeutic response in these cases. Cats with mild pancreatitis also may benefit from a low fat diet, although the potential benefit of such diets is not as clear as in dogs. The use of exogenous pancreatic enzymes is commonly recommended in human beings

*Gastrointestinal Laboratory, Department of Small Animal Medicine and Surgery, 4474 TAMU, College Station, TX 77843-4474. Telephone: 979-862-2861; FAX: 979-862-2864; e-mail: gilab@cvm.tamu.edu; home-page: www.cvm.tamu.edu/gilab

with abdominal pain due to chronic pancreatitis. Exogenous pancreatic enzymes inhibit pancreatic enzyme secretion by a negative feedback mechanism in both dogs and human beings, and this may ameliorate pain in chronic pancreatitis. Although no data are available for cats, trial therapy with pancreatic enzymes should be considered in cats that show either abdominal pain or anorexia attributable to abdominal pain.

The true prevalence of the hepatic fluke *Amphimerus pseudofelineus* in cats is unknown and infestation is usually missed during routine fecal examination. Thus, empiric treatment with praziquantel (see below) may be warranted in cats with chronic pancreatitis.

Prognosis

The prognosis for cats with pancreatitis is directly related to the severity of the disease, the extent of pancreatic necrosis, the occurrence of systemic and pancreatic complications, the duration of the condition, and to the presence of concurrent disease. In a recent report a plasma ionized calcium concentration below 1.00 mmol/L in cats with pancreatitis was a poor prognostic indicator associated with 77% mortality.[11]

As previously mentioned, common concurrent conditions in cats with pancreatitis include hepatic lipidosis, cholangiohepatitis, enteritis, diabetes mellitus, and interstitial nephritis, all of which may negatively influence the overall prognosis of the patient.[12] However, most cats with IBD and concurrent pancreatitis respond well to treatment of IBD.

PANCREATIC PSEUDOCYST

A pancreatic pseudocyst is a common complication of pancreatitis in human beings but has been reported in only one cat to date.[13,14] The clinical signs observed in the cat described were nonspecific and similar to those seen in some cats with pancreatitis. A mass was palpated in the cranial abdomen and a cystic structure in close proximity to the left lobe of the pancreas was identified on abdominal ultrasonography.[13] Surgical correction is the treatment of choice for pancreatic pseudocysts in human beings in cases when they enlarge or do not regress. Surgical correction was also successfully employed in the management of the cat reported.[13]

PANCREATIC ABSCESS

A pancreatic abscess is another common complication of pancreatitis in human beings.[14] A pancreatic abscess is a circumscribed collection of pus, usually in proximity to the pancreas, and contains little or no pancreatic necrosis.[14] To date a pancreatic abscess in a cat has not been described.

EXOCRINE PANCREATIC NEOPLASIA

Pancreatic adenocarcinomas, adenomas, or other primary or metastatic neoplastic lesions have been reported in cats.[15,16] Adenocarcinomas are the most common neoplasia of the exocrine pancreas in cats. They are malignant and usually originate from the duct system but can also originate from acinar tissue.[15]

Etiology and Pathogenesis

Benign neoplastic lesions can lead to transposition of organs of the cranial abdomen, but these changes are subclinical in most cases and the diagnosis is often made as an incidental finding on necropsy examination. In some cases the pancreatic mass can obstruct the pancreatic duct and lead to pancreatic atrophy and clinical signs of exocrine pancreatic insufficiency or to pancreatic inflammation. Malignant neoplastic lesions can cause the same changes but can also be associated with tumor necrosis and pancreatitis. Malignant tumors can also spread to neighboring or distant organs.

Clinical Signs and Diagnosis

Cats with exocrine pancreatic neoplasia present with nonspecific clinical signs. In a report of 58 cases, clinical signs most commonly reported were anorexia (46%), weight loss (37%), lethargy (28%), vomiting (23%), icterus (14%), constipation (9%), and diarrhea (3%).[15] Clinical signs reported in other cases were polyuria, fever, dehydration, a distended cranial abdomen, and voluminous, pale, and soft stools.[16] Obstructive jaundice has also been described in a cat with pancreatic adenocarcinoma. Clinical signs due to metastatic lesions may also be observed and may include lameness, bone pain, or dyspnea. Recently several cases of paraneoplastic alopecia have been reported in cats with pancreatic adenocarcinoma.[17,18] The reported alopecia consisted of generalized alopecia of the ventrum, limbs, and face in most cases, and diffuse zones of alopecia in the remaining cats.[17,18]

Neutrophilia, anemia, hypokalemia, bilirubinemia, azotemia, hyperglycemia, and elevations of hepatic enzymes have all been reported in affected patients, but results of routine blood tests may be unremarkable.[15,16] Serum lipase and amylase activities may be elevated in isolated cases.

Radiographic and ultrasonographic findings in cats with exocrine pancreatic neoplasia are similar to those in dogs with this disease (see previous chapter). As in the dog cytologic evaluation of peritoneal effusion or of fine-needle aspirates are only useful in a small number of cases, but the low invasiveness and cost of these procedures warrant their use. In many cases pancreatic neoplasia is diagnosed at exploratory laparotomy or during necropsy examination.

Therapy and Prognosis

The considerations for treatment of exocrine pancreatic neoplasia in cats mirror those in dogs (see Chapter 232). Overall, the prognosis for cats with pancreatic adenocarcinoma is grave.

PANCREATIC PARASITES

Eurytrema procyonis, the pancreatic fluke of the cat, can be found in the pancreatic ductular system of foxes, raccoons, and cats. Little is known about the life cycle of this parasite. *Eurytrema procyonis* can lead to thickening of the pancreatic duct system and fibrosis. Even though a significant decrease of exocrine pancreatic secretion has been shown to occur in affected animals, cats presenting with clinical signs of EPI secondary to infestation with this parasite are extremely rare.[19] The diagnosis can be made by detection of characteristic dicrocoeliid eggs (average size 34 µm × 50 µm) with a single operculum in fresh feces during routine fecal floatation. Fenbendazole at a dose of 30 mg/kg per os once a day for 6 consecutive days has been recommended for therapy.[20]

The hepatic fluke of the cat, *Amphimerus pseudofelineus*, can also infest the pancreas and can lead to pancreatitis.[21] Infection with this parasite has been reported in cats from Illinois, Iowa, Louisiana, Maryland, Nebraska, Ohio, Texas, and Virginia.[21,22] The life cycle of this parasite is unknown, but it is presumed that similarly to other Opisthorchiidae, mollusces serve as first and freshwater fish as second intermediate host.[22] Diagnosis can be made on fecal examination by formalin-ethyl acetate sedimentation by identification of yellow-brown eggs of approximately 16 µm × 31 µm with a single operculum.[22] Eggs are destroyed during routine fecal floatation and infestation will be missed in those cases. In one report treatment with praziquantel at 40 mg/kg once daily for 3 consecutive days was successful in the management of *Amphimerus pseudofelineus* infestation.[22] Concurrent symptomatic therapy for pancreatitis, as outlined above, also needs to be instituted in these cases. The dose of praziquantel recommended is high when compared with the standard dose recommended for treatment of enteric parasites, but the therapeutic range for praziquantel is wide and the dose recommended is similar to that recommended for treatment of hepatic flukes in human beings.[22]

PANCREATIC BLADDER

A pancreatic bladder is an abnormal extension of the pancreatic duct. Pancreatic bladders can be congenital or acquired. Only a few cats with pancreatic bladders have been described

in the literature. These patients were presented with clinical signs compatible with biliary duct obstruction. Appropriate management has not been studied, but surgical reconstruction may be of most benefit in cases presenting with clinical signs.

NODULAR HYPERPLASIA

As in older dogs, nodular pancreatic hyperplasia occurs quite frequently in older cats. Disseminated small nodules can be found throughout the exocrine portion of the pancreas. Pancreatic nodular hyperplasia can be differentiated from pancreatic adenomas by the absence of a capsule. Nodular hyperplasia does not lead to functional changes, does not cause any clinical signs, and is usually diagnosed incidentally during necropsy examination of older cats.

CHAPTER • 234

Exocrine Pancreatic Insufficiency in Dogs and Cats

Elias Westermarck
Maria Wiberg
Jörg M. Steiner
David A. Williams

CANINE EXOCRINE PANCREATIC INSUFFICIENCY

Chronic diseases of the exocrine pancreas may affect pancreatic function and lead to inadequate production of digestive enzymes, which causes maldigestion and then signs typical of exocrine pancreatic insufficiency (EPI). EPI is a functional diagnosis based on measurement of decreased pancreatic secretion capacity by pancreatic function tests. The exocrine pancreas has a large reserve secretory capacity and clinical signs of maldigestion do not occur until 90% of secretory capacity is lost. In dogs, underlying pathologic processes that may result in clinical signs of EPI are pancreatic acinar atrophy (PAA), chronic pancreatitis, pancreatic hypoplasia, and pancreatic neoplasia. Pancreatic acinar atrophy is reported to be by far the most common cause of severe EPI in dogs.[1,2]

Etiology
Pancreatic Acinar Atrophy
Pancreatic Acinar Atrophy (PAA) results from selective destruction of the digestive enzyme producing acinar cells, which may lead to almost complete loss of secretory capacity. The endocrine function of the pancreas usually is unaffected. PAA has been suggested to be a hypoplastic disease because of the young age of the affected dogs. However, general opinion has been that PAA is a progressive disease and it has been shown that the one dog that developed PAA later in life was born with grossly and histologically normal pancreas.[3]

Only a limited number of studies have been assessed the role of different environmental factors, nonmicrobial or microbial,

in the development of PAA. In one study stress was suggested to be a possible triggering factor preceding the clinical disease.[4]

PAA has been reported in many breeds, but it is most common in German shepherd dogs and rough coated Collies. In both breeds, PAA has been suggested to be inherited.[5-7]

Recent studies in German shepherd dogs and rough-coated Collies have shown that PAA has features typical of autoimmune disease. With these two breeds it has been possible to diagnose the disease in a subclinical phase, before development of total acinar atrophy and the manifestation of clinical maldigestion signs.[8,9,10] Genetic susceptibility of the disease and the marked T-lymphocyte infiltration during the progression of acinar atrophy have been taken as primary evidence of autoimmune nature of the disease. The progression of acinar atrophy was divided into a subclinical phase, characterized by partial acinar atrophy and lymphocytic infiltration. The clinical phase is characterized by severe endstage atrophy. As lymphocytic pancreatitis with active destruction of the acinar structures was shown to precede the end-stage atrophy, the term *autoimmune-mediated atrophic lymphocytic pancreatitis* is preferred to describe pathologic findings. Cellular immune mechanisms were shown to have a major role in the tissue destruction.[8-10]

Other Causes of EPI
Chronic pancreatitis is a common cause of EPI in cats and humans. It has been suggested as an underlying cause of EPI in older dogs, but its prevalence is still unclear. In chronic pancreatitis the clinical signs are usually those of nonspecific gastrointestinal disease. In this situation, the endocrine pancreas

may also be affected. In chronic pancreatitis there can be a progressive destruction of both exocrine and endocrine pancreas, with fibrosis. Congenital exocrine or exocrine and endocrine pancreatic hypoplasia in young puppies is sometimes found. In conjunction with pancreatic neoplasia EPI is a rarely reported clinical sign.[1]

Diagnosis
Diagnosis of exocrine pancreatic dysfunction is based on typical findings in clinical histories and clinical signs. It is confirmed with pancreatic function tests. When it is needed to verify the underlying pathological process causing the clinical signs, morphologic examination of the pancreas is performed.

Clinical History and Clinical Signs
Typical clinical signs of EPI include yellowish or gray feces, increased fecal volume and defecation frequency, weight loss, and flatulence. Other signs include abnormally increased appetite; poorly digested, loose, and pulpy feces; and occasional coprophagia. Nervousness or aggressiveness have also been reported, and these are suspected to result from abdominal discomfort due to increased bowel movements and gas formation. Severe watery diarrhea is usually only temporary. Poor hair coat has also been reported in dogs with EPI.[4] Although these clinical signs are typical for EPI, they are not pathognomonic for the disease, as small intestinal disease may cause similar maldigestion signs.

Clinical Pathologic Evaluation
Results of standard laboratory analysis are usually not helpful in diagnosing of EPI. Some dogs have hypocholesterolemia and increases in serum alanine aminotransferase activities. This may reflect hepatocyte damage secondary to increased uptake of hepatotoxic substances through small intestinal mucosa. Serum amylase and lipase concentrations are of no value in diagnosing EPI.[1]

Pancreatic Function Tests
Various pancreatic function tests have been shown to be valuable in confirmation of the diagnosis of clinical EPI. The value of these tests lies of their ability to distinguish whether the clinical signs are due to exocrine pancreatic dysfunction or to small intestinal disease.[1]

Serum Trypsin-like Immunoreactivity
The measurement of serum canine trypsin-like immunoreactivity (cTLI) by radioimmunoassay has become one of the most commonly used pancreatic function tests to diagnose canine EPI. Serum cTLI measurement is species- and pancreas-specific. It measures only pancreatic trypsin and trypsinogen that has entered the bloodstream directly from the pancreas. The reference range for cTLI in healthy dogs is more than 5.0 to 35 µg/L.

Abnormally low serum cTLI concentrations (<2.5 µg/L), in association with the typical clinical signs of maldigestion, are considered highly diagnostic for severe EPI. Because trypsinogen is not absorbed from the intestinal lumen, intestinal disease does not affect cTLI measurement. Serum cTLI measurement is a practical test since usually only a single sample is needed to confirm the clinical diagnosis of EPI. Fasting samples (8 to 12 hours) are recommended as a postprandial increase of serum trypsinogen levels, even though slight and transient, may occur. Because trypsinogen is eliminated by glomerular filtration, renal dysfunction associated with pancreatic disease can cause a rise in serum cTLI.[11]

Fecal Proteolytic Activity
Low fecal proteolytic activity has been reported in dogs with severe EPI. The reliability of different fecal proteolytic activity tests varies. The X-ray film test is a simple method but not reliable. More valuable, semiquanititative methods for measuring fecal proteolytic activity are the azocasein method and radial enzyme diffusion into agar containing a casein substrate. Fecal proteolytic activity should be measured in repeated samples because of considerable daily variations in results and because healthy dogs may occasionally pass feces with low proteolytic activity. To prevent incorrect abnormal results, fecal proteolytic activity has been measured after giving dogs raw soybean in their food and determining activities by a radial enzyme diffusion method in fecal samples for 3 days (soybean stimulation test).[12]

Fecal Elastase Activity
A new fecal test for diagnosing exocrine pancreatic dysfunction is the measurement of fecal elastase using the ELISA method. Canine fecal elastase is a species- and pancreas-specific test. A single fecal sample is adequate for diagnosing severe EPI and an elastase concentration of less than 10 µg/g in association with clinical signs of EPI is suggestive of severe dysfunction. A drawback of this test is that abnormal results can occasionally be found in normal dogs.[13]

Diagnosis of Subclinical EPI and Partial PAA
Serum cTLI values within the subnormal range of 2.5 to 5.0 µg/L have been shown to reflect decreased pancreatic function and can be used for the early diagnosis of EPI. In breeds predisposed to PAA, cTLI measurement can be used for diagnosis of the subclinical disease. Repeatedly subnormal serum cTLI values in dogs showing no typical signs of EPI indicate subclinical EPI and suggest partial PAA.

Despite low fasting serum cTLI values, the reserve secretory capacity of the pancreas may prevent the appearance of clinical signs. Some of the dogs with a subclinical disease may have cTLI values of less than 2.5 µg/L. To diagnose subclinical disease, repeated cTLI measurements are needed to increase the accurance of the diagnosis. One single subnormal value is not diagnostic for pancreatic dysfunction. In addition overlapping of cTLI results between subclinical and normal dogs is possible. A normal cTLI (>5.0 µg/L) does not exclude mild to moderate pancreatic dysfunction.[8]

Verification of Underlying Pathologic Process
Pancreatic morphologic examination is performed when it is necessary to identify the underlying pathologic process causing pancreatic dysfunction. In dogs with either partial or end-stage PAA, the clinical histories, clinical signs, and results of function tests are usually highly suggestive of the underlying pathologic process. With breeds predisposed to PAA, morphologic examination is rarely needed. Morphologic examination can be useful in atypical cases. The disadvantage of laparotomy and laparoscopy is that they are invasive methods. Further, the morphologic changes in the pancreas are usually unevenly distributed, thus the severity of findings is greatly dependent on the site of biopsy. Pancreatic biopsies can be taken by laparotomy to dissect a small pancreatic sample or by laparoscopy using crushing forceps.[3]

Treatment
Treatment and Prognosis of Subclinical EPI
Asymptomatic dogs with partial PAA and subclinical EPI do not need any treatment. The speed of the progression of atrophy from subclinical to clinical phase is variable, and the factors affecting the speed of progression are not yet identified. Early immunosuppressive treatment to halt the progression of the autoimmune mediated tissue destruction has been considered to prevent the clinical disease.

Long-term follow-up of the dogs with partial PAA and subclinical EPI showed that the value of immunosuppressive treatment in slowing acinar atrophy is questionable. Dogs may stay in the subclinical phase for years or sometimes for life with or without medication. No diagnostic markers predicting which dogs will develop clinical disease have been found, thus immunosuppressive treatment is not recommended.[14] Some dogs with partial PAA may show chronic or intermittent gastrointestinal signs not typical for EPI. The gastrointestinal signs may be due to subnormal pancreatic function or an underlying small intestinal disease or a combination of both. The diagnostic workup and treatment for possible concurrent small intestinal disease is recommended. If no underlying small intestinal disorder is identified, a trial treatment with pancreatic enzymes should be initiated.[14]

Treatment and Prognosis of Clinical EPI

Enzyme replacement therapy When clinical signs of EPI appear, enzyme replacement therapy is indicated. Basic treatment for EPI is supplementation of each meal with enzyme extracts. Various pancreatic enzyme extracts are available. In dogs, the highest enzyme activity in the duodenum has been obtained with nonenteric-coated supplements; like raw chopped pancreas or powdered enzymes. In clinical trials, these two supplements have proved to be equally effective in controlling clinical signs. The choice between the preparations is therefore based on practical properties, availability, and costs. In many countries the use of raw pancreas is not allowed because of possibilities of zoonotic diseases. The maintenance dosage for the powdered enzyme preparation is usually 1 tsp/meal, and for raw, chopped pancreas 50 to 100 g/meal for dogs that weigh 20 to 35 kg. The value of enteric-coated supplements has been demonstrated to be limited in dogs because of the delayed gastric emptying of the preparations.[1,15]

Supportive treatments When the treatment response to nonenteric-coated enzyme supplements and ordinary dog food is not satisfactory, the supportive therapies should be considered.

Orally administered enzymes are largely destroyed by gastric acid and despite accurate enzyme therapy the digestive capacity does not return to normal. In some dogs the increase of enzyme dosage or change to another nonenteric-coated enzyme supplement may be beneficial. Inhibition of gastric acid secretion by H_2-antagonist has shown some positive effects. The routine use of H_2-antagonists is not recommended but is indicated when response to enzyme treatment is poor. Preincubation enzymes in food before feeding and supplementing with bile salts or antacids have been recommended to increase the efficiency of enzyme supplementation, but with no proven efficiency.[1]

Dietary modification Clinical feeding studies have shown controversial results on the actual benefits of using special diets. In general, no dietary modification is needed and the dogs may continue to be fed with their ordinary food. However, special attention should be paid to individual needs and radical dietary changes should be avoided.[1,15]

In those dogs that do not show the satisfactory treatment response, dietary modification may be useful. A highly digestible, low-fiber and moderate-fat diet has shown to be able to alleviate such clinical signs as flatulence, borborygmi, increased fecal volume, and defecation frequency. Highly digestible diets may be of particular value in the initial treatment until nutritional status has improved. A low-fat diet has been considered to be valuable because enzyme supplements alone are unable to restore normal fat absorption. Lipase is most easily destroyed by gastric acid. Fat absorption may be affected also by the bacterial deconjugation of bile salts in a small intestinal disease, producing metabolites, which in turn may result in diarrhea. Dietary sensitivities may be a consequence of EPI. Therefore hypoallergenic diets may benefit some dogs with EPI, especially in the early treatment. No obvious clinical benefits have been demonstrated with adding medium-chain triglycerides to food.

Antibiotics Antibiotics are the most commonly used adjunctive medications in treatment of EPI. Small intestinal bacterial overgrowth is common in dogs with EPI before and during enzyme replacement treatment. An increased amount of substrate for bacteria in the small intestinal lumen, a lack of bacteriostatic factors present in normal pancreatic juice, and changes in intestinal motility and immune functions are possible reasons for an abnormal accumulation of bacteria in the small intestine of dogs with EPI. Antibiotics have particularly been used during initial treatment in cases of poor treatment response to enzymes alone and when clinical signs, such as diarrhea, borborygmus, and flatulence have recurred during long-term treatment. Antibiotics reported to be effective are tylosin, oxytetracyclin, and metronidazole. Usually treatment with antibiotics for 1 to 3 weeks is effective.[1,15]

Cobalamin Cobalamin deficiency is common in dogs with EPI. This deficiency is partly due to an increased uptake of cobalamin by intestinal bacteria and partly because of the lack of pancreatic intrinsic factor, demonstrated to have a major role in the absorption of cobalamin. Enzyme supplementation alone has not been found to be helpful for increasing serum cobalamin levels. Parenteral cobalamin treatment is needed when low serum cobalamin values are detected. The clinical signs of cobalamin deficiency are still poorly documented in canine EPI. The doses for cobalamin recommended are 250 to 500 μg parenterally. The vitamin treatment should be repeated based on the serum levels.[1,15]

Other supportive treatments Malabsorption of fat soluble vitamins may be suspected in dogs with EPI. The clinical importance of vitamin A, D, E, K deficiency in dogs has not been reported. When treatment responses to enzymes and supportive therapies are insufficient, concomitant small intestinal disease and lymphoplasmacytic enteritis should be suspected. To date, no comprehensive studies on EPI and associated small intestinal diseases have been published. Glucocorticoids treatment is not recommended.[1]

Prognosis

Usually a lifelong enzyme treatment is needed. Response to enzyme treatment is usually seen during the first weeks of treatment, with weight gain, decrease in polyphagia and fecal volume, and cessation of diarrhea. The level of treatment response achieved during the initial treatment period seems to remain rather stable. Although some dogs show short relapses of clinical signs, usually no permanent deterioration of clinical condition is seen during the long-term enzyme treatment.[1,15]

During long-term treatment with nonenteric-coated supplements, 50% of dogs are almost totally controlled. However, despite similar treatment regimes, the treatment response has been shown to be variable, and about 20% of EPI dogs have a poor response. Although it is not always possible to eliminate all the signs, good resolution is found especially for more serious signs such as continuous diarrhea and malnutrition. Why some clinical signs are incompletely controlled and others so variable is not completely understood.

About 20% of the dogs diagnosed for EPI are euthanized during the first year after diagnosis. The most common reason for euthanasia is poor response to treatment. Another reason is owner reluctance for expensive and lifelong treatment.[15,16] A rare, but severe complication of EPI is mesenteric torsion.

The etiology of mesenteric torsion remains unclear. Today mesenteric torsion is rare, probably because of the improvement of treatment regimes for EPI.

FELINE EXOCRINE PANCREATIC INSUFFICIENCY

Exocrine pancreatic insufficiency (EPI), although uncommon, does occur in cats and therefore should be considered in the differential diagnosis for weight loss and diarrhea in this species. Although the pathophysiology, etiology, diagnosis, and treatment are similar to those of EPI in dogs, there are some important differences.[17] Chronic pancreatitis is the most common cause of EPI in the cat. Rare cases of EPI without pancreatitis have been reported due to duct obstruction associated with *Eurytrema procyonis* infestation. Adenocarcinomas of the exocrine pancreas can lead to obstruction of the pancreatic duct, followed by atrophy of acinar tissue. Finally, the authors are aware of several reports of pancreatic acinar atrophy (PAA) that is histologically indistinguishable from that so commonly observed in dogs; whether the pathophysiology in such cases is the same as in dogs is not known.[17]

Classical clinical signs include loose, malodorous, and voluminous stools, with poor body condition. Weight loss, even in untreated cases, is rarely as extreme as in untreated dogs. As in dogs, polyphagia is not an invariable sign. It should be emphasized that most cats with polyphagia, weight loss, and diarrhea are ultimately diagnosed as having small intestinal disease associated with severe cobalamin deficiency. These cases are clinically indistinguishable from those with EPI. Indeed, the frequent occurrence of severely subnormal serum cobalamin concentrations, and somewhat less commonly serum folate concentrations, in cats with EPI (abnormalities seen far less often in dogs), indicate that many have severe concurrent small intestinal disease leading to vitamin malabsorption. Cats with EPI may exhibit a greasy, wet-looking and generally unkempt hair coat, especially in the perineal region, which may in part reflect severe cobalamin deficiency.

The differential diagnosis for cats with weight loss, diarrhea, and changes in appetite include chronic small intestinal disease (most commonly inflammatory bowel disease), hyperthyroidism, and diabetes mellitus. In older cats these conditions may be concurrent. Owing to the underlying pathophysiology of EPI in cats, diabetes mellitus is a far more frequent complication of EPI than it is in dogs. It has been reported that more than 50% of cats with diabetes mellitus have pancreatitis. Although it is unknown if this is a cause-and-effect or coincidental relationship, some of these patients do develop EPI.

Results of hematologic and serum biochemical testing, and abdominal radiography or ultrasonography are generally unremarkable, although lymphopenia, lymphocytosis, neutrophilia, eosinophilia, and elevations of hepatic enzymes have been reported sporadically. Many specific tests to evaluate exocrine pancreatic function in cats are either impractical or unreliable, including the bentiromide absorption test, plasma turbidity, microscopic examination of feces for undigested fat, starch, or muscle fibers. Fecal proteolytic activity (FPA) can be determined by either azocasein- or azoalbumin-based methods, or by a radial enzyme diffusion method, and most cats with EPI have undetectable FPA. Unfortunately, this finding is not specific for EPI; FPA is somewhat labile, and few diagnostic laboratories determine FPA using reliable assay methods. Furthermore, the requirement to collect and assay several fecal samples makes this approach expensive and inconvenient. Fortunately, a highly reliable and economical species specific radioimmunoassay for feline trypsin-like immunoreactivity (fTLI) has been developed and validated, and shown to be accurate in the diagnosis of feline EPI.[18,19] Similar to the situation in dogs, severely decreased serum fTLI concentration is diagnostic for EPI in the cats. The fTLI is presently only run at the laboratory directed by two of the authors, but serum fTLI is very stable and samples can readily be shipped worldwide directly to this laboratory. Numerous commercial laboratories will also forward samples to this laboratory on request.

Treatment

Cats with EPI will at least require dietary supplementation with pancreatic enzymes for resolution of clinical signs. It is important to recognize that in most cats, treatments in addition to enzyme supplementation will be required to achieve an optimal response. Dried powdered extracts (give 0.5 teaspoonfuls per meal) of porcine pancreas are available (e.g., Viokase, Pancrezyme, PancreVed). Tablets, capsules, and enteric-coated formulations are usually less effective. Raw pancreas (1 to 2 oz per meal) can also be offered and can be stored frozen for several months prior to feeding. Preincubation of the food with pancreatic enzymes, supplementation with bile salts, or concurrent antacid therapy are unnecessary.[17]

Since cats with EPI almost always have extreme depletion of total body cobalamin stores and undetectable serum cobalamin, it is not surprising that parenteral cobalamin (100 to 250 µg subcutaneously once weekly) is often beneficial. Uncorrected cobalamin deficiency may lead to villous atrophy, intestinal inflammation, and malasborption, with resultant failure to respond to pancreatic enzymes alone. Serum folate concentration is also subnormal in many affected cats, and in some cases serum concentrations can be very low. Oral folate supplementation (400 µg daily orally) will rectify any deficiency. Serum cobalamin and folate concentrations should be routinely evaluated in cats with suspected EPI and periodically assessed following initiation of therapy since deficiencies often recur. Some affected cats also have hypovitaminosis K, and if untreated this can lead to bleeding disorders, which can be fatal if they go unrecognized.

Some cats will not respond appropriately to enzyme supplementation and cobalamin and/or folate supplementation. These cats usually have concurrent small intestinal disease, perhaps associated with abnormal proliferation of bacteria in the upper intestine. In these cases treatment with oral prednisolone (initial dose 5 mg twice daily for 1 to 2 weeks) and/or oral metronidazole (100 mg twice daily for 2 to 4 weeks) is often beneficial. Long-term treatment with either antibiotics nor glucocorticoid is usually not required.

SECTION
XVI

Endocrine Disorders

CHAPTER 235

Acromegaly and Pituitary Dwarfism

Hans S. Kooistra

GROWTH HORMONE

Growth hormone (GH) is a rather large single-chain polypeptide with a molecular weight of approximately 22 kDalton. The amino acid sequence of GH varies considerably between different species. The amino acid sequence of canine GH is, however, identical to that of porcine GH.[1]

Like the other hormones of the pituitary anterior lobe, GH is secreted in a pulsatile fashion. Pituitary GH secretion is regulated mainly by the opposing actions of the stimulatory hypothalamic peptide GH-releasing hormone (GHRH) and the inhibitory hypothalamic peptide somatostatin (Figure 235-1). The GH pulses predominantly reflect the pulsatile delivery of GHRH, whereas GH levels between pulses are primarily under somatostatin control. The release of GHRH and somatostatin is controlled by complex neural regulatory mechanisms. GH release can also be elicited by synthetic GH secretagogues. These GH secretagogues exert their effect on GH release by acting through receptors different from those for GHRH. In 1999 Kojima et al characterized the endogenous ligand for these receptors and called it *ghrelin*.[2] The main source of circulating ghrelin, which also is stimulatory for canine GH[3], appears to be the stomach.

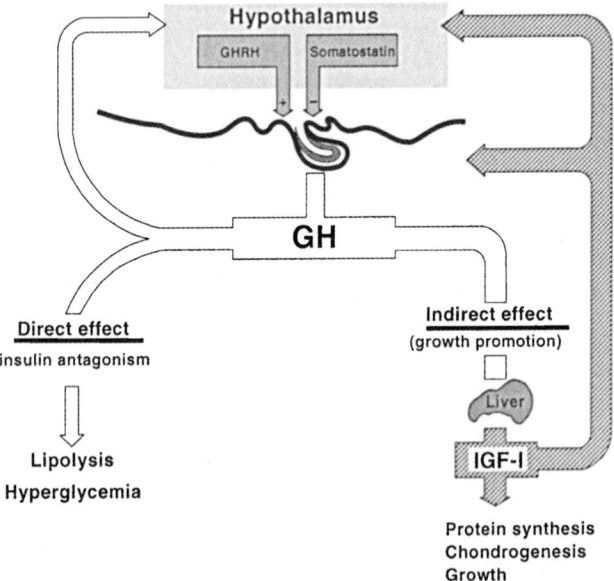

Figure 235-1 The pituitary secretion of GH is under inhibitory (somatostatin) and stimulatory (GHRH) hypothalamic control and is also modulated by negative feedback control of IGF-I and GH itself. The direct catabolic (diabetogenic) actions of GH are shown on the left side of the figure, and the indirect anabolic actions are shown on the right. (Redrawn from Rijnberk A, editor: *Clinical endocrinology of dogs and cats*, Dordrecht, The Netherlands, 1996, Kluwer Academic Publishers.)

In the dog, circulating GH not only originates from the pituitary but also may be of mammary origin. In the 1970s and 1980s it was shown that administration of progestins to dogs could lead to elevated plasma GH levels. These progestin-stimulated plasma GH levels do not have a pulsatile secretion pattern, are not sensitive to stimulation with GHRH or the α-adrenergic agonist clonidine, and are not inhibited by somatostatin, which points to autonomous secretion. Furthermore it was shown that the progestin-induced elevated plasma GH levels do not decrease after hypophysectomy, which indicates that this GH originates from an extrapituitary site. In 1994 Selman et al published that the progestin-induced GH production in the dog originates from foci of hyperplastic ductular epithelium of the mammary gland.[4] It was also demonstrated that mammary GH is biochemically identical to pituitary GH and that the gene encoding GH in the mammary gland is identical to the gene in the pituitary gland.

The pulsatile secretion pattern of GH changes during progression of the luteal phase of the estrous cycle of healthy bitches, with higher basal GH secretion and less GH secreted in pulses during stages with a high plasma progesterone concentration.[5] It is likely that this is caused by a partial suppression of pituitary GH release by progesterone-induced GH production in the mammary gland. This indicates that progestin-induced mammary GH production is not just an aberration but a normal physiologic event during the luteal phase of the estrous cycle in healthy cyclic bitches. The GH-receptor is also present in the mammary gland, which supports the concept that the progesterone-induced mammary GH production may promote the physiologic proliferation of mammary gland tissue and the preparation for lactation during the luteal phase by local autocrine and paracrine effects. High concentrations of GH have also been found in mammary secretions, particularly in colostrum.[6] The high GH levels in colostrum, often 100 to 1000 times higher than plasma GH levels, may be of importance for the gastrointestinal development of neonates. The progestin-induced mammary GH production may also play a role in mammary gland tumor development or tumor progression.[7]

The effects of circulating GH can be divided into two main categories: rapid catabolic actions and slow (long-lasting) hypertrophic actions. The acute catabolic actions are mainly due to insulin antagonism and result in enhanced lipolysis, gluconeogenesis, and restricted glucose transport across the cell membrane. The net effect of these catabolic actions is promotion of hyperglycemia. The slow anabolic effects are mainly mediated via insulin-like growth factors (IGFs). IGFs are produced in many different tissues, and in most of these tissues they have a local (paracrine or autocrine) growth-promoting effect. The main source of circulating IGF-I is the liver. The chemical structure of IGFs has about 50% sequence similarity with insulin. In contrast to insulin, IGFs are bound to binding proteins (IGFBPs). As a result of this binding to carrier proteins they have a prolonged half-life, which is consistent with long-term growth-promoting effects. IGFs are important determinants in the regulation of body size, by stimulating protein synthesis, chondrogenesis, and growth. There is increasing evidence that GH exerts its growth-promoting effect not only via IGFs but also by a direct effect on the cells.

IGF-I exerts an inhibitory effect on GH release, by stimulating the release of somatostatin and by a direct inhibitory influence at the pituitary level. In addition, GH itself has a negative feedback effect at the hypothalamic level (see Figure 235-1).

ACROMEGALY

Pathogenesis

Acromegaly is a syndrome of bony and soft tissue overgrowth and insulin resistance due to excessive GH secretion. The pathogenesis of acromegaly is completely different in dogs and cats. In middle-aged and elderly female dogs, either endogenous progesterone (luteal phase of the estrous cycle) or exogenous progestins (used for estrus prevention) may give rise to GH hypersecretion of mammary origin. In the cat, acromegaly is caused by an acidophilic pituitary adenoma that secretes excessive amounts of GH. The condition is encountered most often in middle-aged and elderly, predominantly male, cats. Progestins may also induce GH expression in mammary tissue in the cat, but the hormone does not seem to reach the systemic circulation.

Clinical Manifestations

Signs and symptoms of GH hypersecretion tend to develop slowly and are characterized initially (particularly in the dog) by soft tissue swelling of the face and the abdomen. In some acromegalic dogs severe hypertrophy of soft tissues of the mouth, tongue (Figure 235-2), and pharynx causes snoring and even dyspnea. Affected dogs may also have polyuria (and sometimes polyphagia). The polyuria is usually without glucosuria, but manifest diabetes mellitus can develop due to insulin resistance. Physical examination may reveal thick skin folds, (especially in the neck), prognathism, and wide interdental spaces. Prolonged GH excess also leads to generalized visceromegaly, which results in abdominal enlargement. Laboratory investigations in dogs with acromegaly may demonstrate hyperglycemia and/or an abnormal glucose tolerance test. Plasma alkaline phosphatase activities may also be increased. This may, in part, be due to the intrinsic glucocorticoid activity of progestins.

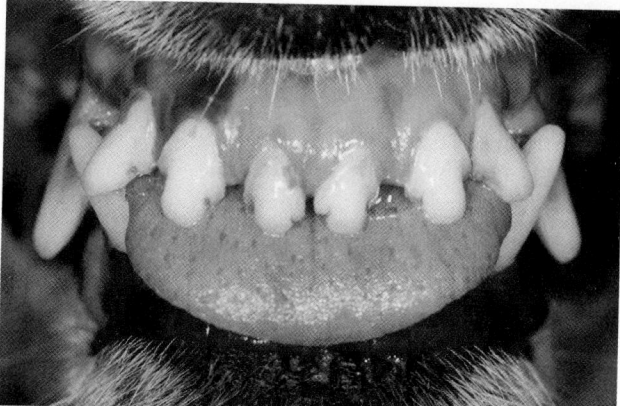

Figure 235-2 The mouth of a 4-year-old beagle dog with progestin-induced GH excess. Note the hyperplasia of the gingiva, the widening of the interdental spaces and the relatively large tongue.

The physical changes in cats tend to be less pronounced than in dogs. The head may also become somewhat massive and may have rather pronounced features. The most common problem in acromegalic cats is (severe) insulin-resistant diabetes mellitus. There may also be proliferative changes that lead to a progressive degenerative arthropathy with lameness. Affected cats may have dyspnea due to hypertrophic cardiomyopathy and subsequent heart failure. Finally, when the pituitary adenoma causing acromegaly becomes large, it may cause neurological signs. For many acromegalic cats the only routine laboratory changes are the hyperglycemia and glucosuria due to the secondary diabetes mellitus.

Diagnosis

Acromegaly is an uncommon condition in diabetic cats. Conversely, insulin resistance or "apparent insulin resistance" is quite common in cats with diabetes mellitus. Thus the diagnosis of acromegaly should be considered only after all other causes for blood glucose concentrations that are persistently increased are eliminated from the differential diagnosis. A complete discussion of feline diabetes mellitus and its management strategy is provided in Chapter 241.

The diagnosis of GH excess can generally be established by measuring basal plasma GH levels. The basal plasma GH level in acromegalic animals often exceeds the upper limit of the reference range (6 µg/L). However, if the disease is mild or just beginning, the basal plasma GH concentration may be only slightly increased. Conversely, a high value may be the result of a secretory pulse in a normal animal. Nonresponsiveness of normal or increased plasma GH concentrations to stimulation may further support the diagnosis.[8] Because of the variation in amino acid sequence of GH in different species, GH should be determined in a homologous radioimmunoassay. Fortunately, feline GH can be measured reliably in a radioimmunoassay developed for the dog.

Measurement of plasma IGF-I concentration may also contribute to the diagnosis. As reviewed, the circulating IGF-I concentration is GH-dependent. Being bound to proteins, the IGF-I concentration is less subject to fluctuation than is GH. However, there is some overlap in plasma IGF-I concentrations between healthy animals and those with acromegaly. In addition, it has been reported that there may be increases in plasma IGF-I levels in diabetic cats unrelated to acromegaly. The amino acid sequence of IGF-I is less species specific than that of GH and therefore IGF-I can be determined in a heterologous (human) assay.

Excessive GH secretion in cats is due to a pituitary adenoma. Consequently, when acromegaly has been demonstrated in a cat, the pituitary should be visualized by computed tomography (CT) or magnetic resonance imaging (MRI) (Figure 235-3).

Treatment

Acromegaly in dogs can be treated easily and effectively by discontinuation of exogenous progestins and/or ovario(hyster)ectomy. The animal may then change dramatically due to the reversal of the soft tissue changes. The bony changes appear to be irreversible but do not seem to cause problems. For dogs in which the GH excess did not lead to complete exhaustion of the pancreatic β-cells, the elimination of the progesterone source by ovario(hyster)ectomy may prevent persistent diabetes mellitus. In case of recent administration of exogenous progestins, synthetic progesterone receptor blockers may be useful, but experience with long-term administration of this class of drugs is lacking. In the end one may even decide for total mammectomy.

In cats treatment should be directed at the pituitary tumor. In principle, there are three options: hypophysectomy, irradiation, and medication. There is little experience with any of

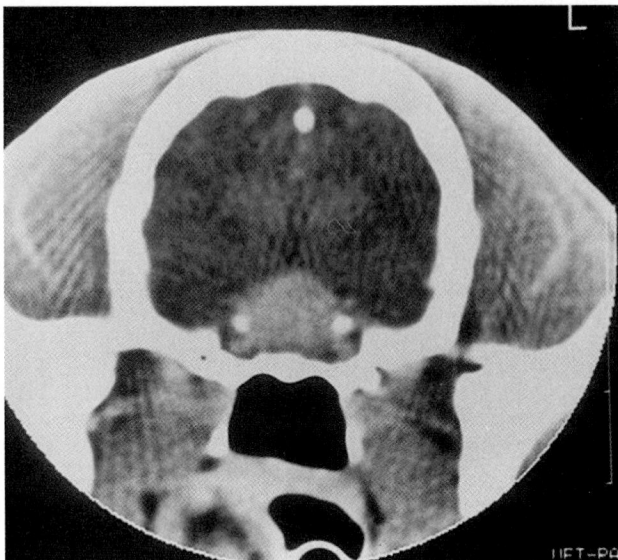

Figure 235-3 Contrast-enhanced CT scanning of the pituitary fossa, in a 10-year-old castrated male cat with diabetes mellitus and acromegaly, showing a large pituitary tumor. (From Rijnberk A, editor: *Clinical endocrinology of dogs and cats*, Dordrecht, The Netherlands, 1996, Kluwer Academic Publishers.)

the three. Medical treatment with drugs such as dopamine agonists does not seem to be effective. Long-acting somatostatin analogues have been shown to lower circulating GH levels in a single cat.[9] In others the drug was not effective. Therefore due to expense and lack of efficacy, it is questionable whether this drug will be used in clinical practice. The development of GH-receptor antagonists such as pegvisomant used in humans may hold promise for dogs and cats with acromegaly. Cobalt irradiation may result in temporary improvement and in (transient) discontinuation of insulin therapy.[10] Transspheniodal hypophysectomy has been performed successfully in cats with hyperadrenocorticism due to a pituitary corticotroph adenoma[11] and may also become an effective treatment option for cats with acromegaly.

PITUITARY DWARFISM

Pathogenesis
Any defect in the organogenesis of the pituitary gland may result in a form of isolated or combined pituitary hormone deficiency. Congenital GH deficiency or pituitary dwarfism is the most striking example of pituitary hormone deficiency. Congenital GH deficiency has been mentioned to occur in cats and different dog breeds.[12] However, the condition is encountered most often as a simple, autosomal recessive inherited abnormality in the German shepherd dog. Inherited pituitary dwarfism in German shepherd dogs is due to combined pituitary hormone deficiency. German shepherd dwarfs have a combined deficiency of GH, TSH, and prolactin together with impaired release of gonadotropins. In contrast, ACTH secretion in German shepherd dwarfs is preserved (Figure 235-4).[13]

Originally, pituitary dwarfism in the German shepherd dog breed has been ascribed to pressure atrophy of the pituitary anterior lobe by cyst formation in Rathke's pouch. Indeed, in most German shepherd dwarfs pituitary cysts are present. However, at a young age German shepherd dwarfs sometimes have no or only a very small pituitary cyst, unlikely to be responsible for pressure atrophy. Also the finding that the ACTH secretion is preserved in German shepherd dwarfs argues against cyst formation in Rathke's pouch as the primary cause of pituitary dwarfism in this breed. It is therefore more likely that the disorder is caused by a primary failure of differentiation of the craniopharyngeal ectoderm into normal tropic-hormone-secreting pituitary cells. In this view in German shepherd dwarfs the cyst formation in Rathke's pouch is rather a consequence of an underlying genetic defect than the cause of dwarfism.

Clinical Manifestations
By 2 to 5 months of age, pituitary dwarfs usually have proportionate growth retardation and an abnormally soft and woolly hair coat (Figure 235-5). The latter is due to retention of lanugo or secondary hairs and lack of primary or guard hairs. The lanugo hairs are easily epilated and there is gradual development of truncal alopecia, beginning at the points of wear. The alopecia typically spares the head and extremities. The skin becomes progressively hyperpigmented and scaly. Secondary bacterial infections of the skin are quite common. In male dwarfs unilateral or bilateral cryptorchidism is common, whereas in female dwarfs persistent anestrus is common. These abnormalities may be ascribed to the impaired release of gonadotropins.

Initially, pituitary dwarfs are usually lively and alert. With time the animals develop inappetence and become less active. This situation is usually reached at the age of two or three years and has been ascribed to secondary hypothyroidism and impaired renal function.[9]

Diagnosis
Although the physical characteristics of pituitary dwarfism may be obvious, other endocrine and nonendocrine causes of growth retardation and alopecia have to be excluded.

Routine laboratory examination usually does not reveal abnormalities, except for an elevated plasma creatinine concentration. GH deficiency is associated with maldevelopment of the glomeruli. In addition, renal function may be impaired due to a functionally decreased glomerular filtration rate as a result of the deficiencies of GH and thyroid hormones. As indicated above (see also Figure 235-4) the combined pituitary hormone deficiency includes secondary hypothyroidism. Consequently, a low plasma TSH concentration in combination with a plasma thyroxine level below the reference range is a common finding in pituitary dwarfs. Plasma IGF-I concentrations are also decreased in pituitary dwarfs, even when age and body size are taken into account. Nevertheless, a definitive diagnosis should rely on measurements of circulating GH concentration.

Since basal plasma GH values may also be low in healthy animals, the definitive diagnosis GH deficiency is based upon the results of a stimulation test. For this purpose GHRH (1 μg/kg body weight) or α-adrenergic drugs, such as clonidine (10 μg/kg body weight) or xylazine (100 μg/kg body weight), can be used. The plasma GH concentration should be determined immediately before and 20 to 30 minutes after intravenous administration of the stimulant. In healthy dogs, plasma GH concentrations should increase at least two- to fourfold after administration of the stimulant. In dogs with pituitary dwarfism there is no significant rise in circulating GH concentrations. Supra-pituitary stimulation with corticotropin-releasing hormone (CRH), thyrotropin-releasing hormone (TRH), and gonadotropin-releasing hormone (GnRH) may reveal the presence of other pituitary hormone deficiencies.

Diagnostic imaging of the pituitary area (CT or MRI) often reveals the presence of pituitary cysts in dogs with congenital GH deficiency. In the majority of young dogs with pituitary

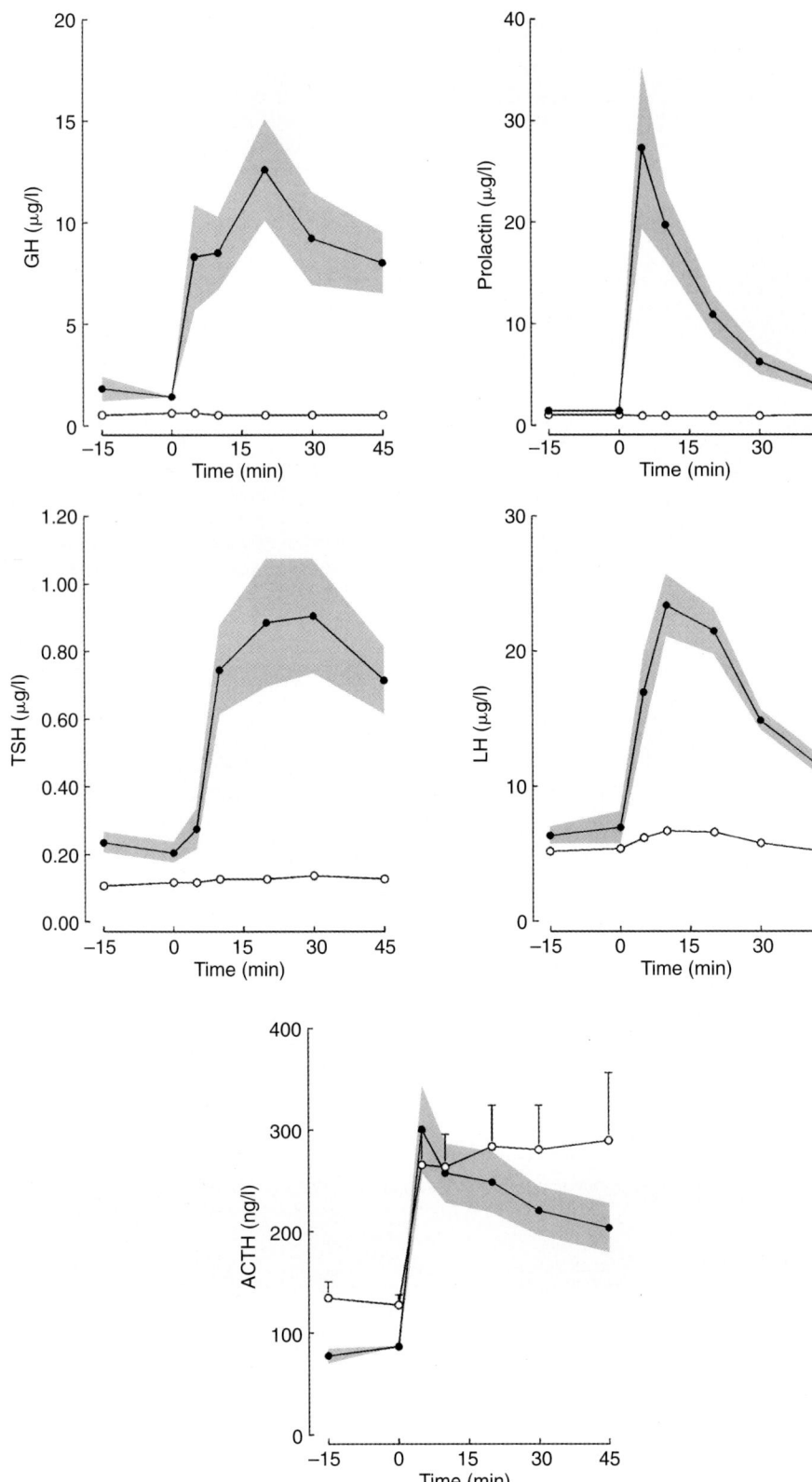

Figure 235-4 Results of a combined pituitary anterior lobe function test (mean and SEM) in eight German shepherd dogs with dwarfism (○) and in eight healthy beagle dogs (●). (From Kooistra HS et al: Combined pituitary hormone deficiency in German shepherd dogs with dwarfism, *Domest Animal Endocrinol* 19:177, 2000.)

dwarfism the pituitary is quite small, in spite of the presence of cysts.[13] This is compatible with pituitary hypoplasia, that is, a lack of endocrine cells in the pituitary anterior lobe. As pituitary dwarfs age the pituitary cysts become larger.[14] It is important to understand that healthy dogs, especially brachycephalic dogs, may have pituitary cysts. Consequently, a definitive diagnosis of pituitary dwarfism cannot be based solely upon the presence of a cyst.

Course

The long-term prognosis of German shepherd dwarfs is usually poor without treatment. By the age of 3 to 5 years

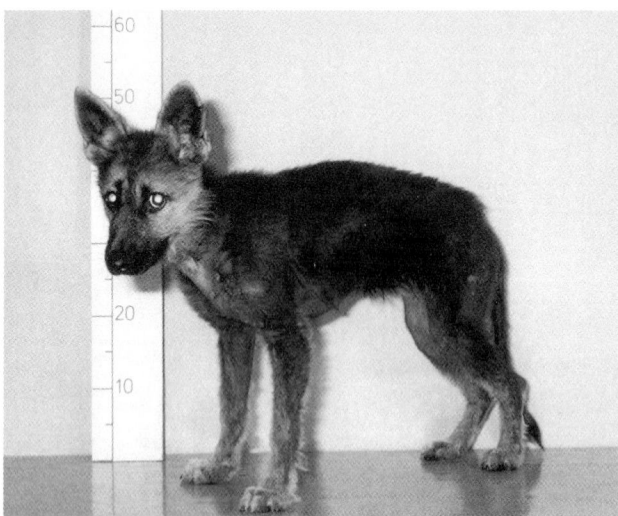

Figure 235-5 A 6-month-old female German shepherd dog with growth retardation, retention of secondary hairs (puppy coat), and lack of primary hairs due to pituitary dwarfism.

the animal has usually become a bald, thin, and dull dog. These changes may be due to (1) progressive loss of pituitary functions, (2) continuing expansion of pituitary cysts, and (3) progressive renal failure. At this stage owners usually request euthanasia for their dog, if they have not done so long before this.[9]

Treatment

The long-term prognosis for German shepherd dwarfs is poor primarily because of the lack of an adequate therapy. Canine GH is not available for therapeutic use and hence there have been attempts to treat dogs that have congenital GH deficiency with porcine or human GH. However, antibody formation precludes the use of biosynthetic human GH.[15] As indicated above the amino acid sequence of porcine GH is

identical to that of canine GH[1], and therefore porcine GH is an option.

The recommended subcutaneous starting dose for heterologous GH is 0.1 to 0.3 IU per kg body weight three times per week for 4 to 6 weeks. This treatment may result in GH excess and consequently side effects such as diabetes mellitus may develop. Weekly monitoring of the plasma concentrations of IGF-I and glucose is therefore of utmost importance. Long-term dose rates after the induction period should also depend on measurements of the plasma concentration of IGF-I. Treatment often does not result in a significant increase in body size, because the growth plates in most dwarfs have already closed or are about to close at the time GH treatment is initiated. The hairs that grow back are primary lanugo hairs; growth of guard hairs is variable.[12]

The demonstration of the ability of progestins to induce the expression of the GH gene in the canine mammary gland and the subsequent release of this GH into the systemic circulation has raised the possibility of treating dogs with congenital GH deficiency with progestins. Treatment of young German shepherd dwarfs with subcutaneous injections of medroxyprogesterone acetate in doses of 2.5 to 5.0 mg per kg body weight, initially at 3-week intervals and subsequently at 6-week intervals, has resulted in some increase in body size and the development of a complete adult hair coat. Parallel with the physical improvements, plasma IGF-I concentrations rose sharply, whereas plasma GH concentrations did rise but never exceeded the upper limit of the reference range.[14] Also treatment of pituitary dwarfs with proligestone has been reported to result in the development of an adult hair coat, increased body weight, and elevated plasma IGF-I concentration.[16]

Treatment of dogs with congenital GH deficiency with progestins may give rise to side effects, such as recurrent periods of pruritic pyoderma and, infrequently, development of mammary tumors. As with the treatment using heterologous GH, monitoring of the plasma concentrations of IGF-I and glucose is important to prevent diabetes mellitus and acromegaly. Bitches should be ovariohysterectomized before the start of the progestin treatment, to prevent development of cystic endometrial hyperplasia. Finally, thyroid hormone replacement should be part of the treatment schedule.

CHAPTER • 236

Diabetes Insipidus

Ad Rijnberk

Diabetes insipidus refers to the passage of large quantities of dilute urine and is actually synonymous with polyuria. In central diabetes insipidus the polyuria results from a lack of sufficient vasopressin to concentrate urine. The disease is characterized by three primary findings: (1) dilute urine despite strong osmotic stimuli for vasopressin secretion, (2) absence of renal disease, (3) a rise in urine osmolality following the administration of vasopressin.

VASOPRESSIN

Vasopressin is released by the posterior lobe or neurohypophysis, which is an extension of the ventral hypothalamus. Together with the other neurohypophyseal hormone oxytocin, vasopressin is synthesized in both the supraoptic and paraventricular nuclei of the hypothalamus, from which axons extend through the pituitary stalk to the posterior pituitary.

The hormones vasopressin and oxytocin are formed by separate neurons and migrate down the axons as part of precursor proteins. They are stored in secretory granules within the nerve terminals in the neurohypophysis and are released by exocytosis into the bloodstream in response to appropriate stimuli. As in most mammals, in dogs and cats arginine-vasopressin (AVP) or antidiuretic hormone (ADH) (in pigs: lysine-vasopressin) plays a vital role in water conservation. Oxytocin stimulates uterine contractions and milk ejection.

The nonapeptide AVP is synthesized as part of a large precursor molecule that is composed of a signal peptide, the hormone, a carrier protein termed neurophysin and a glycopeptide. The major determinant of the release of vasopressin is plasma osmolality. In addition, significant changes in circulating blood volume may influence the setting of the osmoregulation. Specialized neurons called *osmoreceptors* are concentrated in the anterolateral hypothalamus, which is near but separate from the supraoptic nuclei. This area is supplied with blood by small perforating branches of the anterior cerebral arteries. The major role of vasopressin is to regulate body fluid homeostasis by affecting water reabsorption. The antidiuretic effect is achieved by promoting the reabsorption of solute-free water in the distal and collecting tubules of the kidney. The cellular mechanism of AVP activity in the renal tubule involves binding to specific contraluminal V_2-receptor sites, an adenylate cyclase response, and phosphorylation of membrane proteins that lead to transient insertion of water channels in the luminal membrane of the cell. In the presence of these channels water molecules can move passively along an osmotic gradient, that is, from the distal and collecting tubules to the hypertonic renal medulla.

Cations, drugs, and hormones can influence the action of AVP and thereby cause polyuria. Calcium inhibits the adenylate cyclase response to vasopressin. Glucocorticoids also interfere with the action of AVP, although in dogs loss of reactivity of the osmoreceptor system also seems to contribute

to corticosteroid-induced polyuria (Figure 236-1).[1] Even physiologic increases in cortisol inhibit basal vasopressin release in dogs.[2] Although much less pronounced than in the dog, also in humans with hyperadrenocorticism, there is decreased ability to concentrate urine. Interferences of glucocorticoids with vasopressin action, similar to those in dogs, have been reported in man.[3]

PATHOGENESIS

Insufficient AVP release may be caused by defects at several functional sites in the chain of events that regulates discharge of the hormone into the blood. As a result, different forms of central diabetes insipidus can be distinguished. In dogs and cats only two forms have been recognized: complete and partial central diabetes insipidus. In the first type there is very little rise in urine osmolality with increasing plasma osmolality. These animals are essentially devoid of releasable AVP (Figure 236-2). In the second type AVP is released with increasing plasma osmolality but is subnormal in amount (Figure 236-3). In some cases this moderate AVP release only

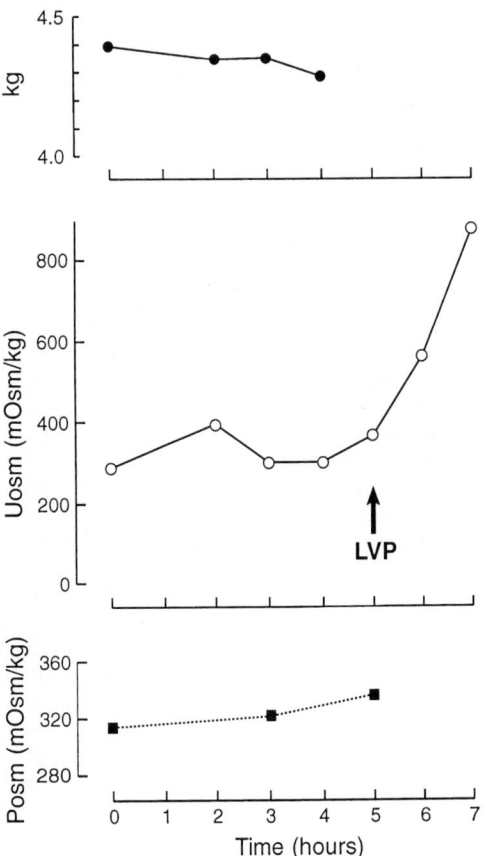

Figure 236-2 The effect of water deprivation on body weight, plasma osmolality *(Posm)* and urine osmolality *(Uosm)* in a 4-year-old castrated male cat with a history of head trauma. The arrow represents an injection of aqueous vasopressin (lysine-vasopressin, LVP). In this case the dehydration-induced rise in Posm did not lead to an increase in Uosm. This in combination with the sharp rise in Uosm following vasopressin administration justified the diagnosis of complete central diabetes insipidus. (Redrawn from Rijnberk A, editor: *Clinical endocrinology of dogs and cats*, Dordrecht/Boston, 1996, Kluwer Academic Publishers.)

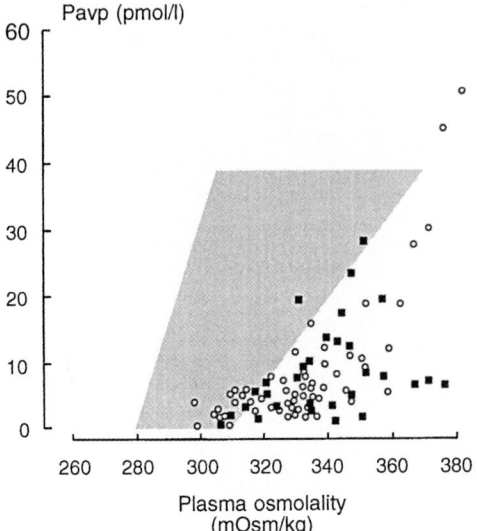

Figure 236-1 Relation of plasma vasopressin *(Pavp)* to plasma osmolality in nine dogs with pituitary-dependent hyperadrenocorticism (○) and six dogs with hyperadrenocorticism due to an adrencortical tumor (■) during hypertonic saline infusion. The gray area represents the range in healthy dogs.[1] (Redrawn from Rijnberk A, editor: *Clinical endocrinology of dogs and cats*, Dordrecht/Boston, 1996, Kluwer Academic Publishers.)

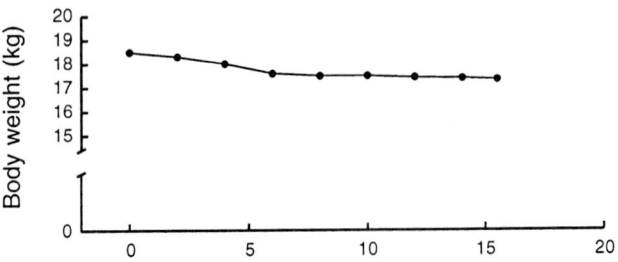

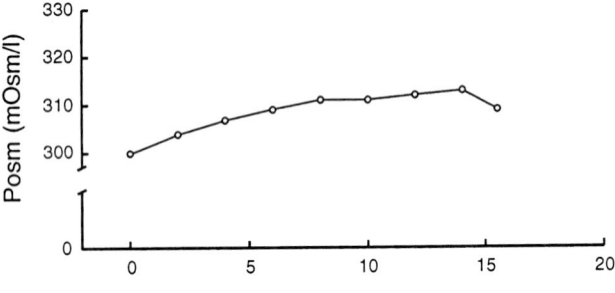

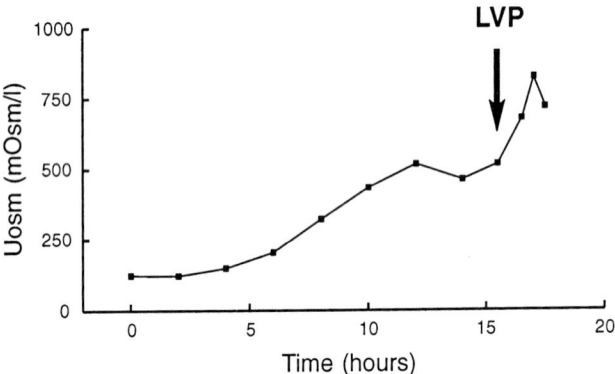

Figure 236-3 In a 5-month-old mongrel dog presented for polyuria, water deprivation led to a slow, subnormal rise in urine osmolality *(Uosm)*. At maximal Uosm, that is, when a "plateau" was reached, vasopressin (lysine-vasopressin, LVP) administration caused a 60% increase in urine osmolality. These observations are compatible with partial central diabetes insipidus. (Redrawn from Rijnberk A, editor: *Clinical endocrinology of dogs and cats,* Dordrecht/Boston, 1996, Kluwer Academic Publishers.)

starts at rather high plasma osmolality values and therefore it may be said that not only is the secretory capacity limited but that there is also a high setting of the osmoreceptor.

Among the lesions leading to impaired vasopressin release, an intracranial tumor is a likely cause in middle-aged and old animals. This is most often a primary pituitary neoplasm, but a craniopharyngioma or a meningioma may also be the causative lesion.[4-7] Metastatic lesions and inflammatory and parasitic lesions may also cause central diabetes insipidus.[8] Severe head injury, usually associated with fractures of the skull, is a rare cause in dogs and cats (see Figure 236-2); spontaneous remission may occur, probably because of regeneration of disrupted axons in the pituitary stalk.[9] There is also a report on a dog with evidence for the combination of anterior pituitary hormone deficiency and diabetes insipidus; in this case the pathogenetic significance of the head trauma at early age was unclear.[10]

An increasingly common cause of central diabetes insipidus is pituitary surgery.[11,12] The diabetes insipidus develops immediately after surgery and in the large majority of cases disappears spontaneously after periods of days to months. When the pituitary stalk is sectioned high enough to induce retrograde degeneration of the hypothalamic neurons, the central diabetes insipidus may be permanent. Finally, there is the possibility of the so-called idiopathic form. This term is used in cases of central diabetes insipidus in which no lesion in the hypothalamic and/or pituitary region can be demonstrated. This diagnosis is most common in young animals, although the course of the disease and/or the autopsy may eventually reveal a lesion that could not be identified initially.[13]

CLINICAL MANIFESTATIONS

The major manifestations are polyuria, polydipsia, and a near-continuous demand for water. These clinical signs may be sudden in onset and the maximum urine flow reached in 1 or 2 days. In severe cases water intake and urine volume may be immense and require micturition almost every hour throughout day and night. However, in the incomplete forms the urine volume may be only moderately increased. In the severe cases the enormous water intake may interfere with food intake and result in weight loss. Animals in which a large neoplasm is the underlying cause may have additional neurologic signs.

The urine concentration will be below that of plasma (specific gravity [SG] <1.010 and urine osmolality [Uosm] <290 mosmol/kg), but in the mild cases higher osmolalities (up to 600 mosmol/kg) may be found. Blood examination usually does not reveal abnormalities except for a slight hypernatremia due to commonly inadequate replenishment of the excreted water. When water is withheld from animals with the complete form of the disease, they develop within a few hours a life-threatening hypertonic encephalopathy (plasma sodium [PNa$^+$] > 170 mmol/l; Posm >375 mosmol/kg), initially characterized by ataxia and stupor. This situation may also be encountered when the causative lesion extends to the thirst center and adipsia develops.[14]

DIFFERENTIAL DIAGNOSIS

Apart from central diabetes insipidus there are in principal only two basic disorders that can account for the polyuria. These disorders are (1) primary polydipsia and (2) nephrogenic diabetes insipidus. Primary polydipsia is said to occur in hyperactive young dogs that are left alone during the day for many hours or have gone through significant changes in their environment. It has been observed that placing of the animal in a completely different environment may stop the problem. In these dogs during serial measurements urine osmolality spontaneously may reach values greater than 1000 mosm/kg. This finding can be regarded as diagnostic and precludes the need for a water deprivation test.[15]

Dogs fulfilling the commonly accepted criteria of primary polydipsia may exhibit abnormalities of vasopressin release. It is not clear whether these changes in vasopressin secretion are the result of the polydipsia and polyuria or may play a causative role.[15]

There are a few individual case reports of congenital nephrogenic diabetes insipidus, the condition in which the kidney tubules are insensitive to the action of antidiuretic hormone. Familial occurrence has been documented in huskies, in which the defect could be ascribed to a mutation affecting the affinity of the V$_2$ receptor for ligand.[16]

However, in addition to these two basic and infrequently encountered differential diagnoses, a wide variety of conditions cause polyuria. In the young animal this may be congenital kidney disease, whereas at all ages acquired kidney disease may lead to polyuria. Especially in the middle-aged and elderly animals endocrine conditions such as diabetes mellitus, hyperadrenocorticism, hyperaldosteronism[17], hyperthyroidism, pyometra, progestin-induced (luteal phase) growth-hormone excess[18], hyperparathyroidism, hypercalcemia of malignancy, tumor-associated polyuria[19], and the syndrome of inappropriate vasopressin secretion[20] have to be considered. In several of these conditions impaired release of vasopressin and/or interference with its action may play a role in the polyuria (see earlier and Figure 236-1). This has been documented for conditions such as hyperadrenocorticism, hepatoencephalopathy, and polycythemia.[1,21,22] In polycythemia it is likely that increased blood volume causes the impairment of vasopressin release. This range of possibilities may make it a difficult task to come to a diagnosis in an animal with polyuria. The algorithm presented in Figure 236-4 may be helpful.

DIAGNOSIS

Urine osmolality (161-2830 mOsm/kg) and urine specific gravity (1.006->1.050) vary widely among healthy pet dogs.[23] In some dogs urine osmolality fluctuates considerably during the day and values close to plasma osmolality may be reached (Figure 236-5). There is experimental evidence that water consumption increases with food intake and exercise.[24] For example, with dry food, dogs consumed 40% of the total daily water intake during 2 hours after food intake. After treadmill running for 30 minutes water intake was higher than the water losses during the excercise.[24] However, it is unlikely that the sometimes strong fluctuations in urine osmolality of pet dogs during the day can be explained solely as an effect of feeding. There may be individual differences in early satiation of thirst, as mediated through oropharyngeal receptors.[23]

Apparently, in most pet dogs, low urine osmolalities are associated with sufficiently high urine osmolalities at other times of the day so that the owners do not perceive their dog to be polydipsic or polyuric. However, in other dogs the situation may be more pronounced and the animals are brought to the veterinarian because of polyuria and polydipsia.[23] Some of these animals may be recognized as having primary polydipsia (see above, section differential diagnosis). Therefore it is advisable to start the evaluation of dogs with polyuria by repeated measurements of urine osmolality and/or urine specific gravity during the day. As in humans, this approach may limit further clinical studies.[25]

The water deprivation test combined with vasopressin administration[26], as exemplified in Figures 236-2 and 236-3, is most commonly used for differentiation of the causes of polyuria. The test is difficult to perform correctly, unpleasant for the animal, relies heavily on the emptying of the bladder, and is indirect because changes in urinary concentration are used as an index of vasopressin release. Furthermore, the stimulus to vasopressin release is a combination of hypertonicity and hypovolemia, especially towards the end of the period of dehydration.

Briefly the procedure is as follows: After 12 hours of fasting, water is withheld and plasma and urine are collected every hour or every 2 hours, depending on the severity of the polyuria. Osmolality is measured in both samples. At each collection, the animal is weighed. When the weight loss approaches 5% of initial body weight, the test should be stopped. When, in the presence of an adequate osmotic stimulus (Posm >305 mOsm/kg), urine concentration is maximal (less than 5% increase in Uosm between consecutive collections), (lysine) vasopressin or a vasopressin analogue such as DDAVP (see below) is administered.

In both nephrogenic diabetes insipidus and central diabetes insipidus Uosm will remain low during water deprivation.

In complete diabetes insipidus Uosm will rise by 50% or more following the administration of vasopressin, whereas in the partial forms of central diabetes insipidus the rise will be greater or equal to 15%, and in nephrogenic diabetes insipidus there will be very little or no rise in Uosm (see Figures 236-2 and 236-3). Probably in part due to the indirect character of the test, the results may not always be conclusive.[27]

A more direct way to differentiate between the three basic causes of polyuria rests on the measurement of plasma vasopressin during osmotic stimulation by hypertonic saline infusion (Figures 236-1 and 236-6).[28] The euhydrated animal is infused for 2 hours through the jugular vein with 20% NaCl solution at a rate of 0.03 mL/kg body weight per minute. Samples for plasma (arginine) vasopressin (AVP) and plasma osmolality are obtained at 20-minute intervals. In the severely polyuric animal there is the risk of inducing critical hypertonicity. The test requires close observation of the animal and monitoring of plasma osmolality. This, and the fact that vasopressin is sensitive to proteolytic breakdown, make it advisable that the test is performed in institutions that have developed experience with the test.[29]

As in humans this approach can improve the diagnostic accuracy. The advantage is not in the severe forms of central diabetes insipidus, as in these conditions the standard indirect test will give a correct diagnosis. In all other categories of polyuria (i.e., in animals that concentrate their urine to various degrees during dehydration), the indirect test may be less reliable. Dogs in which the polyuria had initially been attributed to renal disease or to primary polydipsia proved to have partial central diabetes insipidus in the direct test. However, with regard to primary polydipsia some reservation in the interpretation is needed, as it has been demonstrated for humans that this chronic overhydration downregulates the release of AVP in response to hypertonicity.[28] As indicated above, also in dogs with so-called *primary polydipsia* there are indications for abnormalities in vasopressin release.[15]

The use of this direct approach has been limited so far, but it is worth considering in the few unresolved cases that remain after exclusion of the many other causes of polyuria (see Figure 236-4). It is often a question of whether the animal must endure for many years a life hampered by thirst, a large bladder, and unwanted behavior.

TREATMENT

As for almost all peptides, orally administered vasopressin is ineffective. Aqueous (lysine) vasopressin may be administered subcutaneously in doses of 2 to 5 U. It will act for only about 3 hours. Nevertheless a good response has been reported in one dog, which received 5 U each 48 hours.[6]

The vasopressin analogue desmopressin, (DDAVP, 1-deamino, 9-D-arginine vasopressin)*, provides antidiuretic activity for about 8 hours. One drop (1.5 to 4 µg) placed twice daily in the conjunctival sac sufficiently controls the polyuria in most dogs with central diabetes insipidus. With the administration of three drops a day the urine production usually returns to normal, but some owners (in part for financial reasons) prefer to apply the drug only twice daily. In one report on a cat with partial diabetes insipidus the effect of conjunctivally administered desmopressin was described as poor, which might have been due to incorrect placement because of the cat's struggling.[30] With the injectable preparation (4 µg once a day or every 12 hours) of desmopressin the water consumption could be adequately controlled. The analogue can also be

---

* Minrin, Ferring AB, Malmö, Sweden (0.1 mg DDAVP/mL).

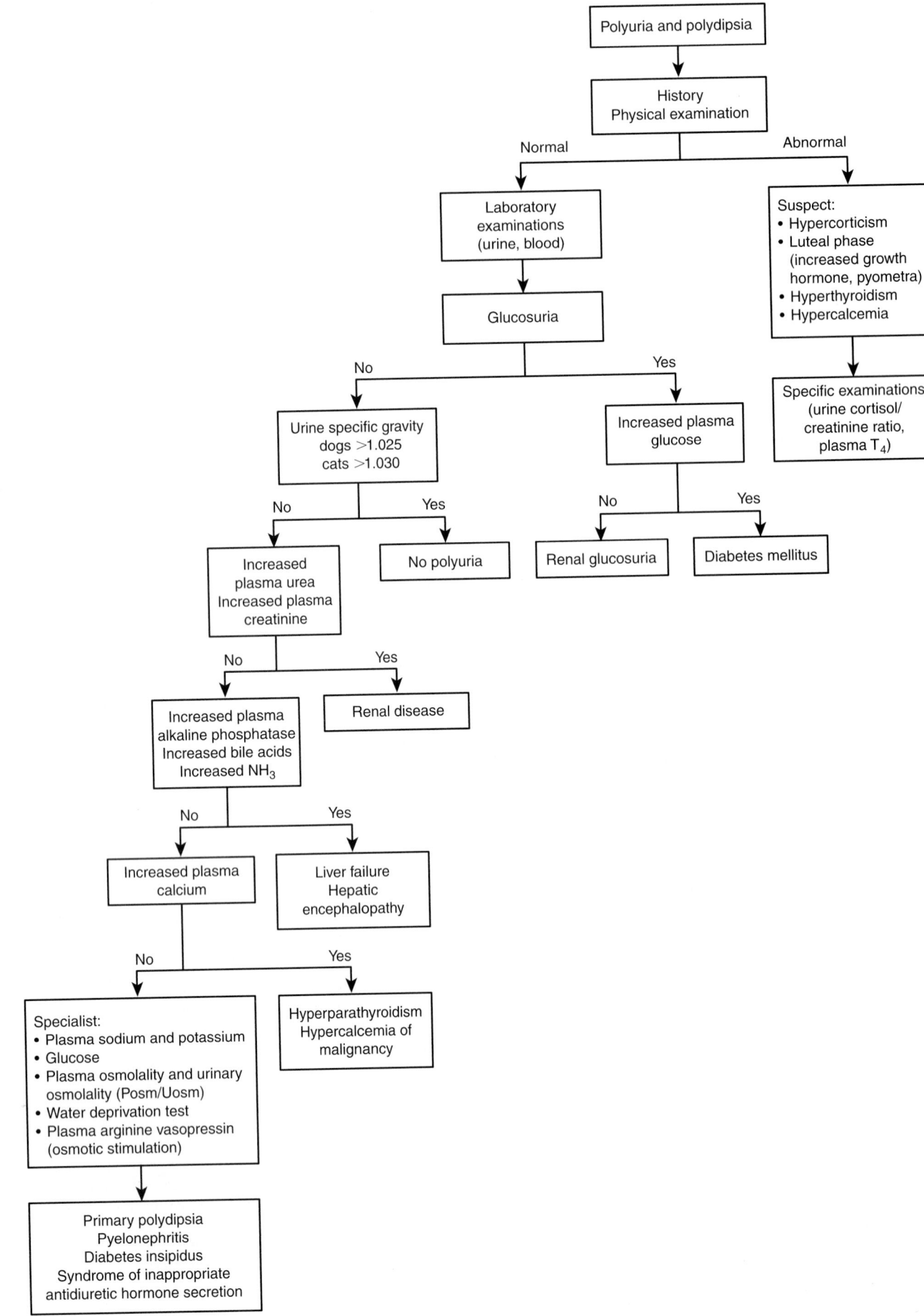

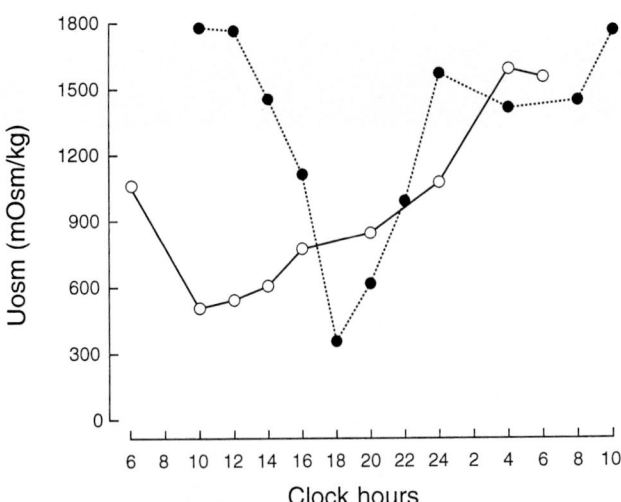

Figure 236-5 Fluctuation of Uosm during the day in a 9½-year-old castrated male Schnauzer (interrupted line) and a female 7½-year-old Belgian Shepherd (uninterrupted line). (Redrawn from Van Vonderen IK et al: Intra- and interindividual variation in urine osmolality and urine specific gravity in healthy pet dogs of various ages, J Vet Intern Med 11:30, 1997.)

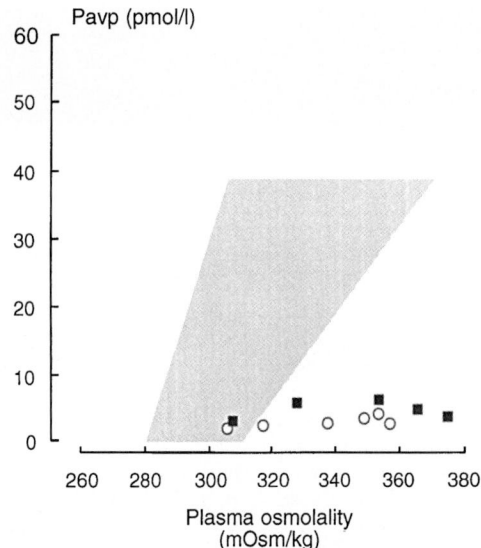

Figure 236-6 Relation of plasma vasopressin with plasma osmolality (Pavp) during hypertonic saline infusion in two dogs with central diabetes insipidus caused by pituitary tumor.[4] See also legend to Figure 236-1. (Redrawn from Rijnberk A, editor: *Clinical endocrinology of dogs and cats*, Dordrecht/Boston, 1996, Kluwer Academic Publishers.)

effective when administered as tablet: one-half tablet of 0.1 or 0.2 mg, two or three times per day, depending on the size of the animal and the effect.

In dogs and cats undergoing hypophysectomy the administration of desmopressin is begun immediately after surgery. In healthy dogs this prevents hypernatremia.[31] In dogs hypophysectomized for pituitary-dependent hyperadrenocorticism mild hypernatremia may occur in the first 24 hours after surgery, despite prophylactic administration of desmopressin. This is probably related to the fact that in these dogs the hypercortisolism-induced vasopressin resistance is insufficiently compensated in the postoperative period by infusions and water intake.[11]

In cases of polyuria, in which all of the above mentioned differential diagnoses have been excluded, including central diabetes insipidus, the suspicion of nephrogenic diabetes insipidus may arise; a rare congenital disorder. Such cases have been treated with thiazide diuretics and a low-sodium diet. Oral administration of hydrochlorothiazide (2 to 4 mg/kg twice daily) and a low-sodium diet may decrease urine volume, albeit probably without significant change in urine osmolality. It is thought that the thiazide diuretic and the low

sodium diet reduce plasma sodium concentration. This would decrease the stimulation of the thirst center and consequently the water intake. This may lead to extracellular volume contraction, a decreased glomerular filtration rate, increased proximal tubular sodium and water reabsorption, and decreased delivery of water to the distal tubule. The net effect is a reduction in urine volume.[32]

PROGNOSIS

In the absence of a neoplastic lesion the long-term prospects for cases with central diabetes insipidus are good. With appropriate treatment the animals become asymptomatic. Untreated animals with the complete form are always at risk of developing life-threatening dehydration when left without water for longer than a few hours. Animals with diabetes insipidus due to a pituitary tumor may lead acceptable lives for many months until the lesion has reached such size that neurologic signs develop.

Figure 236-4 In the first part of this algorithm the approach of the problem polyuria/polydipsia (pu/pd) is based upon the information from history. As a second step urinalysis has been introduced as it may happen that an animal presented with a seemingly convincing history of pu/pd has only pd because the owner has changed the food to dry food. As indicated in the text, it may be advisable at this stage to ask the owner for urine collections at 2-hour intervals. When the routine clinical chemistry has not revealed a specific suspicion, tests such as water deprivation and hypertonic saline infusion with AVP measurements may be needed. (Redrawn from Rijnberk A, editor: *Clinical endocrinology of dogs and cats*, Dordrecht/Boston, 1996, Kluwer Academic Publishers.)

CHAPTER • 237

Disorders of the Parathyroid Glands

Edward C. Feldman

The parathyroid glands and their production of parathyroid hormone (PTH) control serum calcium concentrations. Dogs and cats normally have four glands (two pairs). Two glands are anatomically closely associated with each thyroid lobe. Primary parathyroid gland disorders involve excess secretion of PTH (primary hyperparathyroidism [PHPTH]) or deficiencies of PTH secretion (primary hypoparathyroidism). Both conditions are relatively uncommon, but PHPTH is diagnosed at a much greater frequency than its counterpart. Further, hypercalcemia is diagnosed relatively frequently in dogs, and the first challenge for the veterinarian is appreciating the differential diagnosis for hypercalcemia and then diagnosing the specific condition causing this biochemical abnormality in an individual dog or cat (Box 237-1).

PRIMARY HYPERPARATHYROIDISM AND HYPERCALCEMIA IN DOGS

Cause

The essential disorder in PHPTH is the excessive synthesis and secretion of PTH by abnormal, autonomously functioning parathyroid "chief" cells.[1,2] The cause of this hormonal excess is usually a solitary parathyroid adenoma, but an adenoma of

---

Box • 237-1

Differential Diagnosis of Hypercalcemia

Common
Lymphosarcoma
Hypoadrenocorticism
Primary Hyperparathyroidism
Chronic renal failure

Uncommon
Apocrine gland carcinoma of the anal sac
Multiple myeloma
Vitamin D toxicosis

Uncommon to Rare
Spurious
Hemoconcentration
Carcinomas:
   lung, mammary, nasal, pancreas, testicle, thymus,
   thyroid, vagina
Acute renal failure
Nutritional secondary hyperparathyroidism
Granulomatous disease
   blastomycosis, histoplasmosis, schistosomiasis

---

more than one gland, adenomatous hyperplasia of one or more parathyroid glands, and parathyroid carcinomas have been identified in both dogs and cats. By contrast, other forms of hyperparathyroidism (e.g., renal or nutritional secondary hyperparathyroidism) are usually the result of nonendocrine alterations in calcium and phosphorus homeostasis. Such disturbances indirectly affect the parathyroid glands, causing diffuse hyperplasia. However, in these conditions the secretion of PTH is not autonomous. The "hyperplasia" occasionally diagnosed in the primary condition (PHPTH) is a condition associated with autonomous secretion of PTH. Therefore histologic descriptions may not indicate primary autonomous from secondary secretory patterns. Depending on cause, serum calcium concentrations in secondary disorders may range from low to normal to increased. PHPTH is virtually always associated with hypercalcemia.

Pathophysiology

Calcium-Parathyroid Hormone Feedback System Serum calcium is the major factor in regulation of PTH secretion. In normal animals, an inverse linear relationship exists between serum calcium and PTH concentrations.[3] In other words, as calcium concentrations in the serum decrease, PTH secretion is stimulated to maintain serum calcium concentrations at some specific level. The system functions as if there were a "calciostat" that operates at a serum calcium concentration set point of about 10.5 to 11.5 mg/dL. When serum calcium concentrations decrease below these levels, the rate of PTH secretion increases; when the serum calcium concentration exceeds the set point (as might occur after intake of a high-calcium meal), PTH secretion is suppressed. In PHPTH, normal negative-feedback homeostatic control is lost, and PTH secretion becomes chronically increased. This appearance of "autonomous" secretion may be a change in the "set point." The autonomous secretion of PTH is not suppressible by the increased concentration of calcium perfusing the parathyroid glands. Conversely, in secondary hyperparathyroidism, secretion by the parathyroid glands is normally suppressible by increased concentrations of calcium.

Severe Hypercalcemia Hypercalcemia develops when the entry of calcium into the extracellular fluid (regardless of the source) overwhelms mechanisms that maintain normocalcemia. One such mechanism is suppressed secretion of PTH, a process obviously negated when the cause of hypercalcemia is autonomous secretion of PTH or a molecule with similar biologic activity. In cancer-associated hypercalcemia, the secretion of PTH is suppressed, but the humoral factor that activates osteoclasts is the autonomous secretion of a parathyroid hormone–related protein (PTHrP). PTHrP is a protein with a structure and biologic activity quite similar to that of PTH.[4,5]

In the setting of accelerated bone resorption, the kidney is the principal defense against hypercalcemia.[6] When renal and endocrine function is normal, any tendency for a rise in serum calcium is attenuated by increased urinary excretion of calcium. This process is inhibited by PTH in PHPTH or by

PTHrP in hypercalcemia of malignancy. These hormones induce osteoclast-mediated bone resorption, intestinal absorption of calcium, and renal tubular reabsorption of calcium.[7] This impairs the ability of the kidneys to excrete the increased filtered load of calcium. Thus animals with an excess of PTH lack the first lines of defense against hypercalcemia. The hypercalcemic state also interferes with renal mechanisms for reabsorption of sodium and water, leading to polyuria. This is due to an acquired inability to respond to antidiuretic hormone (ADH)—in essence, a reversible form of nephrogenic diabetes insipidus. In PHPTH, hypercalcemia is enhanced by the increased production of vitamin D and by a decrease in the amount of serum phosphate available to form complexes with serum ionized calcium. The result is a decreased tubular reabsorption of phosphate, hyperphosphaturia, and hypophosphatemia. These actions are responsible for the development of the biochemical triad classic for PHPTH: hypercalcemia, hypophosphatemia, and hyperphosphaturia.

Signalment

Age and Gender PHPTH is typically diagnosed in older dogs and appears to be much less common, or at least less frequently diagnosed, in cats. The mean age of the 187 dogs with PHPTH seen at our hospital is 11.2 years, with a range of 4 to 17 years (Figure 237-1). More than 95% of the dogs are 7 years of age or older. No apparent sex predilection exists.

Breed Reliable information regarding breed predisposition for any disorder requires sophisticated epidemiologic evaluation. To the author's knowledge, such an investigation has not been undertaken with respect to canine PHPTH. Regardless, it is reasonable to point out that the Keeshond is far from being the most popular breed of dog, as opposed to poodles, German shepherds, retrievers, and the like. In spite of this relative lack of popularity, 48 of the 187 dogs (26%) in our series have been Keeshonden. The other breeds represented three or more times in series include Labrador retrievers, German shepherd dogs, Cocker spaniels, golden retrievers, springer spaniels, Shih Tzu, poodles, Australian shepherds, Rhodesian ridgebacks, Doberman pinschers, and mixed breed dogs (Table 237-1). Several of these breeds, however, are simply popular. Whether or not breed predispositions exist awaits epidemiologic evaluation. However, two points should

be made. First, the Keeshond is over-represented; second, dogs of any breed or mixed breeding and any age from 4 years of age and older can be afflicted by this condition.

Hereditary Disease Hereditary neonatal PHPTH was reported in two German shepherd dogs.[8] The incidence of this syndrome in puppies and young dogs must be quite rare because no other report of neonatal disease has appeared in the literature. Our series of dogs with PHPTH does not include any less than 4 years of age.

Anamnesis: Clinical Signs

General Clinical signs due solely to hypercalcemia, when observed by an owner, are mild in most dogs.[9] The only condition that has hypercalcemia as the sole problem is PHPTH. The most common signs associated with PHPTH include polyuria, polydipsia, decreases in appetite, decreases in body weight, decreased activity (muscle weakness?), and signs related to stones or infection within the urinary tract. Other signs reported secondary to hypercalcemia include the gastrointestinal (GI) signs of anorexia, vomiting, constipation, and, rarely, pancreatitis. Signs associated with the central nervous system (CNS) include mental dullness, obtundation, and even coma. One dog with PHPTH had ataxia and circling that resolved after resolution of the PHPTH. Again, clinical signs in dogs with PHPTH are almost always mild or not noticed. When a dog with hypercalcemia has worrisome signs, it almost always has a disease other than PHPTH. These worrisome signs therefore are almost always associated with the underlying cause for the hypercalcemia (e.g., cancer, renal failure, hypoadrenocorticism, toxin).

The mildest form of PHPTH may not be associated with any signs, and the hypercalcemia is identified serendipitously only after a standard biochemical panel has been obtained and reviewed. This is certainly true in humans, in whom *occult* primary hyperparathyroidism is more prevalent than the symptomatic form of the disorder.[10-13] When clinical signs in dogs do develop, they initially tend to be mild, insidious, and nonspecific. Most owners are unaware of specific clinical signs. It is not until their pet has been treated for PHPTH that owners, retrospectively, realize that their dog had signs. It is this concept that resulted in an editorial suggesting that all people with PHPTH be treated, because they may appreciate their illness that they have been ill until their disease has

Table • 237-1

Breed Distribution of 187 Dogs with Primary Hyperparathyroidism

BREED	NUMBER OF DOGS	PERCENT OF DOGS
Keeshond	48	26%
Labrador retriever	18	10%
Cocker spaniel	14	7%
German shepherd dog	14	7%
Golden retriever	12	6%
Springer spaniel	9	5%
Standard poodle	8	4%
Shih Tzu	8	4%
Australian shepherd	7	4%
Rhodesian ridgeback	6	3%
Doberman pinscher	6	3%

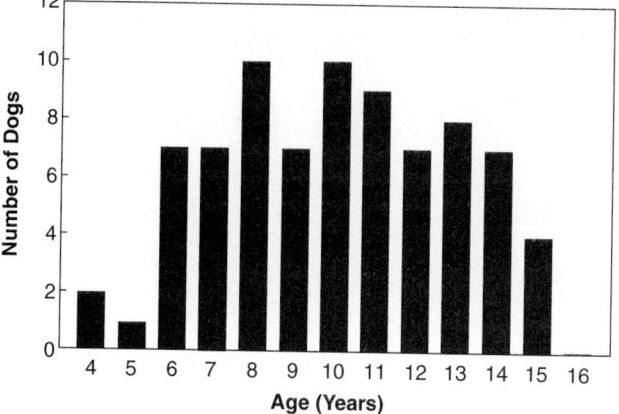

Figure 237-1 Age distribution of 78 dogs with primary hyperparathyroidism. The mean age at the time of diagnosis was 10.5 years. (From Feldman EC, Nelson RW: Canine and Feline Endocrinology and Reproduction, 3rd ed. Philadelphia, WB Saunders Co, 2004.)

Table • 237-2

Duration of Clinical Signs in 168 Dogs with Naturally Occurring Primary Hyperparathyroidism

DURATION (MONTHS)	PERCENT OF DOGS
< 1	19%
1-3	20%
3-6	19%
6-12	24%
>12	18%

Table • 237-3

Frequency of Clinical Signs Reported in 168 Dogs with Naturally Occurring Primary Hyperparathyroidism

SIGN	PERCENT OF DOGS
Polyuria/polydipsia (PU/PD)	81%
Listlessness	53%
Incontinence	47%
Weakness, exercise intolerance	47%
Inappetence	37%
Urinary tract signs (straining, blood, frequency)	29%
Muscle wasting	17%
Vomiting	12%
Shivering	10%
Constipation	6%
Stiff gait	5%

been resolved.[14] In our series of dogs with PHPTH, 35% had clinical signs related to PHPTH for more than 6 months and *all*, either retrospectively or prospectively, had signs for at least 1 month (Table 237-2). The clinical signs attributable to PHPTH and hypercalcemia usually involve one, two, or all three of these organ systems: renal, GI, or neuromuscular (Table 237-3).

Renal: Kidneys, Bladder, and Urethra

Polydipsia, polyuria, or both   The most common clinical signs in dogs with PHPTH (152 of 187 dogs; 81%) are polyuria, polydipsia, and urinary incontinence (see Table 237-3). These signs are a result of impaired renal tubular response to ADH and impaired renal tubular resorption of sodium and chloride. Together, these alterations account for a significant increase in urine volume and are a direct result of hypercalcemia. This acquired and reversible form of nephrogenic diabetes insipidus causes the production of relatively dilute, solute-free urine. Compensatory polydipsia develops to maintain normovolemia. Surprisingly, the polydipsia and polyuria

either are not observed or are thought to be mild by most owners but are obvious on review of randomly obtained urine specific gravities (USGs). These specific gravities were much more dilute than would have been expected from owner comments. Of 187 dogs with PHPTH, 46 (24%) had USGs of 1.001 to 1.007; 69 dogs (38%) had USGs that were in the isosthenuric range of 1.008 to 1.012; 60 dogs (32%) had USGs of 1.013 to 1.020; only eight had values of 1.021 to 1.030 and 4 greater than 1.030. Thus 94% of dogs with PHPTH had USGs less than or equal to 1.020 (Table 237-4).

Urinary tract calculi or infection   Another of the more common causes for owner concern in dogs with PHPTH was

Table • 237-4

Serum BUN, Creatinine, and Phosphate Concentrations and Urine Specific Gravities at the Time of Primary Hyperparathyroidism (PHPTH) Diagnosis in 187 Dogs*

	BUN (mg/dL)			SERUM CREATININE (mg/dL)			SERUM PHOSPHATE (mg/dL)			URINE SPECIFIC GRAVITY (USG)		
Reference range	18-28			0.5-1.6			3.0-6.2			—		
Mean (PHPTH dogs)	17.1			1.0			2.8			1.011		
Range (PHPTH dogs)	4-92			0.3-4.1			1.1-6.9			1.002-1.039		
Breakdown of individual results	Values	# Dogs	% Dogs	Values	# Dogs	% Dogs	Values	# Dogs	% Dogs	Values	# Dogs	% Dogs
	≤10	9	5	≤.5	2	1	<2	20	11	≤1.007	46	24
	11-17	112	60	0.6-0.9	84	45	2.0-2.9	99	53	1.008-1.012	69	37
	18-22	39	21	1.0-1.6	96	51	3.0-3.9	50	27	1.013-1.020	60	32
	23-28	18	10	1.7-2.0	3	2	4.0-4.9	12	6	1.021-1.030	8	4
	29-47	8	4	2.0-3.0	1	0.5	5.0-6.2	5	3	1.031-1.039	4	2
	>47	1	—	>3.0	1	0.5	>6.2	1	—			

*Reference range and mean values from the PHPTH dogs and arbitrary data listed.

observation of clinical signs consistent with urinary tract infection, calculi, or both. These signs included frequency, urgency, incontinence, hematuria, stranguria, or apparent urinary obstruction. At some time in the year preceding diagnosis, 123 of 168 owners (73%) had seen at least one of these clinical signs in their dogs. Sixty-one of 187 (33%) PHPTH dogs had uroliths, and 46 dogs (24%) had a urinary tract infection at the time of diagnosis.

Listlessness, Depression, and Decreased Activity
Listlessness or decreases in activity were observed in 99 (53%) of 187 dogs with PHPTH. Increased serum calcium concentrations depress the excitability of central and peripheral nervous tissue, which may be responsible for this clinical manifestation. Alternatively, these clinical signs may be a reflection of muscle weakness. Humans with this disorder may exhibit nonspecific neurologic abnormalities that include impaired mentation, mental depression, hypoactive deep tendon reflexes, and loss of pain perception.[13]

Weakness and Muscle Wasting Weakness or exercise intolerance was observed in 88 (47%) of 187 dogs with PHPTH. Increased serum calcium concentrations decrease cell membrane permeability in nervous and muscular tissue. In addition, skeletal muscle weakness, primarily of the proximal muscle groups, may result from a primary neuropathy that ultimately causes muscle atrophy. Muscle wasting and weight loss were observed in 32 (17%) of the 187 dogs.

Inappetence Owners observed some degree of reduced appetite in 69 (37%) of 187 dogs with PHPTH. This problem probably developed as a result of hypercalcemia-induced decreased excitability of GI smooth muscle or from direct effects on the CNS. Gastric ulcers, noted in some hypercalcemic people, has not been observed in dogs with PHPTH. Only one dog had concurrent pancreatitis. One common assumption is that hypercalcemia would induce secondary renal failure and tertiary loss of appetite. However, this is quite uncommon.

Shivering, Twitching, and Seizures Shivering and muscle twitching have been observed in hypercalcemic dogs, and seizure activity has been reported in a dog with PHPTH.[15] These signs might result from cerebral microthrombi, vasospasm, or other conditions.

Physical Examination
A thorough physical examination is imperative in any animal with documented hypercalcemia. Physical examinations are usually unremarkable in dogs with PHPTH. When abnormalities exist, they are typically related to the presence of uroliths. Other abnormalities (weakness, muscle atrophy) are usually subtle or nonspecific. Although parathyroid gland tumors are not palpable dogs with PHPTH, tumors have been palpable in four of ten cats with this condition. The most common cause of hypercalcemia in dogs is hypercalcemia of malignancy (Box 237-1). Lymphosarcoma, apocrine gland carcinoma of the anal sac, mammary gland adenocarcinoma, vaginal sarcoma, and multiple myeloma are among cancers capable of causing hypercalcemia that may be identified on examination. The diagnostic approach to a dog with confirmed hypercalcemia is to rule out the presence of malignancy before pursuing the diagnosis of PHPTH (see Figure 237-2). Non-neoplastic causes of hypercalcemia may be suspected after a thorough physical examination. For example, in renal failure, the kidneys may be palpably abnormal. Dogs with Addison's disease may have bradycardia, weak femoral pulses, melena, or a bloody rectal discharge.

Clinical Pathology: Hemogram, Serum Biochemical Profile, and Urinalysis
No typical hemogram abnormalities have been identified in dogs with PHPTH.

Serum Total Calcium Concentration
Results in dogs and humans Hypercalcemia is the hallmark abnormality of PHPTH (Figure 237-3). The mean serum calcium concentration in 187 dogs with PHPTH was 15.3 mg/dL, with a range of 12.1 to 23.0 mg/dL (Table 237-5). This mean value could be arbitrarily inflated because evaluation of hypercalcemia is limited to those animals with serum calcium concentrations greater than 12.0 mg/dL (the upper reference range limit is 11.7 mg/dL). In most dogs, hypercalcemia was initially identified by a referring veterinarian on at least two occasions and then rechecked several times after referral. Of PHPTH dogs, 102 of 187 (55%) had an initial total serum calcium concentration of 12 to 14 mg/dL; 58 (31%) had an initial concentration of 14 to 16 mg/dL; 18 (9%) had an initial concentration of 16 to 18 mg/dL; and nine (5%) had an initial concentration of greater than 18 mg/dL (range of 18 to 23 mg/dL). Of these latter nine dogs with severe hypercalcemia, it is of interest to mention that their mean blood urea nitrogen (BUN) concentration was 22 mg/dL, with only one dog having a BUN above the reference range limit of 28 mg/dL.

Although it is assumed that untreated PHPTH will result in progressively increasing serum calcium concentrations, this has not been the experience in people. A group of 60 "asymptomatic" PHPTH people was not treated for 10 years. Their mean total serum calcium concentration, at the time of diagnosis, was 10.5 mg/dL (reference range 8.4 to 10.2 mg/dL), 5 years later it was 10.6, and a total of 10 years after diagnosis it was 10.3 mg/dL.[13] However, eight developed uroliths during the decade, leaving 52 who remained asymptomatic. Our experience with dogs suggest that hypercalcemia associated with PHPTH remains static or slowly increases with time.

Factors affecting serum calcium concentration Marked lipemia can falsely increase total calcium values determined by some automated analyzers. Hemoconcentration (dehydration) can cause mild hypercalcemia (typically < 13 mg/dL). Hemolysis can also falsely increase the total serum calcium concentration measured with an automated analyzer. Young animals may have mild increases in serum calcium concentration, and postprandial samples may yield false increases. Excess use of oral phosphate binders may cause the serum calcium concentration to increase. Ethylenediamine tetra-acetic acid (EDTA) increases calcium values determined by atomic absorption spectrophotometry and decreases results obtained with other methods. Collecting and storing samples in glassware or plastic containers that have been washed with detergents or exposed to chalk may increase calcium results and also cause spurious values for other electrolytes. Acidosis may decrease plasma protein-binding affinity for calcium and increase ionic calcium concentrations, creating mild physiologic hypercalcemia.

Plasma protein concentrations Calcium in plasma or serum exists in three forms or fractions: ionized (free calcium), complexed or chelated (bound to phosphate, bicarbonate, sulfate, citrate, and lactate), and protein bound. In clinically normal dogs, protein-bound, complexed, and ionized calcium account for approximately 34%, 10%, and 56% of the total serum calcium, respectively.[16,17] Laboratories generally measure these components together and report them as a *total* calcium value. Ionized calcium is the biologically active component, and the protein-bound calcium serves as a "reservoir" or storage pool for the ionized fraction. However, changes in serum concentration of albumin and globulins may alter the

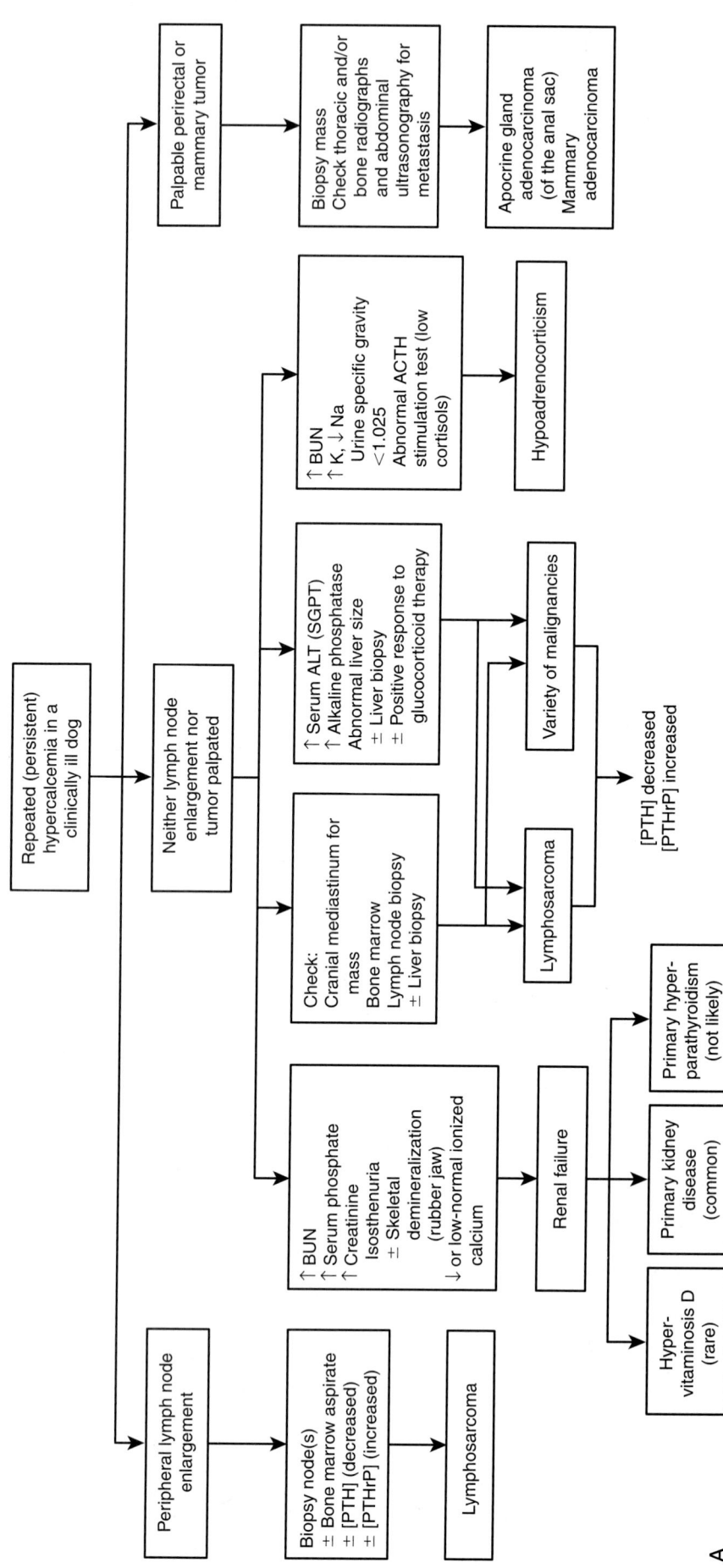

Figure 237-2 **A,** Algorithm for evaluating an ill hypercalcemic dog. **B,** Algorithm for evaluating a dog with hypercalcemia but without serious or worrisome clinical signs. (From Feldman EC, Nelson RW: Canine and Feline Endocrinology and Reproduction, 3rd ed. Philadelphia, WB Saunders Co, 2004.)

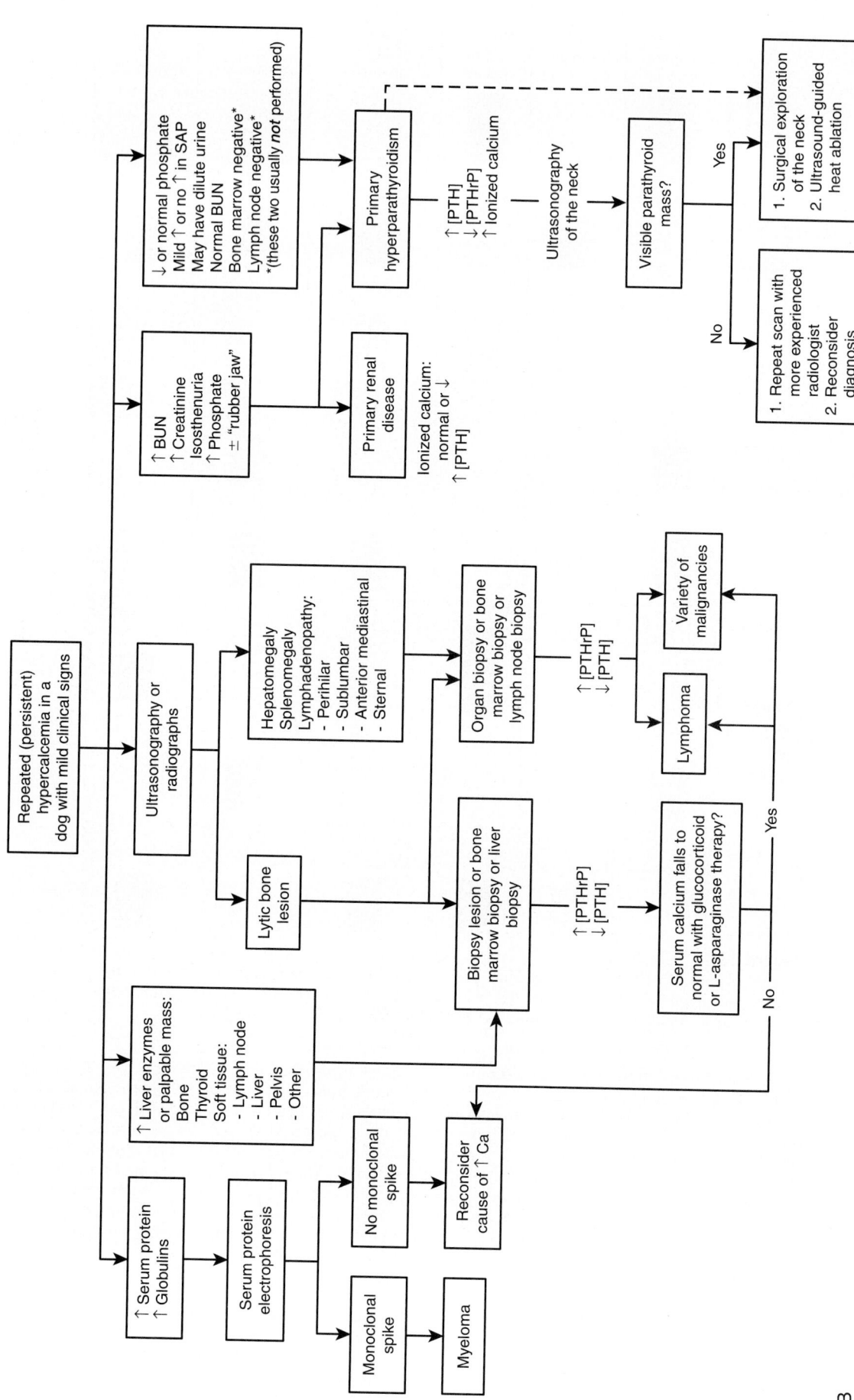

Figure 237-2 Cont'd.

B

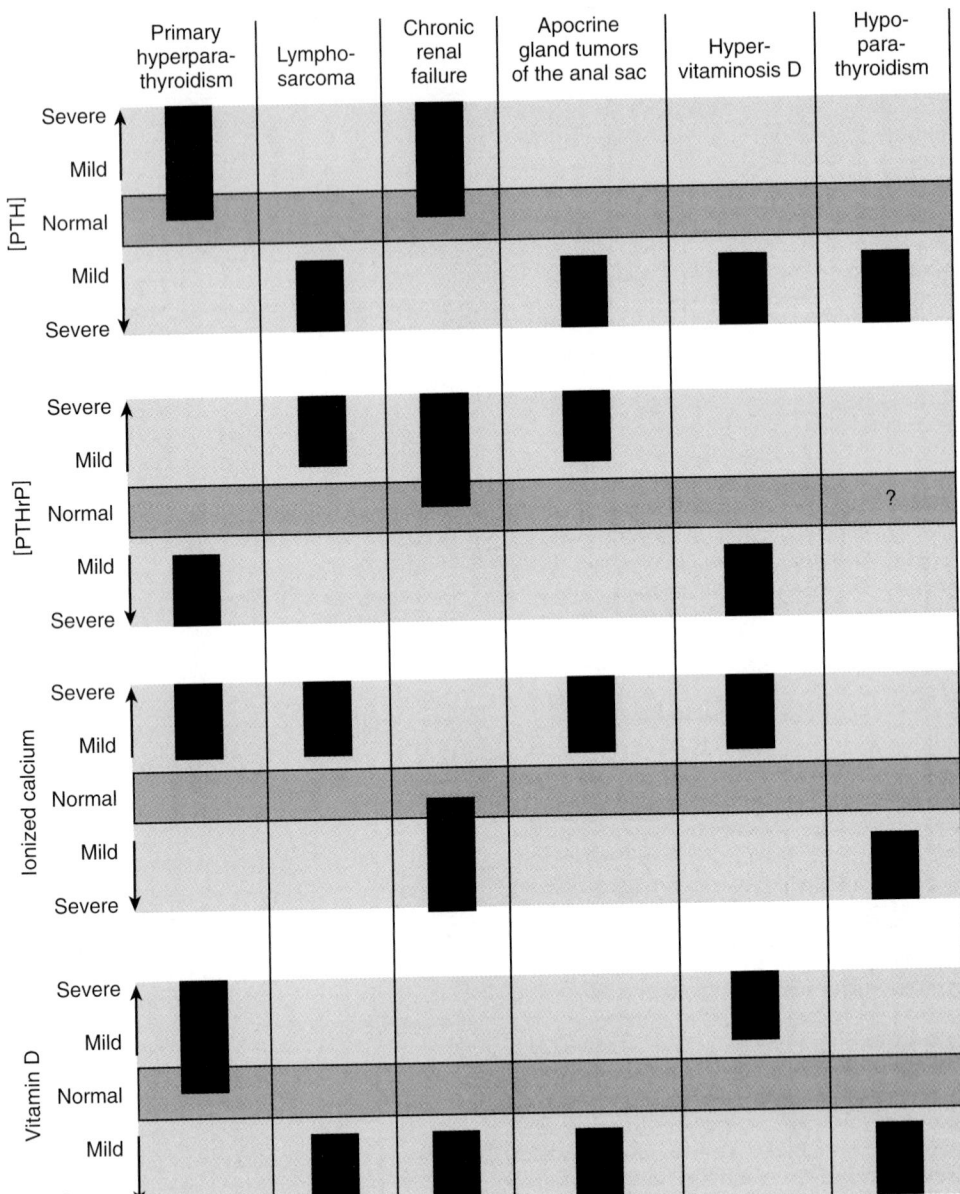

Figure 237-3 Graph showing the serum parathyroid hormone (PTH), parathyroid hormone-related peptide (PTHrP), ionized calcium, and vitamin D concentrations in the most common causes for hypercalcemia of dogs. (From Feldman EC, Nelson RW: Canine and Feline Endocrinology and Reproduction, 3rd ed. Philadelphia, WB Saunders Co, 2004.)

measured *total* serum calcium concentration without altering ionized calcium levels. Despite an alteration in the total amount of plasma calcium resulting from hyperproteinemia or hypoproteinemia, the biologically active *ionized* calcium concentration usually remains within reference limits.

Two formulas were developed for use in dogs to account for changes in the reported serum calcium value attributed to changes in serum protein values.[18] The formulas were of significant value prior to routine availability of ionized calcium assays. These formulas are:

Corrected Total Ca (mg/dL)
    = Measured Total Ca (mg/dL) – albumin (g/dL) + 3.5

or

Corrected total Ca (mg/dL)
    = Measured total Ca (mg/dL) – [0.4 × total protein (g/dL)] + 3.3

Hypoalbuminemia is a common explanation for apparent hypocalcemia. However, this "hypocalcemia" usually causes no clinical signs and is associated with only mild changes from reference ranges. Although correction to normal limits implies that the ionized fraction is normal, the ionized fraction may yet be low. These formulas, developed more than 2 decades ago, were derived from serum albumin concentration results obtained with analytical methods no longer used by modern automated analyzers. At the time, a positive correlation was noted, but only 33% of the variability in serum total calcium concentration could be attributed to serum albumin concentration, and only 17% of the variability could be attributed to serum total protein. There was no association in cats between serum total protein and serum calcium concentrations, and only 18% of the variability in total calcium concentration could be attributed to albumin concentration.[19] In another study, only 17% and 29% of the variability in total serum calcium concentration in dogs and cats, respectively, could be

Table • 237-5

Serum Total (187 Dogs) and Ionized (136 Dogs) Calcium Concentrations, Serum Parathyroid Hormone (PTH) Concentrations (162 Dogs), and Ultrasonographically Identified Parathyroid Masses (98 Dogs, 11 of 98 had Two Masses Each) in Dogs With Primary Hyperparathyroidism

	TOTAL CALCIUM (mg/dL)			IONIZED CALCIUM (mmol/L)			PTH (pmol/L)			ULTRASOUND MASS SIZE (mm)		
Reference range	9.6-11.7			1.12-1.42			2-13			< 4		
Mean (PHPTH dogs)	14.3			1.86			11.9			7		
Range (PHPTH dogs)	12.1-23.0			1.22 - 2.29			3.7-12.1			3-23		
Breakdown of individual results	Values	# Dogs	% Dogs	Values	# Dogs	% Dogs	Values	# Dogs	% Dogs	Size	# Masses	% Masses
	12-14	102	55	1.22-1.42	9	7	3.7-7.9	63	39	3-6	65	60
	14.1-16	5S	31	1.43-1.65	37	27	8.0-13.0	44	27	7-10	29	27
	16.1-18	18	9	1.66-190	64	47	13.1-20.0	25	15	11-l5	9	8
	≥ 18.1	9	5	≥ 1.91	26	19	≥ 20.1	30	19	> 15	6	5

attributed to serum albumin concentration.[20] For these reasons, use of these correction formulas are not recommended.[21]

Serum Ionized Calcium Concentration The ionized fraction of total circulating calcium concentration is the biologically active form. This information (together with the increasing availability of valid assays for ionized calcium and realization that dogs with chronic renal failure tend to have normal to low ionized concentrations versus the increased concentrations in other hypercalcemic conditions) has created a growing interest in results of this parameter in hyper- and hypocalcemic dogs. The mean ionized calcium concentration on initial blood samples in 136 dogs with PHPTH was 1.86 mmol/L, with a range of 1.22 to 2.29 mmol/L (reference range 1.12 to 1.42 mmol/L; see Table 237-5). Nine of the 136 dogs (7%) had a serum ionized calcium concentration within the referee range; 37 (27%) had results of 1.43 to 1.65 mmol/L; 64 (47%) had concentrations of 1.66 to 1.9 mmol/L, and 26 (19%) had concentrations greater than 1.9 mmol/L. In general, there was good correlation between serum total and ionized calcium results. However, no dog with PHPTH had a total calcium concentration within the reference range, whereas 7% had ionized calciums within the reference range. It is suspected that these ionized calcium concentrations within the reference range are the result of external (in vitro) factors (aerobic collection, pH).

Serum Phosphorus Concentration Low or low-normal serum phosphorus concentrations (< 4.0 mg/dL) are typical of PHPTH (see Figure 237-3). Hypophosphatemia is the result of PTH-induced inhibition of renal tubular phosphorus resorption, resulting in excessive urinary loss. In 187 dogs with PHPTH, the mean serum phosphorus concentration was 2.8 mg/dL (< the lower limit of the reference range; 3.0 to 6.2 mg/dL), with a range of 1.5 to 6.8 mg/dL (see Table 237-4). Twenty of 187 dogs (11%) had serum phosphate concentrations less than 2.0 mg/dL; 99 (53%) had results of 2.0 to 2.9 mg/dL; 50 (27%) had results in the low normal range of 3.0 to 3.9 mg/dL; 12 (6%) had values in the mid-normal range of 4.0 to 4.9; 4 (3%) had values 5.0 mg/dL and only one of those four dogs had a serum phosphate concentration above reference limits (6.8 mg/dL). As a point of interest, nine of the 187 dogs had BUN values above the

reference limit of 28 mg/dL. Of those nine dogs, eight had serum phosphate concentrations within the reference range.

The serum phosphorus concentration should always be evaluated relative to the serum calcium concentration and renal function. Hypophosphatemia, when dietary phosphate is adequate and when oral phosphate-binding agents are not being given, is consistent with either PHPTH or hypercalcemia of malignancy (see Figure 237-3). Other causes for hypophosphatemia are less common (Box 237-2). Hyperphosphatemia in the absence of azotemia suggests a nonparathyroid cause for hypercalcemia. When both hyperphosphatemia and azotemia are present, the clinician must rely on the history, physical examination, and other diagnostic tests to determine if the primary problem is hypercalcemia with secondary renal failure (rare) or renal failure with secondary hypercalcemia (common). Determination of the serum ionized calcium concentration can be of value. Dogs with renal failure and increases in total serum calcium concentration usually have ionized calcium concentrations that are normal or mildly decreased, dogs with PHPTH have increases in both fractions.

Blood Urea Nitrogen and Serum Creatinine Concentration BUN (mean: 17 mg/dL) and serum creatinine concentrations (mean: 1.0 mg/dL) are usually within reference limits in dogs with PHPTH (see Table 237-4). Nine dogs (5%) had BUN concentrations less than 10 mg/dL; 112 (60%) had values of 10 to 17 mg/dL; 39 (21%) were 18 to 22 mg/dL; 18 (10%) were 23 to 28 mg/dL; 8 (4%) were 29 to 47 mg/dL, and one dog had a value of 92 mg/dL. Four of the nine dogs with an abnormal BUN had a serum creatinine concentration within the reference range. The two highest serum creatinine concentrations were 2.3 and 4.1, respectively. This is most impressive when considering the mean age of these dogs (11.2 years). The literature strongly suggests that hypercalcemia, especially when chronic, may damage kidneys. However, it would appear that dogs with PHPTH are protected from renal damage, whether this protective effect is due to the low calcium × phosphate product or some other factor.

Urinalysis The mean USG in 187 dogs with PHPTH was 1.011. Forty-six dogs (24%) had a USG on initial evaluation

Box • 237-2

Potential Causes for Hypophosphatemia

Decreased Intestinal Absorption
Decreased dietary intake
Malabsorption/steatorrhea
Vomiting/diarrhea
Phosphate-binding antacids
Vitamin D deficiency

Increased Urinary Excretion
Primary hyperparathyroidism
Diabetes mellitus ± ketoacidosis
Hyperadrenocorticism (naturally occurring/iatrogenic)
Fanconi's syndrome (renal tubular defects)
Diuretic or bicarbonate administration
Hypothermia recovery
Hyperaldosteronism
Aggressive parenteral fluid administration
Hypercalcemia of malignancy (early stages)

Transcellular Shifts
Insulin administration
Parenteral glucose administration
Hyperalimentation
Respiratory alkalosis

---

less than 1.008; 69 (38%) had specific gravities of 1.008 to 1.012; 60 (32%) had values of 1.013 to 1.020; eight (4%) had results of 1.021 to 1.030; and four had concentrations greater than 1.030 (see Table 237-4). Hypercalcemia interferes with ADH action and thereby causes a reversible form of nephrogenic diabetes insipidus. Isosthenuria (or hyposthenuria) may develop from *any* cause of hypercalcemia. Thus the combination of hypercalcemia and dilute urine is considered a "cause-and-effect" phenomenon but is not specific.

Urine Sediment   Hematuria, pyuria, bacteriuria, and crystalluria are identified frequently on urine sediment examination from dogs with PHPTH. Fifty-nine of 187 PHPTH dogs (31%) either had a history of uroliths removed by referring veterinarians within the 12 months preceding examination or were identified as having uroliths with radiographs or ultrasonography at the time of initial evaluation at our hospital. Urinary tract infection had been present or was present on initial examination at the author's hospital in 46 of 187 dogs with PHPTH (24%).

Electrocardiography

Experimentally induced hypercalcemia may increase myocardial contractility, shorten mechanical ventricular systole, and decrease myocardial automaticity. Potential electrocardiographic changes caused by hypercalcemia include a prolongation of the P-R interval and a shortening of the Q-T interval due to a shortened S-T segment. Theoretically, decreases in myocardial conduction velocity and shortened refractory periods could predispose the heart to arrhythmias. However, dogs with PHPTH rarely have abnormalities on electrocardiogram.

Radiology

Thoracic Radiographs   The major purpose of evaluating radiographs in the hypercalcemic dog or cat is to identify abnormalities that would help establish a cause. The anterior mediastinum, perihilar, and sternal lymph nodes should be evaluated for a mass or lymphadenopathy. Dogs with hypercalcemia secondary to lymphosarcoma may have a mediastinal mass. The ribs, vertebrae, and any long bones included in the film can be evaluated for osteolytic areas due to myeloma or other metastatic tumors. Lung fields should be assessed for possible masses that might represent primary or metastatic lesions.

Abdomen and Skeleton   The sublumbar area and mesenteric lymph nodes can be evaluated for enlargements that would support metastatic apocrine gland carcinomas of the anal sac or lymphoma. The liver and spleen can be evaluated for enlargement or irregularities associated with lymphoma. Other than calculi within the urinary system, radiographic abnormalities are not associated with PHPTH.

Ultrasonography

Neck   With continuing improvement in equipment and experience, normal parathyroid glands are now routinely visualized with ultrasonography in dogs.[22] Parathyroid nodules from dogs with PHPTH have been measured to be as small as 2 mm in diameter and as large as 23 mm in diameter. Most adenomas are 4 to 9 mm in diameter and are easily visualized.[23,24] One recent study demonstrated a statistically significant difference in lesion size, comparing hyperplastic parathyroid glands (2 to 6 mm, mean 2.9 mm) to parathyroid adenomas and adenocarcinomas (4 to 20 mm, mean 7.5 mm).[25]

Radiologists have evaluated the cervical area of 98 dogs in our series with confirmed PHPTH. Virtually all these dogs had one or more parathyroid gland (masses) visualized. Eleven of the 98 dogs had two parathyroid nodules each. Thus 109 nodules were identified in the 98 dogs. Sixty-five of 109 parathyroid masses (60%) were 3 to 6 mm in diameter; 29 (27%) were 7 to 10 mm in diameter; nine (8%) were 11 to 15 mm in diameter; and six (5%) were 16 to 23 mm in diameter (see Table 237-5; Figure 237-4). No dog had more than two parathyroid masses identified. Parathyroid masses are usually round or oval, well marginated, and hypoechoic to anechoic compared with surrounding thyroid gland parenchyma (Figure 237-4). However, not every parathyroid nodule is obvious. It is occasionally difficult to distinguish large parathyroid masses from thyroid. Another important issue that must be stressed, is the subjective nature of this tool. In one of our studies, experienced radiologists correctly identified a solitary parathyroid mass in 11 of 11 dogs and two parathyroid masses in another. However, less experienced radiologists identified a parathyroid mass in only four of seven dogs.[26]

The accuracy of cervical ultrasonography in dogs with PHPTH has been similar to that reported in humans: 90% to 95% of parathyroid adenomas and a smaller percentage of hyperplastic parathyroid glands can be visualized.[27] Experienced radiologists identify parathyroid masses with ultrasonography more consistently than surgeons during surgery because of the occasional parathyroid mass located within a thyroid lobe that is neither visible nor palpable to the surgeon. Therefore cervical ultrasonography is potentially an extremely valuable diagnostic aid.

Abdomen   Ultrasonic scanning of the abdomen should also be a routine component of the diagnostic evaluation of hypercalcemic dogs and cats. If the liver, spleen, mesenteric lymph nodes, or other abdominal structures appear abnormal, percutaneous biopsy of that structure should be strongly considered. Ultrasonography has been an excellent tool for identifying uroliths as well. Most are seen within the bladder, but renal, ureter, and urethral stones have also been visualized.

Assays: PTH, PTHrP, Vitamin D (Calcitriol)

Dogs with PHPTH usually have serum PTH concentrations that range from within the reference range to being exceedingly

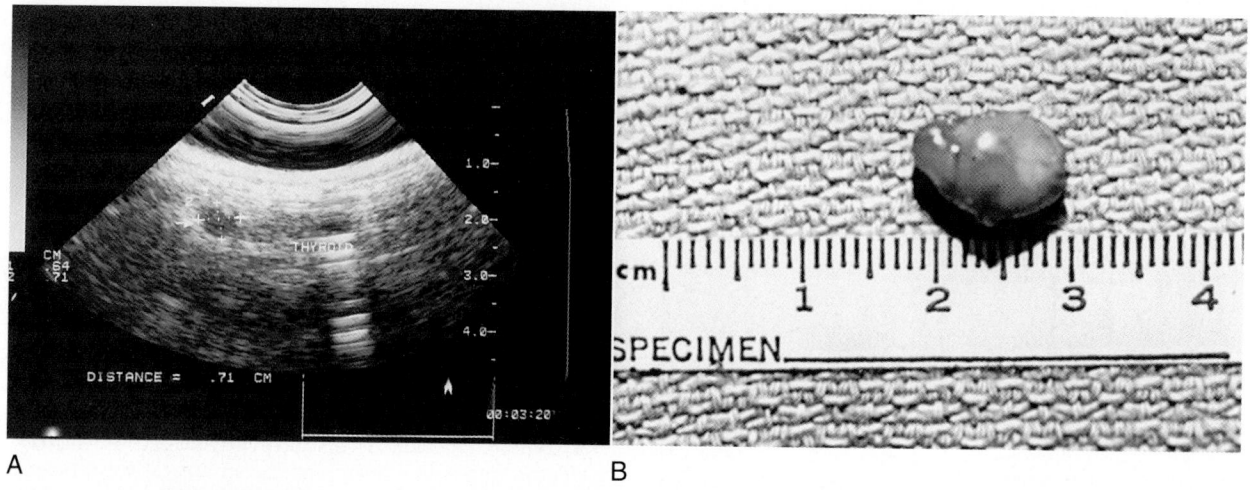

Figure 237-4 **A,** Cervical ultrasonogram from a dog with a functional parathyroid adenoma. The reader should note the right thyroid lobe, in which a well-marginated, hypoechoic mass *(arrows)* is visible at the cranial pole of the thyroid. **B,** Solitary parathyroid adenoma removed from a dog with primary hyperparathyroidism. (Ultrasound courtesy of Dr. Tom Nyland and Dr. Eric Wisner, Davis, Calif.)

increased (see Table 237-5 and Figure 237-3; Figure 237-5). In addition, serum PTHrP concentrations are usually undetectable, whereas calcitriol concentrations (not usually tested) would be normal to increased.[28] Serum PTH concentrations must always be evaluated in the context of the serum calcium concentration. In healthy animals, as the serum calcium concentration increases, the serum PTH concentration decreases. Relative to their hypercalcemia (using total or, preferably, ionized calcium), virtually all dogs and cats with PHPTH have excessive PTH secretion. In other words, serum PTH concentrations within the reference range should be considered "excessive" in a dog or cat with hypercalcemia. Such results are consistent with autonomous secretion of hormone.

The "sandwich" (two-site immunoradiometric [IRMA] assay system) for measuring PTH is considered the most reliable assay system currently available for dogs. At least one serum PTH concentration was obtained from each of 162 dogs with PHPTH (see Table 237-5). Most laboratories have similar PTH reference ranges (2 to 13 pmol/L). The mean serum PTH

concentration in these untreated dogs (11.9 pmol/L) was within the reference range, and 107 of the 162 results (66%) were within that reference range. Sixty-three dogs (39%) had serum PTH concentrations of 3.7 to 7.9 pmol/L; 44 dogs (27%) had values of 8 to 13 pmol/L; 25 dogs (15%) had results of 13.1 to 20 pmol/L; and 30 dogs (19%) had results greater than 20 pmol/L. The availability of both PTH and PTHrP assay results has improved clinicians' ability to identify the specific problem causing hypercalcemia in many dogs. These assays are accessible for practitioners.

Radionuclide Scans
Radionuclide procedures have been used as an aid for detecting and localizing parathyroid adenomas in humans.[29] The most commonly used radionuclide imaging technique uses technetium-99m-sestamibi.[30,31] Two reports suggested that this procedure might be helpful in localizing parathyroid adenomas in dogs with PHPTH.[32,33] In a subsequent study, double-phase parathyroid scintigraphy was evaluated in a group of hypercalcemic dogs, and only one of 10 dogs with PHPTH had a scan that correlated with surgery. The poor sensitivity and specificity achieved with scintigraphy led the authors to conclude that use of this tool could not be recommended.[34]

Selective Venous Sampling
An attempt was made to localize autonomously functioning parathyroid masses using serum PTH assay results from each jugular vein. The hypothesis was that the vein draining the side of the autonomously functioning mass would have greater amounts of PTH. Blood samples were obtained from each jugular vein prior to surgery from dogs with PHPTH caused by a solitary functioning adenoma. Unfortunately, a gradient between samples was only identified in one of 11 dogs, and the conclusion was that selective venous sampling was not reliable.[26]

Diagnostic Approach to the Hypercalcemic Dog or Cat
General The list of differential diagnoses for hypercalcemia is relatively short (see Table 237-1; Box 237-3), allowing a logical approach to identifying its cause. The most common cause in the dog and cat is *malignancy-associated hypercalcemia.* In an attempt to be practical, logical, and cost-effective, the

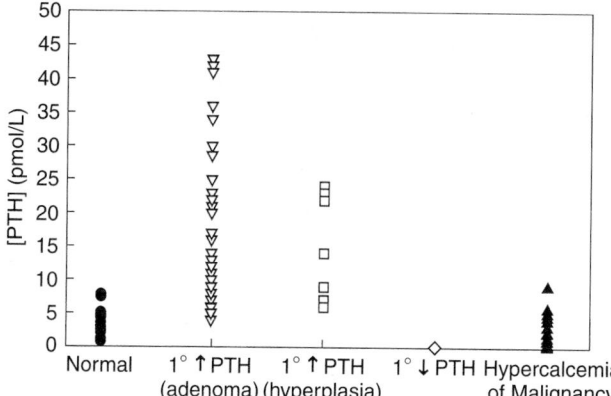

Figure 237-5 Serum PTH concentrations for normal dogs and those with various disorders of calcium homeostasis. The reader should note that some overlap exists in test results. (From Feldman EC, Nelson RW: Canine and Feline Endocrinology and Reproduction, 3rd ed. Philadelphia, WB Saunders Co, 2004.)

Box • 237-3

Differential Diagnosis for Humoral Hypercalcemia of Malignancy

Hematologic Cancers
Lymphosarcoma
Lymphocytic leukemia
Myeloproliferative disease
Myeloma

Solid Tumors with Bone Metastasis
Mammary adenocarcinoma
Nasal adenocarcinoma
Epithelial-derived tumors
Pancreatic adenocarcinoma
Lung carcinoma

Solid Tumors without Bone Metastasis
Apocrine gland adenocarcinoma of the anal sac
Interstitial cell tumor
Squamous cell carcinoma
Thyroid adenocarcinoma
Lung carcinoma
Pancreatic adenocarcinoma
Fibrosarcoma

diagnostic approach should first identify or rule out an underlying malignancy.[35] Only after testing has failed to identify a malignancy should PHPTH be considered.

Review the History and Physical Examination

First steps The diagnostic approach to the hypercalcemic dog or cat should be relatively straightforward (see Figure 237-2, A and B). The first step should be to confirm the presence of hypercalcemia by resubmitting a *second* blood sample for calcium and phosphorus determination, although the second sample virtually always has the same result as the first. Whenever possible, veterinary practitioners would be well served to submit appropriate samples for serum ionized calcium concentration. Such results, if increased, confirm hypercalcemia. If the ionized calcium concentration in a dog with confirmed increases in serum total calcium, is within or below the reference range, chronic renal failure or laboratory error should be considered. Review of the signalment, thorough history, and physical examination often allows the clinician to identify the cause for hypercalcemia or at least develop a likely list of high-priority possibilities. Both the history and physical examination should be repeated after the serendipitous finding of hypercalcemia.

Signalment Signalment (age, gender, breed) is emphasized, in part, because of the remarkable incidence of PHPTH in the Keeshond and in dogs that are 8 years of age or older. Renal failure can occur at any age, but certain breeds are predisposed to familial renal problems (Shih Tzu, Lhasa Apso, Doberman pinscher). Young dogs are more likely to suffer from renal failure, malignancy (lymphosarcoma), or hypoadrenocorticism (especially in the female), whereas apocrine gland carcinoma of the anal sac, and other malignancies occur in older dogs.

History The owner should be questioned about the pet's diet, vitamin-mineral supplementation, and exposure to rat and mouse poisons or houseplants that contain vitamin D analogues. One can attempt to determine if the pet is in pain (lytic bone lesions). Answers to questions regarding the presence of polydipsia, polyuria, appetite, and activity may be important. Generally, the more ill the pet appears the less likely that it has PHPTH (and the more likely it has a malignancy, renal failure, vitamin D toxicosis, granulomatous disease, or hypoadrenocorticism).

Physical examination After assessing hydration status and severity of illness, the physical examination should include careful palpation of peripheral lymph nodes (lymphoma) and the mammary glands (mammary cancer). A thorough rectal and perirectal examination is imperative in the identification of an apocrine gland carcinoma of the anal sac. A digital vaginal examination should also be performed (vaginal tumor). The clinician should gently palpate as much of the skeleton as possible, searching for an area of focal bone pain that could then be pursued with radiographs (multiple myeloma). The kidneys should be palpated in an attempt to identify irregularities.

Initial Data Base

Blood and urine The initial data base should include a hemogram (complete blood count [CBC]), a serum biochemical profile, serum ionized calcium concentration, urinalysis, and thoracic radiographs. The abdomen should be evaluated with ultrasonography, radiography, or both. If the serum phosphorus concentration is normal or low, renal failure, vitamin D toxicosis, and hypoadrenocorticism are less likely (see Figure 237-2, A and B). The serum creatinine, sodium, potassium, and BUN concentrations are extremely valuable in this assessment as well. A sodium-to-potassium ratio less than 27:1 is consistent with, but not diagnostic of, adrenal insufficiency. An ACTH stimulation test should be performed if this disease is possible. Low, low-normal, or normal serum phosphate concentrations are consistent with PHPTH and malignancy-associated hypercalcemia. Striking increases in total protein concentrations, specifically due to a monoclonal spike, are classic for multiple myeloma.

Parathyroid versus primary renal disease A diagnostic dilemma exists when hyperphosphatemia and hypercalcemia coexist with azotemia. The clinician must determine whether the hypercalcemia is the cause or the consequence of renal disease. Other abnormalities in the initial data base may support renal failure as the primary problem. These abnormalities include marked increases in serum phosphorus concentration, low-normal or low serum ionized calcium concentrations, nonregenerative anemia, proteinuria, and palpably or radiographically small and irregular kidneys. The serum ionized calcium in dogs with PHPTH is increased. If the hypercalcemia dissipates with aggressive fluid therapy and diuresis, PHPTH is less likely than primary renal failure or hypoadrenocorticism.

Radiography and ultrasonography Radiography of the thorax and ultrasonography of the abdomen should be evaluated for soft tissue masses, soft tissue calcification, evidence of fungal disease, organomegaly, osteolysis, or osteoporosis. The goal is to identify an abnormal area that could be biopsied to provide a definitive explanation for hypercalcemia. An anterior mediastinal mass is demonstrable radiographically in as many as 40% of hypercalcemic dogs with lymphosarcoma.[36] If hepatomegaly or splenomegaly is identified, histology of a biopsy (obtained percutaneously) taken from either of these organs should be evaluated to help establish a diagnosis. Adenocarcinomas derived from the apocrine glands of the anal sac may appear radiographically as a mass in the pelvic canal. Sublumbar lymphadenopathy due to tumor metastasis is also common. Soft tissue calcification is most frequently observed with hypervitaminosis D or chronic renal failure, although mineralization can be seen with any hypercalcemic disorder in association with hyperphosphatemia and a calcium × phosphorus product greater than 60 to 80.

Discrete lytic lesions in the vertebrae or long bones are suggestive of either myeloma or malignancy-associated hypercalcemia with bone metastasis. Radionuclide bone scans can be performed at specialty centers to identify bone lesions not detected with radiographs. Concurrent hyperproteinemia is supportive of myeloma. Solid tumors with metastasis to bone are more likely if lytic bone lesions and normoproteinemia (especially normal serum globulin concentrations) are present. A core biopsy of a lytic lesion may be necessary to establish a definitive diagnosis.

Ultrasonography of the cervical region has been reviewed. This tool is noninvasive and easily used. Identification of a solitary mass within or near one thyroid lobe supports the diagnosis of PHPTH, if the dog is not in renal failure.[22] This tool requires the 10-MHz transducer and, most importantly, the results are subjective.

Lymph Node and Bone Marrow Evaluations If the initial data base has not established a diagnosis, the next diagnostic steps should include evaluation of lymph nodes, bone marrow, or both. Because lymphosarcoma is the most common neoplasm associated with hypercalcemia in the dog and cat, peripheral nodes should be palpated. Ideally, the largest lymph node (*not* the submandibular node) should be assessed for histologic evaluation. Needle aspirates for cytology are occasionally acceptable, but pathologists may be hesitant to make a definitive diagnosis based on cytology alone. If any abnormalities are found on cytologic evaluation of an aspirate, histologic evaluation of a large biopsy sample or lymph node excision should be obtained to establish or rule out the diagnosis. This step should be omitted in dogs that are relatively healthy, based on an index of suspicion against the diagnosis of lymphosarcoma.

A bone marrow aspirate should also be considered in the hypercalcemic pet because the lymphosarcoma may be associated only with invasion of the marrow by neoplastic cells.[37] As with the peripheral lymph node evaluation, presence of a normal bone marrow aspirate does not definitively rule out lymphosarcoma. We usually omit a bone marrow aspirate when a dog is clinically well and when its CBC is unremarkable.

Serum PTH and PTHrP Concentrations Assay for these hormone concentrations can be quite helpful. Because the evaluation of hypercalcemic dogs tends to be logical, each step has the potential for ruling out causes. The diagnosis of PHPTH can be reached by simple exclusion. In other words, as all other differential diagnoses are eliminated, PHPTH may remain as the only reasonable diagnosis. Treatment of most of the dogs in our series for PHPTH was completed before the results of serum PTH concentrations were available.

Acute Medical Therapy for the Hypercalcemic Dog
Primary Hyperparathyroidism versus (PHPTH) Other Disorders
PHPTH The primary mode of therapy for severe hypercalcemia should be aimed at resolving its underlying cause. Surgical excision of abnormal parathyroid tissue is the most common therapy for dogs and cats with PHPTH. In these animals, however, hypercalcemia is neither an acute problem nor is the calcium × phosphate product greater than 60 to 80. Therefore conditions developing secondary to hypercalcemia (other than uroliths) are not usually a concern in dogs with PHPTH.

Renal failure or vitamin D toxicosis Severity of clinical signs and degree of damage to nephrons appears dependent, in part, on serum phosphorus concentrations via the calcium × phosphate product. Renal damage (nephrotoxicity) induced by metastatic mineralization is thought to correlate with serum Ca × PO₄ product greater than 60 to 80. Thus hypercalcemia associated with PHPTH is less worrisome and dangerous than the hypercalcemia associated with renal failure or hypervitaminosis D. The latter two disorders are almost always accompanied by hyperphosphatemia, a problem that amplifies the potential of soft tissue calcification (see Table 237-6).

Indications
Source of illness versus need for treatment Clinically, both to owners and veterinarians dogs with PHPTH appear relatively healthy. Further, despite having dramatic increases in serum calcium concentration (mean serum calcium concentrations > 14 mg/dL; see Table 237-5), dogs and cats with PHPTH are usually not in need of acute therapy because, in part, their calcium × phosphate products are not worrisome (see Table 237-6). In contrast, dogs with concurrent lymphosarcoma and hypercalcemia often exhibit extremely worrisome clinical signs that are caused by their malignancy rather than the hypercalcemia. Treatment for cancer often indirectly decreases serum calcium concentrations. Dogs that have mild hypercalcemia and renal failure or vitamin D toxicosis also usually have worrisome clinical signs and moderate to severe hyperphosphatemia. They are at risk for tissue mineralization and they benefit from treatment directed specifically at decreasing the calcium × phosphorus product. Dogs with apocrine gland carcinoma of the anal sac or those with "other" malignancies (e.g., multiple myeloma) also tend to be much more ill than dogs with PHPTH.

Indications for symptomatic treatment Because of the deleterious effects of hypercalcemia on renal, cardiovascular, or neurologic function, it may become necessary to treat a dog or cat symptomatically in an attempt to lower the blood calcium

Table • 237-6

Typical Serum Calcium and Phosphate Concentrations for Various Conditions

	TYPICAL SERUM CALCIUM (MG/DL)	TYPICAL SERUM PHOSPHATE (MG/DL)	TYPICAL CALCIUM × PHOSPHATE PRODUCT*
Normal dog	10	4.5	45
Primary hyperparathyroidism	14.3	2.8	40
Lymphosarcoma	15	3.0	45
Apocrine cell carcinoma of the anal sac	15	3.0	45
Chronic renal failure	11.5	10	115
Vitamin D toxicosis	11.5	10	115

*Aggressive therapy is recommended when the product of these two electrolytes exceeds 60 to 80. For most conditions causing hypercalcemia, emergency therapy is not necessary to reduce the serum calcium concentration.

concentration while completing tests to establish a diagnosis. The decision to implement symptomatic therapy should be based on the severity of the pet's clinical signs, the rapidity of progression of these signs, and the status of renal, cardiac, and neurologic function. *No specific serum calcium concentration exists above which therapy must be initiated.*

Therapy for hypercalcemia is indicated when dehydration, azotemia, cardiac arrhythmia, severe neurologic dysfunction, or weakness exists.[6,38] Death or encephalopathy directly attributable to hypercalcemia (except after ingestion of large amounts of rat poison containing vitamin D) is extremely uncommon. Therapy (intravenous fluids ± furosemide) may be indicated in a relatively stable dog or cat in which progressive metastatic calcification of soft tissues is suspected. Tissue mineralization can be assumed when the calcium × phosphorus product exceeds 60 to 80. With a product below 60, no urgent need exists to lower the serum calcium concentration, because the risk for soft tissue mineralization is not great.[39] Several methods have been suggested to control acute or severe hypercalcemia (Box 237-4 and Table 237-7). In dogs and cats, saline diuresis, diuretic therapy with furosemide or ethacrynic acid, and corticosteroids are the most commonly used modes of therapy. As a general rule, diuretic therapy and saline diuresis can be initiated without interfering with the diagnostic evaluation. Because the incidence of hypercalcemia associated with lymphosarcoma is great, glucocorticoids should not be administered unless a specific diagnosis has been confirmed.

Fluid Therapy

Correction of fluid deficits The primary indication for fluid therapy is dehydration. Decreases in fluid intake due to nausea and vomiting, plus an inability to concentrate urine, are common causes for dehydration in hypercalcemic dogs and cats. Dehydration, in turn, impairs calcium excretion by reducing GFR and increasing renal tubular absorption of calcium.[40] Dehydration also causes hemoconcentration, hyperproteinemia, and further increases in total and ionized serum calcium concentrations. Correction of fluid deficits should reduce the severity of hypercalcemia, although it usually does not return serum calcium concentrations to normal except in dogs with hypoadrenocorticism or those that are not, in fact, hypercalcemic. In humans, a rapid fall of 2 to 3 mg/dL in total serum calcium concentration is typical after rehydration.[3]

Saline diuresis Once fluid deficits have been corrected, saline diuresis should promote continuing renal loss of calcium; an effective short-term therapy for any cause of hypercalcemia. Physiologic saline promotes calciuresis because the large amount of filtered sodium competes with calcium for renal tubular resorption.[40] Increased sodium excretion leads to increased calcium excretion. Normal saline given at two to three times the maintenance rate (120 to 180 mL/kg/day) is usually effective. Potassium supplementation is often necessary to prevent hypokalemia. The pet should also be monitored carefully to detect adverse effects (e.g., pulmonary edema) resulting from administration of large fluid volumes. Monitoring body weight, urine output, blood pressure, central venous pressure (CVP), and auscultation of the thorax are recommended.

Diuretic Therapy The use of potent diuretics, in conjunction with saline diuresis, ensures maximal urinary sodium excretion and, in turn, calciuresis. Volume expansion must precede administration of furosemide. Furosemide enhances the calciuric effects of volume expansion by inhibiting calcium reabsorption in the thick ascending limb of the loop of Henle. Furosemide should also prevent severe volume overload.[6] Recommended protocols typically suggest a 5 mg/kg intravenous bolus followed by 2 to 4 mg/kg given twice a day or three times a day.[41] Thiazide diuretics should not be used because they decrease renal calcium excretion and may exacerbate hypercalcemia by enhancing distal tubular reabsorption.[6]

Glucocorticoids The beneficial effects of glucocorticoids in the symptomatic management of hypercalcemia include reducing bone resorption of calcium, decreasing intestinal calcium absorption, and increasing renal calcium excretion. Glucocorticoids are cytotoxic to neoplastic lymphocytes and inhibit growth of neoplastic tissue, accounting for their beneficial effects in lymphoma and multiple myeloma. They counteract effects of vitamin D toxicosis or granulomatous diseases. In general, nonhematologic cancers do not respond to glucocorticoids nor do animals with PHPTH.[42] Administration of glucocorticoids should be delayed until a definitive diagnosis has been established. Lymphosarcoma is the most common cause of hypercalcemia in the dog, but the administration of glucocorticoids may interfere with subsequent ability to confirm this diagnosis. Prednisone or prednisolone (1 to 2 mg/kg twice a day) or dexamethasone (0.1 to 0.2 mg/kg twice a day) can be used in the management of hypercalcemia. These drugs can be given orally, subcutaneously, or intravenously.

Bisphosphonates The bisphosphonates are compounds structurally related to pyrophosphate, a normal metabolic by-product. The chief property of these compounds is their inhibitory effect on osteoclast function and viability.[43] GI absorption is poor (< 10%), but intravenous administration has been effective in treating hypercalcemic humans.[6] Considering the early occurrence of bone resorption and bone loss in humans with multiple myeloma, for example, the benefit of bisphosphonates are impressive, even in humans who have no osteolytic lesions at the start of therapy. These drugs have beneficial skeletal effects and also slow tumor growth by inhibiting the production by osteoblasts of interleukin-6 (IL-6), a growth factor essential to myeloma cells.[44] Three bisphosphonates (etidronate, clodronate, and

---

Box • 237-4

General Treatment of Hypercalcemia

Definitive
Remove underlying cause

Supportive
Initial considerations
  Fluids (0.9% sodium chloride)
  Furosemide
  Sodium bicarbonate
  Glucocorticosteroids
Secondary considerations
  Bisphosphonates
  Calcitonin
Tertiary considerations
  Mithramycin
  Ethylenediamine tetra-acetic acid (EDTA)
  Peritoneal dialysis, homodialysis
Future considerations
  Calcium channel blockers
  Somatostatin congeners
  Calcium receptor agonists
  Nonhypercalcemic calcitriol analogues

Table • 237-7

Specific Treatment of Hypercalcemia (Not Needed in Primary Hyperparathyroidism)

TREATMENT	DOSE	INDICATIONS	COMMENTS
Volume Expansion			
SQ saline (0.9%)*	75-100 mL/kg/day	Mild hypercalcemia	Contraindicated if peripheral edema is present.
IV saline (0.9%)*	100-125 mL/kg/day	Moderate to severe hypercalcemia	Contraindicated in congestive heart failure and hypertension.
Diuretics			
Furosemide	2-4 mg/kg bid to tid IV, SQ, PO	Moderate to severe hypercalcemia	Volume expansion is necessary before use of this drug.
Alkalinizing Agent			
Sodium bicarbonate	1 mEq/kg IV slow bolus; may continue at 0.3 × base deficit × wt in kg/day	Severe hypercalcemia	Requires close monitoring.
Glucocorticoids			
Prednisone	1-2.2 mg/kg bid PO, SQ, IV	Moderate to severe hypercalcemia	Use of these drugs before identification of cause may make definitive diagnosis difficult!
Dexamethasone	0.1-0.22 mg/kg bid, IV, SQ		
Bone Resorption Inhibitors			
Calcitonin	4-6 IU/kg SQ bid to tid	Hypervitaminosis D	Response may be short-lived. Vomiting may occur.
Bisphosphonates			
EHDP-Didronel	15 mg/kg q24h to bid	Moderate to severe hypercalcemia	All are expensive, and use in dogs is limited.
Clodronate	20-25 mg/kg in a 4-hr IV infusion		Clodronate is approved for use in humans in Europe; availability in United States may be limited.
Pamidronate	1.3 mg/kg in 150 mL 0.9% saline in a 2-hr IV infusion, can repeat in 1 week		
Mithramycin	25 µg/kg IV in 5% dextrose over 2-4 hr q2-4 wk	Severe hypercalcemia, refractory HHM	Limited use in dogs and cats. Nephrotoxicity, hepatoxicity, thrombocytopenia.
Miscellaneous			
Sodium EDTA	25-75 mg/kg/hr	Severe hypercalcemia	Nephrotoxicity.
Peritoneal dialysis	Low calcium dialysate	Severe hypercalcemia	Short duration of response. Use in hypercalcemia not reported.

*Potassium supplementation is necessary. Clinician should add 5 to 40 mEq KCl/L depending on serum potassium concentration.
HHM, Humoral hypercalcemia of malignancy.

pamidronate) are approved in western countries for treatment of hypercalcemia in humans. Availability of other potent bisphosphonates (aminohexane bisphosphonate, risedronate, and alendronate) and other inhibitors of bone resorption (gallium nitrate, paclitaxel) open new avenues for more efficient treatment of hypercalcemia and bone disease. Clodronate was used successfully for treatment of lymphoma-induced hypercalcemia in one dog and vitamin D toxicosis in one dog.[45] Pamidronate has been used successfully to reverse vitamin D–induced toxicosis in dogs.[46,47]

Calcitonin Calcitonin reduces osteoclast activity and the formation of new osteoclasts. It may be effective, at least

temporarily, in decreasing serum calcium concentrations in those cases of hypercalcemia associated with excessive osteoclastic activity.[40] In humans, calcitonin has not been uniformly effective in lowering serum calcium concentration, either because the mechanisms of hypercalcemia induced by the disease are nonresponsive to calcitonin or because patients become refractory to its effects. The drug has been described as "weak," short-acting, and having few side effects.[6,48,49]

Salmon calcitonin (Calcimar solution, USV Laboratories, Tarrytown, New York) is the most potent congener available. Reports in the veterinary literature support use of this drug for the treatment of cholecalciferol rodenticide intoxication. Several doses have been reported, but the number of dogs and cats in which the drug has been used is too small for recommendations regarding their effectiveness. Some reported doses in dogs include 4.5 U/kg subcutaneously every 8 hours; 8 U/kg subcutaneously every 24 hours; and 5 U/kg subcutaneously every 12 hours.[50,51] In cats, 4 U/kg intramuscularly every 12 hours was used successfully.[52]

Plicamycin (Mithramycin) Plicamycin (previously termed *mithramycin*) is a cytotoxic compound initially evaluated as a cancer chemotherapeutic agent. This agent is a potent inhibitor of RNA synthesis in osteoclasts and an effective treatment for hypercalcemia. Significant toxicity, including thrombocytopenia, hepatic necrosis, renal damage, and hypocalcemia has been caused by the drug. Clinically significant toxicity was not observed in normal dogs after two IV treatments. Shivering was noted during the infusion, and osteoclastic activity was reduced.[53,54] Two doses have been reported: 25 g/kg and 50 g/kg once or twice weekly, to control hypercalcemia.[55] Effects of this drug on serum total and ionized calcium concentrations were studied in nine dogs with hypercalcemia of malignancy, one dog with PHPTH, and one dog with vitamin D toxicosis. High-dose mithramycin (100 g/kg) caused fatal acute hepatocellular necrosis in two dogs. Low doses (25 g/kg) were effective in normalizing total and ionized calcium concentrations within 24 to 48 hours in six of nine dogs, including a dog with vitamin D toxicosis. The effects were short lived (1 to 3 days) in three dogs and lasted longer (about 7 days) in three dogs. Side effects were mild in dogs treated with the low dose and included mild GI signs in three dogs and reduction in platelet counts in three dogs. The low dose did not cause evidence of hepatic disease, reduce tumor size, or reduce PTHrP concentrations.[54]

EDTA The intravenous injection of sodium EDTA has been used to reduce ionized calcium concentrations immediately in humans with life-threatening hypercalcemia. Infused EDTA forms complexes with ionized calcium that are rapidly excreted by the kidney.[40] A dose of 25 to 75 mg/kg/hr has been suggested as a starting point for the treatment of hypercalcemia in the dog.[21] Unfortunately, EDTA is nephrotoxic, and acute renal failure may be a consequence of its infusion.

Bicarbonate The ionized fraction of serum calcium is determined partly by an animal's acid-base status. Correcting acidosis or creating a slight alkalosis with bicarbonate therapy shifts ionized calcium to the protein-bound fraction, rendering it less harmful.[39] A dose of 1 to 4 mEq/kg has been recommended.[56] A single intravenous dose may last as long as 3 hours in normal cats.[57] The effect of the drug is mild, and it may be helpful when administered with other treatments.

Dialysis Hemodialysis and peritoneal dialysis with calcium-free dialysate solutions have been used effectively in humans to lower serum calcium concentrations when other methods have failed.[3,40] These techniques are particularly effective in patients with severe renal failure because fluid and diuretic therapy depends on enhanced renal excretion of calcium. Significant quantities of phosphate may also be dialyzed from the blood. Because phosphate depletion may aggravate hypercalcemia, serum phosphorous concentrations should be monitored and supplements given as required.

Calcium Receptor Agonist Therapy Medical therapy for PHPTH has been limited, although new approaches have followed discovery of a calcium-sensing receptor on parathyroid cells that down-regulate synthesis and secretion of PTH. Molecules that mimic the effect of extracellular calcium could also activate this receptor and inhibit parathyroid cell function. The Phenylalkylamine (R)-N-(3-methoxy-alpha-phenylethyl)-3-(2-chlorophenyl)-1-propylamine, or R-5658, is one such

calcimemetic compound. The drug did reduce serum PTH and ionized calcium concentrations in postmenopausal women with primary hyperparathyroidism.[58]

Surgical Therapy for Primary Hyperparathyroidism
Assessing the Parathyroid Glands During Surgery

How many glands are involved? Surgical techniques for removing parathyroid tumors are described in various textbooks. It is important to attempt identification and evaluation of all four parathyroid glands before deciding on which gland or glands to remove. However, most dogs with PHPTH only have one obvious gland because the others are atrophied. About 90% of dogs with PHPTH have a solitary, autonomously functioning, parathyroid mass. Virtually all of the remaining dogs have two abnormal glands. Once an ultrasonographer demonstrates competence at identifying parathyroid glands and parathyroid tumors, the clinician should be reluctant to send any dog suspected of having PHPTH to surgery if an abnormal parathyroid mass or masses are not seen via cervical ultrasonography. Visualizing a mass supports the diagnosis and informs the surgeon where abnormal tissue is located. The process of evaluating parathyroid tissue at surgery without prior ultrasound evaluation can be extremely easy or quite difficult. The surgeon may easily visualize enlargement of one (common), two (less common), or more than two glands (rare). However, abnormal parathyroid tissue may not be readily identified. Any enlarged or abnormal tissue should be removed and submitted for histologic evaluation, assuming that three or fewer parathyroids appear enlarged, discolored, or both. The remaining intact gland or glands should prevent permanent hypoparathyroidism, although transient hypocalcemia may develop after surgery due to atrophy of normal glands after chronic suppression by the autonomously functioning abnormal gland or glands. An attempt must be made to ensure that at least one parathyroid gland remains intact to maintain calcium homeostasis and prevent permanent hypocalcemia. If none of the parathyroid glands appear enlarged or if all appear small, the diagnosis of primary PHPTH must be questioned. Uniform enlargement of all four glands should make one suspicious of a secondary condition.

Intravenous methylene blue infusion (3 mg/kg) has been described as a tool for improving a surgeon's ability to recognize abnormal glands. Three dogs with PHPTH were evaluated, and each had a tumor identified after new methylene blue infusion. Two of the three dogs developed anemia, Heinz bodies, and red blood cell (RBC) "blistering" after the procedure.[59] This procedure is not recommended.

The solitary adenoma, hyperplastic nodule, or carcinoma Almost all dogs with PHPTH have a solitary, easily identified, parathyroid adenoma. Fourteen of the 187 dogs with PHPTH in our series had parathyroid masses that at surgery appeared to be typical adenomas but histologically were diagnosed as carcinoma. Another 12 dogs had parathyroid masses that were classified as hyperplasia.[60] Approximately one half of tumors have been identified on the ventral surface of the thyroid glands. If not seen on the ventral surface, careful inspection of the dorsal surface of each thyroid lobe usually reveals the mass as a discrete structure on, or within, the adjacent thyroid tissue (Figure 237-6). "External" parathyroid adenomas have been easily removed without damage to surrounding tissue. Surgeons may choose to remove the entire thyroid-parathyroid structure in dogs with an "internal" parathyroid adenoma. In about 5% of dogs, the surgeon was not able to identify abnormal tissue and removed the thyroid lobe suggested by cervical ultrasonography as containing the parathyroid mass. In each case, that decision was correct.

Enlargement of multiple parathyroid glands When more than one enlarged gland is identified, the concern is primary versus secondary (renal or nutritional) hyperparathyroidism.

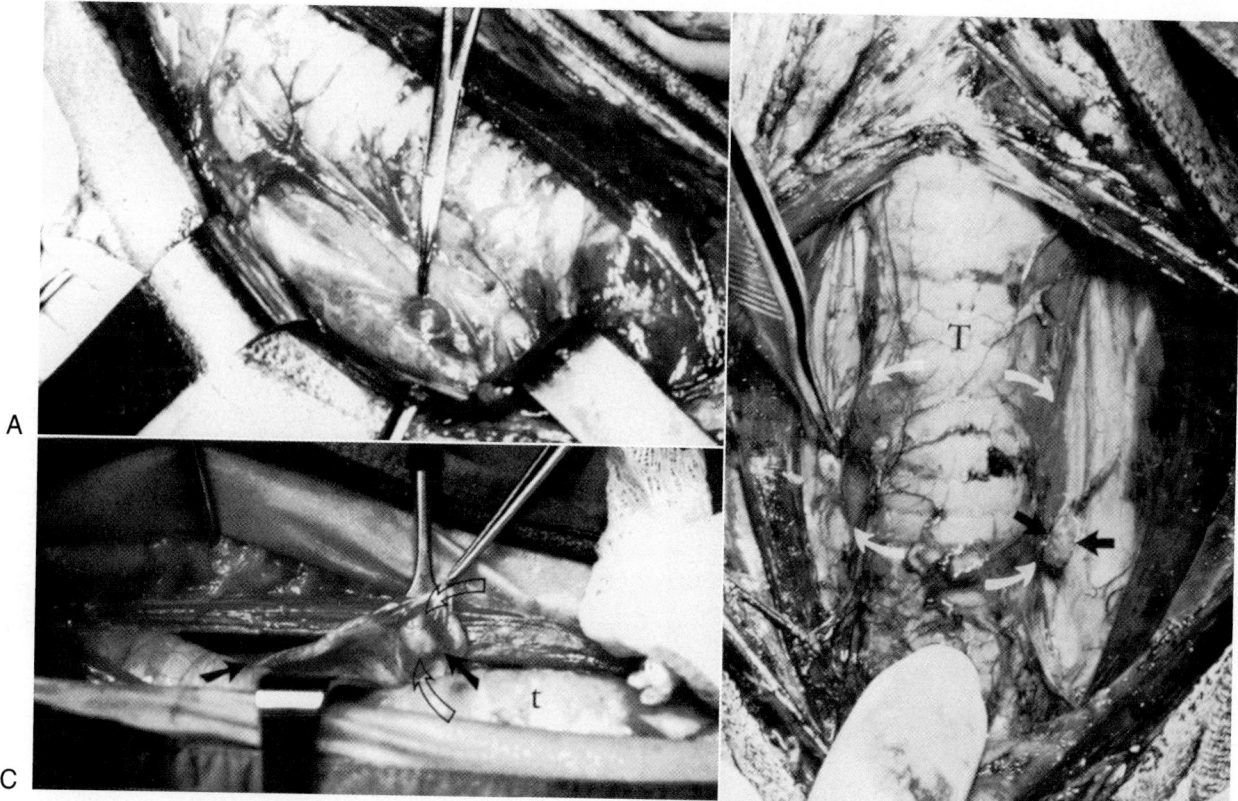

Figure 237-6 **A,** Surgical site during removal of a solitary parathyroid adenoma *(tip of forceps).* **B,** Surgical site during removal of a solitary parathyroid adenoma. White arrows delineate the cranial and caudal poles of the thyroid glands; black arrows point out the parathyroid adenoma. **C,** Surgical site during removal of an "internal" parathyroid adenoma. Solid arrows delineate the cranial and caudal poles of the thyroid, which is being retracted from the trachea to reveal the parathyroid adenoma *(open arrows)* on the dorsal surface of the thyroid. *T,* trachea. (From Feldman EC, Nelson RW: Canine and Feline Endocrinology and Reproduction, 3rd ed. Philadelphia, WB Saunders Co, 2004.)

The presurgical evaluation, as reviewed, should identify or eliminate secondary disease. If the clinician is convinced that primary disease is present, a decision to remove two glands is straightforward. However, if four glands are involved (an extremely rare situation), the decision should be based on clinical status, renal function, and ability of the owner to treat permanent hypoparathyroidism.

Only 14 of 187 dogs with PHPTH (7%) had enlargement of more than one gland each. Of these 14 dogs, each of 13 dogs had two enlarged glands and one had four enlarged glands. Each of three dogs had two "hyperplastic" parathyroids, each of three dogs had two parathyroid adenomas, each of three dogs had one adenoma and one hyperplastic gland, each of two dogs had one hyperplastic gland and one carcinoma, and one of the dogs with two masses had one adenoma and one carcinoma (histologic classification is discussed in a following section). One of the 187 PHPTH dogs had enlargement of all four glands.[60] Each of these four glands were classified histologically as being hyperplastic. Enlargement of all four glands suggests either multiple adenomas or, more likely, parathyroid hyperplasia.

Recurrence of PHPTH Sixteen of 187 dogs with PHPTH in our series had a solitary parathyroid mass removed surgically with resolution and then recurrence of their disease. In each case, resolution of the PHPTH persisted for at least 6 months, and in 13 of the 16 dogs, PHPTH had resolved for 12 to 30 months, whereas in three it lasted 6 to 12 months. Each dog then had recurrence of hypercalcemia caused by a

second solitary, autonomously functioning, surgically removed parathyroid mass. The initial diagnosis in 11 dogs was parathyroid adenoma, three had a parathyroid carcinoma, and two had parathyroid hyperplasia. The histology report after the second surgery was the same in 12 dogs. However, two of the three dogs that initially had a parathyroid carcinoma had an adenoma at recurrence and one dog with an adenoma initially had a carcinoma removed at the second surgery. One dog with hyperplasia initially had an adenoma removed at the second surgery. Thus it is possible for the disorder to recur, suggesting that periodic rechecks of the serum calcium concentration after stabilization would be warranted. Seven of the 16 dogs were Keeshonden, and this breed may warrant more routine evaluations after initial treatment.

No parathyroid mass at surgery If an enlarged parathyroid gland is not identified after thorough inspection of both thyroid areas by an experienced surgeon, careful exploration of the ventral neck should be completed and any abnormal tissue excised. The most likely explanation for not finding a parathyroid mass includes hypercalcemia due to occult neoplasia, PTH production by a parathyroid tumor located outside of the typical cervical region (in the cranial mediastinum), or the presence of a nonparathyroid tumor producing PTH (i.e., ectopic hyperparathyroidism). Presurgical cervical ultrasonography should identify a parathyroid mass. Failure to visualize a parathyroid mass would best be managed by obtaining another ultrasound opinion or delaying surgery for 1 to 3 months and then rechecking the cervical ultrasonography.

We have no experience with surgical exploration of the cranial mediastinum for a parathyroid mass. Such surgeries have inherent technical difficulties. The likelihood of finding ectopic abnormal parathyroid tissue is small. The greater likelihood of malignancy-associated hypercalcemia suggests that the decision to continue surgical exploration be carefully considered. Further diagnostic tests should be undertaken to identify occult neoplasia.

Novel Therapies for Primary Hyperparathyroidism in Dogs

Percutaneous Ultrasound-Guided Ethanol Ablation

Ultrasonography is an excellent method of identifying parathyroid masses in dogs with hypercalcemia secondary to PHPTH. Based on our experience with this tool as a diagnostic aid and studies performed on people with PHPTH,[61] we elected to assess the efficacy of ethanol ablation as a treatment for this disorder.[62] Ethanol causes coagulation necrosis and vascular thrombosis in the parenchyma of exposed tissue. PHPTH was diagnosed in 12 dogs. Their clinical and biochemical evaluation was typical for the disease. Each dog had a solitary hypoechoic round to oval mass near the thyroid gland on cervical ultrasonography. Parathyroid masses were identified on the right side of the neck in eight dogs and on the left in the other four. All the masses were 4 to 10 mm in length, located at the cranial aspect of one thyroid lobe in six dogs, within the caudal pole of a thyroid lobe in three dogs, and in the midbody of the thyroid gland in three dogs. Calculated volume of the parathyroid masses ranged from 0.06 to 0.16 cm[3]. It was assumed that each dog had a mass autonomously secreting PTH.

Each dog was placed under general anesthesia, and the ventral cervical region was clipped and aseptically prepared. The parathyroid mass was identified with ultrasound, and the tip of a 27-gauge needle, with tubing and syringe attached, was guided into the parathyroid using ultrasound (Figure 237-7). The approximate volume of the mass was matched with an equal volume of ethanol placed in the syringe. Ethanol was slowly injected into the mass with continuous ultrasound monitoring. The goal of therapy was to inject enough ethanol to allow complete diffusion throughout the mass. The injection procedure requires a high-resolution transducer (10 MHz frequency) to allow assessment of the superficial tissues of the neck. Because parathyroid masses are small and sometimes in close proximity to nerves and vessels, considerable experience with ultrasound-guided needle placement is necessary.

Ethanol was easily seen with ultrasound during injection because it is hyperechoic (see Figure 237-7). Each parathyroid

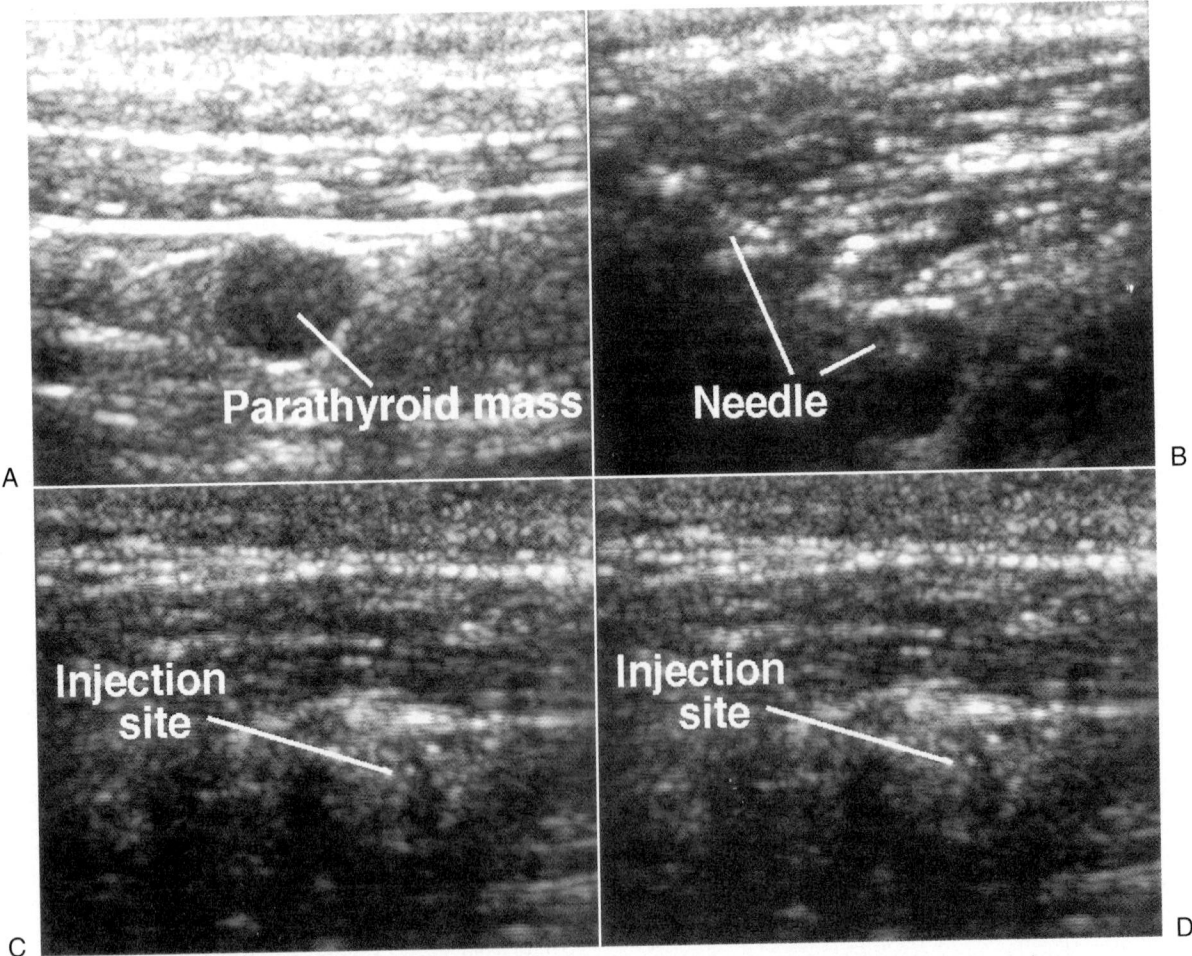

Figure 237-7 Ultrasonographic appearance of chemical ablation of a parathyroid mass in a dog. **A,** Sagittal view of the parathyroid mass prior to treatment. **B,** A 27-gauge needle is inserted into the mass. **C,** A test injection of 96% ethanol is used to confirm placement of the needle inside the mass. The reader should note that the ethanol is hyperechoic in relation to the parenchyma of the mass. **D,** After injection of the target dose of ethanol, the entire mass has an echogenic appearance. (From Long CD et al: Percutaneous ultrasound-guided chemical parathyroid ablation for treatment of primary hyperparathyroidism in dogs. J Am Vet Med Assoc 215:217, 1999, with permission.)

mass was injected with 50% to 150% of the calculated parathyroid volume. No dog was under anesthesia for more than 1 hour, and the mean duration of anesthesia was 38 minutes. A single injection was administered to 11 of the 12 dogs. One dog was injected a second time 48 hours after the first dose failed to decrease the serum calcium concentration into the reference range. All 12 dogs had decreases in serum total calcium concentration into the reference range. In 11 dogs this decrease was documented within 48 hours of injection (10 after the first injection and one after the second injection). One dog did not have resolution of its hypercalcemia until the fifth day post-treatment. One dog had a recurrence of hypercalcemia 30 days after injection and was treated surgically. Each of the other 11 dogs remained normal for more than 18 months. The only adverse side effect was a transient change in the "bark" in two dogs, potentially as a result of transient, unilateral, laryngeal paralysis injection of bilateral masses is not recommended.

The conclusion of this study was that ultrasound-guided ethanol ablation was an efficacious mode of therapy for PHPTH in dogs. The cost of the procedure was considerably less than for surgery. Chemical ablation of parathyroid masses may be more effective in dogs than in humans because canine parathyroid masses are considerably smaller, thus requiring a smaller dose of ethanol for complete ablation.

Percutaneous Ultrasound-Guided Radiofrequency Heat Ablation
Heat destroys tissue by causing thermal necrosis. This form of therapy has several advantages as compared with ethanol ablation. First, radiofrequency damages a discrete quantity of tissue surrounding the noninsulated portion of the needle (no potential for "leakage" exists as with ethanol). Radiofrequency offers the additional advantage of not causing damage to regional vasculature. Vascular blood flow disperses heat from vessel walls. In humans, this treatment modality has a higher success rate than ethanol for ablation of masses, and fewer treatments are required to achieve remission. Radiofrequency heat ablation has been used in the treatment of multifocal hepatic masses and breast and nasal masses.[63,64] The disadvantage of radiofrequency is equipment cost.

Candidates for this procedure must have a parathyroid mass visible with ultrasonography; that mass must be large enough to have a needle inserted into it with ultrasound guidance (usually greater than 3 mm in diameter); the mass can not

be subjectively considered too close to the carotid artery; and the dog should not have cystic calculi to be surgically removed because cervical surgery is a straight-forward addition to abdominal surgery. Since starting to use this treatment, 19 dogs did not meet the criteria for inclusion. An attempt was made to treat two dogs early in the study period, but the capsule could not be penetrated with the needle, and treatment was not attempted. Since then, a different more penetrating needle has been used. In one dog the parathyroid mass was too small for needle placement, and in four dogs the parathyroid mass was considered too close to the carotid artery for safe needle placement. Twelve dogs had cystic calculi that required surgical removal. In each of these dogs, parathyroid surgery and abdominal surgery were performed at the same time.

Between September of 1999 and January of 2003, 33 dogs with PHPTH were treated with percutaneous heat ablation. Each dog had clinical and biochemical features that were typical for PHPTH. A solitary parathyroid nodule was identified by use of cervical ultrasonography in 26 dogs, seven dogs had two nodules each (a total of 40 masses in the 33 dogs). Five of these seven dogs had both nodules on the left side of the neck and two dogs had one nodule associated with each thyroid lobe. The ultrasonic appearance of the 40 masses was similar. All masses were spherical or ovoid and hypoechoic to the surrounding thyroid parenchyma. Length varied from 3 to 20 mm. Each dog with a solitary parathyroid mass was treated once. Each dog with two parathyroid nodules on the same side of the neck had both masses treated during the initial anesthesia. Each nodule was treated separately, 30 days apart, in the two dogs with one nodule on each side of the neck.

Each dog was placed under general anesthesia and the ventral cervical region was clipped and aseptically prepared. The parathyroid mass was identified with ultrasound, and the tip of a 20-gauge, over-the-needle (insulated) catheter, was directed into the mass using ultrasound guidance. An insulated wire connected the needle with the radiofrequency unit (Radiotherapeutics, Inc., Redwood City, California). Initially, 10 watts of energy was applied to the tissue for 10 to 20 seconds. If echogenic bubbles were not sonographically viewed at the needle tip during this time, the wattage was increased. Two-watt incremental increases were continued every 5 to 10 seconds until echogenic foci became apparent (Figure 237-8). Further, if an audible popping sound could be heard, the

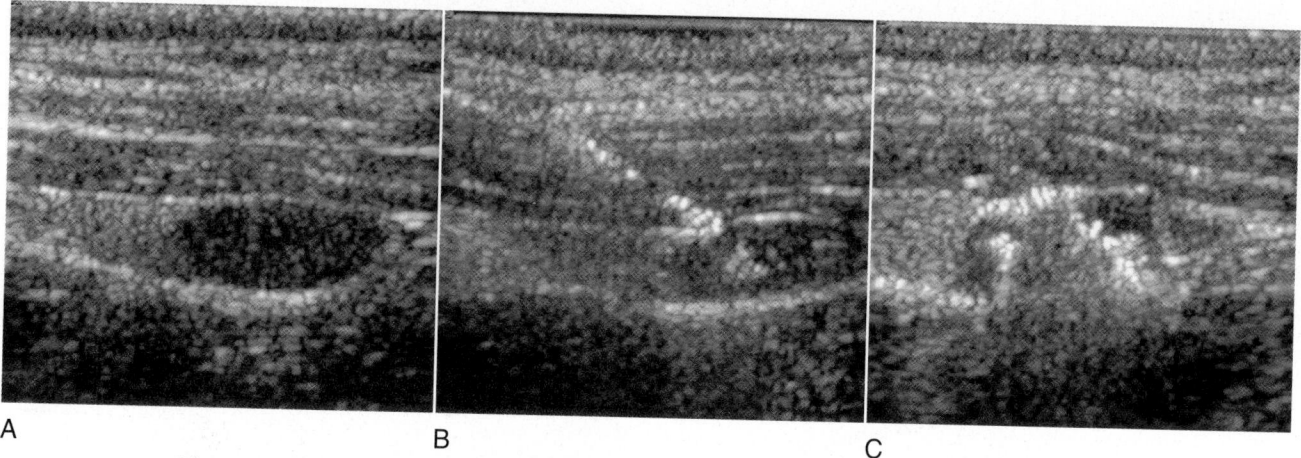

A   B   C

Figure 237-8 Left lateral sonographic images of an oval hypoechoic parathyroid nodule in a dog prior to heat ablation (**A**), with the insulated needle passing through the superficial soft tissues into the cranial aspect of the mass (**B**), and after heat ablation (**C**). The reader should note the hyperechoic foci in the parenchyma of the gland in **C**. (From Pollard RE et al: Percutaneous ultrasonographically guided radiofrequency heat ablation for treatment of primary hyperparathyroidism in dogs. J Am Vet Med Assoc 218:1106, 2001, used with permission.)

maximum heat application was arbitrarily determined to have been reached and additional wattage increases were not made. The needle was arbitrarily redirected multiple times, if necessary, in an attempt to completely ablate each mass. Mean anesthesia time was about 40 minutes, but this progressively decreased as experience with this procedure increased.[65]

The procedure was uniformly successful in these 33 dogs as demonstrated by the dramatic reduction in serum PTH and normalization of both total and ionized calcium concentrations that occurred within days of heat ablation. Serum calcium concentrations have remained within the reference range for more than 1 year. One dog improved for only 1 month and was treated surgically after hypercalcemia recurred. One dog with a unilateral parathyroid mass developed a transient voice change immediately after heat ablation, which resolved within 5 days. It is uncertain whether this voice change was secondary to intubation or the ablation procedure. Signs of pain, swelling, or respiratory distress were not detected in any of the dogs. Fifteen of the dogs required vitamin D therapy for postablation hypocalcemia (see following section). This is currently our preferred mode of treatment for dogs with PHPTH that do not have cystic calculi.

Post-Treatment Management of Potential Hypocalcemia

Background   Normal parathyroid glands atrophy if their function has been suppressed for a prolonged time due to autonomous secretion of PTH by a parathyroid adenoma, carcinoma, or primary hyperplasia. Surgical removal or ablation of this source for PTH results in a rapid decline in circulating PTH concentration (Figure 237-9) and a corresponding decline in serum calcium concentrations. This process typically takes place over a period of 1 to 7 days. Risk of post-treatment hypocalcemia correlates with the duration and severity of hypercalcemia prior to surgery (i.e., the higher the pretreatment calcium and the longer a dog has been hypercalcemic, the greater the risk of hypocalcemia after resolution of the PHPTH). Beginning vitamin D therapy immediately prior to or after surgery does not prevent decreases in serum calcium concentrations to or below the reference range but usually helps to avoid worrisome hypocalcemia or tetany.

Presurgical Serum Calcium Concentration Less than 14 mg/dL
If the serum calcium concentration prior to surgery is less than 14 mg/dL, the risk of postsurgical hypocalcemia is relatively small. Results between 14 and 15 mg/dL

are inconsistent. The recommendation is to hospitalize such dogs for at least 5 days after surgery to monitor total serum calcium concentrations once or twice daily. Hospitalization also reduces a dog's activity by maintaining it in a cage or run. Active hypocalcemic dogs are at greater risk for clinical tetany than those kept quiet. If the total serum calcium concentration remains above 8.5 mg/dL (assuming a lower reference limit of 9 to 10 mg/dL), treatment for hypocalcemia is not recommended. If the serum ionized calcium concentration remains above 0.8 mmol/L (assuming a lower reference limit of about 1.1 mmol/L), treatment is not recommended. The reader should note, however, that these are general recommendations. It would never be incorrect to begin vitamin D therapy if one is concerned about rate of decrease in calcium or simply one wishes to be proactive. If the serum calcium concentrations decline below the limits suggested, or if clinical signs of hypocalcemia are observed (Box 237-5), treatment with vitamin D (± calcium) is suggested.

Presurgical Serum Calcium Concentration Greater than 15 mg/dL
The higher the presurgical serum calcium concentration, the more chronic the hypercalcemic condition, or both, the more likely it is that a dog will become clinically hypocalcemic after resolution of PHPTH. Knowing the duration of hypercalcemia would be valuable but is often not possible in dogs or cats. It can be assumed that dogs with serum calcium concentrations persistently greater than 15 mg/dL due to PHPTH have been hypercalcemic for sometime. It is recommended to prophylactically attempt to avoid hypocalcemia after surgery in this population of dogs by beginning vitamin D (Hytakerol or Calcitriol) ± calcium therapy the evening before or the morning of surgery or immediately after recovery from anesthesia. In some cases we have begun vitamin D therapy 24 to 36 hours *before* surgery because of the known delay in onset of vitamin D action. This becomes important in dogs severely hypercalcemic prior to surgery (>18 mg/dL). Initiation of these treatments has not prevented decreases in serum calcium concentration to or below reference ranges after surgery. Each dog should be kept quiet in the hospital for at least 5 days after treatment. Postsurgical hypocalcemia has been documented as quickly as 12 hours after surgery to as long as 20 days later. Most become hypocalcemic between 2 and 6 days after surgery. Tetany, when it has occurred, is most commonly seen 4 to 7 days after treatment. The serum calcium concentration should be monitored once or twice daily.

The goal of calcium and vitamin D therapy is to maintain the serum calcium concentration slightly low to low-normal (i.e., 8 to 9.5 mg/dL). These serum calcium levels prevent clinical signs of hypocalcemia and minimize risk of hypercalcemia while simultaneously being low enough to stimulate recovery of function in atrophied parathyroid glands. In addition, one should avoid mid- to high-normal or increased serum

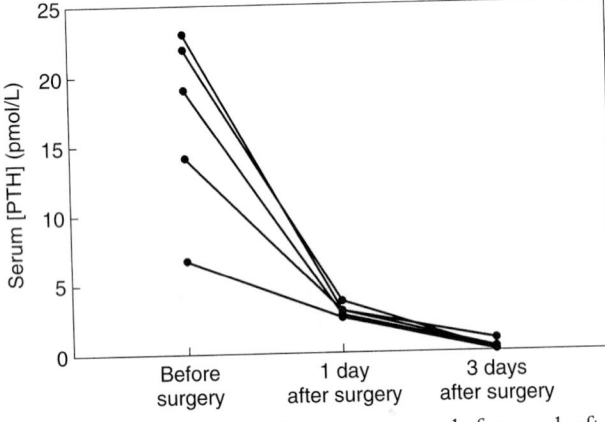

Figure 237-9 Serum PTH concentrations before and after surgery in eight dogs in which a solitary functional parathyroid adenoma was removed. (From Feldman EC, Nelson RW: Canine and Feline Endocrinology and Reproduction, 3rd ed. Philadelphia, WB Saunders Co, 2004.)

Box • 237-5

Clinical Signs Associated with the Acute Onset of Hypocalcemia

Panting
Nervousness
Muscle trembling, twitching
Leg cramping, pain
Ataxia, stiff gait
Facial rubbing
Focal or generalized seizures
Biting of the feet

calcium concentrations. Such levels of calcium are typically associated with increases in serum phosphate concentrations and predispose the dog to tissue mineralization.

As the parathyroid glands regain control of calcium homeostasis, calcium and vitamin D supplements can be gradually withdrawn. This process of returning parathyroid function in remaining glands is predictable, allowing the gradual withdrawal (tapering) of calcium and vitamin D supplements. Once the serum calcium concentration is stabilized and the dog has been returned to the owner, withdrawal of the supplements may be initiated. Vitamin D is usually withdrawn first by gradually extending the time between administration (e.g., twice daily to once daily for 2 weeks; to once every other day for 2 weeks; then once every third day for 2 weeks; then once every fourth day for 2 weeks; and finally once weekly for 2 to 4 weeks). The serum calcium concentration should be checked prior to each downward adjustment in dosing interval to prevent development of occult hypocalcemia. If the serum calcium concentration drops below 8 mg/dL, decreases in vitamin D supplementation should be delayed or the dose increased. The serum calcium concentration should remain above 8 mg/dL to minimize the risk of tetany. Once the vitamin D supplementation has been reduced to once weekly for a period of 2 to 4 weeks, it may be discontinued. If the serum calcium concentration remains within the normal range, the calcium supplements can then be gradually withdrawn. The entire withdrawal process for vitamin D and calcium usually takes 3 to 4 months. The clinician should remember that considerable individual variation occurs in response to therapy; therefore it is impossible to check the serum calcium concentration too frequently.

Vitamin D Resistance Occasionally, dogs (but more often cats) seem resistant to vitamin D in tablet form. This problem is usually resolved by using the liquid form of dihydrotachysterol or by using oral or parenteral calcitriol. It is not common for dihydrotachysterol to begin to have an effect within the first 24 hours of therapy. Rather, vitamin D gradually takes effect during the first several days of therapy and almost always within 4 to 7 days of the first dose.

Pathology
Abnormal, autonomously functioning parathyroid glands from humans, dogs, and cats have been characterized histologically as adenoma, carcinoma, and hyperplasia. Controlled studies of histologic interpretations by pathologists have shown that it is difficult to consistently distinguish adenoma from hyperplasia and that nonmalignant parathyroid tissue may, in some cases, have many of the histologic features of malignancy.[3] Thus histologic classification of parathyroid disease depends, to some degree, on gross features observed during surgery. The surgeon determines the number, size, and appearance of normal versus abnormal glands. The pathologist then determines whether removed tissue is parathyroid. Single-gland involvement (adenoma, carcinoma, or hyperplasia) occurs in about 80% of hyperparathyroid humans and multiple-gland involvement ("hyperplasia") in about 20%.[48,66] It appears that single-gland involvement occurs in about 90% of dogs with PHPTH and multiple glands (almost always two but not more than two) occurs in about 10%. The diagnosis of carcinoma is based on a combination of gross appearance, histology, and, ultimately, biologic behavior of the lesion. Less than 2% of autonomously secreting parathyroid glands in humans are malignant.[67] In dogs, about 5% to 10% of dogs have been assigned the diagnosis of carcinoma. Regardless of the histologic diagnosis, no dog with distant metastasis has been recognized in our of 187 cases, and recurrence rate (10%) is similar, regardless of the histologic diagnosis.

Prognosis
The prognosis in dogs with PHPTH is excellent. With proper monitoring and appropriate supplementation, hypocalcemia may occur after therapy but should be treatable, transient, and should not alter the prognosis. About 33% of the dogs developed clinically significant hypocalcemia after treatment. The routine use of vitamin D (dihydrotachysterol or calcitriol) and calcium supplementation has dramatically decreased the incidence of tetany. Clinicians should avoid overdosing vitamin D, because renal damage is much more likely in this situation than in dogs with PHPTH.

PRIMARY HYPERPARATHYROIDISM IN CATS

Differential Diagnosis for Feline Hypercalcemia
It is fair to state that, in general, the same differential diagnoses for hypercalcemia in dogs applies to cats. In a study of 71 hypercalcemic cats, their mean age at the time of diagnosis was about 9 years and their mean serum total calcium concentration was 12.2 (lower than hypercalcemic dogs). Anorexia and lethargy were the most common clinical signs (70%). Vomiting, diarrhea, or constipation were observed in 27% of the cats; polyuria, polydipsia, or both were observed in 24%; and urinary signs were observed in 23%. Neurologic signs were observed in 14%.[68]

Neoplasia was diagnosed in 30% of the cats. The most common cancers diagnosed included lymphoma and squamous cell carcinoma. Less common neoplasms included leukemia, osteosarcoma, fibrosarcoma, undifferentiated sarcoma, and bronchogenic carcinoma.[68,69] Renal failure was diagnosed in 25% of the cats, and half of those cats had urolithiasis. In a separate study, chronic renal failure in cats was usually associated with total serum calcium concentrations within the reference range, whereas serum ionized calcium concentrations were low-normal to low.[70] Of cats with hypercalcemia, several had urolithiasis without renal failure. Six percent of the cats (four cats) had PHPTH and one had hypoadrenocorticism. Several cats had hyperthyroidism or diabetes mellitus, but it would not seem likely that either of these endocrine problems would contribute to hypercalcemia. Four cats (6%) had infectious or granulomatous disease (feline infectious peritonitis [FIP], toxoplasmosis, actinomyces, and cryptococcosis). Thus the differential diagnosis for hypercalcemia in cats is not dramatically different from that in dogs (see Box 237-1).[68,71] Other differential diagnoses (e.g., vitamin D toxicosis, other neoplastic conditions, various granulomatous diseases) should also be considered.

Idiopathic Hypercalcemia of Cats
Hypercalcemia is less common in cats than in dogs, but an increased frequency of hypercalcemia in cats has been observed in several geographically distinct veterinary centers since about 1990.[21,72,73] It is striking that this hypercalcemia has not been, thus far, explained. Veterinarians are identifying young, middle-aged, and old cats with mild to moderate hypercalcemia and no identifiable cause. Serum total calcium concentrations in some of these cats have been increased for years, often without clinical signs, but some have poor appetites, weight loss, and appear weak. Serum ionized calcium concentrations are also increased, sometimes out of proportion to the increase in total calcium concentration.[21]

Nephrocalcinosis or uroliths may be observed on radiographs or on abdominal ultrasonography in some hypercalcemic cats. It has been estimated that as many as 33% of cats with calcium oxalate urolithiasis have had hypercalcemia. Renal function (based on BUN and serum creatinine concentrations) is initially within reference ranges, but renal failure may develop in some cats. By definition, these cats have had no evidence of a neoplastic condition (including necropsy), and they are feline leukemia virus (FeLV) and feline immunodeficiency virus (FIV) negative. Serum PTH concentrations have been normal or low, PTHrP has not been detectable, and vitamin D concentrations have been within reference ranges.

Venous blood gas analyses have not demonstrated significant abnormalities.[21] Exploratory surgery of the cervical region has not identified any abnormalities, and subtotal parathyroidectomy has failed to resolve the hypercalcemia. A change to high-fiber or to nonacidifying diets may be associated with transient improvement but also failed to permanently resolve the condition. Treatment with prednisone (usually 5 to 10 mg/cat/day) has resulted in long-term decreases in serum calcium concentrations in some but not all afflicted cats. Prednisone, regardless of the effect on serum calcium concentrations, has resulted in improved appetite and weight gain in some but not all cats.

Primary Hyperparathyroidism in Cats

In addition to 10 cats with PHPTH in our series, an additional nine cats with PHPTH have been reported. Thus, only 19 cats with this condition, as compared with a much larger number of similarly afflicted dogs. Seven cats in the author's group of 10 with hypercalcemia due to PHPTH were described in one report, reported four cats were described in one report, two in each of two reports and one in another separate report.[21,74-77] The mean age of these 19 cats was approximately 13 years (range: 8 to 20 years), and various breeds were represented. The most common clinical signs described by owners were anorexia, lethargy, and vomiting. Less common signs were constipation, polyuria, polydipsia, and weight loss. A parathyroid mass was palpable in at least 11 of the 19 cats. The presence of a palpable mass and the owner observations contrast with those of dogs, in which none had a palpable cervical mass and polyuria, polydipsia, and muscle weakness are common.

The only consistent abnormality on CBC and serum biochemical profiles was hypercalcemia (Table 237-8). All afflicted cats had persistent increases in both serum total and ionized calcium concentrations. Several cats had cystic calculi, and a large percentage had abnormalities in BUN and serum creatinine concentrations, findings not typical of their canine counterparts. Cervical ultrasonography was described as "normal" in several cats, but others had visible masses that would be considered huge in a dog. Cervical ultrasonography on two cats revealed parathyroid masses measuring $4.5 \times 2 \times 1$ cm in one cat and $1.7 \times 1.1 \times 1$ cm in the other.[77] Serum PTH concentrations, when measured, ranged from within the reference range (0 to 4 pmol/L) to increased. In one cat, seven separate serum PTH samples were assayed with five results being within the reference range and two being increased.

Most of the 19 cats had surgery and had resolution of the PHPTH after extirpation of the abnormal tissue. It seems that tetany has not been described in any cat treated with surgery, although several became hypocalcemic and were treated with vitamin D and calcium. Of the nine cats we followed after surgery, all lived well beyond 1 year from surgery, although at 1.5 years, one had recurrence of hypercalcemia and at necropsy was demonstrated to have both a parathyroid adenoma and a parathyroid carcinoma. Histologic evaluation of tissue from 13 cats had demonstrated parathyroid adenomas, three had carcinomas, two had hyperplasia (involving all four glands), and one had bilateral cystadenomas.

Table • 237-8

Clinical, Laboratory, and Histologic Findings in 10 Cats with Primary Naturally Occurring Hyperparathyroidism in the University of California, Davis Series

SIGNALMENT	CLINICAL SIGNS	SERUM Ca (mg/dL)	SERUM PO₄ (mg/dL)	BUN (mg/dL)	SERUM CREATININE (mg/dL)	URINE SPECIFIC GRAVITY (USG)	PARATHYROID HISTOLOGY
15 y.o. M/N/, DLH	Anorexia, vomiting	14.6	3.4	35	1.8	1.011	Solitary adenoma
14 y.o. F/S, Siamese	Anorexia, vomiting, muscle fasciculation	22.8	6.6	70	3.2	1.013	Solitary adenoma
1.5 y.o. M/N, Siamese	None	13.5	3.3	21	2.2	1.031	Solitary adenoma
15 y.o. F/S, Siamese	Polydipsia, polyuria	13.3	2.2	31	2.7	1.010	Solitary adenoma
8 y.o. F/S, DSH	Anorexia, weight loss	13.8	1.8	15	1.0	1.015	Solitary adenoma
14 y.o. F/S, DSH	Polydipsia, polyuria, lethargy	15.4	2.5	30	1.2	1.010	Solitary adenoma
9 y.o. F/S, Siamese	Anorexia	17.1	6.2	63	2.6	1.026	Bilateral cystadenoma
9 y.o. M/N, DSH	Anorexia, vomiting, lethargy, dysuria	15.2	2.6	59	3.6	1.015	Solitary carcinoma
14 y.o. M/NDSH	Constipation	13.4	3.7	41	2.2	1.022	Solitary adenoma
12 y.o. M/NDSH	Weight loss, lethargy, constipation	14.1	3.2	27	1.4	1.018	Bilateral carcinomas
Reference values		8.8-11.4	2.4-6.1	10-30	0.8-2.0		

y.o., Years old; *M*, male; *N*, neutered; *F*, female; *S*, spay/ovariohysterectomy; *DLH*, domestic longhaired; *DSH*, domestic shorthaired.

HYPOPARATHYROIDISM AND HYPOCALCEMIA

Background

Several historic landmarks in the understanding of parathyroid physiology, maintenance of homeostasis, and calcium regulation are significant with respect to hypocalcemia. Rickets (hypovitaminosis D) was first described in 1645. More than 200 years later (1884), an association was made between thyroidectomy in dogs and cats and the development of clinical hypocalcemia (tetany). In 1891, Gley proved that the parathyroids must be removed with the thyroids to produce tetany. Shortly thereafter, administration of calcium salts after parathyroidectomy was demonstrated to prevent tetany.

Pathophysiology

Initial Physiologic Alterations Cessation of parathyroid function leads to a decrease in serum calcium concentration and an increase in plasma phosphate concentration. Urinary calcium and phosphate excretion diminishes. These changes are due to loss of PTH effects on mobilization of calcium and phosphate from bone, renal retention of calcium, enhanced renal excretion of phosphate, and increased absorption of calcium and phosphate from intestine.

Neuromuscular Activity Ionized calcium is involved in the release of acetylcholine during neuromuscular transmission. Calcium is essential for muscle contraction, and it stabilizes nerve cell membranes by decreasing their permeability to sodium. Calcium's role as a membrane stabilizer is most obvious during severe hypocalcemia. When the extracellular concentration of calcium ion declines to subnormal levels, the nervous system becomes progressively more excitable owing to increased neuronal membrane permeability. Nerve fibers begin to discharge spontaneously, initiating impulses to peripheral skeletal muscles, where they elicit contractions. Consequently, hypocalcemia causes tetany. Dogs with untreated hypoparathyroidism have serum calcium concentrations consistently below 6.5 mg/dL. The onset of clinical tetany, however, is not entirely predictable.

In hypocalcemic dogs, "latent" tetany probably occurs. Owners mention that sudden excitement, activity, or petting unpredictably causes sporadic muscle cramping, lameness, facial rubbing, pain, irritability, or aggressive behavior. The nontetanic, severely hypocalcemic pet is often described by the owner as having a change in personality. Such signs are vague, but after hypocalcemia is diagnosed, the clinical signs are consistent with those of an animal in latent tetany. The various disturbances are completely and quickly reversible with therapy.

Clinical Features of Naturally Occurring Hypoparathyroidism—Dogs

Signalment In reviewing the records of dogs in our series with naturally occurring primary hypoparathyroidism, the youngest dog was diagnosed at 6 weeks of age, the oldest was 13 years (average was 4.8 years), and 65% were female.[78] The breeds most frequently identified as having primary hypoparathyroidism were poodles, miniature schnauzers, retrievers, German shepherds, and terriers.

Anamnesis

Duration of illness The clinical course usually begins with an abrupt onset of intermittent neurologic or neuromuscular disturbances. Signs may be initiated or worsened by excitement or exercise. Signs associated with hypocalcemia had been observed for only 1 day in some dogs and for as long as 2 years in others. Many had been diagnosed and treated for nonspecific seizure disorders without the benefit of pretreatment laboratory testing. Most owners reported that their pets were "always" tense or nervous. Intense facial rubbing with the paws or on the ground was commonly observed but not usually mentioned by owners until specifically questioned. Additional signs included cramping and tonic spasm of leg muscles. Focal muscle twitching, generalized tremors, fasciculations, or trembling was frequently observed, as was a stiff, stilted, hunched, or rigid gait.

Seizures Grand mal convulsions have been observed in 80% of dogs with primary hypoparathyroidism. Some of this seizure activity was atypical because there was no loss of consciousness and the dogs were not incontinent during the episode.[79] More than 80% of these dogs were observed, by a veterinarian, to have seizures or to be "in tetany." This represents a much higher incidence of veterinarian-witnessed neuromuscular signs than expected with most seizure disorders. The neuromuscular problems became so severe that several dogs, although not having seizures, were not able to stand or walk. Seizure episodes were as brief as 20 to 90 seconds and rarely lasted more than 30 minutes. Most, but not all, generalized seizures spontaneously abated.

Facial rubbing More than 60% of the dogs in our series were observed to paw or rub violently at their muzzles, eyes, and ears, as well as rubbing their muzzles on the ground. These signs are thought to result from the pain associated with masseter and temporal muscle cramping caused by the hypocalcemia or from a "tingling" sensation around the mouth. Classic signs of hypocalcemia in humans include paresthesias—numbness and tingling that often occur around the mouth, in the tips of fingers, and sometimes in the feet.

Physical Examination Other than signs related to hypocalcemia, dogs with primary hypoparathyroidism have no classic abnormalities on physical examination. A few dogs were thin, and several growled when examined. Retrospectively, the growling dogs were in pain or were anticipating that handling would result in pain because, after resolution of hypocalcemia, each became friendly. Cardiac abnormalities were apparent in about 40% of dogs on initial examination. These abnormalities consisted of paroxysmal tachyarrhythmias and muffled heart sounds with weak pulses. About half of the dogs appeared to be extremely tense, with splinted abdomens and stiff gaits. A smaller number had generalized muscle fasciculations, fever, or both. Almost 50% had generalized seizures during their initial examination, and more than 80% had at least one convulsion during the initial 48 to 96 hours of hospitalization.

Clinical Features of Naturally Occurring Hypoparathyroidism—Cats

The clinical features of eight cats reported in the literature to have naturally occurring hypoparathyroidism are much like those reported in dogs. The clinical course for each cat was characterized by an abrupt or gradual onset of intermittent neurologic or neuromuscular disturbances that included focal or generalized muscle tremors, seizures, ataxia, stilted gait, disorientation, and weakness. Other commonly observed abnormalities included lethargy, anorexia, panting, and raised nictitating membranes.[80]

Diagnostic Evaluation—Dogs and Cats

Serum Calcium and Phosphate Concentrations Severe hypocalcemia was a serendipitous finding in each of the dogs and cats with primary natural hypoparathyroidism (Table 237-9). Because therapy for hypocalcemia was quickly instituted, each animal had its serum calcium concentration monitored three to five times during the first 72 hours of hospitalization. In no dog or cat was the serum calcium concentration greater than 6.5 mg/dL until the therapy began to have an effect. Each dog and cat also had a serum phosphorus concentration higher than its calcium concentration, and all had normal BUN concentrations.

Table • 237-9

Pertinent Findings in Dogs with Primary Hypoparathyroidism

DOG	AGE (Years)	GENDER	DURATION OF SIGNS (Days)	SERUM CALCIUM (mg/dL)	SERUM PHOSPHORUS (mg/dL)	SERUM MAGNESIUM (mg/dL)	BLOOD UREA NITROGEN (mg/dL)	SERUM ALBUMIN (mg/dL)	PARATHYROID HORMONE (pmol/L)	PARATHYROID HISTOLOGY
1	5	F/S	3	5.7	7.3	—	14	4.1	—	—
2	5	F/S	30	4.1	5.4	1.9	31	3.1	—	—
3	5	M	30	4.7	6.0	—	8	2.9	—	—
4	4	F	7	4.5	5.9	1.2	17	3.5	—	—
5	10	F/S	1	5.2	7.0	2.1	15	2.9	—	Lymphocytic parathyroiditis
6	11	F/S	3	5.6	8.9	—	4	3.7	—	—
7	1	F	14	4.2	9.8	—	20	3.6	—	—
8	5	M	180	5.7	10.2	—	12	3.1	—	—
9	10	F	3	5.5	7.2	1.9	9	3.5	—	—
10	1	M	1	5.2	7.8	—	19	3.2	—	—
11	10	M	11	4.9	5.9	1.8	10	3.1	1.0	Lymphocytic parathyroiditis
12	10	M	1	6.0	6.3	—	13	4.5	0.1	Lymphocytic parathyroiditis
13	4	F/S	14	3.9	4.9	1.9	16	3.5	1.0	—
14	7	F/S	10	6.0	8.3	2.3	12	3.1	1.0	Lymphocytic parathyroiditis
15	9	M	4	3.6	5.8	—	9	3.3	0.05	—
16	0.5	F/S	2	3.9	8.4	1.9	11	2.6	0.1	—
17	13	M	6	4.2	7.1	—	15	3.6	0.1	Lymphocytic parathyroiditis
18	1	F/S	7	5.1	8.7	1.2	14	2.9	0.1	Lymphocytic parathyroiditis
19	0.5	F/S	7	4.8	10.2	2.0	22	2.5	—	Lymphocytic parathyroiditis
20	2	M	45	4.4	7.4	2.1	16	3.4	0.1	—
21	3	F/S	9	5.1	6.8	—	25	4.1	0.5	—
22	6	M	360	5.1	8.8	2.2	23	3.8	0.1	Lymphocytic parathyroiditis
23	8	M	3	3.9	8.3	1.9	19	3.7	0.5	—
24	12	F/S	2	4.6	8.5	2.3	18	3.7	0.1	—
25	6	M	3	5.5	8.5	2.2	19	4.1	0.7	—
Mean	6	—	30	4.8	7.6	1.9	15.6	3.4	0.3	—
Reference range	—	—	—	8.9-11.4	3.0-4.7	1.8-2.4	12-28	2.3-4.3	2-13	—

M, male; F, female; S, spay/ovariohysterectomy.

The absence of an *absolute* hyperphosphatemia in some of dogs can be explained in part by the broad reference range provided by veterinary laboratories. No other abnormal laboratory findings were common.

Electrocardiogram Hypocalcemia prolongs the duration of the action potential in cardiac cells. The findings most consistent with hypocalcemia included deep, wide T waves; prolonged Q-T intervals; and bradycardia. No obvious ECG findings could explain the arrhythmias, weak pulses, or muffled heart sounds that were noted on several physical examinations.

Serum Parathyroid Hormone Concentration Undetectable serum PTH concentrations in animals that are severely hypocalcemic confirm the diagnosis of primary hypoparathyroidism, assuming that the assay used is reliable and validated. Serum PTH concentrations may be detectable as "low-normal"

in some animals with hypoparathyroidism if the assay used is quite sensitive. However, a low-normal or low value would not be "normal" in a hypocalcemic animal that has healthy parathyroid glands.

Differential Diagnosis for Hypocalcemia

The differential diagnoses for hypocalcemia are presented in Box 237-6 and Figure 237-10.

Parathyroid-Related Hypocalcemia Naturally occurring hypoparathyroidism is a rare condition in dogs and cats. Iatrogenic primary hypoparathyroidism has been recognized in dogs and cats after thyroid, parathyroid, or other surgeries of the neck. Magnesium deficiency can cause hypocalcemia. Severe hypomagnesemia in humans can result in a condition characterized by being refractory to PTH or it inhibits synthesis or secretion of PTH.

Box • 237-6

Differential Diagnosis of Hypocalcemia

Parathyroid-related hypocalcemia
  Primary hypoparathyroidism
    Destruction of glands
      Immune-mediated process
      Iatrogenic: surgical complication
      Any disease in neck causing damage
    Idiopathic atrophy (autoimmune process?)
  Pseudohypoparathyroidism
Chronic renal failure
Hypoalbuminemia
Acute pancreatitis
Puerperal tetany (eclampsia)
Intestinal malabsorption syndromes
Nutritional secondary hyperparathyroidism (rare)
Anticovulsant therapy
Acute renal failure
Ethylene glycol toxicity
Phosphate-containing enemas
Miscellaneous diagnoses
  Laboratory error
  Use of EDTA-anticoagulated blood
  Vitamin D deficiency
  Transfusion using citrated blood
  Soft tissue trauma
  Medullary carcinoma of the thyroid
  Primary and metastic bone tumors
  Cancer chemotherapy

Acute Renal Failure and Ethylene Glycol Toxicity Acute renal failure, such as occurs with urethral obstruction, ureter obstruction, or ethylene glycol poisoning, can result in abrupt and severe increases in serum phosphate concentration. An acute increase in serum phosphate concentration causes a reduction in serum calcium concentration. This hypocalcemia may be exaggerated in acute renal failure, because the rapid progression of these disturbances blunts compensatory mechanisms. Cats with ureteral or urethral obstruction and hyperphosphatemia often have associated hypocalcemia, hyperkalemia, azotemia, and sometimes seizures.[39] Ethylene glycol intoxication can cause severe renal failure, acidosis, and death. The metabolites of this toxin can chelate serum calcium ions and cause tetany.

Chronic Renal Failure, Hypoalbuminemia, and Pancreatitis Chronic renal failure is an extremely common disorder in dogs and cats. This condition is most commonly associated with increases in serum phosphate concentrations with concurrent normal serum calcium concentrations. However, either hypocalcemia or hypercalcemia may occur in animals with chronic renal failure. Serum ionized calcium concentrations from animals with renal failure are often low-normal to low.[81]

Reductions in total serum protein, serum albumin concentrations, or both are encountered in a variety of disorders. Decreased circulating albumin causes a decrease in the protein-bound fraction of circulating calcium. However, ionized calcium concentrations are typically normal. Hypocalcemia, when it occurs in dogs with acute pancreatitis, is usually mild and subclinical. Coexisting pancreatitis and acidosis, which is commonly present, increases the amount of serum calcium that is ionized and further reduces any chance of tetany.

Puerperal Tetany (Eclampsia) Eclampsia is an acute life-threatening condition caused by extreme hypocalcemia in lactating bitches and queens. In most studies, dogs with eclampsia are severely hypocalcemic (< 6.5 mg/dL). Eclampsia is most common in small dogs, being less common in cats and large dogs.

Nutritional Secondary Hyperparathyroidism Dogs and cats fed diets containing low calcium-to-phosphorus ratios, such as beef heart or liver, can develop severe mineral deficiencies. Dietary calcium deficiency results in transient decreases in serum calcium concentration, inducing increased PTH secretion, reduction in bone mass as calcium is removed from bone to replace that lacking in the diet, and diffuse skeletal disorders. Skeletal problems include bone pain and pathologic fractures and are the result of the normal physiologic processes that maintain serum mineral homeostasis. Usually these animals have normal serum concentrations of both calcium and phosphorus. Occasionally, such an animal is hypocalcemic. These dogs and cats should be treated by providing balanced diets and restricting activity until skeletal remodeling is complete. Diagnosis is based on recognizing skeletal disorders in a dog or cat given an improper diet.

Miscellaneous Causes of Hypocalcemia Commercial phosphate-containing enemas may result in acute, marked hyperphosphatemia and, subsequent hypocalcemia after colonic adsorption of the enema solution, especially when administered to dehydrated cats with colonic atony and mucosal disruption. These rare problems include laboratory error, vitamin D deficiency, use of citrated blood, trauma, medullary carcinoma of the thyroid, primary and metastatic bone tumors, and some forms of chemotherapy.

Therapy for Hypoparathyroidism and Hypocalcemia

Emergency Therapy for Tetany When treating a seizing animal without a specific diagnosis, diazepam is the initial drug usually chosen to control the signs. However, if this treatment fails or if a diagnosis is still not obvious, blood should be drawn for glucose, calcium, and any other parameter that may lead to a definite diagnosis. Hypocalcemic tetany improves after replacement of calcium, although these animals usually respond to diazepam. Calcium should be administered intravenously, slowly to effect. The dose is 1 to 1.5 mL/kg or 5 to 15 mg/kg, administered slowly over a 10- to 30-minute period. Calcium gluconate, as a 10% solution (Table 237-10), is recommended because, unlike calcium chloride, calcium gluconate extravasating outside a vein is not caustic. Calcium chloride can cause not only tremendous tissue sloughing but also calcinosis cutis.[82] Electrocardiographic monitoring is advisable. If bradycardia, premature ventricular complexes, or shortening of the Q-T interval is observed, the IV infusion should be briefly discontinued.[40] This rapid emergency therapy is invariably successful, with a response noted within minutes of initiating the infusion. However, the final dose needed to control tetany is somewhat unpredictable. The recommendation is to use the suggested dose (in mg/kg) as a guideline and patient response as the definitive factor in determining the volume administered. Infusion of calcium-rich fluids should proceed with caution in a dog or cat with hyperphosphatemia. The additional calcium could result in mineralization of soft tissue causing further damage to the kidneys in animals with coexisting renal insufficiency or failure.[39]

Fever Fever frequently accompanies tetany. It is not unusual to have a dog or cat in tetany with a rectal temperature above 105° F. There is often temptation to treat both the hypocalcemia and the fever (with ice or alcohol baths; parenteral drugs). It is recommended, however, that with institution of calcium

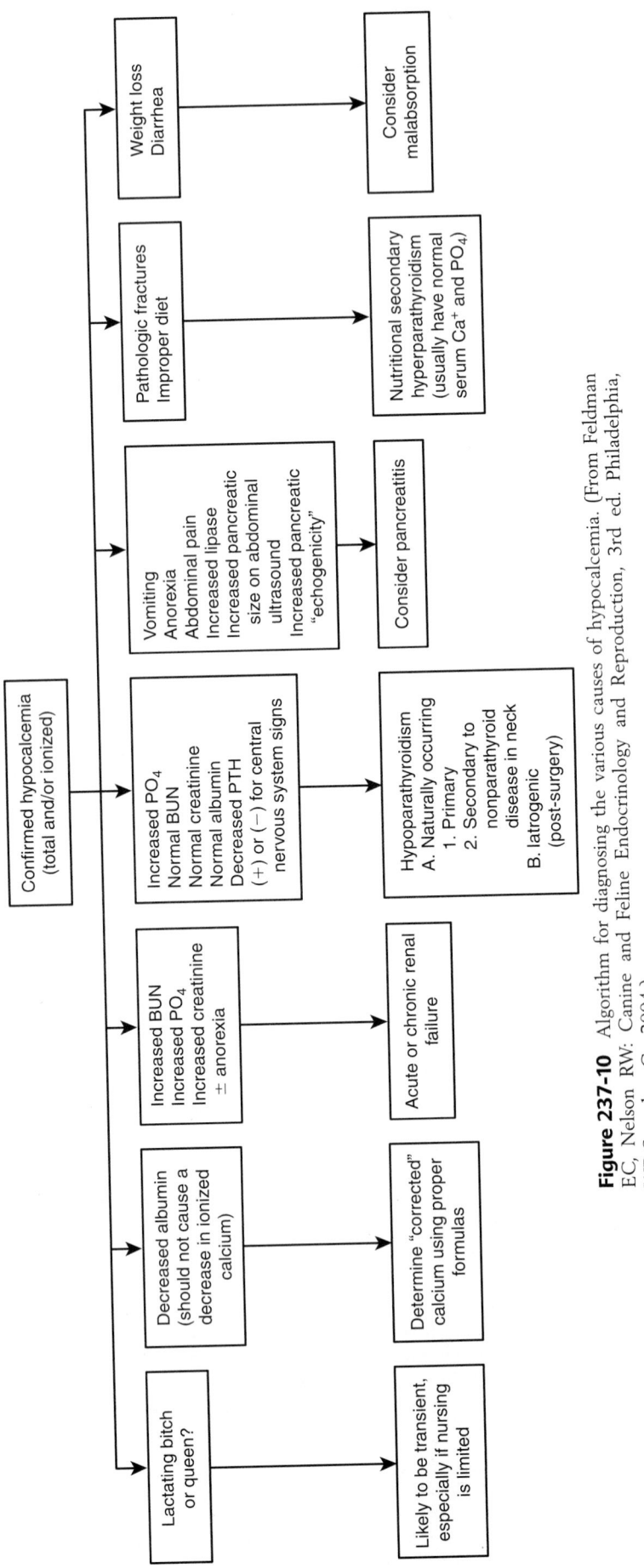

Figure 237-10 Algorithm for diagnosing the various causes of hypocalcemia. (From Feldman EC, Nelson RW: Canine and Feline Endocrinology and Reproduction, 3rd ed. Philadelphia, WB Saunders Co, 2004.)

Table • 237-10

Some Available Calcium Preparations

	PREPARATIONS AVAILABLE	APPROXIMATE CALCIUM CONTENT	DOSE
Oral			
Calcium carbonate/gluconate	Chewable tablet: 700 mg	250 mg Ca/tablet	Cats: 0.5-1 g/day
Calcium gluconate	Tablets: 325 mg	30 mg Ca/tablet	Dogs: 1-4 g/day
	500 mg	45 mg Ca/tablet	
	650 mg	60 mg Ca/tablet	
	1000 mg	90 mg Ca/tablet	
Calcium lactate	Tablets: 325 mg	42 mg Ca/tablet	
	650 mg	85 mg Ca/tablet	
Calcium carbonate	Capsules: 500 mg	145 mg Ca + 155 mg P/capsule	
	650 mg	190 mg Ca + 148 mg P/capsule	
	Tablets: 650 mg	190 mg Ca + 148 mg P/tablet	
	1000 mg	295 mg Ca + 228 mg P/tablet	
Calcium glubionate	Syrup: 360 mg/mL	20 mg Ca/mL	
Injectable			
Calcium gluconate (IV, SQ)	10% solution, 10-mL ampule	9.3 mg Ca/mL	1-1.5 mL/kg: 5-15 mg/kg: slowly
Calcium chloride (IV)	10% solution, 10-mL ampule	27.2 mg Ca/mL	Not recommended
Calcium gluceptate (calcium glucoheptonate) (IV, IM)	22% solution, 5 mL ampule	18 mg Ca/mL	—

Ca, Calcium; *P*, phosphate; *IV*, intravenous; *SQ*, subcutaneous; *IM*, intramuscular.

therapy, one should monitor but not treat fever. Fever usually dissipates rapidly with control of tetany. Additional measures to lower body temperature may result in hypothermia and the development of shock.

Post-Tetany Short-Term Maintenance Therapy

Subcutaneous Calcium Once tetany has been controlled with intravenous bolus calcium gluconate, administration of subcutaneous calcium is effective, simple, and inexpensive. A dose of calcium gluconate equal to that needed for the initial control of tetany can be given subcutaneously every 6 to 8 hours. The calcium gluconate should be diluted in an equal volume of saline. This protocol has effectively supported serum calcium concentrations while waiting for oral vitamin D to take effect. It is a procedure that can be easily taught to owners, further decreasing their expense.

After serum calcium concentrations have been maintained for 48 hours, the frequency of subcutaneous injections should be decreased from every 6 to every 8 hours. If serum calcium concentrations remain stable for the ensuing 48 to 72 hours, the calcium can be tapered to twice daily. This protocol is continued until parenteral calcium has been completely discontinued. Obviously, the tapering process in each animal may not be this smooth, because response to oral Vitamin D therapy is variable. Ideally, the serum calcium concentration should be maintained above 8 mg/dL. Serum calcium concentrations below 8 mg/dL indicate the need to increase the dose of parenteral calcium, serum calcium concentrations of 8 to 9 mg/dL suggest that the current dose should be maintained, and values greater than 9 mg/dL suggest the need to reduce the parenteral calcium dose.

Repeating Intravenous Bolus One alternative to the management of hypocalcemia in the immediate post-tetany period would be intravenous calcium by bolus, as needed. This procedure is not recommended except as required in an emergency.

Calcium Supplementation in a Continuous Intravenous Solution Calcium can be administered slowly, intravenously, via an infusion solution. Calcium gluconate is administered in the infusion to attain a dose of 60 to 90 mg/kg per day (approximately 2.5 mL/kg of 10% calcium gluconate added to the infusion solution and administered every 6 to 8 hours). This calcium should not be added to a bicarbonate-containing solution because of potential precipitation problems. Serum calcium concentrations should be monitored once or twice daily, with the rate of infusion adjusted as needed.

Maintenance Therapy

Vitamin D The need for vitamin D therapy is usually permanent in dogs and cats with primary naturally occurring parathyroid gland failure. Calcium supplementation, however, can often be tapered and then stopped, because dietary calcium is sufficient to meet the needs of the animal. Supplemental calcium in conservative doses, however, ensures that vitamin D, which raises serum calcium by promoting its intestinal absorption, has a substrate upon which to function. Iatrogenic hypoparathyroidism in cats that have had neck surgery is often transient, and lifelong therapy is not always needed. In contrast to treating tetany, when the immediate goal is to avoid recurrence of neuromuscular signs, the aim of long-term therapy is maintaining the serum calcium concentration at mildly low to low-normal concentrations (8 to 9.5 mg/dL). These calcium concentrations are above the level of risk for clinical hypocalcemia and below that which might be associated with hypercalciuria (risk of calculi formation) or severe hypercalcemia and hyperphosphatemia (risk of nephrocalcinosis and renal failure).

Vitamin D₂ (Ergocalciferol) It is recommended that dihydrotachysterol or calcitriol be used for long-term treatment. For some owners, however, these drugs are too expensive. Vitamin D₂ can be given as a less-than-ideal but

Table • 237-11

Vitamin D Preparations

PREPARATION	DOSE FORM	COMMERCIAL NAME (MANUFACTURER)	DAILY DOSE	TIME REQUIRED FOR MAXIMAL EFFECT	TIME REQUIRED FOR TOXICITY RELIEF
Vitamin D_2 (ergocalciferol)	Capsules 25,000 U 50,000 U	Calciferol (Rorer) Drisdol (Winthrop-Breon) Deltalin Lilly	Initial: 4000-6000 U/kg/day	5-21 days	1-18 weeks
	Oral syrup 8000 U/mL IM injectable 50,000 U/mL	Drisdol (Winthrop-Breon) Calciferol (Rorer) Vitadee (Gotham)	Maintenance: 1000-2000 U/kg once daily-once weekly		
Dihydrotachysterol	Tablets 0.125 mg 0.2 mg 0.4 mg	Dihydrotachysterol (Phillips-Roxane)	Initial: 0.02-0.03 mg/kg/day	1-7 days	1-3 weeks
	Capsules 0.125 mg Oral solution 0.25 mg/mL	Hytakerol (Winthrop-Breon) Hytakerol (Winthrop-Breon)	Maintenance: 0.01-0.02 mg/kg q24-48h		
Vitamin D_1 (calcitriol)	Capsules 0.25 μg 0.5 μg	Rocaltrol (Roche) (also generic)	Approximate: 0.03-0.06 μg/kg/day	1-4 days	24 hours-2 weeks
	Vitamin D_3 injectable 1.0 μg/ml	Calcijex (Abbott Laboratories)	Approximate: 0.02 μg/kg/day		1 to 7 days/week

less-expensive alternative. It is a widely available drug (Table 237-11). Initially, large doses are required to induce normocalcemia. Dogs and cats can be given 4000 to 6000 U/kg once daily. These doses are needed to offset the decreased biologic potency of this product in hypoparathyroid animals. Additionally, large doses are required to saturate fat depots, because vitamin D is a fat-soluble vitamin. Effect of the medication is usually obvious 5 to 14 days after beginning therapy. Parenteral calcium can usually be discontinued 1 to 5 days after starting oral treatment.

Dogs and cats receiving vitamin D_2 should be hospitalized, ideally, until the serum calcium concentration remains between 8 and 10 mg/dL without parenteral support. At this time, the pet can be returned to the owner and vitamin D given every other day. Serum calcium concentrations should be monitored weekly, with the vitamin D dose adjusted to maintain a serum calcium concentration of 8 to 9.5 mg/dL. The aim of therapy is to avoid hypocalcemic tetany, but the most common problem with therapy is induction of hypercalcemia. Once the pet appears stable, monthly rechecks are strongly advised for 6 months and then every 2 to 3 months, thereafter.

Dihydrotachysterol The advantages of dihydrotachysterol versus vitamin D_2 are that it raises the serum calcium concentration faster (1 to 7 days) and its effects dissipate faster when administration is discontinued. Therefore the veterinarian has more control over the therapy. Dihydrotachysterol is readily available and is more expensive than vitamin D_2 (see Table 237-11). This product is more potent than vitamin D_2, 1 mg of dihydrotachysterol being equivalent to 120,000 U of vitamin D_2. Dihydrotachysterol is initially given at a dose of 0.03 mg/kg per day for several days or until effect is demonstrated, then 0.02 mg/kg per day for 2 days, and finally 0.01 mg/kg per day. As suggested with the less potent vitamin D, the pet should remain hospitalized until the serum calcium concentration remains stable between 8 and 9.5 mg/dL for

several days. we have seen cats and dogs that appeared to be resistant to the tablet and capsule forms of this drug (0.125, 0.25, 0.4 mg) but responded readily to the liquid (0.25 mg/mL). Rechecks of the serum calcium concentration on a weekly basis allow dose adjustment while avoiding prolonged hyper- or hypocalcemia. As with vitamin D_2, long-term rechecks at two to three month intervals are strongly encouraged. Hypercalcemia (> 12 mg/dL) should be treated by discontinuing vitamin D therapy and, depending on the severity of the clinical signs and biochemistry abnormalities, possibly initiating intravenous fluids, furosemide, corticosteroids, or a combination of these treatments. The period from stopping dihydrotachysterol to noting a fall in the serum calcium concentration is between 4 and 14 days, a much briefer period than that seen with vitamin D_2.

1,25-Dihydroxyvitamin D (Calcitriol) This drug offers the advantages of rapid onset of action (1 to 4 days) and short half-life (less than 1 day). If hypercalcemia results from overdose, it can be rapidly corrected by discontinuing the drug. Because 1,25-dihydroxyvitamin D does not require activation by the kidney, physiologic doses should readily maintain normocalcemia in a pet with hypoparathyroidism, a state in which renal 1-alpha-hydroxylase activity is low. In contrast, relatively larger pharmacologic doses of vitamin D_2 or dihydrotachysterol must be used to overcome this block in renal 1-hydroxylation. We have not used this drug for chronic maintenance therapy of dogs or cats with primary hypoparathyroidism.

Calcium

Initial Approach to Oral Calcium Dietary calcium must be adequate when treating hypoparathyroidism, because the primary mode of therapy is the administration of vitamin D, which acts to increase absorption of calcium present in the intestinal lumen. Usually sufficient calcium is found in commercial pet foods. However, to avoid the catastrophic problems of hypocalcemia, especially early in the course of therapy, oral calcium supplementation is strongly recommended. Oral calcium and vitamin D therapy should be started while tetany is being controlled with parenteral calcium. After 24 to 96 hours, the parenteral calcium administration can often be discontinued while oral therapy is maintained. In this manner, smooth, continuous control is achieved.

Calcium Supplements Supplements can be provided by administering calcium as the gluconate, lactate, chloride, or carbonate salt. Each have disadvantages. Calcium gluconate and lactate tablets contain relatively small quantities of elemental calcium, so relatively large numbers of tablets must be given. Calcium chloride tablets contain large quantities of calcium but tend to produce gastric irritation. Calcium carbonate tablets also contain large quantities of calcium but tend to produce alkalosis, which may aggravate hypocalcemia. Calcium carbonate is 40% calcium. One gram yields 20 mEq of calcium, and gastric acid converts the calcium carbonate to calcium chloride. Calcium lactate is 13% calcium, and 1 g yields 6.5 mEq. Calcium gluconate contains 9% calcium, and 1 g yields 4.5 mEq. Obviously, numerous calcium preparations are available (Table 237-11). Calcium carbonate is the preparation of choice in treating hypoparathyroid humans because of its high percentage of calcium, ready availability in drugstores in the form of antacids, low cost, and lack of gastric irritation.[2] No specific research is available to support recommendations for use of this drug in dogs and cats, although the author's success with calcium carbonate has been excellent.

Treatment Protocol

In cats the dose of calcium is approximately 0.5 to 1 g per day, in divided doses. In dogs, the dose is usually 1 to 4 g per day, in divided doses. These recommendations are approximate, and the primary therapy that determines stability of the serum calcium concentration is the use of vitamin D. As the vitamin D dose reaches a steady level, the dose of calcium can be gradually tapered over 2 to 4 months. This method of treatment avoids unnecessary therapy, considering that dietary calcium should be sufficient to supply the needs of the pet and should decrease the demands of treatment placed on the owner. It must be emphasized that the ideal serum calcium concentration in these animals is 8 to 9.5 mg/dL. Concentrations above 10 are too high, are unnecessary in avoiding tetany, and increase the likelihood of unwanted hypercalcemia.

Parathyroid Histology in Primary Hypoparathyroidism

Animals have been classified as having idiopathic hypoparathyroidism when the clinician finds no evidence of trauma, malignant or surgical destruction, or other obvious damage to the neck or parathyroid glands. The glands are difficult to locate visually and are microscopically atrophied. Approximately 60% to 80% of the glands are replaced by mature lymphocytes, occasional plasma cells, extensive degeneration of chief cells, and fibrous connective tissue. Chief cells are randomly isolated in multiple small areas or bands at the periphery. In the early stages, infiltration of the gland with lymphocytes and plasma cells occurs, with nodular regenerative hyperplasia of remaining chief cells. Later, the parathyroid gland is completely replaced by lymphocytes, fibroblasts, and neocapillaries, with only an occasional viable chief cell. The final interpretation is one of lymphocytic parathyroiditis.[83,84]

Prognosis

The prognosis with primary hypoparathyroidism is dependent, for the most part, on the dedication of the owner and, to a lesser extent, on the experience of the veterinarian. With proper therapy, the prognosis is excellent. Twenty-one of 25 dogs that we observed, lived more than 5 years. However, proper management requires close monitoring of the serum calcium concentration, ideally once every one to three months once the pet is stabilized. The more frequent the rechecks, the better chance the pet has of avoiding extremes in serum calcium concentrations. The chance for a normal life expectancy is excellent with proper care.

CHAPTER • 238

Hypothyroidism

J. Catherine R. Scott-Moncrieff
Lynn Guptill-Yoran

Hypothyroidism is the result of decreased production of thyroxine (T_4) and triiodothyronine (T_3) by the thyroid gland. Naturally occurring hypothyroidism is common in dogs but extremely rare in cats.

PHYSIOLOGY AND METABOLISM

Thyroid hormones are iodine-containing amino acids synthesized in the thyroid gland (Figure 238-1). All circulating T_4, but only 20% of T_3, is derived from the thyroid gland. The majority of T_3 is derived from extrathyroidal enzymatic 5'-deiodination of T_4. In the blood, more than 99% of T_4 and T_3 are bound to plasma proteins, with T_4 more highly bound than T_3. In the dog, the thyroid binding proteins are thyroid hormone-binding globulin (TBG), transthyretin, albumin, and apolipo-proteins, with most T_4 bound to TBG. Dogs have lower avidity of thyroid hormone binding to serum proteins than do humans, which results in lower total serum concentrations of T_4 and T_3, higher free hormone concentrations, and more rapid clearance rates.

Figure 238-1 Synthesis of thyroid hormones. The follicular cells of the thyroid gland concentrate iodide, which diffuses down a gradient into the colloid. Thyroglobulin is synthesized within thyroid follicular cells and secreted into the colloid. Iodide is oxidized and bound to tyrosine residues on the thyroglobulin molecule by thyroid peroxidase. Iodinated tyrosine residues (monoiodotyrosine [MIT] and diiodotyrosine [DIT]) within the thyroglobulin molecule then undergo oxidative condensation to form the iodothyronines (T_3 and T_4), which remain bound to thyroglobulin until secreted. Thyroglobulin is ingested by endocytosis from the colloid; the peptide bonds between the iodinated residues and the thyroglobulin are hydrolyzed; and MIT, DIT, T_4, and T_3, are released into the cytoplasm. MIT and DIT are deiodinated and the iodine is recycled, while T_4 and T_3 are released into the bloodstream. (From Mountcastle VB: *Medical physiology*, ed 14, vol 2. St Louis, 1980, Mosby.)

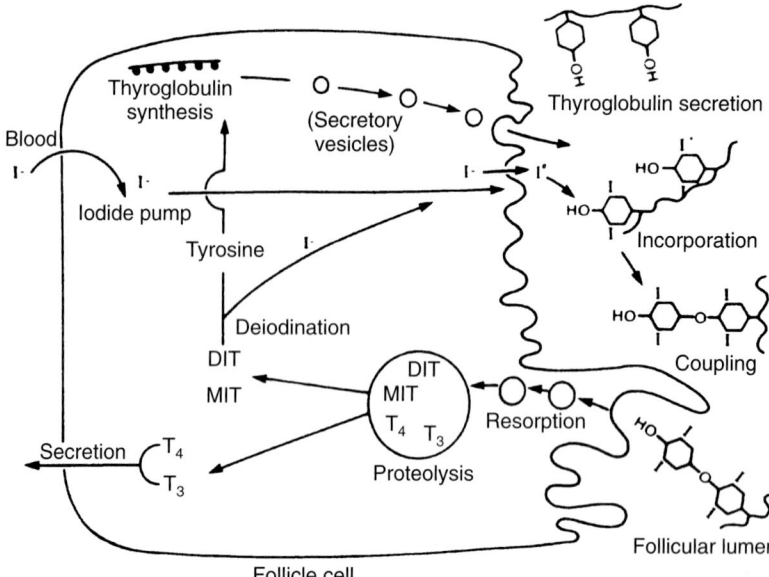

Only free hormone enters cells to produce a biologic effect or a negative feedback effect on the pituitary and hypothalamus. T_3 enters cells more rapidly, has a more rapid onset of action, and is three to five times more potent than T_4. Thyroid hormones bind to receptors in the nuclei; the hormone receptor complex binds to DNA and influences the expression of a variety of genes coding for regulatory enzymes.

Thyroid hormone synthesis and secretion are regulated primarily by changes in the circulating concentration of pituitary thyrotropin (TSH) (Figure 238-2). Thyroid hormones are metabolized by progressive deiodination. Outer-ring deiodination of T_4 produces T_3, whereas inner-ring deiodination results in formation of biologically inactive reverse T_3 (rT_3). Deiodination is regulated by the relative activity of different deiodinase enzymes and is an important regulatory step in thyroid hormone metabolism. Thyroxine and T_3 are both concentrated in the liver and secreted in the bile.

Thyroid hormones have a wide variety of physiologic effects. Thyroid hormones increase the metabolic rate and oxygen consumption of most tissues, with the exception of the adult brain, testes, uterus, lymph nodes, spleen, and anterior pituitary. Thyroid hormones have positive inotropic and chronotropic effects on the heart. They increase the number and affinity of beta-adrenergic receptors, enhance the response to catecholamines, and increase the proportion of alpha-myosin heavy chains. Thyroid hormones have catabolic effects on muscle and adipose tissue, stimulate erythropoiesis, and regulate both cholesterol synthesis and degradation. Thyroid hormones are also essential for the normal growth and development of the neurologic and skeletal systems.

CANINE HYPOTHYROIDISM

Pathogenesis
Hypothyroidism may result from dysfunction of any part of the hypothalamic-pituitary-thyroid axis (see Figure 238-2). Most acquired canine hypothyroidism is the result of lymphocytic thyroiditis or idiopathic thyroid atrophy.

Approximately 50% of canine primary hypothyroidism is due to lymphocytic thyroiditis.[1] Grossly, the thyroid gland may appear normal or atrophic. There is multifocal or diffuse infiltration of the thyroid gland by lymphocytes, plasma cells,

and macrophages.[1] Remaining follicles are small, and lymphocytes, macrophages, and degenerate follicular cells may be found within vacuolated colloid. As thyroiditis progresses, parenchyma is destroyed and replaced by fibrous connective tissue.

Canine thyroiditis is believed to be immune-mediated[2], but the immunologic and molecular pathogenesis has not been well characterized. Antithyroglobulin antibodies are present in 36% to 50% of hypothyroid dogs[3-4], but whether

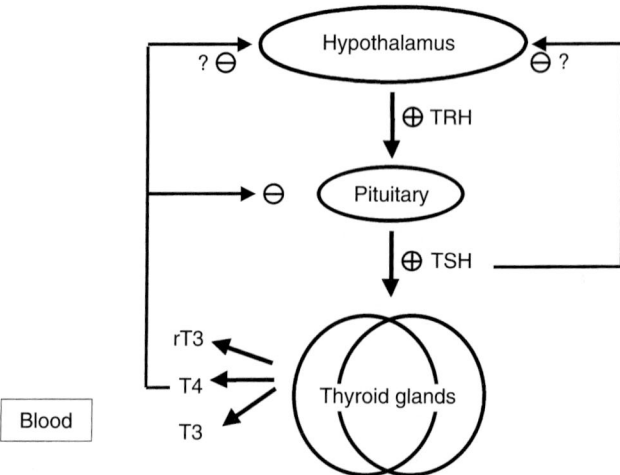

Figure 238-2 Regulation of thyroid hormone concentrations. Thyroid hormone concentrations are controlled by the hypothalamic-pituitary-thyroid axis, which operates as a negative feedback loop. Thyrotropin (TSH) causes synthesis and release of T_4 and lesser amounts of T_3 from the thyroid gland. Intracellular T_3, derived from deiodination of T_4 within the pituitary gland, causes decreased TSH synthesis and secretion and is the main determinant of TSH concentration. Thyrotropin-releasing hormone (TRH), secreted by the hypothalamus, modulates TSH release from the pituitary gland. Increased thyroid hormone concentrations are also believed to decrease TRH synthesis and secretion. Hormones that inhibit TSH secretion include dopamine, somatostatin, serotonin, and glucocorticoids. TRH, prostaglandins, and alpha-adrenergic agonists increase TSH secretion.

these antibodies occur secondary to follicular cell damage from infiltrating T-cells, or are directly involved in the pathogenesis of thyroiditis is unclear. Thyroiditis is heritable in the beagle and the Borzoi.[5-7] The prevalence of antithyroglobulin antibodies varies significantly from breed to breed.[8]

In idiopathic follicular atrophy, there is loss of thyroid parenchyma and replacement by adipose connective tissue.[1] Degeneration of individual follicular cells occurs, with exfoliation of cells into the colloid. Because of the absence of fibrosis or inflammation it is unclear whether follicular atrophy is a distinct syndrome or the final result of thyroiditis.

Less commonly, hypothyroidism is caused by bilateral thyroid neoplasia or invasion of the thyroid by metastatic neoplasia.[9] Dogs with thyroid neoplasia remain euthyroid until at least 75% of the thyroid parenchyma has been destroyed. Lymphocytic thyroiditis has been identified as a risk factor for thyroid neoplasia.[5]

Secondary hypothyroidism (deficiency of TSH) is rarely described in dogs. Causes of acquired secondary hypothyroidism include pituitary malformations and pituitary neoplasia. Histologic changes observed in secondary hypothyroidism include flattening of follicular epithelial cells and distention of thyroid follicles with colloid.[10] Tertiary hypothyroidism (deficiency of thyrotropin releasing hormone [TRH]) has yet to be documented in the dog.

Congenital hypothyroidism (cretinism) is rarely diagnosed in dogs. Reported causes of congenital primary hypothyroidism include iodine deficiency, thyroid dysgenesis, and dyshormonogenesis.[11] Congenital hypothyroidism with goiter due to thyroid peroxidase deficiency was reported as an autosomal recessive trait in toy fox terriers.[12] A genetic test is available to detect carriers of the affected gene. Secondary congenital hypothyroidism due to apparent isolated TSH or TRH deficiency was reported in a family of young giant schnauzers and in a young boxer.[10,13] In both reports, central hypothyroidism was suspected because of increased T_4 secretion and increased uptake of ^{99m}Tc-pertechnetate after repeated administration of TSH. Congenital secondary hypothyroidism is also a feature of panhypopituitarism.

Iatrogenic causes of hypothyroidism include ^{131}iodine treatment, administration of antithyroid drugs, and surgical thyroidectomy. Because of the presence of accessory thyroid tissue, permanent hypothyroidism is rare after thyroidectomy.

Epidemiology
The reported prevalence of canine hypothyroidism is from 0.2% to 0.8%.[14-15] Mean age at diagnosis is 7 years, with a range of 0.5 to 15 years. Golden retrievers and Doberman pinschers are among the breeds reported to be at higher risk for hypothyroidism. Neutered males and females were reported in one study to be at increased risk for developing hypothyroidism compared with sexually intact animals[14]; however, in the most recent study of hypothyroid dogs in the United Kingdom there was no association with breed, gender, or neuter status.[15]

Clinical Signs
Because thyroid hormones influence the function of many organs, hypothyroidism is considered in the differential diagnosis of a wide range of problems. Clinical signs of hypothyroidism may be nonspecific and insidious in onset, and hypothyroidism is commonly misdiagnosed. Common clinical signs attributable to decreased metabolic rate include lethargy, mental dullness, weight gain, unwillingness to exercise, and cold intolerance.[14-15] Obesity occurs in approximately 40% of hypothyroid dogs, but most obese dogs suffer from overnutrition rather than hypothyroidism.

Dermatologic changes occur in 60% to 80% of hypothyroid dogs.[14-15] Common findings include dry scaly skin, changes in

haircoat quality or color, alopecia, seborrhea (sicca or oleosa), and superficial pyoderma. Hyperkeratosis, hyperpigmentation, comedone formation, hypertrichosis, ceruminous otitis, poor wound healing, increased bruising, and myxedema may also occur. Alopecia is usually bilaterally symmetric and is first evident in areas of wear, such as the lateral trunk, ventral thorax, and tail. The head and extremities tend to be spared. The hair is often brittle and easily epilated, and loss of undercoat or primary guard hairs may result in a coarse appearance or a puppy-like haircoat. Fading of coat color may also occur, and failure of hair regrowth after clipping is common. Signs of decreased metabolic rate in conjunction with dermatologic abnormalities should increase suspicion of hypothyroidism.

Hypothyroid dogs are predisposed to recurrent bacterial infections of the skin such as folliculitis, pyoderma, and furunculosis. *Malassezia* spp. infections and demodicosis are associated with hypothyroidism. Pruritus may occur with concurrent infection.

Myxedema (cutaneous mucinosis) is a rare dermatologic manifestation of hypothyroidism characterized by nonpitting thickening of the skin, especially of the eyelids, cheeks, and forehead. It is caused by deposition of hyaluronic acid in the dermis.[16] A rare complication of myxedema is cutaneous mucinous vesiculation.[17]

Female reproductive abnormalities attributed to hypothyroidism include prolonged interestrous interval, silent estrus, failure to cycle, spontaneous abortion, small numbers or low–birth-weight litters, uterine inertia, and weak or stillborn puppies; however, the evidence for this association is weak. Inappropriate galactorrhea apparently due to hyperprolactinemia has been reported in sexually intact hypothyroid bitches.[18] Male reproductive problems attributed to hypothyroidism include low libido, testicular atrophy, hypospermia, and azoospermia. However, a prospective study of six male beagles with ^{131}iodine-induced hypothyroidism showed no decrease in libido or sperm quality over a 2-year period.[19] Decreased testicular size, subfertility, or sterility were reported in association with thyroiditis and orchitis in a colony of beagles.[20]

Both the peripheral and central nervous systems may be affected by hypothyroidism. Peripheral neuropathy is the best documented neurologic manifestation.[21-22] Affected dogs have exercise intolerance, weakness, ataxia, quadriparesis or paralysis, deficits of conscious proprioception, and decreased spinal reflexes. Clinical signs resolve with *l*-thyroxine (T_4) supplementation. A subclinical myopathy also occurs in hypothyroid dogs.[23] Unilateral lameness reported in hypothyroid dogs may be a manifestation of generalized neuromyopathy.[24]

Dysfunction of multiple cranial nerves (facial, trigeminal, vestibulocochlear) and abnormal gait and postural reactions are also reported.[22,25] Hypothyroid dogs with vestibular deficits have abnormal brain stem auditory-evoked responses and some dogs also have electromyographic abnormalities of appendicular muscles. Clinical signs resolve with T_4 supplementation. Because dogs with vestibular disease may have resolution of clinical signs owing to compensation, a causal relationship is less clear.[22] Although laryngeal paralysis and megaesophagus have been reported in association with hypothyroidism, treatment of hypothyroidism does not consistently result in resolution of clinical signs, and a causal relationship has not been confirmed. Myasthenia gravis has been reported in association with hypothyroidism.[26] Concurrent hypothyroidism may exacerbate clinical signs of myasthenia gravis such as muscle weakness and megaesophagus.

Rarely, cerebral dysfunction occurs in hypothyroidism due to myxedema coma, atherosclerosis, or the presence of a pituitary tumor causing secondary hypothyroidism. Seizures, disorientation, and circling may occur due to severe hyperlipidemia or cerebral atherosclerosis.[27-28] In myxedema coma, profound mental dullness or stupor is accompanied by nonpitting edema, hypothermia with a lack of shivering, bradycardia, weakness, and inappetence.[29]

Abnormalities of the cardiovascular system such as sinus bradycardia, weak apex beat, low QRS voltages, and inverted T waves occur in hypothyroid dogs.[14] Reduced left ventricular pump function has also been documented, and hypothyroidism may exacerbate clinical signs in dogs with underlying cardiac disease.[30] Although hypothyroidism rarely causes clinically significant myocardial failure in dogs, dilated cardiomyopathy and hypothyroidism may occur concurrently. A recent case report documented dramatic long-term improvement in cardiac function after treatment with T_4 in two Great Danes with concurrent dilated cardiomyopathy and hypothyroidism.[31]

Ocular abnormalities reported in canine hypothyroidism include corneal lipidosis, corneal ulceration, uveitis, lipid effusion into the aqueous humor, secondary glaucoma, lipemia retinalis, retinal detachment, and keratoconjunctivitis sicca, however a definite causal relationship has not been proven. Dogs with experimentally induced hypothyroidism did not develop ocular changes over a 6-month time period.[32]

Clinical signs of secondary hypothyroidism are similar to those of primary hypothyroidism, but clinical signs related to a deficiency of other pituitary functions may predominate, particularly if a pituitary neoplasm is present.

Congenital hypothyroidism results in mental retardation and stunted disproportionate growth due to epiphyseal dysgenesis and delayed skeletal maturation (Figure 238-3).[33] Affected dogs are mentally dull and have large, broad heads, short thick necks, short limbs, macroglossia, hypothermia, delayed dental eruption, ataxia, and abdominal distention.[10-13] Dermatologic findings are similar to those seen in the adult hypothyroid dog. Other clinical signs may include gait abnormalities, stenotic ear canals, sealed eyelids, and constipation. Affected puppies are often the largest in the litter at birth but start to lag behind their littermates within three to eight weeks. It is likely that many severely affected puppies die without a diagnosis in the first few weeks of life. Vertebral physeal fracture causing tetraparesis was reported in a dog with congenital hypothyroidism.[33]

Clinicopathologic Changes

Results of a hemogram, biochemical panel, and urinalysis often support a diagnosis of hypothyroidism and rule out other disorders. A mild nonregenerative anemia occurs in 30% of hypothyroid dogs.[14] Fasting hypercholesterolemia occurs in 75% of hypothyroid dogs, whereas hypertriglyceridemia occurs in up to 88%.[15] In rare cases hyperlipidemia may lead to atherosclerosis. Less common abnormalities include mild increases in alkaline phosphatase, alanine aminotransferase, and creatine kinase. Mild hypercalcemia has been reported in congenital hypothyroidism.

Hemostasis

Decreased plasma von Willebrand factor antigen (vWf:Ag) concentration was reported in hypothyroid dogs; however, studies have failed to demonstrate a relationship between vWf:Ag or factor VIII activity and thyroid hormone status.[34-36] Canine hypothyroidism is rarely associated with clinical bleeding, and platelet function and bleeding times are normal. Concentrations of vWf:Ag do not consistently increase during treatment of hypothyroid dogs with T_4.[35]

Polyendocrinopathies

Canine hypothyroidism may occur in association with other immune-mediated endocrine disorders such as hypoadrenocorticism and diabetes mellitus.[37-39] Hypothyroidism causes insulin resistance and may mask the classic electrolyte changes of hypoadrenocorticism.

Diagnosis of Hypothyroidism
Patient Selection

Appropriate patient selection is important in evaluation of thyroid function. The positive predictive value of diagnostic tests is highest when the prevalence of the disease is high. A complete history, physical examination and minimum database aid in identification of other diseases and determination of whether thyroid dysfunction is likely. Testing of healthy dogs prior to breeding or of obese dogs with no other clinical signs of thyroid disease increases the chance of false-positive test results.

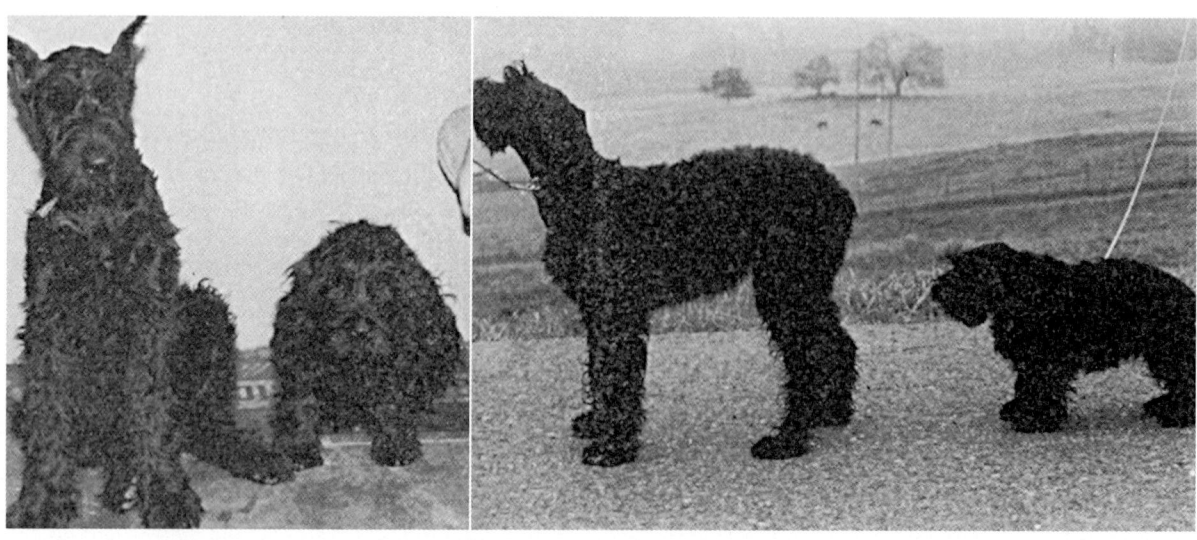

A   B

Figure 238-3 Eight-month-old female giant schnauzer littermates. The dog on the left is normal, whereas the smaller dog on the right has congenital hypothyroidism (cretinism). Note the small stature; disproportionate body size; large, broad head; wide, square trunk; and short limbs in the cretin. (From Feldman EC, Nelson RW: *Canine and feline endocrinology and reproduction,* ed 2, Philadelphia, 1996, WB Saunders, p 83.)

Basal Thyroid Hormone Concentrations

Thyroid hormones commonly measured include total T_4 (TT_4), total T_3 (TT_3), and free T_4 (fT_4). Assays for free T_3 (fT_3) and reverse T_3 (rT_3) are less commonly used. Assays must be validated for the dog. Serum antibodies directed against T_3 and T_4 may interfere with thyroid hormone assays because they compete for hormone with antibodies used in the assay. These antibodies may cause spuriously high or low results, depending on the assay used. Thyroid hormones are stable at 37° C for 5 days, provided the samples are stored in plastic rather than glass.[40] They are also stable when frozen, even with repeated freezing and thawing. Samples should be stored and shipped in plastic tubes.

Total T_4 concentration Total T_4 concentration is an excellent screening test for canine thyroid dysfunction (Figure 238-4). A dog with a TT_4 concentration well within the reference range is euthyroid, unless anti-T_4 antibodies are causing a spurious increase in the TT_4 value. This is uncommon, because anti-T_4 antibodies are detected in less than 2% of samples from dogs with suspected hypothyroidism,[41] and antibody interference most commonly results in TT_4 measurements outside the reference range. Unfortunately, decreased TT_4 concentration is not specific for a diagnosis of hypothyroidism. Decreased TT_4 may be normal for an individual, a result of nonthyroidal illness, or secondary to drug administration. The reference range for TT_4 concentration depends on the laboratory but is usually 1.5 to 3.5 µg/dL. Time of day, age, breed, season, and ambient temperature may influence serum TT_4 concentration. In healthy euthyroid dogs, TT_4 concentration may decrease below the reference range as much as 20% of the time, but there is no predictable diurnal pattern.[42] Serum TT_4 concentrations in neonates are similar to those of young adult dogs; they then increase to more than two to five times the adult concentration by 3 weeks of age. Total T_4 concentrations return to that of the adult dog by 12 weeks of age, then gradually decline with age.[43]

Total T_4 concentrations do not differ significantly between males and females but are higher in small dogs than in medium and large breed dogs.[43] Greyhounds and Scottish deerhounds have lower TT_4 concentrations than other breeds.[44] During diestrus and pregnancy, TT_4 concentration increases owing to changes in thyroid hormone protein binding. Mild increases in TT_4 concentration may also occur in obese dogs.

Free T_4 concentration Protein-bound hormone acts as a reservoir to maintain concentrations of free hormone in plasma despite fluctuations in release or metabolism of T_3 and T_4, or in plasma protein concentrations. Thus free hormone concentrations are less affected by changes in protein concentration and binding than are total hormone measurements. Because only free hormone can enter cells and bind to receptors, measurement of fT_4 should give a more accurate representation of thyroid function. In humans, fT_4 concentration often remains normal during nonthyroidal illness, but this does not always occur in dogs. The standard method for measuring fT_4 is equilibrium dialysis. Because this is expensive and time consuming, single-stage solid phase (analog) radioimmunoassays for human fT_4 are sometimes used for measurement of canine fT_4. These assays depend on the dominance of thyroid hormone binding by TBG, concentrations of which are lower in dogs than in humans. Canine fT_4 concentrations measured by analog methods are lower than those measured by equilibrium dialysis and have no diagnostic advantage over measurement of TT_4. A commercial fT_4 assay that uses an equilibrium dialysis step is more accurate than analog methods and is more sensitive and specific for canine hypothyroidism than is measurement of TT_4.[45,46] This assay is also unaffected by anti-T_4 antibodies and is the most accurate single hormone measurement for diagnosis of hypothyroidism.

Total T_3 concentration Measurement of TT_3 concentration is less accurate than TT_4 measurement for distinguishing euthyroid from hypothyroid dogs, because TT_3 concentrations fluctuate out of the normal range even more than TT_4 concentrations in euthyroid dogs.[42] Spurious results may occur because of anti-T_3 antibodies.

Reverse T_3 and free T_3 concentrations In humans, one mechanism for the euthyroid sick syndrome is decreased 5'-deiodinase activity. This results in a reciprocal relationship between T_3 and rT_3 concentrations. Although this change was documented experimentally in dogs[47], it does not occur predictably in all dogs with nonthyroidal illness. The clinical utility of measurement of rT_3 or fT_3 in dogs has not been demonstrated.

Effect of Drugs on Thyroid Hormone Concentrations

Drug administration can change thyroid hormone concentrations in dogs.[48] Glucocorticoids influence peripheral metabolism of thyroid hormones and inhibit TSH secretion. The effect of glucocorticoids is dependent on the dose and specific preparation. In most studies oral administration of glucocorticoids at immunosuppressive doses (1 to 2 mg/kg q12h) resulted in rapid decreases in TT_4, fT_4, and T_3, but little change in serum TSH.[48] Thyroid hormones return to normal within 1 week after stopping treatment if dosing is for 3 weeks or less. Longer treatment may prolong duration of suppression.

Sulfonamides block iodination of thyroglobulin and can cause clinical hypothyroidism in a dose and duration dependent manner. Trimethoprim-sulfadiazine (15 mg/kg q12h) had no effect on thyroid function but caused clinical hypothyroidism at a dose of 24 mg/kg every 12 hours for 40 days.[48] Trimethoprim-sulfamethoxazole at a dose of 30 mg/kg orally every 12 hours decreased TT_4 and TT_3 concentrations, increased TSH, and decreased response to TSH administration within 4 weeks. Effects are reversible within 2 to 4 weeks of discontinuation of therapy. Phenobarbital administration causes decreased TT_4 and $fT4$ concentrations and mild increases in TSH concentration. Whether dogs treated with phenobarbital have mild clinical signs of hypothyroidism is difficult to assess. Clomipramine results in decreased TT_4 and $fT4$ concentrations but no change in TSH concentration. Other drugs that may affect thyroid hormone concentrations in dogs include androgens, furosemide, heparin, nonsteroidal anti-inflammatory drugs, propranolol, amiodarone, radiocontrast agents, and iodide.[48]

Effect of Systemic Illness on Thyroid Hormone Concentrations

In nonthyroidal illness, thyroid hormone concentrations are often decreased. Changes in hormone binding to serum carrier proteins (e.g., decreased protein concentration, reduced binding affinity, circulating inhibitors of binding), or peripheral hormone distribution and metabolism (e.g., reduced 5'-deiodinase activity), inhibition of TSH secretion, and inhibition of thyroid hormone synthesis may occur. Cytokines such as interleukin-1, interleukin-2, interferon gamma, and tumor necrosis factor alpha decrease TT_4 concentrations.[49] In dogs, TT_4 concentration is more frequently decreased than is TT_3 concentration. The magnitude of decrease depends on disease severity and is a predictor of mortality.[50] Thyroid hormone supplementation does not improve survival in euthyroid humans with decreased thyroid hormone concentrations. Conditions reported to decrease TT_4 concentrations in dogs include hyperadrenocorticism, diabetic ketoacidosis, hypoadrenocorticism, renal failure, hepatic disease, peripheral neuropathy, generalized megaesophagus, heart failure, critical illness or infection, and surgery or anesthesia.[50-54] In 59 euthyroid dogs with concurrent illness, 20% had low TT_4 concentrations and

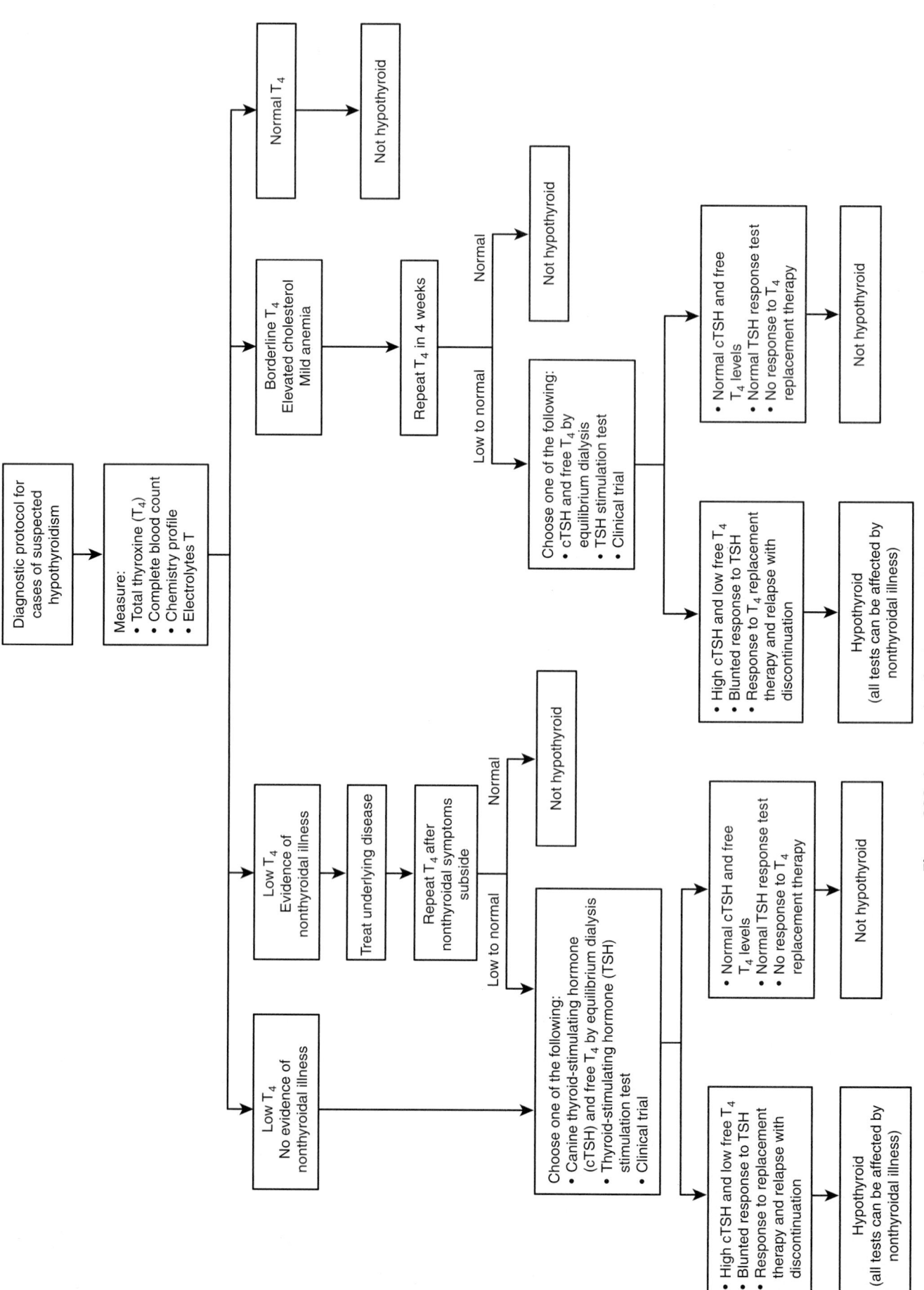

Figure 238-4 Algorithm for diagnosis of hypothyroidism.

17% had low fT_4 concentrations.[51] In 67 critically ill euthyroid animals, 61% had low T_4 concentrations and 56% had low T_3 concentrations.[50] In 42 dogs with hyperadrenocorticism, 38% had low TT_4, 24% had low fT_4, and 39% had low TT_3 concentrations.[52] Dogs with chronic weight loss had decreased TT_4 and TT_3 concentrations regardless of the cause of weight loss.[54]

Basal Thyrotropin (TSH) Concentration

Because of the negative feedback effect of TT_4 on the pituitary gland, measurement of canine TSH concentration should be an accurate indicator of thyroid dysfunction. However, current assays for canine TSH have poor sensitivity for diagnosis of hypothyroidism. From 13% to 38% of hypothyroid dogs have a TSH concentration within the reference range.[45,46,55,56] Possible reasons for a normal TSH concentration in hypothyroid dogs include secondary or tertiary hypothyroidism, fluctuation in TSH concentration, and effect of drugs or concurrent illness. In addition, the TSH assay may not detect all isoforms of circulating TSH. Although some hypothyroid dogs with normal or low TSH concentrations have secondary or tertiary hypothyroidism, it is unlikely that this accounts for most hypothyroid dogs with normal TSH concentrations. Serum TSH concentrations in hypothyroid dogs fluctuate into the normal range, but there is no predictable pattern.[57] In hypothyroid humans, concurrent illness and drugs can decrease TSH concentration toward or into the high-normal range.

Specificity of TSH alone for diagnosis of hypothyroidism is lower than measurement of fT_4 or TT_4 because TSH concentrations are increased in 7% to 18% of euthyroid dogs. Reasons for increased TSH with a normal TT_4 include early hypothyroidism, effects of drugs and recovery from nonthyroidal illness. TSH concentrations remain within the reference range in most euthyroid dogs with concurrent illness.[58] Specificity of TSH for diagnosis of hypothyroidism in dogs with concurrently low TT_4 or fT_4 approaches 100% (Table 238-1).[45,55]

TSH response test The TSH response test is a test of thyroid gland reserve and is the criterion standard for diagnosis of canine hypothyroidism. Clinical use of this test is limited by the availability and expense of medical grade bovine TSH. Life-threatening reactions may occur in some dogs following use of chemical grade TSH. The most widely accepted protocol for the TSH stimulation test is measurement of TT_4 followed by intravenous administration of bovine TSH at 0.1 units/kg (maximum 5 units). A second sample for measurement of TT_4 is collected 6 hours later. Other protocols use a fixed dose of 1 to 5 units per dog; however, lower TSH doses

result in smaller and less prolonged increases in TT_4 concentration and more borderline responses in pets. Recombinant human TSH may also be used at a dose of 25 to 100 µg IV but is expensive.[59] Reconstituted TSH may be refrigerated for up to 3 weeks or frozen at −20°C for up to 6 months.[60,61]

A diagnosis of hypothyroidism is likely if both pre- and post-TSH serum T_4 concentrations are below the reference range (<1.5 µg/dL). A post-TSH T_4 concentration greater than 3 µg/dL indicates euthyroidism.[60-63] Interpretation of intermediate results is more difficult and should take into consideration the clinical signs and severity of concurrent systemic disease. Change in TT_3 before and after TSH administration is of little diagnostic utility. The TSH response test cannot be used to evaluate thyroid function in dogs receiving T_4, because treatment causes thyroid atrophy. Supplementation must be discontinued 6 to 8 weeks before testing.

TRH response test The TRH response test is used in humans to differentiate primary from secondary hypothyroidism. In people with primary hypothyroidism response of TSH to TRH administration is exaggerated, whereas in secondary hypothyroidism there is no response. In contrast, most hypothyroid dogs have a decreased TSH response to TRH compared with euthyroid dogs.[64] The TRH response test is therefore not useful for differentiation of primary and secondary hypothyroidism in dogs.

In dogs, the TRH response test is most commonly used in place of the TSH response test, and change in TT_4 is usually measured. Doses ranging from 0.01 to 0.1 mg/kg of TRH have been evaluated.[63-66] Lower doses cause similar increases in TT4 as do higher doses and are less likely to result in side effects such as salivation, vomiting, urination, defecation, miosis, tachycardia, or tachypnea. A common protocol is administration of 200 µg TRH per dog intravenously with blood collected before and 4 hours after TRH administration.[64] Freshly reconstituted TRH may be frozen at −20°C for at least a week without a loss in potency. Euthyroidism is likely if the post-TRH TT_4 concentration is greater than 2 µg/dL. Euthyroidism is also more likely if there is a relative increase in TSH of greater than 100% at 30 minutes after TRH administration.[64] A diagnosis of hypothyroidism is possible if the post-TRH TT_4 concentration is below the reference range (< 1.5 µg/dL); however, some euthyroid dogs fail to respond to TRH. The TRH response test is therefore less reliable than the TSH response test for diagnosis of canine hypothyroidism.[66]

Scintigraphy Few studies evaluate the use of scintigraphy for diagnosis of thyroid dysfunction in the dog. Dogs with normal thyroid function have a median thyroid: salivary (T:S) ratio of approximately 1 at 20 and 60 minutes after injection of ^{99m}Tc-pertechnetate.[67] Decreased thyroid uptake of pertechnetate is reported in hypothyroid dogs, but increased uptake of pertechnetate was documented in a hypothyroid dog with thyroiditis. Further evaluation of scintigraphic findings in canine hypothyroidism is necessary. Scintigraphy can identify the underlying cause in puppies with congenital hypothyroidism. In puppies with thyroid agenesis, minimal uptake of pertechnetate in the area of the thyroid gland is detected, whereas in those with iodination defects, thyroid lobes are large, with normal or increased T:S ratios. Scintigraphy may also help identify central hypothyroidism. Administration of TSH for 3 days does not alter the thyroid image in dogs with primary hypothyroidism but does result in increased thyroid uptake in dogs with central hypothyroidism.[10] Radioactive iodine uptake and perchlorate discharge tests may also be useful in characterization of dogs with congenital hypothyroidism.[12]

Table • 238-1

Performance of Various Diagnostic Tests for Hypothyroidism in Dogs

	SENSITIVITY	SPECIFICITY	ACCURACY
Total T_4	89% to 100%	75% to 82%	85%
Free T_4	80% to 98%	93% to 94%	95%
TSH	63% to 87%	82% to 93%	80% to 84%
TSH/T_4[†]	63% to 67%	98% to 100%	82% to 88%
TSH/free T_4[†]	74%	98%	86%

*The data are compiled from three published studies of a total of 100 hypothyroid dogs and 164 euthyroid dogs.[45,46,56] Not all studies evaluated all diagnostic tests listed.
[†]A dog was considered to have hypothyroidism only if the T_4 or free T_4 was low and the TSH was high.

Diagnosis of Thyroiditis
Antithyroglobulin Antibody

Antithyroglobulin antibodies (ATA) are found in 36% to 50% of hypothyroid dogs.[3-4] A commercially available enzyme linked immunosorbent assay (ELISA) for ATA is a sensitive and specific indicator of thyroiditis, with false-positive results occurring in less than 5% of dogs with other endocrine disorders.[3] Importantly, a positive ATA titer is not diagnostic of abnormal thyroid function because subclinical thyroiditis may be present for long periods of time before progression to hypothyroidism. In addition, vaccination can result in transient increases in ATA titer.[68] It is unknown whether all dogs with ATA ultimately develop hypothyroidism. In 171 euthyroid dogs with ATA followed for 12 months, 4% progressed to overt hypothyroidism, 13% developed some evidence of thyroid dysfunction, and 15% became antibody negative.[8] It is likely that the natural history of thyroiditis varies from breed to breed. Breeds with increased prevalence of antithyroglobulin antibodies include the golden retriever, great Dane, English and Irish setters, Doberman pinscher, Old English sheepdog, dalmatian, basenji, Rhodesian ridgeback, boxer, Maltese, Chesapeake Bay retriever, Cocker spaniel, Shetland sheepdog, Siberian husky, border collie, and Akita.[8] Measurement of ATA has been advocated for screening breeding stock, with the aim of ultimately eliminating heritable forms of thyroiditis. Whether this is an effective approach has yet to be demonstrated.

Anti-T_3 and -T_4 Antibodies

Antibodies directed against T_3 and T_4 (THAA) also occur in canine thyroiditis, although they are less prevalent than ATA. Because T_3 and T_4 alone are small molecules, these antibodies probably develop against T_3- and T_4-containing epitopes of thyroglobulin. Anti-T_3 antibodies are found in only 5.7% of samples from dogs with clinical signs consistent with hypothyroidism but in 34% of confirmed hypothyroid dogs. Anti-T_4 antibodies are found in 1.7% of samples from dogs with clinical signs consistent with hypothyroidism but are found in 15% of confirmed hypothyroid dogs.[8,41] Because dogs with thyroiditis may still have adequate thyroid reserve, THAA are not diagnostic of hypothyroidism. Prevalence of THAA is highest in younger dogs (2 to 4 years), large-breed dogs, and females. Dog breeds with a high prevalence of THAA include pointers, English and Irish setters, Skye terriers, Old English sheepdogs, boxers, and Maltese terriers.[41]

Thyroid Biopsy

Lymphocytic thyroiditis is readily identified by histopathology, but it is more difficult to determine thyroid function. Thyroid biopsy is rarely indicated for clinical diagnosis of thyroid dysfunction.

Treatment and Therapeutic Monitoring
Hypothyroidism

The initial treatment of choice regardless of the underlying cause of the disease, is synthetic sodium *l*-thyroxine (T_4). Treatment with T_4 preserves normal regulation of T_4 to T_3 conversion, which allows normal physiologic regulation of tissue T_3 concentrations and therefore should decrease the likelihood of iatrogenic hyperthyroidism. Treatment with synthetic T_3 is not recommended because of an increased risk of iatrogenic hyperthyroidism. In addition, T_3 has a shorter half-life and requires administration three times daily. Treatment with T_3 may be indicated if there is inadequate gastrointestinal absorption of T_4. Gastrointestinal absorption of ingested T_3 approaches 100%, whereas oral bioavailability of T_4 is lower, at 10% to 50%. Treatment with T_3 was previously advocated in suspected hypothyroid dogs with a normal T_4 but a low T_3; however, this is no longer recommended. This scenario was thought to be due to a T_4 to T_3 conversion defect, but such a defect has not been documented in dogs. Rather, this

hormone profile likely represents sick euthyroid syndrome, presence of anti-T_3 antibodies, or normal daily fluctuations in plasma T_3 concentration.

The use of desiccated thyroid extract, thyroglobulin, or "natural" thyroid preparations is not recommended because the bioavailability and T_4:T_3 ratio of these compounds is variable, making consistent dosing difficult. In humans, substitution of T_3 for some of the T_4 dose is associated with an improved psychologic state in some studies, possibly because tissues vary in their ability to convert T_4 to T_3.[69] Commercially available combination T_4/T_3 products contain a T_4:T_3 ratio of 4:1, and may predispose to iatrogenic hyperthyroidism because the normal ratio of T_4:T_3 secreted by the thyroid gland is approximately 20:1.

Optimum dose and frequency of supplementation varies among dogs because of variability in T_4 absorption and serum half-life.[70] A dose of 0.02 mg/kg q24h normalizes TSH concentration in most dogs; higher doses (0.04 mg/kg q12h) are required to consistently normalize T_3 concentration,[71-72] but there is little evidence that normalization of T_3 is necessary for a good clinical response. Treatment should be initiated at a dose of 0.02 mg/kg PO q12h and the dose adjusted based on the measured serum T_4 concentration (Figure 238-5). Twice daily treatment with T_4 is initially recommended to improve the likelihood of response to treatment. If clinical signs resolve and T_4 concentrations are within the therapeutic range, the frequency of T_4 administration may be decreased to once daily. It is advisable to use a brand-name product for initial treatment because studies in people have shown large variability in the bioavailability of generic products. Name brand canine and human products appear to have similar bioavailability.[72,73]

Adequacy of therapy should be confirmed by therapeutic monitoring 4 to 8 weeks after beginning supplementation. Serum T_4 concentration should be within the reference range immediately prior to administration of a dose, and at the high end or slightly above the reference range 4 to 6 hours after administration of a dose. This is a clinically effective approach but it may result in over-supplementation in some dogs. Current assays for TSH are not sensitive enough to distinguish a normal from a low TSH concentration and thus cannot distinguish between those dogs that are adequately supplemented and those that are over-supplemented. Dogs are believed to be relatively resistant to development of iatrogenic hyperthyroidism because of the short half-life of T_4 in this species, however the risk of long-term over-supplementation of thyroid hormone in dogs has not been investigated. Serum T_4 concentrations should be measured at 6- to 8-week intervals during the first 6 to 8 months of treatment, because metabolism of T_4 changes as the metabolic rate normalizes. Frequency of serum T_4 measurement may then be decreased to once or twice a year. If the brand of supplement is changed, serum T_4 concentration should be measured 4 to 8 weeks after the change.

The majority of hypothyroid dogs demonstrate good control of their disease at a dose of 0.02 mg/kg T_4 administered orally once daily.[74] However, therapy should be individualized based on clinical response, therapeutic monitoring, and presence or absence of concurrent illness. Improvement in activity should occur within the first 1 to 2 weeks of treatment; weight loss should be evident within 8 weeks.[14] Achievement of a normal hair coat may take several months and the coat may initially appear worse as telogen hairs are shed.[75] Improvement in myocardial function is usually evident within 8 weeks, but may be delayed for as long as 12 months. Neurologic deficits improve rapidly after treatment but complete resolution may take 8 to 12 weeks.[22]

Inadequate supplementation with thyroid hormone results in an incomplete clinical response. It may be difficult to establish what is normal for some dogs, because subtle clinical signs

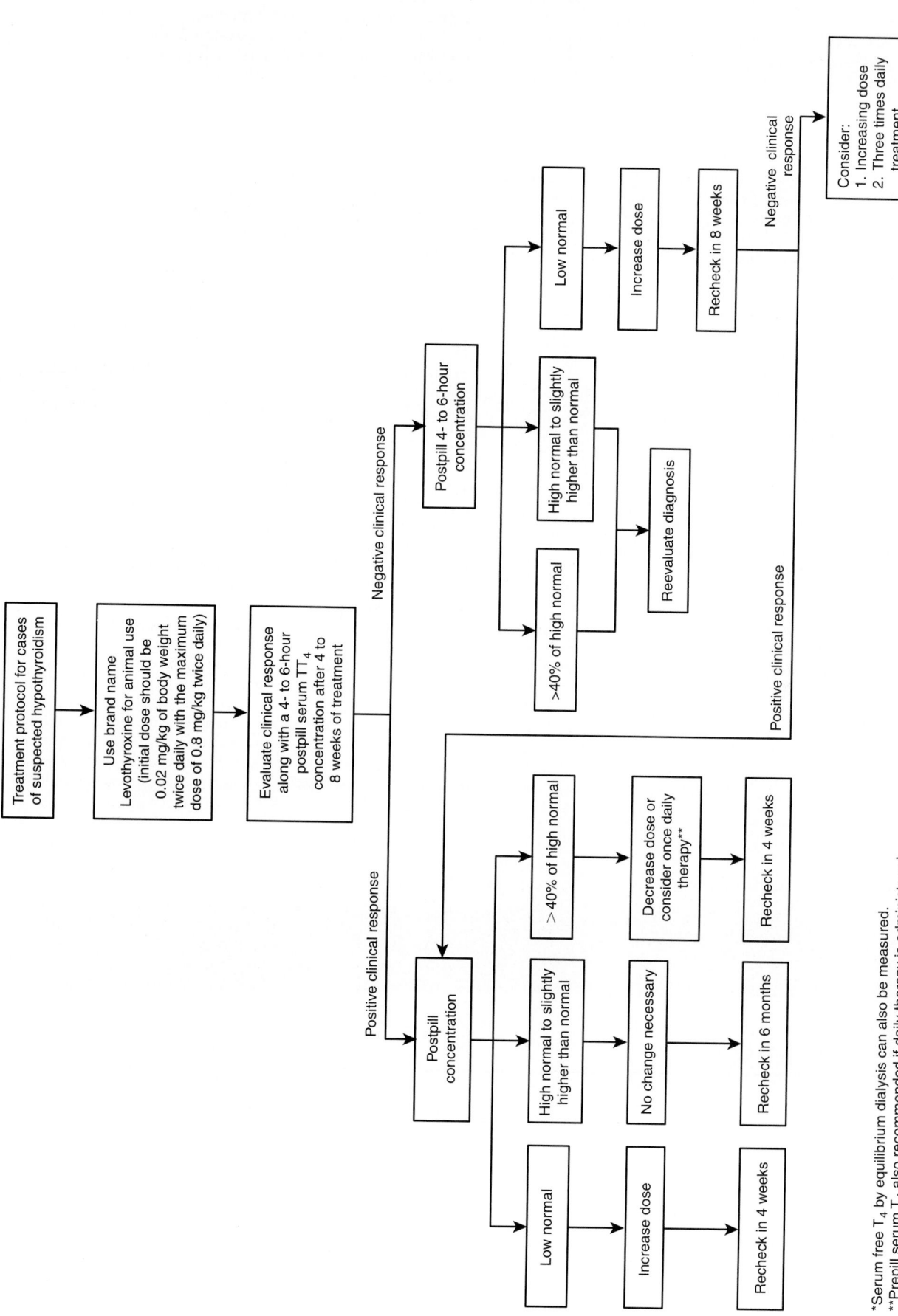

Figure 238-5 Algorithm for treatment of hypothyroidism.

*Serum free T$_4$ by equilibrium dialysis can also be measured.
**Prepill serum T$_4$ also recommended if daily therapy is administered

of hypothyroidism may have been present for so long that the owners do not know what activity level is normal for their dog. This is one reason therapeutic monitoring is important. Some hypothyroid humans do not have complete resolution of clinical signs unless treated with a small amount of T_3 in addition to T_4. Whether this is also the case in some dogs is unknown.

In myxedema coma, T_4 should be administered initially intravenously (5 μg/kg) because of poor gastrointestinal absorption due to hypomotility. Other supportive care including appropriate fluid therapy, passive rewarming, and ventilatory support may also be necessary.

Concurrent Nonthyroidal Illness

Cardiomyopathy In hypothyroid dogs with cardiac disorders, thyroid hormone supplementation increases myocardial oxygen demand and may cause cardiac decompensation. Initial doses of thyroid hormone replacement should be 25% to 50% of the usual starting dose. The dose may then be increased incrementally based on the results of therapeutic monitoring and reevaluation of cardiac function. Because euthyroid dogs with cardiac disease may have decreased thyroid hormone concentrations, it is important to adequately document hypothyroidism to avoid inappropriate treatment.

Hypoadrenocorticism Replacement of mineralocorticoid and glucocorticoid deficiency should be initiated before treatment with T_4, because the increased basal metabolic rate may exacerbate electrolyte disturbances.

Treatment Failure

An incorrect diagnosis of hypothyroidism is the most common reason for treatment failure. Diseases such as hyperadrenocorticism, atopy, and flea hypersensitivity may have clinical signs similar to those of hypothyroidism and often are associated with decreased thyroid hormone concentrations (sick euthyroid syndrome). Other causes include insufficient absorption from the gastrointestinal tract or poor owner compliance. If poor gastrointestinal absorption is suspected, T_3 may be substituted for T_4 (4 to 6 μg/kg q8h).

Prognosis

Prognosis for return to normal function following treatment is excellent in most adult hypothyroid dogs. Prognosis in myxedema coma is dependent on early recognition. Resolution of clinical signs in puppies with congenital hypothyroidism is dependent on the age at which treatment is initiated.

FELINE HYPOTHYROIDISM

Naturally occurring hypothyroidism is rare in cats. The most common cause of low serum TT_4 in cats is nonthyroidal illness. Iatrogenic hypothyroidism occasionally occurs following treatment for hyperthyroidism. Clinical signs of hypothyroidism in cats are similar to those reported for dogs. Causes of spontaneous feline hypothyroidism include congenital hypothyroidism in domestic shorthair cats and Abyssinian cats[76-78] and lymphocytic thyroiditis reported in a 5-year-old cat and in young kittens.[79,80]

Diagnosis of feline hypothyroidism is confirmed by physical examination, history, measurement of serum TT_4 concentration, and results of TSH or TRH stimulation tests. For a TSH stimulation test, TSH is administered at 1 IU/cat intravenously or 2.5 to 5 IU/cat intramuscularly.[81] Blood samples are collected before injection and 4 to 7 hours after intravenous injection or 8 to 12 hours after intramuscular injection. Serum TT_4 concentration should double after TSH administration. The dose of TRH is 0.1 mg/kg given intravenously, with blood collected before and 4 to 6 hours after injection. Serum TT_4 concentration should increase by greater than 50% after TRH administration. Immediate transient side effects following TRH administration include salivation, vomiting, tachypnea, and defecation. A commercial assay for canine TSH has been validated for feline use. A high TSH measured using this assay in conjunction with a low T_4 in the presence of appropriate clinical signs supports a diagnosis of hypothyroidism.

Hypothyroid cats may be treated with T_4 at a dosage of 0.05 to 0.1 mg/cat given orally once daily. Therapeutic monitoring and dosage adjustments should be performed as recommended for dogs.

CHAPTER • 239

Hyperthyroidism

Carmel T. Mooney

FELINE HYPERTHYROIDISM

Hyperthyroidism (thyrotoxicosis) is a multisystemic disorder arising from the excess production of the active thyroid hormones (triiodothyronine [T_3] and/or thyroxine [T_4]) from an abnormally functioning thyroid gland.[1] In cats, this condition was first definitively diagnosed in the late 1970s. Its prevalence has increased significantly such that it is now recognized not only as the most common endocrine disease of the cat but also as one of the more frequently diagnosed disorders in small animal practice.

Etiopathogenesis

Functional adenomatous hyperplasia (or less frequently adenoma) of one (approximately 30% of cases) or, more commonly, both (70% of cases) thyroid lobes is the most common abnormality associated with hyperthyroidism in cats.[1-6] On histologic examination, the normal thyroid follicular architecture is replaced by one or more, well-discernible foci of hyperplastic tissue that can form nodules ranging in size from less than 1 mm to greater than 3 mm, with wide variation in follicular size and architecture both within and between individual nodules.[4] Normal but compressed thyroid tissue is often found surrounding abnormal follicles, but occasionally zones of smooth transition between normal and hyperplastic tissue are present. Thyroid carcinoma, by contrast, is rare, accounting for less than 2% of hyperthyroid cases.[1,7]

Prior to 1979, when hyperthyroidism was first definitively diagnosed, there were a few anecdotal reports of thyroid abnormalities in cats but rarely with clinical signs.[7] However, the frequency with which hyperthyroidism is diagnosed has since increased dramatically.[8] Retrospective necropsy studies reveal few cats with thyroid abnormalities prior to 1979,[7] whereas clinical studies demonstrate a significant increase in cases since that time. In the Animal Medical Center, New York, approximately three hyperthyroid cases per month were seen in 1983; this increased to 22 cases per month in 1993, despite a similar feline caseload.[9] Increased awareness and easier availability of thyroid hormone assays alone is unlikely to account for the dramatic increased frequency of diagnosing this disease, and it has been suggested that it is truly a new disease of cats. However, it remains unclear whether this disorder is simply diagnosed more frequently because of both a general growth in the pet cat population and an overall increase in the longevity of the cat.[9]

Although the disorder and its pathologic lesions have by now been well described, the cause remains obscure. Histologically the disease most closely resembles human toxic nodular goiter, although the fact that bilateral involvement is more common (despite no clear anatomic link between the two thyroid lobes) is reminiscent of human Graves' disease. Graves' disease is an autoimmune disorder in which circulating antibodies (thyroid-stimulating immunoglobulins [TSIs]) bind to thyrotropin (thyroid-stimulating hormone [TSH]) receptors and mimic TSH. Initial studies in hyperthyroid cats suggested that autoantibodies (thyroid microsomal and antinuclear) were common and could be involved in the pathogenesis of the condition.[10] However, four separate studies, using three different techniques, including transfected cells expressing the TSH receptor gene, have failed to identify TSIs in hyperthyroid cats.[11-14] Increased titers of growth-stimulating immunoglobulins have been demonstrated in hyperthyroid cats but their role in the pathogenesis of the condition is unclear.[13]

As in human toxic nodular goiter, adenomatous thyroid tissue from hyperthyroid cats retains its histologic appearance and continues to grow and function when transplanted onto nude mice.[4] Thyroid cells from affected cats, cultured in TSH-free media, also continue to grow and hyperfunction.[15] Somatic mutations of the TSH receptor gene are an important cause of toxic adenoma in humans. However, one research group investigating the possibility of such a cause in cats did not find any corresponding mutations between codons 480 and 640 of the feline TSH receptor gene—the area corresponding to the majority of human disease.[16] Extending such a study to include codons 66 to 530, allowing inclusion of the transmembrane and most of the extracellular part of the TSH receptor, also found no mutations, suggesting that the pathogenesis of hyperthyroidism in cats is unlikely to involve mutations in this gene.[17] After TSH binds to its receptor, signal transduction is cyclic adenosine monophosphate (cAMP)-dependent via a G protein–mediated pathway. Decreased expression of a G protein (specifically G_{i2}) that is normally involved in inhibition of a wide range of G protein–dependent intracellular signaling processes (amongst them the signal to secrete thyroid hormones) has been demonstrated in hyperthyroid cats.[18,19] A more recent study has suggested that mutations in the $G_{s\alpha}$ gene found in some hyperthyroid cats may play a role in the development of adenomatous hyperplasia.[17]

Thyroid tissue from hyperthyroid cats has also been examined immunohistochemically to identify expression of the oncogenes c-ras, bc12, and the tumor suppressor gene p53. Overexpression of the product of c-ras has been demonstrated but without detectable staining for either bc12 or p53. Gain-of-function mutations in this oncogene may therefore play a role in the etiopathogenesis of the feline disease.[20]

Several epidemiologic studies have attempted to uncover risk factors that may be implicated in the pathogenesis of the disease. Two separate studies have reported that two genetically related breeds, the Siamese and Himalayan, are at decreased risk of developing hyperthyroidism.[8,21] Cats fed almost entirely canned food and those using cat litter have an increased risk of developing hyperthyroidism.[8,21] In addition, cats that prefer to eat certain flavors of canned cat food (fish or liver and giblet flavor) have a significantly increased risk of developing hyperthyroidism.[22] Because of this dietary association, iodine has been implicated in the cause or progression of the disease. The iodine content of cat food is extremely variable and often up to 10 times the recommended level.[23,24] It has been postulated that wide swings in daily iodine intake may somehow contribute to the development of thyroid disease. Although serum free T_4 concentrations may be acutely affected by varying iodine intake, more prolonged ingestion has no apparent statistical effect.[25,26] Selenium status could also potentially modify thyroid function. One study found no difference in selenium status in cats from different geographic regions with high and low prevalence of hyperthyroidism but did find that cats had higher circulating selenium concentrations than other species (possibly as a result of increased intake) that may play a role in the pathogenesis of the condition.[27] Many other goitrogenic compounds exist (e.g., phthalates) that can contribute to the development of adenomatous lesions in exposed cats. These may be of particular importance because most are metabolized by glucuronidation, a metabolic pathway particularly slow in the cat. A recent study has shown that the potentially goitrogenic soy isoflavones, genistein, and daidzein, are common constituents of commercially available cat foods and may be present in concentrations sufficient to result in some biologic effect.[28]

Clinical Features

Hyperthyroidism is a disease of middle-aged to older cats, with an average age of onset of 12 to 13 years.[2,6,9,29] Although the reported age range is 4 to over 20 years, less than 5% of cats are younger than 10 years of age at the time of diagnosis.[1] There has been a recent report of hyperthyroidism in an 8-month-old kitten, but thyroid histologic changes were unlike those found in adult cats and are likely to represent a separate disease entity.[30] No sex predisposition exists, and despite the decreased risk of developing hyperthyroidism associated with certain breeds, most large case studies have failed to identify a breed predilection.[2,6,9,29]

Thyroid hormones are responsible for a wide variety of actions including the regulation of heat production and carbohydrate, protein, and lipid metabolism. They also interact with the nervous system, increasing overall sympathetic drive. Consequently, almost any organ can be involved, and a variety of clinical signs are possible in hyperthyroid animals. Table 239-1 lists the most common clinical signs recorded in cats from previous and more recent studies. Both the number and severity of the clinical signs vary in individual cats, depending on the duration of the condition, the ability of the cat to cope with the demands of thyroid hormone excess, and the presence or absence of concomitant abnormalities in other organ systems.[6] The disease is insidiously progressive, and owners may consider the signs, when mild, as part of the generalized aging process. Therefore months may elapse before veterinary attention is sought. Cats are less symptomatic today compared with 10 or 15 years ago, presumably because of increased awareness and earlier diagnosis. It is now not unusual for hyperthyroidism to be confirmed before owners fully realize their cats are ill.[9,31] Although the combination of certain clinical signs (weight loss despite a normal or increased appetite, hyperactivity, intermittent gastrointestinal (GI) signs, palpable goiter, tachycardia, and cardiac murmur) is highly suggestive of hyperthyroidism, the presence or absence of any one sign cannot confirm or exclude the disorder. Clinical signs suggestive of dysfunction of only one organ system may predominate in some cats; as a consequence, hyperthyroidism is considered an important differential for many presenting features in older cats.

General Features   Weight loss is the most common feature of hyperthyroidism occurring in over 80% of cats, resulting in overt cachexia in severe cases.[2,6,9,29] This reflects the overall increase in metabolic rate that may be accompanied by a mild elevation in body temperature or heat intolerance.

Hyperthyroidism is associated with hyperactivity in many affected cats. This may be more noticeable during a physical examination than to the owners, because the cats are often restless, difficult to examine, and may become aggressive,

Table • 239-1

Clinical Findings in 131 Cats (1983 Survey) Compared with 202 Cats (1993 Survey)

FEATURE	NUMBER (%) OF CATS 1983 SURVEY	NUMBER (%) OF CATS 1993 SURVEY
Weight loss	128 (98%)	177 (87%)
Polyphagia*	106 (81%)	99 (49%)
Hyperactivity*	99 (76%)	63 (31%)
Tachycardia*	87 (66%)	85 (42%)
Polyuria/polydipsia*	78 (60%)	73 (36%)
Vomiting	72 (55%)	89 (44%)
Cardiac murmur	70 (53%)	109 (54%)
Diarrhea*	43 (33%)	30 (15%)
Increased fecal volume*	41 (31%)	17 (8%)
Anorexia*	34 (26%)	14 (7%)
Panting*	33 (25%)	19 (9%)
Muscle weakness*	33 (25%)	24 (12%)
Congestive heart failure (CHF)*	16 (12%)	4 (2%)
Increased nail growth	15 (12%)	13 (6%)
Dyspnea	14 (11%)	20 (10%)
Alopecia	9 (7%)	6 (3%)
Ventroflexion of neck	4 (3%)	2 (1%)
Palpable goiter	118 (90%)	167 (83%)

*There was a significant decrease in the prevalence of the finding between the surveys.
Data from Peterson ME et al: Feline hyperthyroidism: pretreatment clinical and laboratory evaluation of 131 cases. J Am Vet Med Assoc 183:103, 1983; Broussard JD et al: Changes in clinical and laboratory findings in cats with hyperthyroidism from 1983 to 1993. J Am Vet Med Assoc 206:302, 1995.

when restrained. Hyperthyroid cats are often described as having an anxious or frantic facial expression and have an impaired tolerance to stress.[2,29,32] In severe cases, stressful events, such as blood sampling, can result in collapse, cardiac arrhythmias, and dyspnea; care should be taken to handle hyperthyroid cats appropriately. Some hyperthyroid cats wander aimlessly, pace, and circle (presumably reflecting a state of confusion, anxiety, and nervousness).[32] Sleep may be abbreviated, and cats may be awakened easily.[32] Focal or generalized seizures characteristic of epilepsy have developed in a few rare cases, with lessening or resolution of the seizures after treatment of the hyperthyroidism.[32]

Muscle weakness and muscle atrophy with fatigability are occasionally described. Owners may describe a decreased ability to jump or fatigue after short bursts of physical activity.[1,2,32] The pathophysiology of muscle weakness is unclear but presumably is related to the thyrotoxicosis-associated weight loss. Severe muscle weakness (exhibited by ventroflexion of the neck) is rarely described and may result from hypokalemia recently reported in hyperthyroid cats.[6,33]

In previous case series, hair and coat changes were common. Shorthaired cats frequently had an unkempt and even matted coat, presumably due to undergrooming, whereas some longhaired cats had alopecia, presumably due to excess grooming.[6,29] Excessive nail growth with increased fragility has also been described.[6,29] These signs are less commonly noted today.

Polyuria and polydipsia reportedly occur in less than 50% of hyperthyroid cats but can be marked in individual cats.[9] Various mechanisms may be responsible, including concurrent primary renal disease (not unexpected in a group of aged cats), increased renal blood flow decreasing medullary solute concentration gradient, electrolyte abnormalities, and primary polydipsia because of a hypothalamic disturbance induced by thyroid hormone excess.[1] Hyperthyroidism could contribute to the development of renal disease in cats. The systemic hypertension accompanying hyperthyroidism could be transmitted to glomeruli, and in the absence of autoregulation, intraglomerular hypertension and glomerular hyperfiltration potentially results.[34] These factors contribute to glomerular sclerosis and progression of renal failure in cats. On the other hand, hyperthyroidism may prove beneficial in maintaining sustainable renal function in cats with pre-existing renal disease. Overt signs of renal dysfunction may be unmasked upon reversal of the hyperthyroid state, and it is this effect that appears to be of greatest concern when considering treatment of affected cats (see Effect of Treatment on Renal Function).

Gastrointestinal Features   While some hyperthyroid cats have no discernible change in appetite, approximately 50% are described as polyphagic.[9] Despite the increased appetite, caloric intake is rarely adequate to compensate for increased energy expenditure, and weight loss generally ensues. Up to 20% of hyperthyroid cats exhibit short periods of anorexia that alternate with longer periods of normal or increased appetite, although the reasons for this are unclear.[6] Cats with apathetic hyperthyroidism usually exhibit partial to complete anorexia (see Apathetic Hyperthyroidism).

Intermittent GI signs of vomiting and, less commonly, diarrhea (increased frequency or volume or steatorrhea) are frequently observed in hyperthyroid cats.[1,2,6,9,29] Rapid overeating may contribute to vomiting, particularly in multicat households; however, direct stimulation of the chemoreceptor trigger zone is also possible.[1,2] Intestinal hypermotility, excess fat intake, and a reversible reduction in pancreatic exocrine function all contribute to the diarrhea associated with hyperthyroidism in humans.[6] Many of these mechanisms have not yet been fully evaluated in cats. However, two separate studies evaluating 10 and 13 hyperthyroid cats each have reported an accelerated orocecal transit time compared with healthy cats and compared with hyperthyroid cats after successful treatment, respectively.[35,36]

Cardiovascular Features Cardiovascular signs are common in hyperthyroidism and are frequently the most significant findings on physical examination (alerting the clinician to the possibility of hyperthyroidism). They include tachycardia, systolic murmurs, a prominent apex beat, and less commonly arrhythmias.[6,29] Systolic murmurs appear to be more commonly recognized than tachycardia in more recent reports.[9] Congestive heart failure (CHF) appears to be uncommon; when it arises it may be associated with a gallop rhythm, coughing, dyspnea, muffled heart sounds, and ascites.[6,9] Hyperthyroidism is usually associated with a form of hypertrophic cardiomyopathy that can result in cardiac failure in the absence of any underlying myocardial abnormalities.[37] Less commonly, a dilated form of cardiomyopathy with severe signs of CHF has been described.[38] Cats with CHF require treatment for both their hyperthyroidism and cardiac failure, using those drugs recommended for the specific form of cardiomyopathy present. While often reversible, cardiomyopathy persists or worsens after treatment in some cats, suggesting a pre-existing cardiac defect or thyroid hormone–induced irreversible structural damage.[39] The exact mechanism for the cardiac abnormalities is unclear but appears to involve a combination of direct action of excess thyroid hormones on the heart, interactions between thyroid hormones and the sympathetic nervous system, and cardiac changes that compensate for altered peripheral tissue function.[2,37]

An early study suggested that mild to moderate hypertension that is reversible after successful induction of euthyroidism is relatively common in hyperthyroid cats.[40] Hypertension in cats has been associated with a variety of ocular abnormalities including retinal detachment, hemorrhage, edema, and degeneration with resultant blindness.[41] However, in most studies of hyperthyroid cats, obvious ocular signs such as blindness are not reported.[42,29] In addition, fundoscopic examination in hyperthyroid cats rarely reveals retinal lesions even in the presence of hypertension.[41-43] A more recent study has suggested that hyperthyroidism, although causing mild increases in systolic blood pressure, is not often a cause of severe hypertension unless accompanied by renal failure.[44]

Respiratory Features Respiratory abnormalities, chiefly tachypnea, panting, and dyspnea have been reported in hyperthyroid cats, although their prevalence, like other clinical signs, have decreased in recent years.[2,6,9,29] Obviously, these signs occur in cats with CHF. However, they may also be seen in cats without overt cardiac disease and in such cases are often precipitated by stressful events such as veterinary intervention. Proposed explanations include varying combinations of respiratory muscle weakness, increased ventilatory drive to breathing, increased airway resistance, diminished lung compliance and even, albeit rarely, tracheal compression due to an enlarged thyroid gland.[29]

Apathetic Hyperthyroidism Apathetic (occasionally called *masked*) hyperthyroidism is an unusual form of thyrotoxicosis that is seen in approximately 10% of cats.[6,29] In such cases, hyperactivity is replaced by depression and polyphagia by anorexia; weight loss continues unabated. Affected animals can be extremely ill. In human medicine, the term *apathetic hyperthyroidism* is usually restricted to those patients with signs (particularly atrial fibrillation and CHF) induced by excess thyroid hormones and does not include those with concurrent disease.[29] In cats this distinction is not always made.

Therefore although many cats are ill as a result of CHF, a significant proportion have concurrent illnesses such as renal failure or neoplasia that account for the majority of their clinical signs. In cats with apathetic signs, a thorough investigation for CHF and other illnesses is indicated because results may alter the therapeutic protocol and eventual prognosis.

Palpable Goiter In healthy cats the thyroid gland is divided into two separate lobes positioned just below the cricoid cartilage. Each lobe extends ventrally over the first five or six tracheal rings and are not normally palpable. Enlargement of one or more thyroid lobes is detectable by palpation in over 80% of cases.[9] With progression of the disease and greater clinician experience, goiter may be detectable in over 95% of cases.[29] Thyroid lobes are loosely anchored to surrounding tissues and as they enlarge tend to migrate ventrally toward the thoracic inlet, occasionally entering the anterior mediastinum. Ectopic thyroid tissue, located anywhere from the base of the tongue to the base of the heart, can also be involved.[45]

Occasionally goiter is visible, but in most cases palpation is required. To palpate for goiter the cat should be restrained by holding its front legs in a sitting position. With the neck gently extended, the thumb and forefingers are placed on either side of the trachea and swept carefully downwards from the larynx to the manubrium. The fingertips should remain within the jugular furrows, but it is important to be gentle and to avoid hyperextension of the neck or the thyroid lobes can become embedded into muscle or deviated retrotracheally. Goiter is usually felt as a mobile subcutaneous nodule or "blip" that slides or slips under the fingertips.[1] When palpation is difficult, clipping the ventrocervical area and moistening the skin with alcohol may help in the visualization of small mobile nodules. More recently a semiquantitative thyroid palpation technique has been described with the clinician positioned behind the cat and the head raised and turned alternatively to the right or left, depending on which side is being assessed.[46] The degree of enlargement is assigned a score between 1 and 6, linked to the severity of hyperthyroidism. Although considered sensitive, such a technique is highly subjective.

The presence of a cervical mass is not always synonymous with hyperthyroidism. Masses can be associated with lymph node enlargement or parathyroid hyperplasia and neoplasia. In addition, goiter may develop in cats without overt hyperthyroidism, although undoubtedly T_4 secretion increases in many of these individuals with time, necessitating careful and regular re-examinations.[47]

Diagnostic Procedures

A variety of procedures have been recommended for evaluating cats suspected of having hyperthyroidism. The results of screening laboratory tests, diagnostic imaging, and electrocardiography may provide supportive evidence of hyperthyroidism or detail extent of cardiac involvement. Screening laboratory tests are also useful in eliminating other diseases with similar clinical signs or in depicting concurrent disorders potentially masked by hyperthyroidism that may be important in treatment decisions and ultimate prognosis. Specific thyroid function tests are necessary for confirmation of the disorder.

Echocardiography and Radiology Evidence exists of mild to severe cardiac enlargement on thoracic radiography in over 50% of hyperthyroid cats.[31] This is accompanied by evidence of pleural effusion and pulmonary edema in cats with CHF.[6,31] The most common echocardiographic abnormalities include hypertrophy of the left ventricular caudal wall (approximately 70% of cats), left atrial and ventricular dilation (70% and 45% of cats, respectively), and hypertrophy of the interventricular septum (40% of cases).[39]

Myocardial hypercontractility, as evidenced by increased shortening fraction and velocity of circumferential fiber shortening, is often found.[39] These abnormalities usually resolve or improve once hyperthyroidism has been effectively treated.[39] Occasionally, hyperthyroidism is associated with a dilated form of cardiomyopathy with echocardiographic evidence of reduced myocardial contractility and marked ventricular dilatation.[38] Thoracic radiographs are necessary in cats suspected of having cardiac failure.

Electrocardiography *Sinus tachycardia* (approximately 60% of cases) and increased R-wave amplitude in lead II (approximately 30% to 50% of cats) were originally the most frequent abnormalities recorded on electrocardiographic examination of hyperthyroid cats.[2,6,48] Other recorded abnormalities included atrial and ventricular arrhythmias, prolonged QRS duration, shortened Q-T interval, intraventricular conduction disturbances, and ventricular pre-excitation.[2,6,48] A more recent study reported a reduced prevalence of tachyarrhythmias, increased R-wave amplitude in lead II, atrial and ventricular arrhythmias, and conduction disturbances, but an increased prevalence of right bundle branch block.[31] The reason for the latter is unclear.

Screening Laboratory Tests In early reports of hyperthyroidism, mild to moderate erythrocytosis and macrocytosis were common.[2,9] In one study of 131 hyperthyroid cats, an increased packed cell volume (PCV), mean corpuscular volume (MCV), red blood cell (RBC) count, and hemoglobin concentration were reported in 47%, 44%, 21%, and 17% of cats, respectively; the prevalence of such changes remained as high in a study undertaken 10 years later.[6,9] Such changes are thought to reflect increased erythropoietin production resulting from increased oxygen consumption or direct thyroid hormone–mediated beta-adrenergic stimulation of erythroid marrow. Erythropoietin excess is also a potential factor in promoting the release of macrocytes into the circulation. However, in a similar study of hyperthyroid cats from the United Kingdom, there were minimal changes in red cell parameters and macrocytes were rare.[29] Although it is difficult to explain the differences between the studies, it is worth stressing that none of the previously mentioned abnormalities, if observed, is clinically important. Anemia appears to be rare.[6,29] When it occurs it is usually associated with severe hyperthyroidism and may result from bone marrow exhaustion, iron, or other micronutrient deficiency.[29] Despite the lack of overt anemia, a significantly higher prevalence of Heinz body formation has been reported in cats with hyperthyroidism compared with healthy cats, although with fewer and smaller Heinz bodies compared with other diseases.[49] Hyperthyroid cats also appear to have higher mean platelet size than healthy cats, but the significance of this remains unclear.[50]

Changes in white blood cell (WBC) parameters are not unusual in hyperthyroidism but are relatively nonspecific. The most frequent changes include leukocytosis, mature neutrophilia, lymphopenia, and eosinopenia, presumably reflecting a stress response.[2,6,9,29] However, eosinophilia and lymphocytosis have also been described and potentially result from a relative decrease in available cortisol because of excess circulating thyroid hormone concentrations.[29]

The most striking biochemical abnormalities observed in hyperthyroid cats are increases in liver enzyme activities. These include alanine aminotransferase (ALT), alkaline phosphatase (ALKP), lactate dehydrogenase (LDH), and aspartate aminotransferase (AST). In more recent and previous reports, at least one of these enzymes is abnormally increased in over 90% of hyperthyroid cats.[2,6,9,29] The elevations in these enzymes can be dramatic. However, at least in one study serum ALKP and total T_4 concentrations were significantly

correlated, and concentrations of ALT and ALKP declined to within reference range with successful induction of euthyroidism.[51,52] As a consequence, the degree of elevation is subtle, if present at all, in early or mild cases of hyperthyroidism. If marked elevation in liver enzyme activities are seen with only mildly abnormal serum thyroid hormone concentrations, concurrent hepatic disease should be suspected and investigated.

Despite the marked increases in hepatic enzyme activities in some hyperthyroid cats, histological examination of hyperthyroid cat livers has revealed only modest and nonspecific change. These include increased pigment within hepatocytes, aggregates of mixed inflammatory cells in the portal regions, and focal areas of fatty degeneration.[2] In more severe cases, centrilobular fatty infiltration may occur together with patchy portal fibrosis, lymphocytic infiltration, and proliferation of bile ducts.[2,6] Suggested explanations for such abnormalities have included malnutrition, CHF, infections, hepatic anoxia, and direct toxic effects of thyroid hormones on the liver. However, several recent reports have examined the possibility of other sources of these enzymes and have shown that both liver and bone contribute to increased ALKP activity in hyperthyroid cats.[51,53,54] The bone isoenzyme contributes approximately 20% to 30% of total ALKP activity; although frequently increased in hyperthyroid cats, a poor correlation is seen with total T_4 concentrations.[51,54]

Hyperphosphatemia, in the absence of azotemia, was originally reported in approximately 20% of cases, and this has more recently been reported in a higher percentage (36% to 43%) of hyperthyroid cats particularly when compared with an age-matched control group.[54,55] This, together with the increase in the bone isoenzyme of ALKP, is suggestive of altered bone metabolism. Circulating osteocalcin concentration, used as a measure of osteoblastic activity and bone remodeling, although variable, has been shown to be increased in hyperthyroid cats.[54] In human thyrotoxic patients, an increased risk of osteoporosis exists because of a direct effect of thyroid hormone on bone. The net bone loss leads to the release of calcium and a tendency toward hypercalcemia, hyperphosphatemia, hypoparathyroidism, and reduced concentrations of activated vitamin D.[6,55] Early reports suggested that despite hyperphosphatemia, circulating calcium concentration was largely unaffected by hyperthyroidism in cats.[6] However, only total calcium was measured. In two separate studies it has been shown that up to half of hyperthyroid cats have serum ionized calcium concentrations below the reference range.[54,55] In addition, hyperparathyroidism appears to be common and has been demonstrated in over 70% of hyperthyroid cats with maximum parathormone (PTH) values approaching 19 times the upper limit of the reference range.[55] Preliminary results suggest that circulating 1,25 Vitamin D concentrations are not suppressed in cats as in humans.[55] The cause of hyperparathyroidism, hyperphosphatemia, and ionized hypocalcaemia remain unclear and warrant further study. In addition, its clinical consequences are unknown, although the increased secretion of PTH necessary to maintain ionized calcium at the low end or below the reference range might contribute to the tendency of some cats to develop hypocalcemia after surgical thyroidectomy.

In early reports of hyperthyroidism, mild to moderate azotemia appeared to be common, occurring in 25% to 70% of cats.[2,6,29] Current figures suggest that just over 20% of hyperthyroid cats are azotemic.[9] Although such prevalence is not unexpected in a group of aged cats, the increase could be exacerbated by the increased protein catabolism, hypertension, and the possible prerenal uremia of thyrotoxicosis.[2,34] In hyperthyroid cats without azotemia, serum creatinine concentration is significantly lower compared with age-matched healthy animals.[55] This may be related to a loss of muscle mass and a reduction in the rate of formation of creatinine rather than any effect of thyrotoxicosis on tubular secretion of creatinine, because this is not considered to occur in cats. Whatever the cause of decreased creatinine concentrations, it is likely that this effect will tend to mask evidence of renal failure in cats. This has implications when assessing renal function in hyperthyroid cats prior to deciding on the best option for treatment (see Effect of Treatment on Renal Function).

A number of other clinicopathologic abnormalities have been described in hyperthyroid cats. Clinically significant hypokalemia has been reported in four hyperthyroid cats, but the cause remains unclear.[33] Blood glucose concentrations may be increased in small number of hyperthyroid cats, presumably reflecting a stress response.[6,9] Hyperthyroidism is also associated with glucose intolerance characterized by delayed clearance of administered glucose from the plasma despite increased secretion of insulin.[56] This is not reversible after treatment, which may be related to weight gain as euthyroidism is achieved. Two separate studies have examined the effect of hyperthyroidism on circulating fructosamine concentration.[57,58] In both studies, serum fructosamine concentration was significantly lower in hyperthyroid compared with healthy cats, presumably as a result of increased protein turnover. Importantly, as many as 50% of cats had values below the respective reference range. Caution is therefore advised in interpreting serum fructosamine concentration in hyperthyroid cats, particularly if concurrently diabetic. Other biochemical parameters such as cholesterol, sodium, chloride, bilirubin, albumin, and globulin are usually within their respective reference ranges in hyperthyroid cats unless affected by a concurrent nonthyroidal illness. Urinalysis is generally unremarkable. The urine specific gravity (USG) is extremely variable, ranging from 1.009 to 1.050, but is generally lower than in an age-matched population, presumably reflecting the effect of hyperthyroidism on renal concentrating mechanisms.[6,9,55]

Thyroid Function Tests The diagnosis of hyperthyroidism is confirmed by the demonstration of increased production of the thyroid hormones or thyroidal radioisotope uptake.

Pathophysiology In cats, T_4 rather than T_3 is the main secretory product of the thyroid gland. However, T_3 is three to five times more potent than T_4. Most circulating T_3 is produced from extrathyroidal 5'-deiodination of T_4 and, as a result, T_4 is often considered as a prohormone, and activation to T_3 a step that is autoregulated by peripheral tissues. Over 99% of circulating T_4 is protein bound, the remainder is free and metabolically active. Overall control of thyroid function is mediated via the negative-feedback effect of circulating T_4 and T_3 on thyrotropin-releasing hormone (TRH) from the hypothalamus and TSH from the anterior pituitary.

Basal circulating thyroid hormone concentrations Increased basal circulating concentrations of total T_4 and T_3 concentrations are the biochemical hallmarks of hyperthyroidism and are extremely specific for its diagnosis. However, since the first reports of the disease, it has been recognized that although circulating total T_4 and T_3 concentrations are highly correlated, measurement of circulating total T_4 is preferable.[6,29] In early studies, a small percentage (< 10%) of cats with elevated circulating total T_4 concentrations had concurrent reference range total T_3 values. This has increased to approximately one third of cats tested in more recent reports (Figure 239-1).[9,59] Severe concurrent nonthyroidal illness may play a role in suppressing T_3 concentration by inhibiting peripheral conversion of T_4 to T_3, as it does in humans, although this appears to be a less common phenomenon in cats.[29] The majority of hyperthyroid cats with total T_3 concentration within reference range are classified as mildly affected, with only mild abnormalities in circulating T_4 concentration. It is

likely that the total T_3 concentration would increase into the reference range if the disorder were allowed to progress untreated.[6]

Early reports suggested that all hyperthyroid cats had elevated total T_4 concentrations with values up to 19 times the upper limit of the reference range.[6,29] However, it has recently been recognized that up to 10% of hyperthyroid cats have reference range circulating total T_4 concentrations (Figure 239-2).[9,59] Such values are usually, but not exclusively, within the mid- to high end of the reference range. Hyperthyroidism, therefore, should not be excluded based on finding a single reference range total T_4 value.

Nonspecific fluctuation of thyroid hormones has been reported in hyperthyroid cats and may account for the reference range total T_4 values found. In cats with markedly elevated serum thyroid hormone concentrations, the degree of fluctuation is of little diagnostic significance.[60,61] However, in mildly affected cats with marginally elevated total T_4 values, the degree of fluctuation can result in reference range values.[61] Increased thyroidal production could result in increased circulating concentration, but because the serum half-life of thyroid hormones is measured in hours, acute decreases presumably reflect fluctuations in binding proteins or other unclear

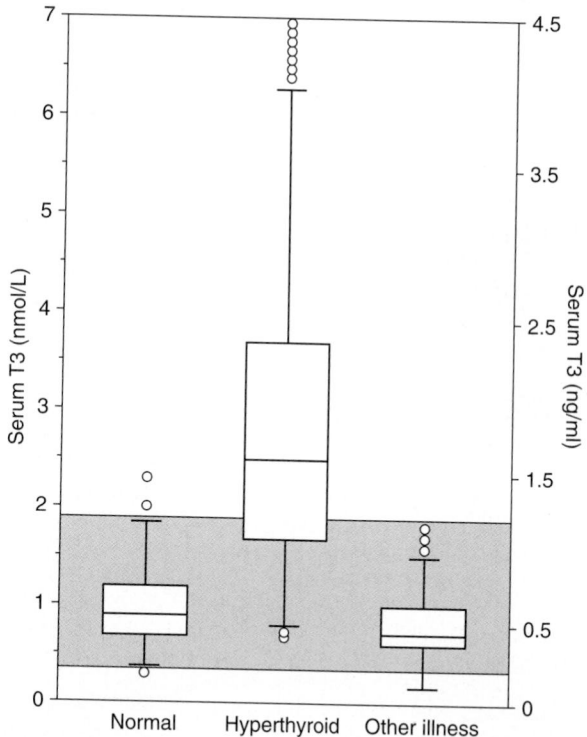

Figure 239-1 Box plots of serum total triiodothyronine (T_3) concentrations in 172 clinically normal cats, 917 cats with untreated hyperthyroidism, and 221 cats with nonthyroidal disease (other illness). The box represents the interquartile range (i.e., 25% to 75% range or the middle half of the data). The horizontal bar in the box represents the median value. For each box plot, the T-bars represent the main body of the data, which in most instances is equal to the range. Open circles represent outlying data points. The shaded area indicates the reference range for serum T_3 concentration. To convert serum T_3 concentrations from nmol/L to ng/dL, one should divide the given values by 0.0154. (From Peterson ME et al: Measurement of serum concentrations of free thyroxine, total thyroxine, and total triiodothyronine in cats with hyperthyroidism and cats with nonthyroidal illness. J Am Vet Med Assoc 218:529, 2001.)

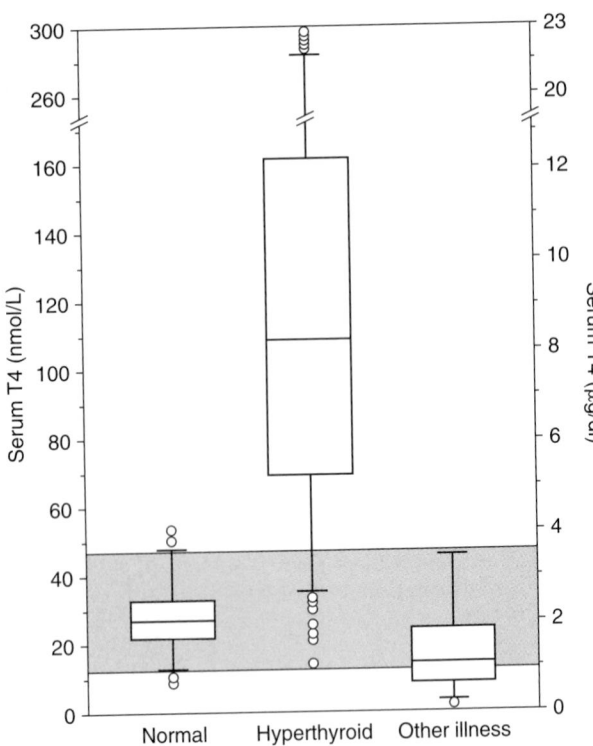

Figure 239-2 Box plots of serum total thyroxine (T$_4$) concentrations in 172 clinically normal cats, 917 cats with untreated hyperthyroidism, and 221 cats with nonthyroidal disease (other illness). Data are plotted (i.e., box plots) as described in the legend of Figure 239-1. The shaded area indicates the reference range for serum T$_4$ concentration. To convert serum T$_4$ concentrations from nmol/L to ng/dL, divide the given values by 12.87. (From Peterson ME et al: Measurement of serum concentrations of free thyroxine, total thyroxine, and total triiodothyronine in cats with hyperthyroidism and cats with nonthyroidal illness. J Am Vet Med Assoc 218:529, 2001.)

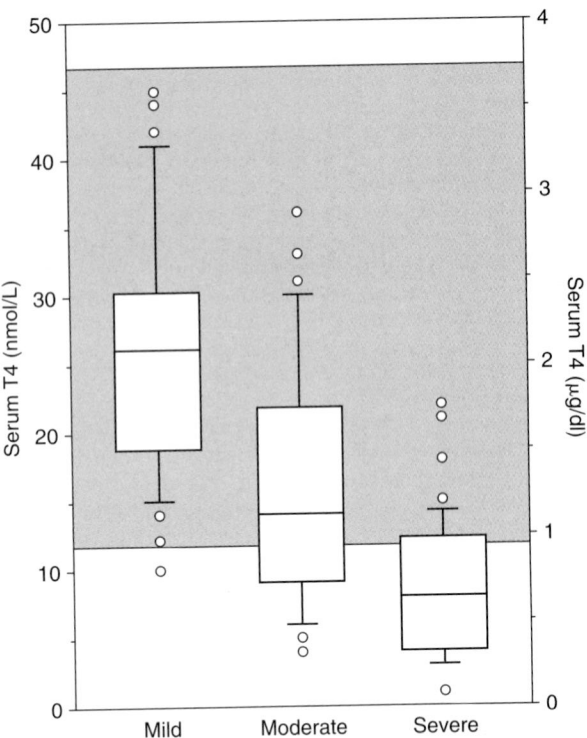

Figure 239-3 Box plots of serum total thyroxine (T$_4$) concentrations in 221 cats with nonthyroidal disease (other illness), grouped according to severity of illness. Of the 221 cats, 65 had mild disease, 83 had moderate disease, and 73 had severe disease. Data are plotted (i.e., box plots) as described in the legend of Figure 239-1. The shaded area indicates the reference range for serum T$_4$ concentration. To convert serum T$_4$ concentrations from nmol/L to ng/dL, one should divide the given values by 12.87. (From Peterson ME et al: Measurement of serum concentrations of free thyroxine, total thyroxine, and total triiodothyronine in cats with hyperthyroidism and cats with nonthyroidal illness. J Am Vet Med Assoc 218:529, 2001.)

hemodynamic changes. If mild hyperthyroidism is suspected in a cat with mid- to high reference range circulating total T$_4$ concentration, a repeat measurement is indicated. Because the degree of fluctuation is greater over a period of days than hours, further sampling should be deferred for 1 or 2 weeks.[1,61]

Nonthyroidal illness is capable of suppressing circulating total T$_4$ concentration in cats as in dogs. The degree of suppression is correlated to the severity rather than the type of illness; because it is inversely correlated to mortality, it can be used as a prognostic indicator (Figure 239-3).[59,62,63] The mechanisms remain unclear but are more likely to involve changes in protein binding or metabolism rather than any effect on the hypothalamic-pituitary-thyroid axis.[62,63] Similar suppression occurs in hyperthyroid cats with concurrent nonthyroidal illness. The degree of suppression has little diagnostic significance in hyperthyroid cats with markedly elevated serum total T$_4$ concentration.[29,62,64] However, in cats with mild or early hyperthyroidism, reference range circulating total T$_4$ concentrations may occur. In the largest study of 917 hyperthyroid cats, a concurrent illness was identified in 17 of 80 (22%) cats with mild hyperthyroidism and reference range serum total T$_4$ concentration.[59] In the majority of affected cats, serum total T$_4$ concentration is within the mid- to high end of the reference range. Occasionally, values are within the mid- to low end of the reference range, but such cats usually exhibit the most severe concurrent illnesses. Other signs, particularly detection of a palpable thyroid nodule, may indicate the need

to further investigate hyperthyroidism in such cats.[59] Serum total T$_4$ values will increase into the thyrotoxic range upon stabilization of or recovery from the nonthyroidal illness.[1,62]

Measurement of circulating free T$_4$ concentration may provide an alternative means of diagnosing hyperthyroidism, particularly in cats with reference range total T$_4$ values. In humans, free T$_4$ measurement is considered a superior diagnostic test for hyperthyroidism because it is less affected by nonthyroidal factors than is total T$_4$ and provides a more accurate reflection of thyroid status.[65] Notably, when serum total T$_4$ concentration is increased, the concentration of free T$_4$ is disproportionately increased. This may be related in part to relative saturation of binding proteins by T$_4$ and subnormal concentration of the principle binding proteins.[65] In addition, serum free T$_4$ concentration remains increased in hyperthyroid patients with nonthyroidal illnesses when total T$_4$ concentration is suppressed into the reference range.[65] Measurement of free T$_4$ concentration has recently been evaluated in a large number of hyperthyroid cats and as in humans, appears to be an extremely sensitive diagnostic test (Figure 239-4).[59] In this study, serum free T$_4$ concentration was elevated in 903 (98.5%) of 917 hyperthyroid cats, whereas corresponding serum total T$_4$ values were elevated in only 837 (91.3%) cases. However, in all cats with an elevated serum total T$_4$ concentration, free T$_4$ concentration is concurrently high.[59] Thus measurement of free T$_4$ concentration offers no further diagnostic information. However, in 205 hyperthyroid cats categorized as mildly affected with or without a concurrent illness, serum total T_4 concentration was only elevated in 125 (61%) cases, whereas corresponding free T_4 concentrations were high in 191 (93.2%) cats (Figure 239-5). Free T_4 analysis is not without disadvantage. It is only reliably measured by methods involving dialysis that increase expense and are not always readily available.[1] In addition, it lacks diagnostic specificity compared with total T_4 measurement. In two separate studies, 6% to 12% of sick euthyroid cats had elevated circulating free T_4 concentrations.[29,59] These cats generally had corresponding total T_4 values in the lower half of or below the reference range. Serum free T_4 concentration should therefore be interpreted with caution if used as the sole diagnostic criterion for confirmation of hyperthyroidism. It is more reliable if interpreted together with a serum total T_4 concentration. A mid- to high reference range total T_4 and elevated free T_4 concentration is consistent with hyperthyroidism.[59] By contrast, low total T_4 and elevated free T_4 values are usually associated with nonthyroidal illness.[29,59]

Identification of concurrent nonthyroidal illness, repeat total T_4 analysis or simultaneous free T_4 measurement usually provides enough evidence to confidently diagnose hyperthyroidism. However, dynamic thyroid function tests have been recommended as helpful in achieving a diagnosis. The methods for performing these tests are outlined in Table 239-2. Realistically they should be reserved for cats with clinical signs suggestive hyperthyroidism when repeated total T_4 concentration remains equivocal and serum free T_4 measurement is unavailable or unhelpful.[65]

Thyroid-stimulating hormone response test

In an early study it was suggested that the TSH response test was useful in confirming a diagnosis of hyperthyroidism because there was little difference in serum concentrations of T_4 before and after exogenous TSH administration.[6] In a larger study of 40 hyperthyroid cats, including those with equivocal total T_4 values, the overall limited T_4 response to TSH stimulation was confirmed.[66] However, it was shown that hyperthyroid cats with equivocal basal total T_4 concentrations exhibit a response indistinguishable from that in healthy cats, suggesting that the

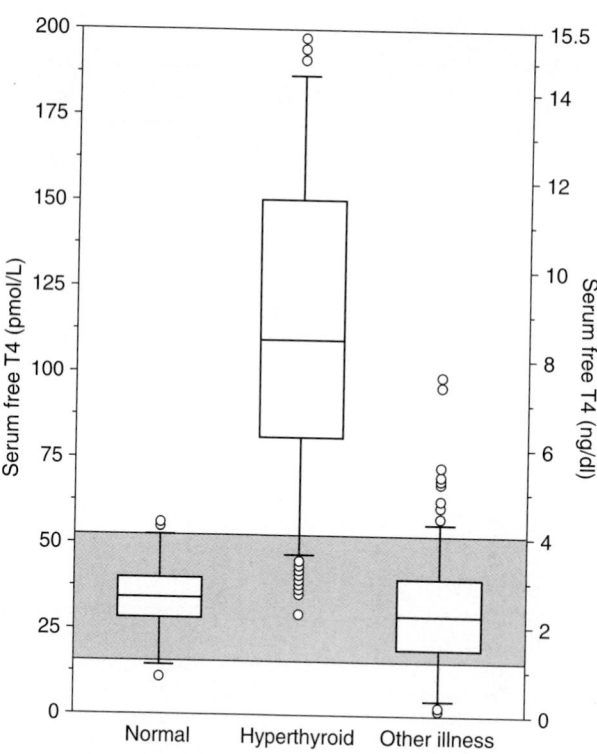

Figure 239-4 Box plots of serum free thyroxine (T_4) concentrations in 172 clinically normal cats, 917 cats with untreated hyperthyroidism, and 221 cats with nonthyroidal disease (other illness). Data are plotted (i.e., box plots) as described in the legend of Figure 239-1. The shaded area indicates the reference range for serum free T_4 concentration. To convert serum free T_4 concentrations from nmol/L to ng/dL, one should divide the given values by 12.87. (From Peterson ME et al: Measurement of serum concentrations of free thyroxine, total thyroxine, and total triiodothyronine in cats with hyperthyroidism and cats with nonthyroidal illness. J Am Vet Med Assoc 218:529, 2001.)

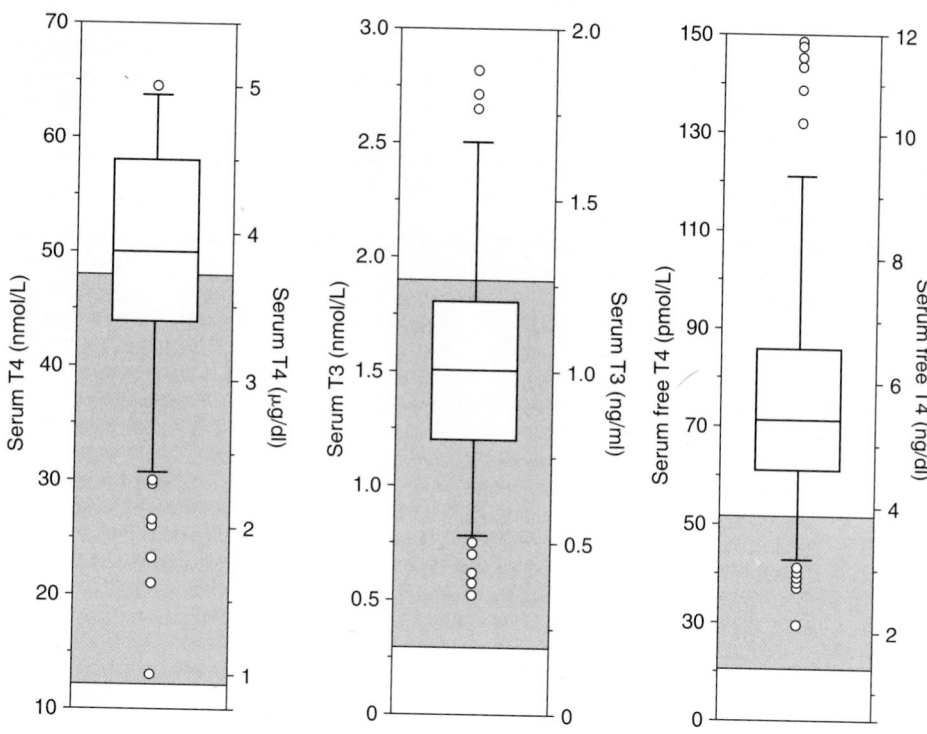

Figure 239-5 Box plots of serum total thyroxine (T_4), total triiodothyronine (T_3), and free T_4 concentrations in 205 cats with mild hyperthyroidism (defined as total T_4 concentration < 66 nmol/L). Data are plotted (i.e., box plots) as described in the legend of Figure 239-1. The shaded area indicates the reference range for each hormone. (From Peterson ME et al: Measurement of serum concentrations of free thyroxine, total thyroxine, and total triiodothyronine in cats with hyperthyroidism and cats with nonthyroidal illness. J Am Vet Med Assoc 218:529, 2001.)

Table • 239-2

Protocols for Dynamic Thyroid Function Tests Used for Diagnosing Hyperthyroidism in Cats

TEST	TSH RESPONSE		TRH RESPONSE	T$_3$ SUPPRESSION
Drug	Bovine TSH	Recombinant human TSH*	TRH†	Liothyronine‡
Dose	0.5 IU/kg	0.025-0.20 mg/cat	0.1 mg/kg	15-25 µg every 8 hours for 7 doses
Route Sampling times	Intravenous Zero and 6 hours	Intravenous Zero and 6-8 hours	Intravenous Zero and 4 hours	Oral Zero and 2-4 hours after last dose
Assay	Total T$_4$	Total T$_4$	Total T$_4$	Total T$_4$ and total T$_3$

*Thyrogen, Genzyme Corporation
†Relefact TRH, Hoechst-Roussel Pharmaceuticals; Thypinone, Abbott Diagnostics
‡Cytomel, Jones Medical Industries
Data compiled from references 66-71.

abnormal thyroid glands do retain the ability to respond to TSH but are producing T$_4$ at maximal rates. Presumably hyperthyroid cats with the lowest basal total T$_4$ concentration have the greatest potential to respond to TSH, although it has been suggested that this response may be related to stimulation of normal thyroid tissue often found within hyperplastic glands.[66] Bovine TSH has traditionally been used for the TSH response test but is no longer commercially available as a pharmaceutical preparation. Recombinant human TSH has been evaluated in euthyroid cats and appears to be a safe and effective replacement for bovine TSH.[67] However, TSH is expensive and because of the difficulties in interpreting the test results, the TSH response test has significant limitations in the evaluation of hyperthyroidism in cats.

Thyrotropin-releasing hormone response test In healthy cats, administration of TRH causes an increase in TSH and, in turn, thyroid hormone secretion. In hyperthyroidism, this pathway is less functional because of chronic TSH suppression from autonomous thyroid hormone production. A significant increase occurs in mean serum total T$_4$ concentration after TRH administration in healthy and hyperthyroid cats and those with nonthyroidal illness.[68] However, the percentage increase in total T$_4$ is considerably less in the hyperthyroid cats compared with healthy cats and those with other diseases. It has been suggested that a relative increase in total T$_4$ of less than 50% is consistent with mild hyperthyroidism, a value greater than 60% is suggestive of euthyroidism, and values between 50% and 60% remain equivocal.[68] Similar to the TSH response test, measurement of total T$_3$ concentration is unhelpful because of the greater variability in response both within and between healthy and sick cats.[66,68] Adverse reactions to TRH administration appear to be common, occurring within minutes of administration. Adverse reactions include vomiting, excessive salivation, tachypnea, and defecation. TRH possibly evokes these effects indirectly, via activation of central cholinergic and cate-cholaminergic mechanisms and directly, via central TRH-binding sites.[1] However, although these reactions are transient and usually resolve within hours, the diagnostic accuracy of the TRH response test has recently been questioned. Results of the TRH response test are largely indistinguishable between sick euthyroid and hyperthyroid cats with concurrent nonthyroidal illness and total T$_4$ concentrations within or below the reference range, thereby limiting its diagnostic usefulness.[69]

Triiodothyronine-suppression test The T$_3$ suppression test relies on the ability of administered liothyronine, through negative feedback, to decrease T$_4$ production by the thyroid gland.

In hyperthyroidism, because excess circulating thyroid hormone concentrations have already suppressed TSH production and secretion, additional T$_3$ has minimal effect on T$_4$ production. Therefore serum total T$_4$ concentration remains significantly higher after liothyronine administration in hyperthyroidism compared with euthyroid (both healthy and sick) cats, and the percentage decrease is consequently significantly lower.[70,71] Although individual laboratories vary, as a general guideline, postliothyronine serum total T$_4$ concentration tends to be greater than 20 nmol/L in hyperthyroid cats and less than 20 nmol/L in euthyroid cats (Figure 239-6). A greater overlap of results is seen in hyperthyroid and euthyroid cats when percentage change in total T$_4$ is calculated. However, suppression of 50% or more is consistent with euthyroidism, whereas hyperthyroid cats rarely have values exceeding 35%. Although the T$_3$ suppression test is a potential aid for confirming the diagnosis of hyperthyroidism, it has been suggested to be most useful in confirming euthyroidism and ruling out hyperthyroidism.[70] Unlike the TRH response test, it is not associated with any adverse reactions. However, it is a relatively prolonged test and highly dependent on good owner compliance in reliably administering liothyronine tablets and adequate GI absorption (necessitating confirmation by pre- and postserum total T$_3$ measurement).[7,70] If a dynamic thyroid function test is deemed necessary to investigate hyperthyroidism in a cat, the T$_3$ suppression test is preferred (given the problems of both the TSH and TRH response tests).

Thyroid radionuclide uptake and imaging Hyperthyroid cats usually exhibit increased uptake of radioactive iodine (as ^{131}I or ^{123}I) or technetium-99m as pertechnetate (^{99m}TcO$_4^-$).[6,72-75] Percentage uptake of ^{99m}TcO$_4^-$ or increased thyroid:salivary ratio at 20 minutes are strongly correlated with circulating thyroid hormone concentrations.[73,75] Preliminary studies suggest that ^{99m}TcO$_4^-$ scans are a more sensitive means of diagnosing hyperthyroidism than basal thyroid hormone analyses or TRH response test results, but further studies are required in this area.[76,77] Care should be taken in interpreting uptake results in cats recently treated with antithyroid drugs. Radioisotope uptake is increased in healthy cats treated with methimazole with significant enhancement after drug withdrawal, and presumably the latter situation may exist in hyperthyroid cats.[78]

Determining percent uptake of radioisotopes is expensive and requires access to sophisticated equipment. However, qualitative scintigraphic imaging remains a useful procedure to determine unilateral or bilateral lobe involvement, alterations in the position of the thyroid lobes, the site of hyperfunctioning

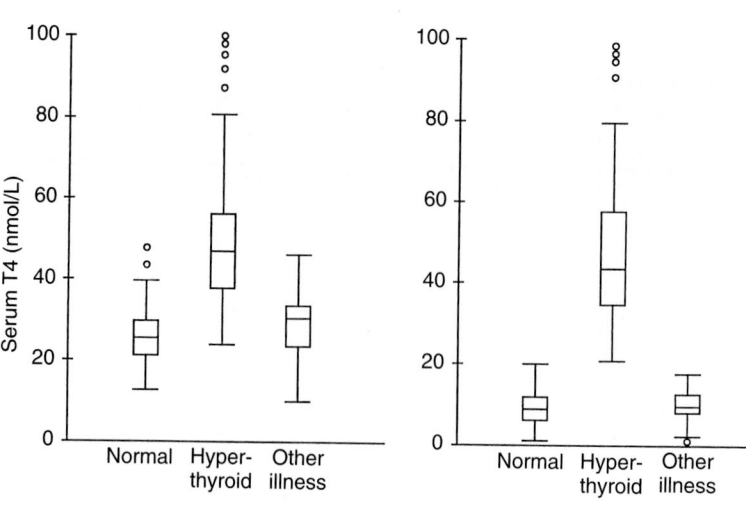

Figure 239-6 Box plots of the serum total thyroxine (T_4) concentrations before (**A**) and after (**B**) administration of liothyronine to 44 clinically normal cats, 77 cats with hyperthyroidism, and 22 cats with nonthyroidal disease. Data are plotted (i.e., box plots) as described in the legend of Figure 239-1. To convert serum T_4 concentrations from nmol/L to ng/dL, one should divide the given values by 12.87. (From Peterson ME et al: Triiodothyronine suppression test. An aid in the diagnosis of mild hyperthyroidism in cats. J Vet Intern Med 4:233, 1990.)

ectopic or accessory tissue, or distant metastases from a functioning thyroid carcinoma.[5] For such imaging $^{99m}TcO_4^-$ is preferred. It has a more rapid uptake and half-life; scanning can commence within minutes rather than hours, allowing for more rapid completion. In addition, higher doses can be used without delivering a high radiation dose, and the quality of the scans is consistently equal or superior to that when radioactive iodine is used.[5]

Treatment

Spontaneous remission of hyperthyroidism does not occur, and prevention is not possible because the cause is unknown. Failure to institute therapy will result in insidious progression to emaciation, severe metabolic and cardiac dysfunction, and ultimately death. However, because of the benign nature of the thyroid lesions, the disease carries a favorable prognosis with effective therapy. Treatment of hyperthyroidism is aimed at removing or destroying abnormally functioning thyroid tissue, pharmacologic inhibition of thyroid hormone synthesis, and release or amelioration of the influence of excess thyroid hormones on peripheral tissue. Surgical thyroidectomy or thyroid ablation using radioactive iodine are the only reasonable curative methods available. Medical management is noncurative; because of this, it is not recommended alone in the rare cases of functioning thyroid carcinoma.

Each treatment method has its own advantages and disadvantages. No one therapy can be recommended above another for all cats. The selection must be individualized for each cat, taking into account several factors including age, severity of thyrotoxicosis, presence of concurrent illnesses, facilities available, potential complications, cost, and the owner's willingness to accept the form of treatment advised.

Antithyroid Drugs and Other Medical Treatments

Numerous pharmacologic agents may be used in the medical management of feline hyperthyroidism. Indications, dose regimens, potential adverse reactions, and contraindications are summarized in Table 239-3. Chronic medical management is a practical treatment option for hyperthyroidism that requires no special facilities, is readily available, easy to implement, and reasonably inexpensive. Almost all cats are potential candidates, because unless it is suspected of thyroid carcinoma, few specific contraindications exist. When thyroid hormone production or secretion is inhibited, generally a rapid return to euthyroidism occurs. Anesthesia is avoided, as are the peri- and postoperative complications associated with surgical thyroidectomy. Unlike radioactive iodine therapy, hospitalization is unnecessary. On the other hand, few drugs are available for long-term control, daily medication is necessary, and a real risk

of poor compliance exists (by the owner, the cat, or both) in regularly administering and accepting the medication. This impinges on efficacy and cost because it necessitates more frequent monitoring. In addition the development of adverse reactions may necessitate drug withdrawal; therefore not all cats initially managed medically can be maintained long-term with this form of therapy. A further consideration is that relapse of hyperthyroidism invariably occurs within 24 to 72 hours after drug withdrawal.[52,79] Although often considered a disadvantage, it may prove beneficial in cats that develop overt renal failure on induction of euthyroidism (see Effect of Treatment on Renal Function).

Pharmacologic intervention is also necessary prior to surgical thyroidectomy to decrease the metabolic and cardiac complications associated with thyroid hormone excess. In addition, it may be desirable to provide some control, at least clinically, while awaiting radioactive iodine administration.

Thioureylene antithyroid drugs The thioureylene antithyroid drugs include propylthiouracil, methimazole, and carbimazole. These drugs are actively concentrated by the thyroid gland and act as general inhibitors of thyroid peroxidase-catalyzed reactions including oxidation of iodide and iodination of tyrosyl residues in thyroglobulin. They also interfere with the coupling of iodotyrosines to iodothyronines via inhibition of thyroid peroxidase or by binding to and altering the structure of thyroglobulin, a reaction more sensitive to inhibition than the formation of iodotyrosines. The trapping of inorganic iodide by, or the release of preformed hormones from, the thyroid gland is not affected by these drugs.[1,52,78,79]

The thioureylene antithyroid drugs are the therapeutic mainstay in the medical management of both human and feline hyperthyroidism because of their consistent effect in lowering serum thyroid hormone concentrations. They are widely recommended to stabilize hyperthyroid cats prior to surgery and are the only drugs that can be used chronically for management of hyperthyroidism. Propylthiouracil is the least potent but is widely available and has an additional advantage of inhibiting peripheral T_3 production. However, it is associated with an unacceptably high incidence of serious hematologic complications in both healthy and hyperthyroid cats; therefore it is no longer recommended for use in this species.[65]

Methimazole is available in the United States (Tapazole, Jones Medical Industries) and is specifically licensed for use in hyperthyroid cats in the United Kingdom (Felimazole, Arnolds Veterinary Products Limited). Elsewhere, methimazole or carbimazole is variably available. Carbimazole is a carbethoxy derivative of methimazole and was originally developed in the

Table • 239-3

Indications, Doses, Adverse Reactions, and Contraindications for the Drugs Commonly Used to Manage Hyperthyroidism

DRUG	INDICATIONS	DAILY DOSE	ADVERSE REACTIONS	CONTRAINDICATIONS
Methimazole and carbimazole	Prior to surgery (2-3 weeks)	5-15 mg divided two or three times daily	Vomiting, anorexia, depression; facial excoriations; hematologic complications; hepatopathy	If adverse reactions occur; at the time of radiotherapy
	Chronic management	5-10 mg once or divided twice daily		
Propranolol	Symptomatic control	7.5-15 mg divided three times daily	Bradycardia, myocardial depression; bronchospasm; diarrhea	Asthma, uncontrolled heart failure; chronic management
Atenolol		6.25-12.5 mg once or twice daily		Chronic management
Propranolol with potassium iodate	Prior to surgery (3 weeks)	7.5-15 mg divided three times daily, days 1-21 63.75 mg divided three times daily, days 11-20	Anorexia, depression, vomiting	Chronic management; immediately prior to ^{131}I therapy
Calcium ipodate	Prior to surgery (up to 14 weeks)	100 mg divided twice daily	None	Chronic management

hope of obtaining a drug with a longer duration of activity than methimazole for human use. Although possessing inherent antithyroid activity, it exerts its antithyroid effect through immediate conversion to methimazole when administered orally.[80] Serum concentrations of methimazole achieved after carbimazole administration are less than after administration of an equal weight of methimazole, reflecting the molar ratio of the two drugs. This conversion results in a 5 mg dose of carbimazole being approximately equivalent to 3 mg of methimazole and may account for the slight differences in dose regimes recommended for the two drugs.[52,79] However, given the reduction in severity of thyrotoxicosis in cats seen currently, such differences have become less noticeable.

Pharmacological studies in healthy cats have shown that methimazole has good oral bioavailability with a serum half-life of between 4 and 6 hours.[81,82] After multiple-dose administration of methimazole, some evidence of drug-induced accelerated metabolism is seen; however, this has not been borne out by clinical studies.[82] Most pharmacokinetic parameters of methimazole in cats are not significantly altered by hyperthyroidism; although a trend toward faster elimination exists, this is not considered to be clinically important.[81]

Initially, methimazole should be administered orally at a dose of 10 to 15 mg/day, in divided doses every eight to 12 hours, depending on the severity of the thyrotoxicosis.[79] Carbimazole has been recommended at an initial oral dose of 15 mg, divided three times daily.[52] Attainment of biochemical euthyroidism is relatively rapid, occurring in a mean of approximately 6 days at least for carbimazole.[52] Not surprisingly the

length of therapy is correlated with the basal serum total T_4 concentration. As cats are diagnosed with hyperthyroidism earlier, the trend toward using only twice-daily administration of low doses (2.5 to 5 mg) of carbimazole or methimazole increases.[83] Once-daily dosing, however, appears less effective in inducing euthyroidism.[83] For practical purposes, the initial dose is prescribed for a period of 2 to 3 weeks, which allows time for more obvious clinical improvement and ensures the attainment of euthyroidism in over 90% of cats.[52,79] At that time, a circulating total T_4 concentration is measured and, if within or below the reference range, surgery can be performed (administering the last dose on the morning of surgery). For severely affected cats, although biochemical euthyroidism is rapidly achieved, a longer course of preoperative therapy may be beneficial before the patient is considered a reasonable surgical candidate. In such cases, the dose is adjusted as in cats in which medical management has been selected as the sole therapy. If euthyroidism is not achieved within this initial period, the duration of therapy is increased or the dose altered in 2.5 to 5 mg increments. Rarely doses as high as 25 to 30 mg of methimazole are required to restore euthyroidism.[1,7,79] Lack of owner or cat compliance should be excluded as a possible reason for failure of therapy. Documenting a decline in the activities of the liver enzymes provides an inexpensive but nonspecific alternative to monitoring serum total T_4 concentration when assessing therapeutic efficacy.[52]

For long-term therapy, once euthyroidism has been achieved, the daily dose is adjusted in 2.5 to 5 mg decrements, aiming for the lowest possible dose that effectively maintains euthyroidism.

Further dose adjustments are based on circulating total T_4 concentrations assessed every 2 to 3 weeks until stable and every 3 to 6 months thereafter or as indicated clinically. Most cats require 10 mg methimazole per day, whereas a few require doses as high as 15 to 20 mg/day or as low as 2.5 to 5 mg/day.[79] Although divided doses are most successful in treating hyperthyroid cats (and despite the relatively short serum half-life), the intrathyroidal residence time may be approximately 20 hours as it is in humans. When owner compliance is problematic, once-daily dosing may prove effective chronically, although this has not been fully evaluated. Further increasing the time between dosing results in recurrent hyperthyroidism.[52,79] Carbimazole appears to be most effective if chronically administered at a dose of 5 mg twice daily.[52]

In many cats, such antithyroid therapy results in serum total T_4 concentrations below the reference range. However, clinical signs of hypothyroidism do not develop, and surgical risks are not increased. Corresponding serum total T_3 concentrations tend to remain within the reference range, and euthyroidism is maintained because T_3 is more metabolically active than T_4.[52] This may result from increased extrathyroidal T_4 to T_3 conversion or increased thyroidal secretion of T_3 because of intrathyroidal iodine deficiency or increased TSH production. In addition, serum free T_4 concentration, representing the active portion of T_4, appears to remain relatively higher than total T_4 concentration during methimazole therapy.[65] As a result, the aim is to suppress total T_4 into the lower half of the reference range; however, if severely depressed, the dose should be adjusted and the cat retested because at least some adverse reactions appear to be dose related.[79]

Methimazole and carbimazole have no effect on the underlying pathologic lesion in hyperthyroid cats. Thus over months to years of treatment, the thyroid nodule or nodules can continue to grow and enlarge. As a result it is common for the daily dose of antithyroid drugs to progressively increase. Some cats may no longer adequately respond to methimazole or carbimazole, and an alternative form of therapy is necessary.[1]

Although antithyroid dugs are routinely administered orally, compliance can be problematic in fractious or inappetant cats; absorption is potentially adversely affected by concurrent intestinal disease, and obvious difficulties exist in cats that vomit. Preliminary studies have shown that methimazole in a pluronic lecithin organogel (PLO) is effective in hyperthyroid cats when applied transdermally. However, subsequent studies of healthy cats have demonstrated poor bioavailability by this route, and further studies are required before widespread recommendation.[84]

Most clinical adverse reactions associated with methimazole or carbimazole occur within the first 3 months of therapy. They include vomiting, with or without anorexia and depression, usually within the first 4 weeks of therapy (occurring in 10% to 15% of cases).[52,79] These effects are more common with methimazole and may be related to its unpleasant bitter taste (compared with carbimazole, which is tasteless). However, these signs are usually transient and rarely require withdrawal of the drug. Self-induced excoriations of the head and neck have been seen in a small number of cats treated with methimazole or carbimazole within the first 3 months of therapy.[65,79] Drug withdrawal is usually required together with glucocorticoid therapy, and an alternative treatment for the hyperthyroidism is necessitated.

Early in the course of therapy, mild hematologic complications of eosinophilia, lymphocytosis, and leukopenia (with a normal differential count but without apparent clinical effect) occur in up to 16% of cases treated with methimazole and only 5% of cases treated with carbimazole.[52,79] More serious hematologic complications occur in less than 5% of cats treated with methimazole and include agranulocytosis and thrombocytopenia, either alone or concurrently, or more rarely, immune-mediated hemolytic anemia (usually occurring within the first 3 months of therapy).[7,79] These are apparently not dose related. While rarely reported for carbimazole, these worrisome problems can and do occur anecdotally. To predict such reactions, complete blood count (CBC) and platelet count is recommended every 2 weeks at least initially.[1,79] However, this is not cost-effective because of their low frequency and unpredictable occurrence. Therefore testing, if and when clinical signs develop, is more appropriate. There may however, be some merit in checking cats prior to surgery, particularly because thrombocytopenia is a potential risk.[1] Hepatic toxicity, exemplified by marked increases in the liver enzymes and bilirubin concentration, has also been described in less than 2% of cats treated with methimazole.[79] Cessation of therapy is required if either serious hematologic or hepatic reactions develop.

Serum antinuclear antibodies develop in approximately 50% of cats treated with methimazole for longer than 6 months, usually in cats on high-dose therapy (> 15 mg/day).[79] Although clinical signs of a lupuslike syndrome have not been reported, decreasing the daily dose is usually recommended. Such studies have not yet been carried out for carbimazole. A bleeding tendency without associated thrombocytopenia has been suggested to occur in cats treated with methimazole.[65] However, methimazole therapy had no effect on prothrombin time (PT) or activated partial thromboplastin time (APTT) after over 12 weeks of therapy, and it had no effect on thrombin clotting time or buccal mucosal bleeding time after 3 to 4 weeks of therapy in hyperthyroid cats.[85,86] However, a prolonged proteins induced by Vitamin K antagonism or absence (PIVKA) clotting time, together with melena, was reported in one cat, and this test is considered a more sensitive indicator of potential or actual bleeding tendencies than either PT or APTT.[86] Acquired myasthenia gravis (MG) and a cold agglutinin-like disease have been described in a few cats treated with methimazole.[1]

Editor's Note: There are numerous protocols for medical management of hyperthyroidism in cats. Our current recommendation is to administer 2.5 mg of methimazole orally once daily (or 2.0 mg of topical methimazole once daily) for 2 weeks. After this 2 week period, if the owners note any improvement or deterioration in their cats' condition, a serum total T_4 (with or without a CBC, serum biochemistry profile and urinalysis) should be obtained 4 to 6 hours after methimazole administration. If the value is within reference limits, that dose should be continued indefinitely. If neither improvement nor deterioration is appreciated or if the serum total T_4 concentration remains abnormally increased, the medication should be given BID for an additional 2 weeks. The cat should then be rechecked and the dose increased in 2 mg (topically) or 2.5 (orally) increments every 2 weeks, as needed. If administered topically, owners should be instructed to thoroughly rub the medication into the skin and then remove all excess vehicle within 30 minutes of each dose. If any abnormalities are detected that could be the result of methimazole, its' use should be discontinued until it can be demonstrated that continued use of the drug is warranted. It is further recommended that topical methimazole be compounded so that each dose is 0.05-0.10 cc this limits the problem of excess vehicle building upon the ears.

Other medical treatments The thioureylene antithyroid drugs are preferred for the treatment of hyperthyroidism, but there may be occasions when alternatives are required either because of the development of adverse reactions or other specific contraindications. However, chronic management is only achieved with methimazole or carbimazole. Beta-adrenergic blockers, stable iodine, and calcium ipodate only provide short-term control, and a more permanent treatment option is subsequently required.

Propranolol (Inderal, Wyeth-Ayerst) and atenolol (Tenormin, ICI Pharma) are the most frequently used beta-blockers in hyperthyroid cats. They are usually used to symptomatically control the tachycardia, polypnea, hypertension, and hyperexcitability associated with hyperthyroidism and to prevent the arrhythmias that may occur when anesthetizing affected cats.[1] Traditionally these drugs were considered to have no direct effect on the thyroid gland or thyroid hormones; however, propranolol, at least, may inhibit peripheral conversion of T_4 to T_3 in cats as in humans.[87] They are usually used in combination with antithyroid drugs when rapid control of the clinical effects is required or with stable iodine to ensure a more effective response.[1,87] Because they do not affect uptake of radioactive iodine, they may be useful while awaiting such therapy or in cats that have a delayed return to euthyroidism after treatment.[1]

Propranolol is a nonselective beta-adrenergic receptor–blocking agent and is therefore contraindicated in cats with asthma or pre-existing uncontrolled overt CHF. Atenolol, as a selective beta1 adrenoceptor–blocking agent is more useful in some of these situations and has the added advantage of a potential once-daily dosing regime. Propranolol is administered initially at a dose of 2.5 to 5 mg every 8 to 12 hours and subsequently titrated based on clinical effects and reduction in heart rate. Hyperthyroidism affects the pharmacokinetic profile of propranolol, and as such, low doses are recommended initially.[88] Atenolol is administered at a dose of 6.25 mg/cat either once or twice daily.

Large doses of stable iodine acutely decrease the rate of thyroid hormone synthesis (Wolff-Chaikoff effect) and thyroid hormone release. The mechanisms are unclear but are presumed to be protective. Its effects on reducing the vascularity and friability of thyroid tissue are controversial. Use of stable iodine has never gained widespread popularity because of its inconsistent, short-lived, and erratic effect in inducing euthyroidism and the potential for escape from inhibition and exacerbation of thyrotoxicosis. In addition, it is contraindicated prior to radioactive iodine administration and is associated with a high incidence of adverse reactions (salivation and partial to complete anorexia), purportedly because of its unpleasant brassy taste.[1,7] However, a recent report has suggested using potassium iodate tablets together with propranolol in a staged regime for 20 days before surgery.[87] Propranolol is administered at a dose of 2.5 mg three times daily for 20 days before surgery, titrated to effect, and potassium iodate is administered at a dose of 21.25 mg three times daily from the tenth to the twentieth day. Using such a regime, serum total T_3 concentration decreases in most cats, and serum total T_4 concentration falls to within reference range in approximately one third of cats. Adverse reactions of potassium iodate are minimized by placing the tablets in a gelatin capsule prior to administration and using a relatively low dose for as short a period as possible. However, despite this, adverse reactions may still occur, albeit less frequently, suggesting a systemic rather than a local effect.[87]

Calcium ipodate, an oral cholecystographic contrast agent, is the only other drug that has been assessed in hyperthyroid cats. Its major effect is to acutely inhibit peripheral T_4 to T_3 conversion. In one study of 12 hyperthyroid cats treated with calcium ipodate at a dose of 100 mg divided twice daily, eight exhibited a good response as indicated by a reduction in serum total T_3 concentration to within the reference range within 2 weeks and an obvious improvement in clinical signs.[89] However, although associated with no adverse reactions, serum total T_4 concentration was unaffected, and cats were not evaluated for longer than 14 weeks. This drug is now of limited availability and further studies are unlikely.

Surgical Thyroidectomy
Surgical thyroidectomy is a relatively simple, quick, and curative procedure and is therefore often considered the preferred treatment option in practice. However, to decrease the cardiac and metabolic complications associated with anesthetizing hyperthyroid cats, prior medical management and control of the thyrotoxicosis is required. Once euthyroidism has been achieved, the main surgical considerations are whether to perform a unilateral or bilateral thyroidectomy, the type of technique to use, and the potential postoperative complications.

It is estimated that both thyroid lobes are affected in over 70% of hyperthyroid cats, thereby necessitating a bilateral thyroidectomy. In many of these cats, both thyroid lobes are palpably enlarged, grossly abnormal (or both) on visual examination. However, as many as 15% of cats with bilateral disease have one thyroid lobe that appears grossly normal and if left in situ results in recurrent hyperthyroidism usually within 12 months.[90] Thyroid imaging is obviously useful in depicting thyroid lobe involvement, but access to nuclear imaging facilities is required.[5] High resolution ultrasonography, capable of assessing thyroid lobe size and parenchymal appearance, is useful in characterizing thyroid tissue when scintigraphy is not available.[91] In the absence of imaging techniques and as surgical experience increases, many practitioners routinely perform bilateral thyroidectomies regardless of the gross appearance of thyroid lobes.[65] If not routinely attempted, both thyroid lobes must be carefully examined at the time of surgery.

Thyroidectomy can be performed by extracapsular or intracapsular techniques. With extracapsular thyroidectomy, the intact thyroid lobe and capsule is removed after ligation of the cranial thyroid artery while attempting to maintain blood supply to the cranial parathyroid gland. This technique is associated with an unacceptably high prevalence of postoperative hypoparathyroidism and is no longer recommended.[92] With intracapsular thyroidectomy, the thyroid capsule is incised, the thyroid lobe removed, and the capsule left in situ, preserving the blood supply to the cranial parathyroid glands. However, this technique is associated with an unacceptably high risk of recurrence.[90,93] Both techniques have by now been modified to minimize the risk of postoperative hypoparathyroidism and recurrent hyperthyroidism.[92-94] The modified extracapsular technique uses bipolar cautery rather than ligatures, minimizing blunt dissection around the cranial parathyroid gland, whereas the modified intracapsular technique involves removal of the majority of the capsule after dissection. No significant difference is seen in the rate of postoperative hypocalcaemia or recurrence between these two methods, and both are considered equally appropriate for bilateral thyroidectomy in cats.[93] In unilateral cases, the choice of technique is not as important providing recurrence is avoided, because only one parathyroid gland is necessary to maintain eucalcemia.

Hypoparathyroidism resulting in hypocalcemia is the most significant potential postoperative complication. It has been suggested that the osteopenic effects of hyperthyroidism, rapidly reversed after surgical thyroidectomy, may exacerbate hypoparathyroidism in cats as in humans. However, the hyperparathyroidism and tendency toward ionized hypocalcemia reported in hyperthyroid cats suggests that such a phenomenon does not occur in this species.[55] While this in itself may play some role in postoperative hypocalcemia, hypoparathyroidism generally arises only if the parathyroid glands are injured, devascularized, or inadvertently removed during the course of a bilateral thyroidectomy. Revascularization of parathyroid tissue can occur even after removal and subsequent implantation to a nearby muscle belly.[95] Staged thyroidectomies (3 to 4 weeks apart) exploit this premise.[90] A more radical staged simplified complete thyroparathyroidectomy with parathyroid autotransplantation has been described in 10 cats with no postoperative hypocalcemia, which may be of particular benefit as a learning tool or if surgical experience is limited by a small throughput of cases.[65,96] However, a risk of simultaneous transplantation of diseased thyroid tissue exists, and increased costs and risk are associated with two general anesthetic procedures.[90,95]

Mild hypocalcaemia develops in most cats after bilateral thyroidectomy, but treatment is not necessary until clinical signs develop.

Hypoparathyroidism is rarely permanent, and recovery of parathyroid function may occur days to months after surgery. In such cases the parathyroid damage is presumed reversible. Alternatively, accessory parathyroid tissue is activated or more likely, calcium homeostasis is maintained through a PTH-independent mechanism.[97] Other potential postoperative complications include Horner's syndrome, laryngeal paralysis, and voice change, but these are rare.[90]

Circulating thyroid hormone concentrations usually fall below the reference range for weeks to months after thyroidectomy. T_4 supplementation is often recommended, particularly after bilateral thyroidectomy.[1] However, it is not strictly necessary because clinical hypothyroidism is a rare sequelae. Presumably, eventual normalization of thyroid hormone production occurs, either because of activation of the contralateral lobe in unilateral cases or accessory thyroid tissue in bilateral cases. Recurrence of hyperthyroidism is always a possibility after thyroidectomy, and cats should be monitored every 6 to 12 months thereafter. If a unilateral thyroidectomy was originally performed, development of lesions in the contralateral gland should pose no additional surgical risk providing parathyroid function is maintained. However, in cases of recurrent hyperthyroidism after bilateral thyroidectomy, postoperative morbidity and mortality is significantly increased and an alternative form of treatment for the hyperthyroidism is indicated.[93]

Radioactive Iodine Administration of radioactive iodine as ^{131}I is considered to be the safest, simplest, and most effective therapy for feline hyperthyroidism. [131]I, like stable iodine, is actively concentrated by the thyroid gland, has a half-life of 8 days, and emits both β-particles and γ-radiation. The β-particles, cause over 80% of damage, but are locally destructive, traveling a maximum of 2 mm with an average path length of 400 μm. Therefore no significant damage occurs to adjacent parathyroid tissue, atrophic thyroid tissue, or other cervical structures. The aim of therapy is to restore euthyroidism with the smallest possible single dose of radiation, while avoiding the development of hypothyroidism or the persistence of hyperthyroidism.

Since its first use, controversy has surrounded the best method to calculate the optimum dose for individual cats. Tracer kinetic studies have been used that allow calculation of percentage iodine uptake, effective half-life, and estimation of thyroid gland weight—all factors known to influence the therapeutic dose.[98,99] The predictive value of tracer studies in estimating a therapeutic dose has been shown to be significantly closer to the therapeutic goal than the hypothetical administration of a fixed low dose (111 MBq).[100] However, this method requires access to sophisticated computerized nuclear medicine equipment, is time-consuming, expensive and can involve repeated sedation of the patient. It is therefore rarely used.

Another method is to use a relatively high fixed dose of between 148 and 250 MBq in all cats regardless of the size of the goiter or severity of the thyrotoxicosis.[101-105] Although this method is successful and simple, it potentially results in the under- or overtreatment of a significant proportion of cats. Extremely high fixed doses (> 1000 MBq) are retained for cats after surgical removal of a thyroid carcinoma.[106]

In most studies examining radioactive iodine therapy, it is recognized that markedly elevated pretreatment serum thyroid hormone concentration, the size of goiter, and the

severity of the clinical thyrotoxicosis all potentially adversely affect the eventual response. The dose administered can be determined based on a scoring system that takes these factors into consideration.[107-109] When such a scoring system is used, doses range from 39 to 222 MBq, allowing titration to each individual cat and avoiding unnecessary under- or overtreatment. It is an extremely simple method that does not require access to sophisticated nuclear medicine equipment. Success is comparable to dose estimation by tracer kinetic studies.

Traditionally, ^{131}I is administered intravenously.[98,102-105,107-109] Oral administration has been attempted, but higher doses are generally required, the risks of radiation spillage are greater, and vomiting may occur.[101,104,110] Subcutaneous administration is equally effective, is simpler to administer, is safer to personnel, is less stressful to cats, and is currently preferred.[108,109,111] Whatever method of dose calculation or route of administration, attainment of euthyroidism is expected in over 90% of cats with a single dose (Figure 239-7). A small percentage of cats remain persistently hyperthyroid, but euthyroidism is eventually attained in some of these animals weeks to months later without further treatment.[108,109] Both hypothyroidism and recurrent hyperthyroidism can develop but appear to be rare, and other side effects are minimal.[112]

Several studies have estimated survival time in cats after treatment with hyperthyroidism. In one study of 66 cats followed for a mean of 13 months, 44 (67%) cats were alive and euthyroid 1 to 33 months after treatment. The remaining cats had died of unrelated causes, including renal failure.[103] In a larger study of 524 cats, median survival time (MST) was

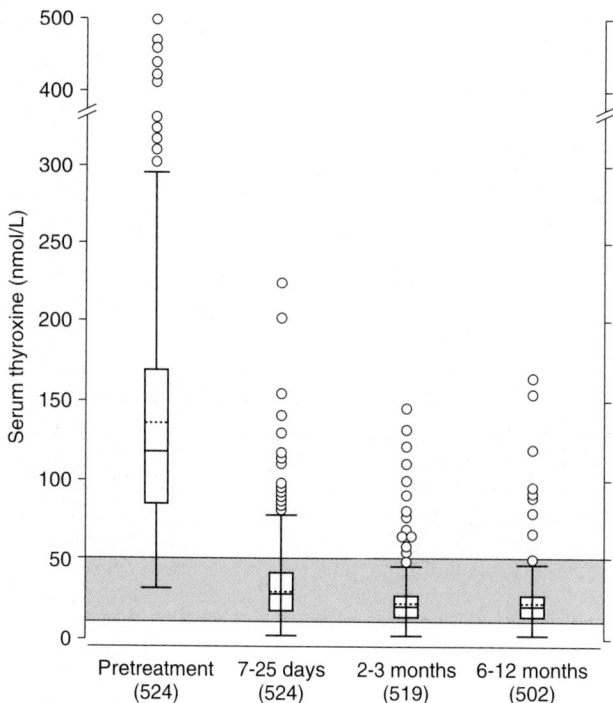

Figure 239-7 Box plots of serum total thyroxine (T_4) concentrations in 524 cats before and at various times after administration of radioiodine for treatment of hyperthyroidism. Data are plotted (i.e., box plots) as described in the legend of Figure 239-1. The shaded area indicates the reference range for serum T_4 concentration. To convert serum T_4 concentrations from nmol/L to ng/dL, divide the given values by 12.87. (From Peterson ME et al: Radioioidine treatment of 524 cats with hyperthyroidism. J Am Vet Med Assoc 207:1422, 1995.)

24 months (range 2 weeks to 7 years).[109] The percentage of cats alive at 1, 2, 3, and 4 years after treatment was 89%, 72%, 52%, and 34%, respectively. The most common causes of death in treated hyperthyroid cats are malignancy and renal disease.[109,113]

The effect of prior medical management on eventual outcome of radioactive iodine therapy is controversial. Obviously prior administration of stable iodine is contraindicated because of its inhibitory effect on the thyroid gland. Beta-blockers are often recommended because they have no effect on the thyroid gland *per se*. However, prior methimazole (and therefore carbimazole) therapy has been suggested to enhance, worsen, or have no effect on radioiodine treatment outcome.[98,109,110,112] Methimazole does not inhibit thyroidal iodine uptake, but current administration adversely affects effective half-life of radioactive iodine and is not recommended.[100] However, iodine uptake is enhanced in healthy cats after recent methimazole withdrawal and this short-term rebound effect is potentially beneficial when treating with radioactive iodine.[78] A more recent study has shown that discontinuing methimazole for less than or greater than 5 days prior to radioactive iodine therapy has no effect on treatment outcome.[105]

The main drawback to widespread use of radioactive iodine is the requirement for special licensing and the isolation of the cat for variable periods after treatment. This can range from several days to several weeks, depending on the dose used and state or local radiation regulations.[1] Cats appear to tolerate these periods of hospitalization well.

Other Therapies Intrathyroidal infusion of ethanol causes tissue necrosis and eventual induction of euthyroidism. Single injections in unilateral cases, preferably using ultrasound guidance, are efficacious in inducing euthyroidism in hyperthyroid cats.[114] Staged injections in bilateral cases are less successful in treating hyperthyroidism.[115] However, percutaneous ethanol injection is associated with a high incidence of adverse reactions such as transient dysphonia, Horner's syndrome, gagging, and laryngeal paralysis and cannot therefore be recommended for treatment of hyperthyroid cats.

Gene therapy could potentially be used to deliver cytotoxicity specifically to abnormally functioning thyroid cells. The feline thyroglobulin promoter has been characterized and its cell type specific activity demonstrated, paving the way for transcriptional targeting of gene therapy. However, a great deal of work is required before any such technology reaches veterinary practice.[116]

Effect of Treatment on Renal Function Despite the potential adverse effect of hyperthyroidism on renal function, its presence can increase glomerular filtration rate (GFR), decrease serum creatinine concentration, and mask underlying renal disease.[34,55,117] Decreased GFR, increased serum urea and creatinine concentration, and development of overt clinical signs of renal disease have all been reported after successful treatment of hyperthyroidism, regardless of therapeutic modality utilized (methimazole, surgical thyroidectomy or radioiodine).[34,118-120] Assessment of GFR before treatment can act as a predictor of post-treatment renal failure with a low GFR in hyperthyroidism, indicating an increased risk for adverse clinical outcome.[119] However, techniques for assessment of GFR are impractical because they typically involve use of radioisotopes. Estimation of GFR is also possible using a plasma iohexol clearance test that requires no special licensing but is technically demanding.[120] In the absence of such estimations, accurate prediction of impending renal failure is difficult. However, serum urea and creatinine concentrations and USG should be carefully evaluated prior to treatment

of hyperthyroidism. If both serum parameters are normal and the urine is concentrated, the risk of developing renal failure after therapy is minimized. Serum creatinine should be evaluated in light of the animal's muscle mass with lower values expected in emaciated cats.[34] If the serum creatinine and urea concentrations are higher than expected and the urine isosthenuric, a risk of developing renal failure exists. In such cases, trial therapy using either methimazole or carbimazole should be attempted and renal function reassessed once euthyroidism is achieved. Initially low and then increasing doses of methimazole have been suggested in suspect cases, but limited scientific evidence exists to support this.[34] If no deterioration occurs after treatment of the hyperthyroidism, then a more permanent therapeutic option may be selected. If renal function declines, therapy should be instituted for renal failure and the dose of antithyroid medication adjusted to maximize renal function while attempting to control clinical signs. Maintenance of a mildly hyperthyroid state may be beneficial in some individuals. Avoidance of hypothyroidism is important because it may have its own detrimental effects on GFR.[34]

THYROID NEOPLASIA AND HYPERTHYROIDISM IN DOGS

Thyroid tumors account for 1.2% to 3.75% of all tumors and approximately 10% to 15% of all head and neck neoplasms in the dog. In pathologic studies, benign adenomas account for approximately 30% to 50% of all thyroid tumors, but these are usually small focal lesions uncommonly detected during life.[121,122] On the other hand, carcinomas, responsible for only 50 to 70% of all thyroid tumors diagnosed postmortem, account for up to 90% of those tumors detected antemortem. All thyroid masses detected during life should, therefore, be presumed malignant until proven otherwise. Carcinomas are usually larger than adenomas, coarsely multinodular, nonmobile, and often have necrotic or hemorrhagic centers or, occasionally, focal areas of mineralization or bone formation. Unilateral involvement is more than twice as common as bilateral involvement; when the latter occurs, the neoplastic process is usually extensive. It is therefore difficult to determine if the tumor arose in both thyroid lobes or if metastases occurred from one lobe to the other. Occasionally, ectopic thyroid tissue (arising from thyroglossal duct remnants) located anywhere from the base of the tongue to the base of the heart becomes neoplastic, and thyroid tumors must therefore be included in a range of differential diagnoses for oral, cervical, and thoracic masses.

Thyroid carcinomas are poorly encapsulated and commonly extend into or around the trachea, cervical muscles, esophagus, larynx, nerves, and blood vessels, although invasion into the esophageal or tracheal lumen is unusual. Metastatic spread to the retropharyngeal and cervical lymph nodes is common. However, early invasion into the cranial and caudal thyroid veins with the formation of tumor cell thrombi leads to multiple pulmonary metastases, often before involvement of regional lymph nodes. Other reported, but rare, sites of metastatic lesions include kidney, adrenal gland, liver, spleen, spinal cord, and bone.

Histopathologically, thyroid carcinomas are usually well differentiated and classified as follicular, compact (solid), mixed, or papillary. The majority of tumors in the dog are mixed, follicular, or less commonly, compact. The correlation between this histopathologic classification and ultimate prognosis is unclear. Undifferentiated (anaplastic) thyroid tumors appear to be highly malignant but are rare. Medullary (parafollicular, C-cell) carcinoma may have a more favorable prognosis, because distant metastatic spread is uncommon and they appear to be well encapsulated and easily resectable at the time of surgical thyroidectomy. However, specific immunocytochemical stains are required for diagnosis.[123] The probability of metastases clearly increases in proportion to the size of the tumor. Dogs with small thyroid tumors (< 20 cm³) have a less than 20% incidence of metastatic disease, whereas nearly all dogs with large tumors (> 100 cm³) have metastases.

Clinical Features

Thyroid tumors occur in middle-aged and older dogs, with an average age at onset of 10 years. Almost all dogs are greater than 4 years old at the time of diagnosis. No sex predilection exists, unlike the situation in humans in which females are more than twice as likely to develop thyroid cancer as males at most ages. Beagles and golden retrievers appear predisposed to the development of thyroid carcinomas and boxers to the development of both adenomas and carcinomas.

Thyroid tumors are occasionally coincidentally found as freely mobile masses when grooming, petting, or during a general health check. However, most dogs have a visible mass in the neck or have its associated consequences (coughing, gagging, dysphonia, dysphagia, retching, regurgitation, and vomiting). The duration of these signs varies from weeks to months. The mass is usually felt in the region of the thyroid gland, below the larynx, but occasionally, larger tumors may descend toward the thoracic inlet. Clinical signs referable to regional (enlarged lymph nodes or cording of local lymphatic and blood vessels) or distant (dyspnea from pulmonary metastases) metastatic spread may be apparent. A few dogs may have the additional clinical signs of hypothyroidism or hyperthyroidism. Dogs with hyperthyroidism exhibit similar clinical signs to those in cats (weight loss, polyphagia, polyuria/polydipsia [PU/PD], restlessness, tachycardia) but tend to be less symptomatic.

In general, canine thyroid tumors are nonfunctional, and euthyroidism is maintained throughout the course of the disease. It has been suggested that up to 30% of dogs with detectable thyroid tumors are hypothyroid.[124] Hypothyroidism may arise because of destruction of all normal thyroid tissue by aggressive bilateral carcinomas. Alternatively, large tumors could potentially produce excessive inactive thyroid hormones capable of pituitary TSH suppression and eventual atrophy of normal thyroid tissue, although this has not yet been substantiated. A diagnosis of hypothyroidism must be approached with caution because of the suppressive effect of nonspecific illness on circulating thyroid hormone concentrations. Hyperthyroidism occurs in approximately 10% to 20% of thyroid carcinomas but is unusual in the rare cases of detectable adenomas.

In humans, thyroid tumors form part of the multiple endocrine neoplasia (MEN) syndromes in which neoplasia or hyperplasia develops in several different endocrine organs simultaneously. MEN syndromes are classified as type 1 or type 2, the latter further divided into type 2A and 2B. The MEN syndromes tend to involve one or more specific polypeptide- and biogenic amine-producing cell types, exhibit a histologic progression from hyperplasia to adenoma and (in some cases) to carcinoma, and each has an autosomal dominant pattern of inheritance. MEN type 1 syndrome involves parathyroid, pancreatic islet, and pituitary hyperplasia or neoplasia. MEN type 2A is associated with the development of bilateral pheochromocytomas, medullary thyroid carcinomas and, less commonly, parathyroid hyperplasia or adenoma. The association of medullary thyroid carcinoma and pheochromocytoma with multiple mucosal neuromas is termed *MEN type 2B*. Some patients do experience unusual manifestations of these syndromes, but these are less well characterized. Although rare, it has been suggested that MEN syndromes

exist in dogs,[124] and a careful clinical evaluation should be carried out in all dogs with thyroid carcinoma.

Diagnosis

The differential diagnoses for large cervical swellings include abscess, granuloma, thyroid tumor, other tumors, and salivary mucocele. Fine needle (21 to 23 gauge) aspiration is helpful in distinguishing many of these. Unfortunately, because of the vascular nature of thyroid tissue, samples are frequently heavily contaminated with blood and exfoliation of neoplastic cells can be poor.[125] Evaluation of wide bore needle biopsies, although of greater diagnostic yield, significantly increases the risk of hemorrhage and should only be carried out under ultrasound guidance. Even with such biopsies there may still be difficulty in distinguishing benign from malignant tumors, and the latter is often only confirmed by demonstration of vascular or capsular invasion in biopsies taken at the time of surgical thyroidectomy.

Results of postmortem studies show that up to 80% of dogs have evidence of distant metastatic spread, although this decreases to just over 60% in clinical cases.[126] Thus it is imperative that once a mass is identified as thyroid, a systematic search for metastatic spread should follow. Routine screening laboratory tests may be helpful in identifying secondary organ involvement or concurrent problems that may ultimately affect the prognosis. Local lymph nodes should be carefully examined and biopsied as necessary. Radiography of the cervical area may help to assess the size of the mass and the extent of local invasion. Thoracic radiography should always be evaluated for evidence of pulmonary spread even in the absence of clinical signs. Abdominal radiography and ultrasonography may be useful in cases where hepatic metastasis is suspected.

As in cats, thyroid scintigraphy using radioactive iodine or technetium may be useful because most thyroid tumors and their metastases retain the ability to trap iodine. Such scans do not provide any information with regard to thyroid function but are helpful in depicting location of the tumor and regional metastases.[127] Some thyroid tumors fail to adequately concentrate radioisotopes, and it has been suggested that these are less likely to respond to radioactive iodine administration.[124] Compared with thoracic radiography, thoracic scintigraphy to depict pulmonary metastases is not considered useful.

Measurement of serum total T_4 concentration is necessary in dogs with appropriate clinical signs of thyrotoxicosis. Elevations are generally moderate, compared with the marked elevations often seen in hyperthyroid cats. Measurement of circulating endogenous TSH concentration is not useful due to the poor sensitivity of currently available assays and their inability to detect suppressed values. However, free T_4 in combination with cTSH measurements will provide the most useful information to support hypothyroidism if clinical signs are suggestive.

Treatment

Currently, several possible treatment options exist for thyroid carcinoma. Clinicians find that the selection of any one option is complicated by poorly defined prognostic indicators, inconsistencies in case selection and reporting criteria amongst the different studies, and the variety and number of treatments attempted in individual patients. However, it is clear that the prognosis is excellent for mobile, nonfixed tumors; that local control may halt metastatic spread; and that metastatic spread may not ultimately affect outcome with certain treatment options. In addition, functional state appears irrelevant and clinical signs of hyperthyroidism can easily be controlled using carbimazole or methimazole at 5 mg orally three times daily initially and subsequently adjusted for effect.

Surgical thyroidectomy is approached as for cats. However, in dogs most tumors are unilateral and therefore it is not necessary to preserve parathyroid glands on the affected side.

In dogs with no evidence of metastatic spread and operable thyroid tumors, resection alone results in long-term control without subsequent development of metastases.[128] However, in many cases extensive local tumor invasion precludes complete removal, and aggressive surgical attempts significantly increase the risk of extensive hemorrhage and damage to the recurrent laryngeal nerves and parathyroid glands. In such cases, surgery alone is only associated with a 25% survival rate at 1 year.[123] Surgical debulking followed by chemotherapy with cisplatin or doxorubicin has been recommended for such cases.[129,130] Administration of radioactive iodine may be helpful if iodine uptake is maintained but generally high, and multiple doses must be used, limiting its value clinically.[124,131] Two recent studies suggest that definitive or palliative radiotherapy may be associated with the best survival.[132,133] In these studies, prior existence of metastatic spread did not appear to alter survival, and there was a decreased risk of metastatic spread with local control of tumor progression.

Standard dose T_4 supplementation is necessary after bilateral thyroidectomy. In addition, T_4 therapy is usually recommended after unilateral thyroidectomy. Receptor affinity and concentration and functional response to TSH are similar in healthy and carcinomatous thyroids.[134] Although it is unclear if TSH has any growth-stimulating properties in thyroid neoplasia *in vivo*, T_4 therapy seems a wise precaution.

CHAPTER • 240

Insulin-Secreting Islet Cell Neoplasia

Rebecka S. Hess

Insulinoma is uncommon in the dog and rare in the cat. This chapter, therefore, focuses on canine insulinoma unless otherwise noted. The first case series documenting successful surgical therapy of insulinoma in human beings was reported by Whipple in 1935. *Whipple's triad* was defined as the presence of neurologic clinical signs associated with a low plasma glucose concentration and relieved by feeding or administration of glucose. Canine insulinoma was first described in 1935.[1]

PATHOLOGY

Insulin-secreting beta cell neoplasia is the most common islet cell neoplasia in the dog. This may be due to the fact that beta cells comprise approximately 70% of cells in the islets of Langerhans. Most canine insulinomas are malignant. In one immunocytochemical report, 17 of 18 insulinomas were carcinomas and only one was an adenoma.[2] About 80% of pancreatic tumors are solitary, and most are located in one of the two limbs of the pancreas rather than in the body.[3-5] Occasionally, no discrete nodule or nodules are apparent during gross examination of the pancreas, and histopathologic evaluation is needed to identify the tumor.

The rate of detected metastatic lesions in 179 dogs from different studies ranged from 45% to 64% and was higher in studies based on necropsy than in those based on surgical biopsies.[3,6,7] Clinical staging of pancreatic tumors according to the World Health Organization's tumor-node-metastasis (TNM) system defines stage I as $T_1N_0M_0$ (presence of a primary tumor and absence of regional lymph node or distant metastases), stage II as $T_1N_1M_0$, and stage III as $T_1N_1M_1$ or $T_1N_0M_1$. Most dogs with insulinoma have stage II or stage III disease.[8] The most common sites of metastases are regional lymph nodes and the liver. Other reported metastatic sites are the duodenum, mesentery, omentum, spleen, heart, and spinal cord.

Although the etiology of insulinoma is unknown, growth hormone production, which is not associated with increased plasma growth hormone concentrations, has been documented in primary and metastatic canine insulinoma lesions. Local growth hormone may affect insulinoma cell proliferation through paracrine or autocrine mechanisms.[9]

Pathophysiology

Proliferation of beta pancreatic cells results in excess secretion of insulin and therefore hypoglycemia. The most important compensatory mechanisms for hypoglycemia are inhibition of insulin secretion and stimulated secretion of counter-regulatory hormones.

Glucose is the primary regulator of insulin secretion. When glucose enters beta pancreatic cells, it is metabolized to adenosine triphosphate (ATP) and closes ATP-sensitive potassium (K^+) channels. Closure of the K^+ channels reduces K^+ efflux and results in depolarization of the beta cell and opening of voltage-sensitive calcium (Ca^{2+}) channels. An increase in the cytoplasmic Ca^{2+} concentration results in insulin exocytosis. In a normal animal, insulin secretion is completely inhibited when the blood glucose concentration is less than 65 to 80 mg/dL. However, insulin secretion from neoplastic beta cells occurs independent of the blood glucose concentration and persists despite a low blood glucose concentration. Therefore the hallmark of an insulin-secreting tumor (insulinoma) is an increased blood insulin concentration despite a low blood glucose concentration.

The four counter-regulatory hormones secreted in response to hypoglycemia are glucagon, catecholamines, growth hormone, and glucocorticoids. Of these hormones, glucagon and catecholamines are most important in increasing the blood glucose concentration.

HISTORY AND CLINICAL SIGNS

The mean age of dogs with insulinoma is 9 years (range, 3 to 15 years). Although any breed can develop an insulinoma, the tumor has been reported mainly in medium to large breed dogs. Controlled studies of breed risk for insulinoma have not been published, and there is no apparent sex predilection for the disease.

Most clinical signs arise from the effect of hypoglycemia on the central nervous system (neuroglycopenia) or from hypoglycemia-induced release of catecholamines. Glucose is the single most important source of energy in the brain, and carbohydrate storage in neural tissue is limited. Brain function, therefore, depends on a continuous supply of glucose. Clinical signs attributable to neuroglycopenia include seizures, collapse, weakness, ataxia, disorientation, mental dullness, and visual disturbances. Clinical signs related to excess catecholamine release and stimulation of the sympathetic nervous system include tremors, hunger, and nervousness.

The severity of clinical signs increases as blood glucose drops, and severe hypoglycemia ultimately can result in coma and death. Clinical signs may also be related to the duration of the hypoglycemia and the rate at which it develops, because a gradual decrease in the blood glucose concentration may be less likely to stimulate catecholamine secretion. Occasionally clinical signs are episodic, because secretion of counter-regulatory hormones elevates the blood glucose concentration and temporarily resolves neuroglycopenic clinical signs. Feeding can result in either alleviation or exacerbation of clinical signs. If feeding restores the blood glucose concentration to normal, the clinical signs resolve. However, feeding may also stimulate insulin secretion and exacerbate the clinical signs. Fasting, exercise, or excitement can worsen clinical signs either by decreasing the blood glucose concentration or by increasing sympathetic stimulation.

Clinical signs reported in 198 dogs from several studies are listed in Table 240-1.[3-5,7,8,10] Although most dogs have more than one of these clinical signs, some dogs have none. The reported duration of clinical signs prior to diagnosis varies from 1 day to 3 years.

Physical Examination

The physical examination is unremarkable in most dogs with insulinoma.[4,6] Dogs may be overweight as a result of the anabolic effects of insulin, and postictal findings may be apparent if the dog has had a recent seizure. A peripheral polyneuropathy, characterized by tetraparesis and decreased or absent appendicular reflexes, has been described in association with insulinoma in 13 dogs.[8,11,12] The etiology of insulinoma-associated peripheral neuropathy is not known. It has been suggested that this polyneuropathy develops as a paraneoplastic immune-mediated disorder that is unrelated to the metabolic changes associated with insulinoma.[12]

DIFFERENTIAL DIAGNOSES

Differential diagnoses for hypoglycemia may be categorized as (1) those associated with excess secretion of insulin or insulin-like factors, (2) those associated with decreased glucose production, (3) those associated with excess glucose consumption, (4) drug-associated causes, and (5) spurious causes. Disorders in which the most important mechanism for hypoglycemia is excess secretion of insulin or insulin-like factors include insulinoma, extrapancreatic tumor, and islet cell hyperplasia. Conditions associated with decreased glucose production include hypoadrenocorticism, hypopituitarism, growth hormone deficiency, liver diseases, glycogen storage diseases, neonates, and toy breeds. Fasting, malnutrition, and

Table • 240-1

Clinical Signs Reported in 198 Dogs from Several Studies[3-5,7,8,10]

CLINICAL SIGN	NUMBER OF DOGS
Seizure	95
Collapse	79
Generalized weakness	74
Shaking/trembling/muscle twitching	40
Ataxia	40
Exercise intolerance	30
Hindlimb weakness	28
Disorientation/bizarre behavior/hysteria	19
Polyphagia	16
Polyuria and polydipsia	16
Stupor/lethargy	12
Focal facial seizures	6
Obesity or weight gain	6
Blindness	5
Anorexia	5
Diarrhea	4
Head tilt	2
Nervousness	2

pregnancy may also result in hypoglycemia. Excess glucose consumption may develop in sepsis or extreme exercise. Some of the many drugs reported to induce hypoglycemia in human beings include insulin, oral hypoglycemics (e.g., sulfonylurea), salicylates (e.g., aspirin), acetaminophen, beta blockers (e.g., propranolol), beta$_2$-agonists, ethanol, monoamine oxidase inhibitors, tricyclic antidepressants (e.g., amitriptyline), angiotensin-converting enzyme inhibitors (e.g., captopril), antibiotics (e.g., tetracycline), lidocaine overdose, and lithium. Factitious hypoglycemia may occur when blood cells are not promptly separated from serum or in cases of severe polycythemia or leukocytosis if serum separation is delayed longer than 1 hour.

Diagnostic Evaluation

A clinical suspicion of insulinoma is established with documentation of appropriate clinical signs, hypoglycemia (blood glucose concentration less than 60 mg/dL), and concurrent hyperinsulinemia (serum insulin concentration greater than 20 µU/mL).[13] Identification of a pancreatic mass with imaging studies may strengthen this suspicion. The diagnosis of insulinoma is confirmed with histologic examination and immunohistochemical staining of the pancreatic mass.

The results of a complete blood count, chemistry screen, and urinalysis are usually unremarkable, aside from the low blood glucose concentration.[4,7] Although hypoglycemia is observed in most dogs with insulinoma, especially if the measurement is repeated twice,[7] it is important to remember that some dogs with insulinoma may have euglycemia on repeated measurements.[14] Mild hypokalemia and increased serum alkaline phosphatase or alanine aminotransferase activities have also been documented.[5,7]

If a dog suspected of having an insulinoma has euglycemia, it should be fasted and the blood glucose concentration should be measured every 1 to 2 hours. In most dogs with insulinoma, hypoglycemia develops within 12 hours of fasting. Blood for measurement of the insulin concentration should be collected when the animal is hypoglycemic, and it should then be fed. However, a small percentage of dogs do not exhibit hypoglycemia, even with repeated measurements and after a prolonged fast (48 to 72 hours).[7] A low fructosamine concentration has been used to strengthen the clinical suspicion of insulinoma in several dogs with euglycemia.[14] The glycosylated hemoglobin A1c concentration has been significantly low in some but not all dogs with insulinoma.[15] Repetition of serum insulin measurements may also aid in the diagnosis. One study of canine insulinoma found that 76% of dogs had an increased serum insulin concentration when it was measured once, and 91% of dogs had an increased serum insulin concentration when it was measured twice.[7]

Other tests have been described as aids in the diagnosis of insulinoma in euglycemic dogs with a normal serum insulin concentration. However, insulin to glucose and glucose to insulin ratios are not recommended because of their low sensitivity, and the amended insulin to glucose ratio is not recommended because of its low specificity. Additional tolerance and stimulation tests have been described but are not advocated because of questionable usefulness and potentially fatal side effects, such as hypoglycemia and seizures.[16]

Most dogs with insulinoma have normal abdominal and thoracic radiographs.[4,6,8,17] According to the combined results of several studies in which abdominal ultrasound scans were performed in dogs with insulinoma, a pancreatic mass was identified in 49 of 87 (56%) dogs, and abdominal metastasis was noted in 17 of 87 (20%).[3,5,8,17] Although abdominal ultrasonography may be helpful in increasing the clinical suspicion of a pancreatic mass and metastases, both false-positive and false-negative results have been described.

Computed tomography (CT) is the most common imaging technique used for identification of pancreatic tumors in human beings; it detects about 50% of tumors greater than 2 cm in diameter and almost none of the smaller tumors.[18] CT has been reported in a small number of dogs with insulinoma, but its sensitivity in dogs has yet to be determined.[8] Intravenous administration of radioactively labeled synthetic somatostatin, followed by whole body scintigraphy, has been shown to be a sensitive and specific tool for pancreatic tumor imaging in humans[18] and has been reported in one dog with insulinoma.[19] Intravenous intraoperative administration of methylene blue was used to characterize pancreatic tumors in five dogs.[20]

TREATMENT

Therapy for insulinoma can be divided into treatment of the acute hypoglycemic crisis and long-term management. During an acute hypoglycemic crisis, dextrose can be given as a slow bolus (0.5 g/kg given intravenously, diluted in 0.9% sodium chloride at a 1:3 ratio). The bolus is followed by an intravenous continuous-rate infusion of dextrose (2.5% to 5% in water). Dextrose must be administered with caution because it can stimulate insulin secretion and cause hypoglycemia. Fluid resuscitation is performed as necessary. In most dogs, neuroglycopenia resolves with administration of dextrose. However, if the animal fails to respond to dextrose administration alone, dexamethasone (0.5 mg/kg given intravenously over 6 hours, every 12 to 24 hours) and a somatostatin analog (20 to 40 μg given subcutaneously every 8 to 12 hours) may be administered. In severe cases the animal may have to be sedated with pentobarbital for several hours while the above treatment is continued and until seizures resolve.[21]

A continuous-rate infusion of glucagon (5 to 13 ng/kg/min with or without a concurrent 10% dextrose infusion) has been reported in one dog with insulinoma-associated hypoglycemia. Clinical signs attributed to the hypoglycemia

resolved within 20 minutes, and the hypoglycemia resolved within 1 hour. Glucagon increases the blood glucose concentration by promoting glycogenolysis and gluconeogenesis. However, glucagon also increases insulin secretion, and animals should be monitored carefully for worsening hypoglycemia.[22]

The long-term treatment of choice for insulinoma is surgical resection of the tumor and gross metastases.[5] Surgical exploration and biopsy of the pancreatic mass also can confirm the diagnosis and may aid estimation of the survival time.[10] When postoperative hyperglycemia develops, it usually is transient and resolves once normal beta cells, which have been suppressed by excess insulin secretion from neoplastic cells, regain their function. However, about 10% of dogs develop diabetes mellitus and require treatment with exogenous insulin for 1 to 37 months.[6,7,10] Other postoperative complications include acute pancreatitis, diabetic ketoacidosis, delayed wound healing, ventricular arrhythmias and cardiac arrest, hemorrhage, sepsis, and leukopenia.[3,5,7]

The discussion of medical therapy is limited to clinically important agents reported as having been used in dogs with spontaneous insulinoma. The use of additional medications is discussed elsewhere.[21] Medical treatment is indicated prior to surgery, postoperatively if needed, and in cases in which surgery is not performed. Medical therapy can be divided into cytotoxic treatment directed at destroying insulin-secreting beta cells and treatment aimed at relieving the hypoglycemia.

Streptozocin is a nitrosourea antibiotic derived from the bacterium *Streptomyces achromogenes*. Streptozocin selectively destroys beta cells in the pancreas or metastatic sites. The drug is nephrotoxic and has been reported to cause acute renal failure and renal tubular atrophy in the dog. Diuresis with saline decreases the drug's contact time with renal tubular epithelial cells and may reduce the risk of nephrotoxicity. Successful use of streptozocin in veterinary medicine is limited to a study of 17 dogs, most of which had surgery with incomplete resection of gross lesions.[8] Dogs were treated with 0.9% sodium chloride (18 mL/kg/hr given intravenously) for 3 hours prior to streptozocin administration, during 2 more hours of streptozocin treatment, and for 2 additional hours after treatment. Streptozocin (500 mg/m^2) was given every 3 weeks. Butorphanol (0.4 mg/kg given intramuscularly) was administered immediately after streptozocin therapy as an antiemetic, but vomiting still occurred in about 30% of treatments. Other side effects included diabetes mellitus, transient hypoglycemia and seizures, transient hyperglycemia, transient increases in alanine aminotransferase activity, azotemia, mild thrombocytopenia, and mild neutropenia. The median duration of normoglycemia in dogs treated with streptozocin was 163 days, which was not significantly different from the median duration in control dogs treated surgically or medically. Further studies are needed to determine whether the benefits of streptozocin treatment outweigh its risks.

The main methods of relieving hypoglycemia include dietary modification and treatment with prednisone, diazoxide, or synthetic somatostatin. Small, frequent meals (every 4 to 6 hours) of a diet high in protein, fat, and complex carbohydrates are recommended, and simple sugars (present in soft, moist dog foods) should be avoided.

Prednisone increases the blood glucose concentration by increasing gluconeogenesis and glucose 6-phosphatase activity, decreasing blood glucose uptake into tissue, and stimulating glucagon secretion. Glucocorticoids can be administered intravenously in the form of dexamethasone during an acute hypoglycemic crisis or can be given orally once the dog is stable. Prednisone, the least expensive and most commonly used drug for the treatment of canine insulinoma, should be administered at a dosage of 0.5 to 4 mg/kg/day given orally, beginning with the lower end of the dosage and gradually increasing if necessary.[10,21]

Diazoxide is a benzothiadiazine derivative, the main action of which is to inhibit closure of ATP-dependent K^+ channels in beta pancreatic cells. This prevents depolarization of beta cells and inhibits opening of voltage-dependent Ca^{2+} channels. Decreased Ca^{2+} influx results in decreased exocytosis of insulin-containing secretory vesicles. Diazoxide also increases the blood glucose concentration in pancreatized dogs by increasing glycogenolysis and gluconeogenesis and by inhibiting tissue uptake of glucose.[23] Diazoxide is administered at a dosage of 10 to 40 mg/kg/day given orally, divided every 8 to 12 hours, beginning at the lower end of the dosage and gradually increasing if needed. Approximately 70% of dogs with insulinoma respond to treatment with diazoxide.[7] Side effects in dogs, which are uncommon, include ptyalism, vomiting, and anorexia. However, in human beings, myocardial ischemia, salt retention, water retention, hyperglycemia, hypotension, and cerebral ischemia have also been reported.

Octreotide is a long-acting synthetic somatostatin analog, and its main mode of action is inhibition of insulin secretion. In human beings, octreotide's action depends on its binding affinity to any of five somatostatin receptor subtypes present in tumors. Dogs have only one somatostatin receptor subtype, and their response to octreotide is variable.[24] The lack of a dependable response to octreotide in dogs may be due to the drug's inhibition of glucagon and growth hormone secretion. If suppression of glucagon and growth hormone secretion is of greater magnitude and duration compared with suppression of insulin secretion, octreotide may actually worsen the hypoglycemia. Also, some canine insulinomas may not have somatostatin receptors. For these reasons, further studies are needed to determine octreotide's efficacy and safety in dogs. Octreotide has been administered to dogs with insulinoma at dosages of 2 to 4 µg/kg given subcutaneously every 8 to 12 hours.[25] Side effects have not been reported in dogs; in humans they are mild and include pain at the site of injection (which can be reduced if octreotide is warmed to room temperature before administration), nausea, vomiting, abdominal pain, constipation, and steatorrhea.

PROGNOSIS

The median survival time of 142 dogs that underwent partial pancreactomy, as reported in several studies, was 12 to 14 months, with a range of zero days to 5 years.[3-5,7,10] Several prognostic factors have been identified. Dogs with clinical stage I disease have a significantly longer disease-free interval, and about 50% are expected to be normoglycemic 14 months after surgery compared with only 20% of dogs with clinical stage II or stage III disease.[6] Young dogs have a worse prognosis.[6] Dogs with postoperative hyperglycemia or normoglycemia have a significantly better prognosis than those with hypoglycemia.[3]

A decreased mitotic rate is strongly associated with survival of human beings with insulinoma. Although a correlation between the number of mitotic figures per high-power field and local invasiveness of the tumor has been documented in dogs, a significantly worse prognosis in dogs with a high mitotic count has yet to be established.[10]

Age, sex, body weight, clinical signs and their duration, ultrasonographic detection of a pancreatic mass, tumor location, gross presence of metastatic disease, and the blood glucose or insulin concentration are not significantly associated with the prognosis.

INSULIN-SECRETING ISLET CELL NEOPLASIA IN THE CAT

Feline insulinoma is rare; it has been reported in five cats that were 12 to 17 years of age. Three of the cats were Siamese, and four were neutered males. The history and clinical signs are similar to those reported for dogs with insulinoma. The diagnosis is based on documentation of an increased serum insulin concentration at the time of hypoglycemia. Care must be taken to use an insulin radioimmunoassay validated for cats. Therapy consists of surgical resection of the pancreatic mass and metastases, followed by prednisone treatment and small frequent meals.[21,26]

CHAPTER • 241

Diabetes Mellitus

Richard W. Nelson

The endocrine pancreas is composed of the islets of Langerhans, which are dispersed as "small islands" in a "sea" of exocrine-secreting acinar cells. Four distinct cell types have been identified in these islets on the basis of staining properties and morphology: *alpha cells*, which secrete glucagon; *beta cells*, which secrete insulin; *delta cells*, which secrete somatostatin; and *F cells*, which secrete pancreatic polypeptide. Dysfunction involving any of these cell lines ultimately results in either an excess or a deficiency of the respective hormone in the circulation. In the dog and cat, the most common disorder of the endocrine pancreas is diabetes mellitus, which results from an absolute or relative insulin deficiency due to deficient insulin secretion by the beta cells. The incidence of diabetes mellitus is similar for the dog and cat, with the reported frequency varying from 1 in 100 to 1 in 500.[1]

CLASSIFICATION AND ETIOLOGY

Overview of Classification

In humans, diabetes mellitus is classified as type 1 or type 2 based on the pathophysiologic mechanisms and the pathogenic alterations affecting the beta cells. Type 1 diabetes is characterized by a combination of genetic susceptibility and immunologic destruction of beta cells, with progressive and eventually complete insulin insufficiency. The presence of circulating autoantibodies against insulin, the beta cell, and/or glutamic acid decarboxylase (GAD) usually precedes the development of hyperglycemia or clinical signs. Type 2 diabetes mellitus is characterized by insulin resistance and "dysfunctional" beta cells; defects believed to be genetic in origin are evident for a decade or longer before hyperglycemia and clinical signs of diabetes develop, and the deleterious effects can be accentuated by environmental factors such as obesity.[2,3] Humans with type 1 diabetes are dependent on insulin for control of the disease (i.e., insulin-dependent diabetes mellitus [IDDM]), whereas control of the diabetic state in humans with type 2 diabetes is usually possible through diet, exercise, and oral hypoglycemic drugs. Insulin treatment may be necessary in some type 2 diabetics if insulin resistance and beta cell dysfunction are severe. As such, humans with type 2 diabetes can have IDDM or non-insulin-dependent diabetes mellitus (NIDDM).

It is more clinically relevant and perhaps more accurate to classify diabetes in dogs and cats as IDDM or NIDDM rather than as type 1 or type 2. The familial history is rarely available in diabetic dogs and cats, and the clinical presentation is usually not helpful in differentiating type 1 and type 2 diabetes, especially in cats. Insulin secretagogue tests are not routinely performed, and their results may be misleading. Autoantibody tests for type 1 diabetes are not readily available.[4,5] Therefore, as clinicians, veterinarians usually classify diabetic dogs and cats as either IDDM or NIDDM based on their need for insulin treatment. This can be confusing, because some diabetics, especially cats, initially can appear to have NIDDM progressing to IDDM, or they flip back and forth between IDDM and NIDDM as the severity of insulin resistance and the impairment of beta cell function waxes and wanes. Apparent changes in the diabetic state (i.e., IDDM and NIDDM) are understandable when one realizes that islet pathology may be mild to severe and progressive or static; that the ability of the pancreas to secrete insulin depends on the severity of islet pathology and can decrease with time; that the responsiveness of tissues to insulin varies, often in conjunction with the presence or absence of concurrent inflammatory, infectious, neoplastic, or hormonal disorders; and that all these variables affect the animal's need for insulin, the insulin dosage, and the ease of diabetic regulation.

Insulin-Dependent Diabetes Mellitus

The most common clinically recognized form of diabetes mellitus in the dog and cat is IDDM. In our hospital, virtually all dogs and 50% to 70% of cats have IDDM at the time diabetes mellitus is diagnosed. Insulin-dependent diabetes mellitus is characterized by permanent hypoinsulinemia and an absolute necessity for exogenous insulin to maintain glycemic control. The etiology of IDDM has been poorly characterized in dogs and cats but is undoubtedly multifactorial (Box 241-1).

In the dog, genetic predispositions have been suggested by familial associations (Table 241-1).[6,7] Common histologic abnormalities in dogs include a reduction in the number and size of pancreatic islets, a decrease in the number of beta cells within islets, and beta cell vacuolation and degeneration (Figure 241-1). In some dogs an extreme form of the disease may occur, represented by a congenital absolute deficiency of beta cells and pancreatic islet hypoplasia or aplasia. Less severe changes of pancreatic islets and beta cells may predispose the adult dog to diabetes mellitus after it has been exposed to environmental factors, such as insulin-antagonistic diseases and drugs, obesity, and pancreatitis. Environmental factors may induce beta cell degeneration secondary to

chronic insulin resistance or may cause release of beta cell proteins that induce immune-mediated destruction of the islets.[8] The results of studies evaluating for anti–beta cell autoantibodies in diabetic dogs have been conflicting; the autoantibodies were identified in newly diagnosed diabetic dogs with IDDM in one study[9] but not in another.[10] Immune-mediated insulitis has also been described in diabetic dogs.[11] Seemingly, autoimmune mechanisms, in conjunction with genetic and environmental factors, may play a role in the initiation and progression of diabetes in dogs.

Common histologic abnormalities in cats with IDDM include islet-specific amyloidosis (see Noninsulin-Dependent Diabetes Mellitus), beta cell vacuolation and degeneration, and chronic pancreatitis (see Figure 241-1).[12] The cause of beta cell degeneration is not known. Still other diabetic cats have a reduction in the number of pancreatic islets and/or insulin-containing beta cells on immunohistochemical evaluation, a finding that suggests that additional mechanisms may be involved in the physiopathology of diabetes mellitus in cats. Although lymphocytic infiltration of islets, in conjunction

---

Box • 241-1

Potential Factors in the Etiopathogenesis of Diabetes Mellitus in Dogs and Cats

Dog
Genetics
Immune-mediated insulitis
Pancreatitis
Obesity
Concurrent hormonal disease
    Hyperadrenocorticism
    Diestrus-induced excess of growth hormone
    Hypothyroidism
Drugs
    Glucocorticoids
Infection
Concurrent illness
    Renal insufficiency
    Cardiac disease
Hyperlipidemia
Islet amyloidosis (?)

Cat
Islet amyloidosis
Obesity
Pancreatitis
Concurrent hormonal disease
    Hyperadrenocorticism
    Acromegaly
    Hyperthyroidism
Drugs
    Megestrol acetate
    Glucocorticoids
Infection
Concurrent illness
    Renal insufficiency
    Cardiac disease
Hyperlipidemia (?)
Genetics (?)
Immune-mediated insulitis (?)

Table • 241-1

Breed Risk for the Development of Diabetes Mellitus*

BREED	CASES	CONTROL	ODDS RATIO
Australian terrier	33	3	9.39
Standard schnauzer	96	14	5.85
Miniature schnauzer	526	88	5.10
Bichon frise	39	11	3.03
Spitz	34	10	2.90
Fox terrier	88	28	2.68
Miniature poodle	712	224	2.49
Samoyed	159	56	2.42
Cairn terrier	61	23	2.26
Keeshond	47	18	2.23
Maltese	42	20	1.79
Toy poodle	186	90	1.76
Lhasa apso	85	47	1.54
Yorkshire terrier	96	57	1.44
Mixed breed	1755	1498	1.00
			(reference group)
English springer spaniel	62	77	0.69
Irish setter	66	84	0.67
Beagle	70	94	0.64
English setter	29	41	0.60
Basset hound	28	43	0.56
Rottweiler	37	62	0.51
Boston terrier	27	45	0.56
Doberman pinscher	103	180	0.49
Labrador retriever	199	375	0.45
Australian shepherd	32	62	0.44
Cocker spaniel	77	186	0.35
Golden retriever	91	274	0.28
Shetland sheepdog	27	109	0.21
Collie	25	104	0.21
German shepherd	68	317	0.18

From Guptill L et al: Is canine diabetes on the increase? *In* Recent Advances in Clinical Management of Diabetes Mellitus, Iams, Dayton, Ohio, 1999, p 24.
*Derived from analysis of the Veterinary Medical Database (VMDB) from 1970 to 1993. The VMDB comprises medical records of 24 veterinary schools in the United States and Canada. VMDB case records analyzed included those from first hospital visits of 6078 dogs with a diagnosis of diabetes mellitus and 5922 randomly selected dogs with first hospital visits for any diagnosis other than diabetes mellitus seen at the same veterinary schools in the same year. Only breeds with more than 25 cases of diabetes mellitus are included.

with islet amyloidosis and vacuolation, has been described in two diabetic cats,[13] this histologic finding is uncommon, and beta cell and insulin autoantibodies have not been identified in newly diagnosed diabetic cats.[14] The role of genetics remains to be determined.

Noninsulin-Dependent Diabetes Mellitus

Clinical recognition of NIDDM occurs more often in the cat than in the dog, accounting for approximately 30% of diabetic cats seen at our hospital. Clinical recognition of NIDDM is uncommon in the dog and is usually associated with a concurrent insulin-antagonistic disease or drug. In humans, obesity, genetics, and islet amyloidosis are important factors in the development of NIDDM. Amyloid is a common pathologic

finding in the pancreatic islets of diabetic cats. Islet amyloid polypeptide (IAPP), or amylin, is the principal constituent of amyloid isolated from the pancreatic tissue of humans with NIDDM and of adult cats with diabetes.[15] The amino acid sequence of human and feline IAPP is similar[16]; immuno-electron microscope studies have identified IAPP in beta cell secretory granules in both cats and humans,[17,18] and amylin is cosecreted with insulin by the beta cell.[19] Stimulants of insulin secretion also stimulate the secretion of amylin. Amylin acts as a neuroendocrine hormone, having several glu-coregulatory effects that collectively complement the actions of insulin in postprandial glucose control. These effects include a slowing of the rate at which nutrients are delivered from the stomach to the small intestine for absorption, sup-pression of nutrient-stimulated secretion of glucagon, and stimulation of satiety.[20,21] Chronic increased secretion of insulin and amylin, as occurs with obesity and other insulin-resistant states, results in aggregation and deposition of amylin in the islets as amyloid (see Figure 241-1). IAPP-derived amyloid fibrils are cytotoxic and are associated with apoptotic cell death of islet cells and a resultant defect in insulin secre-tion.[22-24] If deposition of amyloid is progressive, islet cell destruction progresses and eventually leads to diabetes melli-tus (Figure 241-2). The severity of islet amyloidosis would determine in part whether the diabetic cat has IDDM or NIDDM (Figure 241-3). Total destruction of the islets results in IDDM and the need for insulin treatment for the rest of the cat's life. Partial destruction of the islets may or may not result in clinically evident diabetes, insulin treatment may or may not be required to control glycemia, and transient diabetes may or may not develop once treatment is initiated. If amy-loid deposition is progressive, the cat progresses from a sub-clinical diabetic state to NIDDM and ultimately to IDDM.

The presence and severity of insulin resistance is an impor-tant variable that influences the clinical picture in cats with par-tial destruction of pancreatic islets. Insulin resistance increases the demand for insulin secretion, a demand that may not be met in some cats with partial destruction of islets. The more severe the insulin resistance and the loss of islets, the greater the likelihood that hyperglycemia will develop. Persistent hyper-glycemia can in turn suppress function of remaining beta cells, causing hypoinsulinemia and worsening hyperglycemia (see Transient Diabetes Mellitus). A sustained demand for insulin secretion in response to insulin resistance can also lead to wors-ening islet pathology and a further reduction in the population of beta cells. Any chronic insulin-resistant disorder can have a deleterious impact on the population and function of beta cells and can play a role in the development of NIDDM or IDDM. Examples in the cat include obesity, chronic pancreatitis, acromegaly, hyperadrenocorticism, and chronic administration of glucocorticoids or megestrol acetate. Obesity-induced carbo-hydrate intolerance is the classic insulin-resistant disorder affil-iated with the development of NIDDM in humans and has been identified as a potential causative factor in the develop-ment of diabetes in cats as well.[1,25] Obesity causes a reversible insulin resistance that is a result of downregulation of insulin receptors, impaired receptor binding affinity for insulin, and postreceptor defects in insulin action. Impaired glucose toler-ance and an abnormal insulin secretory response have been doc-umented in obese cats,[26,27] abnormalities that are reversible with correction of obesity.[28,29]

Our current understanding of the etiopathogenesis of dia-betes in the cat suggests that the difference between IDDM and NIDDM is primarily a difference in the severity of loss of beta cells and the severity and reversibility of concurrent insulin resistance. Most cats with IDDM or NIDDM have islet amyloidosis, vacuolar degeneration of beta cells, or islet hypoplasia.[12,30] The more severe the islet pathology, the more likely the cat is to have IDDM, regardless of concurrent

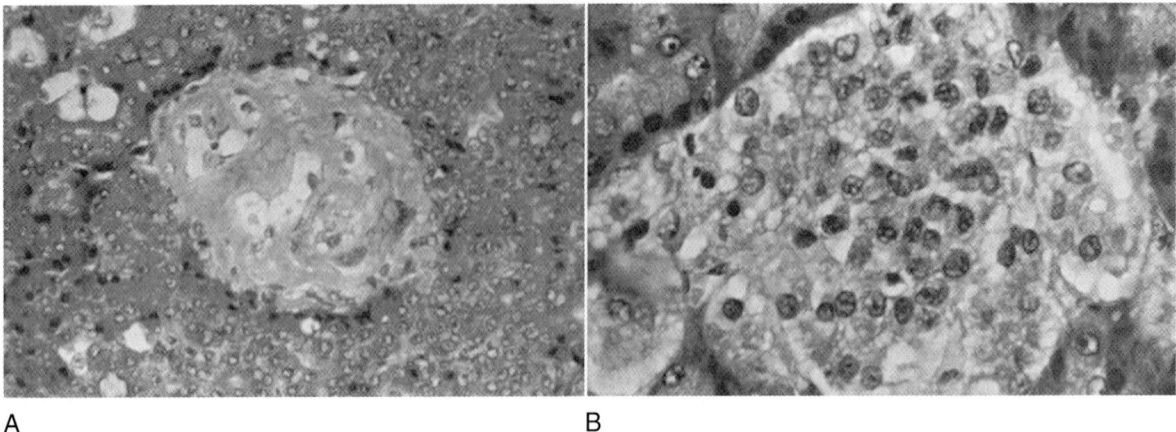

A   B

Figure 241-1 Pancreatic islet cell histology. **A,** Severe islet amyloidosis from a cat with insulin-dependent diabetes mellitus (IDDM) (hematoxylin and eosin stain [H&E], ×100). **B,** Severe islet cell degeneration and vacuolation from a cat with IDDM (H&E, ×200). (From Feldman EC, Nelson RW: Canine and Feline Endocrinology and Reproduction, 2nd ed. Philadelphia, WB Saunders, 1996, p 341.)

insulin resistance (see Figure 241-3). The less severe the islet pathology, the greater the role of concurrent insulin resistance in determining whether the cat has IDDM or NIDDM. The more severe and the less reversible the cause of the insulin resistance, the more likely the cat with mild islet pathology is to be insulin dependent, and vice versa. Fluctuations in the severity of insulin resistance, as occur with chronic pancreatitis, can cause a cat with mild islet pathology

to oscillate between IDDM and NIDDM as the severity of pancreatic inflammation waxes and wanes. Persistent insulin resistance can also worsen islet pathology and cause the diabetic cat to progress from NIDDM to IDDM as the progressive loss of beta cells leads to worsening insulin deficiency.[30,31]

Transient Diabetes Mellitus

Approximately 20% of diabetic cats become "transiently diabetic," usually within 4 to 6 weeks of establishment of the diagnosis of diabetes and initiation of treatment. In these cats, hyperglycemia, glycosuria, and clinical signs of diabetes resolve, and insulin treatment can be discontinued. Some diabetic cats may never require insulin treatment once the initial bout of clinical diabetes mellitus has dissipated, whereas others become permanently insulin dependent weeks to months after resolution of a prior diabetic state. Based on findings from a recent evaluation of a group of cats with transient diabetes mellitus, the author theorizes that cats with transient diabetes are in a subclinical diabetic state that becomes clinical when the pancreas is stressed by exposure to a concurrent insulin-antagonistic drug or disease, most notably glucocorticoids, megestrol acetate, or chronic pancreatitis (Figure 241-4).[30] Unlike healthy cats, those with transient diabetes mellitus have some abnormality of the islets (e.g., amyloidosis, vacuolar degeneration) and a significant reduction in the population of beta cells. Islet abnormalities impair the ability to compensate for concurrent insulin resistance, resulting in carbohydrate intolerance. Insulin secretion by beta cells becomes reversibly suppressed, most likely as a result of worsening carbohydrate intolerance. Chronic hyperglycemia impairs insulin secretion by beta cells and induces peripheral insulin resistance by promoting the downregulation of glucose transport systems and causing a defect in post-transport insulin action; this phenomenon is referred to as *glucose toxicity*.[32] Beta cells have an impaired response to stimulation by insulin secretagogues, thereby mimicking IDDM. The effects of glucose toxicity are potentially reversible upon correction of the hyperglycemic state. The clinician makes a correct diagnosis of diabetes and initiates appropriate treatment for diabetes and identifiable insulin-antagonistic disorders. Treatment improves hyperglycemia and insulin resistance, the suppressive effects of hyperglycemia decrease, beta cell function improves, insulin secretion returns, and an apparent IDDM state resolves. The future requirement for insulin treatment

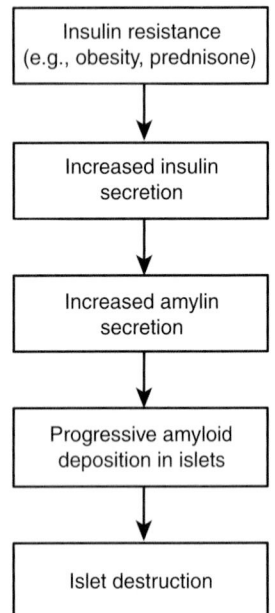

Figure 241-2 Schematic of the interplay between insulin resistance, amylin secretion, and amyloid deposition in the pancreatic islets. Insulin secretion increases to compensate for insulin resistance induced by environmental factors, insulin-antagonistic drugs, and concurrent illness. Because amylin and insulin are cosecreted, amylin secretion also increases in insulin-resistant states. If sustained, increased amylin secretion can lead to amylin aggregation and the formation of amyloid in the islets. (From Feldman EC, Nelson RW: Canine and Feline Endocrinology and Reproduction, 3rd ed. Philadelphia, WB Saunders, 2004.)

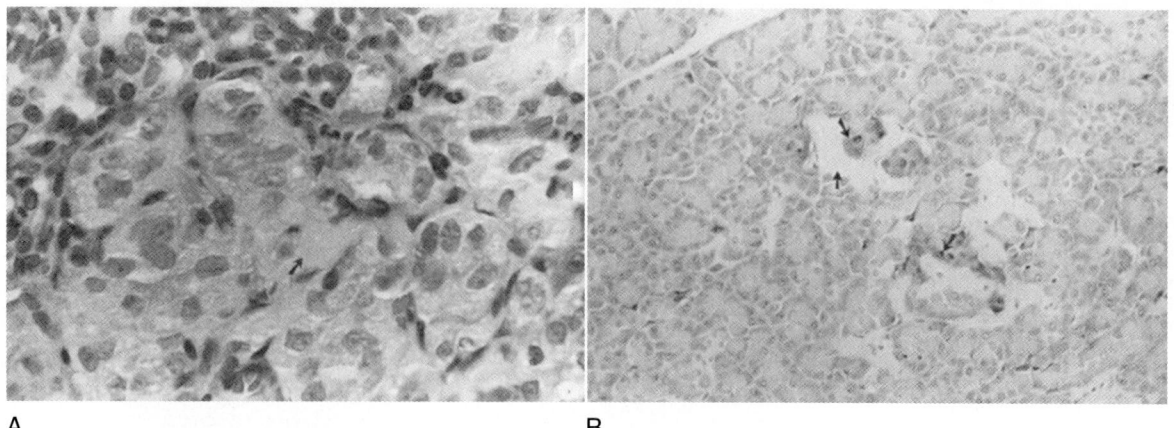

Figure 241-3 Pancreatic amyloidosis. **A,** Mild islet amyloidosis *(arrow)* and vacuolar degeneration in a cat with non-insulin-dependent diabetes mellitus (NIDDM) treated with diet and glipizide (H&E, ×200). **B,** Severe islet amyloidosis *(straight arrow)* in a cat with initial NIDDM that progressed to IDDM. Pancreatic biopsy was obtained during IDDM state. Residual beta cells containing insulin *(curved arrows)* are also present. (Immunoperoxidase stain, ×100). (From Feldman EC, Nelson RW: Canine and Feline Endocrinology and Reproduction, 3rd ed. Philadelphia, WB Saunders, 2004, p 542.)

depends on the underlying abnormality in the islets. If the islet pathology is progressive (e.g., amyloidosis), eventually enough beta cells are destroyed to cause permanent IDDM.

Transient or reversible diabetes is extremely uncommon in dogs and usually occurs in dogs with subclinical diabetes treated with insulin-antagonistic drugs (e.g., glucocorticoids) or in the early stages of an insulin-antagonistic disorder (e.g., diestrus in the bitch, hyperadrenocorticism). Such dogs have a reduced but adequate mass of functional beta cells to maintain carbohydrate tolerance when insulin resistance is not present but are unable to secrete an adequate amount of insulin to maintain euglycemia in the presence of insulin antagonism. Early recognition and correction of the insulin antagonism may re-establish euglycemia without the long-term need for insulin therapy. Failure to correct the insulin antagonism quickly results in progressive loss of beta cells and the eventual development of IDDM.

Diagnosis of Insulin-Dependent versus Noninsulin-Dependent Diabetes Mellitus

Dogs and cats are not usually brought to a veterinarian until clinical signs of diabetes become obvious and worrisome to an owner. As such, at the time of diagnosis, all diabetic dogs and cats have fasting hyperglycemia and glycosuria, regardless of the type of diabetes mellitus that may be present. Once the diagnosis of diabetes has been established, the clinician must consider the possibility of NIDDM and the need for insulin treatment. Dogs should uniformly be considered to have IDDM and treatment with insulin should be initiated unless there is a strong suspicion of diabetes mellitus secondary to a concurrent insulin-antagonistic disorder (e.g., intact bitch in diestrus).

Because of the significant incidence of NIDDM and transient diabetes in cats and the successful treatment of some diabetic cats with diet and oral hypoglycemic drugs, it would be advantageous to be able to prospectively differentiate IDDM from NIDDM in cats. Unfortunately, measurements of the serum insulin concentration at baseline and after administration of an insulin secretagogue have not been consistent aids in the differentiation of IDDM from NIDDM in the cat.[4,5] A fasting serum insulin concentration greater than the normal mean concentration (greater than 12 μU/mL in our laboratory) or any postsecretagogue insulin concentration greater than one standard deviation (SD) above the reference mean (greater than 18 μU/mL in our laboratory) suggests the existence of functional beta cells and the possibility for NIDDM. Unfortunately, cats subsequently identified has having IDDM and many of those with NIDDM have a low baseline serum insulin concentration and do not respond to a glucose or glucagon challenge.[4,5,30] This apparent insulin deficiency in cats subsequently identified with NIDDM is presumably the result of concurrent glucose toxicity (see Transient Diabetes Mellitus). The ultimate differentiation of IDDM from NIDDM is often made retrospectively, after the clinician has had several weeks to assess the cat's response to therapy and to determine the animal's need for insulin. The initial decision between insulin treatment and oral hypoglycemic drugs is based on the severity of the clinical signs, the presence or absence of ketoacidosis, the cat's general health, and the owner's wishes.

PATHOPHYSIOLOGY

Nonketotic Diabetes Mellitus

Diabetes mellitus results from a relative or absolute deficiency of insulin secretion by the beta cells. Insulin deficiency in turn causes decreased tissue utilization of glucose, amino acids, and fatty acids; accelerated hepatic glycogenolysis and gluconeogenesis; and accumulation of glucose in the circulation, resulting in hyperglycemia. Glucose obtained from the diet also accumulates in the circulation. As the blood glucose concentration increases, the ability of the renal tubular cells to resorb glucose from the glomerular ultrafiltrate is exceeded, resulting in glycosuria. In dogs this typically occurs whenever the blood glucose concentration exceeds 180 to 220 mg/dL. The threshold for glucose resorption appears more variable in cats, ranging from 200 to 280 mg/dL. Glycosuria creates an osmotic diuresis, causing polyuria. Compensatory polydipsia prevents dehydration. The diminished peripheral tissue utilization of ingested glucose results in weight loss as the body attempts to compensate for perceived "starvation."

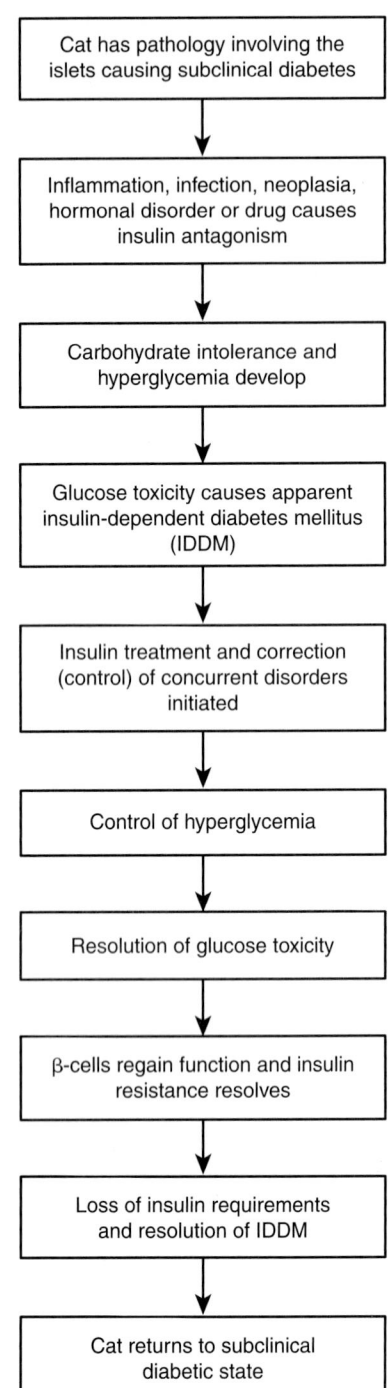

Cat has pathology involving the islets causing subclinical diabetes

↓

Inflammation, infection, neoplasia, hormonal disorder or drug causes insulin antagonism

↓

Carbohydrate intolerance and hyperglycemia develop

↓

Glucose toxicity causes apparent insulin-dependent diabetes mellitus (IDDM)

↓

Insulin treatment and correction (control) of concurrent disorders initiated

↓

Control of hyperglycemia

↓

Resolution of glucose toxicity

↓

β-cells regain function and insulin resistance resolves

↓

Loss of insulin requirements and resolution of IDDM

↓

Cat returns to subclinical diabetic state

Figure 241-4 Sequence of events in the development and resolution of an insulin-requiring diabetic episode in cats with transient diabetes. (From Feldman EC, Nelson RW: Canine and Feline Endocrinology and Reproduction, 3rd ed. Philadelphia, WB Saunders, 2004, p 546.)

The interaction of the "satiety center" in the ventromedial region of the hypothalamus with the "feeding center" in the lateral region of the hypothalamus is responsible for controlling the amount of food ingested.[33] The feeding center, responsible for evoking eating behavior, is chronically functioning but can be transiently inhibited by the satiety center after food ingestion. The amount of glucose entering the cells in the satiety center directly affects the feeling of hunger; the more glucose that enters these cells, the less the feeling of

hunger and vice versa. The ability of glucose to enter the cells in the satiety center is mediated by insulin. In diabetics with a relative or absolute lack of insulin, glucose does not enter satiety center cells, resulting in failure to inhibit the feeding center. Thus these individuals become polyphagic despite hyperglycemia.

The four classic signs of diabetes mellitus are polyuria, polydipsia, polyphagia, and weight loss. The severity of these signs is directly related to the severity of hyperglycemia. As these signs become obvious to the owner, the pet is brought to the veterinarian for care.

Ketoacidosis

Unfortunately, some cats and dogs are not identified by their owners as having signs of disease, and these untreated diabetics may ultimately develop diabetic ketoacidosis (DKA). Ketone bodies (i.e., acetoacetate, beta hydroxybutyrate, and acetone) are derived from oxidation of nonesterified or free fatty acids (FFAs) by the liver and are used as an energy source by many tissues during periods of glucose deficiency. The most important regulators of ketone body production are FFA availability and the ketogenic capacity of the liver.[34] For synthesis of ketone bodies to be enhanced, two major alterations in intermediary metabolism must occur: (1) mobilization of FFAs from triglycerides stored in adipose tissue must be enhanced, and (2) a shift in hepatic metabolism must occur from fat synthesis to fat oxidation and ketogenesis.[35,36] Insulin is a powerful inhibitor of lipolysis and FFA oxidation. A relative or absolute deficiency of insulin "allows" lipolysis to increase, thus increasing the availability of FFAs to the liver and in turn promoting ketogenesis.

Virtually all dogs and cats with DKA have a relative or absolute deficiency of insulin. In most dogs and cats with newly diagnosed DKA, circulating insulin concentrations are low or undetectable. Some dogs and cats have serum insulin concentrations similar to those observed in normal, fasted nondiabetics (i.e., 5 to 20 µU/mL). However, such insulin concentrations are inappropriately low ("relative" insulin deficiency) for the severity of hyperglycemia encountered. Some diabetic dogs and cats develop ketoacidosis despite receiving daily injections of insulin, and circulating insulin concentrations may even be increased. In this group, a "relative" insulin deficiency is also present, presumably because of concurrent insulin resistance caused by an increase in circulating glucose counter-regulatory hormones (i.e., epinephrine, glucagon, cortisol, growth hormone), increased plasma FFA and amino acid concentrations, and metabolic acidosis. With the development of insulin resistance, the need for insulin may exceed the daily injected insulin dose, leading to a predisposition to the development of DKA.

Circulating levels of the glucose counter-regulatory hormones typically are markedly increased in humans with DKA and presumably are in dogs and cats as well.[37] The body increases its production of the glucose counter-regulatory hormones in response to a wide variety of diseases and stress situations, such as pancreatitis, infection, renal insufficiency, and concurrent hormonal disorder. The net effects of these hormonal disturbances are accentuation of insulin deficiency through the development of insulin resistance; stimulation of lipolysis, leading to ketogenesis; and stimulation of gluconeogenesis, which worsens hyperglycemia. Recognition and treatment of disorders that coexist with diabetic ketoacidosis are critically important to the successful management of DKA.

The physiologic derangements that accompany DKA are a direct result of relative or absolute insulin deficiency, hyperketonemia, and hyperglycemia. Increasing plasma ketone concentrations eventually surpass the renal tubular threshold for complete resorption and spill into the urine, contributing to the osmotic diuresis caused by glycosuria and enhancing the excretion of solutes (e.g., sodium, potassium, and magnesium). Insulin deficiency per se also contributes to the excessive renal losses of water and electrolytes. The result is an excessive loss of electrolytes and water, leading to volume contraction, underperfusion of tissues, and prerenal azotemia. As ketones continue to accumulate in the blood, the body's buffering system becomes overwhelmed, and progressively worsening metabolic acidosis results. Further loss of water and electrolytes occurs as a result of repeated bouts of vomiting or diarrhea combined with a lack of fluid intake, problems that often develop as the metabolic acidosis worsens. Excessive loss of electrolytes and water leads to further volume contraction, underperfusion of tissues, and worsening prerenal azotemia and dehydration. Renal excretion of glucose and to a lesser degree hydrogen ions becomes impaired, allowing glucose and ketones to accumulate in the vascular space more quickly. The result is increasing hyperglycemia and ketonemia and worsening metabolic acidosis. The rise in the blood glucose concentration raises the plasma osmolality, and the resulting osmotic diuresis further aggravates the rise in plasma osmolality by causing water losses in excess of the salt loss. The increase in plasma osmolality causes water to be shifted out of cells, leading to cellular dehydration and the eventual development of obtundation and coma. The severe metabolic consequences of DKA, which include severe acidosis, hyperosmolality, obligatory osmotic diuresis, dehydration, and electrolyte derangements, ultimately become life-threatening.

SIGNALMENT

Diabetes mellitus typically occurs in older dogs and cats, with a peak prevalence at 7 to 9 years of age in dogs and 9 to 11 years in cats.[1,12] Juvenile-onset diabetes occurs in dogs and cats less than 1 year of age and is uncommon. In dogs, females are affected about twice as often as males, whereas in cats, diabetes occurs predominately in neutered males.[1,12] Genetic predispositions for or against the development of diabetes have been suggested by familial associations in dogs and by pedigree analysis of keeshonden (see Table 241-1).[6,7] No apparent breed predisposition is seen in cats, although Burmese cats may be over-represented in Australia.[38]

ANAMNESIS

The history in virtually all diabetic animals includes the classic polydipsia, polyuria, polyphagia, and weight loss. Owners often bring a dog to the veterinarian because the pet can no longer make it through the night without having to be let outside to urinate or because it begins urinating in the home. A common complaint of cat owners is the constant need to change the litter and an increase in the size of the kitty litter clumps; problems that reflect the polyuria associated with diabetes mellitus. Additional clinical signs in cats include lethargy; decreased interaction with family members; lack of grooming behavior and the development of a dry, lusterless, unkempt, or matted haircoat; and decreased jumping ability, rear limb weakness, or the development of a plantigrade posture (Figure 241-5). Occasionally a dog owner may be concerned about sudden blindness caused by cataract formation. The classic signs of diabetes mellitus may have gone unnoticed or may have been considered irrelevant by the owner. If the clinical signs associated with uncomplicated diabetes are not observed by the owner, a diabetic dog or cat is at risk for developing systemic signs of illness (i.e., lethargy, anorexia, vomiting, weakness) as progressive ketonemia and metabolic acidosis develop. The time sequence from onset of initial clinical signs to development of DKA is unpredictable, ranging from a few days to several months.

PHYSICAL EXAMINATION

A thorough physical examination is imperative in any dog or cat suspected of having diabetes mellitus, in part because of the high prevalence of concurrent disorders that can affect the response to treatment. Physical examination findings in a dog or cat with newly diagnosed diabetes depend on whether DKA is present and if so, its severity; on the duration of diabetes prior to diagnosis; and on the nature of any other concurrent disorders. The nonketotic diabetic dog or cat has no classic physical examination findings. Many diabetic dogs and cats are obese but are otherwise in good physical condition. Dogs and cats with prolonged untreated diabetes may have lost weight but are rarely emaciated unless concurrent

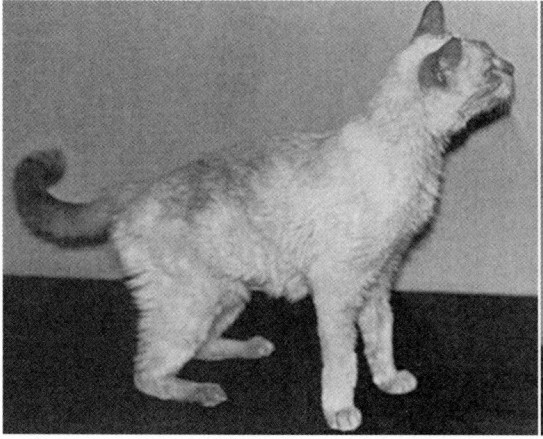 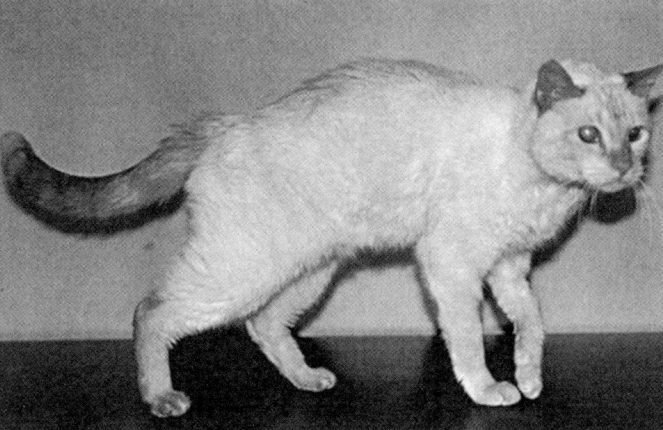

A   B

Figure 241-5 **A,** Plantigrade posture in a cat with diabetes mellitus and exocrine pancreatic insufficiency. **B,** Resolution of hindlimb weakness and plantigrade posture after glycemic control was improved by adjustment of insulin therapy and initiation of pancreatic enzyme replacement therapy. (From Feldman EC, Nelson RW: Canine and Feline Endocrinology and Reproduction, 3rd ed. Philadelphia, WB Saunders, 2004, p 548.)

disease (e.g., pancreatic exocrine insufficiency, hyperthyroidism) is present. Lethargy may be evident. The haircoat of newly diagnosed or poorly controlled diabetic dogs may be sparse, with dry, brittle, lusterless hairs, as well as scales from hyperkeratosis; diabetic cats often stop grooming and develop a dry, lusterless haircoat. Diabetes-induced hepatic lipidosis may cause hepatomegaly. Lenticular changes consistent with cataract formation are another common clinical finding in diabetic dogs. Impaired ability to jump, weakness in the rear limbs, ataxia, or a plantigrade posture (i.e., the hocks touch the ground when the cat walks) may be evident in cats that develop diabetic neuropathy (see Figure 241-5). The distal muscles of the rear limbs may feel hard on digital palpation, and cats may object to palpation or manipulation of the rear limbs, presumably because of pain associated with the neuropathy.

In the ketoacidotic diabetic dog or cat, physical examination findings include dehydration, depression, weakness, tachypnea, and sometimes a strong odor of acetone on the breath. With severe metabolic acidosis, slow, deep breathing (i.e., Kussmaul respiration) may be observed. Gastrointestinal signs of vomiting, abdominal pain, and distention may be present, and dogs and cats that develop severe hyperosmolarity are often extremely lethargic and may be comatose.

ESTABLISHING THE DIAGNOSIS OF DIABETES MELLITUS

A diagnosis of diabetes mellitus requires the presence of appropriate clinical signs (i.e., polyuria, polydipsia, polyphagia, weight loss) and documentation of persistent fasting hyperglycemia and glycosuria. Measurement of the blood glucose concentration using a portable blood glucose monitoring device and testing for the presence of glycosuria using urine reagent test strips (e.g., KetoDiastix; Ames Division, Miles Laboratories, Elkhart, Indiana) allow rapid confirmation of a diagnosis of diabetes mellitus. Concurrent documentation of ketonuria establishes a diagnosis of diabetic ketosis or ketoacidosis.

It is important to document both persistent hyperglycemia and glycosuria to establish a diagnosis of diabetes mellitus, because hyperglycemia differentiates diabetes mellitus from primary renal glycosuria, whereas glycosuria differentiates diabetes mellitus from other causes of hyperglycemia (Box 241-2). Transient, stress-induced hyperglycemia is a common problem in cats and can cause the blood glucose concentration to increase above 300 mg/dL. Unfortunately, stress is a subjective state that cannot be accurately measured, it is not always easily recognized, and it may evoke inconsistent responses among individual cats. Glycosuria usually does not develop in cats with stress hyperglycemia because the transient increase in the blood glucose concentration prevents glucose from accumulating in urine to a detectable concentration. However, hyperglycemia and glycosuria can occur secondary to stress in cats. For this reason, the clinician should always document persistent hyperglycemia and glycosuria when establishing a diagnosis of diabetes mellitus in cats. If doubt exists, the "stressed" cat can be sent home with instructions for the owner to monitor the urine glucose concentration with the cat in the nonstressed home environment. Alternatively, a serum fructosamine concentration can be measured. Documentation of an increase in the serum fructosamine concentration supports the presence of sustained hyperglycemia; however, a serum fructosamine concentration in the upper range of normal can occur in symptomatic diabetic cats if the diabetes developed shortly before the cat was brought to the veterinarian.[39]

Mild hyperglycemia (i.e., 130 to 180 mg/dL) is clinically silent and is usually an unexpected and unsuspected finding. If the dog or cat with mild hyperglycemia is examined for polyuria and polydipsia, a disorder other than clinical diabetes

---

Box • 241-2

Causes of Hyperglycemia in Dogs and Cats

Diabetes mellitus*
"Stress" (cat)*
Postprandial effect (diets containing monosaccharides, disaccharides, and propylene glycol)
Hyperadrenocorticism*
Acromegaly (cat)
Diestrus (bitch)
Pheochromocytoma (dog)
Pancreatitis
Exocrine pancreatic neoplasia
Renal insufficiency
Drug therapy*
    Glucocorticoids
    Progestagens
    Megestrol acetate
    Thiazide diuretics
Dextrose-containing fluids*
Parenteral nutrition*
Head trauma

*Common cause.

---

mellitus should be sought. Mild hyperglycemia can occur up to 2 hours postprandial in some dogs and cats, in "stressed" dogs and cats, in early diabetes mellitus, and with disorders causing insulin resistance. A diagnostic evaluation for disorders causing insulin resistance is indicated if mild hyperglycemia persists in the fasted, unstressed dog or cat. Insulin therapy is not indicated in these animals because clinical diabetes mellitus is not present.

PATIENT EVALUATION

Nonketotic Diabetic Animal

A thorough clinicopathologic evaluation is recommended once the diagnosis of diabetes mellitus has been established. The clinician must be aware of any disease that might be causing or contributing to carbohydrate intolerance (e.g., hyperadrenocorticism), that may result from carbohydrate intolerance (e.g., bacterial cystitis), or that may force modification of therapy (e.g., pancreatitis). The minimum laboratory evaluation in any "healthy" nonketotic diabetic dog or cat should include a complete blood count (CBC), serum biochemical panel, serum thyroxine concentration (cat), and urinalysis with bacterial culture. The serum progesterone concentration should be determined if diabetes mellitus is diagnosed in an intact bitch, regardless of her cycling history. If available, abdominal ultrasonography is indicated to assess for pancreatitis, adrenomegaly, pyometritis in an intact bitch or queen, and abnormalities affecting the liver and urinary tract. Because of the relatively high prevalence of pancreatitis in diabetic dogs and cats, measurement of serum lipase or serum trypsin-like immunoreactivity (TLI) or serum pancreatic lipase immunoreactivity (PLI) should be considered if abdominal ultrasonography is not available. Measurement of the baseline serum insulin concentration or an insulin response test is not routinely done, although it may be considered in cats prior to treatment with oral hypoglycemic drugs (see Diagnosis of Insulin-Dependent versus Noninsulin-Dependent Diabetes Mellitus). Additional tests may be warranted after the history has been obtained, the physical

and correction of acidemia
the intracellular fluid [ICF]
with hypokalemia require a
therapy to replace deficit
life-threatening hypokalemia
The exception to potassiur
hyperkalemia associated witl
supplementation should ini
and cats until glomerular fi
production increases, and hy

Ideally the amount of
actual measurement of the s
an accurate measurement of
40 mEq of potassium should
intravenous fluids (36 mEq
tion). Subsequent adjustmer
should be based on measu
concentration, preferably ev
cat is stable and serum ele
range.

Phosphate Supplementatic
Most dogs and cats with
decreased serum phosphoru
testing. Within 24 hours of
the serum phosphorus con
some levels (i.e., less than
tional effects of fluid th
phosphorus after initiation
renal and gastrointestinal l
primarily the hematologic a
and cats. Hemolytic anemia
can be life-threatening i
Weakness, ataxia, and seizu
hypophosphatemia may be
Phosphate therapy is inc
sis are identified or if the
decreases to less than 1.5 n
by means of intravenous
phosphate solutions contai
4.4 mEq of potassium or
The recommended dosage
0.01 to 0.03 mmol of phos
per hour, preferably admin
fluids (e.g., 0.9% sodium
severe hypophosphatemia
increased to 0.03 to 0.12 1
phosphate needed to rep
response to therapy canr
initially to monitor the
every 8 to 12 hours and
accordingly. Adverse effe
administration include iatr
ated neuromuscular signs,
metastatic calcification. Th
ized) calcium concentratic
time as the serum phosph
phosphate infusion shoul
identified. Phosphorus su
dogs and cats with hypere
uria, or suspected tissue n
tion, phosphorus should n
of renal function and the
are known.

Magnesium Supplement
Hypomagnesemia is comi
often worsens during the i
without treatment as the

---

examination has been performed, or ketonuria has been identified. Potential clinicopathologic abnormalities are listed in
Box 241-3.

Ketoacidotic Diabetic Animal
The laboratory evaluation of apparently healthy dogs and cats
with both glucose and ketones present in the urinalysis is
similar to that for the nonketotic diabetic patient. The healthy
ketotic diabetic can usually be managed conservatively, without fluid therapy or intensive care. In contrast, sick ketoacidotic diabetic dogs and cats are critical metabolic emergencies
that require a much more aggressive therapeutic plan. To aid
in the formulation of an appropriate treatment protocol, a group
of critically important studies must be performed, including
urinalysis, hematocrit, total plasma protein concentration, blood
glucose, venous total carbon dioxide (CO_2) or arterial acid-
base evaluation, blood urea nitrogen or serum creatinine, and
serum electrolytes (sodium [Na], potassium [K], calcium [Ca],

---

Box • 241-3

**Clinicopathologic Abnormalities Commonly
Found in Dogs and Cats with Uncomplicated
Diabetes Mellitus**

Complete Blood Count
Typically normal
Neutrophilic leukocytosis, toxic neutrophils
    (with pancreatitis or infection)

Biochemistry Panel
Hyperglycemia
Hypercholesterolemia
Hypertriglyceridemia (lipemia)
Increased alanine aminotransferase activity
    (typically <500 IU/L)
Increased alkaline phosphatase activity (typically <500 IU/L)

Urinalysis
Urine specific gravity typically >1.025
Glycosuria
Variable ketonuria
Proteinuria
Bacteriuria

Ancillary Tests
Hyperlipasemia (with pancreatitis)
Hyperamylasemia (with pancreatitis)
Serum trypsin-like immunoreactivity
    Usually normal
    Low with pancreatic exocrine insufficiency
    High with acute pancreatitis
    Normal to high with chronic pancreatitis
Serum pancreatic lipase immunoreactivity
    Usually normal
    Low with pancreatic exocrine insufficiency
    High with pancreatitis
Variable serum baseline insulin concentration
    Insulin-dependent diabetes mellitus: Low, normal
    Non-insulin-dependent diabetes mellitus:
        Low, normal, increased
    Insulin resistance induced: Low, normal, increased

---

and phosphate [PO_4]). The results of these tests guide the
proper choice of fluid therapy, as well as corrections that must
be made with respect to electrolyte alterations, acidosis, and
renal function. Additional data, such as radiographs, abdominal ultrasound scans, or further clinical pathologic studies,
may be needed, depending on the results of the history and
physical examination and the nature of concurrent disorders.

THERAPY FOR THE ILL DIABETIC KETOACIDOTIC PATIENT

An aggressive therapeutic plan (Box 241-4) is indicated if the
dog or cat has systemic signs of illness (i.e., lethargy, anorexia,
vomiting); if the physical examination reveals dehydration,
depression, weakness, and/or Kussmaul respiration; if the
blood glucose concentration is greater than 500 mg/dL; or if
severe metabolic acidosis is present, as diagnosed by a total
venous CO_2 or arterial bicarbonate concentration less than
12 mEq/L. The goals of treatment for a severely ill, ketoacidotic, diabetic pet are (1) to provide adequate amounts of
insulin to normalize intermediary metabolism, (2) to restore
water and electrolyte losses, (3) to correct the acidosis, (4) to
identify precipitating factors for the current illness, and (5) to
provide a carbohydrate substrate when required by the insulin
treatment. Proper therapy does not imply forcing as rapid a
return to normal as possible. Because osmotic and biochemical problems can be created by overly aggressive therapy, as
well as by the disease process itself, rapid changes in various
vital parameters can be as harmful as or more harmful than no
change. If all abnormal parameters can be slowly moved
toward normal (i.e., over 36 to 48 hours), the likelihood of
successful therapy is greater.

Fluid Therapy
Initiation of appropriate fluid therapy should be the first step
in the treatment of DKA. Replacement of fluid deficiencies
and maintenance of normal fluid balance are important for
ensuring adequate cardiac output, blood pressure, and blood
flow to all tissues. Improvement of renal blood flow is
especially critical. In addition to the general beneficial aspects
of fluid therapy in any dehydrated animal, fluid therapy can
correct the deficiencies in total body sodium and potassium,
dampening the potassium-lowering effect of insulin treatment.
Fluid therapy can reduce blood glucose concentrations in diabetics even without insulin administration. Unfortunately,
fluid therapy alone does not decrease the concentrations
of acetoacetate and beta hydroxybutyrate or improve the
severity of metabolic acidosis. For these reasons, insulin is
always required.
The type of parenteral fluid initially used depends on the
electrolyte status, blood glucose concentration, and osmolality. Most dogs and cats with DKA have severe deficits in total
body sodium, regardless of the measured serum concentration. Unless serum electrolyte concentrations dictate otherwise, the initial intravenous fluid of choice is 0.9% sodium
chloride with appropriate potassium supplementation. Most
dogs and cats with severe DKA usually are sodium depleted
and therefore are not suffering from dramatic hyperosmolality despite potentially remarkable increases in the blood glucose concentration. Other replacement crystalloid solutions
that can be used if physiologic (0.9%) saline is not available
are Ringer's solution, Ringer's lactated solution, Plasma-Lyte
148 (Baxter Healthcare, Deerfield, Illinois), and Normosol-R
(Abbott Laboratories, Chicago, Illinois). Hypotonic fluids
(e.g., 0.45% saline) are rarely indicated in dogs and cats with
DKA even with severe hyperosmolality. Hypotonic fluids do
not provide adequate amounts of sodium to correct the
sodium deficiency. Rapid administration of hypotonic fluids
can also cause a rapid decrease in plasma osmolality, which

Box • 241-4

Initial Management

Fluid Therapy
Type: 0.9% saline solu
Rate: 60 to 100 mL/kg
Potassium supplement
 KCl to each liter of f
Phosphate supplement
 develops; initial IV i
Dextrose supplementa

Bicarbonate Therap
Indication: Administer
 concentration is les
 then give only once
Amount: HCO₃⁻ (mEq
 unknown, use 10 in
Administration: Add
Retreatment: Only if

Insulin Therapy
Type: Regular crystal
Administration
• Intermittent intra
 concentration app
• Low-dose intraveno
 tered via infusion o
 blood glucose mea
 Decrease the hourl
 hypokalemic at the
Goal: Gradual declir
 less than 250 mg

Ancillary Therapy
Concurrent pancrea
 are indicated.
Concurrent infectio
Additional therapy

Patient Monitorir
Blood glucose meas
 concentration ap
Hydration status, r
Serum electrolyte c
Urine output, glyco
Body weight, packe
Additional monitor

may result in cerebr
eventually coma. H
tonic fluids and jud

Fluid administra
replacement of hyd
tenance fluid need
matched. Rapid re
unless the dog or ca
critical phase, fluic
effort to correct t
manner. As a gener

(Ralston Purina, St. Louis, Missouri) and Science Diet Feline Growth (Hill's Pet Products, Topeka, KS).[56,57] Purina DM is a high-protein, low-carbohydrate, low-fiber diet, and Science Diet Growth is a high-fat, low-carbohydrate, low-fiber diet.

The central theme in dietary studies in diabetic cats has been restriction of carbohydrate absorption by the gastrointestinal tract, by inhibiting starch digestion (acarbose), inhibiting intestinal glucose absorption (fiber), or decreasing carbohydrate ingestion (low-carbohydrate diets). Intuitively, the most effective means of minimizing gastrointestinal absorption of carbohydrates in the diabetic cat is to feed diets that contain minimal amounts of carbohydrate. The beneficial role in the control of glycemia, if any, of the high protein or high fat content of current carbohydrate-restricted diets is not yet known. It is also not known what effect, if any, a high protein intake may have on the development of ketosis or diabetic nephropathy, the induction of satiety, or maintenance of a stable body weight. Similarly, it is not known what effect, if any, a high fat intake may have on the development of obesity, hepatic lipidosis, and chronic pancreatitis or the induction of insulin resistance and increased hepatic glucose production secondary to the generation of nonesterified fatty acids, beta hydroxybutyric acid, and hypertriglyceridemia, especially in older cats that may have decreased lipoprotein and hepatic lipase activity.[58-60] For now, all three diets are considered viable choices for the management of diabetes in cats. Which diet will be most beneficial at improving control of glycemia in any given diabetic cat is unpredictable. As such, the initial diet of choice is based on the veterinarian's personal preferences and experience. If palatability or adverse effects become an issue or if poor control of glycemia persists despite adjustments in insulin therapy, a switch to one of the other diets should be considered.

Exercise

Exercise plays an important role in the maintenance of glycemic control by helping to promote weight loss and by eliminating the insulin resistance induced by obesity. Exercise also exerts a glucose-lowering effect by increasing the absorption of insulin from its injection site, increasing blood flow (and therefore insulin delivery) to exercising muscles, stimulating translocation of glucose transporters in muscle cells, and increasing glucose effectiveness (i.e., the ability of hyperglycemia to promote glucose disposal at basal insulin concentrations).[61,62] The daily routine for diabetic dogs should include exercise, preferably at the same time each day. Strenuous and sporadic exercise can cause severe hypoglycemia and should be avoided. The insulin dose should be decreased in dogs subjected to sporadic, strenuous exercise on days of anticipated increased exercise. The reduction in the insulin dose required to prevent hypoglycemia is variable and is determined by trial and error. The author recommends reducing the insulin dose by 50% initially and making further adjustments based on the occurrence of symptomatic hypoglycemia and the severity of polyuria and polydipsia that develop during the ensuing 24 to 48 hours. In addition, owners must be aware of the signs of hypoglycemia and must have a source of glucose readily available to give their dog should any of these signs develop.

Identification and Control of Concurrent Problems

Concurrent diseases and administration of insulin-antagonistic drugs are both commonly identified in the dog and cat with newly diagnosed diabetes mellitus.[63,64] Concurrent disease and insulin-antagonistic drugs can interfere with tissue responsiveness to insulin as a result of a decreased number of insulin receptors at the surface of the cell membrane, alterations in insulin receptor binding affinity, or impairment in one of several postreceptor steps responsible for the activation of

glucose transport systems. Loss of tissue responsiveness results in insulin resistance, which may be mild and easily overcome by increasing the dosage of insulin, or may be severe, causing sustained and marked hyperglycemia regardless of the type and dosage of insulin administered. Some causes of insulin resistance are readily apparent at the time diabetes is diagnosed, such as obesity and the administration of insulin-antagonistic drugs (e.g., glucocorticoids). Other causes of insulin resistance may not be readily apparent, and identification of these causes may require an extensive diagnostic evaluation. In general, any concurrent inflammatory, infectious, hormonal, or neoplastic disorder can cause insulin resistance and can interfere with the effectiveness of insulin therapy. Identification and treatment of concurrent disease plays an integral role in the successful management of the diabetic dog and cat. A thorough history and physical examination and a complete diagnostic evaluation are imperative in the newly diagnosed diabetic dog or cat.

Oral Hypoglycemic Drugs

In the United States, five classes of oral hypoglycemic drugs have been approved for the treatment of NIDDM in human beings: sulfonylureas, meglitinides, biguanides, thiazolidinediones, and alpha-glucosidase inhibitors. These drugs work by stimulating pancreatic insulin secretion (sulfonylureas, meglitinides), by enhancing tissue sensitivity to insulin (biguanides, thiazolidinediones), or by slowing postprandial intestinal glucose absorption (alpha-glucosidase inhibitors).[65] Although controversial, chromium and vanadium are trace minerals that may also function as insulin sensitizers. Studies have documented the efficacy of sulfonylureas for treating diabetes in cats[4,66] and of alpha-glucosidase inhibitors for improving glycemic control in diabetic dogs (see below).[67,68] The pharmacokinetic properties of the insulin-sensitizing drugs metformin (a biguanide) and troglitazone (a thiazolidinedione) have been evaluated in healthy cats.[69,70] Unfortunately, in one study metformin was ineffective as a sole therapeutic agent in a small number of newly diagnosed diabetic cats and was discontinued in most because of progressively worsening clinical signs or the development of ketoacidosis.[71] The only cat that responded to metformin had a fasting serum insulin concentration greater than 20 μU/mL, a finding consistent with the concept that metformin as an insulin-sensitizing drug is effective only in the presence of adequate blood concentrations of insulin. Similarly, oral chromium picolinate was ineffective in improving control of glycemia in a group of insulin-treated diabetic dogs.[72] Studies evaluating the efficacy of thiazolidinediones for the treatment of diabetes in dogs or cats have yet to be reported.

Sulfonylureas   Glipizide and glyburide are the sulfonylureas most commonly used to treat NIDDM. The primary effect of these drugs is direct stimulation of insulin secretion from the pancreas.[73] Some pancreatic insulin secretory capability must exist for sulfonylureas to be effective in improving glycemic control. Sulfonylurea treatment is ineffective as the sole form of treatment for IDDM and has not been effective in diabetic dogs, presumably because of the high incidence of IDDM in this species. The clinical response to glipizide and glyburide treatment in diabetic cats is variable, ranging from excellent (i.e., blood glucose concentrations decreasing to less than 200 mg/dL) to a partial response (i.e., clinical improvement but failure to resolve hyperglycemia), to no response.[4,66] Presumably, the population of functioning beta cells dictates the clinical response; that is, variation from an absence of functioning beta cells (severe IDDM) to a near-normal population of beta cells (mild NIDDM) results in a response range of none to excellent. Cats with a partial response to glipizide have some functioning beta cells but not enough to reduce the blood glucose concentration to less than 200 mg/dL. These cats may have severe NIDDM or the early stages of IDDM.

No consistent parameters have been identified that allow the clinician to prospectively determine which cats will respond to glipizide or glyburide therapy. Identification of a high preprandial serum insulin concentration or an increase in the serum insulin concentration during an insulin secretagogue test supports a diagnosis of NIDDM, but failure to identify these changes does not rule out the potential for a beneficial response to glipizide or glyburide. Selection of diabetic cats for treatment with glipizide must rely heavily on the veterinarian's assessment of the cat's health, the severity of clinical signs, the presence or absence of ketoacidosis, other diabetic complications (e.g., peripheral neuropathy), and the owner's desires.

Currently, the author administers glipizide (Glucotrol; Pfizer, New York, NY) at a dosage of 2.5 mg per os twice a day in conjunction with a meal, to diabetic cats that are nonketotic and relatively healthy on physical examination (Figure 241-6). The history and complete physical examination findings; body weight and urine glucose/ketone measurements; and several blood glucose concentrations are evaluated 2 weeks after initiation of glipizide therapy. If adverse reactions (Table 241-3) have not occurred after 2 weeks of treatment, the glipizide dosage is increased to 5 mg twice a day and the cat is re-evaluated 2 weeks later. Therapy is continued as long as the cat is stable. If euglycemia or hypoglycemia develop, the glipizide dosage may be tapered or discontinued and blood glucose concentrations re-evaluated 1 week later to assess the need for the drug. If hyperglycemia recurs, the dosage is increased or glipizide is reinitiated at a reduced dosage in cats that previously developed hypoglycemia. Glipizide is discontinued and insulin therapy is initiated if clinical signs continue to worsen; if the cat becomes ill or develops ketoacidosis; if the blood glucose concentration remains greater than 300 mg/dL after 1 to 2 months of therapy; or if the owners become dissatisfied with the treatment. It is important to remember that stress-induced hyperglycemia can artificially elevate the results of blood glucose tests. Therefore, if an owner believes that the drug is effective but the blood glucose concentration remains greater than 300 mg/dL, assessment of the fructosamine or glycosylated hemoglobin level will distinguish the stressed cat from one that truly is not responding to the drug. In some cats, glipizide becomes ineffective weeks to months later, and exogenous insulin is ultimately required to control the diabetic state. Presumably, the transition from glipizide to insulin treatment is due to progression of the underlying pathophysiologic mechanisms (e.g., islet-specific amyloid deposition) responsible for the development of diabetes in the cat. The more rapid the rate of progression, the shorter the beneficial response to glipizide.

One theoretical adverse reaction of chronic glipizide therapy is accelerated loss of pancreatic beta cell function caused by glipizide-induced stimulation of amylin secretion and worsening islet amyloidosis. In a recent study using an induced model of diabetes in cats, mild to moderate islet amyloid deposition and moderate to severe islet vacuolar change were identified in three and one of four cats, respectively, that were treated with glipizide for 18 months and in one and three of four cats, respectively, that were treated with recombinant human NPH insulin for 18 months.[74] The results suggested that glipizide treatment could cause progressive amyloid deposition as a result of glipizide-induced insulin and amylin secretion. Does this mean that glipizide should not be used for the treatment of diabetes in cats? To answer this question, one has to look at the underlying reason for using this drug. Glipizide has no advantage over insulin therapy with regard to cost of treatment, time required to treat, efficacy of treatment, or frequency of re-evaluations by the veterinarian. However, glipizide gives many owners an initially more palatable option (i.e., pills versus injections) for the treatment of their newly diagnosed diabetic cat. Most owners who are unwilling to give insulin injections would euthanize their cat. Many of these people are willing to try oral medication. During the ensuing weeks, many of these owners become willing to try insulin injections if glipizide therapy fails. In the author's opinion, the real advantage of glipizide is that it keeps more diabetic cats alive by giving the owner treatment options in lieu of insulin injections and by not forcing a quick life-and-death decision at the time diabetes is diagnosed.

Alpha-Glucosidase Inhibitors

Acarbose and miglitol are complex oligosaccharides of microbial origin that competitively inhibit alpha-glucosidases (glucoamylase, sucrase, maltase, and isomaltase) in the brush border of the small intestinal mucosa. Inhibition of these enzymes delays digestion of complex carbohydrates and disaccharides to monosaccharides. This inhibition delays absorption of glucose from the intestinal tract and decreases postprandial blood glucose concentrations. Placebo-controlled clinical studies in healthy dogs documented a decrease in postprandial glucose absorption and insulin secretion when the dogs were treated with acarbose, compared with placebo. A decrease in the daily insulin dose and the blood glucose and glycated protein concentrations were documented in diabetic dogs treated with acarbose, compared with placebo.[67,68] Unfortunately, diarrhea and weight loss as a result of carbohydrate malassimilation were common adverse effects, occurring in approximately 35% of dogs. Diarrhea was more prevalent at higher doses of acarbose (i.e., 100 and 200 mg/dog) and typically resolved within 2 to 3 days of discontinuation of the medication. Because of the cost and prevalence of adverse effects, acarbose should be reserved for treatment of poorly controlled diabetic dogs in which the cause of the poor control of glycemia cannot be identified and insulin treatment by itself is ineffective at preventing clinical signs of diabetes. The initial acarbose dosage is 12.5 to 25 mg per dog at each meal. The benefit of this drug depends on its interaction with the meal; it should be given only at the time of feeding. A stepwise increase to 50 mg/dog and, in large dogs (greater than 25 kg), a further increase to 100 mg/dog can be considered in dogs that fail to show improvement in control of glycemia after 2 weeks on the 12.5 to 25 mg/meal regimen. Adverse reactions (especially diarrhea) are more likely to occur at these higher doses.

TECHNIQUES FOR MONITORING DIABETIC CONTROL

The basic objective of therapy is to eliminate the clinical signs of diabetes mellitus while avoiding the common complications associated with the disease. Common complications in dogs and cats include blindness caused by cataract formation (dogs); weakness, ataxia, and a plantigrade stance caused by peripheral neuropathy (cats); poor haircoat from lack of grooming (cats); weight loss; hypoglycemia; recurring ketosis; and poor control of glycemia secondary to concurrent infection, inflammation, neoplasia, or hormonal disorders (see Box 241-5). The devastating chronic complications of human diabetes (e.g., nephropathy, vasculopathy, coronary artery disease) require several decades to develop and are uncommon in diabetic dogs and cats; as such, it is not necessary to establish near-normal blood glucose concentrations in these animals. Most owners are happy and most dogs and cats are healthy and relatively asymptomatic if most blood glucose concentrations are kept between 100 and 250 mg/dL.

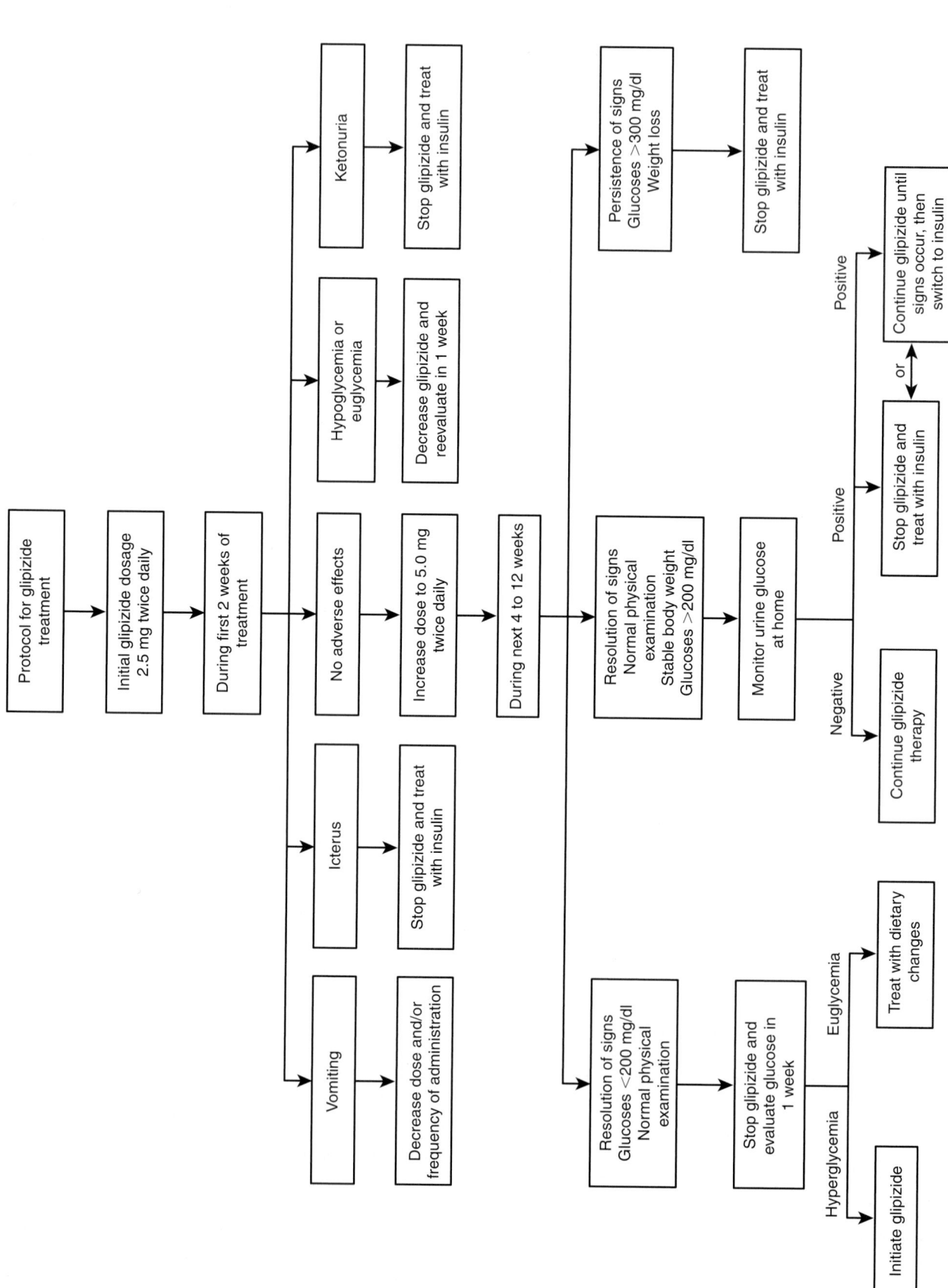

Figure 241-6 Algorithm for treatment of diabetic cats with the oral sulfonylurea drug glipizide. (From Feldman EC, Nelson RW: Canine and Feline Endocrinology and Reproduction, 3rd ed. Philadelphia, WB Saunders, 2004, p 558.)

Table • 241-3

Adverse Reactions to Glipizide Treatment in Diabetic Cats

ADVERSE REACTION	RECOMMENDATION
Vomiting within 1 hour of administration	Vomiting usually subsides after 2 to 5 days of glipizide therapy; decrease dose or frequency of administration if vomiting is severe; discontinue if vomiting persists longer than 1 week.
Increased serum hepatic enzyme activities	Continue treatment and monitor enzymes every 1 to 2 weeks initially; discontinue glipizide if cat becomes ill (lethargy, inappetence, vomiting) or if alanine transaminase activity exceeds 500 IU/L.
Icterus	Discontinue glipizide treatment; reinstitute glipizide treatment at lower dose and frequency of administration once icterus resolves (usually within 2 weeks); discontinue treatment permanently if icterus recurs.
Hypoglycemia	Discontinue glipizide treatment; recheck blood glucose concentration in 1 week; reinstitute glipizide therapy lower dose or frequency of administration if hyperglycemia recurs.

An important factor that affects the monitoring of diabetic cats more commonly than that of diabetic dogs is the propensity to develop stress-induced hyperglycemia as a result of frequent visits to the veterinary hospital for blood sampling. Once stress-induced hyperglycemia develops, it seems to be a perpetual problem, and blood glucose measurements can no longer be considered accurate. Veterinarians must remain wary of stress hyperglycemia in diabetic cats and should take steps to prevent its development. Micromanagement of diabetic cats should be avoided, and serial blood glucose curves should be done only when there is a perceived need to change insulin therapy. The determination of good versus poor control of glycemia should be based on the owner's subjective opinion regarding the presence and severity of clinical signs and the pet's overall health; the cat's ability to jump and its grooming behavior; the findings on physical examination, and the stability of body weight. Generation of a serial blood glucose curve should be reserved for newly diagnosed and poorly controlled diabetic cats unless stress-induced hyperglycemia is suspected. If this phenomenon is suspected, a switch should be made from reliance on serial blood glucose curves generated in the veterinary hospital to reliance on blood glucose results generated by the owner in the less-stressful home environment or on evaluation of sequential serum fructosamine concentrations, in addition to the history and physical examination findings.

History and Physical Examination

The most important initial parameters that should be assessed in the evaluation of control of glycemia are the owner's subjective opinion of the severity of clinical signs and the pet's overall health, the physical examination findings, and the stability of body weight. If the owner is happy with the results of treatment, if the physical examination is supportive of good glycemic control, and if the body weight is stable, the diabetic dog or cat is usually adequately controlled. Measurement of the serum fructosamine concentration can add further objective evidence of the status of glycemic control (see below). Poor control of glycemia should be suspected and additional diagnostics (i.e., serial blood glucose curve, serum fructosamine concentration, tests for concurrent disorders) or a change in insulin therapy should be considered if the owner reports clinical signs suggestive of hyperglycemia or hypoglycemia (i.e., polyuria, polydipsia, lethargy, weakness, ataxia) or peripheral neuropathy (changes in jumping ability, weakness, ataxia, plantigrade stance); if the physical examination identifies problems consistent with poor control of glycemia (e.g., thin or emaciated appearance, poor haircoat); or if the dog or cat is losing weight.[75]

Documentation of an increased blood glucose concentration does not *by itself* confirm poor control of glycemia. Stress or excitement can cause marked hyperglycemia that does not reflect the cat's or dog's responsiveness to insulin and can lead to the erroneous belief that the diabetic dog or cat is poorly controlled. If a discrepancy exists among the history, physical examination findings, and blood glucose concentration or if the cat or dog is fractious, aggressive, excited, or scared and the blood glucose concentration is known to be unreliable, the serum fructosamine concentration should be measured to further evaluate the status of glycemic control.

Serum Fructosamine Concentration

Fructosamines are glycated proteins synthesized after an irreversible, nonenzymatic, insulin-independent binding of glucose to serum proteins. Serum fructosamine concentrations are a marker of the mean blood glucose concentration during the circulating life span of the protein, which varies from 1 to 3 weeks, depending on the particular protein. The extent of glycosylation of serum proteins is directly related to the blood glucose concentration; the higher the average blood glucose concentration during the preceding 2 to 3 weeks, the higher the serum fructosamine concentration and vice versa. Serum fructosamine concentrations increase when glycemic control of the diabetic dog or cat worsens and decrease when glycemic control improves. The erum fructosamine concentration is not affected by acute increases in the blood glucose concentration, as occurs with stress or excitement-induced hyperglycemia, but it can be affected by hypoalbuminemia (less than 2.5 g/dL) and hyperlipidemia (triglycerides greater than 150 mg/dL).[39,76,77]

Fructosamine is measured in serum, which should be frozen and shipped on cold packs overnight to the diagnostic laboratory. In the author's laboratory, the normal reference ranges for serum fructosamine are 225 to 365 µmol/L in dogs and 190 to 365 µmol/L in cats.[39,78] Interpretation of the serum fructosamine level in a diabetic dog or cat must take into consideration the fact that hyperglycemia is common, even in well-controlled diabetic dogs and cats (Table 241-4). Most owners are happy with their pet's response to insulin treatment if the serum fructosamine concentration can be kept between 350 and 450 µmol/L. Values greater than 500 µmol/L suggest inadequate control of the diabetic state, and values greater than 600 µmol/L indicate serious lack of glycemic control. Serum fructosamine concentrations in the lower half of the normal reference range (i.e., less than 300 µmol/L) or below the normal reference range should raise concern that significant periods of hypoglycemia have occurred. Increased serum fructosamine concentrations (i.e., greater than 500 µmol/L) suggest poor control of glycemia

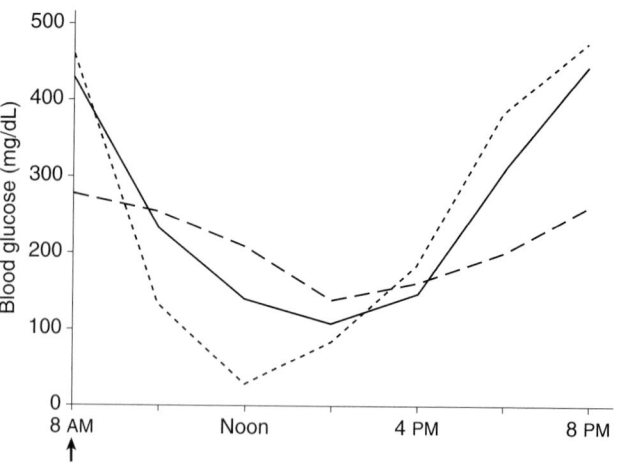

Table • 241-4

Sample Handling, Methodology, and Normal Values for Serum Fructosamine Concentrations Measured in Our Laboratory in Dogs and Cats

Blood sample	1 to 2 mL serum
Sample handling	Freeze until assayed
Methodology	Automated colorimetric assay using nitroblue tetrazolium chloride
Factors affecting results	Hypoproteinemia and hypoalbuminemia (decreased), hyperlipidemia (decreased [dog]), azotemia (decreased [dog]), storage at room temperature (decreased)
Normal range	Dog: 225 to 365 μmol/L
	Cat: 190 to 365 μmol/L
Interpretation in diabetic dogs and cats	
Excellent control	350 to 400 μmol/L
Good control	400 to 450 μmol/L
Fair control	450 to 500 μmol/L
Poor control	>500 μmol/L
Prolonged hypoglycemia	<300 μmol/L

Figure 241-7 Blood glucose concentration curves in a dachshund receiving 0.8 U of recombinant human Lente insulin per kilogram of body weight twice a day *(solid line)*; a miniature poodle receiving 0.6 U of recombinant human Lente insulin per kilogram of body weight twice a day *(broken line)*; and a terrier-mix receiving 1.1 U of recombinant human Lente insulin per kilogram of body weight twice a day *(dotted line)*. Insulin and food were given at 8 AM. Interpretation of the blood glucose curves suggests a short duration of insulin effect in the dachshund, insulin underdosage in the miniature poodle, and the Somogyi effect in the terrier-mix. Note that the blood glucose concentrations were similar in the three dogs at 2 PM and 4 PM and that the glucose results at these times do not establish the diagnosis in any of the dogs. (From Nelson RW, Couto CG: Small Animal Internal Medicine, 3rd ed. St Louis, Mosby, 2003, p 741.)

and a need for insulin adjustment but do not identify the underlying problem.

Urine Glucose Monitoring

In diabetic dogs and cats that have problems with recurring ketosis or hypoglycemia, occasional monitoring of urine for glycosuria and ketonuria in the home environment is helpful for (1) determining whether ketonuria or persistent negative glycosuria, respectively, is present; (2) in cats that have reverted to a non-insulin-requiring diabetic state, for determining whether glycosuria has recurred; (3) in cats treated with oral hypoglycemic drugs, for determining whether glycosuria has improved or worsened; and (4) in cats with suspected stress-induced hyperglycemia, for differentiating transient from persistent hyperglycemia. For cats, a small amount of urine can be obtained by decreasing the amount of litter in the pan; by temporarily replacing the litter with non-absorbable material, such as aquarium gravel; or by assessing the change in the color of urine glucose test squares (Glucotest Feline Urinary Glucose Detection System; Ralston Purina) that have been mixed into the kitty litter. We do not have the owner adjust daily insulin dosages based on morning urine glucose measurements in dogs except to decrease the insulin dose in dogs with recurring hypoglycemia and persistent negative glycosuria. In the author's experience, the vast majority of diabetic dogs develop complications as a result of owners being misled by morning urine glucose concentrations. For both dogs and cats, persistent glycosuria throughout the day and night suggests inadequate control of the diabetic state and the need for a more complete evaluation of diabetic control using techniques discussed in this section.

Serial Blood Glucose Curve

If an adjustment in insulin therapy is deemed necessary after a review of the history, physical examination findings, changes in body weight, and serum fructosamine concentration, a serial blood glucose curve should be generated to provide guidance for the adjustment, unless the blood glucose measurements are unreliable because of stress, aggression, or excitement. The serial blood glucose curve provides guidelines for rational adjustments in insulin therapy. Evaluation of a serial blood glucose curve is mandatory during the initial regulation of the diabetic dog or cat and is necessary in the dog or cat in which clinical manifestations of hyperglycemia or hypoglycemia have developed. Reliance on the history, physical examination findings, body weight, and serum fructosamine concentration to determine when a blood glucose curve is needed helps reduce the number of blood glucose curves generated and the number of venipunctures and also shortens the time the dog or cat spends in the hospital. This may minimize the animal's aversion to evaluations and may improve the chance of obtaining meaningful results when a blood glucose curve is needed.

Blood glucose concentrations are typically determined with either a point-of-care glucose analyzer or a hand-held portable blood glucose monitoring device. Commercially available portable blood glucose monitoring devices provide blood glucose concentrations reasonably close to those obtained with reference methods, although the results often consistently overestimate or underestimate actual glucose values (Figure 241-8).[78,79] The blood glucose values determined by most portable blood glucose monitoring devices typically are lower than the actual glucose values determined by reference methods. This may result in an incorrect diagnosis of hypoglycemia or the misperception that glycemic control is better than it actually is. Failure to consider this "error" could result in insulin underdosage and the potential for persistence of clinical signs despite apparently "acceptable" blood glucose results.

The author prefers to adjust insulin therapy based on interpretation of a single serial blood glucose curve, with the ideal goal of maintaining the blood glucose concentration between

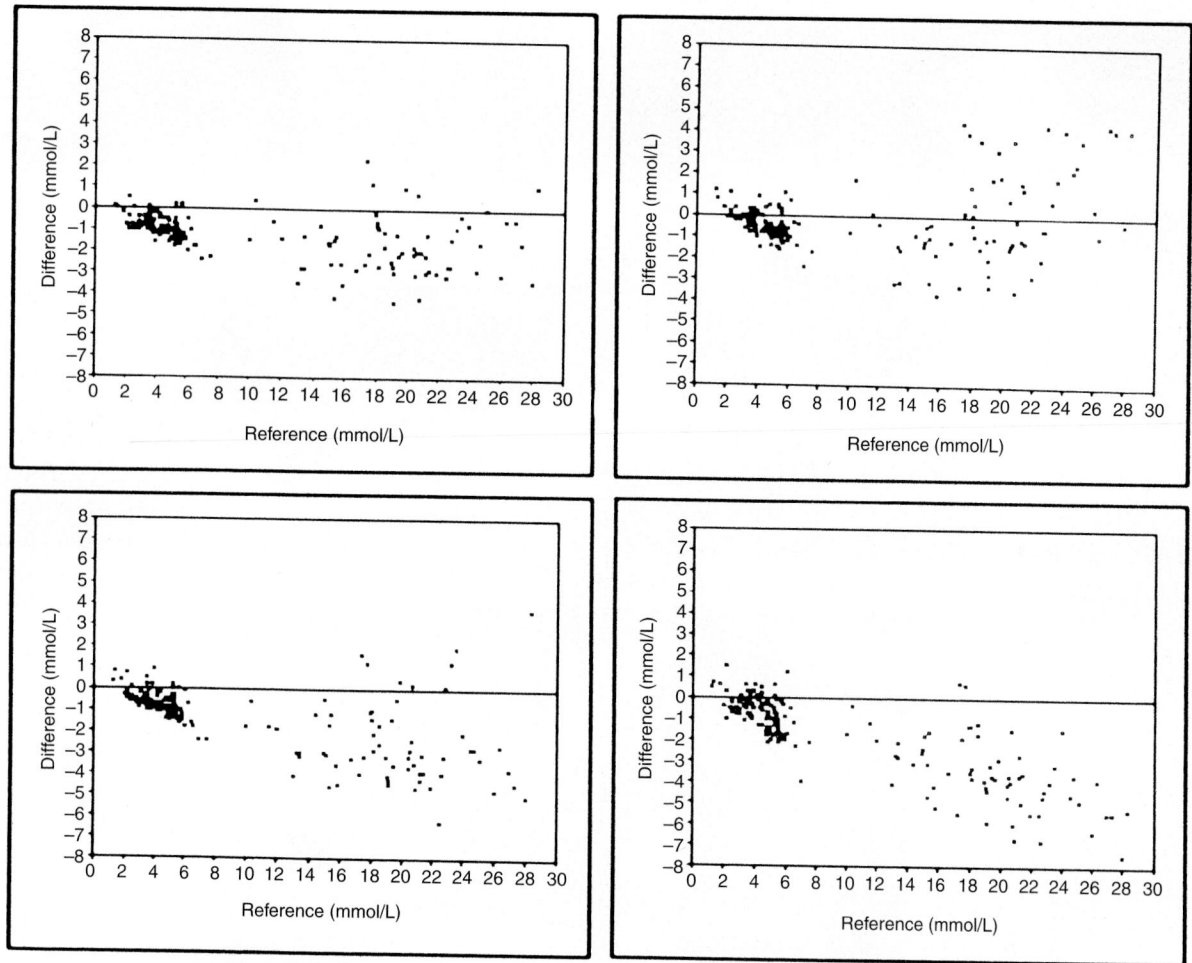

Figure 241-8 Scatterplots of the difference between blood glucose concentrations obtained with four portable blood glucose meters and concentrations obtained with a reference method versus concentration obtained with the reference method for blood samples from 170 dogs. (From Wess G, Reusch C: Evaluation of five portable blood glucose meters for use in dogs. J Am Vet Med Assoc 216:203, 2000.)

100 and 250 mg/dL. We typically relies on owner perceptions of clinical response and the change in the serum fructosamine concentration to initially assess the impact of the insulin adjustment on control of glycemia. If problems persist, we consider repeating the blood glucose curve. We rarely perform blood glucose curves on multiple consecutive days because it promotes stress-induced hyperglycemia. In addition, information gained from a prior serial blood glucose curve should never be assumed to be reproducible on subsequent curves. Variables such as the actual amount of insulin drawn into the syringe and subsequently absorbed from the subcutaneous site of deposition and the interaction among insulin, diet, exercise, stress, excitement, any concurrent disorders, and secretion of the counter-regulatory hormones (i.e., glucagon, epinephrine, cortisol, growth hormone) change with time and affect the reproducibility of serial blood glucose curves. Lack of consistency in the results of serial blood glucose curves creates frustration for many veterinarians. It is important to remember that this lack of consistency is a direct reflection of all the variables that affect the blood glucose concentration in diabetics. Daily self-monitoring of blood glucose concentrations and daily adjustments in the insulin dose are recommended in human diabetics to minimize the effect of these variables on control of glycemia. A similar approach for diabetic dogs and

cats undoubtedly will become more common in the future, as home glucose monitoring techniques are refined. For now, initial assessment of the control of glycemia is based on the owners' perception of their diabetic pet's health combined with periodic examinations by the veterinarian. Serial blood glucose measurements are indicated if poor control of glycemia is suspected. The purpose of serial blood glucose measurements is to obtain a glimpse at the actions of insulin in that diabetic animal and hopefully to identify a reason that could explain why the diabetic dog or cat is poorly controlled.

Generation of the Serial Blood Glucose Curve at Home

An alternative to hospital-generated blood glucose curves for cats is to have the owner generate the blood glucose curve at home using the marginal ear vein prick technique and a portable home blood glucose monitoring device that allows the owner to touch the drop of blood on the ear with the end of the glucose test strip (e.g., Glucometer Elite XL portable blood glucose meter; Bayer Diagnostics, Tarrytown, New York) (Figure 241-9). The marginal ear vein prick technique decreases the need for physical restraint during sample collection, thereby minimizing the cat's discomfort and stress. The accuracy of blood glucose results are similar when blood for

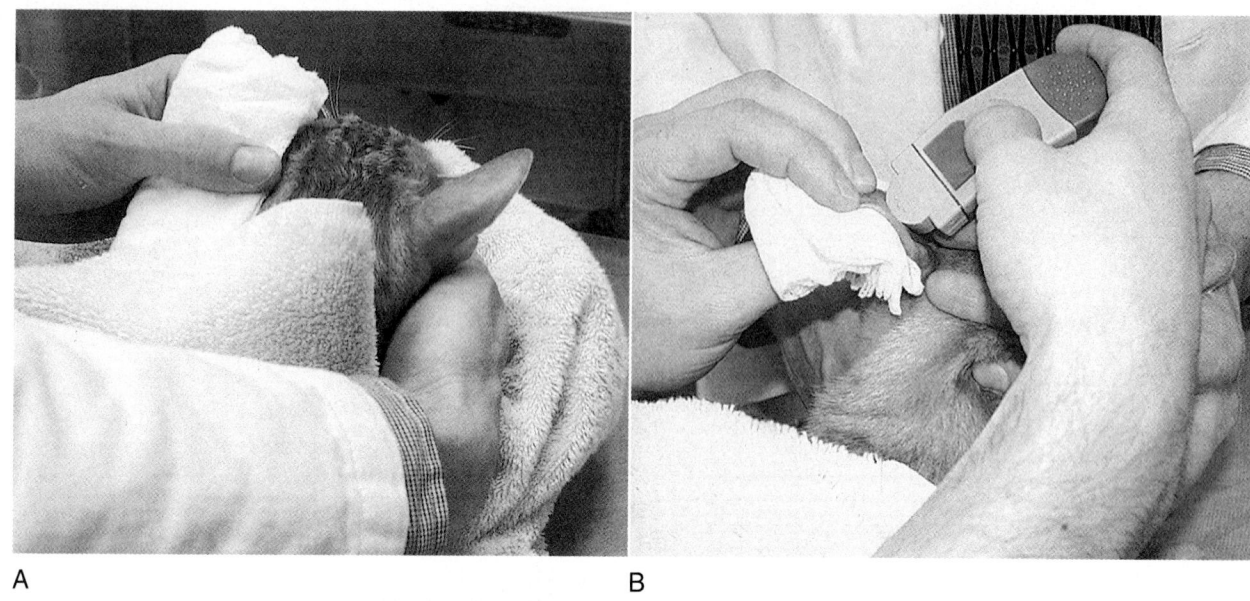

A

B

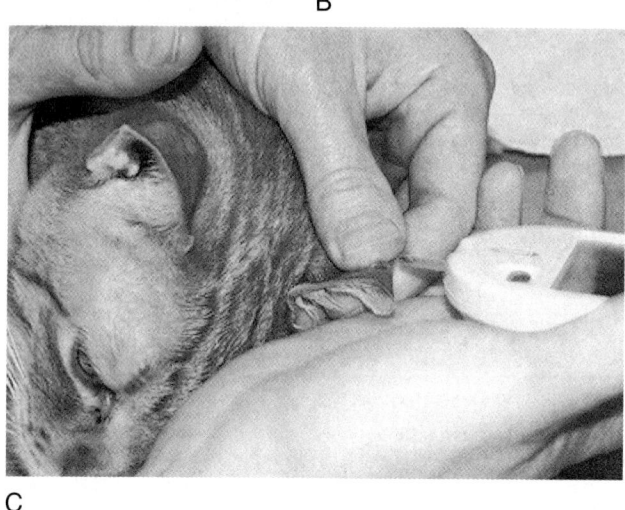

C

Figure 241- 9   Marginal ear vein prick technique for measuring the blood glucose concentration. A, A hot washcloth is applied to the pinna for 2 to 3 minutes to increase circulation to the ear B, The marginal ear vein is identified on the periphery of the outer side of the pinna, and a thin coating of petrolatum jelly is applied to a small spot over the vein; the spot is then pricked with the lancet device supplied with the portable blood glucose meter. Gauze should be placed between the pinna and the digit holding the pinna to prevent pricking of the finger if the lancet's blade accidentally passes through the pinna. Petrolatum jelly is applied to help the blood form a ball on the pinna as it seeps from the lanced site. C, Digital pressure is applied in the area of the lanced skin to promote bleeding. The glucose test strip is touched to the drop of capillary blood that forms and is removed once enough blood has been drawn into the test strip to activate the meter. (From Nelson RW, Couto CG: Small Animal Internal Medicine, 3rd ed. St Louis, Mosby, 2003, p 759.)

glucose determination is obtained by ear prick and venipuncture.[79,80] However, blood glucose results obtained by portable blood glucose monitoring devices may overestimate or, more commonly, underestimate the actual blood glucose values obtained with reference methods, as discussed in the previous section.[81] This inherent error must be considered in the interpretation of blood glucose results obtained by a portable home blood glucose monitoring device. Several web sites on the Internet (e.g., www.sugarcats.net/sites/harry/) explain in detail the marginal ear vein prick technique in lay terms and provide information on owner experiences with the technique and with different portable home blood glucose meters.

At the time diabetes is diagnosed, the author provides this web site URL to clients and asks them to read the information to decide if they would be interested in monitoring blood glucose concentrations at home. We spend time teaching the technique to individuals willing to give it a try, advise them on how often to perform a blood glucose curve (ideally no more frequently than one day every 2 to 4 weeks), and how often to measure the blood glucose concentration on the day of the curve (typically at the time of insulin administration and 3, 6, 9, and 12 hours later). We have had excellent results using the marginal ear vein prick technique in cats. Stress has been significantly reduced, and the reliability of the blood glucose results has improved immensely. The biggest problem has been overzealous owners who monitor blood glucose concentrations too frequently. A similar approach can be used in diabetic dogs, using either the ear or lip prick technique. However, the author does not push home glucose monitoring for dogs as much as for cats, primarily because stress-induced hyperglycemia is not as significant a problem in diabetic dogs.

For the marginal ear vein prick technique, the cat is allowed to remain in sternal recumbency with restraint only as needed to keep the animal stationary. The marginal ear vein is identified, and a damp cloth or gauze sponge previously warmed in water is applied to the vein for 15 to 30 seconds to increase perfusion. A thin film of petrolatum is placed over the sampling site to allow a drop of blood to form without dissipating into the fur, the pinna is immobilized with a digit, an automatic lancing device (e.g., Microlet automatic lancing device; Bayer Diagnostics) is placed over the vein, the ejected needle is used to nick the ear vein and, if necessary, the pinna in the region of the nick site is gently squeezed to promote formation of a drop of blood. A glucose test strip previously inserted into the blood glucose meter is applied to the drop of blood to measure the blood glucose concentration (see Figure 241-9). Digital pressure is then applied at the marginal ear vein prick site until bleeding stops. The skin puncture is rarely painful, and the puncture sites are barely visible even after numerous blood collections. Application of a thin film of petrolatum is critical for formation of the drop of blood. A small amount of padding, such as a cotton ball or gauze sponge, between the pinna and the digit used to stabilize the pinna helps prevent inadvertent pricking of the finger if the lancet goes through the pinna. Dehydration can interfere with the ability to obtain a drop of blood; a problem that occurs in some poorly controlled cats with marked hyperglycemia and severe polyuria and polydipsia. Administration of subcutaneous fluids may improve circulation to the ear. Only portable home blood glucose monitoring devices that allow the end of the glucose test strip to touch the drop of blood formed on the pinna while the strip is in the glucose monitoring device are used.

Evaluation of Aggressive, Excitable, or Stressed Diabetic Cats or Dogs

Hyperglycemia induced by stress, aggression, or excitement is the single biggest problem that affects the accuracy of the serial blood glucose curve. Stress can over-ride the glucose-lowering effect of the insulin injection, causing high blood glucose concentrations despite the presence of adequate amounts of insulin in the circulation, leading to a spiraling path of insulin overdosage, hypoglycemia, Somogyi phenomenon, and poor control of glycemia. The primary factors that induce stress hyperglycemia are hospitalization and multiple venipunctures. An alternative to hospital-generated blood glucose curves is to have the owner generate the blood glucose curve at home, as discussed above. Alternatively, serum fructosamine concentrations can be used to assess control of glycemia and the effectiveness of adjustments in insulin therapy in aggressive, excitable, or stressed diabetic cats or dogs. If a change in insulin therapy is deemed necessary, the clinician must make an educated guess as to where the problem lies (e.g., low insulin dose, short duration of insulin effect), adjust the insulin dose, and rely on the change in subsequent serum fructosamine measurements to assess the benefit of the change. The author measures serum fructosamine concentrations prior to and 2 to 3 weeks after changing insulin therapy. If the change has improved control of glycemia, the serum fructosamine concentration should decrease. If the serum fructosamine concentration is the same or has increased, the change was ineffective at improving glycemic control, another change in therapy can be tried, and the serum fructosamine measured again 2 to 3 weeks later.

COMPLICATIONS OF INSULIN THERAPY

Hypoglycemia

Hypoglycemia is a common complication of insulin therapy and is most apt to occur after sudden large increases in the insulin dose; with excessive overlap of insulin action in dogs and cats receiving insulin twice a day; during unusually strenuous exercise (dogs); after prolonged inappetence; after sudden decreases in insulin resistance; and in insulin-treated cats that have reverted to a non-insulin-dependent state. In these situations severe hypoglycemia may occur before glucose counter-regulation (i.e., secretion of glucagon, epinephrine, cortisol, and growth hormone) is able to compensate for and reverse the hypoglycemia. Signs of hypoglycemia include lethargy, weakness, head tilting, ataxia, seizures, and coma. The occurrence and severity of clinical signs depends on the rate of blood glucose decline and the severity of hypoglycemia. Symptomatic hypoglycemia is treated with glucose administered as food, sugar water, or intravenous dextrose. Whenever signs of hypoglycemia occur, the owner should be instructed to stop insulin therapy until glycosuria recurs. The adjustment in the subsequent insulin dosage is somewhat arbitrary; as a general rule, the insulin dosage initially should be reduced 25% to 50%, and subsequent adjustments in the dosage should be based on clinical response and blood glucose measurements. Failure of glycosuria to recur after a hypoglycemic episode suggests reversion to a non-insulin-dependent diabetic state or impaired glucose counter-regulation.

Stress Hyperglycemia

Transient hyperglycemia is a well-recognized problem in fractious or frightened cats. Hyperglycemia develops as a result of an increase in catecholamines and, in struggling cats, lactate concentrations and presumably increased hepatic glucose production.[82,83] Blood glucose concentrations typically exceed 200 mg/dL in these cats, and values in excess of 300 mg/dL are common. Diabetes mellitus may be inadvertently diagnosed in such cats if the diagnosis is based solely on the blood glucose concentration. Stress hyperglycemia can also significantly increase blood glucose concentrations in diabetic cats despite administration of insulin, an effect that seriously interferes with the clinician's ability to judge the effectiveness of exogenous insulin accurately. Induction of stress hyperglycemia is variable but usually starts during a venipuncture procedure and begins earlier and earlier on subsequent visits to the veterinarian, until eventually stress hyperglycemia is induced by hospitalization and ultimately by the car ride to the veterinary hospital. Blood glucose concentrations can remain greater than 400 mg/dL throughout the day, despite administration of insulin (Figure 241-10), when stress hyperglycemia develops prior to the first venipuncture of the day. Failure to recognize the effect of stress on blood glucose measurements may lead to the erroneous perception that the diabetic cat is poorly controlled, and insulin therapy is invariably adjusted, often by increasing the insulin dosage; repetition of this cycle eventually culminates in the Somogyi phenomenon, clinically apparent hypoglycemia, or referral for evaluation of insulin resistance.

Stress hyperglycemia should be suspected if the cat is visibly upset or aggressive or struggles during restraint and the venipuncture process. However, stress hyperglycemia can also be present in diabetic cats that are easily removed from the cage and do not resist the blood sampling procedure. These cats are scared, but rather than become aggressive, they remain crouched in the back of the cage, often have dilated pupils, and usually are flaccid when handled. Stress hyperglycemia should also be suspected when (1) a disparity exists between assessment of glycemic control based on the results

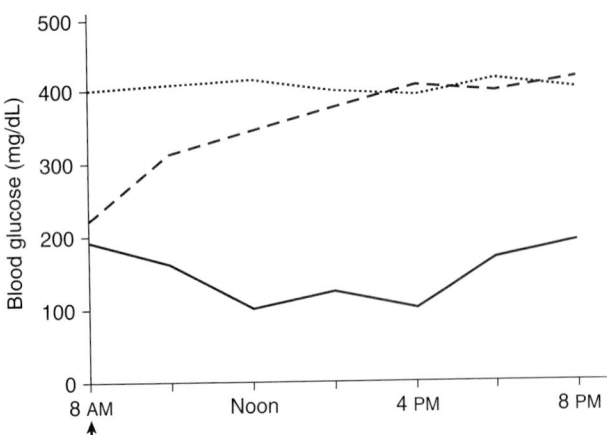

Figure 241-10 Blood glucose curves in a 5.3 kg male cat receiving 2 U of recombinant human Ultralente insulin *(solid line-solid circles)* 2 weeks after initiation of insulin therapy; 2 U of recombinant human Ultralente insulin *(broken line)* 2 months later; and 6 U of recombinant human Ultralente insulin *(dotted line)* 4 months later. The insulin dosage had been gradually increased based on the blood glucose curve results. The owner reported minimal clinical signs regardless of the insulin dosage, the cat had maintained its body weight, and the blood glycosylated hemoglobin concentration was 2.2% at the 4-month recheck. The cat became progressively more fractious during each hospitalization, supporting a finding of stress-induced hyperglycemia as the reason for the discrepancy between the blood glucose values and other parameters used to evaluate glycemic control. ↑, Subcutaneous insulin injection and food. (From Feldman EC, Nelson RW: Canine and Feline Endocrinology and Reproduction, 3rd ed. Philadelphia, WB Saunders, 2004, p 569.)

of the history, physical examination, and stability of body weight and assessment of glycemic control based on the results of blood glucose measurements, or (2) the initial blood glucose concentration measured in the morning is in an acceptable range (i.e., 150 to 250 mg/dL), but subsequent blood glucose concentrations increase steadily throughout the day (see Figure 241-10). Once stress hyperglycemia develops, it is usually a perpetual problem, and blood glucose measurements can no longer be considered accurate.

Recurrence or Persistence of Clinical Signs

Recurrence or persistence of clinical signs of diabetes is the most common "complication" of insulin therapy in diabetic dogs and cats. Recurrence or continuing clinical signs suggest insulin ineffectiveness, which is usually caused by problems with the biologic activity of the insulin or by owner technique in administering the insulin; problems with the insulin treatment regimen; or problems with responsiveness to insulin caused by concurrent inflammatory, infectious, neoplastic, or hormonal disorders (i.e., insulin resistance). The most common problems with the insulin treatment regimen in the dog are insulin underdosage, the Somogyi phenomenon, short duration of effect of Lente insulin, and once a day insulin administration. The most common problems with the insulin treatment regimen in the cat are insulin overdosage, causing the Somogyi phenomenon; inadequate absorption of longer acting insulin preparations; short duration of effect of intermediate-acting insulin preparations; and once a day insulin administration.

Discrepancies in the parameters used to assess glycemic control, resulting in an erroneous belief that the diabetic dog or cat is poorly controlled, should also be considered. This situation

usually is caused by erroneously high blood glucose concentrations that suggest insulin ineffectiveness; these high values may be stress induced and do not reflect the animal's responsiveness to insulin. In the evaluation of a diabetic dog or cat for suspected insulin ineffectiveness, it is important that all parameters used to assess glycemic control be critically analyzed, most notably the owner's perception of how the pet is doing in the home environment, physical examination findings, and changes in body weight. If the history, physical examination, change in body weight, and serum fructosamine concentration suggest poor control of the diabetic state, a diagnostic evaluation to identify the cause is warranted, beginning with evaluation of the owner's insulin administration technique and the biologic activity of the insulin preparation.

Insulin Underdosage

Control of glycemia can be established in most dogs and cats using less than 1 U of insulin per kilogram of body weight administered twice each day. An inadequate insulin dosage in conjunction with once a day insulin therapy is a common cause of persistence of clinical signs. In general, insulin underdosage should be considered if the insulin dosage is less than 1 U/kg and the dog or cat is receiving insulin twice a day. If insulin underdosage is suspected, the insulin dose should be gradually increased by 1 to 5 U per injection in dogs (depending on the size of the dog) and 0.5 to 1 U per injection in cats, per week. The effectiveness of the change in therapy should be evaluated by the owner's perception of clinical response and measurement of serum fructosamine or serial blood glucose concentrations. Other causes of insulin ineffectiveness (most notably the Somogyi phenomenon) should be considered if the insulin dosage exceeds 1 to 1.5 U/kg/injection, if insulin is being administered every 12 hours, and if control of glycemia remains poor.

Insulin Overdosage and Glucose Counter-Regulation (Somogyi Phenomenon)

The Somogyi phenomenon results from a normal physiologic response to impending hypoglycemia induced by excessive insulin. When the blood glucose concentration declines to less than 65 mg/dL or when the blood glucose concentration decreases rapidly regardless of the glucose nadir, direct hypoglycemia-induced stimulation of hepatic glycogenolysis and secretion of diabetogenic hormones, most notably epinephrine and glucagon, increase the blood glucose concentration, minimize signs of hypoglycemia, and cause marked hyperglycemia within 12 hours of glucose counter-regulation (Figure 241-11). The marked hyperglycemia that occurs after hypoglycemia is due in part to inability of the diabetic dog or cat to secrete sufficient endogenous insulin to dampen the rising blood glucose concentration. By the next morning, the blood glucose concentration can be extremely elevated (400 to 800 mg/dL), and the morning urine glucose concentration is consistently 1 to 2 g/dL as measured with urine glucose test strips. Unrecognized short duration of insulin effect combined with insulin dosage adjustments based on morning urine glucose concentrations is historically the most common cause of the Somogyi phenomenon in dogs.

Clinical signs of hypoglycemia are typically mild or are not recognized by the owner; clinical signs caused by hyperglycemia tend to dominate the clinical picture. The insulin dose that induces the Somogyi phenomenon is variable and unpredictable. The Somogyi phenomenon is often suspected in poorly controlled diabetic dogs for which the insulin dosage is approaching 2.2 U/kg/injection but can also occur at insulin dosages less than 0.5 U/kg/injection. Toy and miniature breeds of dogs are especially susceptible to development of the Somogyi phenomenon with lower than expected doses of insulin. In cats, the Somogyi phenomenon can be induced

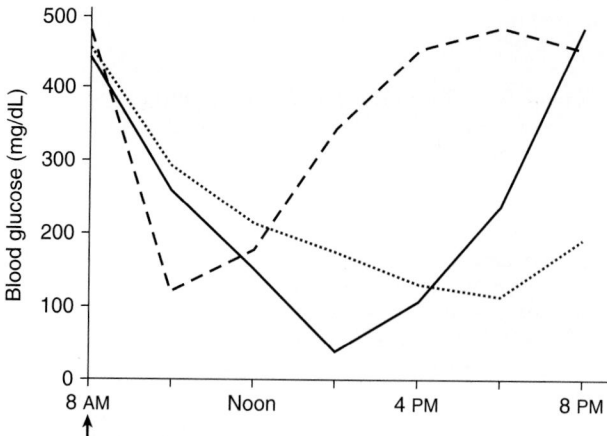

Figure 241-11 Blood glucose concentration curves from three dogs with poorly controlled diabetes that were treated with recombinant human Lente insulin twice a day, illustrating the typical blood glucose curves suggestive of the Somogyi phenomenon. In one dog *(solid line)*, the glucose nadir is less than 80 mg/dL and is followed by a rapid increase in the blood glucose concentration. In another dog *(dashed line)*, a rapid decrease in the blood glucose concentration occurs within 2 hours of insulin administration and is followed by a rapid increase in the blood glucose concentration; the rapid decrease in the blood glucose concentration stimulates glucose counter-regulation despite maintenance of the blood glucose nadir above 80 mg/dL. In the third dog *(dotted line)*, the blood glucose curve is not suggestive of the Somogyi phenomenon per se. However, the insulin injection causes the blood glucose level to decrease by approximately 300 mg/dL during the day, and the blood glucose concentration at the time of the evening insulin injection is considerably lower than the 8 AM blood glucose concentration. If a similar decrease in the blood glucose occurs with the evening insulin injection, hypoglycemia and the Somogyi phenomenon would occur at night and would explain the high blood glucose concentration in the morning and the poor control of the diabetic state. (From Nelson RW, Couto CG: Small Animal Internal Medicine, 3rd ed. St Louis, Mosby Inc, 2003, p 745.)

with insulin doses of 2 to 3 U per injection; as a result, cats may receive 10 to 15 U of insulin per injection because veterinarians, interpreting the persistence of clinical signs and the high blood glucose and serum fructosamine concentrations as underdosage, increase the insulin dose, thereby perpetuating the problem.

Diagnosis of the Somogyi phenomenon requires demonstration of hypoglycemia (a serum glucose concentration less than 80 mg/dL) followed by hyperglycemia (a serum glucose concentration greater than 300 mg/dL) after insulin administration. The Somogyi phenomenon should also be suspected when the blood glucose concentration decreases rapidly regardless of the glucose nadir (e.g., a drop from 400 to 100 mg/dL within 2 to 3 hours). If the duration of insulin effect is greater than 12 hours, hypoglycemia often occurs at night after the evening dose of insulin, and the serum glucose concentration is typically greater than 300 mg/dL the next morning (see Figure 241-11). Unfortunately, diagnosis of the Somogyi phenomenon can be elusive, partly because of the effects of the diabetogenic hormones on blood glucose concentrations after an episode of glucose counter-regulation. Secretion of diabetogenic hormones during the Somogyi phenomenon may induce insulin resistance, which can last 24 to 72 hours after the hypoglycemic episode. If a serial blood glucose curve is obtained on the day glucose counter-regulation occurs, hypoglycemia can be identified and the diagnosis

established. However, if the serial blood glucose curve is obtained on a day when insulin resistance predominates, hypoglycemia will not be identified, and the insulin dose may be incorrectly increased in response to the high blood glucose values. A cyclic history of 1 or 2 days of good glycemic control followed by several days of poor control should raise suspicion for insulin resistance caused by glucose counter-regulation. Serum fructosamine concentrations are unpredictable but are usually increased (greater than 500 μmol/L); these results confirm poor glycemic control but do not identify the underlying cause.

Establishment of the diagnosis may require several days of hospitalization and serial blood glucose curves, an approach that eventually leads to problems with stress-induced hyperglycemia. An alternative approach, which the author prefers, is to arbitrarily reduce the insulin dosage 1 to 5 U and have the owner evaluate the dog's or cat's clinical response over the following 2 to 5 days. If clinical signs of diabetes worsen after a reduction in the insulin dosage, another cause of the insulin resistance should be pursued. However, if the owner reports no change or improvement in clinical signs, the clinician should continue to reduce the insulin dosage gradually. Alternatively, glycemic regulation of the diabetic dog or cat could be started over, using an insulin dosage of 0.25 U/kg (dogs) or 1 U/injection (cats) given twice daily.

Short Duration of Insulin Effect

Short duration of insulin effect (i.e., less than 10 hours) is a common problem in diabetic dogs, and especially diabetic cats, despite twice a day insulin administration. In some diabetic cats, the duration of effect of NPH and Lente insulin is less than 8 hours. As a result, significant hyperglycemia (blood glucose concentration greater than 300 mg/dL) occurs for several hours each day, and the owners of these pets usually mention continuing problems with persistence of clinical signs or weight loss, or weakness caused by the development of peripheral neuropathy. Diabetic dogs with short duration of insulin have persistent morning glycosuria (greater than 1 g/dL on urine glucose test strips). If the owners are adjusting the daily insulin dosage based on the morning urine glucose concentration, they usually induce the Somogyi phenomenon, because the insulin dosage is gradually increased in response to the persistent morning glycosuria. Serum fructosamine concentrations are variable but typically greater than 500 μmol/L. The diagnosis of short duration of insulin effect is made by demonstrating recurrence of hyperglycemia (blood glucose concentration greater than 250 mg/dL) within 6 to 10 hours of the insulin injection; also, the lowest blood glucose concentration is maintained above 80 mg/dL (see Figure 241-7). The clinician must evaluate multiple blood glucose concentrations obtained throughout the day to establish the diagnosis. The use of one or two afternoon blood glucose determinations consistently fails to identify the problem. Treatment involves changing to a longer acting insulin given twice a day (e.g., switching to PZI [cats], Ultralente, or insulin glargine) or increasing the frequency of insulin administration (i.e., initiating three times a day therapy) if the duration of effect is less than 8 hours.

Prolonged Duration of Insulin Effect

In some diabetic dogs and cats, the duration of effect of Lente insulin or PZI is greater than 12 hours, and twice a day insulin administration creates problems with hypoglycemia and the Somogyi phenomenon. In these dogs and cats, the glucose nadir after morning administration of insulin typically occurs near the time of the evening insulin administration, and the morning blood glucose concentration is usually greater than 300 mg/dL (see Figure 241-11). Gradually decreasing blood glucose concentrations measured at the time of sequential insulin injections are another indication of prolonged duration of insulin effect. The effectiveness of insulin in lowering the blood glucose concentration varies from day to day, presumably because of varying concentrations of diabetogenic hormones, the secretion of which was induced by prior hypoglycemia. Serum fructosamine concentrations are variable but typically greater than 500 µmol/L. Effective treatment depends in part on the duration of effect of the insulin. A 24-hour blood glucose curve should be generated after administration of insulin once in the morning and with the dog or cat being fed at the usual times of the day. This allows the clinician to estimate the duration of effect of the insulin. If the duration of effect is less than 16 hours, a shorter acting insulin given twice a day or a lower dose of the same insulin given in the evening, compared with the morning insulin dose, can be tried. If the duration of effect is 16 hours or longer, switching to a longer acting insulin administered once a day or administering Lente insulin in the morning and regular crystalline insulin at bedtime (i.e., 16 to 18 hours after the morning insulin injection) can be tried. When different types of insulin are used in the same 24-hour period, the goal is to have the combined duration of effect of the insulins equal 24 hours. Differences in the potency of intermediate- and long-acting insulins versus regular crystalline insulin often necessitate the use of different dosages for the morning and evening insulin injections; regular crystalline insulin is more potent, and less is required to achieve the same glycemic effect, compared with Lente, NPH, PZI, and Ultralente insulins.

Inadequate or Impaired Insulin Absorption

Slow or inadequate absorption of subcutaneously deposited insulin is most commonly observed in diabetic cats receiving Ultralente insulin, a long-acting insulin that has a slow onset and prolonged duration of effect.[84,85] In approximately 25% of cats evaluated at our hospital, Ultralente insulin is absorbed from the subcutaneous site of deposition too slowly for it to be effective at maintaining acceptable glycemic control. In these cats, the blood glucose concentration may not decrease until 6 to 10 hours after the injection or, more commonly, it decreases minimally despite insulin doses of 8 to 12 U/cat given every 12 hours. As a consequence, the blood glucose concentration remains greater than 300 mg/dL for most of the day. We have had success in these cats by switching from Ultralente to Lente or PZI given twice a day.[85] When a change is made in the type of insulin, the insulin dosage is decreased (usually to amounts initially used to regulate the diabetic cat) to avoid hypoglycemia. The duration of effect of the insulin becomes shorter as the potency of the insulin increases, which may create problems with short duration of insulin effect (Figure 241-12). We have not yet identified similar problems with insulin glargine in diabetic cats, although our experience with this form of insulin is limited.

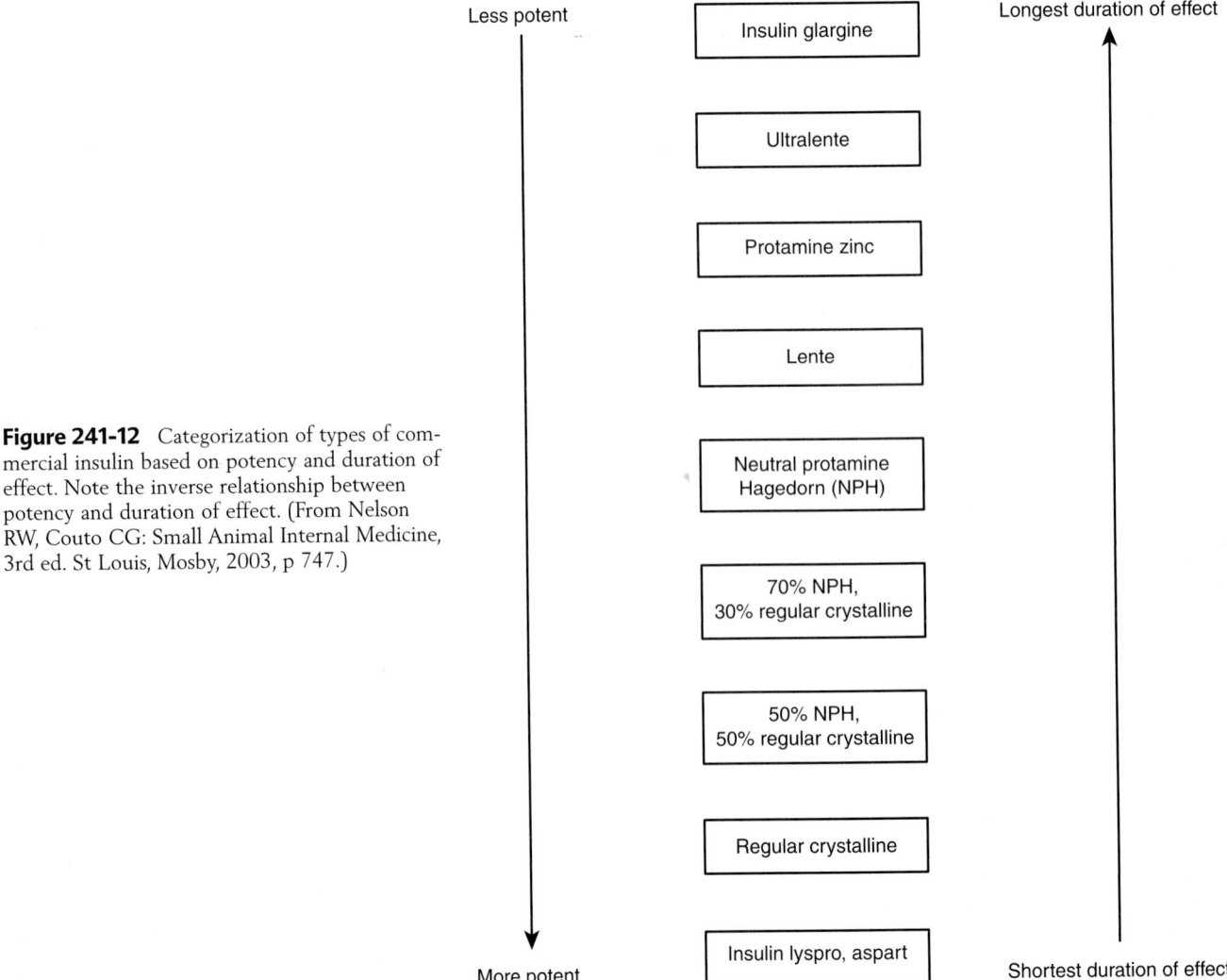

Figure 241-12 Categorization of types of commercial insulin based on potency and duration of effect. Note the inverse relationship between potency and duration of effect. (From Nelson RW, Couto CG: Small Animal Internal Medicine, 3rd ed. St Louis, Mosby, 2003, p 747.)

Impaired absorption of insulin may also occur as a result of thickening of the skin and inflammation of the subcutaneous tissues caused by chronic injection of insulin in the same area of the body. Rotation of the injection site helps prevent this problem.

Circulating Insulin Antibodies

Insulin antibodies result from repeated injection of a foreign protein (i.e., insulin). The structure and amino acid sequence of the injected insulin relative to the native endogenous insulin influences the development of insulin antibodies. Conformational insulin epitopes are believed to be more important in the development of insulin antibodies than differences in the linear subunits of the insulin molecule per se.[86] The more divergent the insulin molecule from the species, the greater the likelihood that significant or worrisome levels of insulin antibodies will develop. Canine and recombinant human insulin are similar, and the development of insulin antibodies is uncommon in dogs treated with recombinant human insulin.[87] In contrast, canine and beef insulin differ, and serum insulin antibodies have been identified in 40% to 65% of dogs treated with beef/pork or beef insulin.[10,86,87] In the author's experience, the presence of serum insulin antibodies is often associated with erratic and poor control of glycemia, frequent adjustments in the insulin dose to improve control, and the occasional development of severe insulin resistance. Dogs treated with recombinant human insulin have more stable control of glycemia for extended periods compared with dogs treated with beef insulin. Although uncommon, insulin antibodies can develop in dogs treated with recombinant human insulin and should be suspected as the cause of poor glycemic control when another cause cannot be identified. Documentation of serum insulin antibodies should use assays that have been validated in diabetic dogs. A switch to porcine source insulin or to a purer form of insulin (i.e., regular crystalline insulin), or both, should be considered if insulin antibodies are identified in a poorly controlled diabetic dog.

Fortunately, insulin antibody formation is not common in diabetic cats treated with exogenous human insulin despite the differences between human and feline insulin.[88] Two studies identified an approximately equal frequency of positive serum insulin antibody titers in diabetic cats treated with beef insulin compared with diabetic cats treated with recombinant human insulin.[14,89] In the author's experience, insulin antibody titers are weakly positive in most cats, the prevalence of persistent titers is low, and serum insulin antibodies do not appear to affect control of glycemia. Overt insulin resistance caused by insulin antibody formation occurs in fewer than 5% of cats treated with recombinant human insulin. Switching from recombinant human insulin to beef/pork source PZI may improve control of glycemia if insulin antibodies are the suspected cause of insulin ineffectiveness.

Concurrent Disorders that Can Cause Insulin Resistance

Insulin resistance is a condition in which a normal amount of insulin produces a subnormal biologic response. Insulin resistance may result from problems occurring before the interaction of insulin with its receptor, at the receptor, or at steps distal to the interaction of insulin and its receptor. Prereceptor problems reduce free metabolically active insulin concentrations; such problems include an increase in insulin degradation or in insulin-binding antibodies. Receptor problems include alterations in the insulin-receptor binding affinity and concentration and the development of insulin-receptor antibodies. Postreceptor problems are difficult to differentiate clinically from receptor problems, and the two types often coexist. In dogs and cats, receptor and postreceptor abnormalities are usually attributable to obesity or to a disorder that causes excessive secretion of an insulin-antagonistic hormone (e.g., cortisol, glucagon, epinephrine, growth hormone, progesterone, or thyroid hormone).

No insulin dose clearly defines insulin resistance. For most diabetic dogs and cats, control of glycemia can usually be attained using 1 U or less of intermediate- or long-acting insulin per kilogram of body weight given twice daily. Insulin resistance should be suspected if control of glycemia is poor despite an insulin dosage in excess of 1.5 U/kg, when excessive amounts of insulin (i.e., greater than 1.5 U/kg) are necessary to maintain the blood glucose concentration below 300 mg/dL, and when control of glycemia is erratic and insulin requirements must be constantly changed in an attempt to maintain control of glycemia. Failure of the blood glucose concentration to decrease below 300 mg/dL during a serial blood glucose curve is suggestive of but not definitive for insulin resistance. An insulin resistance–type blood glucose curve can also result from stress-induced hyperglycemia, the Somogyi phenomenon, and other problems with insulin therapy (Box 241-6), and a decrease in the blood glucose concentration below 300 mg/dL can occur with disorders that cause relatively mild insulin resistance. Serum fructosamine concentrations are typically greater than 500 μmol/L in animals with insulin resistance and can exceed 700 μmol/L if resistance is severe.

In general, any concurrent inflammatory, infectious, hormonal, or neoplastic disorder can cause insulin resistance and can interfere with the effectiveness of insulin therapy (see Box 241-6). In the author's experience, the conditions or disorders that most commonly cause insulin resistance in dogs are treatment with diabetogenic drugs (glucocorticoids), severe obesity, hyperadrenocorticism, diestrus, chronic pancreatitis, renal insufficiency, oral and urinary tract infections, hyperlipidemia, and the development of insulin antibodies in dogs treated with beef insulin. The disorders that most commonly cause insulin resistance in cats are severe obesity, chronic pancreatitis, renal insufficiency, hyperthyroidism, oral infections, acromegaly, and hyperadrenocorticism. Obtaining a complete history and performing a thorough physical examination constitute the most important step in identifying these concurrent disorders. Abnormalities identified on the physical examination may suggest a concurrent insulin-antagonistic disorder or an infectious process, which gives the clinician direction in the diagnostic evaluation of the animal. If the history and physical examination findings are unremarkable, other diagnostic tests should be pursued to further screen for concurrent illness, including a complete blood count, serum biochemical analysis, serum thyroxine concentration (cat), serum progesterone concentration (intact female dog), abdominal ultrasound scan, and urinalysis with bacterial culture. The use of additional tests depends on the results of the initial screening tests (Box 241-7).

CHRONIC COMPLICATIONS OF DIABETES MELLITUS

Complications resulting from diabetes or its treatment are common in diabetic dogs and cats and include blindness and anterior uveitis resulting from cataract formation (dogs), peripheral neuropathy of the hind limbs, causing weakness, inability to jump, a plantigrade stance and ataxia (cats), chronic pancreatitis, recurring infections, hypoglycemia and ketoacidosis (see Box 241-5). Most of the devastating chronic complications of human diabetes (e.g., nephropathy, vasculopathy, and coronary artery disease) require 10 to 20 years or longer to develop and therefore are uncommon in diabetic dogs and cats. Diabetes mellitus is a disease of older dogs and cats, and most do not live beyond 5 years from the time of diagnosis.[12]

Box • 241-6

Recognized Causes of Insulin Ineffectiveness or Insulin Resistance in Diabetic Dogs and Cats

Cause: Insulin Therapy
Inactive insulin
Diluted insulin
Improper administration technique
Inadequate dosage
Somogyi effect
Inadequate frequency of insulin administration
Impaired insulin absorption (especially with Ultralente insulin)
Anti-insulin antibody excess

Cause: Concurrent Disorder
Diabetogenic drugs
   glucocorticoids
   megestral acetate
   progestagens
Hyperadrenocorticism
Diestrus (bitch)
Acromegaly (cat)
Infection (especially of the oral cavity or urinary tract)
Hypothyroidism (dog)
Hyperthyroidism (cat)
Renal insufficiency
Liver insufficiency
Cardiac insufficiency
Glucagonoma (dog)
Pheochromocytoma
Chronic inflammation (especially pancreatitis)
Pancreatic exocrine insufficiency
Severe obesity
Hyperlipidemia
Neoplasia

Box • 241-7

Diagnostic Tests to Consider in the Evaluation of Insulin Resistance in Diabetic Dogs and Cats

Complete blood count (CBC), serum biochemistry panel, urinalysis
Bacterial culture of the urine
Serum lipase and amylase activities (pancreatitis)
Serum trypsin-like immunoreactivity, pancreatic lipase immunoreactivity (exocrine pancreatic insufficiency, pancreatitis)
Adrenocortical function tests
  Adrenocorticotropic hormone (ACTH) stimulation test (spontaneous or iatrogenic hyperadrenocorticism)
  Low-dose dexamethasone suppression test (spontaneous hyperadrenocorticism)
Thyroid function tests
  Baseline serum total and free thyroxine (hypothyroidism or hyperthyroidism)
  Endogenous thyroid-stimulating hormone (TSH) (hypothyroidism)
  TSH stimulation test (hypothyroidism)
  Thyroid-releasing hormone stimulation test (hypothyroidism or hyperthyroidism)
  Triiodothyronine suppression test (hyperthyroidism)
Serum progesterone concentration (diestrus in intact female dog)
Plasma growth hormone or serum insulin—like growth factor I concentration (acromegaly)
Serum insulin concentration 24 hours after discontinuation of insulin therapy (insulin antibodies)
Serum triglyceride concentration (hyperlipidemia)
Abdominal ultrasonography (adrenomegaly, adrenal mass, pancreatitis, pancreatic mass)
Thoracic radiography (cardiomegaly, neoplasia)
Computed tomography or magnetic resonance imaging (pituitary mass)

In the author's experience, owners are usually willing to undertake the care of a diabetic pet once the fears related to chronic complications seen in human diabetics are alleviated.

Cataracts

Cataract formation is the most common chronic complication of diabetes mellitus in the dog. A retrospective cohort study on the development of cataracts in 132 diabetic dogs referred to a university hospital found cataract formation in 14% of dogs at the time diabetes was diagnosed and a time interval of 25%, 50%, 75%, and 80% of the study population to develop cataracts of 60, 170, 370, and 470 days, respectively.[90] The pathogenesis of diabetic cataract formation is thought to stem from altered osmotic relationships in the lens induced by the accumulation of sorbitol and fructose; these sugars are potent hydrophilic agents that cause an influx of water into the lens, leading to swelling and rupture of the lens fibers and the development of cataracts.[91] Cataract formation is an irreversible process once it begins, and it can occur quite rapidly. Diabetic dogs that are poorly controlled and that have problems with wide fluctuations in the blood glucose concentration seem especially at risk for rapid development of cataracts. Blindness may be eliminated by removal of the abnormal lens. Vision is restored in approximately 75% to 80% of diabetic dogs that undergo cataract removal. Factors that affect the success of surgery include the degree of glycemic control and whether retinal disease or lens-induced uveitis is present.

Lens-Induced Uveitis

During embryogenesis, the lens is formed within its own capsule, and its structural proteins are not exposed to the immune system; consequently, immune tolerance to the crystalline proteins does not develop. During cataract formation and resorption, lens proteins are exposed to local ocular immune systems, resulting in inflammation and uveitis. Uveitis that occurs in association with a resorbing, hypermature cataract may decrease the success of cataract surgery and must be controlled before surgery. Treatment of lens-induced uveitis focuses on reduction of the inflammation and prevention of further intraocular damage. Topical ophthalmic corticosteroids are the drugs most commonly used to control ocular inflammation. However, systemic absorption of topically applied corticosteroids may cause insulin antagonism and thus interfere with glycemic control of the diabetic state, especially in toy and miniature breeds. An alternative is topical administration of nonsteroidal anti-inflammatory agents (e.g., 0.03% flurbiprofen) or cyclosporine.

Diabetic Neuropathy

Diabetic neuropathy is the most common chronic complication of diabetes in cats, with a prevalence of approximately 10% of cats with IDDM, but it is infrequently recognized in the diabetic dog. The cause of diabetic neuropathy is not known, although an alteration in polyol pathway activity may play a role in cats. The polyol pathway consists of two consecutive reactions: glucose first is reduced to sorbitol by aldose reductase and sorbitol subsequently is oxidized to fructose by sorbitol dehydrogenase. Aldose reductase is present in the Schwann cell, and accumulation of polyols (e.g., sorbitol, fructose) has been implicated in the pathogenesis of diabetic neuropathy. In a recent study, the severity of neurologic clinical signs and electrophysiologic abnormalities was best related to the blood glucose concentration; nerve water content was significantly elevated in diabetic versus healthy cats, nerve glucose and fructose were increased eightfold and twelvefold in diabetic versus healthy cats, respectively, and nerve myoinositol content in diabetic cats was reduced to 80% of the levels in healthy cats.[92] Myoinositol is a key element in many nerve cellular functions, and myoinositol depletion correlates with reduced nerve conduction velocity in diabetic nerves.[93,94] The role, if any, of other metabolic derangements, such as glycosylation of myelin, in the pathogenesis of diabetic neuropathy in cats remains to be determined.

Clinical signs of diabetic neuropathy include hindlimb weakness; impaired ability to jump; a plantigrade posture, with the cat's hocks touching the ground when it walks (see Figure 241-5); muscle atrophy, especially of the distal pelvic limb; depressed limb reflexes; deficits in postural reaction testing; and irritability on manipulation of the hindlimbs and feet.[92] Clinical signs may progress to include the thoracic limbs. Abnormalities on electrophysiologic testing, which are consistent with demyelination at all levels of the motor and sensory peripheral nerves, include decreased motor and sensory nerve conduction velocities in the pelvic and thoracic limbs and decreased muscle action potential amplitudes.[92,95] Electromyographic abnormalities are usually absent but when identified are consistent with denervation. The most striking abnormality detected on histologic examination of nerve biopsies from affected cats is Schwann cell injury; axonal degeneration is identified in severely affected cats.

Currently, there is no specific therapy for diabetic neuropathy in cats. Aggressive glucoregulation with insulin may improve nerve conduction and reverse the posterior weakness and plantigrade posture in some diabetic cats (see Figure 241-5). However, the response to therapy is variable, and the risks of hypoglycemia increase with aggressive insulin treatment. Generally, the longer the neuropathy has been present and the more severe it is, the less likely improvement in glycemic control is to reverse the clinical signs.

Diabetic Nephropathy

Renal insufficiency and diabetes mellitus are common geriatric diseases that often occur concurrently, especially in older cats. Abnormal renal function may result from the deleterious effects of the diabetic state (i.e., diabetic nephropathy), or it may be an independent problem that develops in conjunction with diabetes in the geriatric pet. Histopathologic findings in diabetic nephropathy depend on the duration of the disease prior to evaluation of the dog or cat and on the degree of glycemic control; these findings include membranous glomerulonephropathy with fusion of the foot processes, glomerular and tubular basement membrane thickening, an increase in the mesangial matrix material, the presence of subendothelial deposits, glomerular fibrosis, and glomerulosclerosis. The pathogenic mechanism of diabetic nephropathy is unknown but is undoubtedly multifactorial. Clinical signs depend on the severity of glomerulosclerosis and the functional ability of the kidney to excrete metabolic wastes. Initially, diabetic nephropathy is manifested as severe proteinuria, primarily albuminuria, as a result of the glomerular dysfunction. As the glomerular changes progress, glomerular filtration becomes progressively impaired, resulting in the development of azotemia and eventually uremia. With severe fibrosis of the glomeruli, oliguric and then anuric renal failure develops. No specific treatment is available for diabetic nephropathy, apart from meticulous metabolic control of the diabetic state, conservative medical management of the renal insufficiency, and control of systemic hypertension.

PROGNOSIS

The prognosis for dogs and cats diagnosed with diabetes mellitus depends in part on the owners' commitment to treating the disorder, the ease of glycemic regulation, the presence and reversibility of concurrent disorders, and the avoidance of chronic complications associated with the diabetic state. The mean survival time for diabetic dogs and cats is approximately 3 years from the time of diagnosis, although survival time is somewhat skewed because dogs and cats are usually 7 years or older at the time of diagnosis, and the mortality rate during the first 6 months is relatively high because of concurrent life-threatening or uncontrollable disease (e.g., ketoacidosis, acute pancreatitis, renal failure).[12] Diabetic dogs and cats that survive the first 6 months can easily maintain a good quality of life for longer than 5 years with proper care by the owners, timely evaluations by the veterinarian, and good client-veterinarian communication.

CHAPTER 242

Hyperadrenocorticism

Claudia E. Reusch

HYPERADRENOCORTICISM IN DOGS

In 1932 Dr. Harvey Cushing, a neurosurgeon, documented the presence of small, basophilic pituitary adenomas in human patients with clinical signs of adrenocortical hyperfunction. Years later, it was found that these tumors produced excess adrenocorticotropic hormone (ACTH), with resultant bilateral adrenocortical hyperplasia. In humans as well as in dogs and cats, pituitary ACTH hypersecretion (Cushing's disease) is now recognized as the most common cause of naturally occurring hyperadrenocorticism (Cushing's syndrome). This condition must be distinguished from other natural causes, such as non-ACTH-dependent adrenocortical tumors and ACTH-secreting nonpituitary tumors (ectopic ACTH syndrome). The latter disorder has not been described in dogs and cats. It is also necessary to differentiate naturally occurring hyperadrenocorticism from iatrogenic causes, which result from chronic glucocorticoid therapy and probably constitute the majority of cases of hyperadrenocorticism.

HYPOTHALAMUS–ADENOHYPOPHYSIS–ADRENAL GLAND AXIS

Neurotransmitters from the central nervous system (CNS) modulate the release of hypophysiotropic hormones, such as corticotropin-releasing hormone (CRH) and arginine vasopressin (AVP), from neurons in the hypothalamus. Both CRH and AVP are considered the predominant stimulating neurohormones for ACTH secretion *in vivo*.[1] CRH consists of 41 aminoacids, and its structure is identical in humans, dogs, rats, and horses.[2] CRH and AVP are released into the hypothalamohypophyseal portal blood system and travel to the corticotropic cells in the anterior pituitary, where they stimulate the release of ACTH. ACTH is a single-chain polypeptide comprising 39 amino acids. The amino acid sequence of ACTH is highly conserved. In all mammals studied thus far, the first 24 amino acids are identical. Canine ACTH differs from human ACTH by only one amino acid residue, at position 37. It is synthesized from a well-characterized precursor molecule, pro-opiomelanocortin (POMC), which also gives rise to a variety of other peptides coreleased with ACTH.

In contrast to humans, the adenohypophysis of dogs and cats has a pars distalis and a discrete pars intermedia (Figure 242-1). The processing of POMC and the regulation of ACTH secretion differ between these two parts. The pars distalis produces mainly ACTH and beta lipotropin (beta-LPH). The pars intermedia contains two cell types and processes alpha melanocyte-stimulating hormone (alpha-MSH) and corticotropin-like intermediate lobe peptide (CLIP) in the predominant A cells. The B cells of the pars intermedia resemble the corticotrophs of the pars distalis, and cleavage of POMC is mainly into ACTH and beta-LPH (Figure 242-2). In the pars intermedia, the release of POMC-derived peptides is largely regulated by tonic dopaminergic inhibition.[3] It has long been assumed that the pars intermedia does not actively secrete ACTH into the circulation. However, the results of a recent study in dogs suggest that the pars intermedia may contribute to circulating ACTH concentrations.[4] The physiologic function of peptides processed from POMC is an exciting area of neuroendocrine research that requires further investigation.

In the adrenal cortex, ACTH stimulates the synthesis and secretion of several hormones, specifically glucocorticoids and androgenic steroids in the zona fasciculata and zona reticularis and mineralocorticoids in the zona glomerulosa. The effect of ACTH is rapid; within minutes, plasma levels of these hormones rise. Because aldosterone is mainly regulated by the renin-angiotensin system and plasma potassium concentrations and because the amount of androgens produced is small, ACTH exerts its most important effect on glucocorticoids. The synthesis and release of glucocorticoids are almost exclusively controlled by ACTH. Cortisol is the major glucocorticoid, and this is the term used to describe glucocorticoids in the following section. Cortisol in turn inhibits ACTH release.

In summary, cortisol secretion is closely regulated by ACTH, and plasma levels of cortisol parallel those of ACTH.

Four mechanisms effect neuroendocrine control:
- Secretion of ACTH in an ultradian pulsatile fashion, which is influenced by the hypothalamus. The number of pulses ranges from six to 12 per 24-hour period.
- Stress responsiveness of the hypothalamus–adenohypophysis–adrenal gland axis. ACTH and cortisol are secreted within minutes after the onset of stress. Stress originates in the CNS and causes increased release of CRH and AVP.
- Feedback inhibition of ACTH by cortisol. Cortisol acts at multiple target sites, two of which have been identified: neurons in the hypothalamus that produce CRH and AVP, and corticotropic cells in the anterior pituitary. Two kinds of feedback are discussed: *fast feedback*, which occurs rapidly and inhibition of which affects stimulated but not basal secretion, and *slow feedback*, which depends on steroid levels and leads to a decrease in ACTH synthesis. Inhibition of slow feedback affects both basal and stimulated ACTH release.
- Release of interleukin-1, interleukin-6, tissue necrosis factor, and other cytokines associated with infection, which activates the hypothalamus–pituitary–adrenal gland axis.

ETIOPATHOLOGY

Cushing's Disease (Pituitary-Dependent Hyperadrenocorticism)

Approximately 80% to 85% of dogs with naturally occurring hyperadrenocorticism suffer from pituitary-dependent hyperadrenocorticism (PDH), which is characterized by overproduction of ACTH (Figure 242-3). In many cases the

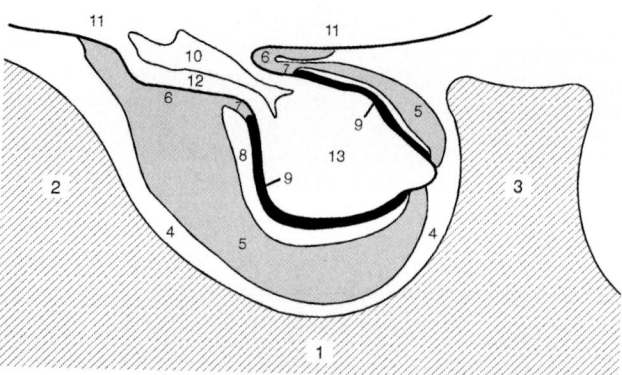

Figure 242-1 Schematic illustration of a median sagittal section through the canine pituitary gland. (Left is rostral, right is caudal.) *1*, Sphenoid bone; *2*, tuberculum sellae; *3*, dorsum sellae; *4*, pituitary fossa; *5*, pars distalis adenohypophysis; *6*, pars infundibularis adenohypophysis; *7*, transitional zone; *8*, hypophyseal cleft or cavity; *9*, pars intermedia adenohypophysis; *10*, third ventricle; *11*, hypothalamus (median eminence); *12*, pars proximalis neurohypophysis; *13*, pars distalis neurohypophysis. (From Meij B: Hypophysectomy as a treatment for canine and feline Cushing's disease. Vet Clin North Am Small Anim Pract 31:1021, 2001.)

pituitary lesions are small adenomas, although in some dogs large tumors, usually adenomas, are found. Pituitary carcinomas, which appear to be rare in dogs, may invade surrounding structures.[5] In a small percentage of dogs with ACTH-dependent disease, corticotropic cell hyperplasia occurs rather than a tumor. Whether hyperplastic lesions occur exclusively or small pituitary tumors are missed during histopathologic examination is a matter of debate.

In about 70% of dogs with PDH the tumors originate in the pars distalis, whereas in about 30% they arise either from the A cells or the B cells of the pars intermedia.[6]

Two hypotheses have been proposed for the pathogenesis of PDH. According to one hypothesis, the disease results from a defect at the hypothalamic level. Secretion of ACTH from the pars intermedia is controlled by tonic dopaminergic inhibition, and some evidence indicates that dopamine affects the pars distalis of the adenohypophysis. A decrease in the central dopamine concentration has been proposed to result in dysregulation of the hypothalamic–adenohypophysis–adrenal gland axis and, in turn, overproduction of ACTH and possible tumor formation.[7] According to the other hypothesis, PDH is caused

by a primary pituitary defect, and increasing evidence substantiates this, such as the monoclonal character of corticotropic adenomas,[8] the occurrence of secondary adrenal insufficiency after selective resection of tumors,[9] and the low CRH concentration in the cerebrospinal fluid of dogs with PDH.[10] The current view is that corticotropic adenomas are the result of a complex, multistage process of tumorigenesis. The earliest stage may be an inherited aberration that plays an initiating or promoting role. A report of the occurrence of PDH in a family of seven Dandie Dinmont terriers supports the role of genetic factors.[11] Clonal expansion of the genomically altered cell may be caused by an intrinsic mutation that results in activation of cell replication; by extrinsic factors, such as intrapituitary growth factors; or by both these mechanisms.[12]

Some reports have addressed pituitary tumor size in dogs. The most extensive tumor proliferation was encountered in dogs with a strong resistance to dexamethasone, therefore it was postulated that a pituitary tumor's growth potential depends on the degree of insensitivity to glucocorticoid feedback.[13] Whether large tumors are more likely to arise from the pars intermedia than the pars distalis has long been the subject of debate. Because the pars intermedia lacks glucocorticoid receptors and extensive tumors appear to be resistant to glucocorticoids, tumors originating in the pars intermedia may grow larger than those in the pars distalis. However, it has also been stated that pituitary tumors do not always maintain the characteristics of the cells of origin and that PDH cannot be simply divided into either pars distalis or pars intermedia type by plasma alpha-MSH levels or dexamethasone resistance.[14]

Another characteristic of corticotropic adenomas is their ability not only to produce ACTH but also to release excessive amounts of ACTH precursors. In dogs with PDH, the ACTH precursor concentration is significantly higher in animals with large pituitary tumors compared with those with small tumors.[15] It is important to be aware of this phenomenon as a clinician. ACTH precursors have low biologic activity, therefore dogs with (large) pituitary tumors may have only subtle or no clinical signs of hyperadrenocorticism.

PDH is also associated with alterations in the release of several pituitary hormones. It generally is agreed that glucocorticoids inhibit the release of AVP in dogs. A recent study found that, compared with controls, dogs with PDH had higher basal plasma levels of prolactin, lower levels of growth hormone (GH), and similar levels of luteinizing hormone (LH) and thyroid-stimulating hormone (TSH).[16]

Functional Adrenocortical Tumor

Among dogs and cats with naturally occurring hyperadrenocorticism, 15% to 20% have a functional adrenocortical tumor (FAT), which secretes cortisol independent of pituitary control.

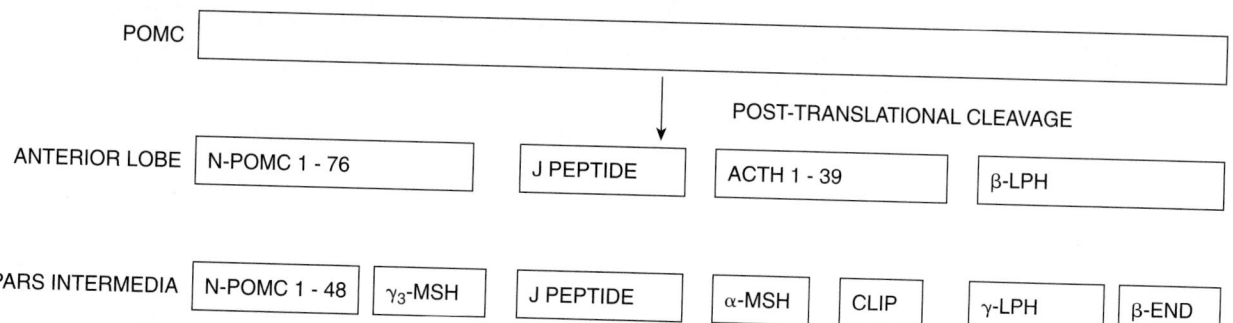

Figure 242-2 Processing of pro-opiomelanocortin (POMC) in the anterior lobe and in the pars intermedia of the pituitary gland. *J Peptide*, Joining peptide; *LPH*, lipoprotein; *MSH*, melanocyte-stimulating hormone; *CLIP*, corticotropin-like intermediate lobe peptide; *END*, endorphin.

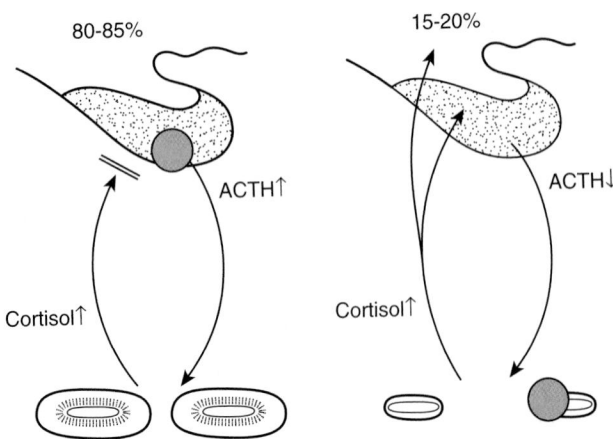

80-85%   15-20%

ACTH↑   ACTH↓

Cortisol↑   Cortisol↑

Figure 242-3 Simplified schematic of the pituitary-adrenal axis in dogs with pituitary-dependent hyperadrenocorticism *(left)* and with functional adrenal tumor *(right)*.

Cortisol in turn suppresses CRH in the hypothalamus and ACTH in the pituitary gland. The result of this chronic negative feedback is cortical atrophy of the uninvolved adrenal gland and atrophy of all normal cells in the involved adrenal gland (see Figure 242-3).

For many years it was assumed that adrenocortical tumors produced large amounts of hormone, more in fact than hyperplastic adrenal glands of dogs with PDH. However, the opposite appears to be true; in many dogs with an FAT, the hormone excess and subsequent clinical signs are only moderate. Therefore, even though adrenocortical tumors usually greatly exceed the size of the normal adrenal gland, the tumor tissue is only moderately active, and the neoplastic transformation results in a decreased degree of function per unit of volume.[17] It is also possible that the cortisol synthesis pathway in dogs with an FAT is not intact. In humans, adrenal carcinomas tend to produce large amounts of intermediates in the biosynthesis of cortisol, and a partial or complete deficiency of 11-beta-hydroxylase is common. The existence of a similar phenomenon in dogs has recently been suggested.[18]

In dogs with an FAT, the right and left adrenal glands are affected with equal frequency. Usually a unilateral, solitary adrenal mass is seen, although bilateral tumors are found in approximately 10% of cases.

Information in the literature on the incidence of adenomas and carcinomas varies, but the two tumor types probably occur with equal frequency. As with other endocrine tumors, it is difficult to distinguish between adrenal adenomas and adrenal carcinomas. Differentiation of adrenocortical tumors and pheochromocytoma may require a pathologist with experience in special immunohistochemical staining techniques. In some cases adrenocortical tumors that initially had been diagnosed as benign turned out to be malignant when metastases were discovered later.

Histologic differentiation between benign and malignant tumors is straightforward only when capsular or vascular invasion by the tumor has occurred. Otherwise, it is difficult to establish the biologic nature of the tumor, and distant metastasis may not occur.[19] Interestingly, it is not uncommon for adrenocortical tumors to be associated with pheochromocytoma.[17]

Simultaneous Occurrence of Pituitary and Adrenocortical Tumors

The co-existence of pituitary and endocrine tumors was recently described in 17 dogs with hyperadrenocorticism. Necropsy or surgery demonstrated unilateral adrenocortical adenoma with contralateral adrenal hyperplasia in 10 dogs; bilateral adrenal cortical adenoma in four dogs; and adrenal carcinoma with contralateral hyperplasia in three dogs. Pituitary lesions included a chromophobe microadenoma in 12 dogs; pituitary macroadenoma in four dogs; and pituitary carcinoma in one dog.[20] Two years later the study was revised, and it was speculated that some of these dogs actually may have had a condition similar to macronodular adrenal hyperplasia in humans.[21]

Adrenocortical Nodular Hyperplasia

In humans, bilateral nodular hyperplasia with hyperadrenocorticism has been identified as a sequel to several pathophysiologic conditions. Long-standing ACTH hypersecretion may result in nodular enlargement of the adrenal gland. Over time, these nodules may become autonomous or semiautonomous. Another type of nodular hyperplasia has been called *massive macronodular adrenal hyperplasia*. This type is ACTH independent and is characterized by bilateral large nodules that secrete excessive amounts of cortisol. This condition suggests that non-ACTH factors may induce cortisol secretion.[22] Recent studies indicate that receptors for various hormones may be abnormally expressed by the adrenal glands; for example, ectopic expression of the gastric inhibitory polypeptide receptor has been convincingly demonstrated.[23] This polypeptide stimulates the release of cortisol *in vivo* and *in vitro*. It is assumed that adrenocortical nodular hyperplasia also exists in dogs, although studies currently are lacking.

Clinical Findings

Hyperadrenocorticism, or Cushing's syndrome, is one of the most common endocrinopathies in dogs. The clinical signs and laboratory results in dogs with hyperadrenocorticism are largely attributable to chronic glucocorticoid excess and, to a much lesser extent, overproduction of adrenal androgens. In a few cases, symptoms are due to tumor growth, local invasion of tumors, or metastases.

Signalment

Dogs with naturally occurring hyperadrenocorticism are usually 6 years of age or older (the average age is 9 to 11 years). Of 100 dogs with Cushing's syndrome diagnosed in our clinic, only five were younger than 6 years, and all had PDH: two of the dogs were 5 years old (a German shepherd and a dachshund), one was 4 years old (a cocker spaniel), and two were 2 years old (a weimaraner and a puli). Dogs with an FAT tend to be older than dogs with PDH.[24]

A number of different breeds and mixed breeds with hyperadrenocorticism have been reported. The most commonly represented breeds are poodles, dachshunds, beagles, boxers, and various terrier breeds. Approximately 75% of dogs with PDH weigh less than 20 kg.[24] FAT most often occurs in poodles, German shepherds, dachshunds, Labrador retrievers, and various terrier breeds. Approximately 45% to 50% of dogs with an FAT weigh more than 20 kg.[24] Between 55% and 60% of dogs with hyperadrenocorticism are female.[24]

History and Physical Examination

Dogs with hyperadrenocorticism may have a number of dramatic clinical signs, although affected animals are usually in stable condition. Severe apathy, vomiting, diarrhea, muscle pain, and anorexia are not characteristic symptoms of Cushing's syndrome, therefore these signs indicate another disease or complications of hyperadrenocorticism (see below).

The clinical signs of hyperadrenocorticism are the sequelae to the combined gluconeogenic, immune-suppressive, anti-inflammatory, protein catabolic, and lipolytic effects of glucocorticoids exerted on various organ systems. PDH cannot be distinguished from FAT on the basis of the type or duration of symptoms.

Clinical signs, which may vary from mild to severe, depend on the duration of the disease and the degree of cortisol excess. Usually the course of hyperadrenocorticism is insidious and slowly progressive. Rarely, clinical signs are intermittent, with periods of remission and relapse in dogs with mild disease.[25] Fewer dogs are presented with severe clinical signs today than in years past, probably because of today's owners' heightened awareness of their pets' problems. Consequently, diagnosis of the disease may be more difficult in dogs with mild symptoms.

Typical symptoms include polydipsia, polyuria, polyphagia, truncal obesity or abdominal enlargement (due to hepatomegaly, muscle wasting and/or intra-abdominal fat accumulation), thin haircoat, failure to regrow shaved hair, alopecia (may or may not be bilaterally symmetric, usually sparing the head and extremities), thin skin, pyoderma, panting, muscle weakness, muscle atrophy and lethargy. Less common signs are heat intolerance, seborrhea, comedones, hyperpigmentation, calcinosis cutis, bruising, testicular atrophy, failure to cycle, clitoral hypertrophy, and facial paralysis (Table 242-1). In rare cases (five out of 800 dogs),[26] affected dogs develop a characteristic stiff gait, most often restricted to the pelvic limbs, called *myotonia* or *myotonia-like syndrome.*

It is important to note that the number and severity of these signs vary remarkably. Dogs with Cushing's syndrome may have only one sign or may have almost all the signs listed. In our clinic, 30% of the dogs with hyperadrenocorticism had only polydipsia and polyuria, and 10% had only dermatologic problems (Figure 242-4).

Dogs that develop Cushing's syndrome during the first year of life show weight gain and growth retardation in addition to more typical signs (i.e., polydipsia, polyuria, and alopecia).[26]

Clinicopathologic Findings

When the results of the clinical examination lead to a presumptive diagnosis of Cushing's syndrome, further diagnostic testing is required, including hematology, a biochemical profile, urinalysis, radiography and, when applicable, ultrasonography. These tests detect typical abnormalities associated with hyperadrenocorticism and rule out other diseases with similar signs, such as chronic renal failure, diabetes mellitus, liver diseases, hypothyroidism, diabetes insipidus, and the side effects of anticonvulsant drugs. Concomitant problems, such as urinary tract infection, can also be investigated. A definitive diagnosis of Cushing's syndrome necessitates specific tests.

Hemogram Under the influence of increased glucocorticoids, most dogs develop a so-called stress leukogram, which is characterized by neutrophilia without a left shift, lymphopenia, eosinopenia, and monocytosis. Neutrophilia does not imply greater resistance to infection in affected dogs, because cell function is impaired. Not all changes are present in dogs with hyperadrenocorticism, but lymphopenia and eosinopenia are the most consistent abnormalities. It should be emphasized that a stress leukogram is a nonspecific finding that occurs in many sick dogs. In our clinic, 87% of the dogs with hyperadrenocorticism have thrombocytosis, with counts ranging from 403,000 to 1,140,000 platelets/μL.

Biochemical profile About 85% to 95% of dogs with hyperadrenocorticism show increases in serum alkaline phosphatase (ALP) activity. This is partly due to the induction of a glucocorticoid isoenzyme, which is unique to the dog and is a hyperglycosylated form of the intestinal isoenzyme.[27] Some maintain that determination of the levels of this isoenzyme is a valuable test in the diagnosis of hyperadrenocorticism. Several methods, such as levamisole inhibition[28] and heat inactivation,[29] have been described. Although these tests

Table • 242-1

Clinical Signs in Dogs with Hyperadrenocorticism

CLINICAL SIGN	INCIDENCE (% OF CASES)
Polydipsia/polyuria	80-91
Alopecia	60-74
Pendulous abdomen	67-73
Hepatomegaly	51-67
Polyphagia	46-57
Muscle weakness	14-57
Anestrus	54
Muscle atrophy	35
Comedones	25-34
Panting	30
Hyperpigmentation	23-30
Testicular atrophy	29
Calcinosis cutis	8-15
Facial nerve paralysis	7

Modified from Ling et al 1979; Peterson ME: Hyperadrenocorticism. *In* Peterson ME (ed): The Veterinary Clinics of North America, Small Animal Pracitce—Endocrinology. Philadelphia, WB Saunders, 1984, p 731; and unpublished data from the author. Not all symptoms were mentioned in all three studies, therefore the number of dogs varies among the symptoms. The total number of dogs in the three studies was 457.
*From the history and physical examination.

have a high sensitivity, their lack of specificity makes them unsuitable as diagnostic tests. The increase in ALP activity may be dramatic; levels above 1000 U/L are frequently seen. However, no correlation exists between ALP activity and the severity of hyperadrenocorticism, the response to therapy, or the prognosis.[26]

In 50% to 80% of dogs, a mild increase in alanine aminotransferase (ALT) activity is seen (less than 400 IU/L), which is attributed to hepatocellular leakage associated with cell swelling or minor necrosis. Mild to moderate increases in the cholesterol and triglyceride concentrations are common (50% to 90% of dogs) and are believed to be the result of increased lipolysis. Often affected dogs have alterations in glucose metabolism, although only about 10% of dogs develop overt diabetes mellitus. Mild fasting hyperglycemia may be seen in 30% to 40% of dogs. The blood urea nitrogen and creatinine concentrations are low as a result of diuresis in about 30% to 50% of cases. Hypophosphatemia has been described in 38% of 300 dogs with hyperadrenocorticism.[30] Mild increases in the sodium concentration and mild decreases in the potassium concentration occur in few dogs with Cushing's syndrome.

Serum bile acids may be mildly elevated in up to 30% of cases.[31] When primary liver disease is considered a major differential diagnosis, this finding, together with an elevation in liver enzymes, may be confusing (Table 242-2).

Urinalysis Urinalysis is an important part of the diagnostic workup. It is recommended that owners obtain a urine sample for determination of the specific gravity at home. Collection of a urine sample in hospitalized dogs with Cushing's syndrome is not recommended, because water intake often is decreased in a stressful environment. Most water-deprived dogs with hyperadrenocorticism are able to concentrate the urine, with specific gravities reaching 1.025 to 1.035. In 85% of dogs with Cushing's syndrome, the urine specific

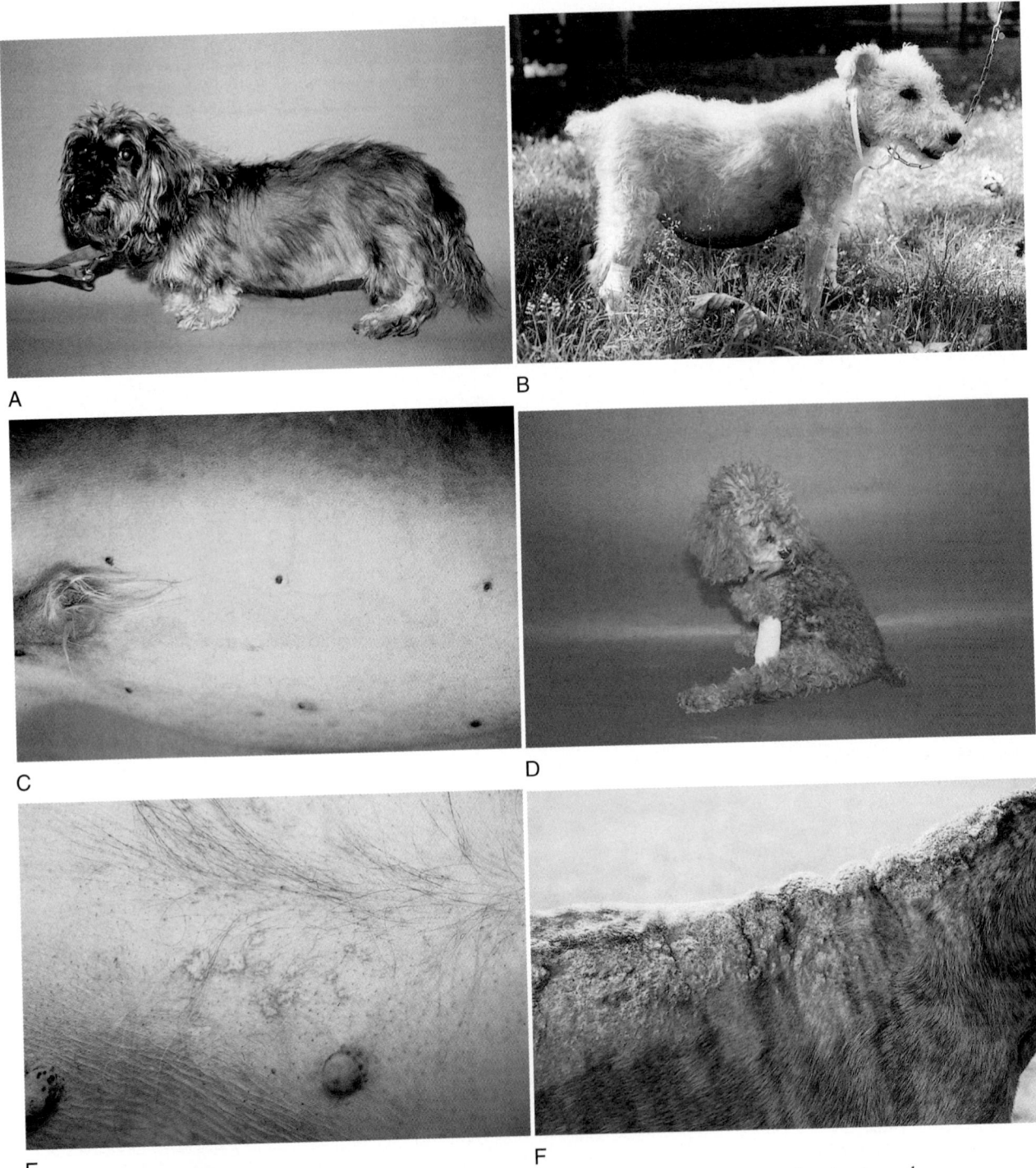

Figure 242-4 **A,** Dachshund with pituitary-dependent hyperadrenocorticism showing truncal obesity, truncal alopecia, and sparse, fine remaining hair. **B,** Fox terrier with a functional adrenal tumor showing truncal obesity and truncal alopecia; the latter is less pronounced than in the dog in A. **C,** Terrier cross with pituitary-dependent hyperadrenocorticism showing ventral alopecia, thin skin, and prominent vasculature. **D,** Poodle with pituitary-dependent hyperadrenocorticism showing a stiff gait involving the pelvic limbs. This abnormality, called *myotonia-like syndrome*, occurs in only a few dogs. **E,** Dachshund with pituitary-dependent hyperadrenocorticism showing mild calcinosis cutis. **F,** Boxer with pituitary-dependent hyperadrenocorticism showing severe calcinosis cutis.

Table • 242-2

Frequently Encountered Clinicopathologic Abnormalities in Dogs with Hyperadrenocorticism

CINICOPATHOLOGIC FINDINGS	INCIDENCE (% OF CASES)
Increased ALP	85-95
Hyperlipidemia	50-90
Increased ALT	50-80
Decreased BUN	30-50
Fasting hyperglycemia*	30-40
Hypophosphatemia	38
Urine specific gravity <1.015-1.020	80
Proteinuria (UPC >1.0)	60-80
Urinary tract infection	40-50
Glucosuria	10

From Peterson ME: Hyperadrenocorticism. *In* Peterson ME (ed): The Veterinary Clinics of North America, Small Animal Practice—Endocrinology. Philadelphia, WB Saunders, 1984, p 731; Feldman EC, Nelson RW: Canine and Feline Endocrinology and Reproduction, 2nd ed. Philadelphia, WB Saunders, 1996, p 187; and from unpublished data from this author.
*Only about 10% of dogs develop overt diabetes mellitus.
ALP, Alkaline phosphatase; *ALT*, alanine aminotransferase; *BUN*, blood urea nitrogen; *UPC*, urine protein concentration.

gravity of samples obtained at home is less than 1.015 to 1.020.[26] Glucosuria occurs in dogs with overt diabetes mellitus. Glucose is not found in the urine of dogs with hyperglycemia below the renal threshold. Many dogs with hyperadrenocorticism have proteinuria, which in some may be due to urinary tract infection. The urine protein/creatinine ratio in dogs with Cushing's syndrome usually ranges from 1.0 to 6.0 (normal is less than 1.0).

Long-term administration of glucocorticoids results in glomerular lesions and proteinuria in dogs.[32] The mechanisms by which glucocorticoids cause glomerular disease are not yet fully understood. Glucocorticoids may enhance the development of antigen excess by delaying clearance of immune complexes. Glomerular damage may also be caused by hypertension; many dogs with hyperadrenocorticism are hypertensive, and a relationship between hypertension and proteinuria has been postulated.[33] Proteinuria in dogs with hyperadrenocorticism does not lead to hypoalbuminemia.

Almost 50% of dogs with hyperadrenocorticism have a urinary tract infection,[34] and bacterial culture of a urine sample obtained by cystocentesis should be performed in all such dogs. As a result of immunosuppression and/or dilution, urinary sediment frequently is inactive despite bacterial infection, therefore sediment examination must not replace urine culture.

Thyroid function tests More than 50% of dogs with hyperadrenocorticism have a total serum thyroxine (T$_4$) concentration below the reference range. Free T$_4$ is low in about 25% of cases.[35] Possible mechanisms include alterations in serum thyroid hormone binding and/or alterations in peripheral hormone metabolism. Glucocorticoids may also suppress TSH release from the pituitary. In dogs with clinical signs suggestive of both hyperadrenocorticism and hypothyroidism (alopecia, weight gain, lethargy), diagnosis may be difficult, and misdiagnosis may occur if the endocrine tests are not carried out in the correct order. In such cases, hyperadrenocorticism must be ruled out before tests for hypothyroidism

are performed. Determination of the circulating thyroid-stimulating hormone (cTSH) concentration is not always helpful; although dogs with Cushing's syndrome usually have normal or decreased cTSH concentrations, about one third of dogs with hypothyroidism have low-normal cTSH concentrations.[36-38] Thyroid hormone supplementation is thought to be unnecessary because thyroid hormone concentrations return to normal after successful treatment of hyperadrenocorticism.

Diagnostic imaging

Thoracic radiographs Radiographic manifestations of hyperadrenocorticism include mineralization of the tracheobronchial tree and pulmonary parenchyma. Although these abnormalities appear to be significantly more common in dogs with hyperadrenocorticism, they are considered nonspecific.[39] Even though the clinical consequences have not been fully elucidated, pulmonary mineralization may contribute to the hypoxemia seen in dogs with hyperadrenocorticism.[40]

In dogs with an adrenal tumor, thoracic radiographs should be examined for metastases. Pulmonary thromboembolism is a potential complication of hyperadrenocorticism (see below). In dogs with sudden onset of dyspnea, radiographs should be carefully evaluated for abnormalities.

Abdominal radiographs Radiographic findings associated with Cushing's syndrome are hepatomegaly, obesity, and good contrast and mineralization of the adrenal glands and other soft tissue structures. However, it was recently shown that hepatomegaly, obesity, and osteopenia are nonspecific and also may be seen in dogs with diabetes mellitus or hypothyroidism. The same study also reported that adrenal mineralization and calcinosis cutis were rarely seen and only in dogs with hyperadrenocorticism.[39] Approximately 50% of adrenal tumors are calcified, which allows good radiographic visualization. No difference is seen between adenomas and carcinomas regarding calcification; approximately 50% of both types undergo calcification.[41]

Ultrasonography An increase in experience among radiologists and improved resolution of imaging equipment have made visualization of the adrenal glands possible in almost all healthy dogs. However, a systematic approach is necessary for accurate identification and evaluation of the glands. Measurement of the dorsoventral dimension (thickness) appears to be the most accurate means of assessing size. Normal thickness has been reported to be 3 to 7.5 mm.[42,43] In dogs with PDH, the adrenal glands have a bilaterally symmetric appearance. It is important to remember that the absolute adrenal thickness is of limited diagnostic value because reference ranges have been established with limited numbers of dogs; different breeds may have different reference ranges; diseases other than hyperadrenocorticism may cause adrenomegaly (possibly stress related); and the measurement may be within the reference range of a dog population but may be enlarged for an individual dog. Ultrasonography, therefore, should not be used to diagnose Cushing's syndrome but rather to differentiate PDH from FAT. The shape and echogenicity of the adrenal glands in dogs with PDH are usually normal although focal areas of increased echogenicity and loss of the bilayer appearance are possible.

In comparison, the affected adrenal gland of a dog with an FAT often has an irregular, rounded shape with mixed echogenicity. In some cases the tumor appears as a homogenous nodule (Figure 242-5). The size and shape of adrenal tumors are variable and do not allow differentiation between adenoma and carcinoma. In a study of a small number of dogs with an FAT, all tumors of a thickness greater than 4 cm were malignant.[44] Therefore the likelihood that an adrenal tumor is malignant may increase as its size increases. Other possible ultrasonographic findings include adrenal mineralization, renal displacement, and compression or invasion of the caudal vena cava (Doppler ultrasonography is a valuable tool for diagnosing compression or invasion). Both adrenal glands should always be visualized, for several reasons: (1) bilateral tumors do occur; (2) in quite a few dogs, the adrenal gland contralateral to an adrenal tumor is not decreased in size, and the diagnosis would be missed if only the normal gland is imaged[45]; and (3) concurrent FAT and PDH are possible.

Ultrasonography is useful for detecting local invasion and distant metastases in dogs with an FAT and for revealing other abnormalities, such as urinary calculi and an enlarged renal pelvis (indicating pyelonephritis). In most dogs with hyperadrenocorticism, the liver is enlarged and has increased echogenicity. As with most diagnostic tools, ultrasonography has its limitations; it is difficult or impossible to differentiate between bilateral nodular hyperplasia and bilateral adrenal tumors, and between an FAT and other adrenal tumors (e.g., pheochromocytoma or metastatic tumor).

Specific endocrine testing   Further diagnostic workup of dogs suspected of having Cushing's disease is a two-step procedure. The first step is to confirm hyperadrenocorticism, and the second is to differentiate between PDH and FAT. Because the treatment protocols and risks are different for PDH and FAT, the second step should always be undertaken. In dogs with a unilateral adrenal tumor, adrenalectomy may be the treatment of choice, although owners should be informed of the risk of metastasis (approximately 50% of FATs are carcinomas). When mitotane is the chosen treatment, the dose usually is higher for dogs with FAT than for those with PDH. Therefore, if the etiology is unknown, dogs that have an FAT may not respond to a dose of mitotane tailored for treatment of PDH. In addition, it is important to diagnose an FAT correctly so that owners can be informed of the risk of tumor growth.

The screening tests used routinely in the diagnosis of hyperadrenocorticism are the urine cortisol to creatinine

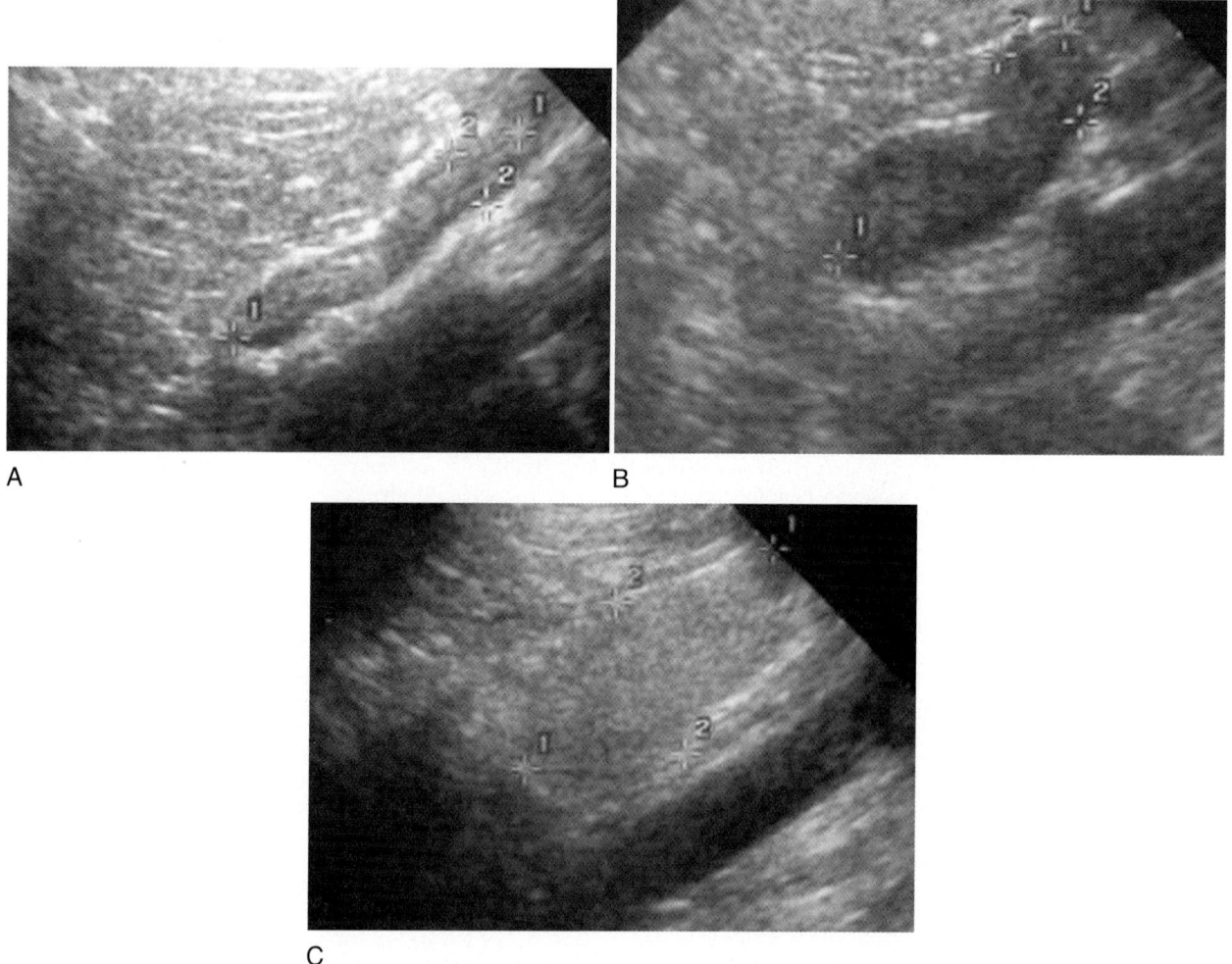

A

B

C

Figure 242-5 **A,** Longitudinal ultrasonographic view of the left adrenal gland of a healthy dog. The adrenal gland is peanut shaped and hypoechoic compared to the surrounding tissue. It is 2.9 cm long and 0.5 cm wide (thick). **B,** Longitudinal ultrasonographic view of the left adrenal gland of a dog with pituitary-dependent hyperadrenocorticism. The adrenal gland is still peanut shaped, but it is plumper than the one shown in **A.** This adrenal gland is 2.4 cm long and 0.8 cm wide (thick). It should be noted that measurements have limited diagnostic value, because the adrenal size of a variety of dogs with pituitary-dependent hyperadrenocorticism falls within reference ranges. **C,** Longitudinal ultrasonographic view of a right-sided adrenocortical tumor. The adrenal gland is seen as a rounded mass with increased echogenicity (length, 2.7 cm; width [thickness], 1.3 cm).

(C:C) ratio, the ACTH stimulation test, and the low-dose dexamethasone test. The question as to which of these is the best screening test is difficult to answer; each has advantages and disadvantages. For a sound interpretation of these tests, their accuracy, sensitivity, and specificity must be considered, as well as the prevalence of the disease. As a general rule, it is extremely important that dogs be carefully selected for testing and that the test be delayed if concomitant disease is a factor. Also, test results should be interpreted in relation to clinical signs.

Differentiating tests for hyperadrenocorticism include the extended low-dose dexamethasone test, high-dose dexamethasone test, extended urine C:C ratio, measurement of the ACTH concentration, adrenal ultrasonography, computed tomography (CT) and magnetic resonance imaging (MRI).

Screening tests

Urine cortisol to creatinine ratio Measurement of the urine C:C ratio is an easily performed test of adrenocortical function. In animals with hyperadrenocorticism, urine cortisol excretion increases as a reflection of augmented adrenal cortisol secretion.[46] Determination of the urine C:C ratio provides an integrated picture of glucocorticoid production by adjusting for fluctuations in plasma levels.[47] Numerous studies on the diagnostic value of the urine C:C ratio[48] have concluded that this test has a high sensitivity (up to 100%) but a low specificity (values as low as 20% are given) (Figure 242-6). Therefore determination of the urine C:C ratio has been advocated as a good test for ruling out hyperadrenocorticism.

Several important points should be considered when the urine C:C ratio is used. Most corticoid measured in the urine is free cortisol. However, depending on the assay used, varying amounts of cortisol metabolites may be detected. It is imperative, therefore, that each laboratory generate its own reference ranges. It is preferable that morning urine samples be submitted, although no consistent diurnal fluctuations have been demonstrated.[46] Also, urine samples for determination of the cortisol/creatinine ratio should be collected at home by the owner to avoid the influence of stress on glucocorticoid secretion.[49]

When the urine C:C ratios of 111 dogs with PDH were compared with those of 49 dogs with an FAT, the highest values were found in dogs with PDH. In dogs with a urine C:C ratio greater than 100×10^{-6} (reference range, less than 10×10^{-6}), the calculated probability of PDH is 90%.[50]

ACTH stimulation test The ACTH stimulation test, which measures the response of the adrenal glands to maximal ACTH stimulation, is a test of adrenal gland reserve. The major function of this test is to diagnose or rule out hypoadrenocorticism. It has a sensitivity of 60% to 85% and a specificity of 85% to 90% (Figure 242-7). The sensitivity is higher (up to 85%) for the diagnosis of PDH than for the diagnosis of FAT (approximately 60%).[48] However, it is not possible to differentiate PDH from an FAT by means of the ACTH stimulation test on an individual case basis.

Several test protocols have been described that use either aqueous porcine ACTH gel (Acthar® Gel, Questcor Pharmaceuticals, Inc., Union City, USA; not available in certain countries) or a synthetic polypeptide containing the first 24 aminoacids of ACTH (Cortrosyn, Synacthen). Plasma samples are obtained before and 2 hours after intramuscular injection of 2.2 IU/kg of ACTH gel to determine the cortisol concentration. With the synthetic preparations, most protocols recommend collection of plasma before and 1 hour after intramuscular or intravenous[51] administration of 250 μg of synthetic ACTH. However, maximal stimulation of the adrenal glands can also be achieved with a dosage of 5 μg of synthetic ACTH per kilogram of body weight.[52] Reconstituted ACTH can be stored in plastic syringes at −20° C for 6 months.[53] The normal baseline cortisol concentration is 0.5 to 6 μg/dL, and the normal post-ACTH cortisol concentration is 6 to 17 μg/dL.

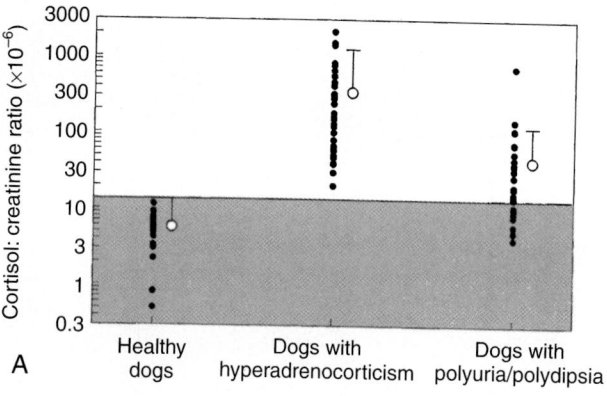

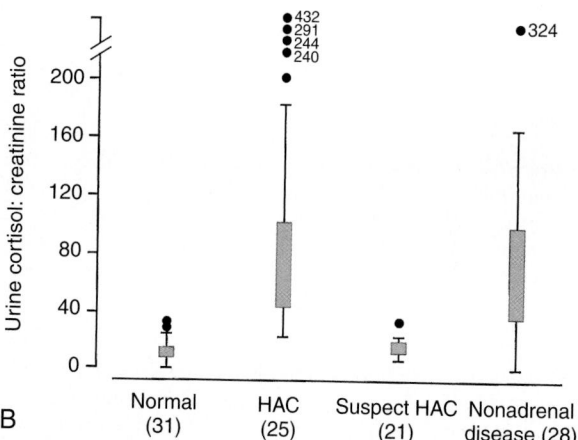

Figure 242-6 **A,** Urine cortisol to creatinine (C:C) ratios from healthy dogs, dogs with naturally occurring hyperadrenocorticism, and dogs with polyuria and polydipsia due to disorders other than hyperadrenocorticism. These values illustrate that the C:C ratio is a sensitive test for Cushing's syndrome, but it is not specific and should not be used as the sole test to confirm a diagnosis. **B,** Box plots of the urine C:C ratios found in normal dogs, dogs with hyperadrenocorticism (HAC), dogs in which hyperadrenocorticism initially was suspected but that did not have the disease (suspect HAC), and dogs with a variety of severe nonadrenal diseases. The number of dogs in each group is shown in parentheses. The box represents the interquartile range from the 25th to the 75th percentile (representing the middle half of the data). The horizontal bar through the box is the median. The "whiskers" represent the main body of data, which in most cases is equal to the range. Outlying data points are represented by the circles (exact values are given for these cases). These data illustrate that the urine C:C ratio is sensitive but not specific for the diagnosis of Cushing's syndrome. (**A** from Feldman EC, Mack RE: Urine cortisol:creatinine ratio as a screening test for hyperadrenocorticism in dogs. J Am Vet Med Assoc 200:1637, 1992; **B** from Smiley LE, Peterson ME: Evaluation of a urine cortisol: creatinine ratio as a screening test for hyperadrenocorticism in dogs. J Vet Intern Med 7:163, 1993.)

Post-stimulation cortisol values between 17 and 22 μg/dL are considered borderline; values above 22 μg/dL are consistent with hyperadrenocorticism.

There are several reasons to use of this test despite its relatively low sensitivity. First, it is the only test to differentiate between iatrogenic and naturally occurring hyperadrenocorticism. Second, because the test is frequently used to monitor medical therapy, it appears helpful to know the stimulation capacity of the adrenal glands prior to treatment. A possible third reason was recently revealed. It has been hypothesized

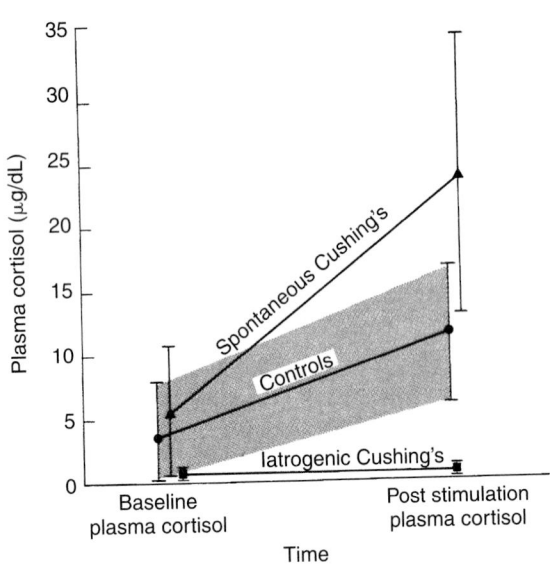

Figure 242-7 Mean radioimmunoassay (RIA) plasma cortisol concentrations (±2 SD) determined before and 1 hour after administration of synthetic ACTH in control dogs, dogs with spontaneous hyperadrenocorticism, and dogs with iatrogenic hyperadrenocorticism.

that some dogs with hyperadrenocorticism that have normal ACTH stimulation results, in fact have a derangement of the steroid synthesis pathway; this would lead to abnormally increased precursor concentrations but normal concentrations of the end product, cortisol. Preliminary evaluations revealed that 17-hydroxprogesterone, one of the precursors, showed an exaggerated response to ACTH stimulation in dogs with Cushing's syndrome, which had abnormal or normal cortisol responses.[54] Further studies are needed to confirm whether the measurement of 17-hydroxprogesterone or other precursor concentrations is helpful in the diagnosis of canine Cushing's syndrome.

Low-dose dexamethasone suppression test Dexamethasone is a synthetic glucocorticoid that does not cross-react with cortisol assays, therefore it can be used to evaluate the pituitary–adrenal gland axis. In normal dogs, the cortisol concentration decreases 2 to 3 hours after administration of dexamethasone and remains low for up to 24 to 48 hours. In dogs with hyperadrenocorticism, the pituitary–adrenal gland axis is abnormally resistant to the suppressive effects of dexamethasone and/or dexamethasone is metabolized more rapidly than normal. For the low-dose dexamethasone suppression (LDDS) test, blood samples are collected before and 4 and 8 hours after intravenous administration of dexamethasone at a dosage of 0.01 mg/kg. Either dexamethasone sodium phosphate or dexamethasone in polyethylene glycol may be used. In normal dogs the cortisol concentration is less than 1.4 μg/dL at 4 and 8 hours after dexamethasone administration. The cortisol concentration 8 hours after dexamethasone administration is used to detect hyperadrenocorticism; a concentration equal to or greater than 1.4 μg/dL is consistent with hyperadrenocorticism. The cortisol concentration at 4 and 8 hours after dexamethasone administration is also used as a differentiating test (see later). For the diagnosis of hyperadrenocorticism, the sensitivity of the test at 8 hours after dexamethasone administration is higher (85% to 95%) than the specificity (70% to 75%) (Figure 242-8).[48]

Misleading results All three screening tests can have false-positive results in dogs suffering from nonadrenal disease,[55] therefore testing of such animals for hyperadrenocorticism

should be avoided if possible. In general, a definitive diagnosis of hyperadrenocorticism should never be made solely on the basis of positive test results; the history and clinical findings should be considered carefully with each dog.

The extent to which phenobarbital treatment affects the results of screening tests is unclear. A review of the literature suggests that test results probably are not affected by this drug.

Glucocorticoid-induced alkaline phosphatase isoenzyme, liver biopsy, and combined dexamethasone suppression and ACTH stimulation tests None of these tests give reliable results, therefore they are not recommended as screening tests for hyperadrenocorticism.

Differentiating tests

Extended low-dose dexamethasone suppression test In dogs with an FAT, pituitary ACTH secretion is suppressed as a result of autonomous secretion of cortisol from the tumor. Administration of dexamethasone has no effect on the pituitary, and cortisol secretion therefore continues. Pituitary tumors have variable sensitivities to feedback inhibition, and the result is different response patterns after dexamethasone application.

The LDDS test can be used to identify dogs with PDH based on three criteria: a 4-hour cortisol concentration of less than 1.4 μg/dL; a 4-hour cortisol concentration of less than 50% of the basal cortisol concentration; and an 8-hour cortisol concentration of less than 50% of the basal cortisol concentration but equal to or greater than 1.4 μg/dL. When one or more of these criteria are met, the dog most likely has PDH.

Approximately 25% of dogs with PDH have a 4-hour cortisol concentration of less than 1.4 μg/dL; 60% have a 4-hour cortisol concentration of less than 50% of the basal concentration; and 25% have an 8-hour cortisol concentration of less than 50% of the baseline value. Overall, approximately 60% of dogs with PDH meet at least one of the three criteria. Dexamethasone resistance (none of the criteria are met) occurs in about 40% of dogs with PDH and in virtually all dogs with an FAT.[56] In such dogs another differentiating test must be used (see Figure 242-8).

A significant positive correlation was found between the size of the pituitary tumor and resistance to dexamethasone using the high-dose dexamethasone suppression test.[13] According to a preliminary study, similar results may be achieved with the LDDS test. Dogs with large pituitary tumors were significantly more often resistant to dexamethasone (according to the criteria cited above) than dogs with small tumors.[57]

High-dose dexamethasone suppression test Traditionally, the high-dose dexamethasone suppression (HDDS) test has been used to differentiate PDH from an FAT. In dogs with an FAT, even large doses of dexamethasone should not suppress plasma cortisol levels. In contrast, administration of a large dose of dexamethasone should suppress ACTH secretion in most dogs with PDH. The test protocol is the same as that for the LDDS test except that a dexamethasone dosage of 0.1 mg/kg is used. Suppression is defined as a cortisol concentration less than 50% of the baseline concentration or less than 1.4 μg/dL at 4 or 8 hours after injection of dexamethasone. Suppression of the cortisol concentration occurs in approximately 75% of dogs with PDH, whereas suppression virtually never occurs in dogs with an FAT. The HDDS test, therefore, is interpreted as follows: If the cortisol concentration is suppressed, a dog most likely has PDH; if no suppression of cortisol levels occurs, a dog may have either PDH or an FAT.

According to the results of one study,[13] if the cortisol concentration is not suppressed in the HDDS test, a dog with PDH may have large pituitary tumors.

Many dogs with PDH that show suppression of the cortisol concentration on the HDDS test also show cortisol

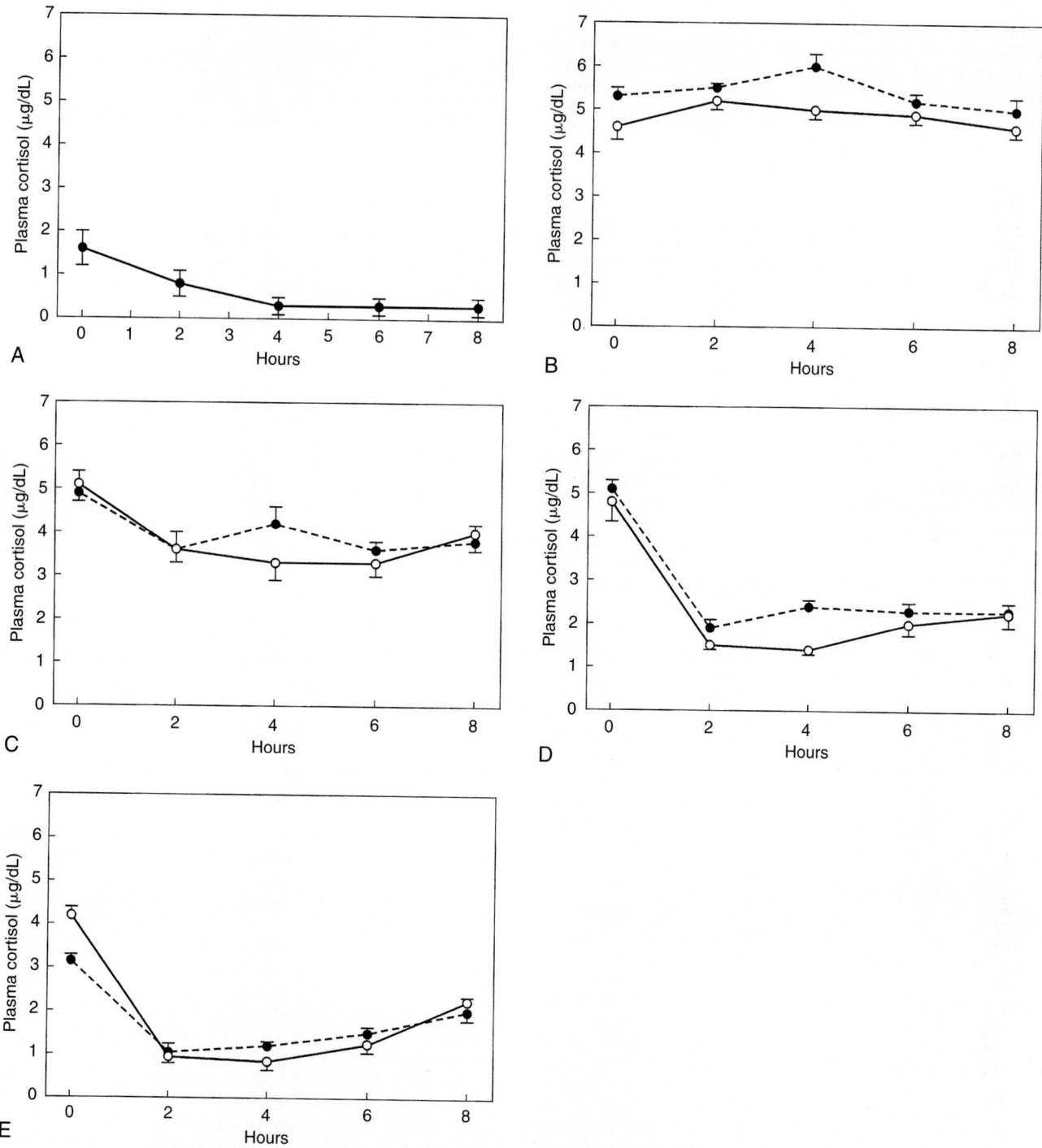

Figure 242-8 Mean plasma cortisol concentrations before and after administration of a low dose of dexamethasone in **(A)** 27 normal dogs; **(B)** 48 dogs with adrenocortical tumors; **(C)** 130 dogs with pituitary-dependent hyperadrenocorticism (PDH); **(D)** the dogs among the 178 with Cushing's syndrome that had at least one plasma cortisol concentration less than 1.4 µg/dL after dexamethasone administration (total, 54; each had PDH); and **(E)** the dogs among the 178 with Cushing's syndrome that, after dexamethasone administration, had at least one plasma cortisol concentration less than 50% of the baseline concentration (total, 95; each had PDH). Note the two curves for graphs **B, C, D,** and **E.** These represent the use of dexamethasone sodium phosphate *(dashed line)* and dexamethasone in polyethylene glycol *(solid line)*. No significant difference in results is seen with these dexamethasone products. (From Feldman EC, Nelson RW: Canine and Feline Endocrinology and Reproduction, 2nd ed. Philadelphia, WB Saunders, 1996, p 227.)

suppression on the LDDS test. In one large study,[56] the HDDS test results provided additional information in only a small percentage of dogs (26 of 216 [12%]). It therefore appears useful routinely to perform an extended LDDS test in dogs suspected of having Cushing's syndrome. In dogs with dexamethasone resistance, rather than a HDDS test, it probably would be more efficient to perform one of the other differentiating tests, such as measurement of endogenous ACTH or adrenal ultrasonography.

Extended urine cortisol to creatinine ratio   The extended urine C:C ratio combines a screening test (urine C:C ratio) with a differentiating test (a special form of the HDDS test). Urine samples are collected at home for 3 consecutive days for determination of the C:C ratio. After the second urine sample has been collected, the owner administers 0.1 mg/kg of dexamethasone, per os, at 8-hour intervals (three times). The mean is calculated from the first two urine samples and is used as baseline urine C:C ratio. Provided the baseline urine C:C ratio is elevated, a diagnosis of PDH is justified if the ratio of the third sample is less than 50% of the baseline value.[17]

The advantage of this test is that it can be performed at home. Disadvantages include the limited specificity of the urine C:C ratio and possible owner error associated with administration of the dexamethasone tablets. Little current information is available regarding the accuracy of this test.

Endogenous ACTH   Determination of the ACTH concentration is a reliable test for differentiating PDH from an FAT. In dogs with an FAT, the ACTH concentration is suppressed through negative feedback, whereas in dogs with PDH, the pituitary tumor secretes ACTH. Rapid processing of the sample is important because the hormone disappears quickly from fresh whole blood. Blood should be collected into a chilled plastic tube containing ethylenediamine tetra-acetic acid (EDTA) and immediately centrifuged at 4° C. The plasma should be stored at –20° to –70° C, then packed on dry ice and shipped to a laboratory. Addition of the protease inhibitor aprotinin (500 kallikrein inactivator units per milliliter of blood) to the EDTA tube may prevent rapid breakdown of ACTH.[58] Not all assays for human ACTH can be used in the dog, therefore validation is imperative.

The reference range for ACTH is 20 to 100 pg/mL. Concentrations of ACTH less than 20 pg/mL are strongly suggestive of an FAT, and concentrations greater than 45 pg/mL are consistent with a diagnosis of PDH. The range between 20 and 45 pg/mL is considered nondiagnostic. It should be noted that reference ranges and cutoff values may differ among laboratories. In one study, approximately 70% of dogs with an FAT had ACTH concentrations less than 20 pg/mL; in the remaining dogs, the ACTH concentration was in the nondiagnostic range.[24] In another study, 85% to 90% of dogs with PDH had ACTH concentrations greater than 45 pg/mL, and in the remaining 10% to 15%, the levels were nondiagnostic.[59] In dogs with a nondiagnostic test result, another sample should be submitted or another differentiating test performed (Figure 242-9).

Ultrasonographic examination of the adrenal glands   Adrenal ultrasonography is an extremely valuable tool for differentiating PDH from an FAT (see Ultrasonography, above).

Advanced diagnostic imaging   Because the adrenal glands can be visualized so well with ultrasonography, advanced imaging techniques usually are not required. However, techniques such as CT and MRI are the only reliable methods of evaluating the size of a pituitary tumor. Survey radiography of the skull does not aid in their diagnosis because pituitary tumors in dogs usually do not erode bone or invade the sphenoid bone.

Because the pituitary lacks a complete blood-brain barrier, contrast medium diffuses freely from the circulation into the

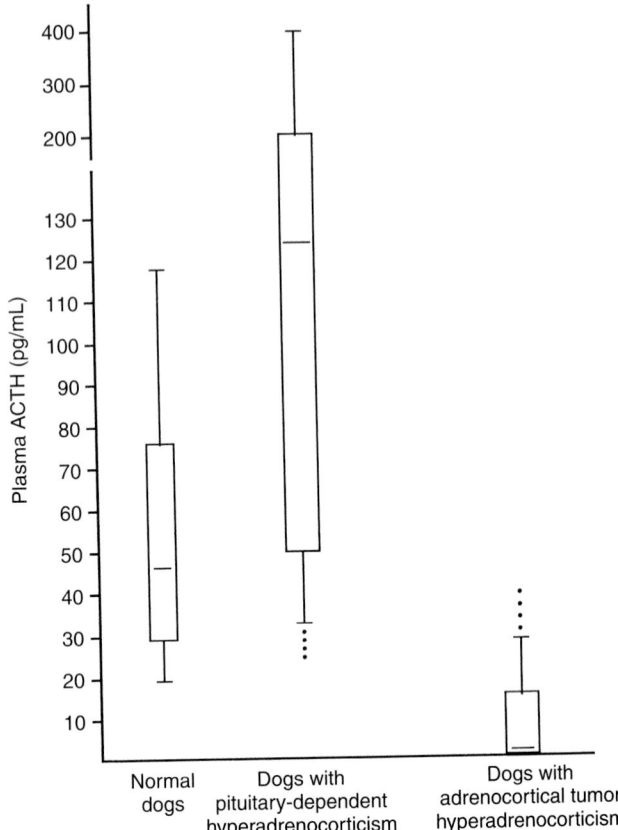

Figure 242-9   Endogenous plasma ACTH concentrations from clinically normal dogs, dogs with functioning adrenocortical carcinomas or adenomas, and dogs with pituitary-dependent hyperadrenocorticism (PDH). Each box represents the interquartile range from the 25th to the 75th percentile (the middle half of the data). The horizontal bar through the box is the median. The "whiskers" represent the main body of data, which in most cases is equal to the range. Outlying data points are represented by the circles. (From Feldman EC, Nelson RW: Canine and Feline Endocrinology and Reproduction, 2nd ed. Philadelphia, WB Saunders, 1996, p 230.)

interstitial space. Contrast enhancement of a pituitary tumor improves its detection and allows delineation of tumor from peritumoral edema and adjacent neural structures.

In dogs, pituitary tumors grow dorsally. The so-called suprasellar tumor extension is partly a reflection of the incomplete diaphragma sella, which provides minimal resistance. Growth may result in invagination into the third ventricle, and the tumor may eventually compress and/or invade the hypothalamus and thalamus and, when large enough, other brain structures. In contrast to humans with pituitary tumors, the optic chiasm in dogs is usually spared because of its more rostral location.

Currently we recommend that CT (or MRI) be performed in dogs with PDH because of the potential risk of a large tumor (see below). However, CT and MRI cannot replace endocrine function tests, because about half of pituitary tumors are not visible. In addition, CT and MRI do not differentiate between a functional and nonfunctional mass (Figures 242-10 and 242-11).

Computed tomography   The size of the pituitary gland varies among different breeds of dogs and among dogs of the same breed. In 35 healthy dogs, CT measurements of the pituitary gland ranged from 3.2 to 5.1 mm for height, 4.2 to

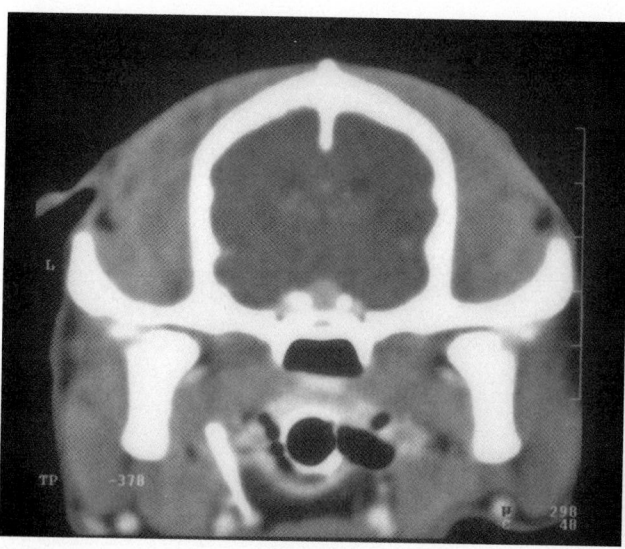
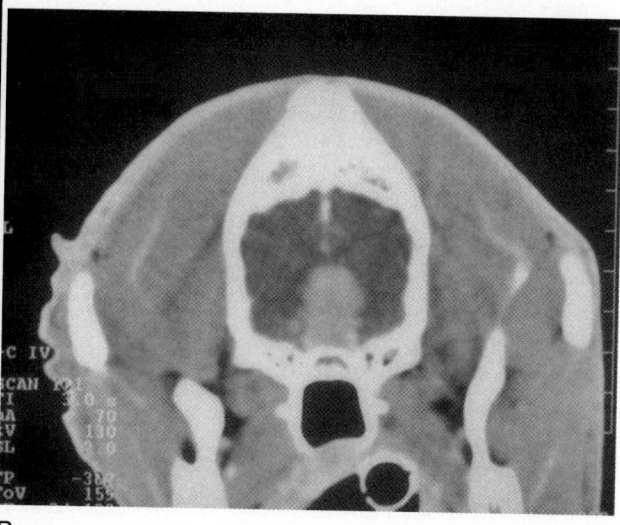

A   B

Figure 242-10 Contrast-enhanced transverse computed tomographic images through the pituitary. **A,** Mixed-breed dog with signs of hyperadrenocorticism but no neurologic signs. The pituitary is enlarged (0.6 cm in height). **B,** Bergamasker with hyperadrenocorticism that had been treated with mitotane for 2 years, after which neurologic signs developed (i.e., disorientation, ataxia, aggressive behavior). The pituitary is grossly enlarged (2.1 cm in height).

6.9 mm for width, and 3.6 to 7.2 mm for length.[60] The first sign of pituitary enlargement appears to be an increase in height (i.e., dorsal extension into the suprasellar region). The pituitary gland is considered to be enlarged when the dorsal contour of the pituitary protrudes above the suprasellar extension of the intercrural cisterns, which are easily recognized on CT images.[13] Alternatively, the ratio of the height of the pituitary gland to the area of the brain measured on an image through the center of the pituitary (P:B ratio) can be used to discriminate between enlarged (P:B greater than 0.31) and normal (P:B less than or equal to 0.31) pituitary glands.[60] Large tumors are easily detected on contrast-enhanced CT images because of their size and altered shape. In rare cases, tumors may be difficult to visualize without contrast. In 50% to 60% of dogs with PDH, a pituitary mass can be detected by CT. In the remaining 40% to 50% of cases, the disease is caused by a small tumor (less than 3 to 4 mm) that is not visible even with contrast. Newer CT techniques, using a series of transverse scans through the center of the pituitary during and after rapid intravenous injection of contrast medium (dynamic CT), reveal a difference in enhancement between the neurohypophysis and the adenohypophysis. This is due to variations in the blood supply; an early, strong enhancement of the central neurohypophysis ("pituitary flush") is seen, as is a slightly delayed, weaker enhancement of the peripheral adenohypophysis. Displacement or distortion of the neurohypophyseal flush may reveal the existence of small tumors.[61]

Magnetic resonance imaging Although CT and MRI are both effective at identifying large pituitary tumors, MRI is superior for defining the full extent and relationship of a tumor to surrounding structures and is probably more accurate in identifying small lesions. The size, signal, and contrast enhancement characteristics of the normal canine pituitary gland using MRI have been described.[62] In one study, in about 50% of dogs with PDH and no neurologic signs, a pituitary tumor was visible on MRI, and the tumors ranged in size from 4 to 12 mm.[63]

Treatment

The method of treatment must be carefully chosen based on the cause of the disease (PDH or an FAT), the age and condition of the dog, and whether concomitant disease is a factor. The cost and availability of treatment methods, as well as the frequency of follow-up evaluations, are also important considerations.

Surgery

Adrenal tumor Surgical removal is the treatment of choice for adrenal tumors. Each dog must be assessed preoperatively for metastases or invasion of the tumor into surrounding tissues. Adrenalectomy is technically challenging and should be performed by a skilled surgeon. Approximately 50% of dogs develop severe postoperative complications, including pancreatitis, pneumonia, pulmonary thromboembolism, acute renal failure, sepsis, and hypoadrenocorticism due to insufficient steroid levels. The reported death rate after adrenalectomy varies greatly; in two large studies the rate was 27% and 34%.[19,26] It is not known whether dogs with an FAT that undergo long-term medical treatment before adrenalectomy have fewer postoperative complications and higher survival rates. In dogs in which tumor removal was incomplete, clinical signs persist, or hyperadrenocorticism recurs weeks to months after surgery.

Autonomous cortisol secretion results in atrophy of the cells of the zona fasciculata and zona reticularis and, in a few dogs, of the aldosterone-producing cells of the zona glomerulosa. Thus glucocorticoid substitution intraoperatively and postoperatively is necessary. Mineralocorticoid treatment is instituted when required.

Intravenous fluids (0.9% sodium chloride [NaCl] or Ringer's solution) should be administered at a maintenance rate at the start of anesthesia and during surgery and the postoperative period. When the tumor is located, dexamethasone should be given at a dosage of 0.1 mg/kg over a 6-hour period. The dose should be repeated two to four times per day, subcutaneously, until oral medication can be started.[59] An alternative to dexamethasone is hydrocortisone, which can be

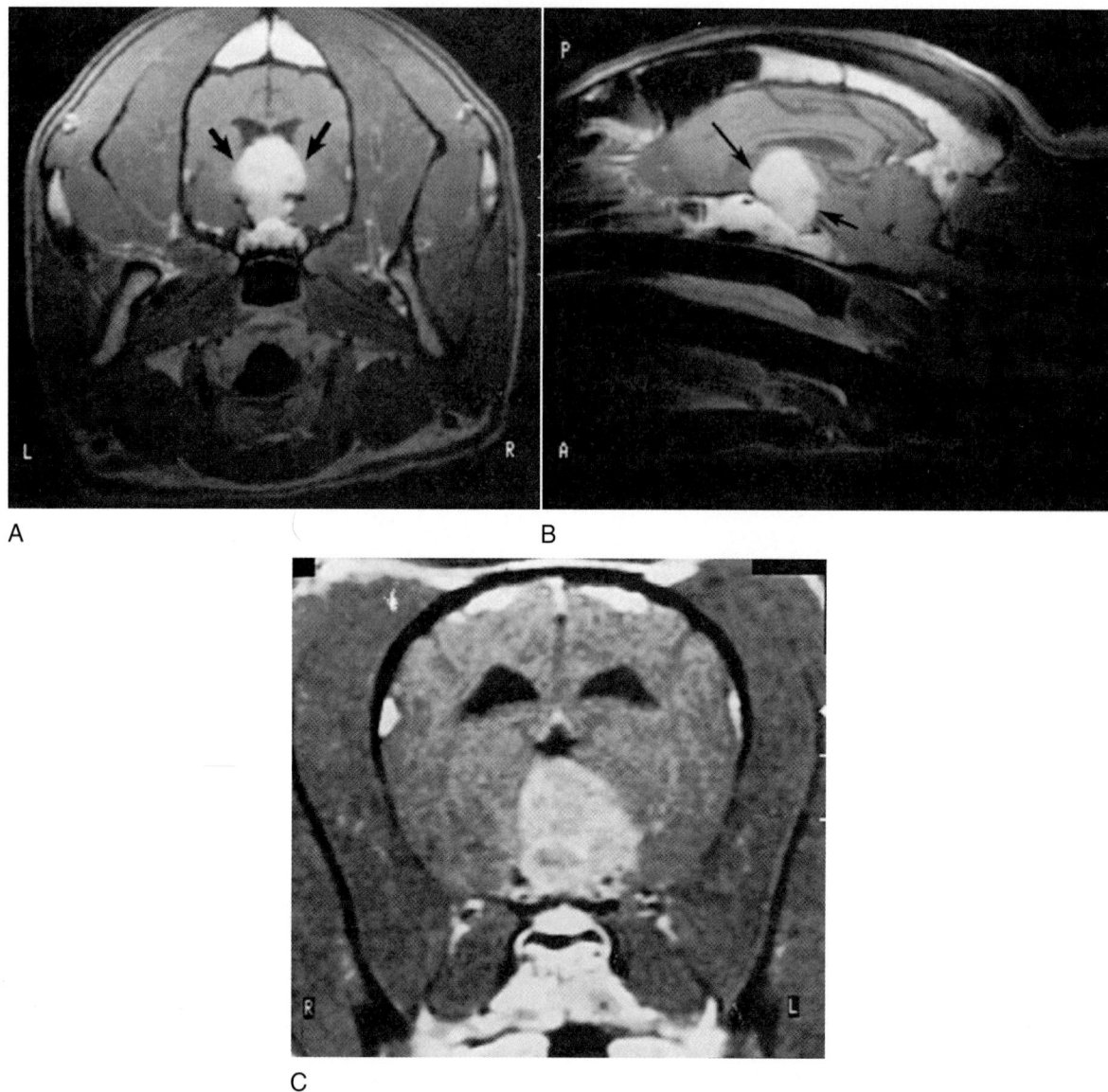

Figure 242-11 **A,** Transverse view of a post-gadolinium MRI scan of a 7-year-old bull terrier with pituitary-dependent hyperadrenocorticism (PDH) caused by a 2.4 cm mass *(arrows)*; the dog developed signs of disorientation and ataxia. **B,** Midline sagittal view of the brain of the same dog (using MRI), showing the densely enhancing mass *(arrows)* arising from the pituitary fossa and causing compression of the floor of the overlying third ventricle. **C,** Post-gadolinium MRI scan of an 8-year-old Boston terrier with PDH and signs of disorientation, ataxia, and circling. (From Feldman EC, Nelson RW: Canine and Feline Endocrinology and Reproduction, 2nd ed. Philadelphia, WB Saunders, 1996, p 237.)

given intravenously during surgery at a dosage of 4 to 5 mg/kg, and thereafter at a dosage of 1 mg/kg given intravenously every 6 hours until oral medication is started. Compared to dexamethasone, hydrocortisone has the advantage of having both glucocorticoid and mineralocorticoid activity. Prednisolone is then administered orally according to the following schedule:

- 1 mg/kg twice daily for 2 to 3 days
- 0.5 mg/kg twice daily for 2 to 3 days
- 0.25 mg/kg twice daily for 3 weeks
- 0.25 mg/kg once a day for 3 weeks
- 0.25 mg/kg every other day for 3 weeks
- 0.25 mg/kg every 3 days

Prednisolone usually can be discontinued after 2 to 3 months. The ACTH stimulation test is helpful for evaluating adrenal function. Intensive postoperative monitoring is essential for preventing or detecting potential complications. If hyperkalemia and/or hyponatremia occur, oral fludrocortisone (0.01 to 0.02 mg/kg/day) or parenteral desoxycorticosterone pivalate (DOCP; 2.2 mg/kg every 25 days) should be given. In most cases these electrolyte abnormalities, which reflect mineralocorticoid deficiency, last only a few days. Antibiotics, pain medication, and heparin should be used routinely. When bilateral adrenalectomy is performed (because of bilateral tumors), the dog needs lifelong supplementation with mineralocorticoids and glucocorticoids.

Pituitary tumor

Hypophysectomy During the past decade, transsphenoidal pituitary surgery has become the treatment of choice for humans with PDH. Although hypophysectomy has been attempted numerous times in dogs, the procedure has only recently become feasible.[60,64] Hypophysectomy in dogs (and cats) is performed by a transsphenoidal approach. Of 84 dogs with PDH that underwent hypophysectomy,[65] six died within 4 weeks of surgery and were considered procedure-related mortalities. In another six dogs, the tumor was incompletely removed. The overall response rate was 86% (i.e., 72 of the 84 dogs went into remission). This compares favorably with the results of dogs with PDH treated medically with mitotane. Perioperative and long-term complications include mild transient hypernatremia, transient reduction or cessation of tear production, diabetes insipidus (persistent in 10% of cases), and secondary hypothyroidism (persistent in all cases). Hyperadrenocorticism recurred in 11 of 72 dogs (15%), 5 to 47 months after surgery. Thus far, only dogs with small or moderate-sized tumors (up to 10 mm in diameter) have been suitable candidates.

Pituitary surgery is possible only in a specialized veterinary institution and requires a team approach involving a neurosurgeon, an endocrinologist, and a radiologist.[65] Transsphenoidal hypophysectomy has the potential to become the treatment of choice for dogs (and cats) with PDH.

Adrenalectomy Removal of both adrenal glands results in complete resolution of the clinical signs of hyperadrenocorticism. However, because the success rate of medical treatment is relatively high and treatment is fairly easy, the risk of surgery seems unwarranted.

Medical Management

Medical management of dogs with Cushing's disease may be questioned, because unlike adrenalectomy or hypophysectomy, it does not result in a cure. No studies have investigated the degree to which medical treatment increases the life expectancy of dogs with Cushing's syndrome. However, uncontrolled hyperadrenocorticism markedly affects the quality of life and can lead to a number of complications, including infection and life-threatening thromboembolism. For these reasons, treatment should be undertaken in most dogs with clinical signs of hyperadrenocorticism. Exceptions include very old dogs and those with concomitant disease in which appetite is sustained by excess cortisol. Dogs with laboratory values consistent with hyperadrenocorticism (increased ALP, positive screening test results) but without clinical signs should not be treated. In cases in which the cause of the abnormal test results (e.g., primary hepatopathy) remains unknown, the dog should be re-evaluated a few weeks or months later.

Mitotane, trilostane and, to a lesser extent, ketoconazole are effective treatments for hyperadrenocorticism.

Mitotane Mitotane (o,p'-DDD, Lysodren) is a potent adrenocorticolytic drug that causes necrosis of the zona fasciculata and zona reticularis (sites of glucocorticoid production). The zona glomerulosa (site of mineralocorticoid production) is less sensitive to this drug. Mitotane is fat soluble and should always be administered with a meal.

Depending on the dosage and duration of treatment, the adrenal cortex may be partly or completely destroyed. Currently, two main treatment regimens are based on this pretext.

Partial adrenocortical destruction The goal of this treatment regimen is to partly destroy the zona fasciculata and zona reticularis so that excess cortisol production is stopped and synthesis is restricted to amounts needed for daily life.

The zona glomerulosa should retain all of its function. Treatment consists of an induction phase and a maintenance phase.

Induction phase For induction, mitotane is administered at a dosage of 50 mg/kg/day, divided, given twice a day at the end of a meal. It is difficult to determine when adrenocortical destruction is adequate to prevent the occurrence of hypoadrenocorticism by further treatment. Daily administration of mitotane should be stopped when (1) the dog's water intake decreases markedly; (2) the dog's appetite is reduced or the dog eats more slowly (thus the meal is offered before administration of mitotane); or (3) the dog has vomiting, diarrhea, or lethargy. For most dogs with Cushing's syndrome, a change in appetite is the most reliable indicator of effective treatment. When a change in the dog's appetite is noted, re-evaluation by the veterinarian and an ACTH stimulation test should be performed. Treatment is considered adequate when the post-ACTH plasma cortisol concentration is 1 to 4 µg/dL. The time required to achieve this varies among dogs. The average length of induction reported in the literature differs. We found that the target concentration of cortisol was achieved after 3 to 4 days of therapy in more than 50% of dogs with PDH.[66] Thus we routinely perform an ACTH stimulation test on the fifth day of treatment. When the post-ACTH plasma cortisol concentration is 1 to 5 µg/dL, maintenance therapy is started. Some dogs may need 1 or more days of induction therapy, and a second ACTH stimulation test may be required.

Another method of monitoring treatment involves daily phone calls by the veterinarian to the owner regarding the dog's condition, particularly appetite.[59] Appetite is the most important aspect of the monitoring of the response to treatment. Dogs with a poor appetite before the start of treatment should be carefully reassessed; either they do not have Cushing's syndrome, or they have concurrent disease, which must be treated first.

Even with careful treatment and monitoring, some dogs experience apathy, weakness, anorexia, vomiting, diarrhea, and/or ataxia. These symptoms may be due to (1) lower than normal plasma cortisol concentrations (overdose), (2) a decrease in plasma cortisol levels to within the normal range (relative glucocorticoid deficiency, or *glucocorticoid withdrawal syndrome*); or (3) mitotane intolerance. With these dogs, owners are told to stop mitotane treatment and to administer prednisolone (or prednisone) at a dosage of 2 mg/kg per os. When the symptoms are attributable to decreased cortisol levels, dogs return to normal within a few hours. An ACTH stimulation test should be performed to differentiate overdose of mitotane from glucocorticoid withdrawal syndrome. In dogs with mitotane overdose (i.e., a post-ACTH cortisol level of less than 1 µg/dL), prednisolone is administered and tapered over 1 to 3 weeks. If the dog's condition is then stable without prednisolone, mitotane treatment can be restarted at a maintenance dosage. In dogs that do not tolerate mitotane, the daily dosage can be divided into smaller portions, or another drug can be used.

A few researchers advocate administration of both mitotane and prednisolone during the induction phase. We feel that mitotane overdose can be more rapidly recognized clinically when that drug is used alone.

Maintenance phase Maintenance therapy starts with administration of about 50 mg/kg of mitotane per week (e.g., given on Wednesday and Sunday); the dose should be divided and given with meals. With time the dosage may need to be altered (some dogs require half the dose; others, double), therefore owners must be told to monitor the dog for signs of hypoadrenocorticism or recurrence of Cushing's symptoms. An ACTH stimulation test should be performed every 1 to 3 months during the early stages of maintenance treatment and then twice yearly. The goal of maintenance therapy is the same as that for induction: a post-ACTH plasma cortisol concentration of 1 to 5 µl/dL. Determination of the urine C:C ratio is not suitable for monitoring treatment, because overlap occurs between well-regulated and overdosed patients.

Mitotane overdosage may occur at any time during treatment and usually manifests as a glucocorticoid deficiency. Rarely, a concomitant mineralocorticoid deficiency with electrolyte abnormalities may be seen. Treatment consists of cessation of mitotane therapy (transient in most cases) and administration of prednisolone. In dogs with complete adrenocortical insufficiency, a mineralocorticoid (fludrocortisone or DOCP) must also be administered. Permanent adrenocortical insufficiency rarely occurs and is seen in about 5% of cases. In a small number of dogs, mitotane induces CNS symptoms, such as apathy, ataxia, blindness, and head pressing. These clinical signs usually occur several months after the start of treatment and, because of their transient nature, disappear a few hours after administration of the drug. Dividing the dosage over multiple administrations is often helpful, but in some cases the dosage must be reduced. Similar symptoms occur with mitotane overdosage or an expanding hypophyseal tumor, therefore careful re-evaluation of the patient is required.

Approximately 50% of dogs have recurrence of symptoms at some point during treatment. The reasons are similar to those for recurrence during the induction phase: (1) the individual animal requires a higher dosage; (2) owner compliance is poor; (3) the drug is not given with food and thus is poorly absorbed; (4) a drug-associated decrease in intestinal fat absorption results in decreased mitotane absorption; (5) the dog has an FAT rather than PDH; (6) increased ACTH secretion by the hypophyseal tumor (possibly supported by a decrease in negative feedback) results in regeneration of the adrenal cortex; and (7) mitotane stimulates induction of microsomal liver enzymes for its own metabolism.

The partial adrenocortical destruction regimen results in a good to excellent response in about 80% of dogs with PDH. It can also be used to treat dogs with an FAT. It is important to remember that compared to hyperplastic cells, tumor cells frequently are more resistant to the cytotoxic effects of mitotane. About 50% of dogs with an FAT require an induction phase lasting longer than 2 weeks. On average, they also require a higher maintenance dosage of mitotane.[67] Because approximately 50% of dogs with an FAT have adrenal carcinomas, we use the following treatment regimen in those that do not undergo adrenalectomy.

Complete adrenocortical destruction   The goal of this treatment regimen is destruction of the entire adrenal cortex, with resultant iatrogenic hypoadrenocorticism, by long-term mitotane administration.[68]

Mitotane is administered at a dosage of 50 to 75 mg/kg/day (divided into three or four smaller doses given with food) for 25 days. Lifelong administration of fludrocortisone (0.01 mg/kg) and cortisone is started on the third day of mitotane administration. The cortisone dosage is 1 mg/kg given twice a day; then, 1 week after the discontinuation of mitotane treatment, the cortisone dosage is reduced to 0.5 mg/kg given twice a day. An equivalent dose of prednisolone (approximately 0.4 mg/kg and then 0.2 mg/kg) can be used instead of cortisone, because it is less expensive. In a number of dogs, daily mitotane administration must be stopped for a short period because of adverse side effects, such as anorexia, vomiting, diarrhea, weakness, and neurologic symptoms. In most dogs, mitotane administration can be resumed after a few days. This treatment regimen is easier to implement than that for partial adrenocortical destruction because it is not necessary to determine when the therapy takes effect. The side effects and complications are similar to those of other regimens using mitotane. However, the risk of unrecognized adrenal insufficiency is lower, because cortisone and mineralocorticoids are substituted.

The necessity of administering daily medication to prevent life-threatening hypoadrenocorticism must be emphasized to owners. The complete adrenocortical destruction regimen should be used only when the diagnosis is certain and owner compliance can be assured. Recurrence of initial symptoms can also occur with this regimen, therefore an ACTH stimulation test should be performed regularly (two to four times a year). Routine electrolyte evaluation (sodium, potassium) is recommended as for dogs with spontaneous Addison's disease. Clinical remission is reported to occur in 86% of dogs with PDH.[69]

We use complete adrenocortical destruction almost exclusively in dogs with inoperable adrenal tumors. In some dogs, this treatment regimen results in complete tumor remission and disappearance of metastases. For these patients, a modified treatment regimen is used: after the 25th day of daily therapy, mitotane is administered at a dosage of 50 to 75 mg/kg, given weekly (divided over two to four days) for life. An ACTH stimulation test is used routinely to ensure complete cessation of cortisol production, as indicated by a pre-ACTH and post-ACTH plasma cortisol concentration below the assay detection level.

For both protocols, the cortisol requirement in times of stress (illness, surgery) is increased and higher than the partly destroyed adrenocortex can produce or that is administered exogenously. Depending on the level of stress, up to 2 mg/kg of prednisolone may be given daily.

Trilostane   The use of trilostane for the treatment of canine PDH was first reported in 1998.[70] Since then the drug has gained wide popularity, especially in Europe. Two prospective studies that evaluated the effects of trilostane were recently published.[71,72] In the United Kingdom, trilostane is officially registered for use in dogs under the name of Vetoryl. The human preparation is available as Modrenal. Trilostane is an orally administered competitive inhibitor of 3-beta-hydroxysteroid dehydrogenase. This enzyme system mediates the conversion of pregnenolone to progesterone in the adrenal gland. Cortisol, aldosterone, and androstenedione are produced from progesterone via various biochemical pathways. Trilostane inhibits progesterone and blocks the synthesis of its end products (Figure 242-12).

We have used trilostane for nearly 4 years in the treatment of PDH and have found that about 80% of dogs have a good to excellent response. The time required for a noticeable response to trilostane is similar to that for mitotane. Improvements include a rapid decrease in polydipsia, polyuria, and polyphagia and a rapid increase in activity level, as well as delayed improvement in the haircoat, skin condition, and abdominal muscle tone. Some dogs may show transient worsening of dermatologic problems before clinical improvement becomes obvious; this may also occur with mitotane. The ACTH stimulation test determines adrenal reserve and therefore is suitable for evaluating the extent of enzyme inhibition during treatment and for calculating dosage adjustments (Figure 242-13).

We currently administer trilostane as follows: dogs weighing less than 5 kg receive 30 mg once a day; those weighing 5 to 20 kg receive 60 mg once a day; and those weighing more than 20 kg receive 120 mg once a day. Re-evaluations, which are performed after 1, 3, 6, and 13 weeks and 6 and 12 months, include the history, a physical examination, and an ACTH stimulation test. It appears important that, for each evaluation, testing be performed at the same time after drug administration. When the ACTH stimulation test is performed 2 to 6 hours after drug administration, the target range of the post-ACTH cortisol level is 1 to 2 µg/dL; this corresponds with the low end of the desired range for dogs treated with mitotane.

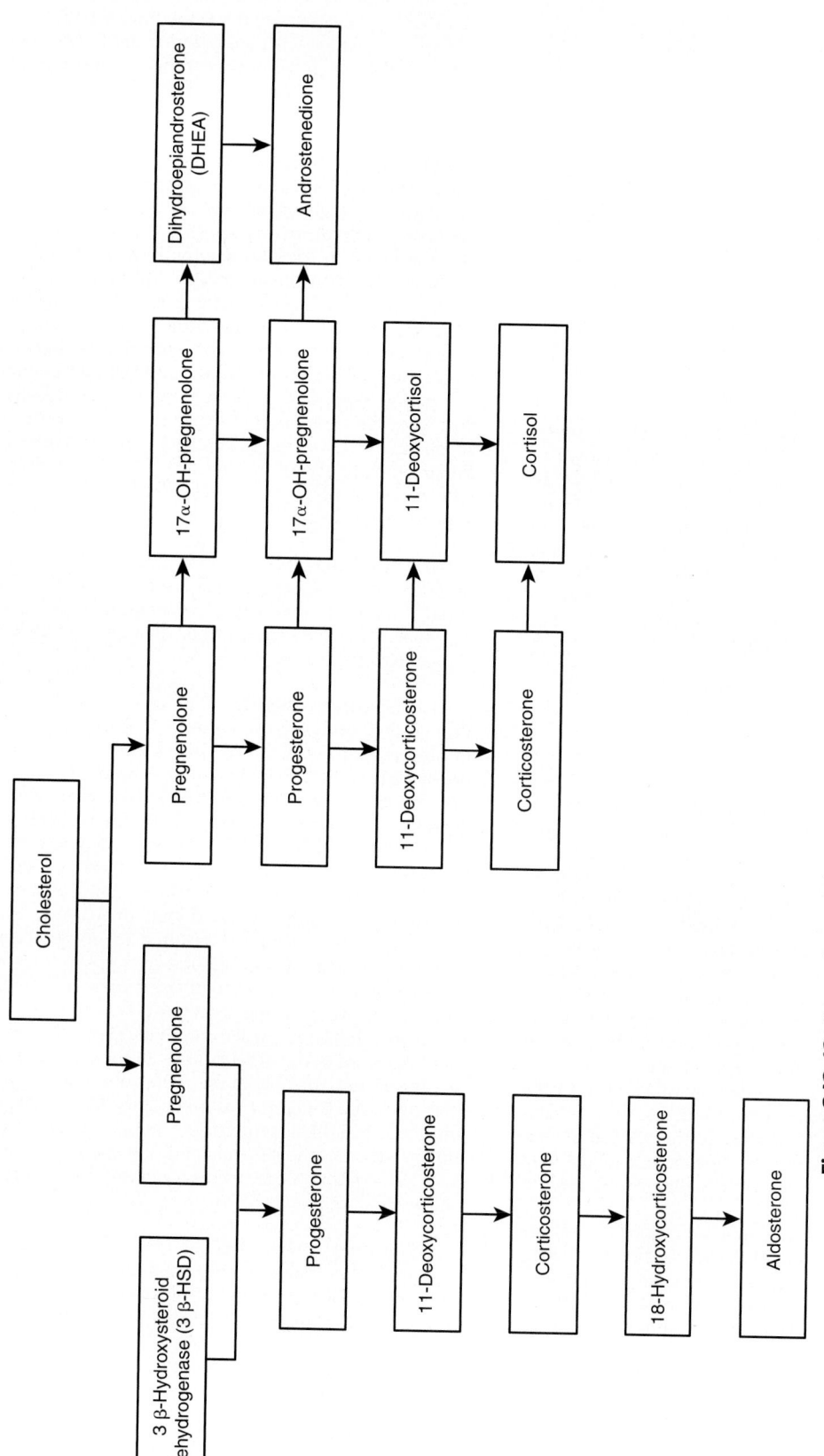

Figure 242-12 Biosynthetic pathways of mineralocorticoids, corticosteroids, and androgens in the adrenal cortex. *3β-HSD*, 3β-Hydroxysteroid dehydrogenase, which converts pregnenolone to progesterone and dehydroepiandrosterone to androstenedione. This enzyme system is blocked by trilostane.

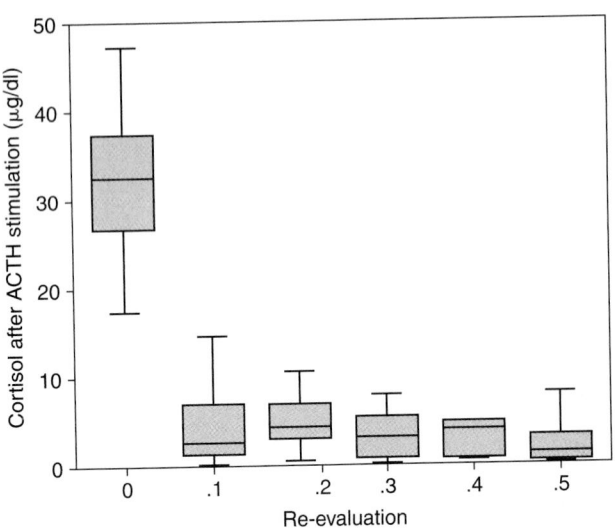

Figure 242-13   Cortisol concentrations after ACTH stimulation in dogs with PDH treated with trilostane. *0*, Prior to therapy; *1* to *5*, re-evaluations at 1, 3 to 4, 6 to 7, 12 to 16 and 24 to 28 weeks after initiation of treatment with trilostane. Data are presented as box plots; the boxes represent values from the 25th to the 75 percentile, the horizontal line in each box is the median, and the "whiskers" represent the range. (From Ruckstuhl NS et al: Results of clinical examinations, laboratory tests, and ultrasonography in dogs with pituitary-dependent hyperadrenocorticism treated with trilostane. Am J Vet Res 63:506-512, 2002.)

Several of our dogs had post-ACTH cortisol levels between 0.5 and 1 μg/dL for months without showing signs of hypoadrenocorticism. Two explanations for this may be that (1) trilostane is known to decrease the cortisol concentration for only a few hours; and (2) steroid precursors, which have accumulated as a result of enzyme inhibition, may have certain glucocorticoid-like effects that prevent signs of hypocortisolism even when the cortisol concentration is low.

Frequent adjustments in the dosage of trilostane (both increases and decreases) are required, particularly during the first few weeks of treatment. Adjustments should be made in increments of 20 to 30 mg/dog. The effective dosage of trilostane differs markedly among dogs with PDH, possibly because of a significant variation among individuals in 3-beta-hydroxysteroid dehydrogenase activity in the adrenal glands. However, the response to treatment appears to stabilize over a period of time, after which dosage adjustments are seldom necessary.

Distinct changes in the ultrasonographic appearance of the adrenal glands were observed in our studies. In almost all dogs, a marked increase was seen in the thickness and echogenicity of the outer zone, which was assumed to be the adrenal cortex. This finding may reflect increased synthesis of precursors arising from an increase in ACTH secretion, or it may be the result of abolition of negative feedback normally exerted by cortisol. Studies are under way to verify this.

Overdosage of trilostane is possible and was assumed to be the cause of adverse symptoms in four of 88 dogs.[71,72] Three of the dogs survived with discontinuation of trilostane and institution of symptomatic treatment. Other problems attributed to the use of trilostane are rare and include lethargy, anorexia, vomiting, and diarrhea. These symptoms are usually mild and self-limiting. In a study of 78 dogs treated with trilostane,[72] it was not known whether the death of two dogs shortly after the start of treatment was related to the drug or to another illness. Postmortem examination of one dog revealed signs suggestive of terminal heart failure.

Our experience with trilostane is limited to treatment of canine PDH, which has entirely replaced mitotane at our hospital. It has been reported that trilostane can also effectively control hyperadrenocorticism caused by an FAT.

Ketoconazole   Ketoconazole, a fungistatic drug, also blocks several P-450 enzyme systems, effectively inhibiting the synthesis of glucocorticoids and androgens. Its effects on mineralocorticoids are negligible. Dogs are started at a dosage of 5 mg/kg given twice a day for 1 week. If the drug is well tolerated (i.e., no decrease in appetite or icterus is seen), the dosage is increased to 10 mg/kg given twice a day for 2 weeks. After this period, an ACTH stimulation test is performed. If the post-ACTH cortisol concentration is higher than the target range of 1 to 4 μg/dL, the dose should be increased to 15 mg/kg twice a day. Most dogs require a daily dose of 30 mg/kg for a long period for good clinical control. The disadvantages of ketoconazole are the expense, the requirement for twice daily administration for life, and the drug's lack of efficacy in up to 50% of cases. Possible side effects include anorexia, diarrhea, and increased hepatic enzyme activity. Hypocortisolism can also occur, but dogs respond rapidly to cessation of ketoconazole administration and administration of glucocorticoids. Before the introduction of trilostane, ketoconazole was primarily used in dogs that did not tolerate mitotane. Today, trilostane rather than ketoconazole would be chosen for such cases.

Selegiline hydrochloride   The use of selegiline hydrochloride (L-deprenyl) for the treatment of hyperadrenocorticism in dogs is controversial. L-deprenyl has been hypothesized to downregulate ACTH by enhancing the dopamine concentration, thereby controlling pituitary hyperadrenocorticism. For a number of years, various reports have described the efficacy of L-deprenyl in dogs with PDH, and aggressive advertising campaigns have been mounted. Interestingly, no scientific data were presented to substantiate these claims. A 6-month controlled clinical study revealed that of 10 dogs with PDH, treatment with L-deprenyl resulted in no clinical improvement in four dogs, worsening of symptoms in four others, and improvement in two. Several of the owners reported that dogs were more lively during treatment; this was assumed to be one reason for good owner compliance and for the improvement reported in the other studies. In those studies, evaluation of clinical signs was based on owner observations and not on scientific data. L-deprenyl is metabolized into substances with amphetamine-like structures, which may explain the improvement in the general condition and behavior of treated dogs. We do not recommend L-deprenyl for the treatment of canine PDH.[73]

Other drugs   A variety of other drugs (bromocriptine, cyproheptadine, metyrapone, aminoglutethimide) have been investigated for the treatment of hyperadrenocorticism; however, they have not produced favorable results.

Complications and Concurrent Disease Associated with Hyperadrenocorticism

Large pituitary tumors   Generally, dogs with PDH have a risk of pituitary tumor growth. Approximately 50% of dogs with PDH have a tumor that is visible on CT or MRI scans at the time of diagnosis, and in approximately 50% of all dogs with PDH, the tumor has a tendency to grow. Neurologic signs caused by expansion of a pituitary tumor are seen in about 15% to 20% of dogs with PDH.[74-76]

Hypophyseal tumors are often categorized, according to their size, as macrotumors (equal to or greater than 10 mm in height) or microtumors (less than 10 mm in height). However, this categorization is useful for neither clinical nor imaging purposes. Tumors as small as 3 to 4 mm can be visualized using advanced imaging techniques. Neurologic symptoms occur in some dogs with tumors less than 10 mm but may not occur in others with tumors 10 mm or larger. It would appear more appropriate to use the term *macrotumor* to describe tumors visible by means of CT or MRI and the term *microtumor* to define masses that cannot be visualized. Pituitary tumors grow dorsally in the dog. The diversity of neurologic signs is due to involvement of different regions of the hypothalamus and thalamus and other brain regions.

The onset of neurologic signs may precede, coincide with, or follow (most often in clinical practice) the diagnosis of hyperadrenocorticism. Clinical signs are usually quite subtle at the start and can be recognized only by someone who knows the dog well. In most cases these signs constitute slight changes in the dog's behavior. Symptoms progress slowly to include dullness, listlessness, restlessness, loss of interest in normal activities, brief episodes of disorientation, anorexia, and weight loss. Later in the course of the disease, symptoms include ataxia, aimless pacing, and stupor. Some dogs may be misdiagnosed with blindness because mental dullness results in inappropriate responses to visual stimuli. Some symptoms, particularly anorexia, resemble those of hypocortisolism caused by medication overdose. For these reasons, careful re-evaluation, including an ACTH stimulation test, is necessary when suspicious symptoms develop.

Diagnosis of a pituitary tumor requires CT or MRI, and good correlation exists between tumor size and the severity of symptoms. In dogs with marked neurologic symptoms, tumors are frequently greater than 10 mm in height, although tumors with a height of only 0.7 to 0.8 mm may occasionally cause symptoms.[76,77] In addition to tumor size, the development of neurologic symptoms probably is related to the tumor growth rate, the size of the skull cavity, and whether peritumoral inflammation or edema is present. Radiation currently is the only treatment available. Most regimens use cobalt-60 teletherapy or a linear accelerator to administer 3.5 to 4 Gy three times a week for 4 to 6 weeks with the animal under general anesthesia. Complications are uncommon, and only rarely do dogs need to be treated with anti-inflammatory doses of steroids because of initial worsening of signs, which probably is related to radiation-associated brain edema. Other problems include graying of hair at the entrance sites of the beam, scalp epilation, and otitis externa.

It is difficult to draw a final conclusion from the few reports available on radiation therapy, and the optimal treatment protocol has yet to be established. In our experience, hypophyseal tumors are relatively sensitive to radiation, and dramatic improvement may occur in some dogs with severe neurologic symptoms. Generally, the prognosis and severity of clinical signs are inversely related.[78] Dogs with severe neurologic symptoms and a tumor larger than 20 to 25 mm have a much poorer prognosis than dogs with mild to moderate symptoms and a tumor less than 20 mm. It is important to remember that some dogs improve during radiation therapy, whereas others require weeks for improvement or normalization. Therefore dogs should not be euthanized during or shortly after radiation treatment because of lack of improvement.

In most dogs, radiation has little or no effect or only a transient influence on the secretory nature of the tumor, and additional medical treatment is required. Recurrence of neurologic signs weeks to years later is possible, and in such cases deterioration may be rapid.

We currently recommend CT or MRI for every dog with PDH. For dogs with dexamethasone resistance (per LDDS or HDDS tests), we strongly recommend pituitary imaging. For dogs with tumors greater than 7 mm, we suggest radiation therapy regardless of whether neurologic signs are present.

Adrenal tumors. Adrenal tumors may invade local tissues and vessels and may metastasize. Traumatic and nontraumatic rupture of the tumor may result in intra-abdominal or retroperitoneal hemorrhage or vena caval thrombosis, causing hindlimb edema.[79-81]

Pulmonary thromboembolism Pulmonary thromboembolism is a potentially life-threatening complication of hyperadrenocorticism. However, because no systematic studies exist and a definitive diagnosis is often difficult, its incidence is not known. Dogs with hyperadrenocorticism that undergo surgery (e.g., adrenalectomy) are at increased risk of developing pulmonary thromboembolism. Thromboembolism may occur in other organs, but this is probably rare. It is generally accepted that hyperadrenocorticism leads to a state characterized by hypercoagulation. In humans with Cushing's syndrome, this state is thought to be related to an increase in plasma clotting factors, especially factor VIII and the von Willebrand factor complex, and to an impairment of fibrinolytic capacity.[82] Similar mechanisms are thought to occur in dogs. Recently it was shown that dogs with hyperadrenocorticism had elevated levels of factors II, V, VII, IX, X, and XII and of fibrinogen. Antithrombin was decreased, whereas thrombin-antithrombin complexes were increased.[83] Conditions such as hypertension and obesity may also play a role in the development of pulmonary thromboembolism.

An acute onset of respiratory distress (tachypnea, dyspnea, cyanosis) is characteristic of pulmonary thromboembolism, which may be difficult or impossible to diagnose definitively in veterinary patients. Pulmonary thromboembolism can result in a variety of radiographic patterns; in fact, a recent study found no radiographic abnormalities in 27% of 29 cases.[84] Therefore an animal with severe respiratory distress in which no radiographic changes are seen should be suspected of having pulmonary thromboembolism. Abnormal radiographic findings include interstitial, alveolar, or mixed patterns; pleural effusion; increased diameter and blunting of pulmonary arteries; and decreased vascularity of affected lung lobes with increased vascularity of unaffected lobes. Echocardiography, including Doppler evaluation, is a helpful diagnostic tool in human medicine but needs further investigation in veterinary medicine. In most dogs, arterial blood gas analysis reveals hypoxemia (partial pressure of oxygen [PO_2] less than 70 mm Hg) and hypocapnia (partial pressure of carbon dioxide [PCO_2] less than 35 mm Hg). However, these are nonspecific findings of inefficient gas exchange and cannot be used alone for diagnosis. A definitive diagnosis may be obtained with pulmonary angiography or ventilation and perfusion scanning with radioisotopes. Because these procedures are either invasive or not widely available, a diagnosis often is made on the basis of clinical signs, radiographic findings, and blood gas analysis results.

Treatment is mainly empirical. In experimental conditions emboli begin to dissolve within hours of formation without treatment, and complete resolution has been documented within days. In naturally occurring disease, however, prothrombic tendencies persist. Therapy consists of general support and administration of oxygen and anticoagulants, such as heparin or warfarin. These drugs have no effect on existing emboli but are used to prevent further clot formation. One of several protocols used for heparin treatment involves an initial dosage of 200 to 300 IU/kg given every 8 hours. The dosage must be modified for each dog to maintain the activated partial thromboplastin time (aPTT) at 1.5 to 2.5 times normal. No information is available on the use of low-molecular-weight heparin. Warfarin is administered initially at a dosage of

0.1 to 0.2 mg/kg given orally every 24 hours. During the first few days, heparin should also be given to combat the initial prothrombic effects of warfarin. The warfarin dosage is then adjusted to achieve an aPTT of 1.5 to 2.5 times normal.

Thrombolytic agents, such as streptokinase, have the potential to dissolve clots. However, their effectiveness in naturally occurring disease has not been critically evaluated, probably because of the expense and the risk of life-threatening hemorrhage.

The prognosis in dogs with pulmonary thromboembolism is guarded to grave. Recovery, if it occurs, usually requires at least 7 to 10 days.

No studies have been done on the success of prophylactic treatment in animals at risk of developing pulmonary thromboembolism. In humans with Cushing's syndrome, it has been shown that thromboembolic complications after surgery can be significantly reduced by anticoagulant prophylaxis.[82] It may be advisable to start low-dose heparin therapy several days prior to surgery in dogs with hyperadrenocorticism and to continue administration for several days afterward.

Diabetes mellitus Dogs with hyperadrenocorticism may develop diabetes mellitus because of insulin antagonism by glucocorticoids. Insulin resistance results either directly, because of a reduction in the number or efficacy of glucose transporters, or indirectly, because of an increase in the glucose concentration and resultant free fatty acid concentration. Approximately 30% to 40% of dogs with Cushing's syndrome show mild elevations in the glucose concentration, but only about 10% develop overt diabetes mellitus. Diagnosis of diabetes mellitus in a dog with previously diagnosed Cushing's syndrome usually is straightforward. However, it is much more difficult to diagnose Cushing's syndrome in a dog with established diabetes mellitus. It often is not possible to make a diagnosis based on clinical signs. Both diseases are characterized by polydipsia, polyuria, polyphagia, hepatomegaly, and sometimes weakness. Also, in dogs with both endocrine diseases, skin and haircoat changes typical of Cushing's syndrome (bilateral symmetric alopecia, skin atrophy) may not occur or may be very mild. It may not be possible to make a diagnosis based on the results of routine laboratory tests, because a stress leukogram and increased hepatic enzyme activities occur in both diseases. The urine specific gravity in most diabetic dogs is greater than 1.025, whereas dogs with both Cushing's syndrome and diabetes mellitus often have hyposthenuria or isosthenuria. Dogs with diabetes mellitus often have false-positive results on screening tests for Cushing's syndrome, therefore the results of these tests must be interpreted carefully. To avoid false-positive results, we recommend that dogs suspected of having Cushing's syndrome and other severe illness not undergo screening tests. Screening tests should be performed only after good glycemic control has been achieved; however, this is difficult to impossible in dogs with Cushing's syndrome. In such cases, therefore, positive results may be due to poor glycemic control or concurrent hyperadrenocorticism. Further management of such dogs must be considered carefully based on all clinical and laboratory findings.

Urinary tract infection, pyelonephritis, and calcium-containing uroliths Nearly 50% of dogs with hyperadrenocorticism have a bacterial urinary tract infection. Dysuria and pyuria may not occur because of the anti-inflammatory and immunosuppressive effects of steroids. Hyperadrenocorticism may also predispose dogs to calcium-containing uroliths, because glucocorticoids increase renal calcium excretion.

Pancreatitis Anecdotal reports indicate that hyperadrenocorticism may predispose dogs to pancreatitis. A recent study found that the risk of developing fatal acute pancreatitis was increased by hyperadrenocorticism, as well as by other factors.[85]

The mechanism for this is unknown, but it may result from disturbed lipid metabolism.

Degenerative and immune-mediated diseases The anti-inflammatory and immunosuppressive effects of cortisol can mask concurrent problems. The most common of these are degenerative arthropathy and skin allergy, which may become apparent once treatment is initiated and cortisol concentrations decrease.

Hypertension and glomerular disease Systemic hypertension occurs in a large percentage of dogs with hyperadrenocorticism. Blood pressure can remain elevated despite resolution of hypercortisolemia. According to a recent study, aldosterone does not appear to contribute to hypertension in dogs with hyperadrenocorticism.[86] The major cause of hypertension may be excess cortisol, which enhances sensitivity to endogenous vasoconstrictors.

Hypertension may cause or contribute to glomerular damage and may lead to glomerulosclerosis. Glucocorticoids may also cause glomerulonephritis (see Chapter 261). Both types of glomerular lesions are associated with proteinuria.

HYPERADRENOCORTICISM IN CATS

Hyperadrenocorticism is an endocrine disorder not commonly recognized in cats. Over a 10-year period, one university clinic diagnosed Cushing's syndrome in more than 800 dogs and in only 34 cats.[26]

Similar to the incidence seen in dogs, 80% to 85% of cats have PDH, and 10% to 15% have an FAT. Adenomas and carcinomas occur with equal frequency. Adrenal tumors may secrete excessive amounts of steroids other than cortisol. Two recent case reports described cats with clinical signs of hyperadrenocorticism caused by a progesterone-secreting adrenal mass.[87,88]

Clinical Findings

Middle-aged to older cats are most commonly affected with hyperadrenocorticism. There does not seem to be a breed predilection; however, approximately 70% of feline cases are female. The most common clinical signs are polydipsia, polyuria, and polyphagia. Most authors have assumed that these symptoms are caused by diabetes mellitus, which develops in approximately 80% of cases, and that they therefore are late signs of hyperadrenocorticism. However, a recent case study described polydipsia and polyuria in two cats with hyperadrenocorticism that did not have concurrent diabetes mellitus and in one cat that had hyperadrenocorticism for 8 months before diabetes mellitus developed.[89] Other frequent findings include pendulous abdomen, generalized muscle wasting, lethargy, and obesity. Many cats have dermatologic symptoms, including hair loss; unkempt haircoat; truncal or patchy alopecia; fragile, thin skin prone to traumatically induced tears (so-called feline fragile skin syndrome); and secondary infections (including demodicosis). Hepatomegaly and weight loss occur less frequently.

Hyperglycemia is the most frequent laboratory abnormality. Only 10% of dogs with hyperadrenocorticism develop overt diabetes mellitus, whereas as many as 80% of cats with Cushing's syndrome are diabetic. Cats seem to be more sensitive to the diabetogenic effects of steroids than dogs, and in many cases it is only after diabetes mellitus has been diagnosed that hyperadrenocorticism is suspected. Insulin resistance is a typical feature of diabetes mellitus caused by hyperadrenocorticism. However, it should be noted that not all cats with Cushing's syndrome and concurrent diabetes mellitus are insulin resistant.

Other findings include hypercholesterolemia and an increase in ALT activity, which may be caused by hyperadrenocorticism or diabetes mellitus. Some cats have elevated ALP activity. Because the activity of a steroid-induced isoenzyme is not increased, this elevation is thought to be associated with diabetes mellitus (and hepatic lipidosis) rather than with hyperadrenocorticism.[90]

Specific Endocrine Testing

A diagnosis of hyperadrenocorticism should be based on the results of one or more of the screening tests (urine C:C ratio, ACTH stimulation test, LDDS test). The endogenous ACTH concentration, an HDDS test, and adrenal ultrasonography can be used to differentiate PDH from an FAT in cats.

Urine Creatinine to Cortisol Ratio

Slightly more than 70% of cortisol (free cortisol and metabolites) is eliminated in the urine in dogs, whereas only 18% is eliminated in the urine of cats. Despite this difference, the urine C:C ratio of cats with hyperadrenocorticism is significantly higher than that of healthy cats, and this test can be used in the diagnosis of Cushing's syndrome.[91] Urine should be collected by the owner at home. It is important to remember that false-positive results may be caused by other disease processes. Goosens et al.[91] reported a reference range of 2 to 36×10^{-6} based on the results of 42 healthy cats. Our reference range, using 31 healthy cats, was 0 to 4×10^{-6}. This discrepancy is possibly due to the different types of radioimmunoassay used. The amount of cortisol metabolites measured varies among assays, therefore it is critical that reference ranges be established for each assay.

ACTH Stimulation Test

In both dogs and cats, the ACTH stimulation test is mainly a test of adrenal reserve, and its major role is to rule in or rule out hypoadrenocorticism. The test's sensitivity is low, and because a variety of nonadrenal illnesses can cause abnormal test results, its specificity is also low. According to the test protocol most often used, blood samples for cortisol determination are taken before and 30 and 60 minutes after intramuscular administration of 125 µg/cat of a synthetic polypeptide containing the first 24 aminoacids of ACTH (e.g., Cortrosyn, Synacthen). The time to maximum peak cortisol response is longer and the maximum cortisol concentration is significantly higher after intravenous administration than after intramuscular administration. Therefore the protocol for intravenous administration is to collect blood samples before and 60 and 90 minutes after administration of ACTH. Because peak effect of cortisol is less consistent in the cat than in the dog, two post-ACTH samples are recommended. Reference ranges for the cat are slightly lower than those for the dog and should be established for the laboratory and protocol used. In our laboratory, the upper limit for the normal post-ACTH cortisol concentration using the intramuscular protocol is 13 µg/dL.[92] We consider levels between 13 and 16 µg/dL to be borderline, and a concentration above 16 µg/dL to be consistent with hyperadrenocorticism.

Low-Dose Dexamethasone Suppression Test

The degree and duration of adrenocortical suppression after dexamethasone administration is more variable in cats than in dogs. It appears that a dosage of 0.1 mg/kg of dexamethasone suppresses cortisol levels in healthy cats and cats with nonadrenal illness more reliably than 0.01 mg/kg of dexamethasone, which is the dosage used in dogs. Currently, the protocol most often used involves collection of blood samples for production of plasma or serum before and 4 and 8 hours after intravenous administration of 0.1 mg/kg of dexamethasone. Cortisol levels of less than 1 µg/dL at 4 and 8 hours are considered normal, levels between 1 and 1.4 µg/dL are borderline, and levels greater than 1.4 µg/dL are consistent

with hyperadrenocorticism. Post-dexamethasone suppression of cortisol concentrations at 4 and 8 hours does not occur in cats with an FAT. Approximately 70% of cats with PDH show no or inadequate suppression.[90]

Measurement of Endogenous ACTH

Healthy cats may have very low ACTH concentrations, therefore the measurement of endogenous ACTH test can be used only after a diagnosis of hyperadrenocorticism has been made. Normal to elevated levels of ACTH support a diagnosis of PDH, and low to undetectable levels indicate an FAT. Sample handling is critical (see discussion earlier in this chapter).

High-Dose Dexamethasone Suppression Test

Compared with dogs, a higher dose of dexamethasone (1 mg/kg) has been advocated to differentiate between PDH and an FAT in cats; however, very limited information is available. Blood samples should be taken before and 4 and 8 hours after administration of dexamethasone. Suppression (less than 50% of baseline or less than 1.4 µg/dL) is consistent with PDH. No or insufficient suppression may be due either to an FAT or to PDH and cannot be used to differentiate between the two conditions.

Adrenal Ultrasonography

High-resolution transducers have made ultrasonographic visualization of the adrenal glands possible in cats, and reference ranges have been reported.[92] Symmetric adrenal glands of normal or enlarged size are suggestive of PDH, whereas unilateral enlargement or an adrenal gland with a masslike appearance suggests an FAT. Detailed information on the ultrasonographic appearance of the adrenal glands in cats with hyperadrenocorticism currently is limited.

Treatment

Hyperadrenocorticism is a debilitating disease in the cat. The deleterious effects of chronic hypercortisolism on skin fragility as well as on immune and cardiovascular function are frequently responsible for the death of untreated cats. Therefore treatment should be pursued, although compared to dogs, options are more limited and medical treatment is not as successful.

Adrenalectomy

Adrenalectomy (unilateral in cats with an FAT, bilateral in cats with PDH or bilateral FATs) appears to be the most successful of the treatment options available.[93] The surgical protocol and the medical management of cats during and after the procedure are similar to those followed in dogs. After discontinuation of intravenous steroids, oral prednisolone (2.5 mg twice daily) should be given. Mineralocorticoids (fludrocortisone, 0.1-0.2 mg/cat) should be administered to cats after bilateral adrenalectomy or to those that have hyperkalemia and/or hyponatremia after surgery. Serum electrolyte concentrations should be evaluated twice daily for several days after surgery. After bilateral adrenalectomy, cats require lifelong supplementation with both mineralocorticoids and glucocorticoids, whereas after unilateral adrenalectomy, supplementation generally can be weaned off over a 2-month period. Postsurgical complications are common and include sepsis, pancreatitis, thromboembolism, and hypoadrenocorticism. Surgery-related death occurs in about 30% to 40% of cases.

Successful adrenalectomy typically results in resolution or marked improvement of clinical signs within 2 to 4 months. In about 50% of cases, diabetes resolves, and in others the insulin requirement decreases.[89,93]

Hypophysectomy

Recently, transsphenoidal hypophysectomy for the treatment of PDH was described in seven cats.[94] Two cats died within

4 weeks of surgery. Remission was achieved in five cats, although relapse occurred in one of these 19 months after surgery. Diabetes mellitus resolved in two of the four cats that had the disease. In the future, transsphenoidal hypophysectomy may be the treatment of choice for cats with hyperadrenocorticism.

Radiation Treatment

The success rate for radiation treatment in cats has been variable at best. However, the number of cats treated with radiation is very small, therefore conclusions are difficult to draw.

Medical Treatment

A number of different medical protocols have been used in cats with hyperadrenocorticism. However, success rates are variable or poor, and long-term results are often disappointing. Medical treatment may be indicated for the presurgical management of hyperadrenocorticism and may improve the outcome of surgery.

Mitotane   The use of mitotane to treat hyperadrenocorticism has been discouraged in the past because of a perceived sensitivity of cats to chlorinated hydrocarbons. In addition, the success rate of mitotane treatment was reported to be poor.[26] One recent report describes successful long-term mitotane treatment in a cat with PDH.[95]

Ketoconazole   Treatment with ketoconazole (15 mg/kg given twice a day) resulted in clinical improvement in some cats and no response in others. Severe thrombocytopenia was reported in one cat and was thought to be due to an adverse drug reaction.

Metyrapone   Metyrapone has been successfully used as a treatment prior to bilateral adrenalectomy.[96,97] The optimal dose was 65 mg/kg given orally every 12 hours.

Trilostane   There are no published reports on the use of trilostane in cats with hyperadrenocorticism.

Prognosis

Hyperadrenocorticism in cats is a serious disease with a guarded to grave prognosis. Medical therapy has limited success, and the outcome of surgery is often hampered by the debilitated condition of the patient.

Hyperaldosteronism

Primary hyperaldosteronism, also called *Conn's syndrome* in human medicine, is a very rare disease in dogs and cats. It is usually caused by a unilateral adenoma or rarely by a carcinoma of the zona glomerulosa of the adrenal gland. Bilateral adrenal hyperplasia in association with hyperaldosteronism has been reported in only one dog.[98] Aldosterone is the principal regulator of sodium and potassium balance and is important in the maintenance of normal intravascular fluid volume. It also plays a role in the control of acid-base equilibrium. In conditions involving excessive autonomous aldosterone secretion, sodium and water are retained, leading to expansion of the extracellular fluid volume and hypertension. The increase in sodium and water is usually limited by an "escape" mechanism. Nevertheless, hyperaldosteronism tends to be associated with extracellular volume expansion and arterial hypertension. The renin system is suppressed. Increased potassium excretion leads to progressive depletion of body potassium, development of hypokalemia, and hypokalemic metabolic alkalosis. Aldosterone also stimulates the excretion of phosphorus and magnesium. Other characteristics of hyperaldosteronism include resistance to vasopressin and disturbed vasopressin release.[99]

Clinical signs consist of weakness, which may be episodic; ventroflexion of the neck (in cats); stiff gait; myalgia; and lethargy. Hypertension may be present and may cause hypertensive retinopathy. Recently polydipsia and polyuria were described as the lead symptoms in a dog with an aldosteronoma.[99] Moderate to severe hypokalemia is the typical and most consistent finding. The sodium concentration may be normal or only slightly elevated. Definitive diagnosis requires demonstration of an inappropriately elevated aldosterone concentration with a low plasma renin concentration. Ultrasonography and CT are useful for localization and staging of the tumor. Initial treatment should be directed at alleviation of hypokalemia. Surgical intervention is the treatment of choice for tumors with no detectable metastases. For animals with metastases or in the rare case of bilateral hyperplasia, potassium supplementation and spironolactone, an aldosterone antagonist, can be given.

CHAPTER • 243

Hypoadrenocorticism

Michael E. Herrtage

Hypoadrenocorticism is a syndrome that results from deficient production and secretion of glucocorticoids and/or mineralocorticoids by the adrenal cortices. Destruction of more than 90% of both adrenal cortices causes a deficiency of all adrenocortical hormones and the resulting clinical condition is termed *primary hypoadrenocorticism* (Addison's disease). Secondary hypoadrenocorticism is characterized by deficient production and secretion of adrenocorticotropic hormone, ACTH, which leads to atrophy of the adrenal cortices and impaired secretion of glucocorticoids. The production of mineralocorticoids, however, usually remains adequate because ACTH has only minor tropic effects on mineralocorticoid production. Primary and secondary hypoadrenocorticism differ not only in their pathophysiology but also in their clinical presentations.

ANATOMY AND PHYSIOLOGY

One adrenal gland is located craniomedial to each kidney, in retroperitoneal fat. The right adrenal gland lies between the medial surface of the cranial pole of the right kidney and the lateral aspect of the caudal vena cava at the level of the thirteenth thoracic vertebra. The right phrenicoabdominal vein crosses the ventral surface of the gland before joining the caudal vena cava. The left adrenal gland is found craniomedial to the border of the left kidney at the level of the second lumbar vertebra. Medially it is bounded by the descending aorta between the cranial mesenteric artery and the left renal artery.

Together, both adrenal glands from normal dogs weigh about 1 g. On cross-section, the adrenal cortex appears pale yellow whereas the medulla is dark brown. The cortex completely surrounds the medulla and consists of three distinct zones: the outer zona glomerulosa (arcuata) makes up about 25% of the cortex, the middle zona fasciculata makes up approximately 60%, and the inner zona reticularis accounts for the remaining 15% of the cortex. The medulla is adjacent to the zona reticularis, which makes up 10% to 20% of the total volume of the adrenal gland.

The adrenal cortex produces about 30 different hormones, many of which are believed to have little or no clinical significance (Figure 243-1). The hormones can be divided into three groups based on their predominant actions: *mineralocorticoids*, which are important in electrolyte and water homeostasis; *glucocorticoids*, which promote gluconeogenesis; and small quantities of sex hormones, particularly male hormones that have weak androgenic activity.

Aldosterone is the most important mineralocorticoid and is produced by the zona glomerulosa. The principal glucocorticoid, cortisol, and the sex hormones are produced in the zonas fasciculata and reticularis. Glucocorticoid and mineralocorticoid release are controlled by separate mechanisms (Figure 243-2).

Regulation of Glucocorticoid Release

Glucocorticoid release is controlled almost entirely by adrenocorticotrophic hormone (ACTH) secreted by the anterior pituitary, which in turn, is regulated by corticotrophin releasing hormone (CRH) from the hypothalamus (see Figure 243-2). CRH is secreted by the neurons in the anterior portion of the paraventricular nuclei within the hypothalamus and is transported to the anterior pituitary by the portal circulation, where it stimulates ACTH release. There is probably an internal or "short loop" negative feedback control by ACTH on CRH. ACTH secreted into the systemic circulation causes cortisol release with concentrations rising almost immediately. Cortisol has direct negative feedback effects on (1) the hypothalamus to decrease formation of CRH and (2) the anterior pituitary gland to decrease the formation of ACTH. These feedback mechanisms help regulate the plasma concentration of cortisol.

Regulation of Mineralocorticoid Release

Aldosterone release is influenced primarily by the renin-angiotensin system and by plasma potassium levels (see Figure 243-2). Renin is secreted into the blood by the cells of the juxtaglomerular apparatus within the kidneys. This apparatus consists of specialized cells in the wall of the afferent arteriole immediately proximal to the glomerulus as well as specialized epithelial cells of the distal convoluted tubule adjacent to that arteriole, the macula densa. Renin release may be stimulated by stretch receptors in the juxtaglomerular apparatus in response to hypotension, reduced renal blood flow, or by sodium and chloride receptors in the macula densa. Renin is also released by sympathetic nerve stimulation and is inhibited by angiotensin II, antidiuretic hormone, hypertension, and increased reabsorption of sodium by the renal tubules.

Renin is a proteolytic enzyme that splits circulating angiotensinogen, an alpha-2 globulin produced by the liver, into the decapeptide, angiotensin I. Angiotensin I is hydrolysed to the octapeptide, angiotensin II by angiotensin converting enzyme found almost exclusively in the pulmonary capillary endothelium. Angiotensin II is a powerful vasoconstrictor that also stimulates aldosterone secretion from the zona glomerulosa. Through its action on the distal convoluted tubule, aldosterone has negative feedback effects on the juxtaglomerular apparatus. Potassium has a direct stimulatory effect on the zona glomerulosa cells to release aldosterone. ACTH and sodium play less significant roles in aldosterone secretion. ACTH is necessary to maintain normal aldosterone output. In the absence of ACTH, the zona glomerulosa partially atrophies, causing mild to moderate aldosterone deficiency compared with almost total atrophy of the other zones.

The main function of aldosterone is to protect against hypotension and potassium intoxication. Aldosterone promotes sodium, chloride, and water reabsorption as well as potassium excretion in many epithelial tissues including the intestinal mucosa, salivary glands, sweat glands, and kidneys. Its main site of action is the renal tubule, where it promotes sodium and chloride reabsorption in the proximal convoluted tubule and sodium reabsorption by exchange with potassium in the distal convoluted tubule. It is one of the complex regulatory systems for the regulation of extracellular fluid electrolyte concentrations, extracellular fluid volume, blood volume, and arterial pressure.

PRIMARY HYPOADRENOCORTICISM (ADDISON'S DISEASE)

Primary hypoadrenocorticism results from progressive destruction of the adrenal cortices, which must involve more than 90% of the function before clinical signs become apparent. The condition is also referred to as Addison's disease, after the English physician, Thomas Addison, who in 1855 described the syndrome in humans. In those days, the most common cause was destruction of the adrenals by chronic tuberculosis.

Primary hypoadrenocorticism is rare in the dog although probably occurs more frequently than is recognized. Hypoadrenocorticism appears to be rare in cats with only one case series and a few case reports published.[1-3] The clinical signs, diagnosis, and treatment of hypoadrenocorticism are similar in the dog and cat.

PATHOGENESIS

Idiopathic Adrenocortical Atrophy

This is the most common cause in the dog and is thought to be the end result of immune-mediated destruction of the adrenal cortices. Immune-mediated destruction of the adrenal cortices is the most common cause of human primary hypoadrenocorticism and 21-hydroxylase (see Figure 243-1) is considered to be the major autoantigen.[4] The presence of antiadrenal antibodies in two dogs and characteristic histopathologic findings in another support the hypothesis of immune-mediated destruction.[5] The increased predisposition of primary hypoadrenocorticism in young to middle-aged female dogs is also suggestive of an immune-mediated disease. An immune-mediated etiology is also suspected in the cat.

In approximately 50% to 60% of humans with primary hypoadrenocorticism, the disease is associated with other immune-mediated disorders such as Hashimoto's thyroiditis, insulin-dependent diabetes mellitus, hypoparathyroidism, primary gonadal failure, and atrophic gastritis. Autoimmune polyglandular disease has also been recognized in the dog

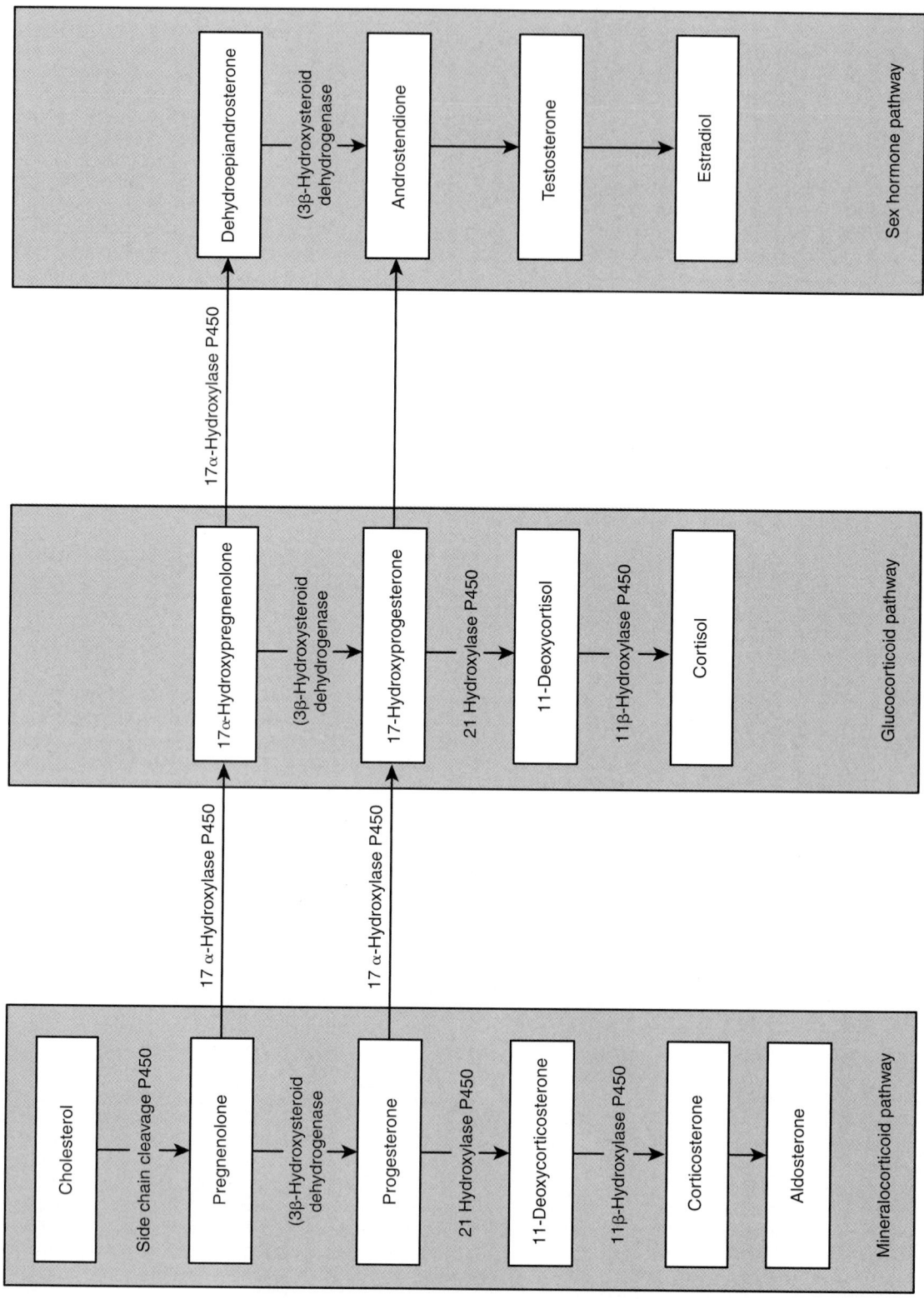

Figure 243-1 Major biosynthetic pathways of adrenocortical steroid production. The zona glomerulosa produces mineralocorticoids. The zona fasciculata and reticularis produce glucocorticoids and sex hormones.

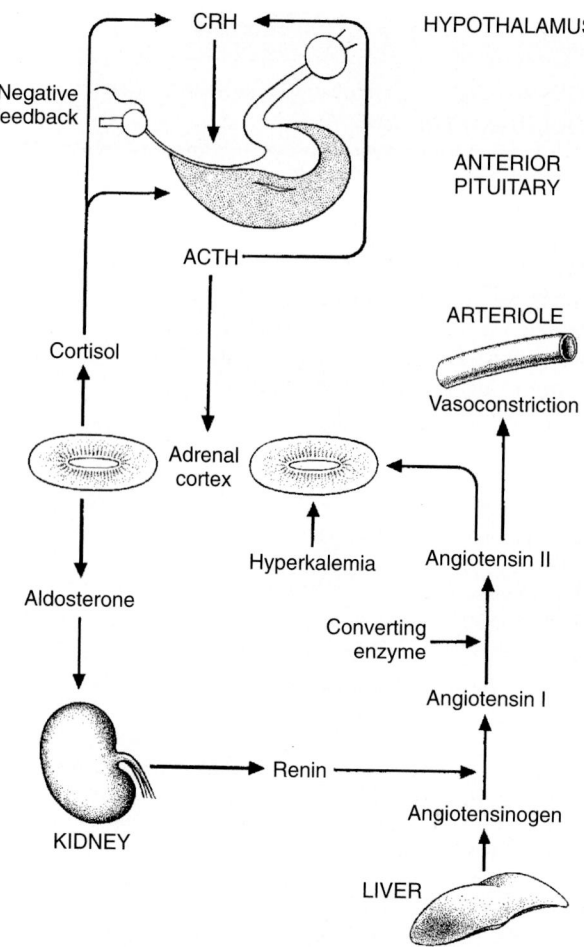

Figure 243-2 Regulation of glucocorticoid and mineralocorticoid release. Corticotrophin releasing hormone (CRH), adrenocorticotrophic hormone (ACTH)

with hypoadrenocorticism and hypothyroidism being the most common combination, but diabetes mellitus and/or hypoparathyroidism may also occur concurrently.[6]

Drug-Induced Adrenocortical Necrosis

Iatrogenic hypoadrenocorticism is a possible complication of mitotane therapy used in the treatment of canine hyperadrenocorticism (see Chapter 242). Although mitotane usually spares the zona glomerulosa and therefore mineralocorticoid secretion, cases of complete adrenocortical failure may occur in as many as 5% of treated dogs. In most of these dogs, the adrenal cortex does not recover when mitotane therapy is withdrawn and permanent mineralocorticoid and glucocorticoid replacement therapy is required. This is a separate entity from transient glucocorticoid deficiency, which may occur following overdosage of mitotane during the induction or maintenance phase of therapy for hyperadrenocorticism.

Adrenocortical necrosis has also been reported following treatment of canine hyperadrenocorticism with trilostane.[7] Since trilostane is a reversible inhibitor the 3β-hydroxysteroid dehydrogenase enzyme system, which blocks adrenal synthesis of glucocorticoids, mineralocorticoids, and sex hormones (see Figure 243-1), this complication is not common. However, awareness of this possible complication is important because prompt treatment is required to correct this life-threatening situation.

Bilateral Adrenalectomy

The surgical removal of both adrenals has been used for the treatment of canine and feline pituitary-dependent hyperadrenocorticism. The surgery is technically difficult and there is a high morbidity and mortality rate even when performed by experienced surgeons. These dogs and cats must be treated for hypoadrenocorticism with replacement hormone therapy for the rest of their lives.

Other Possible Causes

Rarely, canine hypoadrenocorticism can be caused by hemorrhage or infarction of the adrenal glands, granulomatous or neoplastic involvement of the adrenal glands, amyloidosis of adrenal cortices, or following trauma to the adrenal glands.

PATHOPHYSIOLOGY

Adrenocortical pathology leads to mineralocorticoid and glucocorticoid deficiency. Aldosterone is the major mineralocorticoid and promotes sodium, chloride, and water reabsorption as well as potassium excretion in many epithelial tissues, including the intestinal mucosa, salivary glands, sweat glands, and kidneys. Its main site of action is the renal tubule, where it promotes sodium and chloride reabsorption in the proximal convoluted tubule and sodium reabsorption by exchange with potassium in the distal convoluted tubule. Deficiency of aldosterone causes impaired ability to conserve sodium and water and failure to excrete potassium leading to hyponatremia and hyperkalemia. Hyponatremia induces lethargy, depression, and nausea while causing development of hypovolemia, hypotension, reduced cardiac output, and decreased renal perfusion. Hyperkalemia causes muscle weakness, hyporeflexia, and impaired cardiac conduction. Glucocorticoid deficiency causes decreased tolerance of stress, loss of appetite, vomiting, diarrhea, abdominal pain, and lethargy.

SIGNALMENT

Breed

Many breeds of dog have been reported with hypoadrenocorticism, but great Danes, Portuguese water dogs, Rottweilers, standard Poodles, West Highland white terriers, and soft-coated Wheaten terriers appear to be at greater risk of developing hypoadrenocorticism compared with dogs of other breeds.[8] Evidence of familial occurrence and the possibility of an hereditary factor has been suggested in standard Poodles,[9,10] bearded collies,[11,12] and Leonbergers,[13] although the precise genetic mechanism responsible for inheritance of the disease remains undetermined.

No breed predisposition has been identified in the cat. Most reported cases of hypoadrenocorticism have been in domestic shorthaired and longhaired cats.

Age

Hypoadrenocorticism appears to be a disease of the young and middle-aged dog with an age range of 2 months to 14 years and a median age of 4 to 6 years. A similar age range has been noted in cats with hypoadrenocorticism.

Sex

Approximately 70% of dogs with naturally occurring hypoadrenocorticism are female and sexually intact females have been shown to have a significantly higher risk of developing hypoadrenocorticism than spayed females.[8] This is similar to autoimmune Addison's disease in humans and supports the hypothesis of an immune-mediated pathogenesis in most dogs. However, in the bearded collie and standard poodle, in which hypoadrenocorticism is considered to be highly heritable, both sexes are affected with equal probability.[10,12] No sex prediposition has been reported in cats.

CLINICAL SIGNS

The clinical signs of primary hypoadrenocorticism vary from mild to severe with the progression being either acute or chronic. The chronic form of hypoadrenocorticism with clinical signs present for weeks to months is more common than the acute disease in the dog, although the distinction between these two syndromes is not always clear.

Acute Primary Hypoadrenocorticism

The clinical appearance of acute hypoadrenocorticism is that of hypovolemic shock (an Addisonian crisis). The animal is usually found in a state of collapse or collapses when stressed. Other signs include weak pulse, profound bradycardia, abdominal pain, vomiting, diarrhea, dehydration, and hypothermia. Bradycardia is an inappropriate response in a collapsed, hypovolemic patient and warrants immediate investigation. Acute hypoadrenocorticism is rapidly progressive, life threatening, and represents a true medical emergency. Symptomatic therapy with aggressive fluid therapy will help most afflicted dogs and cats by allowing more time to make a diagnosis.

Chronic Primary Hypoadrenocorticism

The clinical signs in the chronic form are often vague and nonspecific and may be exacerbated by stress (Box 243-1). The diagnosis should be considered in any dog or cat with a waxing and waning type of illness or that shows episodic weakness and collapse. The most consistent clinical signs include anorexia, vomiting, lethargy, weight loss, diarrhea, obtundation, depression, shaking or shivering, muscle fasciculations, severe muscle weakness, and polydipsia/polyuria. Less common signs such as regurgitation due to megaesophagus[14], painful muscle cramping[15], and hypoglycemic seizures[16] have been reported. The severity of each sign can vary during the course of the disease and may be interspersed with periods of apparent good health often following nonspecific veterinary therapy, usually consisting of cage rest, glucocorticoid therapy and/or parenteral fluid administration. Hypoadrenocorticism can easily be mistaken for primary renal, gastrointestinal, or neuromuscular diseases.

Common findings on physical examination apart from obtundation and weakness include dehydration, bradycardia, weak femoral pulses, and prolonged capillary refill time. In a few cases, severe gastrointestinal hemorrhage with melena, hematochezia, and occasionally hematemesis can occur, resulting in profound anemia.[17] Since the history and clinical findings are not pathognomonic for hypoadrenocorticism, a high index of suspicion and a careful and critical evaluation of dogs and cats are necessary to arrive at the correct diagnosis.

CLINICOPATHOLOGIC FINDINGS

Hematology

Hematologic changes may include lymphocytosis, eosinophilia and mild normocytic, normochromic, nonregenerative anemia (Box 243-2). However, these findings are not as consistent as those changes seen in hyperadrenocorticism. Normal or increased eosinophil and lymphocyte counts in a sick animal with signs compatible with hypoadrenocorticism are significant, because the expected response to stress would result in eosinopenia and lymphopenia. A mild anemia may not be

---

Box • 243-1
Clinical Signs of Primary Hypoadrenocorticism (Addison's Disease)
Anorexia
Lethargy/depression
Weakness, usually episodic
Vomiting
Waxing and waning illness
Weight loss or failure to gain weight
Dehydration
Diarrhea or occasionally constipation
Polydipsia and/or polyuria
Collapse or syncope
Restlessness/shaking/shivering
Regurgitation
Painful muscle cramps
Melena
Weak pulse
Bradycardia
Abdominal pain

---

appreciated until the dog has been rehydrated because of the hemoconcentration effect of dehydration. Profound anemia (PCV < 20%) is usually found in association with gastrointestinal hemorrhage.

Biochemistry

The most consistent laboratory findings in hypoadrenocorticism are prerenal azotemia, hyponatremia, hyperkalemia, and mild to moderate metabolic acidosis. However, approximately 10% of dogs with primary hypoadrenocorticism have normal serum electrolyte concentrations and these cases are referred to as *atypical Addison's disease*.[18]

Blood Urea, Creatinine, and Urine Specific Gravity

Blood urea nitrogen (BUN) and serum creatinine concentrations are increased secondary to reduced renal perfusion and decreased glomerular filtration rate. Reduced renal perfusion results from hypovolemia, reduced cardiac output and hypotension, which in turn result from chronic fluid loss through the kidneys, acute fluid loss through vomiting, and/or diarrhea and inadequate fluid intake. This prerenal azotemia is often associated with hyperphosphatemia. Increases in BUN also result from gastrointestinal hemorrhage, which is common. This usually explains the discordant moderate-to-severe increase in BUN in a dog or cat with Addison's disease that has only a mild-to-moderate increase in serum creatinine concentration.

Prerenal azotemia is usually associated with concentrated urine (specific gravity >1.030) whereas the urine concentration in dogs and cats with primary renal failure is often isothenuric or only mildly concentrated (1.008 to 1.025). The urine specific gravity in dogs and cats with hypoadrenocorticism is variable but is usually between 1.015 and 1.030, which may cause confusion for the clinician as it is more dilute than would be expected in an animal with prerenal azotemia. This reduction in urine specific gravity develops in hypoadrenocorticism because of impaired concentrating ability secondary to chronic sodium loss reducing the renal medullary concentration gradient.[19] With appropriate fluid therapy, the blood urea and creatinine concentrations in cases of hypoadrenocorticism will usually quickly return to normal confirming that the azotemia is prerenal.

Box • 243-2

Routine Laboratory Findings in Primary Hypoadrenocorticism (Addison's Disease)

Hematology
Lymphocytosis
Eosinophilia
Relative neutropenia
Anemia usually a normocytic, normochromic, non-regenerative anemia, but can be blood loss anemia associated with gastrointestinal hemorrhage

Biochemistry
Azotemia
    Increased blood urea
    Increased creatinine
    Increased phosphate
Hyponatremia (<135 mEq/L)
Hyperkalemia (>5.5 mEq/L)
Reduced sodium: potassium ratio (< 25:1)
Reduced bicarbonate and total CO_2 concentrations
Hypochloremia
Hypercalcemia
Hypoglycemia
Hypoalbuminemia

Urinalysis
Specific gravity variable (usually 1.015 to 1.030)

Box • 243-3

Differential Diagnosis for Significant Hyperkalemia and/or Hyponatremia in Dogs and Cats

Renal or urinary tract disease
    Acute primary renal failure
    Chronic severe oliguric or anuric renal failure (rare)
    Urethral obstruction
    Uroabdomen (ruptured ureter, bladder, or urethra)
    Postobstructive diuresis
    Nephrotic syndrome
Hypoadrenocorticism
Severe gastrointestinal disease
    Parasitic infestations
        Trichuriasis
        Ascariasis
        Ancylostomiasis
    Salmonellosis
    Viral enteritis
        Parvovirus
        Distemper
    Gastric dilatation/volvulus
    Gastrointestinal perforation
    Severe malabsorption
    Idiopathic hemorrhagic enteritis
    Pancreatitic disease
Severe hepatic failure
    Cirrhosis
    Neoplasia
Severe metabolic or respiratory acidosis
Congestive heart failure
Massive release of potassium to the extracellular fluid
    Crush injuries
    Aortic thrombosis
    Rhabdomyolysis
        Heat stroke
        Exertional
    Massive infections
    Massive hemolysis (rare)
Chylous and non-chylous pleural effusions
Pregnancy
Lymphangiosarcoma
Pseudohyperkalemia
    Japanese Akitas and related breeds
    Severe leukocytosis (>100,000/mm³)
    Severe thrombocytosis (>1,000,000/mm³)
Diabetes mellitus
Primary polydipsia
Inappropriate ADH secretion
Drug-induced
    Potassium-sparing diuretics
    Nonsteroidal anti-inflammatory agents
    Angiotensin-converting enzyme inhibitors
    Potassium-containing fluids

Most of these diagnosis/conditions are rarely associated with abnormal electrolyte abnormalities.
References 20 through 25.

Sodium and Potassium Concentrations

The serum sodium concentration is usually less than 135 mEq/L and the serum potassium concentration usually greater than 5.5 mEq/L. However, because of the variability of these two abnormalities, the ratio of sodium to potassium may be more reliable than the absolute values. The normal ratio varies between 27:1 and 40:1, whereas in dogs and cats with hypoadrenocorticism, the ratio is usually less than 25:1 and may be below 20:1. Serum chloride concentration is also reduced in association with sodium and frequently chloride concentrations below 100 mEq/L are found in animals with hypoadrenocorticism.

Concurrent hypovolemia, hyponatremia, and hyperkalemia may develop in other conditions apart from hypoadrenocorticism such as gastrointestinal disease, chronic blood loss, acute and chronic renal failure, chronic hepatic failure, chronic heart failure, repeated drainage of chylous and non-chylous pleural effusions, lymphangiosarcoma, and pregnancy (Box 243-3).[20-22] In a recent review of low sodium:potassium ratios in 34 dogs, renal failure or urinary tract disease leading to decreased urine excretion of potassium accounted for the low ratio in most of the dogs with sodium:potassium ratios of between 19.9 and 15.[23] These low ratios were more strongly associated with high serum potassium concentrations than with low serum sodium concentrations. Four of the dogs in that study had sodium:potassium concentrations ratios of less than 15 and each dog had hypoadrenocorticism. However, although *suggestive* of hypoadrenocorticism, a low sodium:potassium ratio of less than 15 is not *diagnostic* of hypoadrenocorticism. Pseudohyperkalemia, which is defined as a spurious increase in serum or plasma potassium concentration caused by in vitro changes, may be seen in hemolysed blood samples, especially from Akitas[24] and in dogs with thrombocytosis or extreme leucocytosis.[25]

Approximately 10% of dogs with primary hypoadrenocorticism have normal serum electrolyte concentrations at the time of initial examination. It is generally believed that these dogs with atypical Addison's disease have early or mild primary hypoadrenocorticism and that typical electrolyte abnormalities would develop with time. Rarely isolated primary hypocortisolemia has been reported in dogs that never develop serum electrolyte abnormalities.[26]

Calcium Concentration

Mild to moderate hypercalcemia is seen in about a third of dogs with hypoadrenocorticism. Usually these dogs are most severely affected by the disease. The mechanism by which hypercalcemia occurs in hypoadrenocorticism remains to be elucidated, but hemoconcentration, increased renal tubular reabsorption, and decreased glomerular filtration are thought to contribute. The differential diagnosis of hypercalcemia includes neoplasia, primary hyperparathyroidism, chronic renal failure, hypervitaminosis D, and granulomatous disease. In a study of 40 dogs with hypercalcemia, hypoadrenocorticism was the second most common cause and accounted for 25%.[27] In the same study, the degree of hypercalcemia was found to be significantly lower in dogs with hypoadrenocorticism (mean plasma calcium concentration 14.0 ± 1.6 mg/dL) than in lymphoproliferative disease (mean plasma calcium concentration 17.2 ± 2.8 mg/dL).

Blood Glucose Concentration

Theoretically, dogs with hypoadrenocorticism should have a tendency to develop hypoglycemia because glucocorticoid deficiency reduces glucose production by the liver and peripheral cell receptors become more sensitive to insulin. However, hypoglycemia is uncommon.[28] The potential for this complication should remain a concern for the clinician as rarely the severity of the hypoglycaemia may result in clinical signs of ataxia, disorientation, or seizures.[16]

Serum Albumin Concentration

Moderate to severe hypoalbuminemia has been noted in dogs with hypoadrenocorticism. The pathogenesis of hypoalbuminemia in primary hypoadrenocorticism is unknown, but gastrointestinal hemorrhage, impaired intestinal absorption of nutrients, and impaired albumin synthesis may be involved. The major causes of hypoalbuminemia include increased loss (for example, protein losing nephropathy or enteropathy, blood loss, severe exudation, or hemorrhage into body cavities) and decreased production (for example, severe malabsorption, maldigestion, or malnutrition or inadequate production in chronic liver disease). In one study, 39% of dogs with hypoadrenocorticism were found to have hypoalbuminemia.[29] However, other studies have shown the frequency of hypoalbuminemia to be considerably lower, between 6% and 12% of cases.[8,30] Some of the hypoalbuminomic dogs also have hypocholesterolemia, microhepatica, and/or ascites.

Liver Enzyme Concentrations

Mild to moderate increases in liver enzyme activities, such as alanine aminotransferase, aspartate aminotransferase, and alkaline phosphatase, are found in some dogs with hypoadrenocorticism. Although the precise cause of these increases is unknown, reduced cardiac output and poor tissue perfusion probably play a role. Increased liver enzyme activities hypoalbuminemia, and hypoglycemia would raise the suspicion of primary hepatic disease in some dogs with hypoadrenocorticism and clinicians should be aware of this potential confusion.

Acid-Base Balance

Mild to moderate metabolic acidosis is common in dogs with hypoadrenocorticism. Total carbon dioxide concentrations and serum bicarbonate determinations are reduced. Acidosis develops because reduced aldosterone concentrations impair renal tubular secretion of hydrogen ions. Hypotension and poor renal perfusion are likely to contribute to the acidosis.

Electrocardiographic Findings

Hyperkalemia impairs cardiac conduction and may cause life-threatening arrhythmias. These changes can be assessed by electrocardiography (ECG) (Figure 243-3). Although the ECG changes do not correlate precisely with serum potassium concentrations, probably because of the influence of other electrolyte abnormalities particularly the cardioprotective effects of increased calcium, metabolic acidosis, and impaired tissue perfusion, the following guidelines have proved helpful:

>5.5 mEq/L	peaking of the T wave shortening of the Q-T interval
>6.5 mEq/L	increased QRS duration
>7.0 mEq/L	P wave amplitude decreased P-R interval prolonged
>8.5 mEq/L	P wave absent (sinoatrial standstill) severe bradycardia

In some cases, bizarre QRS complexes representing ventricular extrasystoles, paroxysmal ventricular tachycardia, or ventricular fibrillation may be seen and these are most likely the result of hypoxia and/or hyperkalemia.

Electrocardiography can also be used for monitoring the response to treatment. An improvement in the ECG tracing suggests a reduction in serum potassium concentration.

Radiographic Findings

Dogs with hypoadrenocorticism may show radiographic signs of hypovolemia, which include: microcardia, decreased size of pulmonary vessels, reduced size of the caudal vena cava, and

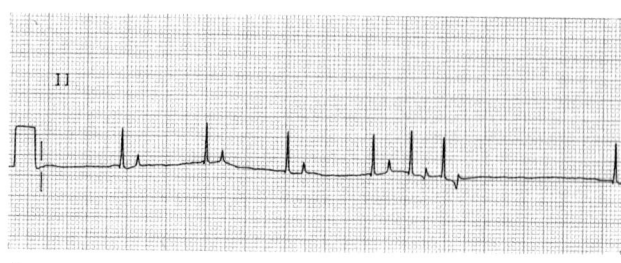

A

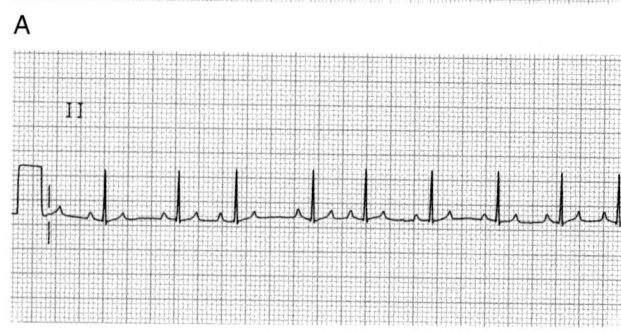

B

Figure 243-3 Electrocardiograms from a 4-year-old bearded collie dog with primary hypoadrenocorticism taken (**A**) before and (**B**) after supplementation with glucocorticoids and mineralocorticoids. Paper speed is 25 mm/sec and sensitivity is 1 cm = 1mV. **A,** The P waves are absent, the T waves are peaked, and there is profound bradycardia. The serum sodium concentration was 138 mEq/L and the serum potassium 9.5 mEq/L. **B,** ECG after treatment showing sinus arrhythmia. The serum sodium concentration was 142 mEq/L and the serum potassium 5.4 mEq/L.

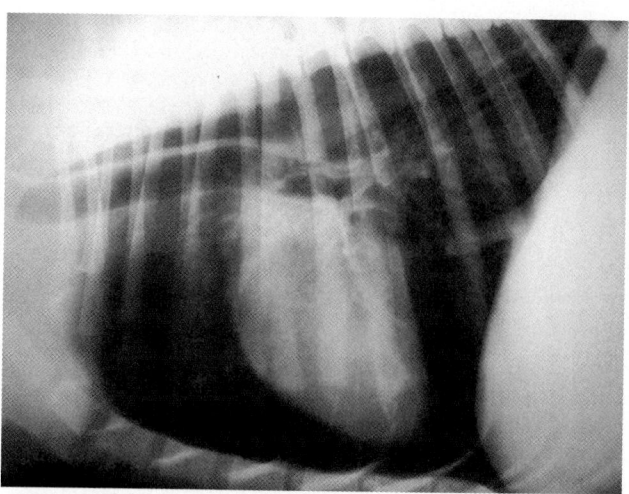

Figure 243-4 Lateral thoracic radiograph of a standard poodle with primary hypoadrenocorticism showing the effects of hypovolemia, including microcardia, decreased pulmonary vasculature, and reduced caudal vena cava. The esophagus is dilated with air in the cranial thorax as evidenced by a dorsal tracheal stripe sign.

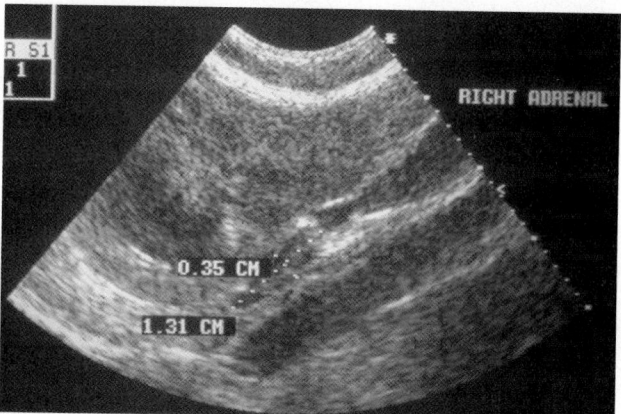

Figure 243-5 A longitudinal sonogram of the right adrenal gland of a Labrador retriever with primary hypoadrenocorticism. The adrenal thickness (3.5 mm) and the adrenal length (13.1 mm) have been measured.

microhepatica (Figure 243-4). These changes, however, are not specific and only represent hypovolemia and dehydration regardless of the cause. The severity of these radiographic findings usually correlates with the degree of hypovolemia.

A few dogs with hypoadrenocorticism develop esophageal dilation or megaesophagus as a result of generalized muscle weakness and this can be seen on thoracic radiographs as an air-filled, dilated esophagus. Image-intensified fluoroscopy, using barium paste or barium mixed with food demonstrates a complete absence of esophageal peristaltic activity. The cause of esophageal dilatation in hypoadrenocorticism remains unclear but was considered to be attributable to the effect of abnormal sodium and potassium concentrations on membrane potential and neuromuscular function.[31] However, in some dogs with hypoadrenocorticism and megaesophagus, abnormal serum electrolyte concentrations were never documented, which suggests that the esophageal dilatation was associated with glucocorticoid deficiency.[14,32] The megaesophagus resolves rapidly with appropriate treatment for hypoadrenocorticism.

Ultrasonography
With high resolution ultrasound equipment, it is possible for an experienced ultrasonographer to image the adrenal glands of most normal and diseased dogs. Ultrasonographic examination of the adrenal glands has been performed in dogs with hypoadrenocorticism, and the adrenal glands were shown to be shorter (median values: left adrenal 12.1 mm; right adrenal 13.1 mm) and thinner (median values: left adrenal 2.4 mm; right adrenal 2.5 mm) than those of healthy dogs.[33] However, there is considerable variation in the normal measurements of canine adrenal glands with maximum dimensions (length × thickness) in the range 10 to 52 mm × 2 to 12 mm.[34,35] There is poor correlation between these dimensions and body weight and there are no published normal adrenal measurements for different breeds of dog. Although ultrasonography could not distinguish between primary and secondary hypoadrenocorticism, the technique was considered to be a useful screening test especially in critically ill animals with acute disease (Figure 243-5).

Blood Pressure
Hypotension is present in nearly all humans with primary hypoadrenocorticism but is an uncommon finding in those with secondary hypoadrenocorticism. No large series of blood pressure measurements in dogs with hypoadrenocorticism have been published, but hypotension has been recorded in individual cases.[36]

Endocrine Tests
ACTH Stimulation Test
The ACTH stimulation test is the gold standard test for providing a definitive diagnosis of hypoadrenocorticism. Intravenous synthetic preparations of ACTH, either cosyntropin (Cortrosyn, Organon) or tetracosactrin (Synacthen, Alliance), should be used. Absorption of depot products such as ACTH gel cannot be relied on, particularly if the animal is collapsed or severely hypotensive. The protocol is described in Box 243-4.

In dogs and cats with hypoadrenocorticism, the resting cortisol concentration will be low or undetectable with a subnormal or negligible cortisol response to ACTH. About 85% of dogs with naturally occurring hypoadrenocorticism have basal and post-ACTH cortisol concentrations of less than 1.0 μg/dL (30 nmol/L) and more than 90% of cases have cortisol concentrations that do not exceed 2.0 μg/dL (60 nmol/L) at any time during the test.[37] Similar low cortisol concentrations have been reported in cats with hypoadrenocorticism. The ACTH stimulation test, however, does not distinguish between primary hypoadrenocorticism and secondary hypoadrenocorticism due to pituitary failure or iatrogenic glucocorticoid administration.

Endogenous Plasma ACTH Concentration
Plasma ACTH concentrations are useful in distinguishing primary from secondary hypoadrenocorticism, but stringent and meticulous sample handling is crucial since the activity of ACTH in the plasma will reduce rapidly resulting in falsely low values and incorrect interpretation (see Box 243-4). Dogs and cats with primary hypoadrenocorticism have extremely increased endogenous ACTH concentrations (>500 pg/mL), due to the lack of a negative feedback of cortisol on the pituitary, whereas those with secondary hypoadrenocorticism have low or even undetectable concentrations of ACTH (<5 pg/mL).

Plasma Aldosterone Concentrations
Basal aldosterone concentrations are of little or no diagnostic value. Plasma aldosterone concentrations should be measured in response to ACTH stimulation (see Box 243-4). Theoretically, plasma aldosterone concentrations should help

Box • 243-4

Box • 243-4

Protocols for Endocrine Tests for Hypoadrenocorticism

The ACTH Stimulation Test

- Collect 2 to 3 mL plasma or serum sample for basal cortisol concentration.*
- Inject 0.25 mg of synthetic ACTH (cosyntropin, Cortrosyn, Oganon: tetracosactrin; Synacthen, Alliance) intravenously to dogs or cats over 5 kg. Use only 0.125 mg in dogs or cats less than 5 kg.
- Collect a second sample for cortisol concentration 30 to 60 minutes later in the dog. In the cat, two samples should be collected at 60 and 90 to 120 minutes to ensure the peak response is measured.

Plasma Endogenous ACTH Concentration

- Blood (3 mL) is collected into a cooled plastic EDTA tube and centrifuged at 4° C immediately.
- The plasma should then be harvested and stored frozen (at less than −20° C) in a plastic tube.
- Samples must be transported to the laboratory frozen and must be kept frozen until assayed.
- Stringent and meticulous sample handling is crucial since hormone activity in the plasma will reduce rapidly resulting in falsely low values and incorrect interpretation.
- The endogenous ACTH assay must be validated for use in dogs and cats, otherwise the test may provide spurious results that could be misleading.

*The recent administration of glucocorticoids such as hydrocortisone, prednisolone, or prednisone may result in elevated cortisol concentrations due to cross-reactivity in many cortisol assays. For this reason glucocorticoids should be withheld for at least 24 hours before testing. There is no cross-reactivity with dexamethasone, but dexamethasone will suppress cortisol concentrations in animals with an intact hypothalamic-pituitary adrenal axis.

differentiate between primary hypoadrenocorticism (with reduced cortisol and aldosterone concentrations) and secondary hypoadrenocorticism (with normal aldosterone and reduced cortisol concentrations). However, aldosterone assays are not widely available and few studies have reported.

After stimulation with ACTH in normal dogs, plasma aldosterone concentrations should double, unless the basal concentration is already in the high-normal range.[38] In dogs suffering from primary hypoadrenocorticism with hypoaldosteronism, the basal aldosterone concentration is low with minimal or no increase in the post-ACTH aldosterone concentration. Some dogs with atypical Addison's disease have basal and post-ACTH aldosterone concentrations below the detectable limit of the assay despite the presence of normal serum sodium and potassium concentrations. Other dogs with atypical Addison's disease may have higher aldosterone concentrations than classical cases of hypoadrenocorticism both before and after ACTH stimulation, but concentrations are still abnormally decreased.

Treatment of Primary Hypoadrenocorticism
Acute Primary Hypoadrenocorticism

Intravenous saline   Hyperkalemia is life threatening in the acute Addisonian crisis but can be reliably treated with aggressive intravenous fluid therapy using normal saline (0.9% sodium chloride) at an initial rate of 60 to 80 mL/kg/hour for the first 1 to 2 hours. This treatment also helps in correcting the hypovolemia, hyponatremia, and hypochloremia. Urine output should be measured and if possible a central venous catheter should be used to monitor central venous pressure during fluid therapy. The response to treatment is often dramatic and other treatments for hyperkalemia such as glucose and insulin therapy or calcium administration are not usually required in animals with hypoadrenocorticism. The serum potassium decreases because of the dilution effect of the saline and the improvement in renal perfusion and glomerular filtration, which encourages further excretion of potassium into the urine. Although most cases respond quickly, generally within 12 hours, a few cases require intravenous fluid therapy over several days to correct the electrolyte imbalance and prerenal azotemia.

Intravenous glucose   If hypoglycemia is suspected, a 50% glucose solution should be added to the normal saline to produce a 5% dextrose solution. If hypoglycemia is known to be present, a bolus injection of 1 mL/kg of 50% glucose should be given intravenously initially before continuing with the 5% dextrose in 0.9% sodium chloride solution.

Glucocorticoid therapy   Glucocorticoid therapy should be used early in the treatment of the acute Addisonian crisis to correct hypocortisolemia. The glucocorticoids of choice in an acute crisis include the following:

hydrocortisone sodium succinate	10 mg/kg IV repeated every 3 to 6 hours or as a constant rate infusion at 0.5 mg/kg/hour[39]
prednisolone sodium succinate	5 mg/kg IV repeated every 3 to 6 hours
dexamethasone sodium phosphate	0.5 to 1.0 mg/kg IV given once

If possible, glucocorticoids should be withheld until after completion of the ACTH stimulation test since hydrocortisone and prednisolone have the potential to cross-react with cortisol in the assay falsely increasing the cortisol concentration. Dexamethasone can be used because it will not interfere with the cortisol assay and is recommended if glucocorticoid therapy cannot be delayed.

Mineralocorticoid preparations are not essential for treating an Addisonian crisis. However, mineralocorticoid therapy is recommended for any dog or cat suspected to have hypoadrenocorticism, once the ACTH stimulation test has been completed. As discussed, intravenous saline should help correct the hypovolemia, hyponatremia, hyperkalemia, and azotemia typical of this condition. No serious adverse reactions are associated with mineralocorticoid administration to non-hypoadrenal animals and the beneficial effects to those with the disease are complimentary to saline administration. Therefore it is recommended that desoxycorticosterone pivalate (DOCP; 2.2 mg/kg, IM) be administered. If the animal has hypoadrenocorticism, the drug will need to be given once again at 25 days, usually subcutaneously. The standard in management of these animals in crisis is administration of saline during completion of the ACTH stimulation test followed immediately by both glucocorticoid and mineralocorticoid therapy. Alternatives to DOCP have been tried. Hydrocortisone has been recommended as it possesses glucocorticoid and mineralocorticoid activities identical to those of endogenous cortisol.[39] Prednisolone also has some mineralocorticoid activity. Neither hydrocortisone or prednisolone have been shown to be superior to dexamethasone, which has no mineralocorticoid activity, in treating an Addisonian crisis (Table 243-1).

Table • 243-1

Relative Potencies of Adrenal Steroids

COMPOUND	GLUCOCORTICOID EFFECT	MINERALO- CORTICOID EFFECT
Cortisol/ hydrocortisone	1	1
Prednisolone/ prednisone	5	0.8
Dexamethasone	37	Negligible
Betamethasone	40	Negligible
Desoxycorticosterone	Negligible	50
Fludrocortisone	10-20	150
Aldosterone	0	500

Chronic Primary Hypoadrenocorticism (Maintenance Therapy)

Mineralocorticoid therapy Dogs and cats with primary hypoadrenocorticism that have the classic electrolyte disturbances of hyponatremia, hyperkalemia, and hypochloremia, require lifelong treatment with mineralocorticoids. Use of mineralocorticoid supplementation in those with atypical Addison's disease, where the electrolyte concentrations are normal, is more complex. In one study, two dogs with atypical primary hypoadrenocorticism were discharged on glucocorticoid supplementation only and both dogs died within 9 days of a presumed Addisonian crisis.[40] However, rarely some dogs with atypical primary hypoadrenocorticism have an isolated glucocorticoid deficiency and normal mineralocorticoid concentrations; these respond well to just glucocorticoid replacement therapy as do those with secondary hypoadrenocorticism.[26] Certainly it is prudent to try and differentiate primary and secondary hypoadrenocorticism or isolated glucocorticoid deficiency with plasma ACTH concentrations and basal and post-ACTH stimulated plasma aldosterone concentrations. While awaiting test results, it is recommended to administer both mineralocorticoid and glucocorticoid replacement therapy to reduce the possibility of an acute Addisonian crisis developing.

There are two preparations used for mineralocorticoid supplementation, fludrocortisone acetate, and desoxycorticosterone pivalate.

Fludrocortisone acetate (Florinef, Squibb) Fludrocortisone is a potent oral synthetic adrenocortical steroid with mainly mineralocorticoid effects, although it retains some glucocorticoid activity. It is available in 0.1 mg tablets. An initial dose of 15 μg/kg of fludrocortisone is administered once daily. The response is monitored and serum electrolytes measured after 5 to 7 days. The dose rate should then be adjusted until the serum sodium and potassium concentrations are within the normal range. Frequently the dose of fludrocortisone has to be increased during the first 6 to 18 months of therapy to maintain normal electrolyte concentrations and in a few of these cases, fludrocortisone may have to be administered twice daily. In one study, the daily maintenance dose of fludrocortisone increased from an initial median dose of 13 μg/kg to a final median dose of 23 μg/kg.[40] In the same study, the final dose of fludrocortisone administered to more than half the dogs ranged from 15 to 30 μg/kg/day.

Adverse effects develop in some dogs, particularly those receiving high doses of fludrocortisone to maintain serum electrolyte concentrations within the normal range. These include mild signs of iatrogenic hyperadrenocorticism (i.e., polyuria, polydipsia, polyphagia, and weight gain) due to the glucocorticoid effects of fludrocortisone (see Table 243-1).

Desoxycorticosterone pivalate (Percorten-V, Novartis) Desoxycorticosterone pivalate is a long acting ester of desoxycorticosterone acetate, a synthetic corticosteroid with only mineralocorticoid activity and no glucocorticoid activity. It is formulated into a microcrystalline suspension for injection. This preparation is not available in all countries, but studies have shown it to be effective in replacing the mineralocorticoid deficiency in dogs with hypoadrenocorticism.[41] It is considered the drug of choice in the United States (editor's note). The recommended dosage is 2.2 mg/kg intramuscularly or subcutaneously every 25 days. In another study, lower doses of between 1.4 and 1.9 mg/kg were found to be effective in controlling electrolyte concentrations and this study also showed that the interval between injections varied among dogs, ranging from 14 days to 35 days.[40]

Signs of iatrogenic hyperadrenocorticism have not been associated with long-term use of desoxycorticosterone pivalate since it possesses negligible glucocorticoid activity (see Table 243-1). However, some dogs developed anorexia and depression in the presence of normal electrolyte concentrations, which resolved promptly with glucocorticoid replacement therapy.

Glucocorticoid therapy The majority of dogs treated with fludrocortisone do not require daily glucocorticoid supplementation for maintenance therapy after the initial period of treatment. Those treated with DOCP should also be given glucocorticoids. Glucocorticoids at replacement dosages are administered for the first 1 to 2 weeks of treatment until the animal is stable and then gradually reduced. If glucocorticoid therapy is discontinued, owners of dogs and cats with hypoadrenocorticism should always be provided with a supply of prednisolone tablets to be given if the pet appears unwell (depressed, anorexic, or vomiting). Prednisolone at a dose of 0.1 to 0.2 mg/kg daily should be sufficient as glucocorticoid replacement for those animals that do require glucocorticoids. Higher doses are more likely to produce signs of iatrogenic hyperadrenocorticism.

Salt supplementation Sodium chloride tablets or salting of the food should be instigated at a dose 0.1 mg/kg/day initially to help correct hyponatremia but can be phased out and is not usually required long-term in most cases. Dogs requiring unusually high doses of fludrocortisone, however, may respond to a lower dose of fludrocortisone if concurrently provided with salt supplementation.

Prognosis

The prognosis with hypoadrenocorticism is excellent when appropriate maintenance therapy has been used together with thorough owner education. In one study, the median survival time for dogs with hypoadrenocorticism was 4.7 years with a range 7 days to 11.8 years.[40] In this study, age, breed, and sex were not shown to influence survival time and no significant difference was found in the survival time of dogs treated with fludrocortisone compared with desoxycorticosterone pivalate. The long-term prognosis also appears to be excellent in cats, although fewer cases have been studied.[2]

SECONDARY HYPOADRENOCORTICISM

Secondary hypoadrenocorticism is associated with a deficiency of glucocorticoids caused by a deficiency in ACTH production and/or release. The production of mineralocorticoids, although reduced, generally remains adequate to control serum sodium and potassium concentrations.

Causes of Secondary Hypoadrenocorticism

Secondary hypoadrenocorticism can be associated with destructive lesions; for example, large nonfunctional tumors in the hypothalamus or pituitary. More commonly, however, it is an iatrogenic condition associated with prolonged suppression of ACTH by drug therapy with glucocorticoids or progestogens such as megestrol acetate.[42,43]

Clinical Signs

The clinical signs are variable, but may include depression, anorexia, occasional vomiting or diarrhea, weak pulse, and sudden collapse when stressed. If the secondary hypoadrenocorticism is associated with glucocorticoid therapy, then clinical signs of iatrogenic hyperadrenocorticism (Cushing's disease) are usually present.

Diagnosis

The diagnosis of secondary hypoadrenocorticism is based on a failure of the plasma cortisol concentrations to respond to ACTH stimulation together with low or undetectable endogenous plasma ACTH concentrations. If measured, the plasma aldosterone concentrations may be reduced, but basal concentrations will increase with ACTH stimulation.

Treatment

Glucocorticoid replacement, using prednisolone at a dose of 0.1 to 0.2 mg/kg daily is indicated for immediate correction of the clinical signs. Further treatment and the prognosis depend on the cause of the disease and whether it can be treated. Management of glucocorticoid therapy and the prevention of iatrogenic hyperadrenocorticism should be considered for all patients on long-term therapy with glucocorticoids or progestogens.

CHAPTER • 244

Gastrointestinal Endocrine Disease

Cynthia R. Ward
Robert J. Washabau

GASTROINTESTINAL ENDOCRINOLOGY

Endocrine, Neurocrine, and Paracrine Activation

A gastrointestinal (GI) hormone is classically defined as a substance that (1) is found in gastrointestinal endocrine cells, (2) is released by physiologic stimuli (e.g., feeding), (3) circulates in blood, (4) binds to a cell receptor at a distant site, and (5) evokes a biologic response.[1,2] However, the characterization of an event as the physiologic result of a hormonal action may be exceedingly difficult. It is now clear that many substances previously classified as gastrointestinal hormones are neither confined to the gastrointestinal tract nor solely bloodborne. For example, many of the peptides localized in GI endocrine cells (e.g., cholecystokinin, substance P, neurotensin, and somatostatin) also may be found in GI neurons and act as neurocrine substances.[3] As enteric neuropeptides, these substances may evoke similar or different biologic responses.

Some of these same peptides (e.g., cholecystokinin, substance P, somatostatin) are also located outside the enteric nervous system in vagal afferent fibers or central nervous system neurons. Thus some GI hormones may also function as enteric or brain neuropeptides. A further complication is that some GI endocrine cells may release peptides into the extracellular fluid from which they diffuse to, and directly act on, neighboring cells. Thus a GI peptide may evoke a biologic response through a paracrine mechanism of activation that operates independent of, or in parallel to, an endocrine mechanism of activation. Finally, some substances (e.g., somatostatin) may evoke biologic responses through endocrine, paracrine, and neurocrine mechanisms: endocrine regulation of gastric acid secretion, paracrine regulation of antral gastrin secretion, and neurocrine regulation of smooth muscle contraction.

Although it is clear that some GI peptides evoke biologic responses through an endocrine mechanism, it is equally clear that other GI peptides activate cells through a multitude of cellular pathways: endocrine, neurocrine, and paracrine. The endocrine, neurocrine, or paracrine status of each well-established gastrointestinal peptide and other bioactive substances is reviewed in this chapter. An overview of endocrine, neurocrine, and paracrine mediators may be found in Table 244-1.

Endocrine Substances and Endocrine Cell Types

Gastrointestinal endocrinology has developed from a small subset of endocrinology consisting of three distinct peptides (secretin, gastrin, cholecystokinin) with local secretagogue effects, to a biologic discipline made up of more than 100 bioactive peptides, all of which are expressed in a controlled cell-specific manner. This chapter reviews only those GI hormones (and enteric neuropeptides and paracrine mediators) for which there are clearly defined biologic functions. Just as knowledge of bioactive peptides has proliferated in recent years, so too has knowledge of the cell types that produce these substances. More than 20 different endocrine cell types have been identified in the GI tract, and the number continues to grow. Differences in cell type and lineage have been addressed in recent reviews.

Gastrointestinal Hormones
Gastrin-Cholecystokinin Family

GI hormones[1,2,4] and related peptides have been divided into structurally homologous families, one of which consists of gastrin and cholecystokinin (CCK). Gastrin and CCK share five basic characteristics: (1) partial sequence homology; (2) similar, but not identical, biologic activities; (3) heterogeneity—each hormone exists in different molecular forms; (4) ubiquity—each hormone is synthesized in different cell types; and (5) differential principality—different molecular forms predominate in different tissues and cells.[1,4,5]

Gastrin Gastrin exists in several molecular forms that contain 34, 17, and 14 amino acids, respectively. G-34, also known as *big gastrin*, is the most abundant form of gastrin in serum. G-17, known as *little gastrin*, is less abundant than G-34 in serum but is much more potent in stimulating gastric

acid secretion. Mini gastrin (G-14) has little biologic effect. Endocrine cells (G cells) in the gastric antrum and duodenum secrete gastrin in response to protein meals and, to a lesser extent, gastric distension.[1,4,5]

The most important biologic action of gastrin is the stimulation of gastric acid secretion by gastric oxyntic (parietal) cells. A substantial fraction of the gastric acid secretory response to protein meals is, in fact, mediated by gastrin. However, interactions between gastrin, acetylcholine (neurocrine stimulant), and histamine (paracrine stimulant) determine the final gastric acid secretory output.[6] Most evidence suggests that the gastrin effect occurs through the binding

Table • 244-1

Overview of Endocrine, Neurocrine, and Paracrine Mediators

SUBSTANCE	PHYSIOLOGIC RELEASE	SITE OF ACTION	EFFECT
GI Hormones			
Gastrin	Intra-gastric peptides, gastric distension	Gastric parietal and chief cells	H^+ and pepsinogen secretion
Cholecystokinin	Duodenal fatty acids, amino acids, H^+	Pancreatic acinar cells Stomach, duodenum, pancreas Gallbladder Sphincter of Oddi Pancreas Stomach	Enzyme secretion Growth Contraction Relaxation Enzyme secretion and growth Inhibition of gastric emptying
Secretin	Duodenal H^+, fatty acids	Pancreatic duct cells, biliary epithelium, duodenum	HCO_3^- and water secretion
Oxyntomodulin GLP-1	Ileal/colonic glucose and lipid Duodenal fatty acids	Gastric parietal cells Pancreatic islet (β) cells	Inhibition of H^+ secretion Stimulates insulin secretion (incretin during euglycemia)
	Ileal fatty acids	Stomach	Inhibition of gastric emptying ("ileal brake")
GLP-2	Carbohydrates, lipids, SCFA	Small intestine, colon	Inhibits gastric emptying (ileal brake) and secretion Crypt cell proliferation, suppression of apoptosis Reduces gut permeability and bacterial translocation
Gastric inhibitory polypeptide	Fatty acids, glucose, amino acids	Duodenum, jejunum, ileum	Inhibition of gastric and intestinal motility Stimulates insulin secretion (incretin during euglycemia)
Somatostatin	Lipids, protein, and bile	Stomach, intestine, pancreas	Inhibition of gastric, intestinal, and pancreatic secretion
Motilin	H^+ and lipids	Stomach, duodenum, jejunum	Increases GES pressure, stimulates propulsive motility Stimulates gastric, pancreatic, and biliary secretion
Neurotensin	Fatty acids	Stomach, pancreas, gallbladder	Stimulation of gastric and pancreatic secretion Gallbladder contraction
Pancreatic polypeptide	Protein, cholinergic reflexes	Pancreas	Inhibition of pancreatic enzyme and fluid secretion

Continued

Table • 244-1

Overview of Endocrine, Neurocrine, and Paracrine Mediators—Cont'd

SUBSTANCE	PHYSIOLOGIC RELEASE	SITE OF ACTION	EFFECT
Peptide YY	H+ and lipids	Ileum and colon	Ileal brake, proliferation of gut mucosa
		Stomach and pancreas	Inhibition of secretion (H+, pancreatic enzyme)
5-Hydroxytryptamine	H+	Intestine and colon	Stimulation of motility and secretion
Ghrelin	Dietary protein	Pituitary	Stimulation of growth hormone secretion
Enteric Neuropeptides			
Substance P	Luminal distension, H+, hyperosmolarity	Stomach, intestine, colon	Sphincteric contractions, intestinal peristalsis
		Pancreas	Stimulation of pancreatic enzyme secretion
Vasoactive intestinal polypeptide	Vagal stimulation	Stomach, intestine, colon	Increased blood flow, stimulation of fluid secretion
		Stomach, intestine, colon	Relaxation of smooth muscle
		Pancreas	Stimulation of fluid and bicarbonate secretion
Opioids	Intestinal distension	Stomach, intestine, colon	Inhibition of longitudinal smooth muscle contraction
			Stimulation of circular smooth muscle contraction
			Inhibition of water and electrolyte secretion
Bombesins (GRP and Neuromedin B)	Vagal stimulation	Stomach	Stimulation of gastric acid secretion
		Pancreas	Stimulation of pancreatic enzyme secretion
		Gallbladder	Stimulation of gallbladder contraction
Somatostatin	Lipids and protein	Stomach, intestine, pancreas	Descending inhibitory reflex of peristalsis
Gastrin/CCK	Intestinal distension	Ileum and colon	Ileal and colonic contractions
Neuropeptide Y	Intestinal distension	Intestine and colon	Inhibition of intestinal motility
5-Hydroxytryptamine	H+ and hypertonic solutions	Stomach, intestine, colon	Regulation of migrating myoelectric complex
Paracrine Mediators			
Histamine	Vagal stimulation	Stomach	Stimulation of gastric acid secretion
Somatostatin	Lipids and proteins	Stomach	Inhibition of gastrin secretion
		Pancreas	Regulation of insulin and glucagon secretion
Prostaglandins	H+, gastric distension	Stomach	Stimulation of bicarbonate and glycoprotein secretion
			Stimulation of epithelial cell renewal and blood flow
			Inhibition of prostanoid receptors

CCK, cholecystokinin; GES, gastroesophageal sphincter; GLP-1, glucagon-like peptide-1; GLP-2, glucagons-like peptide-2; GRP, gastrin-releasing peptide; SCFA, small chain fatty acids.

of gastrin to gastrin receptors on oxyntic cells, although one study suggests that the gastrin effect might be indirectly mediated through gastrin receptors on gastric mucosal immunocytes.[7]

Other important biologic actions of gastrin include stimulation of gastric pepsinogen secretion, gastric mucosal blood flow, antral motility, pancreatic enzyme secretion, and of pancreatic, gastric, and duodenal growth.[1,4,5,8] Pancreatic islet cells (delta cells) are a site of gastrin synthesis and secretion in fetal and neonatal animals.[8] Malignant transformation of these islet cells in adult animals results in functional gastrinomas. All but one of the gastrinomas that have been reported in the dog or cat have been of pancreatic origin (see Gastrinoma).

Cholecystokinin   Cholecystokinin (CCK) also exists in several molecular forms: CCK-63, CCK-58, CCK-39, CCK-33, CCK-12, CCK-8, and CCK-5. The predominant forms in serum are CCK-33, CCK-39, and CCK-58 and probably account for most of the GI hormone responses.[1,2,4] CCK-8 is the predominant form found in neurons and probably accounts for most of the enteric and central nervous system neuropeptide responses. Endocrine cells (I cells) in the duodenum and jejunum secrete CCK in response to intraduodenal fatty acids, amino acids, and H^+ ion.[1,2,4]

As a gastrointestinal hormone, CCK evokes several important biologic responses, most importantly, contraction of the gallbladder and stimulation of pancreatic enzyme secretion. Although CCK receptors have been demonstrated on both gallbladder smooth muscle cells and pancreatic acinar cells, it is now clear that CCK evokes gallbladder contraction and pancreatic enzyme secretion through activation of presynaptic cholinergic neurons at both sites.[4,8]

Other important endocrine actions of CCK include augmentation of pancreatic fluid secretion in the presence of secretin, relaxation of the sphincter of Oddi, inhibition of the gastric emptying of liquids, and stimulation of pancreatic growth.[1,4] Because CCK has trophic effects on pancreatic growth,[8] it has been suggested that canine juvenile pancreatic atrophy might result from CCK deficiency. However, CCK secretory deficiency was not observed in a group of young dogs with exocrine pancreatic insufficiency.[9] CCK has two important biologic actions as an enteric or brain neuropeptide (see Enteric Neuropeptides).

Secretin-Enteroglucagon-Gastric Inhibitory Polypeptide Family

Another structurally homologous group of GI hormones include secretin, enteroglucagon, gastric inhibitory polypeptide (GIP), as well as the enteric neuropeptides vasoactive intestinal polypeptide (VIP) and peptide histidine-isoleucine (PHI).

Secretin   Like gastrin and CCK, secretin exists in several molecular forms: 27-, 28-, 30-, and 71-amino acid polypeptides.[10] Acidification of the duodenum and jejunum by gastric H^+ is the most important stimulus for secretin secretion by endocrine cells (S cells) in the small intestine.[1,4] Intraduodenal lipid may also stimulate secretin release in some species. The most important biologic action of secretin is stimulation of secretion of a bicarbonate-rich pancreatic fluid from pancreatic ductal cells.[8,10] Pancreatic bicarbonate is important in neutralizing gastric acid delivered to the small intestine and in creating an alkaline environment that is close to the pH optimum of pancreatic lipase and co-lipase. Less important biologic actions of secretin are to stimulate secretion of bile bicarbonate and pancreatic enzymes.[1,8] The latter effect is observed only in the presence of CCK. Secretin has also been identified in brain neurons, but a functional role for secretin in these neurons has not yet been elucidated.

Enteroglucagon   Enteroglucagon and pancreatic glucagon arise from the same gene precursor through post-translational processing. Several molecular forms of enteroglucagon have been characterized, including enteroglucagon or oxyntomodulin, a 37 amino acid peptide; glicentin, a 69 amino acid, C-terminal extended form of oxyntomodulin; glucagon-like peptide (GLP)-1; intervening peptide-2; and GLP-2. Endocrine cells (L cells) in the terminal ileum and colon secrete enteroglucagon(s) in response to intraluminal glucose and lipid. The most important gastrointestinal action of the enteroglucagons is the inhibition of gastric acid secretion.[1,4] GLP peptides are also involved in the regulation of insulin secretion and glycemic control. GLP-1 is reported to stimulate proinsulin expression and to delay intestinal glucose absorption through inhibition of gastric emptying[11], thus acting as an incretin hormone during euglycemia to lower blood glucose. GLP-2 is a 33-amino acid peptide hormone released from intestinal endocrine cells following nutrient ingestion.[12] It exerts trophic effects on the small and large bowel epithelium via stimulation of cell proliferation and inhibition of apoptosis. GLP-2 also upregulates intestinal glucose transporter activity and reduces gastric motility and gastric secretion.[13]

Gastric inhibitory polypeptide (GIP)   GIP is a 54-amino acid peptide that exists in a single molecular form.[14] It is secreted by endocrine cells of the proximal small intestine in response to intraduodenal glucose, fatty acids, and amino acids. Two important biologic actions of GIP are inhibition of gastric acid secretion and stimulation of intestinal fluid secretion. The third, and likely most important, biologic action of GIP is the stimulation of pancreatic insulin release during hyperglycemia. It has been suggested that GIP and GLP-1 function as incretins and are the substances responsible for increased glucose disposal and enhanced insulin responses during intestinal absorption of glucose.[1,4,14]

Somatostatin

Somatostatin, or somatotropin release-inhibiting factor was originally isolated from the hypothalamus and found to inhibit growth hormone and thyrotropin release from the pituitary. Somatostatin was subsequently found in gut endocrine cells and gut neurons and shown to have endocrine, neurocrine, and paracrine biologic effects. Two molecular forms of somatostatin have been identified in gut endocrine cells: somatostatin-14 (SS-14), and somatostatin-28 (SS-28). Endocrine cells (D cells) throughout the GI tract secrete somatostatin in response to protein, lipid, and bile. As a GI hormone, somatostatin inhibits gastric acid and pepsin secretion, pancreatic enzyme and fluid secretion, gallbladder contraction, and intestinal amino acid and glucose absorption.[1,4] Synthetic forms of somatostatin (Sandostatin, Sandoz Pharmaceuticals) are available for the treatment of gastric acid secretory disorders.[15] In addition to its role as a gastrointestinal hormone, somatostatin also functions as an enteric neuropeptide (e.g., inhibition of intestinal motility) and as a paracrine substance (e.g., inhibition of gastrin secretion).

Motilin

Motilin is a 22-amino acid peptide found in endocrine cells of the proximal small intestine. Motilin secretion is stimulated by H^+ and lipid during the fed state. However, motilin secretion seems to be most important in the interdigestive (fasting) state. During fasting, motilin is episodically released into the serum and initiates phase III of the migrating motility complex (MMC, or interdigestive motility complex).[16] The MMC is a motility pattern that empties the stomach and small intestine of indigestible solids that accumulate during feeding. The cyclic release of motilin from the small intestinal mucosa during fasting is also thought to coordinate gastric, pancreatic, and biliary secretions with phase III of the MMC.[17] It has been shown that microbially ineffective doses of erythromycin (0.5 mg/lb or 1.0 mg/kg) initiate an MMC pattern that is indistinguishable from that induced by motilin. It has thus been suggested that erythromycin and other macrolide-like antibiotics might be useful gastric prokinetic agents.[18]

Neurotensin

Neurotensin is a 13-amino acid peptide, isolated from dog ileal and jejunal mucosal endocrine cells (N cells), for which no definitive endocrine function has been established. Intraluminal lipid stimulates neurotensin release from these endocrine cells. Neurotensin has been shown to inhibit gastric secretion and emptying, stimulate pancreatic secretion, and stimulate gallbladder contraction. One of the most likely potential roles of neurotensin is that of a physiologic enterogastrone that mediates inhibition of acid secretion after fat ingestion.[1,4]

Pancreatic Polypeptide

Pancreatic polypeptide (PP) is a 36-amino acid peptide that shares sequence homology with the enteric neuropeptide known as neuropeptide Y (NPY). PP is found exclusively in pancreatic islet cells (F cells). PP release is stimulated by protein meals and by cholinergic reflexes. The most important biologic action of PP is the inhibition of pancreatic enzyme and fluid secretion.[1,4] Islet cell PP secretion likely autoregulates acinar and ductal cell secretions because of the islet-acinar portal venous system. Other possible endocrine functions of PP include relaxation of gallbladder smooth muscle, mild stimulation of gastric acid secretion, and initiation of the MMC along with motilin.[17]

Peptide YY

Peptide YY is a 36-amino acid peptide with structural similarities to PP and to NPY. Peptide YY may function as a physiologic enterogastrone similar to neurotensin in inhibiting pancreatic and gastric secretions.[1,4]

5-Hydroxytryptamine

5-Hydroxytryptamine (5-HT or serotonin) is found in endocrine cells (i.e., enterochromaffin cells) and enteric neurons throughout the gastrointestinal tract of most animal species.[1,2,4] In some species, 5-HT is also found in intestinal mucosal mast cells, pancreatic islet cells, and bronchial endocrine cells. 5-HT secreted by enterochromaffin cells may act through an endocrine or paracrine mechanism to stimulate gastrointestinal smooth muscle contraction and intestinal electrolyte secretion.[2] Tumors of these enterochromaffin cells (see Carcinoids) may be associated with hypermotility and secretory diarrhea because of the effects of 5-HT on motility and secretion.

Ghrelin

Ghrelin is a 28-amino acid octanoylated peptide found most abundantly in endocrine cells of the stomach.[18,19] It stimulates pituitary growth hormone (GH) secretion. *Ghre* is the Proto-Indo-European root for the word "growth," and the suffix-*relin* signifies "releasing substances." Ghrelin administration also has been shown to stimulate appetite, body growth, and fat deposition. The post-prandial gastric expression of ghrelin suggests a gastrointestinal-hypothalamaic-pituitary axis that influences GH secretion, body growth, and appetite that is responsive to nutritional and caloric intakes. Ghrelin and leptin may be the "ying and the yang" of a system that relays peripheral information to the brain and directs the body in the appropriate maintenance of energy reserves and nutritional intake.

Enteric Neuropeptides

A substance may be defined as an enteric neuropeptide if (1) it can be demonstrated histochemically in enteric neurons, (2) mechanisms for its biosynthesis exist in enteric neurons, (3) it is concentrated in nerve terminals, (4) it is released from nerve terminals by depolarizing stimuli through a calcium-dependent mechanism, and (5) mechanisms for the breakdown, re-uptake, or removal of the substance exist.[3]

The Tachykinins

The tachykinin family is represented by substance P, substance K, neuromedin K, physalaemin, kassinin, and eledoisin. Substance P is probably the most important enteric neuropeptide of this group. Substance P is distributed in enteric neurons throughout the GI tract and pancreas, and it is released from these neurons in response to luminal distension or depolarization. Substance P has three important biologic actions as an enteric neuropeptide.[3] First, it causes contraction of GI smooth muscle through an indirect effect of mediating cholinergic transmission and a direct effect on smooth muscle during the peristaltic reflex. Second, substance P is located in primary sensory afferent fibers and may be important, along with calcitonin gene-related peptide in pain input to the central nervous system. Finally, substance P neurons stimulate pancreatic enzyme secretion from pancreatic acinar cells.

Vasoactive Intestinal Polypeptide/Peptide Histidine-Isoleucine

The classic enteric neuropeptides VIP and PHI share sequence homology with one another and with the GI hormones secretin, enteroglucagon, and GIP. VIP and PHI have many similar biologic activities and are derived from the same biosynthetic precursor. VIP and PHI are released by vagal stimulation and have four important biologic actions:[3] (1) stimulation of pancreatic fluid and bicarbonate secretion, (2) stimulation of salivary and intestinal fluid secretion, (3) increasing intestinal blood flow, and (4) relaxation of GI smooth muscle. This last property of VIP/PHI is felt to be important in descending intestinal inhibition (along with somatostatin) and in sphincter relaxation. Functional tumors of VIP-producing cells produce a watery diarrhea syndrome (pancreatic cholera or Verner-Morrison syndrome) in humans. This syndrome has not yet been described in dogs or cats.

Opioids

Opioid neurons are distributed throughout the gastrointestinal tract, spinal cord, brain, and adrenal glands. Methionine-enkephalin, leucine-enkephalin, and dynorphin are the most representative members of the opioid enteric neuropeptide family.[3] At least three different types of binding sites for these opioid peptides can be distinguished in the gut (μ, δ, and κ) but there may be others (ϵ and σ). The binding sites for these opioids are located on other neurons, smooth muscle cells, and epithelial cells. Opioid binding results in (1) inhibition of contraction of longitudinal smooth muscle through inhibition of acetylcholine release from myenteric plexus neurons; (2) direct stimulation of circular smooth muscle contraction; and (3) inhibition of intestinal water and electrolyte secretion through inhibition of submucosal plexus neurons. These effects account for the potent antidiarrheal properties of morphine and other opiate alkaloids that have been recognized for centuries.[3]

Bombesins

The bombesins are so-named because of their original isolation from the skin of the frog genus *Bombina*. The mammalian bombesins that have been identified as enteric neuropeptides are gastrin releasing peptide (GRP) and neuromedin B. GRP is released by vagal stimulation, and it stimulates gastrin release from antral G cells. Thus GRP acts a co-transmitter (along with acetylcholine) to stimulate gastrin release.[3,5] GRP also stimulates pancreatic acinar cell enzyme secretion.[3,8]

Somatostatin

In addition to its role as a gastrointestinal hormone, somatostatin (SS-14) has been identified as an enteric neuropeptide in neurons throughout the gastrointestinal tract. Somatostatin inhibits acetylcholine release from myenteric plexus neurons and may be involved in the descending inhibitory reflex of peristalsis.[3] Somatostatin neurons in the submucous plexus have a mucosal projection suggesting a further role for neuronal somatostatin in the control of mucosal function.

Gastrin-CCK

CCK-8 is an important enteric neuropeptide in the ileum and colon, especially in the cat. Intraluminal distension activates CCK-8-containing neurons, which then stimulate the release of acetylcholine from myenteric plexus neurons. CCK-8 thus acts as an excitatory transmitter in stimulating the peristaltic reflex in ileum and colon.[1,3] Brain CCK-8 neurons are involved in mediating the satiety response following feeding. Indeed, it has been suggested that human bulimia nervosa patients do not have normal satiety and have an impaired secretion of cholecystokinin in response to a meal.[20]

Pancreatic Polypeptides

A 36-amino acid peptide, NPY shares structural similarities with the GI hormones PP and peptide YY. Neurons that contain NPY decrease acetylcholine release from myenteric plexus neurons and hence inhibit small intestinal smooth muscle contraction.[3]

5-Hydroxytryptamine (5-HT or Serotonin)

In addition to its role as an endocrine/paracrine substance of the gastrointestinal tract, 5-HT is also found in enteric neurons, where it is believed to regulate the migrating myoelectrical complex and the intestinal peristaltic reflex.[3]

Paracrine Substances

A substance may be defined as having a paracrine mechanism of activation if (1) the substance is found within an effector cell, (2) receptors for the substance exist on an adjacent paracrine target cell, (3) the effector cell and paracrine target cell are in close proximity, and (4) the substance when applied to the paracrine target cell evokes a biologic response.[1,2] Histamine, somatostatin, adenosine, and prostaglandins have been shown to satisfy these criteria.

Histamine

Histamine is formed from the decarboxylation of histidine in mast cells found throughout the GI tract of dogs. In the dog, gastric mucosal histamine stores appear fully accounted for by mast cells, there being no evidence to indicate histamine is stored in endocrine cells.[6] Histamine released from mast cells diffuses into the interstitial milieu and is believed to bind parietal cell H_2 receptors to stimulate H^+ secretion.[6] A large body of evidence has accumulated in support of this idea, although one study suggests that the histamine effect might be indirectly mediated through histamine receptors on gastric mucosal immunocytes.[7] Regardless, H_2 receptor antagonists have been shown to be potent inhibitors of histamine, acetylcholine, and gastrin-stimulated H^+ secretion.

Somatostatin

The endocrine and neurocrine roles of somatostatin were discussed earlier in this chapter. As a paracrine substance, somatostatin has an important role in the inhibition of gastrin release. Somatostatin cells in the gastric antrum have long cytoplasmic processes that terminate adjacent to antral G cells. Paracrine release of somatostatin by these somatostatin cells is postulated to mediate the negative feedback inhibition of H^+ on gastrin release.[21] Somatostatin released from pancreatic islet cells (D cells) may also auto-regulate pancreatic insulin and glucagon secretion through a local paracrine mechanism.[22]

Prostaglandins

Prostaglandins are long chain fatty acids that are distributed throughout the GI tract. The role of prostaglandins as paracrine substances is perhaps best understood in the gastric mucosa, where they bind to inhibitory prostanoid receptors on gastric oxyntic cells. These receptors are coupled to inhibitory G proteins and subsequent inhibition of adenylate cyclase and H^+ secretion.[23] A "cytoprotective effect" of prostaglandins, separate from the direct inhibition of acid inhibition, has also been implied. Gastric prostaglandins, for example, stimulate mucosal bicarbonate and glycoprotein secretion, epithelial cell renewal, and mucosal blood flow. These effects are all central to the barrier properties of the gastric mucosa.[24] Synthetic forms of prostaglandins (Cytotec, Searle) are now available for the therapy of gastric mucosal barrier disorders.[25,26,27]

DISEASES OF THE GASTROINTESTINAL ENDOCRINE SYSTEM

In small animals, the major syndromes of gastrointestinal endocrine pathology are diabetes mellitus, pancreatic islet cell tumors, and intestinal carcinoid. The syndromes of glucagonoma, gastrinoma, carcinoid, and pancreatic polypeptidoma are reviewed.

Glucagonoma

Glucagonoma is a rare tumor of the pancreatic alpha cells in dogs and humans. There are no reports of this disease in the cat. It is characterized by a crusting skin rash, termed *necrolytic migratory erythema* (NME) and glucose intolerance or overt diabetes mellitus (Figure 244-1). Increased serum glucagon concentrations stimulate hepatic amino acid turnover, gluconeogenesis, and glycogenolysis. In dogs, it is definitively diagnosed by immunohistochemistry of excised pancreatic tumor tissue.

Signalment and Clinical Signs

Eight dogs with presumptive or definitively diagnosed glucagonoma have been reported.[28-34] These eight dogs included seven breeds, four females, and four males, and their ages ranged from 5 to 13 years.

In human glucagonoma patients, NME is virtually pathognomonic for the disease. Although NME has been identified in all dogs with glucagonoma, it is more commonly associated with liver disease. Glucose intolerance or overt diabetes mellitus is also found in humans with glucagonoma and is caused by excess gluconeogenesis and glycogenolysis resulting from increased plasma glucagon concentrations. Other clinical signs in people include weight loss, anemia, diarrhea, stomatitis, and thromboembolic disease.

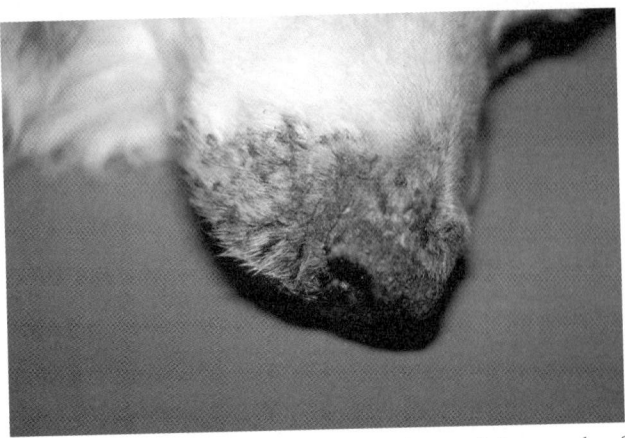

Figure 244-1 Necrolytic migratory erythema of the muzzle of a dog with glucagonoma. (Courtesy William H. Miller, Jr.)

Dogs with glucagonoma had 3-week to 16-month histories of crusting dermatologic lesions with or without ulceration or erosion at the time of presentation. Footpad lesions were present in all dogs with other affected sites including the elbows, hocks, nose, mucocutaneous junctions of the mouth or eyes, prepuce, vulva, scrotum, flank, ventral abdomen, and distal extremities. One dog also had oral ulcerations. Other clinical signs or physical exam findings at the time of initial presentation included lethargy, weight loss, decreased appetite, muscle atrophy, and peripheral lymphadenopathy. One dog also had palpable hepatomegaly.

Laboratory and Imaging Findings

Laboratory abnormalities included hyperglycemia (five dogs), nonregenerative anemia (three dogs), mild to moderately increased ALT activity (four dogs), mild to moderately increased ALP activity (three dogs), decreased albumin (two dogs), decreased globulin (one dog), decreased BUN (two dogs), decreased cholesterol (one dog), and glucosuria (two dogs). Liver function tests, including serum bile acid measurements (six dogs) and ammonia tolerance test (one dog), were normal. One dog had an ACTH stimulation test supportive of hyperadrenocorticism.

One or more imaging studies were performed in all dogs. Abdominal radiographs were unremarkable in all dogs. Abdominal ultrasound was normal in three dogs but revealed liver lesions in four dogs and a possible pancreatic mass in one dog. Liver abnormalities on ultrasound included a small liver with increased echogenicity of the portal and hepatic vein walls, diffuse hyperechogenicity, multiple small hypoechoic foci, and a single well-defined hyperechoic area. A mass in the left pancreatic limb was visualized by computed tomography in one case.

Diagnosis

Diagnosis in people is confirmed by demonstration of increased plasma glucagon concentrations and a pancreatic islet cell tumor that shows positive immunoreactivity for glucagon.

Glucagon measurement Demonstration of increased circulating glucagon concentrations is important to establish the hypersecretion of glucagon by the tumor cells and to associate clinical signs with excess hormone secretion. Plasma glucagon concentrations of more than 1000 ng/L are considered diagnostic of the disease in people. Plasma glucagon concentrations were measured in six of the eight dogs reported in the literature. In all dogs plasma glucagon concentrations were increased, ranging from 1.6 to 10.1 times the upper limit of reference ranges. It is important to note, however, that syndromes other than glucagonoma may be associated with increased plasma circulating glucagon, including acute pancreatitis, hypercortisolism, hepatic failure, and renal failure. Because of the paucity of cases in the veterinary literature, it is difficult to determine plasma glucagon concentrations that are diagnostic of glucagonoma in the dog. The presence of concurrent disease, as noted above, should always be considered.

Plasma amino acid concentrations Hypoaminoacidemia is often found in humans with glucagonoma and is thought to result from increased hepatic conversion of amino acid nitrogen into urea nitrogen by the excess glucagon.[35] Plasma amino acids were measured in three of the dogs reported and were decreased in all three (20 of 24, 13 of 18, and 4 of 5 amino acids determined). Arginine, histidine, and lysine concentrations were consistently decreased, although it must be noted that complete amino acid profiles were not measured in all cases.

Pathology

Most glucagon secreting tumors in people occur singly and are quite large (5 to 10 cm) at the time of diagnosis. Up to 82% are metastatic. In dogs, the diagnosis of glucagonoma has relied on demonstration of a primary pancreatic or metastatic tumor that stains positively for glucagon immunoreactivity. Pancreatic tumors were found in seven of the eight dogs reported. In one animal, serial sections of the pancreas failed to reveal neoplasia; diagnosis was instead based on positive glucagon immunoreactivity of metastatic tissue in the liver in conjunction with hyperglucagonemia. Location of pancreatic tumors included the right lobe (three dogs), left lobe (two dogs), body (one dog). As in the human, metastasis of glucagonoma is common in dogs and occurred in five of the eight cases. The liver was the most frequently affected site (four of the eight dogs) with one dog showing metastasis to a regional lymph node. Lymph node or liver tissue was not obtained in all cases so that the rate of metastasis may be higher than reported.

Glucagon immunohistochemical staining was performed on primary pancreatic and/or metastatic tumors. In most cases, tissue sections were also stained for immunoreactivity to somatostatin, gastrin islet amyloid polypeptide, insulin, pancreatic polypeptide, and/or synaptophysin, a marker for neuroendocrine cells.[36] In accordance with diagnostic criteria, all primary and metastatic tumors stained positively for glucagon immunoreactivity. In five dogs, primary tumor or metastatic tissue stained positively for one or more of above listed peptides. In some cases, metastatic tissue had different immunoreactivity than the primary tumor.

Therapy

Surgical resection or debulking is the treatment of choice for glucagonoma. In people removal of the glucagon-secreting tumor resolves the skin rash and other clinical signs. In the dogs with glucagonoma, four had surgical resection of the pancreatic mass. Two of these animals were euthanized 3 days after surgery because of presumed acute pancreatitis. One dog with metastatic disease of a mesenteric lymph node had surgical resection of both the lymph node and pancreatic mass. Glucagon concentrations decreased into the reference range the day following surgery and remained normal for 3 months. Plasma amino acid concentrations also increased within 30 days, and cutaneous lesions resolved within 45 days of surgery. Nine months after surgery, the dog was euthanized due to the development of new skin lesions. A second dog with metastasis to the liver had mild improvement of skin lesions following surgical resection of the pancreatic mass. Plasma glucagon concentrations, however, remained increased 10 days following surgery, but the dog was well 4 months post surgery.

Medical therapy should be considered as an adjunct for surgical resection in dogs with metastasis or for palliative therapy if surgery is not performed. Long-acting somatostatin analogues such as octreotide have been used to control plasma glucagon concentrations and clinical signs in humans. In one report, somatostatin was administered at a dosage of 6 μg/kg subcutaneously every 8 hours to a dog with metastatic disease, and marked improvement in skin lesions was reported within 14 days.[37] The treatment was not continued due to expense, and the dog was euthanized. Chemotherapeutic agents such as streptozotocin with 5-fluorouracil and dacarbazine have been somewhat successful in human treatment.[38] Intravenous amino acid therapy has also been helpful in some humans for the dermatologic abnormalities. There are no data on use of these agents in dogs.

Humans with glucagonoma often have concurrent diabetes mellitus. Some can be controlled by diet or oral hypoglycemic agents; however, many require insulin therapy.[39] Five of the eight dogs with glucagonoma had mild to moderate hyperglycemia with or without glucosuria. Two of these dogs were treated with insulin, one of which no longer required insulin 10 days after treatment was instituted. No long-term use of insulin in dogs with glucagonoma has been reported.

Prognosis

Because dogs have had metastatic disease at the time of diagnosis, prognosis is poor. Moreover, surgical outcome appears to be further complicated by the occurrence of pancreatitis. NME (also referred to as *superficial necrolytic dermatitis, hepatocutaneous syndrome,* and *metabolic epidermal necrosis*) is found more commonly in dogs with hepatic disease; glucagonoma accounts for less than 10% of the cases of NME. Therefore it is essential to assess liver function in dogs with NME so that a precise etiology may be determined and treatment options and prognosis correctly presented. Serum liver enzyme activities were abnormal in most dogs with glucagonoma; however, liver function tests were normal in all dogs tested.

Abdominal radiography and ultrasonography were found to be poor methods for detecting canine pancreatic glucagonoma. Computed tomography successfully identified the pancreatic glucagonoma in one dog and may prove more useful in the diagnosis of this disease. As clinical awareness and diagnostic testing improve, our understanding of the disease and treatment outcomes will undoubtedly improve as well.

Gastrinoma

In 1955 Zollinger and Ellison described a syndrome in people of gastric acid hypersecretion, severe peptic ulceration, and pancreatic islet cell tumor that was eponymously termed the *Zollinger-Ellison syndrome.* These islet cell tumors were subsequently demonstrated to secrete excessive amounts of gastrin and are now more appropriately called *gastrinomas.* Clinical signs result from excess plasma gastrin concentrations causing gastric acid hypersecretion. Hypergastrinemia and gastric hyperacidity result in gastrointestinal inflammation and ulceration, maldigestion, and hypertrophy of gastric mucosa.

Signalment and Clinical Signs

Gastrinomas are uncommon and have been reported in 30 dogs and in three cats.[40-53] They occur in middle-aged dogs (average age 8.2 years; range 3.5 to 12 years). Cats ranged in age from 10 to 12 years. No breed predilection is noted, and

females may be at slightly greater risk. The most frequent clinical signs have been vomiting and weight loss. Depression, lethargy, anorexia, and intermittent diarrhea are also commonly reported. Less frequent clinical signs include melena, abdominal pain, polydipsia, hematemesis, hematochezia, and obstipation. Physical examination findings are often nonremarkable in the early stages of the disease. However, abdominal pain, fever, tachycardia, pale mucous membranes, and dehydration may occur in extremely sick animals as a result of severe gastrointestinal ulceration or perforation. A palpable abdominal mass was reported in one cat.

Clinical signs result from gastrin-induced gastric acid hypersecretion and gastric mucosal hyperplasia. Hypersecretion and hyperplasia may result in gastric ulceration and gastric outflow obstruction. Gastroesophageal acid reflux may cause severe esophagitis and/or ulceration. Diarrhea and steatorrhea are caused by the large amount of acidic fluid entering the duodenum and jejunum and by the increased circulating concentrations of gastrin that reduce intestinal water and ion absorption.

Laboratory Findings

The CBC may reveal a regenerative anemia presumably due to gastrointestinal bleeding. Gastrointestinal inflammation may elicit a leukocytosis and neutrophilia with or without a left shift. One dog with concurrent myelofibrosis had a nonregenerative anemia. Biochemical abnormalities include hypoalbuminemia, hypoproteinemia, hypokalemia, hypochloremia, hyponatremia, metabolic alkalosis, hyperbilirubinemia, and mild increases in serum liver enzyme activities. Hypoalbuminemia and hypoproteinemia are due to loss of protein through an ulcerated gastrointestinal mucosa. Persistent vomiting in dogs and cats with gastrinoma results in hypokalemia, hyponatremia, hypochloremia, and metabolic alkalosis. Diarrhea and reduced food intake could also contribute to the hypokalemia. Hyper-and hypoglycemia have also been infrequently reported and may be due to concurrent hypersecretion of corticotropin or insulin, respectively; in one dog with hyperglycemia, extracts of the islet tumor revealed adrenocorticotropic hormone in addition to gastrin. Increases in serum liver enzyme activities and bilirubin may reflect tumor metastasis to the liver that is commonly found in these cases.

Imaging Findings

Survey abdominal radiographs are usually unremarkable or they may reveal loss of abdominal detail and/or ascites with gastrointestinal perforation. Contrast-enhanced radiographic studies may show evidence of gastroduodenal ulceration, prominent gastric rugal folds, thickened pyloric antrum, complete pyloric obstruction, or rapid small bowel transit time. Abdominal ultrasound may reveal gastric ulcer, thickened gastric wall or pylorus, or evidence of metastasis in the liver or regional lymph nodes. Gastrinomas are generally small in size and difficult to directly visualize by abdominal ultrasonography. Wider use of other imaging modalities such as endoscopic ultrasound, magnetic resonance imaging, and computed tomography undoubtedly increase diagnostic sensitivity;[54,55] however, no studies have been reported using these techniques on animals.

Endoscopic Findings

Endoscopy was performed on half of the dogs reported. Abnormalities noted were esophageal inflammation or ulceration, thickened gastric rugae, gastric ulceration or hemorrhage, excessive fluid in the stomach, hypertrophied pyloric antrum, and duodenal ulceration. Histological examination of endoscopically derived biopsy samples of thickened gastric mucosa or mural lesions may be relatively normal. In this case surgically obtained, full-thickness biopsy samples should be considered.

Diagnosis

Clinical tests to support a diagnosis of gastrinoma include measurement of basal gastric acid secretion and serum gastrin concentration, provocative tests such as secretin and calcium stimulation, and somatostatin receptor scintigraphy. Demonstration of appropriate histopathological and immuno-histochemical evidence from excised pancreatic tumor or metastatic tissue is necessary to confirm the diagnosis.

Basal gastric acid secretion   This test is commonly performed in humans and is abnormally increased in more than 80% of humans with gastrinoma.[38,56] This test has been performed in four dogs with gastrinoma. Gastric pH was low (pH = 0.99, 1.0, 1.0, 1.5) in all four dogs and was correlated with increased basal acid secretion in two of the dogs.

Basal serum gastrin concentration   This is considered the best screening test for gastrinoma in humans and is abnormal in more than 98% of those with gastrinoma. In dogs and cats with histologic evidence of gastrinoma, measured basal serum gastrin concentrations have been greater than three times the highest value in the reference range. However, other disease syndromes may be associated with increased basal serum gastrin concentrations including renal failure, gastric outflow obstruction, chronic gastritis, liver disease, and drugs that remove the negative feedback inhibition of acid on gastrin secretion, including antacids, H_2 receptor blockers, proton pump inhibitors, and glucocorticoids. Therefore this test cannot be relied upon as a sole diagnostic test, even if these other conditions can be ruled out. In humans with gastrinoma, basal serum gastrin concentrations more than 1000 ng/L combined with gastric pH less than 2.5 is diagnostic for gastrinoma without further testing. Due to the paucity of cases in the veterinary literature, basal serum gastrin concentrations diagnostic for gastrinoma (versus other diseases or drug therapy) have not yet been established.

Secretin stimulation   The preferred provocative test to diagnose gastrinoma in people is secretin stimulation. Secretin will stimulate gastrin secretion in patients with gastrinoma but not in healthy people. This test has been performed in three dogs with gastrinoma and one dog with pancreatic polypeptidoma, and therefore data regarding testing procedure and interpretation is limited. In dogs, serum samples should be collected before and 2, 5, 10, and 30 minutes following intravenous administration of 2 to 4 U/kg of secretin. The 2- and 5- minute samples are thought to be the most diagnostic. In humans a twofold or greater increase in serum gastrin following secretin administration is diagnostic for gastrinoma. In those animals that have been tested, two dogs had a greater than twofold increase in gastrin and one dog had a 1.4-fold increase within 5 minutes of secretin administration. One dog diagnosed with pancreatic polypeptidoma had a transient fasting hypergastrinemia, but no response to secretin stimulation.

Calcium stimulation   Similar to secretin, calcium infusion stimulates an increase in serum gastrin concentrations in humans with gastrinoma, whereas serum gastrin concentrations are unchanged unaffected individuals. This test has been used in two dogs with gastrinoma and one dog with pancreatic polypeptidoma. Calcium is administered as an intravenous bolus of 2 mg/kg over 1 minute. Serum samples are collected before and 15, 30, 60, 90, and 120 minutes after calcium administration. Using this protocol, both of the gastrinoma dogs had a twofold increase in serum gastrin concentration in response to calcium infusion. Such an increase supports a diagnosis of gastrinoma in humans. The dog with pancreatic polypeptidoma, had normal serum gastrin concentrations after calcium infusion. Because of the dangers of intravenous calcium infusion, this test should be used with caution.

Pathology

A definitive diagnosis of gastrinoma requires the findings of hypergastrinemia, histopathologic evidence of pancreatic islet cell neoplasia, and immunohistochemical evidence of gastrin in neoplastic islet cells. The presence of hormones in endocrine tumor tissue alone does not necessarily guarantee their excessive secretion into the circulation. In dogs, gastrin-secreting tumors have been reported most frequently in the right lobe and body of the pancreas. Most animals had solitary nodules, but multiple masses have been reported. At the time of diagnosis, the gastrinoma had metastasized in 85% of cases, usually to the liver. Other metastatic sites included, spleen, lymph nodes, mesentery, omentum, peritoneum, and serosal surfaces of the duodenum and jejunum. The presence of gastrin in the tumors can be documented by immunohistochemistry or by radioimmunoassay of extracts from tumor tissue. Ultrastructural studies to detect unique intracytoplasmic granules can also be used to confirm gastrinoma; however, this requires electron microscopic techniques that may be cost prohibitive. Other pathological findings of dogs and cats with gastrinoma included perforating and nonperforating ulceration (95% of cases) of the esophagus, stomach, duodenum, and jejunum. Gastric hypertrophy, thyroid C-cell hyperplasia, thyroid follicular cell carcinoma, and adrenal hyperplasia have also been reported.

Therapy

Treatment of gastrinoma is directed toward surgical resection or reduction of the gastrinoma and/or metastases and medical control of gastrin secretion from the tumor cells. Adjunct medical therapy includes treatment of gastric acid hypersecretion, gastrointestinal ulceration, and fluid and electrolyte losses.[57]

Treatment directed at tumor cells   Surgical resection of gastrinomas can prove challenging since the primary tumors are small and difficult to localize. Tumor localization with imaging modalities such as endoscopic ultrasound, computed tomography, or magnetic resonance imaging are usually more sensitive than abdominal ultrasound and are used more successfully in humans. Somatostatin receptor scintigraphy, using a somatostatin analogues (e.g., [111]Indium octreotide or pentetreotide) to detect somatostatin receptors present on gastrinoma cells is a sensitive test used to localize tumors and metastases in people. Positive receptor binding can also predict successful medical treatment of gastrinoma with somatostatin analogues. This technique has been reported in one dog in which 2 mCi of the octreotide analogue was used and images successfully generated by gamma camera imaging.[43] Careful digital palpation of the pancreas, liver, and surrounding areas should be performed if the tumor cannot be visualized at surgery; intraoperative pancreatic ultrasound may be beneficial. The pancreas should be handled carefully and pancreatic blood flow should be preserved to avoid postoperative pancreatitis. Because metastasis is common at the time of surgery, the liver, lymph nodes, spleen, duodenum, mesentery, and omentum should be inspected and biopsied as appropriate. Metastatic foci should also be resected, as possible, since this can provide palliation for the patient. As these tumors are slow growing, debulking may provide relief from clinical signs.

Following pancreatic resection or manipulation, the animal should be managed as if it had acute pancreatitis, with fluid support, extensive monitoring, and restriction of food or water by mouth. Administration of octreotide, a somatostatin analogue, pre- and post-operatively has been suggested to decrease pancreatic gastrin and gastric acid secretion.[53]

Somatostatin analogues Somatostatin inhibits gastrin and hydrogen ion secretion in gastrinomas and in gastric parietal cells. A long-acting somatostatin analogue, octreotide, has been used in two dogs with gastrinoma. Doses started at 2 μg/kg twice per day and were increased to 10 to 20 μg/kg three times per day. The dogs were maintained on this therapy for 10 to 14 months. One dog relapsed after the medication was discontinued. The other dog showed marked response to treatment after the dosing was increased to three times per day. At necropsy, one dog showed marked increase of tumor growth and metastasis. Unfortunately, the expense of this drug may limit its use. Successful treatment of gastrinoma with chemotherapeutic drugs has not been reported.

Adjunct medical therapy

Gastric hyperacidity As gastrinomas are slow growing, medical therapy to control the major clinical signs of gastric hyperacidity and gastrointestinal ulceration may provide significant palliation for dogs and cats.[57] Because of the high rate of metastasis, gastrin secretion in most animals remain increased after surgery, and these dogs and cats suffer from continuing gastric hyperacidity. Adjunct therapy should be started immediately to prevent the development of perforating ulcers. The most common agents used to control gastric hyperacidity in veterinary medicine are the H_2 receptor antagonists such as cimetidine (Tagamet), ranitidine (Zantac), famotidine (Pepcid), and nizatidine (Axid). See Box 244-1 for dosages and dosing intervals. They are potent inhibitors of H^+ secretion in dogs and cats. Success with cimetidine therapy has been reported in several dogs and one cat with gastrinoma. It has been suggested that animals unresponsive to standard doses of gastric acid secretory inhibitors may respond to higher doses and/or dual agent therapy.[53]

Omeprazole (Prilosec) is an inhibitor of parietal cell H^+,K^+-ATPase and reduces gastric acid secretion with a long duration of action in normal dogs.[57] Two dogs with gastrinoma have been successfully treated with omeprazole. In one case, omeprazole controlled gastrointestinal signs that were unresponsive to treatment with cimetidine and sucralfate. This dog remained asymptomatic for more than 2 years. Omeprazole may be the better choice for control of gastric hyperacidity either in place of or in addition to H_2 receptor antagonists but it should be emphasized that there is no evidence-based medicine in support of either drug classification.

Gastrointestinal ulceration Treatment of gastrointestinal ulceration includes surgical resection and control of gastric hyperacidity as discussed. The use of diffusion barriers and cytoprotective agents is discussed here. Dosages and dosing regimes are presented in the Drug Index (see Box 244-1).

Sucralfate (Carafate) is an example of a diffusion barrier used to promote ulcer healing. It is a complex of sulfated sucrose and aluminum hydroxide that reacts with gastric acid and binds to necrotic tissue proteins. Misoprostol (Cytotec) is a 16,16-dimethylated synthetic prostaglandin that has cytoprotective properties in addition to its direct acid-inhibitory effect. Synthetic prostaglandins may be useful in restoring the protective properties of the gastric mucosal barrier in ulcer patients, although the beneficial effects of this classification of agents have not yet been unequivocally established in evidence-based medicine type studies.[57]

Box • 244-1

Drug Index

Histamine (H_2) Receptor Antagonists
Cimetidine (Tagamet-SmithKline Beecham), 2 to 4 mg/lb (5 to 10 mg/kg) PO, SQ, IV q6h or q8h
Ranitidine (Zantac-Glaxo), 0.5 to 1.0 mg/lb (1 to 2 mg/kg) PO, SQ, IV q8h or q12h
Famotidine (Pepcid-Johnson & Johnson, Merck Consumer), 0.1 to 0.5/mg/kg PO, IV q12h
Nizatidine (Axid-Eli Lilly), 1.0 to 3.0 mg/kg SQ, IM, IV q8h

H^+, K^+-ATPase Inhibitors
Omeprazole (Losec-MerckSharp & Dohme) 0.35 mg/lb (0.7 mg/kg) PO q24h

Diffusion Barriers
Sucralfate (Carafate-Marion), 1 g q8h for large dogs 0.5 g q8h for smaller dogs 0.25 to 0.5 g q8h to q12h for cats

Synthetic Prostaglandins
Misoprostol (Cytotec-Searle), 2 to 5 μg/kg PO q8-12 h

Somostatin Analogs
Octreotide (Sandostatin-Novartis), 2 to 8 μg/kg SC q8-12h

Prognosis

Long-term prognosis in dogs and cats with gastrinomas is grave since metastatic disease is present in 85% at the time of surgery. In animals that underwent surgery and medical management, survival times ranged from 1 week to 18 months. The prognosis is likely to improve with increased awareness and diagnostic techniques for tumor localization. The availability and affordability of anti-secretory drugs and therapies to reduce gastric hyperacidity and promote ulcer healing will also promote longevity in animals with gastrinoma.

Intestinal Carcinoid

Intestinal carcinoid is a rare tumor arising from enterochromaffin cells that can be found in the tracheobronchial epithelium, pancreatic ducts, biliary tree, genitourinary tract, stomach, and intestine. In people they are classified according to their location and ability to secrete vasoactive amines. People with carcinoid tumors can develop carcinoid syndrome that manifests as facial flushing, abdominal cramping, bronchoconstriction, and diarrhea. Clinical signs are related to the excessive secretion of 5-hydroxytryptamine (serotonin) from the neoplastic enterochromaffin cells.

Carcinoid tumors have been described in 25 dogs and four cats. In dogs this tumor has been found in the liver (15), stomach (1), duodenum (2), cecum (1), ileocecal junction (1), colon (2), rectum (2) and gall bladder (1).[58-64] In cats they have been localized to the stomach, pancreas, intestine, and liver.[65-68] Metastasis was common at the time of diagnosis with sites including liver, lymph nodes, lung, spleen, adrenal glands, and mesentery. A functional carcinoid syndrome as reported in humans has not been recognized in cats and dogs. Most animals had clinical signs relating to structural effects of the tumor or generalized disease related to neoplasia. The most common clinical signs were anorexia, vomiting, weight loss, and gastrointestinal bleeding. Diarrhea was less common.

In veterinary medicine, diagnosis is confirmed by histopathologic and ultrastructural examination of the tumors. Diagnosis in people relies on several factors including measurement of plasma and urinary serotonin levels or its metabolites. Such tests have not been reported in veterinary patients. Most animals were diagnosed upon postmortem examination. Surgical resection was successful in a recent case report in a cat that remained disease free for 4 months before succumbing to an unrelated disease. Although these tumors are slow growing, metastasis is common at diagnosis; therefore prognosis is guarded.

Pancreatic Polypeptidoma

Pancreatic polypeptide is commonly found by immunohistochemical staining in human and canine pancreatic endocrine tumors that secrete other enteric hormones such as gastrin, glucagon, or insulin. The significance of its presence in these cells is unknown, and increased plasma pancreatic peptide concentrations have been documented rarely in humans. These patients do not display a characteristic clinical syndrome; however, secretory diarrhea and a macular rash may be associated with excess pancreatic polypeptide secretion from polypeptidomas. There has been one report in the veterinary literature implicating pancreatic polypeptidoma in clinical disease.[69]

In this case a 7-year-old FS cocker spaniel had chronic vomiting, hypertrophic gastritis, duodenal ulceration, and pancreatic adenocarcinoma with hepatic metastasis. Plasma PP concentrations were extremely high in this dog. Neoplastic tissues obtained at necropsy revealed positive immunohistochemical staining for pancreatic polypeptide and insulin while there was no staining for gastrin, glucagon, or somatostatin. Clinical signs were thought to be due to high plasma PP concentrations since PP decreases pancreatic bicarbonate secretion and mildly increases gastric acid secretion. However, plasma PP may also be elevated in humans with other diseases including inflammatory diseases, renal failure, and laxative abuse; therefore further case reports are needed to characterize this syndrome.

CHAPTER • 245

Pheochromocytoma

Elizabeth McNiel
Brian D. Husbands

Pheochromocytoma is a rare tumor that arises from the chromaffin cells of the adrenal medulla. Unlike the steroidogenic cells of the adrenal cortex, which are derived from mesoderm, chromaffin cells are embryologically derived from the neural crest as a part of the sympathetic autonomic nervous system.[1] The adrenal medulla is essentially a modified sympathetic ganglion that lacks postganglionic processes. In the fetus, chromaffin cells are widely distributed and form paraganglia. With the exception of the adrenal medulla, the paraganglia involute at birth.[1] Tumors arising from remnant paraganglia in adult animals are referred to as *paragangliomas* or *extra-adrenal pheochromocytomas*.

PATHOPHYSIOLOGY

Consistent with the role of the adrenal medulla as a sympathetic ganglion, chromaffin cells are capable of producing, storing, and secreting a variety of neurotransmitters and neuropeptides.[2] Catecholamines are the primary secretary product of the adrenal medullary cells, however. Catecholamines, along with other products including ATP and chromagranin, are stored within cytoplasmic vesicles in the chromaffin cells. When the chromaffin cells are stimulated, vesicles are transported to the cell membrane and the contents are expelled via exocytosis.[3]

Catecholamines are synthesized from the amino acid tyrosine through a series of enzyme modifications (Figure 245-1). The first step in catecholamine synthesis involves the conversion of L-tyrosine to L-DOPA through the action of tyrosine hydroxylase. This hydroxylation reaction is the rate limiting step in the pathway and is subject to negative feedback regulation by norepinephrine.[1] In dogs and humans the end product of catecholamine synthesis in the adrenal medulla is predominantly epinephrine, whereas in the cat it is norepinephrine.[4] Pheochromocytomas may produce any of the catecholamines or other physiologically active peptides.

The half-life of catecholamines in circulation is short (minutes). Two enzymes mediate the catabolism: catecholamine-O-methyltransferase (COMT) and monoamine oxidase (MAO).[1,5] The sequential action of COMT and MAO on catecholamines results in the production of the predominant metabolite, vanillylmandelic acid (VMA)[1] (Figure 245-2). Catecholamines and metabolites are excreted in the urine.

The normal adrenal gland is regulated through a combination of sympathetic innervation and circulating hormones.[2] There is an intricate regulatory connection between the adrenal cortex and medulla. Whereas the peptide products of the adrenal medulla influence steroidogenesis in cortical cells, the steroid hormones influence both differentiation and catecholamine production in the medullary chromaffin cells.[2] One of the hallmarks of neoplastic transformation is the loss of regulatory control, particularly those involved with growth and cell death. For endocrine tumors, such as pheochromocytoma, deregulation may also include loss of normal physiologic control of hormone production and secretion. Thus pheochromocytomas are often associated with increased levels of circulating catecholamines or other physiologically active products.

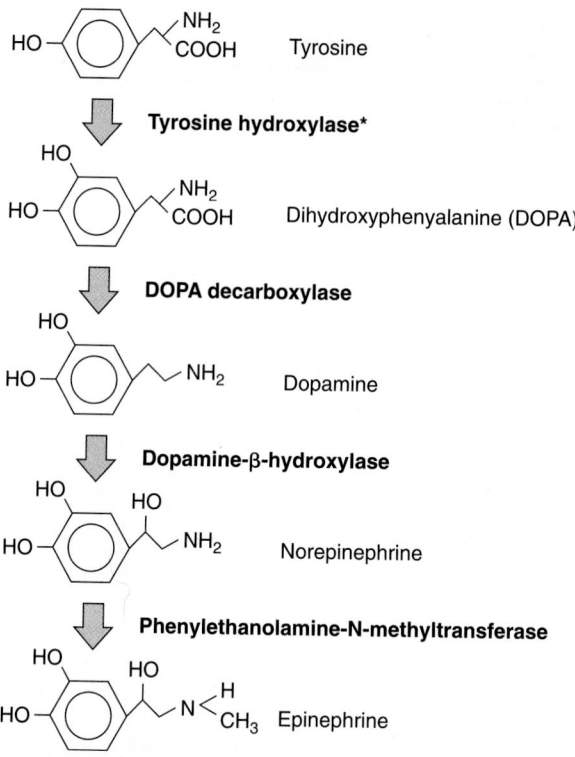

Figure 245-1 Catecholamine synthesis. *Tyrosine hydroxylase is the rate limiting enzyme and is subject to negative feedback control by norepinephrine.

The action of catecholamines is mediated by specific G protein coupled cell surface receptors[3] (Table 245-1). The receptors are subdivided into α and β types, which include the subtypes $\alpha 1$, $\alpha 2$, $\beta 1$, $\beta 2$, and the less prevalent $\beta 3$. The binding

of catecholamines to their receptors initiates cellular increases or decreases in second messengers, which, in turn propagate cellular signaling and affect the cellular response.[3] Epinephrine and norepinephrine have approximately equal affinity for the $\alpha 1$, $\alpha 2$, $\beta 1$ receptors, but epinephrine has higher affinity for $\beta 2$ receptors.[1,3]

ETIOLOGY

Cancer is a genetic disease in that inherited and acquired mutations drive the transformation of a normal cell to a tumor cell.[6,7] The cause of genetic mutations in most cancers is not understood and pheochromocytoma is no exception. Roughly 10% of human pheochromocytomas are considered hereditary, the rest, sporadic. Pheochromocytoma may be a feature of a number of distinct hereditary syndromes including multiple endocrine neoplasia type 2 (MEN-2), von Hippel-Lindau disease (VHL), and neurofibromatosis type I[8,9] (Table 245-2). Additional hereditary forms of pheochromocytoma are distinct from these syndromes. Some of the genes that predispose tumor development in the various hereditary disorders have been characterized[8,9] (see Table 245-2). These genes do not appear to play a role in the development of most sporadic pheochromocytoma. A number of chromosomal loci are consistently mutated in sporadic pheochromocytoma, which suggests that these regions contain genes important for pheochromocytoma carcinogenesis.

The role of genetic factors, hereditary or acquired, has not been evaluated in canine or feline pheochromocytoma. Many canine cancers do have a hereditary basis, however. There are reports of dogs with multiple endocrine tumors including a dog with a syndrome similar to MEN-2.[10,11] In addition, a large proportion of dogs diagnosed with pheochromocytoma also have another malignancy, some of these in endocrine tissue. In a search of the Veterinary Medicine Database (VMDB), which contains medical record data abstracted from 26 North American veterinary colleges, the

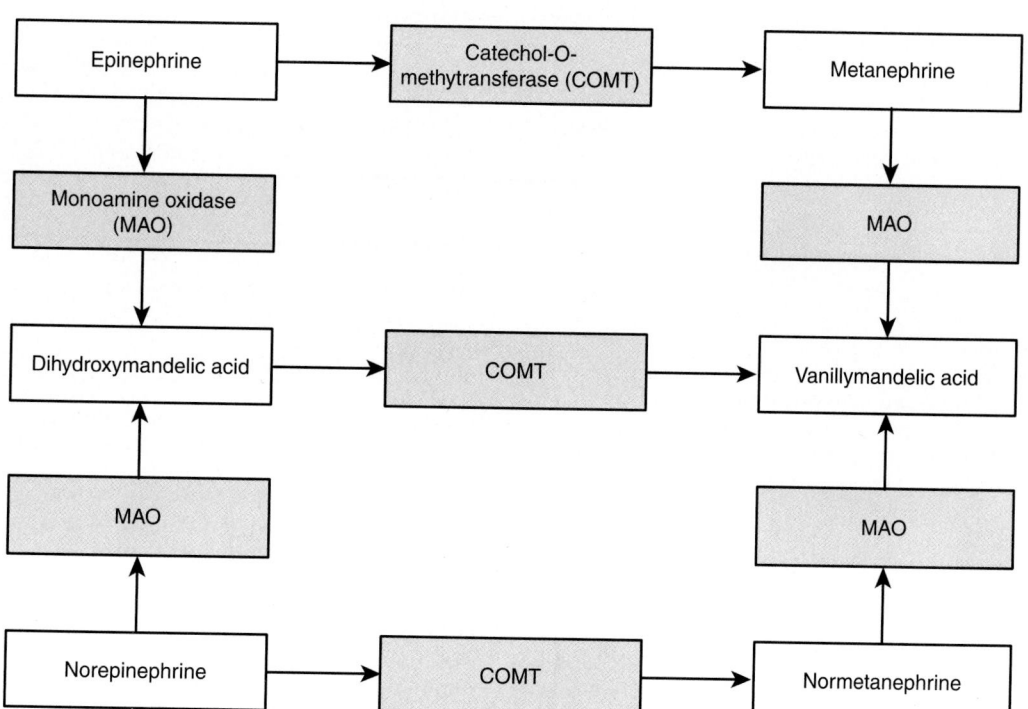

Figure 245-2 Catabolism of catecholamines. *COMT*, catecholamine-O-methyltransferase; *MAO*, monoamine oxidase. Shaded boxes indicate an enzymatic step.

Table • 245-1

The Biochemical Characteristics and Physiologic Effects of Catecholamine Receptors

RECEPTOR TYPE	α1	α2	β1	β2
Biochemistry				
Receptor affinity	Epi ≥ Nor	Epi ≥ Nor	Epi = Nor	Epi >> Nor G_s
G-protein subtype	G_q	G_i	G_s	G_s
Second messenger	↑IP3, DAG	↓cAMP	↑cAMP	↑cAMP
Physiologic Effects				
Ocular	Mydriasis			
Cardiovascular				
Heart			Increase heart rate, contractility, conduction velocity	
Arterioles	Constriction			Dilatation
Veins	Constriction			Dilatation, relaxation
Respiratory				
Bronchial smooth muscle				Relaxation
Gastrointestinal				
Motility	Decrease	Decrease		Decrease
Spincters	Contraction	Contraction		
Liver	Glycogenolysis	Glycogenolysis		Glycogenolysis
Pancreatic acini	Decrease secretion			
Adipose				Lipolysis

ENDOCRINE EFFECTS	ALPHA	BETA
Adrenal cortex	Decreased aldosterone secretion (Both alpha and beta)	
Pancreas		
Alpha cell		Increased glucagon
Beta cell	Decreased insulin	
D cell		Increased somatostatin
PP cell	Increased pancreatic polypeptide	
Gastric antrum		Increased gastrin
Kidney		Increased renin and erythropoietin
Parathyroid		Increased parathyroid hormone
Ovary		Increased progesterone
Testis		Increased testoterone

diagnosis of pheochromocytoma was recorded for only 0.05% of canine patients evaluated between 1990 and 2002.

In the 277 dogs with pheochromocytoma identified in the VMDB, 129 (46%) were diagnosed with other tumors. This finding is consistent with previous reports.[4,12] The presence of multiple tumors in an individual is suggestive of hereditary predisposition.

Fifty-five different breeds were represented among the 277 cases of canine pheochromocytoma in the VMDB. Chi-square analysis comparing the frequency of pheochromocytoma in specific breeds to the frequency of pheochromocytoma in all dogs in the VMDB database revealed significantly increased relative risk of this tumor in seven different breeds of dogs (Table 245-3). Breed predisposition is suggestive of hereditary predisposition, but study of pedigrees is required to confirm this suspicion and to determine the mode of inheritance.

CLINICAL PRESENTATION

The average age of dogs diagnosed with pheochromocytoma is 10 to 11 years, with a range of 1 to 18 years.[4,12,13] Reports indicate that this is a disease of aged cats. No gender predilection is apparent in either species.[14-16] Although certain breeds may be predisposed to pheochromocytoma, any breed can be affected, including mixed breed dogs.

The clinical signs in dogs with pheochromocytomas are complicated by the high frequency of concurrent illnesses, including hyperadrenocorticism, diabetes mellitus, renal failure, and hepatic disease.[4] In humans with pheochromocytoma, the most common complaints include headache, palpitations, and sweating, which are not readily detectable in dogs and cats. In addition, roughly half of the pheochromocytomas diagnosed in dogs are incidental.

Table • 245-2

Familial and Sporadic Pheochromocytoma in Humans[9,22,32]

CLINICAL CHARACTERISTICS		FREQUENCY OF PEOCHROMOCYTOMA	GENES INVOLVED
MEN-2A	Bilateral medullary thyroid carcinoma; Parathyroid hyperplasia;	20% to 40%	RET
MEN-2B	Bilateral medullary thyroid carcinoma, Phenotypic abnormalities: Bony abnormalities, mucosal neuromas, marfanoid habitus, bumpy lips	60%	RET
VHL	Bilateral renal carcinomas and renal cysts; other tumors	18% to 25%	VHL
NF-1	Cafe-au-lait spots of the skin, Neurofibromas, Hamartomas of the iris, macrocephaly, bone dysplasia, learning disability, seizures, CNS tumors, other malignant tumors such as neurofibrosarcomas and leukemia	1%	NF-1
Sporadic	Older than with hereditary syndromes; Unilateral disease	100%	P53, RB, Others?

MEN, Multiple endocrine neoplasia; *VHL*, von Hippel-Lindau disease; *NF-1*, Nuerofibromatosis type 1, *Sporadic*, Nonhereditary.

The most common clinical signs in dogs with pheochromocytoma, in the absence of complicating disease, are weakness and collapse.[4] Other historical complaints may be associated with a variety of systems including gastrointestinal (anorexia, weight loss, vomiting, diarrhea), nervous (restlessness, pacing, depression, seizures), cardiopulmonary (exercise intolerance, lethargy), and miscellaneous complaints such as abdominal distension, polyuria, and polydipsia. In cats with pheochromocytoma, polyuria and polydipsia are consistently reported.[14-16]

Clinical signs associated with pheochromocytoma may be related to increased circulating catecholamines or directly associated with the tumor (Table 245-4). Although most pheochromocytomas occur in the adrenal gland, presentation may differ considerably with paraganglioma in extra-adrenal locations, such as the vertebral canal.[17]

DIAGNOSTIC EVALUATION

Minimum Database

Abnormalities detected in dogs and cats with pheochromocytomas are nonspecific. The presence of concurrent disorders may be reflected in the complete blood count, serum chemistry profile, and urinalysis.[4] Often, the hemogram is normal.[4,13,18] Leukocytosis can be seen secondary to increased circulating catecholamines or stress. Mild anemia may be present secondary to chronic disease or hemorrhage. Thrombocytopenia or thrombocytosis may indicate acute or chronic bleeding, respectively.

Increases in serum liver enzyme activities have been reported in 10% to 25% of pets with pheochromocytoma.[4,13,18] The abnormal serum liver enzyme activities may be secondary to hypertension with changes in hepatic perfusion or can

Table • 245-3

Relative Risk of Pheochromocytoma in Purebred Dogs Identified in the VMDB Database (1990-2002)

BREED	NUMBER OF DOGS WITH PHEOCHROMOCYTOMA	NUMBER OF DOGS WITHOUT PHEOCHROMOCYTOMA	RELATIVE RISK	95% CONFIDENCE INTERVAL
Airedale terrier	6	1950	5.8	2.6-12.9
Basset hound	5	647	14.4	5.9-34.7
English springer spaniel	8	6639	2.3	1.1-2.5
Golden retriever	31	28,246	2.1	1.5-3.1
Puli	2	130	28.1	7.1-111.8
Weimaraner	5	2167	4.3	1.8-10.4
Wire hair fox terrier	6	1569	7.1	3.2-16.0
Mixed breed	70	109,850	1.2	0.9-1.6
All dogs 1990-2002	277	509,751	NA	NA

Table • 245-4

Clinical Signs Associated with Canine Pheochromocytoma[4,12,13,18,33]

EXCESS CATECHOLAMINES	MASS EFFECT
Tachycardia/arrhythmia	Abdominal distention
Polypnea/panting	Weak femoral pulses
Coughing	Hemoabdomen
Ataxia/incoordination	Ascites
Episodic weakness	Pleripheral edema
Seizures	Collapse
Collapse	Budd-Chiari like syndrome*
Blindness (retinal hemorrhages)	
Polyuria/polydipsia	
Anorexia	
Vomiting	
Diarrhea	
Anxiety/pacing	

*Budd-Chiari like syndrome is the mechanical obstruction of the vena cava between the heart and the liver.

occur with concurrent disease such as hyperadrenocorticism. These abnormal liver enzymes do not correlate with the presence of hepatic metastases.[13]

Proteinuria, resulting from hypertensive glomerulopathy or concurrent illness, is observed in as many 50% of dogs and cats with pheochromocytomas.[4,13] Hyposthenuria/isosthenuria may be present due to the inhibitory effect of circulating catecholamines on vasopressin secretion and activity.[4]

Blood Pressure
In dogs with pheochromocytoma, the presence of systemic hypertension (systolic pressure >160 mm Hg) is variable (25% to 86% of patients), which may reflect sporadic secretion of catecholamines resulting in intermittent hypertension.[4,13]

DIAGNOSTIC IMAGING

Imaging techniques are useful for localizing a mass and for determining the extent of disease, including whether the tumor is unilateral or bilateral, is invading local structures, or has metastasized to distant regions.[13] This information is valuable in planning surgical approach and in determining prognosis.

Radiography
Plain abdominal radiographs may reveal a mass or mineralization in the adrenal region.[4,12,13,19] Frequently, the adrenal lesion cannot be detected. Thoracic radiographs may reveal changes consistent with hypertension such as cardiomegaly, pulmonary congestion, or edema.[4,13,18] Contrast studies such as caudal vena cava or nonselective venography and excretory urography may be helpful in detecting caval invasion or thrombosis and renal integrity, respectively.[4,12,13,18,20]

Abdominal Ultrasound
Sonographically, pheochromocytomas appear as mass lesions of the adrenal gland with variable echogenicity.[19,21] Pheochromocytomas cannot be distinguished from other tumors in the adrenal gland based on the sonographic appearance.

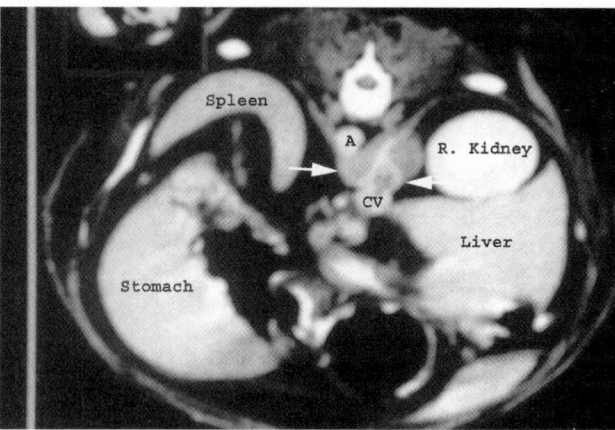

Figure 245-3 Transverse abdominal CT image in the cranial lumbar region of a dog with pheochromocytoma. *A*, Aorta; *CV*, caudal vena cava.

Other findings could include evidence of metastasis, invasion, or vascular involvement.

Computed Tomography
Computed tomography (CT) is sensitive for lesion localization and in assessment for local invasion and metastasis (Figure 245-3).[4,19] Hypertension secondary to intravenous contrast media (diatrazoate sodium meglumine or iothalamate meglumine) has been reported in humans with pheochromocytomas.[19,22] It is suspected that these medications precipitate catecholamine release. In dogs, hypertension subsequent to administration of contrast media has not been reported.

Magnetic Resonance Imaging
Although there are no reports describing the use of magnetic resonance imaging (MRI) in dogs or cats with a pheochromocytoma, this modality is considered highly sensitive in the detection of pheochromocytoma in humans.[19]

Nuclear Scintigraphy
Scintigraphic studies are used frequently in humans and are reported in the dog for localization of pheochromocytoma.[22-25] Radioactive iodine labeled meta-iodobenzylguanidine (MIBG) is structurally similar to norepinephrine and is taken up by chromaffin cells. This technique is less sensitive than CT for identification of pheochromocytoma in humans but is more specific and it may be useful in the identification of metastases.[25] Octreotide is a somatostatin analog that may be radioactively labeled and binds somatostatin receptors on the surface of neuroendocrine cells such as those in pheochromocytomas. Octreotide scanning may detect lesions in patients with normal MIBG scans.[25]

Positron Emission Tomography
Positron emission tomography (PET) using 6-(^{18}F) fluorodopamine has been helpful in humans when conventional testing is equivocal.[22,26,27] The use of this technique for localization of pheochromocytoma in the dog has been reported and shows promise.[26]

BIOCHEMICAL DIAGNOSIS

Catecholamine Measurement
Catecholamines, their metabolites, or other neuroendocrine products may be measured in plasma or urine. These techniques

are infrequently used in dogs or cats because of limited availability, lack of reference ranges, expense, and complicated sample collection and handling.[4,20,26] In addition, the accuracy of these diagnostics is limited. False-positive results are associated with stress, excitement, certain dietary components, and medications. False-negative results are associated with intermittent secretion of catecholamines by the tumor and improper sample handling.[4,20,26]

Provocative Testing
Certain agents, including histamine, tyramine, metoclopromide, and glucagon, cause adrenal catecholamine release and can be used to screen individuals for pheochromocytoma.[4,20] Because of the risk of a hypertensive crisis, these tests are not recommended.

Clonidine Suppression Test
Clonidine is a centrally acting α-agonist that suppresses the release of catecholamines. In all patients, blood pressure and heart rate can decrease after administration. Lack of reduction in plasma catecholamines following administration of clonidine is consistent with pheochromocytoma.

Phentolamine Test
Phentolamine is an α-receptor antagonist, thus administration inhibits α-mediated vasoconstriction. In patients that are hypertensive secondary to excessive catecholamines, phentolamine results in vasodilation and decreased blood pressure within minutes of administration, an effect that lasts about 10 minutes. This test is not recommended due to potential for hypovolemic shock and difficulties in interpretation.

PATHOLOGY

Cytology
Although there is some potential to induce a hypertensive crisis or hemorrhage, fine-needle aspiration can be performed with ultrasound or CT guidance. Cytologic features of pheochromocytoma are consistent with a tumor of neuroendocrine origin. Cytologic misdiagnosis has been documented.[13]

Histopathology
Microscopically, pheochromocytomas are composed of nests of polyhedral cells with lightly eosinophilic, granular cytoplasm that are separated by a fine fibrovascular stroma.[13,23,28] Immunohistochemical techniques may be useful in distinguishing pheochromocytoma from other tumors of the

adrenal gland.[4,28] The distinction between benign and malignant tumors is unclear. In humans, presence of capsular or vascular invasion and nuclear pleomorphism do not correlate with behavior.[23]

TREATMENT

Surgery and Perioperative Management
Surgical excision of pheochromocytoma is the treatment of choice (Figure 245-4). Surgical and anesthetic complications are common, however. The surgical approach to adrenalectomy has been described.[29]

Pre-anesthetic goals include stabilization of hypertension and control of arrhythmias.[30] Treatment with α-receptor antagonists, such as phenoxybenzamine or prazosin, will normalize intravascular volume in individuals with chronic hypertension. Arrhythmias should be treated with β-adrenergic antagonists such as propanolol or esmolol. It may be prudent to normalize blood pressure and rhythm disturbances for 1 to 2 weeks prior to surgery in light of the high complication rate reported in dogs and cats.[18,30,31]

Medications that stimulate release of catecholamines or may precipitate arrhythmias (ketamine, morphine, and halothane) should be avoided. Anesthetic protocols used in humans include the use of thiopental, propofol, isoflurane, or sevoflurane.[30]

Careful monitoring of blood pressure, cardiac rhythm, and red cell volume is essential. Manipulation of a pheochromocytoma can induce catecholamine release with subsequent hypertension. Following resection, hypovolemia may occur as the circulating catecholamine concentrations decrease. Hypotension is best managed by administration of intravenous crystalloids. In dogs that have a poor response to fluid expansion, dopamine may be indicated. Postoperatively, monitoring must continue until the animal is stabilized. In one study of dogs undergoing surgical resection of pheochromocytoma, hospitalization time ranged from 3 to 12 days.[31]

Medical Management
Dogs or cats with nonresectable or metastatic pheochromocytoma may be treated medically. The goals of medical therapy are to control sequelae to elevated catecholamines (hypertension and arrhythmias) and control of the tumor (both primary and metastatic).

Chemotherapy
Chemotherapy has not been evaluated for treatment of pheochromocytoma in dogs or cats. Humans with malignant pheochromocytoma are often treated with protocols combining vincristine, cyclophosphamide, and dacarbazine, which prolongs survival in patients with metastatic disease.[23] In addition to typical chemotherapy related side effects, there is some risk of inducing a hypertensive crisis due to tumor cell lysis with release of stored catecholamines.[23]

Targeted Therapy
Radiolabeled MIBG, in addition to imaging applications, has demonstrated efficacy in the treatment of malignant pheochromocytoma in humans either alone or in combination with chemotherapy. Similarly, octreotide may be useful in people if octreotide scintigraphy demonstrates uptake. Neither of these techniques has been reported in the dog.

PROGNOSIS

Animals with surgically resectable pheochromocytoma can have prolonged survival times. The median survival time for

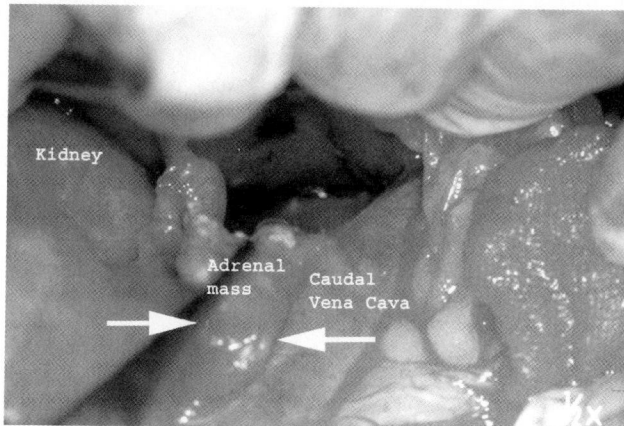

Figure 245-4 Intraoperative photograph demonstrating a noninvasive pheochromocytoma in a dog.

six dogs with surgical resection was 15 months. For dogs surviving the immediate postoperative period, a range in survival from 2 to 40 months has been reported.[4] Prognosis in cats is probably similar. In the few reported cases of pheochromocytoma in cats, only one cat survived postoperatively.

Metastasis has been reported in 13% to 50% of dogs with pheochromocytoma. Sites of metastasis include liver, regional lymph nodes, spleen, lungs, brain, and bone (femur and lumbar vertebral body). Metastasis of feline pheochromocytoma has not been reported.

SECTION XVII

Reproductive System

CHAPTER 246

Estrous Cycle and Breeding Management of the Healthy Bitch

Auke C. Schaeferes-Okkens

THE ESTROUS CYCLE

Onset of puberty in the healthy bitch occurs between 6 and 18 months of age. After each estrous cycle, which has a length of about 3 months, an anestrus with a variable duration occurs. The mean interval from onset of one estrous cycle to the next is about 7 months, with a range of 4 to 12 months. The interestrous interval may be regular or variable within individual bitches. After 8 years of age, the duration and frequency of the cycles become less regular and the interestrous interval increases.[1]

The stages of the estrous cycle are proestrus, estrus, and diestrus (metestrus) (Figure 246-1). The average duration of proestrus is 9 days, with a range of 3 to 17 days. Proestrus is defined as the period when the bitch is sexually attractive while rejecting the male's advances until the first willingness to accept the male. However, early behavioral signs are indistinct. Therefore it is common to use the onset of serosanguineous vaginal discharge and vulvar swelling to mark the first day of proestrus.

On average, estrus (the period of acceptance of the male) has a duration of 9 days, with a range of 3 to 21 days. During estrus the vulva begins to shrink and soften. The discharge usually persists, but generally diminishes. It may remain serosanguineous or turn straw-colored. Diestrus begins when the bitch will no longer accept the dog. It has an average duration of about 70 days if it is assumed to end when the plasma progesterone concentration initially declines to a level of less than or equal to 3 nmol/L (lnmol/L = 0.315 ng/ml). In addition to this behavior-oriented classification of the cycle, it is also possible, and more appropriate, to concentrate on ovarian function and to classify the follicular phase, the phase of preovulatory luteinization and ovulation, the luteal phase and the anestrus (see Figure 246-1).

FOLLICULAR PHASE

As tertiary follicles develop in the ovaries they produce estradiol, leading to peak plasma levels of 180 to 370 pmol/l in late proestrus, 1 to 2 days before the preovulatory luteinizing hormone (LH) surge (Figure 246-2). On laparoscopic

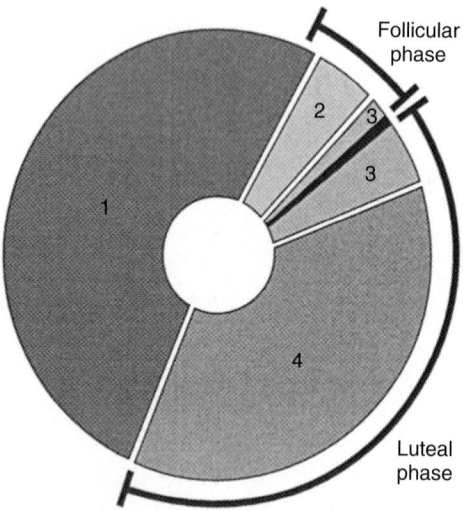

1. Anestrus
2. Proestrus
3. Estrus, ovulation
4. Metestrus or diestrus

Figure 246-1 Diagram of the estrous cycle and anestrus in the dog. (From Schaefers-Okkens AC: The ovaries. In Rijnberk A: *Clinical endocrinology of dogs and cats*. Netherlands, 1996, Kluwer Academic Publishers.)

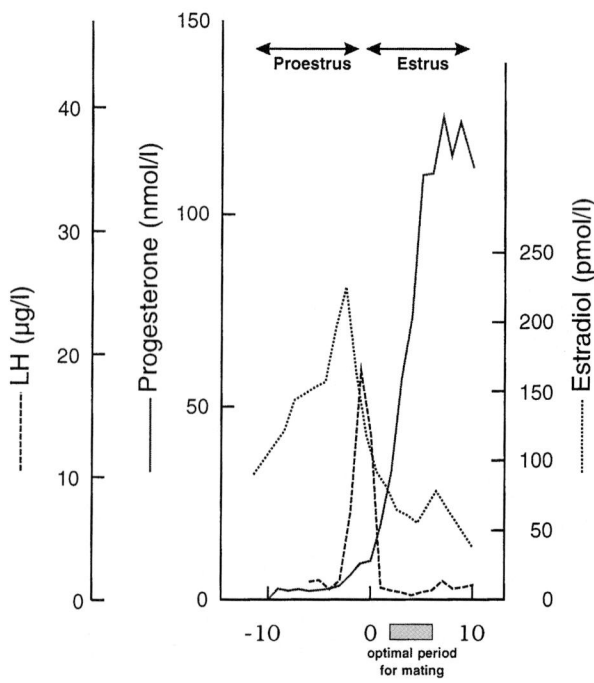

Day of cycle

Figure 246-2 Diagram of estradiol, LH, and progesterone concentrations in plasma in relation to commonly observed estrus behavior of the bitch, and the optimal period for mating. (From Schaefers-Okkens AC: The ovaries. In Rijnberk A: *Clinical endocrinology of dogs and cats*, Netherlands, 1996, Kluwer Academic Publishers.)

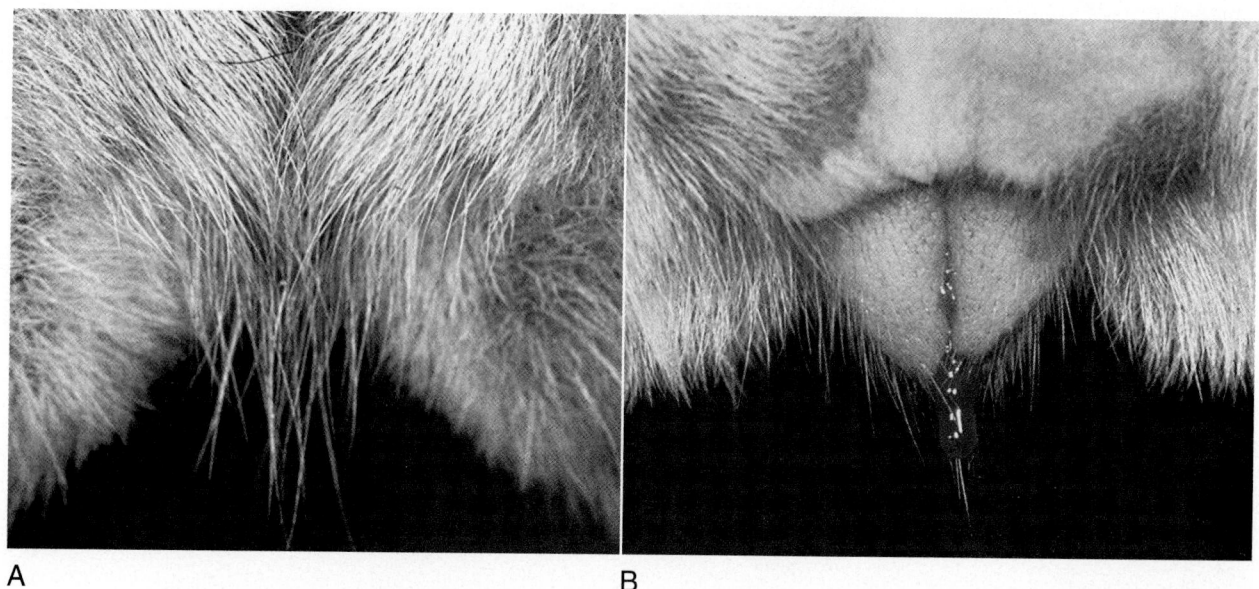

A   B

Figure 246-3 The vulva of a beagle bitch during **(A)** anestrus, and during **(B)** proestrus/estrus. (From Schaefers-Okkens AC: The ovaries. In Rijnberk A: *Clinical endocrinology of dogs and cats,* Netherlands, 1996, Kluwer Academic Publishers.)

inspection, follicle development is not readily apparent on the ovary because of the ovarian bursa. Furthermore, until mid-proestrus, follicular development appears only as clear grayish areas with indistinct boundaries on the ovarian surface. These areas gradually develop into distinct fluid-filled vesicular follicles, which protrude distinctly above the ovarian surface.[2] The external signs of proestrus, such as hyperemia and edema of the vulva and bloody vaginal discharge, are caused by increased concentrations of estradiol (Figure 246-3). This also causes lengthening and hyperemia of the uterine horns, enlargement of the cervix (which can be palpated), and thickening of the vaginal wall.

The percentage of superficial cells in the vaginal smear increases and the percentage of parabasal and small intermediate cells decreases. Erythrocytes are numerous, and leukocytes are seen in the early follicular phase but disappear as cornification progresses (Figure 246-4).

Superficial cells dominate as the follicular phase progresses (Figure 246-5). However, it should be realized that although vaginal cytology gives an indication of the stage of the cycle, it is not reliable for timing the preovulatory LH surge or ovulation.[3]

With vaginoscopy it can be observed that the vaginal mucosal folds are swollen, are pale, and have smooth, rounded surfaces (balloons) (Figure 246-6). The increased concentrations of estradiol frequently cause hypertrophy of the floor of the posterior vagina, just cranial to the urethral orifice and therefore folding over and covering the urethral orifice (Figure 246-7). At the end of the follicular phase that is during the decline in estradiol and the rise in progesterone concentrations in plasma, shrinkage begins in response to reduced estradiol-dependent water retention. These cyclic changes are most marked in the dorsal median fold and precede those of the mid-vaginal mucosa (Figure 246-8).

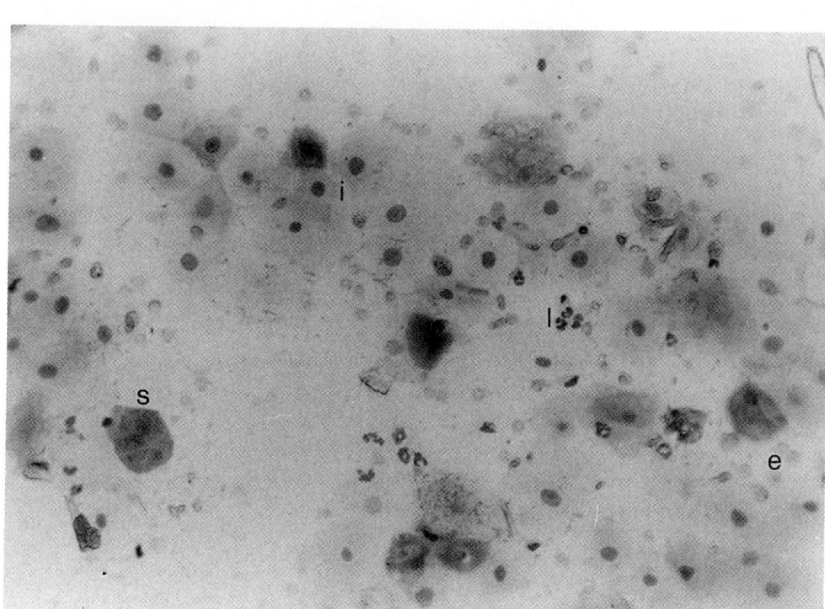

Figure 246-4 Vaginal cytology in the bitch at the onset of the follicular phase, showing primarily intermediate *(i)* cells, some superficial *(s)* cells, erythrocytes *(e)*, and leukocytes *(l)* (May Grünwald Giemsa, original magnification, 200).

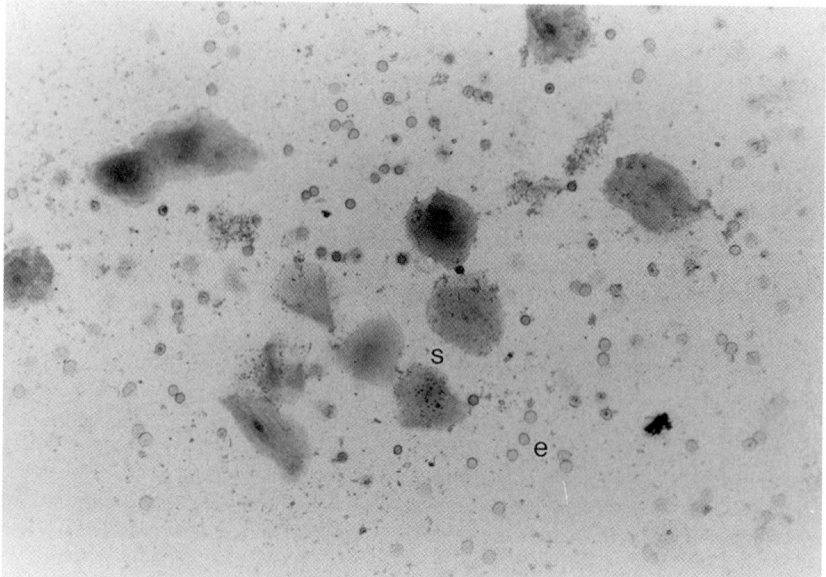

Figure 246-5 Vaginal cytology in the bitch during the second half of the follicular phase, at ovulation, and the onset of the luteal phase. This smear shows superficial cells (s) and erythrocytes (e) (May Grünwald Giemsa, original magnification 200).

The basal plasma follicle-stimulating hormone (FSH) concentration is relatively low during the follicular phase, whereas the basal plasma LH concentration is higher than in different phases of the anestrus (Figure 246-9). The secretory pattern of LH is characterized by frequent increases of short duration.[4] Plasma progesterone concentrations initially remain low but fluctuate and increase during the second half of the follicular phase as a result of partial luteinization of the follicles.

PRE-OVULATORY LUTEINIZATION AND OVULATION

The pre-ovulatory surge of LH lasts 24 to 72 hours. It usually starts shortly after the estradiol peak and coincides with declining estradiol and rising progesterone concentrations in plasma (see Figure 246-2). Rapid and extensive luteinization takes place during the preovulatory LH surge. Ovulating follicles therefore have many of the characteristics of rapidly developing corpora lutea. Most ova in the dog are ovulated in an immature state as primary oocytes. The process of ovulation can take up to 24 hours. In the first 2 to 3 days after ovulation the oocytes mature; that is, they undergo the first meiotic division and the extrusion of the first polar body, after which fertilization can occur.[5]

Plasma progesterone levels are 6 to 13 nmol/L at the time of the LH peak, and 15 to 25 nmol/L at the time of ovulation, 36 to 48 hours later. Concurrent with the LH peak, a pre-ovulatory surge in FSH occurs that reaches peak concentrations 1 to 2 days after the LH peak. Estrus behavior usually starts synchronously with the pre-ovulatory LH peak (see Figure 246-2), but some bitches initially demonstrate estrus behavior days before or after the LH peak.[6] Shrinkage of the vaginal mucosa starts about midway in the follicular phase and continues through the phase of pre-ovulatory luteinization

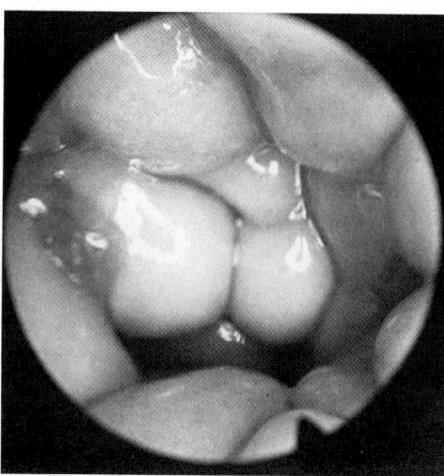

Figure 246-6 Vaginoscopy in the bitch at the onset of the follicular phase. Note the swollen, pale mucosal folds with smooth rounded surfaces (balloons) and the bloody secretion between the folds.

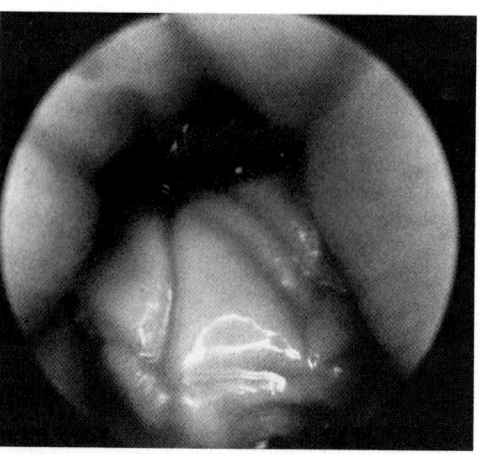

Figure 246-7 A modest vaginal hyperplasia which is observed quite often in the posterior vagina during the estradiol-influenced phase of the cycle (follicular, ovulation, fertilization phase). (From Schaefers-Okkens AC: The ovaries. In Rijnberk A: *Clinical endocrinology of dogs and cats*, Netherlands, 1996, Kluwer Academic Publishers.)

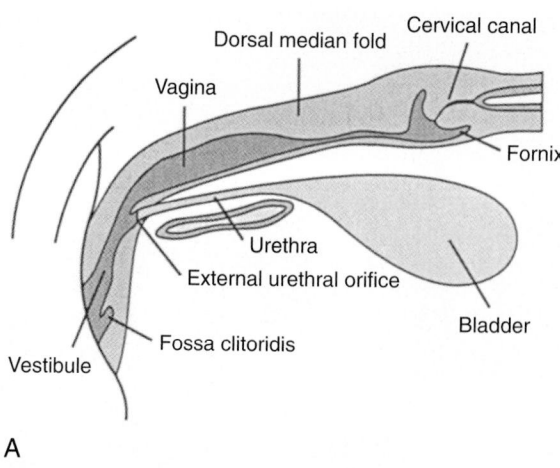

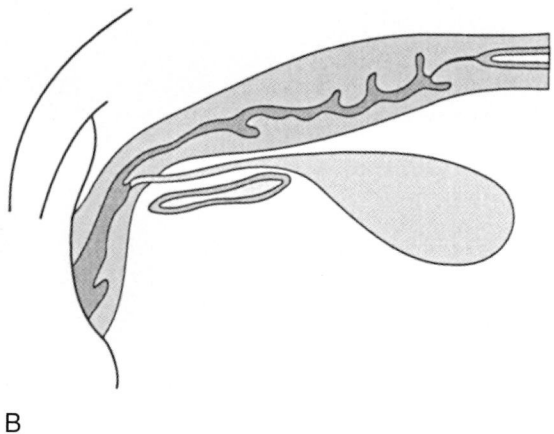

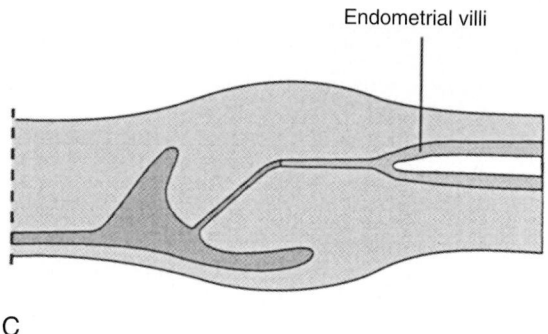

Figure 246-8 A sagittal section through the vestibule, vagina, and cervix of a bitch **(A)** during anestrus and **(B)** during the proestrus/estrus period. In this stage the vaginal wall is extremely folded. **C,** A close up of the cranial part of the vagina and the cervix during the anestrus period. Note the very short cervical canal. (From Schaefers-Okkens, AC: The ovaries. In Rijnberk A: *Clinical endocrinology of dogs and cats,* Netherlands, 1996, Kluwer Academic Publishers.)

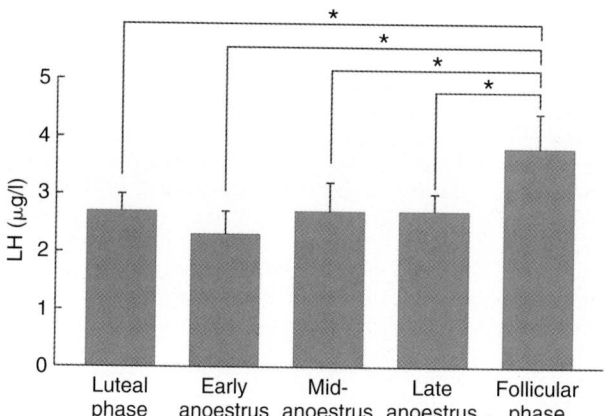

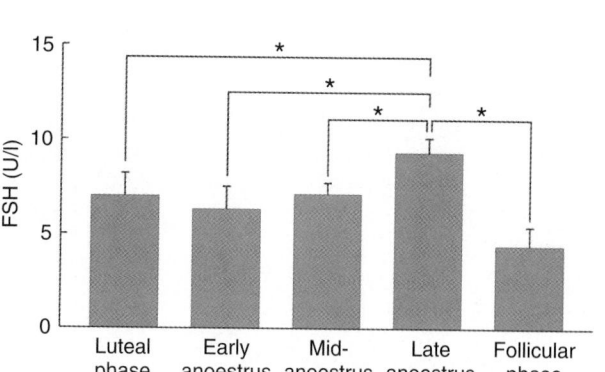

Figure 246-9 The mean (± SEM) plasma FSH and LH concentrations of the smoothed baseline in six beagle bitches during the follicular phase, the luteal phase, and during early, mid-, and late anestrus. *Indicates significant difference. (From Kooistra HS et al: Concurrent pulsatile secretion of luteinizing and follicle-stimulating hormone during different phases of the oestrous cycle and anoestrus in beagle bitches, *Biol Reprod* 60:65, 1999.)

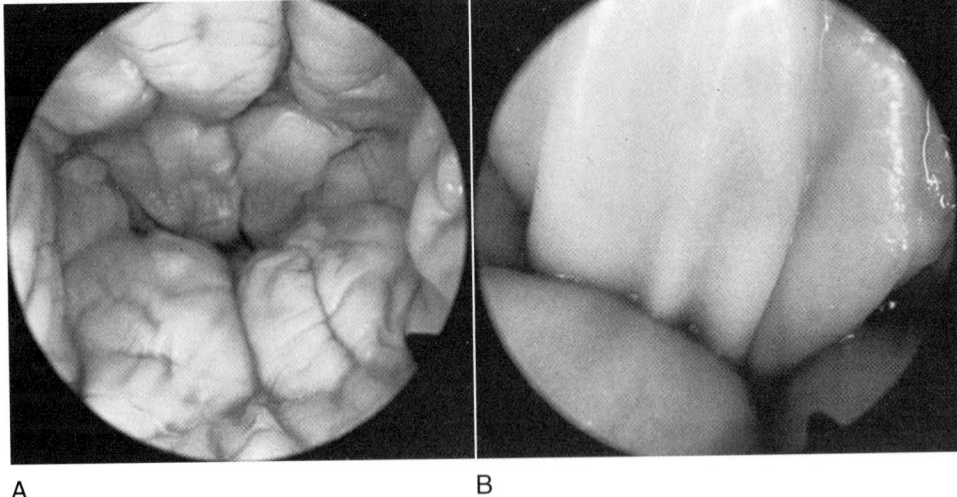

Figure 246-10 Vaginoscopy at the time of ovulation. The plasma progesterone concentration in this bitch was 22 nmol/l. **A,** The mucosal shrinkage leads to longitudinal folds. **B,** Close up of the shrinkage of the longitudinal folds of the dorsal median fold of the cranial vagina. (From Schaefers-Okkens AC: The ovaries. In Rijnberk A: *Clinical endocrinology of dogs and cats,* Netherlands, 1996, Kluwer Academic Publishers.)

A   B

and ovulation, when many longitudinal folds can be observed (Figure 246-10).

LUTEAL PHASE

Plasma concentrations of progesterone originating from the corpora lutea increase during the remainder of the estrus and during the onset of diestrus. Estrus behavior is thus seen during the period of a rising plasma progesterone concentration. Increased progesterone concentrations plateau at 10 to 30 days after the LH peak. Thereafter, in non-pregnant bitches, the progesterone secretion declines slowly and reaches a basal level of 3 nmol/l for the first time at about 75 days after the start of the luteal phase (Figure 246-11).

During the initial part of the luteal phase, the transition from estrus to diestrus takes place. In this period, the cytology of the vaginal mucosa changes from primarily superficial cells to mainly intermediate and parabasal cells and leukocytes (Figure 246-12). This change is an indication that the fertile period has expired. During oocyte maturation, shrinkage of

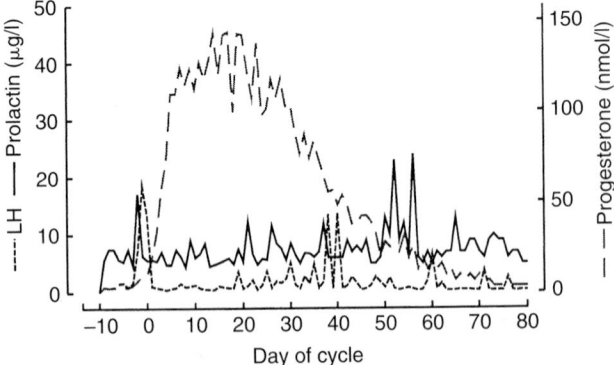

Figure 246-11 Mean LH, progesterone, and prolactin levels in plasma of three dogs during the follicular and luteal phase. The data have been synchronized on day 1, the day after the onset of the follicular phase on which the progesterone concentration in the peripheral blood had reached 16 nmol/l. (From Schaefers-Okkens AC: The ovaries. In Rijnberk A: *Clinical endocrinology of dogs and cats,* Netherlands, 1996, Kluwer Academic Publishers.)

the vaginal mucosa continues and increasing numbers of sharp edged summit profiles appear. In the transition period from estrus to diestrus, the mucosa thins and profiles become round. At the start of diestrus, a patchwork of red and white areas can be seen (Figure 246-13).

The factors that are responsible for initiating the regression of the corpora lutea in the dog are still unknown. Prostaglandin $F_{2\alpha}$ originating from the endometrium is not the causative factor in the bitch as it is in the cow and sheep. This is demonstrated by the fact that hysterectomy does not influence the length of the luteal phase.[7]

Prolactin acts as a luteotropic factor in the second half of the luteal phase.[8,9] During the first half of the luteal phase the corpus luteum functions independent of pituitary support.[10] Thereafter, inhibition of prolactin secretion causes a sharp decrease in progesterone secretion (Figure 246-14). LH concentrations change little during the luteal phase, with the exception of a slight increase in the second half of the luteal phase (see Figure 246-11). There is no proof of direct luteotropic properties for LH in the cyclic bitch.[9,11]

Pseudopregnancy is a syndrome that in greater or lesser degree accompanies the extended luteal phase of all non-pregnant ovarian cycles in the bitch. If the nature of the syndrome is mild, it is generally referred to as a *physiologic* or *covert pseudopregnancy.* In contrast, overt or "clinical" pseudopregnancy includes obvious mammary development, changes that are not distinguishable from the changes of late pregnancy, or lactation are seen (see Chapter 247). Mammary gland development is influenced by prolactin and growth hormone (GH) and their secretion pattern is influenced by progesterone.[12] GH, produced in the mammary gland itself, may promote the physiologic proliferation and differentiation of mammary gland tissue during the luteal phase by local autocrine/paracrine effects, prolactin is important for lobuloalveolar development.[13]

In the start of the luteal phase, a higher basal GH secretion is present, with less GH being secreted in pulses than during the last part of the luteal phase, where the basal GH secretion is lower with more GH being secreted in pulses. This phenomenon may be explained by partial suppression of pituitary GH release by progesterone-induced GH production in the mammary gland (Figure 246-15).[12] In most non-pregnant bitches the decline in plasma progesterone concentrations during the luteal phase is associated with a moderate but significant increase in prolactin secretion (see Figures 246-11 and 246-15).[12] In the overt pseudopregnant bitch, however, the

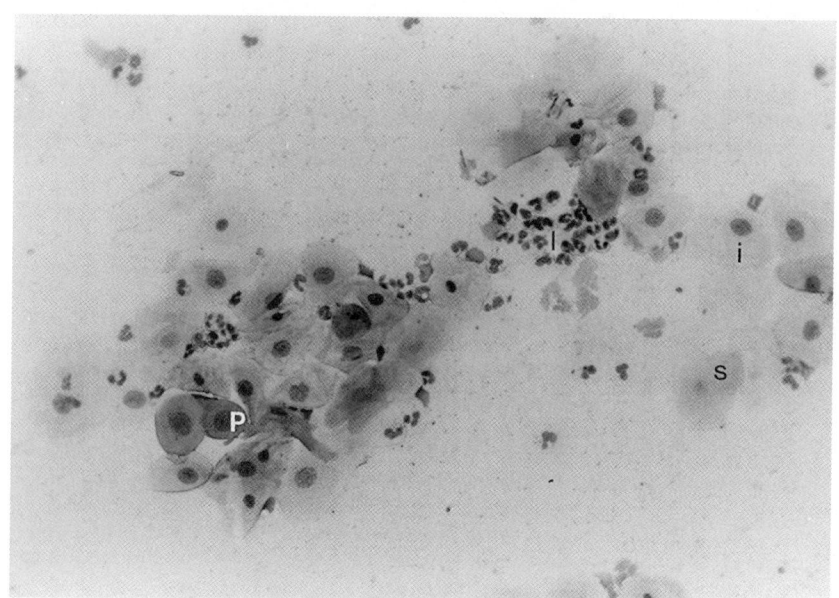

Figure 246-12 Vaginal cytology during diestrus, which starts 6 to 10 days after the preovulatory LH peak. This smear shows intermediate cells *(i)*, parabasal *(p)* cells, and leukocytes *(l)* (May Grünwald Giemsa original magnification, 200).

plasma prolactin concentration may strongly increase, probably corresponding with the degree of "clinical" pseudopregnancy.[14]

ANESTRUS

The time of the onset of anestrus depends on which criteria are being used to define the end of the luteal phase: for example, after 2 to 3 months when mammary development subsides, the first time that the plasma progesterone concentration reaches a level below 3 nmol/L, or the moment that the influence of progesterone on the endometrium is no longer evident. In any case, the transition from the luteal phase into anestrus is gradual and varies considerably among bitches. The transition from anestrus to follicular phase can begin at any time throughout the year and there appears to be little, if any, seasonal influence. Breed differences and strains within breeds can form the basis of variation in mean interestrous intervals. In the Collie, for instance, the mean interval is 36 weeks, and in the Alsatian, it is about 20 to 22 weeks. Some breeds such as the Basenji and Tibetan Mastiff, however, have

a single annual estrous cycle, which may possibly be influenced by a photoperiod. Environmental factors can also affect the interestrous interval: an anestrous bitch placed in close proximity to a bitch in estrus can show an advance of the onset of proestrus by several weeks. Furthermore, bitches housed together often have synchronous estrous cycles.

Progression from early to late anestrus is characterized by a greater amplitude and a higher number of GnRH pulses by the hypothalamus, an increase in the sensitivity of the pituitary to GnRH from early to late anestrus, and an increase in ovarian responsiveness to gonadotropins.[15,16] Furthermore, the increase in the basal plasma FSH concentration should be considered to be a critical event required for the initiation of folliculogenesis (see Figure 246-9).[4,17] In addition, a period of increased LH pulsatility is observed shortly before the onset of proestrus.[4,18,19] There is some evidence that factors that decrease opiodergic activity promote LH release and the termination of anestrus.[18] Finally, during the course of anestrus in the bitch, there is an increase in hypothalamic mRNA encoding for the estrogen receptor and the expression of the gene for P450 aromatase, which catalyzes estrogen biosynthesis.[20,21] Although sporadic elevations are observed, plasma estradiol concentrations are usually low and do not begin to rise until late anestrus.

Apart from these changes in the hypothalamic-pituitary-ovarian axis, there is an involvement of dopaminergic influences in the initiation of a new follicular phase in the bitch. Administration of the dopamine agonists bromocriptine and cabergoline shortens the anestrus and is associated with a decrease in the plasma prolactin concentration, which suggests that the shortened anestrus is the result of the suppression of prolactin secretion.[8,22] However, the anestrus of dogs treated with metergoline, a drug that in a low dose lowers the plasma prolactin concentration via a serotonine-antagonistic pathway, is not shortened, which indicates that not the decrease in the plasma prolactin concentration, but the dopamine-agonistic influence is a critical event in the transition to a new follicular phase.[23] Furthermore, a low dose of bromocriptine, which does not decrease the plasma prolactin concentration, prematurely induces a new follicular phase.[24] In addition, under physiologic conditions low plasma prolactin concentrations are found during anestrus and no obvious changes in the plasma prolactin concentration have been

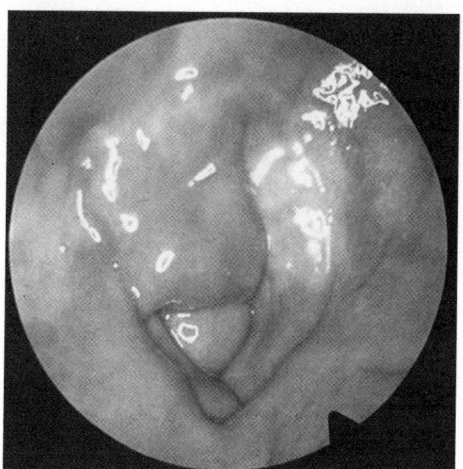

Figure 246-13 Vaginoscopy during diestrus. Note the rounded profiles and the patchwork of red and white areas.

Figure 246-14 Progesterone and prolactin levels in the peripheral blood of one dog, treated with bromocriptine (bar) from ovulation in the first cycle until the onset of the next follicular phase. The luteal phase and especially the anestrus are considerably shortened. (From Schaefers-Okkens AC: The ovaries. In Rijnberk A: *Clinical endocrinology of dogs and cats,* Netherlands, 1996, Kluwer Academic Publishers.)

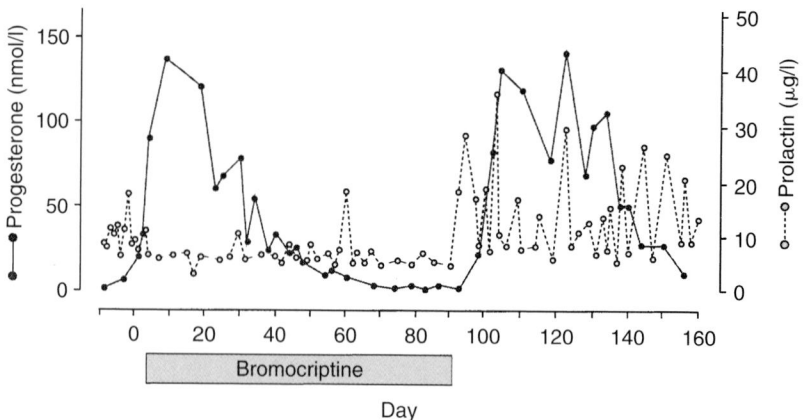

observed in the bitch during the transition from anestrus to the follicular phase (see Figure 246-15).[4,25]

Bromocriptine-induced shortening of the anestrus is associated with a quick rise in the basal plasma FSH concentration without a concomitant increase in the basal plasma LH concentration[26], similar to what is observed during the physiologic late anestrus. This again indicates that in the bitch an increase in the circulating plasma FSH concentration is a critical event in the initiation of ovarian folliculogenesis.[4]

As a consequence of what is described, induction of a follicular phase may take place by pulsatile administration of GnRH. In a study, in which GnRH was administered in pulses of 15 to 500 ng/kg every 90 minutes for 7 to 9 days to 36 anestrous bitches, GnRH pulses resulted in proestrus, estrus, ovulation, and pregnancy in 26, 20, 16, and 12 bitches, respectively. Efficacy was dose dependent.[27] A fertile estrus could also be induced by administering a timed-release GnRH agonist, followed by a GnRH analogue on the first day of induced estrus.[28] Anestrus can also be terminated by treating bitches

with porcine LH. In one study proestrus was induced in all bitches (n = 16). Twelve bitches came in estrus, from which seven ovulated. Bitches, in which proestrus but not estrus occurred, were all treated in early anestrus.[29] The observed rapid increase of plasma estradiol concentration after LH treatment suggests that increased follicle steroidogenesis is a primary effect of LH. On the other hand the insufficient reaction to porcine LH of bitches in early anestrus may be due to a deficiency of FSH or FSH receptors in this stage of anestrus. Follicular aromatase in rats and most other species studied appears to be primarily under up-regulation control by FSH.[30]

Anestrus can thus also be shortened considerably by administration of dopamine-agonists such as bromocriptine and cabergoline.[8,18,22,31] When bromocriptine treatment, twice daily 20 μg/kg, orally, is started during the luteal phase, the interestrous interval can be shortened from 245 days to 100 days (see Figure 246-14).[8] When started during the anestrus 100 days after the ovulation the next proestrus can be expected after a mean period of about 45 days.[31] The fertility

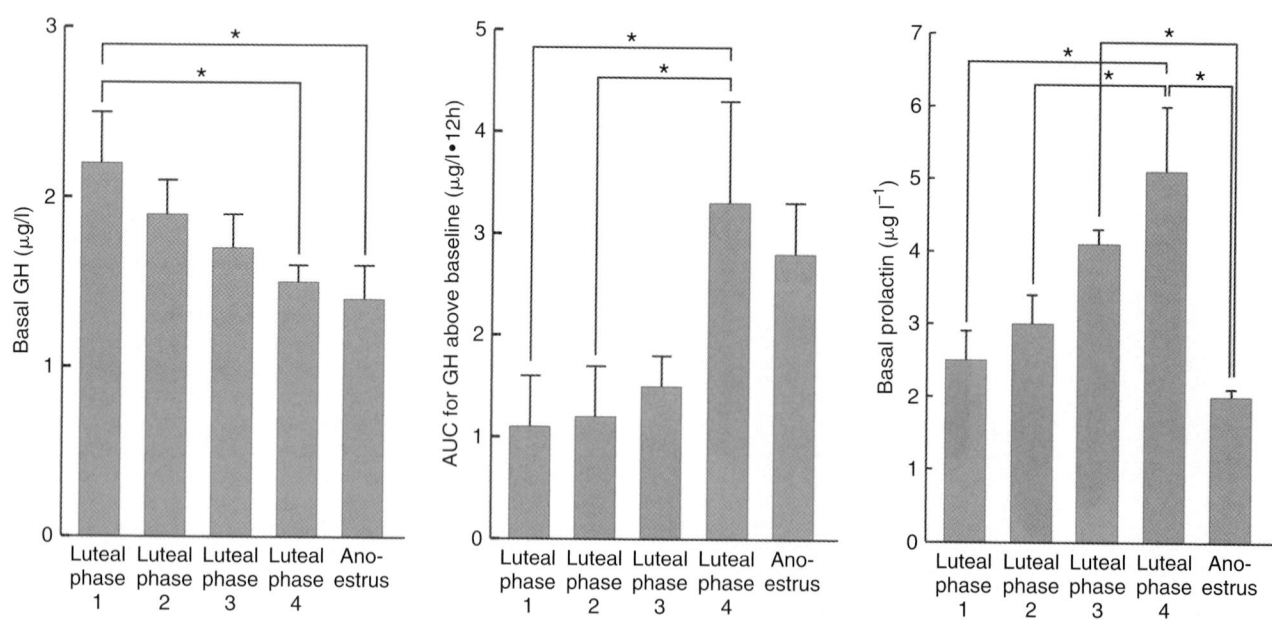

Figure 246-15 The mean (± SEM) basal plasma GH concentration, the mean (± SEM) area under the curve (AUC) for GH above the baseline and the mean (± SEM) basal plasma prolactin concentration in six beagle bitches. Blood samples were collected at 10-minute intervals for 12 hours at four stages of the luteal phase (luteal stage 1 through 4, with mean plasma progesterone concentrations of 123, 56, 20, and 9 nmol/L, respectively) and during mid-anestrus. *Indicates statistically significant difference. (Modified from Kooistra HS, Okkens AC: Secretion of growth hormone and prolactin during progression of the luteal phase in healthy dogs: a review, *Mol Cell Endocrinol* 197:167, 2002.)

of an estrus initiated by bromocriptine treatment appears to be normal.

BREEDING MANAGEMENT OF THE HEALTHY BITCH

Breeding management starts with the determination if the bitch is healthy and if a normal fertility can be expected (Figure 246-16). For that reason the age and the breeding history of both the bitch and the male dog have to be considered. Thereafter, a complete gynecologic examination of the bitch is needed. Recurring examinations should be performed during the follicular phase, ovulation, and pregnancy. A decrease in fertility may be expected with increasing age. One of the reasons for this diminished fertility may be the development of cystic endometrial hyperplasia (CEH; see Chapter 251).

THE HISTORY CONCERNING THE REPRODUCTION DATA

The reproduction history of the bitch must be considered in the breeding management program. The age of the bitch at her first estrus and the length of the interestrous intervals are important. The bitch that has not experienced an estrus by 18 months of age is considered to have a primary anestrus. One of the major causes of primary anestrus is probably true hermaphroditism or pseudohermaphroditism. If a bitch has experienced estrus, an interval of more than 12 months or an interval that is double the usual interestrous interval for that individual bitch is considered to be a prolonged interestrous interval.

One reason for a prolonged anestrus can be hypothyroidism. However, it should be realized that less pronounced cases of hypothyroidism may result in prolonged or abbreviated proestrus or weak estrus symptoms instead of anestrus. Anestrus may also be induced with drugs such as progestagens or glucocorticosteroids. Glucocorticoids probably decrease levels of circulating gonadotropic hormones.[32] In bitches older than 8 years of age, the duration and frequency of the cycles become more irregular and the interestrous interval increases. An apparent prolonged anestrus can be present if the bitch has a silent estrus or if the owner did not observe the estrus properly. Shortened interestrous intervals (intervals of less than 4 months) may be caused by a split heat or are seen in combination with persistent estrus (see Chapter 247).

Attention must also be given to the length of estrous periods. The average length of proestrus and of estrus is 9 days each. The bitch is considered to have a persistent estrus, if ovulation has not occurred after about 25 days from the onset of proestrus. In that case the plasma progesterone concentration will be lower than 16 nmol/L, and estrus symptoms such as sanguineous discharge, estrus behavior, estradiol influence seen during vaginoscopy, and/or the presence of superficial cells in the vaginal smear are present. Plasma estradiol concentrations are not consistently elevated.[33] Persistent estrus can be caused by ovarian tumors and cysts (see Chapter 247).

Attention must also be given to attempts to mate the bitch and/or the results of matings in previous cycles, previous pregnancies and parturitions and how many puppies were born. There are a number of problems that can lead to an unsuccessful mating. One problem can be inexperience or behavioral problems from bitch and/or male dog. Also anatomic disorders may prevent a normal mating. Strictures, adhesions, septa, and hyperplasia, for example, are common in bitches.[34] They can be congenital or acquired as a result of local treatment of vaginitis with irritating drugs (see Chapter 253).

Another important reason for a failure to mate or a missed conception is mating at an improper moment. A large number of fertility problems are the result of inappropriate management of the bitch and are avoidable if a proper breeding program is used. Additionally, CEH or CEH-endometritis or infectious diseases such as canine brucellosis or herpesvirus infection may also lead to breeding problems. Infertility due to CEH without endometritis, in which case the bitch does not show signs of a systemic disease, may be diagnosed during an ultrasonographic examination.

Canine brucellosis is a contagious disease for which the clinical manifestations vary greatly. It is characterized in the bitch by generalized lymphadenopathy and by early embryonic death, abortion (mainly between the 45th and 55th day of gestation), and infertility.[35] Canine brucellosis must be considered whenever there is a history of abortion or poor reproductive performance in either sex. The diagnosis can, however, not be established based on clinical signs alone. Serologic tests are necessary to confirm the diagnosis of canine brucellosis.

Canine herpesvirus can cause a high percentage of dead puppies in the first weeks after parturition. Herpesvirus does not seem to lead to a decrease in fertility.

THE EXAMINATION OF THE BITCH

Breeding management starts with a general examination followed by sequential examinations. During the gynecologic portion of the first examination special emphasis should be given to palpation of the uterus and digital evaluation of the vagina. The following items should be examined every other day, starting 5 to 6 days after onset of proestrus: the vulva (size, swelling), vaginal discharge (quantity, color), and vaginoscopic, and cytologic findings. Furthermore, the owner should be asked to look for behavioral changes consistent with estrus. The start of estrus behavior usually occurs synchronously with the preovulatory LH peak (see Figure 246-2), but the first signs of this behavior can be observed several days before or after the LH peak or may never be seen. Repeated examinations are carried out to determine if the cycle is progressing normally (see Figure 246-16).

Vaginoscopic and cytologic observations not in agreement with the expected stage of the cycle may be a sign of a fertility disorder, which may or may not be serious. For example, a split heat is common in both younger and older healthy bitches. In cases of split heat, the follicular phase stops before ovulation and resumes after a few days or weeks. The vaginal discharge changes from red to brown; the smear shows intermediate cells, parabasal cells, and leukocytes and the swelling of the vaginal mucosal folds diminishes. It is probably caused by prematurely regressing follicles. Ovulation will generally occur if proestrus returns. Treatment is usually not necessary, but close monitoring of the cycle is essential for determining the appropriate mating period.

Sequential examinations should also be carried out to determine the ovulation period. Data concerning vulvar swelling, vaginal discharge, and vaginoscopic and cytologic findings have been described. Because of the variable length of proestrus and estrus, it should be clear that breeding a bitch on preset days of the cycle (e.g., 11 to 13 days after onset of proestrus bleeding) gives inconsistent results. Although breeding in accordance with estrus behavior will give better results, some bitches are nevertheless bred too early and others too late. Determination of the ovulation period is therefore of value. Several methods have been described to determine the ovulation period and the proper period for mating. The principal methods are measurement of the plasma progesterone concentration and vaginoscopy.

Plasma progesterone concentrations should, along with the other examinations, be determined every other day. At the onset of the follicular phase, determined through cytologic and

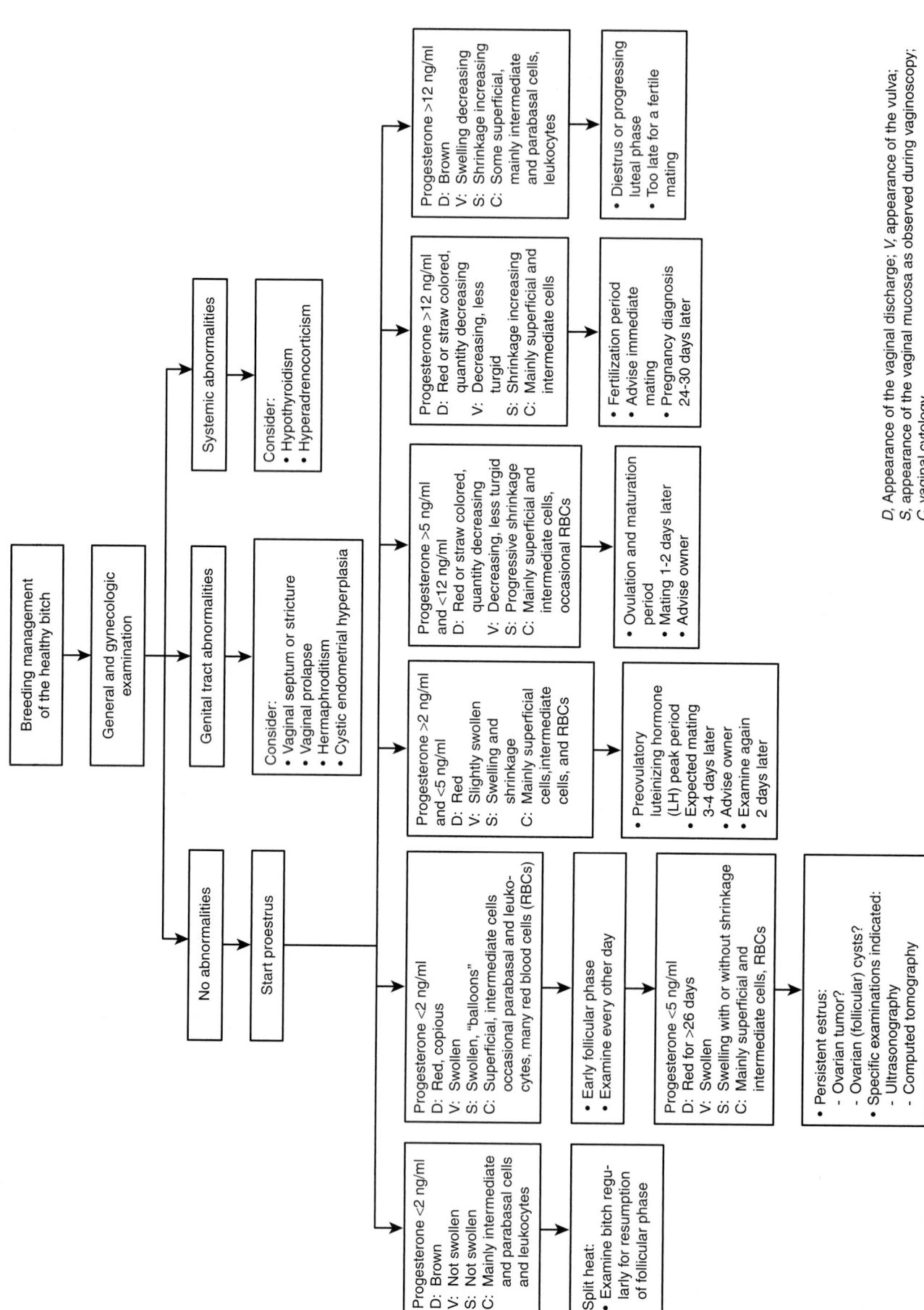

Figure 246-16 Algorithm for the breeding management of the healthy bitch.

D, Appearance of the vaginal discharge; *V,* appearance of the vulva; *S,* appearance of the vaginal mucosa as observed during vaginoscopy; *C,* vaginal cytology.

vaginoscopic findings, the time between two determinations of plasma progesterone may be longer than in the progressing follicular phase. Use of an enzyme-linked immunosorbent assay (ELISA) or enzyme immunoassay kit for plasma progesterone determination may be less accurate, especially in medium (progesterone: >3 nmol/L, <16 nmol/L) plasma progesterone concentrations as compared with a plasma progesterone determination via a radioimmunoassay (RIA).[36,37] The RIA method is therefore the preferred method for progesterone determination. When frozen or chilled extended semen is being used, and sperm life span is expected to be shorter than in fresh semen, it is especially advisable to determine plasma progesterone concentrations by RIA to ensure accuracy in determining the ovulation day and the fertile period, therefore permitting use of a single insemination.

Plasma progesterone concentrations increase slightly at the time of the preovulatory LH peak and rapidly at the onset of ovulation. At this time the plasma progesterone concentration exceeds 16 nmol/L. The onset of the optimal period for mating is 24 hours later and is based on the time needed for maturation of the oocytes, capacitation, and life span of the sperm.[38] With determination of the period for mating using a rapid RIA for the plasma progesterone concentration, it was found that 105 of 112 (94%) bitches with normal fertility became pregnant and 81 of 104 bitches (78%) with suboptimal fertility became pregnant. In the latter group, only 23% of previous matings without proper breeding management had been successful.[39]

Determination of the preovulatory LH peak would also provide an excellent parameter for the estimation of the ovulation time. In-hospital ELISA LH kits are available. However, more frequent blood sampling is required than for progesterone because of the risk of missing the preovulatory LH peak. Vaginoscopy can also be used to try to establish the ovulation period. The mucosal changes are, however, a response to hormonal changes and are therefore secondary changes. Additionally, interpretation of the changes is subjective.

Vaginoscopy is thus a less reliable method of estimation of the ovulation period than measurement of hormone levels. For experienced veterinarians, it can be a useful tool for monitoring the stage of the cycle, but mating advice based on vaginoscopy should include the recommendation to mate at least twice, with an interval of 48 hours. Vaginal cytology is useful in diagnosis of early proestrus, progressing proestrus-estrus, or diestrus. There are, however, no reliable changes in the smear indicative of the preovulatory LH surge or of ovulation.[3] Lastly, ultrasonography is not reliable for ovulation determination.[40]

ADDITIONAL EXAMINATIONS

In bitches with previous fertility problems, vaginal culture may be of use. A mixed bacterial flora, including *Pasteurella*, beta-hemolytic streptococci, and *Escherichia coli*, often inhabits the canine vagina and should not be considered a causative factor for infertility. In an examination of the aerobic bacterial flora of the genital tract of 59 bitches in four breeds during different stages of the cycle and pregnancy (all bitches whelped at least once during this study), culture results were negative in only 5%. Although the cultures in general showed a mixed flora, single species were obtained from 18% of the specimens. The aerobic bacterial flora consisted of common opportunistic pathogens.[41] Therefore bacterial culturing of vaginal swab specimens from bitches without signs of genital disease is of little value. Treatment is indicated in cases of suspected genital inflammation only if there are many bacteria (more than 100 colonies per culture) or the culture reveals only one species. Treatment may be systemic or local, but locally applied drugs alter the vaginal environment, are often spermicidal, and should therefore not be used shortly before breeding.

Pregnancy diagnosis is important within a breeding management program. Between 26 and 32 days after mating, pregnancy may be diagnosed by abdominal palpation. In some bitches an earlier diagnosis can be made depending on the degree of muscular guarding, thickness, and breed. The examination should, however, be repeated in case of a negative finding. In case of a negative or dubious finding, if vesicles of different size and elasticity are palpated, or if only one or two gestational vesicles are found, an ultrasonography is indicated. In the last two instances, fetal resorption has frequently been observed, which may warrant further examinations and sequential ultrasonographic examinations during the rest of the pregnancy. Furthermore, in cases of only one or two gestational vesicles the chance and risk of a prolonged pregnancy have to be discussed with the owner.

CHAPTER • 247

Ovarian and Estrous Cycle Abnormalities

Autumn P. Davidson
Edward C. Feldman

Deviation from anticipated, typical estrous cycle events in a bitch intended for breeding can prompt owners to bring their dogs to a veterinarian for evaluation. The canine reproductive cycle is categorized into four distinct phases, each having particular behavioral, physical, and endocrinologic characteristics. Considerable variation exists within the normal canine reproductive cycle, breeders commonly interpret such variation as an indication that an abnormality exits. The clinician must differentiate bitches having normal estrous cycles with unexpected patterns from those with true abnormalities. Detection of individual variation within the normal range of events in a fertile bitch can be crucial to providing effective counseling concerning breeding management. Additionally, evaluation of the estrous cycle for actual abnormalities is an important component in assessing the apparently infertile bitch. Variations from normal estrous cycle events in the bitch can sometimes be traced to specific ovarian disorders.

THE NORMAL CANINE ESTROUS CYCLE

The interestrous interval normally varies from 4.5 to 10 months in duration, with 7 the average. The anestrus phase of the interestrous interval is marked by reproductive inactivity, uterine involution, and endometrial repair. The normal bitch is neither attractive nor receptive to male dogs. Minimal mucoid vaginal discharge is present, and the vulva is not swollen. Vaginal cytology is scant, characterized by small parabasal cells, with occasional non-toxic neutrophils and may have small numbers of mixed bacteria present. Viewed endoscopically, the vaginal mucosal folds are flat, thin, and pale red. The termination of anestrus (onset of proestrus) follows the pulsatile, hypothalamic gonadotropin-releasing hormone (GnRH) induced secretion of the pituitary gonadotropins, follicle-stimulating hormone (FSH), and luteinizing hormone (LH). Such pulsatile GnRH secretion is a physiologic requirement of gonadotropin release. Following GnRH stimulation during late anestrus, pituitary gonadotrophs release LH in a rapid, transitory pattern and FSH in a slow, sustained pattern. Mean levels of both FSH and LH rise moderately during late anestrus. At the termination of anestrus, the pulsatile release of LH increases, which precedes and likely amplifies ovarian folliculogenesis during proestrus. Estrogen levels are basal (5 to 10 pg/mL) and progesterone levels at nadir (<1 ng/mL) in late anestrus. Anestrus normally lasts from 1 to 6 months.[1,2]

During proestrus, the bitch attracts male dogs but is still not receptive to breeding. She may become more playful or passive concerning the male as proestrus progresses. A serosanguineous-hemorrhagic vaginal discharge of uterine origin is present and the vulva is mildly enlarged and turgid. The microscopic appearance of exfoliated vaginal epithelial cells shifts over a period of 4 to 7 days from small parabasal cells to small then large intermediate cells, superficial-intermediate cells, and finally superficial (cornified) epithelial cells. These changes in the vaginal cells reflect the degree of estrogen influence on the vaginal mucosa. The vaginal wall becomes thickened under the progressive influence of estrogen, in preparation for copulation. Red blood cells are usually but not invariably present on the vaginal smear.

Endoscopically, the vaginal mucosal folds appear edematous, pink and rounded. FSH and LH levels are low during most of proestrus, rising during preovulatory surges. Estrogen rises from basal anestrus levels to peak levels (50 to 100 pg/dl during late proestrus), while progesterone remains basal (<1 ng/mL) until rising (2 to 4 ng/mL) in conjunction with the LH surge. The LH surge generally lasts only 12 to 24 hours in the bitch. Occasionally, more than one LH surge occurs, the one associated with a concurrent rise in serum progesterone level reaching 2 to 3 ng/mL is likely associated with ovulation. Proestrus lasts from 3 days to 3 weeks and averages 9 days. The follicular phase of the ovarian cycle coincides with proestrus and early estrus.[1,3]

During estrus, the normal bitch displays receptive or passive behavior with a male dog, which enables breeding. Serosanguineous to hemorrhagic vaginal discharge diminishes to variable degrees. Vulvar enlargement and edema tends to be maximal but the vulva is soft. Vaginal cytology usually consists of 80% to 100% superficial cells. Red blood cells tend to diminish but may persist throughout estrus. Endoscopically, vaginal mucosal folds become progressively wrinkled or crenulated, the degree correlating with oocyte maturation to a fertilizable stage. Plasma estrogen progressively declines to basal concentrations, achieved as estrus ceases. Progesterone concentrations steadily increase (usually 4 to 10 ng/mL at ovulation), marking the onset of the luteal phase of the ovarian cycle.

Estrus lasts 3 days to 3 weeks, with an average of 9 days. The receptive behavior of estrus may precede or follow shortly after the LH peak. Duration of receptivity is variable and may not coincide precisely with the fertile period. Receptive behavior reflects decreasing estrogen and increasing progesterone concentrations. Ovulation of primary (infertile) oocytes begins approximately 1 to 2 days after the LH surge; oocyte maturation occurs over the following 1 to 3 days. The life span of secondary (fertile) oocytes is 2 to 3 days. The resultant fertile window in the bitch, during which time breeding is most likely to result in conception, is between 3 and 7 days after the LH surge, or after the initial day progesterone reaches 2 to 3 ng/mL.[1-3]

During diestrus, the normal bitch becomes refractory to breeding and gradually less attractive to male dogs. Vaginal discharge diminishes, often becoming mucoid and mildly suppurative and odorous before disappearing, and vulvar edema turgid, then slowly regressing. Vaginal cytology is abruptly altered by the reappearance of parabasal epithelial cells and, frequently, neutrophils. Vaginal cytology on the first day of diestrus has less than 50% superficial cells. Endoscopically, vaginal mucosal folds appear flattened, pink, and flaccid. Plasma estrogen concentrations are low during diestrus, except for a mild rise reported in the pregnant bitch prior to parturition. Plasma progesterone concentrations steadily rise during the first few weeks of diestrus to a plateau of 15 to 80 ng/mL, before progressively declining in late diestrus. Progesterone secretion is dependent on both pituitary LH and prolactin secretion. Proliferation of the endometrium and quiescence of the myometrium occur under the influence of progesterone.

Diestrus usually lasts 2 to 3 months in the absence of pregnancy. Parturition terminates pregnancy 64 to 66 days after the LH peak (or the initial rise in progesterone), or 56 to 58 days after the onset of diestrus as determined by vaginal cytology. Gestational length may be related to litter size and parity.[4] Prolactin concentrations increase in a reciprocal fashion to declining progesterone concentrations as diestrus ends. Prolactin concentrations are higher in pregnant bitches. Mammary ductal and glandular tissues increase in response to prolactin, which makes lactation a normal event even in the non-pregnant state (pseudopregnancy).[1-3]

NORMAL VARIATIONS IN THE CANINE ESTROUS CYCLE

During evaluation of a bitch for estrous cycle abnormalities, the medical history, signalment, and husbandry of a bitch should be taken into account along with the specific reproductive history, physical examination findings, and results of clinical testing. Following the bitch over time, through one estrous cycle, is often necessary to reach a diagnosis.

Delayed Puberty

The onset of the first estrous cycle occurs after a bitch attains 70% of her adult height and body weight. Small breeds generally begin their first estrous cycle between 6 and 10 months of age, whereas large breeds may normally begin as late as 18 to 24 months. Family histories (dam and female siblings) can help predict the onset of reproductive activity. Efforts at differentiating delayed puberty from an actual failure to have reproductive cycles should be postponed until a bitch is at least 2 to 2.5 years old. Bitches with delayed puberty have normal reproductive cycles once initiated.

Silent Heat Cycles

The occurrence of a silent heat cycle needs to be ruled out during evaluation of a bitch for a reported failure to have estrous cycles. Fastidious bitches with minimal vulvar swelling, vaginal discharge, or behavioral changes may have estrous cycles that escape human detection, especially in the absence of a male dog. Estrous cycles tend to become more apparent as the bitch ages. Performing weekly vaginal cytologies, housing the bitch near an intact male, or using white bedding can aid in prospective detection of a silent heat, permitting ovulation timing and breeding. Performing monthly progesterone assays permits retrospective identification of estrus but will not facilitate breeding that cycle. Silent heat cycles need to be differentiated from true primary anestrus. True primary anestrus in the bitch that fails to experience an estrous cycle is most likely due to a disorder of sexual development, and is uncommon.[3]

Split Heat Cycles

Bitches experiencing split heat cycles, in which proestrus and possibly early estrus occur without progression, may be thought to have abnormally short cycles, lack of sexual receptivity, or infertility if breedings were forced or artificial insemination performed. Waves of folliculogenesis with increased estrogen production but without ovulation occur in split heats. Follicular atresia follows, no luteal phase with progesterone production occurs, and normal sexual receptivity fails to develop. These cycles typically occur in young bitches and are characterized by periods of hemorrhagic vaginal discharge typical of proestrus, attractiveness to males, and usually no receptivity. In young bitches, split cycles are thought to be due to immaturity. These cycles may also occur in mature bitches with a history of normal past cycles, usually in association with stress. Increased endogenous cortisol levels associated with stress (travel, shipping, kenneling) may inhibit the LH surge and associated ovulation.

After a period of 2 to 10 weeks, another proestrus typically begins, which may or may not proceed to ovulation. Eventually, most young bitches experiencing split heats progress through a normal estrus to diestrus. The condition is not associated with reproductive pathology in the young or stressed bitch, and no treatment is recommended. Breeding the bitch thought to have been previously stressed in familiar surroundings is advised. Serial vaginal cytology documenting the influence of estrogen on vaginal mucosa early in the cycle, and progesterone assays performed 1 to 2 weeks later (<2 ng/mL) documenting folliculogenesis without ovulation or luteinization confirm the diagnosis of a split heat. Occasionally split cycles occur on a regular basis in mature individual bitches, making them difficult to breed, and likely associated with abnormalities of the hypothalamic/pituitary/ovarian axis.

Management Errors

Bitches examined because they have failed to permit breeding or to conceive after a forced breeding or artificial insemination during the perceived fertile period need to be evaluated for kennel management errors. The timing of receptive and fertile periods during estrus varies significantly among normal bitches and even in individual bitches during different estrous cycles. These periods may not correlate with the handler's choice of predetermined breeding dates, typically between days 10 to 14 after the onset of vaginal bleeding. Ovulation timing protocols utilizing serial vaginal cytology, repeated vaginoscopy, and serum progesterone and LH concentrations are useful in identifying the actual fertile period when breeding

should occur.[5] Behavioral or physical problems can interfere with acceptance of a male for breeding. Dominant bitches exposed to an inexperienced male may not allow breeding even during the appropriate time. Vulvar or vaginal abnormalities such as strictures and septate bands, and vaginal hyperplasia may make natural breeding painful and result in a bitch refusing to permit copulation even when in estrus[6] (Figure 247-1). The pre-breeding veterinary examination permits early detection of such anatomic problems, enabling their correction or adjustment in breeding plans (artificial insemination versus natural) before the onset of proestrus.

PATTERNS OF ABNORMAL ESTROUS CYCLES

Abnormal estrous cycles can be categorized and simplified into several patterns that reflect either a prolongation or abbreviation of a phase of the cycle, or an alteration in the normal sequence of events. An owner's interpretation of a bitches behavior and physical characteristics may not equate with the actual physiologic events, which necessitates prospective documentation of the cycle through vaginal cytology, vaginoscopy, behavioral analysis, and assessment of serum progesterone and LH concentrations.

Prolonged Proestrus or Estrus

Prolonged proestrus or estrus occurs when a bitch displays vaginal bleeding (of uterine origin) for more than 21 to 28 consecutive days, accompanied by attractiveness to males. Greater than 80% to 90% superficial cells are found on vaginal cytology. Such bitches may or may not be receptive to breeding. Prolonged proestrus and/or estrus most likely results from persistent secretion of estrogens with or without small elevations in progesterone secretion. If secreted, progesterone enhances the presence of sexual receptivity.

Endogenous sources of prolonged estrogen exposure in the bitch, with or without progesterone, include ovarian follicular cysts and secretory neoplasias.[7] Secretory, anovulatory follicular ovarian cysts tend to be solitary, lined with granulosa cells and exceed normal preovulatory follicles in size, ranging from 1 to 5 cm in diameter (Figure 247-2). Bilateral follicular cysts may indicate a problem with the hypothalamic pituitary ovarian axis. Follicular cysts tend to occur in bitches less than 3 years of age. Ovarian neoplasias capable of producing

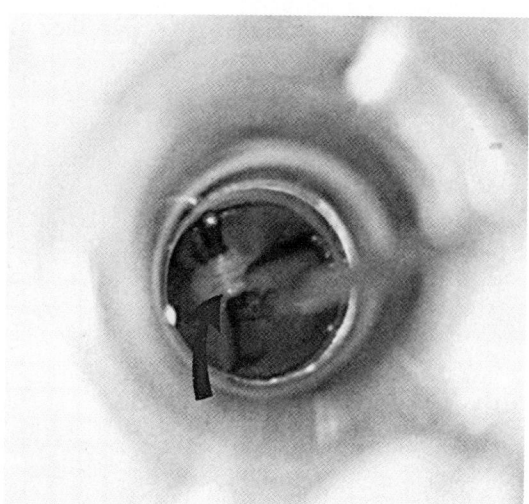

Figure 247-1 Vaginoscopic view of a septate band of tissue in the caudal vaginal of an estrus bitch exhibiting pain during breeding efforts. The band is retracted with a spay hook.

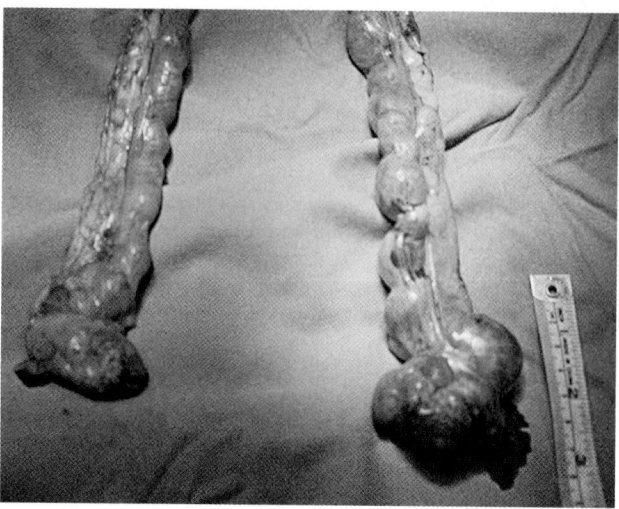

Figure 247-2 Functional, nonovulatory follicular ovarian cysts found in a Mastiff bitch that has been experiencing estrus for greater than 3 months.

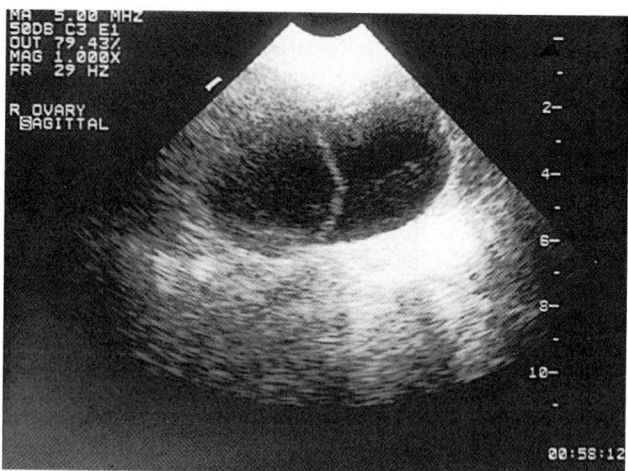

Figure 247-4 Ultrasonographic appearance of a functional, estrogen secreting, nonovulatory ovarian follicular cysts.

estrogen occur and include tumors of epithelial origin (cystadenomas and adenocarcinomas) as well as tumors of gonadal-stromal origin (granulosa-theca cell tumors).[8] Ovarian neoplasia tends to occur in bitches older than 5 years of age. Ovarian tumors can occur unilaterally or, less commonly, bilaterally. Functional ovarian neoplasia and cystic ovarian pathology can occur simultaneously (Figure 247-3). Cysts found in the contralateral ovary, and endometrial hyperplasia that accompany a functional tumor occur most frequently with gonadal-stromal origin tumors.[9]

There are few differential diagnoses for prolonged vaginal bleeding. Vaginal bleeding secondary to infection, inflammation or neoplasia of the genitourinary tract, a vaginal foreign body, or a coagulopathy should be differentiated from prolonged proestrus or estrus. Excessive exogenous administration of estrogen may be encountered when a bitch is treated for urethral sphincter incompetence with diethylstilbestrol (DES), or from attempts to prevent unwanted pregnancy using DES or estradiol cypionate. Recognized sequela to chronic estrogen exposure include bone marrow dyscrasias, predisposition to the cystic endometrial gland hyperplasia/pyometra complex, and the development of ovarian cysts.[7-9]

After confirmation of naturally occurring hyperestrogenism is obtained through vaginal cytologies (they can be

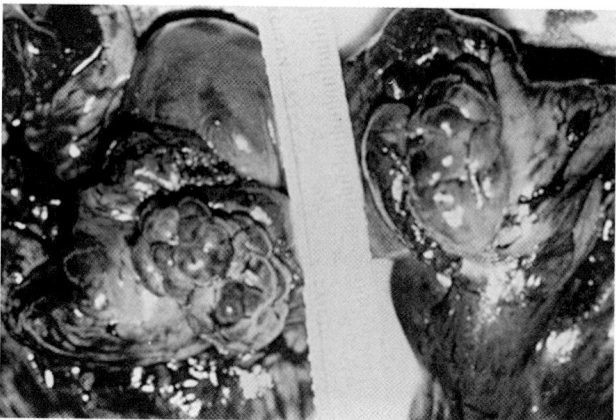

Figure 247-3 Ovarian carcinoma, right ovary (ruler), accompanied by ovarian follicular cysts, left ovary, in a Boxer bitch that has been experiencing estrus for greater than 2 months.

confirmed with serum estrogen level measurement), abdominal ultrasonography is recommended in the attempt to identify an ovarian follicular cyst or functional neoplasia (Figure 247-4). Normal preovulatory follicles measure 4 to 9 mm in diameter, smaller than follicular cysts and most functional neoplasia.[10] Analysis of the estrogen and progesterone levels in fluid from abnormal cystic ovarian structures obtained via ultrasound guidance and histologic analysis of tissues obtained surgically can confirm the diagnosis.

Because follicular cysts may spontaneously undergo atresia or luteinization, not all bitches experiencing prolonged proestrus or estrus require treatment. Progression of the follicular cyst to an atretic follicle or a corpora lutea can be monitored ultrasonographically, via vaginal cytologies, and by serum estrogen and progesterone levels. Therapy aimed at terminating prolonged proestrus or estrus becomes necessary if spontaneous regression fails to occur, vaginal bleeding is a continuing nuisance, estrus behavior and the attraction of males is unacceptable, or other complications develop (blood loss anemia, marrow dyscrasias, vaginal hyperplasia) (Figure 247-5). Medical and surgical options exist for treatment of persistent pathologic follicular cysts. Medical therapies should not place the reproductive health of the bitch at risk. Progesterone treatment of bitches with functional follicular cysts puts the bitch at increased risk for the development of cystic endometrial hyperplasia/pyometra, and is not advised. The use of GnRH (50 to 100 ug/bitch IM q24-48h for up to 3 doses) or human placental gonadotropin (H.C.G.; 11 IU/lb; 22 IU/kg, IM, q24-48h) has been advocated as affective in inducing cyst regression or luteinization, although reported success rates for either vary.[3,7] GnRH does not appear to be antigenic in the bitch and may be the preferred treatment. Successful induction of cyst regression or luteinization is reflected by a reduction in vaginal discharge, change in vaginal cytology reflecting reduced estrogen effect, diminished attractiveness to males, and normalization of behavior. Serum estrogen concentrations fall, and increased progesterone concentrations occur if luteinization results. Ultrasonographic monitoring of ovarian morphology shows regression of hypoechoic structures.

It has been suggested that failure of medical therapies to resolve prolonged proestrus or estrus indicates that ovarian neoplasia is more likely than a follicular cyst; this has not been our experience.[3,6] Medical treatment of prolonged proestrus or estrus is usually unrewarding and surgical removal of the cyst the most expedient means of managing the problem.[3] Removal of the cyst alone is optimal, but resection of the

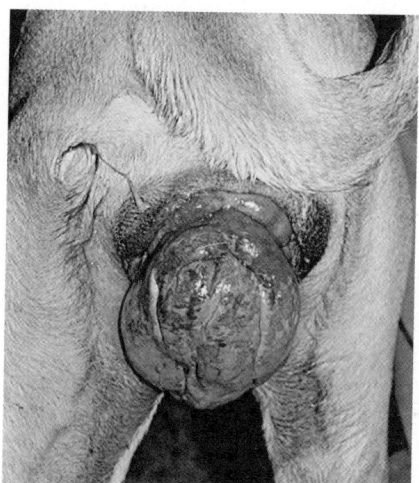

Figure 247-5 Vaginal hyperplasia, present for greater than 3 months in a Mastiff bitch that is experiencing prolonged proestrus/estrus secondary to follicular ovarian cysts.

associated ovary is usually necessary. Histologic evaluation of the removed tissue confirms the diagnosis and, importantly, permits evaluation for evidence of neoplasia that may warrant additional therapy and a much more negative prognosis (Figure 247-6).[11]

Prolonged Interestrous Intervals

Bitches exhibiting prolonged interestrous intervals may have prolongation of either anestrus or diestrus. Prolonged anestrus occurs when no ovarian activity occurs for longer than 16 to 20 months in a bitch having previously experienced estrous cycles (secondary anestrus). An actual failure to continue to cycle must be differentiated from silent heats. Underlying disease and iatrogenic causes for failure to cycle should be ruled out by a careful history, physical examination and database. The mechanism by which anestrus is normally terminated in the bitch is not well understood. Dopamine inhibits prolactin secretion. Prolactin levels decrease from late diestrus to late anestrus. Both FSH and LH have been reported as the hormone initiating proestrus folliculogenesis. Dopamine agonists (cabergoline, bromocriptine) can be used to shorten anestrus in both the normal bitch, and in bitches with secondary anestrus of unknown etiology. The mechanism by which dopamine agonists induce proestrus may be a direct reduction in prolactin levels or a direct dopaminergic action on either the gonadotrophic axis or on ovarian gonadotrophin receptors.[12]

A bitch examined for evaluation of prolonged intervals between heat cycles may be under the influence of increased plasma progesterone concentrations (>2 to 5 ng/mL). When plasma progesterone concentrations remain elevated for longer than 9 to 10 weeks, prolonged diestrus is probable. The clinical behavior of the bitch cannot be differentiated from

one with prolonged anestrus. The value of vaginal cytologies, serial plasma progesterone levels, and the ultrasonographic appearance of the ovaries and uterus becomes important in establishing a diagnosis.

Prolonged diestrus may occur secondary to the presence of a luteinized (progesterone-secreting) ovarian cyst. The progesterone causes negative feedback to the pituitary/hypothalamic axis, preventing the stimulation of normal ovarian activity. Luteinized cysts can be single or multiple, involving one or both ovaries.[3] Abdominal ultrasonography can identify hypoechoic structure(s) within the affected ovary(ies) (Figure 247-7). Abdominal radiography rarely provides diagnostic information because the cysts are relatively small. Serum progesterone levels greater than 2 to 5 ng/mL confirm the diagnosis. Treatment with prostaglandin F2alpha (PGF2α) usually causes only a transient decline in serum progesterone levels, indicating partial luteolysis. Surgical removal of the cyst(s) with histologic analysis is the recommended treatment. Separation of the cyst from the affected ovary is optimal but is technically difficult, necessitating ovariectomy.[3] Acquiring a uterine biopsy to evaluate the presence and extent of accompanying cystic endometrial hyperplasia is advisable, as it can provide valuable information to the owner concerning future fertility of the bitch (see Figure 247-7). Cystic endometrial hyperplasia, if present, may resolve partially after elimination of the cyst.

Nonfunctional ovarian cysts may cause failure to cycle due to their mass effect. Rete ovarii cysts and subsurface epithelial structure cysts are examples of nonfunctional ovarian cysts. Increases in plasma estrogen or progesterone concentrations will not be identified, although these cysts have the potential to produce a wide variety of other steroidal compounds without systemic effect.[3] The diagnosis, initially suspected using abdominal ultrasonography, is confirmed by histologic evaluation of surgically removed tissues.

Premature ovarian failure can result in permanent anestrus. Although the functional longevity of the ovaries of bitches is not known, on average the decline in function would not be expected before 7 to 10 years of age. Prolonged anestrus due to premature ovarian failure could be supported by documentation of markedly increased plasma FSH and LH concentrations as would be seen following ovariohysterectomy. Such increases indicate a lack of negative feedback to the pituitary and hypothalamus, without any other identifiable cause for anestrus.[13] Immune mediated oophoritis, diagnosed by ovarian histopathology, could result in prolonged anestrus. A mononuclear infiltrate predominated by lymphocytes,

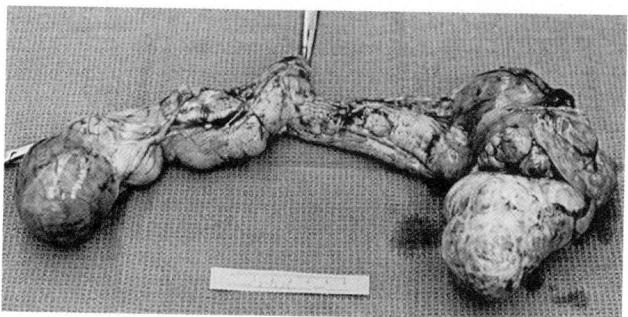

Figure 247-6 Bilateral ovarian neoplasia.

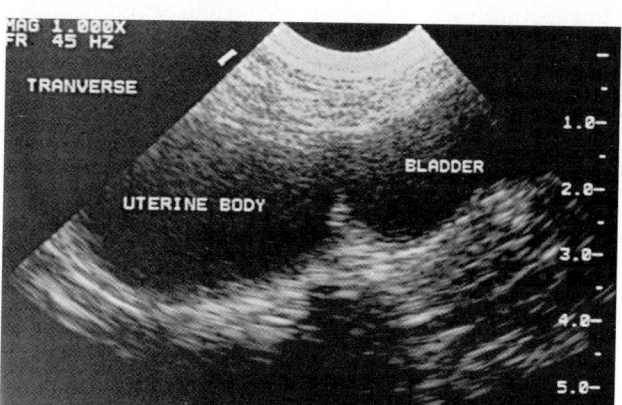

Figure 247-7 Ultrasonographic appearance of cystic endometrial hyperplasia and hydrometra in a Doberman bitch that is experiencing prolonged interestrous intervals, with elevated plasma progesterone concentrations for greater than 4 months, due to a luteinized ovarian cyst.

plasma cells and macrophages has been reported to occur in both ovaries in a bitch experiencing estrous cycle abnormalities.[13] This is an extremely rare disorder.

Hypothyroidism is a potential cause for failure to cycle, but the diagnosis should be well supported by other clinical signs (lethargy, weight gain, bilaterally symmetric alopecia) and clinical pathologic data (hypercholesterolemia, nonregenerative anemia), as well as confirmation of subnormal serum thyroid (total T4 and free T4 by equilibrium dialysis) levels, ideally supported by elevated endogenous TSH levels. Bitches with circulating antithyroid antibodies may have artificially elevated total T4 levels due to cross reactivity. Hypothyroid bitches placed on adequate replacement therapy should begin to cycle within 6 months of becoming euthyroid.[3,14-16] The presence of immune mediated thyroiditis is thought to have a genetic basis in some breeds and may occur with other immune mediated endocrinopathies. The breeding soundness of such bitches should be addressed with clients. Glucocorticoids can feedback on pituitary gonadotrophins FSH and LH, causing a failure to cycle.[16-17] Therefore administration of any steroid medication must be discontinued in a bitch with prolonged anestrus.

Shortened Interestrous Intervals

Bitches with short (less than 4.5 months) interestrous intervals can fail to conceive due to incomplete uterine involution and repair, precluding implantation.[3] Classically, bitches with shortened interestrous intervals are normal in other respects. Ovulation and luteinization occur, the secondary oocyte is fertilized but fails to implant successfully. Documentation of this disorder requires evaluation of serial vaginal cytologies during estrus and diestrus, and plasma progesterone concentrations during the luteal phase of at least two consecutive cycles. Currently, there is no reliable, commercially available, consistent pre-implantation method of confirming fertilization in the dog. The occurrence of folliculogenesis without ovulation (split heat) and hypoluteoidism (premature luteal failure) should be ruled out. Shortened interestrous intervals occur because anestrus is abbreviated. A defect in the hypothalamic-pituitary-ovarian axis may exist, which causes interference with the normal maintenance of anestrus; an imbalance of dopamine versus prolactin levels has been theorized to contribute to this syndrome. Anestrus can be abbreviated clinically in the normal bitch by the administration of prolactin inhibitors such as cabergoline and bromocriptine.

Intervention should not take place unless the bitch is older than 3 years, because these abnormalities may naturally resolve with maturity. One suggested therapy consists of inducing anestrus through the use of mibolerone, a potent synthetic androgen causing negative pituitary and hypothalamic feedback and ovarian inactivity, for 6 months. Mibolerone must be compounded as it has been taken off the market due to the potential for abuse. The compound is started 6 to 8 weeks after the previous estrus. Potential and predictable side effects include clitoral hypertrophy, mucoid vaginal discharge, atrophy of the glandular endothelium, epiphora, and virilized behavior. The bitch should be bred on the first cycle after discontinuation of the drug, which can occur immediately, or be delayed from 6 to 9 months.[3] Unfortunately, many bitches experience infertility during the first cycle after mibolerone administration, likely due to endometrial atrophy, and then begin to cycle frequently again.

No controlled studies exist that document the efficacy of this protocol, and it is not recommended by the authors. The availability of better, reversible birth control medications for the bitch, with fewer side effects, will improve the ability to treat this disorder. A genetic basis is suspected, and bitches experiencing shortened interestrous intervals likely are not good breeding candidates.

Hypoluteoidism

The maintenance of canine pregnancy requires plasma progesterone concentrations of greater than 1 to 2 ng/mL. Hypoluteoidism, primary luteal failure occurring before term gestation is a potential but not documented cause of abortion in dogs.[3,13,17] Induction of abortion follows reduction of plasma progesterone levels below 2 ng/mL.[3,18] The diagnosis of gestational loss caused by premature luteolysis is difficult and requires documentation of inadequate plasma progesterone concentrations prior to abortion for which no other cause is found. Measurement of precise progesterone concentrations, especially in the critical 1 to 3 ng/mL range, is not accurate using currently available rapid in-house ELISA kits.

Plasma progesterone concentrations diminish in response to fetal death, thus documentation of a low value after an abortion does not establish the diagnosis of hypoluteoidism as the cause for reproductive failure. Administration of progesterone to maintain pregnancy in bitches with primary fetal abnormalities, placentitis, or intrauterine infection can cause continued fetal growth with the possibility of dystocia and sepsis. Administration of progesterone to maintain pregnancy in a bitch not actually requiring therapy can delay parturition, which endangers the life of the bitch and her fetuses and may masculinize female fetuses.

Bitches with low plasma progesterone concentrations and historical late term loss of pregnancy with no apparent pathology should be evaluated for premature myometrial activity mid gestation, using uterine monitors. Elaboration of prostaglandins from the endometrium and placenta associated with premature myometrial activity can result in declining progesterone levels. Pharmacologic intervention to decrease myometrial activity may be indicated, using tocolytic agents such as terbutaline. Bitches experiencing premature myometrial activity in one pregnancy may or may not exhibit it during subsequent pregnancies. Exogenous progesterone supplementation for bitches with premature labor (not necessary in the authors' experience with appropriate tocolytic therapy) can interfere with normal parturition, and oral progesterone supplementation can be complicated by causing poor lactation (interference with prolactin production), dystocia, and fetal death.[19,20]

Exaggerated Pseudocyesis (Pseudopregnancy)

Nonpregnant bitches showing overt signs of term pregnancy are frequently brought to veterinarians because of concerns about parturition. Symptoms exhibited during overt pseudocyesis include weight gain, mammary gland hyperplasia and lactation, mucoid vaginal discharge, inappetence, restlessness, nesting, and mothering of inanimate objects. Abdominal palpation and ultrasonography can establish the presence or absence of fetuses. Alternatively, owners may be concerned about bitches showing overt signs of pseudocyesis because they find the behavior or physical symptoms objectionable in a bitch they know is not pregnant.

Pseudocyesis is an exaggeration of the normal physiologic phenomena experienced by any nonpregnant bitch completing the luteal portion of an estrous cycle. These signs are the result of progesterone concentrations declining and prolactin increasing. The clinical expression of pseudocyesis varies from indiscernible to (rarely) potentially serious. Clinical signs of pseudocyesis usually are reported from 6 to 12 weeks after estrus. Signs of pseudocyesis are often reported by owners when giving reproductive histories as if its occurrence indicates a reproductive disorder, when in fact, pseudocyesis probably establishes that the bitch has a normal hypothalamic-pituitary-ovarian axis and estrous cycle.

Bitches that exhibit signs consistent with a diagnosis of pseudocyesis are probably under the influence of prolactin. Similar concentrations can be demonstrated in bitches that have no clinical signs, suggesting that the former may have

Table • 247-1

Drug Appendix

GENERIC	TRADE	DOSAGE	ROUTE	FREQUENCY	DESCRIPTION
GnRH	Cystorelan	50-100 ug	IM	q 24-48h × 3	Hypothalamic releasing hormone
h.c.g.	Gonamone	11 IU/lb (22 IU/kg)	IM	q 24-48h	Placental gonadotropin
PGF2α	Lutalyse	0.05-0.10 mg/lb (0.10-0.20 mg/kg)	SC	q 8h	Natural prostaglandin
Mibolerone	Pseudocyesis:	0.008 mg/lb (0.016 ug/kg)	PO	q 24h × 5	Synthetic androgen
Bromocriptine		0.005-0.05 mg/lb (0.01-0.10 mg/kg)		q 24h	Ergot alkaloid divided
Carbergoline		2.5 ug/lb (5.0 ug/kg)		q 24h or divided bid × 3-5	Ergot alkaloid

increased target organ concentrations or heightened peripheral sensitivity to the hormone.[3] The condition is self limiting, usually regressing in 1 to 3 weeks, and therapy is not recommended unless the signs are unusually prolonged or pronounced, such as causing mastitis. Unusually persistent cases of inappropriate lactation should be evaluated for hypothyroidism, in which excess TRH may, in turn, cause increases in prolactin.

Therapy, when recommended, is usually directed at decreasing or eliminating lactation. Therapy is pursued to reduce the likelihood of mastitis occurring secondary to milk stasis, or to diminish lactation-induced household soiling. Minimal measures are recommended. Mammary stimulation, via licking, mothering behavior, or warm or cold compressing should be discontinued. Dopamine antagonists, of which phenothiazines are a class, enhance prolactin secretion and should not be administered. Mild sedation with a non-phenothiazine tranquilizer may be helpful.[3]

A variety of hormonal and medical therapies have been employed to reduce or stop lactation in pseudopregnant dogs. Side effects, in most cases, outweigh the benefit of these medications. Therapy with gonadal hormones, progesterone, estrogen, or testosterone is not recommended due to complications of repetitive cycles of pseudocyesis, symptoms of proestrus or estrus, and virilization behavior, respectively. The compounded synthetic androgen mibolerone, administered at 0.008 mg/lb (0.016 mg/kg) orally once daily for 5 days, has successfully abbreviated the signs of pseudocyesis in approximately 50% of treated cases, although this medication also may cause virilization.[21] Ergot alkaloids are potent prolactin inhibitors (dopaminergic) and can be used to abbreviate exaggerated pseudocyesis. Bromocriptine can be administered at 0.005 to 0.05 mg/lb/day (0.01 to 0.10 mg/kg/day) in divided doses until lactation ceases. Vomiting, depression and anorexia are commonly reported side effects, usually more problematic than the lactation. Carbergoline, administered at 2.5 ug/lb/day (5.0 ug/kg/day), given divided or once daily for 3 to 5 days effectively decreases prolactin concentrations and diminishes signs of pseudocyesis with fewer side effects, but is expensive and must be compounded for use in all but giant breeds. Permanent avoidance of clinical pseudocyesis requires ovariohysterectomy.

CHAPTER • 248

Abnormalities in Pregnancy, Parturition, and the Periparturient Period

Catharina Linde-Forsberg

PREGNANCY

Physiologic Changes and Clinical Monitoring

Maternal physiologic alterations during pregnancy are due to increased metabolic demands. Blood volume increases by 40%, which provides an adequate reserve to compensate for the large quantities of blood and fluids lost at parturition.

The volume increase is primarily plasma with a resulting hemodilution (the hematocrit is around 30% at term). An increase in cardiac output occurs, caused by enhanced heart rate and stroke volume. The functional residual capacity of the lungs is decreased by anterior displacement of the diaphragm by the gravid uterus, and oxygen consumption during pregnancy increases by 20%. Pregnant animals also have delayed gastric emptying due to decreased gastric motility and displacement of the stomach.

It is recommended to examine bitches and to obtain radiographs at about 45 days of gestation. This allows the veterinarian to assess the health of the bitch, confirm pregnancy, count fetuses, and answer questions. Ultrasound is less exact for determining the number of fetuses but is excellent for assessing fetal viability and can be performed with accuracy from the twenty-fourth day.

Gestation Length   Apparent gestation length in the bitch averages 63 days, with a variation from 56 to 72 days if calculated from the first mating.[1] This surprisingly large apparent variation is mainly due to the long and variable behavioral estrus period of the bitch. Gestation length is quite predictable when instead calculated either from the preovulatory surge of luteinizing hormone (LH) being 65 ± 1 days, from the day of ovulation being 63 ± 1 days, or from the time of fertilization being 60 ± 1 days.[2,3] There exists conflicting data in the literature regarding whether a correlation exists between breed or body weight, and/or litter size and length of gestation.

Prediction of Parturition Day   The ability to determine gestational age and to predict the day of parturition in the bitch is of considerable clinical importance, especially in case of threatening abortion, prolonged gestation, or when the bitch is scheduled for elective caesarean section or suffers from dystocia. B-mode ultrasonography has been used to assess the diameter of pregnancy structures and to estimate fetal size during pregnancy. Inner chorionic cavity diameter on the eighteenth to the thirty-seventh day from ovulation and fetal head diameter on the thirty-eighth day to parturition show the best correlation to gestational age and day of parturition.[4] Other fetal structures used to time pregnancies using ultrasonography are fetal limb buds, first detectable at the thirty-third to the thirty-fifth day; eyes, kidney, and liver at the thirty-ninth to the forty-seventh day; and intestine at the fifty-seventh to the sixty-third day.[1] Using radiography the fetal skeleton is rarely visible before the forty-second day; the skull on the forty-fifth to the forty-ninth day; pelvic bones on the fifty-third to the fifty-seventh day; teeth on the fifty-eighth to the sixty-third day.[1] Serum cortisol levels increase at the time of delivery and remain high for 12 hours to reach basal levels again after 36 hours.[5] Levels of 15-ketodihydro-prostaglandin $F_{2\alpha}$ ($PGF_{2\alpha}$) increase 24 hours before parturition and again at the onset of whelping.[5] In most bitches, parturition occurs 65 ± 1 days from the LH-peak, which coincides with the initial sharp rise in serum progesterone concentrations to greater than or equal to 4.5 nmol/L (≥ 1.5 ng/mL). The accuracy of parturition day prediction within an interval of ± 1, ± 2, and ± 3 days using prebreeding serum progesterone concentrations was 67%, 90%, and 100%, respectively, and was not influenced by body weight or litter size.[6] The fact that serum progesterone levels decrease significantly from 12 to 15 nmol/L (4 to 5 ng/mL) to below 6 nmol/L (2 ng/mL) starting 24 hours before the onset of whelping can also be used to predict parturition in the late gestational stage.

DISORDERS DURING PREGNANCY

Early Fetal Loss and Abortion

The incidence of early embryonic and fetal death (before 45 days of pregnancy) and spontaneous abortion in the bitch is not known and is difficult to determine because resorption of conceptuses may occur until the forty-fifth day of pregnancy without noticeable signs, or the bitch may consume aborted fetuses. However, early pregnancy diagnosis using ultrasonography, which is becoming increasingly popular, indicates that fetal resorption is a frequent occurrence in the bitch.

Infectious Agents

Hemorrhage from the genital tract often precedes abortion caused by a bacterial infection. This may be due to an effect of bacterial toxins on the placenta and a release of $PGF_{2\alpha}$ causing the uterus to contract and expel its contents. The underlying cause of the hemorrhage should be diagnosed. Antibiotics, anti-inflammatory or tocolytic drugs (e.g., terbutaline), or both should be administered in an attempt to prevent the abortion. It should be explained to the owner that the bitch can abort some fetuses but may carry the remainder of the litter to term; therefore the bitch should be examined for the presence of any remaining fetuses after cessation of treatment.

Brucella Canis   Abortion caused by *B. canis* usually occurs between 45 and 55 days of gestation and is accompanied by a highly contagious brown to greenish-gray vaginal discharge that lasts for 1 to 6 weeks. Infected bitches may not exhibit other clinical signs. *B. canis* may also cause conception failure, fetal death, and absorption in early stages of gestation or the birth of weak, infected puppies. The infection is chronic and mostly asymptomatic in adult animals. Infected animals have intermittent bacteremia and shed bacteria through body fluids. Diagnosis is most commonly based on serologic testing, bearing in mind that it can take several months after infection before antibody titers rise and that antibiotic treatment may create false-negative test results. Additionally, surface antigens of *B. canis* cross-react strongly with antibodies to several other nonpathogenic bacterial species. Blood cultures are therefore strongly recommended before declaring an animal infected.

Toxoplasma Gondii and Neospora Caninum   *T. gondii* and *N. caninum* are both tissue cyst-forming protozoan microorganisms that are vertically transmitted to puppies if a bitch is infected during pregnancy. Infected bitches usually remain clinically normal, but the puppies are severely affected. Toxoplasmosis is known to cause fetal death and is a rare cause of abortion in dogs. Premature birth, stillbirth, and the birth of weak puppies have also been reported due to toxoplasmosis. Neosporosis causes fatal encephalomyelitis and polymyositis in neonatal puppies infected in utero and has experimentally been shown to cause fetal death and resorption.[7]

Canine Herpesvirus   The canine herpesvirus is species specific. In experimental studies it has been demonstrated that the effect of an infection is dependent on stage of pregnancy when infection occurs. Infection in early stages causes fetal death and mummification; in midpregnancy it may result in abortion and in later stages premature birth. More common in naturally occurring cases is that the puppies are born apparently healthy but become ill during the first 1 or 2 weeks and succumb within days. Often the whole litter is affected; however, some of the puppies may survive but develop defective vision, deafness, neuromuscular disorders, or kidney malfunction at 7 or 8 months of age. Normally immunity is incurred, and bitches that have lost a litter due to herpesvirus infection subsequently give birth to normal litters. Canine herpesvirus is presumed to be enzootic in dogs all over the world and the seroprevalence is as high as 46% in some European countries, the incidence not being higher in breeding kennels than among nonbreeding dogs.[8] Herpesvirus has been isolated from 67% of infertile and aborting bitches in those countries, but it is not clear whether it is the virus itself or a combination of several agents that cause the disturbances.

Hypoluteodism Inadequate progesterone production by the corpora lutea is a potential cause of fetal death and abortion in some species but has not unequivocally been proven to exist in the dog. A blood sample for progesterone taken at the time of an abortion often will show low concentration due to the luteolytic effects of the prostaglandin release during fetal expulsion; but, if repeated 1 week later, normal for stage levels of progesterone may be found. Any attempts at treating cases of imminent abortion with progestogens should only be done using a short-acting compound, because the bitch cannot deliver a litter when under the influence of high concentrations of progesterone.[1]

Insulin Resistance

The physiologic increased progesterone concentrations typical of diestrus or pregnancy stimulate growth hormone secretion, which in some individuals may cause down-regulation of insulin receptors and inhibition of postreceptor pathways. The condition is typically seen in middle-aged and older bitches that are pregnant or have recently been in estrus. The resulting type II diabetes is usually transient. Once blood progesterone concentration returns to anestrus levels and thus the stimulus for growth hormone secretion declines insulin resistance resolves.

Insulin resistance should be suspected in a bitch with supranormal blood insulin concentrations in the presence of a normal or increased blood glucose concentration.[9] Treatment should be initiated to prevent permanent damage to the pancreas. A poor prognosis exists for the fetuses, which sometimes become undernourished but sometimes instead grow excessively large (due to the excess in glucose), with a poor survival rate. In the bitch, acromegaly may develop as a result of excessive secretion of growth hormone by the progesterone-stimulated mammary gland. Edema, especially of the head, throat, and legs is seen in combination with excessive skin and wrinkling and an increase in interdental spaces. In advanced cases there may be a change of voice, getting coarse from the edema of the throat. The condition may become life threatening for the bitch, and it is often necessary to interrupt a pregnancy.

Hypoglycemia

Preparturient hypoglycemia in the bitch is rare. Some hypoglycemic dogs may be incorrectly diagnosed as hypocalcemic because this is a more common condition and because they respond to treatment with calcium borogluconate. Affected bitches have been reported to be in late gestation and have a short history of muscle weakness, convulsions, or collapse. Blood testing demonstrates the hypoglycemia.[10-12] The condition improves dramatically after treatment with intravenous glucose solutions and resolves after parturition.

Premature Labor

Premature labor may have infectious causes, but can also occur in the clinically healthy bitch. Hypoluteoidism as a cause for premature uterine contractions has not been clearly demonstrated in the bitch. Short-acting progestational compounds may, however, be given in an attempt to maintain pregnancy. To adequately inhibit premature uterine contractions, tocolytic compounds such as terbutaline, a beta-adrenergic receptor antagonist, should also be administered orally or subcutaneously to effect and should be discontinued 48 hours before the anticipated day of delivery.

NORMAL PARTURITION

Litter Size

Litter size in dogs ranges from just one puppy in some of the miniature breeds to 15 or more in some of the giant breeds.

Litter size is smaller in the young bitch and increases up to 3 to 4 years of age, decreasing again as the bitch gets older. A litter size of only one or two puppies predisposes to dystocia and thus fetal death, because of insufficient uterine stimulation and large puppy size (i.e., *single-puppy syndrome*).[13] This can be seen in dog breeds of all sizes. Breeders of the miniature breeds tend to accept small litters but should be encouraged to breed for litter sizes of at least three to four puppies to avoid this complication.

Physiology of Parturition

An understanding of the course and control of normal parturition (eutocia) is necessary for the diagnosis and treatment of abnormal parturition (dystocia). Studies of canine parturition and extrapolations from other species provide information on the physiologic and endocrinologic changes important for normal parturition. Stress produced by the reduction of the nutritional supply by the placenta to the fetus stimulates the fetal hypothalamic-pituitary-adrenal axis, resulting in release of adrenocorticosteroid hormone, and it is thought to be the trigger for parturition. An increase in fetal and maternal cortisol is believed to stimulate the release of $PGF_{2\alpha}$, which is luteolytic (from the fetoplacental tissue), resulting in a decline in plasma progesterone concentration. Withdrawal of the progesterone blockade of pregnancy is a prerequisite for the normal course of canine parturition; bitches given long-acting progesterone during pregnancy fail to deliver.[1] Concurrent with the gradual decrease in plasma progesterone concentration during the last 7 days before whelping, a progressive qualitative change occurs in uterine electrical activity. In addition, a significant increase in uterine activity takes place during the last 24 hours before parturition with the final fall in plasma progesterone concentration to below 6 nmol/L (2 ng/mL).[1,14] The change in the estrogen-to-progesterone ratio is probably a major cause of placental separation and cervical dilation, although in the dog, estrogens have not been unambiguously shown to increase before parturition as they do in many other species. Estrogens sensitize the myometrium to oxytocin, which in turn initiates strong contractions in the uterus when it is not under the influence of progesterone. Sensory receptors within the cervix and vagina are stimulated by the distention created by the fetus and the fluid-filled fetal membranes. This afferent stimulation is conveyed to the hypothalamus and results in release of oxytocin during second-stage labor. Afferents also participate in a spinal reflex arch with efferent stimulation of the abdominal musculature to produce abdominal straining. Relaxin causes the pelvic soft tissues and genital tract to relax, which facilitates fetal passage. In the pregnant bitch, this hormone is produced by both ovary and placenta, increasing gradually over the last two thirds of pregnancy.[15] Prolactin, the hormone responsible for lactation, starts to rise 3 to 4 weeks after ovulation and surges dramatically with the abrupt decline in serum progesterone just before parturition.[1,5]

Signs of Impending Parturition

Relaxation of the pelvic and abdominal musculature is a consistent but subtle indicator of impending parturition. The most consistent change is the drop in rectal temperature caused by the final abrupt decrease in progesterone concentration. The last week before parturition the rectal temperature of the bitch fluctuates to drop sharply 8 to 24 hours before parturition and 10 to 14 hours after the concentration of progesterone in peripheral plasma has declined to less than 6 nmol/L (2 ng/mL).[1,13] To properly assess the prepartum drop in body temperature, measurements should be made every 1 to 2 hours while the temperature decreases and less frequently when the temperature is seen to increase again. The drop in rectal temperature is individual but also may

REPRODUCTIVE SYSTEM

depend on body size. Thus in miniature breed bitches, it can fall to 35° C (95° F), in medium-sized bitches to around 36° C, whereas it seldom falls below 37° C (96.8° F) in bitches of the giant breeds. This difference is probably an effect of the surface area-to-body volume ratio. Several days before parturition the bitch may become restless, seek seclusion, or become excessively attentive, and she may refuse all food. She may exhibit nesting behavior 12 to 24 hours before parturition, concomitant with increasing frequency and force of uterine contractions. Shivering may be an attempt to increase body temperature. In primiparous bitches, lactation may be established less than 24 hours before parturition, whereas after several pregnancies colostrum can be detected as early as 1 week prepartum.

Stages of Parturition

Parturition is divided into three stages, with the last two stages being repeated for each puppy delivered.

First Stage   The duration of the first stage is usually 6 to 12 hours. It may last 36 hours, especially in a nervous primiparous animal; however, for this to be considered normal, the rectal temperature must remain low. Vaginal relaxation and dilation of the cervix occur during this stage. Intermittent uterine contractions, with no signs of abdominal straining, are present. The bitch may appear uncomfortable, and the restless behavior may become more intense. Panting, tearing up and rearranging of bedding, shivering, and occasional vomiting may be seen. Some bitches show no behavioral evidence of first-stage labor. The inapparent uterine contractions increase both in frequency and intensity toward the end of the first stage. During pregnancy the orientation of the fetuses within the uterus is 50% heading caudally and 50% cranially, but this changes during first-stage labor when the fetus rotates on its long axis, extending its head, neck, and limbs, resulting in 60% to 70% of puppies being born in anterior and 30% to 40% in posterior presentation.[16,17] The fluid-filled fetal membranes are pushed ahead of the fetus by the uterine-propulsive efforts and dilate the cervix.

Second Stage   The duration of the second stage is usually 3 to 12 hours (in rare cases 24 hours). At the onset of second-stage labor the rectal temperature rises to normal or slightly above normal. The first fetus engages in the pelvic inlet, and the subsequent intense, expulsive uterine contractions are accompanied by abdominal straining. On entering the birth canal, the allantochorionic membrane may rupture and a discharge of some clear fluid may be noted. Covered by the amniotic membrane, the first fetus is usually delivered within 4 hours after onset of second-stage labor. Normally the bitch will break the membrane, lick the neonate intensively, and sever the umbilical cord. At times the bitch will need some assistance to open the fetal membranes to allow the newborn to breathe, and sometimes the airways will have to be emptied of fetal fluids. The umbilicus can be clamped with a pair of hemostats and cut with a blunt scissors to minimize hemorrhage from the fetal vessels, leaving about 1 cm of the umbilicus. In case of continuing hemorrhage the umbilicus should be ligated.

Diagnosing second-stage labor   It is crucial that the veterinarian is able to determine whether the bitch is in the second stage or still in first stage of labor. Inexperienced breeders tend to get nervous during a bitch's first-stage labor, not fully understanding the function of this preparatory stage of parturition during which uterine contractions, the softening of the birth canal, and the opening of the cervix take place.

Three signs indicate that the bitch has entered into second-stage labor:
1. The passing of fetal fluids (first water bag [allantois], bursts)
2. Visible abdominal straining
3. The rectal temperature returning to normal level

If one or more of these signs have been observed, the bitch is in second-stage labor.

In normal labor the bitch may show weak and infrequent straining for up to 2, and at the most 4, hours before giving birth to the first fetus. If the bitch is showing strong, frequent straining without producing a pup, this indicates the presence of some obstruction, and she should not be left for more than 20 to 30 minutes before seeking veterinary advice.

The bitch should be examined for the following reasons:
- If she has greenish discharge but no pup is born within 2 to 4 hours
- If fetal fluid was passed more than 2 to 3 hours previously, but nothing more has happened
- If she has had weak, irregular straining for more than 2 to 4 hours
- If she has had strong, regular straining for more than 20 to 30 minutes
- If more than 2 to 4 hours have passed since the birth of the last puppy and more remain
- If she has been in second-stage labor for more than 12 hours

Third Stage   The third stage of parturition, expulsion of the placenta and shortening of the uterine horns, usually follows within 15 minutes of the delivery of each fetus. Two or three fetuses may, however, be born before the passage of their placentas occurs. The bitch should be discouraged from eating more than one or two of the placentas because she may develop diarrhea and vomiting, with risk of aspiration pneumonia. Lochia (i.e., the greenish postpartum discharge of fetal fluids and placental remains) will be seen for up to 3 weeks or more but is most profuse during the first week. Uterine involution is normally completed after 12 to 15 weeks.

The bitch should be examined for the following reasons:
- If all placentas have not been passed within 4 to 6 hours (although placental numbers may be difficult to determine because of the bitch eating them)
- If lochia are putrid or foul smelling
- There is continuing continuing severe genital hemorrhage
- If the rectal temperature is higher than 39.5° C (101.3° F)
- If the general condition of the bitch is abnormal
- If the general condition of the puppies is abnormal

Interval Between Births

Expulsion of the first fetus usually takes the longest. The interval between births in normal uncomplicated parturition is from 5 to 120 minutes.[16,17] In almost 80% of cases the fetuses are delivered alternately from the two uterine horns.[16] When giving birth to a large litter a bitch may stop straining and rest for more than 2 hours between the delivery of two consecutive fetuses. The second-stage straining will then resume, followed again by the third stage, until all the fetuses are born.

Completion of Parturition

Parturition is usually completed within 6 hours after the onset of second-stage labor, but it may last up to 12 hours. It should never be allowed to last for more than 24 hours because of the risks involved both for the bitch and the fetuses.

DYSTOCIA

Definition

Dystocia is defined as difficult birth or the inability to expel the fetus through the birth canal without assistance.

Frequency

Dystocia is a frequent problem in the dog. The true average incidence of dystocia in the bitch is probably below 5%, but it may amount to almost 100% in some breeds of dogs, especially those of the achondroplastic type and those selected for large heads.[13,17,18]

Clinical Assessment

When a bitch with possible dystocia is examined, an accurate history and a thorough physical examination are important prerequisites for proper management. The three criteria for being in second-stage labor, namely, (1) passage of fetal fluids, (2) visible abdominal straining, and (3) temperature returned to normal, should be assessed. An evaluation of the bitch's general health status should be made and signs of any adverse effects of parturition noted. Observation should be made of the bitch's behavior and the character and frequency of straining, and the vulva and perineum should be examined, noting color and amount of vaginal discharge. Mammary gland development including congestion, distention, size, and presence of milk should be evaluated. Palpation of the abdomen, roughly

estimating the number of fetuses and degree of distention of the uterus, should be carried out. Digital examination of the vagina using aseptic technique should be undertaken to detect obstructions and determine the presence and presentation of any fetus in the pelvic canal (Figure 248-1). In most bitches it is not possible to reach the cervix during first stage, but an assessment of the degree of dilation and tone of the vagina may give some indication of the status of the cervix and the tone of the uterus. Pronounced tone of the anterior vagina may indicate satisfactory muscular activity in the uterus, whereas flaccidity may indicate uterine inertia.[19] The character of the vaginal fluids also will indicate whether the cervix is closed, with the production of scant fluid volume that is sticky creating a certain resistance to the introduction of a finger. The cervix is likely open when fetal fluids lubricate the vagina, making the exploration easy. When the cervix is closed the vaginal walls also fit quite tightly around the exploring finger, whereas with an open cervix the cranial vagina palpates more open.

Radiographic examination is valuable to assess gross abnormalities of the maternal pelvis and number and location of fetuses, to estimate fetal size, and to detect congenital defects

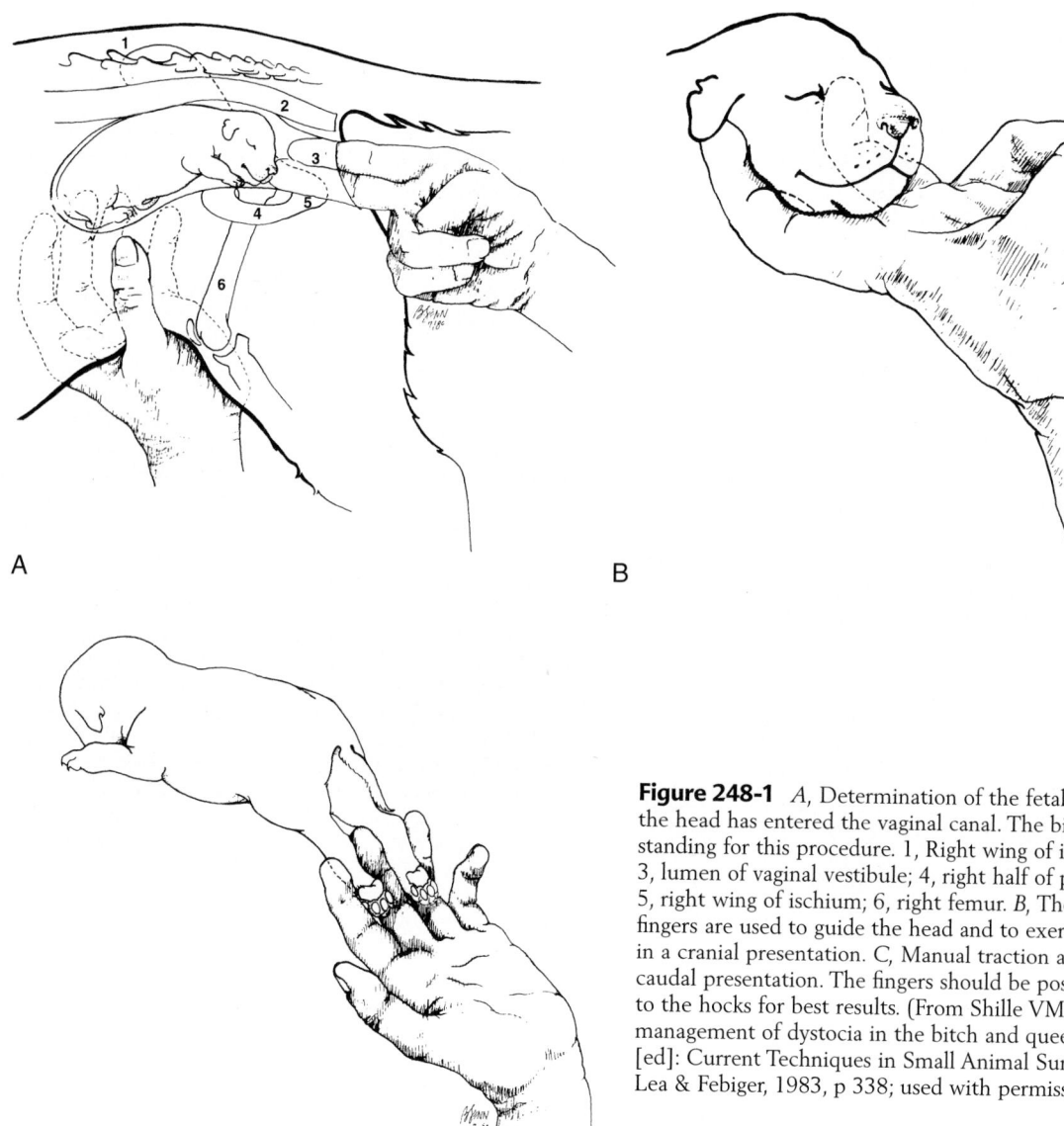

A

B

C

Figure 248-1 *A*, Determination of the fetal disposition when the head has entered the vaginal canal. The bitch should be standing for this procedure. 1, Right wing of ilium; 2, rectum; 3, lumen of vaginal vestibule; 4, right half of pubic symphysis; 5, right wing of ischium; 6, right femur. *B*, The index and middle fingers are used to guide the head and to exert moderate traction in a cranial presentation. *C*, Manual traction as applied in a caudal presentation. The fingers should be positioned proximal to the hocks for best results. (From Shille VM: Diagnosis and management of dystocia in the bitch and queen. *In*: Bojrab MJ [ed]: Current Techniques in Small Animal Surgery. Philadelphia, Lea & Febiger, 1983, p 338; used with permission.)

REPRODUCTIVE SYSTEM

or signs of fetal death. In the dead fetus, intrafetal gas will appear 6 hours after death and can be detected radiographically, whereas overlapping of cranial bones and collapse of the spinal column will not be seen until 48 hours have passed after the death of the fetus. Ultrasound examination will determine fetal viability or distress, with normal heart rate being 180 to 240 beats per minute (bpm), decreasing in the compromised fetus. Some bitches brought to veterinarians for dystocia have already delivered all fetuses or were only pseudopregnant. Pseudopregnancy is most commonly diagnosed as lactation without pregnancy, but it may include abdominal contractions, nesting behavior, and changes in personality that convince an owner that the pet is pregnant.

Diagnosis

The range of normal variations observed in dogs at parturition makes recognition of dystocia difficult, especially for the inexperienced observer. The following criteria for dystocia may assist in making the diagnosis:

- The rectal temperature has been down and returned to normal with no signs of labor.
- A green vulvar discharge is seen, but no fetuses have been delivered. (These discharges emanate from the marginal hematoma of the placentas and indicate that at least one placenta is beginning to become separated from the maternal blood supply. They are normal once birth is underway.)
- Fetal fluids were passed 2 to 3 hours earlier, but no signs of labor are noted.
- Labor is absent for more than 2 hours or is weak and infrequent for more than 2 to 4 hours.
- Strong and persistent nonproductive labor occurs for more than 20 to 30 minutes.
- An obvious cause of dystocia is evident (e.g., pelvic fracture or a fetus stuck in the birth canal and partially visible).
- Signs of toxemia (disturbed general condition, general edema, shock) are noted when parturition should be occurring.

Recently, systems for monitoring labor and delivery in the bitch have become commercially available (Veterinary Perinatal Services, Inc., Wheatridge, Colorado).[20] These systems are intended for use by veterinarians or by breeders at home with veterinary guidance. They consist of a uterine tocodynamometer and a fetal Doppler. Using this device the administration of calcium borogluconate and oxytocin can be monitored based on the individual uterine response of the bitch.

Maternal Causes of Dystocia

Traditionally, dystocia is classified as being of either maternal or fetal origin, or a combination of both (Table 248-1; Figures 248-2 and 248-3).

Uterine Inertia   Uterine inertia is by far the most common cause of dystocia in dogs. It is classified into *primary* and *secondary* inertia. In primary inertia the uterus may fail to respond to the fetal signals because only one or two puppies exist, which provide insufficient stimulation to initiate labor (the single-puppy syndrome), or because of overstretching of the myometrium by large litters, excessive fetal fluids, or oversized fetuses. Other causes of primary inertia may be an inherited predisposition, nutritional imbalance, fatty infiltration of the myometrium, age-related changes, deficiency in neuroendocrine regulation, or systemic disease in the bitch. Primary complete uterine inertia is the failure of the uterus to begin labor at full term. Primary partial uterine inertia occurs when enough uterine activity exists to initiate parturition, but it is insufficient to complete a normal birth of all fetuses in the

Table • 248-1

Causes of Dystocia in Bitches (182 Cases)

	FREQUENCY (%)
Maternal causes	75.3
Primary complete inertia	48.9
Primary partial inertia	23.1
Birth canal too narrow	1.1
Uterine torsion	1.1
Uterine prolapse	—
Uterine strangulation	—
Hydrallantois	0.5
Vaginal septum formation	0.5
Fetal causes	24.7
Malpresentations	15.4
Malformations	1.6
Fetal oversize	6.6
Fetal death	1.1

(From Darvelid AW, Linde-Forsberg C: Dystocia in the bitch: a retrospective study of 182 cases. J Small Anim Pract 35:402-407, 1994.)

absence of an obstruction. Secondary uterine inertia implies that some fetuses have been delivered and the remainder are in utero due to exhaustion of the uterine myometrium caused by obstruction of the birth canal; this condition should be distinguished from primary inertia.

Management   In cases of primary uterine inertia, the owners should initially be instructed to try to induce straining by actively exercising the bitch, for instance, by running the dog around the house or up some stairs. A considerable number of puppies are born in the car on the way to the veterinarian. Most of these would probably have been delivered in the calm and quiet of home had the owners tried to induce straining themselves, thereby giving the puppies a better start in life and possibly also resulting in the whole litter being born without further intervention. Another means of induction of straining in the bitch with insufficient labor is by feathering of the dorsal vaginal wall. Feathering is accomplished by inserting two fingers into the vagina and pushing or "walking" with them against the dorsal vaginal wall, thus inducing an episode of straining (the Ferguson reflex). Feathering can also be effective in initiating labor after correction of the position or posture of a fetus. Nervous voluntary inhibition of labor due to psychologic stress may occur, mainly in a nervous primiparous animal. Reassurance by the owner or administration of a low-dose tranquilizer may remove the inhibition.[21] Once the first fetus is born, parturition will usually proceed normally.

The bitch with complete primary uterine inertia is usually bright and alert, has a normal rectal temperature, and has no evidence of labor. The cervix is often dilated, and vaginal exploration is easy to perform owing to the presence of fetal fluids, but the fetus may be out of reach because of the flaccid uterus. Before initiation of medical treatment of uterine inertia, obstruction of the birth canal must be excluded.

Calcium solutions and oxytocin are the drugs of choice in cases of uterine inertia. Oxytocin has a direct action on the rate of calcium influx into the myometrial cell, essential for myometrial contraction. Many bitches do not respond to oxytocin alone but require prior administration of a calcium solution. Therefore some 10 minutes before the administration of oxytocin, 10% calcium borogluconate, 0.5 to 1.5 mL/kg body weight,

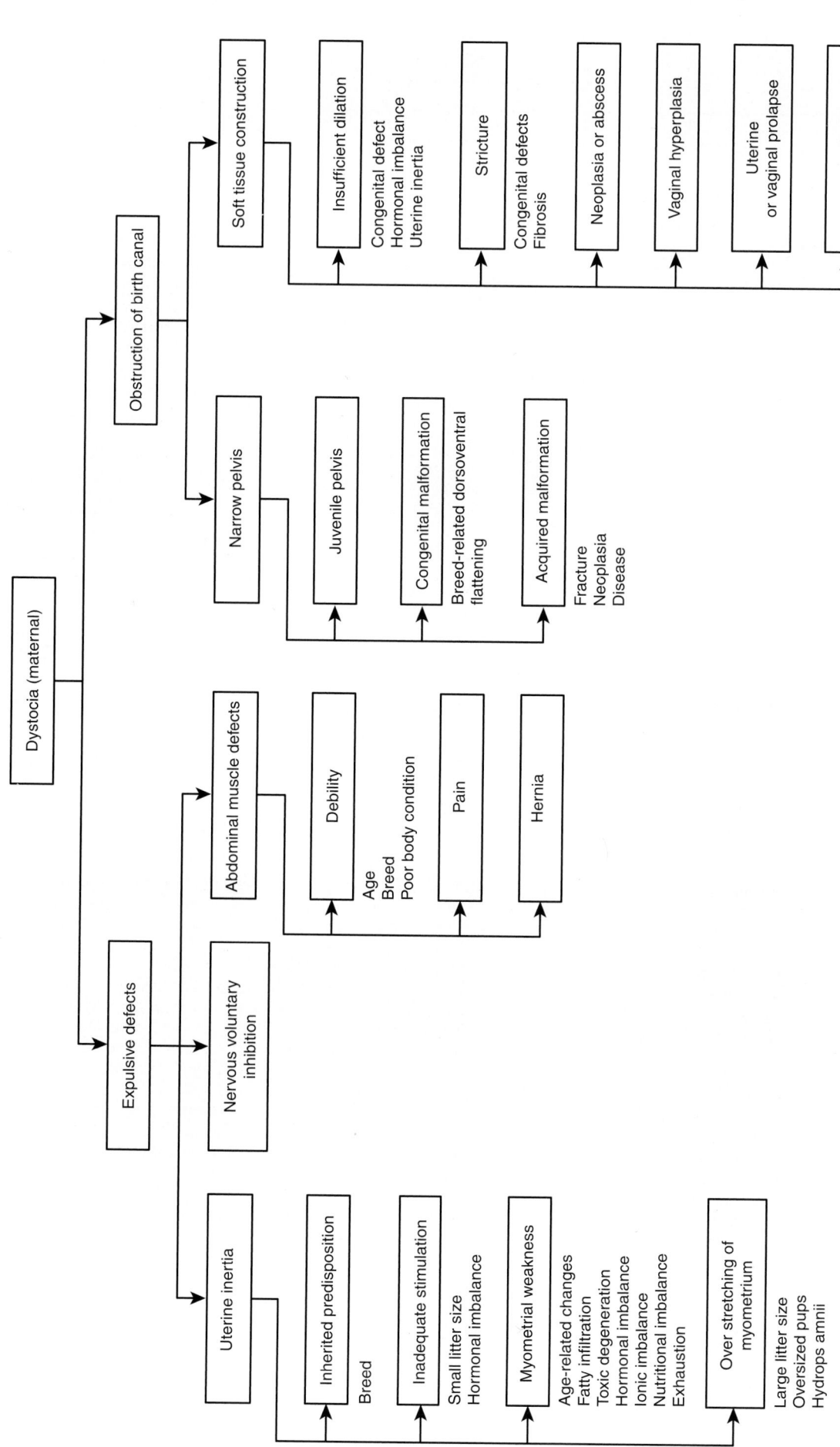

Figure 248-2 Algorithm defining the various maternal causes for dystocia.

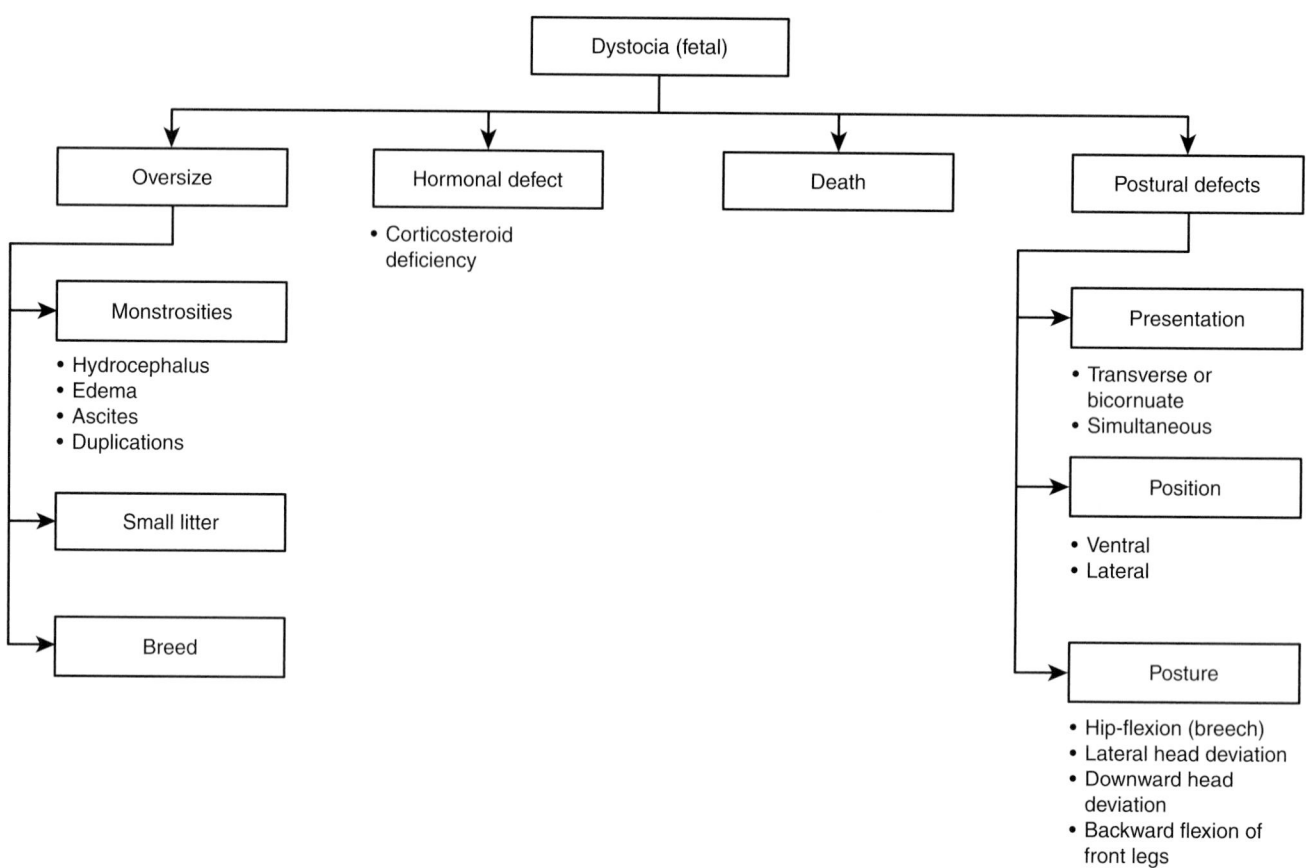

Figure 248-3 Algorithm defining the various fetal causes for dystocia.

should be given by slow intravenous infusion (1 mL/min) with careful monitoring of the heart rate. The calcium can also be administered subcutaneously, which eliminates the risk for arrhythmia but presents a small risk for granuloma formation at the injection site. Small breed bitches may be prone to hypoglycemia, particularly after prolonged straining. In such cases a dilute (10% to 20%) glucose solution can be added to the infusion or given intravenously in doses of 5 to 20 mL. The recommended dose of oxytocin for the bitch is 1 to 5 IU given intravenously or 2.5 to 10 IU intramuscularly, which can be repeated at 30-minute intervals. The response to treatment will be reduced with each repeated administration. Higher doses than recommended or too frequent administration may result in prolonged contracture of the myometrium, preventing fetal expulsion and impeding uteroplacental blood flow. The disadvantages of oxytocin administration include a tendency to cause premature induction of placental separation and cervical closure. If no response to treatment is seen after a second administration of oxytocin, the puppies should be delivered without further delay, either with the aid of obstetric forceps (if only one or two puppies remain and are within easy reach in the uterine corpus) or by cesarean section.

The long-acting ergotamines should never be used in connection with parturition. The treatment regimen includes the following:
• The owner runs with the bitch and feathers the vaginal vault.

• A 10% solution of calcium gluconate is given slowly intravenously while carefully checking the bitch's heart rate.
• The bitch is given 30 minutes to respond to treatment. If straining begins, the treatment can be repeated if necessary or continued with oxytocin.
• If the calcium infusion has no effect within 30 minutes, oxytocin is given intravenously or intramuscularly.
• The bitch again is given 30 minutes to respond to treatment. If straining begins, the treatment can be repeated if necessary, although each additional administration will elicit a weaker response.
• If nothing happens within 30 minutes, it is not likely that further treatment will be successful. The fetuses should be delivered, either by forceps, if only one or two fetuses remain and are within easy reach, or by cesarean section.

Obstruction of Birth Canal   Obstruction of the birth canal may be of maternal or fetal origin. Some maternal causes for obstruction include:
• Uterine torsion and uterine rupture. These are acute, life-threatening conditions that can occur during late pregnancy or at the time of parturition. Sometimes a few fetuses are born before parturition stops, and the condition of the bitch may quickly deteriorate. Surgery is always required, and a quick diagnosis essential for survival.
• Uterine inguinal herniation usually is detected around the fourth week of pregnancy as the fetal uterine enlargements

are growing and the contour of the abdomen is markedly abnormal. Sometimes the early stages may be mistaken for mastitis of the rear mammary glands. The condition is corrected by surgery, whereby the uterine horns are repositioned and the herniation sutured. In cases with circulatory disturbance and advanced tissue damage, the uterus will have to be removed.

- Congenital malformations of the uterus (e.g., partial or complete aplasia or hypoplasia of one or both uterine horns or of the corpus uteri) or the cervix are rare causes of maternal obstructive dystocia. Symptoms depend on the character and degree of the malformation. In cases of unilateral aplasia of an entire uterine horn, small litter size may be the only sign. Retained fetuses behind partial occlusions require surgery, and the final diagnosis is usually made during the operation.

- Soft tissue abnormalities such as neoplasms, vaginal septa, or fibrosis of the birth canal may cause obstructive dystocia. The prepartum relaxation of the vagina will often allow the passage of fetuses. Vaginal septa may consist of remnants from the fetal Müllerian duct system. However, they can also occur secondary to vaginal trauma or infection and, if extensive, may prevent the passage of the fetuses. Often, however, they are not so extensive, and vaginal relaxation may allow the fetuses to pass. Cervical or vaginal fibrosis usually is secondary to trauma or inflammatory processes and in severe cases will cause dystocia. Surgical intervention may save the puppies. Tumors and septa formations may be removed; but in the case of fibrosis, surgery is seldom successful because of new scar tissue formation during the healing process.

- Narrow pelvic canal causing obstructive dystocia may result from previous pelvic fractures, immaturity, or congenital malformation of the pelvis. The normal canine pelvis usually has a vertical diameter greater than the horizontal. Congenitally narrow birth canals exist in some brachycephalic and terrier breeds; in addition, their fetuses have comparatively large heads and wide shoulders. When achondroplasia exists, as in the Scottish terrier, dorsoventral flattening of the pelvis modifies the normal pelvic inlet, which creates a fetal obstruction. In a study using indirect pelvimetry, significant differences were found between Scottish terrier bitches whelping normally compared with those with dystocia owing to a too narrow birth canal, confirming the dorsoflattening and also demonstrating a shortening of the pelvis in the bitches with dystocia. The weight of the puppies was the same in both groups.[17] Boston terrier bitches were also studied, and again a significantly greater inner pelvic height was found in the normally whelping bitches; however, in this breed the size of the puppies was also of importance because the weight of the pup was related with the size of its head. In the bulldog the large, deep chest and pronounced waist causes the gravid uterus to drop down. At parturition, the fetuses are therefore presented at a relatively acute angle to the pelvic inlet. Bulldogs sometimes also have slack abdominal musculature, leading to insufficient uterine contractions and abdominal straining to lift the fetus up into the pelvic cavity.

Fetal Causes of Dystocia

Fetal obstructions may be caused by malpresentations, malorientations, or oversized fetuses as well as monstrosities including hydrocephalus, edema, or various duplications (see Figure 248-3). Simply being oversized is a cause for malpresentation. Fetal death may result in dystocia due to malpositioning or inadequate stimulation for parturition to begin. A healthy fetus is active during expulsion, extending its head and limbs, twisting, and rotating to get through. In most breeds the greatest bulk of the fetus lies in its abdominal cavity, whereas the bony parts (the head and the hips) are comparatively small. The limbs are short and flexible and rarely cause serious obstruction to delivery in the normal-sized fetus.

Oversized Fetuses   A puppy weighing 4% to 5% of the weight of the bitch is considered the upper limit for an uncomplicated birth. In the absence of monstrosities, oversized fetuses are often associated with small litter size. In breeds in which miniaturizing exists, great disparity in fetal size within litters may occur, with some greatly oversized individuals. In brachycephalic breeds like the Boston terrier, dystocia occurs from the combination of a flattened pelvic inlet and puppies having a large head. Obstructive dystocia was found to occur already at pup weights of 2.5% to 3.1% of the adult weight in these breeds.[18] In dystocia due to an oversized fetus, sometimes a portion of the fetus may protrude from the vulva. In anterior presentation the head may be born and the shoulders and chest cause obstruction, whereas in posterior presentation the hind limbs and hips may protrude.

Posterior Presentation   Posterior presentation is considered normal in dogs, occurring in 30% to 40% of fetal deliveries.[14,16,17] Posterior presentations have, however, been related both to higher pup mortality[17] and to a predisposition for dystocia, because mechanical dilation of the cervix may be inadequate, particularly where this involves the first fetus to be delivered. In addition, expulsion is rendered more difficult because the fetus is being delivered against the direction of its haircoat and because the fetal chest, instead of being compressed, becomes distended by the pressure from the abdominal organs through the diaphragm. Occasionally the fetus may have the elbows hooked around the pelvic brim, preventing further expulsion. Should the fetus become lodged in the pelvic canal, pressure on the umbilical vessels trapped between the fetal chest wall and maternal pelvic floor may cause hypoxia and reflex inhalation of fetal fluids.

Breech Presentation   Breech presentation (i.e., posterior presentation with hind legs flexed forward) can be a serious complication, especially in medium- and small-sized breeds. Vaginal exploration will reveal a tail tip, maybe the anus, and the bony structure of the pelvis of the fetus.

Lateral or Downward Deviation of the Head   These are two of the most common malpositionings in the dog. Lateral deviation is most common with long-necked breeds such as rough collies, whereas downward deviation is seen in brachycephalic breeds and long-headed breeds such as Sealyham and Scottish terriers. In lateral deviation, vaginal exploration will demonstrate just one front leg, the one contralateral to the direction of the deviation of the head (i.e., when the head is deviated to the left, the right front paw will be found and vice versa). When the animal has a downward deviation of the head, either both front legs and sometimes the nape of the neck of the fetus can be palpated, or both front legs may be flexed backwards and only the scull of the fetus be reached.

Backward Flexion of Front Legs   This condition is especially common when the fetus is weak or dead and is sometimes seen in combination with deviation of the head, especially downward. For bitches of the larger or even medium-sized breeds, it may be possible to deliver a puppy with one or both front legs flexed.

Transverse or Bicornual Presentation Sometimes a fetus, instead of progressing from the uterine horn through the cervix to the vagina, will proceed into the contralateral uterine horn, possibly due to some obstruction. Another reason may be that the fetus was implanted close to the body of the uterus. These cases always require surgery, because no possibility for manual correction exists.

Two Fetuses Presented Simultaneously Sometimes one fetus from each horn is presented at the same time, jamming the birth canal. When possible, if one is coming backwards, this one should be removed first, because it occupies more space.

Management of Fetal Malpresentations If a fetus is present in the birth canal, manipulation by hand or by obstetric forceps may be attempted. In bitches of the giant breeds it may even be possible to insert one hand through the vagina into the uterus and thus extract the puppy. During natural birth the puppy will almost make a full somersault, emerging from the loop of the uterine horn, progressing upwards to pass through the pelvic canal, and then moving down through the long vestibulum of the bitch to reach the vulva placed some 5 to 15 cm below the level of the pelvic floor. Thus after the fetus is seized, a gentle traction in posteroventral direction is applied.

Fetal position must be assessed. If the fetus has advanced into and partly through the pelvic canal, it will create a characteristic bulge of the perineal region, below the tail. Easing the vulvar lips upward may reveal the amniotic sac and the position of the fetus. Vaginal exploration and radiographic examination will aid in making a diagnosis in the cases when the fetus has not advanced as far.

The narrowest part of the birth canal is within the rigid pelvic girdle. If external manipulation is to be attempted, the fetus that cannot be easily pulled out may have to be pushed forward to in front of the pelvic girdle, where corrections of its position or posture are easier to perform. This should be done between periods of straining of the bitch, never working against the uterine contractions. It should also be remembered that the widest part of the pelvic girdle usually is on the diagonal (see Figure 248-1); thus rotating the fetus 45 degrees may create sufficient room for passage. Generous application of obstetric lubricant (liquid paraffin, Vaseline®, or a sterile water-soluble lubricant) is helpful, especially if the bitch has been in second-stage labor for some time.

Depending on the position and posture of the fetus, a grip should be applied around its head and neck, from above or below whichever is most convenient, around its pelvis, or around the legs. Care should be taken because the neck and limbs of the fetus are easily torn when pulled. Correction of posture may be obtained by manipulation of the fetus through the abdominal wall with one hand and concurrent transvaginal manipulation with the other. A finger may be introduced into the mouth of the fetus to help correct a downward deviation of the head. Should it be necessary to change the postures of the limbs, a finger should be inserted past the elbow or knee and the limb moved medially in under the fetus and corrected.

A gently applied alternating right-to-left traction of the puppy, gently rocking it back and forth or from side to side and possibly twisting it to a diagonal position within the pelvis, will help free the shoulders or the hips one at a time. A slight pressure applied over the perineal bulge may prevent the fetus from sliding back into the uterus again between strainings.

Obstetric forceps should only be used for assisted traction of a relatively oversized fetus when it is likely the rest of the puppies in the litter are smaller or when just one or two fetuses remain. The forceps is guided with a finger and never introduced further than to the uterine body because of the risk of getting part of the uterine wall within the grip, thereby causing serious damage. If the head of the fetus can be reached, the grip should be applied around the neck (Pålssons forceps) or across the cheeks. In posterior presentation the grip should be around the fetal pelvis. If the legs can be reached, the grip should be around those, not around the feet.

Outcome of obstetric treatment A study[13] reporting on treatment outcome shows that digital manipulation, including forceps delivery, medical treatment for dystocia, or both, is successful in only 27.6% of the cases. Around 65% of bitches brought to the clinic because of dystocia thus end up having a cesarean section.

Fetal death increased from 5.8% in bitches brought in within 1 to 4.5 hours after the beginning of second-stage labor to 13.7% in the period between 5 to 24 hours. Overall fetal death was 22.3%.[13] Early diagnosis and prompt treatment is therefore crucial in reducing the puppy death rate in cases of dystocia.

Criteria for Cesarean Section The indications for cesarean section include the following:
- Complete primary uterine inertia that does not respond to medical treatment
- Partial primary uterine inertia that is refractory to medical management
- Secondary uterine inertia with inadequate resumption of labor
- Abnormalities of the maternal pelvis or soft tissues of the birth canal
- Relative fetal oversize, if considered likely to be repeated in several fetuses
- Absolute oversize (single-puppy syndrome or fetal monstrosity)
- Excess or deficiency of fetal fluids
- Fetal malposition unamendable to manipulation
- Fetal death with putrefaction
- Toxemia of pregnancy and illness of the bitch
- Neglected dystocia
- Prophylactic (history of previous difficult deliveries)

Prophylactic cesarean section should be questioned on ethical grounds if it is performed to assist the propagation of a breed line that cannot reproduce successfully without intervention.

Once a decision has been made to deliver the litter by cesarean section, surgery should be carried out without delay. The bitch has often endured hours of more or less intensive labor and may be suffering from physical exhaustion, dehydration, acid-base disorders, hypotension, hypocalcemia, hypoglycemia, or a combination of these symptoms. The prognosis for both bitch and offspring is good if surgery is performed within 12 hours after the onset of second-stage labor; it continues to be fairly good for the bitch after 12 hours but guarded for the fetuses. If more than 24 hours have passed after the onset of second-stage labor, the entire litter is usually dead and further delay compromises the life of the bitch.

POSTPARTURIENT CONDITIONS

It is normal for the bitch to have a slightly elevated rectal temperature, up to 39.2° C (102.56° F), for a couple of days after parturition. It should, however, not exceed 39.5° C (103.1° F). Fever during this period usually emanates from conditions of the uterus or the mammary glands.

Perinatal Loss

Based on a number of surveys, pup losses up to weaning age appear to range between 10% and 35%[17,20,22] and averages around 12%.[22-24] More than 65% of pup mortality occurs at parturition and during the first week of life; few neonatal deaths occur after 3 weeks of age. Inbreeding is said to be associated with a high incidence of fetal and neonatal mortality. Breed differences in pup mortality patterns have been reported.[17] The principal cause of pup mortality has been attributed to fetal asphyxia, accounting for 42.5% of the total mortality. The majority of these pups (82.2%) died during whelping or in the first 24 hours after birth. The death of just over half of these pups could be directly attributed to dystocia. The remaining pups were compromised during what appeared to be a normal whelping.[17]

Uterine Disorders

Hemorrhage Some hemorrhage from the genital tract after parturition is normal, but maternal blood loss should never exceed a scant drip from the vulva. True hemorrhage should be distinguished from normal vaginal postparturient discharge. Excessive hemorrhage after parturition may indicate uterine or vaginal tearing or vessel rupture or may be evidence of a coagulation defect. The hematocrit should be checked, remembering that 30% is normal for the bitch at term. Inspection of the vulva and vagina should be performed in an attempt to locate the source of the bleeding. Oxytocin can be administered to promote uterine involution and contraction of the uterine wall. In more severe cases of uterine hemorrhage, an exploratory laparotomy may be necessary. The bitch should be monitored closely for signs of impending shock, and blood transfusion may be required while attempting to determine the cause of hemorrhage.

Retained Placentas and Fetuses Retained placentas in the bitch may cause severe problems, especially when accompanied by retained fetuses or infection. Clinical signs of retained placenta include a thick dark vaginal discharge. Retained fetuses can be identified by palpation or radiographic or ultrasonographic examination. The examination should also encompass the corpus uteri and the vagina in search for partly expelled fetuses or fetal membranes. A retained placenta is often palpable in the uterus, depending on the size of the bitch and degree of uterine involution. Extraction of retained tissue, by careful "milking" of the uterine horn or by using forceps, is sometimes possible. Treatment with 1 to 5 IU oxytocin per dog subcutaneously or intramuscularly two to four times daily for up to 3 days can help expulsion of retained placentas. The long-acting ergot alkaloids should not be used because they may cause closure of the cervix. Antibiotic treatment is advisable if the bitch is showing signs of illness.

Acute Metritis Acute metritis is an ascending bacterial infection of the uterus in the immediate postpartum period. Dystocia, obstetric manipulation, retained fetuses or placental membranes, or parturition in an unsanitary environment predispose to metritis. Metritis may rarely occur after normal parturition, natural or artificial insemination, or an abortion. Infection usually ascends through an open cervix and is often caused by gram-negative bacteria. Clinical signs include fever, dehydration, depression, anorexia, poor lactation and mothering, and a purulent or sanguinopurulent vaginal discharge. A doughy enlarged uterus may be palpated abdominally. Abdominal radiographic or ultrasonographic examination (or both) is indicated to evaluate the uterine size and uterine contents. A vaginal culture is recommended. Vaginal cytology will show large numbers of degenerate neutrophils, red blood cells (RBCs), bacteria, and debris. The complete blood count (CBC) often shows leukocytosis with a left shift. Therapy consists of immediate administration of intravenous fluids and antibiotics and evacuation of uterine contents. The latter may be accomplished by administering oxytocin or PGF$_{2\alpha}$. One high-dose regimen exists for administration of PGF$_{2\alpha}$ (0.1 to 0.25 mg/kg subcutaneously once or twice daily for 3 to 8 days) and one low-dose regimen (0.025 to 0.05 mg/kg subcutaneously six to eight times daily for 2 to 3 days). The high-dose alternative may cause adverse reactions such as abdominal pain and increases in pulse rate, respiratory rate, and salivary secretions. These reactions appear within 10 minutes of administration and normally disappear again after 30 minutes to 1 hour. It should be remembered, however, that the prostaglandins are not licensed for use in dogs. In more severe cases, ovariohysterectomy (OHE) is the recommended treatment.

Subinvolution of Placental Sites In the postparturient period it is normal for the bitch to have a serosanguineous vaginal discharge for 3 to 6 weeks. Normally the uterine involution is completed within 12 weeks after whelping. Subinvolution of placental sites is suspected if a sanguineous vaginal discharge persists for longer than 6 weeks (Figure 248-4). The cause of this condition is unknown, and the bitch often shows no symptoms of illness. Vaginal cytology shows predominantly RBCs, with syncytial trophoblast-like cells being a useful confirmatory finding. Subinvolution of placental sites almost exclusively affects the young, primiparous animal, and in the majority of cases resolves spontaneously, with the prognosis for future pregnancy being good. Because of increased risk of anemia, secondary bacterial infection, or rupture of the affected placental sites with subsequent peritonitis, the bitch should be monitored until the disorder resolves. OHE is indicated in rare cases of profound permanent bleeding or uterine infection.

Uterine Rupture Uterine rupture should be considered a possible but uncommon cause of illness in the postparturient period. Uterine rupture can occur when prostaglandins or oxytocin have been administered for induction of abortion or treatment of pyometra, metritis, or dystocia. The condition may occur as a result of dystocia or during an apparently normal parturition or may be due to injury occurring in late pregnancy. The clinical signs of uterine rupture include abdominal pain and distention and a rapid deterioration of the condition of the bitch. The diagnosis is confirmed by exploratory laparotomy, and OHE is the usual treatment combined with intravenous fluids and antibiotic therapy.

Uterine Prolapse Uterine prolapse is an uncommon complication during parturition. It occurs in primiparous and multiparous bitches. The prolapse usually occurs immediately or within a few hours after delivery of the last pup. The prolapse can be complete, with both uterine horns protruding from the vulva, or may be limited to the uterine body and one horn. Treatments include manual reposition, reposition by means of laparotomy, and amputation. OHE is usually performed.

Toxic Milk Syndrome The toxic milk syndrome is poorly documented. Pathologic conditions in the uterus of the bitch may cause toxins to be excreted in the milk. Suckling offspring that are affected by toxic milk syndrome become vocal and uncomfortable. Other signs are diarrhea, salivation, bloating, and a reddened anus. Treatment consists of removing the pups from the bitch and the administration of fluid therapy and oral glucose until bloating resolves. If the bitch is successfully treated for the uterine condition, the litter can be returned after 24 to 48 hours, otherwise hand rearing is necessary.

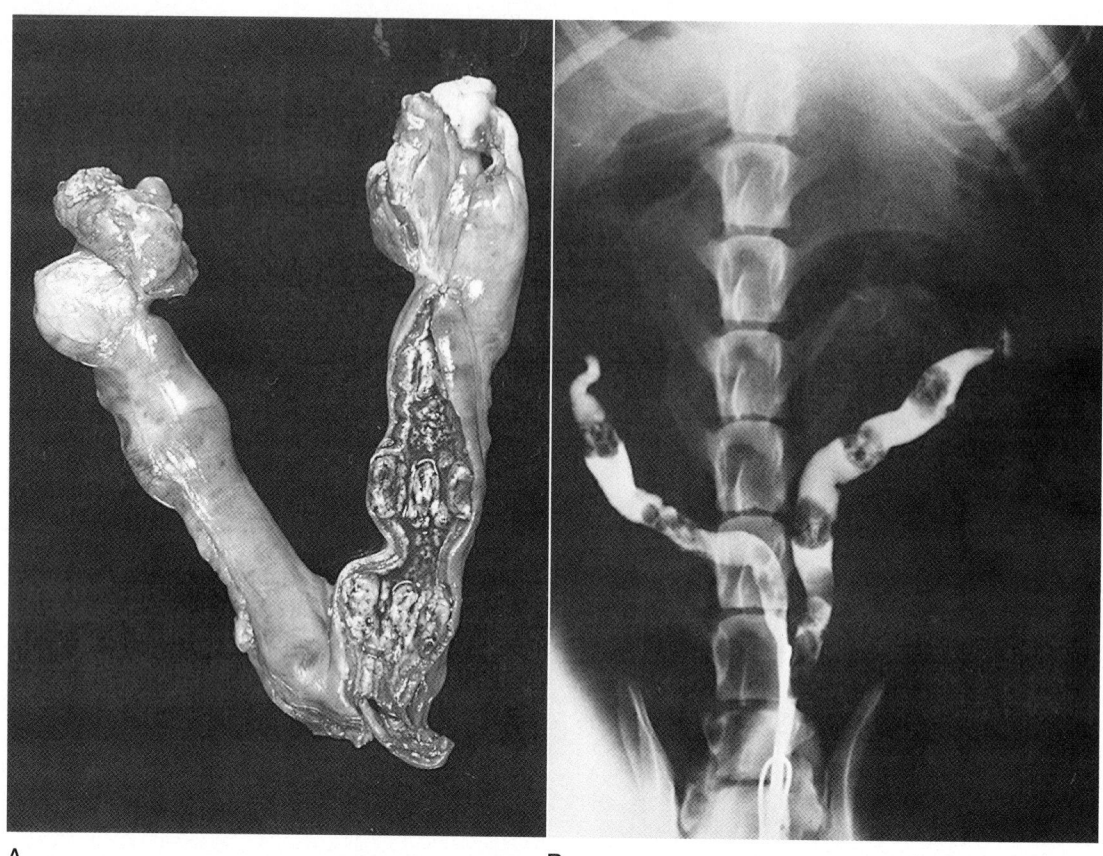

A B

Figure 248-4 *A*, Subinvolution of the placental sites. In the unopened left uterine horn the typical oval swellings of the placental areas can be observed. In the opened horn, the placentation zones and the hemorrhage emanating from those areas can be seen. *B*, A hystographic picture of a bitch with subinvolution of the placental sites, 4 months after whelping. The placentation zones are seen as darker areas. Normal uterine involution is completed within 12 weeks in the bitch.

Mammary Gland Disorders

Agalactia   Agalactia, or absence of milk after parturition, may be due to a failure of milk production or milk letdown. True agalactia, failure of milk production, is uncommon but may occur repeatedly in some bitches. More commonly it may be observed after premature parturitions or cesarean sections. Treatment with metoclopramide 1 to 5 mg/kg subcutaneously or per orally every 6 to 8 hours for a maximum of 5 days may promote prolactin release and milk production in these cases. Failure of milk letdown may occur as a consequence of excessive secretion of epinephrine, resulting from fright or pain, which has a blocking effect upon the release of oxytocin. Oxytocin 0.5 to 2.0 IU per dose can be administered repeatedly for a few days until milk flow has been established. Primiparous, nervous, or confused bitches may experience temporary agalactia. Reassurance by the owner and administration of low doses of acepromazine orally may help the bitch to settle down, and subsequent suckling by the puppies will enhance milk flow. Other causes of agalactia are physical exhaustion, undernourishment, shock, mastitis, metritis, systemic infections, and endocrine imbalances.

Galactostasis   Milk stasis (i.e., galactostasis) causes enlarged and edematous mammary glands that are firm and warm to the touch. The bitch shows signs of discomfort and pain and fails to let down milk. The condition should be differentiated

from mastitis and agalactia. The cause is unknown in dogs, but it usually involves the two most caudal pairs of mammae in bitches with a high milk production, with few puppies, or with both. It can also occur in glands with malformed teats, which the offspring avoid suckling. Another cause can be that nursing comes to an abrupt end owing to death of the litter or sudden weaning. To relieve mammary congestion the owner can apply gentle massage and warm-water compresses to the mammary glands or perform careful milking to relieve some of the pressure. Sometimes it helps to put more aggressively nursing neonates to the bitch. Treatment includes reducing food intake and the administration of a mild diuretic. Neglected galactostasis may lead to mastitis or involution of the mammary gland. Cabergoline (Galastop vet.), a dopamine agonist, at 2.5 to 5 µg/kg/day orally for 4 to 6 days, reduces prolactin secretion and thereby lactation. The use of dopamine agonists should be restricted to bitches that have either lost their litter or have a litter old enough to be weaned.

Acute Mastitis   Acute mastitis in the bitch occurs from hematogenously spread bacterial infections or from bacteria ascending through the teat orifices. Predisposing factors include mammary gland congestion, trauma, and poor sanitary conditions. The mammary glands become hot, painful, and enlarged; the milk shows increased viscosity and changes in color from yellow to brown, depending on the amount of blood and purulent exudate present. Clinical signs include fever, anorexia, and depression in the bitch. The offspring may be restless and crying. Milk cytology reveals the presence of degenerate neutrophils, RBCs, and bacteria. Culture of the milk often shows growth of *Staphylococcus* spp., *Streptococcus* spp., or *Escherichia coli*. Treatment consists of adequate antibiotics, application of warm-water compresses, and massage of mammary glands. If abscessation of the glands occurs, surgical débridement and drainage is essential. Untreated acute mastitis may result in gangrenous mastitis and septic shock. Depending on the severity of the condition, the litter may stay with the bitch or has to be separated and hand reared.

Miscellaneous Disorders

Puerperal Tetany An acute decrease in extracellular calcium concentration is the cause of puerperal tetany (eclampsia). Eclampsia occurs most commonly in dogs of the small breeds, usually within the first 21 days after whelping, but occasionally during late pregnancy or at parturition. Early signs are restlessness, panting, pacing, whining, salivation, tremors, and stiffness. The symptoms aggravate to clonic-tonic muscle spasms, fever, tachycardia, miosis, seizures, and death. Treatment must be instigated immediately and consists of slow intravenous infusion of a 10% calcium borogluconate solution. The dose required varies depending on the degree of hypocalcemia and the size of the bitch. Careful cardiac monitoring for bradycardia and arrhythmias is important. If arrhythmia or vomiting occurs, the infusion must be temporarily halted and then, if necessary, resumed at a slower rate. Because hypoglycemia may follow hypocalcemia, the intravenous administration of a 10% dextrose solution is recommended. The puppies should be removed from the bitch and hand fed a canine milk replacer for 24 hours.

If the litter is 4 weeks old or more, it is advisable to wean them. Oral supplementation of the lactating bitch having experienced eclampsia with calcium carbonate at 100 mg/kg body weight per day, divided with meals, and vitamin D is recommended. Prophylactic calcium treatment during the course of pregnancy of bitches expected to develop eclampsia probably is contraindicated, because it may cause a disturbance of the calcium homeostasis.

Disturbances in Maternal Behavior Maternal behavior involves hereditary factors, several hormones (e.g., estrogens, progesterone, oxytocin, and prolactin), previous experiences as a mother, and the stimulus of the neonate. Good maternal behavior includes nest building, nursing, and protecting. The period during which the bitch will form a bond with a pup is probably less than 24 hours. The bitch should spend most of the time with the litter for at least the first 2 weeks. Most bitches have strong maternal instincts, but their behavior depends strongly upon their hormonal balance, general health, and the environment. In some breeds a higher occurrence of bad mothering exists, and in other species several genes for maternal behavior have been identified. Sublimation (i.e., close emotional attachment to a human) may cause problems at parturition, when the bitch may manifest panic and reject her pups.[21] On the contrary, a bitch may resent human intervention, not accepting assisted birthing and cesarean-delivered offspring, and may sometimes even kill them. Major disturbing factors during and after parturition, mental instability, or pain may cause the mother to kill her neonates. Hypocalcemia should always be ruled out in cases of aggression in lactating bitches. Good health, quiet and familiar surroundings, and most important of all, presence of her young will promote normal maternal behavior.

CHAPTER • 249

Early Spay and Neuter

Margaret V. Root Kustritz

Prepuberal gonadectomy is castration or ovariohysterectomy of puppies or kittens 6 to 14 weeks of age. Performance of neutering of dogs and cats at the more traditional age of 6 months usually also occurs before puberty, so the term *early spay and neuter* is perhaps more correct. Early spay and neuter surgeries have been performed at humane organizations and universities in at least 17 states for as many as 13 years. The procedure is approved by many major veterinary professional and humane organizations, including the American Veterinary Medical Association.[1]

Surgical neutering of young puppies and kittens is of greatest advantage to humane organizations, because it circumvents the problem of noncompliance by adopters with spay and neuter agreements after adoption. It also permits placement of neutered animals while they are still young enough to

benefit from socialization in the new home. Breeders may also benefit from the procedure, which allows placement of neutered pet-quality puppies and kittens while still young, precluding indiscriminate breeding of animals that do not meet the breed standard or that carry hereditary disorders.

In one survey, 57% of humane shelters surveyed could not provide young puppies and kittens that already had been neutered because of unavailability of a veterinarian to perform the surgeries.[2] In 1998 only 48% of 29 North American veterinary colleges responding to a survey reported teaching early spay and neuter surgeries to their students despite 90% having a working relationship with a local humane organization.[2] Students polled at a university after completing a rotation in which early spay and neuter surgeries were performed stated that performance of early spay and neuter surgeries increased their confidence in performing pediatric surgery and anesthesia in general.[3]

Pediatric anesthesia is complicated by the immature physiology and small body mass of the animals.[4] Hypothermia occurs readily in puppies and kittens. Fluids used for surgical preparation should be warm and water based as opposed to alcohol based. The animal should be maintained on a circulating warm-water pad, and anesthesia and surgery time should be minimized to prevent heat loss. Intravenous fluids to be administered intraoperatively also should be warmed.

Hypoglycemia occurs more readily in pediatric than in adult animals because of reduced glycogen stores in skeletal muscle and liver and slower rates of hepatic gluconeogenesis and glycogenolysis. Pediatric animals should be fasted for no more than 3 to 4 hours before anesthesia is induced. Dextrose may be provided in the intravenous fluids intraoperatively.

Pharmacokinetics of drugs administered are altered by immature pediatric renal and hepatic physiology, which do not approach adult levels until the animal is 12 to 14 weeks of age.[4] The overall effect of these physiologic changes is increased availability of anesthetic agents for a longer period of time due to decreased metabolization and slower rate of excretion; drug doses may need to be reduced in pediatric animals.

Anesthetic equipment should be of a size that minimizes resistance and dead space.[5,6] Masks should be tight fitting. Monitoring of anesthesia involves close observation of heart and respiratory rates. Pediatric animals cannot respond to hypoxia with increased stroke volume and do not respond readily to increased concentrations of carbon dioxide in blood with an increase in respiratory rate.[7]

Several anesthetic protocols for early spay and neuter of puppies and kittens have been reported. The optimal reported protocols, defined as those that minimized induction and recovery times and provided the smoothest induction and recovery and best depth of sedation, are listed in Table 249-1.[5,6]

Surgical procedures are as in older animals.[5,8,9] This is an elective procedure and should only be performed on those animals that are in good health, are free of internal and external parasites, and are vaccinated. General principles of surgery on pediatric animals should be observed. These include gentle tissue handling, decreasing surgery time to minimize intraoperative hypothermia, and maintaining meticulous hemostasis.

Castration in puppies is performed as in adult dogs. Both testes are removed through a single prescrotal incision. Both a closed technique, in which the tunic containing the spermatic cord and vessels are left intact, and an open technique, in which

the tunic is opened, have been described.[5,9] Fine absorbable suture or hemostatic clips may be used for ligation of the spermatic cord and vessels. Closure is routine. Either subcuticular closure with absorbable suture or external interrupted or continuous nonabsorbable sutures may be used; external skin sutures have not been reported to bother puppies castrated prepuberally unless they are too tight.[9] Some reports exist of tissue glue used for skin closure after early spay and neuter surgeries, but this is not reported to work well in puppies.

Castration in kittens is performed as in adult cats.[6] Bilateral scrotal incisions are made. Both closed techniques, in which the spermatic cord and vessels within the tunic were either ligated or tied on itself, and an open technique, in which the spermatic cord and vessels were tied to each other, have been described. The scrotal incisions are left open to heal by second intention.

Ovariohysterectomy of puppies and kittens is as in adult animals. Serous fluid in the abdominal cavity is a not infrequent finding and is not associated with any known pathology.[5,8] Use of ovariohysterectomy (Snook) hooks is not recommended.[9] Carmalt clamps, with ridges perpendicular to the tissue enclosed within them, may be preferred to mosquito clamps for compression of the small ovarian vessels and uterine body.[7] Fine absorbable suture material or hemostatic clips may be used for ligation of the ovarian vessels and uterine body. Closure is routine. Subcuticular or external sutures may be used for closure of the skin.

Surgery time should be shorter for early spay and neuter surgeries than for similar surgery in older animals.[10] The animals recover quickly from anesthesia and should be fed a small meal as soon as possible to prevent hypoglycemia. Postoperative pain can be controlled by administration of butorphanol (0.11 to 0.22 mg/kg intravenously, intramuscularly, or subcutaneously);[10] most animals do not require postoperative pain management. External skin sutures can be removed in 10 to 14 days.

It is recommended that all puppies and kittens gonadectomized prior to 16 weeks of age be tattooed to prevent unnecessary surgical exploration to verify intact status later in life. Tattoos are recommended to be ½ to ¾ inches in diameter, and should be placed in the prepubic area of females and the inguinal area of males; the preferred figure is the "male" or "female" symbol with an x across it (Figure 249-1).

A growing body of veterinary literature supports the safety of early spay and neuter surgeries. Short- and long-term complications hypothesized to occur include increased anesthetic and surgical morbidity and mortality, increased prevalence of

Table • 249-1

Optimal Anesthetic Regimens for Early Spay and Neuter Surgeries in Puppies and Kittens*

		PUPPIES		KITTENS
Males	Premed	Atropine (0.04 mg/kg IM) + oxymorphone (0.22 mg/kg IM)	Premed	—
	Induction	Propofol (6.5 mg/kg IV)	Induction	Tiletamine/zolazepam (11 mg/kg IM)
	Inhalant	Isoflurane as needed	Inhalant	Isoflurane as needed
Females	Premed	Atropine (0.04 mg/kg IM) + oxymorphone (0.11 mg/kg IV)	Premed	—
	Induction	Propofol (4.3 mg/kg IV)	Induction	Ketamine HCl (11 mg/kg IM) + midazolam (0.22 mg/kg IM)
	Inhalant	Isoflurane	Inhalant	Isoflurane

*From Faggella AM, Aronsohn MG: Evaluation of anesthetic protocols for neutering 6- to 14-week-old pups. J Am Vet Med Assoc 205:308-314, 1994; Faggella AM, Aronsohn MG: Anesthetic techniques for neutering 6- to 14-week-old kittens. J Am Vet Med Assoc 202:56-62, 1993.

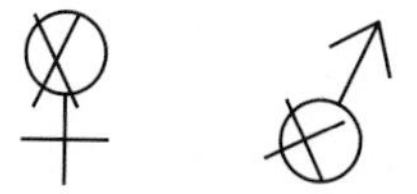

Figure 249-1 Tattoo symbols recommended for placement in the prepubic area of female puppies and kittens and inguinal area of male puppies and kittens after early spay and neuter.

infectious disease, obesity, stunting of growth, increased incidence of feline lower urinary tract disease, behavioral problems, and estrogen-responsive urinary incontinence.

Short-term complications of anesthesia and surgery do not occur more commonly in animals neutered when young compared with those neutered when older. One study evaluating short-term effects of ovariohysterectomy and castration in 1213 dogs and 775 cats on which surgery was performed at less than 12 weeks, 12 to 24 weeks, or more than 24 weeks of age demonstrated that the short-term complication rate was highest in the group neutered at more than 24 weeks of age.[10]

Long-term complications of neutering also are not more common in animals undergoing early spay or neuter than in those animals neutered at more traditional ages, with the possible exception of predisposition to infectious disease in puppies.[11,12] In one study, incidence of parvovirus was higher in dogs neutered at less than 24 weeks of age compared with those neutered at more than 24 weeks of age.[12] This may have been due to the shelter from which the dogs originated, which had an overall higher incidence of parvovirus in young dogs than the other shelters in that study.

Obesity is a multifactorial problem. Retrospective studies have identified neutering as a risk factor for development of obesity. However, a study in dogs did not demonstrate an increase in body weight, food intake, or depth of back fat in those animals gonadectomized either at 7 weeks or 7 months of age, compared with those left intact.[13] That study was concluded when the animals were 15 months of age; predisposition to obesity may have become evident in the neutered animals at an older age. In cats, those neutered at either 7 weeks or 7 months of age had higher body weights and body condition scores and a larger falciform fat pad than did those left intact when evaluated at 24 months of age.[14,15] Metabolic rate has been demonstrated to be decreased in gonadectomized cats, regardless of age at time of surgery.[16]

Stunting of growth does not occur in animals gonadectomized when quite young. Closure of physeal plates is delayed in puppies and kittens gonadectomized at any time prior to puberty with subsequent increase in bone length.[13,14,17] Some question whether the delay in physeal closure may predispose these animals to growth plate fractures; no such correlation has been demonstrated.[18]

Feline lower urinary tract disease (FLUTD) has not been demonstrated to be more prevalent in cats gonadectomized when young. Urethral diameter is not significantly smaller or larger in male or female cats gonadectomized at either 7 weeks or 7 months of age, compared with intact cats at 22 to 24 months of age.[14,19]

Behavior problems have not been demonstrated to be more prevalent in animals gonadectomized when quite young. In addition, these animals are not less likely to be retained in homes after adoption than animals gonadectomized when older.[11,12,20] Service dogs neutered at 7 weeks of age are equally likely as dogs neutered at 7 months of age to be successfully trained and placed.[21]

Estrogen-responsive urinary incontinence has not been demonstrated to occur more commonly in animals gonadectomized when young. Estrogen-responsive urinary incontinence is, in fact, less commonly seen within 3 years of surgery in female dogs ovariohysterectomized before their first estrus than in female dogs ovariohysterectomized after their first estrus, with incidences of 9.7% and 20.1%, respectively.[22,23]

Early spay and neuter surgeries are safe and easy to perform. Performance of early spay and neuter surgeries allows veterinarians to sharpen their general skills regarding pediatric anesthesia and surgery and to provide a service to the humane organizations in their community and to the community at large.

CHAPTER • 250

Contraception and Pregnancy Termination in the Dog and Cat

Bruce E. Eilts

Contraception, or the prevention of pregnancy or estrus, is one of the most frequent requests made to veterinarians. Most often that request is for ovariohysterectomy (OHE), or spay, in the female or neutering (castration) in the male, which results in permanent sterilization. In addition to OHE, a permanent sterilization method is ovariectomy. Temporary estrus prevention has been achieved using several different drugs such as megestrol acetate, mibolerone, and testosterone. Immunologic methods to induce permanent or temporary sterility have been investigated but are not yet perfected. Often a client will request that an unwanted pregnancy be terminated. Pharmaceuticals such as estrogens, prostaglandin, prolactin inhibitors, dexamethasone, antiprogestogens, or combinations thereof have been used successfully in clinical situations to terminate pregnancy (Table 250-1). This chapter will present the most common techniques and drugs, including drug availability and drug cost at the time of writing, that are readily available.

Table • 250-1

Drugs Used to Induce Pregnancy Termination in the Bitch

DRUG	VET. LABEL	DRUG NAME	MFG.	AVAILABILITY	UNIT	PACKAGE SIZE	COST/PACK ($)	MG DOSE	DAYS RX	RX/DAY	COST/ DOSE ($)	COST/ TREATMENT ($)	HOSPITAL	REF
Estradiol cypionate	Yes	ECP	Pfizer	US	2 mg/cc	50 cc bottle	22.66	0.044	1	1	0.099	0.099	No	11
Bromocriptine— oral only?		Parlodel	Geneva	US	2.5 mg tab	30 tab	26.45	0.0622	4	2	0.21	1.75	No	23
Cabergoline— oral only?		Dostinex	Pfizer	US	0.5 mg tab	8 tab/pack	148.57	0.005	7	1	1.857	12.99		24
Cloprostenol	Yes	Estrumate	Schering	US	250 μg/mL	20 mL	14.98	0.025	5	1	0.79	3.95	Yes	20
Dexamethasone		Various	Various	US	6 mg tab	100 tab	2.59	0.22	10	2	0.007	0.14	No	35
Mifepristone (RU 486)		Mifeprix	Danco	US	200 mg tab	3 tab/pack	1.350	2.5	1	1	56.25	56.25	No	29
Prostaglandin PGF$_{2\alpha}$	Yes	Lutalyse	Pfizer	US	5 mg/mL	30 mL	8.79	0.25	9	3	0.145	3.91	Yes	15
Tamoxifen		Taxol	Bristol Meyers	US	10 mg tab	60 tab	59.17	1	10	2	0.99	19.80	No	14
Epostane				Great Britain								0		
Aglepristone		Alizene	Virbac	France	5 mg/mL			100	2	1				

Tab, Tablet; Hospital, Hospitalization required; Ref, Reference; Vet. Label, Veterinary Label Available; Availability Unit, then the drug is packaged.

Techniques using drugs that are not available or in formulations not readily available in the United States will not be presented.

CANINE

Permanent Sterilization

Female The most common contraceptive techniques in the dog are OHE for the female and neutering for the male. Advantages of OHE include permanent sterilization and prevention of estrual behavior, no remaining reproductive tract to incur future pathology, reduced incidence of mammary neoplasia in females, and decreased incidence of some prostatic disease in the male. Disadvantages include permanent sterilization, potential anesthetic complications (4.1% during OHE[1]), intra- and postoperative surgical complications (7.3% for OHE[2]), pathology of reproductive tract remnants, urinary incontinence in the female, and obesity. Clients should be advised about side effects such as obesity and urinary incontinence. Although more females become obese after surgical sterilization than males, the causes of obesity are many and cannot be attributed solely to gonadectomy. Urinary incontinence exacerbated by low estrogen is a common side effect of gonadectomy in the bitch. The exact cause is unknown. The advantages and disadvantages of early spay and neuter are covered in Chapter 249. Although OHE is the most common technique used for permanent female sterilization in the United States, it has been shown that the long-term side effects associated with only performing ovariectomy are no different than when OHE is performed.[3,4] The advantages of performing ovariectomy include shorter surgery time, a smaller incision, and less abdominal trauma. Perhaps North American veterinarians should contemplate the advantages of ovariectomy over OHE. Tubal ligation, although rendering a female sterile, will not alleviate estrus and its associated unwanted behavior or reduce the incidence of mammary neoplasia.

Male Neutering males is the most common technique available to consistently render males permanently sterile. Performing a vasectomy is uncommon. An attempt at intratesticular injections of glycerol to render males permanently sterile was not successful.[5] An intratesticular injection of zinc gluconate neutralized with arginine is now marketed as Neutersol. The company claims 99.6% effectiveness (with the need for anesthesia in only about 24% of dogs) when administered to puppies 2 to 10 months of age.[6]

TEMPORARY CONTRACEPTIVE TECHNIQUES

Before temporary contraceptive drugs are used, the client should be advised that only valuable breeding dogs should be left reproductively intact. Most dogs should have gonadectomies performed to sterilize them and remove sexual behavior. The most commonly available drugs to prevent estrus or pregnancy are megestrol acetate, mibolerone, and testosterone. Megestrol acetate has been marketed as Ovaban. To prevent estrus, the clinician should administer 0.5 mg/kg for 32 days starting at least 1 week before the next anticipated estrous cycle. The manufacturer approves a maximum of 32 days treatment. The next estrus will be in 4 to 5 months if estrus was imminent. If given during diestrus (for example, the client did not know the estrual stage) the next estrous cycle will occur at the regularly anticipated time. To stop estrus when the bitch is in the first 3 days of proestrus, the manufacturer recommends administering 2 mg/kg/day for 8 days. The next estrous cycle will be 4 to 6 weeks earlier than

it normally would have been. It is recommended that the drug not be used during the first estrous cycle and that not more than two consecutive estrous cycles be suppressed. Side effects include increased appetite, weight gain, and (uncommonly) pyometra or mammary neoplasia. However, the drug is contraindicated in bitches with mammary neoplasia, diabetes mellitus, liver disease, uterine disease, or pregnancy. Apparently, it has no effect on post-treatment fertility. Ironically, the drug is not approved for breeding bitches.

Mibolerone was marketed as Cheque drops and is an androgen that blocks LH release, therefore preventing estrus. It is advised not to administer it before the first estrous cycle, because it will cause premature physeal closure. Treatment must be started at least 30 days before the next anticipated estrous cycle at an oral dose of 30 μg/day for dogs 0.5 to 12 kg, 60 μg/day for dogs 12 to 30 kg, 120 μg/day for dogs 25 to 50 kg, and 120 μg/day for dogs greater than 50 kg or German shepherd dogs. The manufacturer has approved administration for a maximum of 24 months, but the drug has been administered experimentally as long as 43 months without apparently causing problems. The next estrous cycle after stopping treatment will reportedly occur in 7 to 200 days (i.e., unpredictable) with normal fertility. If pregnancy does occur during treatment, any female pups will be masculinized. Side effects of mibolereone include clitoral hypertrophy, vaginal discharge, vaginitis, aggressiveness, anal gland inspissations, musky body odor, and epiphora. It is also not recommended for breeding bitches.

Many Greyhound breeders may use testosterone to suppress estrus. Orally, methyl testosterone at 5 mg/wk (or divided, two times/wk) or parenteral testosterone propionate at a dose of 25 mg intramuscularly in the pectorals every 2 weeks prevents estrus. Clitoral hypertrophy or vaginal discharge may be side effects.

Many experimental methods such as antibody formation against GnRH[7] to prevent estrus or antibody formation against conception specific zona pellucida antigens[8] have been investigated; however, none have been consistently successful and none have been marketed.

Nothing that is effective for causing temporary infertility in the male is available. However, administration of leuprolide acetate (a GnRH agonist that down-regulates LH and therefore lowers testosterone concentrations) at a single dose of 1.0 mg/kg subcutaneously suppressed sperm production in 8 weeks and then persisted for 6 weeks.[9] The effects did reverse, leaving the hope that a drug may be available to cause temporary sterility in males.

PREGNANCY TERMINATION

Bitch

Only valued breeding animals should have pregnancy terminated in an effort to preserve future fertility. All other dogs should have an OHE performed to end the pregnancy. Drugs that can be administered during estrus to prevent pregnancy include estrogens and tamoxifen. If a request for pregnancy termination is made for a valued breeding animal, it must be decided if the bitch was actually in estrus and mated. A vaginal cytology examination will quickly determine if the bitch is in estrus. If the vaginal cytology slide is 90% to 100% cornified, the bitch is in estrus; and if the vaginal cytology slide does not contain cornified cells, the bitch is not in estrus (the bitch may have progressed into diestrus). Mating can be confirmed by the presence of sperm cells in the vaginal cytology; however, if no sperm cells are present in the vaginal cytology it cannot be assumed that the bitch was not mated. Sperm cells normally are not evident more than 24 hours after mating when doing routine vaginal cytology examinations. All bitches mated within 24 hours of obtaining a vaginal smear had sperm heads in the sample, and 75% that were mated within 48 hours had sperm heads when the vaginal cytology was prepared in the following manner.[10] A cotton swab moistened with saline is placed in the vagina for 1 minute, and then the tip of the swab is placed in a small tube containing 0.5 mL saline for 10 minutes. After 10 minutes the swab tip is squeezed dry into the tube and the fluid in the tube is centrifuged at $2000 \times g$ for 10 minutes. The sediment is then stained using the same technique as a vaginal cytology.

Few alternatives exist if the client insists on a therapeutic procedure being performed when the bitch is in estrus before a pregnancy examination is performed. The only true mismate drugs available for this time period are the estrogens. The estrogens commonly used for mismate include estradiol cypionate (ECP), estradiol benzoate, and diethylstilbestrol (DES). The administration of DES is not effective as a mismate therapy.[11] Estradiol benzoate when administered at 0.01 mg/kg intramuscularly at 3 and 5 days (and occasionally 7 days) after mating in 358 bitches resulted in 16 (4.5%) of the bitches actually whelping.[12] None of the bitches had bone marrow aplasia reported, but there was a 7.3% incidence of pyometra reported (the "normal" incidence was reported to be 2% to 10% in the study).[12] Using ECP at a dose of 44 µg/kg one time during estrus resulted in no (0/4) bitches becoming pregnant, no pyometras, and no evidence of aplastic anemia at 25 days after treatment.[11] Estrogens must only be used during cytologic estrus and the owner must be warned of potential side effects. If estrogens are administered during diestrus by mistake, or because it is assumed that one must wait 3 to 5 days after mating for administration, then the potential for inducing a pyometra rises considerably.[11] Reports of infertility after estrogen administration[13] are not documented, and in practice situations it is common to see a bitch become pregnant again during the next estrus.

The only other drug that can be used at the time of mismate presentation is tamoxifen citrate (Taxol, Bristol-Meyers, Squibb, New York, NY.). Tamoxifen citrate is normally considered to be an antiestrogen, but in dogs it has estrogenic activity. It has been administered at a dose of 1 mg/kg orally twice a day for 10 days starting either in proestrus, estrus, or the second, fifteenth, and thirtieth days of diestrus.[14] The drug had a 100% (12/12) efficacy for preventing pregnancy when administration began before the fifteenth day of diestrus, but when administered on the fifteenth day of diestrus or later it was not effective at preventing pregnancy. Side effects of the drug included pyometra, endometritis, and cystic ovaries when administered during all stages of the estrous cycle except early diestrus. Half (2/4) of the bitches receiving the drug during proestrus developed pyometra.[14] Because of the poor efficacy and side effects, tamoxifen citrate has not been widely used or accepted as a mismate drug in the dog.

If the client decides to pursue alternative therapies other than OHE or estrogens, it is important to have a pregnancy examination performed before instituting therapy, because 38% of bitches presented for elective pregnancy termination may not actually be pregnant.[15] The pregnancy examination should be performed at least 30 to 40 days after the possible breeding to minimize a false-negative diagnosis caused by an error in calculating the gestation duration from a mating that occurred early in estrus. Pregnancy diagnosis with ultrasound is reliable 25 days after the LH peak (19 days after the first day of diestrus). If a bitch is truly not pregnant, the expense, side effects, and any potential risks associated with pregnancy termination therapy can be avoided (albeit the expense of the pregnancy examination will be incurred). If the bitch is pregnant, the owners may elect to allow the bitch to have that litter and avoid any complications associated with pregnancy termination.

The most common therapies to terminate pregnancy rely on luteal demise, because the bitch requires an ovarian luteal progesterone source to maintain pregnancy. Luteolysis results in a decline in serum progesterone and when serum progesterone drops below 2 ng/mL for 24 hours, abortion occurs.[15] Many clinicians[15-18] have shown prostaglandins to be luteolytic in the bitch. The most common prostaglandin is the natural prostaglandin ($PGF_{2\alpha}$; Lutalyse, Pfizer, New York, NY). A single dose of prostaglandin will not result in luteolysis in the dog. Side effects of prostaglandin therapy include vomiting and diarrhea, but these only last about 30 minutes and tend to wane as the treatment protocol continues. However, it is recommended by some authors that bitches should be hospitalized for the duration of the treatment[19] or for at least 30 minutes after each treatment. To minimize caloric loss it is best to feed the bitches at least 1 hour after treatment so that the food is not vomited and lost on a daily basis. The natural $PGF_{2\alpha}$ is given at a dose of 0.1 to 0.25 mg/kg administered subcutaneously two to three times a day. A protocol found to have the fewest side effects is $PGF_{2\alpha}$ administered at a dose of 0.1 mg/kg subcutaneously every 8 hours for 2 days and then 0.2 mg/kg subcutaneously every 8 hours until abortion is complete.[15] Abortion is usually complete within 9 days,[15] but some bitches will abort fetuses and still have live fetuses after 9 days. It is extremely important to continue the treatments until abortion is complete and to use ultrasound examination to ensure that all the fetuses are expelled. Bitches have had normal litters after abortion with $PGF_{2\alpha}$.[19] The main drawbacks to using $PGF_{2\alpha}$ are the side effects and the duration of treatment. Prostaglandins have not been approved for inducing abortion in the bitch, so it is important to obtain client consent and forewarn them of the potential complications, prolonged treatments, and need for multiple abdominal ultrasound examinations that need to be performed. Because of the side effects of the natural prostaglandins, potent synthetic prostaglandins, with fewer side effects, were developed.

Synthetic prostaglandins have also been used to induce abortion in the bitch. Synthetic prostaglandins available for the bovine include cloprostenol, fluprostenol, and alfaprostol. These synthetic prostaglandins have a much greater affinity for the prostaglandin receptors and have a longer half-life than natural prostaglandins. The synthetic prostaglandins also cause fewer smooth muscle contractions, therefore reducing side effects. It is important to note that the dose of the synthetic prostaglandins is much lower than that of the natural prostaglandin and that an error in dose calculation may be fatal. Cloprostenol has been used at a dose of 1 to 2.5 µg/kg subcutaneously once daily for 4 to 5 days and was 100% effective at inducing abortion after a 4 to 7-day treatment regimen.[20] The once-daily treatments of cloprostenol provide an advantage over treatments with natural prostaglandin, which are required every 8 hours. At the low dose of 1 µg/kg, the side effects of cloprostenol were noted to be minimal to none.[20]

In an attempt to alleviate any side effects associated with prostaglandin administration, other drugs have been added to the treatment regime. These include atropine sulphate at a dose of 0.025 mg/kg, prifinium bromide at a dose of 0.1 mL/kg, and metopimazine at a subcutaneous dose of 0.5 mg/kg.[21] Administration 15 minutes before a 2.5 µ/kg dose of cloprostenol given every 48 hours for three doses prevented side effects in 58% (39/67) of the bitches.[21] After one cloprostenol treatment, 53 of the 67 bitches had aborted, and after a second treatment 2 days later, 62 of the 67 bitches had aborted.

Other drugs that cause serum progesterone to decline are the dopaminergic drugs, which are prolactin inhibitors. Because prolactin is luteotropic during the second half of gestation,[22] lowering the prolactin concentration will cause luteal demise and result in a pregnancy loss. Prolactin inhibitors currently available include bromocriptine (Parlodel, Sandaz, Bloomfield, CO) and cabergoline (Dostinex, Pfizer, New York, NY).

Bromocriptine administered orally at a dose of 62.5 µg/kg twice daily to dogs at 43 to 45 days postovulation resulted in only two of four bitches aborting.[23] Side effects included two episodes of emesis in three of the bitches approximately 3 hours after treatment. Loose stools were also noted. Bromocriptine tabs can be crushed and dissolved in oil to ease dosing (because the compound is inactivated by water). Bromocriptine as a sole abortifacient does not appear to be a good choice in the bitch. It is more commonly used in combination with a prostaglandin product.

Cabergoline administered after 40 days of gestation at 60 µg orally once daily, given to a 32 kg German shepherd dog, resulted in abortion after 7 days with no side effects.[24] In contrast to Europe, only an oral 0.5 mg tablet of cabergoline is available in the United States. Cabergoline may be difficult to administer because the tablets are 0.5 mg and the dose for a 10 kg dog is only 0.05 mg. An oral solution, much like that done with bromocriptine, could be formulated. Expense may be a factor with this drug.

COMBINED STUDIES

In an effort to reduce the side effects and increase the efficacy of prostaglandins and prolactin inhibitors, a combination of the two has been used.[25] Cloprostenol at 1.0 or 2.5 µg/kg/day injected subcutaneously in combination with cabergoline at a dose of 1.65 µg/kg/day subcutaneously daily for 5 days from midgestation was 100% effective (5/5), and side effects were less severe than with cloprostenol alone. In the group treated with the low dose, no adverse side effects were noted.[25]

Oral cabergoline at a dose of 5 µg/kg/day given until 2 days after fetal death (mean: 9 days) combined with cloprostenol at a dose of 1 µ/kg every other day until fetal death (mean: 3 injections) starting at 25 days after the LH peak resulted in 100% (5/5) of bitches resorbing fetuses.[26] Fetal death was documented with ultrasound. There were no side effects of treatment when the cabergoline was administered 1 hour after the cloprostenol, but the bitches did have a serosanguineous discharge that lasted an average of 16 days. Combinations of cabergoline, bromocriptine, and cloprostenol have been used[26] and include treatments of cabergoline administered orally for 10 days at a dose of 5 µg/kg combined with a single subcutaneous injection of 2.5 µg/kg cloprostenol at the start of the treatment; cabergoline administered orally for 10 days at a dose of 5 µg/kg combined with two subcutaneous doses of 1 µg/kg cloprostenol administered on the twenty-eighth and thirty-second day after the LH surge; bromocriptine administered orally at a dose of 30 µg/kg three times a day for 10 days plus a single subcutaneous dose of 2.5 µg/kg cloprostenol; bromocriptine at a dose of 30 µg/kg three times a day for 10 days plus two doses of 1 µg/kg cloprostenol. These combinations were administered to groups of five bitches starting at 28 days after the LH surge, and treatment was successful at inducing fetal resorption without overt abortion in all bitches except one that was administered the cabergoline and 1 µg/kg cloprostenol on the twenty-eighth and thirty-second day after the LH surge. Some bitches that resorbed litters had red cells, neutrophils, and cellular debris in the vaginal cytology smears for 4 to 21 days after treatment. All treated bitches did become pregnant on the subsequent estrous cycle, which occurred sooner than normally anticipated. The side effects of treatment included those commonly seen with prostaglandin when the high dose of cloprostenol was used, but the signs were not seen when the lower dose of cloprostenol was administered.[26] Using either a combination of increasing amounts of bromocriptine

mesylate (15 to 30 µg/kg orally, every 12 hours) and dinoprost tromethamine (0.1 to 0.2 mg/kg subcutaneously, every 24 hours), or bromocriptine mesylate (15 to 30 µg/kg orally, every 12 hours) and cloprostenol sodium (1 µg/kg subcutaneously every 48 hours) resulted in 100% success in inducing abortion in 25 bitches.[27] Side effects included pseudopregnancy and a mucoid sanguineous vulvar discharge for 3 to 10 days.

In an attempt to shorten the treatment period required to induce abortion with PGF$_{2\alpha}$, combination therapy with injectable PGF$_{2\alpha}$ and intravaginal PGE1 (misoprostol) has been used.[28] Prostaglandin was administered at a dose of 0.1 mg/kg subcutaneously three times a day for 2 days and then at a dose of 0.2 mg/kg subcutaneously three times a day to effect. Misoprostol (Cytotec, Pharmacia, Peapack, New Jersey) was administered at a dose of 1 to 3 µg/kg, deposited into the cranial vaginal vault once daily using a cat pilling device. The mean time to complete abortion in nine bitches using this combination was 5 days, as compared with a mean of 7 days previously reported for complete abortion induced with PGF$_{2\alpha}$ as a sole agent.

OTHER DRUGS

Drugs that have been investigated but are not commonly used to induce abortion in practice situations include isoquinolones, progesterone receptor antagonists, progesterone synthesis inhibitors, and progesterone blockers. The antiprogesterone compound mifepristone (Mifeprix, Danco, New York, NY), more commonly known as RU 486 or RU 38486 for its use in preventing human pregnancies, works by preventing the progesterone binding to uterine progesterone receptors and therefore preventing the action of progesterone from occurring. Oral administration of mifepristone at a dose 2.5 mg/kg twice daily for 4.5 days starting at the thirty-second day of gestation resulted in 100% (5/5) of the bitches having a decline in progesterone 2 days after treatment started and pregnancy loss with no side effects around 3 days after treatment initiation.[29] Four pregnancies were terminated in bitches that were at 35 to 39 days gestation using oral mifepristone.[30] Doses as low as 8.3 mg/kg and up to 20 mg/kg were administered orally for one or two treatments and abortion occurred within 2 to 11 days.[30] Mifepristone is available as a 200 mg tablet in the United States but is not labeled to terminate pregnancy in the bitch. Expense may be a factor.

Aglepristone (Alizine) is another progesterone blocker that is available in France, Norway, and Sweden but not the United States to terminate pregnancy in the bitch. Two doses of 10 mg/kg given subcutaneously 24 hours apart from day zero to the twenty-fifth day or on the twenty-sixth day to the forty-fifth day after mating caused uncomplicated abortions within 7 days in 100% (35/35) and 95.7% (66/69) of bitches, respectively.[31] If the bitch was in midpregnancy, a brown mucoid vaginal discharge was seen 24 hours before fetal expulsion. Other side effects included slight depression, transitory anorexia, and mammary gland congestion. A clinical trial using 124 bitches had similar effects, and fetal resorption occurred within 7 days with no subsequent reproductive effects noted.[32] In a subsequent study using the same dose at the thirtieth day of gestation, all (5/5) bitches aborted with no apparent side effects other than a slight mucoid discharge 1 week after administration.[33] A single bitch was bred and became pregnant after treatment.

Epostane inhibits steroid synthesis by inhibition of 3β-hydroxysteroid dehydrogenase and Δ5-4 isomerase, thereby preventing progesterone synthesis.[34] Epostane was 100% (23/23) effective at preventing whelping (compared with a 100% whelping rate for controls) when administered orally for 7 days at doses of 50 or 300 mg (given to beagle bitches

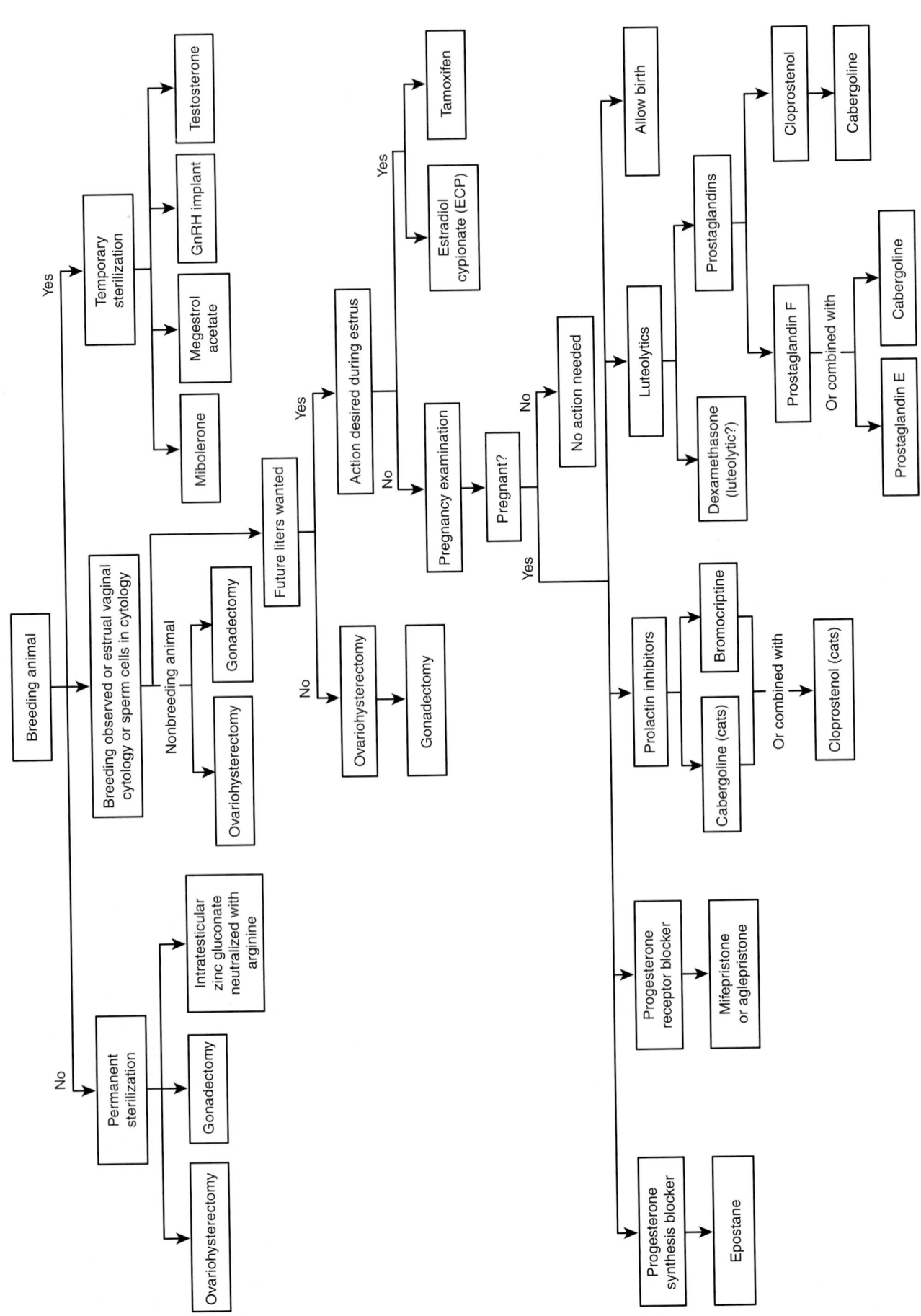

Figure 250-1 Algorithm for breeding.

weighing about 10 kg) starting the first day of diestrus.[34] No side effects were seen, and subsequent fertility was not affected because 94.8% (127/134) of all the bitches treated conceived on the next estrous cycle.[34] Epostane is not available in the United States.

DEXAMETHASONE

Two recent studies have been done using two different dose regimens of oral dexamethasone from 30 to 50 days of gestation.[35,36] The most effective dose regimen was the administration of oral dexamethasone using a 10-day dose schedule as follows: 0.2 mg/kg twice a day for 7 days, 0.16 mg/kg in the morning of the eighth day, 0.12 mg/kg in the evening of the eighth day, 0.08 mg/kg in the morning of the ninth day, 0.04 mg/kg in the evening of the ninth day, and 0.02 mg/kg the morning of the tenth day. A 10-day dose regimen was more effective than a shorter 7.5-day dose regimen in terminating pregnancies. At the author's institution a dose of 0.2 mg/kg twice a day for 10 days is used, with no tapering of the dose. The author and colleagues have observed no more than the anticipated side effects from not tapering the dose.

The initial fetal deaths with dexamethasone treatment were 5 to 9 days after initiation of the treatment; however, live fetuses were seen as long as 8 to 12 days after treatment started.[35] Pregnancies less than 40 days of gestation generally had no fetuses expelled, and the majority had no external signs of pregnancy loss.[36,35] A mild vaginal discharge was seen in only about 20% (26/75) of the bitches that resorbed fetuses. Abortion or resorption was generally complete 10 to 23 days after the treatment was initiated.[35] It is imperative that the pregnancy be re-examined with ultrasound and the drug continued until fetal death is noted. The treatment may fail if a treatment regimen is followed without checking for fetal loss. Although the exact mechanism of action is not known, dexamethasone may have a luteolytic effect. In the few bitches that had progesterone measured, the progesterone concentration fell to less than 1 ng/mL by the fourth day after treatment was initiated. If the initial treatment fails, a second treatment regimen may cause abortion, but most bitches treated a second time carried puppies to term.[35] Clinical failures have occurred using the recommended 10-day dose regimen. In the case of clinical failure, it may be advisable to treat with prostaglandin.

The main side effects of dexamethasone treatment include polydipsia and polyuria.[36,35] The polydipsia and polyuria usually began around 2 to 3 days after treatment started and were maximal 4 to 5 days later. The side effects generally subsided 3 to 4 days after the termination of treatment. Polydipsia and polyuria are not serious side effects but may be undesirable for dogs housed indoors in colder climates.

Successful pregnancies were obtained in 18 of 20 bitches bred during the first estrus after treatment and 2 of 2 on the second estrus. Therefore dexamethasone treatment appears to have no deleterious effects on future pregnancies and oral dexamethasone appears to be a safe, efficacious abortifacient in the bitch. Because dexamethasone is so readily available, inexpensive, has relatively minor side effects reported, does not require hospitalization, and is effective, it is the method recommended. Although not the ideal drug, it offers the most advantages of the ideal mismate drug when compared with all the other products available.

QUEEN

Permanent Sterilization

The same techniques applied to the canine can be applied to the feline, however much less information is available on the effects of OHE or ovariectomy on the queen. Toms are most commonly castrated; however, interest in sterilizing feral cats has led to some research on baited oral contraceptives. No intratesticular injections are approved for cats.

Termination of Pregnancy

The request for mismating or aborting queens is not common. Many of the same drugs can be used for mismate in cats as are used in dogs; however, the list is not nearly as inclusive. Pregnancy in the cat has similar aspects as the dog, in that the ovaries and corpora lutea are needed throughout pregnancy. Any drug altering luteal function will cause a queen to abort. The same strategy for determining pregnancy and the value of OHE can be used in the queen as in the bitch. The following drugs have been investigated for mismate in the queen.

Estrogen

Estrogen can be used shortly after copulation if an unwanted breeding was observed. Estradiol cypionate at a dose of 250 μg intramuscularly administered 6 days after coitus retarded embryo transport in the oviduct and also retarded ova development.[37] A single dose of 0.125 to 0.25 mg/cat of ECP given intramuscularly 40 hours after coitus has been suggested as an effective mismating regimen; however, no data is available on its efficacy.[38] Administration of ECP has the same potentially serious side effects in the queen as in the bitch (such as pyometra or aplastic anemia); however, the incidence is apparently less than the low incidence seen in the bitch.

Prostaglandin

Recent research investigating the period in gestation at which prostaglandin is most successful at inducing abortion in the queen confirmed that greater than or equal to 40 days appears to be a critical time for effectiveness.[39] Prostaglandin administration at doses associated with acceptable side effects before that time does not induce luteolysis. Despite the apparent resistance to abortion seen in other studies before the fortieth day of gestation, daily administration of 2 mg/cat $PGF_{2\alpha}$ subcutaneously for 5 days resulted in 100% (3/3) abortion when administered from the thirty-third day after mating.[40] However, queens exhibited nausea, vomiting, diarrhea, and prostration starting 10 minutes after treatment and continuing for an hour. All queens aborted fetuses within 6 days. This success before the fortieth day of gestation may be related to the timing of gestation from coitus. It is more difficult to measure the exact length of gestation in the queen compared with the dog, because estrus lasts about 8 days, regardless of the day of coitus. A subcutaneous dose of 0.2 mg/kg $PGF_{2\alpha}$ given twice the first day, followed by 0.5 mg/kg twice daily for up to 5 days was given to four queens at 30 days of gestation and four queens at 45 days of gestation.[39] One of four queens at 30 days aborted, whereas 75% (3/4) of queens at 45 days aborted. Queens that aborted had progesterone values less than 1.0 ng/mL, therefore verifying the eventual luteolytic effect of the prostaglandin.

Prolactin Inhibitors

Oral cabergoline at a dose of 5 to 15 μg/kg administered to feral cats 36 to 40 days of pregnancy for 4 to 9 days caused abortion in all (41/41) queens.[41] Combinations of prolactin inhibitors and prostaglandin have also been used to terminate pregnancy in the queen.[42] Cabergoline was administered orally at a daily dose of 5 μg/kg, and cloprostenol was administered subcutaneously every 2 days at a dose of 5 μg/kg starting at the thirtieth day after coitus. All (5/5) queens aborted after an average of 9 days of treatments. No side effects were seen, and queens that were bred subsequently became pregnant.

SUMMARY

Managing a mismate or pregnancy termination must be discussed with the client. Not using drugs and performing an OHE is usually the best alternative. If drugs are to be used, their use must be discussed with the client regarding safety, efficacy, convenience, compliance in treatment, side effects, and cost. As with most treatment regimens, familiarity with one treatment sometimes overrides using a superior method. It is therefore important to be aware of the most current literature available regarding protocols.

CHAPTER • 251

Cystic Endometrial Hyperplasia and Pyometra

Margaret V. Root Kustritz

INTRODUCTION

Pyometra is a chronic disease process with acute manifestation most commonly observed during the luteal phase of the estrous cycle, within 8 weeks of standing heat or ovulation induction.[1,2] Pyometra (from Greek, literally, "pus in the uterus") occurs when bacteria colonize a uterus with progressive hormone-mediated cystic hyperplasia of the endometrium. An inflammatory component is present, but the term *pyometra* is preferred to other published terms including pyometritis, catarrhal endometritis, and chronic cystic endometritis.[2-4] At no time should pyometra be confused with postpartum metritis.[2,5]

Incidence of pyometra in dogs and cats in the United States is poorly described, largely because the majority of bitches and queens are spayed relatively early in life in the United States. Many fewer bitches and queens undergo elective ovariohysterectomy (OHE) in European countries. It was reported in a Swedish study that 23% to 24% of bitches develop pyometra by 10 years of age.[6]

PATHOGENESIS

Pyometra has a two-step pathogenesis. The primary insult is development of cystic endometrial hyperplasia (CEH). The secondary insult is bacterial infection. A recent publication attempting to separate pyometra from CEH was unable to demonstrate independent development of the two entities in clinically ill bitches.[7]

CEH is a hormone-dependent change that develops after repeated estrous cycles in the bitch or queen. This histopathologic change can be induced experimentally with administration of either estrogen or progesterone, with progesterone having a greater effect.[8-10] Experimentally, the condition develops most quickly if progesterone is administered after priming with estrogen, as occurs during the spontaneous estrous cycle in bitches and in queens induced to ovulate.[10] Dogs that develop pyometra have not been demonstrated to have higher endogenous serum progesterone concentrations than normal dogs.[11] However, the normal down-regulation of estrogen receptors in the presence of rising serum progesterone concentrations may not occur in dogs with CEH-pyometra.[12,13] The progesterone-dominated uterus is more susceptible to proliferative and inflammatory changes, as has been demonstrated in studies in which uterine biopsies, scarification of the endometrium, or infusion of bacteria from bitches with pyometra into the uterus of healthy bitches were performed during the luteal phase.[14-17]

Another hormone that may be involved is insulin-like growth factor I (IGF-I). It has been demonstrated that the number of receptors for mitogenic IGF-I is higher in the uterus of bitches with pyometra than in normal bitches.[18] Serum concentration of prostaglandin metabolites also has been demonstrated to be elevated in bitches with pyometra; significance of this is unknown.[19]

Cats are considered to be induced (reflex) ovulators. However, a relatively high incidence of uterine disease in cats housed alone or with no exposure to an intact tom cat has promoted research that has documented apparent spontaneous ovulation to occur in as many as 39% to 40% of queens.[20-22] A tentative diagnosis of pyometra should not be discounted in queens with no known history of coitus.

Administration of exogenous hormones, especially estrogens (diethylstilbestrol [DES], estradiol cypionate [ECP]) and progestins (megestrol acetate, medroxyprogesterone acetate), may hasten development of CEH and subsequent pyometra in bitches and queens.[18,23,24] In one study of eight dogs with CEH-pyometra at the uncommonly young age of less than 3 years, six of eight had received exogenous ECP or megestrol acetate in the previous 6 months.[24]

Secondary bacterial infection is the next step in the pathogenesis of pyometra in bitches and queens. CEH can occur independent of infection or may be associated with formation of sterile intrauterine fluid (hydrometra or mucometra).[25,26] The most common bacterial organism isolated from the infected uterus of bitches and queens is *Escherichia coli*.[4,15,20,27] The biotype of *E. coli* associated with pyometra in a given bitch or queen has been identified to be virtually identical in most cases to that animal's biotype of fecal *E. coli*.[28,29] Other organisms that may be isolated include *Staphylococcus* spp., *Streptococcus* spp., *Proteus mirabilis*, and *Pseudomonas aeruginosa*.[4]

The development of pyometra in bitches and queens transpires thus: (1) development of CEH over repeated cycles; (2) movement of normal vaginal bacterial flora into the uterus during proestrus and estrus[30]; (3) functional closure of the cervix, decreased myometrial contractility, and increased secretory activity of uterine glands during the progesterone-dominated luteal phase; (4) colonization and overgrowth of coliform bacteria or other organisms with secondary endotoxemia (in coliform infections) and renal disease. Studies[15,31] have shown bitches with pyometra to be predisposed to lymphopenia and decreased lymphocyte function, as well as to neutrophil damage with subsequent decrease in phagocytic capacity of PMNs.

Conditions that may develop subsequent to pyometra include septic shock and renal failure. Lipopolysaccharide endotoxins released from the cell wall of Gram negative organisms stimulate release of cytokines, such as tumor necrosis factor (TNF), interleukins (Ils), and platelet activating factor (PAF), which cause vasodilation and subsequent decreased intravascular volume and tissue perfusion.[32] Cardiac arrhythmias may occur in animals with septic shock.[33] Hypoglycemia and hepatocellular damage commonly occur secondary to septicemia.[33]

Renal dysfunction secondary to pyometra is due to decreased renal tubular concentrating ability as the result of endotoxemia and possibly to glomerular changes.[3] Mild tubulointerstitial nephritis and other renal tubular changes have been reported to occur in as many as 38% of bitches with pyometra.[34] Glomerular filtration rate (GFR) has been demonstrated to be decreased in up to 75% of bitches with pyometra and azotemia; glomerular lesions were not demonstrated by histopathology in that study.[35] Other studies have reported glomerulonephritis development secondary to deposition of antigen and antibody complexes in the glomeruli.[2] Renal disease secondary to pyometra usually reverses with successful treatment for pyometra.

SIGNALMENT AND HISTORY

CEH develops after repeated cycles, so CEH-pyometra is usually a disease of older bitches and queens. CEH with minimal to no inflammatory component has been demonstrated to occur at an average age of 7.2 years in bitches.[9] Reported mean age at time of development of pyometra in bitches is 7.8 years, with a reported range of 1 to 15 years and a reported majority in bitches over 6 years of age.[4,24,36,37] Mean age at time of diagnosis of pyometra in queens is 5.3 years, with a majority of cases occurring in queens aged 5 to 6 years or more.[21,24,28]

Reported risk factors include breed, parity, and body condition. Breeds described to be at increased risk in two studies are the golden retriever, rough collie, rottweiler, and Cavalier King Charles spaniel.[6,37] Mongrels are at decreased risk.[37] In several studies, nulliparous animals have been described to be at increased risk of developing CEH-pyometra.[21,37] However, in queens, no correlation was noted between likelihood of developing pyometra and age at first breeding, or occurrence of breeding or queening.[38] One survey in bitches reported that less than 50% of bitches with pyometra were nulliparous.[23] Anecdotal reports suggest that pyometra may be more likely to occur in middle-aged to old queens that are morbidly obese than in older queens with normal body condition.[39]

Bitches with a history of false pregnancy (pseudocyesis) are not at increased risk for development of pyometra. Serum progesterone concentrations do not differ between normal bitches, bitches with a history of false pregnancy, and bitches with pyometra.[11] In a survey of dogs with pyometra compared with age-matched controls, the dogs with pyometra were significantly less likely to have a history of false pregnancy.[36]

Pyometra is usually diagnosed during the luteal (progesterone-dominated) phase of the estrous cycle. Reported mean interval from the last known standing heat in dogs to onset of clinical signs of pyometra is 7.1 weeks, with a range of zero to 15 weeks.[1,4,9,24,40] Reported mean interval from the last known heat in queens to onset of clinical signs of pyometra is 3.8 weeks.[24]

CLINICAL SIGNS

Dogs and cats with uncomplicated CEH or presence of sterile intrauterine fluid (hydrometra or mucometra) may be asymptomatic.[25,26,38] Clinical signs in bitches and queens with pyometra vary depending on patency of the cervix. As might be expected, cervical patency (open cervix pyometra) is associated with presence of vulvar discharge, and cervical impatency (closed cervix pyometra) is more commonly associated with abdominal distension (Table 251-1). Vulvar discharge is usually purulent; it is creamy, red-brown to green in color, and foul smelling. Onset of clinical signs may be acute or gradual; in general, more severe clinical signs are associated with cervical impatency.[5,9]

DIAGNOSIS

Definitive diagnosis of pyometra requires demonstration of presence of purulent fluid within the uterus. A tentative diagnosis is made by demonstration of uterine enlargement in a nonpregnant bitch or queen and usually is associated with clinical signs and physical examination findings of systemic disease and hematologic changes. A complete work-up for dogs and cats with possible pyometra includes a physical examination; radiography or ultrasonography of the abdomen; a complete blood count (CBC), serum chemistry profile and urinalysis; urine culture; and possibly measurement of progesterone in serum. Ancillary tests are performed as needed (e.g., culture of free abdominal fluid in pets with possible peritonitis and a coagulation profile in animals with overtly hemorrhagic discharge).

Physical examination findings often are unremarkable in dogs and cats with uncomplicated CEH. Severity of physical examination findings generally is greater in animals with closed cervix pyometra than in those with open cervix pyometra. Uterine enlargement may or may not be palpable (Table 251-2).

Table • 251-1

Reported Mean Prevalence of Clinical Signs in Bitches and Queens with Pyometra

	BITCHES (%)	QUEENS (%)
Purulent vulvar discharge	87	59
Lethargy	72	32
Anorexia	73	40
Abdominal distension	—	17
Polyuria/polydipsia (PU/PD)	28	9
Vomiting	36	16
Diarrhea	27	—

From Hardy RM, Osborne CA: Canine pyometra: pathophysiology, diagnosis and treatment of uterine and extra-uterine lesions. J Am Anim Hosp Assoc 10:245-268, 1974; Wheaton LG et al: Results and complications of surgical treatment of pyometra: a review of 80 cases. J Am Anim Hosp Assoc 25:563-568, 1989; Kenney KJ et al: Pyometra in cats: 183 cases (1979-1984). J Am Vet Med Assoc 191:1130-1132, 1987.

Table • 251-2

Reported Prevalence of Physical Examination Findings in Bitches and Queens with Pyometra

	BITCHES (%)	QUEENS (%)
Palpable uterine enlargement	31-40	68
Purulent vulvar discharge	75	39
Dehydration	15-28	33
Fever (>102.5° F)	41-43	20
Hypothermia (< 100.0° F)	3	—

From Hardy RM, Osborne CA: Canine pyometra: pathophysiology, diagnosis and treatment of uterine and extra-uterine lesions. J Am Anim Hosp Assoc 10:245-268, 1974; Wheaton LG et al: Results and complications of surgical treatment of pyometra: a review of 80 cases. J Am Anim Hosp Assoc 25:563-568, 1989; Kenney KJ et al: Pyometra in cats: 183 cases (1979-1984). J Am Vet Med Assoc 191:1130-1132, 1987.

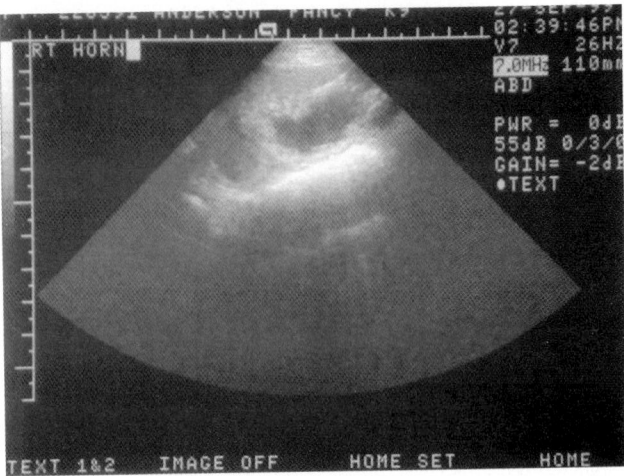

Figure 251-1 Ultrasound image of cystic endometrial hyperplasia (CEH) in a bitch. Reader should note the fluffy, mottled lining of the uterine wall on cross section.

Caution must be used when palpating a potentially friable distended uterus in any animal with possible pyometra.

Cervical patency is inferred from presence or absence of vulvar discharge. A narrow diameter endoscope may be passed the length of the vagina to attempt to see the cervix but usually it is only the appearance of fluid moving into the cranial vagina that allows one to state that the cervix is functionally open.[30]

Nonreproductive abnormalities that may be detected by physical examination in dogs and cats with pyometra include dehydration, which occurs secondary to renal disease, fever, and anorexia; fever due to infection; hypothermia due to septicemia or shock; and abdominal pain, which may be evident in animals with uterine distension or peritonitis due to leakage of purulent material from the uterus (see Table 251-2).[4,24,27,41]

Uterine enlargement that cannot be assessed by physical examination may be detected by abdominal radiography or ultrasonography. Pyometra occurs during diestrus; radiographic demonstration of uterine enlargement prior to 42 to 45 days postestrus may not allow differentiation of pyometra from pregnancy. Abdominal ultrasound is a more definitive diagnostic technique. Ultrasonographically, CEH appears as a fluffy, irregular, mottled thickening of the endometrium on uterine horns viewed in cross-section (Figure 251-1). CEH may not be visible in animals with distension of the uterine horns caused by large volumes of intrauterine fluid. Fluid-filled uterine horns are observed without difficulty in dogs and cats with pyometra and can readily be differentiated from pregnancy by 24 to 25 days postbreeding (Figure 251-2).[2,42]

Hematologic changes reported in dogs and cats with pyometra include changes in white blood cell (WBC) number and anemia. Leukocytosis, often to greater than 30,000 cells/µL, is reported to occur in 62% to 68% of dogs and 66% of cats with pyometra.[24,27,31] A regenerative left shift and monocytosis may accompany the leukocytosis. These changes are characteristic of a suppurative and exudative inflammatory process such as pyometra.[43] Lymphopenia is reported to occur in 8% to 35% of dogs and 5% of cats with pyometra.[24,27,31] Anemia of chronic infection is reported to occur in 25% of dogs and 4% of cats with pyometra.[24,27,43] Thrombocytopenia is rarely reported in dogs with pyometra and may be a component of disseminated intravascular coagulation (DIC).[43] Erythrocyte sedimentation rate is reported to be elevated in bitches with pyometra compared with normal diestrual bitches; usefulness of this change as a diagnostic test is equivocal.[44]

No changes are seen in the serum chemistry profile that are pathognomonic of pyometra in dogs and cats.[44] Azotemia due to dehydration and possible renal dysfunction is reported to occur in 18% to 26% of dogs and 12% of cats with pyometra.[4,27,35] Other changes that are present commonly include hyperproteinemia and increased alkaline phosphatase (ALP) and alanine transaminase (ALT).[2,27]

Urinalysis findings are suggestive of secondary renal disease. Proteinuria may or may not be present, regardless of presence of azotemia.[4,35] Urine specific gravity (USG) varies with hydration status and presence of polyuria due to renal disease subsequent to endotoxemia; in one study of 27 dogs with pyometra, 89% had USG less than 1.035.[35] In that same study, 22% of the dogs had concurrent urinary tract infection.[35]

Increases in serum progesterone concentration promote quiescence of the myometrium and may decrease efficacy of medical therapy. Although dogs and cats generally have clinical signs of pyometra while in diestrus, 16% to 38% of bitches and 20% of queens have been reported to have serum progesterone concentrations of less than 1 ng/mL at the time

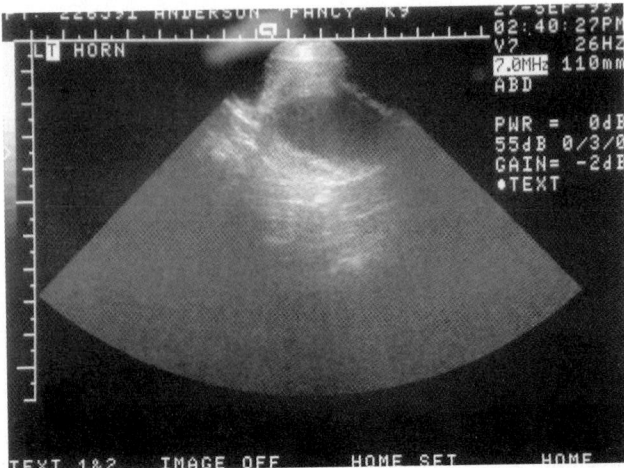

Figure 251-2 Ultrasound image of pyometra in a bitch. Reader should note the uterine horns distended with fluid.

of diagnosis.[15,20,40] This may be due to release of endogenous prostaglandin from the diseased endometrium with subsequent luteolysis. Knowledge of serum progesterone concentration may alter course of treatment.

TREATMENT

OHE is the best treatment of pyometra in dogs and cats. The underlying pathologic change, CEH, cannot be reversed with medical therapy. All animals with CEH are predisposed to pyometra after each subsequent estrus. Recurrence of secondary infection has been demonstrated to occur commonly with the biotype of organism that was causative of pyometra historically in a given animal, suggesting that medical therapy does not clear infection in all cases but rather decreases infection to a subclinical level.[45]

Complete OHE is always recommended. Caution must be used when handling the friable, distended uterus. Ovariectomy alone is reported to cause resolution of clinical signs of pyometra in dogs in 5 to 15 days.[9] This response probably is due to an iatrogenic decrease in serum progesterone concentration and is not a quick enough response to provide relief for critically ill animals.

Other surgical therapies reported involve placement of in-dwelling catheters transcervically to allow flushing of the uterus with antiseptic compounds or mucolytic agents.[4,46] Success with such techniques is not well described, and this mode of therapy is not recommended.

Medical therapy for pyometra is most appropriate for dogs and cats with a patent cervix. Medical therapy for animals with closed cervix pyometra has been reported.[23,43,47] Administration of ecbolic agents cause uterine contractions that propel purulent fluid against the internal cervical os and cause cervical dilation. However, in one survey of 30 dogs with pyometra, 13% had positive bacterial cultures of abdominal swabs despite lack of uterine rupture, suggesting leakage of purulent material through the friable uterine wall or via the uterine tubes.[15] All reported cases of salpingitis (uterine tube inflammation) in dogs were in bitches with pyometra.[2] Finally, with no clear knowledge of viability of uterine tissue, it is impossible to know whether causing uterine contractions may not cause uterine rupture. For these reasons, medical therapy for animals with closed cervix pyometra is not recommended.

All dogs and cats with pyometra, whether treated by OHE or medically, must be treated with antibiotics. An appropriate antibiotic choice is made based on culture and sensitivity testing of vulvar discharge or intrauterine content at the time of OHE. Good empiric choices for use while culture results are pending are ampicillin (22 mg/kg per os three times daily) and amoxicillin-clavulanate (14 mg/kg per os two times daily). Antibiotics should be administered for 2 to 4 weeks after OHE and until vulvar discharge is no longer evident in those animals treated medically. The bacterial infection of pyometra may be difficult to eradicate because of inability of antibiotics to diffuse into the pool of intrauterine fluid and possibly because of spontaneous formation of a glycocalyx biofilm that may bind antibiotics, again preventing ability of the antibacterial agent to reach embedded bacterial cells.[46]

Medical therapy for dogs and cats with pyometra can be considered if (1) the cervix is open, evidenced by presence of vulvar discharge; (2) the animal is still of breeding age, generally 6 years of age or less for dogs and 8 years of age or less for cats; (3) the animal is a valuable component of a breeding program; and (4) no evidence exists of renal disease or other sequelae to the pyometra. The effect of medical therapy may not be evident for up to 48 hours after initiation

of treatment.[5] The author feels it is unethical to prolong the animal's suffering unnecessarily if secondary disease is present.

Antibiotic therapy alone will not affect a cure in dogs and cats with pyometra. An ecbolic agent, which causes uterine contractions and promotes expulsion of the purulent fluid, must be administered concurrently. The best-described ecbolic agent for use in treatment of pyometra in small animals is prostaglandin $F_{2\alpha}$ ($PGF_{2\alpha}$). $PGF_{2\alpha}$ causes uterine contractions when administered once or twice daily and causes luteolysis when given twice daily. Because most animals with pyometra are in diestrus and may have increased serum progesterone concentrations, it may be beneficial to measure serum progesterone concentrations to determine if administration of luteolytic doses of $PGF_{2\alpha}$ is required. Prostaglandins cannot effect luteolysis in the first 5 days of diestrus in dogs at any dose and are not as effective a luteolytic agent in cats as in dogs. Analogues of $PGF_{2\alpha}$ such as cloprostenol, also are ecbolic and luteolytic in dogs and cats, but all doses described here refer to the native compound and should not be used with analogues.

$PGF_{2\alpha}$ is administered subcutaneously, at doses of 0.1 to 0.25 mg/kg.[23,47,48] Some authors recommend a gradual increase in dose over the first 48 to 72 hours of treatment to minimize side effects.[48] The lower end of the dose range generally is recommended for treatment of queens. Infusion of $PGF_{2\alpha}$ into the vaginal lumen also has been described in dogs.[49] $PGF_{2\alpha}$ is administered until the uterus nears normal size, as determined by abdominal palpation, radiography, or ultrasonography. In most cases, less than 7 days of treatment are required.[47]

Side effects of $PGF_{2\alpha}$ are referable to its causing contractions of the gastrointestinal (GI) tract and include hypersalivation, vomiting, and diarrhea. Queens may exhibit excessive grooming and restlessness. Side effects generally occur within 5 to 15 minutes of drug administration, subside within 30 to 60 minutes, and usually lessen in severity with each subsequent injection. The clinician can minimize side effects by using lower doses of $PGF_{2\alpha}$, by diluting the volume of $PGF_{2\alpha}$ to be given with normal saline before administration, and by walking dogs after it is given. Concurrent administration of atropine (500 mg/kg intramuscularly) also may be beneficial.[2] $PGF_{2\alpha}$ is not approved for treatment of pyometra in dogs and cats in the United States.

Progesterone receptor blockers, for example mifepristone and aglepristone, are reported to be efficacious for treatment of pyometra in dogs and cats, with minimal side effects.[50-52] These drugs are not available for veterinary use in the United States. Other compounds described for treatment of pyometra, none of which are recommended, include estrogen, androgens, oxytocin, and ergot alkaloid derivatives.[9,48]

Ancillary supportive therapy to be used includes intravenous fluid therapy and maintenance of normal body temperature. Other ancillary treatments reported for treatment of pyometra in dogs and cats include use of hypertonic saline with 60% dextran to combat septic shock and promote renal blood flow, use of hemoglobin glutamer-200 to enhance tissue delivery of oxygen in animals with poor oxygenation secondary to shock, and treatment with equine-derived antibodies against endotoxin to combat renal disease due to endotoxemia.[32,53,54]

At the subsequent estrus, a sample should be collected from as far forward in the vagina as possible early in proestrus (bitches) or estrus (queens), and appropriate antibiotic therapy should be administered for at least the duration of proestrus and estrus while the cervix is open and the uterus is vulnerable to infection with bacteria ascending from the vagina. Antibiotic therapy is recommended even if the bitch or queen will not be bred during that estrus. Because fertility is compromised and because the bitch or queen still has CEH and a predisposition to pyometra, she should be bred and all desired offspring obtained as quickly as is feasible. The dog or cat should then be spayed as soon as her breeding life is over or if pyometra recurs.

PROGNOSIS

Spontaneous resolution of mild inflammatory changes overlying CEH has been reported to occur subsequent to plasma cell infiltration.[10,55] Animals with pyometra do not recover spontaneously.

Overall reported success rate for treatment of pyometra in dogs ranges from 46% to 100%; reported success rate for treatment of pyometra in one study was 92% in cats.[2] In general, those animals that do not recover have concurrent disease or complications due to sepsis or toxemia.[24]

After medical therapy, reported prevalence of recurrence of pyometra in bitches is 10% to 77% within 27 months of therapy.[2,45] Other reported long-term complications include persistent anestrus, failure to conceive, and spontaneous abortion.[23] In two studies evaluating fertility of bitches after medical treatment for pyometra, reported percentages of dogs bred that went on to whelp were 64% and 87%.[23,48] In the former study, prognosis for future fertility was best in those animals requiring less than 6 days of treatment with $PGF_{2\alpha}$.[23] Prognosis for future fertility generally is better in queens, with a reported queening rate of 90% in those queens bred after medical therapy for pyometra.[2]

UTERINE STUMP PYOMETRA

Pyometra of the uterine stump occurs rarely in dogs and cats. It is assumed to be associated with remnant ovarian tissue or administration of exogenous estrogen or progestins in most cases, because any remnants of endometrial tissue should be quiescent in the absence of hormonal stimulation. Clinical signs are as described for pyometra in intact animals. Diagnosis is best made by abdominal ultrasound; pyometra of the uterine stump appears as a cystic mass near the bladder. Diagnosis of ovarian remnants is described in Chapter 247. Treatment includes systemic antibiotic therapy and surgical removal of the uterine stump and ovarian remnants, if any.

CONCLUSION

CEH is a hormone-mediated gradual change of the uterine lining. Presence of CEH predisposes the uterus to infection; infection overlying CEH with subsequent formation of intrauterine purulent fluid is pyometra. Nulliparous animals may be predisposed; those animals with a history of false pregnancy are not predisposed to pyometra. Diagnosis requires demonstration of uterine enlargement and presence of purulent intrauterine fluid. Neutrophilia with a regenerative left shift and monocytosis often are present. Secondary renal disease may occur subsequent to endotoxemia in dogs and cats with coliform infection. OHE is the treatment of choice in most cases. Medical therapy with $PGF_{2\alpha}$ may be attempted in young, valuable bitches and queens with a patent cervix and no evidence of secondary renal disease.

CHAPTER • 252

Canine Female Infertility

Gary C.W. England

INTRODUCTION

Over recent years there has been increased awareness of canine female infertility, particularly in dogs bred for working and showing purposes. The true extent of infertility is unknown, although reproductive failure is common. It is with increasing frequency that breeders and managers of breeding colonies approach their veterinarian for help with reproductive problems. In some circumstances reduced fertility may not be fully appreciated because breeding is relatively infrequent when compared with other domestic species. In addition, wide breed variations exist (particularly in litter size) that make it difficult to compare animals of different breeds. Certain breeds appear to have an increased incidence of infertility.

The normal expectation of fertility in the bitch is a whelping rate of 70% to 80% after mating to a male with normal semen quality. Variations from this exist, depending in particular upon the age of the bitch. Average peak reproductive efficiency occurs at approximately 3 years of age, and a significant decline occurs in the number of pups born to bitches aged 7 years and older.[1]

The investigation of infertility is complicated by the fact that fertility problems may be difficult to recognize. Failure to conceive does not result in an immediate return to estrus. Furthermore, pseudopregnancy is a normal physiologic event and, in some bitches that do not whelp, the owner may have confused the signs of pseudopregnancy with pregnancy. However, the early diagnosis of pregnancy is now possible using ultrasonography, the detection of acute-phase proteins in serum, and the measurement of serum relaxin concentrations. Early pregnancy diagnosis helps allow prompt investigation into why an individual bitch fails to produce live offspring.

As with other species, the causes of infertility may be classified as structural (including congenital, acquired, and neoplastic diseases), functional (including endocrinologic abnormalities), infectious, or managemental. However, what is most helpful to the clinician is the way in which these cases are presented, namely (1) failure to cycle, (2) abnormal estrous cycles, (3) normal estrous cycles with failure of copulation, (4) normal estrous cycles with copulation (distant from ovulation) and conception failure, (5) normal estrous cycles with copulation (close to ovulation) but conception failure, or (6) normal estrous cycles and conception with subsequent pregnancy failure.[2]

INVESTIGATION OF INFERTILITY

Many cases of "infertility" are caused by a lack of owner understanding of normal canine reproductive physiology. For example, considerable normal variations exist in the onset of puberty between animals and in the timing of ovulation from the onset of proestrus.

The previous breeding history, including parity and litter size, together with information regarding the stud dog, are probably the most important factors (one of the common causes of infertility is related to the male). Additional information concerning the onset of puberty, present cyclicity, general medical history, and the administration of pharmaceutical compounds (steroids in particular) may also be useful. After a full clinical examination to rule out systemic disease, specific examination of the reproductive tract should be performed. This should include inspection of the external genitalia, palpation of the mammary glands, digital examination of the vestibule and caudal vagina, and transabdominal uterine palpation.

Several other techniques are useful for the investigation of reproductive disease, including exfoliative vaginal cytology, vaginal endoscopy, transcervical collection of uterine cells to evaluate uterine disease, and ultrasound imaging of the ovaries and uterus. Laparoscopy and laparotomy may also be valuable for inspection of the uterus, uterine tubes, and ovaries but are infrequently used due to their invasive nature and the requirement for general anesthesia. Measurement of circulating hormone concentration has a number of indications. It can be used to confirm the presence of gonadal tissue, to detect hormone secreting neoplasms and cystic structures, and for the prediction and confirmation of ovulation.

CLINICAL PRESENTATIONS OF INFERTILITY

Failure to Cycle

Failure to cycle may be either primary (no estrus activity before 24 months [i.e., delayed puberty]) or secondary (no estrus activity within 12 months of a previous cycle [i.e., prolonged anoestrus]). In most cases a specific disease process may be responsible for this problem, and careful investigation for an underlying cause is important for appropriate treatment and prognosis. Estrus induction may be attempted with either primary or secondary failure when a specific cause has been identified.

Delayed Puberty   The age at puberty ranges between 6 and 24 months. Most bitches cycle within 1 to 6 months of attaining adult height and weight, and the age of puberty can be influenced by the breed, body weight, and environmental conditions. In general, bitches that do not reach puberty by 2 years of age are considered to have delayed puberty. It is common for there to be few signs associated with the first estrus and therefore some bitches which are thought to have delayed puberty may have simply had an unobserved estrus. Increased serum progesterone concentrations (> 2.0 ng/mL

[6.5 nmol/L]) demonstrates that ovulation has occurred within the last 60 days (i.e., the estrus has been missed).

Investigation of delayed puberty involves collection of information on housing and diet (because poor environmental conditions and nutrition may be associated with failure to cycle) and a thorough clinical examination to rule out chronic debilitating disease.

An underlying chromosomal abnormality may also cause delayed puberty. Many of these bitches are phenotypically abnormal (having a small cranially positioned vulva and developing clitoral enlargement at puberty). A smaller proportion of bitches are phenotypically normal but have an abnormal complement of sex chromosomes that results in ovarian hypoplasia or ovarian dysgenesis. Establishing a karyotype usually demonstrates chromosomal abnormalities such as 77XO, 79XXX, 79XXY, and 78XX/78XY.[3] In normal bitches with no underlying disease, estrus induction can be attempted as described later.

Prolonged Anestrus   The average interestrus interval is 31 weeks; although some variation occurs around this mean value, this has no apparent effect on fertility. Certain breeds, for example the Basenji, cycle only once per year. The reason for these variations is unclear. Prolonged anestrus represents an interestrus interval greater than anticipated for that particular animal (usually more than 12 months from the previous cycle). Failure of normal reproductive cyclicity has several causes. A common problem is the failure of observation of the signs of estrus, particularly in kenneled bitches. This may occur in fastidious bitches, which quickly remove any vulval discharge, or when the discharge is scant. Serum progesterone concentrations greater than 2.0 ng/mL (6.5 nmol/L) indicate a missed estrus and ovulation within the previous 2 months.

Initial investigations should include a thorough history and examination for chronic systemic disease and evaluation of the general body condition. Important factors in the history are any indications of chronic disease and any previous or concurrent treatments or medication. Drug-induced anestrus should be considered when the interestral interval is prolonged; pharmaceutical preparations that have the ability to prevent estrus include glucocorticoids, anabolic steroids, androgens, and progestogens. Investigation of thyroid function may also be useful because some evidence indicates a relationship between thyroid hormone insufficiency and abnormalities of the estrous cycle. Hypothyroidism has been associated with prolonged anestrus and infertility. The mechanism of this abnormality has not been fully established; however, prolactin is released after the injection of thyrotropin-releasing hormone (TRH). Therefore factors that affect endogenous TRH release probably affect prolactin and thyroid function. Low concentrations of serum thyroid hormones and failure to respond to a stimulation test may be used to confirm the condition, although clinically these animals usually have typical clinical signs associated with hypothyroidism. After replacement therapy most bitches return to estrus within 6 months. Interestingly however, hypothyroidism in greyhounds was not shown to be related to poor reproductive function[4] and a consistent relationship between thyroid disease and reproductive function has yet to be established. When no underlying disease is present, estrus induction may be attempted.

Progesterone-producing ovarian cysts have been described in the bitch, producing prolonged interestrus intervals and cystic endometrial hyperplasia. Ovarian cysts may be identified ultrasonographically and the diagnosis confirmed by serial measurement of serum progesterone concentrations. Medical treatment has not been successful, and usually the cystic ovary needs to be surgically removed. These cysts should not be confused with cysts originating from the ovarian bursa that are of no significance.

In some cases, ovarian neoplasms that produce either progesterone or androgens result in a failure to return to cyclical activity. Such tumors are rare and are usually associated with chronic wasting and an abdominal mass effect with ascites. Treatment is surgical removal.

Some bitches have normal cyclical activity, including follicular growth and ovulation, without obvious external signs of proestrus or estrus. This is often called *silent estrus* (silent heat) and is common in certain breeds, greyhounds for example. The condition may be the reason the owner overlooks the signs of estrus. Ovulation may be confirmed by measurement of serum progesterone concentration as described previously. Alternatively, the weekly examination of exfoliative vaginal cytology will allow anticipation and monitoring of estrus.

Premature ovarian failure has been suggested as a rare but permanent cause of anestrus in previously normal bitches.[5] For an accurate diagnosis of these cases, investigation of the karyotype and measurement of serum concentrations of luteinizing hormone (LH), follicle-stimulating hormone (FSH), and thyroid hormone should be undertaken.[3] In valuable breeding animals, estrus induction regimens may be contemplated; however, no information is available concerning the efficacy of these treatments in animals with premature ovarian failure.

Induction of Estrus
Estrus-induction may be attempted when no underlying abnormality has been detected in bitches older than 2.5 years with delayed puberty or in bitches with prolonged anestrus. A variety of agents may be used for this purpose, including prolactin inhibitors (cabergoline or bromocriptine), equine chorionic gonadotropin (eCG) with human chorionic gonadotropin (hCG), gonadotropin-releasing hormone (GnRH), and estrogens. Unlike other domestic species, it is not possible to induce estrus by shortening the luteal phase using prostaglandins because the luteal phase is followed by a variable, but prolonged, period of anestrus.

The most useful method of estrus induction is the administration of prolactin inhibitors (although these may have a variable effect in bitches with delayed puberty). Prolactin plays a role in the regulation of interestrous intervals, possibly by affecting gonadotropin secretion, ovarian responsiveness to gonadotropins, or both. When prolactin inhibitors are administered daily (cabergoline at 5.0 µg/kg/day) during prolonged anestrus, a rapid return to estrus occurs (usually within 30 days). If treatment is stopped once proestrus has begun, a high pregnancy rate usually occurs that is similar to that seen in natural cycles.

For bitches with delayed puberty it may be necessary to attempt estrus induction using gonadotropins, if the administration of prolactin inhibitors fail. Many protocols have used exogenous gonadotropins for the induction of estrus, and commonly low doses of eCG (20 IU/kg for 5 days) with a single administration of hCG (500 IU/bitch on the fifth day) are recommended.

Although several reports document the value of estrogens and GnRH (either in pulses or the use of a superagonist), such regimes are not commonplace in clinical practice because whelping rates are relatively low.

Abnormal Estrous Cycles
Split Estrus A short interval (2 to 12 weeks later) between clinical signs of estrus is often described as a *split estrus*. This occurs most frequently at the pubertal estrus but can occur at any age. An initial phase of follicular growth and estrogen secretion occur, but the follicles regress and signs of estrus disappear. Subsequently a second follicular phase appears. In some cases this may be repeated several times until finally the bitch ovulates normally. This syndrome is confusing because it may be thought that the bitch has failed to ovulate or that fertilization with subsequent resorption or abortion has occurred. The recognition of split estrus syndrome is important to ensure that mating is achieved at the correct time. In some cases, induction of ovulation may be attempted using hCG, although it can be difficult to be certain at which point to administer this preparation. This is most successful when administered at the peak of vaginal epithelial cell cornification.

Ovulation Failure The frequency of ovulation failure is approximately 1% of estrus cycles,[6] and clinicians commonly make the diagnosis by serial monitoring of serum progesterone concentrations. This condition is likely to have a similar cause to those bitches with split estrus (possibly caused by low concentration of LH or LH receptor). Attempts to induce ovulation during estrus using 500 IU/kg hCG between 1 day before to 1 day after the first mating may be successful.

Prolonged Proestrus or Estrus The time at which bitches ovulate after the onset of vulval bleeding is very variable. Usually this is between the sixth and twentieth day after proestrus began. For the average bitch, the surge in serum LH occurs on the tenth day; ovulation follows 2 days later. However, many normal bitches do not ovulate at this time, and most bitches with alleged prolonged proestrus are actually at the extremes of normality; they simply ovulate later in the cycle than anticipated. In some, normal ovulation occurs 30 days after the onset of proestrus.

These animals do not require treatment, but careful assessment of the optimum mating time, usually by evaluation of vaginal cytology or measurement of serum progesterone (see later). It is unlikely that the administration of hCG would produce normal ovulation earlier in the cycle; however, little data is available on such use of this agent.

Estrogen-secreting follicular cysts may produce persistent estrus. These bitches may be brought to a veterinarian because of the inconvenience; however, the persistent elevation of serum estrogen can also lead to bone marrow suppression with anemia and thrombocytopenia.

Ultrasonographically large (8 to 12 mm diameter) fluid-filled follicles may be identified. These must be carefully differentiated from normal follicles and early corpora lutea, both of which have central fluid-filled cavities. Some follicular cysts respond to alternate-day administration of hCG on three occasions. Failing this, cysts may respond to progestogen administration using drugs such as megestrol acetate. With the latter an increased risk of pyometra is seen, because the progestogen is administered after a prolonged period of estrogen priming. Ovariectomy may be required if no response to exogenous hormone therapy is seen. Cyst-like structures are frequently identified around the ovaries at routine surgery. These are often parabursal in origin and have no significance on cyclicity or fertility.

Ovarian Neoplasia Ovarian neoplasms are not common in the bitch, accounting for approximately 1.0% of all neoplasms.[7] The mean age of occurrence is 8 years, although some bitches may develop neoplasia as early as 7 months of age. Tumors that release estrogen may produce signs of persistent estrus and bone marrow suppression, although clinical signs are also often related to a mass effect or ascites. Neoplasia may be most effectively diagnosed at ultrasound examination. The tumors may be germ cell, epithelial, or sex-cord stromal in origin. They do not commonly metastasize. Ovariohysterectomy is the treatment of choice; care should be taken not to rupture neoplasms during surgery because metastatic spread is often by transcoelomic seeding.

Normal Estrous Cycle with Failure of Copulation

Behavioral Problems   Some bitches are frightened and traumatized by attempted breeding and may refuse subsequent mating. Other bitches may be "humanized" or are too familiar with the male and do not exhibit normal estrus behavior. Observation of the bitch at attempted mating should allow identification of typical behavior patterns that may include marked submission or aggression. Careful management of the virgin bitch is important to ensure that behavioral abnormalities do not become established.

Vestibulovaginal and Vestibulovulval Abnormalities
Strictures of the caudal reproductive tract are common. Circular strictures or transverse bands are usually found at the junction of the vestibule and the vagina, although vestibulovulval strictures can also be identified. Vestibulovaginal abnormalities are often first noted during attempted mating when they cause pain or a failure to achieve intromission. Small constrictions and fibrous bands may be manually broken down under general anesthesia when the bitch is in proestrus or estrus. Mating may be allowed later during the same estrus. Surgical exploration via an episiotomy may be required for larger transverse bands.

Vaginal Hyperplasia   Vaginal hyperplasia is an accentuated response of the caudal vaginal floor to normal circulating estrogen concentrations. Usually the vaginal mucosa cranial to the external urethral orifice is involved and becomes edematous and thickened. This mass of tissue may result in pain at coitus in some bitches, and in others it may rapidly increase in size and protrude from the vulva preventing coitus. The latter condition is sometimes referred to as a *vaginal prolapse* (correctly, it is a prolapse of hyperplastic vagina). Occasionally the circumference of the vagina and not just the floor may be involved.

In most bitches the mass decreases in size at the end of estrus, therefore conservative management with local cleansing and lubrication are sufficient. Ovariohysterectomy during the subsequent anestrus will prevent recurrence. In bitches that are required for breeding, artificial insemination may be necessary or submucosal surgical resection of the tissue performed during early estrus before mating. A minority of surgically treated cases recur; however, the use of surgery has been questioned because a familial tendency has been reported in certain breeds.[8] Although rare, true prolapse of the nonhyperplastic vagina has been reported during estrus when it also may prevent mating.

Congenital Anomalies of the External Genitalia
Hypoplasia of the vulva has been described and may be associated with pain at coitus and often a perivulval dermatitis. Considerable breed variation is seen in the normal vulval anatomy; for example, the greyhound has small external genitalia.

Congenital abnormalities including vulvar atresia and vulvar agenesis are rare, and may cause chronic vaginitis.

Vaginal Hypoplasia and Aplasia   Segmental aplasia of the Müllerian duct system may be *partial*, producing vaginal hypoplasia, or *complete*, resulting in vaginal aplasia. The condition is rare and may cause the retention of uterine fluid with signs similar to pyometra. Diagnosis may be made by palpation or positive-contrast radiographic examination of the vagina.

Normal Estrous Cycle with Copulation (Distant from Ovulation) and Conception Failure

The most common reason for failure of conception is inappropriate timing of mating. This is often because mating is planned a set number of days after the onset of proestrus (often the twelfth to the sixteenth day). Although the majority of bitches ovulate between 10 and 14 days after the onset of proestrus, some ovulate as early as the fifth day or as late as the thirtieth day. Therefore should a bitch be mated on the twelfth to the sixteenth day this can be inappropriate and result in failure of conception. A further complication is that bitches are not necessarily consistent in the day on which they ovulate between subsequent estrus cycles. Detecting the time of ovulation is difficult because the behavioral signs of estrus do not always correlate with the changes in peripheral hormones, and often the dog and bitch are not allowed to display normal courtship behavior.

Fertilization Period and Fertile Period   Spontaneous ovulation occurs approximately 48 hours after the surge in serum LH. Eggs are released as primary oocytes that must reach the metaphase of the second meiotic division before fertilization can occur. This maturation takes 48 to 60 hours. Oocytes remain fertilizable for a further 2 to 3 days, therefore the time span over which fertilization may occur, termed the *fertilization period*, is between 4 and 7 days after the LH surge (i.e., between 2 and 5 days after ovulation).

Dog sperm can remain viable and fertile within the uterus and uterine tubes for at least 6 days. Therefore it is possible for matings that take place before the fertilization period to result in conception. A second term is therefore used, the fertile period, which encompasses the fertilization period and the time that sperm survive within the female reproductive tract before ovulation and oocyte maturation. The *fertile period* extends from 3 days before until 7 days after the preovulatory LH surge (i.e., between 5 days before and 5 days after ovulation).

The optimal time for mating is during, or immediately preceding, the fertilization period. The period of peak fertility ranges from 1 day before to 5 or 6 days after the LH surge.

Determination of the Optimal Time of Mating
Clinical and management assessments   In laboratory beagles a close association exists between the time of the LH surge and the onset of standing estrus. However, in many breeding bitches a marked variation exists in this relationship, with the LH surge occurring between 3 days before to 9 days after the onset of estrus. Teasing the bitch has little value in determining the fertile period. Assessment of the volume and color of the vaginal discharge is similarly unreliable.

One clinical assessment that may be useful is the timing of vulval softening. During proestrus, the vulva and perineal tissues become enlarged and increasingly turgid in response to increasing estrogen. At the time of the LH surge, serum estrogen concentrations begin decreasing at the same time that serum progesterone concentrations increase. With this change a reduction is seen in edema of the reproductive tract, with the consequence that a distinct softening of the vulva occurs. In cases where only clinical assessments are available for the determination of the optimum time for breeding, a combination of the onset of standing estrus and the timing of vulval softening may be used. Each of these events occurs on average 1 or 2 days before ovulation. Therefore breeding should be planned commencing on the next day or so for natural mating or commencing 3 days later for preserved semen inseminations.

Hormone measurement   Measurement of peripheral serum concentrations of LH is a reliable and accurate method of determining the optimum time to mate. However, in many countries it is difficult to obtain reliable LH measures in clinical practice, because enzyme-linked immunosorbent assay (ELISA) kits are not always available. Serum progesterone concentrations begin to increase toward the end of proestrus at the time of the LH surge. Luteinizing follicles produce this increase in progesterone; therefore serial monitoring of serum progesterone concentrations allows anticipation of ovulation. Test kits designed to measure progesterone by ELISA are commercially available and have been shown to be useful for predicting the optimum mating time in the bitch. Breeding or insemination should be planned between 4 and 6 days after serum progesterone concentrations exceed 2.0 ng/mL (6.5 nmol/L) (the concentration typically observed at the time of the LH surge). Some reports suggest that breeding should commence 1 day after values exceed 8.0 to 10.0 ng/mL (25.0 to 32.0 nmol/L), which are commonly seen at the beginning of the fertilization period. Progesterone concentration may also be measured in whole blood or vaginal fluid.

Vaginal cytology   The examination of exfoliative vaginal epithelial cells is frequently used to monitor the estrous cycle. During proestrus, increased serum estrogen concentrations cause thickening of the vaginal mucosa, which becomes a keratinized squamous epithelium. Surface vaginal epithelial cells may be collected using either a moistened swab or by aspiration. The relative proportions of different types of epithelial cells can be used as a marker of the endocrine environment. Several methods for staining of cells and various indices of cornification and keratinization have been suggested. In general, the fertile period can be predicted by calculating the percentage of epithelial cells that appear cornified using a modified Wright-Giemsa stain. Breeding should be attempted throughout the period when more than 80% of epithelial cells are cornified. Although this is a useful guide, some bitches reach peak values of only 60% cornification, and in others there may be two peaks of cornification. Neutrophils are generally absent from the vaginal smear during estrus because the keratinized epithelium is impervious to these cells. Their reappearance during late estrus reflects the breakdown of this epithelium. The return of neutrophils to the vaginal smear has been used by some workers as an indicator of the time of optimum fertility.

Some bitches demonstrate poor cellular changes in the vaginal smear; in some, neutrophils may be found throughout estrus (the extent of these variations has not been quantified). Despite these variations, at the Guide Dogs for the Blind Association in the United Kingdom, mating based on vaginal cytology was found to increase the pregnancy rate and litter size of bitches compared with a similar group mated only based on the onset of proestrus.[9] Whelping rates have been consistently maintained above 90% over a 10-year period since the introduction of this technique.

Vaginal endoscopy   Endoscopic assessment of the vaginal epithelial contour and profile, mucosal color, and color of any vaginal fluid may be of use for estimating the time of the fertilization period. Enlarged edematous pink or pinkish-white mucosal folds are present during proestrus and estrus. Progressive shrinking of these folds accompanied by pallor occurs during the preovulatory decline in estrogen. Subsequently, mucosal shrinkage is accompanied by wrinkling of the mucosal folds that become distinctly angulated and dense cream to white in color. These gross changes have been used to assess the fertile period. Jeffcoate and Lindsay[10] proposed a scoring scheme to allow description and recording of the vaginoscopic changes. These clinicians also suggested that vaginoscopy could be used to indicate the end of the fertilization period.

Evaluation of Cervicovaginal Secretions   Many workers have reported changes in the nature of the cervicovaginal secretions in relation to the fertile period. These include changes in electrical resistance, glucose concentration, and mucus crystallization patterns. None of these techniques has been subject to detailed validation or widely used in clinical practice.

Normal Estrous Cycle and Copulation (Close to Ovulation) with Conception Failure

Infertile Male   An important aspect of infertility is the influence of the male. Poor semen quality can reduce the litter size or result in conception failure. Knowledge of a comprehensive breeding soundness examination of the male is mandatory when investigating a female that might be infertile.

Uterine Disease   A common ultrasonographic finding in bitches that fail to become pregnant despite mating to a fertile male during the fertilization period is the presence of cystic endometrial hyperplasia.

Although the exact relationship between this observation and fertility is yet to be proved, the existence of underlying endometrial disease may contribute to infertility by allowing persistence of commensal bacteria within the uterus (after introduction through the open cervix during estrus) or by interfering with normal placental development. Ultrasonographic detection of cystic endometrial hyperplasia is best achieved during the luteal phase. Cystlike lesions are observed most commonly in middle-aged and elderly bitches and anecdotally may precede the development of later pyometra. Treatment regimes to aid fertility have yet to be fully evaluated.

Aplasia of the Tubular Genital Tract   An uncommon cause of infertility is aplasia of one segment of the uterine horn, uterine tube, or both. Frequently this is a unilateral condition that does not influence fertility. Bilateral agenesis is associated with infertility, although the bitch may cycle, ovulate, and mate normally. Diagnosis may be made by positive contrast vagino-uterogram performed during estrus. Laparotomy is a more valuable diagnostic tool.

Normal Estrous Cycle and Copulation with Pregnancy Failure

Habitual Abortion   Some clinicians have implicated progesterone deficiency as a cause of repeated abortion in bitches.[11] Despite this contention, the minimum concentration of progesterone in serum required to support the pregnancy is only 2.0 ng/mL.[12] Measurement of progesterone concentration at the time of an abortion often reveals that concentrations are low; however, this is likely to be the result of the abortion rather than the cause of the abortion. Insufficient luteal function has been demonstrated after estrus induction regimens[13] and in one case of oophoritis.[14] Serum progesterone concentrations of bitches with habitual abortion are usually similar to those of normal pregnant bitches. Progesterone or progestogen supplementation during pregnancy may produce masculinized female pups and cryptorchid male pups, and it may possibly impair or delay parturition resulting in fetal death. Progestogen therapy should therefore be restricted to those cases in which a true luteal insufficiency has been diagnosed.

The majority of cases of abortion and resorption may be documented using real-time B-mode ultrasound. In some cases only a single conceptus is lost and the remaining pregnancy continues normally. Most cases of resorption and abortion are related to an abnormal uterine environment (cystic endometrial hyperplasia, see previous discussion), embryonic and fetal defects, or are the result of infectious agents.

Infectious Causes of Pregnancy Loss

Canine herpesvirus   Canine herpesvirus may cause infertility, abortion, stillbirths, and genital lesions in the bitch.[15] In the pregnant bitch, placental lesions and infection of the fetus occurs. Experimental data suggests that infection during early pregnancy results in fetal death and subsequent mummification, infection during midpregnancy results in abortion, and infection during late pregnancy results in premature birth. The virus has also been recovered from vesicular lesions on the genitalia of bitches, and frequently these lesions are evident at the onset of proestrus, suggesting that venereal transmission is probably important. Viral recrudescence from the vesicular lesions may be stimulated by the stress of pregnancy and parturition. Canine herpes virus infection is becoming increasingly recognized within Europe. As a result of this, a vaccine has recently been licensed for use in breeding animals and is commercially available in France and the United Kingdom.

Brucella canis   This is the only bacterium known to be a specific cause of infertility in the bitch. Infection can produce abortion and infertility. Between 1.5 and 6.6% of dogs in the USA have antibodies to the organism. Brucella can be transmitted by contact with aborted fetal or placental tissue, contact with the vaginal discharge of infected bitches, venereal transmission or congenital infection.

Abortion occurs most commonly between the forty-fifth and fifty-fifth day of pregnancy; however, there may be embryonic resorption or the birth of stillborn or (more rarely) weak pups. The isolation of the bacterium from blood or aborted tissue is diagnostic of the disease; however, there may be prolonged periods when the bitch is not bacteremic, and a negative blood culture does not rule out infection. Fortunately, diagnosis using the plate agglutination test for screening and tube agglutination for confirmation is not difficult. Treatment of the condition with a combination of streptomycin and tetracycline is often effective in clinical cases; however, antimicrobial treatment does not remove the organism from tissues. Because a carrier state can occur and these animals may be potential sources of infection, they are best neutered and removed from the breeding program.

Canine adenovirus   It is well established that infection with canine adenovirus during pregnancy can result in the birth of dead or weak pups that die within a few days after parturition. In most cases, however, the virus is ingested after parturition and causes neonatal mortality. Carrier bitches may act as a source of infection for pups.

Canine parvovirus   Canine parvovirus has been implicated by some breeders as a cause of infertility in their kennels. However, Meunier and colleagues[16] found that the conception rate, incidence of stillbirths, average litter size, or average number of pups weaned per litter did not change after the introduction of canine parvovirus to a kennel. Canine parvovirus may cause an acute generalized infection in pups less than 2 weeks of age, which can occur as a consequence of uterine infection or as a result of exposure to the virus soon after birth.

Canine distemper virus   Experimental exposure of pregnant bitches to canine distemper virus may produce either clinical illness in the bitch with subsequent abortion or subclinical infection of the bitch and the birth of clinically affected pups. Although the latter provides evidence for transplacental transmission, the frequency of this under natural conditions is unknown.

Toxoplasma gondii   Toxoplasma infection of the bitch may cause abortion, premature birth, stillbirth, and neonatal death. Surviving infected pups may carry the infection.

Normal Vaginal Bacterial Flora

A widespread belief exists among breeders and veterinarians that certain bacteria that inhabit the reproductive tract of the dog and bitch cause infertility, vaginitis, and fading puppy syndrome. This arose from the work in the 1930s that concluded that streptococci were responsible for infertility, abortion, anestrus, and weak pups. With the advent of virus isolation techniques, several specific viruses have been identified, and it seems likely that the earlier work overemphasized the importance of the streptococci. These bacteria are now considered to be part of the normal commensal flora and probably invade secondarily to viral damage or are contaminants.

Many aerobic and anaerobic bacteria normally inhabit the vestibule and vagina of the healthy bitch, and the bacterial flora is normally mixed. The aerobic bacteria isolated from normal bitches include *Escherichia coli*, staphylococci, and streptococci, whereas the anaerobic bacteria include *Bacteroides* spp. and *Peptostreptococcus* spp. Mycoplasmas have been isolated from between 30% and 88% of normal bitches.

Several authors have examined the vaginal bacterial flora of normal bitches and compared them with those of infertile bitches. These studies were reviewed by van Duijkeren,[17] who found that the bacterial species cultured from infertile bitches did not differ significantly from healthy bitches. Therefore the results of microbiologic examination of the reproductive tract of the bitch must be treated with caution because the simple isolation of bacteria from the vagina does not constitute a diagnosis of reproductive disease. However, disease may result if the uterine or vaginal defense mechanisms are depressed, thereby allowing overgrowth of the normal commensals. Many of the normal vaginal inhabitants may become pathogens if a breakdown in local immunity occurs.

CONCLUSION

Infertility is an important and increasingly recognized condition in the bitch. Canine female infertility has a number of causes, the most common of which are inappropriate mating time, male factor infertility, and uterine disease. The approach to the infertile bitch should involve a logical investigation to determine the underlying cause, the optimal treatment, and prognosis. After collection of a detailed clinical history and a physical examination, the clinician should determine the typical presentation of the problem, followed by additional investigation to establish the cause. Although specific diseases can be significant causes of infertility, an understanding of the normal anatomy, physiology, and the wide range of variations that can occur is an important aspect of investigating canine female infertility in clinical practice.

CHAPTER 253

Vaginal Disorders

Beverly J. Purswell

ANATOMY

Embryologic Origins of the Posterior Reproductive Tract

In normal sexual development of female dogs and cats, the urogenital sinus, genital tubercle, and genital swellings become the vestibule, the clitoris, and the vulva, respectively.[1] The paramesonephric (mullerian) ducts give rise to the uterine tubes (oviducts), uterus, cervix, and vagina.[2] The caudal end of the vaginal canal opens into the vestibule by joining the urogenital sinus to the distal paramesonephric ducts at the vaginovestibular junction. Although both the paramesonephric ducts and the urogenital sinus probably contribute to the vaginal epithelium, the vaginal squamous epithelial cells are considered to originate from the urogenital sinus.[2] The urogenital sinus also gives rise to the urinary bladder and to the urethra, which enters the vestibule just caudal to the vaginovestibular junction.

Anatomic Relationship of the Vagina and the Vestibule

The *vestibule* is the common external opening of the urinary and reproductive tracts. Cranially, the vestibule ends at the vagina, where the narrowing of the vaginovestibular junction can be palpated digitally. The vestibule has a distinct ventral slope starting at the vaginovestibular junction and extending caudally to the ventral commissure of the vulva (Figure 253-l). The urethral opening is on the ventral floor of the vestibule approximately 0.5 cm distal to the vaginovestibular junction.

The *vagina* extends (caudal to cranial) from the vaginovestibular junction to the cervix. The bitch has a relatively long vagina, which places the cervix in the abdomen, not the pelvic canal. This length makes examination of the vagina in its entirety difficult without special equipment and impossible using only digital palpation. The anterior part of the vagina is quite narrow (5 to 7 mm), which makes visualization of the cervix and its external os difficult even endoscopically.

EXAMINATION OF THE VESTIBULE AND VAGINA

Vaginal Cytology

Vaginal cytology is the technique most widely used to evaluate the distal reproductive tract of the bitch and is valuable in the interpretation of the nature of vulvar discharges. Localization of a disease process may be facilitated by comparing cytology from the vestibule to that of the vagina. Vaginal cytology is indicated any time disease of the reproductive tract is suspected.

Neutrophils in low numbers are seen normally in vaginal cytology at any time except during the peak of the estrogenic phase of the estrous cycle (middle to late proestrus and all of estrus). Large numbers of neutrophils are seen in early diestrus; this influx of neutrophils is not associated with any disease process and is considered a normal phenomenon.

The presence of large numbers of neutrophils during any other stage of the estrous cycle indicates an inflammatory process.

Visual and Digital Examination of the Vagina and Vestibule

Digital examination of the distal reproductive tract is valuable in the diagnosis of a variety of abnormalities. However, the animal's size may limit the examination. Because of the length of the distal reproductive tract, particularly that of the vagina, it is impossible to examine the vagina digitally in its entirety. Only the vulva, vestibule, urethral opening, and vaginovestibular junction can be adequately evaluated with a digital examination. Many of the abnormalities found in this area are best diagnosed with a digital examination and may remain undetected with other forms of inspection.

Vaginoscopy may be performed with an endoscope, a proctoscope, or any fiber-optic equipment long enough (15 to 20 cm) to allow inspection of the entire vagina. The procedure can be performed on the awake, standing bitch with sedation used as needed. Rigid equipment (e.g., proctoscope) tends to allow better visualization of the vagina than the flexible endoscopes because of the collapsing nature of the vaginal folds. When flexible fiber-optic endoscopes are used, insufflation of the vagina with air is necessary for a thorough examination.

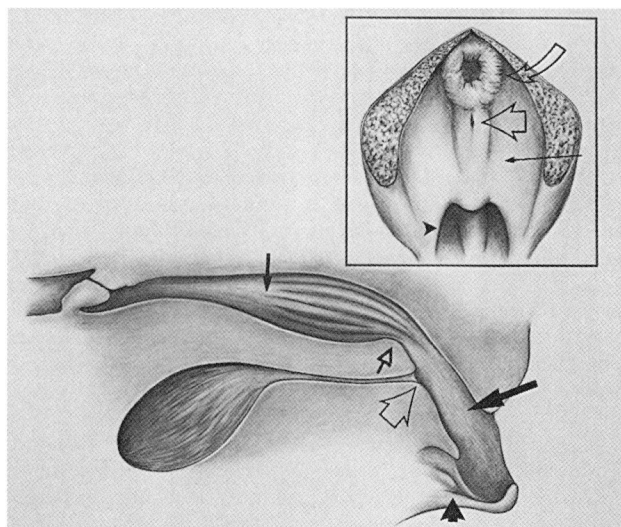

Figure 253-1 Anatomic relationship of the vestibule and the vagina in the bitch. The insert shows the annular stricture at the vaginovestibular junction cranial to the urethral opening. Other structures shown are the urethral opening *(open arrow head)*, the clitoral fossa *(solid arrow head)*, the vaginovestibular junction *(open arrow)*, the vagina *(solid arrow)*, and the vestibule *(large solid arrow)*.

The outside diameter of the endoscope must be 5 mm or less for complete visualization of the anterior vagina and paracervical area.[3] This small diameter may also be helpful for traversing the narrowing at the vaginovestibular junction for examining small bitches (those weighing less than 9 kg). Body size does not always correlate with the vestibular and vaginal diameter, especially in the prepubertal or ovariectomized bitch. Equipment less than 5 cm in length (e.g., otoscopes) provide visualization only of the vestibule.

Vaginal Bacterial Cultures

It has become common practice for clients to request vaginal cultures from bitches prior to breeding. The literature includes reports on vaginal flora in normal bitches and bitches with reproductive tract disease.[4,5] The species of bacteria isolated from the cranial and caudal vagina are similar in these two groups. The aerobic bacterial flora of the bitch's vagina consists of common opportunistic pathogens, the presence of which does not influence fertility.[5] Careful interpretation of culture results is mandatory in the evaluation of an area with normal flora. Culture of the vagina during an overt disease process is valuable in the selection of appropriate therapy. However, isolation of opportunistic aerobic pathogens, anaerobic bacteria, or mycoplasmas in an asymptomatic animal does not constitute evidence of infection.[4] Research shows that prophylactic use of antibiotics in apparently healthy breeding bitches may predispose the vagina to colonization by organisms that are known opportunistic pathogens.[6] Only a guarded swab technique should be used to obtain vaginal cultures.

VAGINAL ABNORMALITIES

Vaginitis

The term *vaginitis* describes an inflammatory process, not necessarily an infectious one. Inflammation can be identified easily with vaginal cytology and vaginoscopy. The clinical signs are those associated with irritation, such as licking, vulvar discharge, and attraction of male dogs. With vaginitis, vaginal cytology shows increased numbers of neutrophils in various stages of degeneration, with or without increased numbers of bacteria. Chronic vaginitis may induce the presence of lymphocytes and macrophages. Vaginoscopy reveals the presence and extent of hyperemia, exudate, and mucosal lesions, such as vesicles, ulcers, and lymphoid follicle hyperplasia. An attempt should be made to differentiate other systemic disorders that cause similar signs. Urinary tract problems should be ruled out as a cause of the vestibular irritation or attraction of male dogs. Lymphoid follicle hyperplasia is a common finding in the vestibule of bitches with urinary tract infections arising from chronic inflammation. Dermatologic lesions may be the cause of a perineal irritation and can prompt excessive licking. Comparison of vestibular cytology with vaginal cytology may aid in localization of the problem.

Juvenile (puppy) vaginitis is a common malady in prepubertal bitches. The most common sign is purulent vulvar discharge. Juvenile vaginitis may respond to systemic antibacterial therapy or to topical douching, but inevitably the signs return when treatment is discontinued. The condition resolves naturally after the first estrous cycle, if not before. Neutering of these animals should be postponed until signs have resolved or the first estrus has occurred. The vulvar area should be kept clean to prevent secondary skin problems. No other treatment is necessary.

Adult vaginitis can be caused by anatomic abnormalities that lead to accumulation of discharge or urine in the vagina. Accumulation of urine in the vagina may cause apparent urinary incontinence, with urine dribbling from the vulva when the bitch changes position. Bacterial or chemical vaginitis occurs secondary to the predisposing cause.

Strictures at the vaginovestibular junction are thought to cause problems in some individuals. Care must be taken to localize the area of inflammation before this diagnosis is made. These vaginovestibular strictures can be easily identified by a digital examination. Digital or surgical dilatation may be required to eliminate the problem, although recurrence is common. Vaginectomy may be required in persistent cases. Vaginoscopy, contrast radiography, or other imaging modalities should be used to rule out foreign bodies, tumors, and uterine stump granulomas as predisposing causes (Figure 253-2). Contrast radiography may be helpful in identifying anatomic abnormalities or concurrent urinary tract disease, including acquired ectopic ureters after ovariohysterectomy.[7] A knowledge of the normal changes that occur in the vagina with the estrous cycle is critical in the interpretation of contrast radiographs (Figure 253-3). When vaginoscopy is performed in an animal with chronic inflammation, care must be taken not to perforate the vaginal wall.

Because systemic disease may predispose a bitch to vaginal infection, the animal's general health should be evaluated. If a predisposing cause is not identified, vaginal cultures should be performed and appropriate antibacterial therapy instituted. In some cases of chronic inflammation without any apparent predisposing cause, glucocorticoids may be useful for eliminating the inflammation. Initial lavage of the vagina may be beneficial for removing accumulated material.

Viral vaginitis has been described in conjunction with canine herpesvirus infection. Genital infections of canine herpesvirus result in diffuse, multifocal, raised vesicular lesions on the vaginal mucosa that characteristically cause no clinical signs in the bitch.[8] No treatment is necessary, but it is advisable to separate the affected animal from any pregnant bitches or neonatal puppies.[9]

Anatomic Abnormalities

A variety of congenital abnormalities of the vagina and vestibule have been described. The exact incidence is unknown, but some of these abnormalities are common. Abnormal embryologic development is responsible for most of these conditions.

A persistent hymen occurs at the junction of the vagina and vestibule where the paramesonephric duct joins the urogenital sinus. Incomplete perforation of the hymen usually causes an annular stricture (see insert in Figure 253-1) or a vertical septum or band. Affected bitches most often have breeding difficulties, chronic vaginitis, or urinary incontinence unresponsive to conventional therapy because of urine pooling. Digital palpation is the preferred method of diagnosing these conditions. Vaginoscopy may bypass the affected area. If these anomalies are incidental findings in an asymptomatic animal, no correction is necessary. Digital dilatation can be attempted in either condition and may be successful, depending on the extent of the tissue involved. An episiotomy may be required to attain adequate exposure of the vaginovestibular junction for surgical manipulation. A vertical band is easily removed surgically, and correction of the presenting signs is usually complete. An annular stricture is more difficult to correct permanently. The stricture may be excised completely, with the mucosa closed perpendicular to the initial incision, in an attempt to enlarge the lumen. Another approach is to make a series of radial incisions perpendicular to the lumen. Both procedures may require frequent and repeated postoperative digital dilatation to prevent stricture recurrence. Clinical signs may persist after attempted surgical correction. Vaginectomy is an alternative therapy that alleviates problems associated with the vagina.

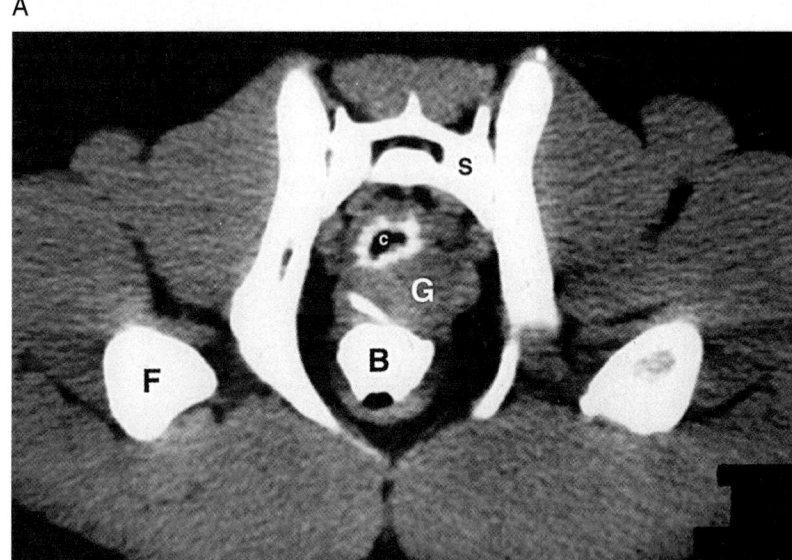

Figure 253-2   Uterine stump granuloma in a 7-month-old spayed bitch presented for urinary incontinence. **A,** Lateral abdominal radiograph obtained after infusion of air into the colon *(C)* and iodinated contrast medium into the urinary bladder *(B)*. The uterine stump granuloma *(G)* is evident as a soft tissue mass compressing the neck of the urinary bladder. **B,** Transverse computed tomographic image obtained at the level of the cranial pelvic canal (sacrum *[S]* and femur *[F]*). The granuloma is compressing the left ureter at the trigone and indenting the left dorsolateral margin of the urinary bladder. (Courtesy Dr. Jeryl C. Jones, Virginia-Maryland Regional College of Veterinary Medicine, Blacksburg, VA.)

Bitches with annular strictures may be bred artificially and re-evaluated immediately prior to parturition. Sufficient relaxation usually occurs to allow normal delivery of the puppies. Cesarean section or an episiotomy may be needed at parturition if relaxation is insufficient to allow whelping.

Vaginal anomalies arise as a result of problems associated with organogenesis of the paramesonephric duct. The external genitalia and vestibule are usually normal in these animals because of their separate embryologic origin. Incomplete fusion of the paramesonephric ducts results in a vertical septum in the vagina (double vagina).[10] Surgery is indicated if the bitch's intended use is breeding or if clinical signs are present. Concomitant anomalies must be ruled out prior to attempted correction of any abnormality. Segmental hypoplasia or aplasia of the vagina has been described in the bitch, and surgical correction is not possible. Vaginal diverticula may occur and can fill with debris, causing local inflammation. Surgical removal of the diverticula is indicated to resolve this condition. Contrast radiography and vaginoscopy are helpful in identifying and defining the extent of the various vaginal anomalies. Ovariohysterectomy may be indicated when the condition is extensive. A partial or total vaginectomy may also be indicated when the condition is causing secondary problems, such as chronic urinary tract infections.

Vulvar anomalies are occasionally identified in a bitch with breeding difficulties. Tight bands at the dorsal commissure are a common cause of painful copulation (dyspareunia) and are easily identified with digital palpation. If necessary, the bitch may be bred artificially and re-examined immediately prior to parturition to assess potential whelping difficulties. Relaxation of the vulva is usually sufficient to allow normal delivery.

Inverted vulvas may be found in prepubertal bitches. The vulva is inverted to the point of being hidden from view by skin folds. Vaginitis, perivulvar irritation, vulvar discharge, or urinary tract disease may occur secondary to the infolding of the vulva and distortion of the vestibule and urethral opening. Neutering of these bitches should be postponed until after the first estrus. Eversion of the vulva normally occurs during the first estrus, and the condition is self-correcting. In bitches neutered prior to puberty, episioplasty may be necessary to alleviate the chronic urinary tract infections and perivulvar dermatitis associated with an inverted infantile vulva.[11,12] Removal of the redundant skin folds around the vulva exteriorizes the vulva, which helps eliminate the perivulvar dermatitis. Exteriorization of the vulva results in less turbulence of urine during voiding, making ascending infections less likely (Figure 253-4).

Faulty urogenital sinus embryogenesis may lead to congenital problems in the vestibule, vulva, and perineum. Open vulvar clefts, perineal dysgenesis, and rectovaginal fistulas have been described in the bitch and require surgical correction.

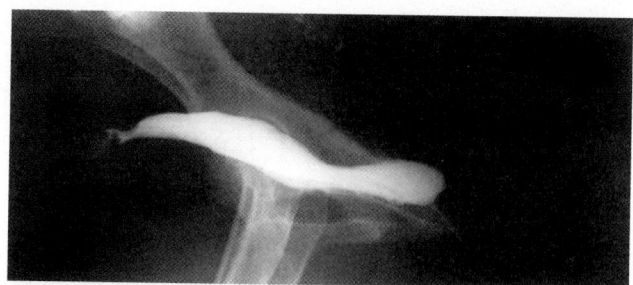

A

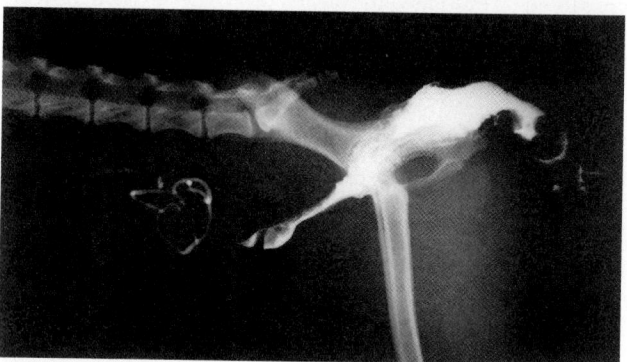

B

Figure 253-3 Variations in the normal appearance of the canine vagina after retrograde positive contrast vaginography. **A,** Anestrus. Note the smooth mucosal margination and absence of filling defects, as well as the closed cervix, which allows no contrast medium to ascend into the uterus. **B,** Estrus. Note the thickened rugae appearing as linear filling defects in the mucosal margins and the open cervix, which allows contrast medium to ascend into the uterus. (Courtesy Dr. Jeryl Jones, Virginia-Maryland Regional College of Veterinary Medicine, Blacksburg, VA.)

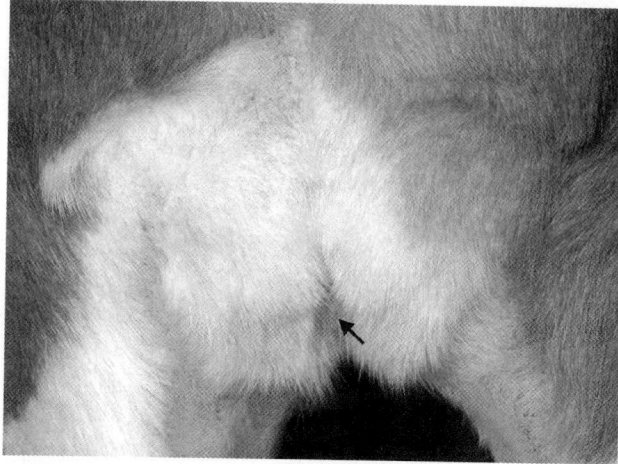

A

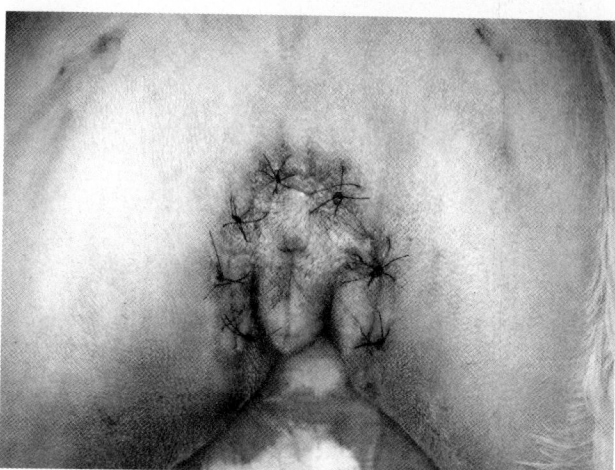

B

Figure 253-4 Episioplasty in a bitch with an inverted vulva, performed as treatment for chronic urinary tract infections and perivulvar inflammation. **A,** Presurgical appearance of the vulva and surrounding skin folds; the arrow indicates the ventral commissure of the vulva. **B,** Postsurgical appearance of the vulva after removal of redundant skin folds.

These distal abnormalities, which can be acquired or congenital, may be associated with other reproductive or urinary tract anomalies. Clitoral anomalies are usually associated with intersex conditions and take the form of clitoral enlargement with penislike anatomy (Figure 253-5). Surgical removal of the clitoris to prevent excoriation is advised if the clitoris protrudes from the vulva.

Vaginal Fold Prolapse, Vaginal Hyperplasia, and Vaginal Prolapse

Under the influence of estrogen, some young bitches develop an edematous ventral fold in the distal vaginal mucosa immediately cranial to the urethral opening (Figure 253-6); this fold may become large enough to protrude from the vulvar opening. Traditionally, this condition has been referred to as vaginal hyperplasia. Histologically, however, this tissue is no more hyperplastic than the rest of the vagina under the influence of estrogen. Pronounced edema is the major histologic lesion, with fibroplasia resulting from the edema. Prolapse of a vaginal fold occurs almost exclusively when the bitch is under the influence of estrogen; this may occur at the first estrus or become evident during later estrous cycles. Once the condition manifests itself, it has a tendency to recur during each subsequent estrus. The condition usually is self-limiting and resolves once the estrogenic influence ends at the onset of diestrus or with ovariohysterectomy. Ovariohysterectomy resolves the condition permanently and is the treatment of choice for animals not intended for breeding. Surgical removal of the prolapsed tissue can be attempted and resolves the condition permanently in some animals. Artificial insemination

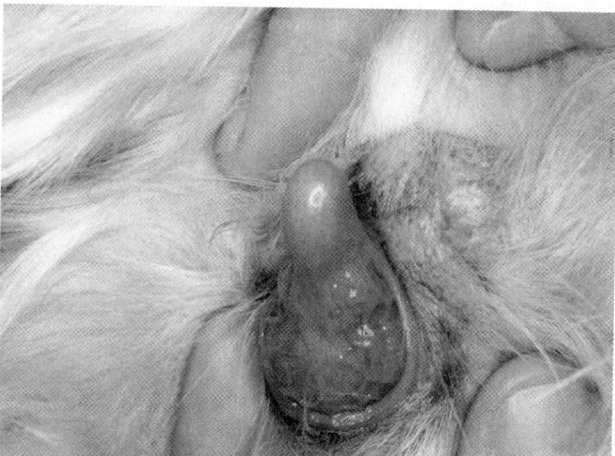

Figure 253-5 Clitoris of a male pseudohermaphrodite, showing penislike anatomy.

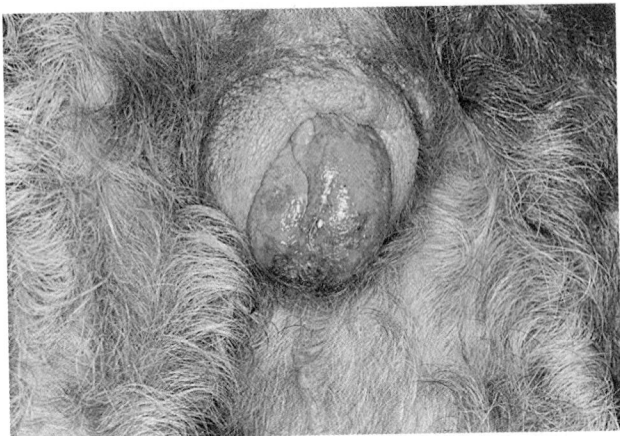

A

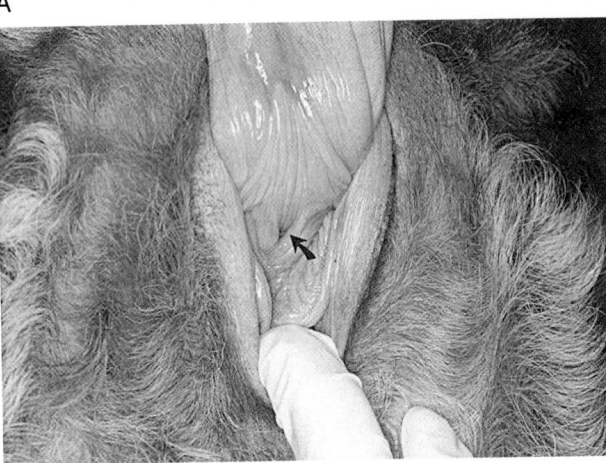

B

Figure 253-6 Vaginal fold prolapse (vaginal hyperplasia) in a bitch. **A,** Vaginal fold prolapse protruding from the vulva; excoriation is evident. **B,** Vaginal fold prolapse originating anterior to the urethral opening (arrow indicates urethral opening).

can be performed in affected bitches, with resolution expected with the onset of diestrus. Occasionally vaginal fold prolapse fails to resolve after estrus, or it recurs at the end of pregnancy, when estrogen levels rise slightly.[13] The condition is not generally thought to be hereditary, although evidence indicates a hereditary predisposition in some family lines and some breeds.

Miscellaneous Vaginal Disorders

Vaginal lacerations can occur during copulation, obstetric procedures, or vaginoscopy. Hemorrhage from the vulva is the primary sign. A bitch that bleeds from the vulva after breeding should be examined for vaginal tears. The decision must be made whether suturing is necessary or possible. Systemic antibiotics should be administered to prevent infections, particularly dissecting pelvic infections.

Vaginal and vulvar neoplasia account for 2.5% to 3% of all canine tumors[14]; 70% to 80% of these tumors are benign. Signs may include perineal enlargement, a mass protruding from the vulva, vulvar discharge, tenesmus, or dysuria. Tumors prolapsing from the vulva must be differentiated from vaginal fold prolapse through evaluation of the stage of the estrous cycle and its relationship to the onset of signs, the location of the mass, and failure of the mass to regress at the onset of diestrus. Leiomyomas are the most common benign tumor and are often pedunculated. Leiomyosarcoma is the most common malignant vaginal tumor. Surgical excision is the treatment of choice for tumors. Transmissible venereal tumors are more common in younger animals and respond readily to chemotherapy. The prognosis for vaginal and vulvar tumors is good provided metastasis has not occurred with the malignant tumors. Ovariohysterectomy is recommended at the time of removal because of the possibility of hormonal influence on the incidence and possible recurrence rate.

Vaginal prolapse rarely occurs in the bitch or queen. It is usually associated with dystocia, tenesmus, or forced extraction of the male during the genital tie in the dog. Uterine prolapse may follow, depending on the cause. Treatment involves replacement of the affected structures. An abdominal approach may be necessary to replace the vagina. An ovariohysterectomy may be performed at the time of correction if so desired.

CHAPTER • 254

Semen Evaluation, Canine Male Infertility, and Common Disorders of the Male

Mushtaq A. Memon
Kaitkanoke Sirinarumitr

SEMEN EVALUATION

The purposes of semen collection and evaluation are to assess an animal for breeding soundness; to perform artificial insemination; to preserve semen; to attempt to localize the site of disorder in some infertile dogs; and to determine treatment response for infertile dogs. Collection of the prostatic fluid

and its submission for cytology and bacterial culture may help differentiate prostatic disorders from other problems. Semen evaluation may be performed before a dog is purchased, before he is first used for breeding, or if he shows signs of infertility. Semen collection and evaluation are relatively easy and can be done at any small animal practice. The results should be recorded on the canine Breeding Soundness

Examination (BSE) form, which was devised by the Society for Theriogenology.

Semen Collection
Equipment

Semen from the dog is easily collected using an artificial vagina (AV), a device composed of a latex rubber cone (Reproduction Resources, Hebson, Illinois) connected to a 15 mL calibrated plastic centrifuge tube. The AV should be washed with plain tap water (no soap, detergent, or other cleansing agent is used), rinsed thoroughly with distilled water, and air dried. Gas sterilization, if available, may be used on the AV. Some dogs may ejaculate into other containers under the pressure of hand massage alone. However, semen is collected successfully from most dogs with an AV because the AV simulates the pressure normally felt by the male during copulation. The calibrated collection tubes used in the procedure should also be washed with tap water, rinsed with distilled water, and sterilized with gas or autoclaved before use to prevent the formation of formaldehyde residues, which are harmful to sperm.[1]

For optimum results, collection should be done in a quiet room with the dog on a nonslip surface and with the owner present. Semen may be collected before other examinations are performed, including the physical examination. For better responsiveness, the semen can be collected in the presence of a teaser bitch in proestrus or estrus. If a bitch in estrus is not available, a commercially available pheromone (Eau d' Estrus, International Canine Genetics, Malvern, Pennsylvania; or methylparaben; Sigma Chemical, Saint Louis, MO) or vaginal swabs from a disease-free estral bitch can be used. The top of the AV should be folded down, and a scant amount of lubricant should be applied to facilitate later removal of the device from the dog's erect penis.

Procedure

The male and female are brought on leashes into a collecting room and allowed to play for a few minutes. The semen collector, if right handed, kneels at the dog's left side and, holding the AV in the left hand, uses the right hand to move the prepuce up and down the penile shaft to achieve protrusion of the penis into the AV. (Left-handed collectors may reverse the sides described above.) As the male begins to thrust the penis into the AV, the collector moves the sheath above the engorging bulbous glandis, keeping firm, steady pressure around the circumference of the penis to maintain the erection (Figure 254-1). Most male dogs ejaculate the presperm (clear) and sperm-rich fractions (cloudy) of the semen during pelvic thrusting; they then dismount and lift one hind leg as though trying to step over the bitch and achieve the tie. At this point the penis should be rotated 180 degrees, so that it is directed caudally, and held still, with tight pressure maintained around the circumference, until the third prostatic fraction of semen has been ejaculated. The prostatic fluid is ejaculated after a short pause in association with anal contractions and rhythmic pulsations of the penile urethra, which the collector can detect. After a few milliliters of prostatic fluid have been collected, the AV may be removed from the penis; the dog may continue to ejaculate prostatic fluid for some time after removal of the AV. The dog should not be kenneled or sent home until the erection has subsided completely and the entire penis is back in the preputial sheath. Normally, this takes about 5 to 10 minutes after semen collection.

Evaluation

Five parameters, in particular, should be evaluated and recorded for each semen collection (Table 254-1): the color and volume of the sample, and the motility, concentration/total number, and morphology of the sperm.

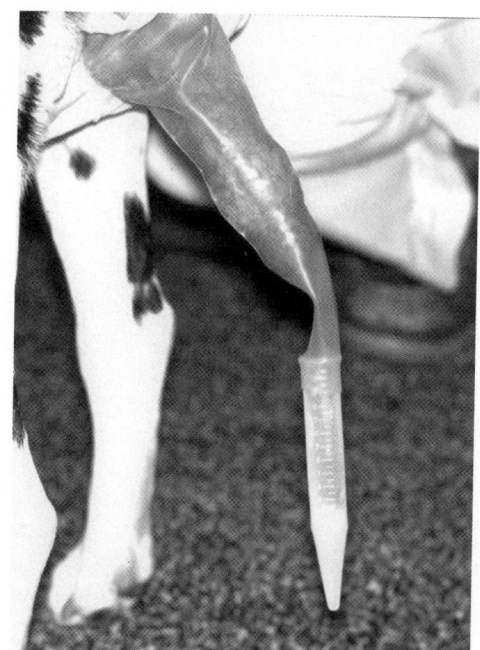

Figure 254-1 Latex rubber cone (artificial vagina) fitted over the penis during semen collection.

Color The color of the sample is observed grossly in the collection tube. The first fraction should be clear, whereas the second (sperm-rich) fraction should be milky white. The third fraction (prostatic fluid) should be clear. Yellow discoloration may indicate urine contamination or the presence of purulent exudate. A red or brown color may indicate prostatic disease, trauma, urethritis, or ulceration.

Volume The volume of semen can be read directly from the calibrated collecting tube. Volume varies among breeds and among individual dogs. Semen volume is not an important parameter with regard to the BSE, but it is necessary for determining the number of sperm per ejaculate. The separate volume for the prostatic fluid need not be recorded, because it varies according to the length of time the prostatic fluid is collected.

Sperm motility Motility testing should be performed immediately after collection. The examiner places a drop of undiluted semen on a slide with a cover slip, examines the

Table • 254-1

Characteristics of Normal Canine Semen

PARAMETER	UNFRACTIONED EJACULATE	SEMINAL FRACTION		
		1	2	3
Color	Opaque to white	Clear	Milky white	Clear
Volume (mL)	~ 30	0.1-2	0.1-4	1-25 +
pH	6.1-7.0	6.2-6.4	—	—
Sperm motility	>80 %	—	—	—
Morphologically normal sperm	>80 %	—	—	—

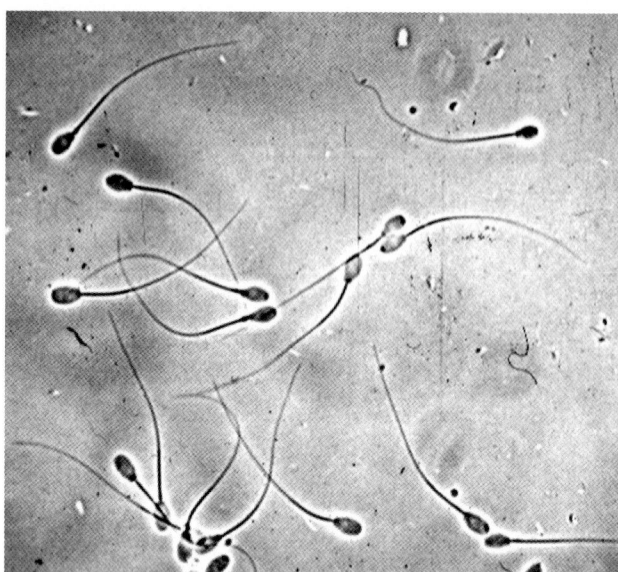

Figure 254-2 Estimation of the percentage of motile sperm (i.e., those moving in a progressive, forward manner) in a semen sample.

specimen at ×100 to ×200 magnification (because canine spermatozoa are resistant to cold shock, the slide need not be warmed), and estimates the percentage of sperm cells moving in a progressive and forward manner across the field (Figure 254-2). Although sperm motility estimation is not precise, it is a quick functional test.

Concentration/total number of sperm The total number of sperm in the ejaculate is more important than the concentration of sperm per milliliter, because the concentration changes dramatically depending on the amount of prostatic fluid collected. The sperm concentration can be measured with a commercial WBC Unopett system (Becton Dickinson, Rutherford, New Jersey) (Figure 254-3). The semen sample is stirred gently, drawn up into the capillary pipette (20 μL) provided with the kit, and dispensed into the diluent-containing reservoir chamber. Diluted semen then is dispensed into both chambers of a Neubauer hemocytometer (Becton Dickinson, Rutherford, New Jersey) (Figure 254-4), and the contents of the grid's 1-mm central square (composed of 25 small squares) are counted on each side of the hemocytometer and averaged.[2] (The central square fills the field of a light microscope when the ×10 objective is used.) The number of spermatozoa in the central square is the concentration in millions of spermatozoa per milliliter of semen. The total number of sperm in the ejaculate equals the concentration multiplied by the volume. The normal total number of sperm[1] ranges from 300 to 2000×10^6; large breed dogs ejaculate more sperm than small breed dogs.[3] (Direct cell counts done with the hematocytometer are time-consuming; quicker methods used to determine the sperm concentration are an electronic blood cell counter or spectrophotometer.) The total number of sperm may be decreased in quite young, old, and inbred dogs.

Sperm morphology Sperm morphology is usually assessed by staining the semen sample and observing the sperm under oil immersion (×1000) objective. Various stain techniques may cause some artifactual changes in sperm morphology. Defects vary with the stain used, but the percentage of morphologically normal sperm should be fairly consistent

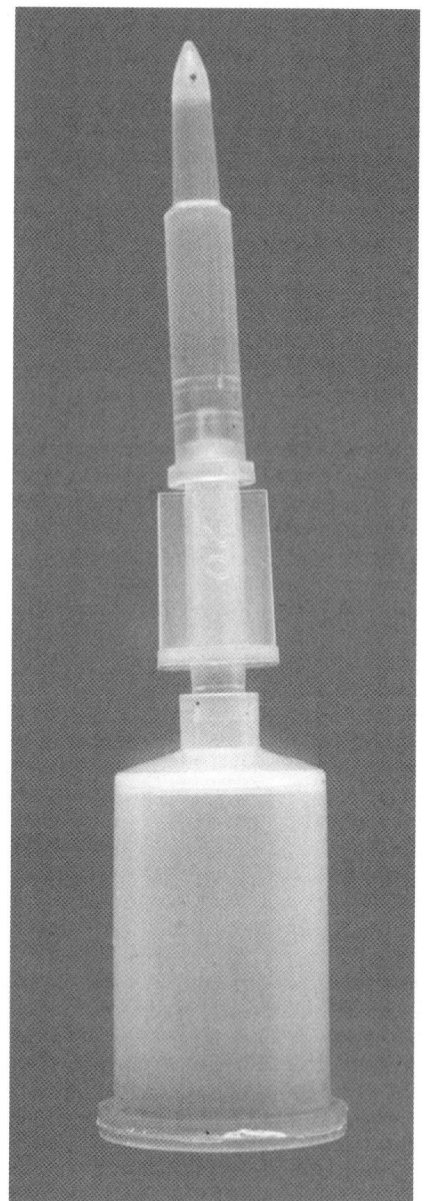

Figure 254-3 WBC Unopett system, used to measure sperm concentration.

regardless of method.[4] Eosin/nigrosin stain and Wright's Giemsa stain (Diff Quik) are the stains most commonly used. For staining with eosin-nigrosin, a drop of semen and a similar-sized drop of stain are placed on one end of a clean glass slide and mixed gently with a wooden applicator. A second slide then is used as a spreader slide. A thin film, similar to a blood smear, is made and air-dried. For staining with rapid Wright's Giemsa stain, the semen smear is made as for a blood smear, air-dried, and immersed in each of the three solutions for 5 minutes each. The slide then is rinsed and allowed to dry. One hundred sperm cells should be examined and the findings recorded, including normal sperm, primary abnormalities (all head defects, proximally coiled tails, proximal cytoplasmic droplets), and secondary abnormalities (detached heads, bent tails, and distal cytoplasmic droplets). Primary abnormalities are abnormalities that occur in the testis during spermatogenesis. Secondary abnormalities occur during epididymal transport or as a result of sample-handling techniques. Most dogs have greater than 80% normal sperm per ejaculation.[5]

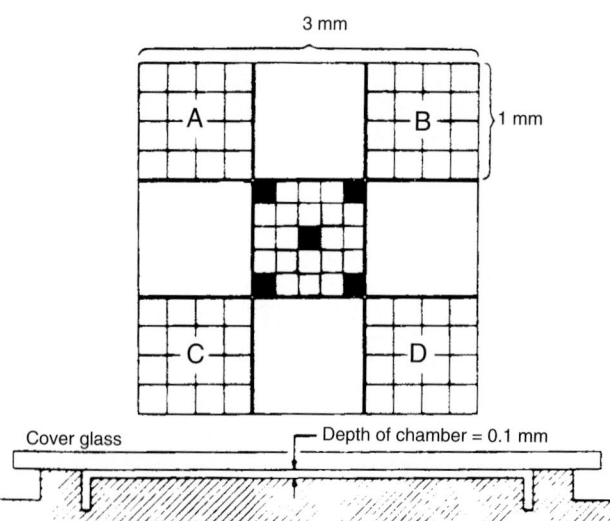

Figure 254-4 Neubauer hemocytometer, which is used to count sperm.

CANINE MALE INFERTILITY

Infertility in the male may result from infections, endocrinopathies, structural abnormalities, neoplasia, illness, or poor breeding management. Abnormalities of the genital tract, which includes the penis, prepuce, testes, epididymis, vasa deferentia, urethra, and prostate gland, may also result in infertility. These conditions may result in reduced libido or failure to achieve normal copulation. A thorough physical examination should be conducted after semen is collected.

History

A complete medical history of the male dog should be obtained, including information on vaccinations, diet, medications, past illnesses, and laboratory results, as well as a complete reproductive history. The record also should include a list of all breedings; the litter size from each breeding; the results of previous semen evaluations; and the breeding history of each bitch, including her estrous cycle, progesterone level, and conception rates from breedings with other males.

Physical Examination

A thorough physical examination should be performed. Abnormalities that may interfere with libido or ability to mount and achieve intromission include a persistent frenulum, hypospadias, disk disease, spondylosis, hip dysplasia, and a luxating patella. Dogs with heritable diseases should not be bred. The penis and prepuce should be inspected and palpated for any abnormalities. The erect penis can be examined after semen collection.

The scrotum and testes should be palpated for consistency and shape. Testicular degeneration, hypoplasia, or atrophy may result in softening of the testis, whereas testicular fibrosis or neoplasia may result in hardness of the testis. Although testicular size varies normally among breeds, the size should be measured with calipers and recorded. An abnormally enlarged scrotum or testis may indicate inflammation. Each epididymis, including the head, body, and tail, should be thoroughly palpated and the results recorded.[5]

The prostate is the major accessory sex gland and is responsible for seminal volume. It is an encapsulated, bilobed, bilaterally symmetric ovoid gland, located at the caudal pole of the bladder, that encircles the proximal urethra.

The prostate should be palpated by digital rectal examination after semen has been collected.

Additional Diagnostic Tests

Infertile dogs may require additional tests, including determination of the seminal plasma pH; aerobic and anaerobic bacterial cultures; culture for mycoplasmas and ureaplasmas; and semen cytology. Seminal fluid from samples that lack sperm should be evaluated for its alkaline phosphatase (ALP) concentration, which comes from the epididymis, to ensure a complete ejaculation.[2] Hormonal assays and epididymal aspiration, testicular biopsy, and chromosomal karyotyping may be considered in dogs with azoospermia. Ultrasonographic examination is a useful diagnostic procedure for detecting some abnormalities of the prostate, testes, and epididymis.

Azoospermia

Azoospermia is the ejaculation of seminal plasma without spermatozoa.[6] The causes of azoospermia may be classified as pretesticular, testicular, and post-testicular. Pretesticular causes in dogs include hypopituitarism, long-term high-dose steroid or antineoplastic therapy, hypothyroidism, inguinal and scrotal hernia, and fever. Testicular causes include intersex, germinal cell aplasia, bilateral cryptorchidism, testicular injury, irradiation, orchitis, autoimmune testicular disorders, and testicular neoplasia.[2,7] Phenotypic male dogs with chromosome abnormalities such as XXY or XX-male syndrome usually have aspermatogenesis. In dogs, XXY karyotype usually causes testicular hypoplasia and hypoplasia of tubular and accessory reproductive organs, along with azoospermia and sterility. Post-testicular causes of azoospermia include obstruction of the collecting ducts, epididymides, or ductus deferens, including epididymal segmental aplasia; sperm granulomas; spermatocele; acute inflammation; neoplasia; and previous vasectomy.[9] Some dogs may have azoospermia as a result of incomplete ejaculation.

Incomplete Ejaculation

Incomplete ejaculation may occur in normal, intact dogs that require the presence of a bitch in proestrus or estrus during semen collection. Some nervous or inexperienced dogs may also have an incomplete ejaculation. The dog may ejaculate only presperm fluid. More than one sample should be collected and evaluated before a diagnosis of azoospermia is made. Seminal fluid should be submitted for ALP measurement. The concentration normally is less than 5000 U/L for dogs that failed to have a complete ejaculation. Dogs with true azoospermia arising from causes other than bilateral blockage of the outflow tract usually have a seminal ALP concentration greater than 5000 U/L. If the seminal ALP concentration is equivocal, another semen collection should be performed and the sample submitted for seminal ALP determination.[2]

Oligospermia

The term *oligospermia* refers to a low total number of spermatozoa in the ejaculate. Oligospermic dogs are not necessarily infertile. Causes of oligospermia reported in dogs include unilateral Sertoli cell tumor, orchitis, epididymitis, prostate diseases, incomplete ejaculation, retrograde ejaculation, overuse, and partial outflow obstruction.[2,9] Reported infectious causes of orchitis and epididymitis in dogs include *Brucella* sp., *Escherichia coli*, mycoplasma, and other aerobic organisms that make up the normal preputial flora.[2] Retrograde ejaculation has been reported in dogs.[10] The diagnosis of retrograde ejaculation may require collection of urine by cystocentesis after ejaculation and comparison of the number of sperm in the ejaculate with the number in the urine sediment. Retrograde flow of semen has been demonstrated in dogs sedated with xylazine.[11] Dogs with idiopathic oligospermia may be treated with a gonadotropin-releasing hormone (GnRH) agonist (1 μg/kg given subcutaneously), with or without subsequent treatment with human chorionic gonadotropin (HCG) (1600 IU given intramuscularly).

Teratozoospermia and Asthenozoospermia

The term *teratozoospermia* refers to a low percentage of morphologically normal sperm (greater than 80% of sperm should be morphologically normal). Congenital causes of teratozoospermia in dogs include fucosidosis, a lysosomal storage disease that affects epididymal epithelial cell function, causing the retention of cytoplasmic droplets. Acquired causes reported are testicular tumors; orchitis; prostatitis; high fever; and obesity, which causes an increase in the intrascrotal temperature due to periscrotal fat. The causes of asthenozoospermia (progressive sperm motility less than 70%) are the same as those for teratozoospermia, as well as infection of the reproductive tract, use of contaminated collection equipment, and immotile cilia syndrome. Water-soluble lubricants, residues from the manufacture of latex or plastic AVs or collecting tubes, urine, and water can reduce the motility of sperm.[2,9] Sperm agglutination and reduced motility may be found in dogs that test positive for *Brucella* infection.

COMMON DISORDERS OF THE MALE DOG

Benign Prostatic Hypertrophy

Benign prostatic hypertrophy (BPH) is a naturally occurring, age-related condition in men and intact dogs. Most dogs with BPH are over 5 years of age. Dogs with BPH are predisposed to prostatic cysts, infections, and prostatic abscessation. An enlarged prostate may compress the descending colon or the rectum, or both.[2]

Pathogenenesis

The pathogenesis of BPH is not completely known. Dihydrotestosterone (DHT), testosterone, estradiol, and some growth factors are involved in prostatic growth.[12] The hormone DHT, a metabolized form of testosterone, plays a major role in the growth of both the stromal and glandular components of the prostate.[13]

Clinical Signs and Diagnosis

Clinical signs of BPH include constipation, dripping of a sanguineous discharge from the tip of the penis, blood-contaminated urine or semen, and difficulty urinating.[13] Dogs with BPH may or may not show any clinical signs related to BPH. Diagnosis of BPH requires determination of prostatic enlargement that is not caused by any other prostatic diseases. The prostate gland of dogs with BPH is symmetrically enlarged and moderately firm, and no signs of pain are associated with rectal palpation.[14] Dogs with BPH that also have a prostatic cyst may have asymmetrically shaped prostatic lobes.

Ultrasonographic examination demonstrates symmetrically enlarged prostatic lobes. The prostatic parenchyma is homogeneous in echogenicity with or without a cavitating cystic lesion. On radiographic films, enlargement of the prostate is suggested if the prostatic diameter on lateral radiographs is greater than 70% of the distance between the sacral promontory and the pubis.

Prostatic volume can be predicted using the following formula:

$$[1/2.6 (L \times W \times D)] + 1.8$$

where *L* is the greatest craniocaudal measurement, *W* is the transverse measurement, and *D* is the dorsoventral measurement of the prostate, as measured using ultrasonography.[15]

The results of a complete blood count in dogs with BPH are normal, and aerobic bacterial culture of prostatic fluid shows less than 10,000 colony-forming units (CFU) per milliliter.[13]

Treatment

The treatment goals for dogs with BPH are to reduce the size of the prostate and alleviate the signs related to BPH. In most dogs, castration is recommended for BPH. Medical treatment is suitable for valuable breeding dogs and for dogs with a high risk of adverse reactions to anesthesia or surgery. The recommended drug for BPH treatment is finasteride (Proscar), administered at a dosage of 0.1 to 0.5 mg/kg (or 1 tablet/dog weighing 1 to 50 kg), given orally every 24 hours for 1 to 4 months.[13] In dogs with BPH that were treated with finasteride, the prostate became involuted through programmed cell death, or apoptosis, rather than necrosis, therefore no inflammatory process arose in the involuted prostate.[16] Finasteride reduces prostatic volume and the serum DHT level but does not adversely affect the semen quality, libido, serum testosterone concentration, or fertility.[13,17,18]

Prostatitis

Bacterial prostatitis is common in sexually intact dogs and can be acute or chronic. The organism most commonly found in dogs with prostatitis is *E. coli*, followed by staphylococci and streptococci.[19]

Clinical Signs and Diagnosis

Clinical signs in dogs with acute prostatitis include fever; pain; depression; straining to urinate or defecate; stiff-legged gait; hematuria; edema of the scrotum, prepuce, or hindlimb; and pollakiuria. During rectal examination of the prostate, dogs with prostatitis show signs of pain. The prostate may be asymmetric if abscessation is present. Dogs with chronic prostatitis may have clinical signs of infertility problems or lower urinary tract disease.[2] Dogs with prostatitis may have leukocytosis. The urine may contain blood, bacteria, and white blood cells. Prostatic fluid collected either by ejaculation or by prostatic massage contains a significant number of inflammatory cells, and the aerobic bacteria count is greater than 10,000 CFU/mL.[2] Prostatic abscesses detected by ultrasonography are usually discrete, hypoechoic or anechoic lesions with or without distant enhancement.

Treatment

Prostatitis with abscessation can be treated medically and/or surgically. Surgical correction of prostatic abscessation may be associated with a high percentage of adverse sequelae. Surgical techniques used include marsupialization, placement of a Penrose drain, drainage with omentalization of the cavities remaining, and partial prostectomy.[2] Medical treatment for prostatitis usually includes appropriate antimicrobial therapy. Finasteride therapy or castration should also be considered. Combination therapy with an antimicrobial and finasteride is more successful than treatment with an antimicrobial alone. Antimicrobial therapy should be based on bacterial sensitivity.

TESTICULAR PROBLEMS

Cryptorchidism

Cryptorchidism is the most common disorder of sexual development. It is defined as a lack of descent of one or both testes into the scrotum by 6 months of age.[8] In normal dogs, the testes usually have descended by 10 days of age. The incidence of cryptorchidism is higher in dogs (0.8% to 9.8%) than in cats (1.7%). The condition is more common in certain breeds (e.g., toy and miniature poodles, Yorkshire terriers,

Chihuahuas, boxers, and miniature schnauzers). Cryptorchidism is considered a hereditary disorder, therefore an animal with this condition should not be used for breeding. The exact mode of inheritance is not known, but it is thought to be a sex-limited autosomal recessive type; therefore both males and females can carry the gene and pass it on to their offspring.

The diagnosis is made on the basis of the physical examination findings. In the cat, the penis should be examined for androgen-dependent penile spines (Figure 254-5).[2,20] The penile spines atrophy by 6 weeks after complete castration. (Retained testes are atrophic and are generally not visible on abdominal ultrasound scans.) An animal with unilateral cryptorchidism (one testis in the scrotum) dog can produce sperm, whereas dogs that are bilaterally cryptorchid usually do not produce sperm. Because cryptorchidism does not affect testosterone production, a cryptorchid animal would show sexual desire and may be able to breed.

Hormonal analysis is the definitive diagnostic test for differentiating bilaterally cryptorchid animals from castrated animals. Baseline serum testosterone concentrations of less than 0.02 ng/mL indicate an absence of retained testicular tissue. In dogs with abdominally retained testes, the serum testosterone concentration usually is 0.1 to 1.2 ng/mL, whereas in adult dogs with one or two scrotal testes, the serum testosterone concentration usually is 1 to 5 ng/mL. However, testosterone is secreted in pulses throughout the day, therefore challenge testing may be more accurate than evaluation of a single sample. A hormonal stimulation test with HCG or GnRH can be used to demonstrate the presence and production of testosterone.[2,20,21] The incidence of Sertoli cell tumors is higher with abdominally retained testes. Although not a common occurrence, torsion of an abdominal testis can occur, leading to sudden abdominal pain. This phenomenon occurs almost exclusively in dogs with testicular tumors.

Treatment of animals with cryptorchidism is limited to castration. In unilaterally cryptorchid dogs, both testes (scrotal and abdominal) must be removed. Medical treatment with hormones such as GnRH or HCG is not effective. Removal of carrier parents from the breeding population would result in a decrease in the incidence of this condition.

Scrotal Hernia

With a scrotal hernia, the abdominal contents pass through the inguinal canal into the scrotum. An incidence of less than

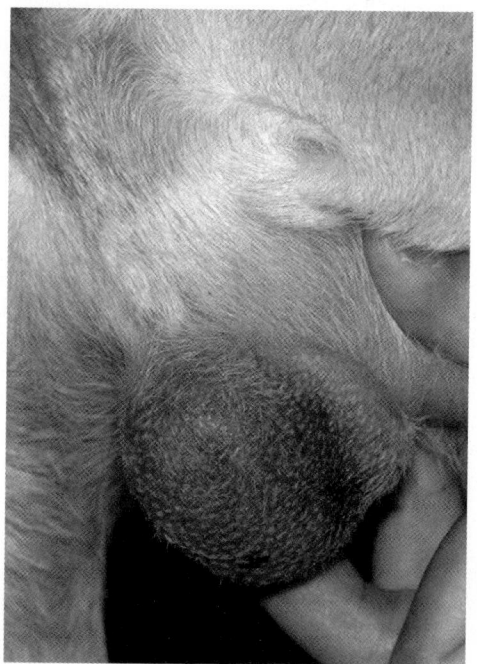

Figure 254-6 Unilateral left side enlargement of the scrotum of a 3-year-old pug with a hernia.

1% is reported, and the condition occurs primarily in young dogs ranging in age from 5 months to 4 years (the average age is 1.73 years).[2]

Differential diagnoses include orchitis, testicular torsion, testicular neoplasia, sperm granulomas, and trauma. On physical examination, a common finding is a fluctuant enlargement of the scrotum; in some cases, unilateral enlargement (Figure 254-6) is associated with ipsilateral inguinal swelling. The definitive diagnosis is made by careful palpation of the scrotum. Ultrasonography of the scrotum provides excellent information on the type of contents (Figure 254-7). Treatment involves surgical removal or replacement of the herniated tissues.

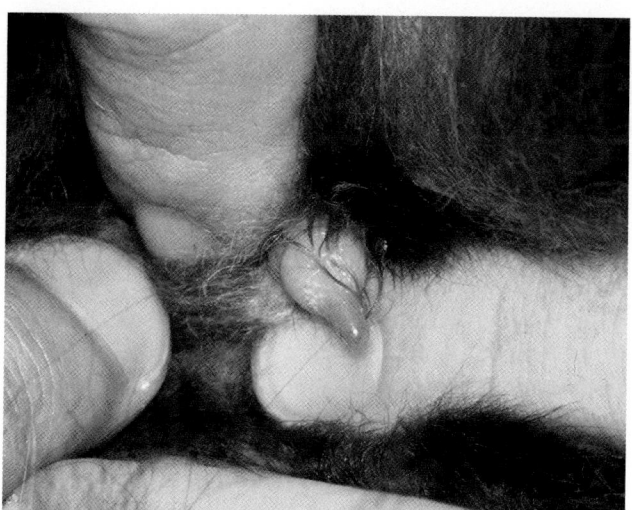

Figure 254-5 Spines on the penis of a cat.

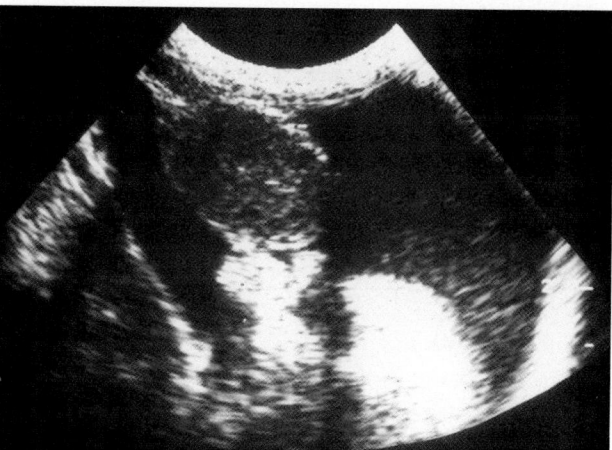

Figure 254-7 Sonogram of the scrotum with a hernia. Note the oval-shaped gray testis. The white areas below the testis are part of the omentum that has herniated from the abdomen. The black area around the testis is fluid, which accumulated in the scrotum. The hernia was corrected by surgery.

Testicular Tumors

Testicular tumors are common in dogs and rare in cats. The three most common types are Sertoli cell tumors, seminomas, and interstitial cell tumors. The reported incidence of testicular tumors is 0.91%, and the age of affected dogs ranges 2 to 19 years. The tumors may be unilateral or bilateral. All three types are equally prevalent in descended testes.

Dogs with testicular tumors most often have testicular enlargement without pain. A presumptive diagnosis is made by digital palpation and/or ultrasonographic examination of the scrotum. A neoplastic testis may or may not be significantly enlarged. Atrophy of the contralateral testis may have occurred as a result of hormone produced by the neoplastic testis or of an increase in the intrascrotal temperature. Nonpalpable tumors may be visualized sonographically, but the tumor type cannot be differentiated with this imaging modality.

Castration is the treatment of choice. Because of the high incidence of bilateral neoplasia and atrophy of the unaffected testis, removal of both testes is recommended. Unilateral orchiectomy may be considered in valuable breeding dogs. Sperm numbers decline 50% immediately after unilateral orchiectomy. Compensatory hypertrophy of the remaining testis, characterized by increased diameter of the seminiferous tubules, may be evident as early as 3 months after surgery.[2]

Sertoli cell tumors (SCTs) are more common in abdominally retained testicles. The scrotal testis that contains a SCT is usually enlarged and firm. Sonographically, the SCT is visible in the testicular parenchyma as a hypoechoic to anechoic area. SCTs commonly are associated with a feminizing paraneoplastic syndrome caused by estrogen secretion, which may lead to estrogen-induced pancytopenia. Feminizing signs are reported in 24% to 39% of dogs with an SCT. The clinical signs of paraneoplastic syndrome include bilaterally symmetric alopecia of the trunk and flanks with hyperpigmentation of the inguinal skin; a dry, easily epilated coat; gynecomastia; a pendulous preputial sheath; attraction of male dogs; and bone marrow hypoplasia with nonregenerative anemia.[2] Signs of feminization resolve within 21 days of surgical removal of the SCT. The prognosis for dogs with bone marrow hypoplasia secondary to SCT is guarded. Exfoliated cytology of the preputial mucosa may be useful for confirming the presence or recurrence of hyperestrogenism in dogs with SCT. The epithelial cells show cornification similar to that seen in the vaginal cells of a bitch in estrus.

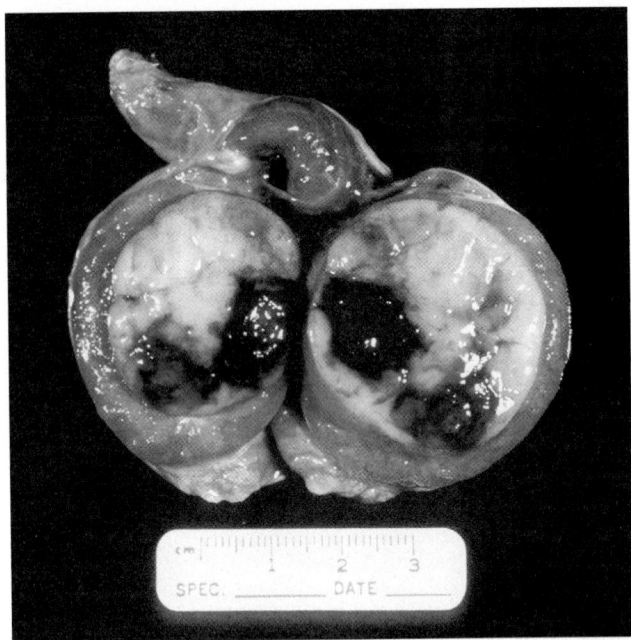

Figure 254-8 Testicular seminoma from an 8-year-old Dalmatian with an enlarged testis. Note the large areas of lobulated neoplasm and the areas of hemorrhage.

Seminomas (SEMs) are tumors of the spermatogenic cells. A higher incidence of these tumors is reported in older German shepherds (those over 10 years of age). Up to 10% of SEMs may metastasize to local or distant sites. Seminomas vary in size from 1 to 10 cm in diameter, are soft on palpation, and grossly are seen as homogenous or ovulated masses that are cream to pink-gray on the cut surface (Figure 254-8).

Interstitial (Leydig) cell tumors (ICTs), also called *interstitial cell adenomas*, arise from the endocrine cells of the testis. These tumors are small, usually less than 1 cm in diameter, and vary in color from yellow to brown on the cut surface. ICTs are the tumor of scrotal testes. Unlike the other two tumor types, ICTs are an incidental finding at the time of necropsy.

CHAPTER • 255

Feline Reproduction

Sophie A. Grundy
Autumn P. Davidson

REPRODUCTIVE TRACT ANATOMY

The Queen
Reproductive Tract

The reproductive tract of the queen is suspended in the abdominal cavity by the broad ligament, an extension of the peritoneum, which consists of the mesovarium, mesometrium, and the suspensory and proper ligaments of the ovary. The ovaries of the queen are mobile, oval, and typically 8 to 9 mm long.[1] The ovaries are attached cranially to the diaphragm by the suspensory ligament, which is attached to the abdominal wall by the mesovarium. The caudal pole of the ovary is attached to the tip of the uterine horn by the proper ligament. The lateral surface of the ovary is covered by an extension of the mesovarium, the mesosalpinx, and the medial surface is covered by the infundibulum of the uterine tube. The mesosalpinx in the queen is small and contains no fat, permitting excellent laparoscopic visualization of the ovary.

The uterine tube (oviduct) in the queen is 4 to 6 cm long and is visible as a tortuous structure within the mesosalpinx near the ovary. The uterus is bicornuate and extends from the uterine tubes cranially to the cervix caudally. The body of the uterus is 2 to 3 cm long, and each horn is 9 to 11 cm long and 0.3 to 0.4 cm wide. The mucous membrane of the uterus, which typically is reddish brown but may be focally pigmented (black), contains wide, spiral, longitudinal folds. Transabdominal palpation of the normal uterus and uterine horns typically is possible only during estrus or pregnancy.

The feline vestibule is 1 to 2 cm long, and the vagina is 2 to 3 cm long. The external urethral orifice is located ventrally at the vestibulovaginal junction. The feline cervix is approximately 45 mm cranial to the vulva. The cervix, vagina, and vestibule of the queen have a horizontal orientation. Examination of the cervix in the queen is difficult, because the vagina is narrower than the vestibule and nondistensible.[2] The intravaginal component of the cervix is papilliform and has the external uterine orifice. The queen has major mucous-producing vestibular glands (Bartholin's glands), 5 mm in diameter, in the lateral aspect of the vestibule.

The vulva of the cat is covered with dense hair and does not vary during different stages of the estrous cycle because it is unresponsive to estrogen. The clitoris is small and protrudes slightly from the shallow fossa clitoridis; it is not normally visible.

Mammary Gland

The typical female cat has eight mammary glands arranged symmetrically in four pairs extending from the ventral thorax to the abdomen. The preferred nomenclature for glandular identification is numeric; from 1 to 4, left and right, with the cranial glands being numbered 1. Each mammary gland consists of multiple lobules drained by four to eight ducts, which open into each teat. The lymphatic drainage of the two caudal teats is the superficial inguinal lymph node, whereas the two cranial mammary glands drain into the axillary lymph nodes. No lymphatic connections exist between the cranial and caudal segments of the mammary glands or across the midline, nor does lymphatic drainage from the mammary gland enter the abdomen or thorax.[3]

Placentation

Implantation occurs 12 to 13 days after ovulation in the cat. Fetuses are usually evenly distributed in the left and right horns as a result of embryo transmigration. The queen exhibits zonary, endotheliochorial placentation resulting from the loss of maternal endometrial epithelium and connective tissue. The fetal chorionic capillary epithelium is in direct contact with the maternal capillary endothelium, and placental transfer of maternal antibodies has been demonstrated in the queen.

The Tomcat

Reproductive Tract

The feline scrotum is ventral to the anus and lies dorsal to the caudally directed penis. The scrotum is densely covered with hair. The testes of the tomcat are ovoid to spherical and approximately 1.5 cm long and are positioned obliquely so that the epididymis is craniodorsal.[4] The epididymis is not normally palpable because of its close attachment to the testes. The spermatic cord and the tubular tunica vaginalis, which covers it, are relatively long due to the distance between the scrotum and the superficial inguinal ring. The feline penis is structurally similar to the canine penis, having proximal cavernous and distal osseous components. The os penis is small (approximately 5 mm long) and is pointed distally. The prepuce is a thick fold with a caudally facing orifice. The penis is usually contained within the prepuce. The base of the penis is studded with six to eight rows of small, cornified, keratinized papilla (spines), which are present only under the influence of testosterone. Penile spines are considered a secondary sex characteristic in the domestic male cat (Figure 255-1).

The tomcat has two accessory sex glands, the prostate and the bulbourethral gland. The prostate of the tomcat is bilobed and consists of the pars compacta and the pars disseminata. The pars compacta, which is approximately 1 cm long,

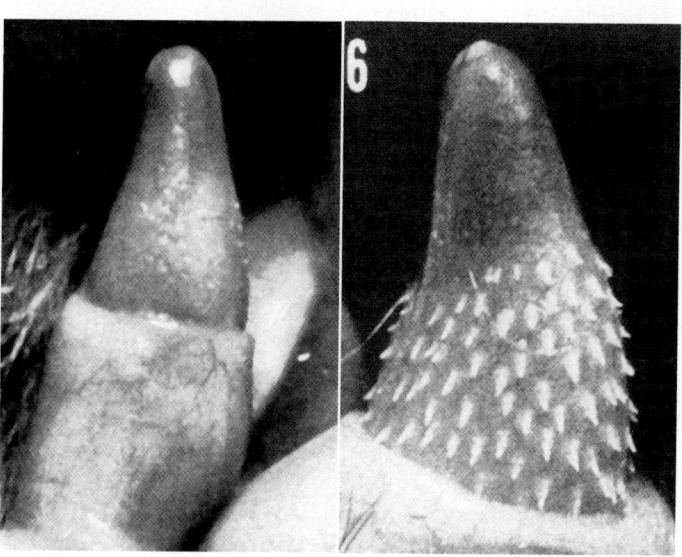

A   B

Figure 255-1 The smooth glands of a castrated male cat and penile spines of an intact male cat. (From Aronson LR, Cooper ML: Penile spines of the domestic cat: their endocrine behavior relations. Anat Rec 157:71-78, 1967.)

surrounds the dorsal and ventral urethra 2 to 3 cm caudal to the bladder. The pars disseminata consists of small lobules in the urethral wall extending from the bladder neck to the bulbourethral gland. The bulbourethral glands are small (5 mm long) and lie dorsolaterally on the urethra at the level of the ischiatic arch.

REPRODUCTIVE PHYSIOLOGY

The Queen

The queen is seasonally polyestrous. Ovarian activity is primarily under the influence of photoperiod and is stimulated by increasing hours of daylight. The true seasonal nature of the reproductive cycle of queens housed strictly indoors may not be evident. Cats maintained strictly indoors and exposed to artificial light for more than 14 hours a day may cycle at any time of the year and do not exhibit the typical seasonal breeding of their free-roaming counterparts. However, if these cats are returned to an outdoor environment, their ovarian activity becomes seasonal in nature. The queen exhibits induced, or reflex, ovulation. However, this is not an absolute phenomenon, and spontaneous ovulation occurs.[5]

Sexual Maturity and Pubertal Estrus

The queen typically reaches sexual maturity at 6 to 9 months of age. Two main factors influence the age of sexual maturity: body weight and exposure to light. The onset of ovarian activity and sexual maturity in the cat occurs as body weight approaches 2.5 kg; exposure to long photoperiod is essential. Queens exposed to outdoor light only typically exhibit estrus at the end of winter as day length increases. If a queen does not reach a body weight and age compatible with sexual maturity until late summer, when day length is decreasing, ovarian activity and sexual maturity most likely will be delayed until the following spring. The impact of breed on sexual maturity in domestic cats is small. As a general rule, oriental breeds are considered to exhibit pubertal estrus at an earlier age compared to long-haired breeds.

Estrous Cycle

In the absence of ovulation or pregnancy, repeated estrous cycles occur every 10 to 14 days during increasing photoperiod. The interval between repeated heat cycles is referred to as the *interestrous interval*. Other than the polyestrous cycle, which results in an interestrous interval, the queen has an estrous cycle that may be considered in four phases, which are similar to those in the dog: proestrus, estrus, diestrus, and anestrus.

Proestrus, the period of follicular development, is characterized by increasing serum estrogen concentrations. Queens do not permit mating during proestrus. The average duration of proestrus in the queen is 1 day. During this time, increased affection may be noted by the observant owner; however, proestrus is difficult to identify clinically. Under the influence of estrogen, the epithelial cells of the vaginal vault become cornified during proestrus and continue to cornify during estrus. In queens that permit vaginal cytology, vaginal smears may aid in the identification of proestrus.

Estrus, the period of sexual receptivity, is associated with follicle maturation and peak circulating serum concentrations of estrogen. In the queen, peak serum estrogen concentrations occur at the same time as maximal vaginal epithelial cornification. During estrus the queen permits copulation. The average duration of estrus in the queen is approximately 7 to 9 days regardless of coitus or ovulation.[6] There are few external physical signs of estrus in the queen. The female cat in estrus exhibits extreme affection, with a marked increase in head rubbing, vocalization, and frequent crouching of the thoracic limbs with rigid extension and treading of the pelvic limbs. Queens in estrus may also exhibit other signs, such as lordosis, and a laterally deviated tail. The presence of a male cat is not required to induce clinical signs of estrus. Queens subjected to stress may not exhibit behavioral estrus.

During copulation the male mounts the female and frequently bites the scruff of her neck. Male thrusting induces vocalization in the queen, which may be attributable to vaginal distention.[2] During the immediate postcoital period, the female exhibits a characteristic rolling and grooms the perineal region. Multiple copulations are common during estrus and may occur as frequently as every 15 to 20 minutes. The queen may exhibit mate preference towards particular tomcats.

After estrus the queen progresses through her estrous cycle, depending on the time of year, whether she experienced coitus, and her fertility. One of two outcomes follows estrus (Figure 255-2). One possible outcome is a nonovulatory cycle. Lack of ovulation typically occurs because of lack of copulation. If a queen does not ovulate, her estrous cycle will be 18 days long. This includes approximately 8 days of proestrus and estrus with a 10 day interestrous interval[5] (Figure 255-3). Anovulatory queens continue to exhibit signs of estrus every 18 days, providing they are exposed to increasing day length.

The other possible outcome is an ovulatory cycle. Estrogen priming of the reproductive tract is required to permit a surge in luteinizing hormone (LH) and ovulation in the queen. Historically, the release of gonadotropin hormone and ovulation in the cat were thought to occur only with stimulation of the vestibule and cervix associated with mating; however, spontaneous ovulation also occurs in the domestic cat.[2,5]

If the queen ovulates and forms functional corpora lutea, the rise in the serum progesterone concentration marks the start of *diestrus*. During diestrus, the serum estrogen concentration returns to baseline, and an increase in the serum progesterone concentration inhibits ovarian follicular development and return to estrus (Figure 255-4).

During an ovulatory nonpregnant cycle, the length of diestrus is determined by the life span of the corpora lutea. In the absence of pregnancy, the corpora lutea spontaneously regress after 35 to 37 days. At this time, the serum progesterone concentration returns to baseline, and the queen exhibits behavioral estrus approximately 10 days later. This results in an interestrous interval of about 45 days.

During an ovulatory pregnant cycle, the life span of the corpora lutea is prolonged and maintains the serum progesterone concentration above baseline for the duration of pregnancy. If the pregnancy is carried to term, gestation length is about 65 days. After queening, lactational anestrus typically delays the return to heat for an additional 45 to 50 days. Lactational anestrus is caused by inhibition of the synthesis of gonadotropin-releasing hormone (GnRH) as a result of sensory input caused by suckling. The ovulatory pregnant interestrous interval in the queen is approximately 120 days if lactational anestrus occurs. Pregnancy loss after 35 days results in a variable interestrous length. Typically, signs of estrus are detected about a week after pregnancy loss.

The interestrous interval is defined as the interval between repeated heat cycles, during which the queen does not exhibit signs of estrus or permit coitus. In the absence of ovulation or pregnancy, the normal interestrous interval in the queen is approximately 10 to 14 days. At the end of the interestrous interval, the onset of behavioral estrus is associated with waves of ovarian follicular activity and increased estrogen production. Each estrus is not necessarily associated with a new follicular wave. Typically, during the interestrous interval, the serum estrogen concentration returns to baseline, and the subsequent estrous behavior is associated with a new follicular wave. However, in some cats, follicular waves may overlap, or

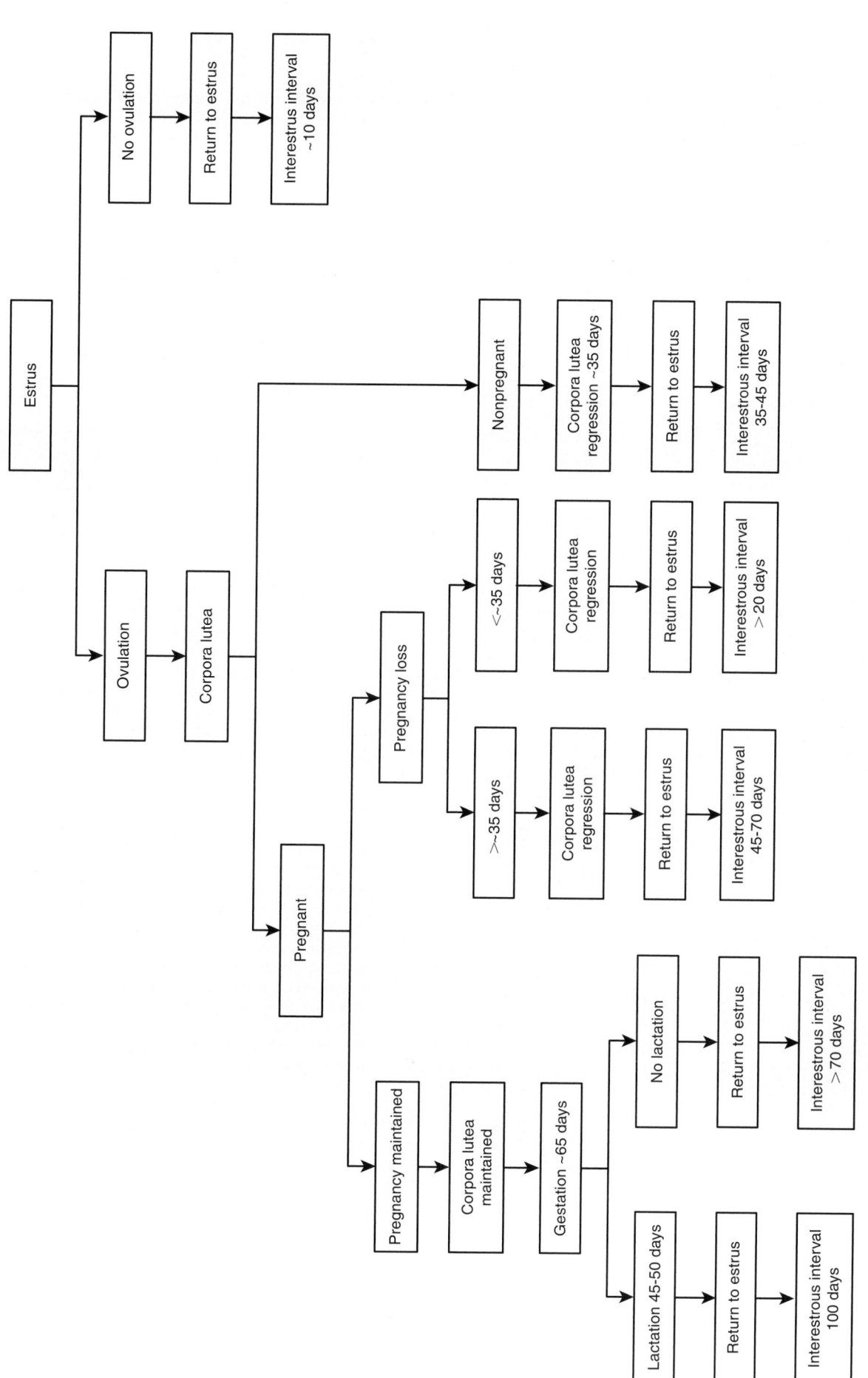

Figure 255-2 Flow diagram depicting the possible outcomes after behavioral estrus in the queen.

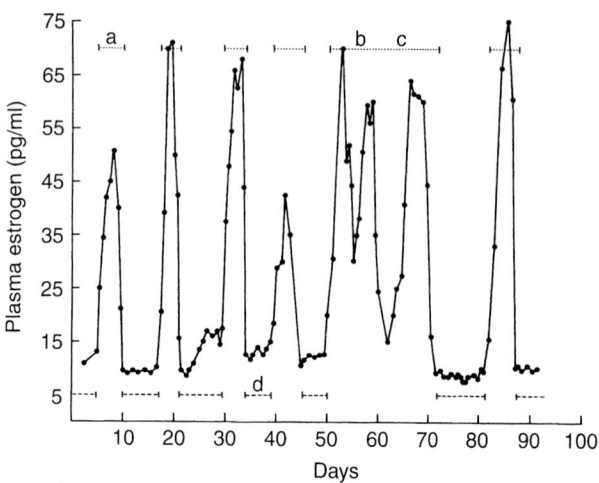

Figure 255-3 Schematic representation of the various estrogen secretion patterns that may occur during the estrous cycle of the cat. (From Feldman EC, Nelson R [eds]: Canine and Feline Endocrinology and Reproduction, 3rd ed. WB Saunders, 2001, pp 744 and 992.)

the serum estrogen level may not return to baseline during the interestrous interval. Clinically, these individuals are identified by persistent behavioral estrus, prolonged estrus, or "nymphomania." This phenomenon is neither typical nor abnormal.

Anestrus is a time of ovarian quiescence, when there is no ovarian follicular activity or functional corpora lutea (CL). In the queen, anestrus occurs in association with a short photoperiod, when females are exposed to less than 4 to 6 hours of light per day. Outdoor queens typically enter anestrus during winter. Indoor queens may exhibit anestrus when exposed to less than 6 hours of light per day. Anestrus also

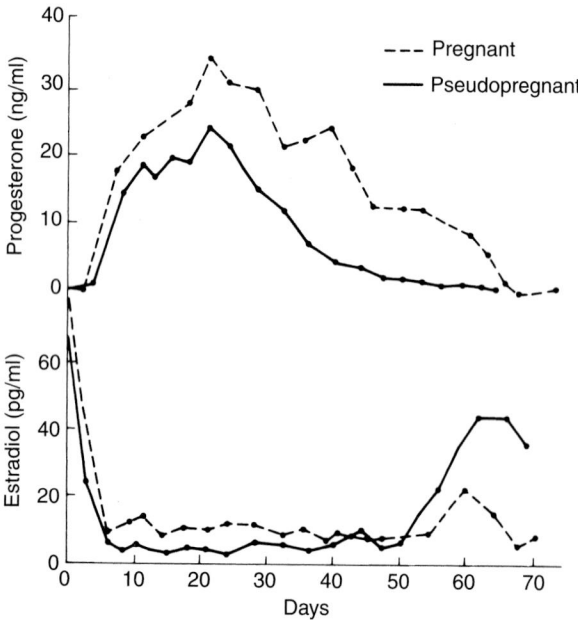

Figure 255-4 Average concentrations of progesterone and estrogen during ovulatory cycles in the queen. (From Feldman EC, Nelson R [eds]: Canine and Feline Endocrinology and Reproduction, 3rd ed. WB Saunders, 2001, pp 744 and 992.)

results from exposure to continuous light due to ovarian hyperstimulation.

Hormone profile of the queen's reproductive cycle
Increased photoperiod is associated with decreased circulating plasma concentrations of melatonin in the queen. Serum prolactin and melatonin concentrations are thought to fluctuate in association with one another. The exact relationship between the serum prolactin and melatonin concentrations and ovarian activity is not well understood; however, during periods of ovarian activity (estrus), serum concentrations of both are low.[7]

Estradiol 17-beta is produced in association with the follicular phase of the ovarian cycle by the developing follicles. The serum estrogen concentration peaks during estrus, often exceeding 80 pg/mL. In the absence of ovulation, ovarian follicles regress, and the serum estrogen concentration typically decreases to baseline (less than 20 pg/mL) during the interestrous interval. As a new follicular wave develops, the cycle continues until cessation of the breeding season or induction of ovulation.

Induction of ovulation in the queen has historically been attributed to vaginal stimulation causing an LH surge. The amplitude and duration of each LH surge are influenced by the intensity and frequency of coital stimulation. An optimal LH surge is reported in association with four copulations within a 2- to 4-hour period. In some instances spontaneous ovulation occurs.

If ovulation occurs, the resulting corpora lutea induce an increase in the serum progesterone concentration within 24 to 48 hours. The serum progesterone level during diestrus may be as high as 60 ng/mL. In the nonpregnant female, the feline corpora lutea exhibit spontaneous regression after 35 to 37 days. A decline in the serum progesterone concentration is noted around day 25, with a return to baseline by day 40. In the pregnant animal, unknown mechanisms result in maintenance of the corpora lutea, with the serum progesterone concentration remaining greater than 2 ng/mL for the duration of gestation. The specific factors responsible for luteotropic support in the cat are unknown, but they may be associated with placental development, fetal development, or other, unidentified factors.

The serum relaxin concentration is detectable only in the pregnant queen. In early pregnancy (until day 25 of gestation), the serum concentration is low. Peak concentration (7 to 9 ng/mL) is reached around day 35 of gestation. During the last 15 days of gestation, a decline is noted, and the serum relaxin concentration is undetectable 24 hours prior to parturition.[8]

In the pregnant queen, the serum prolactin concentration begins to increase at day 35 of gestation and peaks prior to parturition. Prolactin is luteotropic in the pregnant queen and is the hormone responsible for mammary development and lactation. Administration of a dopamine agonist (e.g., cabergoline) results in a decrease in serum prolactin and a decline in serum progesterone. Serum prolactin concentrations are low during estrus.

Vaginal cytology during the estrous cycle Vaginal cytology samples from the cranial vagina may be difficult to obtain in the conscious queen using a cotton tip applicator due to the narrowness of the vaginal vault. As an alternative, a small volume of saline (0.5 mL) can be flushed into and aspirated from the vagina to harvest vaginal epithelial cells. Vaginal cytology varies during the estrous cycle of the queen. During proestrus, the increasing serum estrogen concentration is reflected by an increase in the percentage of cornified vaginal epithelial cells. As queens enter estrus, mucous secretions thin, and debris is less visible in the background of vaginal smears; this is referred to as *clearing*.

An increase in keratinized anuclear squames is also noted on vaginal cytology during estrus in the queen.[7] Vaginal cytology during the interestrous interval is characterized by the predominance of nucleated superficial and intermediate squamous epithelial cells. The diestrus smear in the cat has a predominance of parabasal cells. During anestrus, vaginal cytology is similar to that during the interestrous interval, with a predominance of nucleated superficial and intermediate epithelial cells and much background debris.[7] Red blood cells are not noted during any phase of the reproductive cycle. Clinically, vaginal cytology in the queen may be used to detect the influence of estrogen in queens that fail to exhibit behavioral estrus or in those suspected of having ovarian remnant syndrome. Vaginal cytology is not a useful adjunct for ovulation timing in the queen nor is it useful for determining queening dates.

The Tomcat

The reproductive life span of the tomcat is reported to be more than a decade. In the absence of routine semen evaluation, information about reproductive performance is limited to litter production. Early declines in ejaculate quality typically remain undetected.

Sexual Maturity

Although spermatozoa may be evident in the spermatic cord of tomcats as early as 30 weeks of age, sexual maturity and the ability to mount, complete penile intromission, and ejaculate is rare prior to 12 months of age. Tomcats are typically sexually mature by 24 months of age. Persian and British breeds may mature later (3 years of age). Early characteristics associated with the development of sexual maturity in the tomcat include development of a rounded face and the onset of fighting, marking and mounting behaviors. Testicular descent is usually complete prior to birth. Spermatogenesis occurs in association with testicular weights greater than 1 g as body weight approaches 3 kg. The tomcat is capable of spermatogenesis year round; however, there is evidence of seasonal variation in sperm production and increased spermatozoa concentrations during long photoperiods.

Hormonal Profile of the Tomcat

The basal serum testosterone concentration in the intact male cat varies as a result of the pulsatile nature of the release of LH and follicle-stimulating hormone (FSH) from the pituitary. The serum testosterone concentration is an unreliable indicator of testicular function. In the domestic cat, penile spines develop under the influence of testosterone and provide a clinically useful bioassay for detection of circulating testosterone.

COMMON CLINICAL PROBLEMS

The Queen
Abnormal or Prolonged Estrous Behavior

Estrous behavior in a previously ovariohysterectomized female cat may indicate the presence of ovarian remnant syndrome. Alternatively, abnormalities of the zona reticularis of the adrenal cortex may be associated with sex hormone production. Ultrasonographic examination of the abdomen and evaluation of the serum sex hormone concentrations, along with stimulation of adrenocorticotrophic hormone (ACTH), may be useful for distinguishing between the two syndromes. Abnormal adrenal sex hormone production in the queen is uncommon.

Ovarian Remnant Syndrome

Ovarian remnant syndrome is the presence of functional ovarian tissue in a previously ovariohysterectomized animal. Functional residual ovarian tissue may produce enough follicular activity to trigger clinical signs of estrus in a female cat that had undergone ovariohysterectomy (OHE). Clinical signs of estrus generally occur months to years after OHE but can begin days after the surgery. The residual ovarian tissue is typically not in an abnormal location, and there appears to be no predisposition for the left or right ovary.[9] Accessory ovaries have been reported, but failure to remove ovarian tissue that extends into the mesovarium is more likely. Revascularization of free-floating ovarian tissue has been reported.[10]

The diagnosis of ovarian remnant syndrome is based on observation of appropriate clinical signs and confirmation of the presence of functional ovarian tissue through measurement of the serum estradiol and/or progesterone levels. A serum estradiol concentration greater than 20 pg/mL is associated with clinical signs of estrus. Vaginal cytology is an inexpensive, convenient bioassay that can confirm the influence of estrogen (i.e., cornification of the vaginal epithelium). Provided that no adrenal pathology exists and that exogenous estrogens are not being administered, ovarian remnant syndrome is the most likely cause of cyclic estrous behavior in a cat thought to have been surgically neutered. Various techniques for confirming the presence of ovarian tissue through the use of GnRH or HCG have been described; however, this is seldom clinically justified.[11] An increased serum progesterone level (greater than 2 ng/mL measured 2 to 3 weeks after estrus) may be seen in association with luteinization of ovarian remnants.

Removal of residual ovarian tissue by exploratory celiotomy is curative. Surgery is recommended during estrus or diestrus, because the presence of ovarian follicles or corpora lutea aids the identification of residual ovarian tissue. Medical suppression of follicular ovarian activity with progestational or androgenic compounds is less desirable because of the side effects, such as diabetes mellitus.

Mucometra and Pyometra

Mucometra and pyometra may occur in the queen in association with cystic-endometrial hyperplasia or as separate clinical entities. Under the influence of progesterone, the intrauterine leukocyte response is suppressed, myometrial contractility is reduced, and endometrial gland development is stimulated. Uterine quiescence and endometrial gland secretions create an opportune environment for bacterial proliferation. Intrauterine bacterial contamination may occur via ascending the urogenital tract or by the hematogenous route, resulting in a pyometra. Alternatively, the uterus may become distended with mucus and may remain sterile, resulting in a mucometra. E. coli is the most common intrauterine bacterial isolate in feline pyometra. Exogenous progesterone administration and repeated heat cycles without pregnancy precipitate the development of pyometra.

The clinical signs associated with pyometra in the queen vary with cervical patency. Most queens with pyometra are ill at the time of examination, having clinical signs ranging from anorexia, lethargy, and weight loss to those of septic shock and peritonitis resulting from uterine rupture. Queens with an open-cervix pyometra typically exhibit a moist perineum and purulent vaginal discharge, and owners may report increased grooming behavior. Polyuria and polydipsia may be noted in association with open and closed pyometra as a result of the nephrogenic diabetes insipidus that occurs secondary to the effect of E. coli endotoxins on renal antidiuretic hormone (ADH) receptors.

Clinicopathologic evaluation most often reveals a neutrophilic leukocytosis and hyperglobulinemia. Hypoalbuminemia may be noted in association with sepsis, and a decreased blood urea nitrogen (BUN) may be noted with severe polyuria and polydipsia. The serum progesterone concentration at the time of diagnosis typically is greater than 5 ng/mL. Vaginal cytology is unreliable for the diagnosis of pyometra. However, cytologic specimens containing numerous degenerate neutrophils with intracellular bacteria are consistent with pyometra. Ultrasonographic evaluation of the uterine horns is a reliable method of diagnosing pyometra. The uterine lumen is typically distended with flocculent material of variable echogenicity (Figure 255-5). Cystic ovarian structures may be noted, but the ultrasonographic appearance of the ovary varies.

The treatment of choice for pyometra is medical stabilization with antimicrobials and intravenous fluids, followed by surgical ovariohysterectomy. Medical therapy with natural prostaglandins and antimicrobials may be considered for queens with mucometra or for some cats with pyometra. Successful treatment of mucometra and pyometra with prostaglandin$_2$-α (PGF$_2$-α) (Lutalyse; Pharmacia and Upjohn, Kalamazoo, Michigan) results from the drug's effect on the uterine myometrium, cervix, and corpora lutea. In the queen, the corpus luteum is relatively resistant to the effects of exogenous prostaglandins. Repeated measurement of the serum progesterone concentration is advised prior to and during prostaglandin therapy to identify animals with persistent luteal function. Medical therapy should be considered only if an animal is of reproductive importance. Candidates for medical PGF$_2$-α therapy should be young (less than 6 years of age) and otherwise healthy, with evidence of a patent cervix (i.e., vaginal discharge). Contraindications for medical management of pyometra or mucometra include sepsis, peritonitis, significant organ disease, or old age, which is associated with an increased incidence of cystic endometrial hyperplasia. Concurrent administration of bactericidal broad-spectrum antimicrobials is advised.

PGF$_2$-α should be administered subcutaneously at a dosage of 0.1 mg/kg twice a day for 2 days, and increased to 0.2 mg/kg twice a day until abdominal ultrasound scans reveal no evidence of uterine enlargement, the complete blood count (CBC) has normalized, polyuria has improved, and the serum progesterone level is less than 5 ng/mL. Synthetic prostaglandins are available for use in Europe, and the dosage must be adjusted to account for the variation in potency. Side effects of prostaglandin therapy include restlessness, emesis, salivation, tenesmus, diarrhea, lordosis, and kneading. Administration of the prostaglandin at a reduced dosage for the first 48 hours should reduce the severity of side effects. Breeding at the next estrous cycle is recommended.

Pregnancy Termination
Please refer to Chapter 250.

Abnormal Mammary Development not Associated with Pregnancy
Mammary development in a nonpregnant or spayed female is abnormal. Care must be taken to distinguish between mammary development, which typically involves more than one gland, and formation of a mammary mass. Mammary development occasionally may occur in male or female cats in association with cessation of exogenous progestogen administration; however, the degree of mammary development is usually mild and transient.

In comparison, mammary hyperplasia (also known as *fibroadenomatous mammary hyperplasia*) is associated with dramatic enlargement of multiple mammary glands (Figure 255-6). The glands typically are painless, but they may become necrotic and subject to secondary infection. Usually no milk production occurs in these glands. Mammary hyperplasia is most frequently noted in young animals after their first estrous cycle. The condition appears to be associated with an increase in the serum progesterone concentration, and antiprogestins may be indicated.[12] Surgical mastectomy is indicated with severe necrosis or infection.

Mammary Masses
Mammary tumors are the third most common neoplasia in cats. Early ovariohysterectomy is associated with a decreased risk of mammary neoplasia. Most feline mammary tumors are malignant, and carcinomas are the most common tumor type.[13]

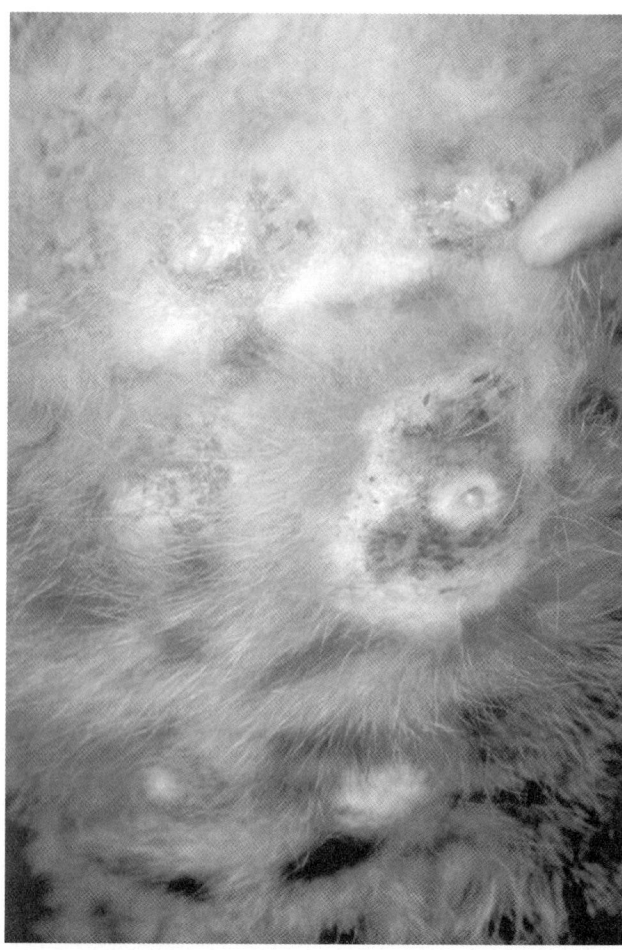

Figure 255-6 Mammary hyperplasia in a cat. (Courtesy Dr. Richard Nelson, University of California, Davis.)

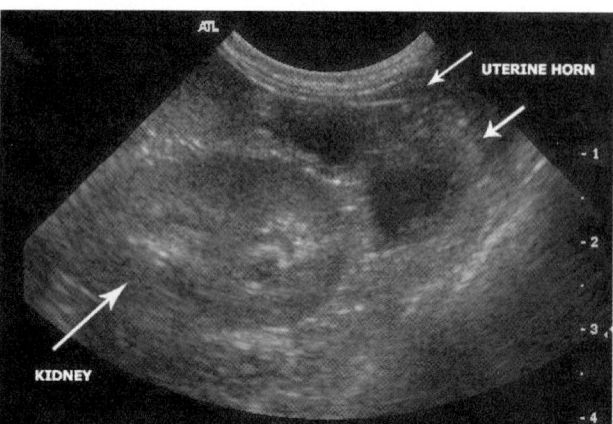

Figure 255-5 Ultrasonographic image of dilated uterine horns in a cat with pyometra. (Courtesy Tom Baker, University of California, Davis.)

Any detected mammary mass in the feline should be surgically removed with wide margins by an experienced surgeon and considered malignant until proven otherwise. Prior to surgical excision, ultrasonographic evaluation of the regional lymph nodes and radiographic evaluation of the thorax are advised to detect metastatic disease.

Subfertility and Infertility

Valuable breeding queens are commonly brought to a veterinarian for evaluation as a result of failure to reproduce at an expected rate. It is essential that, in addition to ensuring that clients have realistic expectations, the clinician take a logical and thorough approach to evaluation of the animal's reproductive performance and health. *Subfertility* in the queen refers to failure to produce an expected number of live kittens successfully; this may occur as a result of failure to breed or conceive or failure to carry fetuses to term. *Infertility* refers to the absolute inability to reproduce. Prior to any examination, cattery and breeding management must be evaluated to ensure that true subfertility or infertility exists. Good husbandry has a significant impact on reproductive performance in any species. Stocking density must be low enough to reduce stress associated with social situations and crowded conditions. Noise pollution should be avoided. Transport of animals between cages, and properties should be minimal. An adequate plane of nutrition should be maintained. Prophylactic techniques for common conditions should be performed on a regular basis, including routine retrovirus evaluation, appropriate vaccinations, grooming, nail trimming, dental care, external and internal parasite control, and appropriate quarantine.

Cattery owners should have a basic understanding of feline reproductive physiology so that estrous behavior, mating, and queening can be accurately recorded. Queens should be mated with a proven tomcat prior to infertility evaluation and ideally should be 1 to 6 years of age.

After ensuring that breeding management is adequate, the clinician should take a complete history and perform a thorough physical examination. The queen should then be further categorized based on her reproductive status.

Failure to cycle A combination of silent heat and spontaneous ovulation may lead an owner to believe that a queen has chronic anestrus. Regardless of whether the owner believes that the queen cycles, evidence for ovarian activity should be obtained. Vaginal cytology provides a convenient bioassay for the influence of estrogen during intervals of increasing photoperiod. Animals that fail to show signs of estrus during appropriate light exposure may be categorized as having prolonged anestrus.

Differential diagnoses for prolonged anestrus should include inadequate light exposure, prior gonadectomy, stress, abnormalities of sexual development, and drug administration. If all differentials have been excluded, attempts can be made to induce estrus by housing a tomcat nearby and increasing the day length. Where appropriate, pharmacologic induction through administration of dopamine agonists or FSH analogs can be attempted.

Prolonged estrus As previously mentioned, overlapping waves of follicular activity in the queen may result in signs of persistent estrus. Other explanations include ovarian follicular cysts and exogenous estrogen administration. Abdominal ultrasound is useful for detecting ovarian cysts. The cysts are typically greater than 4 mm in diameter and are visible in the parenchyma of the ovary; however, they may be difficult to differentiate from follicles. Ovariohysterectomy is curative.

Failure to ovulate Queens with ovulatory failure maintain an interestrous interval of approximately 10 days during the breeding season. Successful ovulation depends on the presence of mature follicles and an adequate LH surge, which is dependent on the frequency and number of copulations (if spontaneous ovulation does not occur). Failure to ovulate indicates that mating was incomplete or that it occurred too infrequently or at the wrong time. Breeding management should be re-evaluated.

Failure to conceive (prolonged interestrous interval) and pregnancy loss An interestrous interval greater than 25 days indicates that ovulation likely occurred. Explanations for failure to conceive include true conception failure and early fetal resorption. Ovulation should be confirmed by measurement of an increased serum progesterone concentration 48 to 72 hours after cessation of mating. Abdominal ultrasonography may also be used to evaluate for implantation. Fetal resorption occurs most commonly in association with congenital defects, which may occur secondary to teratogen exposure. Feline leukemia virus is an important viral cause of embryonic death, fetal death, and abortion in the queen. Other infectious causes of fetal resorption include chlamydia, feline panleukopenia virus, feline coronavirus, and feline respiratory virus complex. *Toxoplasma* infection has been implicated in feline infertility. Bacterial infections (e.g., *Salmonella* spp.) are more likely to result in abortion than resorption.

Uterine monitoring for prevention of early pregnancy loss Uterine monitoring may be used during gestation to evaluate for premature uterine contractions (Figure 255-7). Pregnancy loss as a result of hypoluteoidism has not been documented in the queen. It is more likely that any decrease in serum progesterone associated with premature contractions occurs secondary to endogenous prostaglandin release and destruction of the CL. Clinical signs associated with premature contractions are typically limited to an abnormal vaginal discharge (usually hemorrhagic) prior to term in the pregnant queen. Tocolytic agents (e.g., terbutaline) have been tried successfully in queens to reduce uterine contractions and carry pregnancy to term.

Abnormal sexual behavior Infrequently, queens may exhibit intense dislike for particular males and refuse to allow breeding. Selection of an alternate male or artificial insemination resolves the problem. In queens that fail to show signs of

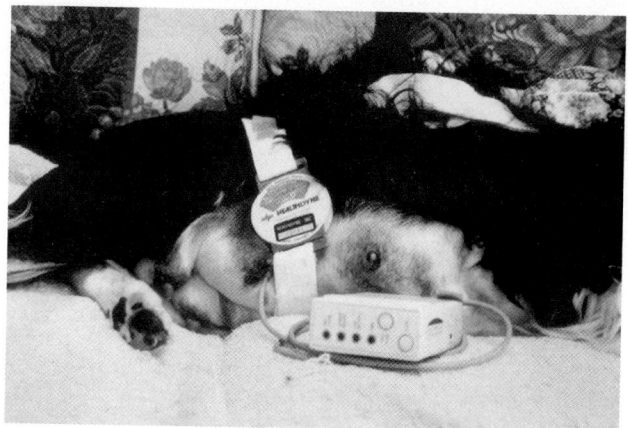

Figure 255-7 Pregnant queen with uterine monitor in place. (Courtesy Karen Copeley, Veterinary Perinatal Services, Colorado.)

estrus or that refuse to permit copulation, induction of ovulation followed by artificial insemination may be required.

Uterine pathology   Cystic endometrial hyperplasia may be associated with infertility in the older queen. Definitive diagnosis requires uterine biopsy. No effective treatment is available.

The Tomcat

Tomcats are not typically brought to the veterinarian for reproductive evaluation unless they have an external abnormality of the genital tract, are exhibiting poor libido, or show evidence of infertility.[14]

Abnormalities of the Genitalia

Trauma   Injury to the external genitalia and other parts of the body is common in tomcats as a result of intermale aggression and fighting behavior. Routine wound management, consisting of cleaning, debridement, and antimicrobial therapy, is appropriate. Animals not intended for breeding should be castrated.

Cryptorchidism   Testicular descent in the tomcat is usually complete at birth. However, because continued movement of the testicles in the inguinal canal is noted until puberty, it is wise to delay evaluation for cryptorchidism in the tomcat until 6 months of age. The incidence of cryptorchidism in the tomcat is low, and there appears to be no predilection for the left or right side. In one retrospective study, cats were more likely to be unilaterally cryptorchid.[15] In the cats with bilateral cryptorchidism, both testicles were in the abdominal cavity. Persian cats were over-represented.[15] Medical therapy for the treatment of feline cryptorchidism cannot be advocated due to suspected heritability. Surgical castration is curative.

There is a single report of estrous behavior in a bilaterally cryptorchid tomcat in association with interstitial cell hyperplasia.[16] Feminizing syndromes in association with cryptorchid testicles and Sertoli cell tumors are extremely rare in the cat.

Testicular hypoplasia   Testicular hypoplasia is rarely reported in the tomcat, because most male cats are castrated. However, it has been detected in association with prepubertal panleukopenia infection, as a result of fever-induced germinal layer destruction, and in association with vitamin A deficiency.

Orchitis   Orchitis is rare in the tomcat and usually occurs secondary to a bite wound. It may also be the result of extension of peritoneal infection through the inguinal ring in association with feline infectious peritonitis. Cats are naturally resistant to *Brucella canis* infection.

Persistent penile frenulum   In the cat, breakdown of the penile and preputial mucosal surface adhesion is an androgen-dependent phenomenon. Persistent penile frenulum is associated with early castration (before 7 weeks of age).

Phimosis, paraphimosis, and priapism   *Phimosis* (constriction of the orifice of the prepuce) and *paraphimosis* (inability to retract the penis into the prepuce) are unusual in cats but may occur secondary to preputial trauma, or to entanglement of the hairs of the prepuce. *Priapism* (persistent erection) is also uncommon but has been reported in association with hemostasis, thrombosis, and failure of detumescence.[17]

Prostatic Disease

The prostate is rudimentary and generally of little clinical concern. However, both bacterial prostatitis and prostatic neo-

plasia have been reported in the cat.[18,19] Clinical signs include dyschezia and intermittent constipation and hematuria.

Urine Spraying and Masturbation

The tomcat sprays urine to identify territory, and this is considered normal behavior for an intact male. Castration resolves urine spraying in 80% of cats.[20] Urine spraying may persist in the castrated cat and is considered undesirable by most owners. It is important for the clinician to distinguish between urine spraying (typically on vertical surfaces) and inappropriate elimination. Selective serotonin reuptake inhibitors and tricyclic antidepressants are commonly used to reduce the occurrence of urine spraying in castrated males. There is a single case report describing the successful use of cyproheptadine for the treatment of urine spraying and masturbation in a tomcat.[20]

Infertility

Evaluation of the tomcat for infertility is uncommon. Limited data are available regarding common problems and their successful management. Reported reasons for reproductive evaluation of the tomcat associated with infertility include lack of libido, behavioral abnormalities, trauma, and infections. Tomcats infrequently undergo semen evaluation because of the reluctance of most owners to permit general anesthesia and electroejaculation to enable semen evaluation and because of the general lack of availability of this service in private practice. Evaluation of infertility in the tomcat should include cattery management evaluation as described for the queen. A complete physical examination should be performed and a routine clinicopathologic and infectious disease database should be obtained, in addition to evaluation of the genital tract for signs of trauma or abnormality.

Lack of Libido

Gonadal abnormalities or sexual immaturity may result in a lack of libido in the male cat. In breeds that are typically late maturing, the evaluation should be delayed until 3 years of age. The penis should be examined to document the influence of testosterone. Testicular palpation and measurement of testicular volume should be performed; however, currently, little published data correlate reproductive performance with testicular volume in the cat. Breeding management should be reviewed to ensure that husbandry or stress is not a contributing factor. If permitted, electroejaculation, semen evaluation, and artificial insemination are advised if the cat appears to be clinically normal and management problems have been excluded. Testosterone supplementation is not recommended in tom cats as it results in negative feedback on endogenous hormone production, thereby exacerbating the problem.

NEOPLASIA OF THE GENITAL TRACT

Please refer to Chapter 188.

PREGNANCY AND PARTURITION

Fertilization takes place in the uterine tube. Morulae enter the uterus approximately 5 days after coitus, and embryos are distributed evenly in the left and right uterine horns. Superfecundation is possible. The hormonal profile during pregnancy reveals increased serum progesterone and relaxin concentrations and a low serum estrogen concentration. The serum prolactin concentration increases in the latter half of gestation. The main source of progesterone support is the corpora lutea. Waves of ovarian follicular activity may

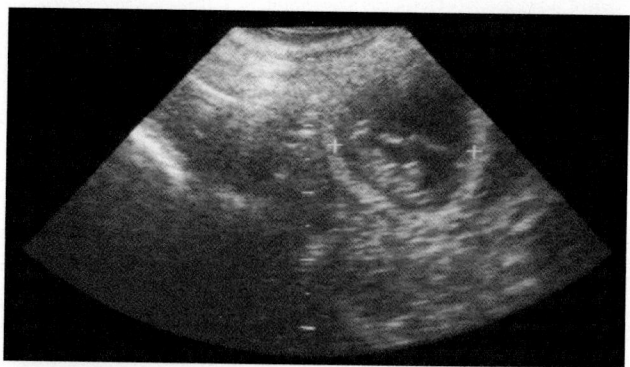

Figure 255-8 Ultrasound image of a gravid uterine horn with an intraluminal fetus and fetal membranes. (Courtesy Tom Baker, University of California, Davis.)

occur during pregnancy, resulting in fluctuations in the serum estrogen concentration, which can result in estrous behavior during gestation.

Pregnancy diagnosis by means of transabdominal palpation in the queen is best performed during the second and third weeks of gestation. During this time, palpation of the uterus reveals grape-sized vesicles. Later in pregnancy, the segmental nature of the uterine lumen is lost, and transabdominal palpation is more challenging. Abdominal ultrasonography is the preferred technique for diagnosing pregnancy in the queen, because it is easy to perform during all stages of gestation and it provides information regarding fetal viability (Figure 255-8). The normal fetal heart rate in the cat exceeds 200 beats per minute, and heart rates are detectable as early as 25 days after mating. Radiographic detection of the fetal skeleton is possible at 45 days after breeding.

A mild, transient increase in the serum estrogen level is noted several days prior to parturition; this is associated with upregulation of oxytocin receptor expression in preparation for parturition.

Care of the Pregnant Feline

Metabolic requirements do not increase until the second half of gestation. The current recommendation is to feed pregnant queens a commercially prepared, AAFCO-approved kitten diet at the time of pregnancy diagnosis; to increase the amount of food by 25% for weeks 5 and 6 of gestation; and to make an additional 25% increase for weeks 7 and 8 of gestation. Food intake may be increased a further 25% in the final week of gestation. Commonly, cat breeders supplement pregnant queens with raw liver during early pregnancy because of concerns about hypovitaminosis A; this is not necessary when queens are fed commercial cat food. Pregnant cats should be weighed once weekly and kept indoors. Weight gains in the range of 5% of body weight are anticipated per week. Routine vaccinations should be avoided because of the risk of cerebellar hypoplasia with the modified-live panleukopenia vaccine. Griseofulvin and glucocorticoids are known teratogens in the queen, and their use should be avoided during pregnancy.

Clinicopathic Changes in the Pregnant Queen

Plasma volume expansion in the queen results in a mild normocytic-normochromic nonregenerative anemia during late gestation. Queens should be given access to a box prior to their anticipated due date. A private cardboard box lined with towels provides the queen with a quiet, dark environment while also permitting observation. Reports of the length of

gestation in the cat vary because of the inability to establish the time of ovulation accurately. As a general rule, parturition occurs 65 days from the first known breeding.

Some queens have a decrease in rectal temperature approximately 12 hours prior to the onset of parturition. Stage one labor (cervical dilatation) commences with the onset of uterine activity and ends with complete cervical dilatation. During this stage, nesting behavior, increased licking of the perineum, and restlessness may be noted. Queens typically choose to stay in the queening box at this time. Some cats that are particularly bonded to their owners may actively seek them.

Typically, visible abdominal contractions indicate the start of stage two labor. This stage is defined by coordinated uterine contractions and expulsion of the neonate. The first delivery should occur within 1 to 2 hours of visible contractions. Clear, blood-tinged fluid is generally expelled from the vulva prior to delivery of the first kitten. It should be noted that posterior presentation of the neonate is common and is not necessarily associated with dystocia. Queening is typically completed within 12 hours. Litter size is breed dependent and ranges from one to 10 kittens per litter.

Dystocia is less common in the queen than in the bitch. Uterine monitoring as described in the bitch has been used successfully in the queen to identify impending labor and to aid in evaluation of dystocia.[21] Medical therapy with oxytocin and calcium gluconate may be attempted without uterine monitoring. Uterine monitoring, when possible, may demonstrate the nature of the problem, and response to therapy can then be accurately judged. Uteroverdin (green discharge) present prior to presentation of a kitten; an interval longer than 1 hour between kittens; a sick queen; or stage one labor that lasts longer than 24 hours without the onset of stage two labor warrants examination of the queen by a veterinarian. The initial evaluation should consist of a physical examination, digital vaginal examination, radiography of the abdomen to establish the presence of kittens, and abdominal ultrasonography to ascertain fetal heart rates. Generally speaking, fetal heart rates less than 150 beats per minute indicate fetal distress, and cesarean section is advised to reduce neonatal mortality and queen morbidity. If available, uterine monitoring may be used to direct medical management of dystocia.

Colostrum is produced as long as 72 hours postpartum. Neonates should nurse within 1 hour of birth. The typical duration of lactation in the queen is 4 to 6 weeks, depending on the time of weaning. Lactational anestrus is typical in nursing queens; however, signs of estrus may occur as early as 2 weeks postpartum.

Care of the Partum Queen

During lactation the metabolic demand doubles. In the immediate postpartum period, many queens are reluctant to leave their kittens and may show transient anorexia. A continuous supply of palatable, easily digestible, calorie-dense food should be available, in addition to an ample supply of fresh water. If possible, the food and water should be placed in the queening box during the first week of lactation to encourage consumption. Postpartum lochial discharge is normal in the queen and should be scant and reddish brown. Nursing queens should be monitored closely for signs of illness, such as excessive or abnormal vaginal discharge (putrid odor, black or green color), fever, inappetence, vomiting, or diarrhea.

Involution in the queen varies between nursing and nonnursing queens. In the non-nursing queen, uterine size and tone return to those of a prepartum queen by 4 weeks postpartum. In the nursing queen, continued hyperinvolution occurs, resulting in a uterus similar in tone and thickness to that seen during ovarian quiescence.[22]

PARTURIENT AND PERIPARTURIENT PRESENTATIONS

Neonatal Care
Please refer to Chapter 256.

Uterine Torsion
There are several reports of uterine torsion in the queen (Figure 255-9). Uterine torsion should be considered a possible problem in any queen seen in late pregnancy or during parturition with dystocia, abdominal pain, or hypovolemic shock.[23] Medical stabilization is essential to reduce mortality. Intravenous colloids may be indicated for blood volume expansion. In addition, pain relief, antimicrobial therapy, and plasma products may be indicated. After stabilization, exploratory celiotomy permits definitive diagnosis, and surgical ovariohysterectomy is curative.

Retained Placenta
Any excessive, malodorous vaginal discharge in the postpartum queen is abnormal. Placental retention should be a considered in any queen with a fever and increased or purulent, foul-smelling vaginal discharge in the immediate postpartum period. The diagnosis of retained fetal membranes is best made by means of ultrasonographic evaluation of the uterus, because owner observations may be unreliable. In these cases, abdominal ultrasonography reveals uterine horn distension and focal hyperechoic intrauterine contents in association with a retained placenta. Medical therapy, consisting of administration of PGF$_2$-α (Lutalyse), 0.1 mg/kg given subcutaneously once a day for 3 to 5 days, is typically effective. Concurrent antimicrobial administration is indicated in queens with a fever or marked leukocytosis.

Metritis
Acute metritis may occur in association with retained fetal membranes or as a result of ascending bacterial infection in the immediate postpartum period. Clinical signs of metritis include anorexia, fever, vomiting, kitten neglect, decreased milk production, and a purulent, sanguineous vaginal discharge. Medical therapy with PGF$_2$-α (Lutalyse) and antimicrobials may be attempted, providing that the queen is stable and the cervix is open.

Prolapsed Uterus
Uterine prolapse has been reported in the queen (Figure 255-10). Queens suspected of having uterine prolapse should be

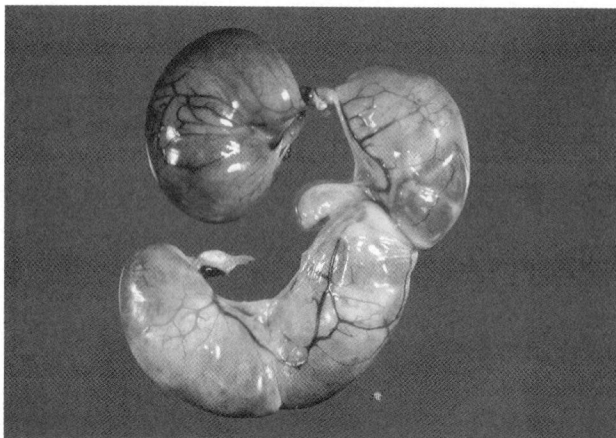

Figure 255-9 Torsion of a gravid uterine horn. (Courtesy Dr. Gerald Ling, University of California, Davis.)

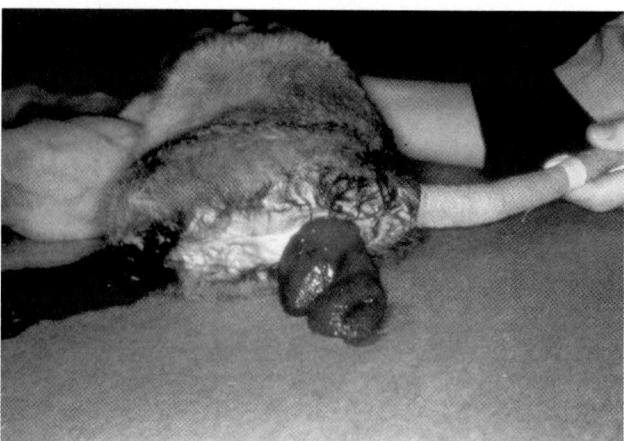

Figure 255-10 Uterine prolapse in a cat. (Courtesy Dr. Richard Nelson, University of California, Davis.)

examined promptly to reduce desiccation and trauma to the exposed tissue. Manual replacement of the uterus can be attempted; however, because repeated prolapse tends to occur, ovariohysterectomy is advised.

Hypocalcemia
Hypocalcemia (eclampsia) may occur early in lactation as a result of the sudden increase in calcium loss associated with milk production. Clinical signs include incoordination, stiff gait, facial pruritus, muscle fasciculation, hyperthermia, and seizure activity. The diagnosis is based on clinical observations in the lactating queen. Immediate medical therapy consists of slow intravenous administration of 2 to 5 mL of 10% calcium gluconate over 5 minutes. Repeated administration may be required to achieve resolution of clinical signs. The electrical activity of the heart should be monitored during intravenous calcium administration to evaluate for arrhythmia. Long-term therapy should include daily calcium carbonate supplementation (TUMS, 500 mg/day). If necessary, kittens should be prevented from nursing and should be hand raised after receiving colostrum.

Mastitis
Inflammation and subsequent bacterial infection of the mammary glands during lactation are common. Clinical signs include anorexia, lethargy, fever, and vomiting. Neonates may have diarrhea. Affected glands appear red and swollen and are warm and painful. Palpation may reveal firm areas associated with inflammation. The milk expressed from the affected glands may be grossly purulent and red or grayish, and the queen's body temperature may be increased. The most common bacterial isolates include *Enterobacter* sp., staphylococci, and streptococci. Medical treatment, consisting of warm compresses, stripping of the affected mammary glands, and administration of broad-spectrum antibiotics usually is curative. In severe cases, when inflammation results in tissue necrosis, surgical debridement may be required.

ASSISTED REPRODUCTION

Electroejaculation
Although male cats may be trained to ejaculate using an artificial vagina, most client-owned cats presented for semen collection are untrained. Semen collection and evaluation in the untrained tomcat are best achieved using electroejaculation techniques with the cat under general anesthesia.

Many drugs commonly used for sedation in the cat interfere with urethral sphincter function. When electroejaculation is performed, urine contamination negatively affects the quality of the ejaculate. The preferred drug combination for electroejaculation in the cat is ketamine and xylazine. An alternate option, in a cooperative tom that permits placement of an intravenous catheter, is a constant-rate infusion of propofol. In a recent study, a propofol infusion was shown to have a minimal impact on urethral sphincter function in dog; however, studies in the cat have not been completed.[24]

Once sedated, tomcats are placed in lateral recumbency, and a well-lubricated rectal electroejaculation probe of appropriate size is inserted into the rectum. The penis should be gently exteriorized and held in the normal caudal orientation for semen collection. For electroejaculation in the carnivore, probes with longitudinal electrodes are preferred.[25] The rectal probe is connected to a standard electroejaculator unit capable of measuring voltage and amplitude. The standard electroejaculation regimen uses a total of 80 electrical stimuli delivered in three series, consisting of 30 (series 1: 10 stimulations at 2, 3, and 4 V), 30 (series 2: 10 stimulations at 3, 4, and 5 V), and 20 (series 3: 10 stimulations at 4 and 5V) stimulations.[25]

Care should be taken to ensure light ventral pressure to maximize ejaculate yield. Semen should be collected in plastic supplies prewarmed to body temperature.

Semen Evaluation
Evaluation of the ejaculate should include determination of the semen volume, pH, and color, as well as the sperm count, percentage motility, progressive motility, gross morphology, and acrosomal integrity.[25] In comparison to the dog, cat ejaculate contains a higher concentration of spermatozoa (1.5 to 2×10^9/mL). Counts are best performed manually using a hemocytometer. The volume obtained varies with the skill of the person performing the electroejaculation; however, an ejaculate volume of 50 to 100 µL per series may be considered normal. The ejaculate should be cloudy. The normal pH of feline ejaculate is 7.4 to 8.3. Urine contamination is suggested by a yellow discoloration and is confirmed by a pH less than 7.4.

Immediately after collection, the ejaculate should be evaluated at body temperature for the percentage motility and progressive motility of sperm. Normal progressive motility of sperm in the cat is 50% to 80%. Sperm morphology is a commonly used indicator of fertility in the male. In general, lower fertility is thought to be associated with a higher percentage of morphologically abnormal spermatozoa and/or a lower percentage motility. However, studies evaluating the percentage of normal spermatozoa required for consistent fertility have not been completed.[26] The gross morphology of feline spermatozoa may be determined by fixing an ejaculate aliquot (20 µL) in 500 µL of glutaraldehyde (1% solution), followed by phase contrast light microscopic evaluation at ×1000.[25] If phase contrast microscopy is not available, morphologic assessment can be performed by staining an air-dried smear of ejaculate with Diff Quick. Some domestic cats consistently ejaculate a high proportion (greater than 50%) of morphologically abnormal spermatozoa without associated infertility.[27]

Evaluation of acrosomal integrity is a useful adjunct to semen evaluation because it is critical to the fertilization process. Examination of the unstained feline acrosome may be challenging because of the small size of spermatozoa (26 µm long). Acrosomal staining prior to evaluation may be done in the cat using the protocol described by Larson and Miller,[28] or it may be completed with phase microscopy if available.

Semen Freezing
Cryopreservation of feline semen is important for the preservation of genetically valuable animals. Although semen freezing in the cat is not routinely performed in private practice, electroejaculation and semen collection and evaluation for the tomcat are not difficult. Numerous protocols have been described for cryopreservation of feline spermatozoa, the details of which are outside the scope of this chapter.[29,30] Of importance is the susceptibility of feline spermatozoa to cold shock. To minimize damage, extreme care must be taken to ensure that everything that comes in contact with feline spermatozoa is at the same temperature as the sperm cells themselves. As a general rule, anything that is added to feline spermatozoa should be added slowly, with gentle mixing. Because of the high incidence of pyometra associated with feline artificial insemination, antimicrobials (commonly penicillin and streptomycin) typically are added prior to insemination.

Induction of Estrus and Induction of Ovulation in the Queen
Infrequently, induction of estrus may be required in the queen for artificial insemination with frozen semen or for queens that fail to exhibit clinically detectable signs of estrus. Induction of estrus in the sexually mature queen has been successfully achieved using exposure to long photoperiod or with administration of exogenous gonadotropins. Various protocols and dosing regimens have been described. Dosing regimens are described per cat, because ovulatory response is not related to body weight. Typically, 100 to 200 IU of equine chorionic gonadotropin (ECG; Sigma Chemical Co., St. Louis, Missouri) is used to stimulate follicular development, and 100 to 150 IU of human chorionic gonadotropin (HCG; Sigma Chemical Co.) is used to stimulate final follicle maturation and ovulation.[31,32] Ovulation occurs approximately 24 to 36 hours after administration of HCG.

The authors' preferred protocol is ECG, 100 to 150 IU, given subcutaneously or intramuscularly on day 1, followed by HCG, 50 to 100 IU, given subcutaneously or intramuscularly 84 hours later. Insemination should be performed 2 to 3 days after HCG administration. Alternatively, cabergoline (5 µg/kg given orally every 24 hours) can be administered for a maximum of 15 days. Insemination should be performed on day 3 of estrus. Ovulation in the cat is compromised by preovulatory anesthesia. If artificial insemination is to be performed, it is important that ovulation occur prior to anesthesia or it may be inhibited. Because of the molecular size of exogenous gonadotropins, repeated administration may be associated with antibody formation and reduced ovarian response. The immunologic consequences of exogenous gonadotropin administration may be minimized by reducing the frequency and number of times they are used during an animal's reproductive life.

Artificial Insemination
Cervical patency varies during the feline estrous cycle. Vaginal insemination is readily achieved using a bulb-tipped, 20-gauge needle and 1 mL syringe. Blind transcervical catheterization under general anesthesia has also been described.[33] The suggested insemination dose for artificial insemination is 50 million progressively motile spermatozoa.

Laparoscopic insemination in felines is well described. The suggested insemination dose is 10 million progressively motile spermatozoa per uterine horn.

CONTRACEPTION

Please refer to Chapter 250.

CHAPTER 256

Care of the Neonate and Fading Pups

Gary C.W. England

The incidence of neonatal death is surprisingly high in domestic dogs born in pet homes and to private breeders. The incidence of stillbirth is 6% to 33% of all births, and the neonatal death rate ranges from 6% to 11%. Some of these cases can be attributed to genetic factors or dystocia, which can be difficult to avoid. However, in many such deaths, inappropriate or poor husbandry practices are the cause or a contributing factor. It is clear, however, that this need not be the case; in a survey of 1342 puppy births at the Guide Dogs for the Blind Association in the United Kingdom, the total rate for stillbirth and neonatal loss (up to 6 weeks of age) was less than 5%.

Understanding the challenges facing the fetus at the end of gestation and during parturition, as well as the normal biology of the neonate, enables the veterinarian and breeder to better deal with neonatal problems. This chapter discusses those challenges and methods that may be used to overcome them.

CHALLENGES TO THE FETUS AND NEONATE

A number of factors may affect the survival of the neonate by challenging (1) the fetus during late gestation, (2) the fetus at parturition, and (3) the neonate immediately after birth.

Fetal Challenges during Late Gestation

Any challenge that adversely affects fetal development and results in the birth of an underweight neonate is likely to influence the newborn's subsequent survival. In humans, low birth weight can result in immaturity of the cardiovascular system and other physiologic functions (Barker hypothesis),[1] and this likely is also true in the dog. Such influences may make the puppy more susceptible to subsequent challenges, such as hypoxia, hypothermia, and neonatal infections.

A small or underweight puppy may be the result of inappropriate nutrition or generalized debility of the dam, the parasite burden of the dam, specific or generalized placental lesions, or infection of the dam with agents that cross the placenta (e.g., canine herpes virus).

Challenges at Parturition

During the change from fetal to neonatal life, a number of significant challenges can arise that may compromise subsequent survival. For example, although uterine contractions are essential to propel the fetus into the birth canal, this process also creates the opportunity for a decrease in the placental blood supply, constriction of the umbilical vessels, and early placental separation. Most, if not all, pups are born with mild to moderate hypoxia and slight to severe acidosis. The acidosis is generally respiratory in origin, but a metabolic component also is often present. In an adult, acidosis usually results in increased respiratory effort to remove the excess carbon dioxide. However, this is not always observed in the neonate (which suggests that carbon dioxide is not such a potent stimulator of respiratory drive in the neonate as it is in the adult).

Also, body temperature declines rapidly after birth, because the wet neonate is born into an environment cooler than the maternal temperature. Although a brief period of hypothermia may actually be useful as a mechanism to protect against the effects of hypoxia, it is clear that persistence of hypothermia contributes to neonatal mortality. In the normal neonate, hypoxia and hypothermia are rapidly reversed and a stable state is reached within 3 to 4 hours after birth. If the acid-base disturbance or hypothermia are maintained beyond this period, a fatal cycle of decline may ensue. Clearly, conditions such as dystocia (including, ultimately, cesarean operation) and poor mothering behavior prolong both hypoxia and hypothermia, resulting in increased neonatal mortality.

Neonatal Challenges

The common challenges met by the neonate are persistence of the previously mentioned hypoxia, as a result of a delay in the removal of fetal membranes or fluid by the dam; persistence of hypothermia, associated with a delay in drying of the neonate; and a cold or drafty environment. Poor mothering behavior by an inexperienced primiparous bitch may be the primary cause of both hypoxia and hypothermia.

Adequate intake of fluid is the next major hurdle for the neonate, not only because of the requirement to absorb colostrum (see discussion below) but also because adequate fluid maintenance is important for recovery from acidosis. Neonates have a relatively higher percentage of fluid in the extracellular space and relatively poorer renal function than do adults. This situation, combined with the neonate's ability to lose fluid because of a high surface area to body ratio, results in a greater susceptibility to changes in fluid balance for neonates compared to adults.

Furthermore, the neonatal immune system is incompletely developed until at least 10 days after birth, which makes newborns susceptible to bacterial and viral infection. The dog has an endothelial-chorial placenta that allows approximately 20% of passive immunity to be acquired by the fetus in the uterus. The remaining 80% of antibodies must be absorbed across the intestine within the first 24 to 48 hours of life. The absorption of immunoglobulin G (IgG) from colostrum decreases markedly after this time, because the ability of the intestinal wall to absorb intact proteins declines. Failure to consume sufficient colostrum during the interval when the intestinal wall is open to the absorption of intact protein seriously compromises the immune status of the neonate.

Neonates have limited reserves of body fat, and their ability to generate energy from precursors is poor. Also, because glycogen reserves are depleted shortly after birth (only limited storage of glycogen occurs), the neonate requires a prompt intake of energy. A short time without food can result in a significant hypoglycemia, particularly in neonates that have been hypoxic or hypothermic. In humans, it has been suggested that anoxia can reduce gut motility and result in abnormal uptake of ingested nutrients. Clearly, food intake can be restricted in its availability from the dam because of illness, poor mothering, poor milk production or letdown, or a large litter size. Several of these factors may occur concomitantly with hypoxia or hypothermia, compounding the problems.

The neonate may also be faced with a number of challenges from potential pathogenic organisms. In many cases these are normally commensal bacteria that become pathogenic in a debilitated animal. In some cases, primary pathogenic organisms are involved (e.g., canine herpes virus, discussed later).

Characteristics of Normal Neonates

Neonatal pups are unable to stand at birth, although they are quite mobile, using their front limbs to crawl. They normally spend 90% of the time asleep and cry only when they are disturbed or hungry. During normal sleep, pups make frequent small movements of the limbs, characteristic of rapid eye movement (REM) sleep.

The normal rectal temperature for the first week after birth is 32° to 34° C. Respiration should be regular and even, usually 15 to 40 breaths per minute. The heart rate is usually 200 to 220 beats per minute (bpm), and heart murmurs may be functional. The capillary refill time is normally 1 to 1.5 seconds.

Normal birth weight varies according to breed, with pups of most medium breeds weighing 200 to 300 g at birth. The birth weight of healthy neonates increases by 5% to 10% per day, and failure to achieve this weight gain may indicate poor health.

Pups are born with their eyes closed; separation of the upper and lower lids, with opening of the eyes, occurs at approximately 10 to 14 days of life.

OPTIMIZING NEONATAL SURVIVAL

It is clear that during late pregnancy, parturition, and the early neonatal period, a number of significant challenges arise that, if not overcome, can result in the ultimate demise of the neonate. Having an understanding of these challenges allows the veterinarian or breeder to manage the pregnant, parturient, and nursing bitch and her litter so as to reduce subsequent mortality.

Care of the Bitch Before and During Pregnancy

Prior to mating, due consideration should have been given to routine anthelmintic treatment, although this does not necessarily reduce the potential for transplacental infection with *Uncinaria* sp. or transplacental and transmammary infection with *Toxocara* organisms. If a significant problem has been identified in a kennel, daily oral administration of 25 mg/kg fenbendazole from day 40 of gestation until 2 days past whelping may reduce transmission to the fetus.

During pregnancy, voluntary food intake usually increases; however, the body condition score of the bitch should be examined to ensure that she is not too fat or too thin. It is normal to increase the amount of food offered in the last 20 days of pregnancy, at which time a diet consisting of at least 30% protein, 18% fat, and 20% to 30% carbohydrate is suitable. At whelping the bitch will be eating 60% more food than usual. Obesity during pregnancy and poor nutrition both can contribute to poor neonatal survival, resulting in fetal oversize or lactational problems and fetal undersize, respectively.

One week prior to anticipated parturition, the bitch should be encouraged to accept a nest in a suitable environment. This should be a warm, clean, draft- and damp-proof room that can be heated. The room is best isolated from the main thoroughfare of the household. Ideally, the bed should

be large enough to allow the dam to stretch, and it should provide sufficient room for a large litter. The sides should be high enough to prevent the puppies from escaping until they are approximately 4 weeks old.

In the last week of pregnancy, it is prudent to record the bitch's rectal temperature at least twice daily to detect the prepartum hypothermia that precedes the onset of parturition by 24 to 36 hours. This decline in body temperature is mediated by a sudden reduction in the serum progesterone concentration. The rectal temperature usually changes from approximately 39° C to less than 37° C.

Care of the Bitch at Parturition

Careful monitoring of the bitch at parturition can reduce neonatal mortality by reducing the risk of hypoxia and hypothermia and ensuring adequate intake of colostrum. Education of the whelping attendant is essential to ensure that this individual understands the normal stages and time sequence of parturition. Uterine activity can be monitored by observation of the bitch's abdomen when she is relaxed, but monitoring is more accurate if external monitoring devices, such as a tocodynomometer, are used.[2]

Prompt veterinary attention should be sought if evidence of any form of dystocia arises. It is not possible to give definitive guidelines for every potential case of dystocia, but veterinary examination is warranted in certain situations, such as when the bitch (1) has exceeded 70 days from the last mating and has no signs of impending parturition; (2) is unsettled and strains forcefully but infrequently; (3) shows signs of straining, which then cease; (4) has a black/green vulval discharge with no signs of parturition; (5) shows a decline in rectal temperature but parturition has not commenced within 48 hours; (6) has been straining ineffectually for 1 hour or longer; (7) has produced the last pup more than 2 hours previously but still is restless; and (8) has produced the last pup more than 2 hours ago, and a larger litter is expected.

Care of the Neonate

The first essential steps after the pup's birth are to establish a clear airway, stimulate respiration, dry and warm it, and encourage it to suck. Normally this is achieved by the dam licking and nuzzling the pup. Young or maiden bitches may need help and encouragement with the immediate licking and cleaning. Failure of this behavior to occur, for whatever reason, can be catastrophic.

It is essential that a clear airway be established as soon as a fetus has been born. If human help is required, this involves removing the surrounding fetal membranes and clearing the mouth and nose of fetal fluid with either a dry towel or a small pipette. Gentle compression of the chest usually establishes respiratory effort. If this does not occur but the heart is beating, respiratory stimulation should continue by means of rubbing of the thorax and removal of more fluid by gently swinging the neonate in a small arc (however, the latter course should be avoided unless absolutely necessary because of the risk of brain trauma). In certain cases, administration of a respiratory stimulant (e.g., doxapram hydrochloride) may be efficacious, as may administration of oxygen. If respiration does not commence, artificial respiration can be attempted. This should be done carefully so as to induce only slight lung expansion and not overinflate the lungs. If the heart is not beating, external cardiac massage combined with artificial respiration may be attempted.

The umbilicus should be cut approximately 3 cm from the fetal abdomen; excessive bleeding can be prevented by application of a ligature.

Once regular respiratory efforts are maintained, the neonate may be placed in a prewarmed box or incubator until it is active, at which point it may be returned to the dam and encouraged to suck. Sucking normally occurs immediately after birth and at intervals of 2 to 3 hours for the first few days.

Hypothermia is a major cause of neonatal mortality, therefore the environmental temperature is a critical factor. Because neonates are unable to regulate their own temperature for the first week of life, they rely on the dam and other neonates for warmth. A chilled neonate does not respond normally or move properly, nor is it able to suck; this may cause the dam to neglect it, exacerbating the problem. The whelping area should be heated to 25° to 30° C for the first few days. This temperature may be almost unbearable for the dam, but it can be safely reduced to approximately 24° C after this time. It is most important that the litter be kept well away from any drafts.

The area where parturition and rearing are to take place is also a concern. Although it is important that this room not be near a thoroughfare, it is beneficial for socialization of the puppies if noise can be heard, such as from a washing machine, a radio, or people talking. The room should be of sufficient size to allow the growing puppies to play and, where possible, to have access to an outside area.

Care of Older Neonates

During the first few weeks of life, the dam normally takes care of the needs of the litter. Nevertheless, the pups should be examined regularly. It is most important to assess for the general demeanor, weight gain, and general characteristics of healthy neonates described previously.

Normally the dam licks the neonate's perineal region to stimulate it to defecate and urinate. After the first 2 to 3 weeks, pups urinate and defecate voluntarily, which increases the amount of soiling in the whelping bed. The environment should always be kept clean, warm, and dry.

An important neonatal assessment is the correct rate of development. At 10 to 14 days, a pup's eyes should open, and it gradually should become able to focus on objects. It also should gain strength and begin to crawl around.

Artificial Rearing of Neonates

For a number of reasons, some or all of the litter may need to be reared artificially; such reasons include the death of the dam, the birth of a large litter, a sick dam, poor mothering ability, eclampsia, or inadequate milk production. When possible, artificial rearing is best avoided. A good alternative is to foster the pups onto another dam, such as a lactating bitch that has just whelped and lost its litter or a bitch with pseudopregnancy. With an excessively large litter, it may be possible to alternate some of the litter between artificial rearing and rearing by the dam. Whenever possible pups should remain in the nest with the dam to ensure normal socialization.

It is essential that all neonates receive colostrum from the dam to ensure an adequate uptake of immunoglobulins. If the dam has died, it may still be possible to express some colostrum from her as long as it is not contaminated with drugs or toxins. Colostrum from a different species may be used as an alternative to bitch colostrum, although the antibody protection offered is limited. Despite this, some nonspecific defense against infectious agents may be afforded by compounds such as lysozyme, lactoferrin, oligosaccharides, and lactoperoxidases.[3] Furthermore, some evidence indicates that the lipid-dependent antimicrobial activity present in bovine milk may be effective in the neonatal puppy.[3] Clearly, the best alternative is to store colostrum for such a possibility by freezing or to purchase a commercially available preparation. Some veterinarians claim reasonable success with the technique of subcutaneously injecting the neonate with serum from vaccinated dogs.[4]

With artificial rearing, consideration must be given to the nutritional requirements of the neonate. An important factor that is often overlooked is the changing composition of mammary secretions during lactation.

The optimum milk protein concentration, total lipid concentration, and milk fatty acid and amino acid composition vary markedly among the different species, and it is not appropriate to substitute milk from another species, at least on a long-term basis. The preferred option is to use a commercially manufactured milk replacer because of the quality and consistency of these products. The milk should be warmed to body temperature (approximately 34° C) and should be fed according to the manufacturer's instructions, with regard to the pup's body weight and age.

Artificial rearing is both demanding and time-consuming, especially if rearing is undertaken entirely without the bitch. Pups normally feed every 2 to 4 hours during the first 5 days of life, after which feeding declines to every 4 hours. Feeding can be achieved by using a commercial feeding kit, which contains a bottle and teat. This encourages normal sucking, but it can be time-consuming. The teat aperture should be large enough to prevent the pup from sucking in air but small enough to prevent the flow of excessive volumes of milk. Feeding can also be done with a dropper bottle or 2 mL syringe. In some cases it may be beneficial to use a stomach tube to feed the pups, especially during the first few days of life. This is especially useful for sick neonates or when the litter is large and the attendant faces time constraints.

As previously discussed, neonates do not voluntarily urinate or defecate until 2 to 3 weeks of age. In the absence of the dam, the perineal region must be stimulated every 3 to 4 hours with a moistened piece of cotton to ensure normal voiding.

SICK PUPPIES

Known Causes of Mortality

Pups may fail to thrive and ultimately die for many reasons, including poor husbandry, maternal factors (e.g., illness and poor nutrition, which usually result in low birth weight pups), congenital defects, problems at parturition (usually dystocia, resulting in anoxia or hypoxia), poor mothering behavior, trauma, immune insufficiency, and infection with viruses, bacteria, or parasites. These causes, most of which were described previously (except for infectious causes), account for approximately 45% of all cases of neonatal mortality.

Infectious organisms are often given much prominence as the cause of neonatal death, although they account only for about 20% of mortality cases, depending on the country. Some infectious agents are specific pathogens, whereas others are opportunistic organisms that can colonize a compromised neonate. Specific examples of agents that can cause neonatal death include canine herpes virus, canine parvovirus, canine distemper virus, and some protozoa.

Exposure of an immunologically naive bitch to canine herpes virus during late pregnancy can result in abortion or in neonatal death, usually 7 to 21 days after birth. Earlier demise of the pups does not occur, and on this ground alone herpes virus infection can be differentiated clinically from true fading puppy syndrome (see below). Canine parvovirus type 1 may cross the placenta if the bitch is exposed in early pregnancy; although such disease is rare, it may result in resorption of the fetuses or in acute neonatal death 7 to 21 days after parturition. Infection with canine parvovirus type 2 may cause myocarditis in neonates, although this now is uncommon. Similarly, congenital infection with canine distemper virus is rarely seen.

Interestingly, a number of bacteria have been isolated from dead pups with peritonitis, pneumonia, pleuritis, and enteritis. These include beta-hemolytic streptococci, staphylococci, *Pasteurella* sp., *Escherichia coli*, *Campylobacter* sp., *Salmonella* sp. and, less commonly, *Ureaplasma* and *Mycoplasma* organisms.

Most of these organisms are part of the commensal flora of the bitch's genital tract, and they cause disease only when the neonate has succumbed to one of the previously mentioned challenges. The inherent vulnerability of a neonate puts it at risk for colonization by these organisms, which may result in rapid death with few initial clinical signs.

Transplacental infection with *Toxoplasma gondii* is uncommon, although experimental infection may result in neonatal death. Similarly, although the incidence of natural transplacental transmission of *Neospora caninum* is unknown, experimental infection results in stillbirth with evidence of myocarditis. *Toxocara canis* infection usually causes disease in pups over 2 weeks of age, by which time the worms have grown large enough to cause gastrointestinal obstruction or to migrate up the biliary tract and cause hepatitis.

Unknown Causes of Mortality (True Fading Puppy Syndrome)

In approximately 55% of pups that die, no specific cause can be determined; these pups are correctly termed *fading puppies*. Such pups usually have a normal birth weight but appear depressed and show poor sucking with persistent crying. The condition progresses to generalized weakness and ultimately to death, usually between day 3 and day 5 after birth.[5] Fading puppies usually have no macroscopic lesions (except often a small liver), no identifiable congenital defects, and no histologic lesions, and they simply have an absence of contents within the large and small intestine. They constitute a distinct category, separate from most other causes of neonatal death. These other "known" causes ultimately result in puppies that "fade," but most often from day 7 after birth onward.

Interestingly, Blunden et al.[6] found that true fading puppies (those with no other known cause) had significantly lower phosphatidylcholine components of lung surfactant than pups that died of known causes. Lung surfactant is required for normal respiratory adaptation and maintenance after birth. A significant reduction of surfactant is observed in sudden infant death syndrome in humans, and the low values in fading puppies suggest that faulty production of surfactant may similarly be involved in the etiology of this condition. In the normal animal, increased respiratory effort tends to stimulate surfactant production; it may be that pups with true fading puppy syndrome are born marginally hypoxic and, because carbon dioxide stimulation of respiration is absent, they do not breathe deeply; they thereby enter a downward spiral of low surfactant, hypoxia, failure to thrive, failure to suck, hypothermia and, ultimately, death.

Despite the clear difference in clinical presentation between true fading puppies and puppies with identifiable causes of disease, it is common for any puppy that becomes ill to enter a downward course of failure to feed, resultant dehydration, and death. Many veterinarians use the term "fading puppy" to describe this demise regardless of its cause.

Clinical Signs of Sick or Fading Puppies

True fading puppy syndrome generally is observed from day 2 after birth onward, and most such pups die between day 3 and day 5. The pups usually show progressive weight loss, depression (or occasionally unusual restlessness early in the disease process), persistent crying, failure to suck, generalized weakness, dehydration, hypothermia and, ultimately, death.

In conditions in which the cause of the illness is identifiable, ill health usually results in frequent crying, restlessness, and hypothermia, progressing to clinical signs of diarrhea and/or dyspnea with resultant dehydration or cyanosis and, ultimately, death, usually later than 7 days after birth. In certain circumstances some neonates are more chronically affected and fail to grow as expected prior to the onset of obvious clinical disease.

Consequences of Disease in Canine Neonates

Whatever the initial challenge, the inherent susceptibility of the newborn results in its ultimate demise. Neonates have poor mechanisms of thermoregulation, which leaves them susceptible to hypothermia. They are unable to shiver and have poor reserves of brown adipose tissue. Puppies have approximately one fifth the glomerular filtration ability of adults and almost twice the water requirement, which makes them susceptible to dehydration. At birth, they have high red and white cell counts, which decline rapidly over the first week, and immature liver enzyme systems. The neonate's ability to regulate blood glucose concentration also is immature, and the newborn relies almost entirely on hepatic glycogen reserves over the first 24 hours. With prolonged parturition or a prolonged interval to feeding, the reserves may be exhausted, and hypoglycemia may complicate hypothermia.

Treatment of the Sick Puppy
Minor Disease

Any neonate with minor signs of disease (lethargy, slowness to feed, lack of weight gain) requires early supplemental feeding. If the intake of colostrum is a concern, a source of frozen-thawed or replacement colostrum should be given, as discussed earlier, preferably before day 3 of life. Thereafter milk supplements should be fed by stomach tube every 2 hours. During this early phase, it is essential that the pup's body temperature be maintained at approximately 34° C and the temperature should be recorded every few hours. The environmental temperature should also be monitored using a thermometer placed adjacent to the neonates and maintained at 25° C to 30° C. Adequate hydration should be ensured and can be estimated from recordings of weight gain (measured three times daily), by evaluation of the skin's elasticity, and by examination of the urine. Because normal neonatal urine is colorless, the presence of color in the urine may be a useful and simple indicator of dehydration. General nursing care also is important and should include regular perineal stimulation to ensure urinary and fecal voiding.

The use of antimicrobials may be considered in an ill neonate, not necessarily because of a primary infectious cause of the illness, but rather because a sick neonate is highly susceptible to colonization from otherwise commensal organisms. A commonly used antibiotic is clavulanic acid–potentiated amoxicillin, administered at a dosage of 12.5 to 25 mg/kg given orally twice daily.

Significant Disease

In a neonate with anything other than mild clinical signs, rapid and aggressive treatment is essential, including oxygen administration, fluid therapy, and administration of broad-spectrum antimicrobial agents.[7] Despite such treatment, the mortality rate can be high. Absence of feeding, dehydration, or other clinical signs are indicators for immediate initiation of aggressive treatment.

If significant disease is suspected, it is important that a regimen of rigorous clinical examination and evaluation every 4 hours be established; it should include recording of the rectal temperature, assessment of the mucous membrane color and capillary refill time, recording of the respiratory and heart rates, and evaluation of skin elasticity and urine color. At specific points in time, evaluation of blood hematology and biochemistry may be useful. Many pups are hypoglycemic, and a rapid evaluation can be done by placing a drop of blood on a glucose reagent stick.

It is important that normal laboratory values be interpreted with respect to the age of the neonate (Table 256-1), because the hematologic and biochemical parameters of neonates differ significantly from those of adults.

An incubator or a homemade oxygen tent system can provide an oxygen-enriched environment for the pup.

Table • 256-1

Normal Hematologic and Biochemical Values for Neonatal Pups (Birth to 8 Weeks Old)

PARAMETER	0 TO 2 WEEKS	2 TO 4 WEEKS	4 TO 8 WEEKS
RBC ($\times 10^6$/uL)	3.4-6	3.5-4.8	4.5-6.8
Hb (g/dL)	9-12.6	8.5-8.9	8.4-9.5
PCV (%)	32-50	25-30	26-40
MCV (fL)	65-90	50-80	65-75
MCH (pg)	21-30	16-25	20-30
MCHC (%)	32-35	32-35	30-33
WBC ($\times 10^3$/uL)	9-25	8-16.5	10-18.9
ALT (IU/L)	20-300	10-30	10-50
AST (IU/L)	20-250	10-50	15-30
ALP (IU/L)	200-10,000	150-500	100-150
TP (g/dL)	3.5-5.5	3.5-4.5	4-5
Alb (g/dL)	1.5-3	1-2	2-3
Glucose (mg/dL)	50-150	60-150	60-250

RBC, Red blood cell concentration; *Hb*, hemoglobin concentration; *PCV*, packed cell volume; *MCV*, mean corpuscular volume; *MCH*, mean corpuscular hemoglobin; *MCHC*, mean corpuscular hemoglobin concentration; *WBC*, total white blood cell concentration; *ALT*, alanine aminotransferase; *AST*, aspartate aminotransferase; *ALP*, alkaline phosphatase; *TP*, total protein; *Alb*, albumin.

Alternatively, a tracheal catheter can be placed, a technique that is especially useful for pups with concomitant upper respiratory tract problems. Oxygen administration can help overcome hypoxia, and artificial ventilation may be useful for reversing acidosis and encouraging the production of lung surfactant.

Pups with pale mucous membranes and a slow capillary refill time (greater than 2.0 seconds) usually are at least 10% dehydrated. This fluid deficit must be replaced, in addition to the ongoing maintenance requirement. Fluid requirements for general maintenance are approximately 60 to 180 mL/kg/day. In a small number of neonates, fluid may be replaced by oral administration of electrolytes; however, in most pups, fluids must be provided by intravenous, intraperitoneal, or intraosseus administration.

Intravenous catheter placement may be difficult in a dehydrated neonate. An over-the-needle catheter should be used whenever possible, because this is the easiest type to keep in position for long periods. However, human neonatal scalp catheters may be technically easier to place in small vessels. It is always worthwhile to spend some time ensuring adequate venous access, and although surgical cut down onto a vein initially may seem to lengthen the procedure, in the long-term it often is the most sensible option. The cephalic vein is most often catheterized, although because of the short length of the neonate's leg, kinking of the catheter is common. Catheterization of the jugular vein is better. With catheter placement, care must be taken to perform appropriate sterile preparation of the site to avoid introducing organisms or providing a focus of infection.

In the consideration of which fluids are most suitable for administration, it is sensible in most cases to assume that acidosis is a factor. The safest fluid replacement, therefore, is lactated Ringer's solution (although the neonate has reduced hepatic function and may be unable to metabolize lactate into bicarbonate), which is given with added maintenance potassium (20 mmol/L). Ideally the acid-base and electrolyte status should be established, although this may be difficult. If the acidosis is likely to be severe, bicarbonate may be given; administration of 2 mmol/kg over 2 to 4 hours is recommended if specific acid-base data are not available.

Once the ideal fluid has been selected, it is important that ongoing maintenance and current deficits be estimated. Normal principles of the estimation of fluid deficit apply; as a rough guide for immediate replacement, 1.5 mL can be administered per 50 g of body weight. In many neonates the total fluid volume to be administered is small, and it may be useful to consider administration via a syringe pump to avoid overhydration. Intraperitoneal administration may be used if venous access is difficult or if ongoing monitoring to ensure successful intravenous administration is likely to be inadequate. The most appropriate intraperitoneal dosing scheme is to provide fluids in three boluses at approximately 8-hour intervals. The risk of accidental puncture of viscera is relatively small, although repeated needle placement poses a risk of sepsis. Despite the relative merits of this technique, intraperitoneal fluids may be relatively slowly absorbed, especially in hypovolemic neonates. In reality, it is preferable to ensure adequate venous access.

If access to a vein is not possible, fluids may be administered by the intraosseus route.[8] In the neonate, access normally is provided via the trochanteric fossa of the proximal femur or the flat medial aspect of the proximal tibia (distal to the tibial tuberosity). The hair should be clipped and the site prepared aseptically. A standard 18- to 20-gauge needle (size and length vary, depending on the pup's size) is used to push longitudinally into medullary cavity. In some cases the cortical bone is sufficiently soft to allow the use of an intravenous over-the-needle catheter. Repeated puncture is not advised, because holes in the cortical bone allow fluid leakage; however the catheter may be left in position for up to 72 hours. Thereafter a new catheter should be placed in a different bone. Fluid and drugs can be administered via the needle at rates similar to those for intravenous infusion.

In some neonates hypovolemia may be complicated by sepsis, and the resultant combination of problems can be catastrophic. Although the use of corticosteroids in neonates with hypovolemic and septic shock remains controversial, short-acting intravenous agents (e.g., methylprednisolone sodium succinate) are the drugs of choice. Septic shock may result in further depletion of glycogen reserves, increased peripheral use of glucose, and decreased gluconeogenesis, resulting in hypoglycemia. In such animals, additional bolus glucose therapy can be provided by using a 5% dextrose solution mixed 50:50 with the lactated Ringer's solution or by giving 1 to 2 mL of 10% glucose intravenously.[9]

In certain circumstances, specific drug therapy may be considered, including administration of vitamin K_1 for pups with signs of hemorrhage, or administration of doxapram hydrochloride for pups with poor respiratory effort (or in an attempt to increase surfactant production). In human neonates, it is common to administer a surfactant (phospholipids, neutral lipids, and hydrophobic surfactant–associated proteins B and C from calf lungs) via the intratracheal route in an attempt to modify alveolar surface tension and thus stabilize the alveoli.[10] This treatment is combined with conventional mechanical ventilation or high-frequency oscillatory ventilation. Because in dogs with true fading puppy syndrome there appears to be an abnormality of lung surfactant composition, a similar treatment may be useful but currently is untested.

Broad-spectrum antimicrobials frequently are administered to neonates with significant illness. In these cases it is not appropriate to wait for culture and sensitivity results; however, it is sensible to collect bacteriologic samples prior to drug administration to allow concomitant processing, which may result in a change in the selected antimicrobial once the results have been obtained. Culture of whole blood is recommended. When drug administration is considered, confusion often arises over products that are given to the dam and excreted in milk. A drug's concentration in milk depends on its lipid solubility, blood protein binding capacity, and pKa; however, in general less than 5% of the maternal dose reaches the milk.

INVESTIGATION OF NEONATAL LOSS

It is important to ensure an accurate diagnosis of neonatal loss. All stillborn pups and those that die shortly after birth should undergo a detailed postmortem examination that includes appropriate bacteriologic, virologic, and histologic testing. The bodies should be chilled rather than frozen and then transported to an appropriate pathology facility.

PREVENTIVE HEALTH CARE PROGRAMS

A preventive health care program should be planned for the differing circumstances of each breeder.[11] In principle, this program should include broad-spectrum anthelmintic therapy, which commences at 3 weeks of age and is repeated 2 weeks later. Fecal examination to determine the parasite burden can modify the subsequent treatment regimen. Immunization of puppies with appropriate vaccines (canine distemper, parvovirus, adenovirus type II, and parainfluenza) should be initiated at 6 to 9 weeks of age. The precise choice of vaccine depends on the preference of the veterinarian and the particular circumstances of the client.

CONCLUSION

Acquiring an understanding of the common challenges facing the neonate may help the veterinarian and breeder to reduce perinatal loss. In the absence of detailed research work into the physiology of birth adaptation, generic management strategies should be followed to ensure the health of the bitch during pregnancy and the care of the neonate during parturition and the first few weeks of life. When neonatal problems occur, rapid and aggressive supportive therapy is mandatory, as is proper investigation of all cases of neonatal mortality.

REPRODUCTIVE SYSTEM

SECTION XVIII

Urinary System

CHAPTER 257

Renal Disease: Clinical Approach and Laboratory Evaluation

Stephen P. DiBartola

DEFINITIONS

Azotemia is defined as an increased concentration of nonprotein nitrogenous compounds in the blood, usually urea and creatinine. *Prerenal azotemia* is a consequence of reduced renal perfusion (e.g., severe dehydration, heart failure), and *postrenal azotemia* results from interference with excretion of urine from the body (e.g., obstruction, uroabdomen). *Primary renal azotemia* is caused by parenchymal renal disease. The term *renal failure* refers to the clinical syndrome that occurs when the kidneys are no longer able to maintain their regulatory, excretory, and endocrine functions, resulting in retention of nitrogenous solutes and derangements of fluid, electrolyte, and acid-base balance. Renal failure occurs when 75% or more of the nephron population is nonfunctional. The term *uremia* refers to the constellation of clinical signs and biochemical abnormalities associated with a critical loss of functional nephrons, including the extrarenal manifestations of renal failure (e.g., uremic gastroenteritis, hyperparathyroidism). The term *renal disease* refers to the presence of morphologic or functional lesions in one or both kidneys regardless of extent.

CLINICAL APPROACH

The clinician should try to answer the following questions:
- Is renal disease present?
- Is the disease glomerular, tubular, interstitial, or some combination of these?
- What is the extent of the renal disease?
- Is the disease acute or chronic, reversible or irreversible, progressive or nonprogressive?
- What is the current status of the animal's renal function?
- Can the disease be treated?
- What nonurinary complicating factors are present and require treatment (e.g., infection, electrolyte and acid-base disturbances, dehydration, obstruction)?
- What is the prognosis?

The diagnosis of renal disease begins with a careful evaluation of the history and physical examination findings.

History

A complete history should be taken, including signalment (age, breed, sex), presenting complaint, husbandry, and review of body systems. The history of the presenting complaint should include information about the onset (acute or gradual), progression (improving, unchanging, or worsening), and response to previous therapy. Information about husbandry includes the animal's immediate environment (indoor or outdoor), use (pet, breeding, show, or working animal), geographic origin and travel history, exposure to other animals, vaccination status, diet, and information about previous trauma, illness, or surgery.

Questions relating to the urinary tract include those about changes in water intake and the frequency and volume of urination. The owner should be questioned about pollakiuria, dysuria, or hematuria. Care must be taken to distinguish dysuria and pollakiuria from polyuria and to differentiate polyuria from urinary incontinence. The distinction between pollakiuria and polyuria is important, because polyuria may be a sign of upper urinary tract disease, whereas pollakiuria and dysuria usually are indicative of lower urinary tract disease. Nocturia may be an early sign of polyuria but also can occur as a result of dysuria. Normal urine output ranges from 20-40 mL/kg/day in dogs and cats.

Information about the initiation of urination and the diameter of the urine stream may be helpful, because animals with partial urethral obstruction may have difficulty initiating urination or may have an abnormal urine stream. If hematuria is present, the owner should be questioned about its timing. Blood at the beginning of urination may indicate a disease process in the urethra or genital tract. Blood at the end of or throughout urination may signify a problem in either the bladder or the upper urinary tract (kidneys or ureters).

Polydipsia usually is more easily detected by owners than polyuria. Water intake should not exceed 60-80 mL/kg/day in dogs and 40 mL/kg/day in cats. It is helpful to describe amounts in quantitative terms familiar to the owner, such as cups (approximately 250 mL) or quarts (approximately 1 liter). The owner should be questioned about exposure of the animal to nephrotoxins, such as ethylene glycol in antifreeze, Easter lily (cats only), aminoglycosides (e.g., gentamicin), and nonsteroidal anti-inflammatory drugs (e.g., flunixin meglumine, ibuprofen). Also, it should be determined whether the animal has received any drugs that could cause polydipsia and polyuria (e.g., glucocorticoids, diuretics).

Physical Examination

A complete physical examination (including fundic and rectal examinations) should be performed. Careful attention should be paid to hydration status and to whether ascites or subcutaneous edema is present, because these may accompany nephrotic syndrome (i.e., glomerular disease). The oral cavity should be examined for ulcers, tongue tip necrosis, and pallor of the mucous membranes (Figure 257-1). The presence of retinal edema, detachment, or hemorrhage or of vascular tortuosity should be noted during fundic examination. Occasionally, severe hypertension secondary to renal disease results in acute onset of blindness due to retinal detachment. Young, growing animals with renal failure may develop marked fibrous osteodystrophy, characterized by enlargement and deformity of the maxilla and mandible (so-called rubber jaw), but this is rare in older dogs with renal failure.

Both kidneys can be palpated in most cats and the left kidney in some dogs. Kidneys should be evaluated for size, shape, consistency, pain, and location. Unless empty, the bladder can be palpated in most dogs and cats. The bladder should be evaluated for degree of distension, pain, wall thickness, and presence of masses, both intramural (e.g., tumors) and intraluminal (e.g., calculi, clots). In the absence of obstruction, a

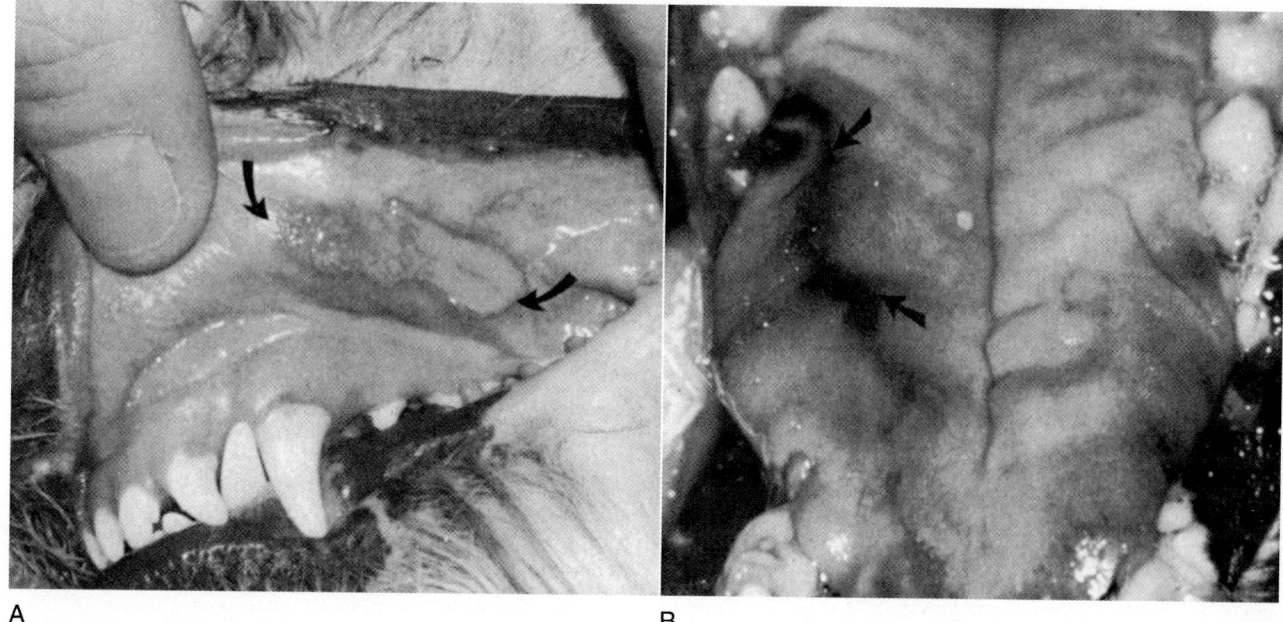

Figure 257-1 **A,** Buccal ulcer. Uremic ulcers often are found in tissue overlying teeth *(arrows).* Oral ulceration is most commonly observed in dogs with primary (intrinsic) renal azotemia. **B,** Tongue margin necrosis. This lesion may occur in dogs with acute or chronic azotemia.

distended bladder in a dehydrated animal suggests abnormal renal function or administration of drugs that impair urinary concentrating ability (e.g., glucocorticoids, diuretics). The prostate gland and pelvic urethra are evaluated by rectal examination. The penis should be exteriorized and examined and the testes palpated. A vaginal examination is performed to evaluate for abnormal discharge and masses and to assess the appearance of the urethral orifice.

Differentiation of Acute from Chronic Renal Failure

Acute renal failure (ARF) sometimes can be difficult to distinguish from chronic renal failure (CRF). However, differentiation is crucial, because ARF potentially is reversible, whereas CRF is not. The history, physical examination findings, renal size, and hematocrit can be helpful in making this distinction. The kidneys are small (but can be normal sized and occasionally even enlarged) in CRF but are normal sized (or slightly enlarged) in ARF. A history of previous polyuria and polydipsia is often (but not always) found in patients with CRF. Physical examination findings such as weight loss and poor haircoat suggest CRF but are not always present. Likewise, nonregenerative anemia often but not always is found in patients with CRF.

Due to the development of renal secondary hyperparathyroidism in CRF, ultrasonography of the parathyroid glands may be helpful in the differentiation of CRF from ARF. In one study, the parathyroid glands of normal dogs and of dogs with ARF and CRF were evaluated using a 10 MHz linear-array, high-resolution transducer.[1] As expected, the maximal measured length of the parathyroid glands in dogs with CRF (3.9 to 8.1 mm) was greater than that for normal dogs (2 to 4.6 mm) and dogs with ARF (2.4 to 4 mm). Although measurements overlapped somewhat among groups, parathyroid gland ultrasonography may be helpful in the differentiation of ARF and CRF. Parathyroid gland size appeared to be related to the body weight of the dog.

Urea can dissociate into isocyanic acid, which in turn can react nonenzymatically with the terminal valine residue of hemoglobin to form carbamylated hemoglobin. The amount of carbamylated hemoglobin present is related to the severity and duration of azotemia. Carbamylated hemoglobin concentrations are higher in dogs with renal failure than in control dogs and higher in dogs with CRF than in those with ARF.[2,3]

LABORATORY EVALUATION OF RENAL FUNCTION

Glomerular Function

Evaluation of glomerular function is an essential part of the diagnostic approach in dogs and cats suspected of having renal disease, because the glomerular filtration rate (GFR) is directly related to functional renal mass. Determinations of the serum creatinine and blood urea nitrogen (BUN) concentrations are commonly used screening tests; the creatinine clearance test is useful in pets suspected of having renal disease that have normal BUN and serum creatinine concentrations. Plasma clearance of radioisotopes and renal scintigraphy are sophisticated techniques that may be used to determine the GFR and obtain information about kidney function but that do not require urine collection. Evaluation of urinary protein excretion allows assessment of primary glomerular disease (e.g., glomerulonephritis, glomerular amyloidosis).

Blood Urea Nitrogen

Urea is synthesized in the liver via the ornithine cycle from ammonia derived from amino acid catabolism. The amino acids used in the production of urea arise from the catabolism of exogenous (i.e., dietary) and endogenous proteins. Renal excretion of urea occurs by glomerular filtration, and the BUN concentration is inversely proportional to the GFR. Urea is subject to passive resorption in the tubules, and this occurs to a greater extent at slower tubular flow rates, which occur during dehydration and volume depletion. Thus urea clearance is not a reliable estimate of the GFR. With significant vascular volume depletion, decreased urea clearance may occur without a decrease in the GFR.

The production and excretion of urea do not proceed at a constant rate. These two processes increase after a high-protein meal, therefore an 8- to 12-hour fast is recommended before measurement of the BUN concentration to avoid the effect of feeding on urea production. Gastrointestinal bleeding can increase the BUN concentration, because blood represents an endogenous protein load. In 52 dogs with hematemesis, melena, or both, the BUN concentrations and BUN to creatinine ratios were significantly higher than in age-matched control dogs; this suggests that gastrointestinal hemorrhage contributes to an increased BUN concentration in dogs as a consequence of increased gastrointestinal absorption of nitrogenous compounds.[4] Clinical conditions characterized by increased catabolism (e.g., starvation, infection, fever) also can increase the BUN concentration. Some drugs may increase the BUN concentration by increasing tissue catabolism (e.g., glucocorticoids, azathioprine) or by decreasing protein synthesis (e.g., tetracyclines), but these effects likely are minimal. On the other hand, the BUN concentration can be decreased by low-protein diets, anabolic steroids, severe hepatic insufficiency, or portosystemic shunting. These nonrenal variables limit the usefulness of the BUN concentration as an indicator of the GFR. The normal BUN concentrations are 8 to 25 mg/dL in the dog and 15 to 35 mg/dL in the cat.

Serum Creatinine

Creatinine is a nonenzymatic breakdown product of phosphocreatine in muscle, and daily production of creatinine in the body is determined largely by the muscle mass of the individual. Young animals have lower concentrations, whereas males and well-muscled individuals have higher concentrations. The serum creatinine concentration is not appreciably affected by diet. Creatinine is not metabolized and is excreted by the kidneys almost entirely by glomerular filtration. Its rate of excretion is relatively constant in the steady state, and the serum creatinine concentration varies inversely with the GFR. Thus *determination of creatinine clearance provides an estimate of the GFR.*

Creatinine is measured by the alkaline picrate reaction, which is not entirely specific for creatinine and which measures another group of substances collectively known as noncreatinine chromagens. These substances are found in plasma, in which they may constitute up to 50% of the measured creatinine at normal serum concentrations, but they normally do not appear in urine. As the serum creatinine concentration increases as a result of progression of renal disease and a declining GFR, the amount of noncreatinine chromagens remains unchanged and contributes progressively less to the total measured serum creatinine concentration. The normal serum creatinine concentrations are 0.3 to 1.3 mg/dL in the dog and 0.8 to 1.8 mg/dL in the cat.

The relationship of the BUN or serum creatinine concentration to the GFR is a rectangular hyperbola. The slope of the curve is small when the GFR is mildly or moderately decreased but large when the GRF is severely reduced (Figure 257-2). Therefore large changes in the GFR early in the course of renal disease cause small increases in the BUN or serum creatinine concentration, which may be difficult to appreciate clinically; on the other hand, small changes in the GFR in advanced renal disease cause large changes in the BUN or serum creatinine concentration. The inverse relationship between the serum creatinine concentration and the GFR is valid only in the steady state.

When nonrenal variables have been eliminated from consideration, an increase in the BUN or serum creatinine concentration above normal implies that at least 75% of the

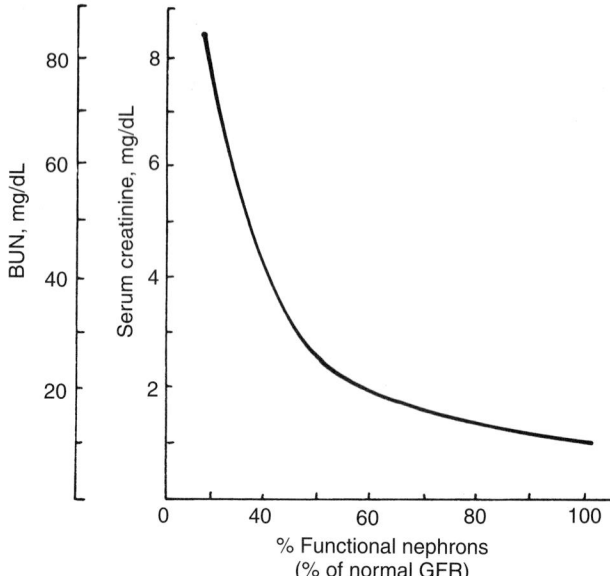

Figure 257-2 Relationship of blood urea nitrogen (BUN) or serum creatinine concentration to percentage of functional nephrons. (From Chew DJ, DiBartola SP: Manual of Small Animal Nephrology and Urology. New York, Churchill Livingstone, 1986.)

nephrons are not functioning (see Figure 257-2). Neither the cause nor the reversibility of this malfunction can be predicted from the increase in the BUN or serum creatinine concentration. Also, the increase in the BUN or serum creatinine concentration cannot be used to predict whether azotemia is prerenal, primary renal, or postrenal in origin, or to distinguish between acute and chronic, reversible and irreversible, and progressive and nonprogressive processes. The BUN/creatinine ratio in prerenal and postrenal azotemia may be increased as a result either of increased tubular resorption of urea at lower tubular flow rates or of easier absorption of urea than creatinine across peritoneal membranes in animals with uroabdomen. A decrease in the BUN/creatinine ratio often follows fluid therapy, reflecting a decrease in tubular resorption of urea rather than an increase in the GFR.

Cystatin C

Cystatin C is a small polypeptide protease inhibitor that is freely filtered by the glomeruli. It does not undergo tubular secretion, and filtered cystatin C is almost completely resorbed by the proximal tubular cells and catabolized to its constituent amino acids. Cystatin C is produced at a constant rate in all tissues, and its excretion is not dependent on age, gender, or diet. As a result, the serum concentration of cystatin C may serve as a useful marker of the GFR. Some concern exists that the serum cystatin C concentration may be affected by the presence of inflammation or neoplasia.

Recently, two studies evaluated normal dogs and dogs with renal failure using an immunoturbidometric assay designed to measure the serum concentration of human cystatin C.[5,6] The serum concentration of cystatin C in normal dogs was found to be approximately 1 mg/dL.

Creatinine Clearance

The renal clearance of a substance is that volume of plasma that would have to be filtered by the glomeruli each minute to account for the amount of that substance appearing in the urine each minute. The renal clearance of a substance that is neither resorbed nor secreted by the tubules is equal to the GFR. For such a substance in a steady state, the amount filtered equals the amount excreted. Thus: $GFR \times P_x = U_x \times V$. Dividing both sides of the equation by P_x gives the familiar clearance formula ($U_x V/P_x$), which in this case is equal to the GFR.

Creatinine is produced endogenously and excreted by the body largely by glomerular filtration, and its clearance can be used to estimate the GFR in the steady state. Numerous studies in the dog and cat have shown that *endogenous* creatinine clearance in these species is 2 to 5 mL/min/kg. Values for glomerular function tests in the dog and cat are presented in Table 257-1.

In chronic progressive renal disease, urinary concentrating ability is impaired after two thirds of the nephron population have become nonfunctional, whereas azotemia does not develop until three fourths of the nephrons have become nonfunctional. Thus the main indication for determination of *endogenous* creatinine clearance is the clinical suspicion of renal disease in a pet with polyuria and polydipsia that has normal BUN and serum creatinine concentrations. The only requirements for determination of *endogenous* creatinine clearance are accurately timed urine collection (usually 12 or 24 hours), determination of body weight, and an assessment of the serum and urine creatinine concentrations. Failure to collect all urine produced erroneously reduces the calculated clearance value.

To eliminate the inaccuracy caused by noncreatinine chromagens, some investigators have advocated use of *exogenous* creatinine clearance. In this procedure, creatinine is administered subcutaneously or intravenously to increase the serum creatinine concentration approximately tenfold and to reduce the relative effect of noncreatinine chromagens. *Exogenous* creatinine clearance values exceed endogenous creatinine clearance values and closely approximate inulin clearance in the dog. In one study, the inulin and *exogenous* creatinine clearances were nearly identical in dogs. The creatinine/inulin clearance ratio was not altered by ablation of 50% to 94% of renal mass and was not affected by gender, dietary protein intake, or duration of time after renal ablation.[7] *Endogenous* creatinine clearance is a reliable estimate of the GFR only when methodology specific for true creatinine is used.[8] In cats, *exogenous* creatinine clearance may be slightly lower than inulin clearance.

Single Injection Methods for Estimating the Glomerular Filtration Rate

Single injection plasma clearance methods using inulin, iohexol, or creatinine have been used in dogs and cats with normal and reduced renal mass to estimate the GFR.[9-14] With these methods, the plasma clearance of a substance that is not bound to plasma proteins and is excreted only by glomerular filtration (e.g., inulin, iohexol, creatinine) is calculated as the quotient of the administered dose divided by the area under the plasma concentration versus time curve. This technique has the advantage of not requiring collection of urine, but its accuracy depends on the pharmacokinetic model used to calculate the area under the curve and the timing and number of samples used to make the calculation. The advantages and limitations of single injection plasma clearance methods for evaluation of the GFR were recently reviewed.[15]

Radioisotopes

Radioisotopes (e.g., ^{125}I-iothalamate or ^{131}I-iothalamate, ^{51}Cr-ethylenediaminetetraacetic acid [EDTA], ^{99m}Tc-diethylenetriamine penta-acetic acid [DTPA]) also have been used to estimate the GFR in dogs and cats using both plasma clearance and dynamic renal scintigraphic methods. The plasma clearance approach has the same advantages and limitations as described above for iohexol or exogenously administered creatinine; procedures involving radioisotopes require technical expertise and equipment available primarily at referral institutions. Methods using ^{99m}Tc-DTPA to estimate the GFR are clinically useful because the short half-life of [99m]Tc (6 hours) allows the animal to be released within 24 to 48 hours after the procedure.

The percentage of an injected dose of ^{99m}Tc-DTPA extracted by the kidneys over a finite period correlates well with inulin clearance (the gold standard for estimation of the GFR). A major advantage of dynamic renal scintigraphy is that it provides information about individual kidney function; however, in dogs with renal disease, this method correlates less well with inulin clearance than does the plasma clearance method.[16] Renal scintigraphy is less accurate than plasma clearance methods for several reasons. A brief sampling period (usually 1 to 3 minutes after injection) is used in dynamic renal scintigraphy to avoid loss of radioactivity as urine is excreted from the kidneys into the ureters and bladder. In a recent study, the ideal time for counting radioactivity during ^{99m}Tc-DTPA renal scintigraphy in normal dogs was found to be 30 seconds to 2 minutes after injection.[17] Data acquired over such a short period may not accurately reflect the animal's steady state GFR. Other factors that contribute to potential inaccuracy include characteristics of the gamma camera itself (e.g., field uniformity, linearity, spatial resolution), the selection of renal and background regions of interest, and renal depth correction.[18] Partial obstruction can delay excretion of the tracer from the kidneys and lead to overestimation of the GFR. Despite these limitations, dynamic renal scintigraphy is helpful in clinical situations when information about individual renal function is important. Nuclear imaging with ^{99m}Tc-DTPA has been used to determine the GFR in normal dogs[19] and dogs with renal disease[20] and in normal cats and cats with renal dysfunction.[21,22]

Quantitative renal scintigraphy[23] and determination of plasma disappearance after single injection[24] using ^{99m}Tc-mercaptoacetyltriglycine have been used to estimate renal plasma flow in dogs. Hepatic uptake of ^{99m}Tc-mercaptoacetyltriglycine in cats may limit the value of this tracer for evaluation of renal plasma flow in this species.[25]

Urine Protein to Creatinine Ratio

In animals with persistent proteinuria on routine urinalysis, the severity of the proteinuria may be assessed by measuring 24-hour urine protein excretion or by performing a urine protein to urine creatinine ratio (U_{Pr}/U_{Cr}). A normal value for 24-hour urine protein excretion in dogs and cats is less than 20 mg/kg/day. Dogs with primary glomerular disease

Table • 257-1

Tests of Glomerular Function in Dogs and Cats

PARAMETER	DOG	CAT
Blood urea nitrogen (mg/dL)	8-25	15-35
Serum creatinine (mg/dL)	0.3-1.3	0.8-1.8
Serum cystatin C (mg/dL)	0.5-1.5	Not available
Endogenous creatinine clearance (mL/min/kg)	2-5	2-5
Exogenous creatinine clearance (mL/min/kg)	3-5	2-4
24-Hour urine protein excretion (mg/kg/day)	<20	<20
Urine protein to urine creatinine ratio (U_{Pr}/U_{Cr})	<0.4	<0.4

(e.g., glomerulonephritis, glomerular amyloidosis) often have markedly increased 24-hour urine protein excretion values, and those with amyloidosis generally have the highest 24-hour urine protein excretion values.[26,27]

Determination of the U_{Pr}/U_{Cr} eliminates the necessity of a 24-hour urine collection and has been shown to correlate closely with 24-hour urine protein excretion in dogs[28] and cats.[29] Its value lies in the fact that, whereas both the urine creatinine and urine protein concentrations are affected by the total urine solute concentration, their ratio is not. The normal U_{Pr}/U_{Cr} in dogs and cats is less than 0.4. In dogs, U_{Pr}/U_{Cr} results are not affected by differences in gender, the method of urine collection, fasted versus fed states, or the time of day of collection.[30,31] Pyuria and marked blood contamination of urine samples can result in an abnormal U_{Pr}/U_{Cr} in the absence of glomerular disease.[32] Consequently, both the urine protein concentration and the U_{Pr}/U_{Cr} must be evaluated in conjunction with urinary sediment findings. Feeding of a high-protein diet or induction of renal failure increased 24-hour urine protein excretion and the U_{Pr}/U_{Cr} in cats,[33] and administration of prednisone to normal dogs increased the U_{Pr}/U_{Cr} from normal to a mean of 1.2 at 30 days and 0.9 at 42 days.[34] Values for 24-hour urine protein excretion and the U_{Pr}/U_{Cr} are presented in Table 257-1.

Dogs with proteinuria on screening urinalysis have been shown to have an increased U_{Pr}/U_{Cr}.[26,28,31,35] A high degree of overlap is found between dogs with glomerulonephritis and those with amyloidosis with regard to 24-hour urine protein excretion and the U_{Pr}/U_{Cr}.[26,27] Therefore renal biopsy remains the only reliable way to differentiate these two diseases.

Microalbuminuria

In humans, microalbuminuria is defined as excretion of 30 to 300 mg of albumin in urine per day, and its presence may be an early indicator of vascular endothelial damage.[36] Microalbuminuria is an established risk factor for progression of renal disease in humans with type 1 or type 2 diabetes mellitus.[37] Whether microalbuminuria is predictive of progressive renal disease in humans with essential hypertension is less certain, but it is associated with adverse cardiovascular events in this population.[38,39] Microalbuminuria in dogs has been defined as a urine albumin concentration of greater than 1 mg/dL but less than 30 mg/dL. Urine albumin concentrations in this range can be detected by an antigen-capture enzyme-linked immunosorbent assay (ELISA) (i.e., ERD-Screen Urine Test; Heska Corp., Fort Collins, Colorado).[40] In recent studies, the prevalence of microalbuminuria in normal healthy dogs was 19%, and the prevalence in a hospital population of dogs was 36%. Microalbuminuria has been detected in heartworm-infected dogs and in those with familial renal disease (e.g., soft-coated wheaten terriers with glomerular disease, male dogs with X-linked hereditary nephritis). The effect of pyuria on detection of microalbuminuria was found to be variable. It remains to be determined whether seemingly normal dogs with microalbuminuria are at increased risk for the development of progressive renal disease. Sequential monitoring of dogs with documented microalbuminuria probably is warranted until this factor's prognostic value in otherwise normal dogs can be determined.

Bladder Tumor Antigen Test

The first-generation Bard bladder tumor antigen (BTA) test (i.e., V-BTA Test; Polymedco, Cortlandt Manor, New York) is a qualitative latex agglutination dipstick test run on voided urine that detects a glycoprotein antigen complex associated with bladder neoplasia in humans. In a prospective study of 65 dogs with transitional cell carcinoma and other urinary tract disorders, the Bard V-BTA Test had a sensitivity of 90% and a specificity of 78%.[41] False positives occurred in urine samples with marked proteinuria or glucosuria and in those with pyuria or hematuria. The high sensitivity of the test and its less reliable performance in the presence of pyuria and hematuria suggest that it would be most appropriately used as a routine screening test in geriatric dogs at risk for the development of transitional cell carcinoma.

In another study, the V-BTA Test reliably differentiated dogs with lower urinary tract neoplasia from normal dogs but did not reliably differentiate dogs with neoplasia from dogs with other abnormalities of the lower urinary tract.[42] The V-BTA Test is commercially available for veterinary use.

Second- and third-generation Bard BTA tests (BTA Stat and Bard Trak, respectively), as well as other tests that use monoclonal antibodies against human bladder tumor antigens, give false-negative results in dogs and should not be used.[41]

Tubular Function

The kidney is an organ of water conservation. Depending on the needs of the animal, the kidney can produce urine that is highly concentrated or quite dilute. Normal urinary concentrating ability depends on the ability of the hypothalamic osmoreceptors to respond to changes in plasma osmolality, the release of antidiuretic hormone (ADH) from the neurohypophysis, and the response of the distal nephron to ADH. In addition, medullary hypertonicity must be generated and maintained by the countercurrent multiplier and exchanger systems of the kidney, and an adequate number of functional nephrons must be present to generate the appropriate response to ADH. Laboratory tests of tubular function are summarized in Table 257-2.

Urine Specific Gravity and Osmolality

The total urine solute concentration is measured either by the urine specific gravity (USG) or the urine osmolality (U_{Osm}). The latter depends only on the number of osmotically active particles, regardless of their size. The *urine specific gravity* is defined as the weight of a solution compared with an equal volume of distilled water. It depends on both the number and molecular weight of the solute particles but has the advantage of requiring only simple, inexpensive equipment for measurement.

Table • 257-2

Tests of Renal Tubular Function in Dogs and Cats

TEST	DOG	CAT
Random urine specific gravity	1.001-1.070	1.001-1.080
Urine specific gravity after 5% dehydration	1.050-1.076	1.047-1.087
Urine osmolality after 5% dehydration (mOsm/kg)	1787-2791	1581-2984
Urine to plasma osmolality ratio after 5% dehydration	5.7-8.9	Not available
Fractional electrolyte clearance (%)		
Sodium	<1	<1
Potassium	<20	<24
Chloride	<1	<1.3
Phosphate	<39	<73

Modified from DiBartola SP: Clinical Evaluation of Renal Function. 16th Annual Waltham/OSU Symposium for the Treatment of Small Animal Disease. Vernon, California, Kal Kan Foods, 1992, p 10.

Normally, urine is composed of solutes of relatively low molecular weight (e.g., urea, electrolytes), and a roughly linear relationship exists between the urine osmolality and the urine specific gravity. The range of urine osmolality that corresponds to a given USG, however, may be relatively wide. If the urine contains appreciable amounts of larger molecular weight solutes (e.g., glucose, mannitol, radiographic contrast agents), these substances have a proportionally greater effect on specific gravity than on osmolality.

The term *isosthenuria* (USG of 1.007-1.015, U_{Osm} of 300 mOsm/kg) refers to urine of the same total solute concentration as unaltered glomerular filtrate. The term *hyposthenuria* (USG less than 1.007, U_{Osm} less than 300 mOsm/kg) refers to urine of lower total solute concentration than glomerular filtrate. Although rarely used clinically, the term *hypersthenuria (baruria)* (USG greater than 1.015, U_{Osm} greater than 300 mOsm/kg) refers to urine of higher total solute concentration than glomerular filtrate. The normal range of the total urine solute concentration for dogs and cats is wide (USG of 1.001 to 1.080). In a study of normal pet dogs, USG values were found to vary widely (from 1.006 to greater than 1.050).[43] Samples obtained in the morning had higher USG values than those obtained in the evening, and urine concentration decreased with age, but no effect of gender on the USG was detected.

Water Deprivation Test

The water deprivation test (WDT) is a useful test of tubular function and is indicated in the evaluation of animals with confirmed polydipsia and polyuria for which the cause remains undetermined after initial diagnostic evaluation. An expedient safe alternative to the WDT is DDAVP (synthetic ADH) trial therapy. Please see Chapter 28 for a discussion on this approach.

The water deprivation test usually is performed in animals with hyposthenuria (USG less than 1.007) that are suspected of having central or nephrogenic diabetes insipidus or psychogenic polydipsia. A dehydrated animal that has dilute urine has already failed the test and should not be subjected to water deprivation. In such an animal, failure to concentrate urine likely is due to structural or functional renal dysfunction or to the administration of drugs that interfere with urinary concentrating ability (e.g., glucocorticoids, diuretics). The water deprivation test also is contraindicated in animals that are azotemic. It should be performed with extreme caution in animals with severe polyuria, because such pets may rapidly become dehydrated during water deprivation if they have defective urinary concentrating ability.

At the beginning of the water deprivation test, the bladder must be emptied and baseline data collected (e.g., body weight, hematocrit, plasma proteins, skin turgor, serum osmolality, urine osmolality, USG). Water then is withheld, and these parameters are monitored every 2 to 4 hours. The urine and serum osmolalities are the best tests to follow, but osmolality results often are not immediately available to the clinician. Thus the USG and body weight assume the greatest importance for decision making during performance of the test. An increase in the total plasma protein concentration is a relatively reliable indicator of progressive dehydration, but increases in the hematocrit and changes in skin turgor are not reliable. The serum creatinine and BUN concentrations should not increase during a properly conducted water deprivation test.

Maximal stimulation of ADH release occurs after the loss of 3% to 5% of body weight. The test is concluded when the dog or cat either demonstrates adequate concentrating ability or becomes dehydrated, as evidenced by loss of 3% to 5% or more of its original body weight. It is important when weighing the animal to use the same scale each time and to empty the bladder at each evaluation.

The time required for dehydration to develop during water deprivation varies. Dehydration usually becomes evident within 48 hours in normal dogs and cats but in rare cases may require a longer time. Dogs with diabetes insipidus and psychogenic polydipsia usually become dehydrated after a much shorter period of water deprivation (less than 12 hours and usually less than 6 hours). By the time dehydration is evident, the USG usually exceeds 1.045 in normal dogs and cats. Failure to achieve maximal urinary solute concentration does not localize the level of the malfunction, and a structural or functional defect may be present anywhere along the hypothalamic-pituitary-renal axis. Furthermore, animals with medullary solute washout may have impaired concentrating ability regardless of the underlying cause of polyuria and polydipsia.

If urine osmolality has increased less than 5% or the USG has changed less than 10% for three consecutive determinations, or if the animal has lost 3% to 5% or more of its original weight, 0.1 to 0.2 U/lb of aqueous vasopressin (Pitressin) (up to a total dose of 5 U) or 5 µg of DDAVP may be given subcutaneously and the parameters of urinary concentrating ability monitored 2 to 4 hours after ADH injection. A further increase in urine osmolality after administration of ADH should not exceed 5% to 10% in normal dogs and cats.

Gradual Water Deprivation

Gradual water deprivation can be performed to eliminate diagnostic confusion caused by medullary solute washout. The owner can be instructed to restrict water consumption to 120 mL/kg/day 72 hours before, 90 mL/kg/day 48 hours before, and 60 mL/kg/day 24 hours before the scheduled water deprivation test. In dogs with psychogenic polydipsia, this promotes endogenous release of ADH, increased permeability of the inner medullary collecting ducts to urea, and restoration of the normal gradient of medullary hypertonicity. An alternate approach is to instruct the owner to reduce water consumption by approximately 10% per day over a 3- to 5-day period (but not less than 60 mL/kg/day). This approach should be used only for animals that are otherwise healthy on initial clinical evaluation, and the owner should provide dry food *ad libitum* and weigh the dog daily to monitor for loss of body weight.

Fractional Clearance of Electrolytes

The extent to which electrolytes appear in the urine is the net result of tubular resorption and secretion. The fractional clearance of electrolytes can be used to evaluate tubular function and is defined as the ratio of the clearance of the electrolyte in question to that of creatinine:

$$FC_x = (U_xV/P_x)/(U_{Cr}V/P_{Cr}) = (U_xP_{Cr})/(U_{Cr}P_x)$$

where FC_x = fractional clearance of X; U_x = urine concentration of X; P_x = plasma concentration of X; U_{cr} = urine concentration of creatinine; P_{cr} = plasma concentration of creatinine; V = urine flow rate.

This ratio usually is multiplied by 100, and the fractional clearance value is expressed as a percentage. The advantage of this measurement is that a timed urine collection is not necessary. In normal animals, the fractional clearances of all electrolytes are much less than 1 (100%), implying net conservation, but values are higher for potassium and phosphorus than for sodium and chloride. Unfortunately, fractional excretion values calculated from "spot" urine samples are variable and do not correlate well with values calculated using 72-hour urine samples.[44]

The fractional clearance of sodium may be useful in the differentiation of prerenal and primary renal azotemia. In animals with prerenal azotemia and volume depletion, sodium conservation should be avid and the fractional clearance of sodium low (less than 1%). In animals with azotemia caused by primary parenchymal renal disease, the fractional clearance of sodium is higher than normal (greater than 1%). Values for fractional electrolyte clearances have been reported for normal dogs,[45] dogs with CRF,[46] normal cats,[47,48] and cats with experimentally induced CRF.[49] Normal values for urinary fractional clearance of electrolytes are summarized in Table 257-2.

ROUTINE URINALYSIS

Urine for urinalysis may be collected by voiding (midstream sample), catheterization, or cystocentesis. Cystocentesis is preferred because it prevents contamination of the sample by the urethra or genital tract, it is simple to perform when the bladder is palpable, the risk of introducing infection is negligible, and it is well-tolerated by both dogs and cats. In animals to be evaluated for hematuria, however, it may be helpful first to evaluate a sample collected by voiding, because other methods of urine collection may add red blood cells to the sample as a result of trauma.

For urinalysis, fresh urine should be examined whenever possible. Refrigerated urine should be warmed to room temperature before the urinalysis is performed. The technique used to collect the sample should be noted, because this may influence the interpretation. Urinalysis is divided into three parts: physical properties, chemical properties, and sediment evaluation.

Physical Properties
Appearance
Normal urine is yellow as a result of the presence of urochrome pigment. Concentrated urine may be deep amber, and dilute urine may be almost colorless. A red or reddish brown color usually is due to red blood cells, hemoglobin, or myoglobin; a yellow-brown to yellow-green color may be due to bilirubin. Normal urine usually is clear. Cloudy urine often contains increased cellular elements, crystals, or mucus. The most common abnormal odor is ammoniac and is due to the release of ammonia by urease-producing bacteria.

Specific Gravity
As mentioned before, the USG reflects the total solute concentration of the urine, and the amount of any substance in urine must be interpreted in light of the specific gravity. For example, 4+ protein in 1.010 urine represents more severe proteinuria than 4+ protein in 1.045 urine. The USG should be obtained before any treatment is given, because fluids, diuretics, or glucocorticoids may alter the specific gravity.

Chemical Properties
pH
Urine pH varies with diet and acid-base balance. The normal pH of urine in dogs and cats is 5.0 to 7.5. Causes of an acidic urine pH include a meat protein–based diet, administration of acidifying agents, metabolic acidosis, respiratory acidosis, paradoxical aciduria in metabolic alkalosis, and protein catabolic states. Causes of an alkaline urine pH include urinary tract infection by urease-positive bacteria, a plant protein–based diet, urine allowed to stand exposed to air at room temperature, postprandial alkaline tide, administration of alkalinizing agents, metabolic alkalosis, respiratory alkalosis, and distal renal tubular acidosis.

Protein
Randomly obtained urine samples from normal dogs contain small amounts of protein (up to 50 mg/dL). Commonly used dipstick methods for protein determination are much more sensitive to albumin than globulin. In the evaluation of proteinuria, it is critical to localize the origin of the protein loss by means of the history, physical examination, and critical evaluation of the urine sediment. Persistent, moderate to heavy proteinuria in the absence of urine sediment abnormalities is highly suggestive of glomerular disease (e.g., glomerulonephritis, glomerular amyloidosis). If the sediment is active and proteinuria is mild to moderate, the possibility of inflammatory renal disease or disease of the lower urinary or genital tract should be considered.

Glucose
Glucose in the glomerular filtrate is almost completely resorbed in the proximal tubules and is not normally present in the urine of dogs and cats. Glucose appears in the urine (glucosuria) if the blood glucose concentration exceeds the renal threshold (approximately 175 to 225 mg/dL in the dog and 250 to 350 mg/dL in the cat). Most dipstick tests use a colorimetric test based on an enzymatic reaction (glucose oxidase) specific for glucose. Causes of glucosuria include diabetes mellitus, stress or excitement in cats, administration of glucose-containing fluids, and renal tubular diseases, such as primary renal glucosuria and Fanconi syndrome. Glucosuria also may be observed occasionally in dogs and cats with chronic renal disease, those with tubular injury caused by nephrotoxins, and in some dogs with familial renal disease.

Ketones
Beta hydroxybutyrate, acetoacetate, and acetone are ketones, the products of exaggerated and incomplete oxidation of fatty acids. They are not normally present in the urine of dogs and cats. The nitroprusside reagent present in dipstick tests reacts with acetone and acetoacetate but is much more reactive with acetoacetate. It does not react with beta hydroxybutyrate. Causes of ketonuria include diabetic ketoacidosis, starvation or prolonged fasting, glycogen storage disease, a low-carbohydrate diet, persistent fever, and persistent hypoglycemia. Ketonuria occurs more readily in young animals, and of the causes listed above, diabetic ketoacidosis is the most important cause in adult dogs and cats.

Occult Blood
Dipstick tests for blood are sensitive but do not differentiate erythrocytes, hemoglobin, and myoglobin. These tests are more sensitive to hemoglobin than to intact erythrocytes; the former causes a diffuse color change, whereas the latter causes spotting of the reagent pad. A positive test result must be interpreted in light of the urine sediment findings (i.e., presence or absence of red blood cells). Free hemoglobin (secondary to hemolysis) is the most common abnormal pigment found in urine. Potential causes of hemolysis include transfusion reaction, autoimmune hemolytic anemia, disseminated intravascular coagulation, postcaval syndrome of dirofilariasis, splenic torsion, and heat stroke. Myoglobinuria is less common but may be present if severe rhabdomyolysis occurs (e.g., status epilepticus, crushing injury). For proper interpretation, the occult blood reaction must be considered together with the urine sediment findings (e.g., hematuria).

Bilirubin
Bilirubin is derived from the breakdown of heme by the reticuloendothelial system. It is transported to the liver, where it is conjugated with glucuronide and excreted in the bile. Only direct-reacting or conjugated bilirubin appears in the urine. The canine kidney can degrade hemoglobin to bilirubin, and the renal threshold for bilirubin is low in dogs. Thus in dogs with liver disease, bilirubin may be detected in the urine before its serum concentration is increased. It is not unusual to find small amounts of bilirubin in concentrated urine samples from normal dogs, especially males. Bilirubin is absent from normal feline urine. The causes of bilirubinuria are

hemolysis (e.g., autoimmune hemolytic anemia), liver disease, extrahepatic biliary obstruction, fever, and starvation.

Leukocyte Esterase Reaction

Indoxyl released by esterases from intact or lysed leukocytes reacts with a diazonium salt and is detected as a blue color reaction after oxidation by atmospheric oxygen. This test is specific for pyuria in canine urine samples but has low sensitivity (produces many false-negative results).[50] In cats, the leukocyte esterase test was found to be moderately sensitive but highly nonspecific (produced many false-positive results) for the detection of pyuria.[51]

Urinary Sediment Examination

Depending on the criteria used for data analysis, as few as 3% or as many as 16% of dogs and cats with normal findings on physical and chemical evaluation of urine may have important urinary sediment abnormalities (e.g., pyuria, bacteriuria, microscopic hematuria).[52] The sediment examination should be performed on fresh urine samples, because casts and cellular elements degenerate rapidly at room temperature. Urine should be centrifuged at 1000 to 1500 rpm for 5 minutes and the sediment then stained with Sedi-Stain (Becton Dickinson, Franklin Lakes, New Jersey) or examined unstained, depending on individual preference. In the evaluation of urine sediment, the method of urine collection must be kept in mind, because it influences the interpretation. The USG must also be kept in mind, because it influences the relative numbers of formed elements. The number of casts is recorded per low power field (lpf), and the numbers of red blood cells, white blood cells, and epithelial cells are recorded per high power field (hpf).

Red Blood Cells

Occasional red blood cells are considered normal in the urine sediment. Normal values are: voided sample, 0 to 8/hpf; catheterized sample, 0 to 5/hpf; and cystocentesis sample, 0 to 3/hpf. The presence of an excessive number of red blood cells in the urine is called *hematuria* (Figure 257-3), which may be microscopic or macroscopic. The causes of hematuria are summarized in Box 257-1.

White Blood Cells

Occasional white blood cells are considered normal in the urine sediment. Normal values are: voided sample, 0 to 8/hpf;

Box • 257-1

Causes of Hematuria in Dogs and Cats

Urinary Tract Origin (Kidneys, Ureters, Bladder, Urethra)
Trauma
  Traumatic collection (e.g., catheter, cystocentesis)
  Renal biopsy
  Blunt trauma (e.g., automobile accident)
Urolithiasis
Neoplasia
Inflammatory disease
  Urinary tract infection
  Feline urologic syndrome (idiopathic feline lower
    urinary tract disease)
  Chemically induced inflammation
    (e.g., cyclophosphamide-induced cystitis)
Parasites
  Dioctophyma renale
  Capillaria plica
Coagulopathy
  Warfarin intoxication
  Disseminated intravascular coagulation
  Thrombocytopenia
Renal infarction
Renal pelvic hematoma
Vascular malformation
  Renal telangiectasia (Welsh corgi)
  Idiopathic renal hematuria

Genital Tract Contamination (Prostate, Prepuce, Vagina)
Estrus
Inflammatory, neoplastic, and traumatic lesions of
  the genital tract

---

catheterized sample, 0 to 5/hpf; and cystocentesis sample, 0 to 3/hpf. The presence of an increased number of white blood cells in the urine sediment is called *pyuria* (Figure 257-4) and, in an appropriately collected urine sample, is indicative of inflammation somewhere in the urinary tract. The presence of white blood cells does not help localize the lesion unless white cell casts are present, indicating renal origin. Urinary tract infection is the most common cause of pyuria, but genital tract contamination also may cause pyuria in voided or catheterized samples (Box 257-2).

Epithelial Cells

Both squamous and transitional epithelial cells may be found in the urine sediment, but they are often of little diagnostic significance. Squamous cells are large, polygonal cells with small round nuclei (Figure 257-5). They are common in voided or catheterized samples because of urethral or vaginal contamination. Occasional squamous cells are normal, and increased numbers may be present during estrus.

Transitional epithelial cells are variable-sized cells derived from the urothelium from the renal pelvis to the urethra (Figure 257-6). Although their size generally increases from the renal pelvis to the urethra, the finding of small transitional cells in the urine sediment does not have localizing value. Caudate cells are transitional cells with tapered ends thought

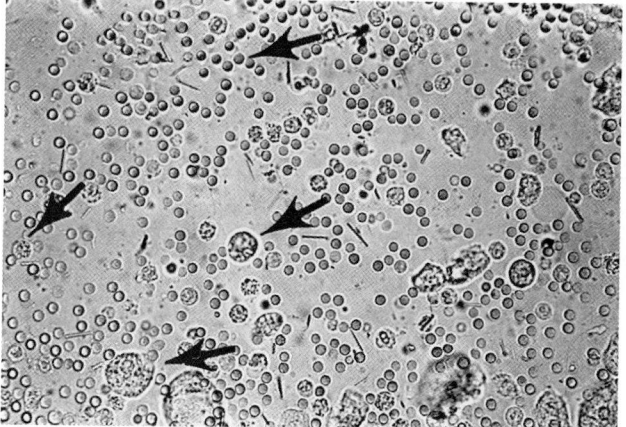

Figure 257-3 Photomicrograph of an abnormal urine sample. Arrow at top indicates red blood cells (RBCs), arrow at left indicates a white blood cell (WBC), and central and bottom arrows indicate two different sizes of transitional epithelial cells. RBCs in urine may resemble those in blood or may shrink or swell in response to variations in urine osmolality.

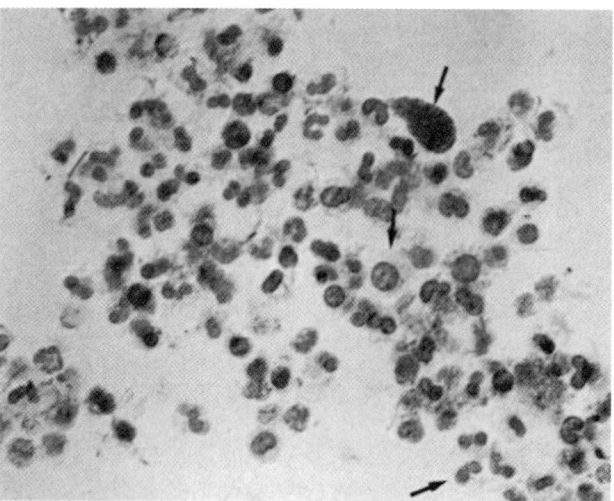

Figure 257-4 Photomicrograph of an abnormal urine sample. White blood cells (WBCs) in urine are subject to degenerative changes that may complicate their identification. They may shrink in concentrated urine or swell in dilute urine. WBCs usually are one and one half to two times the size of red blood cells. Clumps of WBCs often are associated with infection. Occasional transitional epithelial cells also are present in this field. The arrow at bottom right indicates a neutrophil with a swollen cytoplasm and easily identifiable polymorphonuclear nucleus. Occasional transitional epithelial cells also are present *(top arrow).*

to originate from the renal pelvis (Figure 257-7). Occasional transitional cells are normal, and increased numbers may be present with infection, irritation, or neoplasia of the urinary tract. Renal cells are small epithelial cells from the renal tubules, but their renal origin can be determined only if they are observed in cellular casts. Neoplastic epithelial cells are best identified using conventional blood cell stains (e.g., Wright-Giemsa).

Casts

Casts are cylindric molds of the renal tubules composed of aggregated proteins or cells. They form in the ascending limb of Henle's loop and the distal tubule because of the maximal acidity, highest solute concentration, and lowest flow rate in this area. The presence of casts in the urinary sediment

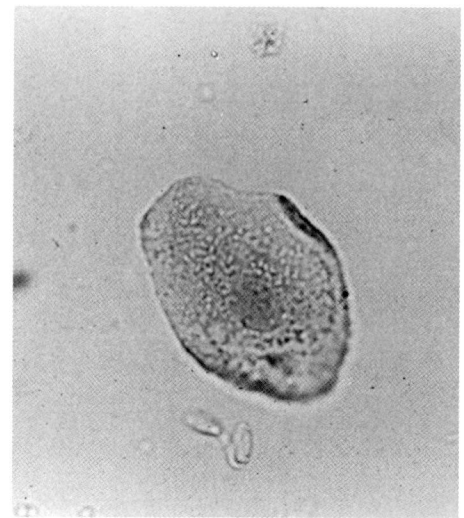

Figure 257-5 Photomicrograph of a squamous epithelial cell in the urine. Note the small nucleus, irregular cell shape, and folding of the cytoplasmic margins in some areas.

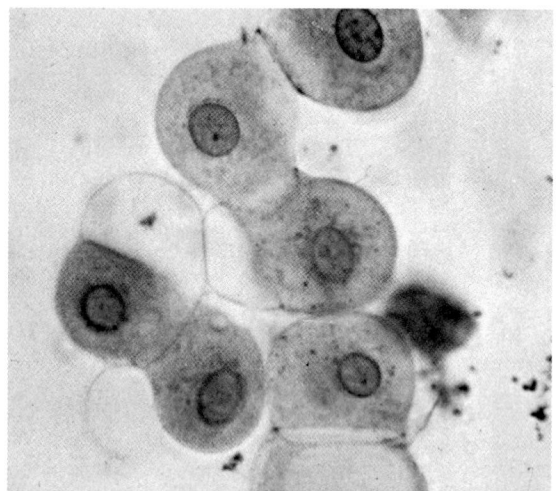

Figure 257-6 Photomicrograph of a raft of transitional epithelial cells in the urine.

Box • 257-2

Causes of Pyuria

Urinary Tract Origin (Kidneys, Ureters, Bladder, Urethra)
Infectious
    Urinary tract infection (e.g., pyelonephritis,
       cystitis, urethritis)
Noninfectious
    Urolithiasis
    Neoplasia
    Trauma
    Chemically induced (e.g., cyclophosphamide)

Genital Tract Contamination (Prostate, Prepuce, Vagina)

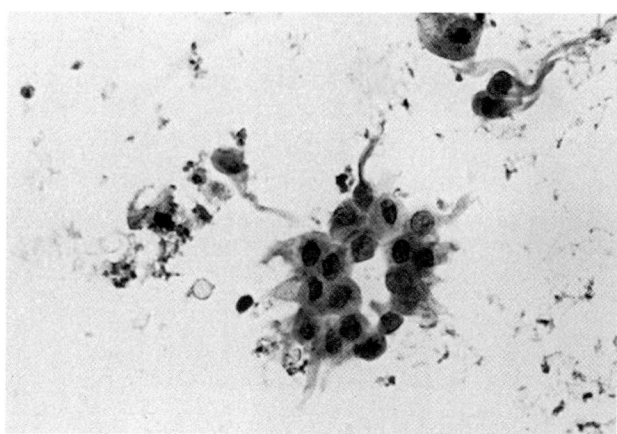

Figure 257-7 Photomicrograph of caudate epithelial cells in urine. The tails on these small epithelial cells suggest that they originated in the renal pelvis.

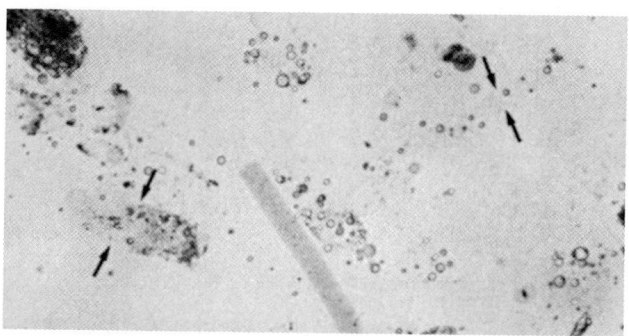

Figure 257-8 Photomicrograph of hyaline casts in urine. Note the transparent nature of these casts *(between arrows)*. The casts are easily missed because their optical density is very low, necessitating low illumination for optimal visualization. The darker cast in the center of the field is a waxy cast. Many lipid droplets are present in the background.

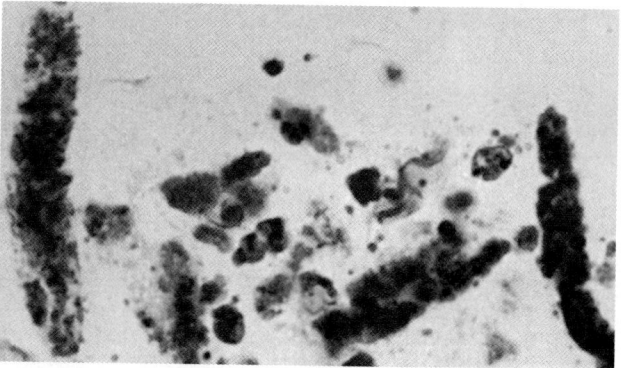

Figure 257-10 Photomicrograph of coarsely granular casts in urine. A "shower" of casts is seen in this field. The cast at the left contains coarse granules; the one on the far right is a cellular cast undergoing degeneration.

indicates activity in the kidney itself and thus is of localizing value. Occasional hyaline (Figure 257-8) and granular (Figure 257-9) casts per low power field are considered normal. No cellular casts should be observed in sediment from normal urine. Excretion of an abnormal number of casts in the urine is called *cylindruria*.

Casts observed in the urine sediment are categorized as hyaline, granular, cellular, or waxy. Hyaline casts are pure protein precipitates (Tamm-Horsfall mucoprotein and albumin). They are difficult to see and dissolve rapidly in dilute or alkaline urine. Small numbers of hyaline casts may be observed with fever or exercise. They are commonly seen in renal diseases associated with proteinuria (e.g., glomerulonephritis, glomerular amyloidosis).

Coarsely (Figure 257-10) and finely (see Figure 257-9) granular casts represent the degeneration of cells in other casts or precipitation of filtered plasma proteins and are suggestive of ischemic or nephrotoxic renal tubular injury. Fatty casts, a type of coarsely granular cast that contains lipid granules, may be seen in nephrotic syndrome or diabetes mellitus. Cellular casts include white cell or pus casts (suggestive of pyelonephritis) (Figure 257-11), red cell casts (fragile and rarely observed in dogs and cats), and renal epithelial cell casts (Figure 257-12) (suggestive of acute tubular necrosis or pyelonephritis).

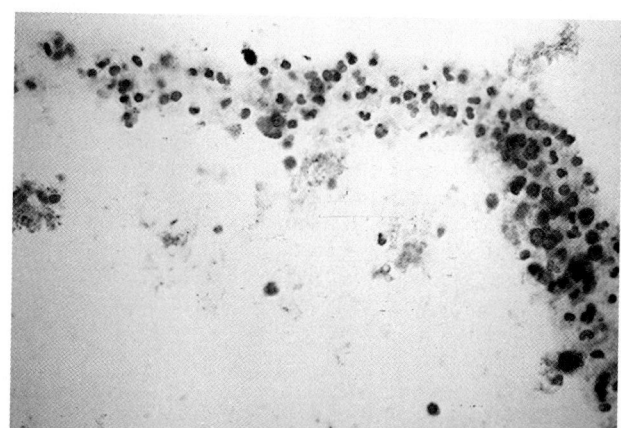

Figure 257-11 Photomicrograph of a white blood cell cast in urine. Neutrophils can be seen within this cast, and their presence suggests renal bacterial infection (i.e., pyelonephritis).

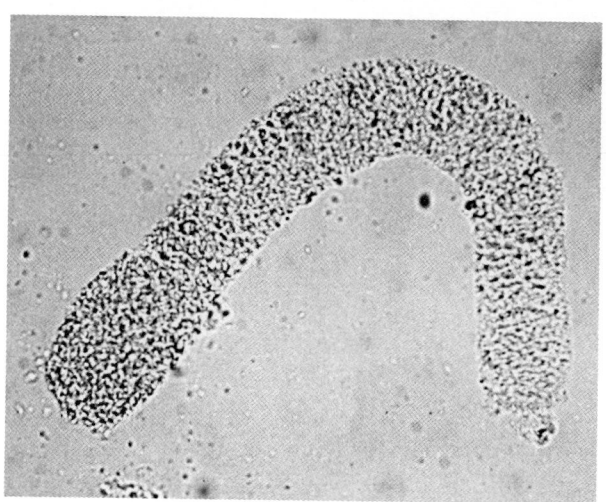

Figure 257-9 Photomicrograph of a finely granular cast in urine.

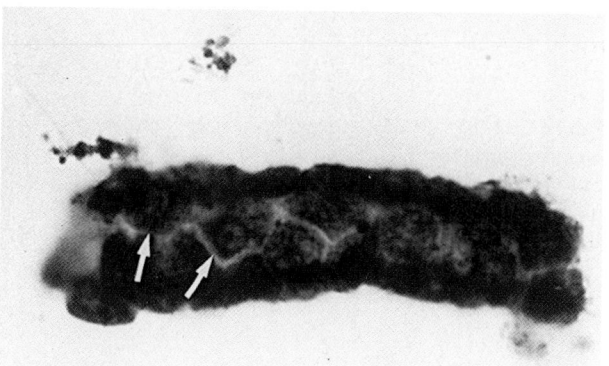

Figure 257-12 Photomicrograph of an epithelial cell cast in urine. Small renal epithelial cells can be identified in this cast *(white arrows)*. (Courtesy Nancy Facklam, nancy.facklam@gov.ab.ca)

URINARY SYSTEM

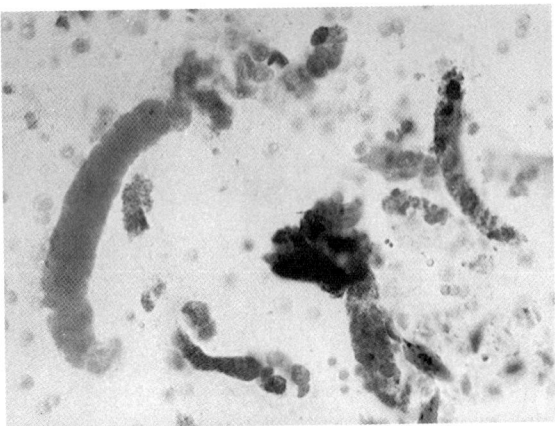

Figure 257-13 Photomicrograph of a urine sample containing waxy and granular casts. The cast at the left is waxy, whereas the others are granular. Note that the waxy cast is translucent, and the hyaline casts are transparent. Waxy casts are brittle and often have cracks or sharply broken ends.

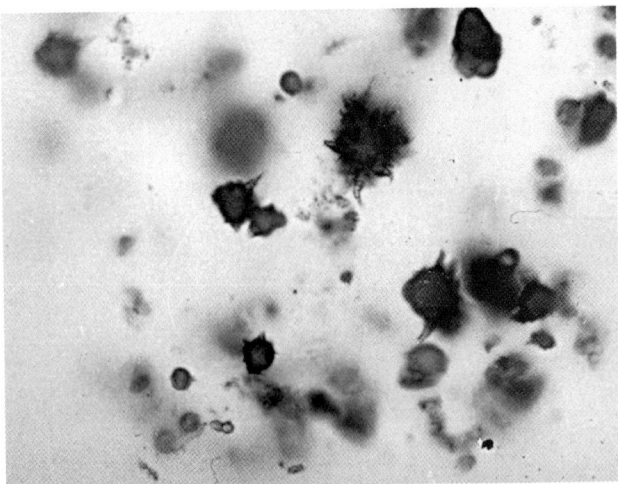

Figure 257-15 Photomicrograph of a urine sample containing ammonium biurate crystals. These crystals may be observed in normal Dalmatian dogs and in dogs with liver disease or portosystemic shunts.

Waxy casts represent the final stage of degeneration of granular casts; they are relatively stable, and their presence suggests intrarenal stasis (Figure 257-13). They often are very convoluted and have cracks and blunt ends.

Organisms

Normal bladder urine is sterile. The distal urethra and genital tract harbor bacteria, and voided or catheterized urine samples may be contaminated with bacteria from the distal urethra, genital tract, or skin. Contamination from the urethra in voided or catheterized specimens usually does not result in large enough numbers of bacteria to be visualized microscopically in the urine sediment. If allowed to incubate at room temperature, however, these contaminants may proliferate. For these organisms to be readily apparent microscopically, there must be more than 10,000 rods or more than 100,000 cocci per milliliter of urine. The presence of large numbers of bacteria in urine collected by catheterization or cystocentesis suggests a urinary tract infection (Figure 257-14). Usually accompanying pyuria is seen. Particulate debris in the sediment may be confused with bacteria and cause false-positive results. Also, the bottle of stain may be contaminated with bacteria. Microscopic absence of bacteria in the sediment does not rule out urinary tract infection. Yeast and fungal hyphae in the sediment usually are contaminants.

Crystals

The solubility of crystals depends on the urine pH, temperature, and specific gravity. Crystals commonly are present in the urine of dogs and cats and often are of little diagnostic significance. Struvite, amorphous phosphates, and oxalates are examples of crystals that may be found in normal urine samples. Uric acid, calcium oxalate, and cystine typically are found in acidic urine, whereas struvite ($MgNH_4PO_4 \cdot 6H_2O$, or so-called triple phosphate), calcium phosphate, calcium carbonate, amorphous phosphate, and ammonium biurate typically are found in alkaline urine. Characteristic crystals also may be found in the urine sediment of animals receiving specific drugs, especially sulfonamides. Bilirubin crystals may be found in concentrated samples of normal dog urine. Urates are commonly observed in the urine of Dalmatians and may be seen in the urine of animals with liver disease or portosystemic shunts (Figure 257-15). Struvite crystals may be observed in the urine of cats with idiopathic lower urinary tract disease, in dogs and cats with struvite urolithiasis, or in

Figure 257-14 Photomicrograph of a urine sample containing bacteria. Chains of bacterial rods are present in this field, as are red blood cells *(arrows)* and a large struvite crystal. Bacteria are most readily identified in urine when they are rods; they often are observed in association with clumped white blood cells or within white blood cells.

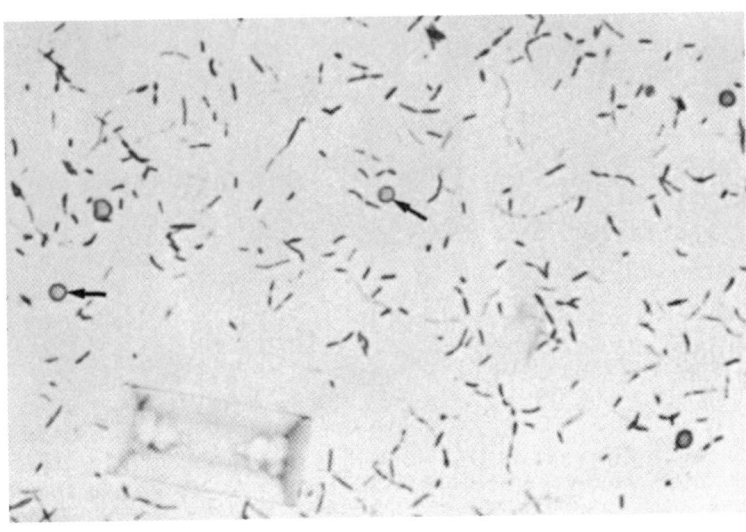

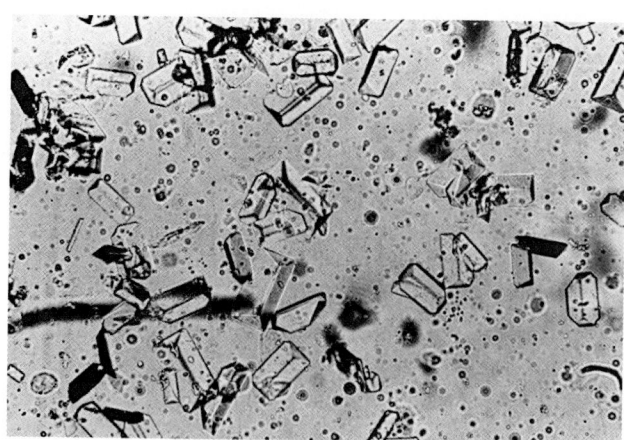

Figure 257-16 Photomicrograph of a urine sample containing struvite crystals. These crystals may be observed in the urine of normal dogs and cats and are common in alkaline urine.

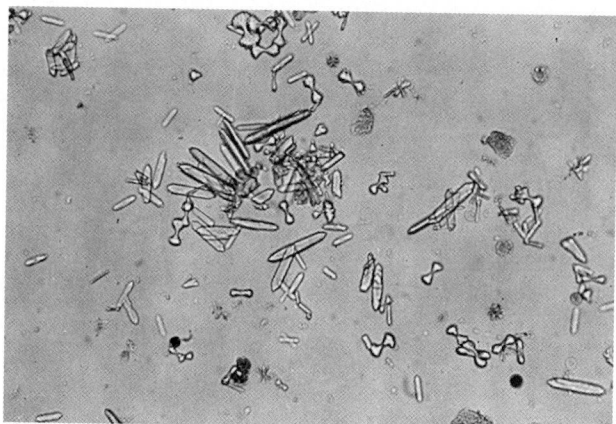

Figure 257-18 Photomicrograph of a urine sample containing calcium oxalate monohydrate crystals. Previously misnamed hippurate, these "picket fence"– and "dumbbell"–shaped crystals may be found in the urine of dogs with acute renal failure caused by ethylene glycol ingestion.

the urine of normal animals (Figure 257-16). In oliguric ARF, the presence of calcium oxalate crystals (Figures 257-17 and 257-18) is highly suggestive of ethylene glycol intoxication. The presence of cystine crystals in the urine of dogs and cats is abnormal and suggestive of cystinuria (Figure 257-19).

Miscellaneous Findings
Sperm commonly are found in urine samples from normal intact male dogs. Rarely, parasite ova of *Dioctophyma renale* or *Capillaria plica* or microfilaria of *Dirofilaria immitis* may be observed in the urine sediment. Refractile lipid droplets may be seen with diabetes mellitus or nephrotic syndrome. They also may be observed in cats as a result of degeneration of lipid-laden tubular cells.

MICROBIOLOGY

Clinical signs and urinalysis findings provide supportive evidence, but microbiology is required to diagnose urinary tract

infection (UTI) conclusively. The kidneys, ureters, bladder, and proximal urethra of normal dogs and cats are sterile, whereas a resident bacterial flora populates the distal urethra, prepuce, and vagina. Urinary tract infection occurs when bacteria colonize areas of the urinary tract that normally are sterile. Aerobic gram-negative bacteria account for most UTIs in dogs and cats, and the remainder are caused by gram-positive organisms. *Escherichia coli* is the organism most commonly implicated in urinary tract infections in dogs and cats. Other organisms isolated include *Proteus* spp., coagulase-positive staphylococci, and streptococci. *Pasteurella multocida* occasionally is isolated from cats with UTI. *Enterobacter* sp., *Klebsiella* sp., and *Pseudomonas aeruginosa* are observed less commonly in dogs and rarely in cats.

Results obtained with bacterial culture of urine depend on the method of urine collection. Voided urine has the greatest potential for bacterial contamination, and catheterization may inoculate the bladder with bacteria from the distal urethra. Urine collected by cystocentesis should be sterile in normal animals. Quantitative bacterial culture of urine allows determination of the number of bacterial colonies (colony-forming units [cfu]) that grow from 1 mL of urine (cfu/mL).

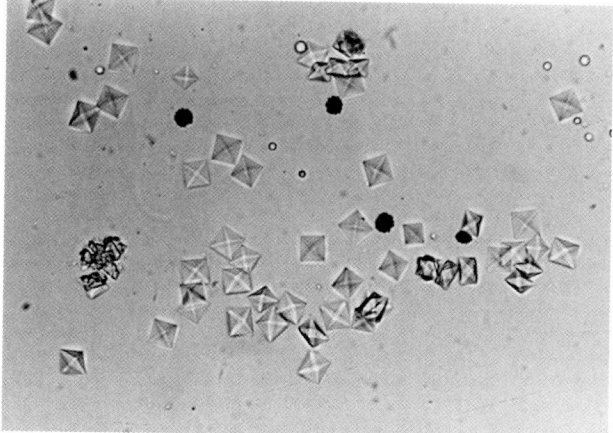

Figure 257-17 Photomicrograph of a urine sample containing calcium oxalate dihydrate crystals. These crystals may be observed in the urine of normal dogs as well as in those with calcium oxalate urolithiasis or acute renal failure caused by ethylene glycol ingestion. Note the typical "Maltese cross" appearance within a rhomboidal structure. These crystals can vary markedly in size.

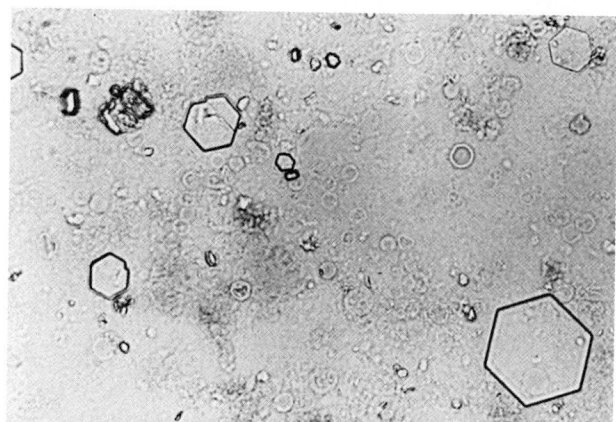

Figure 257-19 Photomicrograph of a urine sample containing cystine crystals. These crystals usually are found in acidic urine and are not present in normal animals. Their presence suggests cystinuria with or without cystine urolithiasis.

URINARY SYSTEM

Ideally, urine should be submitted for culture within 30 minutes of collection. If this is not possible, the sample may be refrigerated for up to 6 hours without significant loss of bacterial growth. Chemical preservation with a solution of boric acid, glycerol, and sodium formate, in combination with refrigeration, effectively maintained bacterial viability in canine urine samples for up to 72 hours.[53]

Bacterial culture of midstream-voided urine samples from normal dogs and cats often results in the growth of less than 1000 to greater than or equal to 100,000 cfu/mL. Therefore culture of voided urine is not recommended in evaluation of patients for UTI. If, however, no growth is obtained from a voided urine sample, UTI can be excluded as a diagnosis. Bacterial growth of greater than or equal to 100,000 cfu/mL may result from culture of urine obtained from catheterization in 20% of normal female dogs. Thus using a measurement of 100,000 cfu/mL as an indicator of UTI in female dogs results in a substantial number of false-positive results. Also, the urethral catheterization procedure itself may cause UTI in 20% of normal female dogs. Consequently, collection of urine by cystocentesis is recommended for establishing a diagnosis of UTI in female dogs. Isolation of bacteria from urine collected by catheterization from male dogs is uncommon, and a measurement of greater than 1000 cfu/mL is recommended for establishing a diagnosis of UTI using these urine samples. In both male and female cats, growth of greater than 1000 cfu/mL in samples collected by catheterization is considered compatible with a diagnosis of UTI.

Urine samples obtained by cystocentesis from normal dogs and cats should yield no growth, because this procedure bypasses the normal bacterial flora of the urethra and genital tract. Consequently, results obtained by cystocentesis are the standard against which results obtained using voided or catheterized samples are compared. A small number of organisms from the skin or environment occasionally contaminate samples obtained by cystocentesis, and growth of less than 1000 cfu/mL may be considered suggestive of contamination. Isolation of bacteria from urinary tissues obtained during surgery indicates UTI regardless of the number. Colony counts used to establish a diagnosis of UTI for different methods of urine collection are summarized in Table 257-3.

Microscopic examination of gram-stained urine smears also may be helpful in the diagnosis of UTI. In one study, one drop of uncentrifuged urine was allowed to dry, gram-stained, and examined under oil immersion. The presence of more than 2 organisms per field correlated with bacterial counts of greater than 1000 cfu/mL, whereas no organisms were visible in specimens with less than 1000 cfu/mL.[53]

RADIOLOGY

Radiography provides precise information about renal size that frequently cannot be obtained from the physical examination. To correct for variation in patient size and radiographic magnification, renal size is evaluated in reference to surrounding anatomic landmarks, usually the second lumbar vertebra (L2) on the ventrodorsal view. The left kidney normally is well visualized in the dog, but the right kidney often cannot be seen as well, especially its cranial pole. In the dog, the left kidney (near vertebra L2 to L5) is located caudal to the right kidney (near vertebra T13 to L3). In the cat, the kidneys lie near vertebra L3, with the right kidney positioned slightly cranial to the left. Renal size in dogs and cats can be assessed radiographically and compared to the length of vertebra L2. On the ventrodorsal view, the kidney to L2 ratio is 2.5 to 3.5 in dogs and 2.4 to 3 in cats.

Excretory urography is performed by taking sequential abdominal radiographs after intravenous administration of an

Table • 257-3

Assessment of Quantitative Urine Culture Results in Dogs and Cats

METHOD OF COLLECTION	SPECIES	SEX	COLONY COUNT INDICATIVE OF URINARY TRACT INFECTION (UTI)
Cystocentesis*	Dog	Male	>10^2 cfu/mL
		Female	>10^2 cfu/mL
	Cat	Male	>10^2 cfu/mL
		Female	>10^2 cfu/mL
Catheterization	Dog	Male	>10^3 cfu/mL
		Female	>10^5 cfu/mL†
	Cat	Male	>10^3 cfu/mL
		Female	>10^3 cfu/mL
Midstream voided	Dog	Male	Unreliable‡
		Female	Unreliable‡
	Cat	Male	Unreliable‡
		Female	Unreliable‡

*Growth of small numbers of a single organism (≤10^2 cfu/mL) from urine samples collected by cystocentesis is suggestive of skin contamination during collection. Growth of large numbers (>10^3 cfu/mL) of multiple organism from urine samples collected by cystocentesis is suggestive of needle puncture of bowel and contamination by intestinal flora.
†This guideline may result in erroneous diagnosis of UTI because >10^5 cfu/mL may be obtained from urine samples collected by catherization in 20% of normal female dogs. Also, the procedure of urethral catheterization itself may cause UTI in 20% of normal female dogs. Collection of urine by cystocentesis is recommended for establishing a diagnosis of UTI in female dogs.
‡Culture of midstream-voided urine samples from normal dogs and cats may result in growth of ≥10^5 cfu/mL. In the absence of prior antimicrobial therapy, a negative result on a voided sample excludes a diagnosis of UTI.

iodinated organic compound. The contrast medium is filtered and excreted by the kidneys, and the quality of the study partly depends on the patient's GFR. Radiographs should be taken at appropriate intervals (e.g., less than 1 minute, 5 minutes, 20 minutes, and 40 minutes) to obtain maximum information about the renal parenchyma and collecting system. Excretory urography is useful for the evaluation of a number of abnormalities, including renal size, shape, or location; filling defects in the renal pelvis or ureters; certain congenital defects (e.g., unilateral agenesis); renomegaly; acute pyelonephritis; and rupture of the upper urinary tract. Excretory urography should not be performed in dehydrated patients or in those with known hypersensitivity to contrast media. Although excretory urography normally is a safe procedure, a decrease in the GFR may persist for several days after intravenous administration of contrast agents to normal dogs, and ARF has been reported in a dog after excretory urography.[54] The general technique and interpretation of excretory urography in dogs and cats have been reviewed elsewhere.[55] Ultrasound-guided percutaneous antegrade pyelography has been used to localize ureteral obstruction in dogs and cats.[56]

Ultrasonography

Renal ultrasonography is a noninvasive imaging technique that does not depend on renal function, has no known adverse effects on the patient, and allows characterization of internal renal architecture. The major advantage of ultrasonography is the ability to discriminate among the renal capsule, cortex, and medulla, the pelvic diverticula, and the renal sinus.[57-60] Normally, the kidney is less echogenic than the liver or spleen. Collagen and fat provide highly reflective acoustic interfaces and account for the observation that the renal capsule, diverticula, and sinus are the most echogenic structures in the kidney. The renal medulla normally is less echogenic than the renal cortex because of its higher water content and fewer acoustic interfaces.[59] The hyperechogenicity of the renal cortex relative to the medulla varies among normal cats and has been attributed to variations in the amount of fat in the proximal tubular cells.[61]

Renal length and volume, as determined by ultrasonography, are linearly related to body weight in dogs.[62,63] In cats, renal length as determined by ultrasonography ranges between 3 and 4.3 cm.[64] Measurements of renal size determined by excretory urography exceed those obtained by ultrasonography.[57,64] This difference is due to osmotic diuresis and radiographic magnification effects during excretory urography and to indistinct renal margins and inaccurate choice of scanning planes during ultrasonography.[62,64]

Renal ultrasonography is useful for differentiating solid from fluid-filled lesions and for determining the distribution of lesions in the kidney (i.e., focal, multifocal, diffuse).[65] A pattern of multiple, anechoic cavitations is highly suggestive of polycystic kidney disease.[66,67] Cysts are smooth, sharply demarcated, anechoic lesions that demonstrate through transmission.[58] The renal pelvis is dilated with anechoic fluid in hydronephrosis, and the kidney is surrounded by an accumulation of anechoic fluid in cats with perinephric pseudocysts.[68,69] Organized hematomas, abscesses, and necrotic nodules present a pattern of mixed echogenicity. Focal or diffuse lesions of mixed echogenicity that disrupt normal anatomy often are tumors.[65] Poorly vascular tumors of homogenous cell type (e.g., lymphosarcoma) may produce hypoechoic lesions that occasionally may be misinterpreted as cysts.[65,66] Diffuse parenchymal renal diseases characterized by cellular infiltration with preservation of normal renal architecture (e.g., chronic tubulointerstitial nephritis) may produce diffuse hyperechogenicity but occasionally have a normal ultrasonographic appearance. Consequently, normal renal ultrasonographic results do not eliminate the possibility of renal disease.

Ethylene glycol intoxication also causes renal hyperechogenicity. Within 4 hours of ethylene glycol ingestion, renal cortical echogenicity exceeds that of the liver and approaches that of the spleen.[70,71] Medullary echogenicity increases to a lesser extent. Increased cortical and medullary echogenicity, with relative hypoechogenicity of the corticomedullary junction and inner medulla, results in a "halo" sign that correlates with the onset of anuria. Renal hyperechogenicity in ethylene glycol intoxication is attributed to deposition of calcium oxalate crystals in the kidneys.

An echogenic line in the outer zone of the medulla and paralleling the corticomedullary junction (so-called medullary rim sign) has been observed in ethylene glycol intoxication but also in acute tubular necrosis, hypercalcemic nephropathy, granulomatous nephritis caused by feline infectious peritonitis, and chronic tubulointerstitial nephritis.[72,73] This lesion also has been observed in normal cats[61] and has been associated with mineralization of tubular basement membranes. In a study of 32 dogs with medullary rim sign, most of the dogs in which this feature was the sole ultrasonographic finding had no evidence of renal dysfunction, whereas those with other ultrasonographic abnormalities (e.g., reduced renal size, increased medullary echogenicity, pyelectasia) had clinical evidence of renal dysfunction.[74]

Intrarenal resistance to blood flow may be assessed during duplex Doppler ultrasonography and evaluated by calculation of the resistive index. The normal value for the renal resistive index in healthy, unsedated dogs is approximately 0.6.[75] Somewhat lower values have been reported in normal, sedated dogs[76] and cats.[77] Other studies have suggested an upper limit of 0.7 for the resistive index in normal, unsedated cats.[78,79] Higher than normal values for the resistive index have been reported in some renal diseases of dogs and cats[80] but not in experimentally induced aminoglycoside nephrotoxicosis.[81]

Renal ultrasonography also has been used to monitor the status of renal allografts in dogs[82] and renal autografts in cats.[78] A rapid increase in renal volume in the immediate postoperative period may signify rejection, but some enlargement normally occurs as a consequence of edema and renal hypertrophy. The renal volume and cross-sectional area, as monitored by ultrasonography, increased by 103% and 83%, respectively, as a result of hypertrophy and rejection by 17 days after allograft transplantation in dogs.[82] Changes in renal width were greater than changes in height or length, which suggests that the cross-sectional area measurement may be a useful parameter to monitor. In cats, renal autografts increased 50% in the cross-sectional area by 13 days after transplantation as a result of postoperative edema and hypertrophy, but no changes were seen in the resistive index.[78]

RENAL BIOPSY

Renal biopsy allows the clinician to establish a histologic diagnosis and should be considered when the information obtained is likely to alter patient management. Examples of such situations include differentiation of protein-losing glomerular diseases, differentiation of ARF from CRF, determination of the status of the tubular basement membranes in ARF, and determination of the patient's response to therapy or the progression of previously documented renal disease. A renal biopsy should not be performed until a thorough clinical evaluation of the patient has been completed.

Before renal biopsy, an intravenous catheter should be placed, and the animal's clotting ability should be evaluated by measurement of the buccal mucosal bleeding time and estimation of platelet numbers. The patient's hematocrit and plasma proteins should be determined before biopsy but after adequate rehydration with parenteral fluids. The hematocrit and plasma proteins may be monitored after biopsy to detect hemorrhage.

Several techniques can be used for renal biopsy, including blind percutaneous, laparoscopic, keyhole, open, and ultrasound-guided approaches. The choice of technique depends largely on the experience and technical skill of the operator, the species to be biopsied, and the sample size required. The blind percutaneous technique works well in cats, because their kidneys can be readily palpated and immobilized. Laparoscopy allows direct visualization of the kidney and detection of hemorrhage but requires special equipment and expertise. The keyhole approach occasionally is used in dogs but is useful only if the operator is experienced with the technique. In one study of renal biopsy techniques in dogs, modifications of the keyhole technique and the use of laparoscopy did not improve the quality of the biopsy specimen obtained or reduce the complication rate.[83]

If the operator is relatively inexperienced with renal biopsy or if a larger sample is required, wedge biopsy by means of laparotomy is recommended. Laparotomy offers the operator the advantages of being able to inspect the kidneys and other abdominal organs visually, to choose the specific biopsy site, to take an adequately sized sample, and to observe the kidney for hemorrhage. Some techniques require general anesthesia for adequate patient restraint and analgesia, but needle biopsy specimens of the kidney can be obtained from dogs and cats under ultrasound guidance using one of several sedation protocols. In one study, the GFR (estimated by ^{99m}Tc-DTPA) was similar in dogs sedated with butorphanol and diazepam, acepromazine and butorphanol, and diazepam and ketamine, and the GFR of sedated dogs was not significantly different from that of awake dogs.[84]

At our hospital, renal biopsy in dogs and cats currently is performed under ultrasound guidance using the Bard® Biopty biopsy instrument (Bard Biopty biopsy system; C.R. Bard, Covington, Georgia) and with the animal sedated with a combination of medetomidine, butorphanol, and atropine. This combination of drugs recen≈tly was evaluated for renal biopsy in dogs (using ^{99m}Tc-DTPA renal scintigraphy as an estimate of the GFR) and was found to have effects on the GFR similar to those observed with saline alone.[85] In another study, needle biopsy of the kidney in normal cats sedated with ketamine and acepromazine had minimal effect on the GFR as evaluated by ^{99m}Tc-DTPA renal scintigraphy.[25] Occasionally, the tissue architecture is less important (e.g., in renal lymphosarcoma and feline infectious peritonitis), and aspiration of the kidney using a 23- or 25-gauge needle may provide useful material for cytology.

The most commonly used biopsy instruments are the Franklin-modified Vim Silverman needle and the Tru-Cut biopsy needle. Excessive penetration of the kidney with the outer cannula of the Franklin-modified Vim Silverman instrument should be avoided to prevent retrieval of an insufficient amount of renal cortex. Care should be taken in directing the angle of the biopsy instrument to avoid the renal hilus and major vessels. Samples containing large amounts of medulla are more likely to contain large vessels and to lead to infarction of renal tissue. It therefore is recommended that the biopsy needle be directed along the long axis of the kidney, solely through cortical tissue (Figure 257-20). In cats, because of the small size of feline kidneys, it is common to obtain relatively large amounts of medullary tissue, and this has been associated with infarction and fibrosis.

After biopsy using the open approach or keyhole technique, the kidney should be digitally compressed for 5 minutes, and after release the abdomen inspected for hemorrhage. The sample may be dislodged from the biopsy instrument with a stream of sterile saline from a syringe or, alternatively, the biopsy instrument may be immersed directly in fixative. For routine histopathology, the sample should be fixed in buffered 10% formalin for at least 3 to 4 hours. For immunofluorescence studies, the sample can be preserved in Michel's transport medium. Immunopathology studies also may be performed by a peroxidase-antiperoxidase method using formalin-fixed samples, without the need for special preservation of the sample.

After renal biopsy, a brisk fluid diuresis should be initiated to prevent clot formation in the renal pelvis. The patient's hematocrit and plasma proteins should be monitored at appropriate intervals over the next 12 to 24 hours to detect serious hemorrhage.

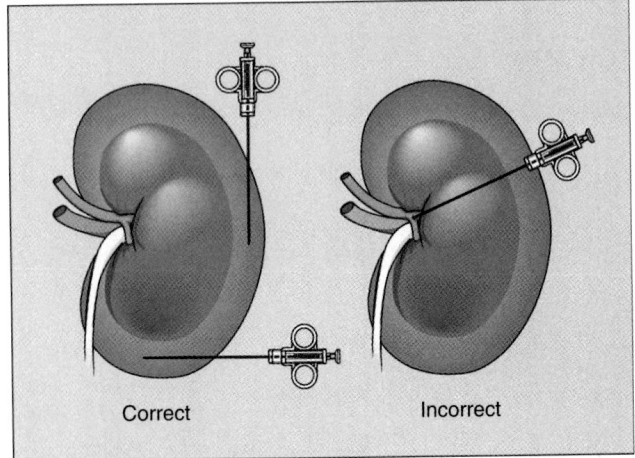

Figure 257-20 Demonstration of renal biopsy technique showing correct and incorrect placement of the biopsy instrument in the kidney. (Drawing courtesy Dr. Shelly Vaden, North Carolina State University, Raleigh.)

The most common complication of renal biopsy is hemorrhage. Subcapsular hemorrhage commonly occurs at the site of biopsy, and many patients experience microscopic hematuria during the first 48 hours after biopsy. Macroscopic hematuria is less common. Severe hemorrhage into the peritoneal cavity is rare and usually is associated with improper technique. Such hemorrhage must be treated aggressively by compression bandage of the abdomen, fresh whole blood transfusion, and exploratory surgery if necessary.

Linear infarcts in the path of the biopsy needle are commonly observed after renal biopsy in both dogs and cats. These are small and superficial when the biopsy is limited to the renal cortex. However, if an arcuate artery is damaged by passage of the biopsy needle through the corticomedullary junction, a wedge-shaped infarct may occur. This complication is more common in cats because of the small size of the kidneys in relation to the length of the biopsy needle.

Hydronephrosis occasionally complicates renal biopsy. If the renal pelvis is penetrated by the biopsy needle, bleeding may occur, and clot formation can lead to obstruction of the kidney and hydronephrosis. This complication should be considered if the biopsy report indicates the presence of transitional epithelium at one end of the biopsy or if progressive renal enlargement is detected after renal biopsy. The risk of this complication can be minimized by limiting the biopsy site to the renal cortex and instituting a fluid diuresis afterward.

Acute Uremia

Larry D. Cowgill
Thierry Francey

Acute uremia is a clinical condition in which the kidneys suddenly and often catastrophically fail to meet the excretory, metabolic, and endocrine demands of the body. This abnormality is induced by rapid hemodynamic, filtration, tubulointerstitial, or excretory injury to the kidneys or outflow system (or both), which results in accumulation of solutes (uremia toxins), metabolic dysfunction, and dysregulation of fluid, electrolyte, and acid-base balance. Acute uremia is, conceptually, a quickly developing disease to intrinsically normal kidneys. However, some animals have prerenal, renal parenchymal, or postrenal events superimposed on a pre-existing chronic renal injury that causes a similar clinical condition.

The term *acute renal failure* (ARF) does not standardize the classification of acute uremia relative to its severity, clinical course, response to therapy, or prognosis for recovery.[1,2] To date no specific biologic markers provide these distinctions. Numerous definitions of acute uremia exist that are based on changes in glomerular filtration rate (GFR), degree of azotemia, or urine production in humans. These criteria, however, are rarely applied to animals because the abruptness of their disease and changes in azotemia or volume of urine production are usually not known. Acute uremia in animals is generally a disease recognized later than in humans and with varying abruptness and azotemia. The diagnosis of ARF is established with high specificity but low sensitivity. Affected animals have a spectrum of functional and clinical deficiencies that should be considered in its classification, management, and outcome.

Acute uremia is associated with a rapid (hours to days) and progressive increase in serum concentrations of urea, creatinine, and phosphate. There may also be variable degrees of hyperkalemia, metabolic acidosis, or both. Progression of azotemia may not be recognized in animals being evaluated for the first time that are already in a late stage of disease or in those without previously obtained serial blood chemistry determinations. After azotemia is demonstrated, the acute condition must be differentiated from functional disturbances (prerenal azotemia) or chronic renal failure (CRF). Oliguria and anuria are characteristic of severe forms of acute uremia, but this feature is unpredictable. Nonoliguric forms of acute uremia are common and must be differentiated from polyuria associated with CRF. In contrast to CRF, acute uremia is potentially reversible if the animal survives until the underlying conditions resolve and natural recovery (repair) of the renal injury takes place. Throughout its progression, therapeutic opportunities exist to alter the outcome of the disease. If the diagnosis is missed or if the injury is too severe, the kidney will be incapable of morphologic repair. Thus delays in initiating therapy or failure to provide appropriate supportive therapy may result in irreversible renal damage and death.

The incidence of acute uremia is lower than that of CRF in both dogs and cats. The clinical signs associated with acute and CRF may be similar, and clinicians must distinguish between these conditions to administer appropriate therapy and render an accurate prognosis. Acute uremia frequently complicates other surgical or medical diseases and must be recognized as a serious complication of any condition.

CAUSE OF ACUTE UREMIA

Acute uremia can be categorized as prerenal azotemia, intrinsic ARF, postrenal azotemia, or some combination of these conditions.

Prerenal Azotemia

Prerenal azotemia is a hemodynamically mediated decline in GFR resulting from decreased renal blood flow, perfusion pressure, or increased renal vascular resistance. It represents a functional alteration in GFR that is completely reversible without morphologic consequences to renal parenchyma. Prerenal azotemia develops as a coordinated neural and humoral response to hemodynamic deficiencies in an attempt to preserve perfusion to vital organs. Filtration failure ensues when the renal perfusion pressure falls below the threshold for renal autoregulation (usually a mean arterial pressure [MAP] < 80 mm Hg).[3,4] As renal compensatory mechanisms are activated in response to hemodynamic failure (cardiogenic, septic, hypovolemic shock) or to decreased functional renal mass, even small additional impairments in renal perfusion or glomerular hemodynamics (nonsteroidal anti-inflammatory drugs [NSAIDs], angiotensin-converting enzyme [ACE] inhibitors, angiotensin receptor blockers) can precipitate severe filtration failure.[5,6] Activation of the sympathetic nervous system (SNS), the renin-angiotensin-aldosterone system, and the release of antidiuretic hormone (ADH) in response to these hemodynamic events promote via salt and water conservation, urine concentration, and oliguria in an attempt to restore blood volume.

Mild azotemia (serum creatinine concentrations < 4 mg/dL, and blood urea nitrogen [BUN] concentrations < 80 mg/dL), increased urine specific gravity [USG], and decreased urine sodium excretion (urine sodium concentration < 20 mEq/L; fractional excretion of sodium < 1%) are hallmarks of prerenal azotemia. These parameters may be masked by the use of diuretics or by underlying conditions (CRF, adrenal insufficiency, hepatic failure, diabetes insipidus) that impair renal concentrating ability. Tubular reabsorption of urea can be increased disproportionately to creatinine at these low urine flow rates, causing variable increases in BUN/creatinine ratio.[7,8] A prerenal component to this azotemia is often superimposed on intrinsic renal failure, causing severe uremia. Prolonged renal hypoperfusion can result in structural alterations secondary to ischemic cellular injury that may induce intrinsic ARF. Vasculitis, pancreatitis, hypoproteinemia, heat stroke, liver failure, and gastric torsion are examples of disease states inducing hemodynamic disturbances with the propensity to cause progressive prerenal azotemia leading to intrinsic ARF.[9]

Intrinsic Acute Renal Failure

Intrinsic ARF is the result of parenchymal damage to the kidney and can be categorized according to the initial site of injury as *primary vascular, glomerular, tubular,* or *interstitial.* This anatomic classification is arbitrary due to multiple interactions between these structures but may be helpful in understanding the pathophysiology of lesions observed in individual dogs and cats (Box 258-1). For clinical purposes, ARF may be categorized based on cause. With this classification, ARF can develop as a continuation of prerenal events, local ischemia (ischemic nephrosis), or as a consequence of exogenous or endogenous nephrotoxins (toxic nephrosis). Using a causative classification, primary renal diseases (pyelonephritis, toxic nephrosis) and systemic diseases with renal manifestations (pancreatitis, ischemic nephrosis) can induce ARF with mixed anatomic involvement.

Ischemia due to prolonged hypotension, hypovolemia, circulatory collapse, or excessive renal vasoconstriction predisposes a dog or cat to filtration failure and acute uremia as an extension of prerenal azotemia. Renal ischemia may also develop after renal arterial thrombosis, disseminated intravascular coagulation (DIC), or septic thrombi.

Box • 258-1

Causes of Intrinsic Acute Renal Failure

Renal Ischemia
Progression of prerenal azotemia
Renal vascular disease (avulsion, thrombosis, stenosis)

Nephrotoxicity
Exogenous toxins
Endogenous toxins
Drugs

Primary Renal Diseases
Infections: pyelonephritis, leptospirosis, infectious canine hepatitis
Immune-mediated disease: acute glomerulonephritis, systemic lupus erythematosus (SLE), renal transplant rejection
Neoplasia: lymphoma
Miscellaneous: "Alabama rot"[26]

Systemic Diseases with Renal Manifestation
Infections: Feline infectious peritonitis (FIP), borreliosis, babesiosis, leishmaniasis, bacterial endocarditis
Pancreatitis
Systemic inflammatory response syndrome, sepsis, multiple organ failure, disseminated intravascular coagulopathy (DIC)
Heart failure
SLE
Hepatorenal syndrome
Malignant hypertension
Hyperviscosity syndrome: polycythemia, multiple myeloma

Nephrotoxins are the primary cause of ARF in dogs. They can be of exogenous or endogenous origin and of diverse chemical classes including organic compounds and solvents, antimicrobials, vasoactive drugs, and miscellaneous therapeutics (Box 258-2).[10-12]

NSAIDs inhibit cyclooxygenase (COX)-dependent synthesis of vasodilatory prostaglandins that regulate renal blood flow when renal perfusion is compromised. Nonselective COX-1/COX-2 inhibitors (flunixin meglumine, ibuprofen, aspirin),[13] promote loss of counter-regulatory vasodilation to an ischemic insult, which intensifies vascular resistance and furthers hypoperfusion of the kidney.[14] Although species differences exist, newer NSAIDs with selective COX-2 inhibition (meloxicam, carprofen, deracoxib) also have the potential to be nephrotoxic.

The principal toxicity associated with NSAIDs use in animals is a nonoliguric ischemic nephrosis. Idiosyncratic tubulointerstitial nephritis, nephrotic syndrome, renal papillary necrosis, and hyporeninemic-hypoaldosteronism have also been described in humans.[15] The nephrotoxicity of NSAIDs is exacerbated in animals with congestive heart failure (CHF), nephrotic syndrome, renal insufficiency, hypertension, cirrhosis, and those undergoing anesthesia in which renal perfusion is compromised and renal vascular tone is increased.[14] Because of the ischemic nature of this nephrotoxicity, the lesions are generally reversible.

ACE inhibitors may induce ARF through alterations in glomerular hemodynamics, renal hypoperfusion, and tubular ischemia. Sodium depletion, diuretic abuse, and CHF may increase the nephrotoxic potential of these drugs. The risks of toxicity are magnified in animals with pre-existing CRF because basal GFR is dependent on increased postglomerular resistance mediated by angiotensin II.[6,16,17] ACE inhibitors with mixed renal and hepatic elimination may prove less toxic in animals with CRF when compared with ACE inhibitors that are excreted only through the kidneys.[18]

Clinicians may prevent ARF induced by NSAIDs or ACE inhibitors with judicious monitoring of serum creatinine concentrations before mitigating treatment, together with early (3 to 5 days) and frequent (biweekly) monitoring of serum creatinine concentrations after the start of therapy. If increased concentrations of serum creatinine are documented, treatment should be stopped or doses reduced. Special precautions should be taken when administering diuretics, ACE inhibitors, NSAIDs, or a combination of these medications concurrently due to their additive hemodynamic effects.

Ethylene glycol toxicosis is one of the most common causes of ARF and one of the most common toxicoses recognized in companion animals.[19] Automobile antifreeze is the usual source of exposure, and the toxicity develops by the direct actions of its metabolites on the tubular epithelium and deposition of calcium oxalate crystals in the tubular lumens and interstitium.

Plant-related intoxications represent a new category of acute uremia in dogs and cats with severe nephrosis. Exposure and ingestion of lilies has been reported to cause severe acute ARF in cats.[20,21] Similarly, ingestion of grapes or raisins has been recently associated with ARF in dogs.[22,23]

Aminoglycosides (gentamicin, amikacin, tobramycin, netilmicin, and neomycin) are potent nephrotoxins causing direct tubular injury or tubular dysfunction associated with wasting of filtered solutes.[24] Further, nearly all antimicrobials (including penicillins, cephalosporins, carbapenems, fluoroquinolones, macrolides, tetracyclines, and sulfonamides) can cause tubular injury, tubular dysfunction, or intratubular obstruction.[15,24,25]

Amphotericin B is a polyene antifungal that complexes with sterol moieties of cell membranes forming pores that disrupt cellular integrity and increase membrane permeability.[26]

Box • 258-2

List of Substances with Nephrotoxic Potential

Therapeutic Agents
Antibacterial drugs
  Aminoglycosides
  Penicillins
  Nafcillin
  Cephalosporins
  Sulfonamides
  Fluoroquinolones
  Carbapenems
  Rifampin
  Tetracyclines
  Vancomycin
  Aztreonam
Antifungal drugs
  Amphotericin B
Antiviral drugs
  Acyclovir
  Foscarnet
Antiprotozoal drugs
  Pentamidine
  Sulfadiazine
  Trimethoprim-sulfamethoxazole
  Dapsone
  Thiacetarsemide
Cancer chemotherapeutics
  Cisplatin, carboplatin
  Methotrexate
  Doxorubicin
  Adriamycin
  Azathioprine
Immunosuppressive drugs
  Cyclosporine
  FK506
  Interleukin (IL)-2
NSAIDS
Ace inhibitors
Diuretics
  Mannitol
Miscellaneous therapeutic agents
  Dextran 40
  Allopurinol
  Cimetidine
  Apomorphine
  Deferoxamine
  Streptokinase
    Aminocaproic acid

Lipid-lowering agents
Methoxyflurane
Penicillamine
Acetaminophen
Tricyclic antidepressants
Radiocontrast agents

Nontherapeutic Agents
Heavy metals
  Mercury
  Uranium
  Lead
  Bismuth salts
  Chromium
  Arsenic
  Gold
  Cadmium
  Thallium
  Copper
  Silver
  Nickel
  Antimony
Organic compounds
  Ethylene glycol
  Carbon tetrachloride
  Chloroform
  Pesticides
  Herbicides
  Solvents
Miscellaneous agents
  Gallium nitrate
  Diphosphonates
  Mushrooms
  Grapes/raisins
  Calcium antagonists
  Snake venom
  Bee venom
  Lily
  Illicit drugs

Endogenous Toxins
Pigment nephrosis
  Hemoglobin
  Myoglobin

Nephrotoxicity is the dose-limiting factor associated with use of this drug, and renal function should be closely monitored throughout its administration. The advent of lipid formulations, and particularly of liposome encapsulated amphotericin B, has markedly decreased the nephrotoxicity associated with amphotericin use and has allowed more aggressive application of this drug.[27-30]

Cisplatin is an alkylating antineoplastic agent concentrated within and excreted primarily by the kidney. Its administration leads to a dose-dependent, progressive, and irreversible non-oliguric ARF. Carboplatin, an analogue of cisplatin, is less nephrotoxic and has largely replaced cisplatin in clinical practice.[15]
  Primary renal diseases include infectious, immune-mediated, neoplastic, or degenerative conditions with primary expression

in the kidney. When peracute or extensive, primary renal diseases produce an acute uremia that must be differentiated from traditional ischemic or nephrotoxic causes. Acute pyelonephritis develops from ureteral reflux of bacteria in the urine of animals with lower urinary tract (LUT) infection. It is an important cause of acute uremia in both dogs and cats.[11,31] The azotemia may be moderate or severe and associated with variable urine output. Suppurative nephritis is an infection arising from hematogenous dissemination of bacteria or septic embolization of the kidneys in animals with bacteremia or septicemia. Predisposing conditions include bacterial endocarditis, discospondylitis, and pyometra.

Leptospirosis is a specific infectious zoonosis of dogs with predominantly hepatorenal manifestation.[32-38] It was a well-characterized syndrome of acute hemorrhagic diathesis, subacute icterus, or subacute uremia caused by *Leptospira interrogans* serogroups *canicola* and *icterohaemorrhagiae*. Widespread use of a bivalent vaccine against these serogroups led to near extinction of leptospirosis in the canine population, until recently.[32,33,35,38] Retrospective studies in the United States and Canada have documented a regional re-emergence of the disease since the 1990s and a change in its epidemiology with *L. pomona*, *L. bratislava*, *L. grippotyphosa*, and *L. autumnalis* as the most commonly identified serogroups. The associated clinical syndrome has also changed, with ARF rather than hepatorenal or coagulation manifestations.[32,33,36,39] Possible explanations for the recently recognized re-emergence and clustering of leptospirosis could include urbanization of the canine population and encroachment of dogs into environments harboring reservoirs of the host species.[32,34,37] New, multivalent vaccines have emerged in response to these epidemiologic trends, but it remains to be seen whether vaccination will change the prevalence or biology of this disease. Because of its growing prevalence as a cause of acute uremia in dogs, leptospirosis should be included routinely in the differential diagnosis of all dogs with ARF, regardless of vaccination status.

A rapidly progressive form of ARF with severe azotemia, proteinuria, peripheral edema, and body cavity effusion has been associated with positive serology for *Borrelia burgdorferi*. This form of the disease is recognized routinely in dogs from endemic areas and, despite aggressive therapy, is invariably fatal.[40]

Systemic diseases including pancreatitis, sepsis, and hemolytic anemia (see Box 258-1) promote intrinsic ARF through secondary mechanisms associated with renal hemodynamics, systemic inflammatory responses, or drug toxicities associated with the underlying disease or diseases (see Pathophysiology, following). The ensuing ARF can exacerbate the course of the primary disease or dominate the clinical presentation of affected animals.

Postrenal Azotemia

Postrenal azotemia occurs with obstruction or diversion of urine and consequent retention of excretory products within the body. The most common causes of postrenal azotemia include partial or complete obstruction of the urethra or bladder by uroliths, mucous plugs, blood clots, or intra- or extraluminal mass lesions. Bilateral ureteral dilation should raise suspicion of a common outflow obstruction at the ureterovesical junction caused by a transitional cell carcinoma in the bladder neck or inadvertent ligation of the ureters during ovariohysterectomy. Bilateral ureteral obstruction or unilateral obstruction in a dog or cat with only one functioning kidney can be caused by calcium oxalate uroliths, solidified blood clots, mucous plugs, inflammatory debris, or stricture. These problems are being recognized with increased frequency as a leading cause acute uremia in cats.[41,42] Rupture of the urinary outflow tract diverts urine into the retroperitoneal space (ureteral), peritoneal cavity (ureteral, bladder, or proximal urethra), or pelvic canal (urethra), with consequent development of oligoanuria and uremia. Correction of the outflow obstruction or rupture may represent a surgical challenge, but if successful it will resolve azotemia without the presence of permanent structural damage to the kidneys.

Protracted outflow obstruction for more than 7 days can result in renal parenchymal damage and intrinsic ARF. At this stage, recovery of renal function is unpredictable and influenced by the severity and duration of the obstruction, completeness of the surgical correction, postobstructive medical complications, and pre-existing renal disease. Intuitively, a successful outcome will be less likely and the animal will be subjected to greater structural damage or death from uremia if correction of the outflow impairment is delayed or incomplete.

PATHOPHYSIOLOGY OF ACUTE UREMIA

Ischemic and toxic insults to the kidney cause a state of acute tubular injury (ATI). At the cellular level, ATI can vary from sublethal cell damage to cellular necrosis or apoptosis. The term *ATI* is often equated with the older term, *acute tubular necrosis*, used to denote ARF; however, the two terms should be distinguished in the pathophysiologic description of the syndrome. The histopathologic changes in some kidneys are more subtle than necrosis, and the tubular injury may be sublethal, making ATI a more appropriate descriptor and providing better correlation between observed structural alterations and clinical correlates of renal dysfunction.[43] With ischemic and nephrotoxic ARF, the tubular injury is characterized by degenerative and less commonly necrotic foci of tubular epithelium distributed heterogeneously throughout the kidneys with minimal evidence of interstitial inflammatory infiltrates. The straight portion of the proximal tubule (S3 segment) shows the most severe degenerative changes after an insult and maximal mitotic activity during recovery. The convoluted proximal tubule (S1 and S2 segments), the segments in the inner medulla, the medullary thick ascending limb, and the collecting tubules are least severely affected or completely spared by ischemic or toxic damage.[43,44]

Phases of Intrinsic Acute Renal Failure

ARF classically proceeds through three clinical phases: (1) initiation, (2) maintenance, and (3) recovery.[45] The late stage of the initiation phase is now recognized as pathophysiologically distinct and this classical progression has been modified recently to include the *extension phase* as indicated in Figure 258-1.[2,46] The initiation phase is the period during which the animal is subjected to the renal insult. At this phase, parenchymal injury evolves, and the tubular epithelium undergoes sublethal but potentially reversible injury.[2,47] Early intervention during the initiation phase will often prevent progression to more severe injury.

During the extension phase the kidney is subjected to alterations in renal perfusion, continued hypoxia, secondary inflammation, and ongoing epithelial and endothelial injury. As a result of these sustained or cumulative insults, the cellular injury progresses to cell death by necrosis or apoptosis. The functional consequences are a progressive decline in glomerular filtration, loss of urine-concentrating ability, and development of oliguria (or nonoliguria) and azotemia. At this critical phase in the pathogenesis, clinical manifestations may not be apparent, but the injury may be unresponsive to therapeutic intervention. The combined initiation and extension phases may last from hours to days but remain unrecognized because the changes in GFR and USG are not clinically apparent.

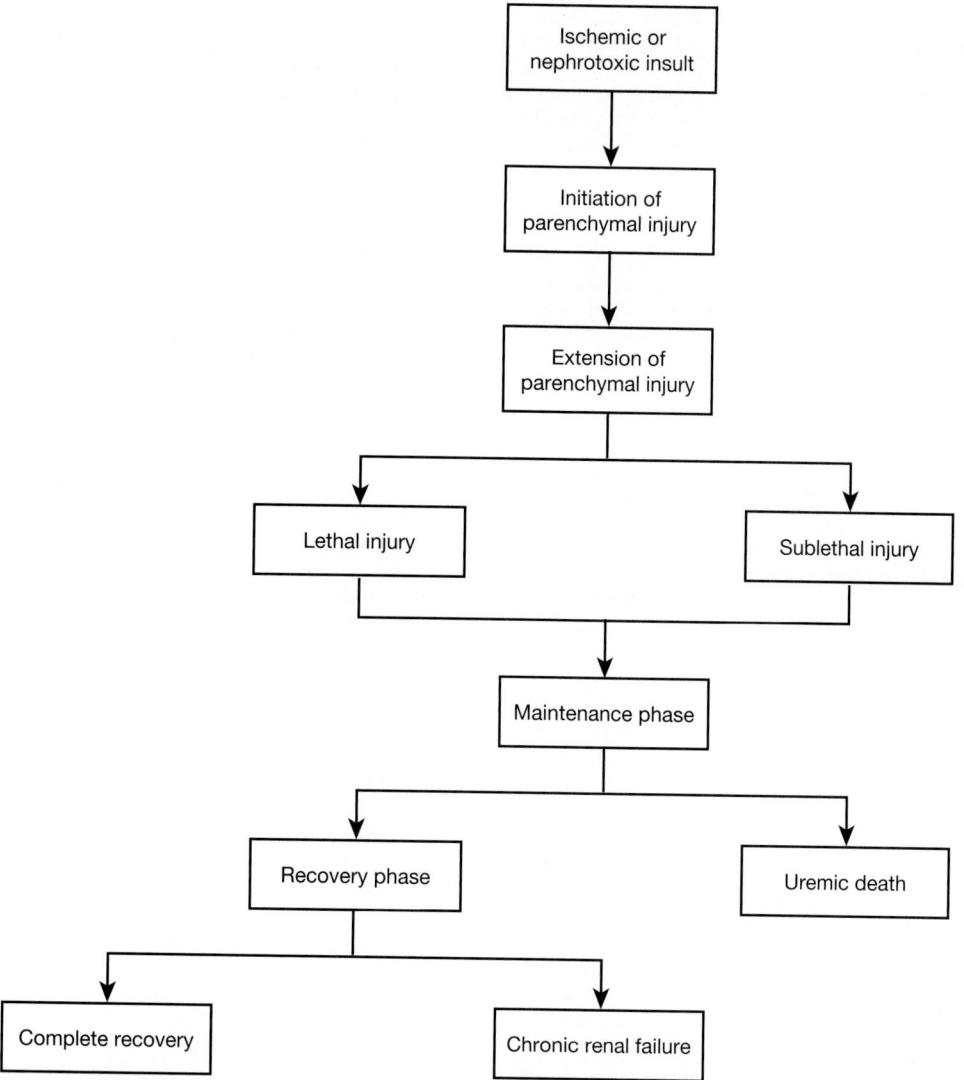

Figure 258-1 Clinical phases of acute renal failure (ARF). In the initiation and extension phases, renal damage and sublethal cellular injury evolve, but renal failure is not evident. In the maintenance phase, the inciting events have ceased, cellular damage is established, and signs of uremia become apparent. The recovery phase involves tubular regeneration and repair and the partial or complete return of renal function.

The maintenance phase ensues after a critical amount of irreversible epithelial damage has occurred. GFR is decreased, the regulation of regional blood flow is altered, urine volume may decrease, and the complications of uremia develop. Elimination of inciting factors at this phase will not alter existing damage or rate of recovery.[17,48] The maintenance phase lasts from days to weeks and when prolonged portends a slower rate of recovery and a likelihood of permanent renal impairment.

The recovery phase is the period where renal tissue undergoes regeneration and repair with restoration of renal function. Recovery may be associated with an increase in urine output and progressive resolution of the azotemia; however, molecular evidence of regeneration may be detected before these signs are apparent.[48] An increase in urine production at this phase may not correspond to meaningful improvement in GFR, so changes in the azotemia may lag behind evidence of

tubular repair. Diuresis is a physiologic response to accumulated water, salt, and osmotically active solutes, immature tubular function, or diuretic therapy. Functional repair follows cellular recovery of the sublethally injured epithelium, removal of intratubular debris, and re-epithelialization of the tubule.[49] The renal injury induces growth factor production and alters gene expression to enable remnants of surviving epithelium to dedifferentiate, re-enter the cell cycle, replicate, repopulate the denuded tubule, and redifferentiate into a functionally mature tubular epithelium. These events are orchestrated by mitogens (stimulate cell proliferation), motogens (stimulate cell mobility), and morphogens (induce changes in multicellular architecture) including insulin-like growth factor-1 (IGF-1), epidermal growth factor (EGF), transforming growth factor (TGF), platelet-derived growth factor (PDGF), fibroblast growth factor (FGF), nerve growth factor (NGF), hepatocyte growth factor (HGF), and vascular endothelial growth factor (VEGF).[50] These same repair factors may also contribute to fibrosis and other deleterious aspects of the pathogenesis and progression of renal damage. The recovery phase may last from weeks to months. With renal repair, some animals recover adequate or even normal renal function after weeks or even months of anuria that follows a severe renal injury like ethylene glycol intoxication.

Outflow Obstruction

Acute urinary outflow obstruction transmits increased hydrostatic pressure to the renal pelvis, the tubular system, and Bowman space. Within glomerular capillaries, the ultrafiltration pressure is dissipated, causing a progressive decline in GFR. The heightened pressure in Bowman capsule and tubular lumen is counterbalanced by ongoing sodium and water reabsorption along the nephron, but this compensation is inadequate to prevent filtration failure. Renal blood flow is progressively altered with initial increases and subsequent decreases due to local vasodilation and increased interstitial hydrostatic pressure, respectively.

Pathogenesis of Acute Renal Failure

Four functional and pathologic alterations have been shown to participate to variable degrees in the initiation, extension, and maintenance phases of ARF on the basis of animal models of ischemic and nephrotoxic ARF: (1) reduction of the glomerular capillary ultrafiltration coefficient (K_f) and permeability, (2) intratubular obstruction, (3) back leak of filtrate across disrupted tubular epithelium, and (4) intrarenal vasoconstriction and renal medullary hypoxia.[45,49,51]

Decreased ultrafiltration coefficient (K_f) reduces GFR by either a decrease in hydraulic conductivity or effective surface area of glomerular capillaries. Transmission and scanning electron microscopy in animal models of ARF demonstrated both loss and fusion of normal foot processes and marked disruption of podocyte architecture.[52] Vasoconstriction initiated by angiotensin II and other vasoactive agents or contraction of the mesangium by ischemia, toxins, thromboxane A_2, endothelin, and platelet activating factor alter K_f by reducing effective glomerular surface area. It is likely that conductivity and surface area are affected by both ischemic and toxic insults.[52-54]

Intratubular obstruction occurs when tubular casts produced by desquamated epithelial cells or cellular debris combine with intratubular proteins.[55,56] Tubular obstruction can also occur by precipitation of filtered heme pigments, crystal deposition (calcium oxalate, sulfonamides), or by extratubular compression (interstitial edema, inflammation). The impediment to tubular fluid flow increases intratubular hydrostatic pressure, decreases net ultrafiltration pressure, and halts single nephron glomerular filtration.

Back leak of tubular fluid across the disrupted epithelium further decreases urine formation and consequently the apparent ultrafiltration rate.[57,58]

Intrarenal vasoconstriction is a common participant in the pathogenesis of either hemodynamic or nephrotoxic injury. The resulting decrease in renal blood flow is transient and may occur in either the initiation or the extension phases. At the same time renal blood flow will be redirected preferentially to the cortex to maximize GFR and solute reabsorption at the expense of perfusion to the outer medulla. The redistribution creates profound hypoxia at the site of this oxygen-demanding segment.[3,51,59,60] Vasoconstriction is induced by altered regulation of competing dilatory and constrictive vasoactive processes that regulate and balance vascular resistance. Up-regulation of the renin-angiotensin system, impairment of renal autoregulatory capacity, enhanced adrenergic activity, and systemic or local release of vasoactive agents (thromboxane A2, leukotrienes C4 and D4, endothelin-1, adenosine, and endothelium-derived prostaglandin E_2) promote enhanced vasoconstrictive forces. The vasoconstriction frenzy is further exacerbated by vascular endothelial dysfunction to cause decreased production and release of vasodilator substances, including nitric oxide and prostaglandins.

Cellular Biology of Intrinsic Acute Renal Failure

Discovery of the cellular responses to ischemic and nephrotoxic injuries have improved our understanding of the clinical course of ARF. An extensive discussion of these mechanisms is beyond the scope of this review but are summarized in Figure 258-2 and reviewed in-depth elsewhere.[17,43,61]

Hypoxia secondary to poor perfusion of the outer medulla causes depletion of energy-dependent mechanisms within cells. Energy depletion alters cytosolic ionic concentrations (Na+, Ca++), loss of cellular polarity and vectorial cellular transport, disruption of tight junctions and the brush border membrane, and detachment of tubular cells from the basement membrane. In addition to these degenerative events, release of inflammatory cytokines (IL-l, TNF-), chemokines, heat shock proteins, nitric oxide, and reactive oxygen species induce a proinflammatory state that further compromises cellular oxygenation. Recognition of these hypoxic and inflammatory interactions provides opportunity for new therapeutic strategies to alter the course of ARF.

The kidney is exposed to high concentrations of endogenous and exogenous toxins, including drugs and their metabolites. This is intensified by regional hemodynamic, reabsorptive, and concentrating processes. In contrast to NSAIDs and ACE inhibitors, which induce ischemic lesions through alterations in blood flow in the glomerulus and the interstitium, other nephrotoxins, like aminoglycosides and ethylene glycol, cause direct epithelial injury and cellular damage (see discussion of cause ARF)[15,19]

CLINICAL CONSEQUENCES OF ACUTE UREMIA

The clinical consequences of acute uremia are the collective result of the excretory (water, potassium, phosphorus, nitrogenous waste products, medications), regulatory (fluid volume, electrolytes, acid-base, divalent cations, blood pressure), and endocrine (calcitriol and parathyroid hormone [PTH], erythropoietin) failure of the kidney. The clinical manifestations of acute uremia are the result of the multisystemic basis of the syndrome. Recent observations in dogs indicate that usually four or more organ systems are affected at presentation and in early stages of management. Ranking of organ system involvement (in percent of uremic dogs) revealed the following: gastrointestinal (GI) (93%), cardiovascular (80%), respiratory (52%), hematologic (40%), and neurologic (36%).[62] The multisystemic features of uremia per se become interspersed with the discrete symptomatology induced by the underlying cause, concurrent diseases, and therapy. An awareness and understanding of these collective manifestations of uremia is necessary to properly direct the therapeutic approach.

Disorders of Fluid Balance

At initial examination most animals are hypovolemic and dehydrated due to GI fluid losses, hemorrhage, and inadequate fluid intake. Dehydration at this stage of disease fosters renal hypoperfusion and leads to a prerenal azotemia. Extended hypovolemia promotes further impairment of renal perfusion, worsens the azotemia, and predisposes the kidneys to additional ischemia injury. Overaggressive fluid therapy predictably leads to hypervolemia and overhydration, causing peripheral and pulmonary edema, pleural effusion, systemic hypertension, and CHF. In dogs referred for severe ARF, nearly 70% were overhydrated when they arrived at the authors' hospital, some in excess of 25% of their body weight.

Serial measurements of body weight and critical assessment of hydration at presentation and at regular intervals during therapy are essential to avoid this iatrogenic complication.

Inadequate Urine Production

Oliguria or anuria is both a hallmark and a critical feature of acute uremia. Whereas anuria constitutes essentially no urine production, no consensus exists on the exact definition of oliguria. Urine production less than 0.27 mL/kg/hr,[63] less than 0.48 mL/kg/hr[64,65] and less than 1 to 2 mL/kg/hr[66] have all been described. The authors interpret urine production less than 1 mL/kg/hr in a rehydrated, euvolemic, or hypervolemic dog or cat on intravenous fluids or receiving diuretics as pathologically oliguric. The concept of pathologic oliguria seems justified by the fact that animals with normal renal function would be expected to produce more than the lower limit of normal urine output under similar clinical conditions. Pathologic oliguria should be differentiated from physiologically appropriate oliguric states associated with prerenal disorders that are responsive to fluid administration.

Approximately one third of dogs with severe ARF are anuric, one third are oliguric, and one third are nonoliguric.[62] Severe renal injuries associated with nephrotoxins have a higher incidence of anuria. Solute retention, overhydration, hyperkalemia, and metabolic acidosis are exacerbated in oligoanuric animals compared with those with nonoliguric disease. Persistent oligoanuria prevents administration of essential therapies associated with large fluid volumes (enteral and parenteral medications, blood products, and nutrition). The conversion from an oliguric to a nonoliguric state may facilitate delivery of these therapies without concurrent improvement in GFR.

Electrolyte and Acid-Base Disturbances

Impaired excretory function of the diseased kidney leads to an array of electrolyte and acid-base disturbances. The most prominent disturbance is hyperkalemia, which can be further aggravated by inappropriate potassium administration in enteral or parenteral fluids and by metabolic acidosis. Hyperkalemia decreases the transmembrane potassium gradient, depolarizes cell membranes, and impairs excitation and conduction. When expressed at the sinus node and on myocardial cells, these perturbations cause classic electrocardiographic abnormalities associated with the severity of hyperkalemia. The cardiac effects lead progressively to bradycardia, atrial standstill, and cardiac arrest as the hyperkalemia worsens. These same electrophysiologic disturbances affecting skeletal muscle, smooth muscle, and peripheral nerves can cause profound weakness, flaccid paralysis, respiratory failure, GI hypomotility, and hyporeflexia. Hyperkalemia is a leading cause of death, failure of conventional therapies, and a specific indication for dialysis.

Abnormalities in serum sodium are frequently iatrogenic and induced by inappropriate fluid therapy and excessive use of sodium bicarbonate. Hyponatremia is an indication of excessive free water administration associated with hyponatric solutions (5% dextrose, TPN, or enteral formulations). Transient dilutional hyponatremia is seen after the administration of mannitol, hypertonic dextrose, or synthetic colloid solutions as free water shifts from the intracellular to the extracellular space. It may also be recognized with excessive losses of sodium associated with vomiting, pancreatitis, adrenal insufficiency, or diuretic administration.

Hypernatremia may be documented at initial examination and indicates excessive free water loss. In hospitalized animals, it is a common complication of isonatric crystalloid administration for maintenance fluid requirements. Hypernatremia is a complication of excessive administration of hypertonic saline or sodium bicarbonate.

Metabolic acidosis is a predictable feature of acute uremia due to the impaired acid excretion, decreased bicarbonate reabsorption, and decreased ammonia generation. Metabolic acidosis is worsened by additional acid loads generated by the underlying disorder (ethylene glycol, salicylate intoxication), decreased perfusion (lactic acidosis), hypercatabolism, and concurrent diseases (diabetic ketoacidosis). These abnormalities are attended by an increased anion gap, decreased serum bicarbonate, acidemia, and hyperkalemia. Severe metabolic acidosis produces tachypnea, Kussmaul's respiration, decreased cardiac contractility, cardiac arrhythmias, hypotension, and pulmonary congestion.[67] Neurologic sequelae include depression, lethargy, stupor, or coma due to impaired volume regulation in the brain.[68] Metabolic acidosis induces insulin resistance and increases protein catabolism, which further contributes to the azotemia and muscle wasting.[69]

Dehydration, intractable vomiting, or sodium bicarbonate therapy will occasionally cause metabolic alkalosis. Mixed acid-base disturbances are common in animals with impaired ventilation (pulmonary edema or hemorrhage, pleural effusion, pneumonia) or hyperventilation (pain, pulmonary thromboembolism).

Uremic Intoxications

Acute filtration failure causes the rapid accumulation of a spectrum of low (< 500 D) and middle molecular weight (500 to 15,000 D) uremia toxins. Collectively, uremia toxins contribute to the multisystemic features of acute uremia in direct proportion to their accumulation in the body. Conversion of urea to ammonia, decreased mucus production, hypergastrinemia, and central effects of uremia toxins contribute collectively to the GI manifestations. The GI signs include anorexia, nausea, vomiting, fetid breath, stomatitis, oral ulcerations, lingual necrosis, xerostomia, reflux esophagitis, gastritis, GI ulcers, hematemesis, GI bleeding, diarrhea, enterocolitis, intussusception, and ileus.[70] As a subcomponent of the collective GI involvement, as many as 10% of dogs with severe ARF develop acute pancreatitis.[11,62]

Toxin-induced bleeding tendencies are promoted by impaired platelet-vessel wall and platelet-platelet interactions. Purpura, petechia, ecchymosis, bruising, bleeding from gum margins and venipuncture sites, epistaxis, and GI blood loss are characteristic. GI bleeding contributes to anemia and on occasion causes acute blood loss. In addition, uremia toxins cause or contribute to hypothermia, uremic pneumonitis, carbohydrate intolerance, and impaired immunity.

Cardiovascular Complications

Volume overload, cardiomegaly, heart failure, cardiac arrhythmias, and hypertension are common cardiovascular complications. Less commonly pericarditis, pericardial effusion, and tamponade may occur.[71] Bradycardia, supraventricular and ventricular premature contractions, and paroxysmal ventricular tachycardia are expected arrhythmias with severe uremia. Approximately 80% of the dogs with severe acute uremia have systemic hypertension. The severity of the hypertension is variably volume dependent and could be exacerbated by fluid therapy. If unresolved it may cause retinal detachment, hyphema, retinal hemorrhage, encephalopathy, and cerebrovascular hemorrhage.[72,73]

Uremic animals are at risk for cardiac arrest due to severe hyperkalemia and the collective metabolic, acid-base, and electrolyte disturbances associated with acute uremia. Bradycardia and vomiting pose additional risks for cardiac arrest secondary to increased vagal tone associated with the gastroenteritis.

Pulmonary Complications

Respiratory disease is seen in approximately half of dogs with severe uremia, is frequently life threatening, and is often

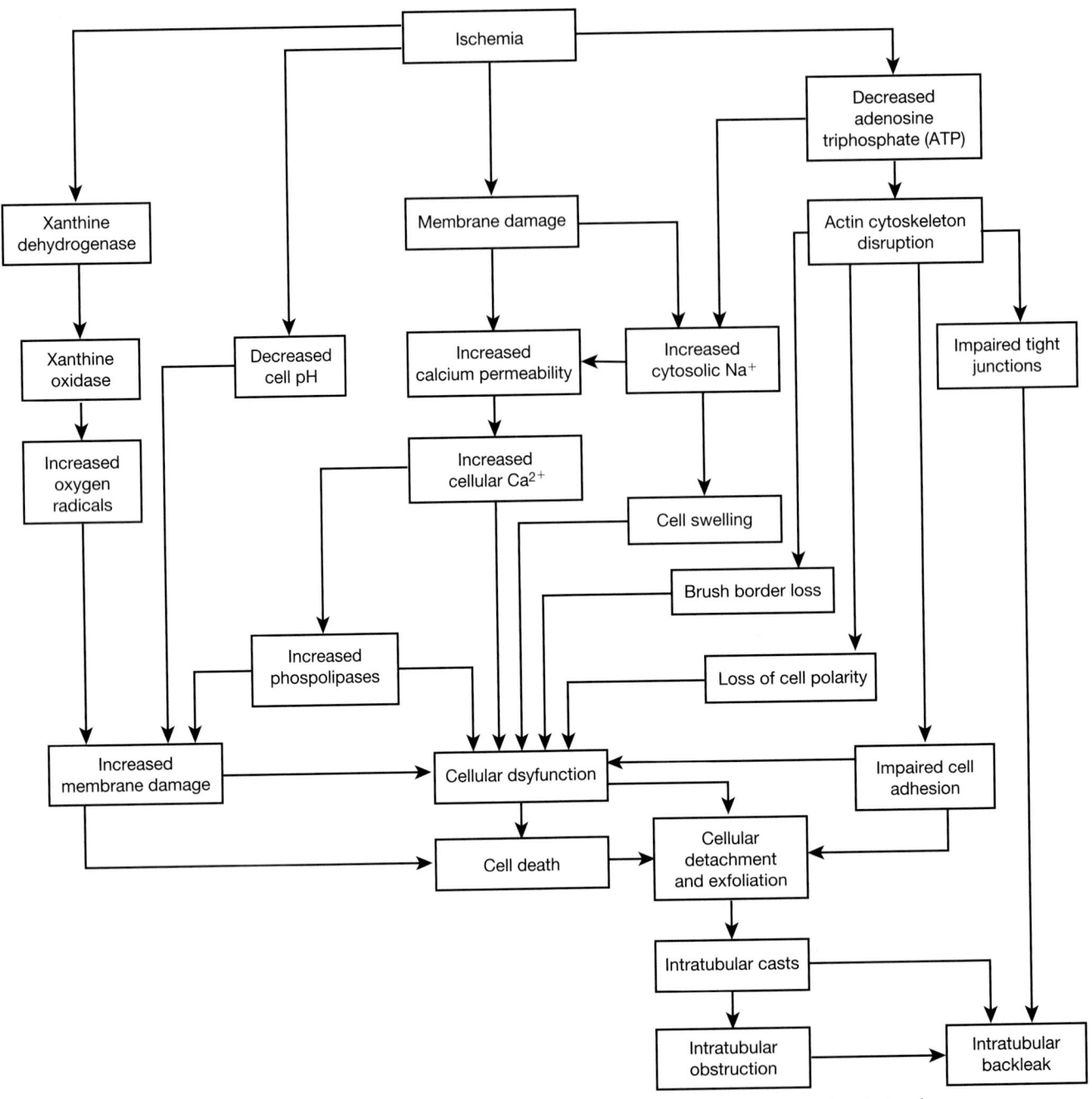

Figure 258-2 Cellular events in renal tubular epithelia in response to an ischemic insult. The diagram illustrates the multifactorial interactions that result ultimately in sublethal cellular dysfunction or cell death.

refractory to conventional therapy. In order of frequency, pulmonary edema, pleural effusion, pneumonia, pulmonary hemorrhage, uremic pneumonitis, and pulmonary artery thromboembolism have been documented. Interstitial or alveolar edema and pleural effusion develop from excessive fluid administration and volume overload. The signs of fluid overload must be distinguished from those of CHF before appropriate therapy can be instituted. Aspiration pneumonia is a common sequelae to protracted vomiting. Severe generalized patchy interstitial to alveolar pulmonary infiltrates and associated pulmonary dysfunction is recognized in some dogs with

leptospirosis.[74] Respiratory arrest may complicate all these respiratory disorders.[75]

Neuromuscular Disorders

The underlying cause for neuromuscular dysfunction is multifactorial but includes intrinsic central nervous system (CNS) pathology (cerebral hemorrhage) and secondary manifestations of the uremic state (electrolyte and acid-base imbalances, hypertension). Resulting clinical signs are diverse and include fatigue, dullness, lethargy, impaired mentation, altered behavior, confusion, stupor, tremors, seizures, coma, peripheral neuropathies, myoclonus, muscular cramps, and muscular weakness. Ethylene glycol toxicosis causes specific CNS dysfunction before the onset of or in concert with the development of overt renal failure. Rapid correction of the azotemia with hemodialysis can induce osmotic shifts of water in the brain, resulting in cerebral edema, seizure, cerebellar and brain stem herniation, coma, and death.

CNS side effects are associated with some medications (H_2 blockers, metoclopramide) when administered at conventional doses to animals with reduced capacity to eliminate such drugs. Animals with acute renal swelling display pain on abdominal palpation due to distension of the renal capsule. Prostration, dullness, or aggressive behaviors are typical manifestations of renal pain, especially in cats.

DIAGNOSIS OF ACUTE UREMIA

The clinical signs of acute uremia vary with the underlying cause and severity of disease, previously administered therapy, and comorbid diseases predisposing or compounding renal injury. A rapid and accurate differentiation of the possible syndromes resulting in acute uremia must be made to direct the therapeutic approach. These possible syndromes are (1) prerenal azotemia, (2) prerenal azotemia complicating CRF, (3) acute (parenchymal) renal failure (ARF), (4) prerenal azotemia complicating ARF, (5) chronic end-stage renal failure, and (6) postrenal azotemia. Each of these disparate azotemic conditions may appear quite similar. Because no specific biologic markers are available to predict the existence, severity, or recovery of renal parenchymal injury, the diagnosis of acute uremia is established from a comprehensive data base (which includes history, physical examination, laboratory testing, diagnostic imaging, histopathology, and special testing).

History
Acute uremia is characterized by a sudden onset of illness of less than 1 week's duration; however, animals with acute uremia secondary to underlying urinary or systemic diseases may have a longer duration of documented illness. Historical signs include listlessness, depression, anorexia, vomiting, diarrhea, and weakness. Less commonly, seizures, syncope, ataxia, and dyspnea may be reported. Potential exposure to nephrotoxic chemicals or plants (lily,[21] grapes or raisins[22,23]), new environmental conditions, ill animals, or traumatic events should be ascertained in the history. Recent surgery, diagnostic testing, travel, newly prescribed medications, or blood loss are potential risk factors for renal injury. Oliguria or anuria are consistent features of acute uremia, but a history of normal or increased urine production does not exclude its consideration. Historical weight loss, polyuria, polydipsia, nocturia or isosthenuria, or laboratory evidence of pre-existing renal insufficiency suggests underlying chronic renal disease. Renal function in animals with asymptomatic chronic renal insufficiency may decompensate suddenly after subtle insults including, fever, concomitant disease, vomiting, diarrhea, CHF, and drug administration, and they may develop a uremic crisis that is seemingly acute.

Physical Examination
Physical examination is an essential component of the diagnostic approach and may define the location and cause of the uremic state. Due to the acute nature of this condition, most animals in ARF have good body and coat condition. They have variable degrees of hydration. Depression, hypothermia, oral ulceration, "uremic breath," bile-stained fur, scleral injection,

cutaneous bruising, discoloration or necrosis of the tongue, tachycardia or bradycardia, tachypnea, muscle fasciculations, and seizures are present in proportion to the severity and duration of the azotemia. Bilaterally enlarged, firm, slightly resilient, or painful kidneys noted on abdominal palpation is indicative of acute nephritis or nephrosis or bilateral ureteral obstruction. Enlarged and firm kidneys on palpation are more suggestive of renal neoplasia, amyloidosis, or polycystic kidney disease. Asymmetry in kidney size is being recognized more frequency in cats with acute uremia due to the increasing incidence of unilateral ureteral obstruction (Figure 258-3). The obstructed kidney is enlarged, and the contralaterally smaller kidney is frequently end-stage and nonfunctional. The size of the urinary bladder is variable on abdominal palpation, depending on the quantity of urine formation and the integrity of the outflow tract. An undetectable urinary bladder indicates profound oliguria or anuria or complete ureteral obstruction. An enlarged, firm, and painful bladder predicts outflow obstruction of the bladder.

In the absence of hemorrhage or hemolysis, mucous membranes are usually pink in dogs and cats with ARF. This is in contrast to the pale mucous membranes observed in animals with CRF. Most animals with ARF have evidence of dehydration when first evaluated, which may underscore prerenal causes or contributions. Prolonged capillary refill time, dry mucous membranes, decreased skin turgor, sunken eyes, tachycardia, poor pulse quality, and hypotension are consistent with the presence of dehydration and hypovolemia. Animals that have been given parenteral fluids may demonstrate signs of overhydration (wet mucous membranes, serous nasal discharge, increased skin turgor, peripheral edema, tachypnea, dyspnea, muffled heart sounds, hypertension, and ascites).

ARF is frequently layered secondarily on other diseases or even CRF. Manifestations of these other conditions may dominate findings of the physical examination and mask its characteristic features. Lameness, icterus, fever, discolored urine, back or flank pain, petechia, and dysuria are associated with some disorders. Uremic animals typically are hypothermic in proportion to the severity of the azotemia. The presence of a normal or slightly elevated body temperature is inappropriate for uremic animals and is consistent with fever associated with an underlying infectious or inflammatory state.

Laboratory Assessment
The initial diagnostic assessment should include a complete blood count (CBC), comprehensive biochemical profile (serum creatinine, urea, phosphate, calcium, bicarbonate, sodium, potassium, chloride, glucose, albumin, globulin, hepatic transaminases, and bilirubin) (Figure 258-4), urinalysis with sediment examination, and urine culture.

CBC results may reflect primary or comorbid conditions of diagnostic relevance. Normal or increased red blood cell (RBC) count, hematocrit, and hemoglobin concentrations are consistent with prerenal azotemia or acute uremia, whereas a nonregenerative anemia suggests CRF. The hemogram may be significantly influenced by the hydration status of the animal and may overestimate the actual RBC mass with dehydration and underestimate red cell mass with over hydration.

Progressive azotemia is part of the definition for acute uremia (Figure 258-4). In humans, the diagnosis is predicated on subtle daily increases in serum creatinine, but this feature is observed rarely in animals. Animals are usually evaluated when the azotemia is well established, and clinical signs are clearly apparent. Both serum creatinine and urea nitrogen will increase in direct proportion to the severity of the renal impairment or completeness of the outflow obstruction. The degree of functional impairment can be broadly categorized

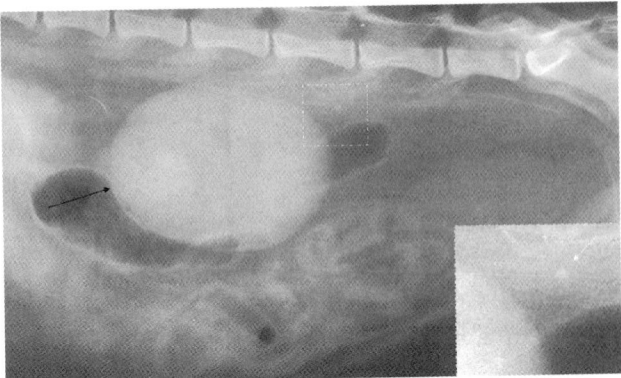

Figure 258-3 Lateral radiographic image of a cat abdomen illustrating extreme asymmetry in renal size characteristic of the "big kidney-little kidney" syndrome associated with ureteral obstruction. The right end-stage kidney *(black arrow)* is superimposed on the enlarged left kidney. The dashed box and insert highlight a radiodense calcium oxalate urolith in the left ureter *(white arrow).*

based on steady-state serum creatinine concentration given the inverse relationship between serum creatinine and renal function (GFR).[76] From this projection, the renal dysfunction can be staged as mild in animals with a serum creatinine concentration less than 2.5 mg/dL (>40% of normal function), moderate for those with a serum creatinine concentration between 2.5 mg/dL and 5.0 mg/dL (between 40% and 20% of normal function), severe for those with a serum creatinine concentration between 5 mg/dL and 10 mg/dL (between 20% and 10% of normal function), and extreme if the serum creatinine concentration is greater than 10 mg/dL (<10% of normal function). Reductions in lean body mass and overhydration can lower the serum creatinine concentration and cause overestimation of true renal function.

Serum urea nitrogen (SUN) concentration also increases inversely with reductions in GFR and contributes to the developing azotemia. Unlike creatinine, urea is influenced by numerous extra renal parameters that make its concentration less specific as a marker of renal function. Urea appearance is closely linked with exogenous and endogenous nitrogen metabolism, hydration status, urine production, and diuretic therapy that make it a useful predictor of the clinical severity of the uremic state. Urea is also used as a surrogate for the production and removal of low molecular weight uremia toxins during dialysis.[77]

For comparable azotemia, animals with acute uremia usually have more profound alterations of serum mineral, electrolytes, and bicarbonate concentrations reflected on the biochemistry profile than animals with CRF (see Figure 258-4). In acute uremia, serum phosphate concentration generally exceeds that of creatinine and may be associated with mild to moderate hypocalcemia. Serum calcium concentration may be less than 5.0 mg/dL in animals with acute antifreeze intoxication. In contrast, serum calcium is usually normal or moderately elevated in proportion to serum creatinine and phosphate in animals with CRF.[78,79] Serum potassium concentration varies with the severity and cause of the uremia, extent of vomiting, and fluid and diuretic administration (see Figure 258-4). Serum potassium typically is increased (between 5.5 mEq/L and 9.0 mEq/L) in proportion to the degree of azotemia. It tends to be higher in animals with anuric ARF or urinary outflow obstruction. Serum bicarbonate concentration decreases with the severity of the renal failure such that bicarbonate deficits of 5, 10, and 15 mmol/L are associated with mild, moderate, and severe degrees of acute uremia, respectively.[80] Profuse vomiting or previous bicarbonate administration may cause metabolic alkalosis that is not consistent for the degree of azotemia.

Distinguishing animals with prerenal azotemia from those with intrinsic ARF can often be made from results of history, clinical findings, and USG. The presence of mild or moderate azotemia, clinical dehydration, hypovolemia or hypotension, and oliguria in conjunction with a concentrated USG or urine osmolality confirms the diagnosis of prerenal azotemia. Therapeutic confirmation of the diagnosis can be made by a rapid resolution of the azotemia and oliguria with restoration of fluid balance and normalization of systemic hemodynamics. Numerous laboratory parameters including BUN/creatinine ratio, urine/plasma sodium (U/P_{Na}), and fractional sodium excretion (FE_{Na}) have also been used to distinguish oliguric animals with a prerenal condition from those with ARF. The discrimination is achieved by the increased reabsorption of urea and sodium in prerenal states compared with ARF. The utility of these tests becomes problematic in animals with coexisting diseases that impair concentration of the urine or after diuretic administration that increases urinary sodium excretion. Additionally, BUN/creatinine ratio has been shown to provide no localizing value in dogs with renal disease but may be more predictive of heightened catabolism or

Figure 258-4 Incidence of serum biochemical changes in 138 dogs with severe ARF at the time of referral. The proportions of dogs with abnormally high (above zero line) and abnormally low (below zero line) values are shown for the following parameters: creatinine (Crea), BUN, sodium (Na^+), potassium (K^+), chloride (Cl^-), total CO_2 (TCO_2), anion gap (AG), calcium (Ca), phosphorus (Phos), total protein (TP), albumin (Alb), globulins (Glob), and glucose (Glu).

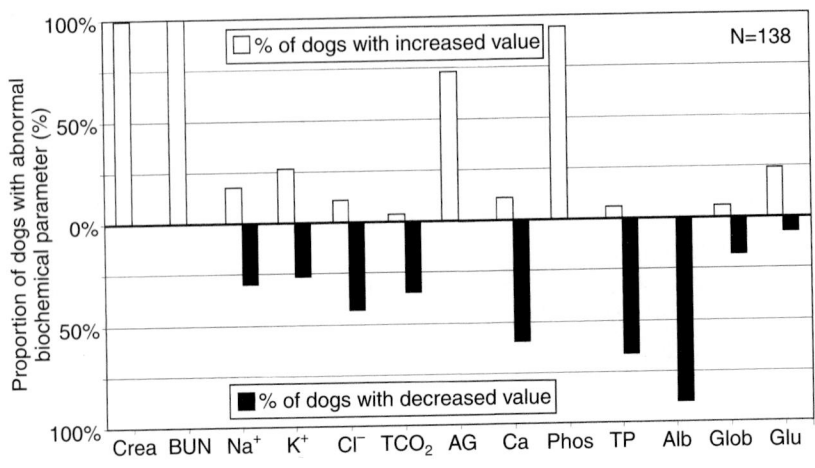

intestinal bleeding.[8,81] More recently, the fractional excretion of urea (FE$_{urea}$) has been shown to be highly sensitive for identification of humans with prerenal azotemia from those with prerenal azotemia and concurrent diuretic administration or others with intrinsic ARF (similar testing may be useful in animals).[82]

The tubular epithelial enzymes, gamma-glutamyl transpeptidase (GGT) and N-acetyl-beta-D-glucosaminidase (NAG), can be measured in urine to predict cellular leakage as an early marker of tubular injury or necrosis.[83-87] Urinary enzymes have shown good sensitivity for early recognition of renal injury, but they have not been adopted widely in veterinary or human diagnostics. Carbamylated hemoglobin is a nonenzymatic and nonreversible reaction product of the urea metabolite, cyanate, with hemoglobin. The concentration of carbamylated hemoglobin reflects time exposure of blood to the azotemia and has been shown to differentiate dogs with acute azotemia from those with CRF.[88,89] Testing for carbamylated hemoglobin is becoming more readily available in human hospitals and is likely to find increased utility in uremic animals.

A complete urinalysis should be performed on every dog or cat with obtainable urine at initial examination prior to instituting therapy. Both renal concentrating and diluting capabilities become impaired in the early phases of intrinsic ARF resulting in a USG that is fixed in the range between 1.008 and 1.018. A USG greater than 1.030 for dogs or greater than 1.035 for cats in the presence of azotemia indicates prerenal filtration failure.[90] A USG between 1.012 and 1.029 (dogs) or 1.012 and 1.034 (cats) associated with azotemia is consistent with a prerenal component superimposed on intrinsic renal insufficiency (*prerenal-on-acute* or *prerenal-on-chronic* disease) or an underlying urine-concentrating defect. Glucosuria in the absence of hyperglycemia is present in 50% of dogs with severe ARF and is an important sign of proximal tubular dysfunction.[62] It predicts tubular necrosis and is a useful discriminator between intrinsic ARF and other types of acute or chronic uremia.[11] Qualitative (dipstick) proteinuria is detected in most uremic animals but has little discriminatory importance.[11] Overt proteinuria associated with a urine protein/creatinine ratio greater than six should alert the possibility of primary glomerular injury.

The urine sediment examination may demonstrate RBCs, white blood cells (WBCs), casts, crystals, yeast, fungi, or bacteria that aid the differential diagnosis and cause of the uremia and should be performed routinely on freshly obtained urine. The presence of granular and hyaline casts document active renal pathology with tubular epithelial shedding or necrosis and glomerular protein leakage. Casts are detected in approximately 30% to 40% of dogs with ARF, but their absence does not exclude a diagnosis of acute parenchymal injury.[11] Calcium oxalate crystalluria is indicative of hyperoxaluria associated with ethylene glycol intoxication and oxalate nephrosis (cats).[19,90-93]

Imaging of the urinary tract with survey radiography and ultrasonography is indicated in the evaluation of all animals with acute uremia. Ultrasonography is complementary to diagnostic radiography and is the preferred imaging modality for urinary disease. Ultrasonography is rapid, noninvasive, and provides greater delineation of renal geometry, intrarenal architecture, parenchymal consistency, and outflow integrity. It provides a more definitive assessment of renal and abdominal pathology, including nephritis and nephrosis, pyelonephritis, urolithiasis, hydronephrosis, outflow obstruction, pancreatitis, abdominal neoplasia, prostatitis, and ascites. Ultrasonic imaging facilitates collection of diagnostic specimens for biochemical analysis, cytology, culture, and histology by incorporation of guided percutaneous needle aspiration or biopsy techniques.[94] Duplex Doppler sonography can be used

to verify segmental blood flow in the kidney and to predict changes in vascular impedance associated with induction and resolution of some forms of renal injury and outflow obstruction.[95,96] The sonographic appearance of the kidneys can provide immediate verification for conditions like antifreeze poisoning, ureteral obstruction, and end-stage renal disease. Ethylene glycol intoxication, for example, is characterized by marked to intense increases in cortical echogenicity with variable degrees of hypoechoic intensity at the cortical medullary junction (halo sign)(Figure 258-5). However, the increased availability and utility of ultrasonography has curtailed the routine use of survey radiography to image the urinary tract. For the diagnosis of ureteral obstruction in cats, survey radiographs may be more sensitive and predictive than ultrasonography, if careful scrutiny is directed to barely perceptible radiodensities in the retroperitoneal space, and they are justified in all cats with acute uremia (see Figure 258-3).

Excretory urography, renal scintigraphy, computed tomography (CT), and magnetic resonance imaging (MRI) may have specific indications in selected animals, but these imaging modalities are not routinely available. Antegrade pyelography incorporating ultrasound-guided pyelocentesis has become increasingly useful to confirm the presence, degree, and location of ureteral obstruction in cats (Figure 258-6). In 20% to 30% of cats with ureteral obstruction, no discrete calcific material is identified with either sonographic or survey radiographic techniques. For these circumstances, and for cases with multiple sites of obstruction or stenosis, antegrade pyelography remains the best aid for identification and localization for surgical intervention.

The cause and course of the acute uremia can be determined for most animals from assessment of the history, physical findings, and contemporary diagnostic testing. Where these features cannot be predicted with certainty, renal histopathology can provide a specific morphologic and potentially causative basis for the disease, its potential reversibility, and chronicity. Details of the techniques, indications, and contraindications for renal biopsy have been described recently.[97,98] Percutaneous or laparoscopic needle techniques can be performed in both dogs and cats with minimal sedation, anesthesia, or invasiveness and obviate the need for surgically obtained renal specimens. Routine biopsy of animals with acute uremia is probably unjustified when balanced against the potential for complications and lack of scientifically documented assessment of risk versus benefit. Renal biopsy should be considered if the definitive cause, extent, and chronicity of the renal injury cannot be established with noninvasive diagnostic methods or if therapeutic decisions would be predicated on this information. Discretion should be used in extrapolating acute morphologic findings from the biopsy to the potential long-term reversibility of the functional deficiencies. The advent of hemodialysis has changed the clinical understanding of reversible and irreversible renal failure. Identification of severe pathology at acute stages of disease may not correspond to an unfavorable outcome if the potential (time) for renal repair is provided with finite periods of renal replacement.

Serologic testing for leptospirosis should be performed on all dogs with acute uremia without a confirmed cause. The evaluation should be expanded to include titers to *L. pomona*, *L. bratislava*, *L. grippotyphosa*, *L. autumnalis*, and *L. hardjo* in addition to *L. canicola* and *L. icterohaemorrhagiae*, because the distribution of infecting serovars differ geographically.* Strict criteria for serologic conformation of an active leptospiral infection have not been established, and the recent introduction

*Referencefs 32, 33, 37, 38, 99, 100.

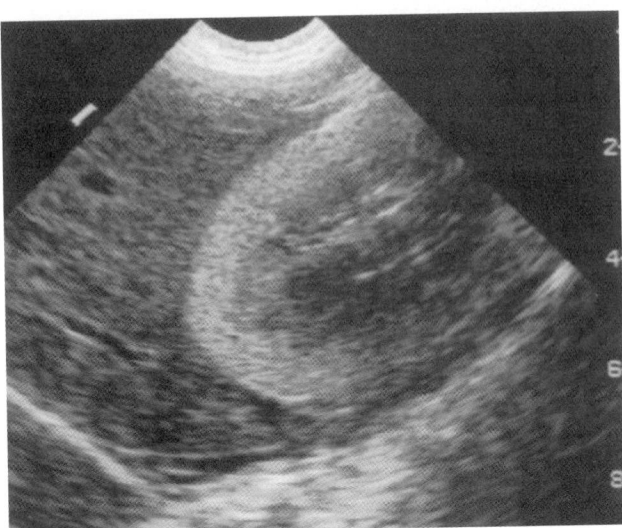

Figure 258-5 Ultrasonographic image of the kidney from a dog acutely poisoned with antifreeze. The renal cortex is markedly hyperechoic, compared with the ultrasonic density of the adjacent spleen. This sonographic feature is a consistent finding with ethylene glycol intoxication.

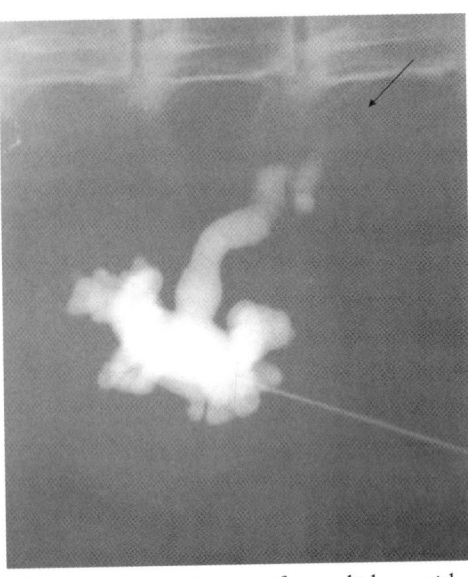

Figure 258-6 Nephropyelogram of a cat kidney with a proximal ureteral obstruction. The figure highlights the ultrasound-placed needle in the renal pelvis and the extensive pelvic and ureteral dilation outlined by the injected contrast. The proximal ureter is dilated, torturous, and ends abruptly *(arrow)*, despite the increased pressure associated with contrast injection. These findings are consistent with a radiolucent structure producing complete ureteral obstruction.

of multivalent vaccines makes interpretation more difficult. A microscopic agglutination titer greater than 1:100 indicates positive serology, and a fourfold or greater rise in titer between paired sera separated by 7 to 14 days predicts active infection.[101,102] Ambiguity in the diagnosis arises when only a single titer is available for analysis. Previous retrospective studies arbitrarily established single titers of greater than 1:800 and greater than 1:3200 to nonvaccinal serovars as criteria for a positive diagnosis of leptospirosis in dogs.[33,34,36] However, laboratory variation, differences in humoral responses to individual serogroups, vaccination, and background (asymptomatic) exposure make strict serologic criteria difficult to assign. Vaccination can produce titers greater than 1:1250 to serogroups, *icterohaemorrhagiae* and *canicola*, in dogs; however, vaccination should not produce titers to nonvaccinal serovars that exceed those of vaccinal agents.[103] A recent survey of nonselected dogs identified a surprisingly high percentage of nonvaccinated dogs with positive serology to leptospirosis serogroups indicating background population exposure.[39] Shedding of leptospiral DNA has also been recognized using a sensitive polymerase chain reaction (PCR) assay in both asymptomatic and symptomatic seronegative dogs.[104] These observations suggest some dogs have delayed seroconversion or fail to seroconvert despite being actively infected. This sensitive diagnostic technique will improve clinicians' ability to diagnose active infections and understanding of renal carriage, shedding, and risks of leptospirosis in the presence and absence of vaccination. Given the limitations of current diagnostic methods, clinical guidelines for a diagnosis of active infection include a single elevated titer (≥ 1:800) to a vaccinal serogroup accompanied by clinical signs consistent with leptospirosis; a single microscopic agglutination titer 1:800 for nonvaccinal serogroups; evidence of seroconversion in paired acute and convalescent sera; and presence of typical clinical signs of leptospirosis followed by a response to appropriate antimicrobial therapy.[32]

A diagnosis of ethylene glycol intoxication can be made presumptively by the presence of an increased serum osmolality, osmolal gap, profound metabolic acidosis, increased anion gap, hypocalcemia, the presence of calcium oxalate crystalluria, and sonographic appearance of the kidneys (see

Figure 258-5).[19,91,93] Confirmation of the diagnosis, documentation of the degree of intoxication, and response to therapy is best performed by chemical analysis of gastric fluid, serum, or urine for the presence of ethylene glycol or its toxic metabolites by commercial laboratories. Blood ethylene glycol and glycolic acid concentrations may persist for days at toxic concentrations despite therapy with alcohol or 4-methylpyrazole in affected animals with severe oliguria or anuria.[104,105]

MEDICAL MANAGEMENT OF ACUTE UREMIA

Medical management of acute uremia in animals remains founded on observations from animal models of ARF and recommendations extrapolated from human therapeutics.[4,106-108] Recommendations are prioritized to prevention of renal injury in predisposed or high-risk animals, to elimination of underlying or ongoing renal insults, and to amelioration of identified biochemical, metabolic and clinical consequences of established uremia. The mechanisms underlying the impaired glomerular hemodynamics, epithelial and vascular disruption, and intratubular obstruction that mediate acute renal injury have been characterized in great detail in recent years (see Pathogenesis of Acute Renal Failure). Cellular energetics, vascular congestion, cytosolic calcium, oxidant stress, necrosis, apoptosis, nitric oxide, epithelial cytoskeleton, and growth promoters are but a few mediators recently recognized to participate in the pathogenesis of ARF. Novel therapies have emerged from each of these areas of discovery to counteract specific pathophysiologic events scientifically crafted in the experimental models. Despite the therapeutic promise of each of these areas of investigation to prevent or ameliorate development of ARF or to accelerate renal repair, none have become established in clinical therapeutics. This is to be expected in animals with naturally acquired disease that possess multifactorial risks and predispositions to acute uremia of diverse cause, severity, duration, and expression.

Thus conventional approaches to management of acute uremia remain supportive for the predicted and documented clinical consequences that develop.

Prevention of Acute Renal Injury

The highest priority for the management of acute uremia is to recognize those dogs or cats highly predisposed to a uremic crisis and to intervene to prevent its development. Pre-existing renal disease, advanced age, dehydration, hypovolemia, hypotension, sepsis, fever, prolonged anesthesia and surgery, trauma, systemic disease, use of vasoactive or nephrotoxic drugs, high environmental temperatures, and nephrolithiasis are predispositions that pose an increased risk.[109] Risk factors are cumulative and predispose additive potential for renal injury. When predispositions coexist with ongoing or projected therapies having a potential for renal injury, the following procedures should be reviewed. Exposure to ischemia and toxic insults should be eliminated, and the dose of nephrotoxic drugs should be modified. Hemodynamic adequacy must be established, and life-threatening fluid, electrolyte, and acid-base imbalances corrected. Decontamination procedures (induced vomiting, gastric lavage, administration of activated charcoal, and cathartics) and treatment with specific antidotes should be instituted after acute exposure to known nephrotoxins. Table 258-1 illustrates these points in the therapeutic approach to acute antifreeze poisoning. The correction of existing fluid deficits and attention to ongoing fluid balance offers the best insurance to moderate ATI. Mild to moderate ECF volume expansion with isonatric fluids is beneficial before the administration of known nephrotoxic drugs (aminoglycosides, cisplatin, amphotericin B), anesthesia, or surgical intervention. Mannitol administered (see details, following) prior to exposure to hemodynamic or nephrotoxic insults will promote urine formation and a natriuresis but has shown only limited efficacy to protect against the development of ATI. The preventative use of other therapies has consistently failed to provide any advantage over judicious fluid management.[4,110-113]

Conventional Management of Established Uremia

Strategy for the management of existing ARF includes elimination of known causes of renal injury (see Prevention of Acute Renal Injury) and supportive therapies directed to the life-threatening consequences of acute uremia. Systemic infections such as leptospirosis should be treated aggressively with appropriate antimicrobial therapy, and hemodynamic deficiencies must be resolved rapidly to establish euvolemia and normotension. Animals with mild renal damage may regain adequate function within 3 to 5 days of initiating treatment. This may forestall progression to life-threatening uremia. Animals with moderate or severe renal damage may require weeks to achieve repair of the injury; yet most die from uremia within 5 to 7 days. The disparity between this window for effective medical therapy and the re-establishment of renal function underlays, in part, the high mortality and unfavorable outcome associated with ARF.

Systemic Hemodynamics and Body Fluids

Alterations in body fluid composition are classic causes and consequences of acute uremia. Fluid therapy remains the foundation of medical management. The fluid plan must restore deficiencies in fluid volume, correct abnormalities in fluid composition, and promote urine formation. Replacement fluids should mimic as closely as possible the composition of fluid deficits. Priority is given to restoration of intravascular and interstitial volume, normalization of arterial blood pressure and renal perfusion, and compensation for ongoing fluid losses. At *initial* examination most animals with ARF are dehydrated and hypovolemic due to active fluid losses (vomiting, diarrhea,

Table • 258-1

Therapeutic Approach to Acute Antifreeze Poisoning

THERAPEUTIC PLAN	THERAPEUTIC OPTIONS
Prevent ongoing exposure (< 2 hours)	1. Induce vomiting 2. Perform gastric lavage 3. Administer activated charcoal
Correct ECF fluid deficits Correct dehydration	1. Correct ECF volume deficits (saline, lactated Ringer's) 2. Correct metabolic acidosis (if present) 3. Correct hypocalcemia if present) 4. Initiate maintenance fluids/ongoing losses
Document urine production/promote diuresis	1. Establish urinary catheter, monitor urine output 2. Administer mannitol, furosemide, or both after rehydration
Administer antidote Eliminate toxin/metabolites	1. Ethanol (20%): 5.5 mL/kg IV q4h-5 Rx, then (dogs/cats) 5.5 mL/kg IV q6h-4 Rx or 2. Ethanol (30%): 1.3 mL/kg IV bolus, then (dogs/cats) 0.42 mL/kg/hr IV for 48 hours 3. 4-methyl pyrazole: 20 mg/kg IV, then (dogs) 15 mg/kg IV @ 12 & 24 hours, then 5 mg/kg IV @ 36 hours 4. Hemodialysis at earliest opportunity (dogs/cats)
Manage ARF/oliguria	1. Conventional medical therapy 2. Hemodialysis

and possibly hemorrhage). The fluid deficit should be corrected with 0.9% sodium chloride or balanced crystalloid solutions (lactated Ringer's) administered intravenously to replete vascular volume. The initial replacement volume (milliliter) to correct the extracellular deficit is calculated from clinical estimates of dehydration according to the formula:

$$\text{Volume Replacement (mL)} = [\text{body weight (kg)}] \times [\text{estimated deficit (\%)}] \times 1000$$

The estimated deficit is a value between 5% and 15% determined from history, physical examination, and laboratory information or computed from known deviations from historical body weight. The rate at which the deficits are corrected is predicated on the hemodynamic stability of the animal and its tolerance for fluid administration. Mild or moderate fluid deficits (5% to 8%) in hemodynamically stable animals can be replaced within 6 to 8 hours. Moderate or severe fluid deficits (>8%) associated with evidence of hypovolemia must be corrected more aggressively. The hypovolemic component of the deficit should be administered as bolus infusions within

30 minutes to restore intravascular volume and prevent prolonged hypoperfusion of kidneys. The remainder of the deficit can then be delivered over 6 to 8 hours to correct the dehydration.

Aggressive fluid replacement must be tempered in animals with cardiovascular disease to prevent circulatory congestion and heart failure. Serial monitoring of central venous pressure (CVP) can facilitate safe and efficient fluid administration. An increase in CVP of 5 to 7 cm H_2O above baseline or an absolute CVP greater than 10 cm H_2O indicates an excessive rate or volume of fluid administration. Five percent dextrose in water or maintenance formulations (including half-strength saline and dextrose solutions) are not appropriate choices to replete the initial deficits and should be reserved to compensate insensible or maintenance losses later in the course of treatment.

Fluid deficits associated with profound hypovolemia and hypotension or severe blood loss must be replaced more rapidly with crystalloid solution (up to or greater than 90 mL/kg/hr) or with fluids targeted for blood volume expansion. Synthetic colloid solutions (Dextran-70 or Hetastarch) administered at 20 mL/kg will expand blood volume immediately by 17% to 24% and by approximately 35% within 60 minutes of administration.[114] Synthetic colloid solutions provide no replacement of extravascular volume necessitating concurrent administration of crystalloid solutions to replete the interstitial compartment. These solutions may be rational choices for support of vascular volume in clinical settings where oxygen-carrying capacity is less critical than volume restoration. Hypovolemia secondary to blood loss or hemorrhage may require administration of compatible whole blood, blood components, or synthetic hemoglobin products (Oxyglobin®, BioPure, Cambridge, Massachusetts).[115,116]

The production of urine at greater than 1.0 mL/kg/hr with fluid volume replacement suggests a significant prerenal contribution to the oliguria and azotemia. Failure to induce a significant diuresis after volume replacement indicates either that parenchymal damage is severe or that initial fluid deficits were underestimated. Additional fluid may be administered taking care to promote only mild volume expansion without overhydration.

After correction of the initial fluid deficits, subsequently administered fluid must reflect maintenance requirements and ongoing losses. Maintenance fluid should be limited to 5% dextrose in water to replace insensible free water losses (20 to 25 mL/kg/day) and balanced electrolyte solutions to replace measured or estimated urine, GI, and other sensible losses. Commercial maintenance formulations can be supplied if insensible and urinary losses are approximately equal. Animals that are provided only isonatric solutions (saline, lactated Ringer's) become depleted of free water and develop hypernatremia within 3 to 4 days. The severity of the hypernatremia may be amplified in animals with appreciable free water loses in the urine during the diuretic phase of ARF, post obstructive diuresis, or subsequent to treatment with osmotic diuretics like mannitol. In oliguric animals, the urinary replacement should be negligible and not prescribed at the same rate as in animals with normal urine production. Urinary losses should be measured or accurately estimated in nonoliguric animals to prevent underestimation of the urinary replacement. Nonoliguric animals in the diuretic phase of ARF or after relief of postrenal obstruction may produce greater than 10 mL/kg/hr of urine that will not be matched by estimates of normal urine production.

Supplementation of potassium in replacement or maintenance fluids must be prescribed on an individual case basis. Fluids containing supplemental potassium are generally contraindicated in oliguric animals or during rapid fluid replacement. If the supplemental load of potassium has no effective elimination route, it will quickly promote hyperkalemia. Animals in the diuretic phase of ARF may excrete excessive amounts of potassium and require supplementation to prevent potassium wasting; but potassium supplementation should always be provided cautiously and only with monitoring of daily serum potassium concentrations.

Fluids must be administered conscientiously to oliguric or anuric animals. Hypervolemia is a common complication of overzealous fluid administration or improper monitoring of fluid balance. Sixty to 70% of animals with moderate to severe acute uremia are overhydrated when referred to the authors' emergency service, or they become hypervolemic during the initial hospitalization period. Failure to induce an effective diuresis (>1 mL/kg/hr) once the fluid deficits are replete predicts further fluid loading will be unproductive and predispose the animal to overhydration. Weight gain, tachypnea, harsh breath sounds, increased skin turgor, chemosis, serous nasal discharge, peripheral or pulmonary edema, circulatory congestion, ascites, and systemic hypertension are consistent indicators of overhydration and hypervolemia. The presence of dry oral mucous membranes in uremic animals does not reflect hydration status due to decreased salivary secretion (xerostomia). This finding may cause underestimation of true hydration and inappropriate fluid administration.

An excessive fluid load may be difficult or impossible to correct in animals with marginal urine formation. At the first evidence of overhydration, all fluid delivery should be curtailed appropriately or discontinued, and attempts should be made to induce a diuresis (see following). If the fluid burden cannot be managed successfully with diuretic administration, no medical options are available to resolve the overhydration and therapy must be directed to consequences of circulatory overload (systemic hypertension, peripheral and pulmonary edema, pleural effusion, CHF, and ascites). For life-threatening overhydration, fluid removal with hemodialysis or peritoneal dialysis is the only available therapeutic option (see Renal Replacement Therapy, following).

Cross-linked polyelectrolyte sorbents offer a promising and clinically applicable oral solution for overhydration in uremic animals. These materials can adsorb up to 50 times their intrinsic weight in GI water, providing an effective alternative for fluid elimination. At typical doses, orally administered sorbets could eliminate up to 1 L of daily fluid accumulation in a 30 kg dog. Additionally, these polymers can adsorb solutes dissolved in intestinal water, providing an alternative clearance for urea, creatinine, and potassium. Prototype materials have been used successfully in a uremic dog and are being developed for human administration.[117]

Inadequate Urine Production

The conversion from oligoanuric to nonoliguric renal failure has been a long-standing goal in the management of acute uremia. The routine use of diuretics and vasodilators has been advocated when fluid therapy alone is ineffective to promote diuresis.[4,110,111,118] Management benefits of an induced diuresis include (1) disclosure of less severe renal injury, (2) better regulation of fluid and electrolyte balance, (3) opportunity to provide parenteral nutrition, (4) increased toxin clearance, and (5) optimism for attending clinicians. Despite conventional endorsement of diuretic therapy in the management of ARF, this practice is losing credibility due to a lack of documented efficacy of pharmacologic agents to alter the course, morphology, or outcome of ARF. Empiric use of these drugs impose recognized risks.[4,107,110-112,118-121] A recent cohort evaluation of diuretic administration in human patients with ARF documented an increased risk of death and failure to recover renal function with diuretic use compared with its nonuse.[112,122] If delayed beyond a few hours from the initiation phase of the insult, the efficacy of diuretics becomes negligible. Their use should never supplant judicious fluid and hemodynamic support.[4,110,111,118,123]

Hypertonic mannitol (an osmotic diuretic) is used commonly for the prevention and management of oliguric forms of ARF. Therapeutic effects include decreased vascular resistance and cellular swelling; increased renal blood flow (RBF), GFR, and solute excretion; protection from vascular congestion and erythrocyte aggregation; increased osmotic tubular fluid flow with dispersion of tubular debris, casts and obstructions; and scavenging of toxic free radicals.[4,110,124-126] Its use to promote urine formation in the early stages of acute oliguric renal failure has been recommended in animals but lacks evidence-based justification.[9,106,127] Mannitol (20% to 25% solution) is administered to fluid replete animals as a slow intravenous bolus at 0.25 to 1.0 g/kg. If an effective diuresis results within 30 to 60 minutes, a CRI at 1.0 to 2.0 mg/kg/min or intermittent boluses of 0.25 to 0.5 g/kg intravenously, every 4 to 6 hours, can be given to continue the diuresis for 24 to 48 hours. If an adequate diuresis is not established by 60 minutes, an additional 0.25 to 0.5 g/kg intravenous bolus can be repeated cautiously, but further administration is contraindicated due to the risks of volume expansion, hemodilution, hypervolemia, and mannitol toxicity.[9,106,127-129] Mannitol should not be given to animals with severe fluid overload, pulmonary edema, or CHF. The more established the onset of uremia, the lower the expectation mannitol will promote a diuresis or influence the course of the disease.

Furosemide is less effective than mannitol at improving renal function in experimental renal injury, but these observations have not been verified in clinical trials or in dogs and cats with naturally occurring forms of disease. Furosemide inhibits active sodium and chloride reabsorption in the distal nephron causing diuresis, natriuresis, and kaliuresis. It increases tubular fluid flow and osmolar clearance, similar to the effects of mannitol. Additionally, it causes vasodilation, increased RBF, and decreased tubular oxygen consumption in hypoxia-sensitive tubular segments.[4,110,126]

Overhydration, hyperkalemia, and toxin elimination are the established indications for the use of furosemide in animals or humans with ARF.* Furosemide is given initially at 2 to 6 mg/kg intravenously after existing fluid deficits have been corrected. If an adequate diuresis of greater than 1 mL/kg/hr is not achieved within 30 minutes, the initial dose can be repeated. If a diuresis is achieved, the dose can be repeated every 6 to 8 hours or given as a CRI at 0.25 to 1.0 mg/kg/hr to extend the diuresis for 24 to 48 hours. Diuretics should always be administered cautiously. The animal's fluid and electrolyte balance must be monitored to prevent depletion of ECF volume that might precipitate additional prerenal insults on the existing renal injury. Like mannitol, the diuresis induced by furosemide may not improve renal morphology or change the outcome or clinical course of animals with ARF. Predictable adverse effects are development of ECF volume contraction, sodium wasting, deafness, and delay to referral.

Dopamine is a catecholamine with diuretic properties caused by PGE_2-mediated renal vasodilation, increased RBF, increased GFR, decreased tubular sodium and water reabsorption, and decreased tubular oxygen consumption. The pharmacologic effects of dopamine are dose dependent and differentially mediated through dopaminergic and adrenergic receptors. In dogs, "renal" doses of dopamine between 0.5 to 3 µg/kg/min promote these responses primarily by activating dopamine-specific D_1-like and D_2-like receptors in the kidney and postganglionic sympathetic nerves. Doses between 5 and 7 µg/kg/min activate β_1-receptors to increase cardiac output; whereas higher doses stimulate alpha receptors causing

undesired vasoconstriction, tachycardia, cardiac arrhythmias and potential for myocardial, intestinal and renal ischemia.[4,110,111,118,130] At doses between 0.5 to 3 µg/kg/min, dopamine may increase urine formation and facilitate conversion from an oliguric to a nonoliguric state. Higher doses promote renal vasoconstriction, tachycardia, cardiac arrhythmias, and are contraindicated in ARF. Problems arise with overlap in dose effects, variable dopamine elimination, and individual animal sensitivity and binding affinities. These variables predispose critical animals to untoward and unpredictable effects to standard dosing.

Studies in anesthetized cats document a different spectrum of dopaminergic effects that suggest a lack of dopamine-specific receptor activity in the kidneys of this species.[130-132] Low-dose dopamine infusion (1 to 3 µg/kg/min) causes no significant changes in mean arterial blood pressure, heart rate, urine output, or sodium excretion.[131,132] Only at doses greater than 10 µg/kg/min did dopamine infusion results in dose-dependent increases in urine output and sodium excretion; however, the diuretic response was coupled with variable decreases in GFR, renal vasoconstriction, and inconsistent changes in mean arterial blood pressure and renal blood flow most consistent with α-adrenoreceptors effects.[131] These differences in the actions of dopamine predict it is conceptually inappropriate for use in cats with oligoanuric ARF. Recently, D_1 receptors with a high affinity to fenolodopam were identified in the kidney cortex of cats, suggesting alternative drug strategies to promote diuresis.[130]

Despite the early observational benefits ascribed to dopamine that have fostered its contemporary use, essentially no documented benefits exist to support its continued use in acute uremia, except for pressor control.[4,110,111,113,119] Dopamine has no propensity to improve renal function or alter outcome and can no longer be patently endorsed.

Management of Electrolyte and Acid-Base Disorders

Hyperkalemia is a common and life-threatening electrolyte disorder in animals with acute uremia. Severity of hyperkalemia and its associated cardiac and neuromuscular disturbances dictate therapeutic approach. Options for the management of hyperkalemia are to antagonize the increased resting potential in cardiac myocytes, redistribute potassium from the extracellular to the intracellular fluid compartments, and eliminate the potassium load from the body (Table 258-2).

Severe hyperkalemia (> 8 mmol/L) is associated with life-threatening cardiac arrhythmias and conduction disturbances that are accentuated by rapid increases in serum potassium and the degree of hyponatremia. To immediately resolve these threats, calcium gluconate (10 % solution) can be administered at 0.5 to 1.0 mL/kg as a slow intravenous bolus over 10 to 15 minutes to increase the threshold potential for cardiac excitation (see Table 258-2).[133-135] Calcium chloride is not an appropriate substitute because of its potency, acidifying tendency, and irritation if injected extravascularly. Rapid injection of calcium solutions may cause hypotension and cardiac arrhythmias; therefore arterial blood pressure and electrocardiogram (ECG) monitoring should be established during calcium administration. The infusion should be halted temporarily if S-T segment elevation, Q-T interval shortening, progressive bradycardia, or hypotension is observed. The effects of calcium infusion on the myocardium are rapid in onset but short lived (approximately 25 to 35 minutes), and it has no effect on serum potassium concentrations. Calcium infusion should be regarded as a *stopgap* to counteract conduction disturbances until longer-lasting controls can be initiated.

Once the cardiotoxicity has been controlled, transient lowering of serum potassium can be achieved by promoting

---

*References 4, 9, 106, 112, 119, 121, 122, 126-128.

Table • 258-2

Management of Hyperkalemia in Acute Renal Failure

THERAPY	MECHANISM OF ACTION
Mild Hyperkalemia (< 6.0 mEq/L)	
IV fluids (0.9% saline, lactated Ringer's)	Plasma volume expansion, dilutes K+, and increases GFR and renal potassium excretion
Kayexalate 2g/kg in 3-4 divided doses PO with 20% sorbitol; may also be given as retention enema without sorbitol	Exchanges K+ for Na+ across the intestinal mucosa
Moderate Hyperkalemia (6.0 to 8.0 mEq/L)	
Sodium bicarbonate 1-2 mEq/kg IV slowly over 20 minutes	Translocates K+ to intracellular space in exchange for H+
Dextrose (20%-50%) 1.5 g/kg IV bolus	Stimulates insulin release, which promotes transcellular entry of K+ into cells
Regular insulin and dextrose (20%-50%) Insulin @ 0.1-0.25 U/kg plus Dextrose @ 1-2 g/U IV	Promotes transcellular entry of K+ into cells
Severe Hyperkalemia (> 8.0 mEq/L)	
Calcium gluconate (10%) 0.5-1.0 mL/kg over 10-15 minutes; monitor the ECG during administration	Specific antagonist of the cardiotoxic effects of K+
Hemodialysis/peritoneal dialysis	Whole-body clearance of excessive potassium load

its translocation from the extracellular to the intracellular fluid compartment with sodium bicarbonate or insulin and glucose administration. During these temporary reprieves from the hyperkalemia, additional measures must be initiated to provide long-term regulation of serum potassium.

Moderate hyperkalemia (6.0 to 8.0 mmol/L) may resolve naturally after induction of diuresis. If diuresis cannot be established or serum potassium cannot be controlled with furosemide administration, all potassium-containing parenteral fluids should be replaced with solutions devoid of potassium. Sodium bicarbonate should be given to correct any existing deficit. Sodium bicarbonate can be administered empirically at 1 to 2 mmol/kg intravenously over 20 minutes in the absence of serum bicarbonate measurements (see Table 258-2). Therapeutic effects begin within 10 minutes and may persist for 1 to 2 hours.[133-135] Bicarbonate administration increases extracellular pH, which translocates potassium into cells in exchange for hydrogen ions.[133,134] Sodium bicarbonate is contraindicated in animals with metabolic alkalosis and is risky in overhydrated animals. Sodium bicarbonate administration may lower serum calcium concentration and precipitate a hypocalcemic crisis in animals with pre-existing hypocalcemia. Recent studies have shown equal efficacy for either hypertonic sodium chloride or sodium bicarbonate to reduce serum potassium and cardiac toxicity in dogs with artificially induced hyperkalemia.[136,137]

Hypertonic (20%) glucose can be administered at 0.5 to 1.5 g/kg intravenously as an alternative to sodium bicarbonate. Glucose stimulates insulin release and promotes the transcellular uptake of potassium. Alternatively, regular insulin can be given at 0.25 to 1.0 U/kg intravenously in combination with intravenous glucose at 1 to 2 g/U of administered insulin.[133,134] The effects of bicarbonate and glucose and insulin are more sustained than the effects of calcium but must be repeated as clinical circumstances dictate until the potassium load is alleviated.

Mild hyperkalemia (<6.0 mmol/L) is rarely problematic but should be monitored at 8- to 12-hour intervals. Mild hyperkalemia generally resolves with initial (potassium free) replacement fluids and routine furosemide or bicarbonate administration (or both). For long-term control in pets with refractory hyperkalemia, sodium polystyrene sulfonate resin (Kayexalate) may be given orally at 2 g/kg in 3 to 4 divided doses as a suspension in 20% sorbitol (to prevent constipation). The resin can also be used as a retention enema suspended in water in animals unable to tolerate oral administration. The resin exchanges sodium for potassium secreted into the intestinal lumen to promote increased intestinal potassium clearance. Exchange resins are effective at controlling low-grade hyperkalemia, but have little efficacy in the management of the associated cardiotoxicity. The acceptability of these preparations is low due to persistent side effects including nausea, constipation, GI ulceration, and necrosis.

If conventional therapy fails to provide an immediate or lasting resolution for the hyperkalemia, peritoneal or hemodialysis is indicated as alternative therapies (see Renal Replacement Therapy).

Hypokalemia

Hypokalemia may develop during the diuretic stage of ARF if renal potassium losses exceed potassium intake. The use of diuretics, inadequate dietary intake, vomiting, and diarrhea contribute to its development. Hypokalemia is usually asymptomatic, but clinical signs may be noted if the serum potassium concentration is less than 2.5 mmol/L. Muscle weakness, fatigue, vomiting, anorexia, GI ileus, and cardiac arrhythmias may become apparent. Ventroflexion of the neck is observed commonly in cats.

Oral potassium supplementation at 1 to 3 mmol/kg/day is usually sufficient in animals that are able to eat. Guidelines for parenteral potassium supplementation are based on the severity of hypokalemia. Serum potassium rarely is less than 2.0 mmol/L in animals with acute uremia, and maintenance fluids containing potassium concentrations between 20 and 30 mmol/L are usually sufficient to restore normokalemia. Potassium supplementation, including that in maintenance fluids, should be provided cautiously in uremic animals. Serum potassium should be evaluated frequently to avoid hypokalemia or hyperkalemia.

Acid-Base Imbalances

Metabolic acidosis is the most common acid-base disorder in uremic animals. Mild metabolic acidosis (serum bicarbonate >16 mmol/L) will often resolve after fluid replacement and the onset of diuresis. Moderate to severe metabolic acidosis (serum bicarbonate <16 mmol/L) should be treated with intravenous sodium bicarbonate. Initial treatment should be directed at correcting serum pH and serum bicarbonate to approximately 7.2 and 14 to 16 mmol/L, respectively. The initial bicarbonate replacement dose (mmol) = [body weight (kg) × 0.3 × bicarbonate deficit (desired bicarbonate – measured bicarbonate)]. One half of the calculated replacement is administered intravenously over 20 to 30 minutes, and the remainder is provided with intravenous fluids over 2 to 4 hours if arterial pH is less than 7.2 after distribution (30 to 60 minutes) of the initial bolus.[108,134,138]

Full equilibration of the initial bicarbonate dose requires 2 to 4 hours, but most uremic animals have an ongoing requirement for sodium bicarbonate of approximately 80 to 90 mg/kg/day to offset production of metabolic acids. Consequently, bicarbonate should be reassessed after administration of the initial replacement dose and at least once daily to determine if therapy has been adequate or additional therapy to normalize serum bicarbonate concentration is required. Excessive sodium bicarbonate administration can promote metabolic alkalosis, volume overload, pulmonary edema, and hypertension. Serum potassium and ionized calcium concentrations may decrease precipitously with overcorrection of the acidemia causing secondary hypoventilation, hypercapnia, shift in oxyhemoglobin dissociation, reduced tissue oxygen delivery, and paradoxic cerebral acidosis after rapid increases in serum pH.[108,134,138] Alternative alkalizing agents, including sodium acetate, sodium lactate, sodium or potassium citrate, and calcium carbonate, require hepatic metabolism to generate bicarbonate and offer no advantage to that of sodium bicarbonate.

Mild to moderate metabolic alkalosis (serum bicarbonate >26 and <35 mmol/L) resolves with administration of normal saline or balanced electrolyte solutions to correct the ECF fluid volume and chloride deficits and with the onset of diuresis. Protracted vomiting must be controlled with antiemetics to prevent persisting metabolic alkalosis. Respiratory acid-base disorders are seen in animals with concurrent pulmonary complications. Management of the respiratory component requires correction of the underlying pulmonary or pleural disease (or both) and appropriate regulation of ventilation and oxygenation. Sodium bicarbonate is not an appropriate therapy for the acidemia of respiratory origins.

Uremia Intoxications

Uremia toxins must be removed from the body by restoration of excretory function, intensive fluid diuresis, or dialysis to resolve the signs attributable to the azotemia. Immediate recovery of excretory function is rarely possible in advanced forms of acute uremia, and symptomatic therapies must be provided to ameliorate the uremic intoxications (Table 258-3).

Oral and Gastrointestinal Complications Oral hygiene, uremic stomatitis, and oral ulcerations can be improved dramatically by rinsing the oral cavity every 6 to 12 hours with solutions or gels containing 0.1% to 0.2% chlorhexidine. This therapy reduces the bacterial contamination of the oral cavity, helps prevent and heal oral ulcers, and relieves the discomfort associated with the stomatitis and lingual necrosis. Pain from lingual necrosis or severe ulceration can be managed further with topical lidocaine preparations.

Antiemetic therapy is required to manage fluid and electrolyte imbalances, nutritional needs, and the discomfort associated with protracted vomiting. All oral fluids, medications, and food should be discontinued until vomiting ceases for 12 to 24 hours. H_2-receptor antagonists such as cimetidine, ranitidine, and famotidine have become mainstays for the management of gastritis, vomiting, and gastric ulceration (see Table 258-3).[70,139] They reduce gastric acid production by blocking the histamine receptor on gastric parietal cells and also reduce pepsin production, which may promote gastric ulcer formation. H_2-receptor antagonists undergo 50% to 70% renal elimination, and dosing should be reduced in proportion to the degree renal failure to prevent side effects. Omeprazole is a potent inhibitor of gastric acid secretion and acts by irreversible inactivation of H^+/K^+-ATPase activity to prevent secretion of hydrogen ions into the stomach.[139] Omeprazole reduces acid secretion in the dog for up to 24 hours; however, expense may limit its widespread application.

Oral antacids are of limited value to reduce gastric acidity due to their frequent dosing requirement. Their usefulness is limited further in animals with protracted vomiting. Sucralfate is a basic aluminum salt of sucrose octasulfate used to manage gastric ulceration. It binds tightly to exposed protein in gastric ulcers to form a protective barrier against pepsin, acid, bile, or pancreatic secretions. Sucralfate also stimulates mucus and bicarbonate secretion and mucosal prostaglandin production to improve microvascular integrity and mucosal blood flow. The efficacy of sucralfate is limited in animals that cannot tolerate oral medications. Medical therapy is typically continued for 2 to 3 weeks but may need to be extended in animals with severe gastritis after antifreeze ingestion or severe uremia. Management of the gastritis generally controls vomiting if excretory function can be restored quickly and the azotemia resolved.

Centrally acting antiemetic therapy should be considered if vomiting cannot be controlled by restricted oral intake and treatment of the gastritis (see Table 258-3). Metoclopramide is a D_2-dopaminergic antagonist that directly suppresses the chemoreceptor trigger zone.[139] It also has prokinetic effects on the stomach to promote gastric emptying, which is often delayed in uremic animals. Metoclopramide can be provided by either oral or parenteral routes and is most effective when administered as a constant intravenous infusion (see Table 258-3). Metoclopramide is excreted by the kidneys, and the dose needs modification in animals with severe uremia. Phenothiazine derivative antiemetics (chlorpromazine, prochlorperazine, acepromazine) suppress vomiting through antagonism of α-adrenergic receptors at the CRTZ and the

Table • 258-3

Therapeutic Agents Used in the Management of Gastrointestinal Uremic Intoxications*

AGENT	INDICATION/MECHANISM	CONVENTIONAL DOSE
Chlorhexidine (CHX-Guard®)	Stomatitis, oral ulceration Bacteriocidal agent	
Cimetidine† (Tagamet® *Smith Kline French*)	Esophagitis, gastritis, gastric ulceration/hemorrhage H_2-receptor antagonist	5-10 mg/kg PO, IM, IV q4-6h (dog) 5-10 mg/kg PO, IM, IV q6-8h (cat)
Ranitidine† (Zantac® *Glaxo*)	Esophagitis, gastritis, gastric ulceration/hemorrhage H_2-receptor antagonist	0.5-2.0 mg/kg PO, IV q 8-12h
Famotidine† (Pepcid® *Merck Sharp Dohme*)	Esophagitis, gastritis, gastric ulceration/hemorrhage H_2-receptor antagonist	0.5-1.0 mg/kg PO, IM, IV q 12-24h
Omeprazole (Prilosec® *Merck Sharp Dohme*)	Esophagitis, gastritis, gastric ulceration/hemorrhage $H+/K+$ -ATPase proton pump blocker	0.5-1.0 mg/kg PO q24h
Sucralfate (Carafate® *Marion*)	Esophagitis, gastritis, gastric ulceration/hemorrhage Cytoprotective agent	0.5-1.0 g PO q 6-8h (dog) 0.25-0.5 g PO q 8-12h (cat)
Misoprostol (Cytotec® *Searle*)	Esophagitis, gastritis, gastric ulceration/hemorrhage Cytoprotective agents-PGE, analogue	1-5 g/kg PO q6-12h
Chlorpromazine (Thorazine ® *Smith Kline French*)	CRTZ, emetic center antiemetic α_2-adrenergic, D_2-dopaminergic, H_1-histaminergic, M_1-cholinergic antagonists	0.2-0.5 mg/kg IM, SQ q6-8h
Prochlorperazine (Compazine® *Smith Kline French*)	CRTZ, emetic center antiemetic α_2-adrenergic, D_2-dopaminergic, H_1-histaminergic, M_1-cholinergic antagonists	0.1-0.5 mg/kg IM, SQ q8-12h
Acepromazine (PromAce® *Fort Dodge*)	CRTZ, emetic center antiemetic α_2-adrenergic, D_2-dopaminergic, H_1-histaminergic, M_1-cholinergic antagonists	0.01-0.05 mg/kg IM, SQ q8-12h
Ondansetron (Zofran® *Glaxo Wellcome*)	$5-HT_3$ receptor antagonist CRTZ, peripheral vagal nerve	0.1 mg/kg PO q12-24h 0.1-0.3 mg/kg IV q8-12h
Dolasetron (Anzemet® *Hoechst Marion Russel*)	$5-HT_3$ receptor antagonist CRTZ, peripheral vagal nerve	0.5 mg/kg PO, SQ, IV q24h
Metoclopramide† (Reglan® *Robins*)	CRTZ antiemetic, prokinetic agent D_2-dopaminergic antagonist, $5HT_3$-serotonergic antagonist	0.1-0.5 mg/kg PO, IM, SQ q 6-8h 0.01-0.02 mg/kg/hr CRI
Cisapride (Propulsid® *Jansen Pharmaceutica Inc*)	Prokinetic agent $5-HT_4$ receptor agonist, $5-HT_1$/$5-HT_3$ receptor antagonist	0.1-0.5 mg/kg PO q8-12h

*Most of these drugs have not been approved for use in the dog or cat.
†Agent undergoes renal excretion and the dose must be adjusted accordingly to prevent toxicity.
CRTZ, Chemoreceptor trigger zone; *5-HT,* 5-hydroxytryptamine.

emetic center. They are effective antiemetics in uremic animals but prone to sedative and hypotensive side effects. They should be considered for animals with intractable vomiting in which the adverse effects can be accepted. Serotonin receptor antagonists (ondansetron and dolasetron) provide central antiemetic effects at both the CRTZ and emetic center. They are highly effective for chemotherapy-induced vomiting and may be effective in acute uremia. Prokinetic agents can be used to treat delayed gastric emptying, uremic gastric paresis, and the persistent vomiting.

Uremic bleeding can be fatal if associated with CNS hemorrhage but more commonly causes GI bleeding and anemia. Uremic bleeding improves with resolution of the azotemia after intensive diuresis or dialysis. Transfusion of packed RBCs is indicated for animals with severe anemia and active bleeding and may reduce bleeding time through indirect effects on platelet function.[140] Transfusion of platelet-rich plasma will not improve platelet function or reduce bleeding time, because function of the transfused cells is altered upon exposure to uremic plasma.

Impaired Immunity Uremia imposes increased susceptibility to infection due to accumulation of toxins that impair immunity and cellular host defenses.[141,142] The deficiencies in host defenses are compounded by widespread breaches of mucosal integrity associated with GI ulceration, intravenous and bladder catheterization, parenteral medications and feeding, and intervention with hemodialysis, peritoneal dialysis, and immunosuppressive drugs.[141] Infection may be difficult to identify because uremia dampens the febrile response. Strict asepsis during catheter placement and meticulous catheter site care are mandatory for uremic animals. If infection is suspected, blood, urine, and catheter tip cultures should be obtained, and broad-spectrum antibiotic therapy initiated pending culture results. Prophylactic use of antibiotics may foster bacterial resistance or "superinfections" and should be prescribed with caution.

Pulmonary Signs Respiratory complications arise mostly from overhydration, infection, and aspiration of gastric fluids during vomiting. Overhydration is treated by cessation of fluid delivery and diuretic administration to achieve an appropriate dry weight. Animals with severe pulmonary edema and oliguria may require removal of the fluid burden by peritoneal or hemodialysis. Bacterial pneumonia is managed with antibiotics and supportive pulmonary care. Aspiration pneumonia should be treated aggressively with antiemetic therapy, parenteral broad-spectrum antibiotics, and supplemental oxygen or ventilatory support, if required. Uremic pneumonitis is a complication of severe azotemia resulting in a respiratory distress syndrome, noncardiogenic pulmonary edema, and respiratory compromise or failure.[75] Uremic pneumonitis is treated supportively with supplemental oxygenation or mechanical ventilation. It has potential to improve with resolution of the azotemia and is an indication for dialysis. Dogs with leptospirosis frequently develop radiographic and clinical signs consistent with uremic pneumonitis that is independent of the severity of the azotemia. The lesions are induced by endothelial damage and vasculitis.[74]

Nutritional Management of Acute Renal Failure

Protein-calorie malnutrition is a component of the acute uremic syndrome. This includes impaired immune function, increased susceptibility to infection, delayed wound healing, decreased strength, and poor quality of life. The imposed catabolism exacerbates the hyperkalemia, hyperphosphatemia, acidosis, and azotemia. It increases morbidity and mortality.[143,144] Anorexia, nausea and vomiting, comorbid diseases, uremic toxins, insulin resistance, and hyperparathyroidism contribute to the nutritional inadequacies. Metabolic acidosis is a major stimulus for breakdown of muscle protein and amino acid oxidation and contributes to the ongoing catabolism.[145,146]

An accurate assessment of nutritional status is necessary to guide nutritional therapy. Change in body weight is the simplest parameter to assess. This can be flawed by changes in hydration status, lean body mass, or fat stores. Body condition scoring is a useful index to document sequential changes in body composition, but it is only qualitative and subject to hydration errors and experience of the evaluator.[147,148] Bioelectrical impedance analysis is a new, safe, noninvasive, and reproducible method to precisely quantitate changes in total body water, extracellular fluid volume, and body cell mass with potential application in uremic animals.[149,150] Goals of nutritional therapy are to meet the energy and nutrient requirements of the animal; alleviate the azotemia; prevent

alterations in fluid, electrolyte, vitamin, mineral, and acid-base balance; and aid the renal repair. The optimal nutritional regime for dogs and cats with ARF has not been defined, but a high-energy and moderate protein, potassium and phosphate formulation as prescribed for CRF is logical. Sufficient energy must be supplied to prevent catabolism of endogenous protein, spare lean body mass, and minimize azotemia. The illness energy requirement for animals with acute uremia is determined as the resting energy requirement times a stress factor (1.2 to 1.4 for uremic dogs and 1.2 for uremic cats). RER is determined according to the following formulae:

$$RER\ (kcal/day) = 70(Wt_{kg})^{0.75}$$

or

$$RER\ (kcal/day) = 70 + (30 \times Wt_{kg})$$

(where Wt_{kg} is the body weight in kilograms[151])

Carbohydrate and fat provide the nonprotein sources of energy required in the diet. Commercial diets, liquid enteral formulations, or parenteral solutions designed for the management of renal failure can be used. These formulations contain a relatively high fat content to increase energy density, and they should be introduced slowly to prevent GI complications, especially pancreatitis.

The optimal protein requirement for animals with acute uremia is not known and is likely to be influenced by underlying and coexistent clinical conditions. Consequently, the minimum protein requirements for normal dogs (1.25 to 1.75 g/kg/day; approximately 8% to 10% protein on a ME basis) and cats (3.8 to 4.4 g/kg/day; approximately 20% to 25% protein on a ME basis) are generally adopted for uremic animals. This degree of restriction may not be necessary or desired in animals with mild or moderate azotemia or greater catabolic stresses, where more liberal protein prescriptions may be needed. Phosphorus, sodium, potassium, and magnesium intake should be restricted to prevent accumulation of these minerals; however, intake must be modified according to the clinical and biochemical dictates of the animal.

Delivery of adequate nutrition is constrained by inappetence and the GI complications of uremia. Oral or enteral feeding may not be possible or recommended in the initial stages of ARF due to gastritis, pancreatitis, or uncontrolled vomiting. Peripheral parenteral nutrition or total parenteral nutrition is indicated under these circumstances to provide interim nutritional support.[152] Peripheral parenteral nutrition is formulated with isotonic solutions administered through a peripheral vein. However, complete nutritional requirements cannot be met by this technique. It should only be used as an adjunct to oral intake or to supply partial nutritional support not to exceed 5 days. Total parenteral nutrition is formulated to provide all essential nutrients for indefinite periods but requires central venous administration due to the hypertonicity of the nutrient solutions.

Oral or enteral tube feeding is recommended in animals that are not vomiting but fail to achieve caloric requirements. The indications, complications, and technical aspects of enteral feeding have been reviewed recently.[151] Esophageal feeding tubes or percutaneous gastrostomy tubes are invaluable aids for the long-term nutritional support of animals that are likely to have prolonged recovery times. Caloric and protein requirements can be met readily by the intermittent or continuous administration of blended therapeutic diets or liquid enteral preparations formulated for the management of renal insufficiency.[151] The clinical benefits of enteral or parenteral nutrition cannot be overemphasized, but it may not be possible to supply the volume required to achieve the nutritional requirements in oliguric animals without dialysis to alleviate overhydration.

URINARY SYSTEM

Renal Replacement Therapy

ARF is the most common indication for dialytic intervention in dogs and cats, and modern dialysis equipment and procedures are well suited for uremic animals.[77,104,105] Medical therapies cannot approach the efficacy, efficiency, and clinical benefits that dialysis provides. Without dialysis, animals with severe uremia generally die within 5 to 7 days precluding sufficient opportunity for regeneration or repair of the renal injury. Dialysis extends the life expectancy of uremic animals facilitating their potential for recovery. Peritoneal dialysis uses the peritoneal lining as a dialytic exchange surface across which diffusive and osmotic forces transfer toxic wastes and excessive fluid from the blood to a dialysate solution instilled in the abdominal cavity.[104,108,153] It is a conceptually simple technique applicable in both general and specialty practice but can be a deceptively intensive and fraught with technical and clinical complications.[104,154] Continuous renal replacement therapy (CRRT) is a noninterrupted extracorporeal procedure using hemofiltration for solute and fluid removal. CRRT is less demanding technically than intermittent hemodialysis. It is generally provided in intensive care settings for patients with profound clinical and hemodynamic instability.[121,155] The technical and clinical lure of CRRT has captured the interest of veterinary critical care specialists for the management of acute uremia. Intermittent hemodialysis is the standard extracorporeal therapy for acute uremia in humans and animals. The fluid, electrolyte, and acid-base abnormalities are corrected, and the accumulated uremia solutes are removed from the body by diffusive and convective gradients between blood and the dialysate solution in the artificial kidney.[77,104,105] Hemodialysis has become a routine therapy for severe uremia in both dogs and cats.

Immediate renal replacement therapy is indicated when the clinical consequences of the azotemia, inadequate urine production, and the fluid, electrolyte, and acid-base disturbances cannot be managed with medical therapy alone. General guidelines for patient selection and indications for dialytic therapy are outlined in Box 258-3. Hemodialysis (and peritoneal dialysis and CRRT therapies) can resolve virtually all excretory deficiency of acute uremia.

To date, failure to recover renal function after 1 to 4 weeks of conventional medical support have been used as benchmarks to predict irreversible from reversible renal failure in animals. However, these criteria have been redefined with the advent of hemodialysis, and many animals with seemingly irreversible disease at the outset of medical management can recover renal function if supported by dialysis beyond the 4-week limit.

Azotemia Even severe azotemia can be corrected completely with just a few hemodialysis sessions, but the expediency of its resolution must be tempered by the tolerance of the animal to rapid changes in serum solute concentrations. Both peritoneal dialysis and CRRT procedures produce a more gradual and continuous resolution of the azotemia throughout the first 2 to 3 days of therapy. For animals that do not recover within this time period, CRRT must be transitioned to intermittent hemodialysis for long-term support.

Electrolyte Disturbances Dialysis is indicated in patients where medical treatments provide only transient resolution of the hyperkalemia and no relief of the excessive potassium load for long-term control. Life-threatening conduction disturbances are frequently corrected within minutes of starting hemodialysis despite the absence of perceptible changes in peripheral blood potassium concentration, thus providing both an immediate and prolonged solution to hyperkalemia.

Abnormalities of other electrolytes or minerals resulting from the uremia, comorbid diseases, or therapy, can be corrected by formulating the dialysate to approximate the serum concentration desired for each solute at the end of the dialysis session. The bicarbonate concentration of the dialysate can be increased above reference values to promote accrual of depleted buffer reserves and to supplement impaired renal bicarbonate generation.

Correction of Fluid Excesses

Excessive fluid load can be removed readily by ultrafiltration using intermittent hemodialysis or CRRT, or by osmotic gradients with peritoneal dialysis. Slow rates of ultrafiltration between 5 to 10 mL/kg/hr generally are tolerated. Increased rates of fluid removal are possible but require careful assessments of the animal's hemodynamic condition and use blood volume monitoring equipment.

Acute Intoxications

Hemodialysis should be considered for the immediate management of acute poisoning when the toxin is dialyzable, when antidotal therapy has been delayed, or when no specific antidote to the intoxication is available. Hemodialysis is indicated specifically for the treatment of common poisonings including ethylene glycol, methanol, salicylate, lithium, ethanol, phenobarbital, acetaminophen, theophylline, aminoglycosides, tricyclic antidepressants, and possibly metaldehyde.[77,104,105] Peritoneal dialysis and CRRT procedures may be capable of removing a variety of toxins, but these treatments are less efficient than hemodialysis and do not represent satisfactory substitutes.

Hemodialysis will rapidly eliminate ethylene glycol and its metabolites from animals poisoned with antifreeze (Figure 258-7). It should be initiated without any delay as the principal therapy to resolve the intoxication and to support the accompanying fluid, electrolyte, and acid-base disorders associated with the toxicosis.[77] For acute poisoning (within 5 to 6 hours), it is possible to remove all the toxin

---

> **Box • 258-3**
>
> ***Indications for Dialytic Therapy in Animals***
>
> **Acute Uremia:**
> 1. Anuria
> 2. Failure of fluid administration or diuretic therapy to initiate an adequate diuresis
> 3. Failure of conventional therapy to control the azotemia or the biochemical and clinical manifestations of acute uremia
> 4. Life-threatening fluid overload
> 5. Life-threatening electrolyte or acid-base disturbances
> 6. BUN > 100 mg/dL; serum creatinine > 10 mg/dL
> 7. Clinical course refractory to conservative therapy for 12-24 hours
>
> **Miscellaneous:**
> 1. Severe overhydration; pulmonary edema; congestive heart failure (CHF)
> 2. Acute poisoning/drug overdose

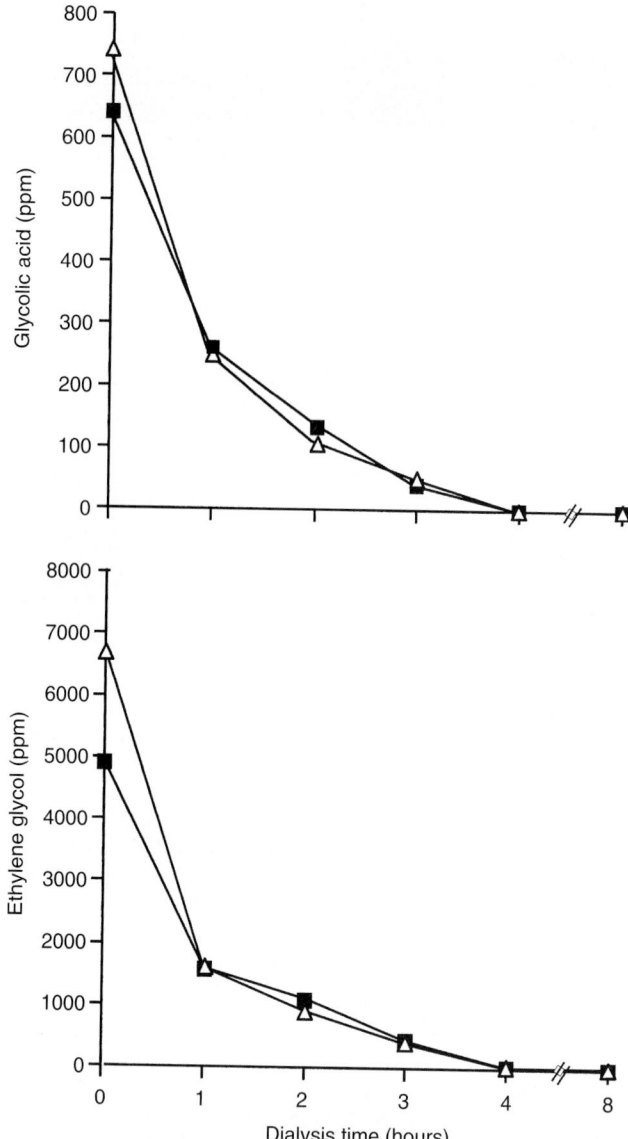

Figure 258-7 Changes in serum glycolic acid *(upper panel)* and ethylene glycol *(lower panel)* concentrations in two dogs treated with hemodialysis after simultaneous exposure to antifreeze 4 to 6 hours before presentation. Despite the extremely high initial concentrations of these toxins, both dogs recovered uneventfully with no evident renal injury after a single dialysis treatment.

and prevent development of renal injury with a single dialysis treatment.[77,112] If the treatment is delayed beyond this window, renal injury may be expected, and a series of dialysis treatments must be provided to support the uremia and renal repair.

Transplantation of renal allografts from unrelated dogs and cats has become more successful in the past 10 years and provides an alternative renal replacement option for animals that sustain irreparable renal injury.[156-159] Transplantation early in the course of severe renal injuries (antifreeze poisoning) may prove more cost-effective than a protracted course of dialysis.

Outcome and Prognosis

The prognosis for recovery from acute uremia depends on the cause, extent of damage, comorbid diseases, multiple organ involvement, and availability of diagnostic and therapeutic services. Little documentation exists in the veterinary literature to accurately predict the importance of these independent variables. A recent review of 99 cases of ARF in dogs produced by the usual causes documented a mortality of nearly 60% from death or euthanasia.[11] Nearly 60% of the surviving dogs subsequently developed CRF, and only 44% recovered normal renal function. Severity of the azotemia, hypocalcemia, anemia, proteinuria, specific cause (ethylene glycol intoxication), and comorbid systemic disease (DIC) were associated with failure to survive. In this series, 92% of dogs with a history of ethylene glycol ingestion died or were euthanatized due to the poor prognosis. In another series of 37 dogs with confirmed ethylene glycol intoxication, greater than 95% of those with initial azotemia died, whereas all nonazotemic dogs survived.[160] Survival for dogs with hospital-acquired ARF was reported as 38%, with age and initial urine production as significant predictors of mortality.[161]

In contrast to these outcomes in dogs, 9 of 15 (60%) cats with severe ARF secondary to pyelonephritis and ethylene glycol intoxication that were managed with hemodialysis or transplantation recovered with partial or normal renal function.[31] One hundred percent of cats with acute pyelonephritis survived. In these animals, as in other series, the magnitude of the azotemia at presentation did not predict survivability. Similar to previous reports, a recent review of 138 cases of severe ARF in dogs requiring hemodialysis revealed an all-cause mortality of nearly 60% from death or euthanasia.[62] For the majority of surviving dogs, renal function had been substantially recovered by the time of discharge. Survival from infectious (80%) and hemodynamic and metabolic causes (40%) is more favorable than survival from toxic causes (20%).[62] The outcome for dogs with acute leptospirosis is particularly favorable, with survival approaching 90% with either severe (dialysis dependent) or milder forms (medically managed) of ARF.[85]

ARF is a serious and frequently fatal disease in both dogs and cats. Recovery is best for animals with infectious causes and worst for animals with nephrotoxic causes or multiple organ failure. Early recognition, appropriate fluid therapy, and extended support with dialysis offer the greatest opportunity for a favorable outcome.

URINARY SYSTEM

CHAPTER • 259

Renal Transplantation

Cathy E. Langston
Lori L. Ludwig

Chronic renal failure is a progressive, debilitating, and terminal disease. Medical management, although effective initially, is not sufficient for cats with end-stage renal failure. Kidney transplantation offers an avenue of therapy when medical management fails. The first clinical feline renal transplantation was performed in 1987. Several centers now offer this procedure.

CANDIDATE SELECTION

Ideally, a feline candidate for kidney transplantation should have no medical problems other than kidney failure. Renal diseases appropriately treated with transplantation include acquired conditions (e.g., chronic interstitial nephritis, toxic nephropathy, membranous glomerulonephropathy) and congenital disorders (e.g., renal dysplasia, polycystic kidney disease). Amyloidosis, pyelonephritis, and obstructive nephropathy from calcium oxalate nephrolithiasis are relative contraindications because of potential effects on the transplanted kidney. To avoid injury to the transplanted kidney, cats with ethylene glycol–induced renal failure should not be considered for transplantation until the ethylene glycol and its metabolites have been completely eliminated from the body. Hemodialysis may be necessary to ensure elimination of these metabolites.

An extensive diagnostic evaluation (Box 259-1) should be performed prior to transplantation to identify contraindications to the procedure. These tests commonly are performed locally, especially if significant travel to a transplantation center otherwise would be necessary, to avoid needless travel and expense for the owners of cats that turn out to be poor candidates.

The immunosuppression necessary to prevent graft (renal) rejection in an animal that previously has had pyelonephritis, a bacterial urinary tract infection (UTI), or an indwelling catheter may "reactivate" a latent infection. Infection may cause pyelonephritis in the transplanted kidney and activation of the rejection process.[1] Also, these animals are predisposed to overwhelming systemic infection. Such cats therefore are not ideal candidates, and a 1- to 3-week "test" course of cyclosporine (CyA) and prednisone prior to transplantation is recommended.[2] If urine culture results are positive after such a trial, transplantation should not be performed.

Another potential contraindication to kidney transplantation is inflammatory bowel disease (IBD). The variability of absorption of CyA in cats with IBD increases the risk of rejection. Inflammatory bowel disease may also heighten immune system activation, making immunologic attack on the transplanted kidney more likely.[1] Cats infected with the feline leukemia virus (FeLV) or the feline immunodeficiency virus (FIV) should also be excluded as candidates because of their increased susceptibility to infection.

The immunosuppression associated with renal transplantation has resulted in activation of *Toxoplasma* tissue cysts and clinical disease in several cats. An attempt should be made to assess carefully both the donor and the recipient for toxoplasmosis. A positive toxoplasmosis titer does not determine whether active infection is present. A serologically positive recipient must be considered at higher risk. A seropositive donor should not be used for a seronegative recipient.

A thorough cardiac evaluation, including thoracic radiographs, an electrocardiogram (EKG), and an echocardiogram, should be performed prior to transplantation surgery. Because of the shortened anticipated life span associated with significant cardiac disease, cats with congestive heart failure or diffuse hypertrophy are eliminated as candidates. Intolerance of aggressive fluid therapy or focal hypertrophy are relative contraindications and must be evaluated in light of the entire clinical picture.[2]

Other conditions likely to affect renal function or patient longevity, including uncontrolled hyperthyroidism, diabetes mellitus, or neoplasia, should exclude any cat from consideration for renal transplantation. Hypertension affects about 30% of feline transplantation candidates.[3] Prior to transplantation, antihypertensive therapy should be titrated to control blood pressure.[2] Intensive handling is necessary, particularly in the immediate postoperative period, therefore fractious cats should not undergo transplantation, because they will not tolerate the level of care necessary for a good outcome.

Transplantation is appropriate when medical management fails to maintain the cat in satisfactory condition. It can be difficult to determine the point of decompensation, but good guidelines include weight loss, the development of anemia, or worsening azotemia. Some programs suggest transplantation when a certain creatinine level has been exceeded (e.g., 4 mg/dL). Despite the uncertainty involved in determining the best time for transplantation, a lengthy delay from decompensation to transplantation must be avoided. Severe debilitation with excessive weight loss (greater than 25%) and chronic uremia reduces the success rate of transplantation. Transplantation is not a salvage operation, and cats that are severely debilitated should not be considered for it. Attempts to reverse the debilitation in these cats with enteral nutrition via a feeding tube have been disappointing.[1] Hemodialysis to control azotemia and uremic symptoms has been quite successful, but peritoneal dialysis is not advised because of frequent complications, including peritonitis.

DONORS

Because sufficient renal function can be provided even by a portion of just one kidney, unilateral nephrectomy for kidney donation does not diminish the quality of life or life span of the donor.[4] Kidney donors should be young cats that have been screened to ensure their general health (i.e., complete blood count [CBC], chemistry panel, urinalysis, and urine culture) and lack of infectious disease (FeLV, FIV, toxoplasmosis).

Box • 259-1

Diagnostic Testing for Candidates for Renal Transplantation

The following diagnostic tests should be performed for any animal being considered for renal transplantation:

- Complete blood count (CBC)
- Chemistry panel
- Thyroid level determination
- Feline leukemia virus (FeLV) and feline immunodeficiency virus (FIV) testing (cats)
- Blood typing
- Electrocardiogram (EKG) and echocardiogram
- Thoracic radiographs
- Abdominal ultrasonography
- Toxoplasmosis titer
- Urinalysis and culture
- Blood pressure measurement

An intravenous pyelogram allows evaluation of renal structure. Donor cats ideally are the same size or bigger than the recipient, but no more than 0.5 kg smaller. Most programs require the recipient family to adopt the donor cat.

PREOPERATIVE MANAGEMENT

The cat that is to receive a new kidney (the recipient) should be admitted to the hospital several days prior to the scheduled transplantation surgery. The recipient is cross-matched to several potential donors, and any further evaluation of the donor or recipient should then be completed. Intravenous fluids are given at a rate that maintains hydration or that provides diuresis if the blood urea nitrogen (BUN) is greater than 100 mg/dL. If anemia has not been corrected by previous erythropoietin therapy, blood transfusions can be given to achieve a target packed cell volume (PCV) of 30% or higher. Cyclosporine (NeOral, 3 to 4 mg/kg given orally twice daily) is administered starting 1 to 2 days before surgery. Prednisone (1 mg/kg given orally twice daily) is started the day of surgery. Enteral nutrition is provided by feeding tube if the recipient cat is not eating voluntarily. Blood samples for determination of CyA concentrations are submitted the morning of surgery.

DONOR SURGERY

If kidney preservation methods are not used, anesthesia is induced in the donor cat approximately 30 minutes before induction in the recipient. The donor is given mannitol (0.25 to 1 g/kg) intravenously prior to harvesting the kidney to protect against acute tubular necrosis associated with warm ischemia.[5] The left kidney is preferred for transplantation because of the longer renal vein. If two renal veins are present, the smallest is ligated and the largest prepared for anastomosis. Kidneys with two renal arteries are usually avoided in cats because both would need to be preserved to ensure adequate renal blood flow. Preservation and anastomosis in dogs with two renal arteries has been reported.[6]

Once the recipient vessels have been prepared, the donor kidney is removed and flushed with ice-cold heparinized saline solution. The surgical team working with the donor closes the abdominal incision while the team working with the recipient performs the vascular anastomosis. If preservation methods are used, the donor kidney is removed, flushed with a storage medium, and stored in solution on ice until the recipient has been prepared. Hypothermic preservation of the harvested kidney has been reported in cats with storage times of up to 7 hours.[7] The advantages of cold preservation include the need for only one surgical team, the additional time available for vessel preparation after kidney harvest, and the longer time before ischemic injury occurs during anastomosis.[5,7]

RECIPIENT SURGERY

Magnification (×3 to ×10) is required for anastomosis of the vessels and ureters in small dogs and cats. In dogs, the left common iliac vein is sutured to the renal vein in an end-to-side manner, and the iliac and renal arteries are sutured end-to-end. This technique was also initially reported for use in cats; however, it has been associated with neuropraxia and lameness of the pelvic limb on the side of the anastomosis.[9] The technique currently preferred in cats is an end-to-side anastomosis of the renal vein to the caudal vena cava and of the renal artery to the aorta. The time from occluding blood flow to the kidney for harvesting to release of the vascular clamps after anastomosis (warm ischemia time) should be kept to less than 60 minutes.[8]

Several techniques have been described for implantation of the donor ureter into the recipient bladder. A drop-in technique initially was used in cats, because the small diameter of the feline ureter (0.4 mm) makes primary anastomosis technically difficult.[10] With this intravesical technique, a ventral cystotomy is performed, and the ureter is brought into the bladder through a small incision in the dorsal bladder wall. The distal end of the ureter is either attached to the inside of the bladder with a single suture or left free in the bladder lumen. Obstruction of the ureter by granulation tissue was a frequent complication of this technique, therefore it has been replaced by the mucosal appositional technique.[11]

For mucosal apposition, an operating microscope is used to allow visualization of the distal end of the ureter, which is incised longitudinally and then sutured to the bladder mucosa in a simple interrupted pattern. Ureteral obstruction is less common with this technique; however, partial obstruction may still be seen in the immediate postoperative period. An extravesical technique was recently described and may reduce the incidence and severity of postoperative obstruction. With this procedure, a seromuscular incision is made in the ventral surface of the urinary bladder, avoiding a large cystotomy, and a small incision is made in the mucosa at the caudal aspect of the seromuscular incision. The ureteral mucosa is sutured to the bladder mucosa, and the seromuscular layer is closed. In dogs either the intravesical or extravesical mucosal appositional technique can be used.[6]

Before the abdomen is closed, the transplanted kidney is stabilized to the body wall by suturing of the kidney capsule to a pocket in the retroperitoneal membrane or to a muscle flap created in the transversus abdominis muscle.[5,8] This helps prevent graft torsion and vessel avulsion in the postoperative period. In dogs, the native kidneys are usually removed to minimize systemic hypertension unless delayed graft function is suspected.[6] The native kidneys are usually preserved in cats. In all recipients, biopsy of one of the native kidneys should be performed.

PERIOPERATIVE MANAGEMENT AND COMPLICATIONS

Postoperative treatment should include fluid therapy, immunosuppressive drugs, analgesia, and careful monitoring of the hematocrit, electrolyte balance, and cardiovascular status.

Blood pressure should be monitored every 1 to 2 hours after surgery for the first 48 hours. Hypotension in the postoperative period is dangerous to graft function because of decreased renal blood flow and an increased risk of vessel thrombosis. Hypertension is also dangerous in the postoperative period because it has been associated with central nervous system (CNS) disorders, including seizures.[12] The urine specific gravity and serum BUN and creatinine concentrations should be monitored daily, and these parameters usually improve within 12 to 72 hours after surgery.[8]

Complications seen in the immediate postoperative period may include vessel torsion, hemorrhage, or thrombosis; ureteral leakage or obstruction; malignant hypertension; neurologic abnormalities; and delayed graft function.[12,13] Delayed graft function associated with ischemia-reperfusion injury or partial ureteral obstruction results in lack of improvement in kidney function after surgery. If improvement is not seen within a few days of surgery, abdominal ultrasonography should be performed to assess blood flow in the renal vessels and to evaluate the transplanted ureter for dilatation, which may indicate obstruction. Complete ureteral obstruction or leakage of urine from the ureteroneocystostomy site would require additional surgery to correct the abnormality. Intestinal intussusception has been reported in dogs after transplantation.[6]

IMMUNOSUPPRESSION

Cyclosporine is a calcineurin inhibitor that blocks the transcription of interleukin-2 (IL-2), impairing T-helper and T-cytotoxic lymphocytes. CyA is not myelosuppressive and has no effect on nonstimulated lymphocytes, thus preserving nonspecific host resistance to infection. The decrease in IL-2 also results in a decrease in other mediators that cause rejection. Prednisone and CyA are synergistic and inhibit T-cell proliferation.

CyA is available as a microemulsified form (NeOral, Novartis Pharma AG, Switzerland; Gengraf, Sangstat Medical Corp., Cambridge, MA). The bioavailability of this formulation is greater and less variable than that of the nonmicroemulsified formulation (Sandimmune, Norvartis), primarily because of more reliable gastrointestinal (GI) absorption. These forms are not interchangeable. The oral form is bitter and should be put in a gelatin capsule. CyA is also available as an intravenous formulation. All forms of CyA must be protected from light.

CyA is cleared by the cytochrome p-450 system. Drugs that induce p-450 enzymes (e.g., phenobarbital) reduce CyA levels. Drugs that compete for clearance by p-450 (e.g., cimetidine, ketoconazole, erythromycin) increase CyA levels. Ketoconazole increases blood levels of CyA twofold in cats and twofold to threefold in dogs.[14,15] Although this reduces the dosage of CyA needed to maintain therapeutic levels, the individual variations in effect and the risk of hepatotoxicity are undesirable. Certain drugs, such as ranitidine, aminoglycosides, trimethoprim, or sulfamethoxazole, can potentiate renal damage.

Because of variations in absorption and metabolism and because the therapeutic window is relatively narrow, CyA blood levels must be closely monitored. The appropriate target range depends on the methodology, sample type, and time after transplantation. Whole blood levels are generally higher than plasma levels, because CyA is extensively bound to the red blood cells. High-performance liquid chromatography (HPLC) provides the most reliable results. Other methods, including immunoassays that use polyclonal or monoclonal antibodies, measure the parent compound and metabolites, which vary in their immunologic effect. Trough levels of 400 to 600 ng/mL as measured by HPLC in whole blood are recommended for the first month. After the first

1 to 3 months, the CyA dosage can be reduced to achieve trough levels of 350 to 450 ng/mL. Fluorescent immunoassay (TDx-FLx assay) yields whole blood levels 1.5 to 4.2 times higher.[5] If HPLC is not readily and reliably available, comparison of HPLC to TDx-FLx values in a minimum of three samples in an individual cat can provide a conversion relationship that allows correct clinical decisions to be made in many cats.[16]

An excess of circulating CyA can cause nephrotoxicity. In humans, values above 1000 ng/mL are associated with azotemia, but many cats tolerate higher levels (up to 3000 ng/mL) before renal toxicity becomes apparent.[17] In contrast, some cats have developed CyA nephrotoxicity at trough levels of 700 to 800 ng/dL.[5] The serum creatinine concentration rarely exceeds 2 to 3 mg/dL from CyA toxicity. Increases in the serum creatinine concentration usually occur 1 to 2 days after the CyA level reaches high values and normally decline within 1 to 2 days of a decrease in the drug to acceptable levels.[5] Adverse effects of CyA in cats include mild GI signs. Dogs may exhibit gastrointestinal irritation, weight loss, gingival hypertrophy, papillomatosis, shedding, and hypertrichosis.

Prednisone is a standard component of transplantation immunosuppression. It inhibits production of some cytokines (IL-1, IL-6, gamma interferon) that are essential for T-cell production and function. Prednisone also inhibits production of local chemotactic factors, prostaglandins, thromboxanes, and leukotrienes. By 1 month after surgery, the initial dosage of 1 mg/kg given every 12 hours can be reduced to 0.5 to 1 mg/kg given orally every 24 hours. Other immunosuppressive drugs are rarely used in feline renal transplant recipients. Azathioprine (0.3 mg/kg given orally every 3 days) has been used in a few cases, but myelosuppression is a potential problem associated with this drug. In dogs, azathioprine has been used successfully with CyA and prednisone, but hepatotoxicity and pancreatitis are noted side effects. Leflunomide analogs are showing promise, but the expense makes this drug unlikely to become the first-line drug of choice.

MONITORING

Weekly examination is recommended for the first month after transplantation. At each examination the BUN, creatinine, cyclosporine levels, PCV, and body weight are evaluated. The owner should bring in a urine sample for assessment of the urine specific gravity; cystocentesis and urinary catheterization should be avoided to reduce the risk of inducing urinary tract infection. Each examination should be arranged so that a trough CyA level can be drawn. The owner should administer the next dose immediately after blood sampling to maintain the dosing schedule.

As the cat clinically improves and the CyA levels stabilize, examinations are reduced to every 2 weeks for a month, then monthly for 3 months. At that point, quarterly examinations are usually sufficient. Urine culture, complete chemistry panel, and CBC are performed two to four times a year, and a cardiac consultation should be done yearly. Monthly measurement of antibody titers to *Toxoplasma gondii* for the first 6 months has been recommended.[18]

COMPLICATIONS

Rejection

Hyperacute rejection from preformed antibodies occurs in the first several hours after transplantation and has not been reported in clinical cases. In the absence of immunosuppression, acute rejection results in destruction of the kidney in 5 to 8 days. Acute rejection is typically reported within the first

2 to 3 months or at any time CyA levels decline to subthera-peutic values. Early clinical signs, which may be vague, include general malaise, vomiting, anorexia, and depression; the serum creatinine concentration may not be elevated in early rejection. Aggressive antirejection therapy should be started with any suspicion of rejection to reduce the damage to the kidney. Intravenous CyA is administered over 4 to 6 hours (i.e., 6.6 mg/kg given every 24 hours, or 4 mg/kg given twice daily diluted in 20 to 100 mL of 0.9% saline or 5% dextrose).[1,5] Intravenous prednisolone sodium succinate (10 mg/kg given every 12 hours) is also administered. Intravenous fluid therapy is administered to maintain hydration. The BUN and creati-nine concentrations should improve within 24 to 48 hours. Once these concentrations have normalized and the cat is taking food, intravenous medications can be changed to the oral form.

Chronic allograft nephropathy can be caused by chronic rejection or nonimmunologic factors. Arterial hyperplasia, which leads to graft ischemia, is the predominant lesion of chronic allograft nephropathy. Nonimmunologic factors, such as glomerular hyperfiltration due to small kidney size and a reduced number of nephrons, hypertension-induced vascular injury, and cyclosporine toxicity, have not been recognized as major problems in feline transplantation. Graft survival in cats with chronic allograft nephropathy is about 3 years.

Ureteral Obstruction

Ureteral obstruction caused by stricture formation occurs most commonly 7 to 14 days after surgery. Signs include an increase in the creatinine concentration, a decrease in the urine specific gravity, and a dilated renal pelvis and/or ureter on abdominal ultrasonography. Surgical revision of the neoureterostomy site is indicated. Use of a mucosal apposition surgical technique has markedly reduced the incidence of this complication. Obstruction secondary to retroperitoneal fibrosis, an uncommon cause, occurs at 1½ to 5 months after surgery.

Neurologic Signs

A variety of neurologic signs can be encountered in the post-operative period, including seizures, disorientation, obtunda-tion, or coma.[19] In humans, several potential causes have been identified, including infection, hypertension, CyA toxicity, hypomagnesemia, uremic encephalopathy, erythropoietin therapy, and underlying neurologic disease.[12] Cyclosporine has been associated with postoperative neurologic signs, although CyA levels have not been consistently increased in cats that showed neurologic abnormalities. An immediately function-ing graft has been proposed to decrease solute concentrations rapidly, as in dialysis disequilibrium syndrome, a neurologic complication associated with rapid osmolar shifts. A BUN concentration greater than 100 mg/dL and a serum creatinine concentration greater than 10 mg/dL increase the risk of CNS disease by tenfold; preoperative hemodialysis should be considered in this population.[12] Control of hypertension post-operatively reduces neurologic signs, making hypertensive encephalopathy a plausible cause of such signs.[3]

Hypertension

Severe hypertension that occurs in the first 48 hours after surgery can lead to neurologic signs, ataxia, stupor, seizures, blindness, ocular hemorrhage, or retinal detachment. The exact reason for the development of postoperative hyper-tension is unknown. Preoperative hypertension does not pre-dict postoperative hypertension, although volume expansion during surgery may play a role. Vasoactive substances gener-ated in the transplanted kidney during the warm ischemia time may be released when the vascular clamps are opened, resulting in hypertension. Pain associated with the surgery

may exacerbate the hypertension. Diligent blood pressure monitoring for at least 48 hours after surgery is advised. If hypertension develops, treatment with a fast-acting antihy-pertensive agent is indicated (e.g., hydralazine, 2.5 mg given subcutaneously).[3]

Infection

The immunosuppression necessary to prevent rejection pre-disposes recipients to infection. Over 50% of human trans-plant recipients develop infection in the first year, and bacterial UTI is the most common type. In humans, common infections (UTI, surgical wound infection, pneumonia) tend to occur more often in the first month, corresponding to the highest levels of immunosuppression. In cats, bacterial UTI, viral upper respiratory infections, toxoplasmosis, and a variety of fungal infections have been reported.

Because CyA primarily interferes with cell-mediated immunity, unusual infections may arise. Toxoplasmosis has caused fatal infections in three cats and one dog.[18] Infections occurred 3 weeks to 6 months after surgery and were associ-ated with administration of increased immunosuppressive medications in three of the four cases. Transmission of toxo-plasmosis from the donor to the recipient was suspected in one case; reactivation of latent infection was suspected in the three with high levels of immunosuppression. Close monitor-ing of seropositive recipients after surgery is recommended, and treatment with clindamycin is advised if titers rise. Transplant recipients should avoid situations that might expose them to large numbers of other cats, including boarding kennels.

Neoplasia

Human renal transplant recipients on long-term immuno-suppressive therapy have a higher rate of neoplasia compared to the general population. The rate of *de novo* cancer in feline renal transplant recipients is 9.5% to 14%. Lymphosarcoma is the most common neoplasm. Other reported malignancies include squamous cell carcinoma, malignant round cell tumors, hepatic carcinoma, bronchogenic adenocarcinoma, transitional cell carcinoma, and intestinal adenocarcinoma.[5,20]

Miscellaneous Complications

A variety of other complications have been reported. A hemolytic-uremic–like syndrome was reported in three cats[21]; it was characterized by hemolysis, thrombocytopenia, and thrombotic microangiopathy. Intrarenal thrombosis leads to renal cortical necrosis. In children, this syndrome is typi-cally caused by *E. coli* O157:H7 endotoxin; other causes in renal transplant recipients include acute vascular rejection, malignant hypertension, and nephrotoxicity arising from CyA, tacrolimus, or antilymphocyte antibody administration. In cats, the outcome has been graft failure and death. Retroperitoneal fibrosis, characterized by the development of fibrous tissue around the ureter and renal capsule, has been encountered. Surgical debulking of this tissue can relieve ureteral obstruction and renal compression.[22] Hypercalcemia was reported in one cat as a result of primary hyperparathy-roidism.[23] Prednisone and CyA have been implicated in the development of post-transplantation diabetes mellitus, which has been recognized in cats.[24]

OUTCOME

The outcome after transplantation has improved as veterinary surgeons have gained more experience with the procedure. Perioperative mortality is approximately 25%. For cats discharged from the hospital, the 6-month survival rate is 60% to 70%. Mortality is highest in the first 6 months after surgery.

URINARY SYSTEM

Older age at surgery (over 10 years) predicts a worse outcome, particularly in the first 6 months, but in one study these deaths were not attributed to age-related diseases.[12] The overall 3-year survival rate is 40% to 50%.[5,12] In one study, one third of deaths were due to allograft rejection.[12] CNS disease, neoplasia, viral upper respiratory infection, hemolytic-uremic syndrome, gastrostomy tube peritonitis, and a variety of other causes of death have also been reported.

CANINE TRANSPLANTATION

Renal transplantation is not as well established in dogs as in cats. Problems with the efficacy and toxicity of immunosuppressive drugs in dogs make sufficient immunosuppression more difficult. Unacceptable GI toxicity of many immunosuppressive drugs precludes their routine use. Long-term survival in unrelated dogs using rabbit antidog antithymocyte serum, CyA, azathioprine, and prednisone have been reported, but antithymocyte serum is not commercially available.[6] Protocols involving leflunomide, CyA, and prednisone, or CyA, azathioprine, and prednisone are undergoing evaluation in unrelated dogs that are haplotype mismatched.

SUMMARY

Renal transplantation provides a method of treating end-stage renal disease in cats. Successful long-term outcomes are possible, with improved quality of life in addition to prolonged longevity. Careful patient selection is advised. Long-term immunosuppression is necessary. Multiple complications have been encountered, but improvements in surgical technique, management, and monitoring are gradually extending the average survival time of transplant recipients. The procedure is becoming more widely available, and more clients are requesting evaluation and referral of their pets.

CHAPTER • 260

Chronic Kidney Disease

David J. Polzin
Carl A. Osborne
Sheri Ross

OVERVIEW OF CHRONIC KIDNEY DISEASE

Chronic kidney disease (CKD) is the most common kidney disease in dogs and cats. Regardless of the cause or causes of nephron loss, CKD is characterized by irreversible structural lesions. After correcting any reversible primary diseases and prerenal or postrenal components of renal dysfunction, further improvement in kidney function should not be expected in patients with CKD, because compensatory and adaptive changes designed to sustain kidney function have largely already occurred. However, unless additional kidney injury occurs or CKD is very advanced, rapid deterioration of intrinsic kidney function is also unusual. The magnitude of kidney dysfunction typically remains stable or slowly declines over months to years.[1,2] However, it may not be necessary for the disease process responsible for the initial kidney injury to persist for progressive dysfunction to occur. Therefore irrespective of underlying causes, CKD is often described as an irreversible and progressive disease.

Patients with CKD often survive for many months to years with a good quality of life. Although as yet no treatment can correct existing irreversible kidney lesions of CKD, the clinical and biochemical consequences of reduced kidney function can often be ameliorated by supportive and symptomatic therapy. In addition, therapy may be designed to interrupt mechanisms that contribute to the self-perpetuation of progressive CKD.

Chronic Kidney Disease—Defined
Kidney disease is defined as the presence of functional or structural abnormalities in one or both kidneys. It is recognized by reduced kidney function or the presence of kidney damage. Kidney damage is defined as either (1) microscopic or macroscopic renal pathology detected by kidney biopsy or direct visualization of the kidneys or (2) markers of renal damage detected by blood or urine tests or imaging studies (Box 260-1).[3] The severity and clinical implication of kidney disease varies greatly depending on the magnitude of kidney involvement.

CKD is defined as (1) kidney damage that has existed for at least 3 months, with or without decreased glomerular filtration rate (GFR), or (2) a reduction in GFR of more than 50% from normal persisting for at least 3 months. The authors recommend that a duration of at least 3 months be used as the benchmark criterion for confirming the diagnosis of CKD based on the observation that renal compensatory hypertrophy and improvement in renal function may continue for up to 3 months after acute loss of nephrons.

Terms and Concepts Related to Kidney Disease, Kidney Failure, and Uremia
Use of the terms *kidney disease, kidney insufficiency, kidney failure, azotemia,* and *uremia* as synonyms may result in misdiagnosis and formulation of inappropriate or even contraindicated therapy. In addition, it may result in misinterpretation of

Box • 260-1

*Markers of Kidney Damage**

Blood Markers
Elevated blood urea nitrogen (BUN) concentration
Elevated serum creatinine concentration
Hyperphosphatemia
Hyperkalemia or hypokalemia
Metabolic acidosis
Hypoalbuminemia

Urine Markers
Impaired urine-concentrating ability
Proteinuria
Cylinduria
Renal hematuria
Inappropriate urine pH
Inappropriate urine glucose concentration
Cystinuria

Imaging Markers—Abnormalities in Kidney
Size
Shape
Location
Density
Number

*Markers must be confirmed to be of renal origin to be evidence of kidney damage.

epidemiologic data. For example, in the past, confusion has occurred in the interpretation of statistics about the frequency of kidney lesions reported by pathologists. Some investigators misinterpreted data regarding the frequency of morphologic evidence of kidney disease and suggested that all cases with kidney disease had kidney failure.

Kidney disease should not be used synonymously with *kidney failure* or *uremia*. Depending on the quantity of renal parenchyma affected and the severity and duration of lesions, kidney disease or diseases may or may not cause kidney failure or uremia. The clinical relevance of the difference between kidney disease and kidney failure is emphasized by the fact that symptomatic and supportive therapies designed to correct fluid, electrolyte, acid-base, nutrient, and endocrine imbalances in patients with kidney failure typically are not appropriate for patients with kidney disease without kidney dysfunction.

Kidney disease may affect glomeruli, tubules, interstitial tissue, and vessels. Some kidney diseases may be associated with dysfunction (e.g., some forms of nephrogenic diabetes insipidus and some forms of renal tubular acidosis) or biochemical abnormalities (e.g., cystinuria) without detectable morphologic alterations. Others may be associated with morphologic kidney disease (anomalies, infections, endogenous or exogenous toxin-induced lesions, immune-mediated lesions, damage caused by hypercalcemia and other mineral imbalances, traumatic lesions) that affects one or both kidneys with variable effects on kidney function. The specific cause or causes of kidney disease or diseases may or may not be known; however, quantitative information about kidney function (or dysfunction) is not defined or implied by the term *kidney disease*.

Kidney function *adequate* for homeostasis does not require that *all* nephrons be functional. The concept that adequate kidney function is not synonymous with normal kidney function is of importance in understanding the difference between kidney disease and kidney failure; formulating meaningful prognoses; and formulating therapy. The term *kidney failure* is analogous to liver failure or heart failure in that a level of organ dysfunction is described rather than a specific disease entity. Similarly, the term *kidney insufficiency* implies kidney dysfunction, but at a level that is less severe than kidney failure. The kidneys perform multiple excretory, regulatory, and biosynthetic functions including selective elimination of waste products of metabolism from the body, maintenance of fluid, acid-base and electrolyte homeostasis, and synthesis of a variety of hormones. Failure to perform these functions may not be an *all or none phenomenon*. For example, in slowly progressive kidney diseases, failure to appropriately concentrate or dilute urine according to body need typically precedes failure to eliminate waste products of metabolism of such magnitude that it causes azotemia. In turn, laboratory detection of impaired ability to eliminate waste products of metabolism (such as urea and creatinine) and to maintain electrolyte and nonelectrolyte solute balance within normal limits typically precedes the onset of polysystemic signs of kidney dysfunction. Clinical signs and polysystemic disorders caused by abnormalities of water, electrolyte, acid-base, endocrine, and nutrient balance are not invariably present in patients with primary kidney failure (i.e., not all patients with primary kidney failure are uremic). This is related, at least in part, to the reserve capacity of the kidneys and the ability of unaffected nephrons to undergo compensatory hypertrophy and hyperplasia.

In dogs, acute loss of two thirds or more of functional nephrons is associated with loss of adequate urine-concentrating ability, whereas acute loss of three fourths or more of functional nephrons results in azotemia. However, over the subsequent weeks to months, urine-concentrating ability and excretory function improve as a consequence of compensatory hypertrophy and hyperplasia of surviving nephrons. As a consequence, 3 months after loss of three fourths of functioning nephrons, renal concentrating ability is often adequate and azotemia is no longer present. Chronic renal insufficiency therefore implies a 75% reduction in GFR that typically corresponds to a loss of substantially more than 75% of the functional nephrons.

Azotemia is defined as an abnormal concentration of urea, creatinine, and other nonprotein nitrogenous substances in blood, plasma, or serum. Azotemia is a laboratory finding with several fundamentally different causes. Because nonprotein nitrogenous compounds (including urea and creatinine) are endogenous substances, abnormally elevated concentrations in serum may be caused by an increased rate of production (by the liver for urea; by muscles for creatinine), or by a decreased rate of loss (primarily by the kidneys). Because azotemia may be caused by factors that are not directly related to the urinary system and by abnormalities of the lower urinary tract (LUT) not directly related to the kidney, *azotemia* should not be used as a synonym for kidney failure or uremia. Although the concentrations of serum urea nitrogen (SUN) and creatinine are commonly used as crude indices of GFR, meaningful interpretation of these parameters depends on recognition and evaluation of prerenal, primary renal, and postrenal factors that may reduce GFR.

Uremia is defined as (1) abnormal quantities of urine constituents in blood caused by primary generalized kidney disease *and* (2) the polysystemic toxic syndrome which occurs as a result of abnormal kidney function. When the structural and functional integrity of both kidneys has been compromised to such a degree that polysystemic signs of kidney failure are clinically manifested, the relatively predictable symptom complex called *uremia* appears, regardless of underlying cause. In some instances, uremic crises may suddenly be precipitated by prerenal disorders or, less commonly, postrenal disorders in patients with previously compensated primary kidney failure. Uremia is characterized by multiple physiologic and metabolic alterations that result from impaired kidney function.

In summary, kidney disease may precede kidney insufficiency and failure, and likewise, kidney insufficiency and failure may precede uremia. In some situations, kidney disease may not progress to kidney insufficiency or failure. In others, prerenal events may precipitate a uremic crisis in patients with chronic kidney insufficiency or failure. In untreated patients with kidney disease, uremia is always accompanied by kidney failure and azotemia.

Staging Chronic Kidney Disease

Patients with CKD can be categorized into stages along a continuum of progressive kidney disease.[4] The value of staging CKD is to facilitate application of appropriate clinical practice guidelines for diagnosis, prognosis, and treatment. The International Renal Interest Society (IRIS) has proposed a four-tier system for staging CKD in dogs and cats (Box 260-2 and 260-3; Figures 260-1 and 260-2). Although the specific values used to categorize patients with CKD into these stages are inherently arbitrary, staging is nonetheless useful for establishing prognosis and managing patients with CKD.

The stage of CKD is assigned based on the level of kidney function. The level of GFR is accepted as the best measure of overall kidney function in health and disease.[3] Ideally, the stage of CKD would be assigned based on measured GFR values. However, because of technical and economic constraints, GFR is usually estimated in dogs and cats by serum

---

> ## Box • 260-3
>
> ### Stages of Feline Chronic Kidney Disease
>
> **Stage 1 (Nonazotemic)**
> Markers of renal disease present
> Creatinine < 1.6 mg/dL (< 140 µmol/L)
> Proteinuria: Classify—P/NP/BP
> Hypertension: Classify—Hc/Hnc/NH/BH/HND
>
> **Stage 2 (Mild Renal Azotemia)**
> Markers of renal disease present
> Creatinine 1.6-2.8 mg/dL (140-250 µmol/L)
> Proteinuria: Classify—P/NP/BP
> Hypertension: Classify—Hc/Hnc/NH/BH/HND
>
> **Stage 3 (Moderate Renal Azotemia)**
> Creatinine 2.8-5.0 mg/dL (251-440 µmol/L)
> Proteinuria: Classify—P/NP/BP
> Hypertension: Classify—Hc/Hnc/NH/BH/HND
>
> **Stage 4 (Severe Renal Azotemia)**
> Creatinine > 5.0 mg/dL (> 440 µmol/L)
> Proteinuria: Classify—P/NP/BP
> Hypertension: Classify—Hc/Hnc/NH/BH/HND

P, Proteinuria; *NP*, nonproteinuria; *BP*, borderline proteinuria; *Hc*, hypertension with complications; *Hnc*, hypertensive with no complications; *NH*, nonhypertensive; *BH*, borderline hypertensive; *HND*, hypertension not determined.

> ## Box • 260-2
>
> ### Stages of Canine Chronic Kidney Disease
>
> **Stage 1 (Nonazotemic)**
> Markers of renal disease present
> Creatinine < 1.4 mg/dL (< 125 µmol/L)
> Proteinuria: classify—(P/NP/BP)
> Hypertension: classify—(Hc/Hnc/NH/BH/HND)
>
> **Stage 2 (Mild Renal Azotemia)**
> Markers of renal disease present
> Creatinine 1.4-2.0 mg/dL (125-180 µmol/L)
> Proteinuria: classify—(P/NP/BP)
> Hypertension: classify—(Hc/Hnc/NH/BH/HND)
>
> **Stage 3 (Moderate Renal Azotemia)**
> Creatinine 2.1-5.0 mg/dL (181-440 µmol/L)
> Proteinuria: Classify—(P/NP/BP)
> Hypertension: Classify—(Hc/Hnc/NH/BH/HND)
>
> **Stage 4 (Severe Renal Azotemia)**
> Creatinine > 5.0 mg/dL (> 440 µmol/L)
> Proteinuria: Classify—(P/NP/BP)
> Hypertension: Classify—(Hc/Hnc/NH/BH/HND)

P, Proteinuria; *NP*, nonproteinuria; *BP*, borderline proteinuria; *Hc*, hypertension with complications; *Hnc*, hypertensive with no complications; *NH*, nonhypertensive; *BH*, borderline hypertensive; *HND*, hypertension not determined.

(or plasma) creatinine concentration. Limitations on specificity and sensitivity of serum creatinine concentration as an estimate of GFR can lead to misclassification. Ideally, two or more serum creatinine values obtained when the patient is fasted and well hydrated should be determined over several weeks to stage CKD. Further, variations between laboratories, patient-specific characteristics (e.g., breed, age, gender, body condition, and lean body mass) and transient prerenal and postrenal events may influence serum creatinine values. Reduced muscle mass, a common manifestation of advanced CKD, may result in a substantial reduction in serum creatinine concentration relative to true GFR. Greyhounds reportedly have higher serum creatinine concentrations, presumably due to their athletic nature.[5] Because of these variations, published reference ranges for serum creatinine are often exceedingly broad. Using the staging system described here, some patients classified as having mild renal azotemia (stage 2) may have serum creatinine values within published reference ranges. As a consequence, the patient's overall clinical status should be considered when interpreting serum creatinine concentration and other laboratory tests and when planning patient management.

Stage 1 CKD includes dogs and cats with CKD that are not azotemic, whereas stage 2 CKD includes dogs and cats that are mildly azotemic (see Boxes 260-2 and 260-3). Patients in these stages of CKD typically do not have clinical signs of kidney dysfunction with the exception of polyuria and polydipsia. Occasionally cats with stage 2 CKD may have weight loss or selective appetites. However, patients may have clinical signs resulting from their kidney lesions (e.g., acute pyelonephritis, nephrolithiasis). Patients with marked proteinuria or systemic hypertension due to CKD may have clinical signs related to these aspects of kidney disease. Renal function is often stable for an extended period in nonproteinuric, nonhypertensive (NH)

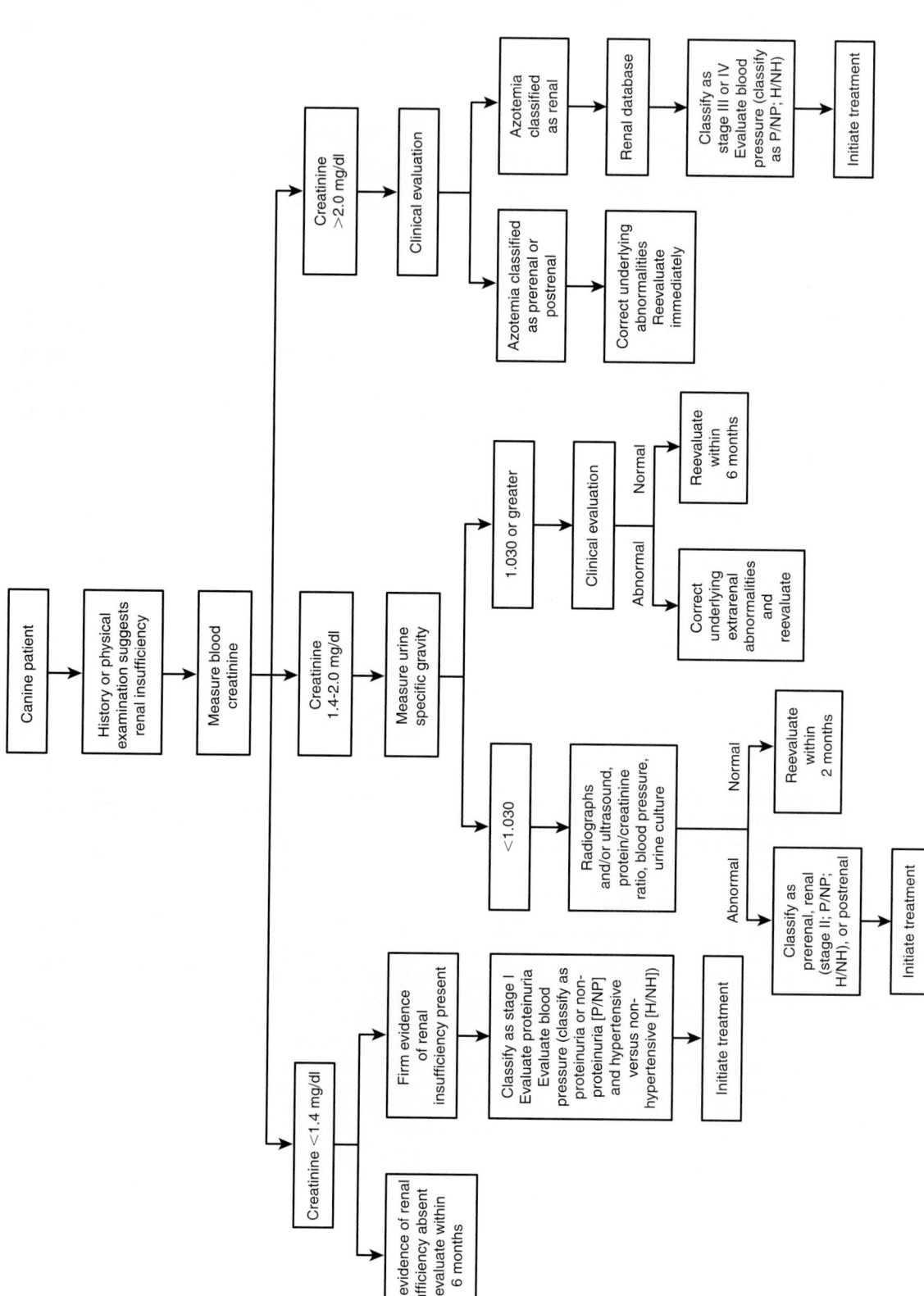

Figure 260-1 Classification of canine chronic kidney disease (CKD) based on serum creatinine concentrations. Firm evidence of renal disease in stage 1 would generally be morphologic, such as abnormal renal architecture on survey radiographs, abnormal renal ultrasound findings, or biopsy diagnosis of renal disease. Classification of prerenal azotemia (generally due to dehydration or renal ischemia) or postrenal azotemia (generally due to ureteral obstruction, urethral obstruction, or a rupture of a portion of the urinary tract) is based on careful evaluation of the history and physical examination and other clinical or imaging findings. This determination may require additional tests. Classification of azotemia as renal is based on the presence of azotemia with no identifiable prerenal or postrenal causes and urine specific gravity (USG) less than 1.030. (Developed by the International Renal Interest Society, www.iris-kidney.com. Used with permission.)

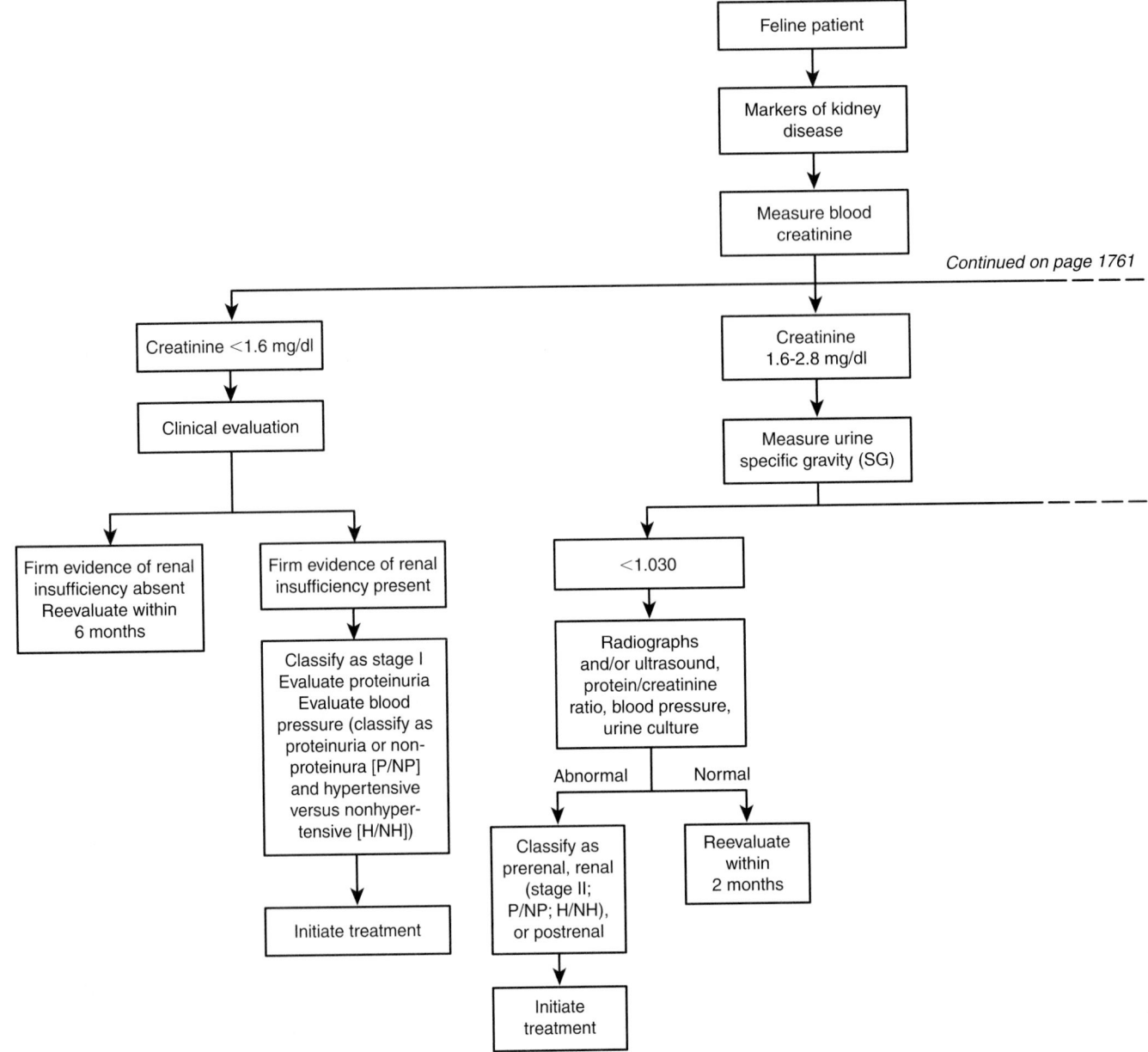

Continued on page 1761

Figure 260-2 Classification of feline chronic kidney disease (CKD) based on serum creatinine concentrations. Firm evidence of renal disease would generally be morphologic, such as abnormal renal architecture on survey radiographs, abnormal renal ultrasound findings, or biopsy diagnosis of renal disease. Classification of prerenal azotemia (generally due to dehydration or renal ischemia) or postrenal azotemia (generally due to ureteral obstruction, urethral obstruction, or a rupture of a portion of the urinary tract) is based on careful evaluation of the history and physical examination and other clinical or imaging findings. Classification of azotemia as renal is based on the presence of azotemia with no identifiable prerenal or postrenal causes and urine specific gravity (USG) less than 1.040. (Developed by the International Renal Interest Society www.iris-kidney.com. Used with permission.)

dogs and cats with stages 1 and 2 CKD. However, when progression does occur in this group of patients, it may occur largely as a consequence of their primary kidney disease.[4] Patients with stages 1 and 2 CKD should be evaluated with the goals of identifying and providing specific treatment for their primary kidney disease. In addition, renal function should be monitored to assess for possible progression of their kidney disease.

Patients with moderate azotemia are classified as stage 3 CKD. Patients in this stage may have clinical signs referable

to their loss of kidney function; however, with appropriate treatment, they typically do not have clinical signs of overt uremia. Patients with stage 3 CKD may progress due to inherent mechanisms of spontaneous progression, as well as their underlying kidney disease. Therefore in addition to identifying and treating primary kidney disease, therapy designed to modify factors promoting progression of renal disease may be of benefit to these patients.

Stage 4 CKD includes dogs and cats with severe azotemia (serum creatinine values greater than 5.0 mg/dL). This stage

Continued from page 1760

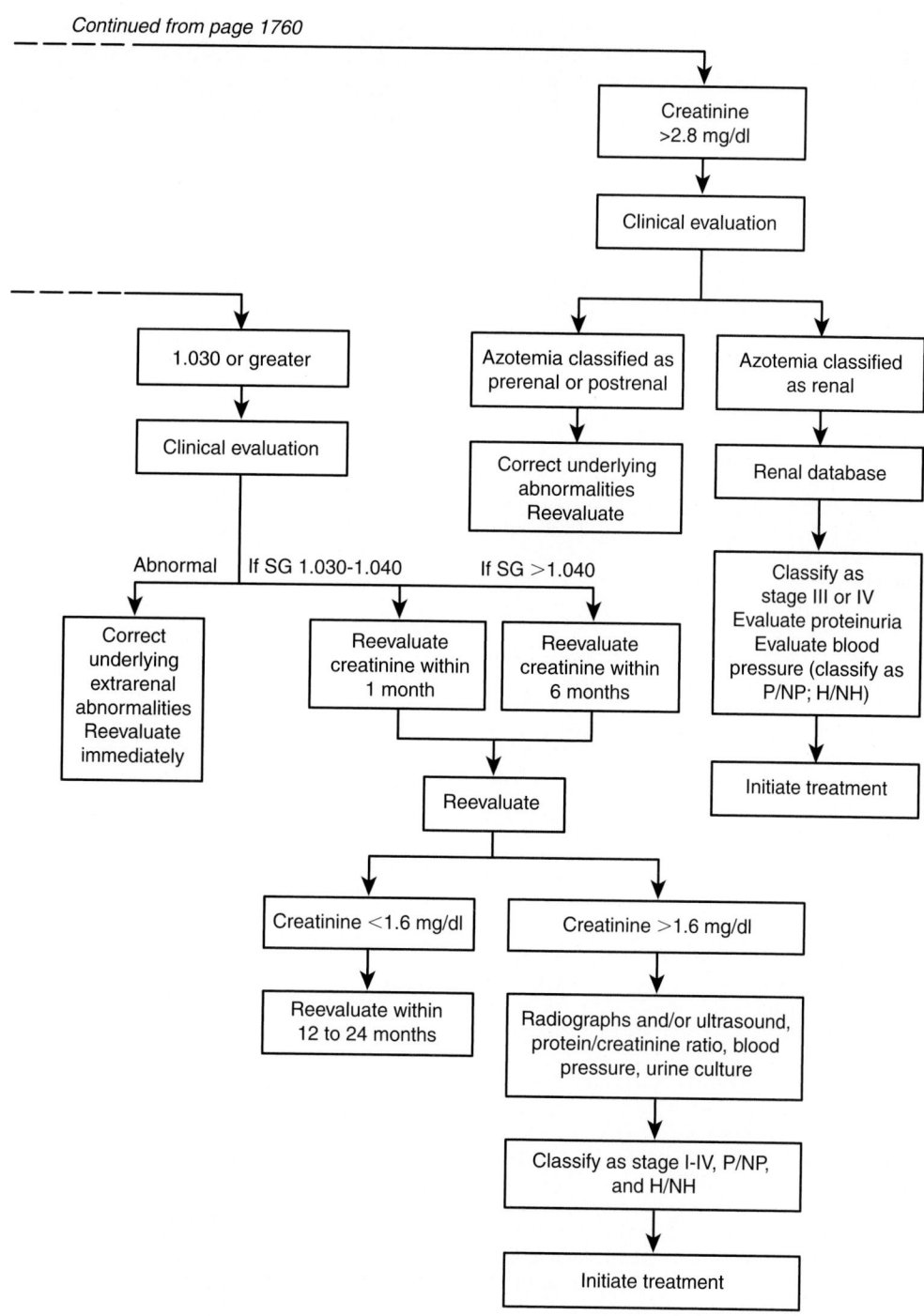

URINARY SYSTEM

is also called *chronic kidney failure* and is frequently associated with clinical signs that occur as a consequence of loss of kidney function. Diagnostic and therapeutic initiatives in this stage include those appropriate for stage 3 patients, as well as therapy designed to prevent or ameliorate signs of uremia.

It is useful to further subclassify patients according to their urine protein loss and systemic blood pressure. Proteinuria and hypertension may influence prognosis and may be amenable to therapeutic intervention. Classification of patients as proteinuric necessitates eliminating hemorrhage, inflammation, or both as the cause for proteinuria and determination of the urine protein/creatinine ratio. For both dogs and cats, patients are classified as proteinuric (P) when their protein/creatinine ratio exceeds 1.0. Values between

0.5 and 1.0 are classified as borderline proteinuric (BP). Values less than 0.5 are classified as nonproteinuric (NP). Patients with borderline proteinuria should be re-evaluated after 2 months to reassess classification. In some patients, classification of proteinuria may change due to the natural course of their disease or in response to therapy. The role of microalbuminuria in this classification scheme remains to be determined.

The lack of consensus as to what blood pressure values constitute hypertension in dogs and cats obfuscates any classification of patients as to their hypertension status. It is likely that "normal" blood pressure values for dogs and cats will change as more data become available. The IRIS has proposed the following hypertension classification system for dogs and cats: Patients may be classified as hypertensive with no complications (Hnc) when their systolic blood pressure exceeds 160 mm Hg and no extrarenal evidence of hypertension exists (i.e., ocular, neurologic, or cardiac changes consistent with hypertensive injury). Patients may be classified as hypertensive with extrarenal complications (Hc) when their systolic blood pressure exceeds 150 mm Hg and extrarenal evidence of hypertension is present. Patients may be classified as borderline hypertensive (BH) when their systolic blood pressure is between 150 mm Hg and 180 mm Hg and no extrarenal evidence of hypertension exists. Patients may be classified as NH when their systolic blood pressure is less than 150 mm Hg. If blood pressure has not been determined, the patient should be classified as hypertension not determined (HND).

Affected Population

CKD is a common cause for illness and death in dogs and cats. It is among the most common diseases recognized in older cats. The prevalence of kidney disease has been estimated to range between 0.5%[6] and 7%[7] in dogs and between 1.6%[6] and 20%[7] in cats.

Although frequently considered a disease of older animals, CKD occurs with varying frequency in dogs and cats of all ages. In a retrospective study of cats with CKD, 53% of affected cats were over 7 years old, but animals ranged in age from 9 months to 22 years.[8] In a study on age distribution of kidney disease in cats based on data submitted from 1980 to 1990 to the Veterinary Medical Data Base at Purdue University, 37% of cats with renal failure were less than 10 years old, 31% of cats were between the ages of 10 and 15, and 32% of cats were older than 15 years of age.[9] Similarly, in a study of cats with CKD reported in 1988, their mean age was 12.6 years with a range of 1 to 26 years.[10] Mean age among 45 control cats in this study was 10.0 years. During 1990, the prevalence of kidney disease among cats of all ages was reportedly 16 cases for every 1000 cats examined. During the same year, the prevalence of kidney disease among cats 10 years of age or older was 77 per 1000 cats examined, and among cats older than 15 years, 153 per 1000.[8] Maine coon, Abyssinian, Siamese, Russian blue, and Burmese cats were disproportionately reported as affected.

Although renal failure apparently occurs less commonly in dogs than cats, its incidence increases similarly with age. Based on data submitted from 1983 to 1992 to the Veterinary Medical Data Base at Purdue University, 18% of dogs with renal failure were less than 4 years old, 17% of dogs were between the ages of 4 and 7, 20% of dogs were between the ages of 7 and 10, and 45% of dogs were older than 10 years of age. During this period, the prevalence of renal failure among dogs of all ages was nine cases for every 1000 dogs examined. The prevalence of renal failure among dogs 7 to 10 years of age was 12.5 per 1000 dogs examined; among dogs 10 to 15 years, 24 per 1000, and among dogs older than 15 years, 57 per 1000.

Causes of Chronic Kidney Disease

CKD may be initiated by a variety of different familial, congenital, or acquired diseases (Box 260-4). In a study of biopsy findings in 37 dogs with primary renal azotemia, chronic tubulointerstitial nephritis was observed in 58%, glomerulonephropathy occurred in 28%, and amyloidosis was observed in 6%.[11] In cats, tubulointerstitial nephritis was observed in 70%, glomerulonephropathy occurred in 15%, lymphoma was observed in 11%, and amyloidosis occurred in 2%. Unfortunately, the initiating cause or causes of CKD often cannot be identified at the time of diagnosis. The initiating causes of diseases thought to originate in the tubulointerstitium have been especially elusive. Although bacteria can cause tubulointerstitial lesions, in the authors' experience, a

---

Box • 260-4
Disorders That May Cause Chronic Renal Failure

Familial or Congenital
  Dogs
    Amyloidosis in Shar Pei and beagle dogs
    Cystadenocarcinoma in German shepherd dogs
    Renal dysplasia in Shi Tzu, Lhasa apso, golden
      retrievers, Norwegian Elkhounds, Chow Chows,
      and others
    Glomerulopathy in English cocker spaniels,
      Doberman pinschers, bull terriers,
      soft-coated Wheaton terriers, Samoyeds
    Fanconi syndrome in Basenjis
    Polycystic disease in Cairn terriers
  Cats
    Amyloidosis in Abyssinian cats and oriental
      shorthair cats
    Polycystic disease in Persian and Himalayans
Acquired
  Infectious
    Bacterial
    Mycotic—blastomycosis
    Leptospirosis
    Leishmaniasis
    Feline infectious peritonitis (FIP)
  Immune complex glomerulopathy
    (Consult Chapter 261 on glomerulopathies)
  Amyloidosis
  Neoplasia
    Lymphosarcoma
    Renal cell carcinoma
    Nephroblastoma
    Others
  Sequela of acute renal failure
  Bilateral hydronephrosis
    Spay granulomas
    Transitional cell carcinoma—bladder trigone location
    Nephrolithiasis
  Polycystic
  Hypercalcemia
    Malignancy
    Primary hyperparathyroidism
  Idiopathic

---

bacterial urinary tract infection (UTI) is more often a sequela of the immunocompromised condition associated with renal failure than the cause. In one retrospective study of renal failure cats, bacterial UTI was detected in 20% of the patients.[9] Glomerulonephropathies have been linked to a variety of neoplastic, metabolic, and infectious and noninfectious inflammatory processes.[12] Periodontal disease has been linked to microscopic renal lesions in dogs, but a cause-and-effect relationship has not been established.[13] Feline immunodeficiency virus (FIV) has been linked to renal disease in cats, although few cats with CKD are FIV positive.[14,15] Subcutaneous administration of feline herpesvirus 1 (FHV-1), calicivirus, and panleukopenia virus vaccines grown in feline tissue culture systems to kittens have been shown to induce production of antifeline renal tissue antibodies in serum (Lappin and colleagues).[16] This observation prompts the question as to whether repeated vaccinations play a role in development of chronic renal disease.

Difficulty in detecting the inciting cause of CKD is associated with three phenomena related to the evolution of progressive renal diseases. First, various components of nephrons (glomeruli, peritubular capillaries, tubules, and interstitial tissue) are functionally interdependent. Second, the functional and morphologic responses of tissues comprising the kidneys to different causative agents are limited. Third, after maturation of nephrons, which occurs at approximately 1 month of age, new nephrons cannot be formed to replace others irreversibly destroyed by disease. Progressive irreversible lesions initially localized to one portion of the nephron are eventually responsible for development of lesions in the remaining but initially unaffected portions of nephrons. For example, progressive lesions (such as amyloid or immune complex disease) confined initially to glomeruli will subsequently decrease peritubular capillary perfusion. Reduced peritubular capillary perfusion will in turn result in tubular epithelial cell atrophy, degeneration, and necrosis. Recent studies suggest that tubular epithelial cells may also be damaged as a consequence of glomerular proteinuria. Secondary tubular damage may be related, at least in part, to excessive tubular cell uptake of filtered proteins or protein-bound substances.[17] Studies showing that the rate of disease progression correlates with the amount of proteinuria, and that therapy designed to reduce proteinuria retards progression, support the concept that glomerular proteinuria damages tubules. The secondary processes of inflammation and fibrosis amplify these processes. An influx of T cells and macrophages into the interstitium may cause further tubular injury, and macrophages in particular produce profibrotic substances. Ultimately nephron destruction initiated by glomerular disease will simulate repair by substitution of functioning nephrons with nonfunctional connective tissue.

Similarly, generalized progressive interstitial disease initially caused by bacteria eventually destroys tubules and glomeruli and stimulates inflammation and fibrosis. Thus irrespective of the initiating cause, replacement of the majority of the damaged nephrons with collagenous connective tissue results in overall reduction in kidney size and impaired renal function.

Because of the structural and functional interdependence of various components of nephrons, differentiation of different progressive renal diseases that have reached an advance stage is often difficult. Functional and structural changes prominent during earlier phases of progressive generalized renal diseases may permit identification of a specific cause and localization of the initial lesion to glomeruli, tubules, interstitium, or vessels. With time, however, destructive changes of varying severity (atrophy, inflammation, fibrosis, and mineralization of diseased nephrons), superimposed on compensatory and adaptive morphologic and functional of remaining partially and totally viable nephrons, provide a functional and morphologic similarity to the findings associated with these diseases.

Despite the irreversibility of generalized renal lesions associated with CKD, it is important to formulate diagnostic plans to try to identify the underlying cause and to determine if it is still active. Although specific therapy directed at eliminating or controlling the primary cause will not substantially alter existing renal lesions, it is important in the context of minimizing further nephron damage. Renal diseases potentially amenable to specific therapy include bacterial pyelonephritis, chronic urine outflow obstruction, nephrolithiasis, renal lymphoma (particularly in cats), hypercalcemic nephropathy, and some immune-mediated diseases.

Acute onset of nonurinary disorders, especially those that interfere with compensatory polydipsia, may precipitate a uremic crisis in patients with asymptomatic CKD (so-called acute-on-chronic uremic crisis). However, if acute decompensation of CKD has been caused by reversible factors, correction of them will often result in recompensation of the CRF.

Prognosis of Chronic Kidney Disease

Cats with stages 2 and 3 CKD commonly survive 1 to 3 years, whereas dogs with stage 3 CKD typically survive about 6 to 12 months. However, many survive much longer. A host of factors influence prognosis of CKD, both favorably and unfavorably. Included among these factors are the quality of medical care provided to the patient and the level of owner commitment. The estimate of prognosis often influences the owner's decisions about treatment options in complying with recommendations for management of the patient. A comprehensive evaluation of the patient is the best way to establish a reasonably accurate prognosis.

Prognosis for patients with CKD is usually subcategorized according to the probability of immediate survival (short-term prognosis) and survival over the subsequent months to years (long-term prognosis). A guarded prognosis indicates that the chances for recovery are unpredictable. Fair, good, or excellent prognoses indicate varying degrees of probable recovery, whereas poor or grave prognoses indicate that recovery is improbable or hopeless. Loss of renal function is irreversible in patients with CKD. In this context, recovery refers to improvement of biochemical deficits and excesses and amelioration of clinical signs rather than recovery of renal function.

Factors to be considered in establishing meaningful prognoses for patients with CKD include (1) the nature of the primary renal disease, (2) severity and duration of clinical signs and complications of uremia, (3) probability of improving renal function (reversibility—primarily of prerenal, postrenal, and newly acquired primary renal conditions), (4) severity of intrinsic renal functional impairment, (5) rate of progression of renal dysfunction with or without therapy, and (6) age of the patient. In addition, blood pressure and the magnitude of proteinuria are risk factors influencing prognosis in dogs with CKD.[18]

Severity of uremic signs is often a relatively good predictor of short-term prognosis. Patients with stable CKD without clinical signs of uremia usually have a good short-term prognosis. Untreated patients with severe clinical signs of uremia typically have a guarded to poor short-term prognosis. However, it is best to determine whether renal function and clinical signs can be therapeutically improved in such cases before establishing the short-term prognosis. A uremic crisis often occurs in patients that present with CKD as a consequence of superimposed acute renal failure or prerenal or postrenal conditions. Although CKD is an irreversible condition, improvement of renal function is potentially possible when uremia results from the sum effects of CKD and a potentially reversible cause of azotemia. If treatment results in improved renal function and ameliorates clinical signs of uremia, the short-term prognosis often becomes guarded to good.

Severity of renal dysfunction as determined by serum creatinine concentration or measurement of GFR provides a less accurate means of assessing short-term prognosis than does the clinical condition of the patient. The relationship between magnitude of renal dysfunction and clinical signs of uremia is often unpredictable. Therefore short-term prognosis should not be established based on a single measurement of the severity of renal dysfunction. In addition, a single determination of renal function is unreliable as an index of the potential for improvement in renal function.

Assessment of the severity of renal dysfunction is typically more useful in establishing long-term prognoses. In general, severe renal dysfunction is associated with shorter long-term survival and, often, a lower quality of life. This generalization is supported by findings of a recent study of cats with spontaneous CKD.[2] For cats with CKD without apparent clinical signs and having a mean plasma creatinine concentration of 2.6 mg/dL, mean survival was 397 days. For cats with CKD with one or more clinical signs attributable to CKD and a mean plasma creatinine concentration of 3.6 mg/dL, mean survival was 313 days. Uremic cats with a mean plasma creatinine concentration of 10.3 mg/dL survived less than 3 days. However, in a recent clinical trial in dogs with spontaneous CKD, mean serum creatinine concentration did not appear to influence survival when dogs were fed a renal diet. Median survival for 21 dogs with a mean serum creatinine concentration of 3.3 mg/dL was 615 days. Median survival for a subpopulation of dogs in this group with serum creatinine values between 2.0 and 3.1 mg/dL was also 615 days. However, among 17 dogs fed a maintenance diet in this study, median survival for dogs with a mean serum creatinine of 3.7 mg/dL was 252 days, whereas survival for the subpopulation with serum creatinine values between 2.0 and 3.1 mg/dL was 461 days. In summary, the prognosis should be established in the context of the clinical condition of the patient, rate of progression of renal dysfunction, response to therapy, cause of the underlying renal disease (if known), and other complicating factors (e.g., UTI, nephrotic syndrome).

Systemic hypertension has been linked to progression of CKD in humans for decades.[19] Increased systolic blood pressure has been shown to increase risk of uremic crises and death in dogs with spontaneous CKD.[18] In this study, systolic blood pressure values determined at the time of initial patient evaluation were compared with long-term outcome. Increased risk of developing a uremic crisis and of death was observed in the patients with the highest blood pressure values. In addition, a greater decline in renal function over time was observed in these dogs. Although this study was not designed to prove a cause-and-effect relationship between hypertension and progressive renal disease, it does indicate that initial blood pressure values should be considered in formulating a prognosis for dogs with CKD. The prognostic significance of blood pressure values in cats with CKD has yet to be established.

Results of a clinical trial from the University of Minnesota Veterinary Medical Center revealed that proteinuria is a risk factor for uremia and death in dogs with spontaneous kidney disease.[20] In this study, the risk of death associated with CKD increased by 60% for each unit of urine protein/ creatinine ratio above 1.0. Whether proteinuria conferred this adverse risk as an independent mediator of renal injury or as a consequence of the biologic behavior of glomerular diseases is unclear. In dogs, glomerulopathies have been associated with poor long-term prognoses.[12] This may be related to the observation that proteinuria has been implicated in promoting progressive renal injury.[21] Therapeutic amelioration of proteinuria using angiotensin-converting (ACE) inhibitors may stabilize renal function in humans and dogs with glomerular disease, further suggesting a likely role for proteinuria in the progression of CKD.[22]

Compared with the rate of progression of CKD in middle-aged to older dogs with acquired renal disease, CKD often progresses at a much slower rate in dogs with congenital and familial nephropathies such as renal dysplasia. A comparably slower rate of progression has also been observed in young dogs with acquired CKD (e.g., after nephrotoxin exposure). Many of these patients appear remarkably resistant to developing clinical signs of uremia despite substantial elevations in serum creatinine and urea nitrogen concentrations.

CLINICAL CONSEQUENCES OF CHRONIC RENAL FAILURE

Uremia

Uremia is the clinical state toward which all progressive, generalized renal diseases ultimately converge. Diverse clinical and laboratory findings characterize uremia and emphasize the polysystemic nature of CKD (Box 260-5). The term *uremia* was adopted originally because of the presumption that all of the abnormalities result from retention in the blood of end-products of metabolism normally excreted in the urine. However, uremia involves more than renal excretory failure alone. A variety of metabolic and endocrine functions normally performed by the kidney are also impaired, resulting in anemia; malnutrition; impaired metabolism of carbohydrates, fats, and proteins; defective use of energy; alterations in immunity; and metabolic bone disease.

Urea, once thought to be "the" uremic toxin, is not a major cause of uremic toxicity, although it may contribute to some of the clinical abnormalities, including anorexia, malaise, and vomiting. Numerous nitrogenous compounds with a molecular mass of 500 to 12,000 D (so-called middle molecules) are retained in CKD and appear to contribute to morbidity and mortality in uremic subjects.[23] In addition to impaired excretion, many middle-sized molecules along with various cytokines and growth factors accumulate in CKD because the kidney's capacity for catabolizing many substances is also impaired. Further, plasma levels of many polypeptide hormones, including parathyroid hormone (PTH), insulin, gastrin, glucagon, luteinizing hormone (LH), and prolactin, increase in patients with CKD because of impaired renal catabolism and enhanced glandular secretion.

Gastrointestinal Consequences

Gastrointestinal (GI) complications are common and prominent clinical signs of uremia. Anorexia and weight loss are nonspecific findings that may precede other signs of uremia in dogs and cats. The patient's appetite may be selective for certain foods, and it may wax and wane throughout the day. Factors promoting weight loss and malnutrition include anorexia, nausea, vomiting and the subsequent reduction in nutrient intake, hormonal and metabolic derangements, and catabolic factors related to uremia, particularly acidosis.

Anorexia appears to be multifactorial in origin. Recent research, using a rodent model, has suggested that an *anorectic factor* in the plasma of uremic patients that can suppress appetite.[24] It appears to be a middle molecule in size and may

---

Box • 260-5

Complications and Comorbid Conditions in Chronic Kidney Disease

Complications of Chronic Kidney Disease (CKD)
Anemia
Arterial hypertension
Dehydration
Hyperparathyroidism
Hyperphosphatemia
Hypocalcemia and hypercalcemia
Hypokalemia
Malnutrition
Metabolic acidosis
Uremic signs

Comorbid Conditions
Cardiac disease
Degenerative joint disease
Dental and oral diseases
Hyperthyroidism (cats)
Nephroliths and ureteroliths
Urinary tract infections (UTIs)

be a peptide. Elevated serum leptin concentrations have also been implicated as a factor contributing to anorexia.[25]

Vomiting is a frequent, but inconsistent finding in uremia. It results from the effects of as yet unidentified uremic toxins on the medullary emetic chemoreceptor trigger zone and from uremic gastroenteritis. The severity of vomiting correlates crudely with the magnitude of azotemia. Because uremic gastritis may be ulcerative, hematemesis may occur. Vomiting may be a more frequent complaint in uremic dogs than cats. Nonetheless, vomiting is reportedly found in one quarter to one third of cats with clinical signs of uremia.[2] Vomiting may impair compensatory polydipsia, enhancing the risk of dehydration and exacerbating prerenal azotemia and clinical signs of uremia.

Uremic gastropathy is characterized microscopically by glandular atrophy, edema of the lamina propria, mast cell infiltration, fibroplasia, mineralization, and submucosal arteritis. Elevated gastrin levels have been implicated in development of uremic gastropathy.[26] Gastrin induces gastric acid secretion directly by stimulating receptors located on gastric parietal cells and by increasing histamine release from mast cells in the gastric mucosa. Enhanced histamine release may also promote GI ulceration and ischemic necrosis of the mucosa through a vascular mechanism characterized by small venule and capillary dilatation, increased endothelial permeability, and intravascular thrombosis.[27] Because up to 40% of the circulating gastrin is metabolized by the kidneys, reduced renal function may promote hypergastrinemia.

Elevated gastrin levels have been documented in cats with spontaneous CKD.[26] Although the prevalence of hypergastrinemia appeared to increase as renal dysfunction became more severe, there was great variability of gastrin levels among cats with similar degrees of renal dysfunction, suggesting that additional factors (in addition to the degree of renal impairment) likely affect serum gastrin levels in CKD.

Gastrin-induced gastric hyperacidity may lead to uremic gastritis, GI hemorrhage, nausea, and vomiting. Back diffusion of hydrochloric acid and pepsin into the stomach wall may lead to hemorrhage, inflammation, and release of histamine from mast cells. Thus the cycle may be perpetuated as mast cell–derived histamine causes further stimulation of parietal cells to produce hydrogen ions. However, gastric hyperacidity is not universally found with uremic gastritis. Some human uremic patients have hypochlorhydria. Thus hypergastrinemia is not the only reason for uremic gastritis. Other factors implicated in the genesis of uremic gastropathy include psychologic stress related to illness, an increase in proton back diffusion caused by high urea levels, erosions caused by ammonia liberated by bacterial urease acting on urea, ischemia caused by vascular lesions, decreased concentration and turnover of gastric mucous, and biliary reflux due to pyloric incompetence (which may be an indirect consequence of elevated gastrin levels).

In a recent study of 80 cats with spontaneous CKD, dysphagia and oral discomfort occurred in 7.7% of uremic cats and 38.5% of cats with end-stage renal failure.[2] Periodontal disease was observed in 30.8% of uremic and 34.6% of end-stage CKD cats in the same study. Halitosis was reported in 7.7% of cats in both groups. Moderate to severe CKD may result in uremic stomatitis characterized by oral ulcerations (particularly located on the buccal mucosa and tongue), brownish discoloration of the dorsal surface of the tongue, necrosis and sloughing of the anterior portion of the tongue (associated with fibrinoid necrosis and arteritis), and uriniferous breath. The mucous membranes may also become dry (xerostomia). Degradation of urea to ammonia by bacterial urease may contribute to many of these signs. Poor oral hygiene and dental disease may exacerbate the onset and severity of uremic stomatitis.

Uremic enterocolitis, manifested as diarrhea, may occur in dogs and cats with severe uremia, but it is typically less dramatic and less common than uremic gastritis. Owners of 80 cats with spontaneous CKD did not report diarrhea.[2] However, when present, uremic enterocolitis is often hemorrhagic. Considerable GI hemorrhage may initially escape clinical detection. Intussusception may occasionally complicate uremic enterocolitis. Constipation is a relatively common complication of CKD, particularly in cats. Primarily it appears to be a manifestation of dehydration, but it can occur as a complication of intestinal phosphate-binding agents.

Impaired Urine-Concentrating Ability, Polyuria, Polydipsia, and Nocturia

Among the earliest and most common clinical manifestations of CKD is onset of polyuria, polydipsia, and sometimes nocturia due to reduced urine-concentrating ability. Polydipsia was the single most commonly reported clinical sign reported in a study of 80 cats with CKD. Cat owners recognized polydipsia over twice as often as polyuria. Although urine specific gravity (USG) values of cats in stages 2, 3, and 4 CKD are usually below 1.035, the authors have seen cats that have remained persistently (up to 18 months) azotemic prior to losing adequate concentrating ability (i.e., specific gravity > 1.040).

A decrease in adequate urine-concentrating ability results from several factors including increased solute load per surviving nephron (solute diuresis), disruption of the renal medullary architecture and counter-current multiplier system by disease, and primary impairment in renal responsiveness to antidiuretic hormone (ADH). Loss of renal responsiveness to ADH may result from an increase in distal renal tubular flow rate, which limits equilibration of tubular fluid with the hypertonic medullary interstitium. Additionally, ADH-stimulated adenyl cyclase activity and water permeability in the distal nephron may be impaired in uremia.[28] Polydipsia is of course a compensatory response to polyuria. If fluid intake fails to keep pace with urinary fluid losses, dehydration will ensue because of the inability to conserve water by concentrating urine. Dehydration subsequent to inadequate fluid intake is a common problem in cats with CKD.

Arterial Hypertension and Cardiovascular Consequences

Hypertension may be either a cause or consequence of CKD. When present, it may adversely affect long-term prognosis.[18] It is a common complications of CKD, reportedly occurring in up to 66% of cats with CKD.[29] Although one recent study suggested that hypertension may be unusual in dogs with CKD,[30] other studies have reported incidences of from 30% to 93% of dogs with CKD.[18,30] Dogs with glomerular diseases are at increased risk for hypertension.

The pathophysiology of arterial hypertension and its complications is described in Chapters 129 and 130.

Neuromuscular Consequences

Encephalopathies and Neuropathies Metabolic encephalopathies and peripheral neuropathies may occur in dogs and cats with uremia.[31,32] It is reported that as many as 65% of dogs and cats with primary renal insufficiency or renal failure have neurologic manifestations. Of dogs with neurologic signs, altered consciousness (31% of patients) and seizures (29% of patients) were the most common signs.[32] In the authors' experience, acute onset of altered mentation is an important neurologic finding in dogs and cats with CKD that typically heralds a poor short-term prognosis. Other common signs include limb weakness, ataxia, and tremors. Patients may develop what has been described as the *twitch-convulsive* state, wherein the simultaneous combination of tremor, myoclonus, and seizures is seen. In advanced CKD, patients may have neurologic signs that are cyclical and episodic, varying from day to day. The severity and rate of progression of neurologic signs appears to vary directly with the rapidity with which uremia develops.

The pathogenesis of uremic neurologic signs remains unclear, but important roles for PTH and the uremic environment are suspected.[31] Both the sodium potassium adenosine triphosphate pump and several of the calcium pumps are altered in uremia. Alterations in the calcium pumps have been thought to be due at least in part to PTH acting through monophosphate-independent pathways. Calcium pumps are particularly suspected of playing a role in uremic encephalopathy because they mediate neurotransmitter release and information transfer at nerve terminals. Clinical signs of tremors, myoclonus, and tetany may develop due to hypocalcemia. Arterial hypertension may also lead to neurologic signs in patients with otherwise well-controlled renal failure. Clinical signs are acute in onset and may include seizures, behavioral changes, dementia, isolated cranial nerve deficits, and death. In the authors' experience, many of the patients with acute onset of neurologic signs also had hypertension.

Imbalances of neurotransmitter amino acids within the brain have also been implicated in uremic encephalopathy. Analysis of cerebrospinal fluid (CSF) in humans with uremic encephalopathy has shown decreased levels of glutamine and GABA, as well as increased levels of glycine, dopamine, and serotonin.

Myopathies Hypokalemic polymyopathy is occasionally observed in association with CKD, primarily in cats. Because of the influence of potassium on resting cell membrane potentials, potassium imbalances typically manifest clinically as neuromuscular dysfunction. Hypokalemia increases the magnitude (i.e., increases electronegativity) of the resting potential, thereby hyperpolarizing the cell membrane, making it less sensitive to exciting stimuli. The cardinal and most dramatic sign of hypokalemia, regardless of cause, is generalized muscle weakness. In hypokalemic polymyopathy, muscle weakness and pain present clinically as cervical ventroflexion and a stiff, stilted gait.[33] Mild cardiac rhythm disturbances may also occur. Serum creatinine kinase and other muscle enzyme activities may be elevated, and in severe instances, rhabdomyolysis may occur.

Muscle dysfunction unrelated to serum potassium concentrations may also occur in uremia. In humans with CKD, accumulation of a dialyzable uremic toxin derived from dietary protein has been shown to promote abnormalities in sarcolemma ion flux leading to reduced muscle membrane potential.

Hematologic Consequences

Anemia The anemia of renal failure is usually characterized by normochromic and normocytic red blood cells (RBCs). Usually hypoplasia of the erythroid precursors in the bone marrow occurs, with little or no interference with normal leukopoiesis and megakaryocytopoiesis. On blood smears, spiculed and deformed red cells (burr cells or echinocytes) may be noted. Although affected by the patient's age, species, specific renal diagnosis, and concurrent diseases, the severity and progression of the anemia correlates with the degree of renal failure and worsens with progressive renal failure in both dogs and cats.[34]

The hematocrit may become profoundly low. At these low hematocrits, compensatory mechanisms such as increased levels of 2,3 DPG; lowered peripheral vascular resistance; and an elevated cardiac output (in the absence of previous cardiac disease) help maintain tissue oxygenation. Clinical signs of anemia include pallor of the mucous membranes, fatigue, listlessness, lethargy, weakness, and anorexia.

Anemia in patients with CKD is multifactorial and may be exacerbated by concurrent illness. Although experimental and clinical evidence exists for the supporting roles of shortened red cell life span, nutritional abnormalities, erythropoietic inhibitor substances in uremic plasma, blood loss, and myelofibrosis, erythropoietin deficiency has clearly emerged as the principal cause of anemia in humans and animals with CKD. The peritubular fibroblasts of the renal cortex appear to be the major source of erythropoietin synthesis. It may also be produced by renal interstitial fibroblasts. The kidneys synthesize erythropoietin on demand in response to intrarenal tissue hypoxia due either to decreased oxygen-carrying capacity (anemia) or decreased oxygen content (hypoxia). Many CKD patients have a relative, rather than absolute, erythropoietin deficiency in that plasma levels exceed the normal range.[35] However, when compared with equivalently anemic but nonuremic patients, plasma erythropoietin concentrations are lower. Anemic CKD cats have been reported to have plasma erythropoietin concentrations similar to normal cats.[36] Erythropoietin deficiency of CKD has been hypothesized to result from decreased renal mass resulting in an insufficient cellular capacity for new hormone synthesis.

Other clinically important causes for anemia in dogs and cats with CKD are iron deficiency and chronic GI blood loss. In most patients, iron deficiency can only be detected by measuring serum iron, staining bone marrow biopsy samples for iron content, or through response to iron supplementation. Chronic GI hemorrhage may occur even in the absence of characteristic color changes in the feces. It can be suspected based on a hematocrit level that is unexpectedly low relative to the magnitude of renal dysfunction, and an elevation in the SUN/serum creatinine ratio.

Hemorrhagic Consequences of Uremia Uremia may be associated with a hemorrhagic diathesis that is characterized by bruising, GI hemorrhage with hematemesis or melena, bleeding from the gums, or hemorrhage subsequent to venipuncture. GI hemorrhage can be an important route of blood loss leading to anemia and exacerbating azotemia and uremia. In renal failure, bleeding results from an acquired qualitative platelet defect, abnormalities in the interaction of platelets and the vessel wall, and biochemical and rheologic abnormalities in the blood itself.[37] Uremic platelet dysfunction appears to be multifactorial in origin. The platelet count is usually within the normal range or mildly decreased. Abnormal platelet aggregability, diminished thromboxane-A$_2$ production, abnormal intracellular calcium mobilization, and increased intracellular cAMP have been described in uremic platelets.[37] Abnormal glycoprotein function may impair platelet adhesiveness to the subendothelium. In addition, uremia may be associated with increased release of prostacyclin and nitric oxide, which may also impair adhesion of platelets to the endothelium. The largest polymers of von Willebrand's factor, which predominate in the platelet adhesion process, are decreased in uremia. Uremic toxins have also been implicated in impairing platelet function. For example, elevated levels of plasma guanidinosuccinic acid, interfere with activation of platelet factor III by ADP, thus leading to abnormal platelet function. Administration of desmopressin acetate (DDAVP) has been shown to shorten bleeding times and improve clinical bleeding in uremic humans.[37] DDAVP is thought to stimulate release of large multimeric von Willebrand's factor complexes from endothelial cells and platelets.

Unfortunately, development of tachyphylaxis often limits usefulness of DDAVP after 2 or 3 doses. Alternative therapies have included administration of cryoprecipitates or conjugated estrogens, which may have similar effects. Increasing hematocrit values to above 30 by transfusion or administration of erythropoietin has also been shown to improve bleeding times in humans. Increasing hematocrit may improve bleeding times by a rheologic effect or by increasing hemoglobin concentrations that may in turn inactivate the platelet-inhibiting effects of nitric oxide.

Renal Secondary Hyperparathyroidism

Incidence and Pathophysiology In a recent study of cats with spontaneous CKD, the overall prevalence of renal secondary hyperparathyroidism was 84%.[38] Hyperparathyroidism occurred in 100% of cats with end-stage CKD and 47% of asymptomatic cats with only biochemical evidence of CKD. Hyperparathyroidism was even detected in some cats with normal serum calcium and phosphorous concentrations. Plasma PTH concentrations have been reported to increase as serum creatinine concentrations increase.[39]

The pathogenesis of hyperparathyroidism in CKD is multifactorial. Renal secondary hyperparathyroidism occurs in association with phosphorous retention, hyperphosphatemia, low circulating 1,25-dihydroxyvitamin D (calcitriol) levels, reduced blood ionized calcium concentration, and skeletal resistance to the calcemic action of PTH. However, in early to moderate renal failure, it is difficult to dissect out the specific factors responsible for hyperparathyroidism because the increase in PTH serves to prevent hypocalcemia, hyperphosphatemia, and the decrease in calcitriol formation.[40] Phosphorous retention and hyperparathyroidism develop early in CKD, although serum calcium and phosphorus concentrations remain within normal limits.[41] Phosphorous retention is intimately related to development of secondary hyperparathyroidism.[42,43]

Relative or absolute deficiency of calcitriol has been hypothesized to play a pivotal role in development of renal secondary hyperparathyroidism.[44] Calcitriol, the most active form of vitamin D, is formed by 1α-hydroxylation of 25-hydroxycholecalciferol in renal tubular cells. PTH promotes renal 1α-hydroxylase activity and formation of calcitriol. In turn, calcitriol limits PTH synthesis by feedback inhibition. Phosphorous retention inhibits renal 1α-hydroxylase activity. Early in the course of CKD, the inhibitory effects of phosphorus retention on renal tubular 1α-hydroxylase activity limits calcitriol production. Because calcitriol normally inhibits PTH synthesis, reduced calcitriol synthesis promotes renal secondary hyperparathyroidism. Initially, the resultant hyperparathyroidism increases 1α-hydroxylase activity despite continued phosphorous retention, thereby restoring calcitriol production toward normal. However, normalization of calcitriol production occurs at the expense of persistently elevated plasma PTH activities—a classic example of the *trade-off hypothesis*. As renal failure progresses, loss of viable renal tubular cells ultimately limits renal calcitriol synthetic capacity and calcitriol levels subsequently remain low. Deficiency of calcitriol leads to skeletal resistance to the action of PTH and elevates the set point for calcium-induced suppression of PTH secretion. Skeletal resistance to PTH limits skeletal release of calcium, whereas elevating the setpoint for PTH secretion allows hyperparathyroidism to persist even when plasma ionized calcium concentrations are normal or elevated.[39,44]

Recent evidence suggests that phosphorous retention may also play a primary role in promoting hyperparathyroidism. Phosphorous has been shown to stimulate PTH secretion in parathyroid cell cultures.[45] Further, phosphorous restriction in dogs and humans with CKD has been shown to decrease PTH secretion without changing serum calcitriol levels.[46,47] In untreated human patients with mild to moderate CKD (serum creatinine concentration ≤3.0 mg/dL), serum phosphorus concentrations correlated directly with PTH, independent of serum calcium and 1,25-dihydroxyvitamin D levels.[48] Interestingly, this correlation was present despite the fact that most patients had serum phosphorous concentrations within the normal range. Notably, in both humans and cats, overt hyperphosphatemia may not be a prerequisite for phosphorous

to have an effect on PTH secretion.[38,48] It has been suggested that high phosphorous intake may accentuate uremia-induced abnormal phosphorous metabolism causing increased parathyroid cell phosphorous concentration.[48] *In vitro* studies have suggested that parathyroid glands exposed to elevated phosphorous levels respond by increasing PTH secretion.[45] Reduced 1,25-dihydroxycholecalciferol may have a permissive effect, may have an additional direct effect on PTH secretion in this setting, or it may have both.[48]

In more advanced renal failure, only serum calcium concentration correlated with serum PTH activity.[48] Impaired intestinal absorption of calcium due to low serum calcitriol levels likely plays an important role in hyperparathyroidism in these advanced renal failure patients. Blood ionized calcium concentrations are often reduced in cats with spontaneous CRF; in one study, over 50% of cats with advanced end-stage CKD were hypocalcemic.[38]

Clinical Consequences Although renal secondary hyperparathyroidism and renal osteodystrophy, are well-documented effects of CKD, clinical signs associated with renal osteodystrophy are uncommon in dogs and cats. In dogs, it most often occurs in immature patients, presumably because metabolically active growing bone is more susceptible to the adverse effects of hyperparathyroidism. For unexplained reasons, bones of the skull and mandible may be the most severely affected and may become so demineralized that the teeth become moveable and fibrous changes are obvious, particularly in the maxilla. Marked proliferation of connective tissue associated with the maxilla may cause distortion of the face. Jaw fractures can occur but are uncommon. Other possible but uncommon clinical manifestations of severe renal osteodystrophy include, cystic bone lesions, bone pain, and growth retardation.

Although excessive levels of PTH affect bones and kidneys, it affects the function of other organs and tissues, including brain, heart, smooth muscles, lungs, erythrocytes, lymphocytes, pancreas, adrenal glands, and testes as well.[49] Toxicity of PTH appears to be mediated through enhanced entry of calcium into cells with PTH or PTH2 membrane receptors. Sustained PTH-mediated calcium entry leads to inhibition of mitochondrial oxidation and production of ATP. Extrusion of calcium from cells is reduced because of the impairment in ATP production and disruption of the sodium-calcium exchanger. Persistently increased basal cytosolic calcium levels promote cellular dysfunction and death.[39]

Potential nonskeletal clinical consequences of hyperparathyroidism include mental dullness and lethargy, weakness, anorexia, and an increased incidence of infections due to immunodeficiency.[39] Hyperparathyroid-induced cellular dysfunction may lead to carbohydrate intolerance, platelet dysfunction, impaired cardiac and skeletal muscle function (due to impaired mitochondrial energy metabolism and myofiber mineralization), inhibition of erythropoiesis, altered red cell osmotic resistance, altered B cell proliferation, synaptosome and T cell dysfunction, and defects in fatty acid metabolism.[39,50] Excess PTH levels may also promote nephrocalcinosis and consequent progressive loss of renal function.[39]

Renal secondary hyperparathyroidism may be associated with substantial enlargement of the parathyroid glands. This finding may be of clinical importance in cats because of frequent coincident hyperthyroidism that may be suggested by the presence of a thyroid nodule palpable in the cervical region. In a recent report, hyperplastic parathyroid glands were palpable as paratracheal masses in 11 of 80 cats with spontaneous CKD.[2] Care should be taken to confirm hyperthyroidism prior to treatment because both hyperparathyroidism and hyperthyroidism can lead to paratracheal masses.

URINARY SYSTEM

Plasma PTH concentrations should be determined by methods that measure intact PTH using a two-site immunoradiometric or immunochemiluminometric assay. The two-site method uses antibodies directed against two different regions of the intact PTH molecule. A commercially available two-site immunoradiometric assay (Allegro Intact PTH, Nichols Institute Diagnostics, San Juan Capistrano, CA) has been validated for use in dogs and cats. Only intact PTH will be recognized because it will be the only form of the peptide to have both determinants. Older PTH assays typically detect those species of hormone that contain amino acids located in the midregion (43 to 68) of the PTH molecule.

However, because renal insufficiency and failure results in reduced renal clearance of the nonbiologically active midregion PTH fragments, these methods do not accurately reflect parathyroid glandular secretion. Thus renal secondary hyperparathyroidism is best monitored by use of a two-site assay for intact hormone.

Laboratory Findings

Metabolic Acidosis Metabolic acidosis is a common manifestation of CKD. It results primarily from the limited ability of failing kidneys to excrete hydrogen ions, because of reduced ammoniagenesis, decreased filtration of phosphate and sulfate compounds, and decreased maximal renal tubular proton secretion.[51] Impaired renal tubular reabsorption of filtered bicarbonate may also contribute to acidosis. Bicarbonate wasting and chloride retention results in hyperchloremic (normal anion gap) acidosis. When phosphorous and organic acid (uric acid, hippuric acid, lactic acid) retention is sufficient, high anion gap acidosis results.

A combination of tubular reabsorption of filtered bicarbonate and excretion of hydrogen ions with ammonia and urinary buffers, primarily phosphorous, maintains normal acid-base balance. As renal function declines, hydrogen ion excretion is maintained largely by increasing the quantity of ammonium excreted by surviving nephrons. However, at some level of renal dysfunction, the capacity to further increase renal ammoniagenesis is lost and metabolic acidosis ensues. Decreased medullary recycling of ammonia due to structural renal damage may also contribute to impaired ammonium excretion.

Chronic metabolic acidosis may promote a variety of adverse clinical effects including anorexia, nausea, vomiting, lethargy, weakness, muscle wasting, weight loss, and malnutrition. Alkalization therapy is often of value in reversing these signs. In addition, chronic mineral acid feeding to dogs has been shown to increase urinary calcium excretion and progressive bone demineralization, the magnitude of which depends on age and dietary calcium levels. Studies on the effects of dietary acidification in cats have revealed that chronic metabolic acidosis can cause negative calcium balance and bone demineralization or negative potassium balance, which may in turn promote hypokalemia, renal dysfunction, and taurine depletion.[52]

Severe acidemia may result in decreased cardiac output, arterial pressure, and hepatic and renal blood flows and centralization of blood volume.[53] Centralization of blood volume results from peripheral arterial vasodilatation and central venoconstriction. Decreases in central and pulmonary vascular compliance may predispose patients to pulmonary edema during fluid administration, an effect that may be particularly important in patients with acute uremic crises requiring intensive fluid therapy. Acidemia also promotes re-entry arrhythmias and a reduction in the threshold for ventricular fibrillation. Severe acidosis may also influence carbohydrate and protein metabolism, serum potassium concentrations, and brain metabolism.

Chronic acidosis may promote protein malnutrition in patients with CKD. Protein catabolism is increased in patients with acidosis to provide a source of nitrogen for hepatic glutamine synthesis, glutamine being the substrate for renal ammoniagenesis.[54] The combined effects of reduced protein synthesis due to uremia and accelerated proteolysis due to acidosis promote elevations in blood urea nitrogen (BUN), increased nitrogen excretion, and negative nitrogen balance typical of uremic acidosis. Altered branched chain amino acid metabolism appears to be involved. Chronic metabolic acidosis increases the activity of muscle branched chain keto acid dehydrogenase, the rate-limiting enzyme in branched chain amino acid catabolism. This is important in that branched chain amino acids are rate limiting in protein synthesis and play a role in regulation of protein turnover. Alkalization therapy effectively reverses acidosis-associated protein breakdown. Clinicians speculate that changes in intracellular pH accompanying acidosis lead to alterations in gene transcription which increase the activity of the cytosolic, ATP- and ubiquitin-dependent protein degradation pathway. Severe chronic metabolic acidosis has the potential to induce a cycle of progressive protein malnutrition and metabolic acidosis. Excessive protein catabolism may lead to protein malnutrition despite adequate dietary intake. This process may then accelerate breakdown of endogenous cationic and sulfur-containing amino acids, thus promoting further acidosis.

Acidosis poses a particularly vexing problem for CKD patients consuming protein-restricted diets. Dietary protein requirements appear to be similar for normal humans and humans with CKD unless uremic acidosis is present. When acid-base status is normal, adaptive reductions in skeletal muscle protein degradation protect patients consuming low-protein diets from losses in lean body mass. Metabolic acidosis blocks the metabolic responses to dietary protein restriction in two ways: (1) it stimulates irreversible degradation of the essential, branched chain amino acids; and (2) it stimulates degradation of protein in muscle.[54] Thus acidosis may limit the ability of patients to adapt to dietary protein restriction. Metabolic acidosis also suppresses albumin synthesis in humans and may reduce the concentration of serum albumin. These findings have not yet been confirmed in dogs and cats.

Azotemia Azotemia is defined as an excess of urea or other nonprotein nitrogenous compounds in the blood. Loss of renal function leads to accumulation of a wide variety of nonprotein nitrogen-containing compounds, including urea and creatinine. Many waste products of protein catabolism are excreted primarily by glomerular filtration. Thus patients with primary renal failure have impaired ability to excrete proteinaceous catabolites because of marked reduction in GFR. Retention of metabolic waste may be further aggravated by impaired tubular secretion, and by extrarenal factors that promote renal hypoperfusion and increased catabolism of body tissues. Although accumulation of wastes is largely the result of decreased renal excretion or increased protein catabolism, production of some compounds may also be increased (e.g., guanidine). Because these compounds are derived almost entirely from protein degradation, their production increases when dietary protein increases.

Urea is synthesized using nitrogen derived from amino acid catabolism. Urea may be excreted by the kidneys, retained in body water, or metabolized to ammonia plus carbon dioxide by bacteria in the GI tract. Ammonia produced in the GI tract is recycled to urea in the liver yielding no net loss of nitrogen or urea. Regardless of whether urea per se is toxic, BUN concentrations are typically directly related to the protein content of the diet. Further, in patients with renal failure, BUN concentrations tend to correlate reasonably well with clinical signs of uremia. For practical purposes, BUN may thus be viewed as a marker of retained *uremic toxins*.

In addition to increasing protein intake and declining renal function, BUN concentrations may also be increased by

GI hemorrhage, enhanced protein catabolism, decreasing urine volumes (due to prerenal factors such as dehydration), and certain drugs (e.g., glucocorticoids). Urea nitrogen concentrations may decline with portosystemic shunts, hepatic failure, and low protein diets. Reduced BUN concentration may also indicate protein calorie malnutrition. Because many extrarenal factors may influence BUN concentration, creatinine is often used as a more reliable measure of GFR in patients with CKD.

BUN concentrations should be interpreted with knowledge of simultaneously obtained serum creatinine values, particularly in patients consuming reduced protein diets. The ratio of BUN/serum creatinine concentration should decline when dietary protein intake is reduced. In patients consuming reduced protein diets, an increase in the ratio of BUN/serum creatinine concentrations may suggest poor dietary compliance, enhanced protein catabolism, GI hemorrhage, dehydration, anorexia or declining muscle mass.

Hyperphosphatemia The kidneys play a pivotal role in regulating phosphorus balance because they are the primary route of phosphorus excretion. Renal phosphorus excretion is the net of glomerular filtration less tubular reabsorption of phosphorus. If dietary phosphorus intake remains constant, a decline in GFR will lead to phosphorus retention and ultimately hyperphosphatemia. However, during the early stages of renal failure, serum phosphorus concentrations typically remain within the normal range because of a compensatory decrease in phosphorous reabsorption in the surviving nephrons. This renal tubular adaptation is largely an effect of renal secondary hyperparathyroidism. Increased PTH levels promote renal excretion of phosphorous by reducing the tubular transport maximum for phosphorous reabsorption in the proximal tubule via the adenyl cyclase system. When GFRs decline below about 20% of normal, this adaptive effect is no longer able to prevent hyperphosphatemia.

In dogs with CKD, serum phosphorus concentrations typically parallel SUN concentrations. Thus hyperphosphatemia is common in azotemic patients but unexpected in patients with nonazotemic renal disease. The primary consequence of hyperphosphatemia is development and progression of secondary hyperparathyroidism. Increases in serum PTH activities in dogs and humans with CKD are closely associated with the degree of hyperphosphatemia.[39,48] Hyperphosphatemia was found to be 72% efficient in predicting hyperparathyroidism in cats with CKD.[38]

The combination of hyperphosphatemia and a normal plasma calcium concentration produces an elevated calcium-phosphate product ($Ca \times PO_4$ in units of mg/dL). If the calcium-phosphate product exceeds approximately 70, a tendency exists for calcium phosphate to precipitate in arteries, joints, and soft tissues. This process is commonly called *metastatic calcification*. Calcification is especially prominent in proton-secreting organs, such as the stomach and kidneys, in which basolateral bicarbonate secretion results in an increase in pH that promotes calcium hydrogen phosphate (brushite) precipitation.[55] However, myocardium, lung, and liver are also commonly mineralized in patients with CKD.

Hyperphosphatemia has been directly linked to increased mortality in humans and dogs with CKD.[56,57] In humans with CKD receiving hemodialysis therapy, the adjusted relative risk of mortality was stable in patients with serum phosphorous concentrations below 6.5 mg/dL, but increased significantly above this level.[56] Patients with serum phosphorous in the 6.6 to 7.8 mg/dL range had 13% higher mortality than patients in the reference range (4.6 to 5.5 mg/dL). Patients in the 7.9 to 16.9 mg/dL range had a relative mortality risk 34% higher than patients in the reference range. Mild hyperphosphatemia (5.0 to 6.5 mg/dL) was not associated with an elevated mortality risk.

The calcium × phosphorous product showed a mortality risk trend similar to that seen for phosphate with patients with $Ca \times PO_4$ products greater than 72 having a relative mortality risk of 1.34 relative to products between 42 and 52 mg^2/dL^2.[56] Mortality risk associated with hyperphosphatemia appeared to be independent of elevated PTH levels, which alone appeared to have only a weak association with mortality. However, the statistical association between PTH and mortality may have been impaired by use of multiple methods for PTH assay in the patients studied. Analysis of calcium revealed no correlation with relative risk of death.[2]

Hypercalcemia, Hypocalcemia, and Hypermagnesemia
Hypocalcemia is a common disorder of calcium found in patients with renal failure. In a recent report, ionized hypercalcemia was detected in 6% and ionized hypocalcemia in 26% of 80 cats with spontaneous CKD.[38] Further, mean blood ionized calcium concentration was significantly lower in CKD cats in this study than in normal control cats, and over half of the cats with advanced end-stage CKD were hypocalcemic. However, when these same 80 cats were evaluated using total serum calcium concentrations, hypercalcemia was found in 21% of the cats, whereas hypocalcemia was detected in only 8%. Clearly, serum total calcium concentrations do not reliably reflect ionized calcium concentrations in cats with CKD. Similar discrepancies have been observed in dogs with CKD.[58] The mechanism of serum total hypercalcemia in the face of normal to reduced blood ionized calcium concentrations is unclear but may be related to increased concentrations of calcium complexed to retained organic and inorganic anions such as citrate, phosphate, or sulfate.

In patients with hypercalcemia, it is important to ascertain whether hypercalcemia is the cause, rather than result of CKD. Hypercalcemia due to malignancy or hypervitaminosis D is most likely to induce renal failure. One way of discriminating the cause-and-effect relationship between hypercalcemia and renal failure is to determine the patient's blood ionized calcium concentration. Only ionized hypercalcemia promotes renal failure. However, true ionized hypercalcemia may occur in patients with CKD as a consequence of excessive doses of calcitriol or calcium-containing intestinal phosphate-binding agents or in patients with severe renal secondary hyperparathyroidism with marked hyperplasia of the parathyroid glands. The authors have also observed small increases in ionized calcium concentrations in dogs with early to moderate CKD that are not receiving calcitriol or calcium therapy and do not have advanced hyperparathyroidism. The mechanism of ionized hypercalcemia in these dogs is unclear.

Hypermagnesemia is common in CKD because the kidneys are primarily responsible for magnesium excretion.[38] Typically in CKD, the protein binding of magnesium is normal, complexed magnesium is usually increased, and ionized magnesium may be increased, normal, or decreased. Although the homeostatic mechanisms involved in the control of magnesium are not well documented, they appear to rely on the bone, gut, and kidney, as found with calcium and phosphorous control.

Hypokalemia An association between CKD and hypokalemia has been recognized in cats by several investigators.[59,60] In contrast, hypokalemia appears to be an uncommon finding in untreated dogs with CKD, occurring primarily as an iatrogenic complication of fluid therapy in this species. A particularly intriguing concept is that hypokalemia may be a cause of CKD in cats, rather than simply a consequence of it. In a recent uncontrolled study of the long-term effects of feeding a potassium-restricted, acidifying diet, evidence of renal dysfunction developed in three of 9 cats; renal lesions consisting of lymphoplasmacytic interstitial nephritis and interstitial fibrosis were observed in five of the 9 cats.[60] However, it is not

URINARY SYSTEM

clear whether potassium depletion or hypokalemia preceded the onset of renal failure. In another study, four of seven cats with induced CKD fed a diet containing 0.3% potassium developed hypokalemia, whereas four cats with normal renal function fed the same diet did not develop hypokalemia.[61] Interestingly, muscle potassium content decreased in normokalemic cats with spontaneous CKD, indicating that a total-body deficit of potassium may develop well before the onset of hypokalemia.[62] These findings support the concept that reduced renal function precedes development of hypokalemia.

The mechanism of hypokalemia in cats with CKD has remained elusive, but inadequate intake and increased renal losses appear to be likely candidates. Inadequate intake of potassium could reflect decreased appetite or insufficient dietary potassium content. Dietary risk factors for hypokalemia include acidifying ingredients, reduced magnesium content, and high protein content. It has yet to be established that renal potassium wasting occurs in cats with CKD.

Normally the kidneys closely regulate potassium. Although large quantities of K^+ appear in glomerular filtrate, essentially all is reabsorbed before reaching the distal tubules. The majority of potassium appears in urine as a result of potassium secretion from tubular cells into the lumen in the distal nephron. Potassium excretion in these segments of the nephron is sensitive to tubular flow rates; rapid urine formation promotes potassium secretion, whereas slow urine formation limits potassium secretion. Distal potassium secretion is modulated by potassium reabsorption by the intercalated cells in the cortical and outer medullary collecting tubules. Thus in potassium depletion, net potassium absorption rather than secretion may occur in the distal nephron.

In patients with CKD, the residual nephrons maintain potassium balance by increasing distal tubular secretion of potassium. GI secretion of potassium (primarily in the colon) also appears to increase in CKD and may play an important role in modulating potassium balance. Because of these adaptations, most dogs and cats with CKD are able to tolerate normal dietary potassium intake (about 0.6% dry matter) until renal dysfunction is very severe. However, the ability to rapidly excrete a potassium load may be impaired in CKD resulting in transient hyperkalemia.

Although hypokalemia continues to be detected with some regularity in cats with CKD, its neuromuscular manifestations are uncommon. Presumably this change is the result of an increase in the potassium content of feline diets that has occurred over the past decade in response to the problem of hypokalemia in cats with CKD.

Although generalized muscle weakness has been described as the cardinal sign of hypokalemia, decreased renal function and anorexia are probably more common manifestations of hypokalemia in cats with CKD. In many cats with CKD and hypokalemia, renal function improves after potassium supplementation and restoration of normokalemia, suggesting that hypokalemia may induce a reversible, functional decline in GFR. Recently, renal function was shown to be adversely affected in normal cats when an acidified, potassium-restricted diet was fed.[63] Potassium depletion and acidosis appeared to have additive effects in impairing renal function in this study. Based on these results, it was hypothesized that in cats with CKD, a self-perpetuating cycle of excessive urinary potassium losses and whole-body potassium depletion may develop that is likely to further decrease in renal function. Feeding acidified diets or dietary acidifiers to cats with CKD was suggested to exacerbate their tendency develop potassium depletion.

Potassium imbalances may disrupt a variety of cell functions. Hypokalemia-impaired protein synthesis has been hypothesized to promote weight loss and poor hair coat.[33] Marked potassium depletion has also been linked to polyuria resulting from decreased renal responsiveness to ADH. This antagonism to ADH appears to be due to interference with generation and action of cyclic AMP and to impairment of the countercurrent mechanism. Locally generated prostaglandins may mediate at least part of this effect.

Progression of Chronic Kidney Disease

A progressive decline in kidney function typically occurs over months to years in dogs and cats with naturally occurring kidney diseases.[64] It is logical to assume that CKD progresses as a consequence of continuing renal damage induced by the disease process that initiated CRF. Although this assumption may be at least partially correct for some patients, the initiating cause cannot be identified at the time of diagnosis of CKD in most patients. Instead, renal lesions observed in progressive nephropathies of diverse origins typically include focal segmental glomerulosclerosis and tubulointerstitial lesions (including tubular dilation and interstitial inflammation and fibrosis). Glomerular lesions accompanied by varying levels of proteinuria are typical of progressive kidney diseases including primary tubulointerstitial diseases. In humans, both the decline in GFR and long-term prognosis are more closely related to the extent of associated tubulointerstitial lesions than glomerular lesions.[65]

In rodents, loss of a critical mass of functional renal tissue invariably leads to failure of the remaining nephrons, suggesting that CKD may progress through mechanisms independent of the initiating cause.[66] For example, removal of approximately three quarters or more of the nephrons in rats by surgical resection, infarction, or a combination of these techniques, results in a syndrome of progressive azotemia, proteinuria, arterial hypertension, and eventually death due to uremia. Lesions that develop in the remaining kidney remnant include focal segmental glomerulosclerosis and tubulointerstitial lesions, including tubular dilation and interstitial inflammation and fibrosis. Progressive renal injury and loss of renal function occurs in this rodent model of kidney failure, despite the fact that the remaining kidney remnant was initially normal.

Numerous studies have been performed in an attempt to determine if findings obtained in partially nephrectomized rodents are relevant in dogs and cats. Reducing renal mass in dogs and cats resulted in mild proteinuria, glomerulopathy, and tubulointerstitial renal lesions.[61,67,68] Although these findings are consistent with observations in rats, reducing renal mass by seven eighths or less did not consistently result in a progressive decline in GFR. In studies performed at the University of Georgia, progressive decline in GFR was detected in dogs in which renal mass had been reduced by fifteen sixteenths.[57] These findings confirm that progressive renal disease develops in dogs; however, a marked reduction in renal mass may be necessary to initiate this process in an otherwise normal remnant kidney.

The preponderance of clinical and experimental evidence suggests that in dogs and cats with stages 3 and 4 CKD, progression of renal disease may result, at least in part, from factors unrelated to the activity of the inciting disease.[4,69,70] These factors may include intraglomerular hypertension, glomerular hypertrophy, hypertension, proteinuria, tubulointerstitial disease, and intrarenal precipitation of calcium phosphate.

Intraglomerular Hypertension and Glomerular Hypertrophy

Long-term elevations in intraglomerular pressure, resulting from transmission of systemic pressures, glomerular hemodynamic processes, or both, appear to be deleterious over time. Intraglomerular hypertension, with consequent glomerular hyperfiltration, occur as a compensatory event designed to maintain the total GFR as nephrons are lost to disease. In glomerular diseases, intraglomerular hypertension may also occur as a compensatory adaptation to reduction in permeability of the glomerular capillary wall to small solutes and water. In this setting, the fall in GFR is minimized by elevating intraglomerular pressure. Primary renal vasodilatation may occur in some diseases such as diabetes mellitus. A compensatory increase in glomerular size may also occur in all of these settings.

The mechanisms by which intraglomerular hypertension and hypertrophy injure glomeruli are incompletely understood, because multiple factors are involved. Intraglomerular hypertension may directly injure endothelial cells of the glomerular capillaries. In addition, increased glomerular diameter and increased capillary wall stress may cause detachment of glomerular epithelial cells from the glomerular capillary walls. The consequent focal areas of denudation permit increased flux of water and solutes through the glomerular capillary wall. However, macromolecules cannot cross the glomerular basement membrane and are trapped in the subendothelial space.

The result is formation of characteristic *hyaline deposits* in glomeruli that progressively narrow the capillary lumens, thereby decreasing glomerular perfusion and filtration. Increased strain on mesangial cells can stimulate them to produce cytokines and extracellular matrix. The release of cytokines, such as transforming growth factor-β (TGF-β) and platelet-derived growth factor, may mediate the rise in matrix synthesis.[71] The consequent expansion of mesangial matrix further encroaches on the capillary surface area.

Although these effects lead to the characteristic glomerular lesions of progressive nephropathies, intraglomerular hypertension also impairs glomerular permselectivity leading to proteinuria. Proteinuria is thought to be an important pathophysiologic link between glomerular injury, tubulointerstitial injury, and progression of renal disease.

Systemic Hypertension
In humans, the association between systemic hypertension and kidney disease is well established. The Multiple Risk Factor Intervention Trial (MRFIT) identified systemic hypertension as a significant risk factor for development of end-stage kidney disease.[72] A similar association has recently been identified in dogs.[18] Further, in the Modification of Diet in Renal Disease (MDRD) study, the level of systemic blood pressure was linked to progression of kidney disease among black and proteinuric human CKD patients.[73]

Systemic hypertension leads to progression of kidney disease, at least in part, through unopposed transmission of systemic hypertension to the glomerular capillary bed resulting in glomerular injury. This event occurs particularly in patients with CKD because autoregulation of blood flow, which normally protects glomerular capillaries from excessive pressure, is impaired. Studies in dogs and cats have confirmed that reduced kidney function is associated with an adaptive preglomerular vasodilatation that permits transmission of systemic hypertension to the glomerular capillaries.[70,74]

Proteinuria
Proteinuria itself may contribute to progressive renal injury.[20] Proteinuria is a strong, independent risk factor for progression to end-stage CKD in humans.[75] Studies performed at the University of Minnesota Veterinary Medical Center have shown proteinuria to be a risk factor for uremia and death in dogs with naturally occurring CKD. Proteinuria has also been reported to be related to progression of renal disease in dogs with induced renal failure.[69] A relationship between proteinuria and progression of renal disease has not yet been established in cats. Proteinuria may promote progressive renal injury in several ways. Some proposed mechanisms include mesangial toxicity, tubular overload and hyperplasia, toxicity from specific proteins such as transferrin containing iron, and induction of proinflammatory molecules such as monocyte chemoattractant protein-1. Excessive proteinuria may injure renal tubules via toxic or receptor-mediated pathways or via an overload of lysosomal degradative mechanisms.

Abnormally filtered proteins accumulate in the renal proximal tubular lumens where, after endocytosis into proximal tubular cells, they contribute to renal tubulointerstitial injury through a complex cascade of intracellular events. These events include up-regulation of vasoactive and inflammatory genes such as the endothelin-1 (ET-1) gene, the monocyte chemoattractant protein-1 (MCP-1) gene, which encodes for an inflammatory peptide involved in macrophage and T-lymphocyte recruitment, and the RANTES (regulated on activation, normal T cell expressed and secreted) that encodes for a chemotactic molecule for monocytes and memory T cells.[76] Formed in excessive amounts, these molecules are secreted toward the basolateral side of tubular cells and incite an inflammatory reaction. In addition, complement components escaping through glomerular capillary walls may initiate interstitial injury. Small lipids bound to filtered proteins may also be liberated during resorption. Inflammatory or chemotactic properties of these lipids may promote tubulointerstitial disease. Finally, inspissation of filtered proteins due to tubular reabsorption of water in the distal nephron may lead to formation of casts that obstruct nephrons.

Tubulointerstitial Disease in Glomerulopathies
In humans, primary glomerular diseases are typically associated with varying degrees of tubulointerstitial lesions. Remarkably, it is the intensity of the accompanying or evolving injury in the tubulointerstitium, rather than injury in glomeruli, that is the most reliable overall predictor of decline in renal function.[77] In contrast, primary tubulointerstitial diseases as a group are the more indolent and slowly progressive of all human nephritides. Although the etiopathogenesis of canine and feline nephropathies is often uncertain, current evidence suggests that a substantial portion of canine CKD results from primary glomerulopathies, whereas the majority of feline CKD appears to be of tubulointerstitial origin.[11,78] The indolent course of CKD commonly observed in cats may be related to the tubulointerstitial origin of their disease, whereas many dogs experience a more aggressive decline in renal function, perhaps as a consequence of the glomerular origin of their primary renal disease.

Glomerular diseases have the capacity to incite tubulointerstitial disease. Although the mechanisms underlying the development of tubulointerstitial disease in this setting are not incompletely understood, multiple factors have been hypothesized to contribute.[77] As described previously, proteinuria is an important factor.[79] Additional factors include tubular ischemia related to decreased postglomerular blood flow; loss of tolerance with subsequent tubulointerstitial damage secondary to immune mechanisms of glomerular injury; seeping of inflammatory mediators from inflamed glomeruli; renal deposition of calcium phosphate; and enhanced tubular ammoniagenesis leading to complement-mediated injury of the tubulointerstitium.[77] Evidence indicates that an active immunologic process may be involved in the tubulointerstitium of patients with glomerulonephritides beginning early in the course of disease. In some instances this process appears to represent an extension of the inflammation in glomeruli.[77] In some models of renal disease, corticosteroids or other immunosuppressive therapy can ameliorate the tubulointerstitial damage without effect on glomeruli.[80]

Intrarenal Precipitation of Calcium Phosphate
Phosphate retention begins early in the course of CKD and has been implicated in promoting progressive renal injury in several species, including dogs and cats.[57,70,81] A role for phosphorus in promoting progressive CKD is based on the observation that dietary phosphorus restriction limited renal-related mortality in dogs and renal mineralization in cats. Phosphorus may promote progression of CKD, at least in part, by precipitation with calcium in the renal interstitium. This renal

mineralization may then initiate an inflammatory reaction, resulting in renal interstitial fibrosis and tubular atrophy.

Other Factors

Lipids and progression   Experimental studies in rodents indicate that hyperlipidemia may promote progression of renal disease.[82] This association is based on the observation that cholesterol loading enhanced glomerular injury, whereas reducing lipid levels with drugs such as lovastatin slowed the rate of progressive injury. Factors responsible for these effects are incompletely understood. Exposing glomerular and tubular cells to low-density lipoprotein and its oxidized variant stimulates their proliferation, induces injury and apoptosis, and stimulates them to produce extracellular matrix contributing to fibrosis.[19] An additive effect of hyperlipidemia and proteinuria has been described in humans with CKD.[83] Although hypercholesterolemia is common in dogs and cats with CKD, the clinical applicability of these findings in other species is unclear. Evidence that lipid reduction is beneficial in humans with CKD is conflicting. However, a meta-analysis of 13 prospective controlled studies indicated that lipid reduction was associated with a lower rate of decline in kidney function and decreased proteinuria.[84]

Metabolic acidosis   Metabolic acidosis has been theorized to enhance progression of renal failure by activation of the alternative complement pathway as a result of enhanced renal ammoniagenesis.[77] In human patients with CKD, reducing renal ammoniagenesis and renal tubular peptide catabolism was accompanied either by reduced renal tubular injury or by tubular hyperfunction. However, recent studies in rats have failed to confirm a role for acidemia and enhanced renal ammoniagenesis in renal injury and progression of renal failure.[85] Longer-term studies have suggested that effects initially attributed to enhanced renal ammoniagenesis may have been transient or related to the timing of therapeutic intervention in the previous study. These researchers concluded that metabolic acidosis neither causes nor exacerbates chronic renal injury. Further, the renal protective effect of alkali therapy is unproven in humans with CKD. Studies performed by the authors in cats with induced CKD have likewise failed to identify an adverse effect of chronic acidosis on renal structure or function.

Chronic hypoxia   It has been hypothesized that chronic oxygen deprivation to the tubulointerstitial compartment contributes to scarring in the tubulointerstitium.[86] Chronic hypoxia is thought to result from compromise of blood flow to the interstitial capillary network downstream from inflamed glomeruli. Concurrently, the peritubular capillary network downstream from other vasodilated glomeruli may be damaged subsequent to transmission of systemic blood pressures to this normally low-pressure capillary network. The resultant tubulointerstitial hypoxia is hypothesized to promote fibrosis by regulating gene expression of a broad spectrum of molecules including growth factors, hormones, vasoactive compounds, and enzymes. For example, *in vitro* studies have indicated that hypoxia is a profibrotic stimulus for tubular epithelial cells, interstitial fibroblasts, and renal microvascular endothelial cells. Hypoxia has been shown to induce a wide variety of growth factors, including many implicated in the pathogenesis of progressive renal disease, such as TGF-β1 and platelet-derived growth factor (PDGF).

The apparent beneficial role for ACE inhibitors in minimizing progressive renal diseases is consistent with the proposed role for chronic hypoxia. In theory, ACE inhibition could protect the kidneys by enhancing interstitial oxygen delivery through dilating the efferent arterioles, reducing vascular resistance, and improving microvascular flow through the interstitium.

DIAGNOSTIC EVALUATION

Patients with CKD should be evaluated to determine their diagnosis (type of kidney disease), severity, complications, comorbid conditions (concurrent diseases unrelated to CKD), and risk for continued loss of kidney function.[3] Morphologic diagnoses usually require evaluation of kidney biopsy samples. However, renal biopsies are indicated only when the benefits of renal biopsies (e.g., the results are likely to substantially change the prognosis or treatment) outweigh the associated risks.

Severity of CRD is classified based on the level of renal function. Serum creatinine concentration is the most commonly used measure of severity of renal dysfunction and is the basis for staging CKD (see Box 260-2). To optimize accuracy of staging of CRD, serum creatinine concentrations used to stage CRD should be evaluated when the patient is well hydrated. Multiple measurements are desirable to establish accuracy and stability of renal dysfunction. However, renal function may be more accurately measured using plasma clearances of iohexol, inulin, or other substances excreted exclusively by glomerular filtration.[87-91] Plasma clearance studies are indicated in at least three settings. First, they provide an accurate measure of renal dysfunction in stages 1 and 2 patients where serum creatinine determinations may be insensitive.

Second, they provide a basis for dose adjustments for drugs that are potentially toxic and are excreted primarily by the kidneys. Third, they are an excellent means of assessing progression of CKD. Because body muscle mass commonly declines as CKD progresses through stages 3 and 4, endogenous production of creatinine from muscle creatine may decline, confounding interpretation of serial serum creatinine values.

Appropriate management of complications and comorbid conditions may improve patient quality of life, as well as short- term and long-term survival (see Box 260-5). Diagnostics necessary to identify complications and comorbid conditions associated with CKD are outlined in Box 260-6. The prevalence of complications of CKD is mainly related to the level of renal function as reflected in the stage of CKD. CKD is typically characterized by alterations in a variety of kidney functions in addition to impaired GFR. These may include impairment of the (1) filtration barrier for plasma proteins (resulting in albuminuria and proteinuria), (2) reabsorption or secretion of water or specific solutes, and (3) various endocrine functions (anemia due to erythropoietin deficiency, calcitriol deficiency, and renal secondary hyperparathyroidism). These functional derangements are the basis of most complications of CKD.

Comorbid conditions are concurrent diseases other than CKD. Because patients with CKD are typically middle-aged to older, they often have a substantial number of comorbid conditions. Comorbid conditions of particular frequency and concern for dogs and cats with CKD include UTIs, urolithiasis, urinary obstruction, degenerative joint diseases, dental and other oral diseases, and cardiac disease. In addition, hyperthyroidism and upper urinary tract uroliths are common and important comorbid conditions in cats with CKD. In a survey of 48 cats with CKD, the authors found that 27 had upper urinary tract stones. Comorbid conditions may have an important influence on prognosis and treatment.

The level of kidney function tends to decline over time for most patients with CKD. It is important to assess the risk for loss of kidney function so that therapy may be designed to minimize progressive decline in GFR can be initiated. The risk of progression of kidney disease is affected by diagnosis and by modifiable and nonmodifiable factors. Some of these factors can be assessed even before the decline in GFR (Box 260-7). Therapies designed to slow progression of CKD may be specific

Box • 260-6

Problem-Specific Data Base for Patients with Chronic Renal Failure

1. Medical history including medication review
2. Physical examination including retinal examination
3. Urinalysis with urine sediment
4. Quantitative urine culture
5. Complete blood count (CBC)
6. Urine protein/creatinine ratio (if indicated by urinalysis)
7. Serum urea nitrogen (SUN) concentration
8. Serum creatinine concentration
9. Serum (or plasma) electrolyte and acid-base profile including:
   a. Sodium, potassium, and chloride concentrations
   b. Blood gas analysis or total serum CO_2 concentrations
   c. Calcium, phosphorus, and albumin concentrations
10. Arterial blood pressure
11. Kidney-bladder-urethra survey radiographs
    a. Kidneys—size, shape, location, number
    b. Uroliths or masses affecting kidneys, ureters, or urethra
    c. Urinary bladder—size, shape, location, uroliths
12. Clinician should consider:
    a. Additional imaging studies as indicated (clinician should rule out urinary obstruction, renal uroliths, pyelonephritis, renal cystic disease, perinephric pseudocysts, and renal neoplasia):
       i. Renal ultrasound
       ii. Intravenous urography
    b. Determining glomerular filtration rate (GFR)
       i. Plasma clearance of iohexol, inulin, creatinine, or other
       ii. Classical clearance methods or scintigraphic methods
    c. Determining parathyroid hormone (PTH) and ionized calcium levels for managing renal secondary hyperparathyroidism
    d. Skeletal radiographs for evidence of renal osteodystrophy, measurement of carbamylated hemoglobin concentration, or parathyroid gland ultrasonography when the distinction between acute and chronic kidney disease (CKD) remains unresolved
    e. Renal biopsy
    f. Prior to initiating therapy, clinician should consider freezing aliquots of serum (or plasma) and urine for additional diagnostics that may be desired later

Box • 260-7

Risk Factors That May Promote Progression of Renal Failure

Risk Factors for Acute Decline in Renal Function:
Volume depletion
Urinary obstruction
Potentially nephrotoxic drugs:
  Antibiotics
  Nonsteroidal anti-inflammatory drugs (NSAIDs)
  Angiotensin-converting enzyme (ACE) inhibitors and angiotensin-2 receptor blockers
  Intravenous radiographic contrast agents

Risk Factors for Long-Term Decline in Renal Function
Active renal disease
Urinary tract infection (UTI)
Nephrolithiasis and ureterolithiasis
Systemic hypertension
Proteinuria
Inappropriate diet

kidney function, management of comorbid conditions, and therapy designed to slow loss of kidney function.[3] To this end, a clinical action plan should be developed for each patient based on their diagnosis, stage of CKD, existing complications and comorbid conditions, and risk factors for progression of their kidney disease.

Specific therapy for CKD is based on a renal diagnosis. Treatment is directed at the etiopathogenic processes responsible for the patient's primary renal disease. Because the renal lesions of CKD are irreversible, they cannot be completely reversed or eliminated by specific therapy. Nonetheless, progression of renal lesions may be slowed or stopped by therapy designed to eliminate active renal diseases. Specific therapies are described in the chapters of this text on glomerular diseases, bacterial infections, familial renal diseases, and renal tubular disease. Unfortunately, a renal diagnosis amenable to specific therapy is not obtained for most patients.

Treatment directed at the complications of decreased kidney function is often termed *conservative medical management*. It consists of supportive and symptomatic therapy designed to correct deficits and excesses in fluid, electrolyte, acid-base, endocrine, and nutritional balance thereby minimizing the clinical and pathophysiologic consequences of reduced renal function. Conservative medical management also includes therapy designed to limit the progressive loss of renal function.

The goals of conservative medical management of patients with chronic primary renal failure are to (1) ameliorate clinical signs of uremia; (2) minimize disturbances associated with excesses or losses of electrolytes, vitamins, and minerals; (3) support adequate nutrition by supplying daily protein, calorie, and mineral requirements; and (4) modify progression of renal failure.[92] These goals are best achieved when recommendations regarding conservative medical management are individualized to patient needs based on clinical and laboratory finding. Because CRF is progressive and dynamic, serial clinical and laboratory assessment of the patient and modification of the therapy in response to changes in the patient's condition is an integral part of conservative medical management.

for the diagnosis (e.g., antibiotics for bacterial pyelonephritis), whereas others are supportive (e.g., dietary intervention, antihypertensive therapy and angiotensin-converting enzyme [ACE] inhibitors).

TREATMENT OF CHRONIC KIDNEY DISEASE

Overview of Treatment

Treatment of CKD should generally include specific therapy, prevention and treatment of complications of decreased

Dietary Therapy

Dietary Modifications in Renal Failure

Diet therapy has been a mainstay in the management of canine and feline CKD for decades and it continues to be the most commonly recommended treatment for these patients. In the past, the emphasis has been on reducing protein content. Although protein content continues to play an important role in diet formulation, other diet modifications are also important in managing renal failure patients. Diets recommended for dogs and cats with renal failure are modified from typical maintenance diets in several ways, including reduced protein, phosphorus, and sodium content; increased B-vitamin content and caloric density; and a neutral effect on acid-base balance. Feline renal failure diets are typically supplemented with additional potassium. Canine renal failure diets may have an increased omega-3/omega-6 polyunsaturated fatty acid (PUFA) ratio. Diets may also have added fiber designed to enhance GI excretion of nitrogenous wastes. Of these diet modifications, only phosphate, omega-3 PUFA, and protein have been extensively examined.

Diet phosphate   Renal diets are limited in phosphorus content to limit phosphorus retention, hyperphosphatemia, renal secondary hyperparathyroidism, and progression of renal disease. Phosphate balance results largely from the interaction between dietary intake and renal excretion. Ingested phosphate is cleared from blood by glomerular filtration, and then total excretion is adjusted by modifying proximal tubular reabsorption. As renal function declines, renal tubular reabsorption of phosphorus declines (increasing renal excretion) in an attempt to compensate for the reduction in glomerular filtration, thereby maintaining phosphorus balance. However, if phosphorus intake continues unabated, the renal adaptive capacity soon becomes overwhelmed and phosphorus retention and hyperphosphatemia develop.

Although phosphorus retention and hyperphosphatemia probably do not cause clinical signs, they may promote renal secondary hyperparathyroidism and renal mineralization that enhances progressive decline in renal function. Dietary phosphorus restriction has been shown to enhance survival and a slow decline in renal function in dogs with induced renal failure.[57] In cats, dietary phosphorus restriction has been shown to limit renal mineralization.

Available evidence supports a recommendation for dietary phosphate restriction for dogs and cats in stages 3 and 4 CKD. Because protein is a major source for phosphate, it is usually necessary to limit dietary protein to limit diet phosphate content.

Omega-3 polyunsaturated fatty acid   Dietary supplementation with omega-3 PUFA have been shown to be beneficial in dogs with induced CKD. Compared with dogs fed diets high in saturated fats or omega-6 PUFA, dogs consuming a diet supplemented with omega-3 PUFA had lower mortality, better renal function, fewer renal lesions, less proteinuria, and lower cholesterol levels.[93] In dogs fed the omega-3 PUFA diet, renal function actually increased and remained above baseline over 20 months of study. Lesions of glomerulosclerosis, tubulointerstitial fibrosis, and interstitial inflammatory cell infiltrates were also diminished in dogs fed the omega-3 PUFA diet. A variety of effects attributed to omega-3 PUFA supplementation may have contributed to the favorable renal effects observed, including their tendency to reduce hypercholesterolemia, suppress inflammation and coagulation (by interfering with the production of proinflammatory, procoagulant prostanoids, thromboxanes, or leukotrienes), lower blood pressure, favorably influence renal hemodynamics, provide antioxidant effects, or limit intrarenal calcification. A subsequent study supported possible roles for altered lipid metabolism, glomerular hypertension and hypertrophy, and urinary eicosanoid metabolism in the beneficial renal effects of omega-3 PUFA.[94]

Available evidence supports a recommendation for dietary supplementation with omega-3 PUFA for dogs in stages 3 and 4 CKD. The optimum quantity of omega-3 PUFA supplementation and ratio of omega-3/omega-6 PUFA appropriate for renal diets have not been conclusively established. Additional omega-3 PUFA supplementation may not be appropriate for dogs already consuming a renal diet enhanced with omega-3 PUFA. Currently, no evidence supports a recommendation for or against omega-3 PUFA supplementation for cats with CKD.

Diet protein   Although the ideal quantity of protein to feed dogs and cats with CKD remains unresolved, a general consensus of opinion supports the fact that reducing protein intake ameliorates clinical signs of uremia in CKD and is therefore indicated for stage 4 CKD. BUN can be used as a crude measure of compliance with dietary recommendations because it declines as dietary protein intake is reduced. Although not generally regarded as an important uremic toxin, BUN is a surrogate marker for retained nonprotein nitrogenous waste products and typically correlates better with clinical signs than serum creatinine concentration.

The concept of reducing dietary protein intake in CKD patients that do not have clinical signs of uremia has been questioned. Limiting protein intake has been advocated for these patients to slow progression of CKD. This suggestion derives from studies in rats indicating that dietary protein restriction limits glomerular hyperfiltration and hypertension and slows the spontaneous decline in kidney function that follows reduction in kidney mass.[66] Studies in humans have supported the concept that protein restriction slows progression of CKD, albeit this effect may be small.[95] In contrast, multiple studies have failed to confirm a beneficial role for protein restriction in limiting progression of kidney disease in dogs or cats.[92] When not excessive, limiting protein intake does not appear to have any adverse effects, and it may be easier to initiate treatment with renal diets before the onset of clinical signs of uremia. In addition, protein restriction may delay onset of clinical signs of uremia as renal disease progresses. Although a role for protein restriction in slowing progression of canine and feline CKD has not been entirely excluded, available evidence fails to support a recommendation for or against protein restriction in patients with stage 3 CKD.

Diet Therapy—Evidence from Clinical Trials

The effectiveness of diet therapy in minimizing uremic episodes and mortality in dogs with naturally occurring stage 3 and stage 4 CKD has been established in a double-masked, randomized, controlled clinical trial.[1] The study compared a renal diet to a prototypical canine maintenance diet. The renal diet was characterized by reduced quantities of protein, phosphorus, and sodium compared with the maintenance diet, and it was supplemented with omega-3 PUFA. In this study the risk of developing an uremic crisis was reduced by approximately 75% in dogs fed the renal diet compared with dogs fed an adult maintenance diet, and the median interval before development of uremic crisis in dogs fed the renal diet was twice as long as that observed in dogs fed the maintenance diet. Further, the risk of death irrespective of the cause was reduced by at least two thirds when dogs were fed the renal diet, and renal death risk was reduced by 70%.

Dogs fed the renal diet survived at least 13 months longer than dogs fed the maintenance diet. In addition, owners of dogs fed the renal diet reported significantly higher quality of life scores for their dogs than owners of dogs consuming the maintenance diet. The delay in development of uremic crises and reduced mortality observed in dogs fed renal diet was associated, at least in part, with reduction in the rate progression of renal failure.

The effectiveness of diet therapy in cats has been tested in a prospective study comparing a renal diet characterized by protein and phosphorus restriction to no diet change.[64] Cats that would not accept the renal diet, either due to pet or owner issues, continued to eat their regular diet. Therefore this study was neither randomized nor blinded, but it nonetheless yielded results similar to those observed in the canine study. Cats fed the renal diet (median survival time [MST], 633 days) survived substantially longer than cats that continued to consume their regular diet (MST, 264 days). In addition, plasma urea nitrogen, phosphorus, and PTH concentrations were reduced in cats that consumed the renal diet.

Indications for Diet Therapy In the past, criteria for timing of dietary intervention in dogs and cats with spontaneous CKD have been based on empiric observations. An often-cited guideline has been to initiate dietary therapy when serum creatinine exceeds 2.5 mg/dL or the SUN exceeds 60 to 80 mg/dL. More recently, one investigator recommended a staged approach whereby dietary phosphorus restriction and omega-3 PUFA dietary supplementation be implemented in dogs with serum creatinine values below 4.0 mg/dL with dietary protein restriction recommended only in dogs with serum creatinine values exceeding 4.0 mg/dL.[4] However, the clinical trial data available to date have demonstrated a benefit of dietary intervention in both stage 3 and stage 4 CKD. In a randomized, controlled clinical trial in dogs with naturally occurring CKD, diet therapy significantly reduced the risk of uremic crises and death in dogs with serum creatinine concentrations between 2.0 and 3.0 mg/dL.[1] These studies did not selectively determine the benefits of modifying individual dietary components, but rather report the results of a *diet effect*. Although studies on individual dietary components have been reported in dogs and cats with induced renal failure, the potential interactions between components have not been examined, nor have the results of these studies been confirmed in clinic patients.

Currently available data supports recommending therapy with appropriately modified diets in dogs and cats in stages 3 and 4 CKD. The value of diet therapy in stages 1 and 2 CKD has not been established; therefore no evidence supports a recommendation for or against diet therapy in these patients.

Drugs—Medication Review and Dose Modification
A review of current medications should be performed at each clinic visit, including dose adjustment based on level of kidney function, detection of potential adverse effects on kidney function or complications of CKD, detection of drug interactions, and, where indicated, therapeutic drug monitoring.[3] The clinician should ensure that all current medications are still necessary and that new medications have specific indications and do not pose a risk of drug interaction.

Because the kidneys are responsible for elimination of many drugs from the body, renal drug clearance is reduced as renal function declines, causing the half-life of the drug to be prolonged. In addition, distribution, protein binding, and hepatic biotransformation of drugs may be altered. For example, two protein-binding defects are seen in renal failure.[50] One group of primarily acidic drugs shows decreased binding leading to increases in free, active drug fractions in plasma (e.g., theophylline, methotrexate, diazepam, digoxin, salicylate). The effect of this change in binding is that lower doses of drugs are required to achieve therapeutic levels, but conventional doses may result in toxic levels. Basic drugs, such as propranolol or cimetidine, have increased binding leading to a decrease in free drug levels, thus diminishing the therapeutic effect. Increased total drug levels may be required to achieve the desired therapeutic effect with these drugs. However, these effects may be complicated by decreased renal clearance of the drugs.

Further, accumulation of active drug metabolites may augment drug potency or toxicity.

The sum effect of these changes is that for many drugs normally excreted by the kidneys, a tendency exists for drugs to accumulate in patients with renal failure. Excessive drug accumulation promotes an increased rate of adverse drug reactions and nephrotoxicity. If drugs requiring renal excretion must be administered to patients with renal failure, dose regimens should be adjusted to compensate for decreased organ function. However, dose adjustments may not be appropriate for drugs that are administered to a physiologic endpoint or effect such as antihypertensive agents.[96]

Because drug accumulation in patients with reduced kidney function is primarily a result of reduced renal drug clearance, dose adjustments should be made according to changes in drug clearance. Net renal excretion of a drug is a composite of glomerular filtration, tubular secretion, and tubular reabsorption. Generally it is assumed that these three factors all decline in parallel. Therefore drug clearance may be estimated by measuring GFR, either by plasma disappearance rate (e.g., iohexol disappearance rate) or classical clearance studies. Drug dose may then be adjusted according to the percentage reduction in GFR (i.e., the ratio of patient GFR/normal GFR), also known as the dose fraction (K_f):

$$K_f = (\text{patient GFR/normal GFR})$$

Dose regimens can be adjusted by increasing the normal dose interval or decreasing the normal dose in direct proportion to K_f.[97] The interval extension method is particularly useful for drugs with wide therapeutic ranges and long plasma half-lives in patients with renal impairment. Interval lengthening will result in wide swings of the plasma drug concentrations from peak to trough levels. If the range between the toxic and therapeutic levels is too narrow, either toxic or subtherapeutic plasma concentrations may result. For drugs excreted 100% unchanged by the kidneys, a precise increase in dose interval may be calculated by dividing the normal dosing interval by K_f:

$$\text{Modified dose interval} = (\text{normal dose interval}/K_f)$$

For example, if a drug is normally administered every 8 hours and the patient's GFR is 25% of normal (i.e., $K_f = 0.25$), then the appropriate dosing interval is (8 hrs ÷ 0.25) or 32 hrs. The calculated dose interval should be rounded to a convenient time schedule.

Alternatively, the size of the individual doses can be reduced while maintaining the normal time interval between doses. Decreasing the individual doses reduces the difference between peak and trough plasma concentrations. This effect is important for dugs with narrow therapeutic ranges and short plasma half-lives in patients with renal dysfunction and is recommended for drugs for which a relatively constant blood level is desired. Dose reduction may be determined by multiplying the normal dose by K_f:

$$\text{Modified dose reduction} = (\text{normal dose} \times K_f)$$

For example, if the normal dose is 10 mg/kg given every 8 hours and the patient's GFR is 25% of normal (i.e., $K_f = 0.25$), then the appropriate dose is (10 mg/kg × 0.25) or 2.5 mg/kg given every 8 hours. Even using the reduced dose, normal interval method, the first dose of drug should be administered at the usual dose to initiate therapeutic drug concentrations in tissues and blood.

There have been no controlled clinical trials to establish the efficacy of the two methods for drug dose alteration in patients with CKD. Prolonging the dose interval is usually more convenient and less expensive. A combination of interval prolongation and dose size reduction may also be convenient and effective.

Dose of antimicrobial drugs may be modified according to three general patterns, depending on the fraction of the drug eliminated by the kidneys (Table 260-1): (1) doubling the dosing interval or halving the drug dose in patients with severe reduction in renal function, (2) increasing the dose interval according to ranges of creatinine clearance values, and (3) precise dose modification as described previously. Drugs in the first category are relatively nontoxic. The second class includes drugs requiring dose modification according to GFR values because they are more likely to be toxic. For drugs in this class, dosing interval is increased twofold when GFR is between 1.0 and 0.5 mL/min/kg, threefold when GFR is between 0.5 and 0.3 mL/min/kg, and fourfold when GFR is less than 0.3 mL/min/kg. Drugs in the third class include relatively toxic antimicrobial drugs that are excreted solely by glomerular filtration (particularly aminoglycoside antibiotics). They require precise dose modification according to K_f. For these drugs, increased interval, fixed dose regimens appear to result in less nephrotoxicity than reduced dose, fixed

Table • 260-1

Drug Dose Modifications for Patients with Renal Insufficiency and Failure

DRUG	ROUTE(S) OF EXCRETION*	NEPHRO-TOXIC?	DOSE ADJUSTMENT IN RENAL FAILURE[†]
Amikacin	R	Yes	Pr
Amoxicillin	R	No	D/I
Amphotericin B	O	Yes	Pr
Ampicillin	R, (H)	No	D/I
Cephalexin	R	No	C_{cr}
Cephalothin	R, (H)	No (?)	C_{cr} or D/I
Clindamycin	H, (R)	No	N
Chloramphenicol	H, (R)	No	N, A
Cyclophosphamide	H, (R)	No	N
Corticosteroids	H	No	N
Dicloxacillin	R, (H)	No	N
Digoxin	R, (O)	No	Pr
Doxycycline	GI, (R)	?	N
Enrofloxacin	R	No	I
Furosemide	R	No (?)	N
Gentamicin	R	Yes	Pr
Heparin	O	No	N
Kanamycin	R	Yes	Pr
Neomycin	R	Yes	C/I
Nitrofurantoin	R	No	C/I
Orbaloxacin	R	No	I
Penicillin	R, (H)	No	D/I
Propranolol	H	No	N
Streptomycin	R	Yes	C_{cr}
Sulfisoxazole	R	Yes	C_{cr}
Tetracycline	R, (H)	Yes	C/I
Tobramycin	R	Yes	Pr
Trimethoprim/sulfamethoxazole	R	Yes	C_{cr}, A

*Routes of excretion: R, Renal; H, hepatic; GI, gastrointestinal; O, other (minor route in parentheses).
[†]Dose modification: N, Normal; D/I, half dose or double dose interval (in severe renal dysfunction); C_{cr}, adjust according to C_{cr} (see text); Pr, precise dose modification (see text—clinician should adjust it according to K_f); C/I, contraindicated; A, clinician should avoid in advanced renal failure.

interval methods. A combination of dose reduction and interval extension has been recommended for animals with markedly reduced kidney function (GFR < 0.7 mL/min/kg).

Although GFR is the preferred measure of renal dysfunction for modifying drug therapy, serum creatinine concentration is a more universally available measure of renal dysfunction. A regression equation relating serum creatinine concentration to GFR in dogs has been established.[98]

Although the relationship between serum creatinine concentration and GFR is not linear, the reciprocal of serum creatinine concentration may be used to approximate GFR when serum creatinine concentration is less than 4 mg/dL. This rule of thumb will overestimate GFR when serum creatinine concentration exceeds 4 mg/dL. Despite increased expense and effort involved, it is recommend that GFR be used as the basis for modifying drug dose schedules whenever possible. This recommendation is particularly relevant when a potentially nephrotoxic drug must be administered.

Patients with preexisting renal disease and renal failure may also be predisposed to nephrotoxicity. For this reason, nephrotoxic drugs and drugs requiring renal excretion should generally be avoided in patients with renal failure. Where possible, less nephrotoxic drugs should be chosen. If nephrotoxic drugs are unavoidable, therapeutic drug monitoring and serial evaluation of renal function is essential.

So-called complementary medications (sometimes called herbal medicines, naturopathic remedies, and phytomedicines) are becoming increasingly popular. The potential for interactions with prescribed medications or simple adverse consequences in patients with reduced kidney function should be considered for patients receiving these medications. Herbal products that should be avoided in patients with renal dysfunction include aristolochic acid, barberry, buchu, Chinese herbal drugs, juniper, licorice, and noni juice.[96]

Phosphorus Retention, Hyperphosphatemia, and Renal Secondary Hyperparathyroidism

Serum phosphorus concentrations represent the net balance between dietary intake and renal excretion of phosphorus. Therefore maintaining serum phosphorus concentrations within the normal range as renal function is lost requires modification of phosphorus intake. In theory, optimum control of hyperphosphatemia would be achieved by reducing dietary phosphorus intake in proportion to the decrease in GFR.

Without treatment, phosphorus retention, hyperphosphatemia and renal secondary hyperparathyroidism occurs in most dogs and cats with stage 3 or stage 4 CKD.[39,99] Although hyperphosphatemia has been linked to pruritus, conjunctivitis, renal osteodystrophy, and soft-tissue calcification in humans, hyperphosphatemia per se is rarely linked to clinical signs in dogs and cats with CKD. Rather, minimizing phosphorus retention and hyperphosphatemia is an important therapeutic goal in patients with CKD because it appears to limit renal secondary hyperparathyroidism and prolong survival.[57,99]

The first step in correcting hyperphosphatemia is to restore hydration and correct prerenal hyperphosphatemia. Minimizing long-term phosphorus retention and hyperphosphatemia may be accomplished by limiting dietary phosphorus intake, oral administration of agents that bind phosphorus within the lumen of the intestines, or a combination of these methods. The usual approach is to start with diet therapy and add phosphorous binding agents if diet therapy alone fails to normalize serum phosphorous concentrations. Diet therapy with or without phosphate-binding agents normalizes serum phosphorus levels in most patients. However, phosphorus restriction alone appears to be insufficient to normalize serum PTH levels in some patients.[39,99] In such patients, a combination of limiting phosphorus intake combined with administration of calcitriol has been recommended.[39] Nagode and colleagues[39] have suggested that normalization of PTH levels using calcitriol therapy may provide clinical benefits that cannot be achieved by phosphorus restriction alone, including amelioration of many clinical signs associated with CKD. However, clinical trials of long-term calcitriol therapy are needed to establish the value of this therapy in dogs and cats with CKD. Calcitriol therapy is described later in this chapter.

Dietary Phosphorus Restriction Dietary phosphorus restriction is an important and effective intervention for normalizing phosphorus balance. It may be effective in normalizing serum phosphorus concentrations in most stage 3 and some stage 4 CKD patients. It will also decrease the dose of intestinal phosphorus-binding agents needed to bind dietary phosphorus in patients with more severe hyperphosphatemia. Dietary phosphorus restriction is clearly indicated for patients with hyperphosphatemia. However, because phosphorus retention and hyperparathyroidism may occur before serum phosphorus concentrations exceed normal limits, and because fasting serum phosphorus concentrations may not accurately reflect overall phosphorus balance, phosphorus restriction may be indicated before the onset of overt hyperphosphatemia.[100]

Because proteins are a major source of dietary phosphorus, manufactured and homemade renal diets are usually restricted in both protein and phosphorus content. Typical commercial dog foods contain approximately 1% to 2% phosphorus on a dry matter basis and provide about 2.7 mg/kcal or more phosphorus. Modified protein diets designed for dogs with renal failure may contain as little as 0.13% to 0.28% phosphorus on a dry matter basis and provide about 0.3 to 0.5 mg/kcal of phosphorus. Typical commercial cat foods contain from 1% to 4% phosphorus on a dry matter basis and provide about 2.9 mg/kcal or more phosphorus. Modified protein diets designed for cats with renal failure may contain as little as 0.5% phosphorous on a dry matter basis and provide about 0.9 mg/kcal of phosphorus.

Phosphorus retention in CKD appears to occur in multiple compartments. As dietary phosphorus restriction reduces serum phosphorus levels, phosphorus leaches out of tissues, delaying the overall reduction in serum phosphorus concentration. Thus the overall efficacy of dietary phosphorus restriction in reducing serum phosphorus concentrations may not occur until the patient has been consuming the phosphorus-restricted diet for several weeks. In a study in cats with renal insufficiency and failure, the effect of restricting dietary phosphorus intake was apparent after 28 to 49 days.[99] Samples obtained for determinations of serum phosphorus concentration should be collected after a 12-hour fast to avoid postprandial effects. Sample hemolysis should be avoided because canine RBCs contain substantial quantities of phosphorus.

The minimum goal of therapy is to bring serum phosphorus concentration to within the normal range, although concentrations between 4.0 and 6.0 mg/dL may be preferred. Although PTH levels generally decline as serum phosphorus levels decline, normalization of serum phosphorus concentrations is not always accompanied by normalization of PTH concentration. In a recent clinical study of cats with chronic renal insufficiency and failure, dietary phosphorus restriction was associated with a normal serum phosphorus concentration in 12 of 13 cats, whereas PTH concentration was normalized in only eight of these 13 cats.[99] It is unclear whether further reducing serum phosphorus concentration within the normal range or using normalization of PTH levels as the preferred therapeutic endpoint would be of any clinical benefit.

Hypercalcemia was reported to develop in two cats managed with dietary phosphorous restriction.[99] The significance of the relationship, if any, between dietary phosphorus restriction and hypercalcemia in these two cats is unclear.

Unfortunately, as renal failure becomes more advanced, dietary phosphorus restriction alone may be insufficient to prevent hyperphosphatemia. When hyperphosphatemia persists despite dietary phosphorus restriction, administration of intestinal phosphorus-binding agents should be considered.

Intestinal Phosphorus-Binding Agents Phosphorus-binding agents should be used in conjunction with dietary phosphorus restriction when dietary therapy alone fails to reduce serum phosphorus concentrations to the normal range. Dietary phosphorus intake should be reduced before initiating therapy with intestinal phosphorus-binding agents to minimize the quantity of phosphorus that must be bound. High dietary phosphorus content may greatly limit the effectiveness of phosphorus-binding agents or substantially increase the dose required to achieve the desired therapeutic effect.[101] Administration of 1500 to 2500 mg of aluminum carbonate to dogs with moderate CKD failed to consistently correct hyperphosphatemia when dogs were fed diets containing greater than 1.0% phosphorus on a dry matter basis.[102]

Currently available phosphorus-binding agents include aluminum-based and calcium-based exchange compounds that liberate varying amounts of their associated cation (e.g., aluminum, calcium) as dietary phosphorus is bound. Factors that may influence selection of a specific phosphorus-binding agent include availability, palatability, and the associated cation. Aluminum-based binding agents have generally been preferred for dogs and cats because they are effective, inexpensive, and seemingly have few side effects. However, concern about the potential toxic effects of aluminum in humans has caused many aluminum-containing drugs to be removed from the market. Encephalopathies, microcytic anemia, and bone disease (particularly osteomalacia) related to aluminum toxicity have been extensively reported in human patients treated with these drugs. The potential for toxicity of aluminum salts in dogs and cats has been confirmed, but little evidence suggests that use of these drugs leads to clinically important aluminum toxicity in dogs and cats. Calcium-based drugs have the potential to promote hypercalcemia, particularly when administered between meals or used in combination with calcitriol.

Aluminum-containing intestinal phosphorus-binding agents include aluminum hydroxide, aluminum carbonate, and aluminum oxide. Initial doses of 30 to 100 mg/kg/day have been recommended for these aluminum-based phosphorus-binding agents. They are available over-the-counter in liquid, tablet, or capsule forms from most pharmacies as antacid preparations. In humans, capsules and tablets are less effective than liquids, but liquid preparations may be unpalatable to some dogs and cats. Sucralfate, a complex polyaluminum hydroxide salt of sulfate used primarily for treatment of GI ulcerations, may also be effective in binding phosphorus within the intestine.

Calcium-based phosphorus-binding agents include calcium acetate, calcium carbonate, or calcium citrate. Because calcium-based products may promote clinically significant hypercalcemia, it is recommended that serum calcium concentrations be monitored intermittently when using these drugs. They should not be used in hypercalcemic patients. When indicated, they may be used between meals as a source of additional dietary calcium. Calcium supplementation may increase the efficacy of phosphorus restriction in normalizing renal secondary hyperparathyroidism.

Reduced doses of calcium carbonate and calcium acetate may be used concurrent with aluminum-based binding agents to limit risks of both hypercalcemia and aluminum toxicity. However, calcium citrate may promote absorption of aluminum and should therefore not be used in concert with aluminum-based binding agents. Calcium acetate is the most effective calcium-based phosphorus-binding agent and the agent least likely to induce hypercalcemia because it releases the least amount of calcium compared with the amount of phosphorus it binds.[101] Initial doses of 60 to 90 mg/kg/day have been recommended for calcium acetate and 90 to 150 mg/kg/day for calcium carbonate. Some calcium carbonate preparations may not be effective because they fail to dissolve well in the GI tract; clinicians may investigate this by examining the stool or obtaining radiographs of the abdomen for evidence of radiodense tablets that have failed to dissolve.

The most recent addition to the phosphorus-binding armamentarium is the cationic polymer agent sevelamer hydrochloride (Renagel® Tablets and Capsules, Genzyme Corp., Cambridge, MA). The primary advantage of this drug is that it does not promote hypercalcemia or absorption of aluminum. However, it is more expensive than older phosphorus-binding agents. In addition, concerns have been raised over its potential for inducing vitamin-K deficiency and hemorrhage. In preclinical studies in rats and dogs, sevelamer hydrochloride reduced vitamin D, E, K, and folic acid levels when given at doses of six to 100 times the recommended human dose. In clinical trials in humans, no evidence of reduction in serum levels of vitamins was seen; however, patients in this study were receiving vitamin supplements. Scant information exists on the safety, effectiveness, or dose of sevelamer in dogs and cats. Based on extrapolating the recommended dose from humans, an initial dose of 30 and 135 mg/kg per day divided and given with meals may be considered. Because the contents of Renagel® (Genzyme Corp.) expand in water, the manufacturer recommends that tablets and capsules should be swallowed intact and should not be crushed, chewed, broken into pieces, or taken apart prior to administration. Sevelamer reportedly lowers total and low-density lipoprotein cholesterol concentrations and elevated high-density lipoprotein cholesterol levels in humans.[103] Consideration should be given to monitoring clotting ability using the prothrombin time (PT) if this drug is used in dogs or cats with CKD.

Intestinal phosphorus-binding agents render ingested phosphorus and the phosphorus contained in saliva, bile, and intestinal juices unabsorbable. Because the primary goal is limiting absorption of phosphorus contained in the diet, administration of phosphorus-binding agents should be timed to coincide with feeding. These agents are best administered with or mixed into the food, or just prior to each meal. It is particularly important that calcium-based phosphorus-binding agents be administered with meals both to enhance the effectiveness of phosphorus binding and to minimize absorption of calcium and the risk of hypercalcemia.

Dose of phosphorus-binding agents should be individualized to achieve the desired serum phosphorus concentration. The effectiveness of therapy should be assessed by serial evaluation of serum phosphorus concentrations at about 2- to 4-week intervals. Dose of calcium-based phosphorus-binding agents should be decreased if serum calcium concentrations exceed normal limits; additional aluminum-based agents should be used in these patients if hyperphosphatemia persists.

Dehydration

Fluid balance in patients with polyuric renal failure is maintained by compensatory polydipsia. If water consumption is insufficient to compensate for polyuria, dehydration is the result. This may occur as a consequence of lack of intake or lack of access to fresh, clean, unadulterated water. Cats and some dogs with chronic kidney disease (CKD) fail to consume sufficient water to prevent chronic or recurrent dehydration. In addition, acute GI fluid losses resulting from renal or non-renal causes may lead to extracellular fluid volume depletion.

Dehydration and volume depletion promote renal hypoperfusion and prerenal azotemia that may exacerbate the clinical and laboratory abnormalities of chronic renal insufficiency and failure. In addition to prerenal azotemia, dehydration may be associated with electrolyte disturbances such as hyperphosphatemia, hyperkalemia, and metabolic acidosis. Clinical signs characteristic of dehydration include decreased appetite, lethargy, and constipation. In some patients, prerenal azotemia may precipitate uremic crisis. Further, if dehydration and decreased renal blood flow are allowed to persist, additional ischemic renal damage may occur.

Patients that develop recurrent episodes of signs consistent with dehydration are candidates for intermediate- to long-term subcutaneous fluid therapy to be administered at home by the owner. The principal benefits of subcutaneous fluid therapy include improved appetite and activity and reduced constipation. The decision to recommend administration of subcutaneous fluids should be made on a case-by-case basis. Not every patient with chronic kidney disease and failure requires or will benefit from fluid therapy. Although a substantial number of cats with CKD appear to benefit from subcutaneous fluid therapy, proportionately fewer dogs require fluid therapy. In addition, home administration of subcutaneous fluids is not appropriate for all owners. Although it is inexpensive, it does require time and may cause stress on the owner-pet relationship. It also has the potential to promote hypokalemia, hypertension, and fluid overload. Although a risk of subcutaneous infections exists, this appears to be an uncommon complication when owners are taught proper technique.

Normal saline or lactated Ringer's solution are the fluids most commonly used for home subcutaneous fluid therapy. They are well tolerated by most cats and dogs and appear to be reasonable choices for most patients. However, chronic administration of lactated Ringer's solution or normal saline as the principal maintenance fluid source may cause hypernatremia because they fail to provide sufficient electrolyte-free water. Ideally, fluids selected for chronic parenteral administration should provide free water and electrolytes for maintenance. A solution containing 0.45% saline and 2.5% glucose supplemented with 20 mEq/L of potassium chloride meets these requirements. Unfortunately, fluids containing dextrose may be irritating when administered subcutaneously, and their use should be discontinued if the patient indicates discomfort when they are given. A typical cat or small dog receives approximately 75 to 150 mL of fluids given daily or as needed. Chronic subcutaneous fluid therapy can result in fluid overload in some patients, particularly when fluid volumes in excess of those recommended here are used. The authors have seen several cats have severe dyspnea due to pleural effusion given large quantities of fluid (200 to 400 mL/day). This condition can usually be avoided by reducing the volume of fluids administered.

Response to long-term subcutaneous fluid therapy should be monitored by serially assessing hydration status, clinical signs, hematocrit, total serum protein concentrations, blood pressure, and SUN, creatinine, phosphorus, potassium, total CO_2, sodium, and chloride concentrations.

Hypokalemia and Potassium Depletion

Potassium depletion and hypokalemia are common in cats with CKD. Estimates of the prevalence of hypokalemia in this population of cats are in the range of 20% to 30%.[2,8,9] Total body potassium depletion is likely to be even more common than hypokalemia.[62] In contrast, hypokalemia is rarely recognized as a complication of canine CKD. The mechanisms underlying development of hypokalemia in cats with CKD remain unclear, but inadequate potassium intake coupled with increased urinary and fecal losses (or both) have been hypothesized to play a role.

Although increasing the potassium content of renal diets has reduced the incidence of overt clinical signs of hypokalemia, hypokalemia remains a common laboratory finding in cats with renal insufficiency and failure. The antihypertensive agent amlodipine may promote hypokalemia in cats with chronic renal insufficiency and failure.[104]

Hypokalemia and potassium depletion may affect the kidneys or muscles of cats with CKD. Diets low in potassium and high in acid content have been implicated in impairing renal function and promoting development of lymphoplasmacytic tubulointerstitial lesions in cats.[33,60-63] Potassium depletion may result in reduced renal blood flow and GFR as a consequence of angiotensin II and thromboxane-mediated renal vasoconstriction. In addition, hypokalemia may promote polyuria by impairing renal responsiveness to ADH and by stimulating the brain thirst centers through increased levels of angiotensin II. Hypokalemic polymyopathy, characterized by generalized muscle weakness and cervical ventroflexion, is a well-recognized complication of chronic renal insufficiency and failure in cats.

Oral supplementation of potassium has been recommended for cats with renal insufficiency and failure to treat or prevent renal and muscular consequences of potassium depletion and hypokalemia. Although a consensus of opinion suggests that cats with hypokalemia should receive potassium supplementation, the justification for *prophylactic* potassium supplementation in normokalemic cats is not well established. Although potassium supplementation is unlikely to be medically harmful to polyuric, normokalemic cats, administration of an oral medication may impose an unnecessary burden on both the cat and the cat owner. Patient acceptance may be a limitation due to the unpleasant flavor of potassium salts that is difficult to mask.

Oral replacement is the safest and preferred route for administering potassium. Parenteral therapy is generally reserved for patients requiring emergency reversal of hypokalemia or for patients that cannot or will not accept oral therapy. Potassium chloride may be added to fluids administered subcutaneously up to 30 mEq/L.

Potassium may be supplemented orally as the gluconate or citrate salts. Potassium chloride is not recommended because of its lack of palatability and acidifying nature. Potassium gluconate may be administered orally as tablets, flavored gel, or in a palatable powder form (Tumil-K, Virbac Corp., Fort Worth, TX). Depending on the size of the cat and severity of hypokalemia, potassium gluconate is given initially at a dose of 2 to 6 mEq per cat per day. Acidosis is a major risk factor for development of hypokalemia and therefore should be rectified early in the management of hypokalemia. Potassium citrate solution (Polycitra®-K Syrup, Baker Norton, Miami, FL) is an excellent alternative that has the advantage of providing simultaneous alkalinization therapy. Potassium citrate is initially given at a dose of 40 to 60 mg/kg/day divided into two or three doses. If muscle weakness is present, it usually resolves within 1 to 5 days after initiating parenteral or oral potassium supplements. Potassium dose should thereafter be adjusted based on the clinical response of the patient and serum potassium determinations. Serum potassium concentration should initially be monitored every 7 to 14 days and the dose adjusted accordingly to establish the final maintenance dose. In patients with hypokalemic polymyopathy, it may be necessary to monitor serum potassium concentrations every 24 to 48 hours during the initial phase of therapy. It is unclear whether all cats require long-term potassium supplementation; however, preliminary evidence suggests that such therapy is likely to be required by at least some older cats with chronic kidney disease.

Routine supplementation of low oral doses of potassium (2 mEq/day) has been recommended for all cats with chronic kidney disease.[59] This recommendation appears to be based on the as yet unproved hypothesis that in some cats with CKD, hypokalemia and potassium depletion might promote a self-perpetuating cycle of declining renal function, metabolic acidosis, and continuing potassium losses. It is proposed that supplementation may stabilize renal function before potassium depletion exacerbates the disease. Some investigators have observed positive responses to potassium supplementation in several normokalemic cats that had chronic renal insufficiency and failure. However, results of a recent clinical trial suggested that in cats with chronic renal insufficiency and failure that initially had normal serum potassium concentrations, daily supplementation for 6 months with 4 mEq of potassium gluconate was not demonstrably superior to providing sodium gluconate in restoring muscle potassium stores.[62] However, there were only a small number of cats enrolled in this clinical trial. In addition, median muscle potassium content did increase in the potassium supplemented cats from 328 to 402 mEq/kg, a value close to the value of 424 mEq/L established for normal cat muscle. Thus although the value of providing supplemental potassium to cats with chronic kidney disease having normal serum potassium concentrations has not been established, it is clear that muscle potassium, and probably total body potassium stores, are likely to be reduced in cats with chronic kidney disease, increasing the risk for developing hypokalemia. Further, evidence from this study indicates that chronic supplementation of 2 to 4 mEq/day of potassium is unlikely to be associated with significant adverse events. Based on current data, a recommendation cannot be made for or against routine supplementation of potassium.

Diets that are acidifying and restricted in magnesium content may promote hypokalemia. Therefore they should generally be avoided in cats with CKD. Intensive fluid therapy during uremic crises, particularly with potassium-deficient fluids, may promote hypokalemia in cats or dogs that were not previously hypokalemic. Therefore serum potassium concentrations should be monitored during fluid therapy, and maintenance fluids should be supplemented with potassium chloride to prevent iatrogenic hypokalemia (concentrations of 13 to 20 mEq/L are appropriate for maintenance fluids). Potassium given intravenously should not be administered at a rate exceeding 0.5 mEq/kg/hr.

Metabolic Acidosis

Alkalinization therapy designed to correct metabolic acidosis plays an important role in management of patients with CKD. Potential benefits of alkalinization therapy in these patients include (1) ameliorating signs of uremic acidosis, including anorexia, lethargy, nausea, vomiting, muscle weakness, and weight loss; (2) minimizing the catabolic effects of metabolic acidosis on protein metabolism[54]; (3) enhancing the patient's capacity to adapt to additional acid stress resulting from such factors as diarrhea, dehydration, or respiratory acidosis; (4) limiting skeletal damage (demineralization and inhibited skeletal growth) resulting from bone buffering; and (5) rectifying adverse effects of severe acidosis on the cardiovascular system (impaired myocardial contractility and enhanced venoconstriction).[105]

Although data are unavailable for dogs, a recent study in cats with chronic renal insufficiency and failure indicated that metabolic acidosis occurred in less than 10% of cats with stage 3 CKD, but it approaches 50% of cats in uremic crisis.[2] Based on this data, it appears that only a minority of cats with clinically stable CKD are likely to benefit from routine alkalinization therapy. Thus the decision to intervene with alkalinization therapy should be based on a laboratory assessment of the patient's acid-base status. Unfortunately, no clinical data provides an obvious intervention threshold for treating metabolic acidosis in dogs and cats. However, in studies performed at the authors' research center, clinicians have been unable to demonstrate any adverse clinical effects of mild to moderate chronic metabolic acidosis in cats with induced chronic renal insufficiency and failure. In absence of clear clinical data, the authors recommend considering alkalinization therapy for dogs and cats with stable chronic renal insufficiency and failure when blood gas analysis confirms plasma bicarbonate values remain below 15 mmol/L on more than one determination. However, for patients with metabolic acidosis associated with a blood pH below 7.10, immediate parenteral intervention with sodium bicarbonate should be considered to increase the blood pH above this value.[105]

Because serum total CO_2 measurements are of questionable accuracy and yet remain the most common tool for establishing acid-base status for most dogs and cats, the authors recommend that blood gas analysis be performed to confirm metabolic acidosis whenever total CO_2 declines below 15 mmol/L. Low serum or plasma total CO_2 values obtained by autoanalyzer techniques should be confirmed by blood gas analysis because falsely low total CO_2 readings may occur when blood collection tubes are not fully filled or are exposed to air while awaiting analysis.[106] In addition, there may be a substantial systematic difference between blood bicarbonate concentrations determined by blood gas analysis and serum total CO_2 concentrations determined on autoanalyzers due to inherent differences in the analytic methods. Appropriate reference ranges are equipment and method specific.

Treatment options for alkalinization therapy include diet, sodium bicarbonate, and potassium citrate. Most renal diets are neutral to slightly alkalinizing in effect and are an appropriate first step in mitigating metabolic acidosis. When several weeks of diet therapy alone fails to ameliorate the metabolic acidosis, alkalinization therapy should be considered.

Oral sodium bicarbonate is the most commonly used alkalinizing agent for patients with metabolic acidosis of chronic renal insufficiency and failure. Because the effects of gastric acid on oral sodium bicarbonate are unpredictable, the dose should be individualized for each patient. A suggested initial dose of sodium bicarbonate is 8 to 12 mg/kg body weight given every 8 to 12 hours. Unfortunately, many dogs and cats find sodium bicarbonate distasteful unless given as tablets. Sodium bicarbonate is available as 5- and 10-grain tablets.

Potassium citrate may offer the advantage, especially in cats, of allowing for the simultaneous treatment of both hypokalemia and acidosis with a single drug. Metabolic acidosis, when accompanied by potassium depletion or magnesium depletion, may respond poorly to alkali therapy alone. However, in that potassium doses required for adequate correction of hypokalemia may exceed the citrate dose required to correct acidosis, a risk exists for excessive alkalinization. Starting doses of 40 to 60 mg/kg every 8 to 12 hours are recommended.

Regardless of the alkalinizing agent chosen, administration of several smaller doses is preferred to a single large dose to minimize fluctuations in blood pH. The patient's response to alkalinization therapy should be determined by performing blood gas analysis 10 to 14 days after initiating therapy. Ideally, blood should be collected just prior to administration of the drug. Dose of the alkalinizing agent should be adjusted to maintain blood bicarbonate concentrations within the normal range. Because urine pH is often insensitive as a means of assessing the need for or response to treatment, it is not recommended for this purpose.

Arterial Hypertension

Rationale for Treatment CKD is the most common recognized cause for arterial hypertension in dogs and cats. In these species, hypertension has been linked to renal, ocular, neurologic, and cardiac complications. In dogs with naturally occurring chronic renal insufficiency and failure, higher initial blood pressure has been reported to be a risk factor for uremic crisis and mortality.[18] In addition, retinopathy and hypertensive encephalopathy were detected in three of 14 dogs with blood pressure values exceeding 180 mm Hg in this study. However, firm evidence that pharmacologically lowering blood pressure will prevent or ameliorate the renal and extrarenal complications of arterial hypertension in dogs is lacking.

Lethargy, blindness, retinal hemorrhage and detachment, cerebral hemorrhage, seizures, stupor, and ventricular hypertrophy have been reported in cats with hypertension.[107-109] Although it is likely that elevated blood pressure promotes progressive renal injury in cats, as yet no reported evidence confirms this relationship. However, in contrast to dogs, studies exist that support the clinical value of therapeutic intervention for hypertension in cats. Subcutaneous administration of the antihypertensive drug hydralazine was reported to reduce the prevalence of seizures that developed as a consequence of hypertension after renal transplantation.[108] In a recent study using a surgically induced model of hypertensive renal insufficiency, only two of 10 cats receiving the antihypertensive agent amlodipine developed evidence of hypertensive retinal lesions, whereas these lesions developed in seven of 10 cats receiving placebo.[107]

Indications for Treatment Unless evidence for hypertension-related organ injury is seen (e.g., retinal lesions, neurologic signs) or the systolic blood pressure is greater than 200 mm Hg, the decision to initiate antihypertensive therapy is not an emergency. Before initiating therapy for arterial hypertension, the patient's blood pressure should be established based on blood pressure determinations performed at three successive clinic visits. Every effort should be made to minimize the risk that measured elevations in blood pressure represent a transient "white coat" effect, rather than a sustained elevation in blood pressure.[110]

Patients with blood pressure values exceeding 160/100 mm Hg should be considered for treatment. Although specific values for diagnosis of arterial hypertension have not been established for dogs and cats, current evidence suggests that concurrent CKD may place them at increased risk for sustaining additional renal injury or developing complications associated with elevated blood pressure.[18,107-109] Findings in two studies suggested that ocular lesions associated with elevated blood pressure occurred in cats with systolic blood pressure values exceeding about 160 mm Hg. Similarly, in a study in dogs with naturally occurring CKD, the risk for uremic crises and increased mortality was reported to be increased in a group of dogs with systolic blood pressure values above 160 mm Hg.[18] However, this cut off point was arbitrarily chosen in this study and therefore should not be interpreted as defining the lower limit of hypertension.

General Goals and Guidelines for Treatment The optimum endpoint for antihypertensive therapy has not been established for dogs and cats with CKD. In the absence of such information, treatment for arterial hypertension should be initiated cautiously with the goal of reducing blood pressure to at least below 160/100 mm Hg. Except in patients with acute, severe ocular or neurologic lesions, rapid reduction in blood pressure is not necessary. Particularly in dogs, it may take weeks to months to achieve satisfactory blood pressure control.

ACE inhibitors, such as enalapril and benazepril, and calcium channel blocking (CCB) drugs, such as amlodipine, have potential renoprotective benefits and are therefore appropriate options for renal patients with hypertension.[111] ACE inhibitors generally produce a relatively small reduction in blood pressure.[112,113] However, because of their beneficial role in altering intraglomerular hemodynamics, proteinuria, and the profibrotic effects of the intrarenal renin-angiotensin system, ACE inhibitors may have renoprotective effects even in absence achieving adequate blood pressure control. In a recent study the ACE inhibitor, enalapril, reduced the severity of renal lesions that develop in dogs with surgically reduced renal mass.[112] Further, in dogs with naturally occurring glomerulopathies, enalapril significantly reduced proteinuria and may have been beneficial in stabilizing renal function.[22] Based on this, they appear to be the preferred antihypertensive agent for dogs with CKD. However, the role of the renin-angiotensin-aldosterone system (RAAS) and ACE inhibitor therapy in cats with CKD and hypertension is more controversial.[114-117] Evidence that activation of the RAAS is consistently central to the genesis of hypertension in cats is contradictory, and ACE inhibitors have not been found to be consistently effective in lowering blood pressure in cats with CKD. Therapy using either benazepril or enalapril may be initiated in dogs or cats with CKD at a dose of 0.5 mg/kg given orally every 24 hours.

Calcium channel blockers preferentially antagonize preglomerular vasoconstriction, which theoretically, should not reduce glomerular hypertension. However, CCBs appear to have additional renoprotective properties.[111] They may prevent renal injury by limiting renal growth, by reducing mesangial entrapment of macromolecules, and by attenuating the mitogenic effects of diverse cytokines and growth factors (e.g., PDGF, platelet-activating factor). In addition, amlodipine inhibits the in vitro proliferation of mesangial cells. However, clinical trials in humans have provided conflicting results as to the renoprotective effect of CCB beyond their antihypertensive effects. Controlled studies on the renoprotective effects of amlodipine in dogs and cats have not been published. In the authors' clinical experience, CCBs have been effective antihypertensive agents in dogs and cats with CKD. Because it is usually highly effective, has few side effects, and has a relative rapid onset, the long-acting dihydropyridine calcium antagonist amlodipine is the antihypertensive of choice for most cats with CKD. Amlodipine is prescribed at a dose of 0.625 mg for cats less than 4 kg and 1.25 mg for cats greater than 4 kg. In cats with CKD, amlodipine typically reduces systolic blood pressure by about 30 to 50 mm Hg within the first 1 to 2 months of therapy.[107,118] General principles of management of hypertension are described in Chapter 130, Hypertension.

Treatment of Anemia of Chronic Renal Failure
General Guidelines for Minimizing Anemia An obvious but often overlooked consideration is minimizing iatrogenic blood loss. Iatrogenic loss is especially likely to occur in hospitalized cats and small dogs because of repeated sampling for diagnostic tests and monitoring. Therefore the quantities of blood collected from these patients should be recorded and monitored.

Chronic low-grade GI blood loss can also result in moderate to severe anemia in patients with CKD that would otherwise have sufficient endogenous erythropoietin production to maintain their hematocrit values in the low-normal range. These patients may lack overt GI signs or melena. Iron deficiency, microcytosis and an elevation in BUN/creatinine ratio above what is expected in context of the patient's diet may provide indirect evidence of occult GI blood loss. Because of difficulty in confirming GI hemorrhage, a therapeutic course with histamine H_2-receptor antagonists and sucralfate may be considered. Improvements in hematocrit, appetite, or both indicate a positive response.

Iron deficiency is a relatively common problem in dogs and cats with CRF. In a recent study, the serum iron concentrations

of 3 of 6 CRF dogs and 3 of 7 CRF cats were below the reference range (transferrin saturations less than 20%).[119] Whether this is related primarily to inadequate intake and absorption of iron or increased losses of iron due to GI blood loss is unclear. Unfortunately, iron status can be difficult to assess in dogs and cats. Serum iron levels can be used to screen for both iron deficiency and anemia of chronic inflammatory disease as contributing factors in the diagnostic evaluation of anemia. In dogs, serum iron levels may not reflect body iron stores in that normal values can occur in patients with iron deficiency. However, determining stainable iron content in bone marrow is helpful in assessing body iron stores and may detect problems not identified by serum iron levels or transferrin saturation. When low serum iron levels reflect true iron deficiency, bone marrow stainable iron levels will be low; in those with anemia of chronic inflammatory disease, bone marrow levels will be normal or high reflecting sequestration. The distinction is important because anemia of chronic inflammatory disease will not improve in response to iron supplements and may even result in iron overload. It is necessary to identify and remove the concurrent inflammatory disease to treat anemia of chronic inflammatory disease. Transferrin saturation (estimated by dividing serum iron by total iron binding capacity) may be useful for assessing the ability of the mobilizable iron stores (perhaps independent of total tissue iron stores) to meet the demands of erythropoiesis and, thus is particularly useful in evaluating patients during periods of increased erythropoiesis such as during recombinant human erythropoietin (rHuEPO) therapy.

Oral supplementation with ferrous sulfate is the preferred therapy for treatment of iron deficiency anemia and also for prevention of iron-deficient erythropoiesis in patients starting erythropoietin replacement therapy. Alternatively, iron dextran may be administered by intramuscular injection. However, parenteral administration of iron is associated with a small risk of anaphylaxis, shunting of iron to reticuloendothelial storage, and iron overload. Although serum iron levels and transferrin saturation should be monitored to adjust therapy, starting doses of iron sulfate of 50 to 100 mg/day for cats and 100 to 300 mg/day for dogs have been recommended. Oral iron supplements may be associated with GI upset and diarrhea, so small divided doses may be preferable.

In addition to iron deficiency, other nutritional abnormalities may contribute to anemia in patients with CKD. Protein malnutrition and its attendant changes in plasma amino acid and hormone concentrations is known to cause suboptimal erythropoiesis and anemia. Similar changes occur in human patients and may reflect mild protein/calorie malnutrition commonly present in advanced CKD. Although they have not been examined in dogs and cats, deficiencies in riboflavin (vitamin B_2), cobalamin (vitamin B_{12}), folate, niacin, or pyridoxine (vitamin B_6) might theoretically induce nutritional anemia. Vitamin status cannot be easily determined in dogs and cats; however, deficiencies should be suspected in patients with persistent anorexia, protein and calorie malnutrition, or GI malabsorption. In addition, some drugs may predispose the patient to nutritional anemia even when dietary intake is normal. For example, therapy with trimethoprim or methotrexate may interfere with cellular folate metabolism. Hypersegmentation of the polymorphonuclear leukocytes may provide a clinical indication of vitamin B_{12} or folate deficiency.

Risk of nutritional deficiencies can be minimized through timely initiation of proper diet modifications and, if necessary, use of dietary supplements. In addition to minimizing renal anemia, preventing protein and calorie malnutrition may reduce morbidity. B vitamins, folate, and niacin can be provided as an oral supplement often with iron.[33] Care must be taken with multivitamins not to oversupplement the fat-soluble vitamins A and D.

RBC life span is decreased in advanced CKD. Proposed mechanisms for this mild hemolytic tendency include a malfunctioning of the membrane Na^+-K^+-ATPase pump and impaired regeneration of reduced glutathione needed to prevent hemoglobin oxidation. Cat hemoglobin appears to be especially prone to oxidative stress as evidenced by the frequent observation of Heinz bodies in their RBCs. Cats with CKD having large numbers of Heinz bodies tend to be more anemic. Drugs and foods (e.g., onions, propylene glycol, methylene blue, sulfonamides) that promote formation of Heinz bodies should be avoided in uremic pets whenever possible.

PTH has been postulated to play a role in the pathogenesis of anemia of CRF. PTH inhibits growth of all bone marrow cell lines in vitro. However, leukopenia and thrombocytopenia are not characteristic of CKD, arguing against an important role for PTH-induced bone marrow suppression. In a clinical series of canine CKD patients with anemia, the authors found no correlation between PTH levels and the degree of anemia.[34]

It has been postulated that increased serum phosphorus leads to increased intracellular red cell phosphorus. This in turn increases red cell 2,3 DPG levels, a noteworthy finding in anemic CRF patients.[34] Increased 2,3 DPG levels cause a rightward shift in the oxyhemoglobin dissociation curve, improving tissue oxygenation and decreasing the stimulus for erythropoietin synthesis.

Anabolic Steroids Anabolic steroids were at one time the mainstay of therapy for anemia associated with CKD. Although controlled safety and efficacy studies in dogs and cats are lacking, clinical experience with anabolic steroids has been disappointing. With the advent of rHuEPO therapy, androgens have largely fallen out of favor for treatment of renal anemia in human and veterinary medicine. Based on studies in human patients and clinical experience with veterinary patients, androgens appear to work in only a small percentage of patients (usually those mildly affected), have a long delay to onset of action, and may be associated with undesirable side effects. Administration of anabolic steroids for treatment of dogs and cats with anemia of CKD should probably be limited to those patients with symptomatic anemia in which all other factors adversely affecting erythropoiesis (nutritional deficiencies, blood loss, hemolysis, concurrent disease) have been eliminated and other treatment options (erythropoietin, transfusion) are unavailable or have been exhausted.

Blood Transfusion Transfusions of packed RBCs or whole blood may be indicated for anemic CKD patients who need rapid correction of their anemia, as in preparation for surgery. For some patients, repeated transfusions can be used for long-term maintenance of hematocrit. However, several drawbacks have limited the use of this therapy in dogs and cats, including lack of availability and expense of blood products, increasing risk of transfusion reactions with multiple transfusions, risk of immunosuppression, risk of transfer of infectious agents, and decreased life span of transfused cells in uremic patients. Even for the first transfusion, only compatible blood products (as determined by cross-matching) should be used in both dogs and cats. The post-transfusion target hematocrit should be the low end of the normal range. This should be adequate to reverse the anorexia and fatigue associated with the anemia while minimizing the complications of too rapid an increase in blood volume and viscosity such as circulatory overload, hypertension, and seizures.

Hormone Replacement Therapy Hormone replacement therapy using rHuEPO has become the treatment of choice for anemia of CKD in cats and dogs when hematocrit values decline below about 20% and clinical signs are attributable to the anemia. Administration of rHuEPO causes a dose-dependent increase in hematocrit.[119] Correction of hematocrit to low normal takes approximately 2 to 8 weeks, depending on the starting hematocrit and dose given. As the anemia is corrected, most clients report that their pets show increases in appetite, body weight, energy level, and sociability.[119] Initially, erythropoietin is usually administered at a dose of 50 to 150 U/kg subcutaneously three times weekly. Most dogs and cats should be started at 100 U/kg administered three times weekly. Hematocrit is monitored weekly or biweekly until a target hematocrit of approximately 30% to 40% for cats and 37% to 45% for dogs is achieved.[119] When anemia is severe (hematocrit < 14%) but does not require transfusion, daily therapy with 150 U/kg may be preferred for the first week. In the presence of hypertension or when anemia is not severe, a dose of 50 U/kg three times per week may help to prevent increases in blood pressure and iron-deficient erythropoiesis. When a hematocrit at the low end of the target range is reached, the dosing interval should be decreased to twice weekly. Most animals require 50 to 100 U/kg two to three times weekly to maintain their hematocrit in the target range; however, the dose and dosing interval required to maintain individual patients in the normal range is highly variable.

Ongoing monitoring of hematocrit will be necessary to allow adjustments in dose and dosing interval. Animals requiring more than 150 U/kg three times weekly should be evaluated for erythropoietin resistance. Because of the lag time between dose adjustment and effect on hematocrit, patience must be exercised so as not to adjust the dose too frequently. Frequent dose adjustments will result in rapid, unpredictable changes in hematocrit and an inability to find a stable dosing regimen. In general, dose should not be changed any more often than once monthly. Avoiding iatrogenic polycythemia is especially important.

The basis for individual differences in response to rHuEPO is incompletely understood. Several causes of blunted response or failure to resolve renal anemia with rHuEPO therapy have been identified, including functional or absolute iron deficiency, anti-rHuEPO antibody formation, ongoing GI blood loss or hemolysis, concurrent inflammatory or malignant disease, and aluminum overload (not documented in veterinary patients). Owner errors related to drug storage, handling, or administration may account for some instances of poor response to rHuEPO therapy.

The demand for iron associated with stimulated erythropoiesis is high, and human patients without pre-existing iron overload will exhaust iron storage during rHuEPO therapy. The same appears true of dogs and cats. Iron supplementation is therefore recommended for all patients receiving rHuEPO therapy.

Adverse effects related to rHuEPO therapy in dogs and cats may include systemic hypertension, seizures, local reactions at the injection site, and development of antibodies directed at erythropoietin.[119] Hypertension may develop or increase in severity with rHuEPO therapy. Increased peripheral vascular resistance secondary to improved oxygen delivery and reversal of the vasodilation induced by chronic hypoxia may contribute to this effect. Increased blood viscosity associated with the increased hematocrit is thought to be only a minor contributor. Seizures have been observed in human, canine, and feline patients being treated with rHuEPO that have no prior history of a seizure disorder.[119] In dogs and cats, they have been reported in the setting of moderate to severe azotemia. Although hypertension, anemia, and uremic encephalopathy may be contributory, in humans, seizures are thought to be related to compensatory adaptations to increases in RBC mass. Seizures are not thought to be directly related to rHuEPO.

Allergic reactions, including cutaneous or mucocutaneous reactions or cellulitis sometimes with fever and arthralgia, were uncommonly observed in both dogs and cats early in the course of rHuEPO therapy.[119] Lesions generally resolved within a few days and some did not recur when therapy was reinstated.

The most important complication associated with use of rHuEPO is refractory anemia and hypoplasia of the erythroid bone marrow associated with formation of neutralizing anti-rHuEPO antibodies.[119] In some affected patients, the severity of anemia was worse than before initiation of rHuEPO treatment. This observation suggested that the anti-rHuEPO antibodies were effective in interfering with the erythropoietin effects of rHuEPO and endogenous erythropoietin. The rHuEPO protein appears to be immunogenic in many, but not all, dogs and cats with antibody titers developing at variable times from several weeks to months after the onset of therapy. After cessation of therapy, antibody titers declined. In the absence of a widely available anti-EPO antibody assay, bone marrow myeloid/erythroid ratios provide the best method to ascertain if rHuEPO resistance is due to antibody formation. After therapy is stopped and antibody titers decline, suppressed erythropoiesis may be reversible and pretreatment levels of erythropoiesis are attained.

The relatively high prevalence of anti-rHuEPO antibody production prompts the question of when to initiate rHuEPO therapy. Premature initiation of erythropoietin therapy with subsequent development of antierythropoietin antibodies may deprive the patient of the clinical benefits of this therapy when clinical signs of anemia eventually do develop and rHuEPO can be of greatest clinical benefit. When hematocrit values are below 20%, anemia likely contributes to adverse clinical signs characteristic of uremia. In addition, degree of azotemia, expected rate of progression of kidney failure, appetite and willingness to eat therapeutic diets, and rate of progression of anemia must all be considered in the risk-benefit analysis of when to start therapy. The advantages and disadvantages of rHuEPO therapy should be discussed with the owners when anemia appears to be contributing to the patient's deteriorating quality of life. Many pet owners may consider quality of life to be as or more important than quantity of life.

Future Treatment Directions Future options for treatment of anemia of CKD may include development of species-specific erythropoietin and gene therapy.[120] Although not commercially available, recombinant canine and feline erythropoietin have been developed.[121] They offer the hope of erythropoietin replacement therapy in dogs and cats without concern for antierythropoietin antibody formation. If concern for antibody formation can be eliminated, erythropoietin therapy could be initiated earlier in the course of chronic renal insufficiency and failure. It also has been demonstrated that gene therapy can be used to induce extrarenal production of erythropoietin in cats.[122]

Calcitriol Therapy
Rationale for Calcitriol Therapy An undesirable consequence of reduced renal production of calcitriol is renal secondary hyperparathyroidism. Calcitriol (1,25-dihydroxyvitamin D), the most active metabolite of vitamin D, results from renal hydroxylation of 25-hydroxyvitamin D. Normally, calcitriol inhibits PTH synthesis and release and parathyroid gland growth, an effect mediated by the vitamin D receptor in the parathyroid gland. As functioning renal mass declines, renal production of calcitriol declines. In addition, phosphorus retention also inhibits renal hydroxylation of 25-hydroxyvitamin D to calcitriol and directly stimulates PTH release. By reducing PTH levels, calcitriol therapy minimizes abnormalities associated with renal secondary hyperparathyroidism. The effectiveness of calcitriol therapy in reducing PTH levels in dogs and

cats with CKD is well established.[39] Although PTH has been proposed as a potential uremic toxin responsible for many constitutional signs or uremia, the clinical benefits of reducing PTH levels have not been conclusively documented. Nagode and colleagues[39] published results of a survey of veterinarians that use calcitriol in management of dogs and cats with CKD. Results of this survey reveal a high level of enthusiasm for calcitriol among veterinarians using the drug. Clinical impressions concerning use of calcitriol in dogs and cats suggest that patients seem (1) to be brighter and more alert and interactive with owners, (2) to have an improvement in appetite, (3) to be more physically active than before treatment, and (4) to have longer life spans. Further, these authors provide pathophysiologic support for the purported benefits of calcitriol therapy through referenced studies from multiple species. In contrast, Finco and colleagues,[123] using parathyroidectomy combined with an experimental model of renal failure, concluded that increased PTH levels do not contribute importantly to clinical signs of uremia in dogs. However, this study was not designed to directly address the effectiveness of calcitriol therapy in managing clinical signs of dogs and cats with CKD.

Despite reported favorable impressions concerning use of calcitriol, its role in managing dogs and cats with CKD should be confirmed by randomized, controlled clinical trials. Routine clinical practice is never *blind*, because owners and veterinarians know when active treatment is being received. Interpretation of uncontrolled studies is confounded by the desire of pet owners and clinicians for success, as well as the placebo effect, which can cause both parties to overestimate efficacy. In addition, calcitriol has the potential to promote hypercalcemia and renal injury if improperly used. A recommendation for or against routine use of calcitriol awaits results of properly designed controlled clinical trials.

Guidelines for Using Calcitriol The primary goal of calcitriol therapy is to prevent or correct renal secondary hyperparathyroidism and its consequences. However, the decision to use calcitriol must be made with caution because hypercalcemia is a potentially serious complication. Sustained calcitriol-induced hypercalcemia will likely result in reversible or irreversible reduction in GFR. Although hypercalcemia reportedly occurs in 30% to 57% of humans treated with calcitriol, hypercalcemia appears to be an uncommon side effect in dogs treated with doses in the range of 2.5 to 3.5 ng/kg/day.[44] Hypercalcemia is likely to occur when calcitriol therapy is combined with calcium-containing phosphorus-binding agents, particularly calcium carbonate.

Serum phosphorus concentrations must be reduced to 6.0 mg/dL or lower before initiating calcitriol therapy (see discussion of management of hyperphosphatemia in this chapter). Serum phosphorus concentrations greater than 6.0 mg/dL may inhibit the effectiveness of calcitriol therapy and enhance the tendency for calcitriol to promote renal mineralization and injury. In addition, phosphorus restriction and calcitriol therapy are likely additive in reducing plasma PTH activities. Thus serum calcium and phosphorus concentrations should be carefully monitored in patients receiving calcitriol.

Calcitriol rapidly and effectively suppresses renal secondary hyperparathyroidism. An important advantage of calcitriol over other forms of vitamin D therapy in CKD is that calcitriol does not require renal activation for maximum efficacy. Dogs and cats appear to require much lower doses of calcitriol than those recommended for humans calculated on the basis of body weight.[39] Nagode and colleagues[39] have recommended a dose of 2.5 to 3.5 ng/kg body weight per day given orally to dogs and cats with CKD. The optimum maintenance dose for calcitriol must be determined for each patient based on serial evaluation of serum calcium and phosphorus and plasma PTH concentrations. The recommended endpoint of calcitriol therapy is normalization of PTH activity in absence of hypercalcemia. When the dose of calcitriol necessary to normalize PTH levels is associated with hypercalcemia, the daily dose may be doubled and given every other day. This approach is thought to be less likely to induce hypercalcemia because the effect of calcitriol on intestinal calcium absorption is related to the duration of exposure of intestinal cells to calcitriol.

When plasma PTH concentration is markedly elevated or when standard therapy with calcitriol fails to normalize plasma PTH levels, pulse calcitriol therapy has been recommended.[39] In this approach, patients are given 20 ng/kg of calcitriol twice per week in the evening on an empty stomach. Pulse therapy is usually used no longer than 1 to 2 months to suppress resistant hyperparathyroidism. If successful, calcitriol is then given at the standard daily dose. Because it enhances intestinal absorption of calcium and phosphorus, calcitriol should not be given with meals. Custom-made capsules or liquid preparations containing appropriate doses of calcitriol for use in dogs and cats are available from compounding pharmacies. Compounded calcitriol preparations should contain appropriate preservatives to prevent oxidation.

Early detection of hypercalcemia is indicated to limit the extent of renal injury. However, the onset of hypercalcemia after initiation of vitamin D therapy is unpredictable (i.e., it may occur after days to months of treatment). Therefore continued monitoring of serum calcium, phosphorus, and creatinine concentrations is necessary to detect hypercalcemia, hyperphosphatemia, or deteriorating renal function before irreversible renal damage ensues. Serum calcium, phosphorus, urea nitrogen, and creatinine concentrations should be monitored 1 week and 1 month after initiating calcitriol therapy, and monthly to bimonthly thereafter. The product of serum calcium and phosphorus concentrations should not exceed 60; the goal is to attain values between 42 and 52.[48] Calcitriol's rapid onset (about 1 day) and short duration of action (half-life less than 1 day) permits rapid control of unwanted hypercalcemia. If hypercalcemia develops, it is advisable to stop treatment completely rather than reduce the dose. Therapy may be reinstituted with a reduced dose when serum calcium concentration returns to normal and serum phosphorus concentration is less than 6.0 mg/dL.

Minimizing Progression of Renal Failure

All patients with CKD are at risk for progressive kidney disease. Progression may occur as a consequence of their primary renal disease, in association with a variety of secondary factors that may promote progressive renal disease, or both. An important therapeutic goal for managing patients with CKD is to minimize or prevent progressive loss of renal function. Treatment designed to limit progression of kidney disease may involve a variety of interventions including diet therapy, controlling hypertension, minimizing proteinuria, and modulating the renin-angiotensin-aldosterone system.

Clinical and experimental evidence indicates that dietary intervention may be effective in preserving renal structure and function and prolonging survival. In a randomized controlled clinical trial in dogs with naturally occurring CKD, dietary intervention significantly prolonged survival and slowed decline in renal function.[1] Dogs consuming the renal diet survived an average 593 days, whereas dogs consuming a maintenance diet survived an average 188 days. This beneficial effect applied over a range of serum creatinine values encompassing both stages 3 and 4 CKD. Renal function declined in both groups, but the decline was significantly greater in the dogs consuming the maintenance diet. The specific mechanisms underlying the beneficial effects of the diet were not determined. However, it is likely that at least dietary phosphorus restriction and omega-3 PUFA supplementation contributed to the favorable effect.[1,57,93,94] It is also likely that

once the dogs progressed to a more advanced level of renal dysfunction, dietary protein restriction provided an additional period of symptomatic relief, thereby prolonging survival further.

Similarly, in a nonrandomized clinical trial, cats fed a renal diet survived significantly longer than cats that continued to consume their usual diet (633 days versus 264 days).[64] It was not possible to establish the differences between diets used in this study, but the therapeutic renal diet was reduced in protein and phosphorus content. The renal diet was shown to be beneficial in lowering serum phosphorus and PTH concentrations, and it was suggested that the beneficial effect of the diet may have been related to this effect.[99]

Treatments designed to limit hypertension and proteinuria may also be of value in slowing progression of kidney disease and kidney failure. Hypertension and proteinuria are a well-established risk factors for progression of renal disease in humans.[19,124] Similarly, studies at the University of Minnesota Veterinary Medical Center have shown that elevated blood pressure and proteinuria are risk factors for uremic crises and increased mortality in dogs with stages 3 and 4 CKD.[18] The effects of blood pressure and proteinuria on progression of feline CKD have not been established.

Experimental and clinical evidence has confirmed the beneficial effect of blood pressure control on slowing progression of diabetic and nondiabetic nephropathies in humans.[19,125] In one large clinical trial, the renoprotective effect of antihypertensive therapy was further enhanced by maintaining blood pressure below the usual target value.[126] As a consequence, the "ideal" blood pressure to attain using antihypertensive therapy in human patients with CKD remains unresolved. Patient factors such as the presence or absence of proteinuria may also influence the goals of therapy. Antihypertensive therapy was most effective in limiting progression of kidney disease in patients with proteinuria. A greater reduction in blood pressure appears to be necessary for equivalent renoprotection in patients with greater levels of proteinuria.[19,126] Further, independent of blood pressure control, reducing proteinuria has been shown to have a favorable influence on kidney disease progression.[127]

Evidence supporting the renoprotective value of antihypertensive therapy in dogs and cats with naturally occurring CKD is lacking. However, studies performed in dogs with induced CKD indicate that administration of the ACE inhibitor, enalapril, limited glomerular and systemic hypertension, proteinuria, and glomerular and tubulointerstitial lesions.[112] Interestingly, enalapril was renoprotective in this study, despite the fact that the dogs had only mild hypertension and relatively modest proteinuria. Enalapril has also been reported to ameliorate proteinuria and stabilize renal function in dogs with naturally occurring glomerulopathies with protein/creatinine ratios greater than 3.0.[22] Enalapril therapy was associated with a reduction in proteinuria of over 50%. Over the 6 months of study, serum creatinine increased by more than 0.2 mg/dL in 13 of 14 dogs receiving placebo, but only three of 16 dogs receiving enalapril. In this study, enalapril significantly reduced systolic blood pressure from a mean of 154+/−25 before therapy to 142+/-19 after 6 months of treatment.

In humans, ACE inhibitors are generally considered to be the antihypertensive drugs of choice in patients with CKD, particularly when proteinuria is evident, because they lower both systemic and intraglomerular pressures and proteinuria.[19] Further, ACE inhibitors are indicated for patients with proteinuric CKD for the purpose of reducing proteinuria, regardless of whether the patient is hypertensive. It appears appropriate to consider ACE inhibitor treatment for dogs with CKD when systolic blood pressure values are proven to remain above 160 mm Hg and when the urine protein/creatinine values exceed 1.0.

ACE inhibitors reduce blood pressure and proteinuria in cats; however, their unique renoprotective value has yet to be established in this species.[113] As a consequence, recommendations concerning use of ACE inhibitors in cats with CKD remain unresolved. The dihydropyridine calcium-channel blocker amlodipine is the antihypertensive drug of choice for most cats. However, in humans, dihydropyridine calcium-channel blockers appear to be associated with a greater risk of progression of kidney disease.[126] Although clinical impression suggests this is not the case in cats with CKD, the effect of amlodipine on progressive renal disease has not been critically examined in cats. It has been suggested that combining amlodipine with an ACE inhibitor might have greater renal-sparing potential. Studies into the clinical value of this drug combination are needed in cats with spontaneous renal failure.

The renoprotective effects of ACE inhibitors cannot be explained entirely by their effects on blood pressure. It is likely that renoprotection results in part from suppressing renal levels of angiotensin II. Angiotensin II may adversely affect the kidneys in several ways (Box 260-8).[125] Because of the role of angiotensin II in progression of CKD, angiotensin receptor blockers have also been considered for humans with CKD.[128] Angiotensin receptor blockers and ACE inhibitors differ in the mechanism by which they inhibit angiotensin II. The ACE inhibitors block conversion of angiotensin I to angiotensin II. However, angiotensin II formation is not completely inhibited because it can also be generated by a nonACE-dependent pathway such as by the enzyme chymase. In addition, because bradykinin is normally degraded by ACE, ACE inhibitor therapy is associated with elevated bradykinin levels. Bradykinin is a vasodilator that may have renoprotective effects by stimulating nitric oxide production. Angiotensin receptor antagonists block the type 1 receptor but leave type 2 receptor effects unopposed, which appears to be important in vasodilation. In rats with nephropathy, angiotensin II antagonism has been reported to normalize proteinuria, eliminate inflammatory cell infiltration, and ameliorate glomerular and tubular structural changes.[129] A combination of an angiotensin receptor antagonist and ACE inhibitor has been suggested as a way to maximize blockade of the renin-angiotensin system by affecting both the bioavailability of angiotensin II and also by affecting its activity at the receptor level.[130] Each type of drug has been shown to be effective in reducing proteinuria and slowing progression of renal disease. However, in experimental models and clinical models in humans, combination therapy has proven more effective than either drug alone.[128] In humans there does not appear to be an increase in toxicity or adverse events with combination therapy.[125]

Whether combination therapy is safe, effective, and provides a therapeutic advantage needs to be determined for dogs and cats with CKD.

Blockade of the renin-angiotensin system limits both angiotensin II and aldosterone while retarding progression of renal disease. Recent studies have implicated aldosterone as an important pathogenic factor in this process.[131,132] Selective blockade of aldosterone, independent of renin-angiotensin blockade, reduces proteinuria and glomerular lesions in rats with experimental kidney disease. Where blockade of the renin-angiotensin system ameliorates proteinuria and glomerular injury, selective reinfusion of aldosterone restores proteinuria and glomerular lesions despite continued blockade of the renin-angiotensin system. This observation suggests an independent pathogenic role for aldosterone as a mediator of progressive renal disease. Aldosterone appears to promote progressive renal injury through both hemodynamic effects and direct cellular actions.[131] It appears to have fibrogenic properties in the kidneys, perhaps in part by promoting production of the profibrotic cytokine TGF-β.[132] Experimental studies have shown that the aldosterone-receptor antagonist eplerenone may attenuate proteinuria and renal damage, independent of its effect on blood pressure. Although ACE inhibitors initially cause an acute reduction in aldosterone concentration, this effect is not sustained. It has been proposed that use of aldosterone-receptor antagonists in addition to ACE inhibitors will have additional benefits toward protecting the kidneys.[131] However, the role of this form of therapy has yet to be established.

Vasopeptidase inhibitors are agents that inhibit both ACE and neutral endopeptidase, an enzyme involved in the breakdown of natriuretic peptides, adrenomedullin, and bradykinin. They decrease angiotensin II production and increase accumulation of the previously mentioned vasodilators. In experimental renal disease, they appear to have a greater renoprotective effect than ACE inhibitors.[133] Studies on these agents have not been reported in dogs and cats with CKD.

Inflammation is a prominent feature of progressive renal diseases. Future therapies are likely to include novel inhibitors of specific profibrotic or proinflammatory cytokines and growth factors. The immunosuppressive agent mycophenolate mofetil has been shown to be renoprotective in remnant kidney rats.[134] Pirfenidone, an antifibrotic agent, has been shown to attenuate renal fibrosis.[135]

PATIENT MONITORING

Response to treatment should be monitored at appropriate intervals so that treatment can be individualized to the specific and often changing needs of the patient. The data base obtained before initiating therapy or after correcting an overt uremic crisis should be used as a baseline for comparison of the patient's progress. This evaluation should be repeated at appropriate intervals. Evaluations every 2 to 4 weeks are suggested until the initial response to therapy can be established. However, the frequency of evaluation may vary depending on severity of renal dysfunction, complications present in the patient, and response to treatment. Patients receiving therapy with erythropoietin or calcitriol require frequent, life-long monitoring. After the initial response to therapy has been established, dogs and cats in stages 1 and 2 CKD may require evaluation as infrequently as every 6 to 12 months. However, patients with substantial proteinuria may require monitoring much more frequently, depending on the course of their disease. Cats and dogs in stages 3 and 4 CKD should be re-evaluated about every 2 to 4 months, depending on the stability of their renal function. Specific recommendations for monitoring are described in the various treatment sections.

Box • 260-8

Potential Adverse Effects of Angiotensin II on the Kidneys

Glomerular hypertension
Impaired glomerular permselectivity
Mesangial cell proliferation
Induction of TGF-β, thereby increasing production of extracellular matrix
Increased aldosterone production
Macrophage activation; activation of inflammation-related transcription factors
Increased production of plasminogen activator inhibitor-1

Modified from Rosenberg ME: Chronic kidney disease: progression. NephSAP 2(3):94, 2003.

CHAPTER 261

Glomerular Diseases

Shelly L. Vaden

Glomerular diseases are a leading cause of renal disease and renal failure in dogs.[1] In randomly selected dogs, the incidence of glomerular lesions is as high as 43% to 90%,[2] and the incidence appears to increase with age.[3] Glomerular diseases also occur in cats, although they are less common. It has been accepted that amyloidosis and glomerulonephritis are the most common glomerular diseases of dogs and cats (Box 261-1). However, to make progress toward improved diagnosis and management of dogs and cats with glomerular disease, veterinarians must come to consider the different forms of glomerulonephritis as specific entities: membranous glomerulopathy, membranoproliferative glomerulonephritis and proliferative glomerulonephritis (including the subclass of IgA nephropathy). The proposed pathogenesis of each entity is somewhat different; in humans this leads to different clinical features and specific treatment recommendations for each disease.[4,5] Hereditary nephritis and minimal change disease are less common glomerular diseases in dogs and cats.

NORMAL GLOMERULAR STRUCTURE AND FUNCTION

The glomerulus is a modified capillary bed that functions as a filter, across which an ultrafiltrate of the plasma is formed.[4,5] The filtration barrier is composed of three layers: the fenestrated endothelium, the glomerular basement membrane (GBM), and the visceral epithelial cells, or *podocytes* (Figure 261-1). This complex structure is freely permeable to water and small dissolved solutes but retains cells and most macromolecules, such as proteins. The major determinant of passage into the filtrate is molecular size. Small molecules, such as inulin (5000 daltons), pass freely through the filter. Substances are retained with increasing efficiency as they increase in size to approximately 60,000 to 70,000 daltons; only small amounts of substances larger than this are filtered. Although the issue currently is a matter of dispute, many believe that ionic charge also influences filtration, and that negatively charged proteins are retained to a greater extent than would be predicted by size alone.[6] The podocyte foot processes and the slit diaphragms between them, as well as the basement membrane and the endothelium, are rich in negatively charged glycoproteins, creating this charge barrier. These polyanions are believed to play an important role in the maintenance of normal glomerular permeability and visceral epithelial cell shape. Albumin, a negatively charged protein with a molecular weight of 69,000 daltons, is normally largely excluded from the filtrate.

Despite this complex filtration system, small amounts of albumin and other proteins are normally found in the filtrate. Substantial degradation of these proteins occurs, resulting in excretion only of peptide fragments, which are not detected by routine total protein assays. Proteins and peptide fragments may also undergo resorption in the nephron distal to the glomerulus.[6]

CLINICAL FINDINGS IN GLOMERULAR DISEASE

Signalment

Glomerular disease can develop in a dog of any age but appears to be most common in middle-aged to older dogs. The prevalence of microalbuminuria, a marker of increased glomerular permeability, increases as dogs age, with more marked increases seen beyond 6 years of age.[7] The average age of 375 dogs with a variety of glomerular diseases reported in five studies was 8.3 years.[1,8-11] Male and female dogs were equally represented. However, the average age and gender predilection seen with specific glomerular diseases varies somewhat from the overall averages. Glomerular diseases often occur secondary to another disease process. Infectious and noninfectious inflammatory diseases may be more likely in young and middle-aged animals, whereas neoplasms are more common causes of glomerular disease in older patients. Familial glomerular diseases often are manifested at an early age. Several breeds of dogs are known to have familial glomerular diseases (Table 261-1). Labrador retrievers and golden retrievers may have a higher incidence of glomerular disease; however, the possibility that this increased representation reflects the popularity of these breeds requires further evaluation.[8,12]

History

The clinical signs associated with glomerular disease vary considerably, depending on the severity of proteinuria and the

---

Box • 261-1

Glomerular Diseases Described in Dogs and Cats

Amyloidosis
Focal segmental glomerulosclerosis
Glomerulonephritis
    Crescentic type (rare)
    Membranoproliferative form
        Type I (mesangiocapillary)
        Type II (dense deposit disease)?
    Proliferative glomerulonephritis (mesangial and endocapillary)
IgA nephropathy
Glomerulosclerosis
Hereditary nephritis
Lupus nephritis
Membranous glomerulopathy*
Minimal change glomerulopathy

*Membranous glomerulopathy is the most common glomerular disease in cats; other glomerular diseases appear to be uncommon in cats.

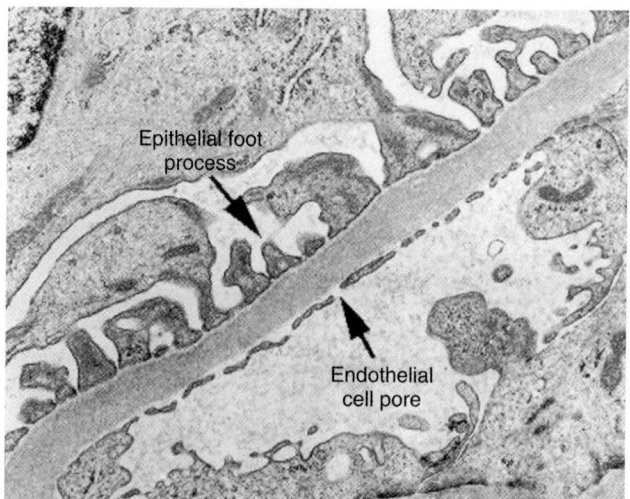

Figure 261-1 Electron micrograph of a glomerular capillary wall showing the filtration barrier composed of the fenestrated endothelium, the glomerular basement membrane, and the visceral epithelial cell (podocyte). (Courtesy J.C. Jennette, Chapel Hill, NC, School of Medicine, University of North Carolina.)

presence or absence of renal failure.[8,9,13] Many animals with glomerular disease are asymptomatic, and proteinuria is detected during routine health screening. Alternatively, animals may manifest specific signs related to an underlying inflammatory, infectious, or neoplastic condition (Boxes 261-2 and 261-3). Signs of glomerular disease may be nonspecific (e.g., weight loss, lethargy) or consistent with chronic renal failure or uremia (polyuria, polydipsia, anorexia, vomiting, and malodorous breath). Acute renal failure is a less common presentation for animals with glomerular disease. When urinary protein losses are severe, signs of fluid retention (e.g., abdominal enlargement consistent with ascites, peripheral edema) or thromboembolism (e.g., dyspnea, loss of limb function) may be present.

Table • 261-1

Breeds of Dogs with Familial Glomerulopathies

BREED	GLOMERULAR DISEASE
Beagle	Amyloidosis
Bernese mountain dog	Mesangiocapillary glomerulonephritis
Bull terrier	Hereditary nephritis
Cocker spaniel (especially English)	Hereditary nephritis
Dalmatian	Hereditary nephritis
Doberman pinscher	Glomerulosclerosis, cystic glomerular atrophy
English foxhound	Amyloidosis
Greyhound	Glomerular vasculopathy and necrosis
Newfoundland	Glomerulosclerosis
Rottweiler	Atrophic glomerulopathy
Samoyed (rare)	Hereditary nephritis
Shar Pei	Amyloidosis
Soft-coated wheaten terrier	Proliferative and sclerosing glomerulonephritis

Box • 261-2

Diseases Reported in Association with Glomerular Disease in Dogs

Systemic Disease (Glomerular Disease)
Infectious
Bacterial
Borreliosis (MPGN)
Bartonellosis (G)
Brucellosis (G)
Endocarditis (G)
Pyelonephritis (A)
Pyometra (A, G)
Pyoderma (A, G)
Other chronic bacterial infections (A, G)
Protozoal
Babesiosis (MPGN)
Hepatozoonosis (G)
Leishmaniasis (A, MPGN, MN, P-E and M)
Trypanosomiasis (G)
Rickettsial
Ehrlichiosis (G)
Viral
Canine adenovirus type 1 (P-M)
Parasitic
Dirofilariasis (A, MPGN, MN)
Fungal
Blastomycosis (A)
Coccidioidomycosis (A, G)
Inflammatory
Chronic dermatitis (A, G)
Inflammatory bowel disease (G)
Pancreatitis (A, G)
Periodontal disease (A, G)
Polyarthritis (A, G)
Systemic lupus erythematosus (A, MPGN, MN, P-E and M)
Other immune-mediated diseases (G)
Neoplastic
Leukemia (G)
Lymphosarcoma (A, G)
Mastocytosis (G)
Primary erythrocytosis (MCD?)
Systemic histiocytosis (G)
Other neoplasms (A, G, MN)
Miscellaneous
Corticosteroid excess (G)
Trimethoprim-sulfa therapy (G)
Hyperlipidemia (?)
Chronic insulin infusion (A)
Congenital C3 deficiency (MPGN)
Cyclic hematopoiesis in gray collies (A)
Familial (see Table 261-1)
Idiopathic (A, G, MPGN, MN, MCD, P-E or M)

A, Amyloidosis; *G*, glomerulonephritis, uncharacterized; *MPGN*, membranoproliferative (mesangiocapillary) glomerulonephritis; *MN*, membranous nephropathy; *MCD*, minimal change disease; *P*, proliferative (*E*, endocapillary or *M*, mesangial).

URINARY SYSTEM

Box • 261-3

Diseases Reported in Association with Glomerular Disease in Cats

Systemic Disease (Glomerular Disease)
Infectious
Bacterial
   Chronic bacterial infections (G)
   Mycoplasmal polyarthritis (G)
Viral
   Feline immunodeficiency virus (G)
   Feline infectious peritonitis (MN)
   Feline leukemia virus (G, MN)
Inflammatory
   Pancreatitis (G)
   Cholangiohepatitis (G)
   Chronic progressive polyarthritis (G)
   Systemic lupus erythematosus (MN)
   Other immune-mediated diseases (G)
Neoplastic
   Leukemia (MN)
   Lymphosarcoma (MN)
   Mastocytosis (G)
   Other neoplasms (G)
Miscellaneous
   Acromegaly (?)
   Mercury toxicity (MN)
Familial (MN)
Idiopathic (MN)

G, Glomerulonephritis, uncharacterized; *MN*, membranous nephropathy.

Hypertensive damage to the central nervous system, eyes, or heart may induce a variety of clinical signs.

Physical Examination Findings

The physical examination is often unremarkable in dogs with glomerular disease.[8,9,13] Nonspecific evidence of systemic disease may be present, such as poor body condition or poor haircoat. Dogs with advanced renal failure may have oral ulcerations, pale mucous membranes, or dehydration. Subcutaneous edema or ascites, or both, is sometimes noted. Occasionally dogs have physical evidence of thromboembolic disease, such as dyspnea or a decreased or absent peripheral pulse. Evidence of a predisposing inflammatory, infectious, or neoplastic process may be detected during the physical examination. The kidneys of affected animals are variable in size. Animals with chronic renal failure often have small, firm, irregularly shaped kidneys, whereas those with milder disease often have normal-sized or, occasionally, enlarged kidneys.

Clinicopathologic and Imaging Findings

Proteinuria is the hallmark of glomerular disease and is discussed in Chapter 32. A urine protein to creatinine ratio (UPC) greater than 0.5 in a urine sample free of evidence of inflammation and macroscopic hematuria is abnormal. With respect to the UPC, no magic number or range of numbers is diagnostic for any one renal disease, and the overlap in expected ranges is too broad to be clinically reliable. In general, dogs with amyloidosis or membranous nephropathy have the highest UPCs, and those with tubulointerstitial disease have lower values.[14] Glomerular lesions have been identified in dogs

without proteinuria.[15,16] In three studies of urine albumin in canine models of glomerular disease, microalbuminuria was detected prior to increases in the UPC, and the magnitude of microalbuminuria increased over time in dogs that eventually developed an increased UPC.[17-19] It therefore seems reasonable to conclude that a dog with persistent microalbuminuria of increasing magnitude should be assessed as having an injurious process to the glomerular filtration barrier and may eventually develop overt proteinuria.

Isosthenuria is a variable finding in dogs and cats with glomerular disease. In one study of dogs with glomerulonephritis, 37% had urine specific gravities in excess of 1.035, and isosthenuria was detected in only 29%.[9] However, dilute urine (i.e., a urine specific gravity less than 1.016) was more common in dogs with amyloidosis, occurring in 63% of dogs, whereas only 5.1% were able to concentrate above 1.035.[13] The presence of renal azotemia and an intact concentrating ability, called *glomerulotubular imbalance*, is indicative of glomerular disease. Cylindruria is common in dogs with glomerular disease; casts are most often hyaline but can be granular, waxy, or fatty. It is believed that proteins are packaged into casts to protect the renal tubular epithelium from their damaging effects. Renal hematuria develops with glomerular injury in humans and is more common in specific diseases (e.g., IgA nephropathy, mesangial proliferative glomerulonephritis), but it appears to be less common in dogs with glomerulopathies.[5] Erythrocytes that have passed through the abnormal glomerular capillary bed are often misshapen; the morphology of urine erythrocytes can be used to differentiate hematuria of glomerular origin from that due to other causes.

Hypoproteinemia due to hypoalbuminemia develops in many dogs and cats with glomerular disease and is more likely in animals with heavy proteinuria. Hypoalbuminemia occurred in 60% and 70% of dogs with glomerulonephritis or amyloidosis, respectively.[9,13] Azotemia, hyperphosphatemia, and metabolic acidosis, consistent with renal failure, may be present in dogs with severe disease. Of dogs with glomerulonephritis or amyloidosis, 53% and 26% respectively, were not azotemic.[9,13] Nonregenerative anemia that develops secondary to renal failure or to a systemic disease is observed in many affected animals. Other hematologic abnormalities also may reflect concurrent and possibly underlying systemic diseases. Thrombocytosis and hyperfibrinogenemia are common findings in dogs with glomerular disease.

The nephrotic syndrome of hypoalbuminemia, proteinuria, hypercholesterolemia, and edema, although pathognomonic for glomerular disease, was present in only 15% of dogs with glomerulonephritis in one study.[9] Incomplete nephrotic syndrome (i.e., without edema or ascites) was more common, occurring in 49% of the dogs.[9] Nephrotic syndrome is expected to occur more commonly in dogs with amyloidosis, membranous nephropathy, hereditary nephritis, and minimal change disease because of the heavy proteinuria associated with these diseases.[5,14]

On abdominal radiographs, the kidneys may appear normal or small and irregular. Some animals may actually have enlarged kidneys. Similar changes in shape and size can be seen with ultrasonographic scans, on which increased echogenicity of the cortex and loss of corticomedullary distinction may also be noted. The renal pelvis may be mildly dilated if polyuria is present or if fluids are being administered.

Dogs and cats with proteinuria should be thoroughly evaluated for underlying infectious, inflammatory, or neoplastic diseases (see Boxes 261-2 and 261-3). This evaluation should include a thorough physical examination, and diseases of the oral cavity and skin should not be overlooked as potential underlying diseases. Aspiration cytology should be performed on all cutaneous and subcutaneous masses. Serologic testing for regional infectious diseases, as well as antinuclear antibody testing, should be performed. During radiographic or ultrasonographic evaluation of the abdomen, attention should be given to other organs to detect any other disease process. Thoracic radiographs should also be evaluated in middle-aged to older dogs.

Histologic Diagnoses

Renal biopsy provides a definitive diagnosis of glomerular disease but may not be needed if treatment of a potential underlying disease leads to resolution of the proteinuria or if end-stage renal disease is already present. When evaluated appropriately, renal biopsy specimens can provide important clinical information about the type and severity of lesions in dogs and cats with glomerular disease. In fact, obtaining an accurate histologic diagnosis may be one of the more important factors in successful management of the dog or cat with glomerular disease. Clinical decisions regarding the diagnosis, treatment, and prognosis can be made from the information obtained through renal biopsy.

Procurement and Processing of the Renal Biopsy Specimen

The procedure used to obtain a renal biopsy specimen is discussed in Chapter 84. When a specimen is to be used for evaluation of glomerular disease, only cortical tissue should be obtained, because biopsy of the medulla is not needed and is associated with a greater risk of hemorrhage, infarction, and fibrosis. The use of general anesthesia is associated with an ability to obtain better quality specimens. An adequate sample of cortex has a minimum of five glomeruli when examined by light microscopy, although one glomerulus may be all that is needed to make a definitive diagnosis.

If a percutaneous method is used to obtain a renal biopsy specimen from a patient with glomerular disease, at least two quality samples of renal cortex should be obtained, using either a 16- or 18-gauge needle. A dissecting microscope can be used to verify that two adequate biopsy samples have been obtained. One sample should be placed in formalin, and the other should be divided into two smaller pieces containing glomeruli. One piece is put into a fixative suitable for electron microscopy (EM) (e.g., 4% formalin plus 1% glutaraldehyde in sodium phosphate buffer), and the other piece is frozen for immunofluorescent microscopy (IFM). An alternative to freezing is to immerse the tissue in ammonium sulfate-N-ethylmaleimide fixative (i.e., Michel's solution), which preserves tissue-fixed immunoglobulins. Wedge biopsies should be divided in a similar fashion; tissue for EM should be minced appropriately.

Thin sections (2 to 4 μm) of paraffin-embedded tissue should be used for light microscopy because standard sections of 5 to 6 μm are too thick for adequate assessment of glomerular cellularity and capillary loop thickness.[4] Hematoxylin and eosin staining can be used for initial assessment of the general appearance of the specimen. However, periodic acid–Schiff (PAS), which stains glycoproteins, is the preferred stain of many nephropathologists and is particularly useful for demonstration of interstitial and glomerular scarring and for assessment of the GBM. Methenamine silver specifically stains the basement membrane of the tubules, glomeruli, and Bowman's capsule. Trichrome is useful for evaluation of the mesangium and is also the best light microscopic stain for visualization of immunoglobulins. Congo red can be used to demonstrate the presence of amyloid.

EM of renal biopsy specimens has not been used frequently enough in dogs and cats to determine the diagnostic merit in groups of patients with varying presentations; however, in humans, EM appears to be most helpful in the evaluation of individuals with renal hematuria, a familial history of renal disease, or proteinuria with normal renal excretory function. Nevertheless, a sample should be collected for EM in nearly all dogs and cats undergoing renal biopsy, because the exact diagnosis is most likely unknown. IFM or immunohistochemistry should include at a minimum stains for immunoglobulin M (IgM), IgG, IgA, and C3.

Evaluation of the Renal Biopsy Specimen

Whenever possible, specimens should be evaluated by a pathologist with expertise in nephropathology. Renal biopsy specimens from proteinuric dogs and cats should be evaluated by light microscopy, EM, and IFM. Limiting the evaluation to light microscopy alone often allows for only a subjective interpretation of the glomerular lesion, leaving too much room for error. Although many reports have described glomerular lesions in dogs and cats, the use of different nomenclature and different morphologic criteria among pathologists sometimes makes interpretation and comparison of the data difficult at best. A standard classification system for the characterization of glomerular lesions in dogs and cats needs to be embraced. The World Health Organization (WHO) criteria for the classification of human glomerulopathies have proved to be applicable to glomerular diseases in dogs.[11] General acceptance of this system would lead to a better understanding of the natural history, pathogenesis, and response to treatment in the various glomerular diseases in dogs and cats.

The normal glomerulus contains four to eight lobules, each composed of capillaries supported on a centrilobular core of mesangial matrix (Figure 261-2).[4,5] The GBM is thin, delicate, PAS-positive, and argyrophilic. The glomerular capillary lumen is normally widely patent and lined with eosinophilic endothelial cell cytoplasm (Figure 261-3). There should be only one or two nuclei per mesangial cell region. Parietal epithelial cells, visceral epithelial cells, endothelial cells, and mesangial cells comprise the normal glomerulus and can easily be identified by EM (see Figure 261-1). The flattened parietal epithelial cells line the inner surface of Bowman's capsule. The visceral epithelial cells (podocytes) line the outer surface of the capillary loops and rest on the GBM. The podocytes, which are characterized by their foot processes, form the outermost layer of the capillary wall. The endothelial cells line the inner surface of the capillary loops, with the nuclei disposed centrilobularly, toward the mesangium. The fenestrations of the endothelial cell cytoplasm can be visualized easily.

Normal Glomerular Capillary

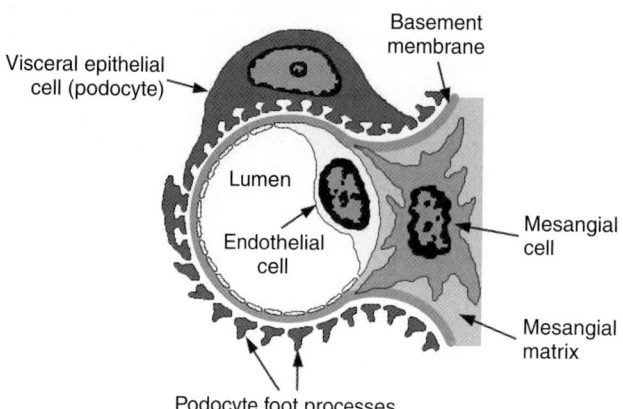

Figure 261-2 Schematic diagram showing the composition of each lobule in a normal capillary. (Courtesy J.C. Jennette, Chapel Hill, NC, School of Medicine, University of North Carolina.)

URINARY SYSTEM

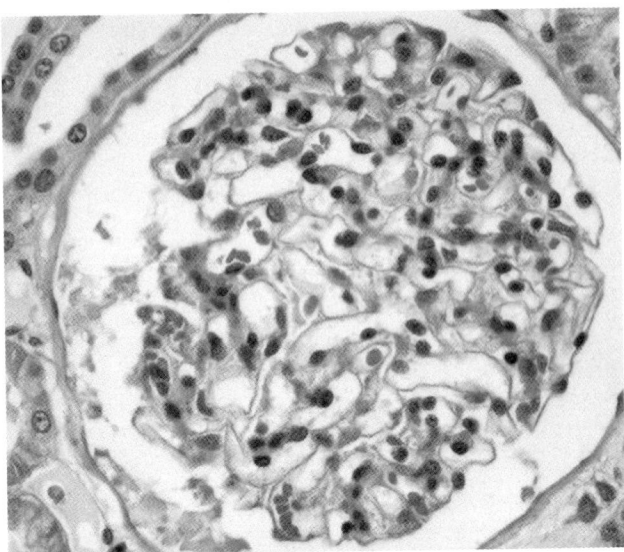

Figure 261-3 Normal glomerulus from a dog. Note that the capillary lumens are widely patent and the capillary loops are thin, often appearing discontinuous. Hypercellularity is not present.

The normal GBM should be approximately the same thickness as the base of a foot process turned 90 degrees.

When glomerular lesions are present, if nearly all of the glomeruli are affected, the disorder is *generalized*. The disorder is *focal* if less than half of the glomeruli are affected. When evaluating individual glomeruli, if the entire glomerulus is affected, the pattern is *diffuse*, or *global*. The lesion is *segmental* or *local* if only a few lobules within affected glomeruli are involved. Descriptions of each of the pathologic findings in the varying glomerular diseases are provided below. Lupus nephritis can be associated with several glomerular lesions and, when active, may have an interstitial infiltrate of mixed inflammatory cells and acute damage to the tubules.[5] *Crescents* can loosely be defined as two or more layers of cells in Bowman's space and are suggestive of severe injury. Crescentic glomerulonephritis, which is diagnosed when crescents are present in 50% or more of the glomeruli, appears to be uncommon in dogs and cats.

Immunofluorescent staining should be positive in dogs or cats with either *in situ* immune complex formation, as is believed to occur with primary membranous glomerulopathy, or with deposition of circulating complexes, as may occur with type I membranoproliferative glomerulonephritis and proliferative glomerulonephritis.[4,5] Because true anti-GBM GN has not been documented in the dog or cat, the expected immunostaining pattern is discontinuous, occurring either in the capillary loops or in the mesangium. The mesangium plays a role in the clearance of macromolecular debris from the glomerular capillary wall. As such, it is possible that some of the immunoglobulin present in the glomeruli of some dogs is not specific in nature and not associated with clinically relevant immunologic injury. Therefore the prevalence and relevance of positive immunofluorescent staining in dogs without glomerular disease needs further investigation.

GLOMERULAR DISEASES

Many glomerular diseases affect dogs; fewer appear to affect cats. Many of these diseases historically have been lumped under the umbrella of "glomerulonephritis" (see Box 261-1). As a profession, veterinary medicine needs to move beyond this generalization and begin to characterize each disease as a separate entity. The historical approach of combining diseases characterized as glomerulonephritis into one group has led to limited information on the natural history and effective treatment of the individual diseases in dogs and cats. In human medicine, the characterization of each glomerular disease as a specific entity has led to an advanced understanding of the pathogenic events leading to the specific glomerular disease. This enhanced understanding is forging the way to the development of optimized and specific therapeutic approaches for the individual glomerular diseases and to more clearly defined prognoses.[4,5] This section outlines what is known about the individual diseases in dogs and cats, with additional information garnered from the wealth of knowledge on these diseases in humans.

Acquired glomerular injury is the result of damage sustained after immune complex formation or deposition (e.g., membranous nephropathy, membranoproliferative glomerulonephritis, proliferative glomerulonephritis) or of damage caused by systemic factors that affect the glomerulus (e.g., amyloidosis, focal segmental glomerulosclerosis, minimal change disease). Although the effects of systemic factors vary, some general statements can be made regarding the pathogenesis of the immune complex–mediated glomerulonephropathies.[20] Immune complexes that are deposited in the glomerulus or that form *in situ* initiate glomerular damage. Cell-mediated immune mechanisms also take part in the pathogenesis of glomerular inflammation. Once glomerular damage has been initiated, other processes contribute to glomerular injury, including activation of complement and of the coagulation cascade and resident cells; influx of neutrophils, monocytes, and platelets; release of proteolytic enzymes; synthesis of cytokines or other growth factors; generation of proinflammatory lipid mediators; and alteration of hemodynamic factors. The mechanisms that determine whether progressive renal damage or resolution of the process occurs are unclear.

Membranoproliferative Glomerulonephritis

Membranoproliferative glomerulonephritis (MPGN) may be the most common glomerular disease in dogs, accounting for 20% to 60% of dogs in various studies.[1,21] However, glomerular lesions are most likely to be called MPGN when they have not undergone thorough evaluation, including the use IFM and EM; the incidence of MPGN is most certainly overestimated in dogs. On the other hand, MPGN is more common in humans living in underdeveloped countries, where exposure to harmful environmental agents, including infectious disease, may be greater than in those living in developed countries.[5] MPGN therefore may be the glomerular lesion expected to be most common in dogs, but it probably is less common than currently reported.

Clinical Features

The mean age of dogs with MPGN in one study was 10.5 years.[11] Males and females appear to be equally affected. Even though the disease is common, no thorough study of MPGN as a distinct glomerular disease has been done in dogs. In humans the disease is characterized by a slowly progressive course, and about 50% of those affected develop nephrotic syndrome.

MPGN has been identified as a familial disease in Bernese mountain dogs. A unique, rapidly progressive form of MPGN that is accompanied by tubular necrosis and interstitial inflammation and is uniformly fatal has been reported in association with *Borrelia burgdorferi* infection in dogs.[12] The average age of affected dogs was only 5.6 years. Labrador retrievers and golden retrievers were significantly predisposed to developing this lesion.

Pathogenesis

There are two types of MPGN.[4,5] Type I MPGN, also called mesangiocapillary GN, is often induced by infectious diseases and is characterized by immune complex accumulation on the subendothelial side of the GBM. The intramembranous dense deposits that characterize type II MPGN, also called *dense deposit disease*, are not immune deposits but are of undefined origin; type II MPGN is not associated with infectious diseases and seems to be uncommon in dogs. Renal lesions appearing to be type I MPGN have been associated with a variety of infectious diseases in dogs (see Box 261-2 and Box 261-3). The accumulation of immune complexes or dense deposits leads to cytokine-mediated activation and expansion of the mesangium and an inflow of leukocytes. In type II MPGN, activation of the alternate pathway of complement predominates, whereas in type I MPGN activation of the classic pathway occurs.

In humans with MPGN, hypocomplementemia is so common that this disease is sometimes called *hypocomplementemic GN*. Hypocomplementemia appears to develop either from increased consumption secondary to immune complex activation of the classic pathway or from the presence of anticomplement autoantibodies known as *nephritic factors*. Interestingly, type I MPGN also occurs in Brittany spaniels and in humans with congenital C3 deficiency.[15] The pathogenic role of hypocomplementemia is not understood.

Histopathologic Characterization

MPGN is diagnosed when both thickened capillary loops and mesangial hypercellularity (more than three nuclei per mesangial region) are present (Figure 261-4).[4,5,11] The glomerulus may become enlarged and segmented or lobular in appearance. The activated mesangium expands the capillary walls and extends into the subendothelial space, causing the double contour, or "railroad," appearance of the GBM that can be seen with light microscopy. With IFM, immune complex deposition can be identified in type I MPGN as granular deposits of C3 in combination with IgG, IgM, or IgA, or combinations thereof, in the GBM or mesangium or both. With EM, type II MPGN can be differentiated from type I by the

identification of intramembranous dense deposits. EM also is used to identify the immune deposits in type I MPGN.

Specific Treatment

Effective treatment of the underlying infectious, inflammatory, or neoplastic disease is the cornerstone of management of patients with MPGN. Because activation of platelets appears to be involved in the pathogenesis of this disease, antiplatelet drugs also should be given.[5]

Prognosis

Specific data regarding the prognosis of MPGN in dogs is lacking. In people, azotemia, severe proteinuria, systemic hypertension and marked tubulointerstitial lesions at presentation are the most significant predictors of an unfavorable outcome.[5]

Membranous Nephropathy

Membranous nephropathy (MN) is probably the second most common glomerular disease in dogs, accounting for up to 10% to 45% of reported cases.[2,11,22-24] It is the most common glomerular disease of cats, in which other forms of glomerular disease are uncommon.[25,26] Because there is rarely evidence of an inflammatory response in the glomeruli or interstitium, the disease is more correctly called a glomerulopathy or nephropathy, rather than glomerulonephritis.

Clinical Features

As in humans, MN appears to be more common in male dogs and cats (approximate male to female ratios are 1.75:1 in dogs and 6:1 in cats). The mean age of affected dogs from four studies was 8 years, but there was considerable range (1 to 14 years). The disease is more common in younger cats, with an approximate mean age of only 3.6 years (range, 1 to 7 years).[25] There does not appear to be any breed predilection, although a preponderance of Doberman pinschers was seen in one report. Interestingly, four of five of these Dobermans were 3 years of age or younger, which may suggest a familial pattern.[23]

Proteinuria in animals with MN may be massive, often as high or higher than that which occurs in dogs with amyloidosis.[14] Because of this heavy proteinuria, many animals present with nephrotic syndrome. Microhematuria is reported in 30% to 40% of humans with MN but has not been systematically studied in dogs and cats.[5] Cats and dogs with MN may present with signs of renal failure. Many cats have normal to enlarged kidneys at presentation.

Membranous nephropathy has four ultrastructural stages that correlate with the temporal evolution of the disease and the clinical presentation in dogs, cats, and humans.[4,5,23,25] There is some suggestion that these stages also correlate with therapeutic outcomes in humans with MN, in that people may be more likely to respond to appropriate management if they are in one of the first two stages. More advanced stages in cats and dogs have been shown to correlate with more severe azotemia, whereas animals with milder disease were more likely to have nephrotic syndrome.[23,25]

Pathogenesis

In humans, MN is considered to be either primary (i.e., idiopathic) or to occur secondary to another disease process; primary disease is most common.[5] In primary MN, immune complexes are found mainly in the subepithelial spaces of the capillary loops. Secondary MN can be distinguished from the primary form by the presence of immune complexes in the mesangium and subendothelial space (or both) and in the subepithelial space. The finding of antibodies on the subepithelial side is unique to MN and suggests that binding occurs on the urinary side of the GBM. The subsequent activation of

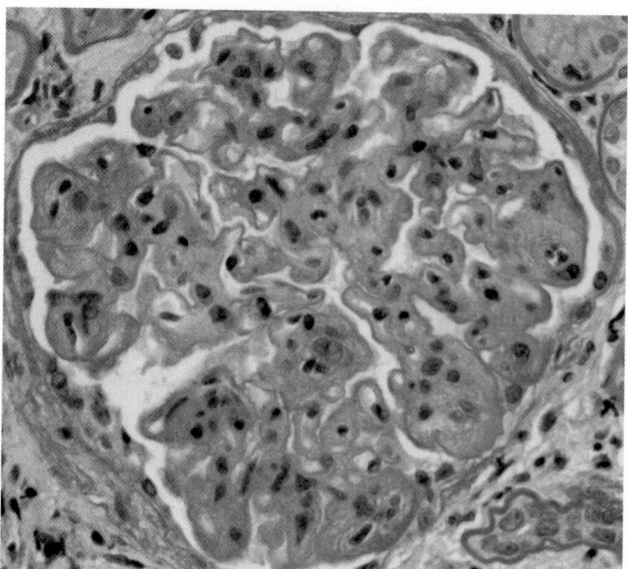

Figure 261-4 Glomerulus from a dog with membranoproliferative (mesangiocapillary) glomerulonephritis. Note the thickened capillary loops and the mesangial hypercellularity, which result in the segmented and lobular appearance.

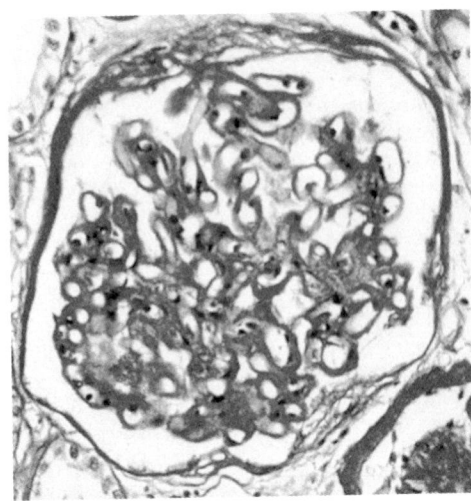

Figure 261-5 Glomerulus from a dog with membranous nephropathy. Note the thickened, rigid-appearing capillary loops and the lack of hypercellularity. (Courtesy of J.L. Robertson, Blacksburg, VA, Virginia Maryland Regional College of Veterinary Medicine.)

complement and cytokine responses may be reduced, because the site of reaction is distant to the circulation, which contributes to the lack of inflammation associated with MN.

Although the exact pathogenesis of this disorder is unknown, it is considered to be an immune complex–mediated disease. There is evidence to support both *in situ* formation of immune complexes and trapping of circulating immune complexes. However, in humans with primary MN, the weight of evidence supports the *in situ* reaction of unbound antibody with fixed antigens, perhaps intrinsic GBM or glomerular visceral epithelial cells antigens. In this regard, primary disease may be a true autoimmune disorder.

Circulating immune complexes most likely play a larger role in patients with secondary disease. Proteinuria probably develops through a complement-dependent mechanism, independent of inflammatory cells. The terminal complement complex (C5b-9 membrane attack complex) has been implicated in the pathogenesis of this disease. Increased urinary concentrations of the membrane attack complex have been demonstrated in some, although not all, individuals with MN. Demonstration of this complex may be more likely early in the disease process, when active immune deposit formation occurs. Myriad immune system irregularities have been reported in association with MN in humans (e.g., altered CD4+ to CD8+ ratio, Fc receptor dysfunction, and impaired lymphocyte and suppressor cell function), which supports a pathogenic role for an underlying immunologic defect. These irregularities are perhaps based on a genetic susceptibility, a theory supported by familial clustering of MN in humans.[4,5]

Histopathologic Characterization

The normally lacey-appearing GBM becomes uniformly thickened and more rigid as a result of the deposition of immune complexes in the subepithelial spaces in MN (Figure 261-5).[4,11]

New basement membrane material accumulates around the immune deposits. Because the deposits do not become impregnated with silver, "spikes" may be identified on the outside of the GBM when an appropriate silver stain is used. Advanced cases may show irregular thickening and distortion of the capillary walls with occasional widening of the mesangium. Immunofluorescent microscopy is useful in determining the site of immune complex deposition. Staining of the immune complexes produces a beaded appearance along the GBM and can be so heavy that it may be difficult to differentiate from a linear pattern. In secondary cases, the mesangial spaces are also positive. In dogs with MN, IgG and C3 have most commonly been identified, although there have also been reports of finding IgM and IgA.[11,21] Several studies have reported affected dogs and cats in which positive staining was identified only in the glomerular capillary loops, which suggests the presence of primary, or idiopathic, disease in these animals.[21-23,25]

Electron microscopy should be used to confirm the location of the immune deposits and to characterize the stage of disease progression (Figure 261-6).[4,23,25] Deposition of immune complexes, progressive engulfment of the complexes by the surrounding GBM, and eventual resolution of the deposits characterize the stages. Stage I is characterized by subepithelial dense immune deposits without adjacent projections of basement membrane material and only minimal thickening of the GBM. Projections of adjacent GBM material, or spikes, are identified in stage II. In stage III, these projections surround the immune deposits. In stage IV, the GBM is markedly thickened, and electron-lucent zones have replaced some or all of the electron-dense deposits. In advanced stage IV disease, sometimes referred to as stage V, there is variable thickening of the GBM and apparent resolution of the electron-dense deposits. In some affected animals, staging is difficult because several stages of disease may be present simultaneously.

Specific Treatment

In addition to identification of potentially inciting disease processes and nonspecific management of proteinuria, immunosuppressive therapy may be warranted in dogs or cats with persistent proteinuria caused by MN, particularly if they appear to have idiopathic, or primary, disease and are not azotemic. Affected humans with similar clinical pictures may respond to immunosuppressive therapy with corticosteroids combined with an alkylating agent (i.e., cyclophosphamide or chlorambucil).[5] The approach that has proven most beneficial is alternation of methylprednisolone and chlorambucil every other day for 6 months. Cyclosporine is considered a valid therapeutic option for patients not responding to corticosteroids and alkylating agents. Even when treatment is effective, relapses may occur. The use of immunosuppressive therapy in dogs and cats with membranous nephropathy needs to be studied more carefully.

Prognosis

Although MN appears to be progressive in some dogs and cats, the progression may be slow enough that many animals can lead relatively normal lives. In a study of 24 cats with MN, four (17%) survived 4 to 10 months and eight (33%) had

Figure 261-6 Ultrastructural stages in the progression of membranous nephropathy. (Courtesy J.C. Jennette, Chapel Hill, NC, School of Medicine, University of North Carolina.)

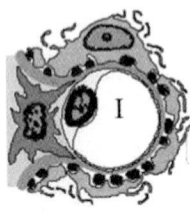 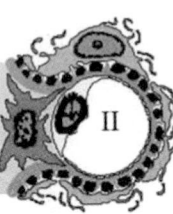 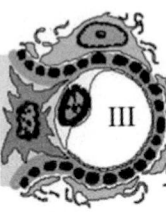 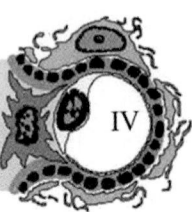

long-term survival of 2.5 to 6 years; clinical remission occurred in seven (29%) of the cats. Corticosteroids were administered to three of the eight long-term survivors. However, 11 cats (46%) died or were euthanized due to nephrotic syndrome or renal failure shortly after diagnosis.[26] Long-term survivors had only IgG deposition, C3 deposition, or both; cats that also had deposition of IgM or IgA had a shorter survival period. Stage III and stage IV disease, defined by the presence of intramembranous deposits, was associated with a poorer prognosis.[26]

Survival data for dogs is more difficult to extract from prior reports, although it appears to be similar to what has been reported in cats. Survival in dogs has ranged from 4 days to greater than 3 years.[23] Spontaneous remissions have been reported. Spontaneous remission occurs in 20% to 30% of humans with MN, whereas 20% to 40% of cases progress to renal failure.[5] The risk of progression in humans appears to correlate with the magnitude of proteinuria and renal function impairment; patients with the highest degree of proteinuria and azotemia are more likely to have more rapid progression compared with other patients.

Proliferative Glomerulonephritis
Proliferative glomerulonephritis, caused by endocapillary or mesangial proliferation, accounted for 2% to 16% of glomerular lesions in dogs in two studies.[11,21] In humans a complete pathologic diagnosis requires both a morphologic description (e.g., focal mesangial proliferative glomerulonephritis) and a specific disease designation (e.g., IgA nephropathy, lupus glomerulonephritis).[4,5] With the exception of IgA nephropathy, proliferative glomerulonephritis in dogs has not included the specific disease designation.[27,28] It therefore is difficult to correlate the diseases that have been described in dogs with the wealth of information regarding pathogenesis and treatment known for the specific diseases in humans.

Clinical Features
Dogs with proliferative glomerulonephritis reported in two studies were on average between 7 and 9 years of age.[11,10] Proteinuria and renal failure are the most common presenting signs in affected dogs. Renal failure may be mild or moderate and acute or chronic. Humans with mesangial proliferative glomerulonephritis often have microscopic or macroscopic hematuria; the presence of hematuria has not been thoroughly evaluated in dogs.[5]

Pathogenesis
Proliferative glomerulonephritis is an immune complex–mediated disease. Anti-GBM disease causes proliferative glomerulonephritis in humans but has not been described in the dog or cat. Postinfectious glomerulonephritis of humans, characterized by endocapillary proliferation, most commonly occurs after a streptococcal infection but has also been identified with other infections (e.g., staphylococcal infection).[5] Interestingly, this pattern of disease is usually caused by infections of limited duration that often have resolved prior to the emergence of clinical signs of glomerular disease. Persistent infections are more likely to cause MPGN or MN.[4]

Histopathologic Characterization
Mesangial proliferative glomerulonephritis is characterized by mesangial cell hyperplasia, defined as four or more cells per mesangial area.[4,11] This is often accompanied by an increase in mesangial matrix (Figure 261-7). Endocapillary proliferative glomerulonephritis occurs with a proliferation of glomerular endothelial cells and may be accompanied by an increase in mesangial cellularity. An influx of mononuclear cells accounts for some of the increase in cellularity. Evaluation by IFM reveals fine granular deposits of IgG or IgM or both in the

GBM and mesangium. EM can be used to characterize further the location of the immune complexes. Because the proliferative glomerulonephropathies often develop secondary to systemic diseases, immune complexes are often identified in the mesangium, although some complexes may be found in the capillary walls. Subepithelial "humps" can be identified in humans with postinfectious glomerulonephritis.[4]

Specific Treatment
Because this category probably encompasses several disease entities, there are no specific treatment recommendations. The potential source of immune complexes should be removed, and nonspecific management of glomerular diseases should be followed.

Prognosis
The prognosis for this specific group of diseases has not been evaluated in dogs. The presence of chronic renal failure or the formation of crescents, or both, is most likely associated with a poorer prognosis.

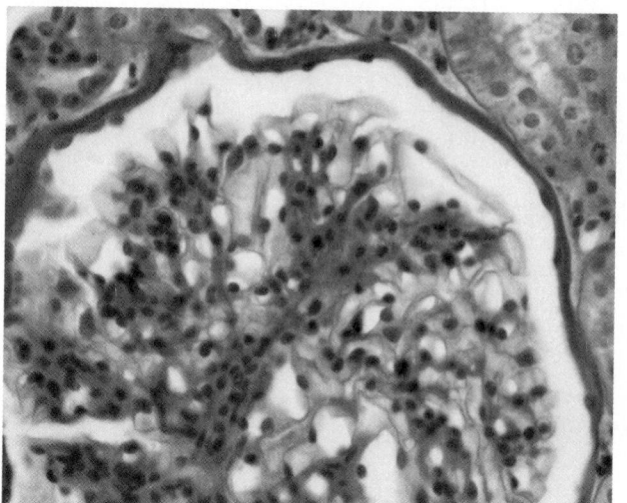

A

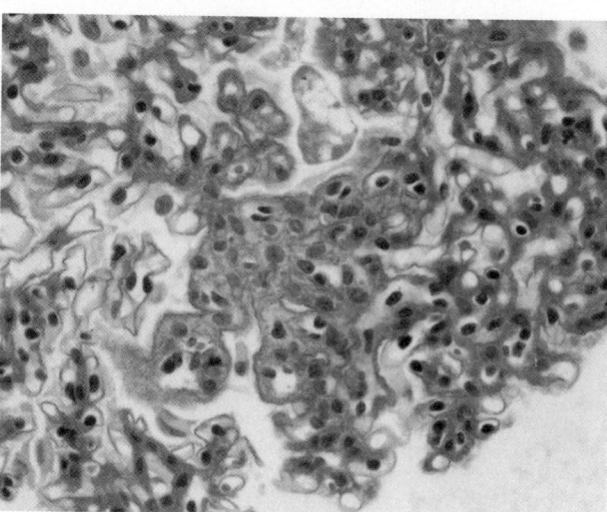

B

Figure 261-7 Glomeruli from dogs with proliferative glomerulonephritis. **A,** Focal mesangial proliferative glomerulonephritis. **B,** Endocapillary proliferative glomerulonephritis.

Immunoglobulin A Nephropathy

In several studies of canine glomerular disease, IFM has demonstrated mild to moderate frequency of IgA positivity, suggestive of IgA nephropathy.[27,28] However, because IgA is predominantly polymeric in dogs, it may be nonspecifically trapped in the mesangium, more so than monomeric IgA, the predominant form in humans. The diagnosis of IgA nephropathy requires a predominance of IgA positivity on IFM evaluation; codeposits of IgG, IgM, or C3 may be present but should be less intense than IgA. Mesangial proliferative glomerulonephritis is the expected light microscopic lesion; some humans do not have any apparent glomerular lesions. In one study of clinically normal dogs with glomerular lesions, 85% had IgA deposits.[16] In another study of 100 dogs with and without renal disease, 47 had IgA deposition, and in six dogs IgA was the only immunoglobulin detected.[28] Increased deposition of IgA was associated with increased cellular proliferation. Dogs with enteric or hepatic diseases had the highest incidence of IgA deposition. Excessive IgA immune complex formation due to enteric disease or decreased clearance of IgA complexes in association with liver disease have been proposed in the pathogenesis of secondary IgA nephropathy in humans.[5]

In people, IgA nephropathy is more common in young adults, with males outnumbering females; the prevalence varies substantially throughout the world.[5] In a report of three dogs with apparent IgA nephropathy, the dogs were male and young to middle aged (4 to 7 years).[27] The dogs had episodes of microscopic and macroscopic hematuria, as well as proteinuria and varying degrees of renal failure. Although the dogs were housed together in a blood donor facility, predisposing environmental factors were not identified. The dog most severely affected had uncontrolled hypertension and codeposits of IgG or IgM, both of which are negative prognostic indicators in humans.

Treatment of patients with secondary IgA nephropathy should be directed at treatment of the associated systemic disease. Control of hypertension should be considered a cornerstone of therapy. Fish oil rich in omega-3 fatty acids administered to affected humans resulted in slowed progression of renal disease but did not lead to a reduction in proteinuria.[5]

Amyloidosis

The term *amyloidosis* refers to a diverse group of diseases that have in common the extracellular deposition of fibrils formed by polymerization of proteins with a beta-pleated sheet conformation.[29] Several different proteins may be deposited to form amyloid in humans, but the number of proteins involved in domestic animals appears to be limited. Many of these proteins display specific tissue tropisms that lead to characteristic clinical syndromes. The dog is the domestic animal most commonly affected by amyloidosis. With the exception of the Chinese Shar Pei, amyloid is deposited primarily in the glomeruli of affected dogs.[13,30] In fact, amyloidosis is one of the most common glomerular diseases in dogs, accounting for 23% of dogs with glomerular disease in one study.[8]

Clinical Features

Reactive amyloidosis is the most common form of amyloidosis in dogs and cats. Renal amyloidosis is more common in older dogs. The mean age of affected dogs was 9.2 years in one study, in which 85% of affected dogs were 7 years of age or older.[13] Females appear to be affected more often than males (the male to female ratio is 1:1.7). Beagles, collies, and Walker hounds may be at increased risk for amyloidosis.[13] Renal amyloidosis may be familial in beagles and English foxhounds.[31]

The most common clinical signs of renal amyloidosis in dogs are those common to other glomerular diseases. Because proteinuria associated with amyloidosis may be massive, many

animals brought to the veterinarian are in nephrotic syndrome. In one study of proteinuria, six of seven dogs with amyloidosis had nonselective proteinuria, suggesting a marked loss of the size-selective properties of the glomerular capillary wall.[16] Although other organ systems may be involved (liver, spleen, adrenal glands, gastrointestinal tract), clinical signs associated with amyloid deposition in these organs are rare in dogs. Chronic infectious and noninfectious inflammatory diseases and neoplasia have been reported in association with reactive amyloidosis in 32% to 53% of affected dogs; however, many dogs and cats with reactive amyloidosis do not have an identifiable inflammatory process at the time of presentation.[8,13]

Renal amyloidosis in the Shar Pei develops at an earlier age (mean age 4.1 years) than in other dogs with amyloidosis, but like other breeds, the disease is more common in females (male to female ratio of 1:2.5).[13] In Shar Peis, amyloid is most commonly deposited in the renal medulla; only 64% of Shar Peis had glomerular involvement in one report.[30] As a result, as few as 25% to 43% of affected Shar Peis have proteinuria. Affected dogs may have signs of involvement of other organs, particularly the liver. Many Shar Peis have a history of recurrent fever and swelling of the tibiotarsal joints (commonly called *Shar Pei fever* or *Shar Pei swollen hock syndrome*) prior to the development of renal amyloidosis. Affected Shar Peis may be an animal model of familial Mediterranean fever in humans.

Amyloidosis is relatively uncommon in the cat, with the exception of Abyssinians and Siamese (especially the Oriental shorthair color variant).[32] In Abyssinians, amyloid is deposited primarily in the medulla, although glomerular involvement has been described. This pattern of deposition results in medullary fibrosis and papillary necrosis and leads to chronic renal failure as the most common clinical manifestation; marked proteinuria is not common. Siamese and Oriental shorthair cats have a predilection for deposition of amyloid in the liver, leading to hepatic rupture and hemorrhage. Diagnosis of renal amyloidosis in affected cats is based on a high index of suspicion and exclusion of other renal diseases or on postmortem examination; biopsy of the renal medulla is associated with too high a degree of risk to be warranted.

Pathogenesis

The primary protein involved in the formation of amyloid deposits in dogs and cats is amyloid A protein (AA), which is formed by the polymerization of the amino terminal portion of serum amyloid A protein (SAA), an acute-phase reactant.[29] SAA is synthesized and released by hepatocytes after they have been stimulated by macrophage-derived cytokines (e.g., interleukin-1 (IL-1), IL-6, tumor necrosis factor). Because of the association of amyloid A with inflammatory diseases, this form of amyloidosis has been termed *reactive*, or *secondary*, amyloidosis.

Concentrations of SAA increase 100- to 1000-fold after tissue injury. Although concentrations decrease to baseline by 36 to 48 hours after removal of the inflammatory stimulus, they remain increased if inflammation persists.[29] Chronic inflammation and persistent or prolonged increases in SAA concentrations are required for the development of reactive amyloidosis. Humans with familial Mediterranean fever, a disease similar to that reported in Shar Peis, have defective formation of pyrin, a protein involved in the downregulation of mediators of inflammation.[33] Because only a small percentage of animals with chronic inflammation develop amyloidosis, other factors must be involved in the pathogenesis.[29] There are multiple polymorphs of SAA, and certain polymorphs perhaps are more amyloidogenic. There may be inherited and acquired variations in the ability to degrade SAA, a two-step process that involves cell surface–associated proteases contained in monocytes. A defect in the second step of this process may predispose some individuals to the development of amyloidosis. It has been demonstrated that the AA-degrading property of normal serum is decreased in humans with reactive amyloidosis. This activity correlated with serum albumin concentrations; hypoalbuminemia associated with the inflammatory process or amyloidosis may contribute to decreased AA-degrading activity. Increased concentrations of other acute-phase reactants that are protease inhibitors (e.g., antitrypsin and antichymotrypsin) also may contribute to the pathogenesis of amyloidosis.

SAA concentrations are increased during the predeposition phase, before the appearance of tissue amyloid deposits, but may persist during the deposition phase. Abyssinians with renal amyloidosis have increased SAA concentrations.[29] Chinese Shar Peis with renal amyloidosis have increased serum concentrations of IL-6, a cytokine that stimulates SAA synthesis and release.[34] The deposition phase, during which amyloid deposits appear in the tissue, is subdivided into two phases. The rapid phase is characterized by rapid increases in the amount of amyloid, whereas the plateau phase is a time when little net change occurs in tissue deposition.

Histopathologic Characterization

The beta-pleated conformation is responsible for the characteristic staining properties of the amyloid deposits.[4] When the kidney is evaluated by conventional light microscopy, amyloid deposits in the glomeruli appear as acellular material that expands the mesangium and glomerular basement membranes and stains homogeneously eosinophilic with hematoxylin-eosin (Figure 261-8). Glomerular deposits are most often diffuse and global but occasionally are focal and segmental. Deposits sometimes can be found in the walls of small blood vessels, tubular basement membranes, and interstitial tissues. When stained with Congo red and evaluated by conventional light microscopy, amyloid deposits take on various shades of red, depending on the amount of amyloid and the thickness of the section. Deposits stained with Congo red and evaluated by polarizing microscopy are birefringent and have an apple green color (Figure 261-9). Reactive amyloidosis can be confirmed by decolorization of the Congo red–stained amyloid deposits by potassium permanganate oxidation. Electron microscopy is not needed to confirm a diagnosis of amyloidosis.

Specific Treatment

The beta-pleated sheet configuration of amyloid fibrils leads to their insolubility and resistance to proteolysis, making

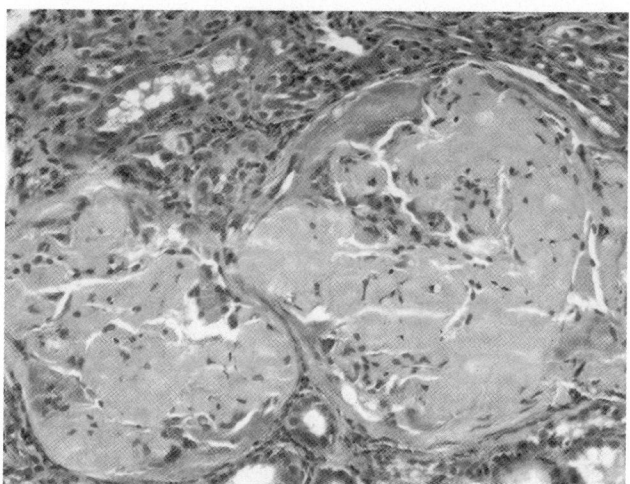

Figure 261-8 Glomerular amyloidosis in a canine renal biopsy section stained with hematoxylin-eosin. (Courtesy S.P. DiBartola, Columbus, OH, College of Veterinary Medicine, Ohio State University.)

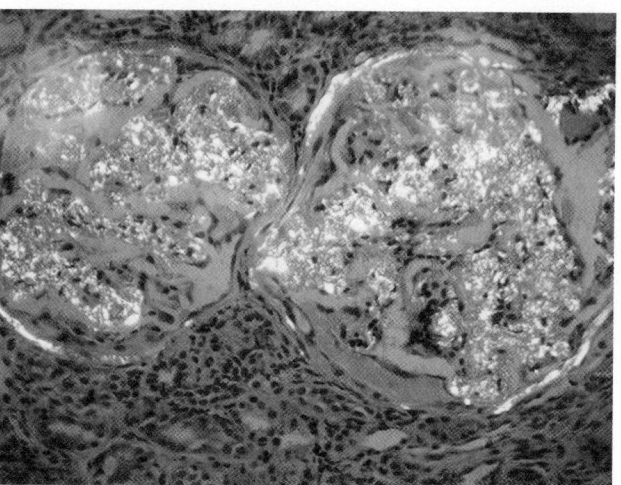

Figure 261-9 Section stained with Congo red, showing typical birefringence of glomerular amyloid deposits. (Courtesy S.P. DiBartola.)

specific treatment relatively ineffectual. In humans with familial Mediterranean fever, colchicine prevented the development of renal amyloidosis even in patients who continued to have recurrent febrile episodes.[33,35] This led to the recommendation that colchicine be used in the management of Shar Peis with renal amyloidosis. Ideally this drug is administered during the predeposition phase, which in Shar Peis is presumably characterized by recurrent fevers and swollen hocks. However, colchicine administration may lead to remission of proteinuria even after the appearance of amyloid deposits. No evidence supports the effectiveness of colchicine once amyloidosis has resulted in renal failure. Although the effects of the drug in the treatment of amyloidosis are not fully known, colchicine does impair the release of SAA from hepatocytes by binding to microtubules and preventing secretion. In addition, colchicine may prevent the production of amyloid-enhancing factor. The dosage of colchicine used is 0.01 to 0.03 mg/kg given orally every 24 hours. Gastrointestinal upset is the primary side effect.

Dimethylsulfoxide (DMSO) has been shown to be beneficial in a limited number of dogs with renal amyloidosis, although the exact benefit remains controversial.[35] If given during the rapid deposition phase, DMSO leads to a decrease in SAA concentrations and resolution of tissue deposits. However, the amount of amyloid deposited in the kidneys of humans was unchanged after DMSO administration, which lends support to the current belief that DMSO does not solubilize amyloid fibrils. The anti-inflammatory effects of DMSO may account for some of the beneficial effects. Reduction of interstitial fibrosis and inflammation may lead to improved renal function and reduced proteinuria. DMSO has an unpleasant odor that may lead to poor owner compliance. Furthermore, this drug may contribute to signs of nausea and anorexia seen in some dogs. The recommended dosage is 90 mg/kg given orally or subcutaneously three times weekly. DMSO should be diluted 1:4 with sterile water before injection to limit the pain associated with injection. Neither DMSO nor colchicine is effective once the plateau phase of deposition has been reached.

Prognosis

The prognosis for dogs and cats with renal amyloidosis is generally poor. In one study of dogs with amyloidosis, 58% died or were euthanized at the time of diagnosis. In the remaining dogs, survival ranged from 2 to 20 months; survival of a year or longer was reported in only 8.5%.[29] The longest survival was observed in a dog treated with DMSO.

Hereditary Nephritis

The term *hereditary nephritis (HN)* refers to a diverse group of inherited glomerular diseases that are the result of a defect in basement membrane collagen (type IV).[36] These diseases are discussed in Chapter 264. A brief discussion of hereditary nephritis is included in this chapter because it should be considered as a differential diagnosis for any dog presenting with proteinuric renal disease, particularly if the dog is young.

Clinical Features

Hereditary nephritis has been reported in several breeds of dogs. An autosomal recessive form of the disease occurs in English cocker spaniels, whereas bull terriers and Dalmatians develop an autosomal dominant form.[36-39] An X-linked dominant form of HN has been described in Samoyeds and mixed-breed dogs; carrier females may have mild disease.[37] The report in the Samoyeds is of a single kindred; the disease is not considered to be common in this breed. HN is characterized by proteinuria, renal hematuria, and progressive glomerular disease. Concurrent hearing and ocular abnormalities, as described in humans with HN, appear to be uncommon in affected dogs, with the exception of anterior lenticonus, which occurs in some bull terriers.[38]

Pathogenesis

HN is the result of a genetic mutation or deletion in type IV collagen, the primary protein constituent of the GBM.[4,36] The presence of defective collagen leads to premature deterioration of the GBM and progressive glomerular disease.

Histopathologic Characterization

Prior to electron micrographic studies of English cocker spaniels, the renal lesions were described as renal cortical hypoplasia or membranoproliferative or sclerosing glomerulonephritis. Electron microscopy is required to make the diagnosis of HN. Multilaminar splitting and fragmentation of the GBM are seen, often with intramembranous, electron-dense deposits.

Specific Treatment

No specific treatment is available for affected dogs. Use of a diet formulated for renal failure and administration of angiotensin-converting enzyme (ACE) inhibitors have proved beneficial in affected dogs. Early detection of HN through screening of dogs of relevant breeds for microalbuminuria allows early therapeutic intervention, which may slow disease progression.[17]

Prognosis

The rate of progression is predictable in Samoyeds and English cocker spaniels, with terminal renal failure generally developing before 2 years of age.[36] However, disease progression is more variable in bull terriers and Dalmatians, with some dogs surviving for as long as 10 years.[38-39]

Minimal Change Disease

Although uncommonly described in dogs and cats, minimal change disease (MCD) is a common cause of nephrotic syndrome in humans, especially children.[5,40] Because EM is required for diagnosis, the disease most likely is underdiagnosed in dogs and perhaps in cats. In humans this disease is sometimes referred to as *nil disease, lipoid nephrosis,* or *idiopathic nephrotic syndrome.*

Clinical Features

There have been isolated reports of dogs that appear to have MCD; we have seen a few dogs in which we suspected this disease at North Carolina State University College of Veterinary Medicine. However, there is only one well-described case report of MCD in a dog presenting with nephrotic syndrome.[40] Proteinuria is likely to be of heavy magnitude with this disease, and nephrotic syndrome is common.

Pathogenesis

In humans, MCD is usually idiopathic, although secondary disease also occurs. Increased production of lymphokines by dysfunctional T cells is believed to be responsible for an increase in GBM permeability.[5] The primary change is loss of anionic charge in the glomerular capillary wall, leading to collapse of the podocyte foot processes. This loss of charge selectivity is the crucial event leading to proteinuria. The resultant proteinuria is highly selective; albumin is the primary protein lost.

Histopathologic Characterization

Animals with MCD have a lack of light microscopic lesions in the glomerulus.[4] Occasionally, slight hypercellularity is present, as evidenced by three or four nuclei in the mesangial region. Some lipid droplets may be present in the renal tubules, but there should not be any evidence of tubular atrophy or interstitial fibrosis. With IFM, immunoglobulin deposition is absent; however, there may be increased staining of vimentin, a marker for visceral glomerular epithelial cells. The diagnosis is confirmed with EM by identification of marked foot process effacement (Figure 261-10). MCD belongs to the WHO classification of minor glomerular abnormalities. In one study of glomerular lesions in dogs, 28 of 115 dogs fell into this classification, but only one of these dogs had MCD.[11] Therefore identification of only minor glomerular abnormalities in a dog or cat with proteinuria does not make a diagnosis of MCD.

Specific Treatment

An important reason to include MCD on the list of differential diagnoses for dogs with nephrotic syndrome is the disease's seemingly exquisite response to corticosteroids; the expected response rate in humans with MCD is 80% to 90%.[5]

Prognosis

The prognosis for MCD in dogs is unknown. One or more relapses are seen in 75% to 85% of affected humans.[5]

Glomerulosclerosis

Glomerulosclerosis often develops as an end-stage lesion in response to glomerular injury.[4] Focal or global sclerosis may be a primary or concurrent lesion in animals with

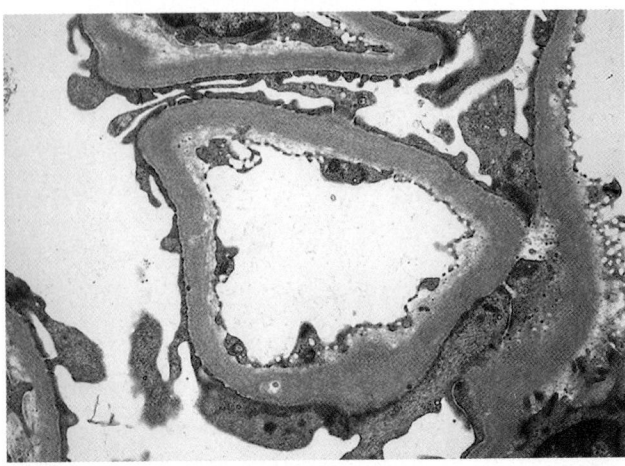

Figure 261-10 Electron micrograph of a glomerular capillary loop in a dog with minimal change disease. Effacement of the foot processes has occurred.

glomerular disease. The incidence of glomerulosclerosis increases with age, although the percentage of glomeruli expected to be sclerotic in dogs of advancing age groups has not been fully characterized. Glomerulosclerosis is a common finding in diabetic nephropathy of humans. Although glomerulosclerosis and proteinuria can develop in dogs with diabetes mellitus, the clinical relevance of this is unknown. Glomerulosclerosis can also develop after hypertensive renal damage.

Focal segmental glomerulosclerosis (FSGS) is a specific glomerular disease that has been identified, but poorly characterized, in dogs (Figure 261-11).[4,11] FSGS is a common glomerular disease in humans, accounting for up to 35% of nephrotic syndrome in adults. The disease is most likely underdiagnosed in dogs and often mischaracterized as MPGN. FSGS was the diagnosis rendered in 10% of dogs with glomerular disease in one study.[11] Males and females were equally represented, and the average age was 8.5 years. FSGS is diagnosed in the proteinuric patient that has segmental glomerulosclerosis in a glomerulus that is otherwise normal, without other glomerular lesions present to explain the sclerosis. IFM evaluation should be negative in affected patients; however, nonspecific trapping of immunoglobulins and C3 can occur in sclerotic areas.

Five subtypes of this disease have been described in humans: perihilar, cellular, tip, collapsing and "not otherwise specified."[4] The clinical features of these subtypes vary somewhat, but the course is generally one of progressive proteinuria and renal failure. Permeability factor, a transferable circulating factor that promotes increased *in vitro* glomerular permeability to albumin and other plasma proteins, has been implicated in the pathogenesis of FSGS in humans.[5] Although the exact identify of this permeability factor is unknown, it is not an immunoglobulin or an immune complex. It is likely that several factors eventually will be identified that are capable of inducing increased glomerular permeability and eventual sclerotic lesions.

Tubulointerstitial Lesions Associated with Glomerular Disease

Proteinuria induces tubular damage, leading to progressive nephron loss.[41] Evidence in support of this includes the

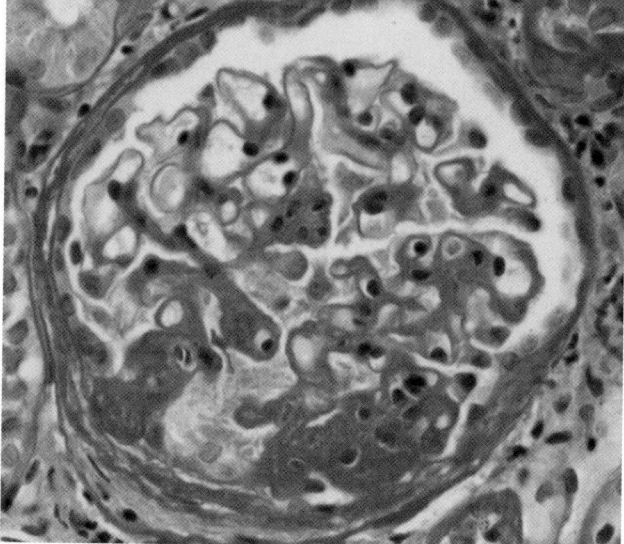

Figure 261-11 Glomerulus from a dog with a lesion resembling focal segmental glomerulosclerosis. Note the relatively normal appearance of the glomerular sections that are not sclerotic.

correlation between heavy proteinuria and a negative patient outcome in humans with various glomerular diseases; also, rodents with albumin-induced overload proteinuria develop renal injury and fibrosis, and the urine of proteinuric humans shows mediators of renal inflammation and fibrosis, some of which are produced by renal tubules exposed to various proteins.[41] However, albumin may not be the culprit. Rodents with albumin-induced overload proteinuria develop altered glomerular permselectivity, with urinary loss of proteins in addition to albumin. Rats and humans with highly selective proteinuria appear to be at lower risk of eventual tubulointerstitial damage.

Some damage occurs secondary to obstruction of the tubules by protein casts.[42] However, the proteins themselves are also toxic to the tubular epithelial cells and lead to increased interstitial inflammation, fibrosis, and cell death. Proteinuria necessitates increased resorption of proteins through tubular cells by means of lysosomal processing. Ruptured lysosomes lead to cytoplasmic damage. Interstitial inflammatory cells, initially recruited in response to injury, contribute to the development of interstitial fibrosis. Other factors that may be involved in the genesis of interstitial inflammation and fibrosis induced by proteinuria include osteopontin, monocyte chemoattractant protein-1, urinary iron, endothelin-1, transforming growth factor-β, and tumor necrosis factor-alpha.[42] A direct link has not been established between proteinuria and progressive renal damage in dogs, but it probably exists to some extent. Because proteinuria may be a major factor responsible for progressive renal failure in patients with glomerular disease, aggressive management of the proteinuria should be considered a cornerstone of the treatment of dogs and cats with glomerular disease.

NONSPECIFIC MEDICAL MANAGEMENT OF GLOMERULAR DISEASE

In addition to specific management that might be implemented with the various glomerular diseases, nonspecific management is indicated. This therapy can be divided into three major categories: (1) treatment of potential underlying diseases processes, (2) reduction of proteinuria, and (3) management of uremia and other complications of generalized renal failure (discussed in Chapter 260).

Many glomerulopathies in dogs are believed to develop secondary to a systemic infectious, inflammatory, or neoplastic disease process. However, the inciting agent may not be obvious at first presentation because the offending disease is no longer present or is occult. Continued observation and scrutiny are necessary, because the causative disease process may become obvious in the ensuing months after presentation. The initial step in the management of a persistently proteinuric dog or cat is to treat and eliminate, if possible, any potential predisposing diseases. The dog should be subsequently evaluated for resolution of the proteinuria, which may occur slowly over a period of months. If proteinuria does not resolve or worsens, a renal biopsy to determine the specific glomerular disease present may be warranted.

Enalapril significantly reduced proteinuria and delayed either the onset or the progression of azotemia in dogs with glomerulonephritis.[43] Treatment of dogs with glomerular diseases with ACE inhibitors is now considered a standard of care.[43] ACE inhibitors may reduce proteinuria and preserve renal function by several possible mechanisms. The decreased efferent glomerular arteriolar resistance effected by ACE inhibitors leads to decreased glomerular transcapillary hydraulic pressure and decreased proteinuria. Other proposed mechanisms include reduced loss of glomerular heparan sulfate, decreased size of the glomerular capillary endothelial pores, improved lipoprotein metabolism, slowed glomerular mesangial growth and proliferation, and inhibition of bradykinin degradation.[43] Typically enalapril (0.5 mg/kg given orally) is administered once a day. If no reduction in proteinuria is seen after 2 to 4 weeks, the frequency should be increased to twice daily (approximately half of the dogs may eventually need twice daily administration).[43] Although the serum creatinine concentration should be monitored, it is uncommon for dogs to have worsening of azotemia due to enalapril administration alone. Adequate blood pressure control of hypertensive dogs may also lead to a reduction in proteinuria and slow the progression of disease. Because ACE inhibitors are relatively weak antihypertensive agents, additional antihypertensive agents (e.g., amlodipine) may be needed if hypertension (i.e., systolic blood pressure greater than 170 mm Hg) persists after the initiation of ACE inhibitor therapy.

Platelets and thromboxane may play an important role in the pathogenesis of glomerulonephritis. Thromboxane is an inducer of platelet aggregation and a chemotactic factor for neutrophils. Neutrophils induce damage to the GBM through release of proteolytic enzymes. Thromboxane release may lead to a reduction in the glomerular filtration rate by inducing vasoconstriction and mesangial cell contraction. Thromboxane synthetase inhibitors have been shown to decrease proteinuria in dogs with experimentally induced glomerulonephritis.[44] Aspirin is a nonspecific cyclo-oxygenase inhibitor that may be used to reduce glomerular inflammation and inhibit platelet aggregation, which may have an added benefit of preventing thromboembolism. In theory, very low doses of aspirin (0.5 mg/kg given orally once or twice daily) may selectively inhibit platelet cyclo-oxygenase without preventing the beneficial effects of prostacyclin formation.

Dietary protein restriction may be useful in the management of dogs with glomerulopathies. Humans and rats with glomerular disease demonstrate a reduction in proteinuria without a change in serum albumin concentrations with restriction of dietary protein. Diets should not be supplemented with protein, because this aggravates urinary protein losses. The enhanced omega-3 to omega-6 polyunsaturated fatty acid ratio and restriction in salt and phosphorus found in canine renal diets may also be of benefit to dogs with glomerulopathies. Omega-3 fatty acid supplementation has been shown to be renoprotective in dogs with renal failure and to mitigate hypertension and reduce serum triglyceride and cholesterol concentrations in humans with nephrotic syndrome.[45] These positive effects are in part mediated through generation of the 3-series prostaglandins. Sodium restriction is beneficial in the control of hypertension and fluid retention. Provision of adequate exercise may help reduce the formation of edema or ascites. Because plasma volume is often reduced in animals with hypoalbuminemia and edema, the use of diuretics should be avoided unless these drugs are needed to control respiratory distress.

The use of immunosuppressive drugs in the treatment of both dogs and humans with glomerular disease is controversial. No controlled study has been done on the use of corticosteroids in dogs with glomerular diseases. Proteinuria has been demonstrated in dogs with corticosteroid excess and may induce glomerular lesions.[9,46] Furthermore, prednisolone administration was shown to reversibly increase proteinuria in dogs with hereditary nephritis.[47] The use of immunosuppressive agents is generally limited to dogs that have developed glomerulonephritis secondary to a steroid-responsive disease, such as systemic lupus erythematosus, but it should also be considered in animals with primary membranous nephropathy or MCD. Cyclosporine, the only drug that has been studied prospectively in dogs with glomerular disease, was found to be

of no benefit.[48] However, dogs with idiopathic disease were included in this study regardless of which specific glomerular disease they had. In the future, the use of immunosuppressive drugs needs to be systematically studied in dogs with primary membranous nephropathy, MCD, or lupus nephritis. Until the results of such a study are available, immunosuppressive agents should be used only with caution and careful patient monitoring.

The UPC, urinalysis, body weight, body condition score, and serum albumin and creatinine concentrations should be evaluated monthly whenever modifications in the therapeutic plan are being made, or every 3 to 6 months if the dog's clinical signs are stable and therapeutic changes are not being made. Slight day-to-day variations in the UPC can occur; changing proteinuria is most accurately measured by assessing trends in the UPC over time. The systemic blood pressure should be measured at least every 3 to 6 months and more frequently if hypertension is unregulated. If the dog no longer has the ability to produce concentrated urine, a urine sample should be submitted for bacterial culture and susceptibility testing every 6 months. Because histologic lesions do not necessarily resolve even though renal function may improve, repeat biopsies generally are not needed. A reduction in proteinuria (ideally greater than 50%) as measured by the UPC without an increase in the serum creatinine concentration indicates improvement or response to therapy.

COMPLICATIONS OF GLOMERULAR DISEASE

Complications of severe proteinuria include edema formation, systemic hypertension, hypercoagulability and thromboembolism, hyperlipidemia, increased risk for infection, altered pharmacokinetics, malnutrition, muscle wasting, and endocrine abnormalities.[42] Edema formation, systemic hypertension, and hypercoagulability are the complications most frequently recognized in dogs, and less commonly in cats, with glomerular disease.

Edema Formation
Several factors contribute to the formation of edema in patients with nephrotic syndrome.[42] In severe forms of nephrotic syndrome, decreases in the plasma oncotic pressure allow for transudation of fluid into the interstitial spaces. The resultant decrease in effective plasma volume leads to increased renin-angiotensin-aldosterone activity and retention of water and sodium and worsening of edema. However, most humans with nephrotic syndrome do not have reduced blood volumes or increased plasma renin or aldosterone activities. Thus primary sodium retention must also be involved in the pathogenesis of edema in these patients. Proposed mechanisms in primary renal sodium retention include a reduced single nephron glomerular filtration rate with enhanced proximal tubular resorption and cytokine-induced modification of distal resorption, leading to resistance to natriuretic factors, including atrial natriuretic peptide. In humans it is believed that mechanisms of primary renal sodium retention are the most important determinants of edema formation until the serum albumin concentration decreases below 2 g/dL. Below this concentration, the plasma oncotic pressure is sufficiently reduced to allow for transudation of fluid from the vascular compartment into the interstitial space.[42] Dogs may be more resistant to the formation of edema, which does not generally occur until the serum albumin concentration is below 1.5 g/dL. Plasma volume may be reduced at this point, making the use of diuretics in the management of edema relatively ineffective and also dangerous because of the increased risk of acute renal failure and thromboembolism.[42]

Hypertension

Systemic hypertension has been reported in up to 80% of dogs with glomerular disease. The frequency of hypertension in each form of glomerular disease has not been established in dogs but does vary in humans. Hypertension appears to be most common in people with FSGS and membranoproliferative glomerulonephritis, whereas it is uncommon in association with MCD and does not occur higher than control populations in humans with membranous nephropathy.[5] The primary mechanism of hypertension in association with nephrotic syndrome is believed to be expansion of the plasma volume in association with primary renal sodium retention. However, generation of several vasoactive factors (e.g., renin, angiotensin II, endothelin) is increased in human patients with nephrotic syndrome and may contribute to hypertension. Nitric oxide deficiency may also play an important role in the development of hypertension.[42]

Target organs of hypertensive injury include the kidneys, the central nervous system, the eyes, and the heart. Blindness may be the presenting complaint in animals with hypertension, most commonly due to retinal detachment. However, retinal hemorrhage, edema, vessel tortuosity, and degeneration; hyphema; and secondary glaucoma may also occur. Hypertensive encephalopathy may be manifested as lethargy, altered mentation, altered behavior, seizures, or balance disturbances. Cardiac changes in dogs and cats with hypertension include systolic murmurs, gallop rhythms, and left ventricular hypertrophy. The blood pressure should be measured in all dogs and cats with glomerular disease, because uncontrolled hypertension is a risk factor for progressive renal injury.

Thromboembolism

Thromboembolism, perhaps the most serious complication of glomerular disease, was reported in 5% of dogs with glomerulonephritis, 14% of dogs with amyloidosis, and 13% of dogs with all forms of glomerular disease.[8,9,13] Because emboli may be difficult to detect, the prevalence of thromboembolism in dogs with glomerular disease may be higher than indicated by these studies. The risk of thromboembolism is highest in dogs with diseases most likely to cause nephrotic-range proteinuria (e.g., membranous nephropathy, amyloidosis). Pulmonary thromboembolism is most common, but emboli may also lodge in other arteries (e.g., mesenteric, renal, iliac, brachial, coronary) or the portal vein.

Although urinary loss of antithrombin III (AT III) has gained the most attention in veterinary medicine, the pathogenesis of the hypercoagulable state is multifactorial.[42] AT III is a serine protease inhibitor that modulates fibrin generation; heparin catalyses these reactions. AT III (65,000 daltons) is similar in charge and size to albumin (69,000 daltons); serum AT III activity closely correlates with the serum albumin concentration. This close correlation allows one to predict an increased risk of thromboembolism in patients with a serum albumin concentration less than 2 g/dL, when serum AT III activity would be expected to be less than 75% of normal.[8] However, AT III activity levels do not always correlate with the development of thromboembolism; other factors are involved.

Albumin binds to arachidonic acid, which, if unbound, would stimulate platelet aggregation through the generation of prostaglandins (i.e., thromboxane B_2); hypoalbuminemia is associated with increased platelet aggregation.[42] Hypercholesterolemia contributes to platelet hypersensitivity by influencing the membrane-associated enzyme and receptor activity through alteration of the membrane composition. The role of platelet hypersensitivity in the development of hypercoagulability may be enhanced by thrombocytosis, which occurs in many animals with glomerular disease. Increased fibrinogen

concentrations (i.e., above 300 mg/dL), which are often present in patients with nephrotic syndrome, lead to increased fibrin complex formation and platelet hyperaggregation. The risk of thromboembolism may be further enhanced by increased concentrations of alpha$_2$ macroglobulin; alpha$_2$ antiplasmin; procoagulant cytokines; coagulation factors V, VII, VIII, and X; increased plasma viscosity and interstitial pressure; decreased plasma plasminogen concentrations; decreased plasma volume and blood flow; endothelial injury; and infections.[42]

Coumadins and aspirin have been used in the prevention of thromboembolism in at-risk dogs. However, warfarin is highly protein bound. It is very difficult to titrate the dose adequately to prolong the prothrombin time appropriately (i.e., 150% of baseline) in dogs with hypoalbuminemia, and its use is not recommended. Alternatively, low-dose aspirin is inexpensive, easy to administer, and has the added benefit of potentially reducing proteinuria.

Hyperlipidemia

Hypercholesterolemia was reported in 79% of dogs with glomerulonephritis and 86% of dogs with amyloidosis.[9,13] Cholesterol concentrations as high as 749 mg/dL have been reported, although the mean concentration was 312 mg/dL in 69 dogs with glomerulonephritis and 350 mg/dL in 23 dogs with amyloidosis.[8,9] Increases in total plasma cholesterol, very-low-density lipoprotein (VLDL), and low-density lipoprotein (LDL) occur.[49] Hyperlipidemia is variably seen in humans with nephrotic syndrome and has not been fully studied in dogs. The pathogenesis of hyperlipidemia in association with nephrotic syndrome is complex.[49] Hypoalbuminemia stimulates hepatic protein synthesis, including the synthesis of lipoproteins, leading to hypercholesterolemia.[42] The serum albumin concentration and plasma oncotic pressure inversely correlate with the magnitude of hypercholesterolemia. It is unclear whether hypoalbuminemia or the decreased plasma oncotic pressure, or both, induce the increased synthesis. Alterations in lipid catabolism also contribute to the development of hyperlipidemia. Orosomucoid, which plays an important role in the maintenance of glomerular permselectivity, is lost in the urine of patients with glomerular disease. Urinary losses of orosomucoid exacerbate proteinuria but also contribute to hyperlipidemia by indirectly causing decreased hepatic production of heparin sulfate, a cofactor needed in normal lipoprotein lipase function.[49]

Some evidence supports the theory that uncontrolled hyperlipidemia contributes to glomerular and tubulointerstitial injury. LDL and oxidized LDL may alter mesangial cell function and increase the synthesis of mesangial matrix, thereby accelerating the formation of glomerulosclerosis.[42] Glomerular and tubulointerstitial lipoprotein deposition and lipoprotein-induced cytotoxicity also contribute to renal injury. Interestingly, glomerular lesions have been identified in cats with lipoprotein lipase deficiency and in miniature schnauzers with hyperlipidemia.[50]

PROGNOSIS FOR GLOMERULAR DISEASE

The prognosis for dogs and cats with glomerular disease is variable and probably based on a combination of factors. The prognosis is expected to differ with the various diseases, as discussed earlier in the chapter. Although progressive disease can be expected to occur in a large percentage of animals with glomerular disease, spontaneous remission and response to specific therapy can also be expected. Furthermore, disease progression can be slow enough for the animals to lead relatively normal lives, especially when the diagnosis is established early in the disease process. In humans, azotemia, severe proteinuria, systemic hypertension, and marked tubulointerstitial lesions at presentation are the most significant predictors of an unfavorable outcome in most forms of glomerular disease. Clinical impressions would suggest that these same variables affect the prognosis in dogs and cats.

Dogs with glomerulonephritis that were azotemic at first evaluation survived less than 3 months.[9] The median survival of 53 dogs with glomerulonephritis and amyloidosis that were not dead or euthanized shortly after presentation was only 28 days, although individual dogs survived for more than 3 years; survival times did not correlate with any biochemical parameter in these dogs.[8] Both of these studies are inherently biased toward death by the inclusion of dogs from which renal tissue samples were collected during postmortem examination. More study is needed to characterize the natural history and prognosis of the various glomerular diseases in dogs and cats.

CHAPTER • 262

Urinary Tract Infections

Joseph W. Bartges

A urinary tract infection (UTI) develops when a breach (either temporary or permanent) occurs in host defense mechanisms and a virulent microbe in sufficient numbers is allowed to adhere, multiply, and persist in a portion of the urinary tract. UTIs typically involve bacteria, although fungi and viruses also may infect the urinary tract. Infection may predominate at a single site, such as the kidney (pyelonephritis), ureter (ureteritis), bladder (cystitis), urethra (urethritis), prostate (prostatitis), or vagina (vaginitis), or it may be present at two or more of these sites. Because a UTI may involve more than one location, it may be relevant to identify the infection anatomically; that is, upper urinary tract (kidneys and ureters) or lower urinary tract (bladder, urethra, and prostate or vagina). UTIs may or may not produce clinical signs.

The reported incidence of bacterial UTI in dogs and cats is variable. Bacterial UTI is estimated to affect 14% of all dogs during their lifetime,[1] and it is more common in females.[2-5] In cats, bacterial UTIs occur more often in animals older than 10 years, and the incidence increases with age.[6-9] Fungal UTI is believed to be uncommon.[10-13] The incidence of viral UTI is unknown, but viruses have been implicated as a cause of lower urinary tract disease in cats (see Chapter 266).[14-18]

The pathogenesis of urinary tract infections represents a balance between uropathogenic infectious agents and host resistance. UTIs should be treated with antimicrobial agents; however, the status of host defense mechanisms is important in the development, treatment, and prevention of these infections.

DEFINITION OF CONCEPTS AND TERMS

Urinary Tract Infection

A *urinary tract infection* is defined as adherence, multiplication, and persistence of an infectious agent in the urogenital system. Infections often involve a bacterial organism that is present normally in the distal urogenital tract.

Microburia

Microburia refers to the presence of microbes, typically bacteria, in the urine.

Bacteriuria

Bacteriuria refers to the presence of bacteria in the urine. However, identification of bacteria in the urine is not synonymous with UTI. The presence of bacteria may represent contamination of a urine sample, particularly if the sample was collected by voiding or catheterization. Bacteria in the distal urogenital tract may appear in urine collected by these methods, or the urine may be contaminated after collection. *Significant bacteriuria* is the term used to describe bacteriuria that represents a UTI. A high bacterial number in a properly collected and cultured urine sample is indicative of a bacterial UTI. Small numbers of bacteria obtained from untreated pets usually indicate contamination. *Asymptomatic bacteriuria* refers to significant bacteriuria that is not associated with clinical signs of UTI. This often occurs in animals with compromised host defenses, such as those with glucocorticoid excess, diabetes mellitus, or feline immunodeficiency virus infection.

Funguria

Funguria refers to the presence of fungi in the urine. Fungi are not normally present in the urogenital system, and identification of these organisms indicates the presence of an infection, regardless of whether clinical signs are seen.

Pyuria

Pyuria refers to the presence of white blood cells (WBCs) in the urine. Pyuria is defined as (1) more than 3 to 5 WBCs (neutrophils) per high-power field in urine sediment prepared from a 5 mL aliquot of urine collected by cystocentesis, or (2) more than 5 to 10 WBCs per high-power field in urine sediment prepared from a 5 mL aliquot of urine collected by catheterization or voiding. Pyuria is not synonymous with UTI; it only implies inflammation.

Inflammation versus Infection

The presence of inflammation is not synonymous with UTI. Many disease processes result in urinary system inflammation, characterized by hematuria, pyuria, and/or proteinuria. The presence of one or more of these conditions does not indicate the etiology or location of the disease process in the urogenital system. To identify the etiology of the inflammation, additional testing must be performed, such as imaging studies, urine culture, renal function tests, endoscopy, urodynamic studies, or biopsy.

ETIOPATHOGENESIS

Normal Host Defenses

Most UTIs are the result of ascending migration of pathogens from the distal urogenital tract into otherwise normally sterile locations. A resident population of bacteria that is normally present in the lower urogenital tract may decrease establishment of an uropathogen or may emerge as a uropathogen if normal host defenses are altered (Table 262-1).

Although the urinary tract communicates with the microbe-laden external environment, most of the urinary tract is normally sterile, and all of it is resistant to infection. Mechanisms of host resistance to UTIs may be divided into two categories: (1) natural inherent resistance factors and (2) acquired or induced resistance factors activated by the onset of a UTI (Box 262-1). Systemic host defenses play a role in the prevention of hematogenous spread of pathogens to and from the urinary tract; however, local host defense mechanisms are the initial defense in the prevention of ascending infection (Box 262-1).[19] There also appears to be a difference in host defense mechanisms between the upper and lower urinary tracts. For example, induction of diuresis is beneficial for preventing experimental induction of bacterial pyelonephritis in rats[20]; however, dilute urine appears to increase the susceptibility of animals to bacterial infection of the lower urinary tact.[7,21]

Table • 262-1

Bacteria Detected in the Urogenital Tract of Normal Male and Female Dogs

GENUS	DISTAL URETHRA OF MALES	PREPUCE	VAGINA
Acinetobacter		+	+
Bacteroides			+
Bacillus		+	+
Citrobacter			+
Corynebacterium	+	+	+
Enterococcus			+
Enterobacter			+
Escherichia	+	+	+
Flavobacterium	+	+	+
Haemophilus	+	+	+
Klebsiella	+	+	+
Micrococcus			+
Moraxella		+	+
Mycoplasma	+	+	+
Neisseria			+
Pasteurella		+	+
Proteus		+	+
Pseudomonas			+
Staphylococcus	+	+	+
Streptococcus	+	+	+
Ureaplasma	+	+	+

From Barsanti JA, Johnson CA: Genitourinary infections. *In* Greene CE (ed): Infectious Diseases of the Dog and Cat, 2nd ed. Philadelphia, WB Saunders, 1990, pp 157-183.

Box • 262-1

Natural and Acquired Host Defenses of the Urinary Tract

1. Normal micturition
   a. Adequate urine volume
   b. Frequent voiding
   c. Complete voiding
2. Anatomic structures
   a. Urethral high-pressure zones
   b. Surface characteristics of urothelium
   c. Urethral peristalsis
   d. Prostatic secretions (antibacterial fraction and immunoglobulins)
   e. Length of urethra
   f. Ureterovesical flap valves
   g. Ureteral peristalsis
   h. Glomerular mesangial cells (?)
   i. Extensive renal blood supply and flow
   j. Others (?)
3. Mucosal defense barriers
   a. Antibody production
   b. Surface layer of glycosaminoglycans
   c. Intrinsic mucosal antimicrobial properties
   d. Exfoliation of urothelial cells
   e. Bacterial interference by commensal microbes of distal urogenital tract
   f. Others (?)
4. Antimicrobial properties of urine
   a. Extreme high and low of urine pH
   b. Hyperosmolality
   c. High concentration of urea
   d. Organic acids
   e. Low-molecular-weight carbohydrates
   f. Tamm-Horsfall mucoproteins
   g. Others (?)
5. Systemic immunocompetence
   a. Cell-mediated immunity
   b. Humoral-mediated immunity

From Osborne CA, Lees GE: Bacterial infections of the canine and feline urinary tract. *In* Osborne CA, Finco DR (eds): Canine and feline nephrology and urology. Baltimore, Williams & Wilkins, 1995, pp 759-797.

Microbial Factors

Not all microbes, particularly bacteria, are pathogenic. For example, of the more than several hundred serotypes of *Escherichia coli*, fewer than 20 account for most bacterial UTIs.[22] Because *E. coli* is the most common bacterial uropathogen in humans, dogs, and cats, its virulence (uropathogenicity) has been studied extensively.[22-33] Less is known about the uropathogenicity of other pathogens (Box 262-2). Uropathogens typically have more than one virulence factor, therefore the absence of one factor does not necessarily result in loss of uropathogenicity. Likewise, bacteria that are nonpathogenic in a normal pet may become pathogenic in one with altered host defenses.

Microbial Isolates

The bacteria that commonly cause UTIs are similar in dogs and cats. Infections caused by *E. coli* are most common, and

Some Factors That May Enhance the Virulence (Uropathogenicity) of Bacteria Causing Urinary Tract Infection

1. *Escherichia coli*
   a. Certain O (somatic) antigens
      i. Outer polysaccharide portion of bacterial envelope
      ii. Smooth colony morphology on culture plate
      iii. Indirect marker of virulence (human studies)
   b. Certain K (capsular) antigens
      i. Capsule surrounds bacterium.
      ii. May inhibit phagocytosis and complement-mediated bactericidal activity
      iii. Increased resistance to inflammation favors persistence of bacteria in tissue.
   c. Adhesive fimbriae (pili)
      i. Proteinaceous filamentous organelles that protrude from the surface of the bacterium
      ii. Specific types of fimbriae (p-fimbriae) enhance the ability of a bacterium to remain adherent to uroepithelium despite cleansing action of urinary system.
   d. Hemolysin
      i. Increases amount of free iron available for bacterial growth
      ii. May cause tissue damage
   e. Aerobactin
      i. Iron-binding protein
      ii. Facilitates bacterial growth
   f. R-plasmids
      i. Promote resistance to antimicrobial agents
   g. Resistance to serum bactericidal activity
   h. Short generation time in urine
2. *Proteus, Staphylococcus,* and some *Klebsiella* spp.
   a. Adherence factors
   b. Urease
      i. Bacterial enzyme that hydrolyzes urea to ammonia
      ii. Ammonia directly injures uroepithelium.
      iii. Urease fosters production of magnesium ammonium phosphatase uroliths.
   c. R-plasmids
3. *Pseudomonas* sp.
   a. Heavy mucoid polysaccharide capsule
      i. Prevents antibody coating
   b. R-plasmids

this pathogen accounts for one third to one half of all organisms isolated from urine. Gram-positive cocci are the second major group of uropathogens. Staphylococci, streptococci, and enterococci account for one fourth to one third of isolates recovered. Bacteria that cause the remaining one fourth to one third of bacterial UTIs include *Proteus, Klebsiella, Pasteurella, Pseudomonas, Corynebacterium,* and *Mycoplasma* spp.; however, infection caused by any of these bacteria is uncommon.[6,7,11,34-37]

Approximately 75% of bacterial UTIs in dogs are caused by a single species of pathogen, approximately 20% are caused by two species, and approximately 5% are caused by three species.[11] A similar pattern is found in cats.[7,8]

Routes of Infection

The majority of UTI occur as a consequence of ascending migration of pathogens through the genital tract and urethra to the bladder, ureters, and one or both kidneys. Rectal, perineal, and genital bacteria serve as the principal reservoirs for infection.[38-42] Although the intrinsic motility of some bacteria, including *E. coli* and *Proteus* spp., may aid their retrograde migration from the distal urogenital tract, brownian movement is the primary mechanism for ascending infection.[41] In addition to gaining access to the urinary tract, microbes must adhere to and colonize the urothelial surface. Thus the establishment of a UTI depends on the number and virulence of microbes and their interaction with host defenses.

The upper urinary tract is most commonly infected by ascending microbes rather than through hematogenous seeding caused by systemic infection.[44-46] Because blood must pass through glomerular capillaries in the renal cortex before it reaches the medulla, most hematogenous bacteria do not reach the renal medulla. Apparently, renal cortical tissue is more resistant to infection than medullary tissue. Urinary tract obstruction or trauma increases the risk of hematogenous seeding of the urinary tract by interfering with the renal microcirculation.[47]

CLINICAL FINDINGS

Historical Information and Physical Examination Findings

Dogs and cats with UTI may or may not be symptomatic. Clinical signs associated with UTI are variable and depend on the interaction of (1) the virulence and numbers of the uropathogen, (2) the presence or absence of predisposing causes, (3) the body's compensatory response to infection, (4) the duration of infection, and (5) the site or sites of infection (Table 262-2). Pollakiuria, stranguria, dysuria, and inappropriate urination may be observed with lower urinary tract infections. Animals with upper urinary tract infections may show pain localized to one or both kidneys, hematuria, septicemia, or renal failure (with resultant clinical signs if both kidneys are infected). If the UTI is associated with a predisposing condition (e.g., diabetes mellitus, hyperadrenocorticism, or bladder neoplasia), clinical signs associated with that condition usually predominate. Female dogs with abnormalities of the vulva, perivulvar dermatitis, or vaginal stenosis may have an increased risk for UTI.[48] Male cats with perineal urethrostomies also have an increased risk for UTI.[49] Some animals may have infection of both the upper and lower urinary tracts, especially if renal failure is present.

Laboratory Results

Unless septicemia or renal failure is present, the results of complete blood cell counts are normal. If septicemia is present, leukocytosis and a left shift may be seen. Lower urinary tract infection does not cause changes in blood work unless another disease process is present. With upper urinary tract infections, serum biochemical analysis may be normal or may indicate renal failure (if both kidneys are diseased). If the UTI is associated with another disease, changes in laboratory parameters may reflect the associated condition. In cats, feline leukemia virus and feline immunodeficiency virus infections increase the risk of UTI.[7]

Results of Imaging Studies and Endoscopy

In many dogs and cats with a UTI, the results of imaging studies are normal. Survey abdominal radiography may reveal

Table • 262-2

Abnormalities that Help Localize Urinary Tract Infections

SITE OF INFECTION	HISTORY	PHYSICAL EXAMINATION FINDINGS	LABORATORY FINDINGS	IMAGING STUDIES
Lower urinary tract	Dysuria, pollakiuria Urge incontinence Signs of abnormal detrusor reflex (overflow incontinence, large residual volume) Gross hematuria at end of micturition Cloudy urine with abnormal odor No systemic signs Recent catheterization or urethrostomy	Small, painful, thickened bladder Palpable masses in urethra or bladder Flaccid bladder wall, large residual volume Abnormal micturition reflex ± Palpation of uroliths	Complete blood count (CBC): Normal Urinalysis: Pyuria, hematuria, proteinuria, bacteriuria Urine culture: Significant bacteriuria	Normal kidneys Structural abnormalities of lower urinary tract ± Urocystoliths and/or urethroliths ± Thickening of bladder wall and irregularity of mucosa Rarely, intraluminal gas formation (emphysematous cystitis)
Upper urinary tract	Polyuria, polydipsia ± Signs of systemic infection ± Renal failure	± Detectable abnormalities ± Fever and other signs of systemic infection ± Abdominal (renal) pain Kidney(s) normal or increased in size	CBC: ± Leukocytosis Urinalysis: Pyuria, hematuria, proteinuria, bacteriuria, white blood cell or granular casts Impaired urine concentration ± Azotemia and other findings of renal failure	Renomegaly ± Abnormal kidney shape ± Nephroliths, ureteroliths ± Dilated renal pelves, dilated pelvic diverticula ± Evidence of outflow obstruction
Acute prostatitis or prostatic abscessation	Urethral discharge independent of micturition Signs of systemic infection ± Reluctance to urinate or defecate	± Fever and other signs of systemic infection ± Painful prostate and/or painful abdomen ± Prostatomegaly or asymmetric prostate	CBC: ± Leukocytosis Urinalysis: Pyuria, hematuria, proteinuria, bacteriuria Prostate cytology: Inflammation and infection	± Indistinct cranial border of prostate ± Prostatomegaly ± Prostatic cysts ± Reflux of contrast medium into prostate
Chronic prostatitis	Recurrent urinary tract infections Urethral discharge independent of urination ± Dysuria	Often no detectable abnormalities ± Prostatomegaly or asymmetric prostate	CBC: Normal Urinalysis: Pyuria, hematuria, proteinuria, bacteriuria	± Prostatomegaly ± Prostatic cysts ± Prostatic mineralization

URINARY SYSTEM

uroliths, renomegaly, or small kidneys, or other defects that may predispose the animal to the development of a UTI. Some dogs may have pelvic displacement of the urinary bladder (so-called pelvic bladder), which can be associated with urinary incontinence and UTI, although it also is observed in dogs without disease.[50] If no abnormalities are found by survey abdominal radiography, ultrasonography or contrast radiography should be performed. The upper urinary tract may be evaluated by excretory urography, and the lower urinary tract may be evaluated by contrast cystourethrography, double contrast cystography, and contrast vaginourethrography. A potential complication of contrast radiography of the lower urinary tract is induction of a UTI. Ultrasonography is a noninvasive technique that is useful for evaluating the echotexture and architecture of the urinary tract except for the distal urethra. In humans, nuclear scintigraphy using technetium-99m–labeled dimercaptosuccinic acid (DMSA) may be useful for evaluating for pyelonephritis; however, this diagnostic aid has not been used in dogs.[51,52]

Endoscopy of the lower urinary tract may be useful for identifying mucosal and intraluminal lesions that may predispose an animal to UTI. In one cat, a urolith not visible by survey radiography was visualized by cystoscopy.[53] Disadvantages of cystourethroscopy include induction of anesthesia to perform the procedure, contamination of and trauma to the lower urogenital tract, and difficulty performing the procedure in male cats.

DIAGNOSIS

Urinalysis

A urinalysis should be performed as a routine part of a minimum database. A complete urinalysis involves determination of the urine specific gravity (USG) using a refractometer, chemical analysis using analytic test pads on dipsticks, and sediment examination. Cystocentesis is the best method of collecting urine when evaluating a dog or cat for UTI. If infectious prostatitis or vaginitis is suspected, these anatomic areas should be evaluated using different techniques (see Chapters 253 and 263).

With urinary tract infection the USG is variable, depending on whether the infection involves the upper urinary tract or an associated disease. Dipstick analysis often, but not always, reveals hematuria and proteinuria. Leukocyte esterase (WBCs) and nitrite (bacteria) test pads are not reliable in dogs and cats and should not be used.[54]

Examination of urine sediment should be a routine part of a complete urinalysis. The presence of a significant number of WBCs (more than 0 to 5 per high-power field) associated with hematuria and proteinuria in a properly collected urine sample suggests inflammation. Detection of significant microburia with pyuria indicates active inflammation associated with an infection. Bacteria and fungi may be difficult to identify in dilute urine, making a diagnosis of UTI problematic. UTI, especially a bacterial UTI, may be present without concurrent inflammation if host defenses are compromised (e.g., as in hyperadrenocorticism or feline leukemia virus infection).[7,12,55-59]

Rod-shaped bacteria may be identified in unstained preparations of urine sediment if more than 10,000 bacteria/mL are present, but they may not be consistently detected if present in fewer numbers. Cocci are difficult to detect in urine sediment if their numbers are less than 100,000 bacteria/mL.[2] Although detection of bacteria on urine sediment examination suggests bacterial UTI, this finding should be verified by urine culture. Urine sediment may be stained with Gram's stain or new methylene blue to aid in detection of microbes; however, urine culture is the gold standard for confirmation of UTI. Failure to detect bacteria on examination of urine sediment does not exclude their presence or rule out a UTI.

Urine Collection

For urine culture, urine should be collected by cystocentesis. With lower urinary tract disease, collection of a sample by this method may be difficult, and it may be necessary to collect urine by catheterization or, less desirably, voiding. These techniques require cleansing of the pet's external genitalia, and the perivulvar fur may require clipping to prevent contamination. Although urinary catheterization of dogs is usually accomplished without chemical restraint, cats require sedation or anesthesia. A sterile catheter and collection container (a syringe or a collection cup with a tight-fitting lid) are used. If the results of quantitative culture of urine samples obtained by catheterization or midstream voiding are equivocal after serial cultures, urine should be collected by cystocentesis.

The presence of bacteria, even in low numbers, in urine collected aseptically by cystocentesis indicates a UTI; however, false-positive results may occur if a loop of intestine is penetrated with the hypodermic needle during the procedure or if the sample is contaminated during handling. Contamination usually involves recovery of more than one organism.

Urine Culture

As mentioned previously, urine culture is the gold standard for diagnosis of a UTI. A diagnosis of UTI based only on clinical signs, hematuria, and/or urinary tract inflammation is a misdiagnosis that may result in inadequate or inappropriate treatment. Under some circumstances, antimicrobial therapy may be initiated without first obtaining the results of urine culture (see Empiric Antimicrobial Treatment, below); however, samples for urine culture should be collected before drug therapy is started. If antimicrobial therapy has been started, it should be discontinued for 3 to 5 days prior to performance of a urine culture to minimize inhibition of microbial growth.

A urine culture is the most definitive means of diagnosing a bacterial UTI. Fungal culture should be considered when yeast or fungi are identified on urine sediment examination. Care must be taken to collect, preserve, and transport the urine sample so as to avoid contamination, proliferation, or bacterial death.[60] Urine specimens for aerobic bacterial culture should be transported and stored in sealed, sterilized containers, and processing should begin as soon as possible. If laboratory processing is delayed by more than 30 minutes, the specimen should be refrigerated at 4°C.[61] At room temperature, bacterial counts may double every 20 to 45 minutes. Multiplication or destruction of bacteria may occur within 1 hour of collection.

If samples cannot be processed immediately for urine culture, several alternatives are available. Blood agar and MacConkey's agar plates may be inoculated and incubated for 24 hours. A calibrated bacteriologic loop or a microliter mechanical pipette that delivers exactly 0.01 or 0.001 mL of urine to the culture plates should be used. The urine is streaked over the plates by conventional methods. Blood agar supports the growth of most aerobic uropathogens, and MacConkey's agar provides information that aids the identification of bacteria and prevents "swarming" of *Proteus* spp. The plates are incubated or placed under an incandescent light.[62] If bacterial growth occurs on the plate after 24 hours, the plates may be submitted for identification and determination of antimicrobial sensitivities, or antimicrobial susceptibility may be determined using the agar disk diffusion method.[62,63] If no growth occurs after 24 hours, the plates may be discarded.

Commercially available urine culture collection tubes containing preservative, combined with refrigeration, may be used to preserve specimens for up to 72 hours.[64] More recently, in-house urine culture and susceptibility kits have become available (IndicatoRx; IDEXX Laboratories, Westbrook, Maine).

Qualitative urine culture   A qualitative urine culture involves the isolation and identification of bacteria in urine; it does not include quantification of bacterial numbers. Although urine in the bladder is normally sterile, urine that passes through the distal urogenital tract often becomes contaminated with resident flora (see Table 262-1). Therefore the presence of bacteria in urine collected by catheterization or voiding is often difficult to interpret, even with quantification of bacteria (Table 262-3). For this reason, a diagnostic urine culture should include quantitation of bacterial numbers in addition to identification of the organism and antimicrobial susceptibility.

Quantitative urine culture   A quantitative urine culture includes isolation and identification of the organism and determination of the number of bacteria (i.e., colony-forming units [cfu] per unit volume). Quantitation allows interpretation of the significance of bacteria present in a urine sample. However, caution should be exercised in the interpretation of quantitative urine cultures obtained by midstream voiding or manual expression of the bladder. Although urine obtained from most dogs without a UTI is either sterile or contains less than 10,000 cfu/mL (see Table 262-3), counts of 100,000 cfu/mL or higher have occurred with sufficient frequency to make collection of urine by midstream voiding or manual expression unsatisfactory.[65] The definition of significant bacteriuria in cats involves lower numbers of organisms, because cats appear to be more resistant to UTI than dogs.

Antimicrobial Susceptibility Testing

Administration of antimicrobial agents is the cornerstone of treatment for UTI. The antimicrobial agent selected should be (1) easy to administer, (2) associated with few, if any, side effects, (3) inexpensive, (4) able to attain tissue or urine concentrations that exceed the minimum inhibitory concentration (MIC) for the uropathogen by at least fourfold, and (5) unlikely to affect the pet's intestinal flora adversely.[2] The antimicrobial agent chosen should be based on antimicrobial susceptibility testing.

Agar disk diffusion technique   Antimicrobial susceptibility testing is often done using agar disk diffusion (Kirby-Bauer technique),[66] which is adequate for most bacterial UTIs.

The agar disk diffusion method consists of Mueller-Hinton agar plates that have been inoculated with a standardized suspension of a single uropathogen. Paper disks impregnated with different antimicrobial drugs are placed on the plate. After 18 to 24 hours' inoculation at 38° C, antimicrobial susceptibility is estimated by measuring zones of inhibition of bacterial growth surrounding each disk. The zones of inhibition are then interpreted in light of established standards and recorded as resistant, susceptible, or intermediately susceptible. Because of differences in the ability of various antimicrobials to diffuse through agar, the antimicrobial disk surrounded by the largest zone of inhibition is not necessarily the drug most likely to be effective. Also, because the concentration of antimicrobial (except nitrofurantoin) in the paper disks is comparable to the typical serum concentration of the drug, drugs that are found to be resistant by the agar disk diffusion method may be effective in the urinary tract if they are excreted in high concentrations in urine (e.g., ampicillin and cephalexin).

Antimicrobial dilution technique   Antimicrobial dilution susceptibility tests are designed to determine the minimum concentration of an antimicrobial drug that will inhibit the growth of the uropathogen (i.e., the MIC). After inoculation and incubation of uropathogens into wells containing serial twofold dilutions of antimicrobial drugs at concentrations achievable in tissues and urine, the MIC is defined as the lowest antimicrobial concentration (or highest dilution) that allows no visible bacterial growth. The MIC is several dilutions lower than the minimum bactericidal concentration of drugs. In general, the antimicrobial agent is likely to be effective if it can achieve a concentration four times that of the MIC (Table 262-4). Many antimicrobial drugs that are excreted through the kidneys reach concentrations in urine that are 10 to 100 times greater than the serum concentration.

TREATMENT

Prevention

Normal host defense mechanisms are effective in preventing UTIs; however, they are not impenetrable. For example, normal host defenses may be overwhelmed if large quantities of a virulent uropathogen are introduced into the urinary tract during diagnostic and therapeutic procedures. Iatrogenic UTI is a common complication of indwelling urinary catheters, especially if an open-ended system is used. Bacterial UTI

URINARY SYSTEM

Table • 262-3

Interpretation of Quantitative Urine Cultures in Dogs and Cats

	SIGNIFICANT		SUSPICIOUS		CONTAMINANT	
SAMPLE TYPE	DOGS	CATS	DOGS	CATS	DOGS	CATS
Cystocentesis	≥1000	≥1000	100 to 1000	100 to 1000	≤100	≤100
Catheterization	≥10,000	≥1000	1000 to 10,000	100 to 1000	≤1000	≤100
Midstream voiding	≥100,000†	≥10,000	10,000 to 90,000	1000 to 10,000	≤10,000	≤1000
Manual compression	≥100,000†	≥10,000	10,000 to 90,000	1000 to 10,000	≤10,000	≤1000

From Lulich JP, Osborne CA: Bacterial urinary tract infections. *In* Ettinger SJ, Feldman EC (eds): Textbook of Veterinary Internal Medicine, 4th ed. Philadelphia, WB Saunders, 1999, pp 1775-1788.
*Values are given in colony-forming units per milliliter of urine (cfu/mL). Data represent generalities. Occasionally, bacterial UTI may be detected with fewer organisms (i.e., false-negative results).
†Because the contamination level of midstream samples may be 10,000 cfu/mL or higher (i.e., false-positive result), these samples should not be used for routine diagnostic culture.

Table • 262-4

Average Canine Urine Concentrations of Some Antimicrobial Agents

DRUG	DAILY DOSAGE (mg/kg)	ROUTE OF ADMINISTRATION	MEAN URINE CONCENTRATION (± SD)
Amikacin	5	SQ	342 ± 143 µg/mL
Amoxicillin	11	PO	202 ± 93 µg/mL
Ampicillin	26	PO	309 ± 55 µg/mL
Cephalexin	18	PO	500 µg/mL
Chloramphenicol	33	PO	124 ± 40 µg/mL
Enrofloxacin	5	PO	40 ± 10 µg/mL
Gentamicin	2	SQ	107 ± 33 µg/mL
Hetacillin	26	PO	300 ± 156 µg/mL
Kanamycin	4	SQ	530 ± 151 µg/mL
Nitrofurantoin	4.4	PO	100 µg/mL
Penicillin G	36,700 U/kg	PO	295 ± 211 µg/mL
Penicillin V	26	PO	148 ± 99 µg/mL
Sulfisoxazole	22	PO	1466 ± 832 µg/mL
Tetracycline	18	PO	139 ± 65 µg/mL
Trimethoprim/sulfadiazine	13	PO	55 ± 19 µg/mL
Tobramycin	2.2	SQ	66 ± 39 µg/mL

From Ling GV: Therapeutic strategies involving antimicrobial treatment of the canine urinary tract. J Am Vet Med Assoc 185(10):1162-1164, 1984; and Lulich JP, Osborne CA: Bacterial urinary tract infections. *In* Ettinger SJ, Feldman EC (eds): Textbook of Veterinary Internal Medicine, 4th ed. Philadelphia, WB Saunders, 1999, pp 1775-1788.
SD, Standard deviation; *SQ*, subcutaneous; *PO*, per os (by mouth).

developed in 20% of healthy adult female dogs after intermittent catheterization; in 33% of male dogs during repeated catheterization; and in 65% of healthy male cats within 3 to 5 days of open indwelling catheterization. In a clinical study, bacterial UTI developed in 52% of dogs and cats with indwelling urinary catheters; the risk of UTI increased with the duration of catheterization.[67] The use of indwelling urinary catheters during diuresis or corticosteroid administration is particularly dangerous, and the problem is compounded if the dog or cat has preexisting urinary tract disease.

Iatrogenic UTI may be prevented by (1) avoiding indiscriminate use of urinary catheters, (2) using a closed collection system for indwelling urinary catheters, (3) using indwelling urinary catheters cautiously when pets are undergoing diuresis, (4) avoiding the use of indwelling catheters in immunosuppressed pets or those receiving immunosuppressive medications (e.g., glucocorticoids), (5) appropriately using antimicrobials with urinary catheterization, and (6) using diagnostic and therapeutic techniques that minimize trauma and microbial contamination of the urinary tract.[2] Although it would seem logical to administer antimicrobial agents while an indwelling urinary catheter is in place so as to decrease the chance of iatrogenic UTI, the practice is discouraged. Concomitant oral or parenteral administration of antimicrobial agents during indwelling urethral catheterization reduces the frequency of development of a bacterial UTI; however, it promotes the development of UTI caused by multidrug-resistant bacteria.[67]

Eradication of Underlying Causes
Although antimicrobial agents are the cornerstone of treatment of UTI, they should be used in a logical fashion. Overuse and misuse of antimicrobial agents may result in the emergence of resistant organisms, a situation that has implications for veterinary and human health. A UTI occurs in association with compromise of host defense mechanisms, which may be transient or permanent. Transient compromise often results in the development of a simple, uncomplicated UTI; however, permanent compromise results in the development of complicated UTI. Evaluation for and correction or control of the compromise or compromises in host defense mechanisms are important in the treatment of UTI, especially if these infections are recurrent (Figure 262-1). For example, recurrent bacterial UTI may occur in female dogs with a recessed vulva; vulvoplasty may help prevent future infections.[68,69]

Bacterial Urinary Tract Infection
Uncomplicated UTI Uncomplicated UTIs are those in which no underlying structural, neurologic, or functional abnormality is identified. Dogs and cats with an uncomplicated UTI are usually successfully treated with a 10- to 14-day course of an appropriate antimicrobial agent (see Figure 262-1). If the proper antimicrobial is chosen and administered at the appropriate dosage and frequency, clinical signs should resolve within 48 hours. Also, the results of a complete urinalysis should improve within this same time frame. If possible, a urine culture should be performed 5 to 7 days after cessation of antimicrobial therapy.

Empiric antimicrobial treatment Treatment of uncomplicated bacterial UTI of acute onset may be undertaken without the results of antimicrobial susceptibility testing, provided (1) that the dog or cat has not been given antimicrobial agents within the last 4 to 6 weeks and (2) that this is an initial or infrequent occurrence. In such situations, the antimicrobial should be chosen for its known properties and with knowledge of bacteria that commonly cause UTI (Table 262-5). Identification of bacteria on examination of urine sediment, especially if Gram's staining is performed, increases the likelihood of empirically choosing an appropriate antimicrobial. For example, *E. coli* is the most common cause of bacterial UTI in dogs and cats and is a gram-negative rod associated with aciduria.

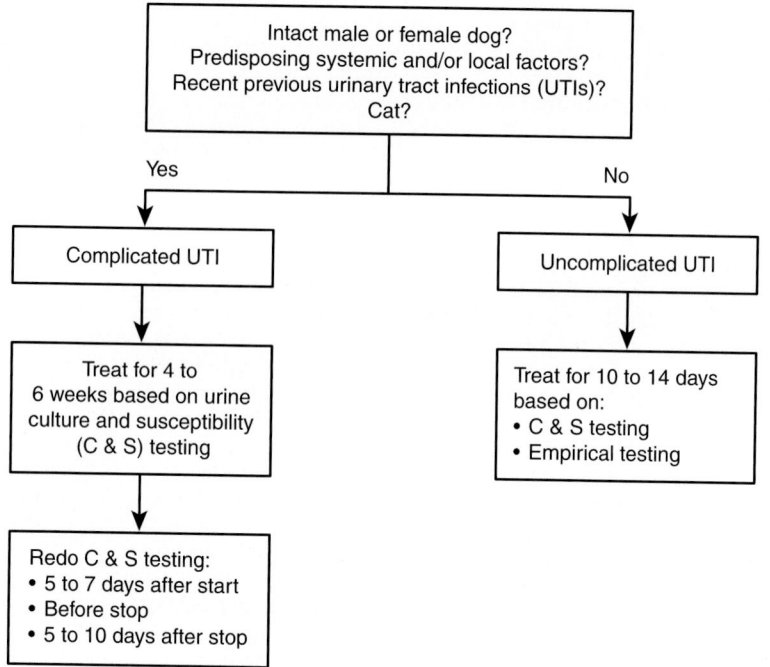

Figure 262-1 Algorithm for treatment of urinary tract infection (UTI) in dogs and cats. *C & S,* Urine culture and susceptibility testing.

Staphylococci, on the other hand, are gram-positive cocci associated with alkaluria because they produce urease, which metabolizes urea to ammonia, resulting in an alkaline urine pH.

The use of fluoroquinolones for empiric treatment of bacterial UTI is discouraged because of the inherent resistance of many gram-positive organisms and the developing resistance of many gram-negative organisms, especially *E. coli,* to this class of antimicrobials.[26,70]

Complicated UTI Reproductively intact dogs, all cats, and animals with identifiable predisposing causes for UTI (e.g., renal failure, hyperadrenocorticism, and diabetes mellitus) should be considered to have a complicated UTI (see Figure 262-1). Pyelonephritis and prostatitis are examples of complicated UTI. Treatment with antimicrobials for longer than the routine 10 to 14 days may be indicated, and the drugs are usually administered for 4 to 6 weeks.

Table • 262-5

Estimate of Susceptibility of Uropathogens to Commonly Used Antimicrobial Agents

UROPATHOGEN	DRUGS OF CHOICE	ALTERNATIVES
Enterobacter spp.	Trimethoprim-sulfadiazine	Cephalosporins (first and second generation), gentamicin, nitrofurantoin
Escherichia coli*	Trimethoprim-sulfadiazine	Cephalosporins (first and second generation), fluoroquinolones, gentamicin
Klebsiella spp.*	Cephalosporins (first generation)	Amikacin, gentamicin, trimethoprim-sulfadiazine, cephalosporins (second and third generation)
Mycoplasma,* *Ureaplasma*	Fluoroquinolones	Tetracyclines
Proteus spp.*	Amoxicillin, ampicillin, amoxicillin-clavulanate	Cephalosporins (first and second generation), gentamicin, nitrofurantoin, trimethoprim-sulfadiazine
Pseudomonas aeruginosa*	Fluoroquinolones	Tetracyclines, gentamicin, cephalosporins (first, second, and third generation)
Staphylococcus spp.*	Amoxicillin, ampicillin, amoxicillin-clavulanate	Cephalosporins (first generation), nitrofurantoin, trimethoprim-sulfadiazine
Streptococcus spp., *Enterococcus* spp.	Amoxicillin, ampicillin, amoxicillin-clavulanate	Cephalosporins (first generation), nitrofurantoin, trimethoprim-sulfadiazine

From Osborne CA, Lees GE: Bacterial infections of the canine and feline urinary tract. *In* Osborne CA, Finco DR (eds): Canine and feline nephrology and urology. Baltimore, Williams & Wilkins, 1995, pp 759-797.
*Prior treatment with antimicrobials may alter the susceptibility of uropathogens to these drugs.

The urine should be evaluated in the first week of treatment for response to therapy and also before discontinuation of therapy. Prophylactic antibiotic treatment may be necessary to control bacterial UTIs that are difficult to eradicate or that recur frequently.

Recurrent UTI

Relapse　A *relapse* is defined as recurrence of a UTI caused by the same organism. Relapses usually occur within days to weeks of discontinuation of antimicrobial therapy. Possible causes of relapse include use of an inappropriate antimicrobial agent; administration of an appropriate antimicrobial agent at an inappropriate dosage, frequency, or duration; and complicating factors. A urine culture should be evaluated prior to reinstitution of antimicrobial therapy, and further diagnostic evaluation for predisposing causes is indicated.

Reinfection　Reinfection is defined as infection with a different organism than that initially present. Reinfections usually occur some time after cessation of antimicrobial therapy. Although predisposing risk factors may be present, many animals that become reinfected do not have identifiable risk factors. If reinfection occurs infrequently, each episode may be treated as an uncomplicated UTI. However, if reinfection occurs more often than three times a year, the animal should be treated as having a complicated UTI. Additionally, prophylactic antimicrobial therapy may be indicated.

Superinfection　A *superinfection* occurs when a second bacterial organism is isolated while an animal is receiving antimicrobial therapy. This organism often displays a high degree of antibiotic resistance. A UTI that occurs in animals receiving antimicrobial therapy that also have an indwelling urethral catheter is an example of a superinfection.[67]

Prophylactic antimicrobial treatment　No good studies have evaluated prophylactic antimicrobial therapy in animals that have frequent reinfections. When prophylactic therapy is undertaken, urine culture and susceptibility testing should be done to ensure that the bacterial UTI has been eradicated. A drug should be selected that is excreted in high concentration in the urine and that is unlikely to cause adverse effects. Often a fluoroquinolone, cephalosporin, or beta-lactam antimicrobial is chosen. The antimicrobial should be given at approximately one third the therapeutic daily dose immediately after the pet has voided, and when the drug and its metabolites will be retained in the urinary tract for 6 to 8 hours. This is typically done at night. The drug is administered for a minimum of 6 months. Urine samples are collected, preferably by cystocentesis (not by catheterization, because this may induce a bacterial UTI) every 4 to 8 weeks for urinalysis and quantitative urine culture. If no evidence of bacterial UTI is found, prophylactic therapy is continued. If a bacterial UTI is identified, the active (break-through) infection is treated as a complicated bacterial UTI. If a break-through bacterial UTI does not occur after 6 months of prophylactic antimicrobial therapy, the therapy may be discontinued and the pet monitored for reinfection.[71,72]

Ancillary therapy　Many forms of ancillary therapy have been developed to aid in the treatment of UTI. Ancillary therapy includes urinary acidifiers, urinary antiseptics, local instillation of antimicrobial agents into the urinary bladder, alteration of urine volume, and the use of pharmacologic agents to affect the storage and voiding phases of micturition. Although the activity of antimicrobial agents is affected by the urine pH, rarely is alteration of the urine pH undertaken in an effort to increase activity. An exception is induction of aciduria when methenamine, a urinary antiseptic, is used.

Instillation of antimicrobial agents into the urinary bladder is ineffective and may be associated with complications. For example, instillation of gentamicin into a compromised urinary bladder may result in absorption and attainment of toxic serum levels. If antimicrobial therapy is required, antimicrobials should be administered orally or parenterally. An instance when instillation of a pharmacologic agent into the urinary bladder may be beneficial is the use of a cystostomy catheter. A cystostomy catheter is inserted directly into the urinary bladder and exits the ventral abdominal wall. Instillation of Tris-EDTA through the cystostomy catheter into the urinary bladder after the bladder has been emptied of urine may decrease the incidence of bacterial UTI.[74]

Fungal Urinary Tract Infection

Fungal UTIs are rare in dogs and cats. They often are associated with glucosuria of diabetes mellitus but may also occur in animals that do not have diabetes. In one study of 20 dogs and cats with *Candida* spp. UTI, concurrent diseases or nonantifungal drugs administered within 1 month of isolation included antibiotics, corticosteroids, diabetes mellitus, nonurogenital neoplasia, and noncandidal urogenital disease. All animals had sources of local or systemic immune compromise that likely predisposed to infection.[12] Treatment of animals with a fungal UTI involves correction or control of the predisposing cause or causes, urinary alkalization, and administration of antifungal drugs. In animals without clinical signs, administration of urinary alkalinizing agents (e.g., potassium citrate or sodium bicarbonate) or the use of diets that induce alkaluria may result in successful eradication of the fungal UTI.[10] Fungal growth is inhibited in an alkaline medium. In animals with active disease, however, antifungal drugs that are excreted renally in an active form should be administered. Although amphotericin B is renally excreted and achieves high concentration in urine, it is not often used because it is parenterally administered and is nephrotoxic. Fluconazole is a good choice and is orally administered. Itraconazole may also be a good choice, but it has not been evaluated for the treatment of fungal UTIs in dogs and cats. Antifungal agents must be administered for several months in association with induction of alkaluria. Correction and/or control of the predisposing underlying disease is paramount in the treatment and prevention of fungal UTI.

Viral Urinary Tract Infection

Although viruses are associated with urinary tract disease in humans, their role in urinary tract disease in dogs and cats is unknown.[75,76] Viral infection of the lower urinary tract may be a cause of lower urinary tract disease in cats.[15,16]

CHAPTER 263

Prostatic Diseases

Michelle A. Kutzler
Amy Yeager

DEVELOPMENT AND ANATOMY

The embryologic development of the prostate begins from multiple outgrowths of the urethral epithelium.[1] During fetal development, testosterone secreted from the testes is reduced to dihydrotestosterone (DHT) in cells in the urogenital sinus, stimulating the formation of the prostatic lobes in the retroperitoneal space caudal to the urinary bladder (Figure 263-1).[2,3] Age, androgenic stimulus, disease, and the degree of urinary bladder distention affect the prostate's position. The gland is intra-abdominal in fetuses and pups less than 2 months old because of the urachal attachment that maintains the bladder in a cranioventral position.[4] The urachal remnant breaks down at about 2 months of age, at which time the prostate moves into an intrapelvic position.[3] Beginning about 8 months of age, androgenic stimulation arising from sexual maturity results in prostatic enlargement; the prostate is repositioned cranially over the pelvic brim as it increases in size, to a total or partial intra-abdominal position.[4] After castration, the prostate atrophies and returns to the intrapelvic position. The degree of urinary bladder distention also affects the prostate's position; specifically, a full bladder displaces the prostate intra-abdominally, whereas an empty bladder facilitates an intrapelvic position.[5]

The prostate is a bilobed, musculoglandular organ that completely encircles the proximal urethra between the membranous portion of the urethra and the neck of the urinary bladder. A capsule surrounds the prostate, and a prominent median septum divides the gland into two ovoid lobes that are dorsally flattened, with the ventral surface covered in a layer of fat.[3] Well-developed arrays of smooth muscle fibers from the capsule extend down into the parenchyma to blend with the smooth muscle of the urethra.[6] Numerous ducts open into the prostatic urethra at the colliculus seminalis, a central portion of the dorsal longitudinal urethral crest.[1] The deferent ducts enter the craniodorsal surface of the prostate and continue caudoventrally to open on each side of the colliculus seminalis.[1]

The urogenital artery, a branch of the internal pudendal artery, supplies blood to the prostate via several prostatic branches through the dorsolateral surfaces (see Figure 263-1).[7] Several prostatic branches originate from the urogenital artery and enter the prostate gland at the dorsolateral surfaces. These branches tunnel beneath the capsule and further divide into smaller parenchymal arteries.[7] Venous drainage occurs via the urethral vein that accompanies the urethra or through small venules that follow the capsular arteries.[7] Lymphatic drainage is to the middle iliac lymph nodes.[3] The hypogastric and pelvic nerves provide sympathetic and parasympathetic innervation to the prostate (see Figure 263-1).[3] Parasympathetic stimulation during erection increases the rate of prostatic fluid production, and sympathetic stimulation during ejaculation ejects the fluid into the prostatic urethra.[8]

PHYSIOLOGY

In the dog, the prostate is the only accessory sex gland, and its secretory function is androgen dependent. Although both testosterone and DHT stimulate prostatic glandular activity, DHT is far more biologically active in that it binds to the androgen receptor with two times the affinity of testosterone

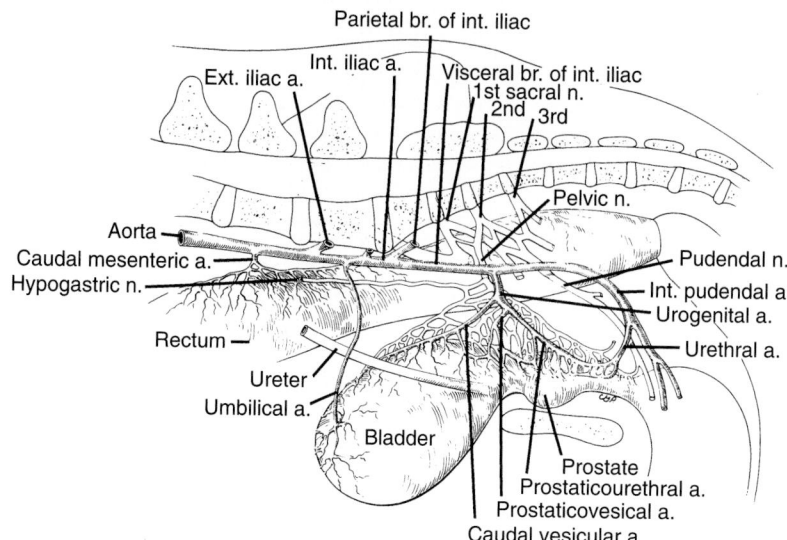

Figure 263-1 Diagram of the normal anatomic relationship of the prostate to other structures in the caudal abdomen. (Adapted from Miller ME et al: Anatomy of the Dog. Philadelphia, WB Saunders, 1964.)

and has a fivefold slower rate of dissociation.[9] In sexually mature dogs, the prostate comprises the compound tubular alveolar glands that radiate from the urethral duct openings.[10] In castrated and sexually immature dogs, the prostate comprises a branching ductular system with poor alveolar development.[10] Elimination of the androgenic stimulus, either pharmacologically or by castration, results in glandular and parenchymal atrophy of the prostate.[11] In addition to androgens, locally produced growth factors (i.e., endothelin-1, basic fibroblast growth factor, transforming growth factor-beta, interleukin-6, and interleukin-8) act to modulate prostatic alveolar development and function.[12]

Prostatic fluid makes up the first and third fractions of the ejaculate; it increases the volume of the ejaculate and possibly aids in sperm transport.[1] Prostatic fluid accounts for greater than 97% of the total ejaculate volume.[13] When neither micturition nor ejaculation is occurring, prostatic fluid is constitutively secreted and expelled into the prostatic urethra, from which it drains into the urinary bladder. Normal prostatic fluid is thin and clear. The major secretory product of the prostate is arginine esterase, which constitutes greater than 90% of the protein in the seminal plasma.[14] Prostate-specific antigen (PSA), the major seminal plasma protein in humans, is not detectable in canine serum or seminal plasma.[15] However, arginine esterase and PSA are both serine proteases and have similar molecular weights and hormonal regulation.[16] The canine prostate also secretes prostatic acid phosphatase.[15]

SIGNALMENT AND CLINICAL SIGNS

Most prostatic diseases are associated with prostatomegaly. Prostatic size correlates with body weight and age[17] (Table 263-1) as well as breed.[18] Scottish terriers are reported to have prostates four times larger than those of dogs of other breeds of similar weight and age.[18] Doberman pinschers and German shepherds were the breeds most commonly represented in a review of 177 cases of prostatic disease.[19]

Clinical signs associated with prostatic disease vary, depending on the degree of prostatomegaly and the specific disorder. Prostatic enlargement is common in dogs more than 5 years old. The most common clinical signs associated with prostatic disease are urethral discharge, hematuria, and tenesmus. However, patients with prostatic disease may be asymptomatic. The urethral discharge may be clear, purulent, or hemorrhagic. In a 14-year retrospective study of prostatic disease, hemorrhagic urethral discharge, which could be exacerbated by sexual arousal, was the only clinical sign observed in 23% of cases.[20] The source of the hemorrhage may be dilated prostatic urethral veins, which can be visualized with cystoscopy.[21] Greatly increased vascularity associated with hyperplasia, infection, or neoplasia in the prostatic parenchyma may be an additional source of hemorrhage.[22] Although widely described as a clinical sign associated with prostatic disease, tenesmus is present only when the prostate is morbidly enlarged. In one report, constipation developed after mineralization of a grossly enlarged paraprostatic cyst.[23] Additional clinical signs associated with prostatic disease include fever, cachexia, abnormal hindlimb gait, and caudal abdominal pain.

EXAMINATION OF THE PROSTATE AND PROSTATIC FLUID

Prostate

A cursory examination of the prostate can be performed by concomitant rectal and abdominal palpation. Rectal palpation permits examination of only the dorsal or dorsocaudal aspect of the prostate.[24] Concomitant abdominal palpation not only allows examination of the cranial aspects of the prostate, it also facilitates better palpation per rectum because the prostate can be pushed into or near the pelvic canal.[1] During palpation, the prostate should be evaluated for size, symmetry, surface contour, movability, and pain. The normal prostate is bilobed, symmetric, smooth, movable, and pain free.

Transabdominal ultrasonography is the best imaging modality for evaluation of the prostate because it is a safe, noninvasive method that allows for precise measurements as well as evaluation of the prostatic parenchyma. Dogs can be imaged in dorsal, dorsal oblique, or lateral recumbency. Because the haircoat is thin in the suprapubic area, clipping usually is not necessary. However, hair may be clipped from the ventral abdomen between the cranial aspect of the prepuce and pubic bone from the midline to the inguinal fold to facilitate imaging. Alcohol and/or coupling gel is applied to the skin to improve contact. A 5 to 10 MHz convex or sector transducer is recommended because of its 90-degree or greater field of view and because the transducer head can follow the body contour of the caudal abdomen better than that of a linear array transducer. To image the prostate, the transducer is placed against the ventral abdominal wall cranial to the pubis. The prostate should be imaged in both the sagittal (longitudinal) and transverse planes to ensure that all areas of the prostate are visualized. The true sagittal plane can be confirmed by observation of the hypoechoic urethral tract.

Prostate dimensions should be measured on both the sagittal and transverse planes (Figure 263-2). Prostate length and

---

Table • 263-1

Formula for Calculation of Maximum Prostatic Measurements from Ultrasonographic Examination of Healthy Male Intact Dogs

DIMENSION	DEFINITION	FORMULA
Length	Diameter along urethral axis	$(0.055 \times BW) + (0.143 \times A) + 3.31$
Width	Diameter perpendicular to axis of height^T	$(0.047 \times BW) + (0.089 \times A) + 3.45$
Height^S (H^S)*	Diameter perpendicular to axis of length	$(0.046 \times BW) + (0.069 \times A) + 2.68$
Height^T (H^T)†	Diameter along line separating two lobes	$(0.044 \times BW) + (0.083 \times A) + 2.25$
Volume	$[1/2.6 \times (Length \times Width \times [(H^S + H^T)/2])] + 1.8 \text{ cm}^3$	$(0.867 \times BW) + (1.885 \times A) + 15.88$

Modified from Ruel Y et al: Vet Radiol Ultrasound 39:212, 1998; and from Kamolpatana K et al: Vet Radiol Ultrasound 41:73, 2000.
*Height as measured from the sagittal view.
†Height as measured from the transverse view.
BW, Body weight; *A*, age.

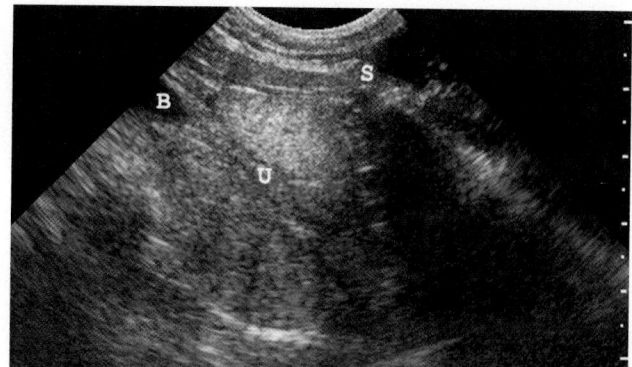

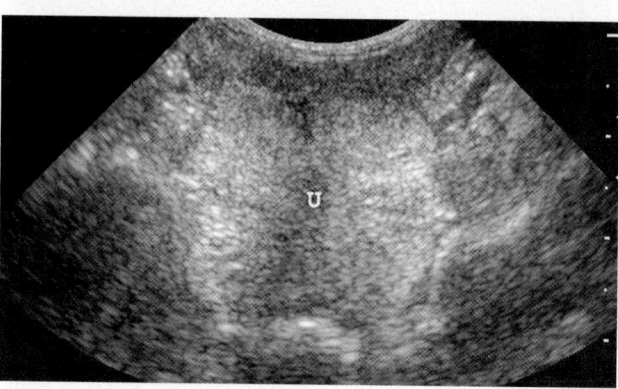

Figure 263-2 Sagittal **(A)** and transverse **(B)** ultrasonographic images of a normal prostate from an intact dog. The prostatic parenchyma is uniformly of medium texture and is moderately hyperechoic compared with surrounding structures, and the prostatic urethra *(U)* is hypoechoic. Note the anechoic bladder neck *(B)* and pubic bone shadow *(S)* on the sagittal image.

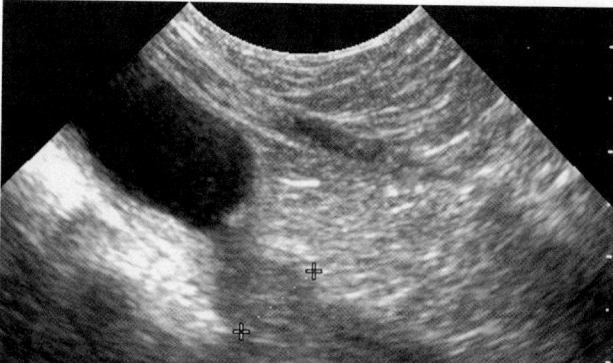

Figure 263-3 Sagittal ultrasonographic image of a normal prostate from a castrated dog. Note the small size of the prostate (0.92 cm) and the slightly hypoechoic parenchyma compared with adjacent structures.

height should be measured on the sagittal images. Length is defined as the maximum prostatic diameter along the urethral axis, and height is defined as the maximum prostatic diameter perpendicular to the axis of the length. The transverse image of the prostate is then obtained by rotating the transducer 90 degrees. From the transverse image, height is defined as the prostatic diameter separating the two lobes, and width is defined as the maximum prostatic diameter perpendicular to the axis of the height. In a study of 100 healthy, intact male dogs, the maximum prostatic dimensions were reported, and the maximum predicted values of prostate size were found to vary by age and body weight.[25] Formulas for calculating the maximum prostatic dimension in a normal, intact dog are presented in Table 263-1. Normal prostatic height on sagittal plane views for a dog castrated before 1 year of age is about 1 cm (Figure 263-3).

The ultrasonographic appearance of a prostate from a normal, intact dog should be uniformly fine-medium texture and moderately hyperechoic, an appearance similar to that of the spleen, with a capsule that is echoic and has smooth margins.[26] The urethra, which runs lengthwise through the middle of the two lobes, generally is hypoechoic compared with the prostatic parenchyma. In contrast, the ultrasonographic appearance of a prostate from a castrated dog is slightly hypoechoic compared with surrounding fat and adjacent structures, such that the urethra is more difficult to visualize (see Figure 263-3). The echogenicity within the prostate should be assessed for focal, multifocal, or diffuse changes in echotexture. Increased echogenicity and coarse echotexture is associated with hyperplasia, inflammation, infection, and neoplasia. A more echogenic, butterfly-shaped hilar region may be imaged in the center of the prostate in the intact male dog (see Figure 263-2); this corresponds to collagen and epithelial tissue in the wall of the prostatic urethra and periurethral ducts.[27] The hilar echo may be masked by increased echogenicity caused by hyperplasia, inflammation, infection, and neoplasia. However, imaging of the hilar echo may be unreliable because of technical artifact.

Ultrasonography also allows the examiner to determine whether cysts are present (or absent) in the prostate. The size, number, and location of the cysts should be characterized. The relative echogenicity of the luminal contents of the cysts should be characterized as hypoechoic or anechoic. Parenchymal mineralization may also be observed and is frequently associated with neoplasia. However, mineralization occasionally may develop with chronic inflammation.

Although ultrasonography can detect enlargement and changes in the internal prostatic architecture, these features are not pathognomonic for a specific disease. The ultrasonographic appearance of the prostate does not correlate well with culture results, nor does the presence and number of cysts factor into the incidence or type of infection encountered.[28] However, compared with radiography, ultrasonographic imaging is more sensitive for assessing focal or regional parenchymal disease.[29,30] Ultrasonography has also proved to be a useful technique for evaluating the response to pharmacologically induced prostatic involution.[31]

Ultrasonographic evaluation for prostatic disease should include evaluation of adjacent structures, including the urethra and urinary bladder. Primary urinary tract disease (e.g., infection, calculi, transitional cell carcinoma) may complicate or mimic prostatic disease. The sublumbar (medial iliac and hypogastric) lymph nodes should be evaluated. Enlargement and/or altered echogenicity may represent extension of prostatic disease into the regional lymph nodes. In addition, the smooth contour of the caudal lumbar vertebrae may become irregular with metastasis of prostatic neoplasia, which may be more accurately diagnosed with a radiograph. In rare cases, when prostatic disease extends beyond the capsule, adjacent fat may become hyperechoic from edema, inflammation, fibrosis, or necrosis. Peritoneal fluid may be visible, and if so, analysis of the fluid may aid in the diagnosis of treatment.

The location, size, and contour of the prostate can be evaluated with caudal abdominal radiography. A normal prostate does not displace the colon and bladder from their normal positions.

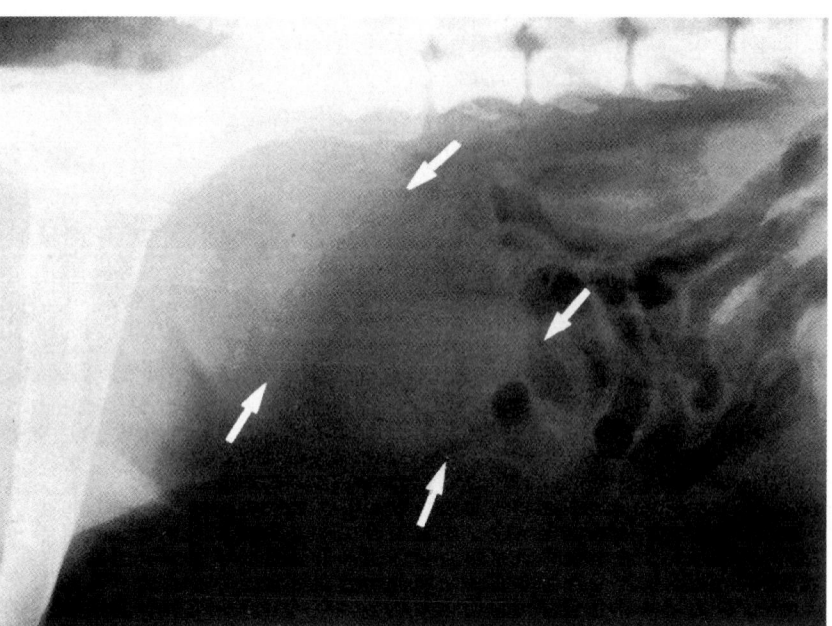

Figure 263-4 Lateral radiograph of the caudal abdomen of a dog with marked prostatomegaly. The bladder is indicated by the cranial arrows and the prostate by the caudal arrows. (From Barsanti JA, Finco DR: Canine prostatic diseases. *In* Ettinger SJ [ed]: Textbook of Veterinary Internal Medicine, 3rd ed. Philadelphia, WB Saunders, 1989, p 1864.)

Radiographically, the prostate has a soft tissue opacity, and its identification is influenced by the differential subject opacity of surrounding tissues. Radiographic diagnosis of prostatomegaly can be made when the prostate dimensions exceed 70% of the pubic-promontory distance on a lateral radiograph (Figure 263-4)[30] or 50% of the width of the pelvic inlet on a ventrodorsal radiograph.[32] However, neither of these methods accounts for the effects of age on prostate size. Often the exact dimensions of the prostate cannot be determined because of superposition of osseous structures or because of lack of abdominal serosal detail as a result of lack of fat, the presence of ascites, or focal peritonitis associated with prostatitis.[33] The ability of radiography to identify parenchymal changes associated with disease is limited to identification of mineralization, which may be insignificant or may be indicative of neoplasia or, less frequently, chronic inflammation. With caudal abdominal radiography, enlargement of sublumbar lymph nodes (medial iliac and hypogastric lymph nodes) may be observed, because it would cause ventral displacement of the colon. In addition, obvious lytic bone lesions involving the lumbar vertebral bodies and pelvic bones may be identified (Figure 263-5).

Distention retrograde contrast urethrocystography (DRCU) has been described as a method for determining prostatic integrity. In a normal prostate, minimal positive contrast is identified in the prostatic parenchyma near the urethra (urethroprostatic reflux) (Figure 263-6).[34] However, accumulation of larger volumes of contrast material in the prostatic parenchyma (intraprostatic reflux) has been reported with all types of prostate diseases.[1] Irregularity or an undulant pattern to the prostatic urethral surface has been associated with

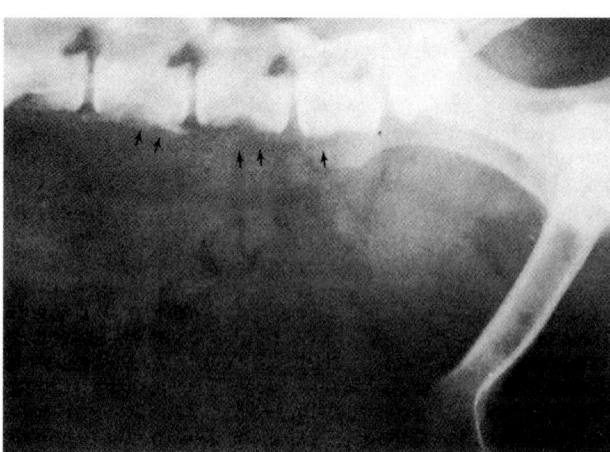

Figure 263-5 Early radiographic changes caused by prostatic adenocarcinoma. Proliferative changes *(arrows)* are indicative of early metastasis (L5-L7). (From Greiner TP, Johnson RG: Diseases of the prostate gland. *In* Ettinger SJ [ed]: Textbook of Veterinary Internal Medicine, 2nd ed. Philadelphia, WB Saunders, 1983, p 1474.)

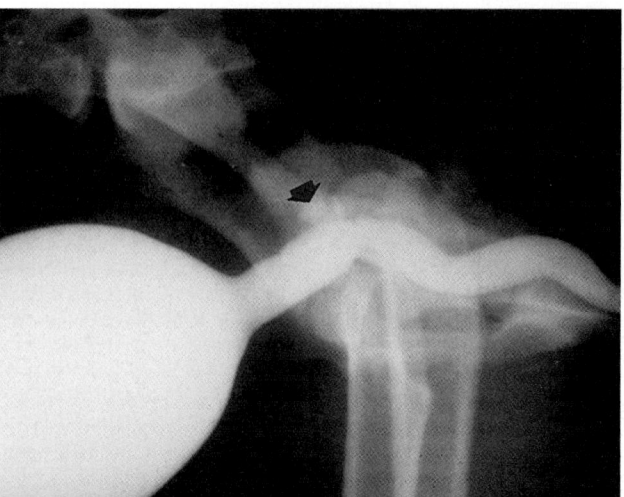

Figure 263-6 Distention retrograde contrast urethrocytogram from a normal dog. Note the small quantity of urethroprostatic reflux *(arrow)*. (From Root Kustritz MV, Klausner JS: Prostatic diseases. *In* Ettinger SJ, Feldman EC [eds]: Textbook of Veterinary Internal Medicine, 5th ed. Philadelphia, WB Saunders, 2000, p 1689.)

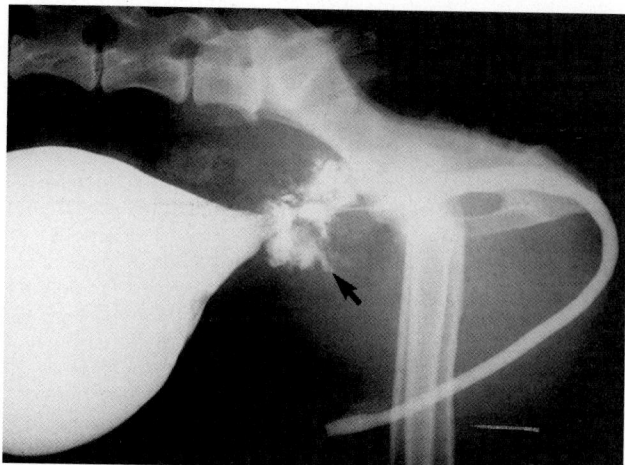

Figure 263-7 Distention retrograde contrast urethrocytogram from a dog with adenocarcinoma. Note the prostatomegaly and intraprostatic reflux of contrast agent (arrow). (From Root Kustritz MV, Klausner JS: Prostatic diseases. *In* Ettinger SJ, Feldman EC [eds]: Textbook of Veterinary Internal Medicine, 5th ed. Philadelphia, WB Saunders, 2000, p 1695.)

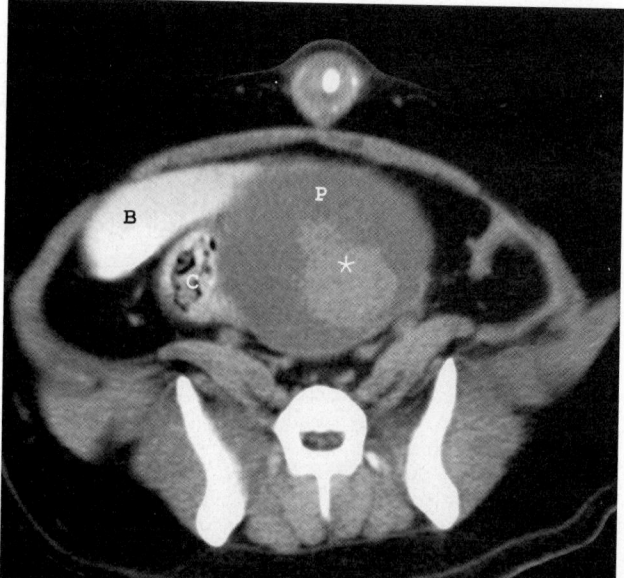

Figure 263-8 Transverse computed tomograph of the caudal abdomen of a dog with profound prostatomegaly *(P)* displacing the colon *(C)* and bladder *(B)*. Positive contrast was introduced into the bladder prior to examination. Note the irregular, high attenuating mass in the prostate *(*)*.

benign prostatic hyperplasia, chronic bacterial prostatitis, and neoplasia (Figure 263-7).[30] Narrowing of the prostatic urethral diameter during DRCU has been reported to occur in association with benign prostatic hyperplasia, prostatic abscessation, and neoplasia.[30] Because the prostatic urethral diameter varies among normal dogs with the degree of bladder distention, changes in prostatic diameter must be interpreted cautiously.[35] In addition, the absence of positive results on contrast studies does not rule out the presence of prostatic disease.[30] In most cases, ultrasonography is a better method than DRCU for imaging prostatic integrity.

Computed tomography (CT) (Figure 263-8) and magnetic resonance imaging (MRI) are excellent modalities for imaging both the prostate and adjacent structures, where metastasis may be a concern. In humans, MRI is an accurate means of assessing changes in prostatic volume that is highly correlated with the weight of the excised prostate.[36] However, the veterinary literature has little information about the value of CT or MRI in the diagnosis of prostatic disease in the dog. Both of these imaging modalities are expensive, and both require immobilization of the dog with general anesthesia. Bone scintigraphy may be helpful for imaging osseous metastatic lesions before they can be identified by radiography.[37]

Prostatic Fluid

With any dog suspected of having prostatic disease, the prostatic fluid should be assessed by cytologic evaluation and quantitative bacterial culture. Prostatic fluid may be obtained either by ejaculation (collection of the third fraction) or by prostatic wash; the former method is preferred, especially when bacterial infection and concomitant cystitis are suspected. To ejaculate a dog, the prepuce is retracted caudally, and digital pressure is applied to the base of the penis, proximal to the bulbus glandis (Figure 263-9). Intense pelvic thrusting occurs with ejaculation. Prostatic fluid can be collected aseptically by ejaculation as long as care is taken (1) to change collection containers after the combined first and second fractions have been collected and (2) to ensure that the tip of the penis does not touch the inside of the sterile collection container. The combined first and second fraction

sample should be saved for semen evaluation if indicated. Cytologic evaluation of the prostatic fluid aids in the determination of whether contamination occurred during ejaculation; specifically, the presence of squamous epithelial cells with gram-positive cocci in conjunction with an absence of neutrophils indicates that contamination occurred during collection.[38]

If the dog will not ejaculate, a prostatic wash should be performed (see Chapter 84). Using aseptic technique, the bladder is catheterized, and urine is removed. The bladder

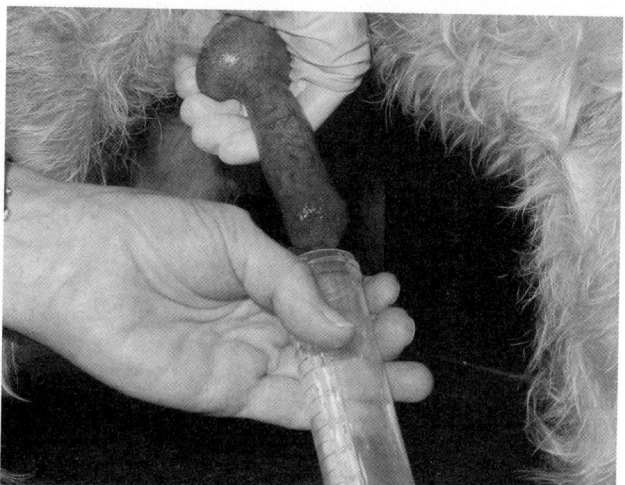

Figure 263-9 Collection of prostatic fluid (third fraction) by means of ejaculation.

then is flushed with 5 mL of sterile saline, and this sample is saved (PM-1).[38] The catheter subsequently is retracted so that the tip is distal to the prostate. The prostate then is massaged per rectum for about 1 minute to express a quantity of prostatic fluid into the urethra, where it can be collected with a urinary catheter. Sterile saline (5 mL) is slowly injected while the urethral orifice is occluded. The catheter is advanced into the bladder as aspiration is performed, and the sample (PM-2) is collected. The prostatic wash sample should be fixed on a glass slide, stained with hematoxylin-eosin, and evaluated for cellularity (Figure 263-10). Comparison of the cytologic examination and quantitative bacterial culture results from both prostatic wash specimens (PM-1 and PM-2) allows the precise location of the problem to be determined.[1] If lower urinary tract infection is present, before the prostatic wash is performed, the dog should be treated with an appropriate antibiotic (e.g., ampicillin) that does not penetrate the prostate. After the infection has been successfully treated, the wash may be performed. Prostatic massage is not without risks. In cases of acute prostatitis or prostatic abscess, there is a risk of creating a septicemia by forcing bacterial organisms into the blood stream or of causing peritonitis.[1] Also, uncertainty exists as to whether prostatic fluid has been expressed.

Fine needle aspiration may also be used for collecting prostatic fluid samples.[1] For this technique, the skin surface through which the needle is to be inserted should be clipped and surgically scrubbed. Once the needle enters the prostate, aspiration should be performed as the needle is redirected several times within the gland. Negative pressure is then slowly released, and the needle is withdrawn. In some cases, fine needle aspirate samples are nondiagnostic. If prostatic neoplasia is suspected, a prostatic biopsy, rather than a fine needle aspirate, may be necessary.[39] In one study, complications associated with fine needle aspiration included hematuria and periprostatic hemorrhage.[38,40] In another report, a sterile intraprostatic cyst was aspirated and developed into a prostatic abscess.[41] Fine needle aspiration therefore may pose an increased risk of complications in febrile animals or those with leukocytosis or before examination of prostatic fluid obtained by ejaculation or prostatic massage.[1]

Cytologic examination of prostatic fluid can identify inflammation but cannot be used in place of bacterial culture to identify infection.[42] Low numbers of neutrophils (fewer than 5 per high-power field) can normally be found in voided urine and in an ejaculate.[1] Prostatic inflammation and infection are well correlated with the appearance of macrophages in prostatic fluid.[42] However, the severity of inflammatory infiltrate is well correlated with the type or number of bacteria present.[28] Quantitative bacterial cultures yielding equal to or greater than 2 $\log_{10}$ of one or more bacterial species in prostatic fluid samples, compared with the number of colonies of the same species in paired urethral or urine samples, is indicative of prostatic infection.[43] Urine bacterial culture results are

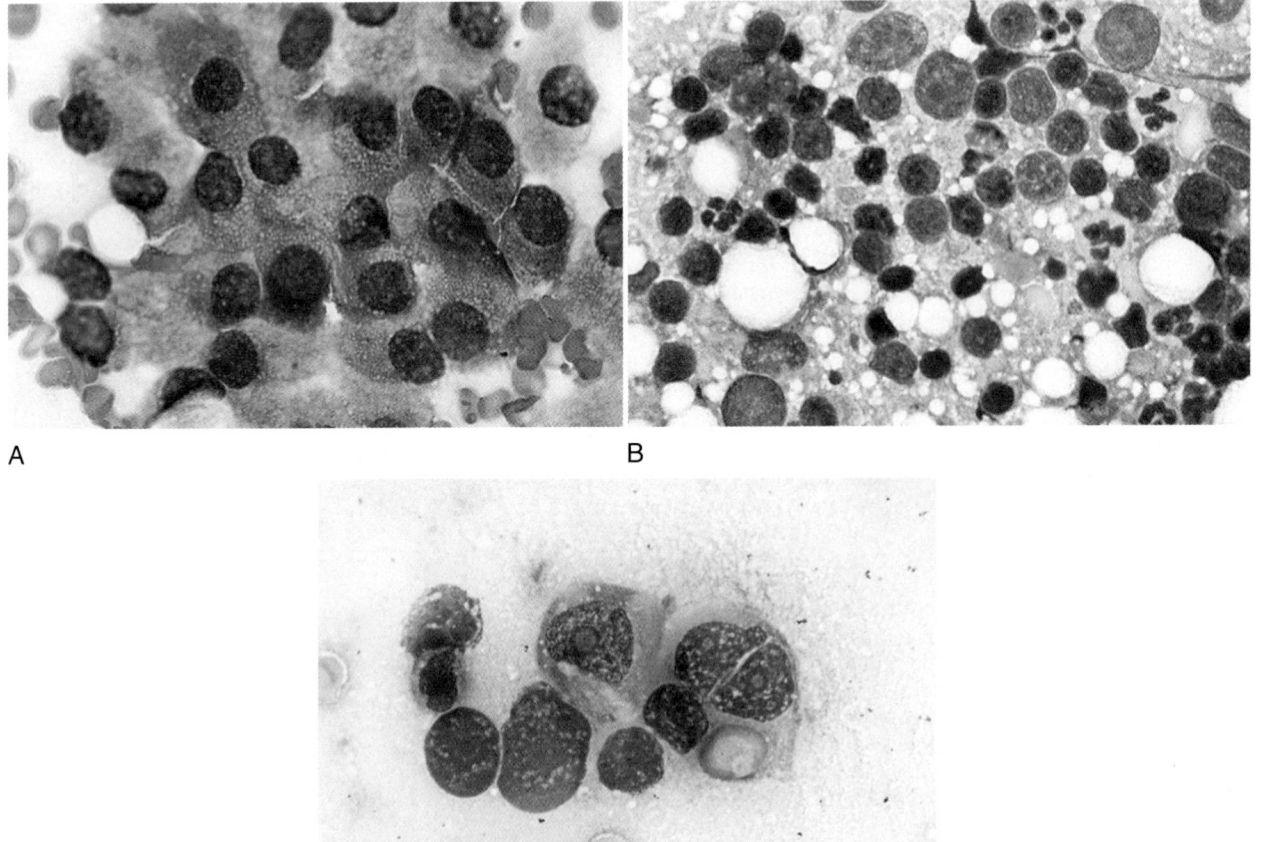

Figure 263-10 Prostatic wash samples from a normal dog (**A**), a dog with adenocarcinoma (**B**), and a dog with transitional cell carcinoma (**C**). (×100 magnification.)

well correlated with prostatic fluid culture results, such that cystocentesis is a safer alternative than fine needle aspiration of the prostate if prostatic fluid cannot be collected by ejaculation or prostatic wash.[42]

The prostatic fluid pH in dogs with experimental prostatic infection (pH 6.3) did not significantly differ from that in dogs without infection (pH 6.25).[42] It is unclear whether prostatic fluid arginine esterase levels would be useful in the diagnosis prostatic disease. In one study, serum arginine esterase levels were significantly higher in dogs with benign prostatic hyperplasia compared with normal dogs, dogs with bacterial prostatitis, and dogs with prostatic neoplasia.[44] In another study, although dogs with benign prostatic hyperplasia had higher arginine esterase levels than normal dogs, the levels were not significantly different from those in dogs with bacterial prostatitis or prostatic neoplasia.[15] Serum and seminal acid phosphatase levels showed no difference when normal dogs were compared with those with prostatic diseases or among different prostatic disorders.[15]

Careful selection and preparation of dogs for biopsy are essential. Prostatic biopsies are not recommended if bacterial prostatitis is suspected unless neoplasia is also suspected or the existence of chronic bacterial prostatitis can not be confirmed by other tests.[1] Antibiotics should be started 48 hours before a prostatic biopsy is performed if bacterial infection is suspected. A fluid- or air-filled urethral catheter can be passed before prostatic biopsy samples are taken to avoid damage to the prostatic urethra.[40] The biopsy site should be clipped and prepared aseptically. "Blind" prostatic biopsies are not recommended. Ultrasonographic guidance should be used for a prostatic biopsy because it provides continuous, real-time imaging of biopsy instrument placement; this reduces the risk of postbiopsy complications (hematuria, dissemination of infection, laceration of major blood vessels, urethral fistulation, orchitis, inadvertent puncture of adjacent organs).[1] In addition, ultrasonographic guidance increases the diagnostic yield of the biopsy sample, because the needle can be directed into what appears to be diseased tissue. The ultrasound transducer should be covered with a sterile sleeve, and sterile acoustic coupling gel should be used (Figure 263-11). The biopsy instrument can be introduced with a clip-on ultrasound guide or by freehand. The clip-on guide ensures that the needle remains in the plane of the sound beam. However, the guide limits the maneuverability of the biopsy instrument

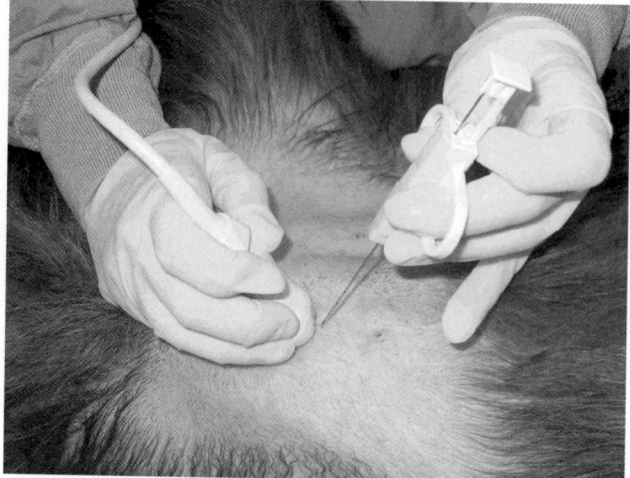

Figure 263-11 Ultrasonographic guidance during biopsy minimizes the risk of complications and maximizes the diagnostic value of the sample.

and may itself be awkward. The biopsy instrument should be directed tangentially to avoid the central prostatic urethra.[45] We prefer to use the spring-loaded Tru-Cut biopsy instrument.

BENIGN PROSTATIC HYPERPLASIA

Benign prostatic hyperplasia (BPH) is the most common prostate abnormality in intact male dogs and is estimated to occur in 100% of old, intact dogs.[6] Androgens are essential for the development and maintenance of BPH. However, with age, a modest decrease in the serum testosterone concentration, combined with no change in the serum estradiol-17-beta concentration, results in a relative decrease in the serum androgen to estrogen ratio.[10] This altered hormonal milieu is believed to contribute to the pathogenesis of BPH by increasing androgen receptor expression.

Histologic evidence of BPH develops at an early age. In a study of beagles, 16% had evidence of BPH at 2 years of age, and 50% had evidence of BPH at 4.1 to 5 years of age.[46] Electron microscopic analyses revealed that the volume densities of rough endoplasmic reticulum and secretory granules were significantly lower in the prostatic epithelial cells from dogs less than 1.5 years of age compared with older dogs.[47] After 4 years of age, intraparenchymal cyst formation may accompany BPH as a result of obstruction of parenchymal ducts that causes accumulation of prostatic secretions. In intact male dogs with no clinical evidence of urologic problems, the prevalence of intraparenchymal cyst formation is 14%.[25,48] The histologic pattern of BPH with intraparenchymal cyst formation shows areas of glandular hyperplasia, foci of atrophy, and chronic inflammation (lymphocytes and plasmocytes) in the stroma.[10] Intraparencymal cyst formation may predispose the prostate to bacterial infection.

The diagnosis of BPH is made indirectly by elimination of other types of prostatic disease. A definitive diagnosis of BPH requires histopathologic confirmation.[19] However, it is difficult to justify a prostatic biopsy when the results of less invasive methods strongly support the diagnosis of BPH and the absence of more sinister prostatic diseases.[38] A presumptive diagnosis of BPH is based on the history, clinical signs, prostatic imaging, and prostatic fluid cytology and culture. Clinical signs associated with BPH include hemorrhagic urethral discharge, hematuria, hemospermia, and tenesmus. In one study in which hemorrhagic urethral discharge was the only sign of prostatic disease, 95% of the dogs had only BPH.[20] However, it is important to mention many dogs with BPH show no clinical signs. In a study on prostatic disease in 177 dogs, nearly half of the histologically confirmed cases of BPH had no clinical signs.[19] BPH may only become a clinical problem once it results in pressure on the colon or if it encroaches on the muscles and nerves in the pelvic canal.

On palpation, BPH produces a symmetrically enlarged prostate with a normal contour, although intraparenchymal cyst formation may result in some degree of asymmetry.[49,50] The ultrasonographic appearance of a prostate from a dog with BPH typically is moderately enlarged with symmetric, smooth margins and normal to slightly increased echogenicity.[51] The central hilar echo may be absent, and small, anechoic cysts in the parenchyma may be present.[52] (See Figure 243-12.) Cytologic evaluation of prostatic fluid from dogs with BPH reveals epithelial dysplasia without significant inflammation or any neoplastic changes.[53] If inflammatory cells are present, most of them (greater than 80%) are mononuclear cells (lymphocytes and plasmocytes).[54] Quantitative bacterial culture from prostatic fluid should be fewer than 100 bacteria per milliliter.[15]

For nonbreeding males, the recommended treatment for BPH is castration. Prostatic size significantly decreases within

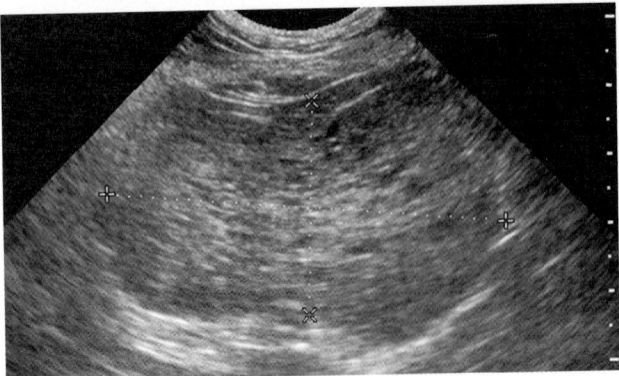

Figure 263-12 Transverse ultrasonographic image of a prostate with benign hyperplasia. Note the enlarged size, absence of hilar echo, and presence of many small cysts (too numerous to count) with anechoic luminal contents.

7 to 10 days after castration.[55] Medical treatments are not as effective as castration in reducing prostatic size,[20,56] but they do offer an alternative for owners who decline surgery. Finasteride (Proscar®, Merck), a 5-alpha-reductase inhibitor, prevents conversion of testosterone to DHT[57,58] and produces a dose-dependent regression in prostate size.[59] At a daily oral dose of 0.1 to 0.5 mg/kg (5 mg of Proscar® per 10 to 50 kg body weight), finasteride reduces prostatic volume and secretory function by 43% in 16 weeks without adversely affecting semen quality.[60] However, the effects of finasteride are reversible within less than 8 weeks of discontinuation of treatment.[61] Finasteride is potentially teratogenic to male fetuses if pregnant females are exposed to the drug during the first third of gestation.

Several antiandrogenic drugs (chloradinone acetate,[58] osaterone acetate,[62] delmadinone acetate,[53] flutamide,[31] and megestrol acetate[50,63]) are effective at reducing prostatic size but can adversely affect gonadal function and are not recommended for use in breeding animals. Estrogens have also been used to treat BPH; however, because of the risk of myelosuppression and prostatic abscess formation, they are no longer a recommended treatment. The liposterolic extract of saw palmetto plant berries or the American dwarf palm tree *(Serenoa repens)* reportedly improves urinary flow rates in humans with BPH. However, treatment with *S. repens* for 91 days had little effect (positive or negative) in dogs.[64] In humans, BPH originates from the transition zone, a unique inner region of the prostate to this species, where its growth can impinge upon the urethra.[65] This differs from dogs, in which BPH is a diffuse process that develops from the peripheral terminal glands, expanding away from the urethra,[66] which may explain the differences observed with *S. repens* therapy.

CHRONIC BACTERIAL PROSTATITIS

Chronic bacterial prostatitis (CBP) is the second most common prostate disorder in intact male dogs. It often occurs in conjunction with BPH. Bacterial infection of the prostate may arise by extension of bacteria from the urethra or by a hematogenous route. The pathogenic agent is usually common to the distal urinary tract (e.g., *Escherichia coli, Pseudomonas* and *Proteus* spp., staphylococci, and streptococci). *Brucella canis* may also cause CBP. However, gram-negative enteric organisms, particularly *E. coli*, are the most common cause.[67]

Clinical signs associated with CBP include recurrent urinary tract infection, hematuria, purulent or sanguineous urethral discharge, tenesmus, and constipation. Recurrent urinary tract

infection caused by the same pathogen is a hallmark of CBP, because the pathogen persists in the prostate during antimicrobial therapy for the bacteriuria. Although the urine can be sterilized and the signs controlled during therapy, discontinuation of treatment leads to reinfection of the urine and recurrence of clinical signs.[68] Constant or intermittent dripping of sanguineous or purulent exudate from the penis independent of urination, another common finding with CBP, is attributed to an increase in the secretory rate of prostatic fluid induced by infection.[1] Constipation may occur secondary to CBP, because the dog may attempt to avoid pain induced by defecation.[1]

The diagnosis is based on the history, clinical signs, prostatic imaging, and prostatic fluid cytology and culture. The ultrasonographic appearance of a prostate from a dog with CBP (i.e., coarsely hyperechoic throughout the parenchyma) may be indistinguishable from that of BPH.[51] Regions of heterogenous echotexture and dystrophic mineralization, caused by fibrosis and chronic inflammation, may be indistinguishable from neoplasia.[52] Cytologic evaluation of prostatic fluid reveals degenerative neutrophils. Quantitative bacterial culture results show more than 10,000 bacteria of a single species per milliliter of seminal plasma.[15] In contrast to humans, the prostatic fluid pH, specific gravity, and cholesterol zinc concentrations are not reliable indicators for CBP.[69]

Chronic bacterial prostatitis is difficult to treat because most antimicrobial agents useful against the pathogens diffuse poorly into prostatic fluids (blood-prostate barrier). If left untreated, CBP can extend through the capsule into the abdomen, resulting in peritonitis.[33] In the absence of a specific secretory or active transport mechanism, an antimicrobial's ability to cross an epithelial membrane depends on its pKa and its lipid solubility (Figure 263-13). The pKa is the pH at which a drug exists equally in both ionized and nonionized forms. Only nonionized forms can cross epithelial membranes. Basic drugs (e.g., trimethoprim-sulfamethoxazole, erythromycin, clindamycin) diffuse easily from blood (pH 7.4) to prostatic fluid (pH less than 7.0).[42,68,70] Both chloramphenicol and enrofloxacin readily cross epithelial membranes; however, ciprofloxacin does not penetrate the prostate well.[71] Drugs with low lipid solubility do not cross epithelial membranes (e.g., ampicillin, penicillin, cephalothin). Antibiotics should be continued for 4 to 6 weeks, regardless of earlier disappearance of clinical signs. Prostatic fluid should be recultured 3 to 7 days

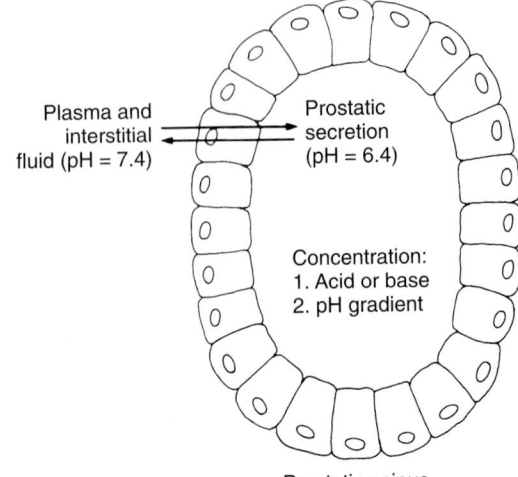

Figure 263-13 Factors determining the diffusion and concentration of antimicrobial drugs across the prostatic acinar epithelium. (From Stamey TA: Pathogenesis and Treatment of Urinary Tract Infections. Baltimore, Williams & Wilkins, 1980.)

after discontinuation of the antibiotics. Adjunctive treatment for CBP includes elimination of BPH. In one study in which CBP was experimentally induced with *E. coli*, castrated dogs cleared the infection within 4.2 weeks, compared with 9.5 weeks for intact dogs.[72] Because 5-alpha-reductase inhibitors also reduce prostate size and secretory function, medical treatment with finasteride should be included if owners decline surgery.

PROSTATIC CARCINOMA

Prostatic carcinoma arising from the glandular or ductal epithelial cells occurs in intact and castrated dogs and is the most common prostate disorder in castrated dogs.[6] Castration at any age has not shown a sparing effect on the development of prostatic carcinoma[73]; however, the influence of early age castration (less than 8 weeks of age) has not been evaluated. Prostatic carcinoma is seen primarily after 6 years of age. Benign prostatic neoplasia has not been reported, and metastasis is common, usually developing in the sublumbar lymph nodes, lumbar vertebral bodies (see Figure 263-5), and lungs.

The diagnosis of prostatic carcinoma is made based on the history, clinical signs, and results of prostatic imaging, fluid analysis, and histopathology. Clinical signs of prostatic carcinoma were reported from 76 dogs and included hematuria, stranguria, and incontinence (62%); tenesmus associated with prostatomegaly (30%); musculoskeletal system involvement (36%); and weight loss and anorexia (42%).[74] In intact dogs, prostatic carcinoma is not always associated with prostatomegaly. However, in castrated dogs, prostatomegaly is highly associated with prostatic carcinoma (Figure 263-14). On palpation, the prostate may be normal in size but may feel firm and asymmetric and adhered to the pelvic canal. Ultrasonographically, a prostate from a dog with prostatic neoplasia typically appears large and irregularly shaped with hyperechoic and heterogenous foci (Figure 263-15).[51,52] Additional ultrasonographic findings from prostatic neoplasia may include areas of mineralization, parenchymal cysts (Figure 263-16), involvement of the bladder neck, capsular disruption with extension into adjacent fat and the peritoneal cavity, irregular contour of caudal lumbar vertebral bodies, and large, heterogenous sublumbar lymph nodes (Figure 263-17). The appearance of neoplastic cells on prostatic fluid cytologic examination is diagnostically significant, but not finding neoplastic cells does not eliminate the possibility of neoplasia.

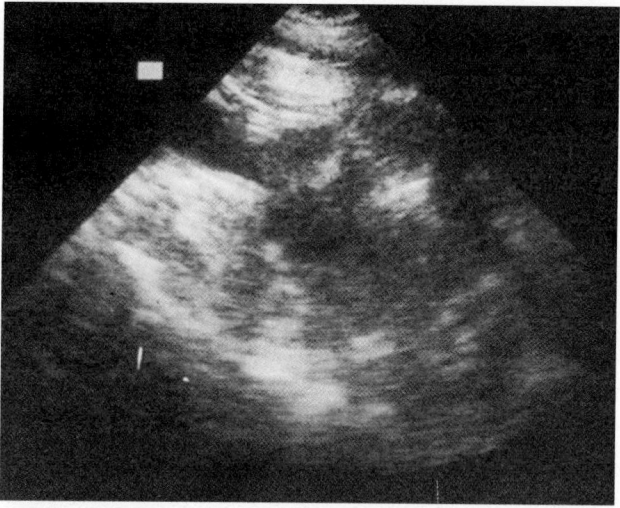

Figure 263-15 Sagittal ultrasonographic image of a prostate with adenocarcinoma. Note the hyperechoic and hypoechoic areas and irregular capsule typical of this lesion. (From Root Kustritz MV, Klausner JS: Prostatic diseases. *In* Ettinger SJ, Feldman EC [eds]: Textbook of Veterinary Internal Medicine, 5th ed. Philadelphia, WB Saunders, 2000, p 1696.)

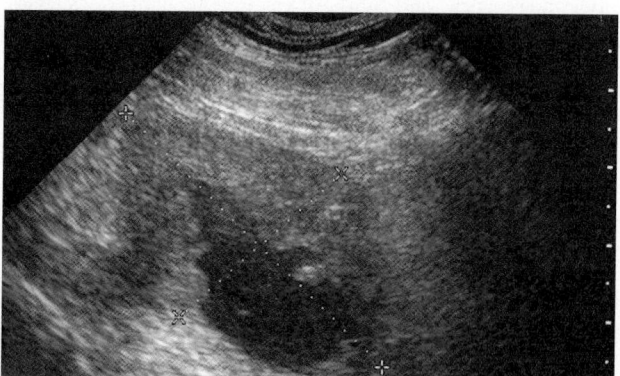

A

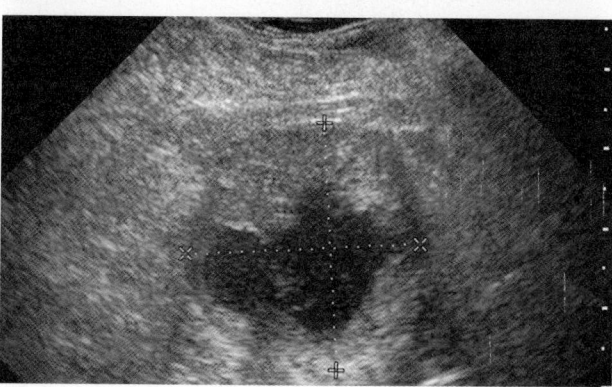

B

Figure 263-16 Sagittal (A) and transverse (B) ultrasonographic images of a prostate with adenocarcinoma. Note the enlarged size of the prostate for a castrated male dog, and the increased echogenicity and presence of large, coalescing cysts with hypoechoic luminal contents. The ultrasonographic appearance of a prostatic cyst or abscess may be similar to that of a prostatic carcinoma, and the diagnosis should be confirmed by prostatic fluid analysis and/or prostatic biopsy.

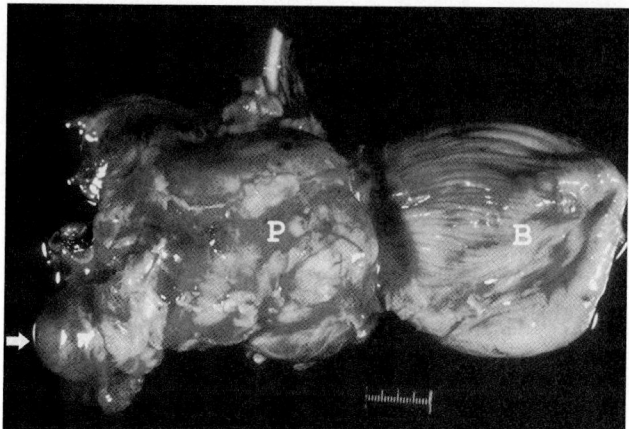

Figure 263-14 Necropsy specimen of a prostate *(P)* and bladder *(B)* with adenocarcinoma. Note the irregular contour and cyst formation *(arrow)*.

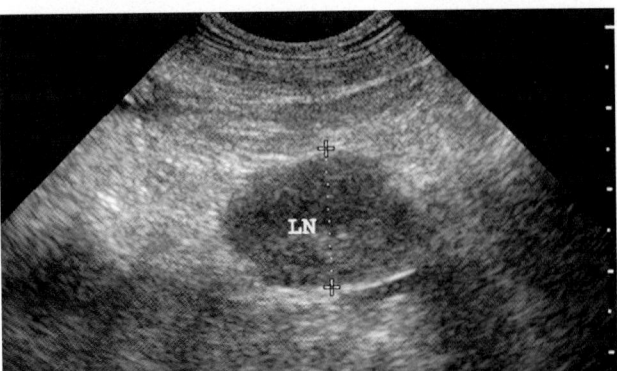

Figure 263-17 Sagittal ultrasonographic image of a mildly enlarged and abnormally hypoechoic medial iliac lymph node *(LN)* from the dog in Figure 263-13 with prostatic adenocarcinoma.

Adenocarcinoma is the most frequent histologic type of prostatic neoplasia, although more than half show intratumoral heterogeneity.[74] Histologic features of prostatic carcinoma include variation in glandular acinar size, shape, and spacing, with acinar cells containing enlarged nuclei and prominent nucleoli (see Figure 263-18).[74] Prostatic intraepithelial neoplasia (PIN), a common precursor prostatic neoplasia in humans, has been reported in the prostates of older dogs with and without neoplasia.[75] In dogs with prostatic neoplasia, the occurrence of PIN (7% to 66% of dogs with prostatic neoplasia) is too variable to be clinically useful.[74-76] Tumor markers frequently used in human medicine, such as PSA and prostatic acid phosphatase, are not useful in the diagnosis of prostatic neoplasia in the dog.[77]

The prognosis for dogs with prostatic neoplasia is poor. Treatment is primarily palliative and includes complete or partial resection of the prostate. There is no evidence that canine prostatic neoplasia is androgen dependent. Castration is recommended, however, because BPH can occur concurrently and may contribute to clinical signs associated with prostatomegaly.

Intraoperative orthovoltage radiotherapy (radiation therapy to surgically exposed prostate tumors) is currently the best adjunctive treatment for dogs without evidence of metastases, because it has the longest survival times (longer than 9 months).[78] Daily treatments (Monday through Friday) with

external beam radiation therapy (43 to 54 Gy in 2.7 to 3.3 Gy fractions for 19 to 28 days) are reported to have limited success, with the complication of colitis developing in 56% of cases.[79] The use of radiation potentiators, such as cisplatin (OPLA-Pt), in conjunction with external beam radiation therapy reportedly increases survival times.[79]

Piroxicam, a specific cyclo-oxygenase-1 (COX-1) inhibitor, administered at a dosage of 0.3 mg/kg given orally once a day, has been used successfully to reduce the size of several canine carcinomas.[80-82] In one study, combining cisplatin treatment (60 mg/m^2 given intravenously every 21 days) with piroxicam therapy resulted in complete or partial tumor remission in 71% dogs, compared with no tumor remission with cisplatin therapy alone.[83] *In vitro* experiments suggest that piroxicam treatment will be effective in the treatment of prostatic adenocarcinoma.[84]

Treatment options currently under investigation include endothelin receptor antagonists and tyrosine kinase inhibitors. Atrasentan, a selective endothelin A receptor antagonist, significantly delayed the progression of metastatic, androgen-refractory prostatic neoplasia in humans at a dosage of 10 mg given orally once a day.[85] Tyrosine kinase inhibitors (CEP-751, CEP-701) inhibit the growth of prostatic neoplasia in rats regardless of androgen sensitivity and metastatic ability.[86] Another potential treatment option for prostatic carcinoma is photodynamic therapy (PDT). Researchers have investigated the biologic responses of the prostate and adjacent vital structures to two photosensitizers, meso-tetra-(m-hydroxyphenyl) chlorin and aluminum disulfonated phthalocyanine, but the completeness of treatment and long-term therapeutic effectiveness in prostate cancer have yet to be determined.[87]

ACUTE BACTERIAL PROSTATITIS AND PROSTATIC ABSCESS

Acute bacterial prostatitis and prostatic abscesses are uncommon in dogs. The occurrence of prostatic abscesses has been associated with BPH[88] and administration of estrogen.[1] Clinical signs associated with acute bacterial prostatitis and prostatic abscesses include anorexia, fever, depression, vomiting, gait abnormalities, and caudal abdominal pain. Neutrophilia with a left shift is also seen. The ultrasonographic appearance of acute bacterial prostatitis is that of a normal-sized prostate with a hypoechoic parenchyma containing small cysts, whereas the ultrasonographic appearance of a prostatic abscess is that of prostatomegaly and one or more large anechoic cysts.[52]

Although the clinical signs may be similar, therapeutic differences between these two diseases make the treatment of acute bacterial prostatitis and prostatic abscess distinctly different. Acute bacterial prostatitis can be treated with an appropriate antimicrobial, as determined by culture and sensitivity, because the prostatic-blood barrier has been breached by infection.[89] Prostatic abscesses, on the other hand, do not resolve with antimicrobial treatment alone. Traditionally, prostatic abscesses have been treated by drainage through a capsulectomy incision via celiotomy. Marsupialization through the abdominal wall has been described but is associated with many complications, including prolonged recovery time, recurrent abscessation, dysuria, urinary incontinence, and septic peritonitis. Alternatives to marsupialization, reportedly associated with a lower risk of complications, include a modified Penrose drain technique[90] or omentalization (inserting omentum through the capsulectomy).[91,92] Surgery texts should be consulted for a more complete description of the techniques. Nonsurgical methods for treating prostatic abscesses have also been reported, with results showing varying efficacy. Antimicrobial therapy in conjunction with castration has been ineffective at resolving prostatic abscesses.[91]

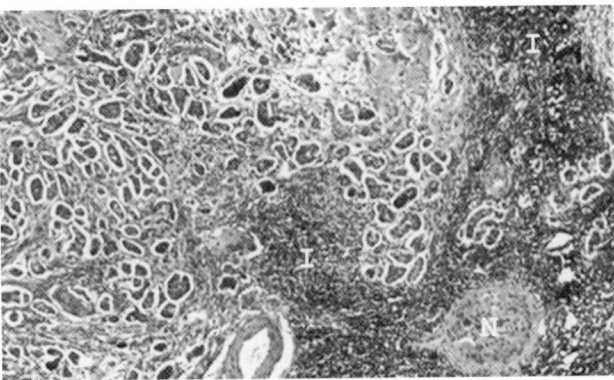

Figure 263-18 Histopathology from the prostate in Figure 263-14. Note that, compared with the normal prostatic epithelial cells *(N)*, the neoplastic epithelial cells are irregularly arranged and are not bordered by a basement membrane. Inflammatory infiltrate *(I)* is also evident.

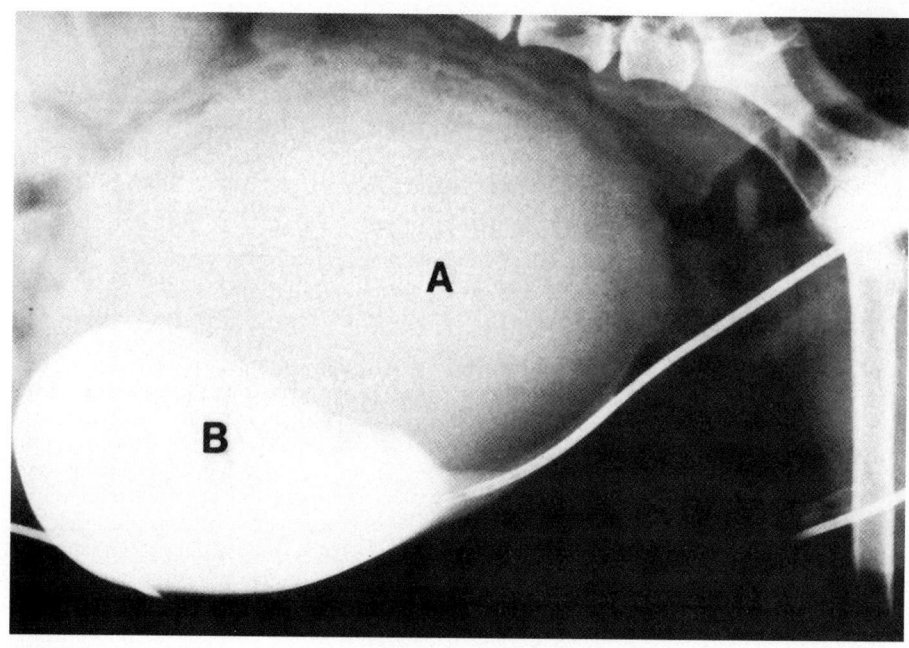

Figure 263-19 Large paraprostatic cyst *(A)* demonstrated with use of contrast material to outline the bladder *(B)*. (From Greiner TP, Johnson RG: Diseases of the prostate gland. *In* Ettinger SJ [ed]: Textbook of Veterinary Internal Medicine, 2nd ed. Philadelphia, WB Saunders, 1983, p 1477.)

However, percutaneous, ultrasonographically guided drainage followed by alcoholization of the cavity was effective at resolving a prostatic abscess in one dog.[88]

PARAPROSTATIC CYST

The etiology of paraprostatic cysts is unknown. These large cysts, located outside the prostatic parenchyma, have a stalk that connects to the prostate. They may result from dilated paramesonephric duct remnants or from retention cysts.[26] Paraprostatic cysts are uncommon and are often not clinically discernible until their size is sufficient to impinge on the colon or urethra, or unless secondary infection occurs and an abscess develops.[93] Paraprostatic cysts vary in size, shape, and location. Most cysts are located cranial or dorsal to the prostate and urinary bladder.[93] The ultrasonographic appearance of a paraprostatic cyst is that of a well-circumscribed, ovoid structure with anechoic or hypoechoic contents.[93] However, a pyometra of the uterine masculinus can occur secondary to infection without hormonal influence and appears as multiple, convoluted, tubular cavitations.[52] Radiographically, a paraprostatic cyst appears as a "second" bladderlike structure (Figure 263-19). Occasionally, paraprostatic cysts have calcified walls. Fine needle aspiration of a paraprostatic cyst yields fluid varying from clear and yellow to turbid and brown.[1] The recommended treatment for paraprostatic cysts that cause symptoms of prostatic disease is surgical removal.[94]

CHAPTER • 264

Familial Renal Disease in Dogs and Cats

Stephen P. DiBartola

Most familial renal diseases result in chronic renal failure at a young age (less than 5 years), but some are characterized by renal tubular defects (e.g., Fanconi syndrome in the basenji) or morphologic abnormalities that result in hematuria (e.g., renal telangiectasia in Pembroke Welsh corgis). A *familial* disease is one that occurs in related animals with a higher frequency than would be expected by chance. *Congenital* diseases are present at birth and may be genetically determined or may result from exposure to adverse environmental factors during development. In many familial renal diseases of dogs, the kidneys are thought to be normal at birth but undergo structural and functional deterioration early in life. Some familial renal diseases of dogs probably are examples of renal dysplasia. The term *renal dysplasia* refers to disorganized development of renal parenchyma as a result of abnormal differentiation; the condition is characterized by the presence of structures in the kidney inappropriate for the stage of development of the animal. Lesions suggestive of renal dysplasia include asynchronous differentiation of nephrons (indicated by persistence of immature or "fetal" glomeruli) and persistent mesenchyme (usually in the medullary interstitium).[1] Persistent metanephric ducts, atypical tubular epithelium, and dysontogenic metaplasia are observed less frequently.

Many familial renal diseases are variable in severity and rate of progression among individual animals. Most of these diseases are progressive and ultimately fatal, and therapy usually is limited to conservative medical management of chronic renal failure. The mode of inheritance and specific pathogenesis for many of these diseases are unknown. The primary nature of the renal disease and its mode of inheritance, when known or suspected, are listed in Table 264-1.

SIGNALMENT

Familial renal disease has been reported in many dog breeds (see Table 264-1) and may occur sporadically in mixed-breed animals. The clinician should consider the possibility of familial renal disease whenever chronic renal failure occurs in immature or young adult animals. In cats, familial amyloidosis has been characterized in Abyssinian, Siamese, and Oriental shorthair cats, and polycystic kidney disease (PKD) is common in the Persian breed.

In most of these diseases there is no clear sex predilection. In Samoyeds, however, hereditary glomerulopathy arises from an X-linked dominant trait. The age of onset of familial renal disease usually is 6 months to 5 years, with many animals developing signs before 2 years of age. Renal amyloidosis in beagles and English foxhounds, suspected glomerular basement membrane disease in beagles,[2] and telangiectasia of the Welsh corgi occur in older dogs (≥ 5 years), whereas PKD in cairn and West Highland white terriers is detected at a young age (5 to 6 weeks).

HISTORY AND PHYSICAL FINDINGS

The most common historical findings in dogs and cats with chronic renal failure due to familial renal disease are anorexia, lethargy, stunted growth or weight loss, polyuria and polydipsia, and vomiting. Other less common client complaints are poor haircoat, diarrhea, foul breath, and nocturia. In the Pembroke Welsh corgi with renal telangiectasia, the most common client complaints are hematuria, dysuria, and apparent abdominal pain. Hematuria also has been reported in German shepherds with multifocal renal cystadenocarcinomas.[3]

Dogs and cats with chronic renal failure due to familial renal disease may be thin and dehydrated. On oral examination, pallor of the mucous membranes, foul odor, and uremic ulceration may be noted. The kidneys usually are small and irregular, with the exception of cairn and West Highland white terriers and Persian cats with PKD, in which the kidneys often are markedly enlarged. Signs of fibrous osteodystrophy, such as "rubber jaw" or pathologic fractures, usually are detected in young growing dogs with renal failure. Signs of renal osteodystrophy rarely are apparent in older dogs with renal failure. The blood pressure should be measured and a fundic examination performed to evaluate for complications of hypertension (e.g., retinal hemorrhage, retinal detachment).

LABORATORY FINDINGS

The most common laboratory findings in dogs with familial renal disease resulting in chronic renal failure are azotemia, hyperphosphatemia, isosthenuria, and nonregenerative anemia.

The serum calcium concentration in dogs may be normal, decreased, or increased. Hypercalcemia may be more common in young versus older dogs with renal failure. Compensated metabolic acidosis also may be observed. The presence of hypercholesterolemia and proteinuria should lead to suspicion of primary glomerular disease. Beagles with glomerular amyloidosis and Bernese mountain dogs with membranoproliferative glomerulonephritis develop nephrotic syndrome and proteinuria; however, proteinuria is variable and depends on the extent of glomerular involvement in Shar Peis and Abyssinian cats with familial amyloidosis. Glucosuria is found in Norwegian elkhounds and basenjis with primary renal tubular disorders.

Juvenile renal disease in the basenji is an animal model of Fanconi syndrome and is characterized by glucosuria, proteinuria, isosthenuria, and amino aciduria. Affected basenjis may also have decreased fractional resorption of phosphate, sodium, potassium, and urate. They may develop hypokalemia and metabolic acidosis with a normal anion gap (hyperchloremic metabolic acidosis). In Welsh corgis with renal telangiectasia, the major laboratory finding is hematuria, but urinary tract infection may also be present. Blood loss anemia is more common than nonregenerative anemia because of the large amounts of blood that may be lost in the urine. Affected Welsh corgis may develop nephrocalcinosis and calculi, and hydronephrosis may occur if a blood clot or calculus obstructs the ureter.

PATHOLOGIC FINDINGS

Familial renal disease is characterized by the presence of primary dysplastic lesions, compensatory lesions, and degenerative lesions.[1] In many cases the secondary degenerative lesions overshadow the underlying primary dysplastic lesions, making correct diagnosis difficult. Primary dysplastic lesions that have been observed in some familial renal disease of dogs include immature or "fetal" glomeruli, hyperplasia or adenomatoid proliferation of the medullary collecting ducts, and persistent mesenchyme in the renal medulla. Such changes are most prominent in the Lhasa apso, Shih Tzu, soft-coated wheaten terrier, standard poodle, chow chow, and miniature schnauzer. Juvenile renal diseases in the Samoyed, English cocker spaniel, and bull terrier result from abnormalities of type IV collagen in glomerular basement membranes and represent animal models of X-linked dominant, autosomal recessive, and autosomal dominant hereditary nephritis in humans, respectively.

Secondary degenerative lesions commonly observed in familial renal disease include interstitial fibrosis, interstitial infiltration by mononuclear inflammatory cells, dystrophic mineralization, and cystic glomerular atrophy.

The pathologic features of several individual familial renal diseases are presented below.

Abyssinian Cat

Abyssinian cats with familial amyloidosis usually develop clinical signs between 1 and 5 years of age. Male and female cats are affected. Amyloid deposits first appear in the kidneys between 9 and 24 months of age, and in many cats amyloid deposition leads to chronic renal failure within the first 3 years of life. Amyloid deposition in the kidney may be mild, and some affected cats may live to an advanced age without detection of the amyloid deposits. Proteinuria is a variable clinical finding and reflects the severity of glomerular involvement. Difficulty determining the mode of inheritance arises from the variability in severity and progression of amyloidosis among affected Abyssinian cats, but the disease appears to be inherited as an autosomal dominant trait with variable penetrance. Amyloid deposits in the kidneys of affected Abyssinian cats contain amyloid protein AA.[4]

Table • 264-1

Familial Renal Diseases of Dogs and Cats

BREED	DISEASE	AGE AT PRESENTATION	INHERITANCE	PROGRESSIVE RENAL FAILURE?
Beagle	Amyloidosis	5 to 11 yr	Unknown	Yes
English foxhound	Amyloidosis	5 to 8 yr	Unknown	Yes
Shar Pei	Amyloidosis	1 to 6 yr	Unknown	Yes
Abyssinian cat	Amyloidosis	1 to 5 yr	Autosomal dominant (incomplete penetrance)*	Yes
Oriental shorthair cat	Amyloidosis	<5 yr	Unknown	Variable; also, severe liver involvement
Siamese cat	Amyloidosis	<5 yr	Unknown	Variable; also, severe liver involvement
Basenji	Tubular dysfunction (Fanconi syndrome)	1 to 5 yr	Unknown	Variable
Norwegian elkhound	Tubular dysfunction (renal glucosuria)	Not reported	Unknown	No
Beagle	Unilateral renal agenesis	Incidental finding	Unknown	No
Bull terrier	Basement membrane disorder	<1 to 10 yr	Autosomal dominant	Yes
Doberman pinscher	Basement membrane disorder	<1 to 6 yr	Unknown	Yes
English cocker spaniel	Basement membrane disorder	<2 yr	Autosomal recessive	Yes
Samoyed	Basement membrane disorder	<1 yr	X-linked dominant (males)	Males
NAV dogs†	Basement membrane disorder	<1 yr (males) 1 to 3 yr (females)	X-linked dominant	Males and females
Bernese mountain dog	Membranoproliferative glomerulonephritis	2 to 5 yr	Autosomal recessive*	Yes
Brittany spaniel	Membranoproliferative glomerulonephritis (C3 deficiency)	4 to 9 yr	Autosomal recessive	Variable
Rottweiler	Glomerular disease	≤1 yr	Unknown	Yes
Norwegian elkhound	Periglomerular fibrosis (primary lesion unknown)	<1 to 5 yr	Unknown	Yes
Soft-coated wheaten terrier	Glomerular disease (membranoproliferative glomerulonephritis)	2 to 11 yr	Unknown	Yes
Beagle	Glomerular disease (basement membrane disorder?)	2 to 8 yr	Unknown	Yes
Cairn terrier	Polycystic kidneys	6 wk	Autosomal recessive*	Not reported
West Highland white terrier	Polycystic kidneys	5 wk	Autosomal recessive*	Not reported
Bull terrier	Polycystic kidneys	<1 to 2 yr	Autosomal dominant	Yes; also, valvular heart disease
Persian cat	Polycystic kidneys	3 to 10 yr	Autosomal dominant	Yes

*Suspected.
†Dogs from Navasota, Texas.

The principal pathologic lesions in the kidneys of Abyssinian cats with familial amyloidosis are medullary amyloid deposits, papillary necrosis, chronic tubulointerstitial nephritis characterized by lymphoplasmacytic infiltration and fibrosis, and variable glomerular amyloid deposits. Glomerular amyloidosis is mild and often difficult to detect in many affected cats but occasionally can be severe. Medullary amyloid deposition was found in all affected Abyssinians, whereas glomerular deposits were found in 75%.[5] Medullary interstitial amyloid deposits interfere with blood flow to the renal papilla, resulting in papillary necrosis and secondary interstitial medullary fibrosis and mononuclear inflammation.[6]

URINARY SYSTEM

Amyloid deposition is not restricted to the kidneys in Abyssinian cats with amyloidosis; deposits frequently are found in other organs (e.g., adrenal glands, thyroid glands, spleen, stomach, small intestine, heart, liver, pancreas, and colon).[5] However, amyloid deposits in these other organs do not appear to make an important contribution to the clinical syndrome, which is that of chronic renal failure. In Siamese and Oriental shorthair cats, however, severe deposition of amyloid in the liver can result in hepatic rupture and hemoabdomen. The amino acid sequence of the amyloid AA protein in affected Siamese cats differs slightly from that found in affected Abyssinian cats, and this difference may explain the predilection for hepatic deposition in affected Siamese cats.[7,8]

Alaskan Malamute
Chronic renal failure in three sibling malamute pups (4 to 11 months of age) was associated with histologic evidence of renal dysplasia.[9] The lesions observed included immature ("fetal") glomeruli, cystic glomerular atrophy, glomerular sclerosis, periglomerular fibrosis, adenomatoid hyperplasia of tubules, and persistent mesenchymal tissue.

Basenji
Histologic findings in the kidneys of basenjis with Fanconi syndrome are not consistent. Nonspecific findings include tubular atrophy and interstitial fibrosis. One morphologic marker for this disease may be enlarged, hyperchromatic nuclei in renal tubular cells (renal tubular cell karyomegaly). Affected animals may deteriorate rapidly and die of acute renal failure with papillary necrosis or pyelonephritis.

Beagle
A family of adult beagles developed glomerular amyloidosis and nephrotic syndrome characterized by proteinuria, hypercholesterolemia, and renal failure.[10] Some dogs had mild medullary deposition of amyloid. The amyloid deposits were sensitive to permanganate oxidation, suggesting the presence of amyloid protein AA. In another study, a family of beagles with proteinuria, late-onset renal failure, and multilaminar splitting of the glomerular basement membranes was described.[2]

Bernese Mountain Dog
Membranoproliferative glomerulonephritis resembling membranoproliferative glomerulonephritis type I in humans was described in young (2- to 5-year-old) male and female Bernese mountain dogs.[11,12] Affected dogs had typical laboratory abnormalities of renal failure, as well as marked proteinuria, hypercholesterolemia, and hypoalbuminemia. Pedigree analysis suggested an autosomal recessive mode of inheritance. Ultrastructural lesions included a double-layered glomerular basement membrane and electron-dense deposits, primarily in a subendothelial location. Immunoglobulin M and the third component of complement were identified by immunofluorescence in glomeruli of affected dogs. Most of the dogs had high serologic titers against *Borrelia burgdorferi*, but the organism could not be detected immunohistochemically in the tissues of affected dogs. Membranoproliferative glomerulonephritis also has been reported in Brittany spaniels with deficiency of the third component of complement.[13]

Bull Terrier
Familial renal disease leading to chronic renal failure has been reported in bull terriers 1 to 8 years of age.[14,15] Both male and female dogs are affected, and the disease is inherited as an autosomal dominant trait.[16] It may represent an animal model of the dominant form of Alport syndrome in human beings.[17] Proteinuria, an early manifestation, correlated with underlying glomerular lesions in affected bull terriers.[18] Repeated urine protein to creatinine (UPC) ratios greater than 0.3 are considered supportive evidence of the disease in suspect bull terriers over 2 years of age that do not have overt evidence of renal failure.[15,18]

Light and electron microscopy of affected bull terriers shows thickening and splitting of glomerular basement membranes and involvement of tubular basement membranes.[14,16,18,19] Familial PKD that occurs in association with nodular thickening of the mitral and aortic valves and mitral dysplasia also has been reported in bull terriers.[20] Affected dogs did not have hepatic cysts.

Cairn and West Highland White Terriers
Autosomal recessive polycystic disease in the cairn terrier is characterized by the presence of multiple cysts throughout the liver and kidneys. Autosomal recessive PKD also has been reported in young (5-week-old) West Highland white terriers.[21]

Chow Chow
Chronic renal failure in six young, related chows chows (five male and one female) was suggestive of renal dysplasia.[22] Renal failure developed in four dogs by 6 months of age and in two dogs after 1 year of age. Renal dysplasia was suspected based on the presence of immature ("fetal") glomeruli and pseudostratified columnar epithelium in the renal tubules of some dogs.

Doberman Pinscher
Diffuse thickening or multifocal irregular thickening with lamellation of the lamina densa has been observed in the glomerular basement membranes of Doberman pinschers with glomerulopathy.[26] Occasionally, deposits of immunoglobulins have been detected in the glomerular capillary wall, but these are thought to result from nonspecific trapping of immune complexes in basement membranes with some underlying structural defect. Unilateral renal aplasia has been observed in some affected female Doberman pinschers. Additional glomerular lesions include lobular accentuation of glomerular capillary loops, increased mesangial matrix, hypercellularity, intraglomerular adhesions, fibroepithelial crescent formation, and periglomerular fibrosis.[26]

English Cocker Spaniel
Juvenile renal disease in the English cocker spaniel is an animal model of autosomal recessive hereditary nephritis in humans.[23-25] Mutations have been identified in genes for the alpha-3 (COL4A3) and alpha-4 (COL4A4) chains of type IV collagen on chromosome 2 in affected human patients, and these loci are candidate genes for the disease in the English cocker spaniel.

The disease affects both male and female English cocker spaniels and manifests itself between 6 and 24 months of age. The earliest detectable abnormality (5 to 8 months of age) is proteinuria followed by reduced growth rate, impaired urinary concentrating ability, and azotemia (7 to 17 months of age).[24] The primary lesion is thickening and multilaminar splitting of the glomerular basement membrane. This lesion is identical to that observed in Samoyeds with X-linked hereditary nephritis and is similar to lesions observed in bull terriers with hereditary nephritis. The disease ultimately leads to diffuse glomerular sclerosis and periglomerular fibrosis with secondary tubulointerstitial disease; it is invariably fatal.

English Foxhound
Renal amyloidosis was reported in related adult English foxhounds.[27] The disease was associated with acute illness, renomegaly, and papillary necrosis in some affected dogs. Amyloid deposits were sensitive to permanganate oxidation, suggesting the presence of amyloid protein AA.

German Shepherd

German shepherds with bilateral, multifocal renal cystadeno-carcinomas are usually 5 to 11 years of age when they develop nonspecific signs such as anorexia, weight loss, polydipsia, and gastrointestinal disturbances.[3,28,29] The renal lesions are accompanied by cutaneous and subcutaneous nodules (dermatofibrosis) and multiple uterine leiomyomas in affected female dogs. The disorder is thought to be inherited as an autosomal dominant trait.

Golden Retriever

Chronic renal failure has been reported in young golden retrievers (less than 3 years of age).[30,31] Hypercholesterolemia was a common finding despite lack of other evidence of primary glomerular disease in most affected dogs. Hypercalcemia also was common and was attributed to an increased serum complexed calcium concentration. Cystic glomerular atrophy and periglomerular fibrosis were common histologic lesions, whereas immature ("fetal") glomeruli were uncommon. Adenomatoid proliferation of the collecting ducts suggestive of primitive metanephric ducts, observed in several dogs, supports a diagnosis of renal dysplasia. Pyelonephritis occasionally complicates the disease in affected dogs.

Lhasa Apso and Shih Tzu

In the Lhasa apso and Shih Tzu, microscopic findings include a reduced number of glomeruli, glomerular atrophy, and small, immature ("fetal") glomeruli that are hypercellular and that have inconspicuous capillary lumens. Tubular changes include atrophy, dilatation, and epithelial hyperplasia. Interstitial fibrosis is particularly severe in the renal medulla, but interstitial inflammation is minimal. To a certain extent, increased interstitial medullary tissue may be persistent mesenchyme and, along with the immature glomeruli, is evidence of a primary renal dysplasia.

Miniature Schnauzer

Chronic renal failure suggestive of renal dysplasia was reported in eight related miniature schnauzers ranging in age from 4 months to 3 years.[32] Immature ("fetal") glomeruli, glomerular sclerosis, and severe interstitial fibrosis were observed.

Norwegian Elkhound

In the Norwegian elkhound, periglomerular fibrosis is an early histologic lesion that may be detected in some dogs before the onset of azotemia. Pathologic findings in dogs with more advanced disease consist of generalized interstitial fibrosis with glomerular sclerosis and atrophy. Hyperplasia of the collecting ducts also has been observed and may represent a primary dysplastic change, but immature ("fetal") glomeruli have not been observed. Norwegian elkhounds may also develop primary renal glucosuria that is not associated with chronic renal failure.

Persian Cat

PKD is inherited as an autosomal dominant trait in Persian cats.[33,34] The prevalence of PKD has been observed to be 35% to 57% in Persian cats surveyed by ultrasonography.[35-37] Cysts originate from both the proximal and distal tubules, they occur in both the renal cortex and the medulla, and they increase in number and size over time.[38] They can be detected by ultrasonographic examination of affected kittens as early as 6 to 8 weeks of age, but the absence of cysts at this early age does not preclude their development at a later age. In one study, ultrasound examination had a sensitivity of 75% and a specificity of 100% when performed at 16 weeks of age and a sensitivity of 91% and specificity of 100% when performed at 36 weeks of age.[34] Although common in human patients

with PKD, hypertension has been absent or mild in cats with PKD that have been evaluated.[39,40] Affected Persian cats usually do not develop renal failure until later in adult life (average, 7 years), and renomegaly may be an incidental finding on physical examination. Occasionally, cysts may be found in the liver.[41,42]

Rottweiler

Chronic renal failure was reported in four related rottweilers (three females and one male) ranging in age from 6 to 12 months.[43] Hypercholesterolemia and an abnormally increased UPC ratio were consistent with a diagnosis of primary glomerular disease. Histologically, cystic glomerular atrophy and irregular thickening of glomerular basement membranes were observed.

Samoyed

Male Samoyeds with hereditary nephritis develop proteinuria, glucosuria, and isosthenuria by 2 to 3 months of age and azotemia by 6 to 9 months of age; death from renal failure usually occurs by 12 to 16 months of age.[44] Mesangial thickening, glomerular sclerosis, and periglomerular fibrosis are observed by light microscopy in affected males by 8 to 10 months of age.[45] Affected females develop proteinuria at 2 to 3 months of age but remain clinically normal, other than failing to achieve normal adult body weight. This difference in the clinical course is a consequence of the X-linked dominant inheritance pattern and results from normal random inactivation of one X chromosome in each cell of the female embryo during development.[46]

Juvenile renal disease in the Samoyed is a hereditary glomerulopathy arising from a single nucleotide substitution in the gene (COL4A5) for the alpha-5 chain of type IV collagen on the X chromosome.[47] At birth, the glomerular basement membranes of affected male Samoyeds are morphologically normal, but reduplication and bilaminar splitting of the lamina densa are detected by electron microscopy at 1 month of age and progress to multilaminar splitting, thickening, and glomerular sclerosis by 8 to 10 months of age.[48] Affected females have only focal splitting of glomerular basement membranes and do not develop progressive disease.

Proteinuria and progressive renal disease presumably result from damaged glomerular basement membranes weakened by abnormal cross-linking of type IV collagen.[49] Deterioration of basement membranes and the onset of renal failure in affected males can be delayed but not prevented by feeding a diet low in protein and phosphorus beginning at 1 month of age.[50] Treatment of affected dogs with angiotensin-converting enzyme (ACE) inhibitors[51] or cyclosporine[52] has slowed progression of the disease. An X-linked dominant form of hereditary nephritis also has been described in dogs from Navasota, Texas (NAV dogs).[53] This disorder was characterized by earlier onset of renal failure in affected females, and alpha-3, alpha-4, and alpha-5 chains of type IV collagen were absent from the glomerular basement membranes in affected dogs. However, no mutation was found in exon 35 of the COL4A5 gene in affected dogs; consequently, this disease appears to result from a different mutation in the COLA5 gene.

Shar Pei

Familial amyloidosis resulting in chronic renal failure at a young age (mean, 4 years) occurs in male and female Shar Peis.[54] Proteinuria and laboratory evidence of nephrotic syndrome (e.g., hypoalbuminemia, hypercholesterolemia) may be present, depending on the severity of glomerular involvement. Some affected Shar Peis had a previous history of episodic joint swelling (usually the tibiotarsal joints) and high fever that resolves within a few days, regardless of treatment.[55,56] Recurrent fever and joint swelling that culminate in renal failure due to reactive systemic amyloidosis in young Shar Peis may represent an animal model of familial Mediterranean fever in humans. Some evidence indicates that amyloidosis in the Shar Pei is inherited as an autosomal recessive trait.[57]

Affected Shar Peis have moderate to severe renal medullary deposition of amyloid, but only two thirds have glomerular involvement. These findings are similar to those seen in Abyssinian cats with familial amyloidosis. The remaining renal lesions are those of end-stage renal disease. Amino acid sequence analysis has demonstrated that the amyloid deposits in affected Shar Peis contain amyloid A protein.[58] In addition to the kidney, amyloid deposits may be observed in many other organs (e.g., liver, spleen, gastrointestinal tract, thyroid gland). Icterus, hepatomegaly, and occasionally hepatic rupture with hemoabdomen may occur in Shar Peis with severe deposition of amyloid in the liver.[59]

Soft-Coated Wheaten Terrier

Pathologic findings in some soft-coated wheaten terriers (SCWTs) with juvenile renal disease are suggestive of renal dysplasia.[60,61] Histologic lesions include interstitial fibrosis, periglomerular fibrosis, cystic glomerular atrophy, decreased numbers of glomeruli, and the presence of immature ("fetal") glomeruli. Adenomatous proliferation of the collecting duct epithelium also is a prominent feature.

SCWTs also are predisposed to protein-losing enteropathy (PLE), protein-losing nephropathy (PLN), or both.[62] Food hypersensitivity and increased gut permeability presumably lead to immune complex glomerulonephritis that progresses to end-stage renal disease. The results of gastroscopic food sensitivity testing and dietary challenge support the hypothesis of food hypersensitivity,[63] but gluten hypersensitivity does not seem to be involved.[64] The disease is thought to be present in 10% to 15% of SCWTs and affects middle-aged to older dogs, with a slight predilection for females. The mode of inheritance is uncertain. Clinical findings include polyuria, polydipsia, vomiting, and weight loss in dogs with PLN; proteinuria, hypoalbuminemia, hypercholesterolemia, azotemia, hyperphosphatemia, and nonregenerative anemia are common laboratory findings. Hypertension occasionally develops, and thromboembolism complicates the disease in 12% of SCWTs with PLN.[62] Renal lesions consist of membranous to membranoproliferative glomerulonephritis that progresses to glomerular sclerosis, periglomerular fibrosis, and chronic interstitial nephritis. Mesangial deposition of immunoglobulin A (IgA), IgM, and complement has been detected by immunofluorescence, which suggests that renal disease in the SCWT may be an animal model of IgA nephropathy or IgM mesangial nephropathy.[65] The disease is progressive, treatment is palliative, and the prognosis is poor. Thus familial renal disease in the SCWT may take the form of renal dysplasia or membranoproliferative glomerulonephritis.

Standard Poodle

In affected standard poodles, cystic glomerular atrophy and large numbers of immature ("fetal") glomeruli are observed, especially in dogs presented at 3 to 4 months of age. The cortical interstitium contains segmental areas of fibrosis, whereas more diffuse lesions occur in the medulla.

Welsh Corgi

Welsh corgi dogs with renal telangiectasia have red to black nodules in the kidneys, especially in the renal medulla adjacent to the corticomedullary junction. Clotted blood often is identified in these lesions and in the renal pelvis. Hydronephrosis (presumably caused by ureteral obstruction) occurs in almost half of affected dogs. Similar nodular lesions may be identified in other tissues, including the subcutis, spleen, duodenum, anterior mediastinum, thoracic wall, retroperitoneal space, and central nervous system. Histologically these lesions are cavernous, blood-filled spaces lined with endothelium, and thrombosis is a frequent finding in the sinuses. These sinuses, with their simple endothelial linings, may represent vascular malformations rather than benign tumors of vascular origin.

CHAPTER • 265

Renal Tubular Diseases

Marie E. Kerl

The renal tubules are responsible for absorption of various components of the blood that has been filtered through the glomerulus. Among the filtered components that are reabsorbed into the blood are glucose, amino acids, and electrolytes. The tubules are also responsible for secretion of drugs and electrolytes, regulation of acid-base balance, and maintenance of fluid balance. Tubular defects occur regionally or globally and are either congenital or acquired. The glomerular filtration rate (GFR) is the main determinant of renal function, but the tubules are responsible for the final composition of the urine. Indicators from biochemical profiles, blood gas analysis, and urinalysis can be monitored to assess tubular function.

The renal tubules can be described according to function and anatomic location. The proximal convoluted tubule, loop of Henle, distal convoluted tubule, collecting tubule, and collecting duct are each responsible for various functions. The proximal tubule receives ultrafiltrate from Bowman's space and reabsorbs 60% to 65% of the filtrate. Absorption is accomplished by active transport of sodium (Na^+), which in turn promotes passive resorption of other solutes. The proximal tubule also actively secretes some solutes (e.g., organic anions, cations, and hydrogen ions [H^+]).[1] Solutes are not reabsorbed uniformly; virtually all filtered glucose and amino acids are reabsorbed, whereas lesser amounts of bicarbonate (HCO_3^-), Na^+, and chloride are reabsorbed. The loop of Henle, with the characteristic hairpin configuration central to the kidney's ability to excrete concentrated urine, is divided into four segments, having different absorption characteristics. The main function of the loop of Henle is to reabsorb approximately 30% of filtered sodium chloride (NaCl) against a concentration gradient to create an ultrafiltrate that is hyposmolar to plasma.[2] The distal tubule and the collecting tubule and duct are responsible for fine control of electrolytes including Na+, potassium, and calcium; final regulation of acid-base balance; and water resorption to produce a concentrated urine.[3] Clinical manifestations of renal tubular disorders include formation of cystic calculi, metabolic acidosis, glucosuria, aminoaciduria, electrolyte disorders, and failure of urine concentration.[4,5]

CYSTINURIA

Cystinuria is caused by an inherited proximal tubular defect in which resorption of particular amino acids fails. Of these amino acids, cystine is relatively insoluble in urine, resulting in the formation of cystic calculi in acidic urine.[6-8] Plasma concentrations of cystine are normal in affected animals. The exact nature of the defect remains unknown; some breeds have cystine loss only, whereas other breeds fail to reabsorb a variety of amino acids.[7]

Many dog breeds have been reported with cystinuria, and occasional reports have been made for cats.[9,10] Commonly affected dog breeds include English bulldogs, Australian cattle dogs, dachshunds, mastiffs, basset hounds, Newfoundlands, Staffordshire bull terriers, and French bulldogs. Mixed-breed dogs are also affected.[8,11,12] The mode of inheritance in various breeds is sex linked or autosomal recessive, but cystinuric dogs do not always develop calculi.[8] The mean age of calculus formation is 4.5 years. The degree of cystinuria can vary among individuals and may decrease with age.[6] Males are over-represented for clinical cystine calculi, but cystinuria without calculi formation has been reported in females. Newfoundlands appear to have a more severe form of cystinuria, with calculi formation occurring in both males and females and at a younger age than for other breeds.[8]

Clinical signs associated with cystine calculi formation include stranguria, pollakiuria, and hematuria. Male dogs may develop secondary urethral obstruction. Evaluation of urine sediment reveals cystine crystalluria in some affected dogs, but a complete blood count and serum biochemical analysis do not aid diagnosis. Imaging studies may identify calculi, but the size, shape, and radiographic density of calculi vary. The radiographic density of larger calculi is similar to that of soft tissue, which allows them to be visualized on plain film radiographs; small calculi may not be visualized by this technique. Ultrasonography and contrast cystourethrography may be diagnostic if plain film radiography is unrewarding.[8]

Treatment involves mechanical removal or medical dissolution of calculi and long-term medical management to prevent recurrence. Surgical management is indicated in animals with urethral obstruction. Quantitative calculi analysis provides a definitive diagnosis. Bacterial urinary tract infection should be resolved with appropriate antibiotic therapy. Dissolution and prevention strategies include exclusive feeding of protein-restricted diets. Cystine is twice as soluble at a pH of 7.8 as at 6.5, therefore urinary alkalization is desired.[5] Some protein-restricted diets (Prescription Diet Canine u/d, Hill's Pet Nutrition, Topeka, Kansas) result in the formation of an alkaline urine, but if dietary therapy does not maintain the urine pH at the desired level, oral potassium citrate is recommended.[8] Induction of diuresis (e.g., by feeding canned, low-protein food or adding water to dry food) is likely to be beneficial.[6,8]

Drug therapies to reduce the formation of cystine calculi include the thiol drugs D-penicillamine and 2-mercaptopropionylglycine (2-MPG). Cystine is formed by a disulfide bond between two cysteine molecules. Thiol drugs form a disulfide bond with cysteine to form a more soluble cystine-thiol drug complex. Although both drugs are effective, metal chelation and gastrointestinal side effects of D-penicillamine make it a less desirable choice.[7] 2-MPG, administered at a dosage of 30 to 40 mg/kg of body weight, divided and given orally twice daily, is the treatment of choice, in combination with dietary modifications for dissolution and prevention of cystine calculi.[6-8,13]

CARNITINURIA

Carnitine is a sulfur-containing nonessential amino acid that functions as an enzyme cofactor necessary to transport energy-generating fatty acids from the cytosol to the mitochondrial matrix. Continued deficiency, which has been reported in dogs with dilated cardiomyopathy, may result from defective biosynthesis, defective tissue uptake or retention, or excessive renal excretion.[14,15] Carnitinuria has been reported in dogs with cystinuria.[16] Although high-fat, low-protein diets are recommended for the management of cystinuria, high-fat diets increase renal carnitine excretion in humans. Healthy dogs that consume low- and high-fat diets excrete similar amounts of carnitine; however, cystinuric dogs with altered amino acid resorption might excrete an excessive amount of carnitine if they consume a high-fat diet.[15] Chronic carnitine excretion in these animals eventually may result in carnitine deficiency, leading to cardiomyopathy.

HYPERURICOSURIA

Abnormal purine metabolism or excretion accounts for hyperuricosuria in dogs of certain breeds or those with underlying hepatic disease. The purine portions of nucleic acids undergo metabolism to form hypoxanthine and xanthine, which are oxidized to uric acid by xanthine oxidase (XO). Uric acid is hepatically metabolized by the enzyme uricase. Most mammals excrete allantoin almost exclusively, but humans and higher apes excrete mostly uric acid.[17]

Two subsets of dogs commonly develop purine urolithiasis: Dalmatians and dogs with primary hepatic disease. Dalmatians are intermediate between dogs of other breeds and humans with regard to purine metabolism, excreting approximately one half to two thirds as much allantoin as urate. Differences exist between Dalmatians and non-Dalmatian dogs in both hepatic and renal management of urates. The enzyme uricase, which converts uric acid to allantoin, is stored in hepatic peroxisomes.[18] Uric acid must be transported into hepatocytes before conversion to allantoin can occur. Dalmatians have normal amounts of uricase compared with non-Dalmatian dogs, but Dalmatians have abnormal uric acid transport across the hepatic membrane.[19] Also, both Dalmatians and non-Dalmatian dogs secrete and reabsorb urates in the proximal tubules, but Dalmatians appear to have less proximal tubular resorption. In addition, they have active distal tubular secretion of urates as a result of a membrane transport defect.[17,20,21] Although all Dalmatians have high urine uric acid levels, only a small percentage develop calculi. Certain breeds, such as English bulldogs, have been reported to have an increased frequency of urate calculi without obvious hepatic disease. These dogs might have a metabolic defect that predisposes to urate calculi formation, but the mechanism is unknown.[20,22]

Dogs with primary hepatic disease have reduced conversion of uric acid to allantoin and of ammonia to urea. These metabolic defects cause hyperuricuria and hyperammonuria.[23] Portal vascular anomalies and hepatic microvascular dysplasia have been most commonly associated with urate calculi formation, although any severe hepatic dysfunction could predispose to calculi formation.[24] Cats have been reported with urate urolithiasis.[10]

The clinical signs of urate urolithiasis are consistent with lower urinary tract disease. Male dogs can develop urethral obstruction. Young to middle-aged dogs are more commonly affected than older dogs.[25] For Dalmatians, males are more frequently affected with urinary calculi than females. Dogs with primary hepatic disease have no gender predisposition for calculi formation. Definitive diagnosis of cystic calculi depends on calculi retrieval and quantitative analysis. Urate calculi are radiolucent on plain film radiography. Abdominal ultrasonography or double-contrast cystography is helpful for identifying calculi. Hepatic function studies are appropriate for non-Dalmatian dogs and for cats. Urate calculi are typically small and smooth and vary in color from yellow to green to black.[20]

Treatment consists of calculi removal or dissolution, followed by long-term medical management to prevent recurrence. Dissolution therapy includes a calculolytic diet, medication with XO inhibitors, alkalization of the urine, elimination of secondary infections, and induction of isosthenuria.[20] A purine-restricted diet that is low in claculogenic minerals (e.g., Prescription Diet Canine u/d; Hill's Pet Nutrition, Topeka, Kansas) is recommended.[20,21,26,27] The synthetic XO inhibitor allopurinol is used to treat and prevent urate urolithiasis because it can reduce the serum and urine uric acid concentrations.[28] Allopurinol should be administered only to dogs consuming a purine-restricted diet to avoid the formation of xanthine calculi.

Urine alkalization reduces renal tubular production of ammonia, thereby diminishing the production of urinary ammonium ions that complex with urate to form calculi. Alkalizing agents (e.g., oral sodium bicarbonate [$NaHCO_3$] and potassium citrate) should be administered at a dosage that maintains the urine pH near 7.0 to 7.5.[20,27] Dilute urine production is accomplished by feeding protein-restricted diets that reduce renal medullary concentrating ability.

Mechanical calculi removal should be considered in animals with urethral obstruction or in those that do not respond to dissolution therapy. The average time to dissolution of urate calculi is approximately 3.5 months (range, 1 to 18 months).[20,27] Dissolution sometimes occurs with definitive repair of a portovascular anomaly, but calculi do not resolve without resolution of underlying hepatic defects.[23] Because the causes of urate stones differ, allopurinol therapy is not recommended for dogs with hepatic defects.[20,23]

The prognosis is fair to guarded for calculi recurrence in Dalmatians and depends on the owner's commitment to ongoing management and expense. In dogs with underlying liver disease, the prognosis is good if definitive therapy for the liver disease exists but guarded in dogs with irreparable liver disease.

HYPERXANTHINURIA

Xanthine calculi are rare. Xanthine is derived from dietary purines and is metabolized to uric acid by activity of XO. Reduced enzymatic conversion increases urinary excretion of xanthine, which has a solubility similar to that of uric acid in urine.[29] Most dogs that form xanthine-containing calculi are receiving allopurinol, an XO inhibitor, for urate calculi.[22,25,29] Congenital xanthinuria has been reported in a family of Cavalier King Charles spaniels and in a wirehaired dachshund.[30,31] Prevention consists of monitoring for xanthine crystalluria in dogs receiving allopurinol to prevent urate calculi.

RENAL GLUCOSURIA

Under normal conditions, glucose is freely filtered at the glomerulus and reabsorbed in the proximal tubules by facilitated diffusion in a cotransport mechanism with Na^+.[1] The transport mechanism has a maximum capacity, which is exceeded at a blood glucose concentration of 180 to 220 mg/dL in dogs and 260 to 310 mg/dL in cats.[4] When hyperglycemia (e.g., stress hyperglycemia, diabetes mellitus) exceeds the transport maximum, glucosuria occurs. Proximal tubular defects caused by tubular damage or inherited disorders can result in glucosuria in the absence of hyperglycemia.[32,33]

Primary renal glucosuria is rare but has been reported in Scottish terriers, basenjis, Norwegian elkhounds, and mixed-breed dogs.[4,34] Persistent glucosuria typically causes polyuria and polydipsia from osmotic diuresis, although some dogs are asymptomatic. Evaluation of serial blood glucose measurements or the serum fructosamine concentration should be considered to diagnose renal glucosuria definitively by ruling out hyperglycemia as a cause for glucosuria.[35] Because bacterial or fungal urinary tract infections occur frequently with persistent glucosuria, regular monitoring and appropriate antibiotic therapy are important. There is no cure for primary renal glucosuria, but the long-term prognosis is good with appropriate fluid intake and control of urinary infections. In some dogs, renal glucosuria is the initial sign of Fanconi syndrome.

FANCONI SYNDROME

In humans, Fanconi syndrome is an inherited proximal tubular defect that results in glucosuria, aminoaciduria, proteinuria, phosphaturia, and hypophosphatemia. Fanconi syndrome has also been reported in dogs, and basenjis are most commonly affected. Fanconi syndrome is thought to be inherited in 10% to 30% of all basenjis, but the mode of inheritance is uncertain. Idiopathic and inherited Fanconi syndrome has been reported rarely in other dog breeds.[4,32] Acquired Fanconi syndrome has been reported in association with gentamicin administration, ethylene glycol toxicity, and primary hypoparathyroidism.[4,33]

Fanconi syndrome causes abnormal fractional excretion of many solutes.[36] Abnormal glucose absorption, resulting in glucosuria and osmotic diuresis, is the most obvious sign. Amino acid resorptive abnormalities vary from one individual to another but generally include abnormal absorption of cystine. Abnormal absorption of bicarbonate, sodium, potassium, and urate also occur. Isosthenuria sometimes occurs prior to glucosuria and osmotic diuresis as a result of nephrogenic diabetes insipidus.[4,36]

The onset of clinical signs in affected basenjis typically occurs by 4 to 8 years of age, with females outnumbering males 3:1.[32] Clinical signs typically include polyuria, polydipsia, weight loss, poor haircoat, weakness, and dehydration. Diagnostic testing reveals glucosuria, euglycemia, and isosthenuria. As the disease progresses, hyperchloremic metabolic acidosis and renal failure occur. Clinically significant hypokalemia might contribute to muscle weakness. Progression is variable; some affected dogs develop renal failure within a few months of the onset of clinical signs, whereas others remain stable for years.[4]

Treatment is supportive, because there is no cure for the tubular defects. Monitoring for metabolic acidosis, urinary tract infections, and azotemia should be performed regularly. Veterinarians are frequently asked to participate in a management protocol developed by basenji breed enthusiasts. This protocol involves oral administration of sodium bicarbonate to manage chronic metabolic acidosis, which exacerbates bicarbonaturia. Urinary alkalization with potassium citrate does not cause bicarbonaturia and provides potassium supplementation. The goals of alkalization should be to maintain the serum HCO_3^- concentration above 12 mEq/L and the potassium concentration at 4 to 6 mEq/L.[4] Renal failure should be managed with dietary protein restriction, fluid therapy, histamine-2 receptor antagonists, and treatment of hypertension. Treatment for acquired Fanconi syndrome should be directed at resolving the underlying cause of the disorder and providing supportive care. The prognosis for short-term management is guarded to good, depending on the severity of azotemia at the time of diagnosis. The long-term prognosis is guarded to poor.

RENAL TUBULAR ACIDOSIS

The renal tubules regulate acid-base homeostasis through two processes: (1) resorption of 80% to 90% of filtered HCO_3^- in the proximal renal tubule, and (2) excretion of acids by means of titration of urinary buffers and excretion of ammonium in the distal renal tubule.[37] The term *renal tubular acidosis (RTA)* describes rare tubular disorders that lead to hyperchloremic metabolic acidosis. Various types of RTA have been described based on the area of the affected renal tubules. Proximal RTA (type II) occurs as a result of inability of the proximal tubules to prevent loss of HCO_3^-, and distal RTA (classic, or type I) occurs as the result of inability of the distal tubule to excrete H^+. Type IV RTA is distal RTA and hyperkalemia secondary to hypoaldosteronism or aldosterone deficiency. Unique diagnostic criteria exist for each type of RTA.[38]

A defect in the basolateral membrane Na^+-HCO_3^- cotransporter, with leakage of HCO_3^- into the tubular lumen, results in proximal RTA.[39] This disorder can occur alone or as part of another clinical tubular defect (e.g., Fanconi syndrome).[38] Ongoing loss causes a reduced plasma bicarbonate concentration, but the associated metabolic acidosis is self-limiting because of the distal tubule's ability to excrete acid. If oral sodium bicarbonate ($NaHCO_3$) is prescribed to normalize the plasma bicarbonate concentration, the amount of HCO_3^-

presented to the distal tubule increases and overwhelms the distal buffering system, resulting in marked bicarbonaturia.[38]

The diagnosis of proximal RTA is based on an acid urine pH and hyperchloremic metabolic acidosis, with a normal GFR but increased urine pH and fractional excretion of HCO_3^- (greater than 15%) after normalization of the plasma HCO_3^- concentration with alkali administration. Identification of concurrent proximal tubular defects (e.g., euglycemic glucosuria, aminoaciduria) also helps localize proximal RTA.[38] Bicarbonate wasting makes metabolic acidosis from proximal RTA difficult to correct, and alkali therapy exacerbates potassium wasting. Potassium citrate is better suited for chronic use than sodium bicarbonate.[38] One 540 mg tablet of potassium citrate provides 5 mEq of potassium and 1.7 mEq of citrate, and its metabolism yields 5 mEq of HCO_3^-.[5]

Distal RTA causes impairment of urinary acidification as a result of impaired H^+ secretion in the distal tubule.[37,38] Consequently, the kidneys are unable to maximally acidify urine in response to systemic metabolic acidosis. Under normal conditions, the distal tubule is able to excrete H^+ ions against a steep concentration gradient because of a hydrogen ion–adenosine triphosphatase (H^+-ATPase) pump. These tubular segments have tight junctions that resist backleak of acid, and they are able to generate ammonia to capture H^+ ions by forming ammonium ions, which are subsequently excreted.[39]

Type IV distal RTA is associated with hypoaldosteronism or aldosterone antagonism. Acidosis most likely results from loss of aldosterone stimulation of H^+-ATPase and decreased distal Na^+ absorption. This syndrome has not been characterized in veterinary medicine but should be considered in animals with hyperchloremic metabolic acidosis and hypokalemia.[37,38]

Characteristics useful in the diagnosis of distal RTA include hyperchloremic metabolic acidosis with an increased urine pH (greater than 6.0). In contrast to proximal RTA, with relatively mild systemic metabolic acidosis, distal RTA can have a more severe metabolic acidosis, because the distal tubule does not provide buffering ability. Clinical characteristics seen in humans with distal RTA include nephrolithiasis, nephrocalcinosis, bone demineralization, growth retardation, and hypokalemia.[37,39] Distal RTA has been reported in cats

URINARY SYSTEM

Table • 265-1

Clinical Features of Proximal and Distal Renal Tubular Acidosis (RTA)

FEATURE	PROXIMAL RTA	DISTAL RTA
Hypercalciuria	Yes	Yes
Hyperphosphaturia	Yes	Yes
Urinary citrate	Normal	Decreased
Bone disease	Less severe	More severe
Nephrocalcinosis	No	Possible
Nephrolithiasis	Not usually	Yes
Hypokalemia	Mild	Mild to severe
Potassium wasting	Worsened by alkali therapy	Improved by alkali therapy
Alkali required for treatment	>11 mEq/kg/day	<4 mEq/kg/day
Other defects of proximal tubular function*	Yes	No
Reductions in plasma bicarbonate (HCO_3^-)	Moderate	Variable
Fractional excretion of HCO_3^- with normal HCO_3^- concentration	>15%	<15%
Urine pH during acidemia	<6.0	>6.0
Urine pH after ammonium chloride administration	<6.0	>6.0

From Bartges JW: Disorders of renal tubules. *In* Ettinger SJ, Feldman EC (eds): Textbook of Veterinary Internal Medicine, 5th ed. Philadelphia, WB Saunders, 2000, p 1704.
*Decreased resorption of sodium, potassium, phosphate, uric acid, glucose, and amino acids.

with pyelonephritis and in one cat with hepatic lipidosis.[4,38] The diagnosis may be made by failure to acidify urine with an ammonium chloride challenge test. This test is performed by measuring the urine pH before and at hourly intervals for 6 hours after oral administration of 110 mg/kg of ammonium chloride. Normal dogs should acidify to a urine pH of 5.0, and cats to a pH of 5.5.

Treatment for distal RTA consists of administration of an alkali source. A combination of potassium and sodium citrate, at a dosage range of 1 to 5 mEq/kg/day, orally, divided into 2 doses, may be preferred over HCO_3^- as the alkali source. Characteristics of proximal and distal RTA are presented in Table 265-1.[5,38]

NEPHROGENIC DIABETES INSIPIDUS

The term *nephrogenic diabetes insipidus (NDI)* describes any disorder in which the urinary concentrating mechanism is unable to respond to antidiuretic hormone (ADH) to produce concentrated urine. ADH is produced in the hypothalamus in response to hyperosmolarity or hypovolemia. Upon release, it attaches to receptors at the basolateral membrane of the collecting tubules and collecting ducts, causing the tubular luminal surface to become permeable to free water and resulting in the formation of urine that is more concentrated than plasma. Acquired NDI is a common cause of polyuria, because it can result from receptor interference caused by toxins (e.g., *Escherichia coli* endotoxin), drugs (e.g., glucocorticoids, chemotherapeutics), metabolic conditions (e.g., hypokalemia, hypercalcemia), tubular injury or loss (e.g., renal cystic disease, bacterial pyelonephritis), or alterations in the medullary concentration gradient (e.g., medullary washout).[40]

Congenital NDI is a rare disease caused by a deficiency of ADH receptors. Clinical signs, apparent soon after birth, include severe polydipsia and polyuria and a hyposthenuric urine (specific gravity of 1.001 to 1.005; osmolarity less than 200 mOsm/kg). The diagnosis is based on failure to concentrate urine after modified water deprivation testing, failure to respond to exogenous ADH, and exclusion of more common causes of NDI.[4]

Treatment for acquired NDI should be directed at resolving the underlying cause. Congenital NDI therapy consists of free-choice water consumption, dietary sodium and protein restriction, and/or thiazide diuretics (chlorothiazide, 20 to 40 mg/lb given orally every 12 hours; or hydrochlorothiazide, 2.5 to 5 mg/lb given orally every 12 hours). Dietary sodium and protein restriction reduces the amount of solute presented to the kidney that must be excreted in the urine each day, further reducing obligatory water loss.[41] The addition of diuretic therapy to dietary restrictions results in mild dehydration, increased fluid and sodium uptake in the proximal tubule, and 20% to 50% reduction of urine output.[41] If medical management is not an option for the client and polyuria can be tolerated, the animal can be maintained on free-choice water consumption alone.

CHAPTER • 266

Feline Lower Urinary Tract Diseases

Jodi L. Westropp
C.A. Tony Buffington
Dennis Chew

The terms *feline urologic syndrome* (FUS) and *feline lower urinary tract disease* (FLUTD) have served as shorthand descriptions for the well-known signs of straining, hematuria, pollakiuria (frequent passage of small amounts of urine), and periuria (urinations in inappropriate locations) in cats.[1] In 1925 an accurate clinical description of cats with lower urinary tract (LUT) signs described the disorder as common.[2] The roles of confinement and highly nutritious food were discussed, and the common occurrence of the problem in Persian cats was identified. In 1970, the term *FUS* was coined by Osbaldiston and Taussig[3] to describe a problem, "characterized by dysuria, urethral obstruction, urolithiasis (although no stones were reported), and hematuria." During the 1980s, Osborne and colleagues[4] suggested that FUS should be considered synonymous with FLUTD.

No diagnosis for the clinical signs of irritative voiding can be determined in approximately two-thirds of cats with LUT signs, and they are classified as having feline idiopathic cystitis (FIC). If a cystoscopy is performed and characteristic submu-cosal petechial hemorrhages are seen,[5] a diagnosis of feline interstitial cystitis can be made (Figures 266-1 and 266-2). This term was chosen because of the similarities between cats and humans with interstitial cystitis, an idiopathic pelvic pain syndrome that is characterized by difficult, painful, and frequent urinations without a diagnosable cause. Two forms of interstitial cystitis exist in humans: (1) nonulcerative and (2) ulcerative.[5] Cats with FIC generally have the nonulcerative form, however, the "classic Hunner's ulcers" have been described rarely in cats.[6] The name *FIC* will be used in this chapter for cats with idiopathic lower urinary tract disease. The term *LUT signs* will be used when referring to all possible causes of LUT disorders.

Approximately 4 million cats are destroyed annually in the United States for "elimination problems," the majority of which are related to the urinary tract.[7] Estimates of the prevalence of LUT signs were approximately 1.5% when private practices were evaluated.[8] Results of university-based studies during the past 40 years suggest that most (55% to 69%) cats

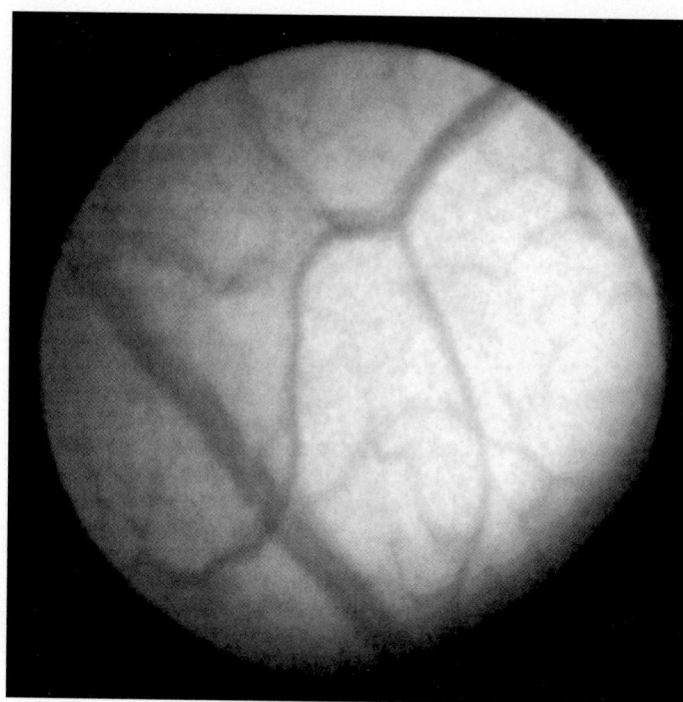

Figure 266-1 Cystoscopic appearance of blood vessels in a normal bladder from a healthy cat using liquid distention to 80 cm water pressure.

presented for evaluation of nonobstructive LUT disorders have FIC; some 13% to 28% have uroliths.[9,10] Other less common problems such as urinary tract infections (UTIs), anatomic defects, behavioral problems, neoplasia, and obstructive uropathy (reflex dyssynergia) account for most other definable disorders referable to the LUT.

When cats present for periuria (but not spraying) as the only reported clinical sign, it can be difficult to decide if they should be classified as FIC or a behavioral problem. On cystoscopy in cats with only periuria, more than half had abnormalities in their bladder such as increased vascularity, edema, or glomerulations (submucosal petechial hemorrhages).[10] Cats with FIC may have a behavioral component simultane-

ously, and as many as 40% of cats with periuria have had a previous diagnosis of cystitis.[11] Regardless of the presence or absence of cystoscopic lesions, we believe that cats with periuria should be treated like cats with FIC.

EPIDEMIOLOGY

The ratio of LUT cases to all cases seen in a clinic or hospital is called the *proportional morbidity rate*. Proportional morbidity differs from incidence because its denominator is biased toward sick animals owned by clients who are willing and able to bring their pets to a veterinarian, as well as the clinical

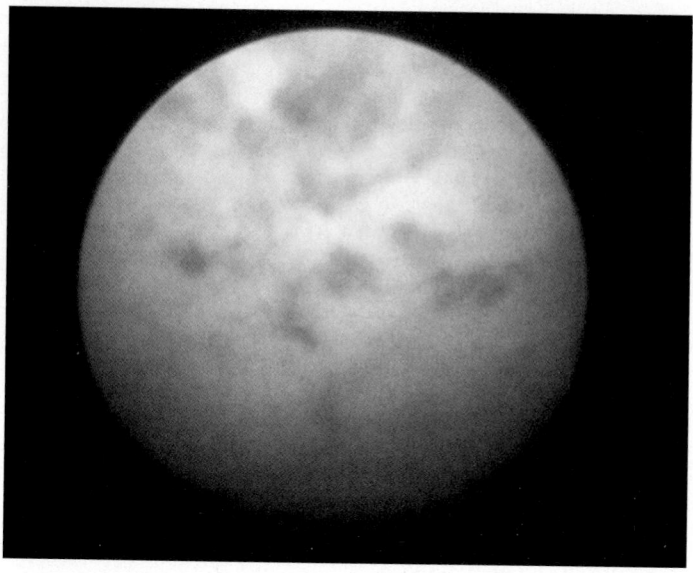

Figure 266-2 Cystoscopic appearance of a bladder from a cat with feline idiopathic cystitis (FIC). Multiple small submucosal petechial hemorrhages (glomerulations) are present, as well as edema.

URINARY SYSTEM

interests of veterinarians involved in the study. Proportional morbidity estimates of LUT signs in cats have ranged from 1% to 6%,[12] and a recent study reported a rate of approximately 1.5%.[8] Recurrence rates for LUT signs are high. In one study, 45% of male cats experienced recurrence within 6 months of an initial episode of LUT obstruction.[13] In another study, the recurrence rate for affected cats without obstruction was 39% within 1 year.[14] A slightly higher recurrence rate (approximately 55%) was reported in another study.[15]

A case-control study of cats with LUT signs was conducted recently in New Zealand (1991 to 1993).[16] One hundred ninety-three affected cats were compared with 189 case-matched (sex and age) and 189 random control cats from 13 private veterinary practices. No difference in age, gender or neuter status was identified between cases and controls. Increased risk of LUT signs was found for use of a litter tray only for elimination (cat unable to leave the house to eliminate), confinement indoor greater than or equal to 21 hours per day, sleeping inside, a move to a new house during the past 3 months, *ad libitum* feeding of dry cat food, and dry cat food feeding with low fluid intake. An increased incidence occurred during winter months, and further analysis identified a highly significant association with rainy days during the previous month. Access to outdoor prey was found to be protective.

Other studies have also reported an increased risk for LUT signs in cats fed exclusively dry food. A recent analysis of these data suggested increased risk with increased dry food consumption.[12] We found a 1-year recurrence rate of 39% in nonobstructed cats with FIC fed the dry formulation of a commercial food, whereas the recurrence rate in cats fed the canned formulation was 11%.[17] In another study, risk increased with the number of meals fed per day and was greater with periodic feeding than with *ad libitum* feeding.[12]

These studies support previous studies that found the risk for LUT signs to be highest in indoor-restricted cats that predominantly eat dry food.[12] Risk factors, however, must be kept in perspective. The proportional morbidity of LUT signs in the cat population is approximately 1.0%, although many cats are kept indoors and fed dry food exclusively.[18] The reformulation of many commercial cat foods (based on earlier epidemiologic studies) apparently has not reduced the role of dry food as a risk factor for LUT signs in cats. This circumstance suggests that environmental factors may unmask an underlying predisposition to LUT signs in some cats. The exact nature of this predisposition remains to be determined. The identification of differences in breed susceptibilities suggests that internal and environmental factors can influence disease risk in cats. Willeberg,[12] in a 1984 review, concluded that Siamese cats had a reduced risk of LUT signs, whereas Persians were at an increased risk. Jones and colleagues[16] reported an increased risk of LUT signs among long-haired but not purebred cats.

LUT signs can occur at any age but are unusual in cats less than 1 year of age and most frequent in cats 2 to 6 years of age. When clinical signs are considered without regard to obstruction, no difference in risk between males and females is observed. Adjustment for age is important because both neutering and LUT signs are age related. When adjusted for age, risk is greater for castrated males and spayed females than for intact cats,[12] but the age at neutering does not seem to be important.[19]

Excessive body weight and decreased activity have been associated with increased risk for LUT signs in some studies. When evaluating husbandry, the data concerning risk for LUT signs are mixed, indicating variously no effect[12,16] or increased risk.[20] If an increased risk exists in multiple-cat households, it could be associated with feeding and husbandry practices, territorial conflict, or horizontally transmitted infectious agents that could play a role in the development of LUT signs.

Lack of a difference between affected and control cats in upper respiratory disease and the increase in risk associated with increasing amounts of time spent *indoors* seem to argue against infection as a causative factor in LUT signs of cats.[16]

FELINE IDIOPATHIC CYSTITIS

Pathophysiology

A variety of abnormalities have been found in the bladders, nervous system, hypothalamic-pituitary-adrenal axis, and other body systems in cats with FIC. FIC in cats is similar to interstitial cystitis in human beings. Humans serve as a useful model for cats with FIC, and vice versa.[5] Cats are classified as having *feline interstitial cystitis* if cystoscopy is performed and characteristic glomerulations are seen. Cats with feline interstitial cystitis meet all inclusion and exclusion criteria for diagnosis of interstitial cystitis that can be applied to animals.[21] Thus (allowing for species differences), cats with feline interstitial cystitis meet the National Institutes of Health (NIH) criteria for humans. Feline interstitial cystitis primarily resembles nonulcer interstitial cystitis in humans, although ulceration and inflammatory infiltrates occasionally have been observed in cats. Abnormalities of local bladder factors, sensory (afferent) neurons, central nervous system (CNS), and sympathetic (efferent) neurons occur in cats as they do in humans.[22]

Gender distribution seems to be different between affected males and females of cats and humans. In cats, both genders are affected roughly equally, whereas 90% of humans are women.[23] One reason for the gender discrepancy may be related to differences in diagnoses rather than diseases. Men with irritative voiding symptoms are more likely to be diagnosed with nonbacterial prostatitis than with interstitial cystitis. Miller and colleagues[24] reported that eight of 20 men evaluated for nonbacterial prostatitis had cystoscopic findings compatible with interstitial cystitis, and "perhaps…should be given the diagnosis of IC." If only half of the reported cases of nonbacterial prostatitis are the same disease as interstitial cystitis, the difference in gender distribution between humans and cats would disappear. For further details, the reader is referred to a recent review on similarities between cats and humans and to other models of interstitial cystitis.[21]

Both humans with interstitial cystitis and cats with FIC seem to excrete smaller amounts of both total urinary glycosaminoglycan[25] (GAG) and a specific GAG (GP-51)[26,27] than do normal individuals. GAG and GP-51 contribute to the surface mucus covering the urothelium that is believed to inhibit bacterial adherence and urothelial injury from the constituents of the urine. A defective GAG layer or damaged urothelium could permit hydrogen, calcium, potassium ions, or other constituents of urine to come into contact with sensory neurons innervating the urothelium. These ions can stimulate local release of neurotransmitters and result in neurogenic bladder inflammation[28] (Figure 266-3). Sensory neurons reach the bladder via the pelvic and hypogastric nerves, and the central processes of these nerves synapse in the dorsal horn of the sacral and lumbar spinal cord, respectively.[29] These neurons include unmyelinated nociceptive fibers, commonly referred to as C *fibers*. In one study of normal cats, only ~2.5% of C fibers responded to bladder distention. However, more than 10% of these fibers responded after infusion of an irritant into the bladder lumen. This increase was attributed to activation of normally "silent" C fibers, which respond only to noxious stimuli.[30]

Histologic changes associated with FIC are generally nonspecific and may include an intact or damaged urothelium with submucosal edema, dilation of submucosal blood vessels

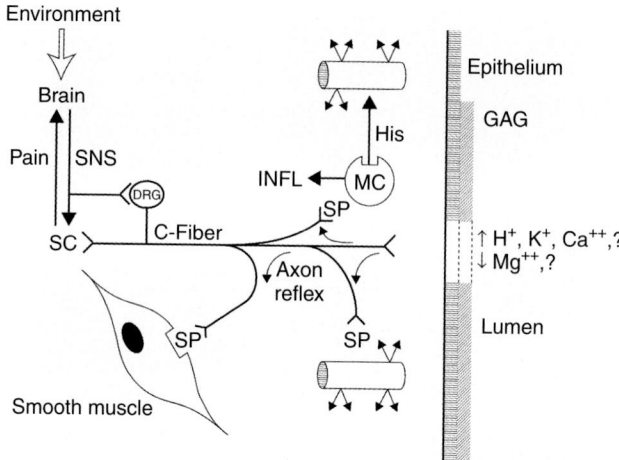

Figure 266-3 Conceptual model of bladder response to noxious stimuli. Damage of malfunction of glycosaminoglycan *(GAG)* layer or urothelium may permit urine constituents to activate sensory neurons *(C fiber)* in submucosa, which transmit action potentials to the spinal cord *(SC)* that are perceived as painful by the brain. Sensory fibers can also generate local axon reflex without propagating action potential. Axon reflex results in release of peptide neurotransmitters, such as substance P *(SP)*, by nerve endings. Interaction of SP with receptors on vessel walls results in vascular leakage, which can be augmented by SP-induced release of histamine *(HIS)* by mast cells *(MC)*. These actions may give rise to submucosal petechial hemorrhages observed at cystoscopy. SP receptors also occur on smooth muscle, which when activated stimulate muscle contraction. In addition to luminal insults, increased vascular permeability and desquamation of superficial cells of urothelium can also results from systemic and environmental stimuli, and activate C fibers and mast cells. *SNS,* Sympathetic nervous system; *INFL,* inflammation; *DRG,* dorsal root ganglia.

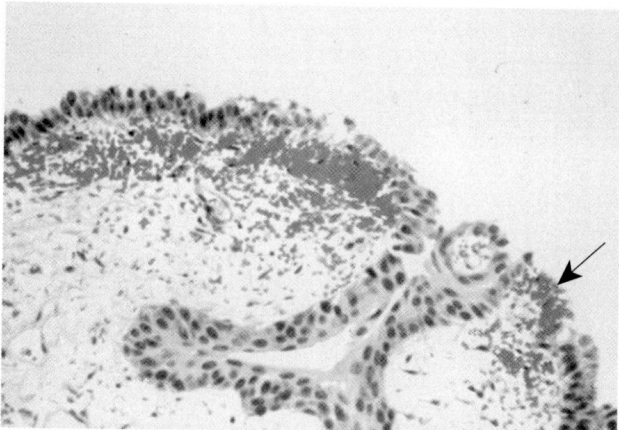

Figure 266-4 Histopathologic section of a bladder biopsy from a cat with feline idiopathic cystitis (FIC). Usually, cats with this disease have a very mild cellular infiltrate. Blood and edema can "pool" under the urothelium, and breaks in the urothelium can be seen. Submucosal hemorrhages would appear as a glomerulations when viewed cystoscopically. (H&E; ×40.)

with marginated neutrophils, submucosal hemorrhage, and sometimes increased mast cell density[5] (Figure 266-4). Bladder mastocytosis appears to be involved in the pathogenesis of interstitial cystitis in some human patients and also in some cats with FIC[31-33] (Figure 266-5). Scanning electron microscopy of bladders in cats with FIC revealed patches devoid of superficial epithelial cells (so-called umbrella cells of the urothelium)[34] and disruption of tight junctions that worsened after hydrodistention (Figure 266-6). No correlation between histology, cystoscopic lesions, and clinical signs appears to exist in cats. In fact, owners have reported complete remission of LUT signs in cats with FIC, but visualization of their bladder revealed glomerulations and other abnormalities.[35] Similar studies have been documented in humans with interstitial cystitis.[36] Because of these findings, the authors do not routinely use cystoscopy or histopathology to monitor response to therapy.

Studies in cats with FIC have shown increased leakage of ions across the urothelium and urea leakage in nonhydrodistended bladders. Marked increases in permeability after hydrodistention were also present.[34] Bladder permeability is reported to be increased in cats with FIC. Bladder permeability to sodium salicylate was increased in an *in vivo* study of cats with FIC.[37] Additionally, *in vitro* bladder epithelial urea permeability was significantly increased from normal in both undistended and distended bladders, water permeability was

significantly increased in distended bladders, and transitional cell desquamation was identified in cats with FIC.[34] Cyclophosphamide-induced cystitis in rats and other animal models of cystitis have increased bladder permeability.[38] Therefore it is likely this finding is not specific to FIC but an underlying problem that might affect the nerves in the urothelium causing a perpetuation of clinical signs.

Substance P (SP), an 11 amino acid peptide neurotransmitter, has been identified in the bladder C fibers of cats with FIC. The authors have observed a modest increase in SP immunoreactivity (IR) in the bladder of cats with FIC.[39] Significant increases in the SP receptor density (NK-1 receptors) in the bladder of humans with interstitial cystitis and cats with FIC also have been reported.[41,42] Unfortunately, clinical trials of the analgesic properties of SP antagonists in

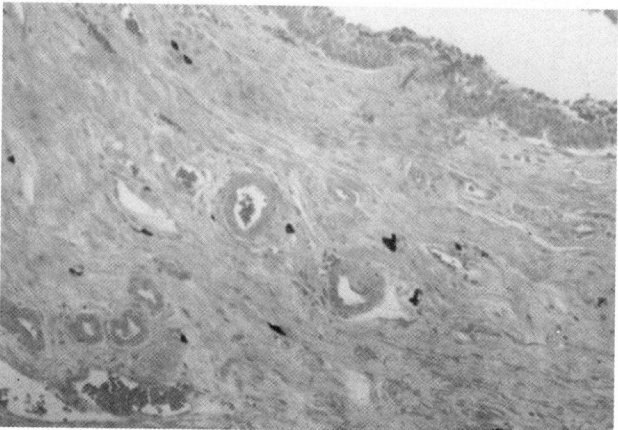

Figure 266-5 Histopathologic section of a bladder from a cat with feline idiopathic cystitis (FIC) stained with toluidine blue to visualize mast cells. Bladder mastocytosis may contribute to the pathophysiology of FIC in some cats, but mast cell stabilizing drugs do not appear to be beneficial in most cases.

URINARY SYSTEM

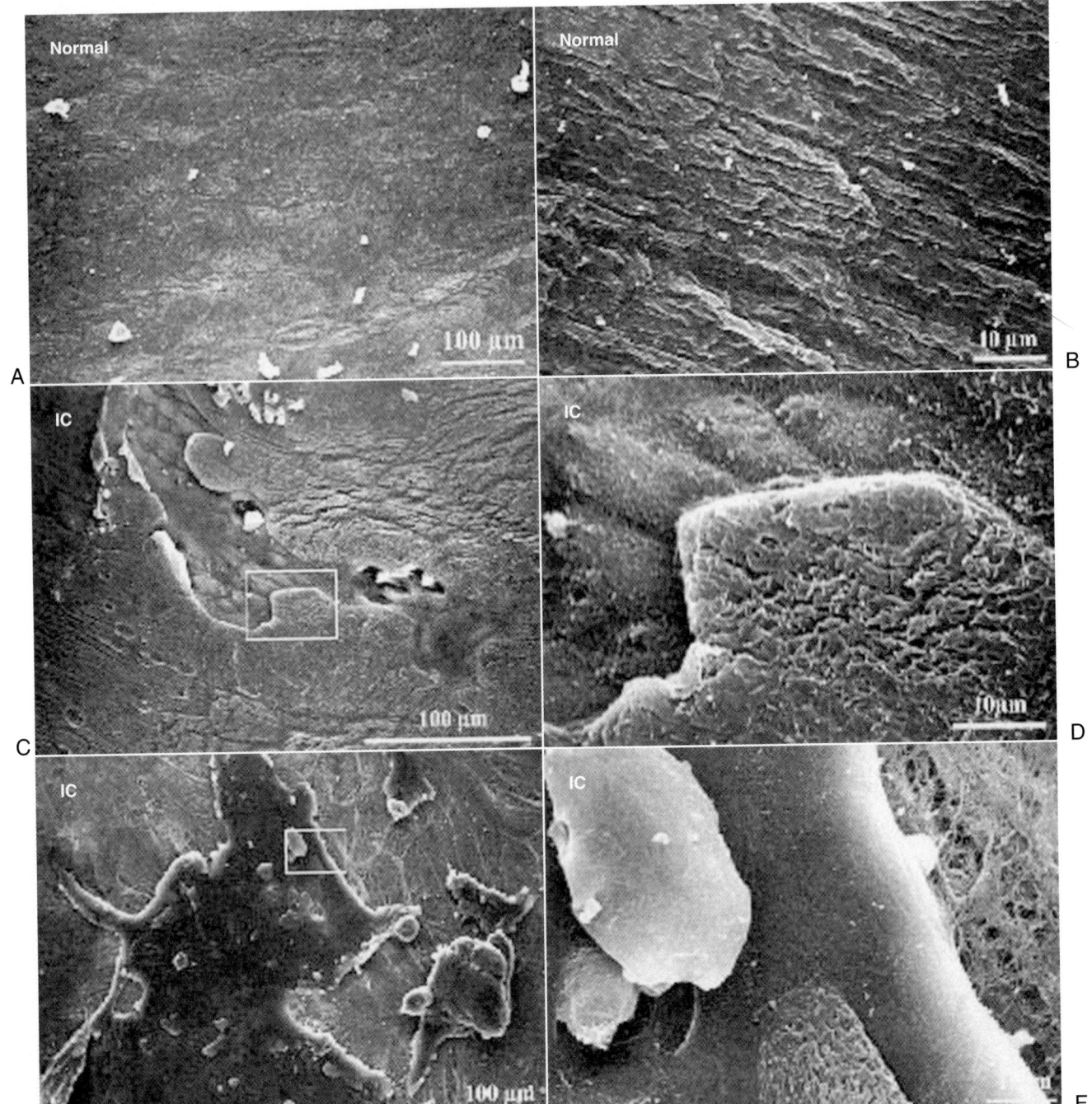

Figure 266-6 Scanning electron microscopy analysis of hydrodistended bladders from normal and feline idiopathic cystitis (FIC) cats. **A,** Low-magnification view of control bladder. **B,** High-magnification view of control bladder showing individual umbrella cells. **C,** Low-magnification view of FIC bladder demonstrating region where umbrella cell layer is disrupted. **D,** Close-up of area enclosed by box in **C. E,** Low-magnification view of FIC bladder showing regions where the urothelium is denuded from the underlying connective tissue. **F,** Close-up of area enclosed by box in **E.** (From Lavelle JP et al: Urothelial pathophysiological changes in feline interstitial cystitis: a human model. Am J Physiol Renal Physiol 278(4):540-553, 2000. Used by permission.)

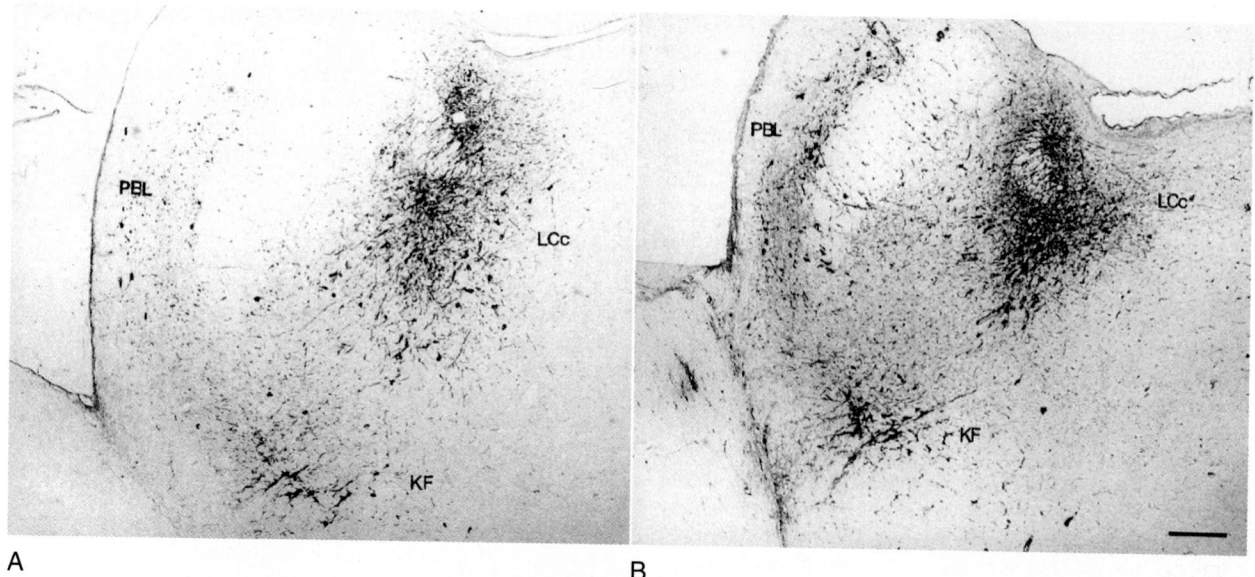

A

B

Figure 266-7 Photomicrographs of coronal sections of locus coeruleus *(LC)* of normal cat **(A)** and a cat with FIC **(B)**, immunostained for tyrosine hydroxylase *(TH)*. Reader should note increased staining density in LC complex *(LCc)*, parabrachial lateral *(PBL)*, and Kolliker-Fuse *(KF)* nuclei of cat with FIC compared with normal cat. Scale bar: 20 μm.

humans have been disappointing.[43,44] SP antagonists have not been investigated in cats with FIC.

A significant increase in tyrosine hydroxylase (THIR) has been identified in the locus coeruleus (LC)[45] and in the paraventricular nucleus of the hypothalamus in cats with FIC[46] (Figure 266-7). TH is the rate-limiting enzyme of catecholamine synthesis. Bladder distention stimulates neuronal activity in the LC, and the LC (Barrington's nucleus) is the origin of the descending excitatory pathway to the bladder.[47] Moreover, chronic stress can increase TH activity in the LC,[48] with accompanying increases in autonomic outflow.[49] The LC contains the largest number of noradrenergic neurons and is the most important source of norepinephrine (NE) in the feline and human CNS. It is involved in such global brain functions as vigilance, arousal, and analgesia and appears to mediate visceral responses to stress.[50] The increased THIR observed in the LC of cats with FIC may provide a clue to the observation that clinical signs of FIC follow a waxing and waning course, and that they can be aggravated by environmental stressors.[28,51]

In addition to increased LC activity, cats with FIC also have increased plasma NE concentrations.[52] Increased plasma and CSF catecholamine concentrations and their metabolites compared with healthy cats have been measured during stressful situations. The stress studies included removing food 12 hours prior to testing, moving the cats to different cages, and abruptly changing their diets. As the healthy cats acclimated to the stress, their plasma catecholamine concentrations decreased, whereas cats with FIC demonstrated even higher concentrations of plasma NE, epinephrine, and their metabolites.[53] Enhanced stimulus-induced local NE release from the bladder,[61] and functional desensitization of central alpha-2 adrenoceptors (α-2 AR) have been reported in cats with FIC.[56] In the LC, α-2 agonists inhibit NE release, whereas in the spinal cord they inhibit transmission of nociceptive input to the brain.[56,57] Although spinal α-2 AR activation can inhibit nociceptive input acutely, the receptors can become desensitized or down-regulated after chronic stimulation (i.e., by continuously elevated NE).[58,59]

In the bladder, α2-ARs are found primarily in the urethral submucosa and bladder mucosa (not the muscle), suggesting a role in the regulation of blood flow and urethral lubrication.[60] In this study, no α2-ARs were found in the bladder muscle, implying these receptors are not involved in bladder contraction. However, the α2-ARs can modulate NE outflow and may alter bladder contractility. Decreased sedation after clonidine administration intramuscularly and decreased mydriasis after medetomidine, a more selective α2 agonist, was found in cats with FIC, suggesting decreased α2-AR responsiveness *in vivo*. The reason for this is unclear, but it could be caused by receptor down-regulation due to persistent elevation in NE. In the presence of elevated NE, presynaptic α2-ARs could become down-regulated and unable to inhibit NE release. Electrical field stimulation studies of bladder strips from FIC cats revealed that atipamezole, an α2 antagonist, did not alter the relaxing effect of NE, further suggesting that α2-ARs are down-regulated in this disease.[61]

Based on history, physical examination and clinical signs, pelvic pain is a feature in cats with FIC. Abnormalities in the α2-ARs could be detrimental to patients because postsynaptic spinal α2-ARs possess antinociceptive properties and the α2a-AR subtype has been documented to play the major role in the control of spinal nociceptive responses.[62]

In addition to the sympathetic nervous system (SNS), abnormalities in the hypothalamic-pituitary-adrenal axis (HPA) have also been observed in cats with FIC. After a high dose (125 μg) of synthetic adrenocorticotropic hormone (ACTH) was administered, cats with FIC had significantly decreased serum cortisol responses compared with healthy cats.[64] Using computed tomography (CT) and gross histopatholgic evaluation, the adrenal volume (both absolute and per kilogram body weight) were significantly lower in FIC cats, but no correlations could be found between adrenal size and cortisol production.[65] Although no obvious histologic abnormalities were identified, the areas consisting of the zonae fasciculata and reticularis were significantly smaller in sections of glands from cats with FIC than from healthy cats. Therefore it appears that although the sympathoneural system is fully activated in this disorder, the HPA axis is not. Other chronic inflammatory and noninflammatory conditions in humans[66] appear to have an apparent "dissociation" of the SNS from the HPA axis as well. The significance of this finding is not known.

Based on the identified sensory abnormalities in cats with FIC, the authors have begun to measure response to acoustic startle. These studies are designed to evaluate the observed anxiety-related behaviors. The acoustic startle response (ASR) is a brain stem reflex that responds to unexpected, loud stimuli. The magnitude of the response can be altered by a variety of experimental manipulations and is affected by many pathologic conditions. These attributes have led to use of the ASR to study neurologic dysfunctions of sensorimotor information processing. Given the role of neural abnormalities in cats with FIC,[52] it was speculated that their ASR responses might be abnormal, and initial results revealed the magnitude of ASR to 105 dB averaged more than double that of healthy cats.

The pathophysiology of FIC is not fully understood and may involve complex interactions between a number of body systems. Abnormalities are not localized just to the bladder, but are present in the nervous,[52] endocrine,[65] and cardiovascular systems.[67] How these systems communicate and manifest as FIC in some cats but not in others remains to be determined. To better treat their patients, it is important for clinicians to understand that this syndrome is not just a "bladder disease" amenable to simple diet or drug therapies.

Approach to the Patient

In humans with interstitial cystitis, various assays for urine markers have been evaluated to attempt to properly identify a marker unique to this disease.[68] Of all the factors evaluated, the recently identified *antiproliferative factor* had the least crossover with healthy controls and could be used to aid in the diagnosis of this disease. This and other assays have not been studied and are not readily available for human or feline patients. Therefore the diagnosis of FIC still remains a *diagnosis of exclusion*. An algorithm to aid clinicians in the diagnostics and treatment of FIC is presented in Figure 266-8. Because some two thirds of cats with LUT signs have FIC, and it appears that approximately 85%[69] of cats with FIC resolve their clinical signs in 2 to 3 days without treatment, it is debatable whether any diagnostics should be performed for a young cat in its first presentation of LUT signs. The basic tests are listed, and the clinician must decide based on the cat's signalment and clinical signs which tests will yield the most benefit for each individual patient.

Radiography A plain abdominal radiograph that includes the entire urinary tract (including urethra) can be a useful diagnostic tool in cats with LUT signs. Approximately 15% of cats with stranguria, hematuria, pollakiuria, or a combination of these conditions will have radiographic evidence of cystic calculi. If only one diagnostic test can be performed, survey abdominal radiography is likely to provide information that is most clinically relevant. Contrast studies of the bladder and urethra in cats with FIC are usually unremarkable, though 15% have diffuse or asymmetrical thickening of the bladder wall.[70] A contrast cystogram and urethrogram can be helpful to evaluate for nonradiopaque calculi and other lesions such as mass lesions, blood clots, and strictures in cats with recurrent episodes. Contrast studies are especially indicated in elderly cats (> 10 years of age) where FIC is not as likely.

Urinalysis and culture Less than 2% of young (< 10 years of age) cats have true bacterial cystitis, so urine culture is a low-yield test.[1,10] Quantitative urine culture should be performed in all cats with recurrent (> 2 episodes) LUT signs. The possibility of a UTI increases with age, perineal surgery, cystic calculi, or dilute urine.[71] A quantitative urine culture should be performed in cats with LUT signs older than 10 years of age, with a urine specific gravity (USG) less than 1.030, which has undergone perineal urethrostomy, or after a urinary catheter has been placed.

Urinalysis findings such as hematuria, proteinuria, and crystalluria are not specific for any particular type of bladder disease or even a specific stone type. For example, one can see pyuria if a true UTI is present, but mild pyuria can also be present in sterile cystitis upon occasion. Crystalluria can be found in many cats with no signs referable to their LUT. A baseline urinalysis is valuable to exclude polyuria. If submaximal urine concentration is present (< 1.035 for cats eating solely dry food; < 1.025 for cats eating primarily canned foods), it is possible that increased urine volume contributed to the condition. Therefore a serum biochemical profile and thyroid evaluation should be obtained.

When radiographic findings are negative and a urine culture reveals no growth in cats with no other identifiable abnormalities, the diagnosis of FIC is likely. However, if clinical signs persist after proper environmental and drug therapy have failed, the veterinarian should consider a referral to a specialty clinic for cystoscopy.

Cystoscopy Cystoscopy is performed at referral practices when LUT signs fail to resolve after standard therapy in those cats with negative findings from radiography and urine cultures. This tool allows one to visualize the urethra and bladder at low and high pressures. Small cystic calculi, urachal diverticula, ectopic ureters, and small polyps all can be visualized (Figures 266-9 and 266-10). The authors do not use cystoscopy to "rule in" FIC, but rather to exclude less common diseases. If none of these are seen, the authors generally still "grade" the amount of edema, glomerulations (pinpoint hemorrhages) and debris that might be suspended in the lumen or peeling from the bladder wall. In humans, no good correlation exists between cystoscopic bladder lesions and symptom severity,[36] and the same appears to be true in cats. Furthermore, glomerulations are not specific for interstitial cystitis in women.[72] Increased vascularity and glomerulations have been observed in stressed, otherwise healthy cats. Such lesions may remain in affected cats without clinical signs after treatment.[35]

Treatment of Feline Idiopathic Cystitis

Having the proper tools to help owners understand FIC is important in maintaining client satisfaction when beginning any treatment regimen. It is not yet possible to predict which cats with FIC will relapse, so clients should be told what they can do to help decrease the risk of another episode. Clinical signs resolve spontaneously in as many as 85% of cats within 2 to 3 days, regardless of treatment. About 40% to 50% of these cats will have another episode within 12 months.[15,73] Some cats will have multiple recurrences, whereas a smaller population will never have complete resolution of clinical signs.

The underlying cause of this disorder is unknown, so current treatment recommendations must be tentative. The current goals of therapy for cats with FIC are not to "cure" them, but to decrease the severity of signs and to increase *interepisode* intervals, especially for severely affected cats.

Enhanced stress response system activity seems to be central to maintaining the chronic inflammatory process. Any treatment strategy to decrease SNS outflow may be important in reducing inflammation. Reduction of the noxiousness of urine or normalizing bladder permeability may also prove useful. An overarching premise is that FIC is not just a bladder disorder but involves complex interactions of the nervous and endocrine systems.[65] The development of chronic FIC

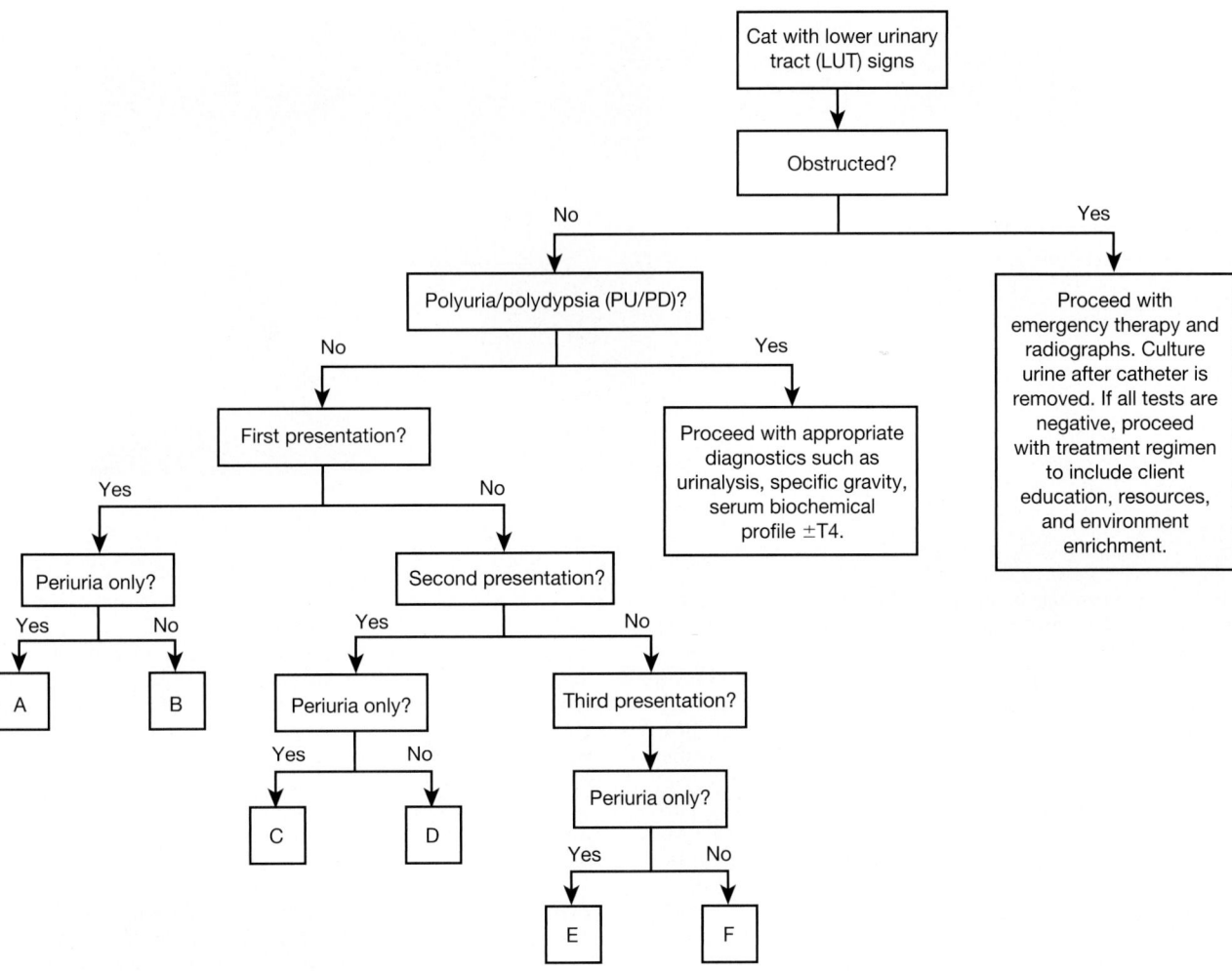

A Diagnostic: None are usually necessary.
Treatment: Litter box management and cleaning of soiled areas should be addressed.
Medications: No medications are recommended.

B Diagnostic: A radiograph should be considered, especially if hematuria is present.
Treatment: If the radiograph is negative, therapy should include analgesia for 2 to 3 days during the acute episode. Litter box management and cleaning of soiled areas should be addressed.
Medications: No medications are recommended.

C Diagnostic: A urinalysis is recommended. If submaximal urine-specific gravity is present, then appropriate diagnostics are needed.
Treatment: If diagnostic tests are negative, then the resource checklist should be reviewed and additional areas that were not previously addressed should be incorporated.
Medications: Phermonotherapy is recommended.

D Diagnostic: A radiograph, urinalysis, and urine culture are recommended.
Treatment: If all tests are negative, analgesia should be provided for 2 to 3 days during acute episode. Canned food is encouraged for the cat in addition to litter box management and cleaning of soiled areas. The cat's urine-specity gravity is monitored for 3 to 4 weeks to assess the cat's water intake.
Medications: Phermonotherapy is recommended.

E Diagnostic: A urinalysis should be performed if it has not already been done. Radiographs, urine culture, and biochemical profile are also recommended.
Treatment: If all tests are negative, then the resource checklist is formally reviewed and those areas that have not already been addressed should be incorporated. Further information for cleaning soiled areas should be provided. Additional resources (web sites, books) on how to provide an enhanced indoor environment for cats should be provided to clients. Intercat conflict issues should also be addressed.
Medications: Phermonotherapy should be used in conjunction with behavior-altering medications such as tricyclic antidepressants (TCAs) or buspirone. The medication should be taken for 4 weeks; if no improvement is seen, a referral for further diagnostics and consultation should be considered.

F Diagnostic: A radiograph, an urinalysis, and a urine culture should be performed. A complete blood count (CBC) and biochemical profile should also be submited. If all tests are negative, a contrast study or abdominal ultrasound of the bladder and urethra should be condered to rule out nonradio-opaque calculi and other mass lesions.
Treatment: If all diagnostics are negative, analgesia should be provided for 2 to 3 days during acute episode. In addition to canned food, the sheet on "Increasing your cat's water intake" should be reviewed. Water should be viewed as a "drug," and the cat's urine-specific gravity should be monitored to evaluate water intake. The resource checklist should be formally reviewed, and those areas that have not already been addressed should be incorporated. Additional resources (web sites, books) on how to provide an enhanced indoor environment for cats should be provided to clients. Intercat conflict issues should also be addressed. Follow up and support for clients are essential.
Medications: Phermonotherapy should be used in conjunction with behavior-altering medications such as TCAs or anxiolytics. Medication should be taken for 4 weeks; if no improvement is seen, a referral for further diagnostics such as a cystoscopy should be considered.

Figure 266-8 Algorithm for lower urinary tract signs in the cat.

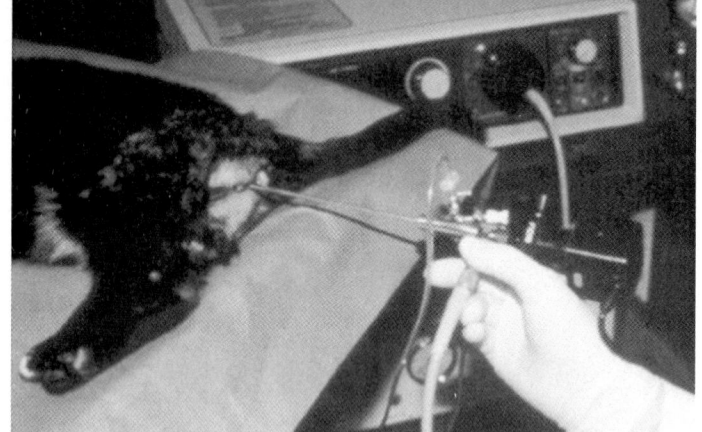

Figure 266-9 Cystoscopy of an anesthetized female cat using a 9F rigid cystoscope.

requires the presence of a susceptible cat in a provocative environment. The challenge is to identify what is provoking the susceptible cat in hopes of preventing future bouts. Analgesia, changes in diet and water intake, discussion of feeding practices, litter box management, cleaning of soiled areas, restoration of normal cat behaviors and activities, and drug therapy all are considered as part of the authors' current approach to therapy.

Using strategies from the literature,[74] the authors have found that clients will report a positive outcome (regardless of how well their cat responds to recommended therapies) if the client feels:
1. Listened to.
2. They receive an explanation for the problem that makes sense to them.
3. They feel care and concern being expressed by the caregivers and others in the clinic.

4. They gain an enhanced sense of mastery or control over the cat's illness or its symptoms.

Because FIC can be a chronic, frustrating disease, the authors have found that keeping these four points in mind when communicating with clients benefits the client, pet, and clinician. The authors have also established a technician program whereby staff members follow a cat's progress as often as necessary to be sure that problems are explained thoroughly and that client gains enough understanding of the disease process to feel comfortable with managing the cat's disease.

Provisional Recommendations (Environmental Changes and Resources Available for Cats with FIC)   A list of necessary resources for indoor-housed pet cats has not yet been validated, but some recommendations are available.[75-78] Cats appear to benefit from appropriate access to resources,

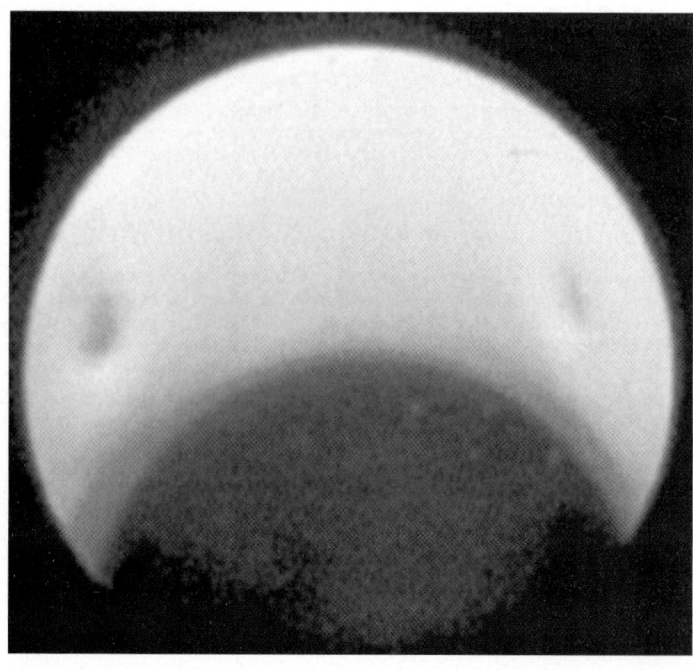

Figure 266-10 Cystoscopic view of the right and left ureteral openings in a cat. They often appear to be in the proximal urethra when the bladder is not fully distended.

control of interactions with owners, and a tolerable level of conflict with other animals. The authors have assembled a provisional list for use by owners to guide consideration of some of these parameters (Box 266-1).

The following tentative recommendations are organized to follow Box 266-1; more comprehensive suggestions are available in the many available publications about pet cats. Owners should try to institute environmental modifications slowly, one at a time, and in such a way that the cat can express its like or dislike for the change.[79] The clinician should follow a staged approach to therapy that begins with client education and environmental enrichment. If a cat relapses, these topics are thoroughly reviewed and pheromonotherapy or drug therapy may then be instituted in conjunction with environmental strategies.

There should be enough litter boxes in different locations throughout the house. A rule that many find helpful is 1 + 1: *one* for each cat of a household plus *one*—and placing litter boxes in quiet, convenient locations. If different litters are provided, it may be preferable to offer them in separate boxes, because individual preferences for litter type have been documented.[80] Cats with a history of LUT problems reportedly prefer, unscented clumping litter.[11] Litter boxes should be cleaned regularly and replaced; some cats seem quite sensitive to dirty litter boxes. Litter box size and whether or not it is open or covered also may be important to some cats.[81]

Research has demonstrated that blowing an innocuous puff of air into a cat's face while it eats can lead to behavioral abnormalities.[82] This suggests that cats should be fed individually in a quiet location where they will not be startled by other animals, sudden movement, or activity of an air duct or appliance that may begin operation unexpectedly. Although canned food may be preferable for cats with FIC due to the increased water content, some cats may prefer dry foods;[83] offering choices in separate, adjacent containers rather than replacing the usual food with a new food permits cats to express their preferences. Feeding behavior also includes predatory activities. These may be simulated by hiding small amounts of food around the house, or by putting dry food in a container from which the cat has to extract individual pieces[84] or move to release the food pieces (if such interventions appeal to the cat).[77] Cats also seem to have preferences for water that can be investigated. Consideration may be given to freshness, taste, movement (water fountains, dripping faucets, or aquarium pump–bubbled air into a bowl), and shape of container (some cats seem to resent having their vibrissae touch the sides of the container when drinking). Food and water bowls should be cleaned regularly unless individual preference suggests otherwise.

The physical environment should include opportunities for climbing, scratching, hiding, and resting. Cats seem to prefer to monitor their surroundings from elevated vantage points; provision of climbing frames, hammocks, platforms, raised walkways, shelves, or window seats have been recommended.[77,78] Playing a radio to habituate cats to sudden changes in sound and human voices also has been recommended,[85] and videotapes to provide visual stimulation are available.[77]

Some cats may prefer to be petted and groomed, whereas others may prefer play interactions.[86] Play interactions with cats may include lures or laser pointers.[76,77] Cats also may enjoy playing with toys, particularly those that are small, move, and that have characteristics of natural prey.[87,88] For cats that prefer novelty, a variety of toys should be provided and rotated or replaced regularly.[87]

In multicat houses, cats also interact with each other. Because cats housed in groups do not appear to develop distinct dominance hierarchies or conflict-resolution strategies, they may attempt to circumvent agonistic encounters by avoiding others or decreasing their activity.[89] Unrelated cats housed together in groups appear to spend less time interacting with one another than related ones.[83] These cats may prefer to have their own separate food and water sources, litter boxes, and resting areas to avoid competition for resources and to avoid unwanted interactions.[89] Published guidelines for introducing new cats into a home are available and may be recommended to clients adding cats to their households.[76] Because of the dearth of controlled trials, it is not currently possible to prioritize the importance of these suggestions or to predict which would be most appropriate in any particular situation.

Dietary Treatment   Dietary modifications may reduce the risk of recurrence of LUT signs in affected cats. Struvite crystals do not appear to damage normal urothelium, and efforts to acidify the urine to reduce struvite crystalluria by dietary modification are often *not* necessary. Efforts to acidify the urine using dry foods have no demonstrated value in treatment of FIC. Clinical experience suggests that diet change can result in recurrence of FIC signs in some cats. Moreover, with the advent of many similarly formulated prescription and commercial foods marketed for use in cats with urolithiasis or to "promote urinary tract health," changing diets can still result in recurrence of signs associated with FIC. No known benefit exists for acidifying the urine or restricting magnesium in cats with FIC. It is not recommended to frequently change diets. It is encouraged to increase water intake, and consumption of a canned food is one way to accomplish this. To avoid the potential stress of being confronted with an unfamiliar diet, it is recommended to begin feeding new canned food alongside the original diet.

In studies from the United States and New Zealand, cats with idiopathic cystitis were significantly more likely to be fed dry food exclusively.[10-16] LUT signs recurred in only 11% of affected cats during 1 year of feeding canned formulation of a dietary product. Recurrence occurred in 39% of cats fed the dry formulation of the same food, suggesting that both constancy and consistency (i.e., increased water intake) may be important. Both diets contained similar potential renal solute load and resulted in a similar urine pH. The average USG of cats fed the dry formulation was 1.050, whereas that of the cats fed the canned formulation was 1.030. It appears that the canned form protected nearly 90% of cats against recurrence of LUT signs for up to 1 year, constancy of diet protected about 60%, and 10% were offered no protection from recurrence by diet. In addition to water contained in food, the suggestions the authors provide owners to encourage increased water intake by their cats are presented in Box 266-2 and 266-3.

Pheromonotherapy   Pheromones are fatty acids that seem to transmit highly specific information between animals of the same species. Although the exact mechanisms of action are unknown, pheromones reportedly induce changes in both the limbic system and the hypothalamus that alter the emotional state of the animal.[90] Five facial pheromones have been isolated from the cat (Table 266-1). A cat deposits the F3 fraction of facial pheromones on prominent objects (including humans) by rubbing their head against the object when the cat feels safe and at ease.[90] Feliway® (Ceva Sante Animale, Libourne, France), a synthetic analogue of this naturally occurring feline facial pheromone, was developed in an effort to decrease anxiety-related behaviors of cats. Although not specifically tested in cats with FIC, treatment with this pheromone has been reported to reduce the amount of anxiety experienced by cats in unfamiliar circumstances, a response that may be helpful to both cat and owner. Increased grooming and food intake in hospitalized cats[91] also has been

Table • 266-2

Drugs Commonly Used to Treat and Manage Cats with Lower Urinary Tract Disease

DRUGS COMMONLY USED FOR ANALGESIA	CLASS	MECHANISM OF ACTION	INDICATION FOR USE	DOSE	POTENTIAL SIDE EFFECTS
Butorphanol (Torbugesic® or Torbutrol®)	Synthetic partial opiate agonist	Kappa and Sigma receptor agonist; analgesic effects in the limbic system	Analgesia for acute episode of FIC	0.2-0.4 mg/kg PO, SQ BID-TID	Sedation
Buprenorphine (Buprenex®)	Synthetic partial opiate agonist	Partial mu receptor agonist	Analgesia for acute episode of FIC	0.01-0.02 mg/kg BID-TID; 0.015 mg/kg PO BID to TID (anecdotal)	Sedation
Fentanyl (Duragesic®)	Opiate agonist	Mu and opiate agonist	Analgesia for acute episode of FIC	25 µg/hr	Respiratory depression; bradycardia

Drugs Commonly Used To Alter Bladder/Urethral Contractility

	CLASS	MECHANISM OF ACTION	INDICATION FOR USE	DOSE	POTENTIAL SIDE EFFECTS
Acepromazine (PromAce®)	Phenothiazine neuroleptic agent	Block postsynaptic central dopamine receptors; varying degrees of anticholinergic, antihistaminic, antispasmodic and alpha-adrenergic blocking capabilities	For sedation and antispasmodic for urethral obstruction	0.05 mg/kg SQ BID-TID	Hypotension; sedation
Prazosin (Minipress®)	Alpha-adrenergic antagonist	Inhibits α-1 adrenergic receptors	For sedation and antispasmodic for urethral obstruction	0.5 mg/kg PO BID	Hypotension; sedation
Phenoxybenzamine (Dibenzyline®)	Alpha-adrenergic antagonist	Inhibits α-adrenoceptors	For sedation and antispasmodic for urethral obstruction	2.5 mg PO BID	Hypotension; sedation
Bethanechol (Urecholine®)	Synthetic parasympathomimetic	Stimulates primarily muscarinic receptors	Detrusor atony	2.5-5.0 mg PO BID	Vomiting, diarrhea, and salivation

Drugs Commonly Used for the Treatment of FIC

Drug	Class	Mechanism	Indication	Dose	Side effects
Amitriptyline (Elavil®)	Tricyclic antidepressant (TCA)	NE reuptake inhibition; central and peripheral anticholinergic activity; antagonism of the H1 receptor; 5-HT reuptake inhibition; glutamate and Na channel receptor antagonist	Chronic FIC	5.0–12.5 mg PO SID-BID	Sedation; weight gain; urine retention; urolith formation
Clomipramine (Anafranil® [human], Clomicalm® [veterinary])	TCA	NE and serotonin reuptake inhibition	Chronic FIC; urine spraying	0.5 mg/kg PO SID	Sedation; anticholinergic effects
Buspirone (BuSpar®)	A nonbenzodiazepine anxiolytic agent	Mixed dopaminergic agonist/antagonist; other mechanisms not well understood	Chronic FIC; urine spraying; anxiety	2.5–5.0 mg PO BID	Rare, but sedation or other neurologic effects
Fluoxetine (Prozac®)	Antidepressant	Selective serotonin reuptake inhibitor	Chronic FIC; urine spraying	1 mg/kg PO SID	Decrease food intake; vomiting and lethargy rare
Pentosan polysulfate sodium (Elmiron®)	GAG replacer	Unknown	Chronic FIC	50 mg PO BID	Diarrhea and vomiting rare
F3 fraction of feline facial pheromone (Feliway®)	Synthetic pheromone	Alter the emotional state of the animal via the limbic system and hypothalamus	Anxiety related behaviors; chronic FIC	1 spray in affected area SID or room diffuser	None reported

Drugs Commonly Used to Manage Urolithiasis

Drug	Class	Mechanism	Indication	Dose	Side effects
DL-methionine	Sulfur-containing amino acid	Methionine metabolized and sulfate excreted in urine as sulfuric acid, thereby acidifying urine	For urine acidification when dietary management fails	0.5–1.0 g PO on food once daily	Gastrointestinal (GI) distress; metabolic acidosis

(Continued)

URINARY SYSTEM

Table • 266-2

Drugs Commonly Used to Treat and Manage Cats with Lower Urinary Tract Disease—Cont'd

DRUGS COMMONLY USED FOR ANALGESIA	CLASS	MECHANISM OF ACTION	INDICATION FOR USE	DOSE	POTENTIAL SIDE EFFECTS
Ammonium chloride	Acid forming salt	Administration results in a decrease in serum bicarbonate and decrease in blood and urine pH	For urine acidification when dietary management fails	20 mg/kg PO BID	Metabolic acidosis; GI distress
Potassium citrate (Uracit-K®)	Alkalinizing salt	Citrate oxidized to bicarbonate; citrate chelates calcium, forming a more soluble salt	To reduce risk of calcium oxalate formation	100-150 mg/kg/day	GI
Allopurinol	Xanthine oxidase inhibitor	Inhibits the enzyme xanthine oxidase, which is responsible for the conversion of oxypurines to uric acid	For prevention/dissolution of ammonium urate stones	9 mg/kg/day	Xanthine stones; rarely used in cats so side effects and safety unknown
2-MPG	Sulfhydryl compound related to penicillamine	Undergoes thiol-disulfide exchange with cystine to form a more water-soluble compound	For prevention and treatment of cystine urolithiasis	No studies performed in cats	No information available in cats; anemia in dogs is reported

FIC, feline ideopathic cystitis; SQ, subcutaneously; BID, twice a day; TID, three times a day; PO, oral administration

least invasive approach for the cat should be attempted first, so routes of medication should be tailored for individual cats.

We have used amitriptyline, (a tricyclic antidepressant [TCA]) in uncontrolled trials to successfully decrease clinical signs of severe, recurrent FIC.[35] Amitriptyline (Elavil®), may provide analgesia by inhibition of NE reuptake at noradrenergic nerve terminals[95] and possibly due to inhibition of a wide range of nociceptive neurons in the spinal trigeminal nucleus.[96] The beneficial effects of amitriptyline treatment on pain appear to be independent of its effect on depression in human beings.[97] This point is important when considering this drug for cats, because analgesia can occur at lower doses, which potentially could decrease the unwanted side effects such as weight gain and lethargy. Other actions of amitriptyline include the ability to stabilize mast cell membranes (by antagonism of the H1 receptor), serotonin (5-HT) reuptake inhibition, and antagonism of both glutamate receptors and sodium channels.[98] Urine retention through anticholinergic effects of the TCAs may result. Findings in a series of cats with severe FIC showed that the clinical signs of some cats were reduced during amitriptyline treatment during a 12-month period. Improvement in clinical signs was not always accompanied by improvement in the cystoscopic appearance of the bladder. Controlled studies of the safety and efficacy of amitriptyline in cats with FIC are not available, but it has been used with apparent safety by animal behaviorists for more than 10 years.

The drug should be given orally once daily before the owner retires for the night. The dose should then be adjusted to produce a barely perceptible calming effect on the cat (usually 2.5 to 12.5 mg). The reduction in severity of clinical signs can be dramatic in some cats; but in others little or no beneficial effect is observed. If no improvement is seen within 2 to 4 months, the medication should be gradually tapered and then stopped.

Clomipramine hydrochloride (Clomicalm®, veterinary label; and Anafranil®, human label) is also a tertiary amine like amitriptyline, but has more selectivity for blocking the reuptake of 5-HT. It has been reported to provide a beneficial effect (in combination with environmental strategies) for psychogenic alopecia in cats.[99] The authors have prescribed this in recurrent cases of FIC with anecdotal improvement in some cats. Complete blood count (CBC) and serum biochemical profile are recommended before treatment and at 1 and 3 months to ensure no untoward effects of therapy during the use of any TCA.

The selective serotonin reuptake inhibitor, fluoxetine (Prozac®),[100] has been reported to help cats with inappropriate urinations with variable success rates. Fluoxetine was used to help decrease the rate of urine marking after environmental alterations such as litter box hygiene and appropriate cleaning strategies. The nonbenzodiazepine anxiolytic, buspirone (BuSpar®) has been used to decrease high arousal and reduce anxiety in intercat aggression.[101] Because cats with FIC have exacerbation of clinical signs associated with stressful situations, buspirone can be used for this disease with some success. Diazepam (Valium®) is a benzodiazepine that is used for behavioral disorders and has sedative, anticonvulsant, and anxiolytic effects. The most serious side effect encountered with the use of oral diazepam in cats is that of idiosyncratic hepatic necrosis,[102] which removes this drug from consideration for long-term therapy. Other benzodiazepines such as alprazolam and temazepam have not been reported to be associated with hepatic toxicity,[103] but experience with the use of these drugs in cats with FIC have not been reported.

We do not recommend amitriptyline for acute treatment of FIC because it has been shown to have minimal to no benefit in the short-term resolution of signs.[15] The authors reserve all the TCAs and the selective serotonin reuptake inhibitors for recurrent, severe cases. These drugs need to be used only after environmental strategies, diet changes (if necessary), and behavior modifications have failed. Furthermore, it is the authors' opinion that these drugs should then only be used in conjunction with the previously mentioned therapeutic strategies for optimal effects.

Amitriptyline (and TCAs) should not be discontinued abruptly, but tapered slowly over 2 to 3 weeks to avoid any possible withdrawal responses that cause exacerbation of clinical signs. The TCAs are extensively metabolized by the cytochrome P450 enzyme system and, although specific drug interactions and safety trials have not been evaluated in animals, caution is recommended when prescribing TCAs with other drugs known to affect drug metabolism.[103]

The act of medicating a cat can be stressful for some cats and owners. Transdermal delivery systems for drugs are available that make the administration of the drug much easier, but no clinical trials compare the plasma concentration, safety, and efficacy of the transdermal preparations to their oral counterparts. The authors are reluctant to recommend transdermal preparations until the pharmacokinetics and pharmacodynamics of compounds administered by this route have been investigated in affected cats.

Glycosaminoglycans GAG replacement treatment has been used with some success in humans with interstitial cystitis[104] but usually does not provide long-term relief. The untested assumption is that exogenous GAG will attach to the defective urothelium, thereby decreasing bladder permeability. In addition, GAG can exert analgesic and anti-inflammatory effects that might prove useful. A study in humans reported that pentosanpolysulfate, a synthetic, branched polysaccharide that resembles the natural proteoglycan chondroitin sulfate, appeared to inhibit allergic and nonimmune mast cell stimulation and decrease intracellular calcium ion concentrations, which suggests another alternative for the benefit of this drug in some human patients.[105] However, there may be differences in the relative efficacy of the various available GAG. GAG replacers, such as Elmiron® can be tried. Side effects in humans can include gastrointestinal (GI) side effects (diarrhea) and hematologic abnormalities. Other veterinary marketed GAG replacers such as Cosequin® and Adequan® can be tried, but no evidence exists as to their efficacy in FIC.

UROLITHIASIS, URETHROLITHS, AND URETHRAL PLUGS

Urethral Obstruction

Urethral plugs are the most common cause of obstruction in male cats. In one series from the 1980s,[9] urethral plugs occurred in 60% of cats, no cause was found in 30%, uroliths alone were documented in only 10%, and uroliths with bacterial UTI were observed in 2%. Occasionally stricture and rarely neoplasia cause the obstruction. Urethral obstruction due to calcium oxalate urethroliths appears to be more common currently as compared with the early to mid-1980s.

It is unlikely for the urethra of female cats to become obstructed, but male cats have a narrow penile urethral lumen and are predisposed to obstruction with a urolith or urethral plug. Currently, it is unknown what causes the matrix of urethral plugs to form and is probably the outcome of several mechanisms. Many urethral plugs are composed of struvite with a proteinaceous matrix[9] (Figure 266-11). Struvite urethroliths were the sole type reported in cats from the 1980s, but calcium oxalate urethroliths occur more commonly now.

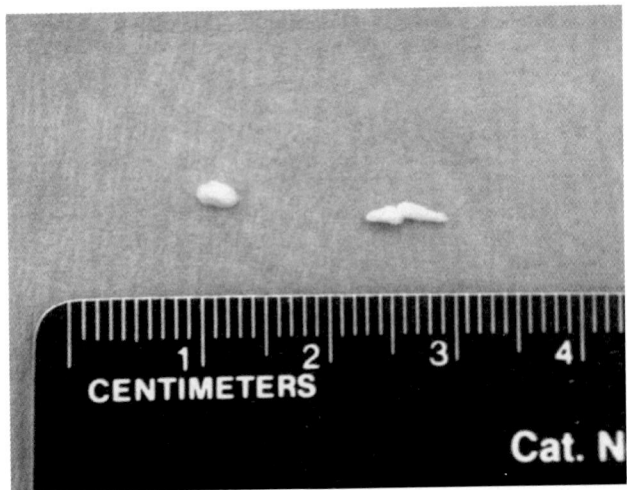

Figure 266-11 Fragments of urethral plugs obtained in a male cat after digital manipulation of the distal urethra and manual compression of the bladder.

It has been hypothesized that the concomitant occurrence of UTIs and crystalluria may lead to formation of matrix-crystalline plugs that obstruct various portions of the urethra, especially in male cats.[106] It was hypothesized that Tamm-Horsfal mucoprotein (THP) is contained within urethral plugs. Once this coalesces together with the crystals, white blood cells (WBCs), and red blood cells (RBCs), it can be surrounded by amorphous material and then obstruct the urethra. No evidence of THP in urethral plugs obtained from obstructed cats was identified in one group of cats we evaluated. However, the eletrophoretic pattern of some plugs resembled that of albumin and its degradation products, suggesting that the plug resulted from precipitated serum proteins. The authors hypothesize that vasodilatation and leakage of plasma proteins from the suburothelial capillary plexus (*bladder weeping*) and secondary urethritis, which can be seen cystoscopically in cats with FIC, may trap crystals within the lumen of the male cat urethra and may result in obstruction. It is likely that oozing of plasma proteins into urine during active inflammation increases the urinary pH that contributes to the precipitation of struvite crystals that participate in urethral plug formation. Though conventional wisdom indicates that urethral plugs form in the urethra, the authors have observed with cystoscopy what appear to be plugs in the bladder. It is interesting that the mineral components of urethral plugs continue to be predominantly composed of struvite despite the apparent increase in frequency of calcium oxalate urolithiais. This may be due to the narrow range of *metabolic supersaturation* of struvite in urine. These and other hypotheses are not mutually exclusive, and plugs may form by different mechanisms, depending on a variety of factors present at any particular instance.

Regardless of the underlying cause or causes, relief of obstructions, re-establishment of urine flow, and correction of fluid, electrolyte, and acid-base imbalances associated with obstruction and postrenal azotemia are the first steps in proper management. Decompressive cystocentesis is a recommended first step, prior to attempts to pass a urinary catheter. A small (22- or 23-gauge) butterfly needle inserted into the lateral bladder wall midway between the apex and urethral outflow works well for this procedure and aids in the removal of urine without reinsertion of the needle. Alternatively, if a longer needle is necessary, it can be attached to an extension set and urine removed with a syringe in a similar manner.

The bladder should be continuously palpated during the drainage and further pressure exerted on the bladder to allow nearly complete evacuation of urine. Complications are rare but include extravasation of urine into the peritoneal cavity and damage to the bladder wall.

Cats with urethral obstruction should be managed aggressively with medical treatment unless recurrent obstructions occur. A perineal urethrostomy surgery may be needed to prevent future episodes of urethral obstruction. This surgery carries some risks or complications such as bacterial UTIs and postoperative strictures.[107] Furthermore, clients need to be made aware that this surgery does not correct the underlying problem. Recurrent uroliths and FIC episodes can still occur. It is reported that the frequencies of feline urethrostomies performed at the University of Minnesota Veterinary Teaching Hospital has declined over the past 20 years, which is due, in part to a decrease in urethral plugs that are diagnosed.[108] The 50% decrease in occurrence of urethral obstruction could be due to the widespread use of urinary acidifying diets because struvite is the most common component to the urethral plug. Other factors that could have contributed to the decrease in perineal urethrostomy surgery could include more such surgeries done by private practitioners in primary or referral practices. Although the decline in urethral obstructions was halved, the frequency of urethrostomies decreased by 90%, suggesting that clinicians at this institution are now managing urethral obstruction successfully by nonsurgical methods.

For most obstructed cats (other than neurogenic obstruction), medical management with analgesics, antispasmodics (α1 adrenoceptor antagonists), and appropriate fluid therapy can be rewarding. Serum biochemistry, CBC, and urinalysis should be obtained, though is not necessary to evaluate such results prior to obstruction relief. Cats that are moribund should be resuscitated with intravenous fluids and correction of serious electrolyte and acid-base disturbances before anesthesia for placement of a urinary catheter. Specific rescue from the cardiotoxic effects of severe hyperkalemia (calcium salts, glucose, or insulin + glucose) may be necessary even before specific values for serum potassium return from the laboratory. An electrocardiagraphic assessment of all systemically ill cats with urethral obstruction should be performed. Only 12% of cats with urethral obstruction had severe hyperkalemia (> 8.0 mmol/L) in one recent report.[109]

Anesthesia is needed to allow proper manipulation of the cat's penis and passage of the urinary catheter. Isoflurane gas anesthesia can be administered by facemask to provide sedation and urethral relaxation. Alternatively, propofol infusion can be given for anesthesia. The combination of ketamine and Valium given intravenously to effect has been used for many years but does not provide adequate relaxation for some cats. After decompressive cystocentesis, the clinician should relieve the obstruction by catheterization and retropulsion with hydraulic forces using a sterile physiologic solution. Any urethral plug or urolith that is retrieved should be submitted for quantitative analysis. An indwelling catheter is not always needed once the obstruction is removed but is advised for cats with pronounced azotemia, those with a poor urine stream after advancing a catheter, and for those with an extremely large bladder volume at the time of obstruction relief because they are more likely to develop detrusor atony.

Urine output should be monitored frequently in severely ill cats. Cats recovering from severe postrenal uremia often have substantial postobstructive diuresis. Urine output is expected to be greater than 2.0 mL/kg/hr shortly after relief of obstruction and intravenous infusion of rehydration fluid volumes. Urine output can be marked, making it essential to ensure the amount of intravenous fluid volume infused is adequate to replace urine volume lost. Diuresis usually subsides as the waste products are excreted, which typically lasts 2 to 5 days. In some instances, the amount of intravenous fluids administered continues to drive the diuresis. The intravenous fluid infusion rate may be decreased by 25% to see if urine volume declines in concert. If so, continued tapering of intravenous fluids is recommended. Tapering of intravenous fluids can also be initiated after there has been resolution of azotemia. The magnitude of postobstructive diuresis is usually parallel to the magnitude of azotemia. Cats with minimal azotemia are not expected to have much, if any, diuresis.

Nearly all cats treated for urethral obstruction at a university referral hospital survived initial treatment and stabilization.[109] Death can occur due to consequences of severe dehydration, hyperkalemia, metabolic acidosis, and hypocalcemia. Rarely, cats have a ruptured bladder secondary to long-standing urethral obstruction. Prognosis for survival in these cats is much worse.

Analgesics such as butorphanol, hydromorphone, and fentanyl (patches) can be used to alleviate pain. α-adrenoceptor antagonists (e.g., phenoxybenzamine, prazosin) and the phenothiazine derivative, acepromazine, can be used to help prevent smooth muscle urethral spasms that can occur after obstruction relief. Urethral spasms are a primary reason for cats to reobstruct once a plug or urethrolith has been removed. Preemptive therapy with antispasmodic medications may help prevent the recurrence of obstruction and help avoid need for perineal urethrostomy surgery. If detrusor atony is suspected, bethanechol can be added to the regimen provided the urethra is patent. After the cat has been successfully managed in the short term, care similar to that given to cats with FIC should be given.

Uroliths

Uroliths are organized concretions found in the urinary tract that contain primarily organic or inorganic crystalloid (ionic component of crystals) and a much smaller amount of organic matrix. When 70% or more of the urolith is composed of one type of crystal it is named for that crystal. Secondary crystalloids can comprise up to 30% of the total weight. Urine is commonly supersaturated with crystalloids, and observation of individual crystals in the urine does *not* mean the cat is at risk for urolithiasis. Crystalluria is not a disease, and no particular treatment is necessary unless a urolith is present, or a urolith or urethral plug has formed in the past. Supersaturation of urine with crystalloids depends on the interaction of dozens of crystalloid species formed by common mineral elements in the urine derived from the amount of each solute ingested and excreted in the volume of urine produced.[110] Moreover, these complex calculations do not take into account potential organic molecule contributions, such as protein inhibitors or promoters of crystallization.[111] Urine pH also affects crystal formation. Struvite, calcium carbonate, and calcium phosphate are less soluble in alkaline urine; cystine and uric acid are less soluble in acid urine, but urate is less soluble in alkaline urine. Urine pH *per se* does not appear to have a major effect on the solubility of calcium oxalate; however, most calcium oxalate stones occur in cats with acid urine. Factors that predispose to urinary stasis play an important role in urolithiasis, because crystals must reside in the urinary tract for a sufficient time for a urolith to form.

Struvite Urolithiasis

The chemical composition of struvite is $MgNH_4PO_4 \cdot 6H_2O$. Calcium phosphate (apatite) sometimes is present in small amounts (2% to 10%). The presence of three cations (Ca^{2+}, Mg^{2+}, and NH_4^+) detected by earlier qualitative methods led to the name *triple phosphate* previously used for these stones. Struvite uroliths are spherical, ellipsoidal, or tetrahedral in shape and may be present singly or in large numbers of varying sizes. The bladder is the most common site of struvite uroliths, although they may occur at any site in the urinary tract. In cats, struvite stones usually form in sterile urine. More than 90% of dogs, in contrast, have struvite stones associated with a urease-producing bacterial infection. Struvite solubility is reduced in urine of pH greater than 6.7. Struvite urolithiasis and urethral obstruction have been induced experimentally in healthy cats by feeding diets containing three to ten times the amount of magnesium found in commercial cat foods.[112] These studies led to the conclusion that magnesium was a primary cause of naturally occurring struvite urolithiasis in cats. It subsequently was learned that struvite stones in the bladder of healthy cats fed large quantities of magnesium dissolved when the urine pH was reduced to approximately 6.0.[112] These results suggested that magnesium's effect on struvite formation depended on the urine pH—an idea supported by the finding that the form of magnesium used in previous studies had increased the urine pH.[113] Therefore factors that may be associated with alkaline urine (e.g., family history of struvite stones, diet based on vegetable proteins [rare in cats], distal renal tubular acidosis) should be considered.

Lekcharoensuk and colleagues,[114] evaluated the association between dietary factors and struvite formation (Table 266-3). They reported that diets low in sodium or potassium or formulated to maximize urine acidity had a decreased risk for struvite urolith formation. Diets with the highest magnesium, phosphorus, calcium, chloride, or fiber contents, moderate protein content, and low fat content were associated with increased risk of magnesium ammonium phosphate urolith formation. However, these differences may also have been confounded by the many correlations between the dietary components and is compatible with the nutrient profile of relatively low-quality cat foods. In addition to nutrients, ingredients, and their combinations, breed, age, sex, body condition, and living environment were also significantly different between case and control cats (which were adjusted for in the multivariate logistic regression). The many interacting variables demonstrate the complexity of the process of stone formation.

It has been reported that spayed female cats have a higher risk of developing struvite uroliths,[115] but a more recent study[116] found a slightly higher risk only for *male* cats. When reproductive status was evaluated in this same study, neutered animals were three and a half times as likely to develop struvite uroliths compared with sexually intact cats. Cats with struvite uroliths were significantly younger than cats with calcium oxalate uroliths in the same study; however, when evaluating age, cats 4 years of age or older and 7 years of age or less had the highest risk for developing struvite urolithiasis. Breeds at risk were reported to be the Foreign Shorthair, Ragdoll, Chartreux, Oriental shorthair, domestic shorthair (DSH), and Himalayan. The Rex, Burmese, Abyssinian, Russian blue, Birman, Siamese, and mixed breed cats had a significantly lower risk of developing struvite uroliths.

Management of Urolithiasis Patients who have had cystic calculi initially should be monitored every 2 to 3 months for recurrence. It is ideal to obtain a radiograph for a quick *stone check*. Uroliths larger than 3 mm will usually be evident with a plain abdominal radiograph. A double-contrast study or abdominal ultrasound may also be necessary for stones that are not radiodense (e.g., urate). If "sand and debris" or even very small stones (3 to 5 mm) are seen in the urinary bladder, surgery may not be necessary and voiding urohydropropulsion may be used to remove the stones (Figure 266-12, *A* and *B*). For a complete review of this technique, the reader is referred to the literature.[117] Stones as large as 5 mm can sometimes be removed from female cats by this method, but one should be

Table • 266-3

Differences in Content of Various Dietary Components and Predicted Urine pH for Diets Fed to Cats With Calcium Oxalate (CaOx) or Magnesium Ammonium Phosphate (MAP) Uroliths and to Control Cats Without Any Urinary Tract Diseases

	DIFFERENCE FROM CONTROL		COMPONENT RANGES*		
	CaOx	MAP	UNITS	CaOx	MAP
Protein	6% ↓	1% ↓	g/100 kcal	8.0-8.8; 10.5-13.8	
Carbohydrate	13% ↑	12% ↑	g/100 kcal	-	-
Fat	2% ↓	9% ↓	g/100 kcal	-	5.0-5.2
Fiber	4% ↑	7% ↓	g/100 kcal	-	Avoid > 0.3
Calcium	11% ↓	7% ↑	mg/100 kcal	-	Avoid > 205
Phosphorus	12% ↓	10% ↑	mg/100 kcal	-	Avoid > 176†
Magnesium	11% ↓	15% ↑	mg/100 kcal	-	Avoid > 26
Sodium	9% ↓	12% ↑	mg/100 kcal	78-370	Avoid >77†
Potassium	5% ↓	5% ↑	mg/100 kcal	181-320	Avoid >181‡
Chloride	5% ↓	6% ↑	mg/100 kcal	-	Avoid >167
Water	33% ↓	11% ↓	%	10.1-81.2	-
pH	1% ↓	1% ↑	pH	6.3-6.9	Avoid >6.5§

*Ranges over which significant differences in risk for affected cats were identified by multivariate analysis. Ranges with increased risk are denoted by "avoid." Reader should see reference for details and limitations of such interpretations.
†May be related to phosphorus salt used.
‡Not considered biologically significant by authors.
§Urine pH less than 6.3 could result in metabolic acidosis.
Data from table obtained from Lekcharoensuk C et al: Association between dietary factors and calcium oxalate and magnesium ammonium phosphate urolithiasis in cats. J Am Vet Med Assoc, 219:1228, 2001.

prepared for surgical removal of stones that are not successfully removed with voiding urohydropropulsion.

Once a urolith has been removed, the cat should be fed a canned diet, if possible, to decrease the urine concentration of stone mineral precursors. If a cat will not accept the new diet, water intake can be increased by the use of drinking fountains, flavored juices (e.g., ham, tuna), and the addition of ice cubes to the cat's water (see Box 266-1 for further suggestions).

Increasing water consumption is the cornerstone of therapy for urolithiasis in human[118] and veterinary medicine. When a urolith is diagnosed, the cat should be encouraged to consume enough water in canned or moistened foods to increase the urine volume until the USG is decreased to less than 1.030. Clients are advised that the urine should be clear, colorless, and odorless. USG should be monitored at periodic re-evaluations.

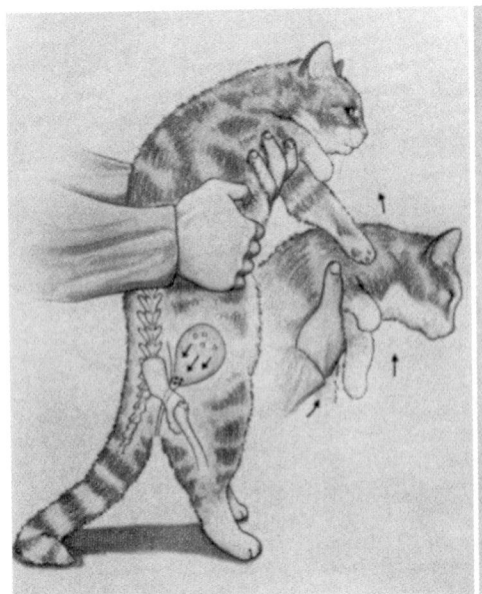
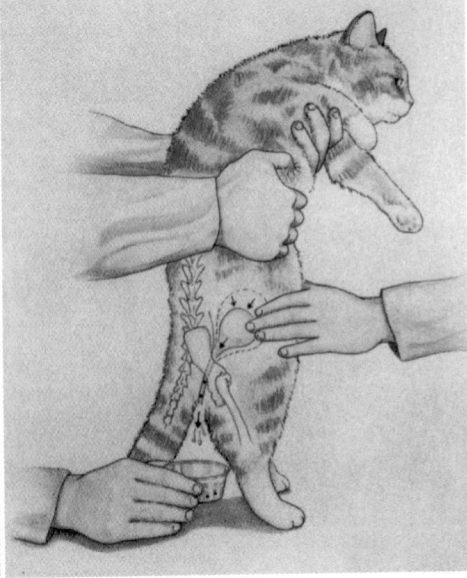

A   B

Figure 266-12 A and B, To remove urocystoliths by voiding urohydropropulsion, the patient is positioned so that the longitudinal axis of the vertebral column is approximately vertical. As a result, uroliths move from the ventral portion of the urinary bladder to the bladder neck. To expel urocystoliths, voiding is induced by applying steady digital pressure to the urinary bladder. (From Lulich JP, Osborne CA: Management of urocystoliths by voiding urohydropropulsion. Disorders of the feline lower urinary tract II. Diagnosis and therapy. Vet Clin North Am 26(3):631-632, 1996. Used with permission.)

Struvite Urolithiasis Management In cats with struvite urolithiasis without a UTI, urinary acidifiers played a more important role until most commercial cat foods were reformulated to reduce urine pH. Urine acidifiers should only be given to cats with urine pH greater than 6.5 measured under *ad libitum* feeding conditions. Ideally, urine should be collected from the cats in their own environment, and the sample brought to the hospital for assessment of pH and specific gravity. A urinary pH meter is reported to be more accurate than urine dip strips.[119] Although the addition of D,L-methionine and ammonium chloride decreases the struvite activity product and sediment in the urine of healthy cats, this supplementation failed to reduce the urinary concentration of the HCL-insoluble fraction that may be a candidate for the matrix of struvite uroliths.[120] Ingestion of large quantities of urinary acidifiers can cause anorexia and systemic acidosis. A number of veterinary diets to help prevent the recurrence of struvite stones are available (Table 266-4 and Box 266-3); although these diets may be of benefit, none have evidence-based outcomes documenting their effectiveness in prevention of recurring struvite urolithiasis. Feeding patterns also may influence the development of struvite uroliths due to an increase in pH (postprandial alkaline tide) that may occur after a meal in meal-fed cats, depending on diet composition.[121] Therefore *ad-libitum* feeding in cats with struvite uroliths seems prudent.

If a struvite urolith was diagnosed with a recurrence, feeding a canned form of a calculolytic diet has been reported to induce dissolution of struvite calculi in female cats.[122] Calculoylysis usually occurs within 1 month. Caution should be observed when considering use of calculolytic diets; the diets should not be fed to growing kittens or to pregnant or lactating queens.

Calcium Oxalate Urolithiasis

Calcium oxalate stones are the most common stone type in people, and their incidence has been increasing in cats during the past 15 years.[114] These stones are composed of calcium oxalate monohydrate (whewellite) or calcium oxalate dihydrate (weddelite). Oxalate frequently is not detected by qualitative analysis, and quantitative analysis is necessary for diagnosis. Calcium oxalate calculi usually are white and hard. They often have sharp, jagged edges and may be single or multiple in number (Figure 266-13). Although they are found most often in the bladder and urethra, when stones appear in the kidneys they are most likely calcium oxalate. Calcium oxalate uroliths frequently

Table • 266-4

Restricted Mineral Diets for Cats

Cat Diet	Mfg.	Weight g	Energy kcal/can	Protein g	Fat G	CHO g	Fiber g	Ca mg	P mg	Na mg	K mg	Mg mg	Cl mg	pH range
CANNED														
Average Values*				11	6	3	0.4	325	280	200	180	20	260	NA
Struvite	0													
c/d-S	HIL	156	164	9.9	5	6	0.5	143	114	133	191	13	286	6.2 -6.4
s/d	HIL	156	215	8.8	7.1	3.3	0.4	130	109	181	196	9	348	5.9 - 6.1
Low pH/S	IAM	170	198	9.5	6.2	3.5	0.2	242	190	95	181	21	138	5.9 - 6.3
UR	PUR	156	217	8.6	7.6	3.4	0.02	190	170	90	200	10	290	5.9 - 6.3
S/O Control pH	WAL	165	175	7.5	8	1.9	0.2	170	210	210	210	15	180	6.3 - 6.5
Oxalate	0													
c/d-Oxl	HIL	156	162	9.5	4.5	7.4	0.2	154	125	67	202	20	115	6.6 - 6.8
Mod pH/O	IAM	170	198	9.1	5.9	3.2	0.2	233	173	99	267	21	147	6.3 - 6.9
S/O Control pH 0	WAL	165	175	7.5	8	1.9	0.2	170	210	210	210	15	180	6.3 - 6.5
Diet DRY	Mfg.	Weight g	Energy kcal/cup	Protein G	Fat G	CHO g	Fiber g	Ca mg	P mg	Na mg	K mg	Mg mg	Cl mg	pH range
Average Values *				8.5	3.8	10	0.6	280	260	180	105	25	180	NA
Struvite														
c/d-S	HIL	76	285	8.5	4.1	10.3	0.2	197	184	106	210	15	258	6.2 - 6.4
s/d	HIL	122	521	7.4	5.8	6.6	0.2	233	165	151	193	16	329	5.9 - 6.1
Low pH/S	IAM	102	441	7.8	3.9	8	0.4	236	203	112	198	18	191	5.9 - 6.3
UR	PUR	227	366	8.3	2.7	10.7	0.3	260	200	60	200	20	260	5.9 - 6.3
S/O Control pH	WAL	NA	390	8.8	4.7	8.3	0.5	170	210	220	230	15	510	6.3 - 6.5
Oxalate														
c/d-Oxl	HIL	76	286	8.5	4.1	10.2	0.3	196	162	85	209	20	244	6.6 - 6.8
Mod pH/O	IAM	105	451	7.6	3.9	8	0.4	238	205	104	305	19	151	6.3 - 6.9
S/O Control pH	WAL	NA	390	8.8	4.7	8.3	0.5	170	210	220	230	15	510	6.3 - 6.5
SEMI-MOIST		g	kcal/cup	g	G	g	g	mg	mg	mg	mg	mg	mg	range
Struvite														
UR Formula	PUR	42	120	9.7	3.7	6.5	0.3	370	400	60	190	30	130	5.8 - 6.2

Diets listed in alphabetic order by manufacturer. Common veterinary diets restricted in mineral contents and formulated to be acidifying or maintain a neutral pH. Although dry foods are listed for completeness, canned food is recommended for cats with a history of urolithiasis.
*Average values of commercial and specialty foods. *Mfg*, Manufacturer; *HIL*, Hills Pet Food Company; *IAM*, Iams Company; *PUR*, Nestle's Purina Petcare Company; *WAL*, Waltham; *CHO*, carbohydrate.

Box • 266-3

Suggestions to Help Clients Change their Cats' Diets

Changing a cat to a new food may not seem easy or convenient at first, but it may be necessary for some cats with feline idiopathic cystitis (FIC) and urolithiasis. To help clients and their cats through this process, the authors offer the following suggestions, collected from clients and cats that have successfully made the change.

1. Before starting to change diets, be sure that the cat is at home, feeling better, and eating its usual diet normally. Never begin the recommended diet while the animal is still hospitalized.

2. A simple way to start is to offer the new food in the cat's usual feeding bowl next to the old diet in a different bowl. Putting both foods in similar bowls can make the change somewhat easier. If the cat eats the new diet readily, then old food can be removed. If the cat does not eat the new diet after 1 hour, take it up until the next feeding. At the next feeding, repeat the process, always providing fresh new food. Once the new diet becomes familiar to the cat (usually in 1 or 2 days), it should start eating it readily. When this occurs, start to decrease the amount of the old diet offered by a small amount (about 25%) each day until the change is complete. Using this strategy, the change should be completed over a period of 1 to 2 weeks.

3. If necessary, small quantities (less than a tablespoon per cup or can of food) of the cat's favorite food, or meat or fish juices can be mixed with the new food initially to make it more appealing.

4. Cats should be fed in a quiet environment where it will not be distracted or startled by humans or other pets.

5. If a cat has food available all the time and refuses the new diet, it may be easier to start by changing its feeding schedule to meal feeding by only leaving food out for 1 hour at each feeding time. If the cat does not eat all its food every day, this may be normal. No more than a 10% loss of weight should occur during this transition. If the inappetence continues, offer the cat's regular favorite diet once again. After 3 to 4 weeks a different diet may be tried once again. Fortunately, several diets are available for certain diseases, and certain cats might prefer one over the other.

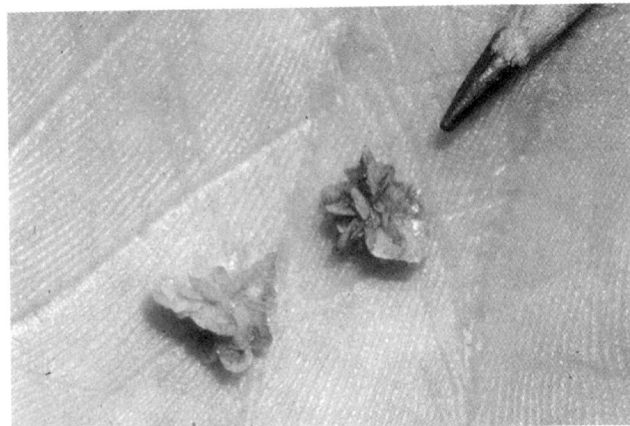

Figure 266-13 Calcium oxalate stones obtained from a cat after a cystotomy.

pH reciprocally increased risk of calcium oxalate uroliths.[114] Other dietary risk factors for cats with calcium oxalate urolithiasis were evaluated in this study, and the reader is referred to Table 266-3.

Results have shown that differences in breed, age, sex, and reproductive status did not contribute to the apparent reciprocal relationship between occurrences of calcium oxalate and struvite uroliths in cats.[116] Indoor housing has also been reported to be an independent risk factor for calcium oxalate urolithiasis.[121] It has been suggested that indoor cats could void less often and allow a longer period for urolith-forming products to aggregate in the bladder.

Although urinary acidifiers can enhance the solubility of struvite crystals in cats, they also promote release of calcium carbonate from bone, resulting in hypercalciuria.[124] Acidosis may be associated with decreased urinary citrate excretion and thus may predispose to calcium oxalate stone formation in humans.[125] Citrate forms a soluble complex with calcium and may normally be an inhibitor of calcium oxalate formation in humans, but this has not been studied in cats. Oxalate is derived both from the diet and endogenously from the metabolism of ascorbic acid (vitamin C) and the amino acid glycine. In human beings, increased dietary oxalate, increased colonic absorption of oxalate secondary to fat malabsorption, vitamin B_6 deficiency, and inherited defects of oxalate metabolism may predispose to the formation of calcium oxalate stones. What, if any, role these and other diet-related factors play in naturally occurring oxalate urolithiasis in cats is not known.

Breeds reported to be at risk for calcium oxalate uroliths include ragdoll, British shorthair, foreign shorthair, Himalayan, Havana brown, Scottish fold, Persian, and exotic shorthair cats. The Birman, mixed breed, Abyssinian, and Siamese cats had significantly lower risks for developing calcium oxalate uroliths.[116] As mentioned previously, cats with calcium oxalate urolithiasis are generally older than cats with struvite urolithiasis. Cats 7 to 10 years of age are reported to be 67 times as likely to develop calcium oxalate uroliths as cats between the ages of 1 and 2 years.[116] Male cats were reported to be one and a half times as likely to develop calcium oxalate uroliths and neutered cats were seven times as likely compared with sexually intact cats.

Cats with calcium oxalate uroliths should have their serum analyzed to evaluate for the presence of hypercalcemia, a risk factor for stone formation. Correction of hypercalcemia is important to prevent recurrent stone formation. Early intervention could prevent subsequent complications,

recur. If a UTI is present, it is usually a complication rather than a predisposing factor to oxalate urolithiasis.

The research implicating magnesium as a potential cause of struvite urinary stone disease in cats seems to have led cat food manufactures to restrict the magnesium content of diets, and add ingredients to promote more acidic urine in an attempt to minimize the struvite-promoting potential of their products. Unfortunately, an increase in the frequency of calcium oxalate urolithiasis appears to have occurred since these modifications began. Between 1984 and 1995 the proportion of calcium oxalate stones submitted to the University of Minnesota Urolith center increased from 2% to 40%.[123] Studies assessing the diet risk factors in cats with urolithiasis have reported that diets formulated to decrease risk of struvite uroliths by reducing

such as renal failure. Altered calcium metabolism may play a role in development of oxalate urolithiasis in some cats. Mild hypercalcemia was reported from the University of Minnesota Urolith Center in 35% of cats with calcium oxalate uroliths.[123] In a recent study of hypercalcemic cats,[126] calcium oxalate urolithiasis was noted in 11 of 16 (69%) with LUT signs. Of these, 73% had calcium oxalate urolithiasis. In a series of case reports, five cats with hypercalcemia and calcium oxalate urolithiasis presented for evaluation of LUT signs also had been fed an acidifying diet or received urinary acidifiers (D,L-methionine).[127] Seven of 20 cats (35%) had urolithiasis in a series of cats with idiopathic hypercalcemia.[128] In four cats that were evaluated, all had elevated urinary fractional excretions of calcium (Figure 266-14). Calcium oxalate urolithiasis has also been reported in a cat with a functional parathyroid adenocarcinoma.[129]

Calcium Oxalate Management

Attempts to dissolve calcium oxalate stones have not been successful, and surgery or voiding urohydropropulsion is required to remove stones. Postoperatively, a diet restricted in calcium and oxalate seems logical, but no evidence-based studies in cats with naturally occurring disease are available to support this recommendation. Moreover, high intake of dietary calcium appears to decrease risk for symptomatic kidney stones in humans, whereas intake of supplemental calcium may increase risk. Thus the timing and association with intake of other nutrients may also influence the role of calcium and other nutrients on stone formation, and these effects may be different in animals with naturally occurring disease than in healthy cats. Reducing only one of these minerals could increase the availability of the other. Dietary phosphorus should not be excessively restricted because reduced phosphorus could result in increased activation of vitamin D_3 to calcitriol by 1-α-hydroxylase in the kidney and cause increased intestinal absorption of calcium. In addition, urinary pyrophosphate derived from the diet may function as an inhibitor of calcium oxalate formation. Magnesium intake should not be restricted because it may serve as an inhibitor of calcium oxalate formation. Caution should be practiced if using dietary salt-supplementation to manage LUT signs (by increasing water consumption), especially in cats with reduced renal function[131] (cardiovascular disease or hypertension). Avoidance of Vitamin C is recommended because ascorbic acid is a metabolic precursor of oxalate, but no stones have been reported to develop in cats due to use of vitamin C.

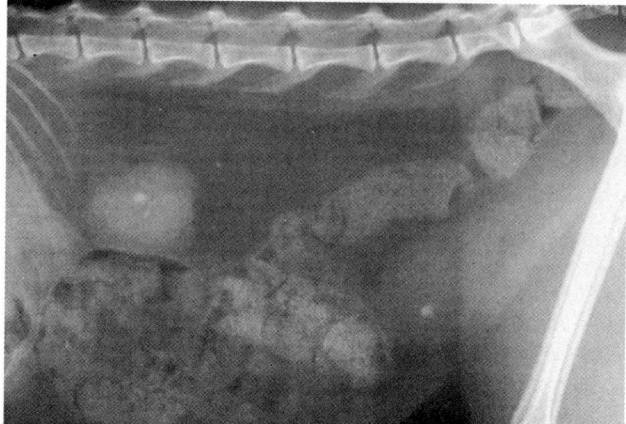

Figure 266-14 Radiograph of a cat with calcium oxalate stones in the renal pelvis and ureter. The cat was subsequently diagnosed with idiopathic hypercalcemia.

Administration of citrate as potassium citrate (Urocit-K®) could be helpful because urinary citrate may act as an inhibitor of calcium oxalate formation, and its alkalinizing effect may reduce bone release of calcium, although no data are available from clinical studies. Beyond this effect, therapeutic manipulation of urine pH is not known to be beneficial because oxalate solubility is relatively unaffected by a wide range of urine pH. The recommended dose of potassium citrate is 100 to 150 mg/kg/day but it is unclear if this dose will actually increase urinary citrate in cats. A number of commercial diets that have been used in attempts to prevent recurrence of oxalate stones are available and listed in Table 266-3, but no evidence-based outcomes of their use have been published.

Urate Urolithiasis

When evaluating mineral composition of 20,343 feline uroliths at the University of Minnesota Urolith Center, only 5.6% were composed of uric acid and urate.[132] Urate stones in cats are composed of uric acid and the monobasic ammonium salt of uric acid (ammonium acid urate). Calcium oxalate may be a secondary component of some urate stones, and those found in cats with portosystemic shunts often contain struvite in addition to urate.[123] Often times, the cause or causes of urate urolith formation are unknown. Urate calculi are small, brittle, spherical stones with concentric laminations. They usually are multiple in number and light yellow, brown, or green in color. They are found most often in the bladder and urethra, and the recurrence rate may be as high as 30% to 50%. When it occurs, UTI is a complication of urate urolithiasis rather than a predisposing cause.

Urate Management Attempts to dissolve urate stones have not been successful, and surgery or voiding urohydropropulsion is required to remove stones. Dissolution and prevention protocols for *dogs* include some combination of urine dilution, low-purine diet, alkalinization of urine, and allopurinol. Dissolution of an ammonium urate stone in a cat was reported to occur using a combination of allopurinol and a diet relatively low in purine precursors.[132] Although allopurinol will reduce the formation of uric acid, xanthine uroliths can occur, and the efficacy and potential toxicity of allopurinol in cats are not known.

Cystine Urolithiasis

When evaluating mineral composition of 20,343 feline urolith at the University of Minnesota Urolith Center, only 0.2% were composed of cystine.[132] Approximately two thirds of the stones were located in the bladder, and slightly more than one fourth of them were voided. Cystine uroliths are usually identified in middle-aged to older cats.[133] Most cats with cystine uroliths are DSH, but Siamese cats appear slightly over-represented. Bacterial UTIs are usually a consequence of cystine uroliths and not a cause. Although the cause of cystine uroliths is unknown, cystinuria results from a hereditable defect in renal tubular transport of cystine and other dibasic amino acids (ornithine, lysine, and arginine). Not all animals with cystinuria develop cystine uroliths; therefore the crystals appear to be a predisposing factor rather than a cause.

Management of Cystine Urolithiasis In addition to increasing urine volume in cats with cystine uroliths, cystine becomes more soluble as the pH increases. Therefore a non-acidifying canned food seems appropriate. (2-mercaptopro-plonyl-glycine) glycine (2-MPG), which decreases the concentration of cystine by a thiol-disulfate exchange reaction resulting in a more soluble compound, has been reported to be of benefit in preventing recurrent cystine uroliths in a cat.[132] No adverse effects were documented in this one cat. Potassium citrate can be used to further alkalinize the urine if necessary.

Sodium bicarbonate is not recommended because dietary sodium may enhance cystinuria.

Bacterial and Viral Cystitis When interpreting the urinalysis, caution should be taken when reporting bacteria from the sediment. These "bacteria" are likely the result of cellular breakdown products in the urine that exhibit brownian motion and look similar to bacteria. Antimicrobials should be administered based on quantitative urine cultures and sensitivities. Bacterial UTIs are rare in cats but are more common in those with defenses that are compromised due to other diseases or treatments. Cats with previous urinary catheterizations, perineal urethrostomies, and tube cystostomies are more susceptible to infections.[71] Cats over 10 years of age with LUT signs have been diagnosed with bacterial UTIs in greater than half of the cases, often in association with renal failure.[134] The bacteria that cause UTIs in cats are similar to other species with *Escherichia coli* being the most common isolate. The gram-positive cocci such as staphylococci and streptococci account for the next most common isolates.[135]

Investigation of viruses as a causative agent of LUT signs began in the 1960s. Virus-like particles (suspected to be calicivirus) were identified in the matrix of urethral plugs from some male cats with urinary obstruction.[123] The isolation of feline calicivirus, bovine herpesvirus 4, and feline syncytia-forming virus from cats with naturally occurring LUT signs has also been reported.[136] Most recently, Rice and colleagues[137] documented feline caliciviruses (FCVs) from one female cat with FIC and one male cat with obstructive FIC in the 40 cats they evaluated. These viruses (FCV-U1 and FCV-U2, respectively) were genetically distinct from other known vaccine and field strains of FCV. What if any relationship viruses play in the etiopathogenesis in LUT sign in cats remains unknown.

CHAPTER • 267

Canine Lower Urinary Tract Diseases

Larry G. Adams
Harriet M. Syme

ANATOMY AND PHYSIOLOGY OF THE LOWER URINARY TRACT

The function of the urinary bladder and urethra is storage and voiding of urine. The urinary bladder acts as a low-pressure reservoir for storage of urine until voiding occurs. The urinary bladder consists of the detrusor muscle (smooth muscle), submucosa, mucosa (composed of transitional epithelium), and serosa. The ureters enter the urinary bladder on the serosal surface and tunnel though the bladder wall obliquely to the mucosal surface. The oblique path of the intramural ureter results in a valvelike effect termed the *vesicoureteral valve*. The vesicoureteral valve, along with ureteral peristalsis and a compliant bladder, promotes unidirectional flow of urine to aid in prevention of ascending infection or urine reflux to the kidneys. A protective glycosaminoglycan layer coats and protects the bladder urothelium, which if defective may increase bladder permeability.[1]

The detrusor muscle is continuous with the smooth muscle of the urethra and helps form the internal urethral sphincter. The internal urethral sphincter is not an anatomically distinct sphincter; rather, it is a functional sphincter involving the proximal urethral and bladder neck.

The innervation of the lower urinary tract (LUT) includes sympathetic, parasympathetic, and somatic innervation. The internal urethral sphincter is innervated by sympathetic (α-adrenergic) innervation from the lumbar spinal cord (L1-L4) via the hypogastric nerve. The external urethral sphincter is composed of skeletal muscle and receives somatic innervation from S1-S3 via the pudendal nerve. The detrusor muscle of the urinary bladder receives parasympathetic innervation from S1-S3 via the pelvic nerve (causing contraction) and sympathetic innervation (β-adrenergic) from L1-L4 via the hypogastric nerve (facilitating relaxation). Afferent (sensory) information from stretch receptors in the bladder wall travels via the pelvic nerve to the spinal cord. Sensory information is also transmitted via the hypogastric nerve when overdistension of the bladder occurs. Afferent information from the urethra is transmitted via the pudendal nerve.

CLINICAL SIGNS OF LOWER URINARY TRACT DISEASE

Dogs with LUT disease most commonly have signs of inflammation or irritation of the bladder and urethra (such as dysuria, pollakiuria, or stranguria), discolored urine (due to hematuria), urinary incontinence, or inability to effectively void urine. Refer to Chapters 29 to 31 for an overview of these clinical syndromes. Dogs with clinical signs that suggest localization to the LUT (e.g., dysuria, pollakiuria and stranguria) may also have disease of the upper urinary tract such as extension of lower urinary tract infection (UTI) to the ureter, renal pelvis, and renal parenchyma.

Animals with rupture of the bladder or urethra often have systemic signs of uremia (anorexia, lethargy, vomiting, and diarrhea), along with indications of fluid accumulation in the abdomen or subcutaneously. Subcutaneous urine leakage may cause tissue necrosis and sloughing of the overlying skin.

DIAGNOSTIC APPROACH TO LOWER URINARY TRACT DISEASE

The reader is referred to Chapter 257 for an overview of the diagnostic approach to dogs with urinary tract disease and

Chapter 188 for neoplasia of the urinary tract. For dogs with signs of LUT disease, the *minimum* diagnostic evaluation should include history, physical examination, and urinalysis. If possible, the initial evaluation should also include urine culture, complete blood count (CBC), serum biochemistry profile, abdominal radiographs, and ultrasound of the urogenital tract. A thorough history should include frequency and volume of urination, estimated daily water intake, color of urine, any abnormal odor of the urine, evidence of straining or pain during urination, and evidence of urinary incontinence including age of onset, when incontinence occurs (awake, asleep, or continuous), and frequency of incontinence. The physical examination of dogs with signs of LUT disease should include abdominal palpation, digital rectal examination, visual and digital examination of the external genitalia, and neurologic examination of the pelvic limbs and perineal region.

Cystoscopy

If a cause of LUT disease has not been determined from routine diagnostic evaluation, transurethral cystoscopy (also termed *urethrocystoscopy*) should be considered. Cystoscopy is becoming an integral part of the diagnostic evaluation of dogs with recurrent or persistent LUT disease.[2] Although minimally invasive, cystoscopy does require general anesthesia to minimize movement. Cystoscopy is more sensitive than excretory radiography for identification of ectopic ureters and associated anatomic defects (Figure 267-1).[3] Cystoscopy is also useful for diagnostic evaluation of dogs with recurrent urinary tract infection (UTI) to evaluate for anatomic defects and to obtain biopsies for cytology, histopathology, and microbiologic culture.

Cystoscopy is useful for documenting the extent and location of LUT neoplasia and for obtaining biopsies for cytology and histopathology from lesions within the bladder or urethra. Using cystoscopy allows the source of gross hematuria to be localized to the genital tract, urethra, bladder, and left or right kidney and ureter with more certainty than by attempting to predict the source of hematuria based on when this is noted during voiding. Box 267-1 lists indications for cystoscopy.[4]

Diagnostic Imaging Abdominal radiographs are an integral part of the diagnostic evaluation of dogs suspected of having LUT disease. Abdominal radiographs should include the

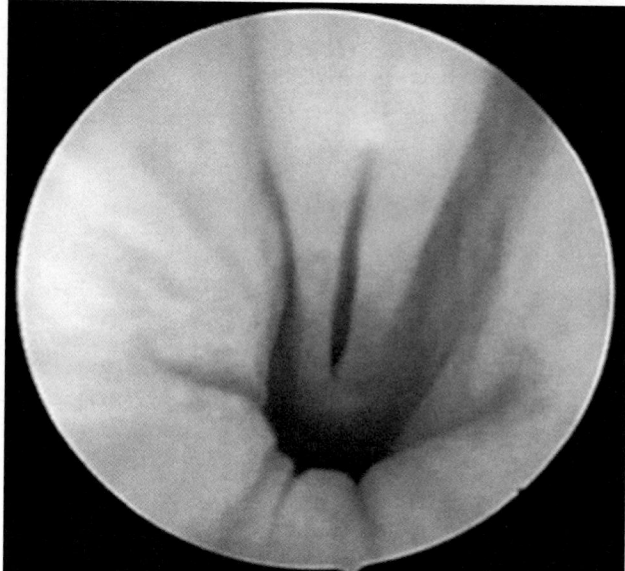

Figure 267-1 Cystoscopy showing an ectopic ureter opening in the proximal urethra along with abnormal urethral confirmation.

Box • 267-1
Indications for Cystoscopy

Localization of source of hematuria
Urinary tract neoplasia
  Determine extent and location of neoplasia
  Obtain biopsy for cytology and histopathology
Recurrent urinary tract infections (UTIs)
  Conduct examination for anatomic abnormalities or uroliths
  Obtain biopsies for cytology, histopathology, and culture
Urinary tract trauma
  Examine for perforations, ruptures, and patency of urinary tract
Urinary incontinence
  Examine for ectopic ureters and/or urethral anomalies
  Give periurethral injection of bulk-enhancing agents for treatment
Urolithiasis
  Confirm and remove small uroliths from bladder or urethra
  Obtain uroliths for quantitative analysis and culture
  Retrieve uroliths from bladder or urethra using stone forceps or stone basket
Fragment urocystoliths with electrohydraulic or laser lithotripsy
Flush bladder using Ellik evacuator to remove small uroliths or urolith fragments

---

entire urinary tract from the diaphragm to the caudal most portion of the urethra. Although the common anatomic landmark for distal collimation of abdominal radiographs is the coxofemoral joint, this is inadequate for evaluation of the urethra caudal to the pelvis, especially in male dogs (Figure 267-2). Failure to include the entire urethra may result in failure to diagnose uroliths in the urethra and potentially ineffective therapy such as incomplete surgical removal of uroliths. Abdominal ultrasound examination of the urogenital tract is a useful complement to abdominal radiographs when available to the practitioner although this modality has the limitation that, unless transrectal ultrasonography is also preformed, the urethra will not be visualized.

Abdominal ultrasound examination of the urogenital tract (combined with cystoscopy) reduces the use of contrast radiographic evaluation of LUT disease. However, contrast radiographs are still required for evaluation of some animals. Positive-contrast urethrocystography is the preferred technique for urethral defects such as delineating the extent and location of urethral strictures or extramural compressive lesions that preclude passage of the cystoscope. Positive-contrast urethrocystography is the preferred technique for diagnosis of pelvic bladder and rupture of the LUT (if cystoscopy is not available). Double-contrast cystography is the preferred technique for evaluation of the bladder for detection of radiolucent uroliths and mass lesions.

Urodynamics Urodynamic evaluation is indicated for evaluation of dogs with refractory urinary incontinence, although urodynamic equipment is only available at selected referral hospitals. Urethral pressure profilometry can confirm a diagnosis

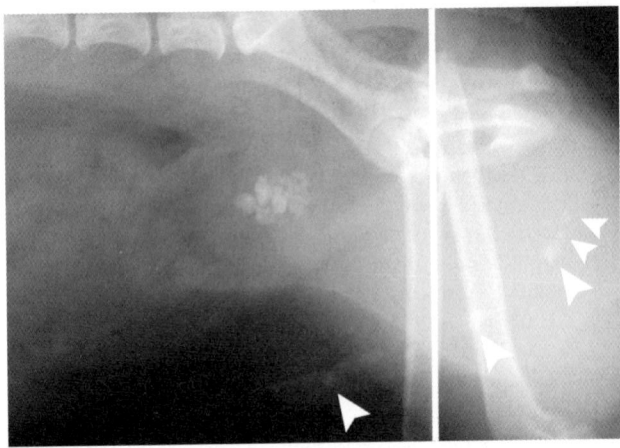

A

B

Figure 267-2 **A,** Abdominal radiographs from a dog with calcium oxalate urocystoliths and urethroliths. Reader should note that if the radiographs were collimated at the coxofemoral joints *(solid white line)*, only one of the five urethroliths *(arrowheads)* would have been detected. **B,** Calcium oxalate uroliths from the dog in **A.** Uroliths were removed by retrograde urohydropropulsion and cystotomy.

of urethral incompetence.[5,6] Cystometrography may be used to diagnose detrusor instability (so-called overactive bladder), which may be due to a variety of inflammatory diseases of the LUT or may be idiopathic.[7] Some dogs with refractory urinary incontinence may have mixed incontinence caused by both urethral incompetence and concurrent detrusor instability. Urodynamic testing allows for identification of the type and severity of urethral or detrusor dysfunction.[5]

UROLITHIASIS

Urolith Kinetics—Formation and Growth of Uroliths

A prerequisite for urolith formation is that urine is supersaturated, at least intermittently, with that compound. The point at which saturation of water with the pure chemical components of the crystal occurs is referred to as the *thermodynamic solubility product* (K_{sp}). However, the concentration of most urolith components in urine is actually greater than this, which can only be accomplished because urine contains inhibitors of crystal formation, which allow higher concentrations of solute to be held in solution. These solutions are described as being metastable (Figure 267-3). As the concentration rises still further, a point is reached at which the substance can no longer be held in solution; this is the formation product for the crystal (K_f). Because the concentrations of most urolith components in urine are in the metastable range, the question we should ask is not why some animals form uroliths, but why most do not. The ability of urine to hold more solute in solution than pure water is due to the many interacting ions that form soluble complexes, effectively reducing the free ionic concentration of each of the components.

Urolith formation is initiated by the precipitation of a submicroscopic crystal nucleus in the form of a mineral lattice. If the crystal forms from a pure solution, this event is termed *homogeneous nucleation*. It is, however, probably more common for heterogeneous nucleation to occur in urine, with the crystal nucleus forming on existing surfaces (such as cell debris, urinary casts, or other crystals) because this requires a lesser degree of supersaturation.[8] If the growth of one type of crystal occurs on the surface of another, this is termed *epitaxial growth*.

Once a crystal nucleus has formed it has the potential to develop into a urolith of the same composition, with direct crystal growth occurring whenever the urine is supersaturated for that substance. Crystal growth requires a lesser degree of supersaturation than crystal nucleation. Direct crystal growth is a relatively slow process and unlikely to account for the development of most uroliths, particularly nephroliths, which must form in the time that it takes the urine to pass along the renal tubule. It is proposed that a combination of crystal growth and crystal aggregation occurs in most humans that develop uroliths.[8] In contrast to direct crystal growth, aggregation of crystals can occur rapidly. Humans that develop nephroliths excrete large crystal aggregates, whereas the urine of nonstone formers contains only small crystals.[9]

A final important factor in the development of uroliths is the retention of crystals or aggregates of crystals within the urinary tract. Crystalluria is a normal phenomenon in dogs; the exit of crystals from the urinary tract must be delayed for uroliths to develop.

In summary, the known causes of urolith formation can be divided into those that favor nucleation; those that promote

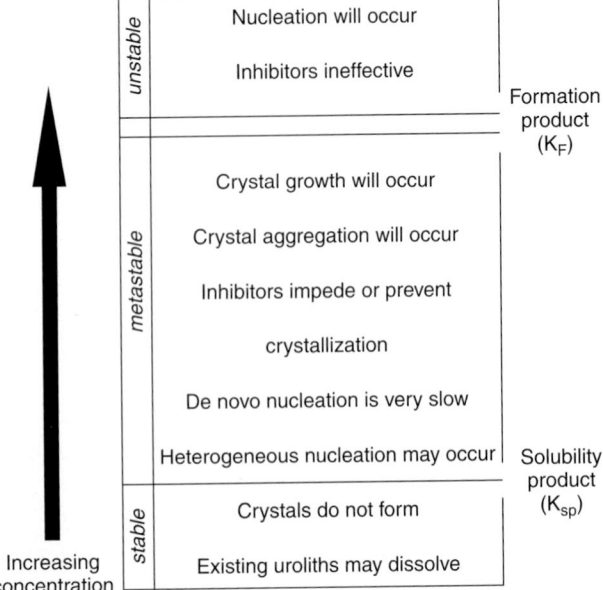

Figure 267-3 States of saturation related to the formation of crystals in urine.

crystal growth, aggregation, or both; and those that retain the urolith within the urinary tract so that further growth may occur. The importance of each of these mechanisms depends on the type of the urolith that is forming. Formation of some types of uroliths occurs principally (although not exclusively) because the concentration of solutes in urine is much higher than normal (e.g., struvite, cystine, and urate uroliths). Prevention of these types of uroliths is primarily directed at reducing the amount of solute excreted and promoting its solubility in urine (e.g., by manipulating urine pH). On the other hand, formation of calcium-containing uroliths (principally calcium oxalate) is much more complex.

Urine is probably always supersaturated with respect to these compounds. Although increased urinary excretion of calcium or oxalate does play a role in the pathogenesis of urolithiasis, factors that complex calcium or oxalate in solution, reducing their effective concentrations (e.g., citrate) and that inhibit growth or aggregation of crystals (e.g., Tamm-Horsfall mucoprotein) are of much greater importance in preventing urolith formation. These individual mechanisms are discussed in more detail in the section on calcium oxalate formation.

Role of Matrix

Uroliths are composed of a crystalline component and variable quantities of matrix. The exact role of matrix in urolith formation in humans and dogs is unknown. Although numerous proteins and glycosaminoglycan have been detected in human nephroliths, it is unknown which ones may contribute to urolith formation versus simply being trapped in layers of the growing urolith. Occasionally, canine uroliths develop that are composed solely of matrix.[10]

In Vitro Assessment of Urolith Formation

The *gold-standard* assessment of dietary or other therapeutic interventions involves a clinical trial measuring the rate of *in vivo* formation or dissolution of uroliths. However, the protracted time course of such trials and the difficulty in studying the effect of a single intervention in isolation has resulted in the development of *in vitro* methods for evaluating the effects of urine composition on urolith formation or dissolution. The two methods that have been used most frequently in veterinary medicine are the determination of relative supersaturation (RSS) and activity product ratios (APRs).

RSS is determined by measuring the concentration of various analytes (including calcium, oxalate, sodium, potassium, magnesium, ammonium, citrate, phosphate, pyrophosphate, and sulphate) in the urine, together with the urine pH, and then entering these values into a computer program that calculates a value for the ion activity product in the urine sample. The ratios of these activity products to the *thermodynamic solubility products* (K_{sp}) of their respective salts yield the RSS values. A RSS value less than one represents a urine sample that is undersaturated, whereas a RSS value greater than one represents a sample that is oversaturated, with respect to the compound being evaluated. Limitations of this method are that the computer program was optimized for calculations using human urine and that influence of promoters and inhibitors of crystal formation, growth, and aggregation on the measured free ion concentration cannot be included in the calculations. This technique has been applied to the analysis of urine from both dogs and cats.[11]

APRs are obtained by calculating ion activity products in the urine using a computer program in a similar manner to that used for determination of RSS. The difference with this method is that the measurements are made before and after incubation, with a seed crystal of the urolith type being investigated. The activity products will increase or decrease with incubation of the seed crystal depending on whether the urine is supersaturated or undersaturated with respect to the mineral being evaluated.[12]

Crystalluria

By convention, microscopic mineral precipitates within urine are called *crystals*, and macroscopic precipitates are called *uroliths* or *calculi*. The presence of crystalluria is not synonymous with disease, although it does signify that the urine is supersaturated with the mineral compound and is evidence that a risk exists for the development of uroliths. However, crystals may be found in the urine of dogs that do not have, and never develop, uroliths. This is particularly true of struvite and calcium oxalate crystals in all breeds and urate crystals in dalmatians. Conversely, some crystal types are not a normal finding and warrant further investigation even in the absence of uroliths. These include cystine, xanthine, and (in breeds other than dalmatians) urate crystals.

Crystals that were not present *in vivo* while the urine was in the excretory pathway, often form *in vitro* as the urine cools below body temperature.[13] Ideally, urinalysis should be performed as soon as possible without refrigeration of the sample when attempting to determine if crystalluria is present.

In dogs with urolithiasis, the type of crystals found in urinalysis may be helpful for predicting the mineral composition of the uroliths, although several caveats exist. If the dog's diet has been changed between the time of urolith formation and diagnosis, the crystals present at the time of diagnosis may be different from the mineral component of the urolith. Likewise, development or resolution of UTI with urease-producing organisms during the urolith formation and growth can change the type of crystal present in the urine.

Diagnosis of Urolithiasis

Uroliths are usually diagnosed based on results from radiography or ultrasonography. Occasionally, dogs have a history of voiding uroliths. Although uroliths may be palpated in the bladder or urethra, palpation is not a sensitive technique for ruling out urolithiasis. When uroliths are detected anywhere in the urinary tract, the entire urinary tract should be imaged with radiographs and ultrasound (or contrast radiography) to determine if uroliths are present in other locations (see Figure 267-2). Palpation of the external portion of the urethra and digital rectal examination of the pelvic urethra should also be performed to examine for urethroliths. Although most uroliths are radiopaque and are visible on survey abdominal radiographs, some uroliths are radiolucent (or strictly speaking have the same radiopacity as the surrounding soft tissues), and some radiopaque uroliths are too small to be detected. In one *in vitro* study, failure rates for detection of uroliths by survey radiography were between 2% and 27%, depending on the size and composition of the uroliths.[14] In contrast, the radiographic procedures with greatest sensitivity were pneumocystography, double-contrast cystography, and ultrasonography using a 7.5 MHz transducer with false-negative results of 11%, 10%, and 6%, respectively.[14] Therefore precise determination of the location, presence or absence of uroliths requires either ultrasonography or contrast radiography. Ultrasonography is preferred, if available, because of relative ease, lack of requirement for urethral catheterization, and it also permits simultaneous evaluation of the upper urinary tract for nephroliths or ureteroliths.

Once the number and location of uroliths is determined, the next step is to attempt to determine the type of urolith present to formulate a treatment plan. Catheter-assisted retrieval of uroliths or mechanical removal during cystoscopy provides urocystoliths for quantitative analysis. Because qualitative analysis methods are unreliable, the preferred quantitative analysis methods are optical crystallography, x-ray defraction, and infrared spectroscopy.[10,15]

If uroliths are not available for analysis (or pending the result of quantitative analysis), the chemical composition can often be correctly predicted from signalment, and results of urinalysis, urine culture, and radiographs (Table 267-1).[16,17]

Table • 267-1

Characteristics of Common Canine Uroliths

COMPOSITION	RADIOGRAPHIC DENSITY	SURFACE CHARACTERISTICS	URINE pH	CRYSTALLURIA	URINARY TRACT INFECTION	COMMONLY AFFECTED BREEDS*	OTHER
Calcium oxalate monohydrate (COM) and/or calcium oxalate dihydrate (COD)	Moderately to markedly radiopaque (see Figure 267-2)	Sharp projections, mulberry shaped or smooth round uroliths (see Figure 267-2); COD may appear jackstone shaped	Acidic to neutral	Calcium oxalate dihydrate crystals (square envelope) or calcium oxalate monohydrate crystals (dumbbell or picket-fence shapes)	None or secondary urinary tract infection (UTI) with common uropathogens	Miniature schnauzer, Lhasa Apso, Yorkshire terrier, Bichon frise, Pomeranian, Shih Tzu, Cairn terrier, Maltese, miniature poodle, Chihuahua	Often multiple small uroliths in bladder; multiple nephroliths if present
Struvite (magnesium ammonium phosphate hexahydrate)	Moderately to markedly radiopaque; larger uroliths appear more radiopaque (see Figure 267-7)	Single—may be smooth or speculated, may assume shape of bladder lumen (see Figure 267-8); multiple—smooth surfaces where uroliths contact each other, often pyramidal shape	Alkaline	Struvite or "triple phosphate" crystals ("coffin lid" appearance)	Urease-producing organisms (Staphylococcus, Proteus, mycoplasma); sterile struvite uroliths in cocker spaniels	Miniature schnauzer, Shih Tzu, Bichon frise, miniature poodle, cocker spaniel, Lhasa Apso	Uroliths >10 cm diameter are likely to be struvite; nephroliths are often staghorn shaped
Urate/xanthine	Radiolucent to faintly radiopaque	Multiple smooth uroliths	Acidic	Ammonium urate crystals (yellow-brown "thorn apple" or spherical shapes) or amorphous urate crystals	None or secondary UTI with common uropathogens; rarely, urease-producing organisms	Dalmatian, English bulldog, miniature schnauzer, Shih Tzu, Yorkshire terrier	PSS or other liver dysfunction; yellow-green urolith color

Type	Radiographic density	Urolith appearance	Urine pH	Crystals	UTI	Breeds	Comments
Cystine	Faintly to moderately radiopaque	Multiple smooth round uroliths in bladder and/or urethra; nephroliths may be staghorn shaped if present	Acidic	Cystine crystals (hexagonal shape) Cystine crystalluria always abnormal	None or secondary UTI with common uropathogens	Mastiff, Australian cattle dog, English bulldog, Staffordshire bull terriers, Newfoundland, dachshund	Positive urine cyanide-nitroprusside test; metabolic screening of urine available; males >> females
Calcium phosphate	Moderately to markedly radiopaque	Hydroxyapatit—multiple small uroliths with variable shape; brushite—multiple smooth round or pyramidal uroliths	Alkaline to neutral pH for hydroxyapatite, acidic for brushite	Amorphous phosphates or calcium phosphate crystals (thin prisms)	None or secondary UTI with common uropathogens	Yorkshire terrier, miniature schnauzer, Bichon friese, Shih Tzu, springer spaniel, Pomeranian, miniature poodle, cocker spaniel	Hypercalcemia is a predisposing factor
Silica	Moderately radiopaque	Classic jackstone appearance	Acidic to neutral	None	None or secondary UTI with common uropathogens	German shepherd, Old English sheepdogs, Labrador retriever, golden retriever, miniature schnauzer, cocker spaniels, Shih Tzus, Bichon frises	Males >> females

The breeds listed are those from which uroliths are most frequently submitted for mineral analysis; due to differences in breed popularity, this is not necessarily the same as the breeds that are at increased risk for stone formation.

URINARY SYSTEM

Two additional imaging approaches for determining urolith composition can be used. Weichselbaum and colleagues[18,19] reported an *in vitro* method of comparing urolith opacity to various concentrations and depths of iodinated contrast solutions to predict urolith composition.

Information from computerized tomography (CT) may eventually provide more objective means of predicting urolith composition in dogs. The peak attenuation measurements (termed *Hounsfield units*) of canine uroliths determined *in vitro* by noncontrast CT was significantly correlated with chemical composition in one study, confirmation of these findings *in vivo* is required.[20] In humans, CT has become the gold standard imaging technique for detection of uroliths,[8] and urolith composition can often be predicted from attenuation values obtained by micro CT scans *in vitro* and helical CT *in vivo*.[21]

Urolith Removal Techniques

Uroliths that may be medically dissolved include struvite, urates, and cystine.[22-24] For dissolution to occur, the urolith should be surrounded by undersaturated urine to allow the crystals to go back into solution. Therefore the location also affects the ability to medically dissolve uroliths; urocystoliths and nephroliths are amenable to dissolution but ureteroliths and urethroliths are not.[24] Urethroliths may be flushed back into the urinary bladder by retrograde urohydropropulsion for medical dissolution or mechanical removal.[25]

Cystotomy   Surgical removal of uroliths by cystotomy is the traditional method of mechanical removal of canine urocystoliths. However, use of newer, nonsurgical techniques for removal of smaller urocystoliths is increasing. It is notable that open surgical removal of uroliths is used in only 0.3% to 4% of human patients.[26]

Laparoscopic-Assisted Cystotomy   A recent report demonstrated that laparoscopic-assisted cystotomy may be used to remove urocystoliths that are too large to pass though the urethra.[27] This approach minimizes surgical trauma and may become more commonly used as veterinarians become more familiar with laparoscopic surgery.

Voiding Urohydropropulsion   Voiding urohydropropulsion is the removal of smaller urocystoliths by inducing voiding while the dog is positioned vertically so that urocystoliths pass with the voided urine (Figure 267-4).[28] Although the technique may be performed with the dog awake, general anesthesia facilitates complete urethral relaxation, preventing development of high intravesicular pressures that could cause iatrogenic trauma to the bladder wall. Cystoscopy may be performed immediately prior to voiding urohydropropulsion to evaluate the urethra for strictures that would interfere with urolith passage. If the bladder is not distended with urine, it is distended with sterile saline via cystoscopy or urethral catheterization. The dog is positioned so that the spine is roughly 25 degrees caudal to a line perpendicular to the effects of gravity, such that a line drawn through the urethra into the bladder is vertical (see Figure 267-4). The bladder is agitated, and time is allowed for the urocystoliths to settle in the trigone. The bladder is palpated, and the intravesicular pressure is gradually increased by manual compression of the bladder to initiate a detrusor contraction. Once voiding begins, the bladder is compressed more firmly to attempt to maintain maximum urine flow rates, dilate the urethra, and flush out the urocystoliths. The bladder is refilled with sterile saline through a cystoscope or urinary catheter and the process is repeated until no urocystoliths are passed with the expelled fluid. Then postprocedural radiographs or cystoscopy are performed to confirm complete removal of the urocystoliths. Although periprocedural antibiotics are sometimes recommended to

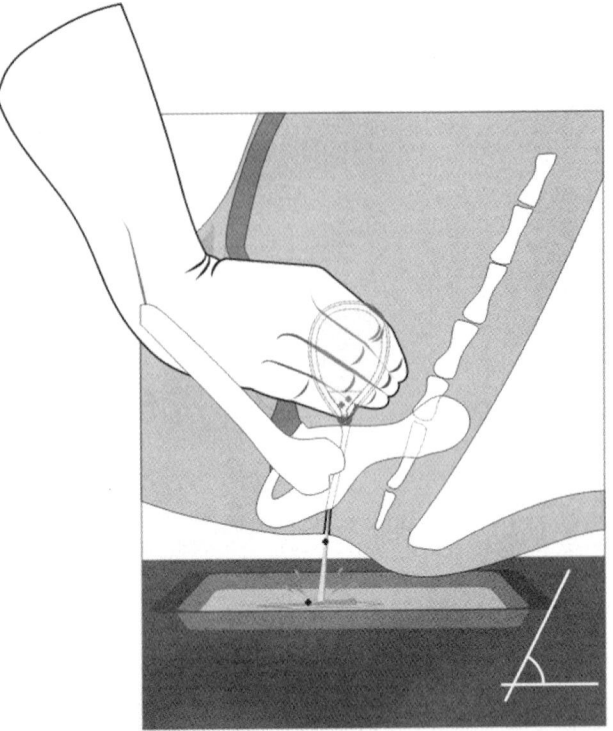

Figure 267-4   Diagram of a dog positioned for voiding urohydropropulsion. Reader should note that the trigone of the bladder is perpendicular to the effects of gravity, whereas the spine is approximately 25 degrees caudal this perpendicular line.

prevent iatrogenic UTI, this is not required provided proper aseptic technique is observed. If significant urethral leakage occurs when the dog is positioned vertically, inadequate bladder distention may prevent effective voiding of the uroliths. If this occurs, a Foley catheter is placed in the urethra with the balloon used to obstruct the trigone and the bladder is distended with saline. After agitation of the bladder to allow the urocystoliths to settle in the trigone, the Foley catheter balloon is deflated, the catheter is removed, and voiding urohydropropulsion is performed as described previously.

Retrograde Urohydropropulsion   Retrograde urohydropropulsion is the flushing of urethroliths into the urinary bladder, usually performed to relieve urethral obstruction.[25] General anesthesia is usually required for successful retrograde urohydropropulsion. If necessary, the dog or cat should be treated by decompressive cystocentesis and fluid therapy to correct acid-base and electrolyte imbalances before anesthesia to minimize the anesthetic risk. If the urinary bladder is overdistended, the bladder is gently decompressed by cystocentesis using a 22-gauge needle connected to a 60 mL syringe by extension tubing and a three-way valve. This lowers the urethral pressures proximal to the urethroliths to allow their retrograde movement. The largest urinary catheter possible is gently passed to the level of the distal calculus. An assistant compresses the urethra against the pubis via rectal palpation. A 2:1 mixture of sterile saline and sterile aqueous lubricant is rapidly flushed into the urethra distal to the obstructive calculus while compressing the urethral orifice around the catheter to prevent fluid leakage from the penis. An estimate of the total volume of flush required is 5 mL/kg of body weight or 60 mL, whichever is less. Once the urethra begins to dilate, the proximal (rectal) compression is released while flushing continues. If the urethroliths pass retrograde, the catheter is gently advanced to the trigone. If the calculus does not move retrograde, the degree of bladder distention should be assessed prior to repeating retrograde urohydropropulsion. If necessary, the bladder may be decompressed by cystocentesis before repeating the process. Subsequent retrograde flushes are done with sterile saline alone, because the urethra is well lubricated from the first attempt and saline can be more rapidly flushed through the catheter. Successful retrograde movement of all urethroliths should be confirmed by cystoscopy or radiography.

The aim of retrograde urohydropropulsion is to flush the uroliths into the bladder, not to push them with the urinary catheter. Pushing against urethroliths with rigid polyethylene catheters may result in excessive mucosal trauma, the catheter being forced through the wall of the urethra, or the catheter being passed round the urolith providing a route for temporary urine drainage but without moving uroliths back into the bladder. Catheter-induced trauma predisposes the dog to future urethral stricture formation.

Catheter-Assisted Retrieval Catheter-assisted retrieval of uroliths may be used to collect small urocystoliths for mineral analysis.[29] A urinary catheter is placed with the tip located within the trigone and the bladder is distended with urine or sterile saline. Next the bladder is vigorously agitated to suspend the smaller uroliths in the urine while rapid aspiration through the urinary catheter results in removal of the suspended uroliths along with the urine. If the dog tolerates urethral catheterization, this procedure may be performed without sedation or anesthesia.

Ellik Evacuator During cystoscopy with a rigid cystoscope the telescope is removed, leaving the cystoscope sheath in place in the urethra with the tip of the sheath just inside the trigone. An Ellik evacuator is attached to the cystoscope sheath, and the bladder is rapidly lavaged to flush sterile saline into and out of the bladder using the bulb attachment. The design of the Ellik evacuator allows the aspirated uroliths to gravitate to the bottom chamber while fluid in the top chamber is flushed into and out of the bladder several times (Figure 267-5). This technique can be used to collect uroliths smaller than the diameter of the cystoscope sheath, and thus it allows for removal of larger uroliths than a standard urinary catheter. This technique may be used to completely remove small uroliths from the urinary bladder or to obtain smaller uroliths for quantitative analysis and culture.

Stone Baskets Stone baskets may be used to remove uroliths from the LUT provided the uroliths are smaller than the dilated urethra. Stone baskets are usually passed through the working channel of the cystoscope, the basket is opened, and once the urolith is engaged in the basket, the basket is closed

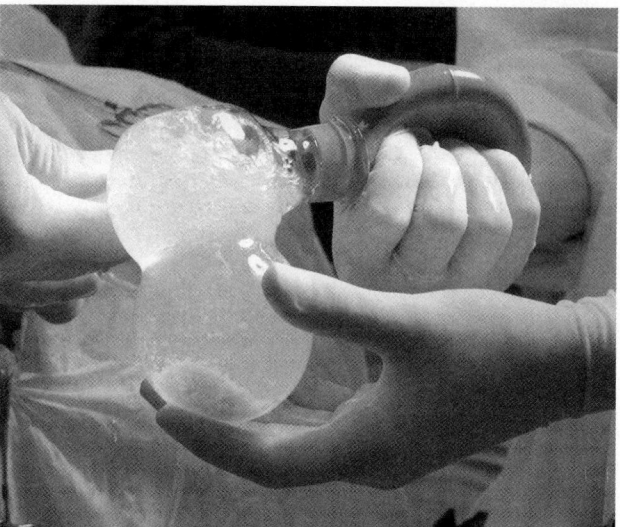

Figure 267-5 An Ellik evacuator attached to a cystoscope sheath used for flushing small uroliths from the bladder. Reader should note the uroliths in the bottom chamber.

around the urolith and positioned at the end of the cystoscope (Figure 267-6, *A*). The cystoscope and basket containing the urolith are then slowly withdrawn through the urethra with direct visualization to ensure the urothelium does not bulge around the urolith edges, which may indicate the urolith is becoming wedged in the urethra. This technique may be safely used to remove some uroliths that will not readily pass during voiding urohydropropulsion; however, caution is required to avoid getting the urolith wedged in the urethra.

Electrohydraulic Lithotripsy Electrohydraulic lithotripsy (EHL), the fragmentation of urinary uroliths with hydraulic shock waves generated within the bladder lumen, has been successfully used to fragment and remove urocystoliths in dogs (see Figure 267-6).[30] The procedure requires an EHL generator and cystoscopic equipment with a 5F working channel for the electrohydraulic electrode. The average treatment time is more than 1 hour to adequately fragment urocystoliths, which are then removed by use of an Ellik evacuator. Large urocystoliths may take several hours to completely fragment by EHL.

Laser Lithotripsy In humans, laser lithotripsy using the holmium laser has become the lithotrite of choice for fragmentation of large bladder calculi, ureteroliths, and nephroliths.[26,31,32] In humans, holmium laser lithotripsy has largely replaced EHL because it is faster and safer than EHL.

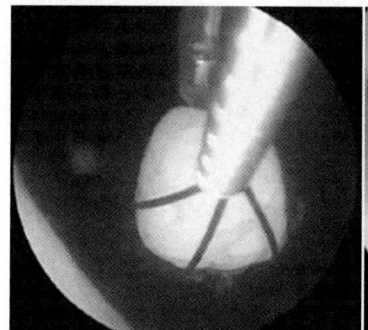
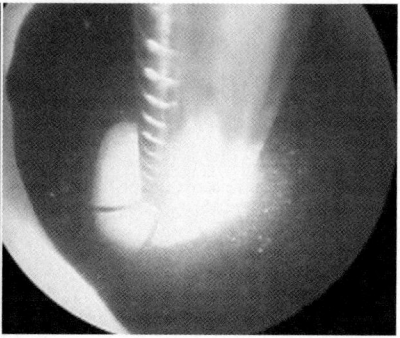

A   B

Figure 267-6 Fragmentation and removal of calcium oxalate monohydrate urocystoliths by electrohydraulic lithotripsy (EHL). **A,** Urocystolith held in a stone basket for fragmentation by EHL. The electrohydraulic electrode is visible dorsal to the basket. **B,** The electrohydraulic electrode has been activated generating a spark on the surface of the urolith.

The holmium laser is absorbed in 0.5 mm of fluid, allowing it to safely fragment uroliths within the urethra or ureter.[26,31] Also, because of the small diameter of the laser fibers, laser lithotripsy can be performed through small-diameter flexible endoscopes. Recent *in vitro* studies confirm that the holmium laser can efficiently fragment uroliths from dogs regardless of chemical composition.[14] Implanted urethroliths in male dogs were safely fragmented by laser lithotripsy using a holmium laser.[8] As holmium lasers become more widely available in veterinary medicine, this technique may replace cystotomy and urethrotomy for removal of uroliths.

Extracorporeal Shock Wave Lithotripsy Extracorporeal shock wave lithotripsy (ESWL) is fragmentation of uroliths using shock waves that are generated outside the body. Although ESWL is better suited for fragmentation of uroliths fixed in one location such as nephroliths or ureteroliths, urocystoliths have been successfully fragmented using ESWL. Because the urocystoliths tend to move out of the focal spot of the lithotriptor, uniform fragmentation does not occur consistently. In treating 14 dogs using ESWL, urocystoliths were fragmented into pieces small enough to be removed through the urethra in 8 of the dogs in one ESWL session. If the fragments are too large to be removed through the urethra, ESWL may be repeated or a secondary procedure may be required to remove larger urocystolith fragments.

CALCIUM OXALATE UROLITHIASIS

Calcium oxalate uroliths are usually composed of 100% calcium oxalate, although some also contain varying amounts of calcium phosphate.[35,36] Calcium oxalate is a common component of many compound uroliths. Calcium oxalate occurs as two crystalline forms: (1) calcium oxalate monohydrate (whewellite) or (2) calcium oxalate dihydrate (weddellite). Calcium oxalate monohydrate occurs more commonly than calcium oxalate dihydrate in canine uroliths. Some dogs have both forms in different layers of the same urolith.[10] The only clinically relevant difference between these forms is that calcium oxalate dihydrate uroliths are more easily fragmented by shock waves than calcium oxalate monohydrate uroliths.[26,37] Calcium oxalate uroliths are radiopaque and often occur as multiple smaller uroliths in the LUT (see Figure 267-2). The surface characteristics vary; uroliths may be smooth, mulberry-shaped, or have sharp projections (see Figure 267-2). Although calcium oxalate uroliths are not caused by infection, they may be associated with secondary UTIs because the presence of uroliths may interfere with host defenses against infection and contribute to recurrent infections. In one study, 52% of female dogs and 32% of male dogs with uroliths that contained calcium oxalate had positive urine or urolith cultures.[38] However, compound uroliths that were made up of less than 50% calcium oxalate were included in the study, and only about half of the uroliths were cultured, which may have resulted in an overestimation of the prevalence of UTI. Other studies do not support an association of calcium oxalate uroliths with UTI.[39]

Epidemiology of Calcium Oxalate Urolithiasis
The percentage of canine uroliths submitted to the Minnesota Urolith Center that are composed of calcium oxalate has increased from approximately 5% in 1981 to 35% in 1997, making it the second most common urolith in dogs.[10,40] This is similar to the increased incidence of calcium oxalate uroliths and decreased incidence in struvite uroliths in cats over the same time period[10] and in humans over the last 50 years.[8] The exact reasons for the shift in prevalence of calcium oxalate uroliths in dogs is unknown. Better medical management of struvite uroliths may be decreasing the percentage of struvite

uroliths, but this does not adequately explain the shift because a concurrent relative increase has not occurred in the percentage other types of uroliths.[10] Alternatively, increased use of diets designed to minimize the risk for struvite uroliths maybe increasing the risk for calcium oxalate uroliths (see section on diet, following). In humans, calcium oxalate uroliths occur most commonly in the upper urinary tract, whereas in dogs and cats they occur much more commonly in the LUT.[8,41]

Calcium oxalate uroliths occur more commonly in male dogs (68% to 71% of calcium oxalate uroliths submitted to two urolith centers) than female dogs (26% to 32%).[40,42] Similarly, in humans, men are affected three times more often than women; this has been hypothesized to be due to estrogen-induced reduction in urinary oxalate and increase in urinary citrate excretion in females.[8] Neutered male dogs have increased risk of calcium oxalate uroliths compared with intact dogs.[43] Obese dogs are more likely to form calcium oxalate uroliths, which is similar to cats and humans.[8,43] Breeds at increased risk for calcium oxalate uroliths include the miniature schnauzer, Lhasa Apso, Yorkshire terrier, Bichon frise, Pomeranian, Shih Tzu, Cairn terrier, Maltese, miniature poodle, and Chihuahua.[42-44] In one study, golden retrievers, German shepard dogs, and cocker spaniels had decreased risk of calcium oxalate uroliths.[43] Dogs that produce lower urine volumes and urinate less often may be more likely to have calcium oxalate urolithiasis.[45]

Etiopathogenesis of Calcium Oxalate Urolithiasis
Excessive urinary calcium excretion (hypercalciuria) or oxalate (hyperoxaluria) results in increased risk of calcium oxalate urolith formation. Calcium oxalate may precipitate on existing surfaces such as epithelial cells, cell debris, or other crystals (e.g., uric acid, calcium phosphate). This process, known as *heterogenous nucleation*, occurs at lower urine saturation for calcium oxalate than is required for homogenous nucleation. In humans, increased uric acid excretion (hyperuricosuria) often contributes to formation of calcium oxalate urolithiasis.

Urinary excretion of uric acid was slightly higher in miniature schnauzers with calcium oxalate urolithiasis than normal beagles[46]; however, because dogs have much lower serum and urine uric acid concentrations than humans (with the exception of dalmatians and English bulldogs),[22] hyperuricosuria is less likely to contribute to calcium oxalate urolith formation in dogs.

Hypercalciuria Increased urinary excretion of calcium (hypercalciuria) is a common contributing factor to calcium oxalate urolithiasis in humans.[8] Hypercalciuria is also a common finding in dogs with calcium oxalate urolithiasis.[46-48] Hypercalciuria is proposed to occur by one of three mechanisms: (1) *absorptive hypercalciuria*, characterized by increased intestinal absorption of calcium; (2) *renal-leak hypercalciuria*, characterized by a primary renal leak of calcium; and (3) *resorptive hypercalciuria*, characterized by increased bone demineralization.[8,49] Humans and dogs with *absorptive hypercalciuria* have increased intestinal absorption of calcium with the excess calcium excreted in the urine (hypercalciuria).[8] The mildly increased serum calcium (from increased intestinal absorption) causes an increased filtered load of calcium in the glomerular filtrate and reduced tubular reabsorption of calcium due, in part, to suppression of parathyroid hormone (PTH) levels by high normal serum calcium concentrations. The combination of increased filtered calcium and reduced tubular reabsorption causes hypercalciuria. The increased intestinal absorption occurs in the jejunum and is accompanied by increased intestinal absorption of oxalate, which contributes to concurrent hyperoxaluria. Approximately 50% of humans with absorptive hypercalciuria have increased concentrations of 1,25-dihydroxycholecalciferol, causing increased intestinal calcium absorption.[8,50] In one study, five of six miniature schnauzers with calcium oxalate urolithiasis were classified as having absorptive hypercalciuria.[46]

Renal-leak hypercalciuria is due to impaired renal tubular reabsorption of calcium.[8] Renal calcium loss reduces the serum ionized calcium, which causes increased PTH and 1,25-dihydroxycholecalciferol. Increased 1,25-dihydroxycholecalciferol causes increased intestinal absorption of calcium (and phosphorus), which returns the serum calcium to normal. The increased PTH also causes increased mobilization of calcium from bone, which could contribute to bone demineralization over time if dietary calcium intake is not adequate. Humans and dogs with renal-leak hypercalciuria have high serum PTH concentrations, normal serum calcium concentrations, and high fasting urinary calcium excretion.

Resorptive hypercalciuria and *hypercalcemic hypercalciuria* are closely related. Resorptive hypercalciuria is a subtle, normocalcemic version of primary hyperparathyroidism, whereas serum calcium is elevated with hypercalcemic hypercalciuria.[8] In humans, the most common cause of hypercalcemic hypercalciuria resulting in calcium oxalate urolithiasis is primary hyperparathyroidism. Other causes in humans include malignancy-associated hypercalcemia, hyperthyroidism and sarcoidosis, and other granulomatous diseases, although these have not been reported associated with calcium oxalate urolithiasis in dogs. In dogs, calcium oxalate uroliths have been reported secondary to primary hyperparathyroidism.[51,52] Dogs with hyperparathyroidism may form calcium phosphate, calcium oxalate, or mixed calcium oxalate and calcium phosphate uroliths.[51,53]

Hyperoxaluria Urinary concentration of oxalate is an important factor in calcium oxalate crystallization and urolithiasis, because on a molar basis, increases in urine oxalate concentration have a greater effect on urinary saturation of calcium oxalate than equivalent increases in urinary calcium concentration.[8,48] Oxalate is freely filtered at the glomerulus and undergoes bidirectional transport in the renal tubules with net tubular secretion. Urinary oxalate is derived mainly from endogenous production in the liver from metabolism of ascorbic acid, glyoxylate, and glycine with lesser amounts from dietary intake of oxalate. Dietary meat protein intake contributes the amino acids hydroxyproline and tryptophan, which are metabolized to oxalate. In humans, rats, and pigs, some of the normal dietary oxalate is degraded in the intestines by normal bacterial flora including *Oxalobacter formigenes*.[8] Some humans with calcium oxalate nephrolithiasis have deceased intestinal *Oxalobacter formigenes*, which may be caused by chronic antibiotic therapy for concurrent medical conditions.[54] The potential role of a paucity of intestinal *Oxalobacter formigenes* in calcium oxalate urolithiasis in dogs has not been evaluated.

Varying degrees of hyperoxaluria is present in up to 50% of humans with calcium oxalate urolithiasis;[8] however, hyperoxaluria has not been detected in dogs with calcium oxalate urolithiasis.[46] Primary hyperoxaluria is a rare genetic disorder of humans that causes either oxalate nephrosis or recurrent calcium oxalate urolithiasis. Primary oxaluria has been reported in both dogs and cats, but was associated with oxalate nephrosis rather than calcium oxalate urolithiasis.[55,56]

Water Source The mineral content of water may be a potential factor in calcium oxalate urolithiasis in humans, although the data are conflicting.[8] It has been proposed that increased sodium or calcium content or absence of trace minerals such as zinc, which chelates calcium, might increase risk of calcium oxalate urolithiasis. In one epidemiologic study in cats, the source of water (e.g., bottled, municipal) did not appear to affect the risk of calcium oxalate urolithiasis.[57] No reports exist on the effects of mineral content of water on calcium oxalate urolithiasis in dogs.

Modifiers of Calcium Oxalate Crystal System In humans the degree of saturation of urine for calcium oxalate overlaps between normal subjects and those who form uroliths. The reason some humans form uroliths and others do not is that urine normally contains several natural inhibitors of urolith formation and growth. Inhibitors are either organic or inorganic substances in urine that inhibit crystal formation, aggregation, or growth and if defective or deficient, may contribute to urolith formation. In humans, inhibitors of calcium oxalate include citrate, magnesium, pyrophosphate, glycosaminoglycans, nephrocalcin, and Tamm-Horsfall mucoprotein.[8] Although little is known about these inhibitors of calcium oxalate in dogs, they may play a similar role in dogs in determining which dogs form uroliths and which do not.

Two important inorganic inhibitors of calcium oxalate are (1) citrate and (2) magnesium. In urine, citrate forms complexes with calcium that are more soluble than calcium oxalate, lowering the ionic calcium concentration. Citrate inhibits both spontaneous and heterogenous nucleation of calcium oxalate crystals.[8] In humans, citrate is filtered by the kidneys and approximately 75% is reabsorbed by the tubules, with the major determinant of the amount reabsorbed being the acid-base status. Metabolic acidosis reduces urinary citrate excretion by augmenting tubular reabsorption of citrate, whereas metabolic alkalosis decreases tubular reabsorption and increases urinary citrate excretion.[8,58] In dogs, urinary citrate excretion is much lower than humans with less than 1% of filtered citrate normally excreted in the urine, although urinary citrate excretion increases dramatically with metabolic alkalosis.[58] Hypocitraturia has been reported in 15% to 63% of humans who form calcium oxalate nephroliths, with metabolic acidosis being the most important cause of decreased urinary citrate excretion.[8,59] In dogs, mean urinary citrate excretion was not significantly different between six miniature schnauzers with calcium oxalate urolithiasis and normal beagles; however, some individual miniature schnauzers appeared to have decreased urinary citrate excretion compared with the normal beagles.[46] Because hypocitraturia only affects 15% to 63% humans with calcium oxalate nephroliths, and because too few dogs have been evaluated to accurately define what level of daily urinary citrate excretion constitutes hypocitraturia in dogs, a role for hypocitraturia in calcium oxalate urolith formation in some dogs is possible, although unproven.

Similar to citrate's role with calcium, magnesium complexes with oxalate, reducing the urine saturation for calcium oxalate.[8] Deficient urinary magnesium concentration results in more oxalate being available to combine with ionic calcium; therefore lower dietary magnesium may predispose to calcium oxalate urolithiasis, a proposal which was supported by two recent epidemiologic studies.[39,60] Citrate and magnesium play complimentary roles by complexing calcium and oxalate respectively and lowering the urine saturation for calcium oxalate.

Pyrophosphate in the urine is another inhibitor of calcium oxalate. The amount of pyrophosphate in the urine is related to dietary phosphorus intake. Although the role of pyrophosphate in canine urine is unknown, diets low is phosphorus have been shown to increase the risk for calcium oxalate urolithiasis in dogs, which could be due to lowering of urinary pyrophosphate along with other factors (see Role of Diet, following).[39,60]

Nephrocalcin, synthesized by renal proximal tubular cells and the medullary thick ascending limb, is a potent inhibitor of calcium oxalate monohydrate crystal aggregation.[61] Urine from humans who form calcium oxalate uroliths contains nephrocalcin that lacks γ-carboxyglutamic acid and is tenfold less effective at inhibiting calcium oxalate monohydrate crystal aggregation than nephrocalcin from normal urine.[61] Lulich and colleagues[40] reported that urine from dogs with calcium oxalate contained different fractions of nephrocalcin than urine from normal beagles, which could also support a role for lack of this inhibitor in the pathogenesis of calcium oxalate urolith formation in dogs.

Tamm-Horsfall mucoprotein, synthesized by the medullary thick ascending limb and the distal tubule, is another potent inhibitor of calcium oxalate aggregation.[8,62] The self-aggregated form of Tamm-Horsfall mucoprotein, which is the predominant form of this protein in the urine from humans with calcium oxalate nephroliths, is a less effective inhibitor of calcium oxalate crystal aggregation and may even promote calcium oxalate crystallization.[63] The role of Tamm-Horsfall mucoprotein in dogs with calcium oxalate uroliths is unknown.

Concurrent Medical Conditions   Hyperadrenocorticism is associated with calcium oxalate urolithiasis in humans and dogs.[8,64] In humans, glucocorticoid excess leads to hypercalciuria secondary to increased mobilization of calcium from bone.[8] Glucocorticoids may also decrease tubular resorption of calcium, resulting in hypercalciuria and increasing the risk of calcium oxalate urolithiasis. Chronic metabolic acidosis may contribute to calcium oxalate urolithiasis in humans and dogs.[8,65] The proposed mechanism is buffering of excess hydrogen ions by bone phosphorus and carbonates. The calcium concurrently released from the bone during buffering is excreted in the urine, resulting in hypercalciuria. Acidosis also reduces the urinary excretion of citrate, a potent inhibitor of calcium oxalate.

Treatment of Calcium Oxalate Urolithiasis

Calcium oxalate uroliths are not amenable to medical dissolution; therefore they must be mechanically removed from the urinary tract (see previous section for details). Once urolith removal is performed, postprocedural radiographs or cystoscopy should be performed to document complete urolith removal so that the efficacy of preventative measures can be accurately assessed. Incomplete surgical removal of uroliths has been reported in up to 20% of dogs in one series.[66]

Prevention of Calcium Oxalate Urolithiasis

Calcium oxalate uroliths tend to recur in most dogs, with recurrence rates of up to 50% within 3 years of initial diagnosis.[67,68] Therefore preventative measures such as diet and medications should be used to reduce the risk of recurrence. Once all uroliths have been removed and before initiation of preventative measures, a baseline database should be obtained, including serum biochemistry profile (to examine for hypercalcemia, metabolic acidosis, or support for concurrent hyperadrenocorticism) and urinalysis (to determine urine specific gravity [USG], pH and crystalluria). Dietary changes should be attempted, and the clinician should add medications if persistence of calcium oxalate crystalluria or recurrence of calcium oxalate urolithiasis is noted.

Role of Diet   Increased water intake though feeding a canned diet or by adding water to the diet may be the most important recommendation to help prevent recurrence of calcium oxalate urolithiasis in dogs.[39,40,42] Increased water intake is also a long-standing recommendation for prevention of urolithiasis in humans.[8] Increased water intake results in dilution of calculogenic substances in the urine and increases the frequency of voiding, which helps remove any free crystals that form in the urinary tract. In normal miniature schnauzers, increasing dietary moisture from 7% to 73% increased net daily water intake and reduced urine calcium oxalate RSS, which is suggested to reflect decreased risk of calcium oxalate urolithiasis.[69] In an epidemiologic study, canned canine diets significantly reduced the risk for calcium oxalate urolithiasis compared with dry diets.[39,60] Addition of water to the diet or changing to a predominantly canned diet should be implemented as the first step in prevention of calcium oxalate urolithiasis in dogs.

The ideal diet for prevention of calcium oxalate urolithiasis in dogs is unknown, and most dietary recommendations have been made based on surrogate end points (such as changes in urine concentration of calcium, 24-hour urinary calcium and oxalate excretion or calcium oxalate RSS), rather than reduction of urolith recurrence rates. The dietary factors thought to contribute to calcium oxalate urolithiasis in dogs are undergoing substantial change, with several conflicting recommendations in the literature. Previously, dietary factors hypothesized to decrease the risk of calcium oxalate urolithiasis in dogs included reduced dietary levels of protein, sodium, and oxalate precursors and higher dietary water, calcium, phosphorus, and potassium content.[16,42] In contrast, recent epidemiologic studies indicate that dietary factors in dogs associated with an decreased risk of calcium oxalate urolithiasis included increased dietary water, protein, calcium, phosphorus, magnesium, sodium, potassium, chloride and decreased dietary carbohydrate content.[39,60] In addition, dry diets that resulted in increased acidification of the urine were associated with an increased risk of calcium oxalate urolithiasis.[39,60] These were epidemiologic studies of commercial diets; thus there may have been significant confounding effects such that an apparent benefit from one factor, such as increased dietary protein, could actually have been due to other factors, such as increased phosphorus or potassium content of the diet rather than the protein content per se, because diets high in protein also tend to be high in phosphorus and potassium. Likewise, these associations do not prove cause and effect.[70]

Although diets designed for dogs with renal failure have been recommended previously for prevention of calcium oxalate urolithiasis, because these diets are phosphorus restricted, the authors do not recommend their use for this purpose. Reduced dietary phosphorus was associated with increased risk of calcium oxalate urolithiasis in dogs.[39,60] Dietary phosphorus restriction promotes increased intestinal absorption of calcium, with the excess calcium excreted in the urine. The increased intestinal calcium absorption occurs because dietary phosphorus binds calcium making it less available for absorption. Deficient dietary phosphorus also increases renal production of calcitriol, which promotes intestinal absorption of calcium and phosphorus.[40] Additionally, increased dietary intake of phosphorus is thought to increase urinary excretion of pyrophosphate, an inhibitor of calcium oxalate crystallization.[40]

Because humans and dogs with absorptive hypercalciuria have reductions in urinary calcium when dietary calcium is restricted, it was previously recommended to restrict dietary calcium. However, recent studies in humans and dogs indicate that dietary calcium restriction actually increases the risk of calcium oxalate urolithiasis.[39,60,71] The proposed mechanism for this apparent paradox is that reduced dietary calcium results in increased dietary absorption of oxalate because less calcium is present in the intestinal lumen to bind oxalate. Increased intestinal oxalate absorption causes greater urinary oxalate excretion, which increases the risk of calcium oxalate urolithiasis. Therefore calcium oxalate preventative diets should not be calcium restricted. Although diets should be replete in calcium, calcium supplements between meals should be avoided because they may promote hypercalciuria and increase the risk of calcium oxalate urolithiasis.[72]

Because dry diets designed to maximize urine acidity were associated with a threefold greater risk of calcium oxalate urolithiasis and some authors have reported an association of acidic urine pH with calcium oxalate urolithiasis,[39,42,60] calcium oxalate preventative diets should not be maximally acidifying. Some diets recommended for prevention of calcium oxalate urolithiasis (e.g. Prescription diet u/d, Hill's Pet Nutrition) contain potassium citrate for the purpose of alkalinizing the urine, whereas other diets do not (e.g., Waltham® Canine S/O Lower Urinary Tract Support Diet, Waltham).

Some authors have recommended targeting a urine pH of 6.5 to 7.5,[42,65] whereas others suggest urine pH of 5.5 to 6.0.[47] The solubility of calcium oxalate is not greatly influenced by urine pH, but because of the potential for acidosis promoting hypercalciuria, the authors currently recommend a target urine pH of at least 6.5 to 7.0. Urine pH greater than 7.5 may promote formation of calcium phosphate uroliths and should be avoided.[53]

Currently the ideal protein content of diets for prevention of calcium oxalate urolithiasis in dogs is not known. Although dietary protein restriction has been recommended in the past,[65] the recent epidemiologic association of higher levels of dietary protein with decreased risk of calcium oxalate urolithiasis has caused re-evaluation of this recommendation.[39,60] The apparent benefit of increased dietary protein could have been due to other factors in the higher protein diets such as higher phosphorus content. In humans, increased dietary protein intake increases the risk of calcium oxalate urolithiasis through increased urinary uric acid excretion and contributes to increased bone buffering of acid derived from catabolism of the excess amino acids, thus promoting hypercalciuria.[8] Because dogs have lower urine uric acid concentrations and because the net acidification of canine diets can be controlled independent of protein content, dietary protein may not have the same effects on recurrence of calcium oxalate urolithiasis in dogs compared with humans.

The ideal dietary sodium content for prevention of calcium oxalate urolithiasis is also controversial. Dietary sodium restriction has previously been recommended based on the hypothesis that minimizing natruresis would concurrently minimize hypercalciuria.[65] However, recent epidemiologic studies associated higher dietary sodium with decreased risk of calcium oxalate urolithiasis.[39,60] In another study using normal dogs, increased dietary sodium (0.3 g of sodium per 100 kcal) reduced urine calcium oxalate RSS, compared with a low sodium diet (0.05 g of sodium per 100 kcal).[47,69] These authors have suggested that calcium oxalate preventative diets should not be sodium restricted or overly sodium supplemented. In a different study in normal dogs, increased dietary sodium increased total urinary calcium and sodium excretion per day, but it decreased the urinary calcium *concentration* because of the diuretic effects of increased dietary sodium.[60] Because crystallization risk is more affected by urinary concentration of calcium and oxalate than the amount excreted per day, the dilutional effects of higher dietary sodium may offset the tendency toward hypercalciuria.

The commercial diets most often recommended to reduce the risk of calcium oxalate urolithiasis include Waltham® Canine S/O Lower Urinary Tract Support Diet and Hill's Prescription diet u/d®.[47,65,67,73] Diets with high fat content such as Prescription diet u/d® should be avoided in dogs with history of pancreatitis, obesity, diabetes mellitus, or hyperlipidemia. An alternative diet suggested for these animals is Hill's Prescription diet w/d® with supplementation of oral potassium citrate to achieve a urine pH of 6.5 to 7.0.[67] Urine RSS was substantially reduced when 17 dogs with calcium oxalate urolithiasis were fed Waltham® Canine S/O Lower Urinary Tract Support Diet.[73] Reduced RSS is suggested to reflect decreased risk of calcium oxalate urolithiasis; however, this is a surrogate end point with the ideal end point being an actual reduction in the urolith recurrence rates. Clinical trials demonstrating reduction of recurrence rates of calcium oxalate urolithiasis are needed to verify efficacy of currently recommended diets.

Medications   Dietary therapy alone will not uniformly prevent calcium oxalate urolith recurrence. If calcium oxalate uroliths recur despite dietary therapy, if calcium oxalate crystalluria is persistent, or if both occur, medications should be considered.

Thiazide Diuretics   Thiazide diuretics are proven to reduce urinary calcium excretion and reduce the recurrence of calcium oxalate urolithiasis in humans.[8,74] In normal dogs, administration of chlorothiazide did not reduce urinary calcium excretion, although these dogs were water loaded, which may have prevented the hypocalciuric effects.[75] In contrast, administration of hydrochlorothiazide decreased urinary calcium excretion and urine calcium concentration in dogs with calcium oxalate urolithiasis.[76] The reduction in urinary calcium was greatest in dogs with the highest pretreatment urine calcium concentrations and when combined with dietary therapy using Prescription diet u/d®.

Hydrochlorothiazide (2 mg/kg orally every 12 hours) should be considered in dogs that have persistence of calcium oxalate crystalluria or recurrence of calcium oxalate urolithiasis despite diet therapy. Thiazide diuretics cause subclinical volume depletion resulting in increased proximal tubular reabsorption of sodium and calcium.[76] This effect may be blunted or prevented by increased dietary sodium content and increased water intake. Therefore the benefit of hydrochlorothiazide needs to be evaluated in conjunction with canned diets with higher sodium content.

Potassium Citrate   Potassium citrate supplementation has been shown to reduce recurrence of calcium oxalate uroliths in humans either when given specifically for hypocitraturia or when done empirically without 24-hour urine collection to determine if hypocitraturia is present.[59] In humans, oral potassium citrate increases urine pH, which causes decreased tubular resorption of citrate, thus increasing urinary citrate excretion.[8]

In the veterinary literature, conflicting opinions exist concerning the utility of potassium citrate for prevention of calcium oxalate urolithiasis in dogs. Potassium citrate supplementation has been recommended at a dose of 50 to 75 mg/kg orally every 12 hours if the urine pH is acidic or if calcium oxalate crystals are still present despite dietary therapy.[42,77] In one study with normal dogs, potassium citrate supplementation did not significantly increase the mean urinary citrate excretion; although in three miniature schnauzers, supplementation did increase urinary citrate excretion and lowered the urinary relative calcium oxalate supersaturation.[78] In another study, potassium citrate also did not increase mean urinary citrate concentration but it did cause a dose-dependent increase in urine pH.[77] Potassium citrate supplementation would be expected to have the greatest effect on urinary citrate excretion in dogs with hypocitraturia or metabolic acidosis; however, this has not been reported. The effectiveness of potassium citrate supplementation for reducing recurrence of calcium oxalate urolithiasis in dogs has also not been reported. Nonetheless, once dietary and hydrochlorothiazide therapy have been implemented, if calcium oxalate crystalluria is persistent or calcium oxalate uroliths recur, the authors recommend potassium citrate given to effect to achieve a urine pH of 6.5 to 7.0 using a starting dose of 50 to 75 mg/kg orally, every 12 hours. If the urine pH is already above 7.0 to 7.5, then potassium citrate should not be added. The serum potassium should be initially monitored monthly during potassium citrate supplementation and the dose reduced if hyperkalemia occurs.

Vitamins   Supplementation of vitamin C or vitamin D should be avoided in dogs with calcium oxalate urolithiasis. Because vitamin C is converted to oxalate, excessive vitamin C may contribute to hyperoxaluria and increased risk of calcium oxalate urolithiasis.[8] Vitamin D supplementation increases intestinal absorption of calcium, thereby promoting hypercalciuria and increased risk of calcium oxalate urolithiasis.[8,67] Although vitamin B_6 has been recommended, no data support any benefit from vitamin B_6 for prevention of calcium oxalate urolithiasis in dogs.

URINARY SYSTEM

Management of Recurrent Calcium Oxalate Urolithiasis
Because calcium oxalate uroliths recur in approximately 50% of dogs within 3 years,[68] appropriate surveillance methods should be used to document recurrences before the uroliths become too large to pass through the urethra. If recurrent urocystoliths are diagnosed early enough, many recurrences may be managed using nonsurgical methods. Although some dogs with recurrent calcium oxalate urocystoliths may be asymptomatic for extended periods of time, removal of urocystoliths is recommended to prevent urethral obstruction.

STRUVITE UROLITHIASIS

Struvite uroliths are usually composed of 100% magnesium ammonium phosphate hexahydrate, although some also contain varying amounts of calcium phosphate (termed *calcium apatite*) or calcium carbonate phosphate (termed *carbonate apatite*).[10,24,79] Struvite uroliths are commonly referred to as *infection stones* or *urease stones* because they are usually caused by UTI with urease producing organisms.[8,24] Struvite uroliths are moderately to markedly radiopaque (Figure 267-7). Although struvite uroliths may assume multiple shapes (e.g., smooth spherical, discoid) or conform to the shape of the bladder or renal pelvis, they are often faceted or pyramidal when multiple urocystoliths are present because the adjacent surfaces are smooth and flattened (see Figure 267-7; Figure 267-8). Large urocystoliths are most commonly composed of struvite. Large solitary urocystoliths may have sharp spiculated projections and assume the shape of the bladder lumen (see Figure 267-8).

Epidemiology of Struvite Urolithiasis
Although the incidence of calcium oxalate urolithiasis in dogs continues to increase, struvite remains the most common urolith type in dogs.[10] In 1997, 45% of all uroliths submitted to the Minnesota Urolith Center were composed of struvite and 35% were composed of calcium oxalate.[10] Struvite uroliths are more commonly located in the LUT (95%) than the upper urinary tract (5%).[24] Struvite uroliths occur more commonly in female dogs (71% to 85% of struvite uroliths submitted to two urolith centers) than male dogs (15% to 29%).[24,42] Female dogs are affected more commonly because they are more likely to have UTIs than males.[24] Breeds most commonly affected with struvite uroliths include mixed breed

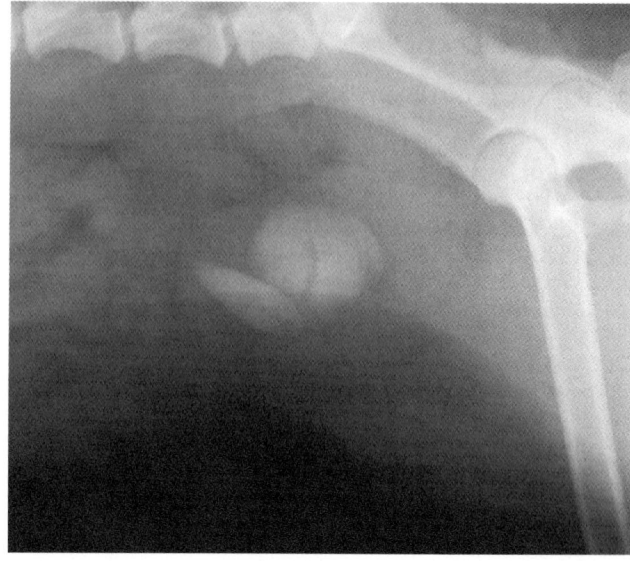

Figure 267-7 Abdominal radiographs from a dog with struvite urocystoliths. Reader should note the smooth surfaces where the urocystoliths contact each other.

dogs, miniature schnauzers, Shih Tzus, Bichon frises, miniature poodles, cocker spaniels, and Lhasa Apsos.[24] It is notable that all of these breeds except cocker spaniels and mixed breed dogs are also predisposed to calcium oxalate urolithiasis.

Etiopathogenesis of Struvite Urolithiasis
Most struvite uroliths in dogs are caused by UTI with urease-producing organisms.[24] Although recurrent, sterile struvite urolithiasis has been reported in related cocker spaniels,[80] sterile struvite uroliths are uncommon in dogs. In dogs, *Staphylococcus* spp. are the most commonly urease-producing organisms causing struvite uroliths, whereas *Proteus* spp. are the most common cause in humans.[8,24] Other urease-producing organisms that infrequently cause struvite uroliths include *Pseudomonas* spp. and *Klebsiella* spp.[24] Urease-producing mycoplasmas (termed *ureaplasma*) such as *Ureaplasma urealyticum* may also cause struvite urolithiasis.[24]

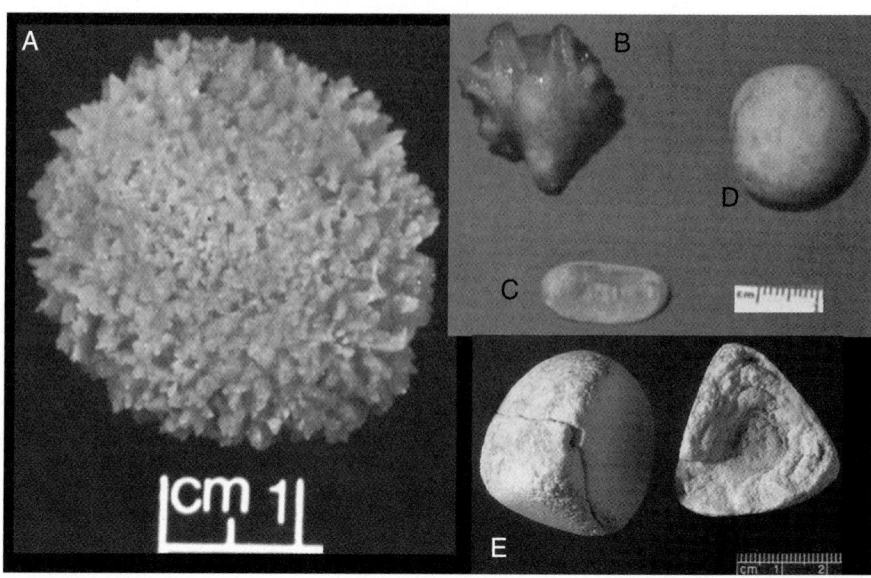

Figure 267-8 Examples of canine struvite uroliths. **A,** Spiculated solitary urocystolith. **B,** Staghorn nephrolith. **C,** Wafer-shaped urocystolith. **D,** Smooth solitary urocystolith. **E,** Pyramidal-shaped urocystoliths with smooth flat adjoining surfaces and distinct layers.

Urease cleaves urea (which is abundant in urine) to form ammonia and bicarbonate. The ammonium is available to combine with magnesium and phosphate, which are normally present in the urine, to form magnesium ammonium phosphate hexahydrate (struvite) crystals. The bicarbonate increases the urine pH, which decreases the solubility of struvite crystals. The ammonium also damages the urothelial glycosaminoglycan coating. This allows struvite crystals and bacteria to attach to the urothelium and may promote production of an organic matrix for crystal-matrix interaction. Attached crystals have more time to aggregate and grow into uroliths before being flushed from the urinary tract with the urine; therefore damage to the glycosaminoglycan layer promotes struvite urolith formation. Increased dietary protein increases the urine concentration of urea and phosphorus. However, unlike in cats where struvite uroliths may occur solely due to diet, UTI with a urease-producing organism is required in most dogs.[24]

Viable bacteria are trapped in the interstices of the layers of infection-induced struvite uroliths as they grow.[8,24] Bacteria have been cultured from the core of struvite uroliths that have been stored in formalin for years.[8] Therefore dissolution or fragmentation of struvite uroliths release viable bacteria into the urinary tract and will cause reinfection unless appropriate antimicrobials are used.[8,24] Antimicrobial penetration into struvite uroliths is limited; therefore as long as struvite uroliths are present anywhere in the urinary tract, resolution of UTI is unlikely and relapses usually occur within days of discontinuation of antibiotic therapy.

Treatment of Struvite Urolithiasis

Treatment options for struvite urolithiasis include medical dissolution or mechanical removal. The reader is referred to the section on urolith removal techniques. It is important that the underlying UTI be controlled with appropriate antimicrobials prior to manipulation or fragmentation of infection induced struvite uroliths to minimize the risk of urosepsis. Medical dissolution of urocystoliths in male dogs is associated with a risk of urethral obstruction once the urocystoliths are small enough to pass into the urethra. Therefore the clinical signs of urethral obstruction should be thoroughly explained to the owner if medical dissolution is used. The risks and benefits of mechanical removal versus medical dissolution should be discussed with the owner before concluding which approach is best for the individual patient.

Medical dissolution of struvite urocystoliths requires a combination of appropriate antimicrobial and calculolytic dietary therapy. Antimicrobial selection should be based on urine culture and antibiotic-susceptibility testing from urine obtained by cystocentesis prior to antimicrobial therapy. Antimicrobial therapy must be given throughout the entire dissolution period because viable bacteria are contained within the interstices of each layer of struvite uroliths. Two commercial calculolytic diets are available for dissolution of struvite uroliths in dogs: (1) Hill's Prescription diet s/d® and (2) Waltham® Canine S/O Lower Urinary Tract Support Diet. Hill's Prescription diet Canine s/d® has been proven to be effective for dissolution of struvite uroliths in dogs.[24] Waltham® Canine S/O Lower Urinary Tract Support Diet was effective for dissolution of canine struvite uroliths in an *ex vivo* model, although *in vivo* efficacy has not been reported.[81] Antimicrobial and dietary therapy should continue approximately 1 month beyond radiographic resolution of struvite urolithiasis because uroliths too small for radiographic detection may still be present.

Five to 7 days after initiation of antimicrobial therapy, urine should be obtained by cystocentesis for urinalysis and culture. Urinalysis should reveal decrease of the urine pH to less than 7.0, and the urine culture should be negative for bacterial growth. If the UTI is persistent, antimicrobial therapy should be changed based on antibiotic-susceptibility testing. Monitoring of dissolution therapy should consist of abdominal radiographs and urinalyses every 4 weeks. If bacteriuria, pyuria, or inappropriate alkaline urine pH are present, the urine should be cultured for aerobic bacteria and mycoplasma. If Hill's Prescription diet Canine s/d® is being fed, several changes on the serum biochemistry profile are common. Because of the low-protein content of this diet, serum urea nitrogen (SUN) concentrations should be low or low-normal, which confirms owner compliance with the dietary recommendations. Mild decreases in serum albumin and phosphorus concentrations are commonly present within 1 month of dietary therapy.[82] Mild increases in serum alkaline phosphatase activity have also been reported in some dogs consuming this diet.[24] These changes in the serum biochemistry profile are not expected with Waltham® Canine S/O Lower Urinary Tract Support Diet.

Average time for dissolution of canine infection-induced struvite urocystoliths is approximately 3 months.[24] Even large struvite urocystoliths may be medically dissolved, although larger urocystoliths take longer to dissolve than smaller uroliths because they have less surface area relative to their volume. Many of the symptoms of LUT inflammation (dysuria and pollakiuria) resolve during the first 10 days of therapy despite the presence of the urolith, which is likely attributable to control of the UTI.[24]

A common cause of failure to effectively dissolve struvite uroliths is inadequate control of the UTI. Therefore if therapeutic attempts fail or cease, urinalysis and urine culture should be repeated. Another common cause of dissolution failure is that if the struvite urolith contains layers of calcium apatite, carbonate apatite, or calcium oxalate, this may prevent dissolution of the struvite component of the urolith.[24,42] If any of the layers of the urolith contain more than 20% of nonstruvite minerals, dissolution is unlikely to occur.[42] Another common cause of failure to dissolve suspected struvite uroliths is that the urolith is composed of another mineral other than struvite.[24,42] If medical dissolution is unsuccessful, mechanical removal of the urolith should proceed with quantitative analysis of the retrieved uroliths.

Sterile struvite urocystoliths in dogs have been successfully dissolved using calculolytic dietary therapy alone or using urinary acidifiers without calculolytic diets.[24,80] Antibiotic therapy is not required for dissolution of sterile struvite uroliths. Sterile struvite uroliths dissolve more quickly (3 to 6 weeks) than infection-induced uroliths.[24,80]

Medications   Acetohydroxamic acid (AHA; Lithostat®) is a competitive and noncompetitive enzyme inhibitor of urease. Inhibition of microbial ureases prevents the breakdown of urea to form ammonium and bicarbonate, thereby lowering the urine pH and the concentration of ammonium. AHA has been used as an adjunct to dietary and antimicrobial therapy to promote dissolution of refractory struvite uroliths at a dose of 12.5 mg/kg orally, every 12 hours. However, AHA commonly causes side effects in dogs including hemolytic anemia, anorexia, vomiting, hyperbilirubinemia, and bilirubinuria.[24] Therefore the authors do not recommend AHA therapy unless mechanical removal of the struvite uroliths also poses a significant risk. Because AHA is renally excreted, it should not be administered to dogs in renal failure. In addition, AHA should not be administered to pregnant dogs because it is teratogenic.[24]

Urinary acidifying agents such as ammonium chloride are not necessary in management of struvite urolithiasis provided a calculolytic diet and antimicrobials are used. Persistence of an inappropriately alkaline pH of the urine is usually due to failure to control the urease-producing bacterial infection. Therefore the addition of urinary acidifying drugs to the dietary therapy is unlikely to reduce the urine pH and may cause metabolic acidosis.

One report exists of dissolution of sterile struvite nephroliths in two dogs using an amino acid preparation, most

URINARY SYSTEM

likely through production of acidic urine pH.[83] Dissolution of struvite urocystoliths in dogs using this amino acid preparation has not been reported.

Prevention of Struvite Urolithiasis

The key to prevention of infection-induced struvite urolithiasis is resolution of the underlying UTI and prevention of recurrent UTI. Antibiotic therapy should be continued for 3 to 4 weeks after mechanical removal or radiographic evidence of urolith dissolution. Then urine culture should be repeated 5 to 7 days after discontinuation of antibiotic therapy. If the urine culture is negative, another urine culture should be obtained 3 to 4 weeks later to confirm resolution of the UTI. If recurrent UTIs occur, prophylactic therapy with antibiotics administered at bedtime may prevent reinfection. The reader is referred to Chapter 262 for treatment of UTI.

The role of dietary therapy for prevention of struvite urolithiasis in dogs is complex. For dogs with sterile struvite urolithiasis, dietary therapy should be used long-term to prevent urolith recurrence; however, sterile struvite uroliths are uncommon in dogs. For dogs with infection-induced struvite urolithiasis, dietary therapy designed to prevent recurrence of struvite is likely unnecessary.[42] Prevention and control of recurrent UTI is usually effective regardless of diet.[42] Many of the breeds predisposed to struvite urolithiasis are also predisposed to calcium oxalate urolithiasis. In these breeds, dietary therapy to prevent struvite urolithiasis that includes urinary acidification and magnesium restriction could potentially contribute to formation of calcium oxalate urolithiasis later in life. Diets currently available for prevention of struvite urolithiasis in dogs include Waltham® Canine S/O Lower Urinary Tract Support Diet and Hill's Prescription diet c/d®. The authors only recommend struvite preventative diets such as Hill's Prescription diet c/d® for approximately 1 month after removal or dissolution of struvite uroliths while the UTI is monitored for recurrence. Once the UTI has been resolved, the dog can be changed to a commercial adult maintenance diet. Alternatively, Waltham® Canine S/O Lower Urinary Tract Support Diet may be fed long-term in breeds predisposed to both calcium oxalate and struvite urolithiasis because it is theoretically designed for prevention of both struvite and calcium oxalate urolithiasis.

Dogs with Calcium Oxalate and Struvite Urolithiasis

Certain breeds of dogs are predisposed to both calcium oxalate and struvite urolithiasis including miniature schnauzers, Shih Tzus, Bichon frises, miniature poodles, and Lhasa Apsos.[24,40,43] Some of these dogs form compound uroliths with different layers composed of both calcium oxalate and struvite. Other dogs form struvite uroliths in one urolith episode and then form calcium oxalate uroliths later in life or vice versa. In both of these situations, the struvite urolith usually forms as a result of UTI with urease-producing bacteria, whereas the calcium oxalate urolith forms due to patient metabolic predispositions such as hypercalciuria. Therefore management of these dogs is by control of the struvite component via control of the UTI and designing the long-term dietary and medication recommendations to prevent calcium oxalate urolith recurrence. It has been hypothesized that these dogs may be deficient in some inhibitors of crystal formation, aggregation, or both, which predisposes them to both urolith types.[24]

PURINE UROLITHIASIS

Naturally occurring canine purine uroliths consist of uric acid (and its various salts) and xanthine. Xanthine and uric acid are successive biodegradation products in the metabolism of purines (Figure 267-9). Purine uroliths may be of pure (100%) composition, or less commonly, may contain varying amounts of other minerals. For the purposes of the following discussion, unless otherwise stated, the term *urate* includes uric acid, ammonium urate, and the other salts of uric acid (principally sodium acid urate, sodium calcium urate, and ammonium calcium urate).

Ammonium urate is, however, by far the most commonly encountered of the urate uroliths, accounting for 86% of these uroliths,[10] and so recommendations for diagnosis, treatment, and prevention are skewed toward the management of this urolith type.

Urate uroliths are typically small, smooth, round or ovoid uroliths that are greenish-brown in color. Frequently multiple urate uroliths are present. Cutting urate uroliths in cross-section reveals concentric laminations. Xanthine uroliths are typically similar in size and shape to urate uroliths; however, they are usually yellow to brown in color. The majority of urate (97%) and xanthine (94%) uroliths that are submitted for analysis have been removed from the LUT[22]; however, nephroliths and ureteroliths may be underrepresented due to the difficulty in removing uroliths from the upper urinary tract. The size and smoothness of purine uroliths explains the relative frequency with which they cause urethral obstruction.

Urate and xanthine uroliths are generally characterized as radiolucent or only slightly radiopaque on survey radiographs (see Table 267-1). Positive-contrast studies may be required to visualize these uroliths: using an *in vitro* model, approximately 20% of ammonium urate and sodium urate uroliths were not detected on survey radiographs, although detection rates were improved if uroliths less than or equal to 1 mm in diameter were excluded from the analysis.[14] Detection rates using high-frequency (5 or 7.5 MHz) sector ultrasound scanning are better than with survey radiographs, although enumeration of uroliths is poor.[14]

Epidemiology of Purine Urolithiasis

Purine uroliths (predominantly ammonium urate) accounted for 8.0% of canine uroliths analyzed at the Minnesota Urolith Center between 1981 and 1997, making it the third most common type of urolith in dogs.[10] Purine uroliths may be retrieved from dogs of any age but are most frequently found in young to middle-aged animals; the average age of dogs with urate uroliths is reported to be approximately 4 years.[22] Naturally occurring xanthine uroliths are rare; most xanthine uroliths are retrieved from dogs that have been treated previously with allopurinol. Urate uroliths are most frequently retrieved from dalmatian dogs, in a recent study 61% of ammonium urate and 91% of sodium and calcium urate uroliths submitted for analysis were from dogs of this breed.[22] Pure urate uroliths occur more often in males than females.[22,35,84] This may at least in part be due to their propensity for causing urethral obstruction; it is possible that some urate uroliths are voided by bitches without being detected.

Etiopathogenesis of Purine Urolithiasis

The solubility of the purine metabolites, uric acid and xanthine, is much lower than that of allantoin. If urine is oversaturated with these substances, uroliths may form. Formation is promoted by a high dietary intake of purines and purine precursors and by the production of acidic urine. Production of alkaline urine decreases the risk of urate urolith formation by two mechanisms; increased solubility of uric acid and decreased production of ammonium ions.[85,86]

In human beings, infection with urease-producing bacteria may promote the formation of urate uroliths, due to the increase in ammonium ion concentration that results from hydrolysis of urea.[87] Although infection with urease-producing bacteria has been reported to occasionally contribute to formation of urate urolithiasis in dogs, in most dogs, UTIs

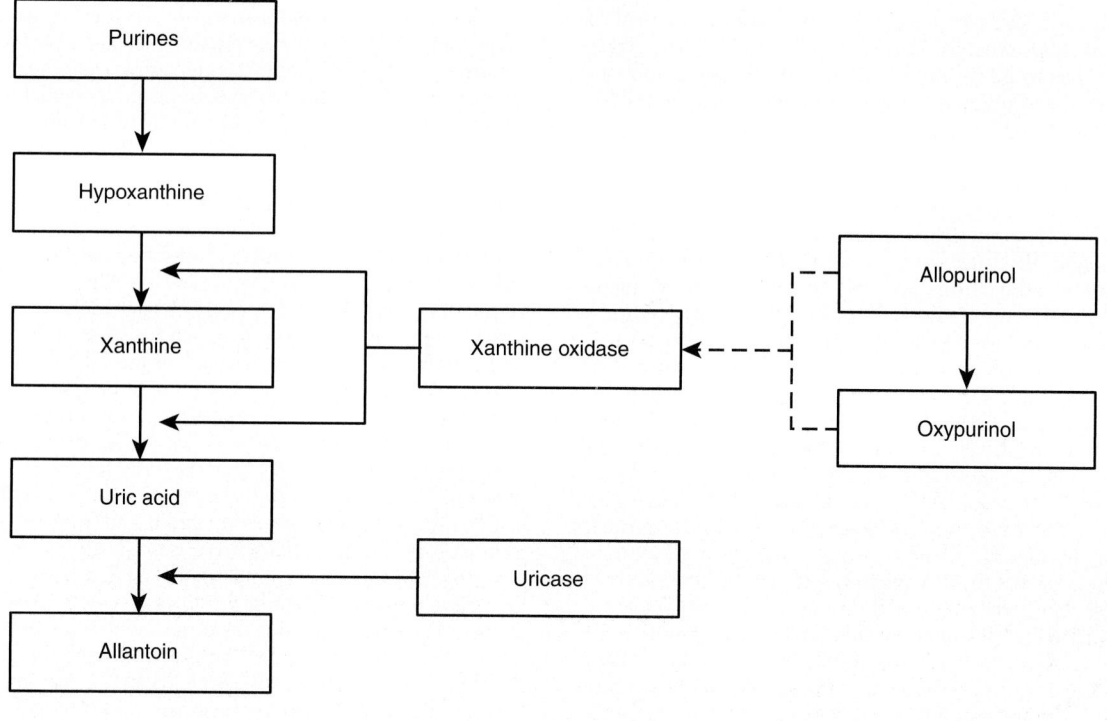

— — — — Inhibition

Figure 267-9 Metabolic pathway of purine degradation to allantoin showing site of action of allopurinol.

probably occur as a result of urolith-induced trauma or as a consequence of urinary catheterization, rather than as the cause of urolith formation.[22]

Dalmatian Dogs
Dalmatian dogs are predisposed to the development of urate urolithiasis due to the reduced rate at which they convert uric acid to allantoin compared with other breeds of dog, which results in 10 to 60 times greater daily urinary excretion of uric acid.[88] The uricase enzyme responsible for conversion of uric acid to allantoin is present in the liver of dalmatians in amounts comparable to those found in other breeds.[89] It is hypothesized that the reduced purine metabolism in dalmatians occurs because of a defective hepatic cell membrane transport system for uric acid.[90] The excretion of uric acid by dalmatians is increased further due to a reduced proximal tubular reabsorption of uric acid compared with other dogs.[91] Although all dalmatians excrete relatively large quantities of uric acid in their urine, not all form urate uroliths. Whether the risk for urolith formation in dalmatian dogs is solely related to the concentration of uric acid in the urine, or whether additional factors such as decreased crystallization inhibitors play a role, has yet to be definitively established. In one study, stone-forming dalmatian dogs had significantly lower urinary concentrations of Tamm-Horsfall protein than dalmatian dogs that had not formed uroliths.[92]

Hepatic Dysfunction
Severe hepatic dysfunction due to any cause may result in urate uroliths formation; however, the incidence of urate urolithiasis appears to be higher in dogs with portal vascular anomalies than with other causes of hepatic dysfunction.[93] Urate urolithiasis has also been reported in three miniature

schnauzers with microvascular dysplasia.[22] The predisposition of dogs with hepatic dysfunction to urolith formation is presumably due to hyperammonuria and hyperuricuria, which result from a reduced ability to convert ammonia to urea and uric acid to allantoin, respectively.

Non-Dalmatian Dogs
Approximately 30% to 60% of urate uroliths submitted for analysis are retrieved from dogs other than dalmatians.[22,44] Many of these dogs do not have detectable hepatic dysfunction, and the reasons for lithogenesis are unknown. The breeds of dogs that, in addition to the dalmatian, are reported to have an increased incidence of urate urolith formation are English bulldogs, miniature schnauzers, Shih Tzus, and Yorkshire terriers.[44,84,94]

Xanthine Uroliths
The most common cause of xanthine uroliths in dogs is therapy with allopurinol, particularly if the dietary consumption of purines is high.[95,96] Xanthine is an intermediary in purine metabolism that is converted to uric acid by the action of the enzyme xanthine oxidase. This enzyme, which also catalyzes the conversion of hypoxanthine to xanthine, is inhibited by allopurinol (see Figure 267-9). Hereditary xanthinuria is a rare disorder that occurs in human beings with a deficiency in xanthine oxidase. Spontaneously occurring xanthine uroliths have been described in Cavalier King Charles spaniels and dachshunds, which were suspected, but not proven, to have a deficiency of xanthine oxidase activity.[97,98]

Treatment of Purine Uroliths
Urate uroliths are amenable to medical dissolution; however, in some circumstances this will not be the most appropriate

mode of therapy, and direct surgical or nonsurgical removal of the uroliths is preferable. Obstruction of the urinary tract (if present) has to be relieved before medical dissolution can be attempted, and owners must be counseled that the risk of reobstruction is high.

Dietary Modification

Dietary modification may promote dissolution of urate uroliths in four ways: (1) decreasing the urinary excretion of uric acid, (2) decreasing the urinary excretion of ammonium ions, (3) urinary alkalinization, and (4) augmentation of urine volume. Reduced excretion of uric acid is achieved by feeding a diet that has a very low content of purine and purine precursors. Diets designed for urate dissolution are therefore restricted in protein content and more specifically contain no fish or glandular organs, which are particularly high in purine content. Protein sources that are relatively low in purine precursors include eggs and dairy products. Restricting protein content also reduces ammonium ion excretion by decreasing the amount of urea generated. In one study in normal beagles, increasing the protein content of the diet by adding casein, a protein source low in purines, doubled the urine saturation with ammonium urate.[99] Diets containing very low-protein content are unsuitable for feeding to growing, pregnant, or lactating animals. Homemade diets[22] and modifications of commercially available diets[100] have been published and may be more appropriate for feeding to growing animals, but the effectiveness of these diets in dissolving urate uroliths has not been systematically evaluated.

Alkaline urine contains very low concentrations of ammonia and ammonium ions, thus reducing the risk of ammonium urate formation. Production of alkaline urine is favored by eating a diet that is low in protein content.[101] The target urine pH for dissolution of urate uroliths is approximately 7.0. To achieve this goal, in addition to consumption of a low-protein diet, urinary alkalinizing agents are generally required. The agents that are most often used are sodium bicarbonate (25 to 50 mg/kg every 12 hours) and potassium citrate (50 to 150 mg/kg every 12 hours) with the dose titrated to produce the desired urine pH. Producing urine that has pH greater than 7.5 is not desirable because this may favor the formation of calcium phosphate uroliths.

For dissolution of urate uroliths, as with all urolith types, feeding a canned diet in preference to dry, or adding supplemental water to the diet is likely to be beneficial due to the resulting increase in urinary volume. Feeding a protein-restricted diet also impairs urine-concentrating capacity by decreasing the medullary concentration gradient (due to the low urea concentration). Other methods for augmenting urine volume are controversial. Adding salt to the diet increases urine output but has not been routinely recommended due to concerns that it increases urinary calcium excretion and may promote the formation of calcium-containing uroliths; however, recent studies refute this view (see the section on calcium oxalate urolithiasis).

Only one commercial diet is marketed specifically for the dissolution of urate uroliths: Prescription Diet Canine u/d®; Hill's Pet Nutrition. This diet has very low-protein content (10% to 13% dry matter, 2.4 to 2.8 g/100 kcal of metabolizable energy) and contains potassium citrate and calcium carbonate for urinary alkalinization, resulting in a urine pH of 7.0 to 7.5. Further alkalinization of this diet is generally not required. In a clinical study of 25 dogs with ammonium urate uroliths fed this diet and treated with allopurinol according to a previously published protocol,[102] complete dissolution occurred in nine dogs (36%), partial dissolution in eight dogs (32%), and no dissolution occurred in eight dogs (32%).[22] Similar results were reported when this diet was used for dissolution of sodium urate uroliths. Feeding of this diet has infrequently been associated with the development of dilated cardiomyopathy in dalmatians.[103]

The risk for development of cardiomyopathy may be increased in some non-dalmatian breeds of dogs, particularly English bulldogs, perhaps through development of carnitine deficiency.[22] Until further information is available, severely protein-restricted diets should only be used cautiously and fed for as short a period as possible in English bulldogs.

Xanthine Oxidase Inhibitors

Allopurinol is a synthetic isomer of hypoxanthine that inhibits the action of xanthine oxidase resulting in decreased uric acid production (see Figure 267-9). Allopurinol has a dose dependent half-life of 2.5 to 3.0 hours in dogs, although its major metabolite, oxypurinol, which is also an effective inhibitor of xanthine oxidase, has a longer half-life of 3 to 5 hours.[104,105] The bioavailability of allopurinol is not altered by administration with food.[104] The recommended dose of allopurinol for the dissolution of urate uroliths is 15 mg/kg every 12 hours.[106] Allopurinol and its metabolites are excreted via the kidney, so the dose should be reduced in patients with renal failure.

A variety of adverse reactions to allopurinol have been reported in humans. These are commonly minor and self-limiting, including gastrointestinal (GI) disturbances, pruritus, and development of a rash, but occasionally a life-threatening hypersensitivity reaction develops, characterized by fever, eosinophilia, hepatitis, renal failure, and erythema multiforme or toxic epidermal necrolysis.[107] Most human patients that develop the hypersensitivity syndrome have evidence of renal impairment prior to treatment with allopurinol, so this drug should be used cautiously in dogs with known renal insufficiency. Rare reports of adverse reactions in dogs receiving allopurinol exist, including hemolytic anemia and trigeminal neuropathy in one dog[108] and cutaneous erythema in a dalmatian receiving allopurinol and ampicillin.[22] Discontinuation of the ampicillin but not the allopurinol resulted in resolution of the skin lesions.[22]

The most commonly reported adverse effect of allopurinol therapy in dogs is development of xanthine uroliths, either in pure form or due to an outer shell of xanthine forming around pre-existing urate uroliths.[96,106] Xanthine urolithiasis is likely to occur if dogs are treated with allopurinol while receiving a nonpurine-restricted diet. Clinicians can sometimes dissolve xanthine uroliths by discontinuing allopurinol and instituting a low-purine diet.[106]

Portal Vascular Shunts

The surgical amelioration of portal vascular anomalies is expected to resolve hyperuricuria and hyperammonuria with the resultant dissolution of ammonium urate uroliths. However, no systematic studies have been performed to determine how frequently dissolution occurs after surgical correction of portovascular shunts. Similarly, although anecdotal reports of dissolution of uroliths in dogs with portovascular shunts fed low-protein diets exist, no controlled studies have determined how frequently dietary therapy alone is successful.

Evaluating Response to Medical Therapy

Owner compliance with dietary therapy can be evaluated by checking urine pH (should be ≥7.0), USG (should be <1.015), blood urea nitrogen (BUN) concentration (<10 mg/dL in previously nonazotemic animals), urine sediment examination (no urate crystals should be seen) and monitoring urolith size and number. Use of urine uric acid/creatinine ratios in randomly collected urine samples is not recommended because the measurements correlate poorly with 24-hour uric acid excretion.[109]

Prevention of Purine Urolithiasis

Urate uroliths recur frequently after urolith removal or dissolution. Preventative therapy after dissolution of uroliths is directed at minimizing the urine concentration of ammonia and uric acid by feeding a low-protein diet and by urinary alkalinization. The risk of urate urolith formation may decline with age. Prophylactic treatment with allopurinol is not recommended routinely due to the risk of xanthine urolith formation.

Although the feeding of prescription diets to all dalmatian dogs in the absence of a documented episode of urate urolithiasis is not recommended, it is prudent to ensure that diets that favor uric acid and ammonium ion excretion (such as those high in protein, particularly fish and meat, or that are acidifying) are routinely avoided in this breed of dog.

CYSTINE UROLITHIASIS

Cystine is composed of two molecules of the amino-acid cysteine, linked by a disulfide bond. Dogs that develop cystine uroliths have cystinuria, a disease in which increased amounts of cystine (and to a variable extent other amino acids), are excreted in the urine. The solubility of cystine in the urine is low; therefore dogs with cystinuria are predisposed to urolith formation. Most canine cystine uroliths are pure, but a few contain other minerals, including struvite, urate, silicate, oxalate, or calcium apatite.[10,110,111]

Cystine urocystoliths are typically ovoid and smooth, and light-yellow to reddish-brown in color. The size of cystine uroliths is variable, but they are often small, and multiple uroliths may be present.[23] Cystine uroliths that are submitted for analysis have generally been removed from the LUT, and this urolith type is relatively frequently associated with urethral obstruction.[23] It is reported that Newfoundlands have a relatively high incidence of cystine nephroliths,[112] although this urolith type does not appear to be over-represented in nephrolith submissions as a whole.[23,113]

Although the *in vitro* radiopacity of cystine uroliths is similar to that of struvite and silica; small cystine uroliths are often difficult to visualize in giant breed dogs. If cystine uroliths are of sufficient size, they can be detected by survey radiography. Small uroliths are detected more reliably by double-contrast cystography or ultrasonography.[14]

Epidemiology of Cystine Urolithiasis
The prevalence of cystine urolithiasis is highly dependent on geographic location. The prevalence in the United States is only 1% to 2%,[10,110] whereas the prevalence in Europe is reportedly as high as 8% in Sweden and 26% in central Spain.[111,114]

Cystine urolithiasis occurs predominantly (98%) in male dogs,[23] although cystinuria may occur in dogs of either gender.[112] The typical age at which cystine uroliths are first diagnosed is 3 to 8 years.[115] Somewhat surprisingly, cystine uroliths are not common in very young dogs.[10] Cystine uroliths have been reported in many breeds of dog, those that are reportedly over-represented include Mastiffs, Australian cattle dogs, English bulldogs, Chihuahuas, Newfoundlands, pit bull terriers, and dachshunds.[84,110] Cystine uroliths are also found frequently in mixed breed dogs, although they are not over-represented.[23,110]

Etiopathogenesis of Cystine Urolithiasis
In the normal animal, cystine is freely filtered at the glomerulus and then actively reabsorbed in the proximal tubules; in cystinuric animals the carrier proteins responsible for reabsorption are defective. The disease in dogs is quite heterogeneous; with differences in both the type and quantity of amino acids excreted in the urine. The dibasic amino acids that may be lost, in addition to cystine, are ornithine, lysine, and arginine (COLA).[116] Although absorption of these amino acids from the intestine may also be reduced, this does not appear to be of any practical consequence, and clinical signs are limited to those of urolithiasis.

The mode of inheritance for cystinuria is reported to be autosomal recessive in Newfoundlands.[112] In Newfoundlands the molecular basis of the defect has been identified as a nonsense mutation in exon 2 of the SLC3A1 (amino acid transport) gene.[117] However, in other breeds of dog with cystinuria this defect was not observed, indicating that the molecular pathogenesis of cystinuria in the dog is heterogeneous, similar to humans. Some forms of cystinuria in humans are incompletely recessive, resulting in a complex pattern of inheritance.

Cystinuria may be suspected by detection of characteristic crystals in urine, which are flat, colorless, and hexagonal, although these are not always present. If the concentration of cystine in urine is sufficiently high, the colorimetric cyanide-nitroprusside test may be used to confirm the diagnosis. The Metabolic Screening Laboratory, Section of Medical Genetics, University of Pennsylvania will perform this test on urine samples and will perform genetic screening in Newfoundlands using ethylenediamine tetra-acetic acid (EDTA) blood samples.

Treatment of Cystine Urolithiasis
Cystine uroliths are amenable to medical dissolution. This may be accomplished by maneuvers to reduce the concentration of cystine in the urine and to increase cystine solubility. As with all uroliths, augmenting urine volume is likely to be beneficial. Additionally, the solubility of cystine can be increased by increasing the urine pH to approximately 7.0 to 7.5, either by dietary therapy or by treatment with potassium citrate.

Feeding of a diet that is markedly protein restricted (Hill's Prescription diet canine u/d®) has been recommended because, among other potentially beneficial effects (alkalinization, sodium restriction, reduced urine concentration), this results in a 20% to 25% decrease in cystine excretion, presumably due to a reduced content of cystine precursors.[23] Feeding high-protein diets, particularly those rich in methionine, a cystine precursor, should be avoided in cystinuric dogs. However, the degree of protein restriction that is advisable is controversial because of the risk of carnitine deficiency and associated dilated cardiomyopathy in cystinuric dogs fed low-protein diets.[118] Dissolution of cystine uroliths has been reported without dietary protein restriction.[115]

Thiol-containing drugs react with cystine, resulting in its conversion to a more soluble compound by a disulfide exchange reaction; essentially, the drug is substituted for one of the cysteine residues of the cystine molecule. The prototypical thiol-containing drug used for this purpose is D-penicillamine, but this is associated with a high incidence of side effects, which effectively limits its use. Instead, the drug N-(2-mercaptopropionl)-glycine (2-MPG, Thiola; Mission Pharmacal Co, San Antonio, Texas), also known as *tiopronin*, is now more frequently used. Treatment with this drug at a dose of 20 mg/kg twice daily resulted in dissolution of approximately 60% of uroliths in one study, with the time required for urolith dissolution ranging from 1 to 3 months.[115] Unfortunately, a relatively high incidence of side effects has also been reported with this drug, including behavioral aggression, myopathy, proteinuria, anemia, thrombocytopenia, elevations of liver enzymes, and dermatologic changes.[23,115]

Prevention of Cystine Uroliths
Cystine uroliths frequently recur after surgical removal, with times to recurrence ranging from 1 to 36 months.[23,115] Recurrence is reportedly more likely to occur if the amount of cystine excreted is particularly high.[115] Treatment with 2-MPG, at a dose of 15 mg/kg twice daily, was successful in preventing the reformation of cystine uroliths in 76 of 88 (86%) of dogs in one study.[115] Urinary alkalinization and moderate protein restriction is likely to also be of benefit in preventing recurrence of cystine uroliths. Preventative therapy may be titrated to maintain a negative cyanide-nitroprusside test result.[23] Because the tendency for cystine uroliths to develop decreases with increasing age, it may be possible to discontinue preventative therapy in older dogs, particularly if it has been several years since uroliths were detected.[23,115]

A few dogs receiving treatment to prevent cystine uroliths reforming have developed struvite uroliths.[115] This possibility should be considered if a urolith forms while a dog is receiving preventative therapy, particularly if it is unresponsive to 2-MPG or if UTI is present.

CALCIUM PHOSPHATE UROLITHIASIS

Most pure calcium phosphate uroliths in dogs are composed of hydroxyapatite; brushite (calcium hydrogen phosphate dehydrate) is less common and whitlockite (calcium orthophosphate) is rare.[53] Hydroxyapatite is also a common component of uroliths predominantly composed of struvite, with the hydroxyapatite either mixed throughout the urolith or as a distinct layer (sometimes an outer shell) within the urolith. Brushite uroliths tend to occur as multiple smaller urocystoliths with either a smooth round surface or a pyramidal shape (see Table 267-1), whereas hydroxyapatite occur as multiple small uroliths with variable surface characteristics. Calcium phosphate uroliths are moderately to markedly radiopaque on abdominal radiographs, thus they can be readily diagnosed with high-quality abdominal radiographs. Because of their size and shape, they often cause urethral obstruction.

Epidemiology of Calcium Phosphate Urolithiasis

Pure calcium phosphate uroliths are uncommon in dogs, comprising only 0.3% to 0.6% of uroliths submitted to the Minnesota Urolith Center per year.[10,53] Breeds most commonly affected with calcium phosphate uroliths include the Yorkshire terrier, miniature schnauzer, Bichon friese, Shih Tzu, Springer spaniel, Pomeranian, miniature poodle, and cocker spaniel.[53] For pure brushite uroliths, male dogs (75%) are more commonly affected than female dogs (24%), whereas with hydroxyapatite, male dogs are only slightly more commonly affected (52%) than female dogs (48%).[53]

Although pure calcium phosphate uroliths are uncommon, calcium phosphate occurs as a part of many uroliths that are predominantly composed (>70%) of struvite or calcium oxalate.[35] Viewed in this manner, calcium phosphate–containing uroliths are the third most common type of urolith.[35] However, the majority of uroliths that contain minor amounts of calcium phosphate are usually classified based on their major crystalline component of struvite or calcium oxalate.[8,10]

Etiopathogenesis of Calcium Phosphate Urolithiasis

Calcium phosphate saturation in the urine is affected by the concentrations of calcium and phosphate, the urine pH, and inhibitors of the calcium phosphate crystal system.[8,53] Alkaline urine pH decreases the solubility of hydroxyapatite and may contribute to calcium phosphate urolith formation. Excessive urinary alkalinization (>7.5) in an attempt to prevent calcium oxalate or other type of uroliths in dogs may contribute to the formation of calcium phosphate uroliths. Excessive urinary excretion of calcium (hypercalciuria) and phosphate (hyperphosphaturia) also results in an increased risk of calcium phosphate urolith formation.

Calcium-containing uroliths have been reported to occur in 30% to 40% of dogs with primary hyperparathyroidism.[51,52] Primary hyperparathyroidism results in hypercalcemia, hypophosphatemia, hyperphosphaturia, hypercalciuria, and alkaline urine pH.[51,52] The combination of increased urinary excretion of calcium and phosphate increases the degree of saturation of calcium phosphate predisposing to urolith formation. The increase in urine pH lowers the solubility of calcium phosphate. Uroliths from dogs with primary hyperparathyroidism may be composed of either calcium phosphate, calcium oxalate, or mixtures of calcium oxalate and calcium phosphate, with calcium phosphate being most common.[51,53]

In humans and cats, chronic hypercalcemic disorders other than primary hyperparathyroidism may cause hypercalciuria, thereby predisposing to calcium oxalate or calcium phosphate uroliths.[8,119-121] However, hypercalcemic disorders, other than primary hyperparathyroidism, that cause hypercalciuria rarely result in calcium-containing uroliths in dogs. Similarly, almost all humans with hypercalcemia who form uroliths have primary hyperparathyroidism.[8] Hypercalciuria in dogs without primary hyperparathyroidism more commonly results in calcium oxalate urolithiasis.

Although renal tubular acidosis is a common contributing factor to formation of calcium phosphate uroliths in humans, this has not been documented in dogs.[8,53,122] Struvite urolithiasis has been reported in two dogs with renal tubular acidosis.[122]

Dogs with urinary tract hemorrhage may develop blood clots that become mineralized with calcium phosphate.[53] These may not be true calcium phosphate uroliths even though the mineral component is composed of calcium phosphate, because they probably do not contain the same matrix proteins or ultrastructure as typical calcium phosphate uroliths.

Inhibitors of Calcium Phosphate Urine contains substances that act to inhibit precipitation or growth of calcium phosphate crystals including pyrophosphates, citrate, magnesium, and nephrocalcin.[53] In urine, citrate forms complexes with calcium that are more soluble than calcium phosphate, lowering the ionic calcium concentration. The reader is referred to Inhibitors of Calcium Oxalate in this chapter for additional information on these inhibitors.

Treatment of Calcium Phosphate Urolithiasis

Calcium phosphate uroliths have been reported to dissolve in a few dogs after parathyroidectomy for treatment of primary hyperparathyroidism.[53] How frequently this occurs is unknown. Because calcium phosphate uroliths are frequently multiple small uroliths, waiting for spontaneous resolution of urocystoliths does carry an inherent risk of urethral obstruction. Therefore urolith removal by surgical or nonsurgical methods should also be considered.

Prevention of Calcium Phosphate Urolithiasis

The emphasis in prevention of calcium phosphate uroliths should initially be to diagnose and treat any underlying or predisposing conditions. The patient should be evaluated for evidence of primary hyperparathyroidism, hypercalcemia, hypercalciuria, hyperphosphaturia, or inappropriately alkaline urine pH. If dietary therapy, potassium citrate therapy, or sodium bicarbonate therapy have been used previously to alkalinize the urine and prevent another type of urolith, a neutral urine pH should be the target. However, the urine should not be acidified because this increases the risk of calcium oxalate urolith formation, which is more common in dogs.

The optimal preventative diet for prevention of calcium phosphate uroliths in dogs is unknown. As with all urolith types, increasing net water intake through feeding a canned diet is likely to be the most important dietary factor. At present, the authors offer similar dietary recommendations to those for prevention of calcium oxalate urolithiasis for dog with calcium phosphate uroliths. The main caution is to avoid excessive alkalinization of the urine, which may occur with some diets used for prevention of calcium oxalate uroliths.

SILICA UROLITHIASIS

Silica (silicon dioxide) uroliths are relatively infrequently diagnosed, accounting for just 0.9% of specimens submitted to the Minnesota Urolith Center.[10] The mean age of affected dogs was 7.2 ± 3.1 years (range 1 to 17 years) and most (93%)

of the affected dogs were male. Silica-containing nephroliths are rarely encountered in dogs from the United States,[10,113,123] although a very high prevalence of silica-containing nephroliths without accompanying cystoliths has been reported to occur in native Kenyan dogs.[124] Although many silica uroliths are pure, some are composed of multiple distinct layers, with oxalate and struvite being the most common additional minerals.[123] This observation has relevance when breed risks are considered; German shepherd dogs and Old English sheepdogs are at increased risk for developing silica uroliths, and when these develop they are typically pure, whereas additional breeds that are over-represented (including the miniature schnauzer, Shih Tzu, Lhasa Apso, and Yorkshire Terrier) are recognized to be at high-risk for development of uroliths generally, and they commonly form uroliths that are multilayered and incorporate other mineral types.[123]

Most silica uroliths have a "jackstone" configuration unless an outer layer of mineral (typically struvite) masks their characteristic appearance.[125] Multiple uroliths are often present. On cross-section, silica uroliths are distinctly laminated. The radiopacity of silica uroliths is similar to that of struvite.[17]

Etiopathogenesis of Silica Urolithiasis

It is proposed that the development of silica uroliths occurs due to an increase in dietary intake of this mineral. Animal protein contains very low concentrations of silica. Therefore dietary sources are likely to be of plant origin or due to ingestion of soil either directly or by contamination of crops during harvesting. The plant sources that have been implicated in the pathogenesis of silica uroliths include rice and soybean hulls, which may be added to diets to provide bulk and thus aid in the management of obesity, and corn gluten feed, which is added to some poor quality pet foods as a cheap source of protein.[125] The high prevalence of silica-containing nephroliths in native dogs in Kenya is proposed to be due to either consumption of maize meal or due to a high silica content in the local groundwater.[124] Silica uroliths develop in humans that consume large quantities of antacids containing magnesium trisilicate, and this has been replicated experimentally in a beagle dog.[125]

Treatment and Prevention of Silica Urolithiasis

Effective protocols for the dissolution of silica-containing uroliths have not been identified. The risk of silica uroliths reforming is not well documented; in one study of silica uroliths, 12% of dogs had had a previous episode of urolithiasis, but in most cases it was not known whether the previous urolith was also composed of silica.[123] The empiric recommendations for reducing the risk of silica uroliths reforming are to change the diet to one in which the vegetable content is limited and to avoid the ingestion of soil.[125] As with all uroliths, increased water intake should be promoted to decrease the resulting concentration of calculogenic material in urine.

UNCOMMON UROLITHS

Drugs and drug-metabolites may form uroliths of pure, mixed, or compound composition. The class of drugs that is most commonly incorporated into uroliths is the sulfonamides, although this is still a rare occurrence.[35,95] In addition, there have been single reported cases of ciprofloxacin, primidone, and tetracycline uroliths developing in dogs receiving these drugs.[95,126] A urolith composed of potassium, magnesium, and pyrophosphate (*perserite*) has been reported in a collie dog and four Persian cats.[127] The composition of this urolith is unexpected inasmuch as inorganic pyrophosphate is generally considered to be an inhibitor of urolith formation. The authors of the report speculate that formation of

pyrophosphate-containing uroliths results from an enzymatic dysfunction similar to the recognized human condition of hypophosphatasia, leading to pyrophosphate supersaturation of the urine.[127]

MIXED AND COMPOUND UROLITHS

Many uroliths are impure. In fact, in one study, only 29% of specimens in females and 61% of specimens in males were composed of a single mineral substance.[35] If uroliths do not contain a predominant mineral (typically defined as >70%), they may be classified as mixed; mixed uroliths comprised 1.9% of uroliths submitted to the Minnesota Urolith Center, with an additional 6.6% of uroliths being described as compound in composition.[10] Compound uroliths are those in which distinct layers are present, with each layer having a different mineral composition. Management of compound uroliths is challenging. In principle, dissolution of compound uroliths may be achieved by first instituting protocols designed to dissolve the mineral that is predicted to form the outer layer of the urolith and then altering the protocol according to the predicted composition of the inner layer or layers. In practice, the probability that the mineral composition of each layer will be successfully predicted, and that all mineral layers will be of a type amenable to medical dissolution is quite low, thus most compound uroliths are treated surgically or removed by other nonsurgical techniques. After removal of a compound urolith, a strategy needs to be implemented to try to prevent recurrent urolithiasis. In general, the strategy is to try to prevent the reformation of whatever mineral composed the core of the removed urolith, because the outer layer or layers may not have formed had there not been a mineral substrate present on which heterogeneous nucleation could occur. Specific strategies designed to prevent the recurrence of compound uroliths of varying composition were reviewed recently.[128] The reader is also referred to the section on compound calcium oxalate and struvite urolithiasis in this chapter.

URETHRAL OBSTRUCTION

Urethral obstruction may occur due to mechanical or functional causes. Functional obstruction results from failure of coordination of urethral relaxation with detrusor contraction (reflex dyssynergia).[129,130] The reader is referred to Chapter 29 for the diagnostic approach to dogs with urinary retention.

Urethral obstruction is life threatening when complete. Dogs with urethral obstruction should be evaluated for hyperkalemia and metabolic acidosis because these may be life threatening. Common causes of urethral obstruction include urethroliths, blood clots, urethral strictures, one-way valve effects from proliferations of the urothelium such as neoplasia or proliferative urethritis, urinary bladder entrapment in perineal or inguinal hernias, and penile fractures.[25,131,132]

Urocystoliths small enough to fit into the urethra may become lodged in the urethra and are termed *urethroliths*. Blood clots causing urethral obstruction may originate from bleeding in the kidney or bladder.[131] Several types of neoplasia may cause urethral obstruction, including transitional cell carcinoma (most common), prostatic adenocarcinoma, leiomyoma, leiomyosarcoma, squamous cell carcinoma, myxosarcoma, and lymphoma.[133-136] The reader is referred to Chapter 188 for additional information.

Urethral strictures may form secondary to previous urethral injury from surgery, urethroliths, external trauma, or iatrogenic trauma from prior urethral catheterization. Firm polypropylene urinary catheters should not be used as indwelling urethral catheters because they often cause

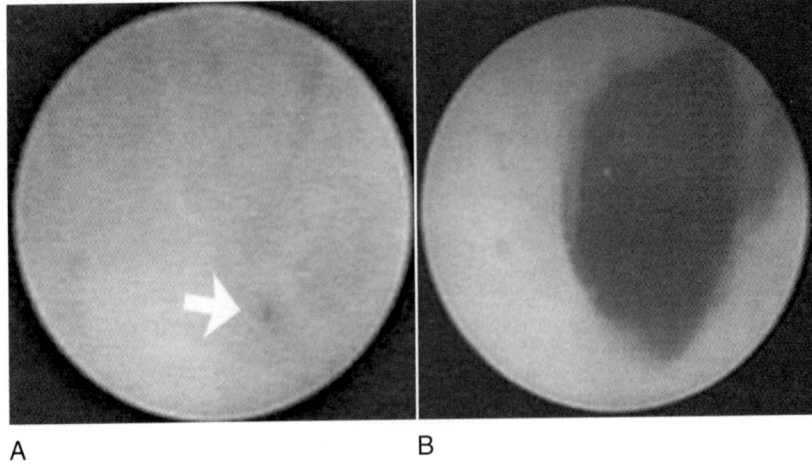

Figure 267-10 Dilation of a urethral stricture. **A,** Cystoscopic view of a urethral stricture in the proximal urethra with a diameter of less than 1 mm *(arrow).* **B,** Cystoscopic view of the proximal urethra after dilation of the stricture to 5 mm.

mucosal trauma and irritation that may lead to stricture formation.[16] Documentation of the site and extent of urethral strictures is best accomplished by positive-contrast urethrography. Although urethral strictures are often treated surgically, they may also be dilated using balloon dilation catheters in male dogs or using urethral or ureteral dilation sets in female dogs (Figure 267-10).

Chronic inflammatory conditions (e.g., UTI, urolithiasis) may cause mucosal thickening and proliferation, which has been termed *granulomatous urethritis* or *proliferative urethritis.*[2,132] Proliferative urethritis is a more accurate description of the disease because the mucosa does not contain a granulomatous inflammatory infiltrate in all dogs, and proliferation of the urethral mucosa is commonly observed during urethrocystoscopy. The mucosal proliferations are often bands of tissue that are connected to the urethral mucosa on each end, unlike the papillary projections of transitional cell carcinoma.[2] The mucosal proliferations cause a one-way valve effect that causes outflow obstruction but often permits retrograde passage of urethral catheters. Digital rectal palpation of dogs with proliferative urethritis reveals a thickened and firm urethra. The site of obstruction can be confirmed by voiding contrast urethrography or urethrocystoscopy. Proliferative urethritis should be differentiated from urethral neoplasia by cytology and histopathology.

Treatment of proliferative urethritis requires effective control of the UTI if this is the underlying cause. If the lesions fail to regress with adequate control of the UTI, immunosuppressive therapy with prednisone (2.2 mg/kg orally, every 12 hours) with or without cyclophosphamide may be added to antimicrobial therapy.[132] However, immunosuppression may exacerbate the underlying infection and is not consistently effective for resolving the lesions. The efficacy of nonsteroidal anti-inflammatory drugs (NSAIDs) for treatment of proliferative urethritis has not been reported. Prognosis is guarded in dogs with urethral obstruction from proliferative urethritis because some dogs fail to respond to the immunosuppressive therapy, and immunosuppression may prevent resolution of the underlying UTI. Urinary diversion via an indwelling urethral catheter or tube cystostomy may be required during initial medical therapy to bypass the urethral obstruction until the dog is able to void urine.[137,138] Surgical resection of a distal urethral obstruction and vaginourethroplasty was successful in treating proliferative urethritis in one dog.[136]

URINARY TRACT TRAUMA

Trauma to the urinary tract may be caused by blunt force (particularly in association with pelvic fractures), accidental incision during celiotomy, penetrating abdominal or perineal wounds, iatrogenic injury from improper cystocentesis technique or from rigid instruments (rigid cystoscopes, polypropylene or metal catheters), or from overdistension of the urinary bladder. Potential types of injury include contusions of the bladder or urethra, urethral tears, rupture or avulsion, urinary bladder rupture, and penile fracture.

Clinical signs of urinary tract trauma depend on the location of the trauma, duration and extent of urinary leakage, and the presence or absence of concurrent UTI. Contusions of the LUT may be asymptomatic or may cause hematuria, dysuria, and pollakiuria. Dogs with bladder or urethral rupture or urethral avulsion may be unable to urinate or may pass small amounts of bloody urine. Persistent intra-abdominal leakage of urine from a ruptured urinary bladder causes chemical peritonitis and postrenal azotemia manifested by lethargy, anorexia, vomiting, dehydration, abdominal distention, or pain on abdominal palpation. Transient urinary leakage caused by cystocentesis of an overdistended bladder, or from small rents in the urinary bladder wall as a result of overdistension during contrast cystography, does not usually cause clinical signs unless concurrent UTI is found. Bacterial peritonitis may result from even transient leakage of infected urine into the abdominal cavity.

The potential for concurrent damage to the urinary tract should be considered in all dogs with abdominal, pelvic, or perineal trauma. Diagnosis of the extent and location of traumatic injury is accomplished by either positive-contrast retrograde urethrocystography or urethrocystoscopy. During contrast urethrocystography, urinary tract rupture is confirmed by either direct visualization of leakage of contrast material from the urinary tract or by increased radiopacity of the abdominal cavity compared with radiographs obtained before injection of contrast (Figure 267-11). Passage of firm polypropylene urinary catheters should be avoided if urethral tears or lacerations are suspected because the catheter tip may enlarge urethral tears. Likewise, the ability to pass a urinary catheter and obtain urine from the bladder is insufficient to rule out urethral or bladder rupture. Urethrocystoscopy allows direct visualization of the location and extent of LUT injury, but the cystoscope should only be advanced under direct visualization of the lumen. If abdominal fluid is present, determination of the creatinine concentration of the fluid and comparison to the serum creatinine concentration is recommended rather than measurement of urea nitrogen concentrations because urea rapidly equilibrates across the peritoneum. Urinary leakage can be confirmed by finding abdominal fluid creatinine concentrations more than one and a half to twofold higher than the serum concentration.

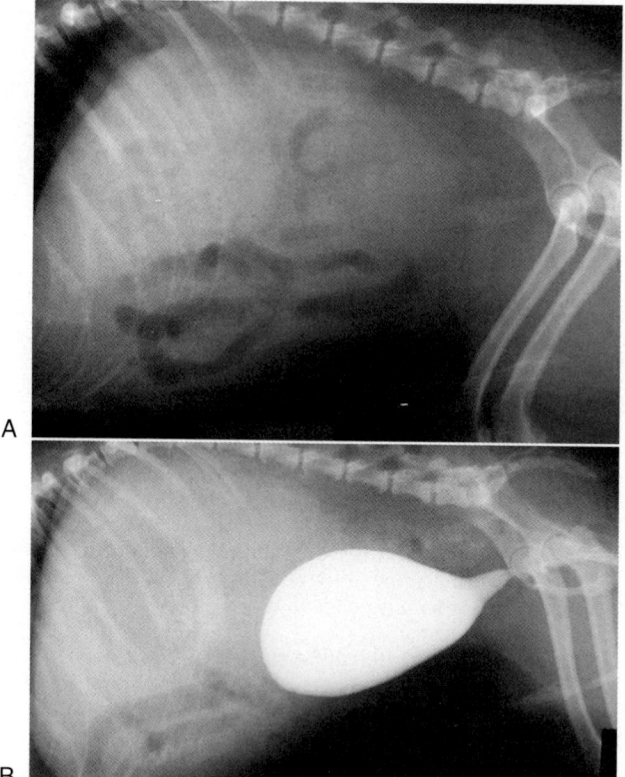

Figure 267-11 Contrast urethrocystography confirming urinary leakage secondary to traumatic cystocentesis of an overdistended urinary bladder. **A,** Abdominal radiographs showing loss of intra-abdominal detail secondary to uroabdomen. **B,** Positive-contrast urethrocystogram failed to demonstrate a leak from the urinary bladder; however, the intra-abdominal fluid is more radiopaque than before filling the bladder with contrast media, confirming urinary leakage.

Surgical repair is required for treatment of large rents in the urinary bladder, urethral avulsion, and large urethral lacerations. Small tears in the urethra or bladder wall may be treated conservatively by urinary diversion using an indwelling urethral catheter or by tube cystostomy.[137,138] Such small tears usually heal within 5 to 10 days. The healing process can be re-evaluated by positive-contrast radiography or urethrocystoscopy. Likewise, contusions of the LUT heal within 3 to 5 days and do not require specific therapy.

INFLAMMATORY CONDITIONS OF BLADDER AND URETHRA

Inflammation of the bladder and urethra are termed *cystitis* and *urethritis*, respectively. Most conditions causing inflammation of the LUT affect both the bladder and urethra. Clinical signs of LUT inflammation include dysuria, stranguria, pollakiuria, and hematuria. By far the most common inflammatory condition of the canine LUT is bacterial infection of the bladder and urethra. (The reader is referred to Chapter 262 for additional information about bacterial UTI.) Dogs with chronic UTI may have follicular cystitis characterized by multiple small mucosal follicles seen in the bladder, urethra, and vaginal vestibule, which are visible during cystoscopy. These follicles contain lymphoid infiltrates and they regress spontaneously with control of the UTI. Follicular cystitis must be differentiated from polypoid cystitis and neoplasia.

Fungal UTI is less commonly diagnosed than bacterial UTI, with the most common isolate being *Candida albicans*.[139] In one study, all affected dogs had concurrent illnesses or received medications that were likely to have predisposed to fungal UTI.[139] Potential reasons for development of fungal UTI in dogs include surgery or instrumentation of the urinary tract, corticosteroid administration or hyperadrenocorticism, chemotherapy, and chronic antibiotic therapy. Persistent funguria should be documented before concluding that fungal UTI is present to exclude the possibility that contamination of the sample occurred *ex vivo*. Spontaneous resolution of fungal UTI occurred in two of 13 dogs in one study.[139] Oral fluconazole, flucytosine, or both may be effective for treatment of fungal UTI caused by *Candida* spp. Although both fluconazole and flucytosine are renally excreted, some stains of *Candida* are resistant to these drugs. Unfortunately, *in vitro* susceptibility testing for antifungal drugs is not readily available. Intravesical infusions of clotrimazole may be required to resolve candidiasis of the LUT in some dogs.[140] Effective management of the underlying condition that predisposed the dog to fungal UTI is required for long-term control of infection.

Polypoid cystitis is a relatively uncommon disease of the bladder characterized by inflammation, epithelial proliferation, and development of a polypoid mass or masses without histopathologic evidence of neoplasia.[141] Polypoid cystitis probably develops due to a hyperplastic inflammatory reaction secondary to chronic irritation of the bladder from recurrent UTI or urolithiasis. Dogs with polypoid cystitis have clinical signs of hematuria or LUT inflammation such as dysuria, stranguria, and pollakiuria. Female dogs are much more commonly affected than male dogs.[141] Ultrasonographic evaluation reveals single or multiple polypoid projections into the bladder lumen without distortion of the layers of the bladder wall (Figure 267-12). Diffuse thickening of the bladder wall may occur in some cases. Cystoscopy reveals polypoid projections in the bladder, which are sometimes difficult to definitively differentiate from transitional cell carcinoma (Figure 267-13). Papillary mucosal proliferative lesions with large blood vessels that extend to the tip of the projection are more characteristic of TCC than polypoid cystitis. Polypoid cystitis occurs more commonly in the cranioventral portion of the bladder, whereas transitional cell carcinoma occurs more commonly in the trigone of the bladder; however, the location and appearance of polypoid masses alone is insufficient for differentiating these diseases. Therefore biopsies of all polyps and papillary masses should be obtained for cytology and histopathology.

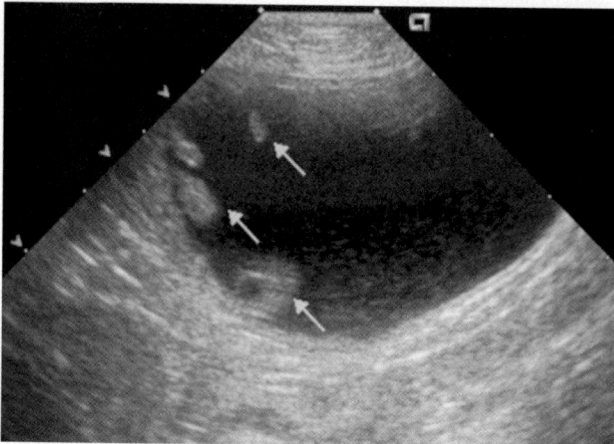

Figure 267-12 Ultrasonographic image of polypoid cystitis in a dog showing multiple polypoid projections *(arrows)* along the cranioventral portion of the bladder.

URINARY SYSTEM

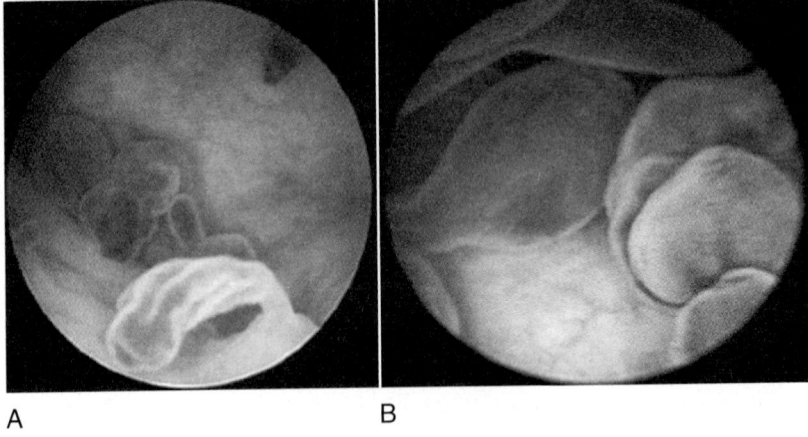

Figure 267-13 Polypoid cystitis and transitional cell carcinoma of the urinary bladder are sometimes difficult to differentiate visually. **A,** Cystoscopic image of polypoid cystitis from the dog in Figure 267-12. **B,** Transitional cell carcinoma of the urinary bladder of a dog.

A   B

Although effective management of UTI may result in spontaneous resolution of polypoid cystitis in a few cases, removal of the polyps by surgery or cystoscopy is required in most dogs. Surgical options include excisional biopsy of the polypoid masses or partial cystectomy of areas that are diffusely affected.[141] Cystoscopic resection of the isolated polyps may be performed using biopsy forceps, electrocautery loops, or the holmium laser.

Emphysematous cystitis is an uncommon form of bacterial cystitis characterized by gas production within the layers of the bladder wall. Emphysematous cystitis usually occurs from intramural gas production from bacterial fermentation of glucose in dogs with UTI and glucosuria. Diagnosis is made based on gas accumulation in the bladder wall visible of abdominal radiographs. Treatment involves effective treatment of the UTI and control of glucosuria.

Cyclophosphamide-induced cystitis is a sterile hemorrhagic cystitis caused by urinary excretion of acrolein, a metabolite of cyclophosphamide. Administration of furosemide concurrently with cyclophosphamide reduces the risk of cystitis developing.[142] Thiazide diuretics should not be used for this purpose because they may potentiate the myelotoxic effects of cyclophosphamide.[142] Treatment consists of discontinuation of cyclophosphamide therapy, short-term symptomatic therapy (e.g., narcotics for analgesia), and treatment of secondary UTI. Parasitic cystitis, caused by mucosal or submucosal invasion by the adult stage of *Capillaria plica*, is an uncommon disease in dogs. Capillariasis may be associated with clinical signs of dysuria, stranguria, and pollakiuria. Capillariasis is diagnosed by identification of the double-operculated ova during urinalysis. Treatment with ivermectin (0.2 mg/kg subcutaneously) eliminates the infection and improves clinical signs. In dogs that cannot be treated with ivermectin, an alternative therapy is fenbendazole (50 mg/kg orally, daily for 5 days).

URINARY INCONTINENCE

Urinary incontinence is defined as loss of voluntary control of urination resulting in leakage of urine from the urinary system to the exterior of the body. Urinary incontinence occurs either when intravesicular pressure is greater than urethral pressures (due to decreased detrusor compliance or poor urethral pressures) or due to anatomic abnormalities that bypass the normal continence mechanisms (e.g., ectopic ureters). Urinary incontinence must be differentiated from inappropriate urination associated with dysuria and pollakiuria. The reader is referred to Chapter 30 for the clinical signs and diagnostic approach to urinary incontinence. Box 267-2 lists common causes of urinary incontinence in dogs.

Urethral Incompetence in Female Dogs

Urethral incompetence (also called *urethral sphincter mechanism incompetence*) is the most common cause of incontinence in adult female dogs and usually occurs months to years after neutering. Congenital anatomic or functional abnormalities of the urethra may also result in urethral incompetence. Urethral incompetence frequently occurs concurrently in dogs with ectopic ureters due to malformation of the urethra (see Figure 267-1) and can result in treatment failure after surgical correction of ectopic ureters.[143]

Urethral incompetence may be confirmed by documenting decreased urethral closure pressure by urethral pressure profilometry; however, urodynamic equipment is only available at some referral hospitals. Although urodynamic confirmation is unnecessary in most cases, urodynamic evaluation should be considered for dogs with urinary incontinence that is unresponsive to standard treatment.[144,145] Alpha-adrenergic agonists (phenylpropanolamine, ephedrine, or pseudoephedrine) or estrogen (diethylstilbestrol or estriol) are recommended for treatment of urethral incompetence in female dogs. Phenylpropanolamine (1.1 to 1.5 mg/kg orally, every 8 hours) is effective in approximately 85% to 90% of female dogs with urethral incompetence.[6,146] Estrogen therapy

---

Box • 267-2
Causes of Urinary Incontinence
Urethral incompetence Ectopic ureters Neurologic disorders Urge incontinence (secondary to urinary tract infection [UTI] or uroliths) Idiopathic detrusor instability Paradoxic (overflow) incontinence Ureterocele Pelvic bladder Ureterovaginal or urethrorectal fistula Patent urachus

increases urethral closure pressure by increasing the density and responsiveness of α-adrenergic receptors in urethral smooth muscle. Estrogen therapy is effective in approximately 50% to 65% of female dogs with urethral incompetence.[147] Excessive doses of estrogen may cause severe bone marrow suppression; therefore owners should be cautioned not to exceed recommended doses and CBCs should be monitored in dogs receiving estrogen therapy. Diethylstilbestrol is administered at 0.1 to 0.2 mg/kg orally, daily (maximum dose 1 mg/dog) for 5 days, followed by the same dose once to twice a week. The maximum maintenance dose of diethylstilbestrol is 0.2 mg/kg/wk. The minimum effective dose should be used for maintenance.

Low-dose daily estrogen using estriol has recently been suggested as an alternative to diethylstilbestrol.[148] Estriol is administered at a dose of 2 mg orally, daily for 1 week, then the dose is reduced at weekly intervals to the minimal effective dose (typically 0.5 to 2.0 mg/dog given daily or every other day). In one study of 129 dogs, there was no evidence of bone marrow toxicity when estriol was administered for 42 days.[148] Although some authors suggest that low-dose daily estrogen therapy may be more effective than weekly therapy with diethylstilbestrol, the long-term safety of low-dose daily estrogen has not been reported.

Because estrogen up-regulates the α-adrenergic receptors that phenylpropanolamine stimulates, combination therapy with these medications is synergistic. Therefore female dogs that are refractory to either medication alone may respond to combination therapy. For dogs that are refractory to combination therapy, urodynamic evaluation is recommended. Alternative therapies for dogs with refractory urinary incontinence due to confirmed urethral incompetence include cystoscopic injections of bulk-enhancing agents (glutaraldehyde cross-linked collagen) or surgical methods to increase urethral resistance.[149-151] Periurethral injection of collagen narrows the urethral lumen and allows for more effective closure of the urethra by existing urethral pressure. Periurethral injection of collagen resolved urinary incontinence in 53% of dogs with an additional 22% that were improved with concurrent administration of phenylpropanolamine.[150] In the authors' experience, repeat cystoscopic injections of collagen are required in some dogs weeks to months after initial injections. Surgical methods for treatment of refractory urinary incontinence include colposuspension and urethropexy.[149,151,152] Surgery resolves incontinence in approximately 50% of dogs, with an additional 25% to 40% being continent with concurrent administration of phenylpropanolamine.[149,151,152] However, improvement may not be sustained with a 1-year response rate of only 14% in one study.[149]

An additional medical treatment for urinary incontinence that has been reported recently is the use of gonadotrophin-releasing hormone (GnRH) analogues.[153] Improved continence was noted for several months after the subcutaneous administration of GnRH depot preparations, even though the bitches that were treated had not responded well to other treatments. This approach was investigated because of the observation that spayed bitches have very high concentrations of luteinizing hormone (LH) and follicle-stimulating hormone (FSH) compared with intact bitches, and the treatment was shown to decrease the concentration of these hormones.

Detrusor Instability and Urge Incontinence

Although urethral incompetence is the most common cause of urinary incontinence, this may also occur due to detrusor contraction during storage of urine or due to low compliance of the detrusor muscle, which may be confirmed by cystometrography.[7,145] When decreased detrusor compliance occurs secondary to inflammatory conditions affecting the LUT (e.g., urolithiasis, UTI), this is termed *urge incontinence* (see Box 267-2). Clinical signs of dogs with urge incontinence may also include pollakiuria, stranguria, and dysuria. If no identifiable cause of decreased detrusor compliance is identified, this is termed *idiopathic detrusor instability*.[7] In one study of 77 dogs with refractory urinary incontinence, 10 dogs had poor bladder storage function alone and 15 dogs had both detrusor dysfunction and concurrent urethral incompetence.[145]

Treatment of detrusor instability is by anticholinergic medications (oxybutynin, imipramine, or dicyclomine) to decrease detrusor contractions during storage of urine.[7,154] Although oxybutynin (0.2 mg/kg orally, every 8 to 12 hours) has been most commonly recommended, dicyclomine appeared to have a greater effect on detrusor compliance in normal dogs than oxybutynin.[154] Clinical effectiveness of dicyclomine has not been reported in dogs with idiopathic detrusor instability. Imipramine is a tricyclic antidepressant medication that has anticholinergic effects to facilitate urine storage and also increases urethral closure pressure. Therefore imipramine may be effective for dogs with mixed incontinence due to detrusor dysfunction and concurrent urethral incompetence.[154]

Urinary Incontinence in Male Dogs

Urinary incontinence occurs much less commonly in male than female dogs and urethral incompetence is a less common cause in male dogs.[155] In one study, only five of 38 incontinent males dogs had urethral incompetence.[156] Surgical procedures involving the proximal urethra and prostate are a common iatrogenic cause of urinary incontinence in male dogs, because the proximal urethra is integral in maintaining continence in male dogs.[155] Urethral incompetence in male dogs may be treated with α-adrenergic medications (phenylpropanolamine: 1.1 to 1.5 mg/kg orally, every 8 hours) or testosterone cypionate (2.2 mg/kg intramuscularly, every 30 days). Testosterone has potential side effects including prostate disease and behavioral aggression; therefore some authors discourage use of testosterone for treatment of urethral incompetence. Unfortunately, less than 50% of dogs with urethral incompetence are responsive to phenylpropanolamine.[155] Therefore surgical correction by vasopexy is recommended in male dogs with urethral incompetence that are unresponsive to phenylpropanolamine.[157] The authors have diagnosed several male dogs with idiopathic detrusor instability that were responsive to oxybutynin; therefore urodynamic evaluation is recommended prior to surgical therapy.

Ectopic Ureters

The reader is referred to the chapter on Diseases of the Ureter for discussion of ectopic ureters. Ectopic ureters are commonly associated with anatomic and functional abnormalities of the bladder and urethra.[3,143,158] Urodynamic evaluation of nine dogs with ectopic ureters revealed that four of nine dogs had decreased detrusor compliance and seven of nine had poor urethral function.[143] Therefore urodynamic evaluation is recommended prior to surgical correction of ectopic ureters to aid in predicting whether the dog will be continent after surgery. Anatomic abnormalities of the urethra and vaginal vestibule are common in dog with ectopic ureters (see Figure 267-1).[3] Ureteral troughs, fenestrations, and the intramural ureter in the dorsal urethral wall may all affect the ability of the urethra to generate adequate closure pressure. Therefore some authors have suggested removal of the submucosal ureteral remnants from the trigone and urethra with reconstruction of the muscular defect caused by the resection in addition to surgical correction of the location of the ureteral opening.[158] Urinary continence is improved by this more aggressive surgical approach in dogs with multiple anatomic abnormalities.[158]

URINARY SYSTEM

ANATOMIC ABNORMALITIES

Ureterocele

A ureterocele is a cystic dilatation of the terminal portion of the ureter which often protrudes into the bladder lumen.[159-161] Ureteroceles are classified as either *orthotopic* (also called *intravesical*), if the ureter opening is in a normal trigonal location, or *ectopic*, if the ureter opening is distal to the normal trigonal position. Ureteroceles may cause a variety of clinical signs depending on their size and whether or not the ureter is ectopic. Urinary incontinence is the most common clinical sign of ureteroceles.[159,160] Ureteroceles may place pressure on the bladder and proximal urethra resulting in functional urinary retention, or they may cause signs of dysuria, stranguria, and pollakiuria. Dogs with ureteroceles may also present for recurrent UTI. Although ureteroceles are congenital abnormalities, some dogs with ureteroceles do not develop clinical signs until later in life.[159] Ureteroceles may be associated with developmental or acquired abnormalities of the upper urinary tract or LUT, including moderate to severe hydroureter and hydronephrosis, ectopic ureters, and urethral anomalies. Ureteroceles are diagnosed by excretory urography or ultrasonography.[160,162]

Treatment of ureteroceles depends on the type and extent of concurrent anomalies and whether or not the ureteral opening is ectopic. Excision of the ureterocele with reimplantation of the ureter is recommended for ectopic ureteroceles or ureteroceles associated with ureteral obstruction.[159] Orthotopic ureteroceles may be incised cystoscopically or by cystotomy; however, this often results in vesicoureteral reflux that could contribute to pyelonephritis if UTI is also present.

Urethral Prolapse

Prolapse of the urethral mucosa through the external urethral orifice is an acquired disease of male dogs, most common in English bulldogs (Figure 267-14).[163] The proposed causes for urethral prolase include excessive sexual excitement or stranguria associated with UTI or urolithiasis.[16,163] Although small urethral prolapses may resolve spontaneously in some dogs,[16] surgical correction is required in most cases. A recently reported urethropexy technique was successful in three of three dogs and is less invasive than surgical resection of the prolapsed tissue with apposition of the urethral and penile mucosa.[163]

Vesicourachal Diverticula

Vesicourachal diverticula are remnants of the urachal canal between the apex of the bladder and the umbilicus. Vesicourachal diverticula usually appear as an out pouching of the bladder wall near the bladder apex that can be diagnosed by contrast cystography or cystoscopy. Dogs with vesicourachal diverticula are predisposed to recurrent UTI, presumably from incomplete emptying of the urine in the dead space of the diverticula.[164,165] Vesicourachal diverticula may resolve spontaneously if the underlying cause can be corrected.[165] Surgical removal of urachal diverticula is recommended for dogs with persistent or recurrent UTIs and for dogs undergoing surgical removal of urocystoliths.

Urethrorectal or Ureterovaginal Fistula

Fistulas between the urethra and the rectum or between the ureter and vagina are uncommon conditions in dogs that may be congenital or acquired.[166-169] Ureterovaginal fistulas usually form as a result of ovariohysterectomy when the ureter is accidentally included in a ligature around the vaginal stump. Urethrorectal fistulas may be congenital or may be acquired after pelvic trauma. Clinical signs of urethrorectal fistulas include passing of urine from the anus during voiding or recurrent infections of the *urogenital tract*.[168,169] Urinary incontinence is the most common clinical sign of ureterovaginal fistulas

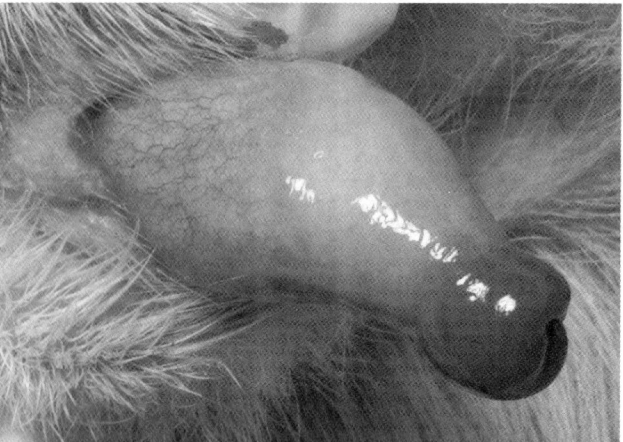

Figure 267-14 Urethral prolapse showing eversion of the distal urethral mucosa.

in dogs.[166,167] Surgical correction of urethrorectal or ureterovaginal fistulas is recommended; however, surgical correction of urethrorectal fistulas may be complicated by intrapelvic location and by concurrent infection. Resolution of secondary UTI is essential after surgical correction of urethrorectal fistulas and may require prolonged antimicrobial therapy.

Persistent Urachus

Persistent urachus is an uncommon congenital abnormality in dogs where the entire urachal canal remains patent from the apex of the bladder to the umbilicus. The clinical signs are dribbling of urine through the umbilicus, and secondary UTI and omphalitis are common sequela. The diagnosis can be confirmed by performing contrast radiography by gently injecting iodinated contrast into the umbilicus. Treatment of persistent urachus is by surgical removal of the urachal canal.

Pelvic Bladder

Pelvic bladder is a term describing urinary bladders that have a blunt-shaped trigone, with the trigone located in an intrapelvic location associated with a shortened urethra.[170] Pelvic bladder is controversial as to whether or not it is a cause of urinary incontinence or an artifact of how contrast urethrocystography is performed.[170-172] The normal urinary bladder trigone tapers and connects to the urethra in an intra-abdominal location. The degree of distention affects the location of the trigone; therefore the bladder should be properly distended during contrast urethrocystography before diagnosing pelvic bladder. Pelvic bladder may also be associated with increased incidence of UTI, although this association has not been definitively proven.[170] Although some dogs with pelvic bladders do not have urinary incontinence[171,172]; other dogs with pelvic bladders have refractory urinary incontinence without any other identifiable cause. [170,173] Diagnosis of pelvic bladder is usually made by contrast urethrocystography, although the abnormal shape of the trigone can also be detected during cystoscopy, raising suspicion of the diagnosis. The authors' approach to dogs with radiographic evidence of pelvic bladder is to rule out other abnormalities that might cause urinary incontinence (e.g., urethral incompetence, ectopic ureters). If concurrent urethral incompetence is present, combination medical therapy with estrogen and α-adrenergic agonists should be attempted prior to surgical intervention. If the dog is refractory to medical therapy, urethropexy or colposuspension are recommended to move the bladder neck cranially.[149,151,152]

CHAPTER 268

Ureteral Diseases

Lori L. Ludwig

ANATOMY AND FUNCTION

The ureters are fibromuscular ducts that carry urine from the renal pelves to the bladder. The course of the ureters is retroperitoneal, adjacent to the caudal vena cava and aorta and ventral to the psoas muscle. The ureters reach the dorsolateral surface of the bladder through the lateral ligaments and turn from a caudal to a cranial direction before they enter the bladder at the cranial border of the trigone. The degree of curvature of the ureters at the trigone depends on the degree of bladder distension. Recognition of this curvature is important in the evaluation of contrast radiographic studies and for catheterization of the ureters during surgery. Upon entering the bladder, the ureters course obliquely in the submucosa toward the bladder neck. This path through the bladder wall facilitates closure of the distal ureter when the bladder is distended with urine, preventing retrograde flow of urine from the bladder (vesicoureteral reflux).

The ureteral wall is composed of an outer adventitial layer, a muscular layer, submucosa, and a mucosa of transitional epithelium. The muscular wall of the ureter consists of an outer longitudinal, middle circular, and inner longitudinal muscle layer except at the ureterovesical junction, where only longitudinal fibers are present. During diuresis, stretching of these muscle layers can result in a seventeenfold increase in the ureteral luminal diameter.[1] The normal width of the ureteral lumen in dogs is reported to be 0.07 times the length of the second lumbar vertebra.[2]

The blood supply to the ureter arises from the renal artery cranially and from the prostatic or vaginal arteries caudally. These vessels anastomose at the level of the adventitia in the ureteral wall. The ureteral veins follow the same path as the arteries. The ureters are innervated by autonomic fibers, but this innervation is not responsible for ureteral peristalsis.[2] Ureteral peristalsis occurs when urine enters the ureter, initiating electrical impulses to be conducted between smooth muscle cells. If the peristaltic activity is initiated in the renal pelvis, urine is propelled toward the bladder. However, if peristaltic waves begin when urine enters the distal ureter because of an incompetent ureterovesical junction, urine moves toward the kidney. Because ureteral peristalsis is myogenic (not neurogenic) in origin, ureteral peristalsis persists with transplantation.

Ureteral contractions in normal dogs occur three to six times per minute.[2] The frequency of contractions increases with diuresis to a maximum point. Once the maximum frequency has been reached, the ureter dilates, and urine stasis occurs. Ureteral peristalsis also is impaired by transection and anastomosis of the ureter. Two weeks after surgery, conduction of peristaltic waves returns across the surgery site.[3] In addition, physical ureteral obstruction and some bacterial toxins can inhibit ureteral peristalsis.[4]

VESICOURETERAL REFLUX

Vesicoureteral reflux is flow of urine in a retrograde direction, from the urinary bladder into the ureters, that occurs when the intraluminal bladder pressure exceeds intraluminal ureteral pressure. This condition may result in transmission of lower urinary tract infection to the kidney.[2] It may also perpetuate lower urinary tract infection, because infected urine from the bladder refluxes into the ureter and then recontaminates the bladder when it returns from the ureter. In addition, renal parenchymal damage may result from increased intrapelvic pressure associated with ureterectasis and transmission of voiding pressure to the renal pelvis during reflux.[2] Vesicoureteral reflux is prevented in normal animals by the long, submucosal/intravesical portion of the ureter (ureterovesical valve), which collapses as pressure in the bladder increases. Factors that may affect the functioning of the ureterovesical valve include the length, diameter, pliability, and ratio of length to width of the intravesical portion of the ureter; ureteral peristalsis, detrusor muscle function, and intraluminal pressure of the ureters or urinary bladder.[2,4]

Primary vesicoureteral reflux occurs in young dogs (7 to 12 weeks old) and may be related to intrinsic maldevelopment of the ureterovesical junction.[2] The process is usually self-limiting, because the submucosal portion of the distal ureter elongates as the dog grows. Primary vesicoureteral reflux is rare in adult dogs. Secondary vesicoureteral reflux is acquired and may occur with inflammation of the vesicoureteral junction, lower urinary tract obstruction, surgical damage, neurogenic disease of the bladder, and ectopic ureters.[2]

Maximum distension and voiding cystourethrography are the techniques most commonly used to diagnose vesicoureteral reflux. A catheter is placed in the membranous or prostatic urethra, and iodinated contrast material is infused into the catheter until the bladder is distended enough to stimulate contraction of the detrusor muscle. Alternatively, external pressure can be applied to the bladder to express urine. Lateral radiographs are taken at the beginning of voiding of the contrast agent from the bladder, or voiding is monitored fluoroscopically. Vesicoureteral reflux may be seen during contrast filling of the bladder, during voiding, or both. Reflux can also be detected cystoscopically by filling the bladder with a colored dye and then watching for this dye to be excreted from the ureters after the bladder is emptied and filled with clear fluid.[2]

Treatment of patients with vesicoureteral reflux should be aimed at eradication of urinary tract infections. Surgery may be indicated to treat predisposing factors such as obstructive lesions or ectopic ureters. Vesicoureteral reflux in young dogs is usually self-limiting and therefore requires no treatment.

CONGENITAL ANOMALIES

Ectopic Ureter

A ureter that enters the bladder distal to the trigone is considered ectopic. Ectopic ureters result from an embryologic abnormality of the ureteral bud of the mesonephric duct. The degree of deviation of the ureteral bud from the normal position determines the location of the ectopic ureteral opening, which can be anywhere along the urethra or in the vagina or uterus. Ectopic ureters may be unilateral or bilateral and extramural or intramural. Extramural ectopic ureters bypass the urinary bladder entirely and insert at a distal location. Intramural ectopic ureters appear externally to enter the bladder at the normal dorsolateral location; however, instead of opening in the trigone, the ureter traverses below the mucosa and opens in the bladder neck, urethra, or vagina. Reported variations to the intramural ectopic ureter include ureteral troughs, double ureteral openings, multiple fenestrated openings, and two intramural ureters opening in a single orifice.[5] Ectopic ureters commonly are associated with other abnormalities of the urogenital tract, including agenesis, hypoplasia, or irregular shape of the kidneys; hydroureter; ureterocele; urachal remnants; pelvic bladder; vulvovaginal strictures; and persistent hymen.[6,7]

The diagnosis of an ectopic ureter is usually made in young females.[5,7] It is possible that males with ectopic ureters remain undiagnosed because the length of the urethra and external urethral sphincter may prevent urine dribbling. Intramural, bilateral ectopic ureters are most commonly reported.[7] A genetic basis for this disease has been suggested by the documentation of ectopic ureters in litter mates and a report of a parent-offspring transmission.[7] Breeds reported to be at greater risk for ureteral ectopia include the Siberian husky, Labrador retriever, golden retriever, Newfoundland, English bulldog, West Highland white terrier, fox terrier, Skye terrier, and miniature and toy poodles.[7] Ectopic ureters have been rarely reported in cats.

Dogs and cats with ureteral ectopia most commonly present with a history of continuous or intermittent incontinence since birth or weaning. The incontinence may be more severe when the animal is in a recumbent position. Normal urine voiding may also occur. On physical examination, the perineum may be soaked or stained with urine, or perivulvar dermatitis may be noted. Male cats may have a constricted preputial orifice with dilatation of the sheath caused by urine accumulation. The results of hematologic studies and a serum biochemistry profile usually are normal unless concurrent renal disease is present. Bacterial urinary tract infections have been reported to occur in 64% of patients with ectopic ureters.[5] These patients may be at greater risk of developing infection as a result of lack or dysfunction of the vesicoureteral valve, impaired ureteral peristalsis, or stasis of urine in the lower urogenital tract.

Several modalities have been used to diagnose ureteral ectopia. Traditionally, contrast radiography has been recommended. Excretory urography allows evaluation of the size and morphology of the kidneys and ureters. To improve the accuracy of evaluation of the ureteral insertion, excretory urography should be combined with pneumocystography. The bladder should be distended with carbon dioxide or room air, which provides negative contrast around the ureter as it enters the bladder. Elevation of the caudal abdomen and oblique or dorsoventral views may be helpful for identifying the ureteral opening. Fluoroscopy can be useful in discriminating the path of the ureter as it enters the bladder. A dilated ureter is the abnormality most frequently detected with excretory urography.[6] Ureteral dilatation may result from obstruction to urine flow caused by a stenotic ureteral orifice or by functional obstruction that occurs with contraction of the urethral sphincter at the site of insertion of the ectopic ureter. In patients with infection, ureteral dilatation may also be a result of inhibition of ureteral peristalsis caused by *Escherichia coli* endotoxin.[6] In addition, a primary neuromuscular abnormality has been proposed as a cause of hydroureter. These changes may not be limited to the affected side, because chronic ascending infection and pyelonephritis may result in dilatation of the contralateral ureter and renal pelvis.

Dilatation of the ureter may not be present if the ureter is only mildly displaced or has a troughlike opening. If the ureter appears to be straight as it enters the bladder, rather than forming the normal J shape, an ectopic location should be suspected.[6] An intramural ectopic ureter may appear to bypass the bladder on these studies and may be confused with an extramural ectopic ureter. Other diagnostic techniques may be required to confirm an ectopic opening because of superimposition of pelvic bones, the gastrointestinal tract, or contrast medium in the bladder and urethra. Lack of opacity of the distal ureter as a result of peristalsis or poor renal excretion may also result in a nondiagnostic study.

Other contrast radiographic procedures that have been described for the diagnosis of ureteral ectopia are retrograde urethrography and vaginourethrography.[4,7] The presence of a catheter in the urethra may obstruct the ectopic ureteral orifice, prohibiting a diagnosis with urethrography. Insertion of a Foley catheter into the vestibule and distension of the vagina and urethra with contrast may result in filling of the ectopic ureter with contrast medium, which confirms the diagnosis.

Ultrasonography has been reported to be an accurate means of determining ureteral anatomy.[4] The ureterovesicular junction is visible as a small, convex structure on the dorsal aspect of the bladder. Flow of urine from this area ("ureteral jet") can be observed in dogs with normally positioned bladders. Distension of the bladder with fluid or administration of a diuretic may aid visualization. Reduced or absent urine flow from the distal ureter into the bladder indicates an ectopic ureter. In addition, dilatation of the ectopic ureter or renal pelvis and thickening of the ureteral wall may be noted. One study that compared ultrasonography to contrast radiography for the diagnosis of ectopic ureters found that both techniques were accurate, with correct identification of 91% of the ectopic ureters.[4]

Direct visualization of the ureteral orifice with vaginoscopy and cystoscopy is a specific means of making the diagnosis of an ectopic ureter and for identifying abnormalities of the vagina and lower urinary tract. The vestibule and vagina can be visualized with a speculum, although ideally a rigid or flexible endoscope is used for complete evaluation of these structures, in addition to the bladder and urethra. Fluid insufflation aids visualization. The normal ureteral opening has a horseshoe-shaped, slitlike appearance when viewed endoscopically. Urine flow should be observed intermittently arising from these openings in the trigone region of the bladder. Inability to identify the normal ureteral openings should raise suspicion of an ectopic ureter. The urethra and vagina should be carefully evaluated for single or multiple ureteral openings and for a submucosal tunnel, which may appear as a slightly raised tube below the mucosal surface.

Cystometrographic studies and urethral pressure profilimetry can be used to identify functional abnormalities of the bladder and urethra in patients with ectopic ureters and may provide prognostic information.[7,8] The urethral pressure profile provides information about the pressures generated along the length of the urethra. This is often combined with the cystometrogram, which evaluates bladder capacity and compliance, and the strength of the detrusor reflex. In one study that evaluated the results of preoperative urodynamic measurements in nine dogs with ectopic ureters, reduced bladder capacity was detected in four dogs and urethral incompetence was found in six dogs.[8] Lack of response of urethral incompetence to phenylpropanolamine treatment before surgery was highly predictive of a poor postoperative outcome.[8]

Surgery is recommended for the treatment of patients with an ectopic ureter. The type of procedure performed depends on the morphology of the ureter and the functioning of the associated kidney. If the kidney is determined to be nonfunctional by preoperative evaluation, it should be removed with the ectopic ureter. Incontinence will likely persist after nephroureterectomy in patients with an ectopic intramural ureter unless the intramural segment is also removed.[7] The traditional treatment for intramural ectopic ureters has been to ligate the distal submucosal ureteral segment and create a new ureteral opening in the trigone of the bladder. Recently it was suggested that the intramural segment of ureter disrupts the functional anatomy of the internal urethral sphincter mechanism.[7] Therefore it has been recommended that the intramural segment be resected from the bladder neck and urethra and that the overlying mucosa and smooth muscle layers be apposed. A neoureterostomy is then performed by suturing the ureteral mucosa to the bladder mucosa in the region of the trigone. This trigonal and urethral reconstruction technique has been reported to result in less postoperative incontinence.[7] Extramural ectopic ureters are treated by ligating the distal end of the ureter at its attachment to the urethra, vagina, or uterus and reimplanting it into the bladder between the apex and the trigone. Because of the frequency of infection in patients with ectopic ureters, a urine culture from the bladder or renal pelvis should also be performed at surgery.

The most common complication after surgical correction of an ectopic ureter is persistent urinary incontinence, which occurs in 44% to 67% of patients.[7,9] Reasons proposed for persistent incontinence include the presence of a submucosal ureteral remnant in the trigone or urethra, primary sphincter mechanism incompetence, other congenital abnormalities of the urogenital tract, or urinary tract infection. Urine culture should be performed in patients with persistent or recurrent incontinence and infection treated based on susceptibility results. Some patients with postoperative incontinence respond to alpha-adrenergic drugs (phenylpropanolamine or ephedrine). Additional procedures that have been proposed for treatment of persistent incontinence include endoscopic submucosal injection of glutaraldehyde cross-linked collagen within the urethra and additional surgical procedures, such as colposuspension and cystourethropexy.[7] Partial or complete resolution of hydroureter and hydronephrosis may be seen after surgical correction of ectopic ureters even if the dilatation was severe before surgery.[10]

Ureterocele

A cystic dilatation of the submucosal segment of the distal ureter near the ureteral orifice is called a *ureterocele*. The proposed embryogenic mechanisms that result in the formation of a ureterocele include persistence of the membrane that separates the ureter from the lumen of the urogenital sinus; stenosis of the ureteral orifice, resulting in obstruction and ureteral dilatation; delayed ureteral migration, resulting in retention of the dilated distal ureteral segment; and embryonic arrest of myogenesis of the distal ureter.[4] Ureteroceles are classified as orthotopic or ectopic, depending on the location of the ureterocele and the associated ureteral orifice. An orthotopic ureterocele is located in the trigone of the bladder with an opening at the normal position of the ureterovesicular junction. Ectopic ureteroceles occur in conjunction with an ectopic ureter and have an opening within or distal to the bladder neck. A grading system for canine ureteroceles was recently proposed.[11] Grade 1 ureteroceles have no evidence of associated upper urinary tract disease. Grade 2 ureteroceles are associated with ipsilateral hydroureter, hydronephrosis, or chronic renal disease, and the condition is bilateral in grade 3 ureteroceles.

Orthotopic ureteroceles may go undiagnosed unless they are large enough to cause obstruction of the urethra or of the ipsilateral or contralateral ureter or unless they are associated with infection. Clinical signs associated with large orthotopic ureteroceles include abdominal pain, hematuria, stranguria,

and pollakiuria. Incontinence is seen if the ureterocele is ectopic. The diagnosis is made with contrast radiography, ultrasonography, or uroendoscopy. Excretory urography combined with pneumocystography may reveal a contrast-filled dilatation of the ureter in the bladder or urethra; this is referred to as the *cobra head sign*.[4] If the kidney associated with the ureterocele has impaired function, a filling defect is seen as contrast accumulates within the bladder or urethra. On ultrasonographic evaluation, the ureterocele appears as a rounded, thin-walled, fluid-filled cystic structure in the bladder.[4]

Cystoscopic incision is commonly used to treat ureteroceles in humans and may also be effective in dogs with orthotopic ureteroceles.[11] In addition, ureteroceles may be treated by open resection. Ectopic ureteroceles should be treated as ectopic ureters by resection of the ureterocele, neoureterocystostomy, and reconstruction of the bladder neck and urethra. Unless renal dysfunction is present prior to surgery, the prognosis for correction of an orthotopic ureterocele is good. Incontinence has been reported to persist in 33% to 50% of patients treated for an ectopic ureterocele.[11,12]

Agenesis or Duplication

Ureteral agenesis results from failure of development of the ureteral bud. Segmental absence of the ureter or lack of a lumen may occur in combination with other congenital abnormalities.[4] Renal agenesis may be associated with ureteral agenesis, because the ureteral bud induces the embryonic metanephric kidney to proliferate and differentiate. Unilateral ureteral and renal agenesis is usually asymptomatic unless the opposite kidney is compromised. Ureteral duplication has also been reported and occurs when more than one ureteral bud develops from the same mesonephric duct or if an abnormality exists in division of the ureteral bud.[13] A duplex kidney results as renal parenchyma is formed around each developing ureter. The ureter draining the lower part of the duplex system enters the bladder in the normal location, whereas the ureter draining the upper part is ectopic, terminating in the urethra.

ACQUIRED DISEASES

Ureteral Trauma

Ureteral injury can result from blunt abdominal trauma, penetrating wounds, or iatrogenic damage during surgery. Trauma to the ureters has been rarely reported in dogs and cats. Ureteral injury resulting from blunt trauma accounted for only 0.01% of the small animal hospital population in a recent report.[14] In humans, ureteral injuries, which usually result from gunshot wounds, are also uncommon, representing 5% of all patients with genitourinary trauma.[15]

The diagnosis of ureteral injury is often delayed for 3 or more days because of the rarity of this condition and the nonspecific clinical signs, which are often masked by hypovolemic shock, pain, and multiple organ injuries caused by the traumatic incident.[13] If the retroperitoneum is intact, urine accumulation is confined to this space, and several days may pass before an increase in the serum creatinine or potassium concentration is detected. Uroabdomen is present if retroperitoneal disruption occurs or with injury at the ureterovesicular junction. Uroabdomen may also result from concurrent urinary bladder rupture. Hematuria is not consistently present in patients with ureteral trauma alone.[14,15] If hematuria, abdominal pain, or uroabdomen is present, further evaluation of the urinary tract is indicated. Although the diagnosis of ureteral injury may not be made for days, this delay in humans has not been associated with increased mortality, loss of renal function, or the necessity for ureteronephrectomy.[15]

Radiography may reveal loss of peritoneal or retroperitoneal detail. Increased density, widening, and streaking of the retroperitoneum are indications of fluid accumulation but are not specific for urine.[4] Excretory urography can be performed if the patient is hydrated, normotensive, and not significantly azotemic. Extravasation of contrast medium from the site of rupture and renal pelvic or ureteral dilatation may be seen in affected animals. One report of ureteral trauma in small animals found excretory urography to be diagnostic in all four animals in which it was used; however, in humans with ureteral trauma, it has been reported to be less than 50% accurate.[14,15] Potential reasons for inaccuracy included poor urine output, a poor quality study, and radiographs taken at only one time period. Ultrasonography may demonstrate fluid accumulation in the retroperitoneal space but does not allow differentiation between a hematoma and extravasation of urine. Additional diagnostic tests that may be helpful include retrograde pyelography, computed tomography (CT), or magnetic resonance imaging. The diagnosis of ureteral trauma can be made at surgery, but direct inspection of the ureters after a traumatic incident is often complicated by the presence of retroperitoneal blood and fluid. Catheterization of the ureter from the bladder may aid identification of the site of ureteral rupture. In addition, intravenous injection of methylene blue increases visualization of urine coming from the proximal ureteral segment; however, this technique should be used with caution, because it has been associated with Heinz body anemia and renal failure. If intraoperative fluoroscopy is available, excretory urography can also be performed at surgery.

The goal of initial treatment should be to stabilize the patient for definitive surgery. Hypovolemic shock, hyperkalemia, and respiratory compromise must be treated prior to administration of anesthesia. If uroabdomen is present and the patient is not stable for surgery, a large-gauge, fenestrated catheter (e.g., peritoneal lavage catheter) can be placed intraabdominally for drainage.

Definitive surgical treatment of the injured ureter depends on the severity and location of the injury and the functioning of the contralateral kidney. Ureteronephrectomy has been reported as the most common treatment in small animal patients.[14] This likely is due to the severity of ureteral damage and the technical difficulties of ureteral surgery. The prognosis with ureteronephrectomy is good if the other kidney is functional; however, ureteronephrectomy is considered a salvage procedure in humans and should not be performed if doubt exists about the function of the remaining kidney.

Successful ureteral anastomosis requires an adequate blood supply, good apposition of ureteral ends, and minimal tension. Urine diversion via a nephrostomy catheter or ureteral stent may also be helpful. A ureteral wound less than 50% the circumference of the ureter seals in 48 hours with adequate urine diversion.[3] Injuries to the proximal one third of the ureter may be treated by primary anastomosis. Injuries to the middle or distal one third may be treated by primary anastomosis or reimplantation of the ureter into the bladder (ureteroneocystostomy). If the ureter is reimplanted, the bladder may be advanced cranially (psoas cystopexy) or the kidney freed and moved caudally (renal descensus) to alleviate tension. Risks of primary repair and reimplantation include urine leakage, dehiscence, and stricture formation. Additional surgical techniques that have been described include bladder flap ureteroplasty and transureteroureterostomy.[13]

Iatrogenic Injury

Injury to the ureters can result from iatrogenic damage, which occurs most commonly during ovariohysterectomy. Inadvertent ligation and transection of the ureters has been reported.[16] The most common location for inadvertent ligation is near the uterine body. This may result in complete obstruction, with associated hydronephrosis, hydroureter, and eventually permanent renal damage if not corrected within 7 days.[13,16]

An additional complication that has been reported to occur as a result of incorporation of the ureter into a uterine or vaginal ligature is ureterovaginal fistula.[17] The fistula may develop within 1 to 2 weeks of ovariohysterectomy and is associated with urinary incontinence. Treatment of ureterovaginal fistula involves ligation of the fistula and ureteral reimplantation into the bladder or ureteronephrectomy. Pyelonephritis is another complication that can occur with ureteral ligation and excision during ovariohysterectomy.

Urinoma

A paraureteral pseudocyst, or urinoma, forms when urine that has leaked from a ureter into the retroperitoneum becomes encapsulated in a thick, fibrous wall. The proposed mechanism of formation involves chronic, low-grade urine leakage from the ureter after trauma or obstruction, which causes necrosis of the surrounding fat and infiltration of round cells.[18] This inflammatory reaction results in the creation of a fibrous capsule over 3 to 6 weeks. A paraureteral pseudocyst was recently reported in a cat 3 weeks after an automobile-related accident.[19] Inadvertent ureteral transection during ovariohysterectomy was also reported to cause urinoma in a dog.[18] A preoperative diagnosis of a paraureteral pseudocyst is made by the identification of contrast accumulation in the pseudocyst during excretory urography or by visualization of hydronephrosis and hydroureter with a fluid-filled cavitary mass on ultrasonography.[4] Ureteronephrectomy has been the reported treatment.[18,19]

Ureteral Obstruction

Ureteral obstruction can result from intraluminal, intramural, or extramural causes. Intraluminal obstruction can occur as a result of a blood clot or calculus. Intramural fibrosis, stricture, or neoplasia may also obstruct urine flow. Extramural compression may occur from a retroperitoneal mass or bladder neoplasm or from a ligature placed inadvertently during surgery. Clinical signs of obstruction may not be apparent unless bilateral obstruction or concomitant infection of the urinary tract is present. Clinical signs may be mild, including dysuria, abdominal pain, vomiting, anorexia, and lethargy. On the other hand, patients with complete, bilateral obstruction are anuric and may be collapsed at presentation. Complete, bilateral obstruction that persists for 3 days or longer is fatal without appropriate treatment.[13]

It may be difficult to distinguish between obstructing and nonobstructing causes of ureteral dilatation. However, this distinction is important, because pyelonephritis may cause ureteral dilatation and would not warrant surgery. Conversely, an obstructing calculus or mass would necessitate early surgical intervention. Obstructing ureteral calculi in cats may be small and difficult to visualize on plain radiographs. Excretory urography is helpful for identifying ureteral dilatation to the point of obstruction and may show a filling defect or stricture if the associated kidney is functional and the patient is not severely compromised. With severe compromise of renal function, opacification of the kidneys and ureters is poor, resulting in a nondiagnostic study.[4] In addition, adverse systemic reactions and the potential for further damage to the kidney make this procedure less than ideal in dehydrated or severely azotemic patients.[4,13]

Percutaneous antegrade pyelography is an accurate diagnostic test for patients in which excretory urography is nondiagnostic, or when concern exists about the adverse effects of systemic contrast administration (Figure 268-1).[20] Fluoroscopy or ultrasonography can be used to guide needle or catheter placement into the dilated renal pelvis. Urine is aspirated from the renal pelvis and submitted for analysis and culture. Iodinated contrast material is then injected into the needle or catheter at a volume equal to one half the aspirated urine volume. The flow of contrast is monitored with fluoroscopy or with radiographs taken

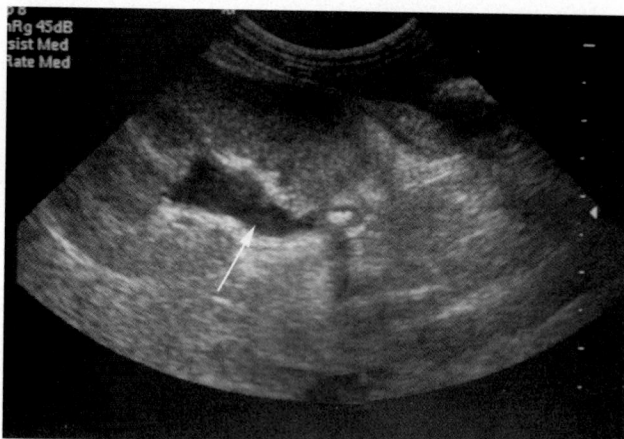

Figure 268-1 Percutaneous antegrade pyelography. Under ultrasound guidance, a needle was placed into the renal pelvis of a cat presenting with azotemia and anuria. Injection of contrast material allowed the diagnosis of complete, bilateral, distal ureteral obstruction by ureteroliths that were not evident on plain radiographs.

immediately after contrast injection. This technique is easily performed and has minimal complications, such as hematuria and leakage of contrast material or urine into the abdomen. Fluid diuresis is recommended with this procedure to prevent blood clot formation, which may result in obstruction.[20]

Ultrasonography is noninvasive, allows limited morphologic assessment of the renal parenchyma, and may allow diagnosis of ureteral obstruction. Although ureteral dilatation alone is not a specific sign of obstruction, visualization of focal hydroureter to the level of obstruction can be diagnostic.[4] In some patients it may be difficult to follow the entire course of the ureter because of its size and because of interference by other organs. In these cases, absence or reduced amplitude and duration of ureteral flow at the ureterovesicular junction can be used as an indirect sign of obstruction.[4] Additional noninvasive imaging that can be used to evaluate patients with ureteral obstruction are CT and renal scintigraphy. Renal scintigraphy allows evaluation of renal function in dogs with ureteral obstruction but does not predict what function will be after the obstruction has been relieved.[21]

Once the diagnosis has been made, rapid surgical intervention is indicated, because recovery of renal function is inversely related to the duration of obstruction.[13] If patency of a completely obstructed ureter is restored within 7 days of obstruction, renal function can return to normal.[13,21] If the obstruction persists for 2 weeks prior to correction, the affected kidney will regain approximately 50% of its preobstruction function. Complete loss of renal function does not occur until complete ureteral obstruction is present for longer than 4 weeks. If the patient is not stable for definitive surgical correction, a nephropyelostomy catheter can be placed to divert urine flow and preserve renal function. If hemodialysis is available, it can be useful for stabilization of severely uremic patients before they undergo long surgical procedures to remove the source of obstruction. The definitive surgical treatment depends on the cause and duration of obstruction.

Calculi

Calcium oxalate calculi are the most common type of uroliths found in the kidneys and ureters of cats.[21] Potential risk factors for the formation of these stones include hypercalcemia, feeding a urine-acidifying diet or a single brand of cat food, an indoor only environment, and being of the Persian breed.[22] Struvite and calcium oxalate calculi most frequently cause ureteral obstruction in dogs.[23] If ureteral calculi are diagnosed by plain radiography and are not associated with significant obstruction, serial radiographs should be taken to monitor calculi movement. Medical dissolution of ureteroliths is unlikely to be successful, because calculi in the ureter are not continually bathed in urine, and calcium oxalate calculi are not amenable to dissolution. Intravenous fluid diuresis, with or without diuretics, may encourage movement of calculi to the bladder. Failure of calculi to progress down the ureter on subsequent radiographs is an indication for surgical intervention. Currently there is no recommendation on the appropriate amount of time for which patients should be monitored for the passage of ureteroliths. An experimental study of artificial calculi in dogs has shown that solid spheres 2.8 mm in diameter become firmly impacted in the ureter; however, spheres 2.3 mm in diameter pass within 1 to 24 hours.[13] A clinical report of 11 cats with ureteroliths found that the calculi did not move toward the bladder in any patient monitored for a mean of 19 days.[21] Furthermore, fibrosis of the ureteral wall and ulcers of the ureteral epithelium at the site of obstruction demonstrated that the stones were immobile in these patients. Because even partial obstruction of the ureter results in decreased renal blood flow, decreased renal function, and potentially irreversible renal damage, early surgical intervention is indicated if there is evidence of obstruction.[21]

Options for surgical treatment of ureteroliths include ureterotomy; retrograde flushing of calculi into the renal pelvis, followed by pyelolithotomy; resection of the affected portion of the ureter, followed by primary anastomosis or reimplantation into the bladder; and ureteronephrectomy. Complications of ureteral surgery include urine leakage, dehiscence, and stricture formation. Placement of a nephrostomy catheter after surgery may be helpful for diverting urine flow until the ureter heals.

Extracorporeal shock wave lithotripsy (ESWL) is an alternative treatment for nephrolithiasis and ureterolithiasis in dogs. ESWL was reported to be effective in two dogs with ureterolithiasis and in one dog that developed ureteroliths after treatment for nephrolithiasis.[23] In humans, ESWL is reported to be less effective for ureteroliths than for nephroliths because of attenuation of shock wave energy by surrounding muscle and bone, difficulty with patient positioning, difficulty identifying ureteroliths by fluoroscopy or ultrasonography, and adherence of the ureterolith to the ureteral mucosa, which prevents fragments from passing during lithotripsy.[23] Disadvantages of ESWL in dogs include lack of availability, the need for general anesthesia, and the potential need for multiple treatments. ESWL is contraindicated in patients with coagulopathies, pacemakers, pregnancy, and obstruction distal to the calculi, which prevents removal of urolith fragments. Lithotripsy was reported to be successful in only one of five cats treated for ureterolithiasis.[21]

Neoplasia

Primary ureteral neoplasia is rare in dogs and has not been reported in cats. Transitional cell carcinoma has been the most frequently reported tumor type and is seen most commonly in females.[24] Other tumor types include leiomyoma, leiomyosarcoma, and benign papillomas.[13,24] In a small number of patients, a good prognosis was reported for ureteronephrectomy of neoplasms confined to the ureter.[24]

SECTION
XIX

Hematology
and Immunology

CHAPTER 269

Problem-Oriented Differential Diagnosis of Autoimmune Skin Diseases

Karen A. Moriello

Immune-mediated skin diseases are uncommon in clinical veterinary practice; they accounted for fewer than 1.5% of all skin diseases seen in a university referral dermatology service (Figure 269-1). Nonetheless, they are problematic to the clinician because they can appear similar to other skin diseases that are more common.

Immune-mediated skin diseases are divided into two major categories: *primary autoimmune diseases*, in which the disease is the result of attack against self-antigens, and *secondary immune-mediated diseases*, in which the disease is the result of an attack against a foreign antigen. The most common foreign antigens are drugs, bacteria, and viruses that trigger an immunologic reaction, causing tissue damage. This chapter provides an overview of the more common autoimmune skin diseases and highlights key features that may narrow the list of differential diagnoses or may answer the question, "Should I be thinking of an autoimmune skin disease?"

CLINICAL CLUES IN THE HISTORY AND PHYSICAL EXAMINATION FINDINGS

Two major clinical presentations are seen in pets with autoimmune skin diseases (ASDs). One is the textbook presentation of the disease, which includes an acute onset of severe lesions. These patients are rarely problematic to the clinician with regard to diagnosis, because suspicion is high from the onset. The clinician suspects something serious, and an aggressive diagnostic evaluation is shortly underway. In the other clinical presentation, the disease manifests itself in a less obvious way, waxes and wanes, partially responds to treatment for a different disease, is a mild form of the ASD, or occurs concurrently with another chronic skin disease (e.g., atopic patients that develop pemphigus). The following points should raise suspicion of a possible immune-mediated skin disease:

Historical Clues
- Any severe skin disease with an acute or rapid onset
- Reports that the lesions wax and wane, especially in relatively short cycles of 7 to 10 days
- Intermittent episodes of depression, fever, and anorexia, especially if they coincide with the development of lesions
- Lack of response to seemingly appropriate therapy. For example:
  - A routine case of otitis externa that does not respond to therapy, with evidence emerging of primary lesions on the inner pinnae
  - Patients that continue to develop pustular lesions despite appropriate antibiotic therapy, especially if therapy has continued for longer than 3 weeks
  - Continued development of oral lesions on gums after appropriate dental therapy
- Difficulty eating or drinking (an early historical finding in dogs with oral ulcers)

Suspicious Physical Examination Findings
- Pruritus (variable in ASD, and its presence does not rule out ASD; evidence of pruritus may come from the history or may be obvious on examination [e.g., excoriations, observed self-trauma])
- Symmetry of skin lesions
- Skin disease (mild or moderate) with concurrent signs of systemic illness (fever, depression, anorexia)
- Large numbers of easily found, intact primary lesions all in the same stage, especially pustules, vesicles, or bullae
  - Intact or recently ruptured pustules on the inner pinnae
  - Intact pustules near the mammae of cats
  - Intact, flaccid pustules spanning several hair follicles, often yellow-green in color
- Thick, adherent crusting on the body
  - Crusting only on the face and/or footpads
  - Crusting that includes the face, footpads, and body
- A strong, offensive odor, with exudation and serum accumulation on the trunk, causing matting of the haircoat, especially if oily seborrhea is not present
- Ulcerations or erosions. For example:
  - Oral ulceration and/or erosions with or without halitosis and drooling
  - Mucocutaneous ulcerations and/or erosions, matting of the haircoat in these areas, and odor (often prominent findings)
  - Ulcerations and erosions in the axillary and/or inguinal region
- Depigmentation of the nose or mucocutaneous junctions

PROBLEM-ORIENTED APROACH TO DIFFERENTIAL DIAGNOSIS

The dermatologic problems most commonly associated with ASD are pustular eruptions, crusting and scaling, mucocutaneous ulcerations, nonmucocutaneous ulcerations, depigmentation, and miscellaneous problems, such as noninflammatory focal alopecia. Box 269-1 presents a problem-oriented list of differential diagnoses for autoimmune skin disorders. Because of the variation in clinical signs, some diseases fit into several categories.

Box 269-2 is a summary of the key diagnostic findings for skin biopsy and immunologic tests in various ASDs that help confirm the diagnosis. Skin scrapings and dermatophyte cultures should be negative in ASD. However, mite infestations and/or dermatophytosis can develop secondary to immunosuppressive disorders and occasionally occur concurrently. Adult-onset demodicosis can precede the development of an autoimmune skin disease. In a "classic" ASD case, bacterial cultures of intact pustules should be reported as "no growth" or "scant" growth. If heavy growth of bacteria is found, this may indicate that the pustular disease is bacterial in origin, that bacteria have

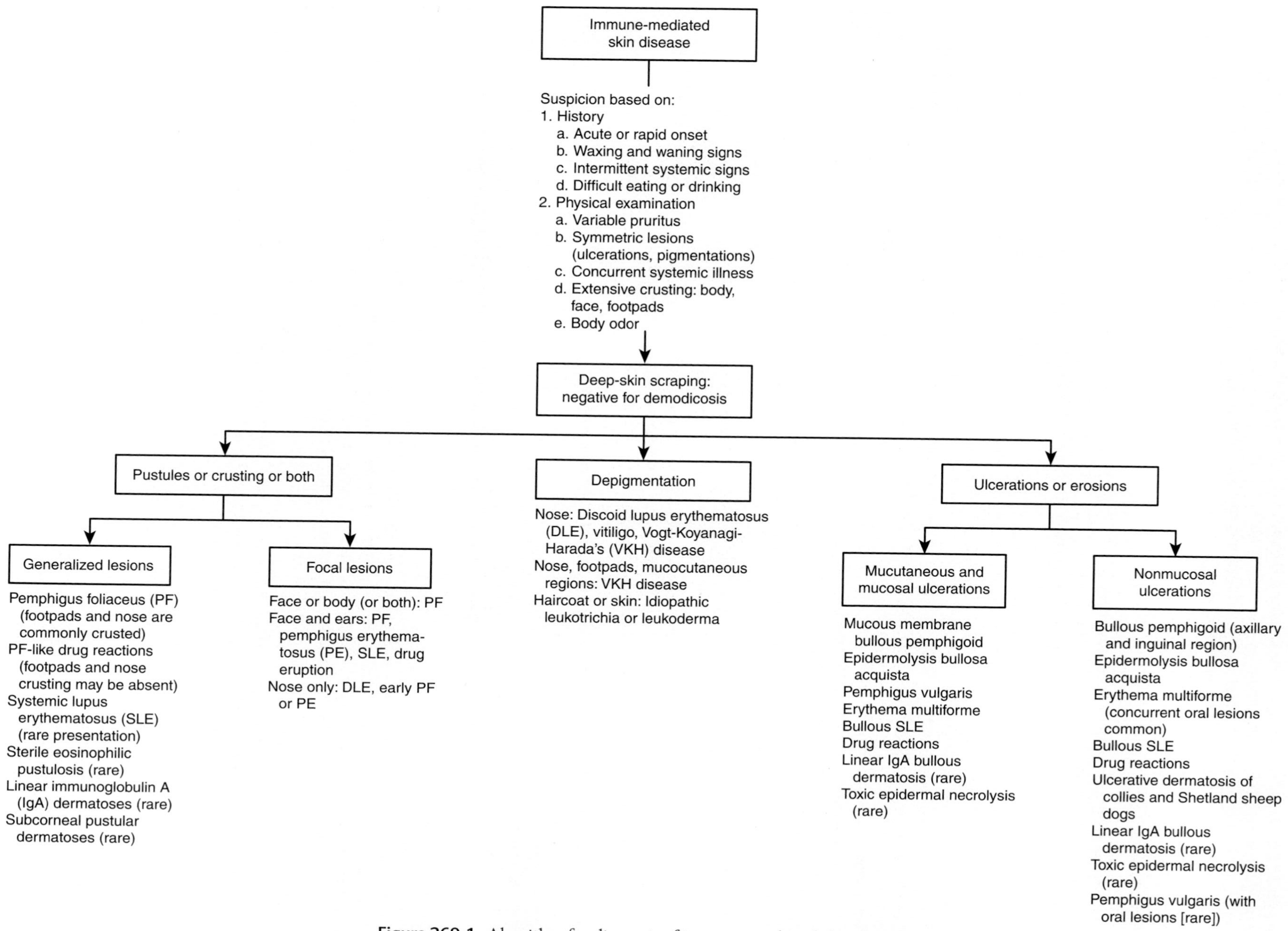

Immune-mediated skin disease

Suspicion based on:
1. History
   a. Acute or rapid onset
   b. Waxing and waning signs
   c. Intermittent systemic signs
   d. Difficult eating or drinking
2. Physical examination
   a. Variable pruritus
   b. Symmetric lesions (ulcerations, pigmentations)
   c. Concurrent systemic illness
   d. Extensive crusting: body, face, footpads
   e. Body odor

Deep-skin scraping: negative for demodicosis

Pustules or crusting or both

Generalized lesions

Pemphigus foliaceus (PF) (footpads and nose are commonly crusted)
PF-like drug reactions (footpads and nose crusting may be absent)
Systemic lupus erythematosus (SLE) (rare presentation)
Sterile eosinophilic pustulosis (rare)
Linear immunoglobulin A (IgA) dermatoses (rare)
Subcorneal pustular dermatoses (rare)

Focal lesions

Face or body (or both): PF
Face and ears: PF, pemphigus erythematosus (PE), SLE, drug eruption
Nose only: DLE, early PF or PE

Depigmentation

Nose: Discoid lupus erythematosus (DLE), vitiligo, Vogt-Koyanagi-Harada's (VKH) disease
Nose, footpads, mucocutaneous regions: VKH disease
Haircoat or skin: Idiopathic leukotrichia or leukoderma

Ulcerations or erosions

Mucutaneous and mucosal ulcerations

Mucous membrane bullous pemphigoid
Epidermolysis bullosa acquista
Pemphigus vulgaris
Erythema multiforme
Bullous SLE
Drug reactions
Linear IgA bullous dermatosis (rare)
Toxic epidermal necrolysis (rare)

Nonmucosal ulcerations

Bullous pemphigoid (axillary and inguinal region)
Epidermolysis bullosa acquista
Erythema multiforme (concurrent oral lesions common)
Bullous SLE
Drug reactions
Ulcerative dermatosis of collies and Shetland sheep dogs
Linear IgA bullous dermatosis (rare)
Toxic epidermal necrolysis (rare)
Pemphigus vulgaris (with oral lesions [rare])

Figure 269-1 Algorithm for diagnosis of immune-mediated skin disease.

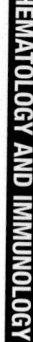

HEMATOLOGY AND IMMUNOLOGY

Box • 269-1

Differential Diagnosis of Autoimmune Skin Diseases

Generalized Pustular Eruptions and/or Crusting Dermatoses (Involving the Body, Head, Face, or Feet)
- Pemphigus foliaceus (PF) (footpad and nose commonly are crusted)
- Pemphigus-like drug reactions (nasal and footpad crusting may be absent)
- Systemic lupus erythematosus (rare presentation)
- Sterile eosinophilic pustulosis (rare disease)
- Linear IgA pustular dermatosis (rare disease)
- Subcorneal pustular dermatosis (rare disease)

Focal Pustular Eruptions and/or Focal Crusting
- Face and/or footpads: PF
- Face and ears only: PF (early), pemphigus erythematosus (PE), drug eruptions, lupus erythematosus
- Nasal only: Discoid lupus erythematosus, PE (early), PE

NOTE: Pustules are quite transient, and many of the generalized pustular diseases also present as generalized, malodorous, crusting dermatoses. The major differential diagnoses here are bacterial pyoderma, dermatophytosis, severe seborrhea, and zinc deficiency. Bacterial pyoderma rarely affects the head, and dermatophytosis is a nonsymmetric skin disease. Most cases occur in young animals (dermatophytosis) or sled dogs (zinc deficiency). Severe, oily seborrhea may also appear as a crusting dermatosis and can mimic PF if nasal and digital hyperkeratosis is present; the major differentiating factor is that primary seborrhea starts out at a young age. Zinc-responsive skin diseases may present as widespread or focal crusting dermatoses and can mimic PF.

Mucocutaneous and Mucosal Ulcerations
- Pemphigus vulgaris (may also have oral ulcerations)
- Mucous membrane bullous pemphigoid
- Epidermolysis bullosa acquisita
- Erythema multiforme (target lesions, cutaneous ulcerations also may be present)
- Bullous systemic lupus erythematosus
- Drug reactions
- Linear IgA bullous dermatosis (rare)
- Toxic epidermal necrolysis (rare)

Note: The primary lesions in these diseases are vesicles and bullae, which are quite transient and rupture, leaving erosions and ulceration. The adjacent haircoat becomes matted and odorous. The major differential diagnoses of concern are candidiasis, ulcerative mucocutaneous bacterial pyoderma, and cutaneous lymphoma.

Nonmucosal Ulcerations (Axillae, Inguina, Pinnae, or Other Haired Areas)
- Bullous pemphigoid
- Epidermolysis bullosa acquisita
- Linear IgA bullous dermatosis
- Bullous systemic lupus erythematosus
- Canine vesicular cutaneous lupus erythematosus (also called idiopathic ulcerative dermatosis of collies and Shetland sheepdogs)
- Erythema multiforme
- Toxic epidermal necrolysis
- Drug eruptions
- Pemphigus vulgaris (with concurrent mucocutaneous lesions)

NOTE: The primary lesions are vesicles and/or bullae, which are quite transient. These patients commonly present with fever, pain, a matted haircoat, and exudation. The major differential diagnoses of concern are deep bacterial pyoderma, deep pyoderma caused by demodicosis, and cutaneous deep and intermediate mycoses.

Depigmenting Skin Diseases
- Nasal only: Discoid lupus erythematosus, vitiligo-like syndrome, uveodermatologic syndrome, early PF or PE
- Nose, footpads, lips, eyelids, and mucocutaneous regions: Uveodermatologic syndrome (these animals have concurrent uveitis)
- Haircoat or skin: Idiopathic leukotrichia or leukoderma

Miscellaneous
- Focal alopecia: Alopecia areata, rabies vaccine, focal vasculitis
- Widespread noninflammatory alopecia: Alopecia areata, pseudopelade
- Erythematous target lesions: Erythema multiforme
- Nodular ulcerative lesions: Nodular panniculitis
- Purpura, hemorrhage, "punched out" lesions: Vasculitis
- Ear margin necrosis, pineal erosions: Vasculitis
- Dependent edema with erythema: Vasculitis

Box • 269-2

Key Diagnostic Findings in Common Autoimmune Skin Diseases

Skin Biopsy
- *Pemphigus vulgaris:* Suprabasilar acantholysis with cleft and vesicle formation; basal cells attachment to basement membrane resembles a row of tombstones.
- *Pemphigus foliaceus:* Intragranular or subcorneal pustules with acantholysis.
- *Pemphigus erythematosus:* Intragranular or subcorneal pustules with acantholysis with a lichenoid reaction.
- *Bullous pemphigoid, epidermolysis bullosa acquisita, linear IgA bullous dermatosis, mucous membrane pemphigoid,* and *bullous systemic lupus erythematosus:* Subepidermal cleft and vesicle formation, no acantholysis, and possible lichenoid reaction.
- *Systemic* or *discoid lupus erythematosus (DLE) (the histologic findings for both systemic and discoid lupus erythematosus are identical, except that pigmentary incontinence may be more prominent in DLE):* Hydropic and/or lichenoid interface dermatitis of the epidermis and possibly of the outer root sheath of the hair follicles, apoptosis of basal cells and, less commonly, subepidermal vesicles.
- *Erythema multiforme (EM) (the histologic findings with EM vary greatly; a key finding is apoptosis of keratinocytes throughout the epidermis):* Interface dermatitis with prominent single cell apoptosis of keratinocytes throughout the epidermis and outer root sheath of the epidermis.
- *Toxic epidermal necrolysis:* Hydropic degeneration of basal cells, full-thickness coagulation necrosis of the epidermis, and minimal dermal inflammation.
- *Uveodermatologic syndrome:* Lichenoid interface dermatitis with large histiocytes, as well as prominent pigmentary incontinence; hydropic degeneration of epidermal basal cells is rare.

Antinuclear Antibody Testing
- *Pemphigus erythematosus:* Weak positive titer may be seen.
- *Systemic lupus erythematosus:* Strong positive titer.

Direct Immunofluorescence Testing
- *Pemphigus complex:* Positive intercellular fluorescence.
- *Pemphigus erythematosus:* Positive intercellular and basement membrane fluorescence.
- *Bullous pemphigoid (50% to 90% of cases), epidermolysis bullosa acquisita, linear IgA dermatosis, mucous membrane pemphigoid, systemic or cutaneous lupus erythematosus (50% to 90% of cases):* Positive basement membrane fluorescence.
NOTE: Direct immunofluorescence testing usually is negative in the other autoimmune skin diseases, however, this is not always the case, and nonspecific staining may be seen.

Indirect Immunofluorescence Testing
- Indirect immunofluorescence testing using a salt split-skin as a substrate is a relatively new method of differentiating the autoimmune subepidermal bullous diseases.

colonized skin lesions caused by the ASD, or that staphylococcal bacteria from the clinician's fingers contaminated the culture. In some cases skin biopsies are diagnostic, and in other cases a trial of antibiotic therapy or a review of previous therapies may answer the question. Cytologic specimens may also show concurrent *Malassezia* overgrowth. It is important to rule out candidiasis in patients with mucocutaneous or ulcerative dermatoses. This is best done by fungal culture at a reference laboratory (a swab is submitted) and by cytologic examination of exudate (unfixed, unstained slides of debris scraped from the lesion margins are submitted).

Cytologic examination of the contents of an intact pustule may be extremely valuable for making a diagnosis. This diagnostic test may be helpful for corroborating a diagnosis of pemphigus foliaceus (PF). Intact pustules are rare in cats, and if found, especially on the inner pinnae and near the mammae, are almost always caused by pemphigus foliaceus.

In dogs, it is rare to easily find large numbers of intact pustules. The pustules of pemphigus are large, flaccid, and filled with a copious amount of pus. The specimen should be stained and examined for acanthocytes, which are round, deeply basophilic epidermal cells often present as rafts (i.e., numerous cells adhered together). In dogs these cells tend to be found in PF and in cases of severe bacterial pyoderma. Cytologic specimens should be carefully examined for eosinophils. In dogs, eosinophils can be seen in pustular specimens from PF. A finding of eosinophils should prompt the clinician to consider other differential diagnoses, such as allergic disease (small numbers of eosinophils), sterile eosinophilic pustulosis (almost pure fields of eosinophils), or parasitic diseases (variable). In cats, a finding of large numbers of eosinophils requires some thought on the part of the clinician, because many allergic skin diseases of cats can mimic ASDs.

CHAPTER 270

Regenerative Anemias Caused by Blood Loss or Hemolysis

Urs Giger

Anemia is not a diagnosis in itself but is a common clinical sign and laboratory test abnormality in companion animals. Thus anemia may indicate a specific erythrocyte problem or can be associated with other organ disorders. Anemia and other hematologic abnormalities occur so frequently that a complete blood cell count (CBC) is generally requested in the diagnostic assessment of any ill dog or cat. Anemia is defined as a decrease in the red blood cell (RBC) mass as expressed by a reduction in number of circulating RBCs, hematocrit, and hemoglobin. Clinical signs of anemia result from decreased oxygen-carrying capacity, reduced blood volume, underlying disease, and the adjustments made to increase the efficiency of the erythron. Severity of clinical signs depends on the rapidity of onset, the degree and cause of anemia, and the extent of physical activity. A logical approach to the cause of anemia is usually fruitful. Anemias are classified by pathophysiologic mechanisms, bone marrow response, and RBC indices. This chapter reviews regenerative anemias caused by blood loss or hemolysis. Non-regenerative anemias will be covered in the next chapter (271) and additional details on hematologic aspects are provided in *Schalm's Veterinary Hematology* and other clinical pathology texts.[1-3]

REGENERATIVE BONE MARROW RESPONSE

The number of circulating erythrocytes is the result of a dynamic equilibrium between the production and delivery of erythrocytes (Figure 270-1) and their destruction or loss. The normal homeostatic mechanisms of the body bring about recovery from anemia by accelerating erythropoiesis. The erythroid bone marrow response is primarily regulated by erythropoietin, a lineage-specific hematopoietic growth factor. Erythropoietin synthesis in the renal cortex is induced by anemia, although the actual sensor measures oxygen tension and renal hypoxia. It acts predominantly on erythroid precursor cells of the bone marrow known as *burst-forming units-erythroid* (BFU-E) and particularly colony-forming units-erythroid (CFU-E). At maximal stimulation, the bone marrow is capable of producing erythrocytes at tenfold to fiftyfold the normal rate. Erythropoietin also contributes to the maturation from the early committed erythroid precursors to fully hemoglobinized erythrocytes, which takes normally approximately 1 week.[1,3]

Reticulocytes
The most useful marker of accelerated erythropoiesis is an increased number of circulating reticulocytes.[1,3,4] Reticulocytes form after extrusion of the pyknotic nucleus from normoblasts and continue to mature, finally to erythrocytes, in the bone marrow and peripheral blood. Reticulocytes normally reside within the marrow for almost 2 days before they are released into the circulation. They continue to synthesize hemoglobin as long as they have functional messenger RNA, which is usually 1 day in circulation. However, during accelerated erythropoiesis, reticulocytes may be released prematurely from the marrow. The so-called stress or shift reticulocytes are macrocytic, less developed, and therefore require a longer time to mature to erythrocytes in circulation. In hemolytic disorders they contain high pyruvate kinase (PK) activity.[4] Because they contain residual RNA, which can be precipitated into a reticulum network and stained by certain supravital dyes, such as new methylene blue or brilliant cresyl blue, reticulocytes can be readily enumerated. The latter stain is particularly suitable as it is relatively free of precipitates. On a stained blood smear, the number of reticulocytes is counted per 500 to 1000 erythrocytes, and the reticulocyte result is reported as a percentage of cells examined (number per 100 cells). Some hematology instruments provide a specific count.

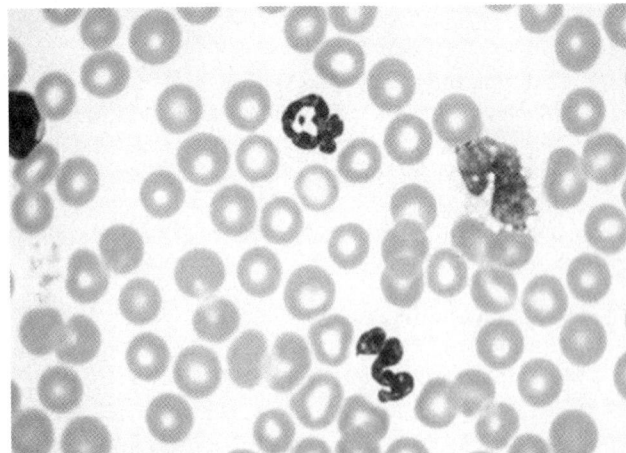

A

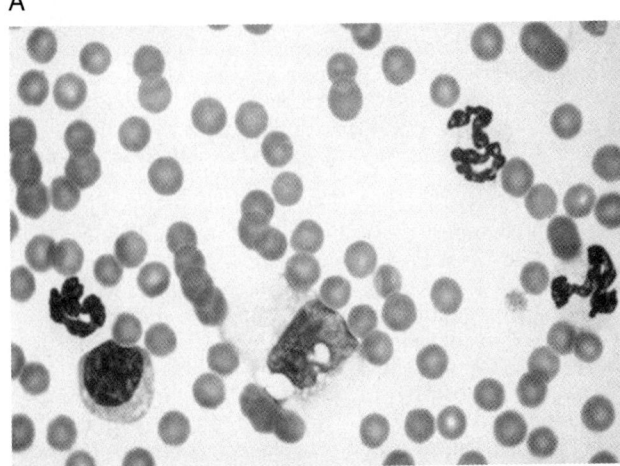

B

Figure 270-1 Normal canine (**A**) and feline (**B**) blood smear, Wright's-Giemsa staining. Reader should note the smaller size of feline erythrocytes.

Because canine reticulocytes contain strong aggregates, they are relatively easy to count (Figure 270-2). In contrast, cats produce two types of reticulocytes: (1) aggregate and (2) punctate. Aggregate reticulocytes correspond to the reticulocytes seen in dogs and indicate an active regenerative response. After a short maturation time of less than 1 day, these aggregate forms become punctate reticulocytes. On a blood smear stained for reticulocytes, they contain up to 10 individual blue dots, which do not coalesce. As punctate reticulocytes circulate over a period of 1 to 2 weeks and represent a cumulative response, they can reach high percentages. It is therefore best to report either the aggregate reticulocytes only, or both separately, in cats.

The upper limit of a normal reticulocyte count is often stated as 1%; however, healthy small animals generally have less than 0.4% reticulocytes per 100 erythrocytes. This number is not only increased by enhanced hematopoiesis but also affected by anemia, because it depends on the number of circulating erythrocytes and the duration of reticulocyte maturation in circulation. Therefore various "adjustments" to reticulocyte counts are used. If the erythrocyte count is available, the absolute reticulocyte count can be calculated and is less than 40,000/µL in a healthy animal:

$$\frac{\% \text{ reticulocytes} \times \text{RBC/µL}}{100} = \text{recticulocytes/µL}$$

The absolute reticulocyte count has now been adopted as the preferred expression of erythroid regeneration. Several automated hematology analyzers have incorporated staining to detect reticulocytes and provide absolute reticulocyte counts; however, some such counts may be falsely increased in the presence of Heinz's bodies, Howell-Jolly bodies, and punctate reticulocytes. If the erythrocyte count is not known, correction for anemia can be made based on the dog or cat's hematocrit compared with the average normal packed cell volume (PCV) value (dogs 45%; cats 37%) and is normally less than 0.4%.

Finally, the reticulocyte production index (RPI) also takes into consideration the extended maturation of stress or shift reticulocytes in circulation. This parameter is no longer applied clinically.

An increase in absolute reticulocyte count or corrected reticulocyte percentage provides the best evidence for a regenerative response. Although not as accurate, other hematologic manifestations such as mean cell volume (MCV) and red cell distribution width (RDW) may be used to indicate increased erythropoiesis when a reticulocyte count is not available. On a blood smear stained with Wright's stain or Diff-Quik, polychromatophilic cells represent erythrocytes recently released from the bone marrow (Figure 270-3). Because their blue-gray tint is due to the presence of RNA, their numbers correlate with the reticulocyte count. When more than one polychromatophilic cell is recognized per microscopic oil immersion field, accelerated erythropoiesis is likely. Polychromatophilic erythrocytes are often macrocytic, which indicates that these cells are released prematurely from the marrow, thereby contributing greatly to the high MCV and RDW, as well as anisocytosis of regenerative anemias. It should be noted that macrocytic anemia is not always regenerative but may indicate a maturation problem such as feline leukemia virus (FeLV) infection or folate deficiency in cats.[5,6]

Nucleated erythrocytes (Figure 270-3) also known as *normoblasts* or *metarubricytes* with variably shrunken nuclei are rarely found in blood of healthy animals (less than 1 per 100 white blood cells [WBCs]). Depending on the hematology instrument, they may not be counted or may be under the WBCs. Large numbers may accompany a marked regenerative response in anemic pets. However, nucleated RBCs may also be seen in animals without reticulocytosis and regenerative response because of a breakdown of the barrier between marrow and vasculature. The highest numbers of normoblasts, for example, are observed in acute lead poisoning in the absence of anemia. Mild to moderate normoblastosis with nonregenerative anemia may be seen with myeloproliferative disorders, dyshematopoiesis, extramedullary hematopoiesis, hemangiosarcoma, and sepsis. Thus, normoblastosis should not be equated with a regenerative marrow response without confirmation by a reticulocyte count.

If an anemia is characterized as regenerative based on a reticulocytosis, bone marrow examination is rarely indicated. In regenerative anemia, the bone marrow cellularity is increased and the ratio of myeloid to erythroid elements in the bone marrow is generally below one. The earliest morphologically recognizable erythroid cell is a pronormoblast. An exponentially increasing number of round erythroid precursors that decrease in size to the pyknotic normoblast and are progressively more hemoglobinized indicate normal maturation. Although the erythropoietin response is lineage specific, independent stimulation of thrombopoiesis (e.g. iron deficiency) or granulopoiesis (e.g. immune-mediated hemolytic anemia [IMHA]) may also be present. Bone marrow examination rarely provides helpful information about an underlying cause

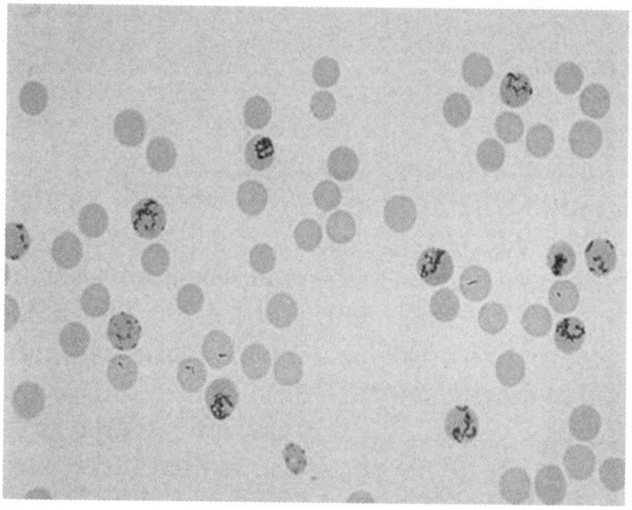

Figure 270-2 Canine reticulocytes as visualized by brilliant cresyl blue stain.

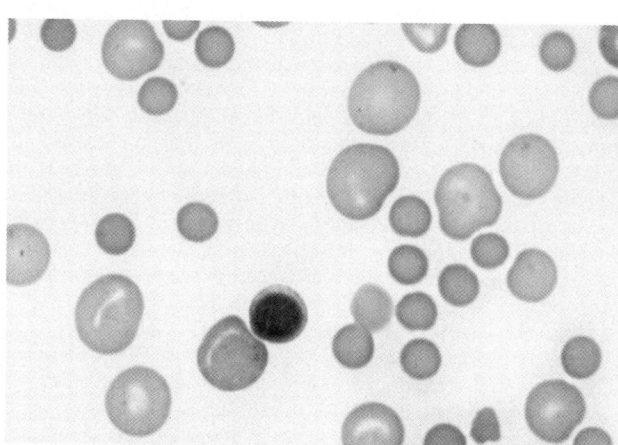

Figure 270-3 Polychromasia and anisocytosis with spherocytes and metarubricytes.

or marrow iron deposition in animals with regenerative anemia that would otherwise remain undetected.

BLOOD LOSS ANEMIA

Blood loss anemia occurs whenever a disease process damages vascular integrity sufficiently for RBCs to escape from the intravascular space. Blood loss may be localized to one site and caused by trauma, surgery, tumor, gastrointestinal (GI) disorders, or parasites. Blood loss may be generalized in association with a hemorrhagic tendency. Surface bleeding such as petechiae and epistaxis suggests a platelet problem, whereas hematomas and cavity bleedings indicate a coagulopathy. These primary and secondary hemostatic disorders are discussed in other chapters (see Chapters 272-274). Regardless of the cause, clinical manifestations of blood loss anemia depend on the volume of blood loss and onset (i.e., whether it is acute or chronic). Both acute and chronic blood loss are regenerative, although in the first few days after acute blood loss and in late stages of severe iron deficiency due to blood loss, such anemias are poorly regenerative.

Acute Blood Loss

Rapid blood loss of major proportions represents a double threat, because it decreases the total blood volume and oxygenation of tissue.[7,8] The total blood volume of dogs and cats is 8-10% and 6-8% of the body weight, respectively. Blood donations for transfusion of 4.4 mL/lb body weight, representing less than 20% of the blood volume of healthy animals, are generally well tolerated. However, when hemorrhage exceeds 20%, cardiovascular signs occur. Initial physiologic adjustments are peripheral vasoconstriction and tachycardia. Regional blood flow to skin and spleen is curtailed to protect perfusion of the brain, heart, and viscera. Thus pallor in acute blood loss anemia is caused not by thinness of blood but by reduced perfusion of the skin and is associated with a prolonged capillary refill time and dry mucous membranes. Besides the redistribution of blood to areas most vulnerable to hypoxemia, the heart rate is increased in an attempt to maintain cardiac output. This high-velocity flow is well tolerated because of the reduced viscosity of anemic blood and vasodilatation in the central and cerebral vascular beds into which most blood is diverted. As the blood loss exceeds 30% to 40% of the original blood volume, cardiac output decreases and hypotension with cardiovascular collapse ensues. The animal becomes immobile and exhibits a rapid, thready pulse, as well as cold skin and extremities. Acute blood loss exceeding 50% of the vascular volume within hours results in shock and eventually death before any changes in hematocrit and plasma protein are observed.[8,9]

If the acute blood loss is gradual, restoration of the plasma volume can occur, which in turn lowers the hematocrit. Unless fluid is administered, plasma volume expansion is a relatively slow process. After a sudden, single hemorrhagic event, albumin-containing fluid is mobilized from the extravascular space over a period of 2 to 3 days. This fluid shift reduces the skin turgor until the fluid deficit is replenished by oral or parenteral fluid intake. Because the associated fall in hematocrit is gradual, the severity of the hemorrhage may be markedly underestimated.

As the anemia is initially normocytic-normochromic and nonregenerative, it could be mistaken for a defective hematopoietic problem. Within a few hours, serum erythropoietin levels are, however, increased and erythropoiesis is stimulated. After 3 days the anemia becomes macrocytic and regenerative. A maximal reticulocyte response is seen within 4 to 7 days. The corrected reticulocyte count may reach 3% to 10% or several hundred thousands per microliter, which is somewhat less than with hemolytic anemias. In acute anemia, adequate iron stores are generally present but the marrow response may be hampered by limited iron mobilization. In cats, the transient rise in aggregated reticulocytes is followed by a marked sustained increase in punctate reticulocytes over a few weeks.

A stress leukogram may also be associated with acute blood loss. Although platelets are being consumed at the site of injury, this does not result in a clinically significant thrombocytopenia; to the contrary, after a slight dip to no less than 60,000/μL, acute blood loss is accompanied by a mild reactive thrombocytosis. In case of external blood loss, a concomitant loss of plasma proteins occurs that includes albumin and globulins. Thus the triad of anemia, hypoproteinemia, and reticulocytosis is considered a hallmark of acute external blood loss. Other test abnormalities depend on the cause of bleeding. Besides typical clinical signs of hemorrhage, examination of a blood smear for platelets and schistocytes and evaluation of an activated clotting time and buccal mucosal bleeding time may suggest a hemostatic defect that can be confirmed by appropriate laboratory tests.

Four main objectives exist in the management of acute blood loss anemia: (1) fluid replacement, (2) prevention of further bleeding, (3) blood transfusion support, and (4) treatment of the underlying disorder. With sudden hemorrhage, the immediate effects of volume depletion are more important than the loss of circulating RBCs. Thus the first requirement is to maintain an adequate blood volume by intravenous infusion of crystalloid fluids (electrolytes), colloid solutions of plasma, hydroxyethylstarch, hemoglobin solution (Oxyglobin®), or whole blood. Fluid choice depends on the clinical setting, particularly the severity and rate of hemorrhage. With major hemorrhage leading rapidly to shock, losses are primarily from the intravascular space with little change in extra- and intracellular fluid compartments. Crystalloid fluids (isotonic saline or Ringer's lactate) are the first choice. Because crystalloids are rapidly distributed between the intra- and extravascular compartments, they need to be infused in a volume of two to four times the estimated loss. An infusion of crystalloids can rapidly restore circulation, thereby normalizing many hemodynamic parameters.

Within days, intra- and extracellular fluids shift into the intravascular space. For adequate resuscitation of a pet with hemorrhagic hypotension and shock, much larger fluid volumes must be given quickly to replete the fluid compartments and restore circulation. Colloid fluids such as 6% hydroxyethylstarch or dextran 70 solutions produce a volume expansion slightly larger than that infused and can maintain this effect for as long as a day. Because species-specific albumin solutions are not available for small animals, plasma, or whole-blood transfusions may be used for replacement therapy. Their use should, however, be discouraged unless clotting factors are needed or, because of anemia due to major blood loss, an oxygen carrier is deemed necessary. A bovine hemoglobin solution (Oxyglobin®) has become commercially available for dogs that provides oncotic pressure and an oxygen transporter. It can prove useful in the emergency management of acute blood loss and lacks immunologically important reactions and in dogs even after repeated administration.[10-12]

The depletion of RBC mass after acute blood loss may be difficult to estimate because of concurrent plasma loss and the hematocrit decreases only after total blood volume returns to normal. Thus the "transfusion trigger" can be particularly difficult to define in a hemorrhaging pet. Although a healthy normovolemic anemic animal at rest may tolerate a hematocrit as low as 5% to 10%, signs of hypoxia develop much earlier in a hypovolemic anemic animal. Thus small animals with precipitous blood loss may be deemed in need of a blood transfusion at hematocrits above 20%. Ten milliliters of whole blood per pound body weight increases the hematocrit by 10%, but fluid shifts and concomitant replacement of fluids may diminish the response. It should be noted that except for isotonic saline, fluids have to be administered through a catheter other than that used for transfusion. If venous access cannot be obtained in severely hypotensive animals, the intraosseous route may be used because RBCs and fluids rapidly reach the intravascular space. Because canine stored blood or packed RBCs have low 2,3-diphosphoglycerate (DPG) concentrations, which may hamper the oxygen release, some clinicians have advocated the use of fresh blood. However, DPGs are rapidly replenished in canine erythrocytes; therefore this may be more of a theoretic concern. Because the hemoglobin-oxygen affinity of feline erythrocytes is not DPG dependent, this is not a problem in cats; however, closed blood collection systems and blood component preparation for storage of feline blood are a problem. When hemorrhage has ceased, the recovery of the red cell mass to normal usually occurs within 1 to 2 weeks. Animals with acute blood loss anemia have adequate iron stores and generally do not require supplemental iron to reach an appropriate erythroid bone marrow response.

Chronic Blood Loss Anemia-Iron Deficiency Anemia

Animals have approximately 9 to 22 mg iron per lb body weight, and most of the iron is located in erythrocytes as hemoglobin (1 mg iron in 2 mL of blood).[3,13] In addition, muscle myoglobin and many important enzymes contain heme iron (e.g., cytochromes). Iron is also stored in various tissues, particularly spleen, liver, and bone marrow, as a soluble mobile fraction (ferritin) or insoluble fraction (hemosiderin), depending on the amount available. Transferrin represents the iron transport protein in the plasma and is normally 20% to 60% saturated with iron. As under physiologic conditions, iron losses through gut, urine, and skin are negligible, amounting to less than 1 mg/day in small animals. Iron balance is regulated by iron absorption. Iron is absorbed in the ferrous (Fe^{2+}) form as heme iron or nonheme iron by the mucosal cells of the proximal small intestine. The exact control mechanisms have not been elucidated, but absorption increases with diminished storage and increased erythropoietic activity. However, the maximal absorption remains rather limited—only a few milligrams per day.[14,15]

Chronic external blood loss is the major cause of iron deficiency anemia in small animals and is associated with a regenerative anemia. Iron deficiency denotes a deficit in total body iron, which occurs in varying degrees. Iron depletion is present when iron stores are depleted but serum iron and blood hemoglobin concentrations remain normal. In iron-deficient erythropoiesis, serum iron levels are also low but the anemia is only mild. *Iron deficiency anemia* refers to the most advanced stage, characterized by absent iron stores, low serum iron concentration, low transferrin saturation, and low hemoglobin and hematocrit values.

Chronic external blood loss may result from GI hemorrhage, parasitism, chronic bleeding neoplasia, and even chronic inflammatory bowel disease (IBD).[16-22] Severe flea infestation can cause substantial blood loss and mortality, particularly in kittens and puppies, because 100 fleas could potentially consume 1 mL of blood daily. Similarly, the quantity of blood loss caused by hookworms and rarely whipworms is proportional to the worm burden and may reach 100 mL/day. Hookworms burrow their heads deeply into the small intestinal wall and suck blood by peristaltic pumping. Chronic or intermittent GI blood loss may also result from hemorrhaging GI neoplasia, including leiomyoma, carcinoma, and lymphoma; bleeding intestinal aneurysm; and ulcerogenic drugs such as glucocorticosteroids, salicylates, and nonsteroidal anti-inflammatory agents. As each regular blood collection (450 mL) removes approximately 200 mg of iron from the body, overzealous blood donations and frequent phlebotomies for diagnostic purposes in small dogs and cats may lead to iron deficiency states.

In young animals the iron needed for growth may exceed the supply available from diet and body stores. Thus they are particularly at risk for developing an iron deficiency anemia. Because milk is low in iron, nursing animals may become iron deficient. However, with the general use of balanced commercial diets for growing animals, iron deficiency related to inadequate intake alone is rare. Intestinal malabsorption syndromes, such as IBD in Shar Peis, can be associated with iron deficiency states.

Iron deficiency anemia develops over weeks and is almost always insidious, allowing remarkably effective adaptation. Clinical signs are nonspecific and depend more on the rate of progression than the extent of anemia. Even when the hematocrit falls below 5% to 10%, clinical signs of anemia, besides pallor, may not be obvious at rest. The animals may become increasingly fatigued and exercise intolerant and, when stressed, may suddenly decompensate and die. Clinical manifestations include extremely pale mucous membranes, bounding pulses, gallop rhythm, and a systolic flow murmur. Reduced blood viscosity, vascular resistance (decreased afterload), and increased left ventricular filling (increased preload) maintain the cardiac output. Thus chronic anemia causes cardiomegaly through cardiac hypertrophy and dilation and may eventually lead to congestive heart failure (CHF).[20] In contrast, tachypnea and dyspnea are not typical features of anemia unless the animal has pulmonary disease that impairs oxygen uptake. Pica, the craving to eat, chew, or lick unusual substances such as dirt, clay, feces, and metal, is a classical manifestation of iron deficiency. Because iron deficiency is most commonly caused by GI blood loss, melena is likely to be present, but occasionally it is intermittent or detected only by the occult fecal blood test. A positive test result for an animal receiving a commercial diet is probably clinically significant. Typical blood sweat and laboratory test abnormalities may provide the first clue to an iron deficiency anemia and possibly an occult intestinal malignancy.

Iron deficiency can produce clinical manifestations independent of anemia because depletion of iron-containing compounds in nonerythroid tissue results in impaired proliferation, growth, and function. These include reduced muscle activity, abnormal behavior, and skin and nail changes.

Severe iron deficiency anemia is characterized by a hypochromic microcytic anemia caused by decreased synthesis of hemoglobin and delayed cell maturation and extra mitosis.[1,7,16,23] On a blood smear the hypochromic cells are readily recognized by the increased central pallor (Figure 270-4) and are reflected by a decreased mean corpuscular hemoglobin concentration (MCHC). In advanced states the red cell corpuscles represent mere rings. Microcytosis is less well appreciated on a blood smear, because cell diameter is less affected than cell thickness; these flat, poorly stained cells are called *leptocytes* and have a reduced MCV. Anisocytosis is also a recognizable

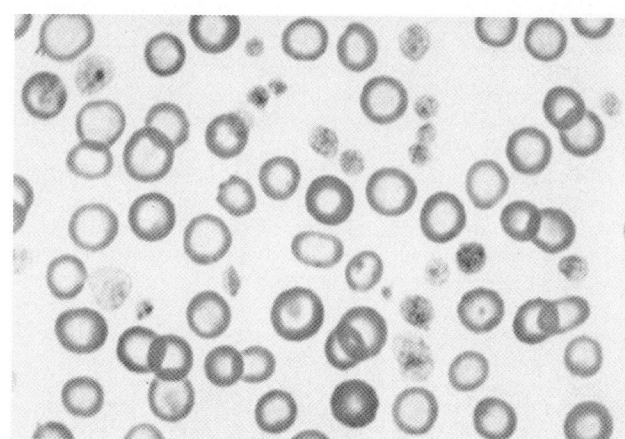

Figure 270-4 Hypochromasia and thrombocytosis in a dog with severe chronic blood loss anemia.

morphologic change and can be quantified by an increased RDW as determined by particle size counters. In addition, iron-deficient erythrocytes appear stiffer and less deformable, presumably because of oxidative damage of membrane proteins. Thus erythrocyte fragmentation, increased mechanical fragility, and accelerated lysis may occur, thereby affecting the various erythrocyte indices. However, in the osmotic fragility test, the red cells may be more resistant to destruction in hypotonic salt solutions because of their increased capacity to expand their volume.[1,14]

In humans, iron deficiency anemia is non- or poorly regenerative[14]; in contrast, iron deficiency in small animals is usually associated with a pronounced reticulocytosis.[16] The reticulocyte counts may reach 500,000/μL (10% corrected), presumably because of their delayed maturation. This reticulocytosis greatly contributes to the degree of anisocytosis and increased RDW.

The leukocytes are usually normal in number, but slight neutropenia may occur, whereas eosinophilia is seen in parasite-induced blood loss anemia. Interestingly, the platelet count is commonly increased to about twice normal, but may exceed $1 \times 10^6/μL$.[9]

Thrombocytosis associated with acute and chronic blood loss is considered reactive, but the exact mechanism remains unexplained. A search for occult blood loss is highly warranted in anemic animals with thrombocytosis. In uncomplicated iron deficiency anemia, the chemistry screening test results are unremarkable except for a low total protein related to concomitant intestinal losses of albumin and globulin.

The bone marrow is characterized by mild to moderate erythroid hyperplasia with nuclear distortions. The normoblasts appear small and have scant cytoplasm. After staining the bone marrow aspirate or biopsy section with Prussian blue, one sees dark-blue granular material scattered throughout the marrow. In iron deficiency anemia, no stainable iron in the form of deep-blue granules is found (hemosiderin appears in the unstained marrow smear as golden refractile granules). However, healthy cats normally store only small amounts of ferritin and hemosiderin in macrophages of their marrow; thus a lack of positive Prussian blue staining is not diagnostic for iron deficiency in cats, but Prussian blue–positive deposits in marrow exclude iron deficiency.

Serum iron concentrations are usually low, ranging from 5 to 60 μg/dL compared with a normal range of 60 to 230 μg/dL, depending to some extent on the method used.[13] However, serum iron concentrations are subject to many variables that may cause normal or even high results, including hemolyzed samples, iron supplementation, and recent transfusions. The iron-binding capacity is a measure of the amount of transferrin in circulating blood and may be slightly increased in iron deficiency states; thus the transferrin saturation is markedly decreased to below 20% (normal 20% to 60%). Serum ferritin concentrations would be expected to be low, but because ferritin is an acute phase protein, values are often increased by coexisting inflammation. Iron parameters can also be affected by transfusions, iron supplements, and glucocorticoid administration.

Management of chronic blood loss anemia is directed toward correction of the anemia, the iron deficiency, and treatment of the underlying disease. Transfusions with packed RBCs or whole blood are indicated only in cases of severe anemia or in preparation for anesthesia and surgery to correct the GI hemorrhage (PCV less than 15% to 20%) and clinical signs of tissue hypoxia. Because these animals are normovolemic and have increased cardiac output, transfusion volumes and rates should be conservative to avoid cardiac failure. Volume overload occurs more commonly in cats than in dogs. Correction of the anemia also results in resolution of cardiomegaly within several weeks. Although ulcerogenic drugs can be withdrawn immediately, control of ecto- and endoparasites

(as well as any surgical corrections) should be undertaken only when the pets has been stabilized. Leiomyomas and leiomyosarcomas are frequent small intestinal tumors in older dogs, and their complete resection is often rewarding.

Once critical care has been provided and the underlying condition has been corrected, iron supplementation should be initiated to replenish iron stores. Iron is highly effective in treating iron deficiency. It has, however, no other legitimate therapeutic use, because it exerts no beneficial effects for other forms of anemia and may be harmful (exception: animals with chronic renal failure may in fact also experience an iron deficiency). Iron can be administered orally and parenterally. The oral route is the safest and least expensive. Ferrous sulfate in tablet or liquid form at a dose of 5 mg/lb daily along with a meal is effective, although the exact iron requirements have not been established for small animals. Iron fumarate and gluconate may be substituted, but other iron preparations are likely not to be effective, may cause gastric irritation, and hence are not recommended. Treatment has to be continued for weeks to months to correct the iron deficiency state, but iron stores may never be completely replenished.

If oral iron replacement is deemed inappropriate or insufficient or a GI disorder prevents iron absorption, parenteral iron may be administered. Iron dextran complex containing 50 mg iron per milliliter can be given intramuscularly. After a small dose is injected deep into the muscle to test for hypersensitivity reaction, a maximal dose of 2 mL is administered daily; two thirds of the iron is absorbed from the injection site within days. Ferrous chloride is potentially available in intravenous form. As 2 mL of blood contains 1 mg iron, blood transfusions also provide an excellent source of iron, but they should be restricted to severely anemic animals.

HEMOLYTIC ANEMIAS

Once the erythrocyte has lost its nucleus and ribosomes, it can no longer synthesize proteins. Nevertheless, it survives hundreds of miles of hazardous travel through large and tiny blood vessels with its limited equipment. It is capable of sustaining adequate energy levels through anaerobic glycolysis, maintaining ionic composition, reducing methemoglobin and oxidized glutathione, and resealing its membrane if portions are lost. Despite these capacities, erythrocytes have a finite life span that may be shortened when the environment becomes hostile or when the cell's ability for self-repair becomes impaired. Accelerated erythrocyte destruction is the major mechanism in hemolytic disorders and plays a minor role in many other common anemias.[24]

The normal life span of erythrocytes averages approximately 100 to 120 days in dogs and 70 to 78 days in cats.[2,3] Although it is rarely done in clinical practice, the erythrocyte life span can be measured directly by two labeling methods. The cohort method depends on the incorporation of an isotopically labeled chemical such as radioactive iron or glycine into newly formed cells. In contrast, the random labeling methods use tracers that bind with all erythrocytes in the circulation and include radiolabeled chromium or cyanate, as well as nonradioactive biotin.[25] Because chromium elutes from cells readily, the apparent half-life is much shorter (i.e., 20 to 30 days instead of 60 days for normal canine erythrocytes and only 6 to 14 days instead of 37 days for feline erythrocytes).[26] If needed, the nonradioactive biotin-labeling method should be considered.

Although the concept of erythrocyte aging and death is well established, the precise mechanisms involved in normal cell senescence are still not clearly defined. No single marker exists to identify aged erythrocytes, but the following factors may contribute to the finite life span of erythrocytes: declining enzyme activities, change in calcium balance, diminished negative membrane charge, repeated oxidative injuries, and binding of complement or naturally occurring autoantibodies against membrane band 3 protein and galactosyl-containing glycolipid.[24,25]

The erythrocyte life span may be shortened as a result of some intrinsic defect, such as an erythroenzymopathy, or because of some extrinsic mechanism that leads to premature erythrocyte removal, such as antibodies against erythrocytes. These can be distinguished experimentally by cross-transfusion studies. When erythrocytes from a healthy animal are transfused to one with an extrinsic cause for hemolysis, the donated cells are destroyed as rapidly as the pet's own cells. However, if an animal's corpuscles are removed from the unfavorable environment, they survive normally. In contrast, erythrocytes with an intrinsic defect would be disposed of rapidly in either the affected animal or a healthy recipient. Such survival studies are generally not required in the evaluation of hemolytic anemias in clinical practice.

Erythrocyte destruction may take place either extra- or intravascularly.[1,3] Extravascular hemolysis predominates and is assumed to be the mode of destruction of senescent erythrocytes in healthy animals. Extravascular destruction refers to erythrophagocytosis by macrophages of spleen, liver, and bone marrow. Damaged or senescent erythrocytes are prone to enhanced sequestration in these organs. Erythrophagocytosis may be either complete (culling) or partial (pitting). In particular, splenic environment with its low glucose concentration, mild hypoxia, hypercapnia, and relatively low pH can be deleterious to erythrocytes. Based on its structure, the canine spleen is more efficient than the feline spleen in removing erythrocytes. Macrophages destroy ingested erythrocytes through proteolytic and lipolytic enzymes.

The heme oxygenase system responsible for hemoglobin degradation is located primarily in phagocytic cells. The globin is broken down to amino acids, which are reused. In heme catabolism, iron becomes liberated, recirculates bound to transferrin in plasma back to the marrow for erythropoiesis, and the protoporphyrin ring opens. Carbon monoxide is split off, exhaled, biliverdin forms, and is subsequently reduced to bilirubin.

Unconjugated bilirubin is then released into the plasma; it is water insoluble and reversibly binds to albumin (indirect-reacting bilirubin). The albumin-bound bilirubin is readily absorbed by hepatocytes. In the liver, bilirubin is conjugated with glucuronic acid to form bilirubin diglucuronide, also known as *direct bilirubin*. The conjugated bilirubin is excreted via the bile canaliculi into the duodenum, but in the presence of massive heme breakdown, conjugated bilirubin leaks back into the plasma and is also excreted in the urine. Intestinal bacteria in the colon convert the bilirubin to urobilinogens. Most of the urobilinogen is excreted in the feces, but a small amount is reabsorbed. The reabsorbed urobilinogen is readily re-excreted by the liver (enterohepatic recirculation), with a small portion lost in the urine.

The serum bilirubin concentration is an important marker of the rate of hemoglobin metabolism and of hepatobiliary function. Normal serum values, measured by colorimetric methods, do not exceed 0.4 mg/dL, and jaundice is not appreciated until the serum bilirubin exceeds 2 mg/dL. One might predict that hemolytic disorders are associated with a greater rise in indirect bilirubin, whereas hepatic failure leads to a larger increase in direct bilirubin. However, because the process to conjugated bilirubin is highly efficient and rapid in small animals, the differential bilirubin determination in serum has not proved helpful in distinguishing hemolytic from hepatic causes of hyperbilirubinemia. Hyperbilirubinemia and hemoglobinemia can affect accurate measurements of serum liver and other chemistry screen parameters. Liver function

tests are often indicated, because hemolysis may be associated with a hepatopathy. Heme can be metabolized by alternative pathways in other tissues (e.g., kidney in dogs). In any case, a rise in heme degradation results in hyperbilirubinuria because of increased urinary excretion of conjugated bilirubin. Bilirubin is readily identified by the diazo-reaction on the urine dipstick. Small amounts of bilirubin are normally found in urine from healthy dogs but not cats. Hemoglobinuria may make the bilirubin readings invalid. Bile pigment gallstones, seen in humans with hemolysis, are not observed in small animals.

Less commonly, erythrocytes are lysed within the systemic circulation as a consequence of membrane permeability changes or cellular fragmentation. With intravascular hemolysis, hemoglobin is directly released into the blood, from which it is removed by several mechanisms. Hemoglobin breaks into two alpha-beta dimers and binds to haptoglobin in plasma or further dissociates into heme to form hemopexin and methemalbumin. After these complexes are taken up by macrophages and hepatocytes, hemoglobin and heme are metabolized as described earlier in relation to extravascular hemolysis. Binding prevents excretion of hemoglobin into the urine, but during intravascular lysis, haptoglobin becomes easily depleted. Unbound plasma hemoglobin and heme may be removed by the liver or excreted through the renal glomeruli.

Proximal tubular cells reabsorb and catabolize most filtered hemoglobin and heme.

Hemoglobinuria ensues when the amount filtered exceeds the limited capacity of the tubular cells to resorb dimers. Although heme pigments may precipitate and form casts in the distal renal tubules, hemosiderinuric tubular necrosis and acute renal failure are rarely observed in small animals with severe or chronic hemoglobinuria.

Intravascular lysis can be readily recognized by the presence of hemoglobinemia, depletion of plasma haptoglobin, and hemoglobinuria. Plasma hemoglobin levels of 10 to 20 mg/dL give plasma an amber coloration, and at 50 to 100 mg/dL the plasma appears reddish. The hemoglobinemia has to be distinguished from artifactual increases in plasma hemoglobin caused by blood collection methods that directly cause hemolysis, as well as delayed plasma separation. Plasma hemoglobin concentrations can be quantitated spectrophotometrically by an accurate and simple hemoglobinometer (HemoCue).[27] Hemoglobinuria imparts a red-brown color to the urine, reflecting both hemoglobin and methemoglobin. Because the urine dipstick identifies only heme (labeled "blood"), hemoglobinuria has to be differentiated from hematuria (whole erythrocytes) by microscopic examination after urine sedimentation. Myoglobinuria associated with massive muscle necrosis can also cause a positive test result but hardly ever occurs in small animals.

Based on the preceding mechanisms of erythrocyte destruction, the clinical features and laboratory test abnormalities of the various hemolytic disorders are similar. Besides the general signs of anemia such as pallor and weakness, characteristic signs of hemolysis are jaundice and pigmenturia. Jaundice is first appreciated on mucous membranes (gingiva and sclera) when serum bilirubin concentration exceed 2 mg/dL, whereas skin becomes icteric at slightly higher concentrations. Milder and chronic forms of hemolysis may not be associated with jaundice. Pigmenturia caused by hemolysis may be due to hyperbilirubinuria and hemoglobinuria. Hyperbilirubinuria persists in dogs with hemolytic disorders, whereas in cats it is not constant. Hemoglobinuria and hemoglobinemia are hallmark features of intravascular hemolysis and often indicate a more severe disorder.

The terms *hemolytic anemia* and *hemolytic disorder* are limited to conditions in which the rate of erythrocyte destruction is accelerated and the ability of the bone marrow to respond to the stimulus is unimpaired. As indicated in the introduction, hemolytic anemias are generally associated with accelerated erythrocyte production that is unrestricted by iron availability. In fact, the highest reticulocyte counts and most severe erythroid hyperplasias are observed in animals with hemolytic anemias. Thus hemolytic anemias are regenerative and macrocytic-hypochromic, although in the early stages and in some complicated acquired forms the erythroid response may be poor (e.g., immune-mediated hemolytic anemia). In addition, a number of common complex anemias related to insufficient erythrocyte production have a component of accelerated erythrocytic destruction such as the previously mentioned advanced iron deficiency anemia.

The division of hemolytic anemias into acute and chronic forms is of limited usefulness, because acute crises may develop during the course of chronic disorders. Classification based on the site of hemolysis, predominantly within the circulation (intravascular) or within tissue macrophages (extravascular), is of some help, because only a few are associated with overt intravascular hemolysis. However, intravascular lysis may occur only transiently; therefore the unique manifestations of hemoglobinemia and hemoglobinuria may be missed. Excessive destruction of erythrocytes may occur either because of an intrinsic defect in the cell itself or because of the action of extrinsic factors on normal erythrocytes. Intrinsic defects are generally inherited and extrinsic are acquired. The division into intrinsic and extrinsic or inherited, and acquired forms is of pathogenic importance and is most useful as hereditary hemolytic anemias gain greater recognition. Furthermore, some hemolytic processes are associated with acquired disorders of other organs and are covered elsewhere.

Inherited Erythrocyte Defects

Several hereditary erythrocyte defects (Table 270-1) have been described in dogs and cats.[19] The mode of inheritance is autosomal recessive for all described erythrocyte defects, with the exception of feline porphyria, in which at least one defect is inherited as a dominant trait. This is a large heterogeneous group of disorders, and most occur rarely. Through inbreeding practices (popular sire, line breeding), some erythrocyte defects have become common in certain breeds. Unless the affected breeds are closely related, a particular disease is probably caused by different mutations of the same gene. Erythrocyte-induced defects vary from mild compensated hemolytic to life-threatening anemia. Accurate laboratory tests are now available for many erythrocyte defects to detect affected and carrier animals.

Some defects represent hematologic curiosities without clinical signs (such as in Akitas and miniature poodles with inconsequential microcytosis and macrocytosis, respectively). Hereditary erythrocyte disorders have been classified into three groups: (1) heme defects and hemoglobinopathies, (2) membrane abnormalities, and (3) erythroenzymopathies.[28] Hereditary production and maturation defects of erythrocytes and other hematopoietic cells are discussed in Chapter 271.

Hemoglobin and Related Disorders

Dogs and cats apparently have embryonic but no fetal hemoglobin.[2] With the exception of some Japanese dog breeds, only one adult hemoglobin has been found in dogs. Historically, two major adult hemoglobins were described in cats with a large variation of the hemoglobin A/hemoglobin B ratios. Later studies, however, revealed only one alpha globin, but six different beta globins were found.[29] With each cat having one to four different beta globins, at least 17 hemoglobin patterns were recognized. In contrast to the common occurrence of thalassemia and sickle cell anemia in humans, no hemoglobinopathies have been documented in anemic dogs and cats.

Physiologically or pathologically generated methemoglobin contains heme in the ferric form (Fe^{3+}) and therefore cannot carry oxygen. It is reduced to the ferrous form (Fe^{2+}) by the methemoglobin or cytochrome b_5 reductase system. Isolated cases of methemoglobinemia associated with methemoglobin reductase deficiency were found among dogs of various breeds and several domestic shorthair cats (DSH).[3,30-32] Affected animals have cyanotic mucous membranes but generally do not exhibit any other clinical signs of hypoxemia unless vigorously exercised. The blood remains dark after air exposure because of the presence of 13% to 52% methemoglobin. In contrast to those with other erythrocyte defects, these animals are not anemic but rather develop a mild erythrocytosis and can have a normal life expectancy. Reducing agents such as methylene blue could be used but are generally not needed.

Defects of heme synthesis known as *porphyrias* have been reported in anemic Siamese cats and nonanemic DSH cats with pigmented and pink-fluorescent teeth and bones.

Erythrocyte Membrane—Related Abnormalities

The erythrocyte membrane consists of a bilayer affixed to a membrane skeleton, which determines cell shape and deformability. Owing to proteolysis, canine and feline erythrocytes lose their Na^+,K^+-adenosine triphosphatase (Na^+,K^+-ATPase) during late maturation in the bone marrow and reticulocytes.[33] Therefore erythrocytes have high-sodium and low-potassium concentrations similar to those of serum electrolyte values. Consequently, hyperkalemia generally does not occur after intravascular hemolysis unless stress reticulocytes are lysed. Erythrocytes from Sheba, Inus, Akitas, and some mongrel dogs in Korea and Japan represent an exception, because they keep their erythrocytic Na^+,K^+-ATPases and therefore have high-potassium and low-sodium concentrations in erythrocytes. Because Akitas' erythrocytes are leaky *in vitro*, pseudohyperkalemia may occur if the plasma and serum are not readily separated from erythrocytes and its clot.[34]

Elliptocytosis and microcytosis related to cytoskeleton protein band 4.1 deficiency has been described in an inbred, nonanemic mongrel dog.[35,36] Other erythrocyte membrane defects are far less well defined but are generally characterized by increased osmotic fragility (Figure 270-5). Stomatocytes are overhydrated, cup-shaped macrocytes that are recognized by a slitlike pallor on a blood film. In the Alaskan malamute, stomatocytosis is associated with a chondrodysplastic dwarfism.[37] Miniature and middle schnauzers with stomatocytosis had no skeletal abnormalities, and both breeds had only mild regenerative anemia on the basis of hemoglobin measurements with high MCV and low MCHC indices[38,39] (Figure 270-6). Furthermore, stomatocytosis and hypertrophic gastritis have been reported in the Drentse partrijshond dog breed (Dutch breed) and a lipid disorder is suspected on the basis of abnormal erythrocyte membrane and plasma phospholipids.[40] A hereditary spherocytosis has been described in some golden retrievers.[41] A marked osmotic fragility of erythrocytes associated with recurrent anemia, severe splenomegaly, weight loss, lymphocytosis, and hyperglobulinemia but a negative Coombs' test has been observed mostly in Abyssinian and Somali cats.[42] Their erythrocytes are so fragile that the lysis is clearly evident once the ethylenediaminetetraacetic acid (EDTA) tube is left in the refrigerator overnight. Although the cause has not been identified, affected cats with marked splenomegaly may benefit from prednisone treatment and splenectomy. This may reduce the degree of *in vivo* phagocytosis of damaged erythrocytes; however, the *in vitro* osmotic fragility of erythrocytes does not appear to improve after treatment. This osmotic fragility has also been seen in Siamese and DSH cats.

Erythroenzymopathies

Devoid of a nucleus and mitochondria, erythrocytes generate energy almost exclusively through anaerobic glycolysis, also

Table • 270-1

Inherited Erythrocyte Defects

DEFECTS	BREEDS	INHERI-TANCE	PACKED CELL VOLUME (PCV) (%) RANGE	RETICULO-CYTE (%) (CORRECTED)	ERYTHROCYTE HALF-LIFE (DAYS)	ERYTHROCYTE MORPHOLOGY	SPECIFIC TESTS	CLINICAL FEATURES
Erythroenzymopathies								
Pyruvate kinase (PK) deficiency	Basenji*, beagle*, West Highland white* and cairn terrier, miniature poodle, dachshund*, toy Eskimo*, pug	AR	11-29	5-95	4-9	Polychromasia, ecchinocytes	DNA test, abnormal M-PK, PK kinetic, stability, and glycolytic intermediates	Hemolytic anemia, myelofibrosis, osteosclerosis
	Abyssinian*, Somali*, DSH cats*	AR	10-33	1-33	U	Polychromasia	DNA test PK activity <20%	Intermittent hemolytic anemia
Phosphofructokinase (PFK) deficiency	English springer spaniel*, cocker spaniel*, mixed breed dog*	AR	11-48	5-23	4	Polychromasia	DNA test PFK activity, 8%-22%	Inducible hemolytic crises, mild myopathy, pigmenturia
Hemoglobin Synthesis Defects								
Hemoglobinopathies	None							
Cytochrome-b_5 reductase (Cb_5R) deficiency	Many isolated cases in dogs and DSH cats	U	High	N	U	Unremarkable	Cb_5R activity, 10%-30%; methemoglobin >10%	Cyanosis, no anemia, but polycythemia, exercise intolerance
Porphyria	Siamese	AD	10-25	U	U	Unremarkable	Porphyrins in urine and erythrocytes	Anemia, discolored teeth
	DSH	AD	N	N to 5	U	Unremarkable	Porphobilinogen deaminase deficiency (?)	Discolored teeth, ± anemia

(Continued)

Table • 270-1

Inherited Erythrocyte Defects—Cont'd

Membrane and Other Abnormalities

DEFECTS	BREEDS	INHERI-TANCE	PACKED CELL VOLUME (PCV) (%) RANGE	RETICULO-CYTE (%) (CORRECTED)	ERYTHROCYTE HALF-LIFE (DAYS)	ERYTHROCYTE MORPHOLOGY	SPECIFIC TESTS	CLINICAL FEATURES
Elliptocytosis (band 4.1 deficiency)	Mixed breed dog*	AR	34	2	16-23	Elliptocytes	Membrane protein electrophoresis	None
Stomatocytosis	Alaskan malamute, miniature & middle schnauzer	AR	N	3-7	6-18	Stomatocytes, macrocytes, polychromasia	Stomatocytes, increased osmotic fragility	Chondrodysplasia in malamutes, none in schnauzers
Increased osmotic fragility	English springer spaniel, mixed breed dogs	U	N	2-5	U	Polychromasia, poikilocytosis	Increased osmotic fragility, unknown	Exercise-induced hyperthermia
Increased osmotic fragility	Abyssinian, Somali	U	8-35	1-4	U	Macrocytosis	Increased osmotic fragility	Intermittent anemia, splenomegaly
High-potassium erythrocytes	Akita, Japanese mongrels	U	N	N	U	Unremarkable	Increased erythrocyte and serum potassium	None, pseudo-hyperkalemia
Nonspherocytic hemolytic disorders	Beagle	AR	29-12	8-23	7-15	Polychromasia	Calcium ATPase pump (?)	None, mild anemia
Poikilocytosis	DSH cats	U	7-12	10-30	U	Severe poikilocytosis	Poikilocytosis	Severe anemia
Familial microcytosis	Akita	U	N	N	U	Microcytosis	Erythrocyte indices	None
Familial macrocytosis and dyshematopoiesis	Poodle (miniature and toy)	U	N	N	U	Macrocytes, hyperseg-mented neutrophils	Macrocytosis, normal osmotic fragility	None, gingivitis

Data collected from references and author's unpublished observations.
N, Normal; *U*, unknown; *AR*, autosomal recessive; *AD*, autosomal dominant; *DSH*, domestic shorthair.
*Molecular defect known.

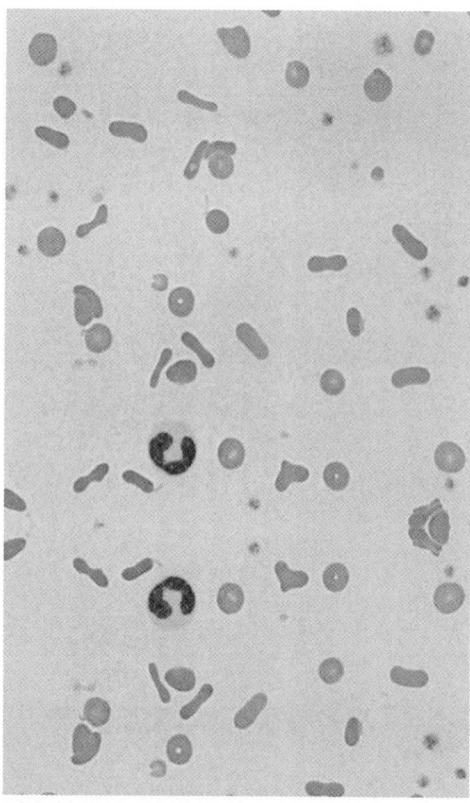

Figure 270-5 Severe hereditary poikilocytosis in a 1-year-old domestic shorthaired (DSH) cat.

known as the *Embden-Meyerhof* pathway. Phosphofructokinase (PFK) and PK are two key regulatory enzymes of this pathway, but their deficiency results in two distinctly different forms of anemia in dogs. The Embden-Meyerhof pathway also plays an important role in an ancillary pathway. The *Rapoport-Luebering* pathway is responsible for the synthesis of DPG, which influences the oxygen affinity of canine but not feline hemoglobin. Erythrocyte DPG concentrations are low in cats.[3,43]

Phosphofructokinase Deficiency (PFK) PFK deficiency is characterized by a chronic hemolytic disorder accentuated by hemolytic crises and an exertional myopathy.[44-47] After episodes

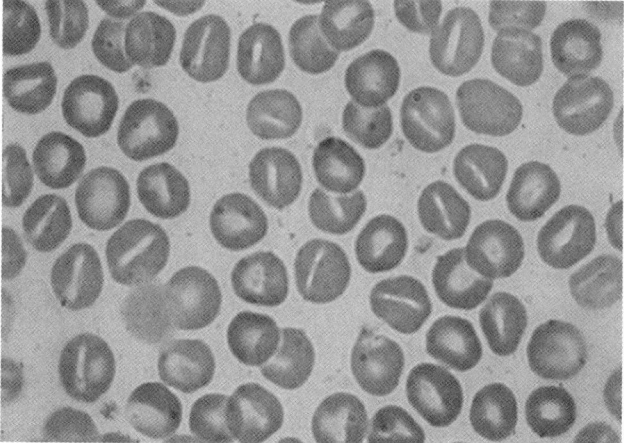

Figure 270-6 Stomatocytosis in a miniature schnauzer without anemia.

of excessive panting and barking, extensive exercise, and high temperatures, affected dogs develop dark brown-red urine because of hemoglobinuria and hyperbilirubinuria. These sporadic events are associated with hyperventilation and elevated body temperature, and the ensuing slight alkalemia results in intravascular lysis of PFK-deficient erythrocytes because these cells are more alkaline fragile than normal canine erythrocytes. During these crises, affected dogs may become severely anemic, icteric, lethargic, anorexic, and develop a fever that usually resolves within days with supportive care. If situations that trigger hemolytic crises are avoided, PFK-deficient dogs may not have problems and can reach a normal life expectancy. However, they have persistent hyperbilirubinuria and reticulocytosis despite a normal hematocrit because of ongoing hemolysis and a high hemoglobin-oxygen affinity because PFK-deficient erythrocytes contain low DPG levels and therefore lead to a relative tissue hypoxia. Furthermore, because affected dogs totally lack PFK activity in muscle, they have a metabolic myopathy characterized by exercise intolerance, occasional muscle cramps, and mildly increased serum creatine kinase activity; thus they perform poorly as field trial dogs.[44]

This glycolytic enzyme deficiency is common in field trial English springer spaniels in the United States, Great Britain, and Denmark, but has also been reported in bench English springer spaniels, as well as a cocker spaniel and a mixed breed dog.[43,48] Although the true prevalence remains unknown, a 1% to 4% prevalence among championed breeding bench and field English springer spaniels has been documented in a randomized survey in the United States.[49] PFK deficiency is caused by a missense mutation of the muscle-type PFK gene that results in truncation and instability of the enzyme, thereby leading to a complete muscle-type PFK deficiency.[50] A simple polymerase chain reaction (PCR)-based DNA test accurately diagnoses PFK-deficient and carrier dogs. A small blood sample, buccal swab, or semen is an appropriate source for DNA testing and requires no special handling or shipping. English springer spaniels (and cocker spaniels) with suspicious clinical signs or before field training and breeding should be DNA tested for PFK deficiency. In other breeds with suspicious signs, an enzymatic PFK test could be performed.

Pyruvate Kinase Deficiency (PK) The classic erythrocytic PK deficiency initially reported in Basenjis is now seen in several other breeds including beagles, West Highland white and cairn terriers, miniature poodles, toy Eskimos, pugs, and dachshunds.[43,44,51-54] Despite a persistent hemolytic anemia, the clinical signs, except for pallor, are often mild. The anemia ranges from about 10% to 32% and is highly regenerative with numerous circulating metarubricytes and reticulocyte counts that can be as high as sometimes approaching 95%. An unexplained progressive myelofibrosis and osteosclerosis of the bone marrow develops at about 1 year of age, although some West Highland white terriers may not show evidence until several years of life. Furthermore, it appears likely that previously described nonspherocytic hemolytic anemia and osteosclerosis in miniature poodles were caused by a PK deficiency.[55] PK-deficient dogs usually die because of anemias and generalized hemosiderosis with associated hepatic failure before 8 years of age. Splenectomy and prednisone treatment appear unhelpful in dogs. Erythrocytes completely lack the adult erythrocyte isozyme form of PK known as *R-PK*. Instead, they express a fetal or leukocyte M-PK form that is dysfunctional in erythrocytes *in vivo*. Molecular genetic screening tests are available for the identification of the PK mutation of affected and carrier Basenjis, beagles, dachshunds, toy Eskimos, and West Highland white and cairn terriers, but not yet for others.[56-58] A cumbersome PK enzyme activity test with isozyme characterization is required to define PK deficiency in other breeds. Carriers do not express the M-PK form and have approximately half-normal PK activity; however, differentiation between carriers and homozygous normal dogs based on enzyme activity may not be accurate.

Feline erythrocytic PK deficiency has also been described in the Abyssinian and Somali breeds and few DSH cats.[59] Affected cats have chronic intermittent hemolytic anemia and mild splenomegaly but no osteosclerosis. The anemia is moderately regenerative and no poikilocytosis is seen. Erythrocyte PK activity is severely reduced, and no M-type PK expression occurs. A deletion caused by a splicing mutation in the R-PK gene has been identified, and a molecular screening test has been made available. Intermittent prednisone therapy and splenectomy appear to ameliorate the clinical signs of intermittent anemia. The oldest living cat reached 13 years of age.

Immune-Mediated Hemolytic Anemia (IMHA)

IMHA arises when an immune response targets erythrocytes directly or indirectly and hemolytic anemia ensues. Until the antierythrocytic antibodies are identified and the pathogenesis is better understood, the nomenclature and classification of IMHA remain imprecise and sometimes confusing.[46,60,61] In primary IMHA no inciting cause can be identified, hence the synonyms *idiopathic IMHA* and *autoimmune hemolytic anemia*. In contrast, secondary IMHA is associated with an underlying condition. "*Alloimmune*" hemolytic anemias such as neonatal isoerythrolysis (NI) and hemolytic transfusion reactions are caused by antierythrocytic alloantibodies.

Immune Mechanisms   Regardless of the underlying cause, IMHA results from a breakdown in immune self-tolerance. The process of clonal deletion for central tolerance is not capable of completely eliminating all potential self-reacting B cell clones *in utero*. Clonal anergy, another central control mechanism, is not totally efficient in the inactivation of B cells designed to respond to self-antigens. Therefore an immune response against erythrocytes may occur.[62] Because some erythrocyte antigens are hidden or cryptic, the appropriate B cell may encounter the antigen only after membrane damage exposes the antigen. An inflammatory or infectious process can also release new antigens into the circulation that cross-react with erythrocyte antigens or attach to the erythrocyte membrane. Furthermore, the appropriate T cell must find the matching B cell and bind via receptor-ligand pairs to activate the respective cell. However, during infection and inflammation, nonspecific activation of lymphocytes can occur, so self-reacting antibodies may be nonspecifically induced. Finally, impairment of the down-regulation mechanisms such as activated B-cell death by apoptosis through a Fas ligand signal from T cells may allow an active autoimmune response to develop.[63-65]

The binding of immunoglobulin G (IgG) or IgM antibodies and complement to the surface of erythrocytes initiates immune destruction of the erythrocytes. Under most clinical circumstances, immune destruction is an extravascular process that depends on recognition of erythrocytes opsonized with IgG, complement, or both by specific receptors on reticuloendothelial cells.

IgG-coated erythrocytes can be destroyed without complement activation because tissue macrophages express receptors that recognize the Fc portion of the IgG molecule. IgG binding by Fc receptors on macrophages can mediate complete phagocytosis, particularly in the red pulp of the spleen. Macrophages with engulfed erythrocytes may be noted by cytologic examination of tissue aspirates. Alternatively, phagocytes remove only a portion of the membrane, leaving erythrocytes with a reduced surface area/volume ratio and thereby forming spherocytes. Because the deformability of spherocytes is impaired, these rigid cells are trapped in the spleen

and are subsequently destroyed. Erythrocyte-bound IgG1 and IgG3 antibodies have a strong affinity for Fc receptors. Erythrocytes that become heavily coated with IgG can also bind complement. In as much as macrophages also have receptors for complement components C3b and iC3b, the attachment of complement component C3b, iC3b, or both via CR1 and CR3 receptors together with IgG enhances the phagocytic process, particularly of hepatic macrophages (Kupffer's cells). In addition, erythrocytes heavily coated with IgG may activate so much complement that intravascular cytolysis occurs.[60,66]

In contrast, macrophages do not have receptors for the Fc portion of IgM, and thus the destruction of IgM-coated erythrocytes is mediated by complement. The pentameric structure of IgM is readily able to induce binding and activation of complement on erythrocytes. High IgM antibody titers can generate the cytolytic complex via the classical complement system and, thereby, intravascular hemolysis ensues. However, the IgM antierythrocyte antibodies are more commonly present in sublytic concentrations, and inhibitory regulatory proteins prevent full complement activation. Nevertheless, some C3b and iC3b are bound to the cell surface, resulting in extravascular destruction of complement-sensitized erythrocytes. Alternatively, erythrocyte-bound complement may be inactivated to C3dg, which no longer impairs erythrocyte survival. Antierythrocytic antibodies inducing hemolysis are generally reactive at body temperature. Only in exceptional cases do cold-acting antibodies (at 4° to 37° C thermoamplitude) contribute to *in vivo* hemolysis and erythrocyte agglutination in cooler, peripheral vasculature.

Underlying Conditions and Predispositions   Historically, in most dogs with IMHA, no underlying condition was ever identified, and thus it was considered to be primary or idiopathic IMHA.[67] However, in later studies of autoimmune hemolytic anemia, probably reflecting more intense clinical investigations, an underlying disease process or trigger could be identified, including drug exposures, emerging infections, bee stings, neoplastic processes, and other immune disorders (Box 270-1).[68-70] Best exemplified in babesiosis and hemobartonellosis, hemolysis is severely exaggerated by immune processes. Many chronic infections including abscesses, discospondylitis, pyometra, and pyelonephritis can induce secondary immune disorders including IMHA. A temporal association between vaccination and onset of IMHA has also been suggested. In a limited retrospective study, one quarter of all dogs with IMHA of unknown cause were vaccinated within 1 month of onset of clinical signs.[71] As this correlation was associated with modified and killed vaccines against common infectious diseases from different manufacturers, it appears likely that vaccines may trigger or enhance a smoldering immune process rather than be the underlying cause. Although a number of anecdotal reports support a temporal relationship between vaccination and IMHA, no significant association was found in a large-scale retrospective survey of animal health insurance records from Britain.[72] The higher rate of IMHA during the warmer months from May through August reported in some studies, but not in others, may also suggest an infectious cause including tick-borne disorders and allergen exposure during the warmer months.[73] The seasonality may vary geographically. The association of IMHA with other immune disorders, including hypothyroidism and immune-mediated thrombocytopenia (ITP), lends support to the hypothesis of a general immune disturbance. IMHA and ITP occurring concurrently are known as *Evans' syndrome*.[52,74] In contrast to humans, IMHA in dogs is often associated with inflammation and necrosis, suggesting again an underlying mechanism to trigger an immune response.

HEMATOLOGY AND IMMUNOLOGY

Box • 270-1

Examples of Underlying Disorders and Triggers of Immune-Mediated Hemolytic Anemia

Infectious

Viral: FeLV, FIV, FIP infection, transient or chronic persistent upper respiratory or gastrointestinal (GI) viral diseases

Bacterial: leptospirosis, hemobartonellosis, various acute and chronic infections (e.g., abscess, pyometra, discospondylitis)

Parasitic: babesiosis, leishmaniasis , dirofilariasis, ehrlichiosis, ancylostoma caninum

Other emerging infectious diseases (e.g., bartonellosis), bee stings

Drugs

Sulfonamides

Cephalosporin

Penicillin

Vaccines

Propylthiouracil (cats)

Methimazole (cats)

Procainamide

Neoplasia

Hemolymphatic: leukemias, lymphoma, multiple myeloma

Solid tumors

Immune Disorders

SLE

Hypothyroidism

Primary and secondary immunodeficiencies

Genetic Predisposition

American cocker spaniel (one third of all cases)

English springer spaniel

Old English sheepdog

Irish setter

Poodle

Dachshund

FeLV, Feline leukemia virus; *FIV,* feline immunodeficiency virus; *SLE,* systemic lupus erythematosus.

IMHA is the most common reason for hemolytic anemias in dogs. A genetic predisposition is evident in some dogs by the breed predilection and familial occurrence. Thus they should no longer be grouped with the idiopathic form.[67,73] American cocker spaniels may represent one third of all dogs with IMHA. In other canine breeds predisposition is less well documented and may vary geographically. Certain histocompatibility leukocyte antigens have been associated with the occurrence of IMHA in humans. The previously reviewed hereditary erythrocyte defects, particularly the common occurrence of PK and PFK deficiency and osmotic fragility problems, should also be considered as an important differential diagnosis whenever IMHA is suspected in breeds documented to have these erythrocytic defects. As with other immune disorders, female dogs appear slightly predisposed, even when spayed. Primary IMHA is relatively rarely documented in cats, but

IMHA may be secondary to FeLV or *Haemobartonella* infections, inflammation, or antithyroidal medication[75,76] No breed, gender, or other association has been found in cats.

Clinical Signs of Immune-Mediated Hemolytic Anemia

IMHA may present at any age but is most commonly encountered in young adult to middle-aged dogs. The clinical history is generally brief and vague. An underlying condition may be identified. A brief episode of vomiting or diarrhea may precede the typical signs of anemia (lethargy, weakness, exercise intolerance, pallor) and hemolysis (pigmenturia, icterus).[59-73] Some animals may be febrile, presumably because of erythrocyte lysis or an underlying infectious or inflammatory disease process. Others develop dyspnea, indicating pulmonary problems either as cause of the underlying disease or as a thromboembolic complication of IMHA.[77] Physical examination may also reveal mild splenomegaly and, less commonly, mild hepatomegaly and lymphadenopathy, which again suggest a secondary cause of IMHA. A normal-sized spleen does not rule out a massive hemolytic process. Furthermore, signs attributable to their underlying disease may predominate, whereas chronic or recurrent signs of IMHA suggest a primary form.

In the rare case of cold-reacting antierythrocytic antibodies, peripheral skin lesions characterized by acrocyanosis and gangrenous necrosis of ear, nose, tail tip, and nail beds may be the obvious problem without any evidence of hemolysis.

Routine Laboratory Test Results

IMHA can be a mild to life threatening condition. The hematocrit may drop precipitously at any time because of active hemolysis. Although a regenerative, macrocytic-hypochromic anemia would be expected, as many as one third of all pets with IMHA have a nonregenerative anemia when first examined.[73,78,79] The disease course may have been peracute, not yet allowing time to mount a regenerative response. Alternatively, antibodies may be directed against erythroid precursors, thereby removing metarubricytes and reticulocytes, or the IMHA disease process may change the microenvironment of the bone marrow and thereby impair erythropoiesis. Evidence of ineffective erythropoiesis and erythrophagocytosis may be found on cytologic examination of a bone marrow aspirate.[80] Autoagglutination of erythrocytes and spherocytosis are typical findings on blood smears (Figures 270-7 to 270-9).

Besides erythroid abnormalities, a leukocytosis is often present and can exceed 100,000/μL, mostly because of a mature neutrophilia, but degenerative left shifts have also been observed. The degree of leukocytosis and toxic neutrophil changes has

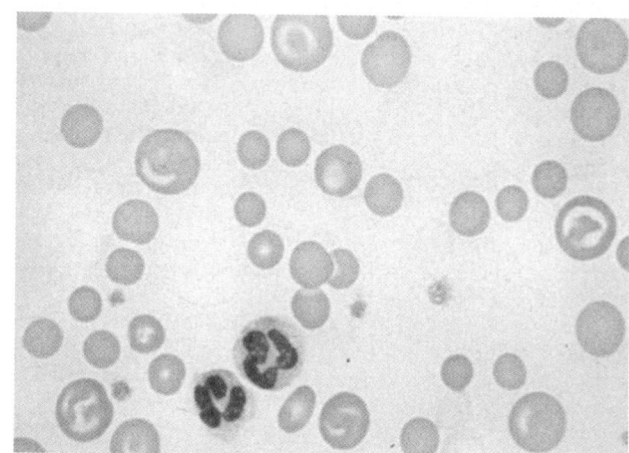

Figure 270-7 Spherocytosis with polychromasia and anisocytosis.

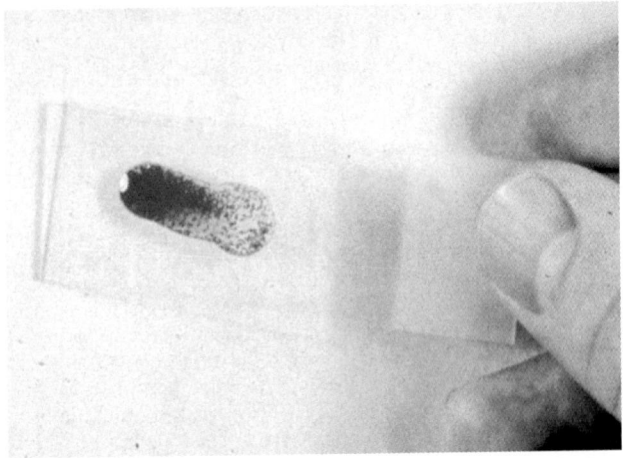

Figure 270-8 Macroscopic agglutination on slide **(A)**. Agglutination of regular and washed blood. Reader should note macroscopic agglutination disappeared **(B)**.

been correlated with the amount of necroses at necropsy.[81] Because high WBC counts are not generally encountered with other forms of anemia, this probably reflects a unique cytokine-mediated response to inflammation and necroses specific for IMHA, but concomitant infection and steroid-induced leukocytosis should also be considered. Thus concurrent hyperplasia of erythroid and myeloid cells may be present in the bone marrow. Furthermore, thrombocytopenia related to a concomitant ITP (Evans' syndrome) or other consumptive processes, such as with disseminated intravascular coagulation (DIC), may occur.[73] Dogs with IMHA often have coagulation test abnormalities with increased plasma fibrinogen and D dimer and FSP concentrations suggesting a DIC like syndrome.[82]

Serum analysis may reveal a hyperbilirubinemia, and a serum bilirubin concentration above 10 mg/dL has been associated with a grave prognosis.[73] However, serum bilirubin values may be only slightly increased in chronic cases, presumably because of highly efficient and accelerated bilirubin metabolism. Thus increased serum bilirubin concentrations could also indicate a concomitant hepatopathy. Dogs with IMHA often have

increased serum liver enzyme activities even before steroid therapy. Pathologic examination has revealed major hepatic and other tissue necroses and inflammation in dogs with severe forms of IMHA.[81] The degree of hemoglobinemia (a sign of intravascular hemolysis) can vary drastically and rapidly and is associated with hemoglobinuria. Hyperbilirubinuria is expected as with any other hemolytic anemia; in cats, any degree of bilirubinuria is considered important, whereas larger amounts of bilirubin are generally present in urine of dogs with IMHA. There may also be evidence of a bacterial cystitis, which may indicate an underlying infectious disease or may occur secondarily because of immunoderegulation or immunosuppressive therapy.

Various imaging studies may be indicated to reveal underlying disease processes, such as neoplasia, and complications of IMHA. Evidence of thromboemboli may be detected on chest radiographs and abdominal ultrasonography, as well as at the site of catheters.[77,82]

Diagnostic Laboratory Test Results A diagnosis of IMHA requires demonstration of accelerated immune destruction of erythrocytes. Thus besides documenting a hemolytic anemia, a search for antibodies or complement or both directed against erythrocytes is required; that is, one or more of the following three hallmarks has to be present to reach a definitive diagnosis of IMHA:

1. Marked spherocytosis
2. True autoagglutination
3. Positive direct Coombs' test

Spherocytosis Spherocytes (Figure 270-3 and 270-7) are spherical erythrocytes that appear microcytic with no central pallor. They result from either partial phagocytosis or lysis. Such cells are rigid and extremely fragile in the erythrocyte osmotic fragility test. Because spherocytes have lost some membrane, they do not have any reserves to expand in hypotonic solution. Large numbers of spherocytes are highly suggestive of IMHA and are present in approximately two thirds of dogs with IMHA, but small numbers may be seen with hypophosphatemia, zinc intoxication, and microangiopathic hemolysis. Hereditary spherocytosis related to various membrane defects in humans has only been reported in one dog. In cats, spherocytes are difficult, if not impossible, to identify owing to the small size and lack of central pallor of normal feline erythrocytes.

Autoagglutination Antierythrocytic IgM and, in large quantities, IgG antibodies may cause direct autoagglutination (Figure 270-8). Agglutination may be visible to the naked eye when blood (at low hematocrit) is in an EDTA tube or placed on a glass slide (macroscopic agglutination) (Figure 270-9), or it may become apparent as small clumps of erythrocytes on a stained blood smear or in a saline wet mount (microscopic agglutination). Autoagglutination has to be distinguished from rouleaux formation (Figure 270-9C), in which erythrocytes stack up on top of each other. For unexplained reasons, canine erythrocytes have a tendency to agglutinate unspecifically in the presence of plasma, particularly at lower temperatures in EDTA. Mixing one drop of blood with one drop of saline may not break up this unspecific form of agglutination. It is therefore important to determine whether the agglutination persists after "saline washing," which has been termed *true autoagglutination*. This is accomplished by adding three times physiologic saline solution to blood (in a ratio of 3:1 to 5:1) after repeated centrifugation and removal of supernatant including the plasma. It should be noted that autoagglutination can interfere with the direct Coombs', crossmatch, and blood typing tests. Thus the simultaneous use of the so-called autocontrols is imperative.

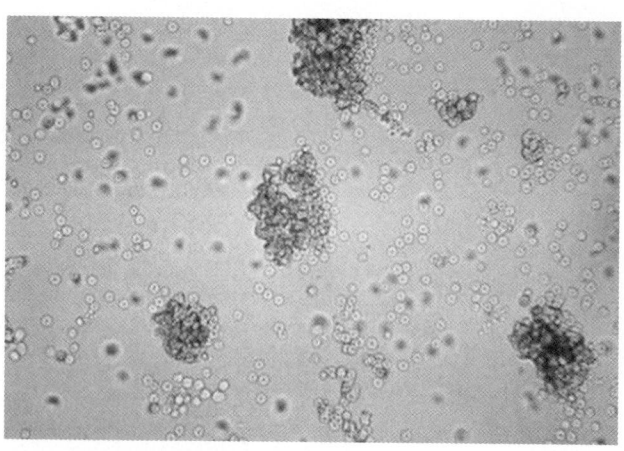

A

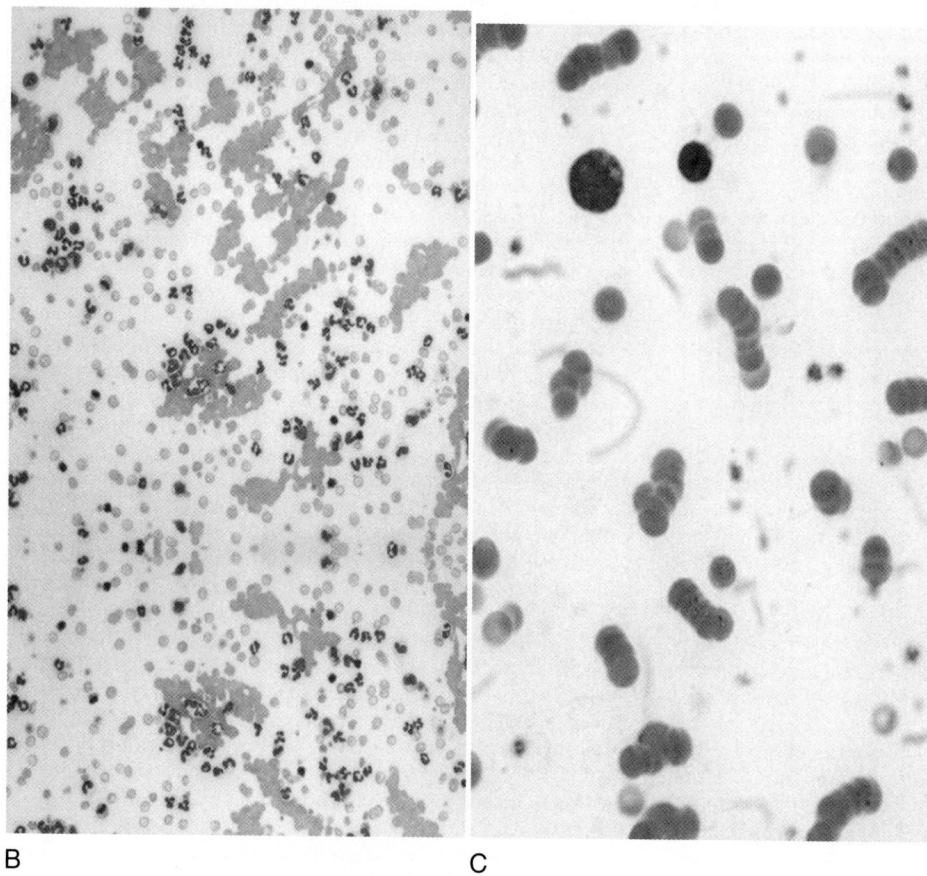

Figure 270-9 Microscopic agglutination wet mount **(A)** and Wright-Giemsa stain **(B)**. Reader should also note leukocytosis. Autoagglutination should not be confused with rouleaux formation **(C)**.

B   C

Direct Coombs test   The direct Coombs' test, also known as the *direct antiglobulin test (DAT)*, is used to detect antibodies, complement on a dog or cat's erythrocyte surface, or both, when the antierythrocyte antibody strength or concentration is too low (subagglutinating titer) to cause spontaneous autoagglutination.[83-85] The so-called incomplete antibodies on erythrocytes, together with species-specific antiglobulins against IgG, IgM, and C3b (Coombs' reagents), allow antibody bridging and thereby agglutination or lysis of coated erythrocytes (or both). Separate IgG, IgM, and C3b, as well as polyvalent Coombs' reagents, are available for dogs and cats. They are added at varied concentrations after washing the patient's erythrocytes free of plasma. The mixture is generally incubated at 37°C, then centrifuged, and supernatant and pellet are analyzed for hemolysis and agglutination, respectively. Performance of the direct Coombs' test at lower temperatures (4° and 20°C) is rarely indicated, because cold agglutinins and hemolysins are rarely strong enough and rarely active at near-normal body temperatures (30°C) to cause hemolysis. Cold agglutinins and hemolysins of clinical importance are generally IgM antibodies at high titer with a thermal amplitude that reaches 30°C. Because the same erythrocyte washing procedure is used in the direct Coombs' test as in the true autoagglutination test and the end point of the Coombs' reaction is agglutination and lysis of erythrocytes, true autoagglutination precludes the performance of a direct Coombs' test.

Positive direct Coombs' test results are reported as +1 to +4 or in the form of dilutions of the Coombs' reagent that cause in vitro agglutination, lysis, or both; the strength of the Coombs' reaction does not necessarily predict the severity of hemolysis seen clinically. Most dogs are IgG positive, some are IgG and IgM positive, and a few are only IgM positive.[86] To reach a definitive diagnosis of IMHA, the direct Coombs' test should be positive, but this does not discriminate between primary and secondary IMHA. Dogs with negative Coombs' test results should be re-evaluated for other causes of hemolytic anemia. However, a small proportion of dogs may have IMHA despite a negative Coombs' test result. False-negative Coombs' test results may occur because of insufficient quantities of bound antibodies on erythrocytes and for many technical reasons (inappropriate reagents or dilutions). Various techniques have been used to enhance the sensitivity of the direct Coombs' test, but none of them have gained wide acceptance in human and veterinary medicine. Furthermore, the test result may be negative in the absence of an inciting agent (e.g., drug). Negative results are also obtained for animals in which the disease is in remission; however, a few days of immunosuppressive therapy are not likely to reverse test results (i.e., in the presence of anemia and hemolysis the Coombs' test should be positive in a dog or cat with IMHA). Some treated animals have positive Coombs' test results long after the hemolytic anemia resolves. False-positive Coombs' test results occur only rarely, for example, early after an incompatible transfusion or because of technical problems. Furthermore, some animals may have a positive Coombs' test result without evidence of hemolysis and anemia; this has also been observed in healthy human blood donors.

Little is known about the usefulness of the indirect Coombs' or antiglobin test in which the presence of antierythrocyte antibodies in the patient's serum is evaluated with random erythrocytes. Clearly, the indirect Coombs' test would remain negative if the antibody is directed against a cryptic or new (drug, parasite) antigen on the erythrocyte surface. Alternatively, a false-positive test result may occur in a dog that has previously been transfused and developed certain alloantibodies.

Therapy of Immune-Mediated Hemolytic Anemia

Because the severity of IMHA ranges from an indolent to a life-threatening disease, therapy has to be tailored for each pet and depends, in part, on whether the IMHA is primary or secondary. Removal of the triggering agent or treatment of the underlying condition can bring the IMHA under control. Thus if the IMHA is thought to be secondary to an infection, treatment with antiprotozoals, antirickettsials, or antibiotics should be instituted. Because of the potential for underlying occult infection and the predisposition to infection related to the immunoderegulation associated with IMHA and immunosuppressive therapy, antibiotic therapy is generally indicated. In addition, surgical correction of abscesses or other infections may be considered. Nonessential drugs, particularly those that might cause an immune reaction, should immediately be withdrawn. Despite these interventions, transfusion and immunosuppressive therapy are probably still required in the initial control of secondary IMHA.

Rehydration of the severely ill animal is pivotal to improve organ perfusion even when it lowers the hematocrit. If hypoxia due to severe anemia and a rapidly dropping hematocrit to critical levels ensues, packed RBC transfusions are beneficial. The increased oxygen-carrying capacity provided by transfused cells may be sufficient to maintain the animal for the few days required for other treatment modalities to become effective. The notion that transfusions are especially hazardous in animals with IMHA has been overemphasized and is not supported by retrospective studies in dogs and humans.

Because the antierythrocytic antibody in IMHA is not an alloantibody, the destruction of transfused cells is no higher than that of autologous erythrocytes. However, autoagglutination may hamper accurate dog erythrocyte antigen (DEA) 1.1 blood typing and cross-matching tests even after RBC washing; hence, only DEA 1.1-negative blood should be transfused in autoagglutinating, untyped dogs. If compatible blood is not available, the ultrapurified bovine hemoglobin solution recently approved by the Food and Drug Administration can be administered and provides increased oxygen-carrying capacity and plasma expansion. In the original randomized study for Food and Drug Administration approval, this hemoglobin solution reduced the need for blood transfusions in the initial management of dogs with severe IMHA.[10] Some retrospective studies, however, suggested that this therapy was not beneficial if it was used as a last effort. With adequate transfusion support, animals with IMHA rarely die because of anemia, but they die because of overwhelming hemolysis and secondary complications such as thromboemboli and infections. Oxygen inhalation therapy is of little benefit unless the animal is suffering from pulmonary disease such as pulmonary thromboemboli.

The main goal in the treatment of IMHA is to control the immune response by reducing phagocytosis, complement activation, and antierythrocytic antibody production.[87] Glucocorticosteroids are the initial treatment of choice for IMHA. They interfere with both the expression and function of macrophage Fc receptors and thereby immediately impair the clearance of antibody-coated erythrocytes by the macrophage system. In addition, glucocorticosteroids may reduce the degree of antibody binding and complement activation on erythrocytes and, after weeks, diminish the production of autoantibodies. Oral prednisone or prednisolone at a dose of 0.5 to 1 mg/lb twice daily is the mainstay treatment. Alternatively, oral or parenteral dexamethasone at an equipotent dose of 0.3 mg/lb daily can be used but is probably not more beneficial. A response reflected by a stabilized or even rising hematocrit, appropriate reticulocytosis, and less autoagglutination and spherocytes can be expected within days. As glucocorticosteroid therapy is associated with well-known side effects, the initial dose is then tapered by reducing the amount by one quarter to one third every 7 to 14 days. Generally the faster the response to treatment the more rapidly the tapering is done. Within weeks to months, a low-dose alternate-day therapy may be reached with minimal steroid side effects. In secondary IMHA with appropriate control of the underlying disease, the tapering can be accomplished more rapidly. Because of the potential for GI ulceration by steroids, treatment with sucralfate or other similar GI drugs may be considered, although none have been documented to be effective.

Despite apparent recovery as judged by reaching a normal hematocrit, animals, particularly those with primary IMHA, may continue to have a positive Coombs' test for weeks to months and could obviously have relapses. Such relapses may be controlled by the same treatment as initially used, but a more gradual tapering regimen may be used in which the animal receives prednisone (preferably every other day) or other immunosuppressive therapy for months.

Other immunosuppressive therapy is warranted when prednisone fails, controls the disease only at persistently high doses, or causes unacceptable side effects. Cytotoxic drugs are usually given with prednisone but may eventually be used independently. These cytotoxic drugs inhibit lymphocytes and thereby suppress the antierythrocyte antibody production only after weeks. They are therefore probably not effective in the acute management of IMHA but may have a place in the long-term control of refractory and relapsing cases.

Cyclophosphamide, an alkylating and potent myelosuppressive agent, has been advocated in cases of fulminant IMHA. However, a randomized limited prospective clinical trial comparing prednisone with a combination of prednisone and cyclophosphamide did not find any beneficial effects of cyclophosphamide in the acute management of IMHA.[88] Retrospective studies with cyclophosphamide, azathioprine (an antimetabolite), or both were similarly disappointing, but overall assessment of these and other immunosuppressive agents is difficult based on retrospective and small case studies.[89-92] In addition to the strong myelosuppressive effects of these cytotoxic drugs, leading to reticulocytopenia, neutropenia, and thrombocytopenia, cyclophosphamide can induce a sterile hemorrhagic cystitis and secondary neoplasia. A potential regimen for the long-term management of dogs with IMHA might include azathioprine at 1 mg/lb once a day or every other day, but dogs need to be carefully monitored for cytopenias.[90] Hence, the risk/benefit ratio should be carefully considered when using these drugs.

Several other immunosuppressive agents have been used on a limited basis in conjunction with prednisone, and anecdotal success has been reported in dogs and rarely in humans. Because some of these agents interfere with antibody action and macrophage function, they can elicit more immediate effects. Cyclosporine, an expensive but potent immunosuppressive agent most commonly used in preventing graft rejection and graft-versus-host disease in transplant patients, may be beneficial in controlling the immune response in dogs with IMHA. A dose regimen of 5 mg/lb once a day may be used initially, but blood concentrations should be monitored periodically to achieve an effective but safe level. Leflunomide and mycophenolate are in a class of agents similar to that of cyclosporine and have been used in a few cases with anecdotal success. Danazol, an androgen derivative, at a dose of 5 mg/lb once a day, may inhibit binding of antibodies and phagocytosis. However, a retrospective study in dogs with IMHA was disappointing; furthermore, danazol is expensive and may be hepatotoxic.[93] Intravenous human immunoglobulin (IVIG) may be helpful in the short-term treatment of dogs with IMHA, although its mode of action remains unresolved.[94-96] IVIG can block Fc receptors on macrophages (thereby reducing Fc-mediated phagocytosis of IgG-coated erythrocytes), interfere with complement action, and suppress antibody production. Human IVIG binds to canine lymphocytes and monocytes and inhibits erythrocyte phagocytosis.[96] A single IVIG dose of 0.25 to 1 g/lb has been beneficial in some refractory cases as indicated by a rising PCV and reticulocytosis within days, but the response has often been only temporary. More recently two 0.5 g/lb doses of IVIG 1 day apart has resulted in good responses. Anecdotally, plasmapheresis has also been used as an adjuvant therapy, but is currently not available for companion animals.[97]

Splenectomy may be considered in IMHA dogs and cats that do not respond to prednisone and other immunosuppressive therapy, that require long-term high-dose therapy to remain in remission, or that have intractable drug-induced side effects. The spleen is a major site of autoantibody production, as well as sequestration and destruction of erythrocytes coated with IgG, but probably does not directly affect the clearance of IgM-coated cells. In addition, histologic examination of the spleen may provide evidence of an underlying disease. The response to splenectomy has recently been described in a few dogs with IMHA, but an objective assessment based on a randomized trial has not been completed.[98] A risk exists of developing overwhelming infections after splenectomy. Splenectomy should not be considered in pets receiving immunosuppressive therapy aside from prednisone.

Thromboemboli and DIC-like syndromes are serious complications of IMHA that greatly contribute to morbidity and mortality. Although the pathogenesis remains unknown, venipuncture, catheters, and glucocorticosteroid therapy represent potential predisposing conditions. No study has documented any successful prevention or management protocol for these life-threatening problems, which represent rare complications in humans with IMHA. Predisposing factors should, whenever possible, be limited. Adequate perfusion and oxygenation of tissue should be provided with fluids and transfusions. Generally, anticoagulant therapy is instituted only after some evidence or suspicion of thromboembolism exists. Heparin at a dose of 5 to 250 IU/lb subcutaneously every 6 hours or by continuous infusion is the most commonly used drug, and other antithrombotic agents are being evaluated.[99] However, none of them have been documented to be effective and safe in dogs or other species in the control of thrombotic complications. Fresh frozen plasma (5 mL/lb every 12 hours) may be administered to replenish dangerously low plasma antithrombin III concentrations, but its efficacy has not been demonstrated.[100] Other complications may also be related to drug therapy.

Despite appropriate implementation of these therapeutic strategies, the mortality rate remains high. An impression exists that the fulminate form of IMHA is more frequently encountered today. Depending on the type of practice (primary to tertiary), mortality rates from 20% to 75% have been reported. Negative prognostic indicators are a rapid drop in PCV, highly increased serum bilirubin concentrations, nonregenerative anemia, intravascular hemolysis, persistent autoagglutination, and thromboembolic complications.[101]

Alloimmune Hemolytic Anemias—Neonatal Isoerythrolysis and Hemolytic Transfusion Reactions

Erythrocyte alloantibodies, also known as *isoantibodies*, are specific antibodies directed against erythrocyte antigens (blood types) from the same species but not from the individual producing the antibody.[2] Depending on the species and blood group system, these alloantibodies occur naturally (cats) or are produced only after sensitization with a mismatched blood transfusion (dog) and are responsible for NI (cats) and acute or delayed hemolytic transfusion reactions (dogs and cats). Additional information can be found in Chapter 127 on transfusion medicine.

In cats, only the AB blood group system has been recognized; it consists of three blood types: type A, type B, and type AB.[2] The inheritance pattern of these blood types is unique and of considerable importance to breeders. The A allele is dominant over the B allele. Thus only homozygous b/b cats express the type B antigen on their erythrocytes. Type A cats are either homozygous (a/a) or heterozygous (a/b).[102] The rare AB blood type, seen in certain families, is inherited separately as a third allele that is recessive to A and codominant with B.[103] Simple in-practice blood typing cards are available, and other methods are being developed. Because a reaction in both test wells could be caused by autoagglutination, type AB test results should be confirmed after saline washing and in a reference laboratory using another method.[104] The prevalence of feline blood types varies geographically and among breeds.[102] Whereas purebred Siamese cats have all type A blood, Turkish Van and Angoras have equal numbers of type A and type B cats. All type B cats develop strong naturally occurring anti-A antibodies with high hemolysin and agglutinin titers (>1:32) after a few weeks of age, whereas type A cats generally develop only weak anti-B antibodies. Type AB cats have no alloantibodies. Thus acute life-threatening hemolytic transfusion reactions occur during the first mismatched transfusion (as little as 1 mL of blood), and NI is seen in type A and AB kittens born to primiparous type B queens.

Feline NI is caused by maternal anti-A alloantibodies that gain access to the circulation and destroy type A and type AB erythrocytes.[2,105-107] Thus type A and type AB kittens from matings between a type B queen and a type A or AB tom are at risk. The proportion of kittens at risk for NI varies from zero to 25%, depending on the frequency of type B cats, and therefore represents a major and now preventable cause of the neonatal kitten complex in purebred cats.[102] The low-titer anti-B alloantibodies of type A queens have not been associated with NI. Cats (and dogs) have an endotheliochorial placenta that is impermeable to immunoglobulins from the mother's serum. However, feline colostrum and milk contains high maternal concentrations of immunoglobulins that pass the GI tract and are absorbed intact only during the first 16 hours of life.

Thus type A or type AB kittens produced by type B queens are born healthy. Upon ingestion of colostrum or milk containing anti-A antibodies, the kittens at risk can develop clinical signs during the first few days of life. They may die suddenly without obvious clinical signs during the first few hours of life. They can develop severe pigmenturia, which is readily visible when stimulating the neonates to urinate with a moist cotton ball. These kittens fail to thrive, are reluctant to nurse, become anemic and icteric, and rarely survive the first week of life. Some kittens at risk may have a subclinical course or slough their tail tip at 1 to 2 weeks of age, presumably because of an agglutinin-induced occlusion. The severity of clinical signs depends on the amount of colostral antibodies ingested before the kitten's ability to digest proteins and closure of the gut to the absorption of intact proteins, which varies from kitten to kitten, between queens and litters, and even within a litter. NI can be confirmed by typing the queen and kitten or the tom if the kitten died with suspicious signs.

Because of the acute disease course, treatment of NI is rarely successful. Foster nursing by a type A queen, who delivered recently, or with milk replacer, transfusion, and supportive care may be attempted. During the first day, when anti-A alloantibodies could still be absorbed, washed type B blood may be preferred, but thereafter type A blood is appropriate and may be best administered by the intraosseous route. However, NI can be readily prevented by (1) blood typing queen and tom and mating type B queens only to type B toms or (2) foster nursing type A and AB kittens born to type B queens for the first 24 hours. This can be accomplished by placing the kittens at risk with a type A queen (exchanged only if the type A queen's kittens are older than 1 day) or feeding a commercial milk replacer at least four times a day. Either all kittens of a litter at risk should be removed from the type B queen, or umbilical cord blood or blood from the jugular vein of the kittens (0.5 mL) can be typed with the typing card or cross-matched with anti-A plasma from the queen, thereby providing an opportunity to leave the type B kittens with the type B queen. Although maternal passive immunity does not appear to be essential in most cattery situations, 1 to 3 mL of serum from a type A cat (which lacks harmful anti-A antibodies) may be given orally during the first few hours of life or intraperitoneally or subcutaneously to kittens receiving a milk replacer.

More than a dozen blood group systems have been described in dogs and are referred to as *DEA* followed by a number.[2,104,108] For all blood groups other than the DEA 1 system, erythrocytes from a dog can be either positive or negative (e.g., DEA 4 positive or negative). The DEA 1 system, however, has at least two subtypes: DEA 1.1 (also known as A_1) and DEA 2 (A_2). Thus the dog's erythrocytes can be DEA 1.1 positive or negative, and DEA 1.1-negative erythrocytes

can be DEA 1.2 positive or negative. The most antigenic and therefore most important blood type is DEA 1.1, for which simple blood typing cards are available. Typing of both blood recipient and donor for DEA 1.1 is recommended. An autoagglutination test card has been added, because autoagglutinating samples appear like DEA 1.1 positive.[104] True autoagglutination precludes typing. Typing for DEA 1.2, 3, 4, 5, and 7 is provided only by Midwestern Blood Services, but this extended blood typing has not be proven helpful in preventing blood type incompatibility reactions. In contrast to cats, dogs do not have clinically important naturally occurring alloantibodies but can develop them after mismatched transfusions, particularly anti-DEA 1.1 antibodies in DEA 1.1-negative dogs. Thus NI is not a clinical problem in dogs unless the bitch has previously received blood products. Similarly, acute hemolytic transfusion reactions are encountered only when a dog receives a blood transfusion 4 or more days after the first transfusion.[108-109] Careful history should indicate prior transfusions. These reactions can be prevented by cross-matching all dogs that have been previously transfused even when using the same donor. Furthermore, delayed hemolytic transfusion reactions characterized by a more rapid than anticipated drop of the hematocrit may be observed 1 to 2 weeks after a (first) transfusion because of the development of new antibodies. Because most reactions are directed against the DEA 1.1 antigen, DEA 1.1-negative (as well as untyped) dogs should never receive any blood products from DEA 1.1-positive donors. The only other acute hemolytic transfusion reactions were documented against a missing common antigen and DEA 4 in a DEA 4-negative dog, thus questioning the term *universal donor* for DEA 4-positive but otherwise negative dogs. However, a matched DEA 1.1 transfusion with crossmatching for a subsequent transfusion is practical and safe. Furthermore, some acute hemolytic reactions may be caused by use of expired, inappropriately stored, and contaminated blood. In case of acute hemolytic transfusion reactions, the transfusion should be stopped immediately and supportive therapy provided. Glucocorticosteroid administration has not been proven to be effective in preventing or treating hemolytic transfusion reactions.

Infection-Associated Hemolysis

Hemolytic anemia may develop after exposure to several parasitic, bacterial, and viral agents because of the direct action of the infectious agent or its products on erythrocytes. Few rickettsial and protozoal organisms are capable of infecting erythrocytes directly and causing severe hemolytic anemia (Table 270-2). Other infectious agents may induce a hemolytic component indirectly along with other major clinical signs. Thus any infection may trigger the production of humoral antibodies against host erythrocytes and together with an activated complement and phagocytic system, the rate of erythrocyte destruction may be markedly accelerated. Cats in particular have an inflammation-associated shortened survival of erythrocytes caused by an abscess, surgery, or trauma.[110] Furthermore, during bacterial (e.g., *Leptospira, Clostridium, Streptococcus, Staphylococcus*) septicemia, specific hemolysins can be produced. For instance, alpha toxin released during clostridial sepsis is a lecithinase that can attack erythrocyte membrane lipids, leading to erythrocyte fragmentation. Additional information on these infectious diseases can be found in Section VIII.

Hemobartonellosis Hemobartonellosis in cats, also known as *feline infectious anemia*, is caused by an epicellular rickettsial organism of erythrocytes.[111,112] *H. felis* is classified in the family Anaplasmataceae, is distinctly different from *Bartonella*, but is genetically similar to *Mycoplasma*. Hence *H. felis* has been renamed as *Mycoplasma haemofelis*, the large and more pathogenic form, and *M. haemominutum*, the small form.

The natural transmission of these mycoplasmas still remains unclear, although bloodsucking ectoparasites are considered to be major vectors. Iatrogenic infection can occur via blood transfusion from carrier cats. In addition, they may be transmitted by oral ingestion of infected blood or from queens to their newborns. Finally, because cat bite abscesses often precede hemobartonellosis by a few weeks, particularly in male cats that roam outdoors, this may represent another form of transmission.

It is considered an opportunistic organism that causes illness only under predisposing conditions. Approximately half of the cats with hemobartonellosis were FeLV positive and infection with both agents exaggerates the severity of the anemia, whereas concurrent infection with feline immunodeficiency virus (FIV) does not appear to worsen the anemia. Although viral infections, abscesses, systemic illnesses, and trauma (including surgery) are apparent predisposing factors, such conditions are not always identifiable.[113,114]

The pathogenesis of hemobartonellosis can be divided into parasitic incubation, acute parasitemia, and recovery or carrier stage.[115] One week to months after infection, cats, when stressed, develop an acute parasitemic phase that results in mild to severe anemia. This stage is characterized by cyclic parasitemia and often lasts for weeks to months unless death caused by massive parasitemia and anemia ensues earlier. Parasitized erythrocytes lose their deformability and elicit an immune response and are therefore rapidly sequestered and phagocytized in spleen and other tissues. However, sequestered erythrocytes may shed the parasites and re-enter the blood circulation. Although cats may recover by mounting an immune response against the parasites, they cannot completely clear the infection and thus they remain carriers indefinitely by harboring organisms in macrophages.

Feline hemobartonellosis is associated with a gradual to precipitous drop in hematocrit that results in clinical signs of anemia. Cats are lethargic, weak, and inappetent, and cyclic fevers occur during the transient periods of parasitemia. Icterus is rare, but pale mucous membranes are common. Splenomegaly and weight loss may develop gradually.

No serologic tests are presently available, but PCR-based tests to detect the mycoplasma-DNA have greatly aided in the detection of these infections.[116] However, not every cat positive for *M. haemominutum* is anemic or experiences hemolysis. These organisms may be incidentally discovered in carrier cats with other diseases. A diagnosis of feline hemobartonellosis can also be made by recognizing the organisms on erythrocytes in a blood smear (Figure 270-10A). Blood needs to be collected before treatment and sometimes repeatedly. Blood smears should be prepared shortly after collection because organisms may detach. Any Romanowsky-type blood stain (e.g., Wright's-Giemsa, Diff-Quik) may be used. Organisms appear as blue-staining ring, rod, or coccoid forms on the surface of erythrocytes. They need to be differentiated from Howell-Jolly bodies, other parasites, basophilic stippling, and staining artifacts. New methylene blue and reticulocyte stains are inappropriate, because organisms may be confused with punctate reticulocytes and Heinz bodies; fluorescent stains provide no advantages. Parasitized erythrocytes become spherical. Erythrophagocytosis by monocytes and tissue macrophages (e.g., bone marrow, splenic aspirates), as well as autoagglutination of parasitized erythrocytes may be observed, and the direct Coombs' test at 37° C is often positive, supporting the major role of immune destruction. Because of the cyclic nature of the parasitemia, absence of organisms does not rule out an infection.

Infected cats should be treated with tetracycline products for 3 weeks.[111] Doxycycline at a dose of 2.5 mg/lb twice a day is the preferred product because it needs to be administered only twice daily and appears to cause fewer side effects such as fever, anorexia, and hepatopathy. Enrofloxacin at a dose of 2.5 mg/lb once a day, orally, alone is a good alternative. Use of the two drugs in combination may be helpful in refractory cats. Parasitemia typically resolves quickly, and a clinical response is seen within days. None of the tetracyclines clear the infection completely; thus treated cats remain carriers, although relapses appear uncommon and have not been documented experimentally. Severely anemic cats may also benefit from blood transfusion from a blood type-compatible donor. Furthermore, because of the immune-mediated mechanism involved, treatment with prednisone at 0.5 to 1.0 mg/lb twice a day is indicated, particularly to inhibit the erythrophagocytosis.

In contrast to cats, dogs rarely have hemobartonellosis. It is caused by *Haemobartonella canis*, which can be transmitted by the brown dog tick (which also serves as a reservoir) and infected blood.[117] Unless dogs are splenectomized or have other serious illness and splenic dysfunction, infected dogs do not develop clinical signs of anemia. On stained blood smears *H. canis* differs from *H. felis* in that *H. canis* often forms chains across the surface of erythrocytes. Infected dogs with anemia are treated as described for cats and probably also remain latently infected.

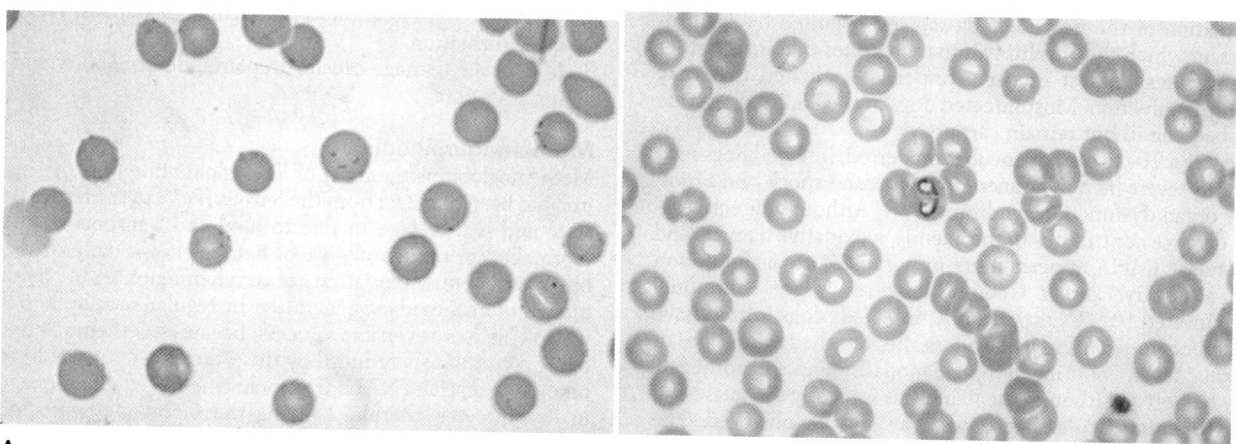

A   B

Figure 270-10 Hemobartonellosis in a cat (A) and babesiosis in a dog (B).

HEMATOLOGY AND IMMUNOLOGY

deformability, and therefore may lyse or be removed from the circulation by macrophages. When passing through the spleen, Heinz body–containing erythrocytes are retained in the meshwork and phagocytized as a whole (culled), or only the Heinz bodies are removed (pitting). However, because of large openings in the venous sinus walls, the feline spleen has poor pitting function. Heinz body hemolytic anemia has been associated with a variety of conditions, many of which also cause methemoglobinemia and membrane injury. Ingestion of dietary onions (raw, cooked, or dehydrated [onion powder]), as well as garlic, usually fed by owners as part of table scraps, can result in up to 90% Heinz body formation within 1 day, followed by hemolysis leading to severe anemia by 5 days.[135-137] Several thiosulfates in onion extracts have been implicated in producing Heinz bodies but only minimal amounts of methemoglobin. Onion and garlic toxicity occurs more commonly in dogs than cats, and the susceptibility appears to vary among individual animals. Administration of various drugs, including methylene blue, DL-methionine, phenacetin, and vitamin K_3 (above 2.5 mg/lb/day) can also lead to Heinz body hemolytic anemia.

Acetaminophen, benzocaine-containing products, and phenazopyridine can induce severe methemoglobinemia and also cause Heinz body formation. Furthermore, increased numbers of Heinz bodies have been associated with various organ disorders in cats. These disorders include hyperthyroidism, lymphoma, other cancers, and diabetes mellitus, particularly in the presence of ketoacidosis.[138]

Membrane Injury Many oxidative agents directly cause membrane lipid peroxidation, cross-linking and clustering of cytoskeleton proteins, and impaired ion transport function. These membrane injuries result in severe intra- and extravascular hemolysis, sometimes without much Heinz body and methemoglobin formation. For instance, naphthalene, the active ingredient in old-fashioned mothballs or crystals and in toilet bowl deodorizers, is an important poison in small animals, causing intravascular hemolysis, vomiting, seizures, and hepatopathy.[139] Hemolytic anemia has also been associated with acute zinc toxicity in dogs that swallowed zinc-containing objects such as zinc nuts and bolts from animal carriers, U.S. pennies minted since 1983 (98% zinc by weight), and zinc oxide dermatologic ointments (Fig. 270-12).[140,142] Because these objects may be retained in the stomach, the gastric acid liberates zinc, which allows absorption. The mechanism by which zinc causes life-threatening intravascular hemolysis

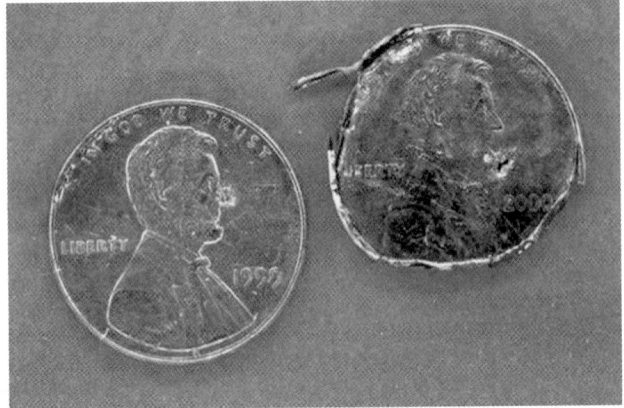

Figure 270-12 Zinc-containing coins eroded in stomach of a dog with hemolytic anemia.

remains uncertain, but few Heinz bodies and spherocytes have been found. Besides identifying the metal object by radiographs, the diagnosis can be confirmed by documenting increased serum zinc concentrations (above 5 parts per million; samples must be submitted in plastic tubes for analysis). Similarly, acute copper toxicosis may result in severe intravascular hemolysis and some methemoglobinemia. It has been associated with fulminant hepatic failure caused by copper storage in Bedlington terriers (see Chapter 227). In contrast, lead toxicity is generally not associated with hemolysis, but large numbers of nucleated RBCs and GI and neurologic signs are observed.

Treatment of oxidative hemolytic anemias includes immediate removal of the oxidative agent, use of antioxidants, transfusion, and supportive care. Vomiting is induced only if the substance has just been ingested and activated charcoal may be administered. Metallic objects such as pennies and nuts are best removed by gastroscopy or gastrotomy. In case of severe anemia, methemoglobinemia, or both, transfusion with packed RBCs is indicated, whereas oxygen therapy hardly improves tissue oxygenation. The anemia nadir is often not reached for several days, but with the commonly observed strong regenerative response, recovery from anemia is swift. Severe methemoglobinemia can be corrected with one slow intravenous injection of methylene blue (0.4 mg/lb). Methylene blue acts as an electron donor for an alternative, otherwise nonfunctional methemoglobin reductase. In cats with acetaminophen intoxication, either oral or intravenous N-acetylcysteine (Mucomyst) at an initial dose of 64 mg/lb followed by seven treatments of 32 mg/lb every 8 hours should be administered. As the drug of choice, N-acetylcysteine, increases the sulfate availability for conjugation of acetaminophen and provides cysteine for glutathione regeneration and metabolism of toxic metabolites of acetaminophen. Treatments with other agents such as sodium sulfate to add sulfide, cimetidine to inhibit cytochrome P-450, and ascorbic acid as weak antioxidants have been proposed, but they have not been shown to provide additional benefit. Because of the effect of oxidative substances on other organ systems including GI tract, liver, and central nervous system (CNS), animals may continue to show clinical signs after correction of the anemia and methemoglobinemia and require additional supportive care. Furthermore, care should be taken to avoid any re-exposure to these and other toxins.

Hypophosphatemia-Induced Hemolysis Severe hypophosphatemia causing hemolysis in dogs and cats has been associated with diabetes mellitus, hepatic lipidosis, enteral and parenteral hyperalimentation (starvation-refeeding syndrome), and oral administration of phosphate-binding antacids.[143-145] During insulin, fluid, and bicarbonate treatment of (ketoacidotic) diabetic animals, serum phosphate concentrations may decrease precipitously. Hypophosphatemia occurs because of intracellular phosphate shifts, enhanced renal loss, and reduced intestinal absorption of phosphate. In addition to myopathy, cardiac dysfunction, neurologic dysfunction, and acute hemolytic anemia (characterized by a rapid drop in PCV and mild intravascular lysis and Heinz body formation) may be observed in animals with hypophosphatemia. Based on experimental data, serum phosphorus concentrations would need to be less than 1 mg/dL (normal 2.9 to 7 mg/dL) to cause hemolysis, but in clinical practice hemolysis occurs with phosphate values less than 2.5 mg/dL. Serum phosphate measurements may underestimate the phosphate depletion in these disease states and can erroneously be higher because of hemoglobinemia and hyperbilirubinemia. The pathogenesis of the hypophosphatemia-induced anemia is probably related to depletion of erythrocytic ATP, DPG (in dogs), and reduced glutathione, which leads to decreased deformability, increased osmotic fragility, and susceptibility to oxidative injury. As discussed in relation to canine erythrocyte PFK deficiency, DPG-depleted erythrocytes are extremely alkaline fragile and have a high hemoglobin oxygen affinity, thereby contributing to intravascular hemolysis and tissue hypoxia in dogs but not in cats. Furthermore, thrombocytopenia and platelet and leukocyte dysfunction have been documented experimentally in dogs.

Hypophosphatemic animals need to receive oral or parenteral phosphate supplementation. Aggressive intravenous phosphate therapy is often needed in severely hypophosphatemic and anorexic or vomiting animals. An initial sodium or potassium phosphate dose of 0.005 to 0.015 mmol/lb/hr (maximum, 0.03) appears safe and effective, but serum phosphorus and calcium concentrations should be measured every 6 hours and the dose adjusted and route switched to oral when appropriate. Potential complications of intravenous phosphate supplementation include hypocalcemia, acute renal failure, and dystrophic soft tissue calcification and should be immediately corrected by stopping the phosphate infusion and initiating infusion of a calcium gluconate. Oral supplementation with a normal balanced diet, skim milk, or commercial phosphate products is preferred in cases of mild hypophosphatemia, and prophylactic phosphorus supplementation should always be considered when treating severe diabetes mellitus or hepatic lipidosis. This can be easily accomplished by supplementing potassium using both chloride and phosphate solutions.

Microangiopathic Hemolytic Anemia

A large variety of conditions may cause physical damage to erythrocytes that leads to cell fragmentation and intra- and extravascular hemolysis.[146] In case of water intoxication

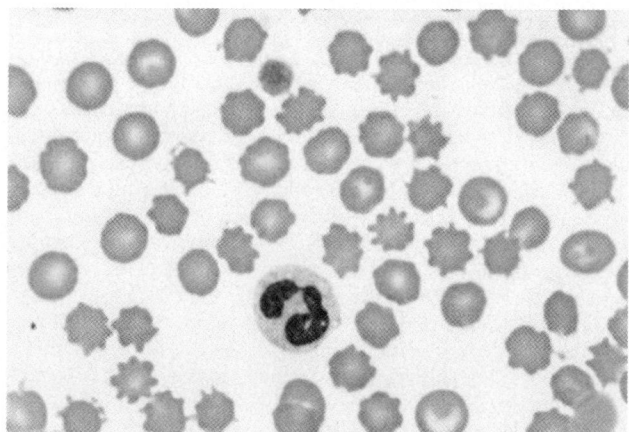

Figure 270-13 Acanthocytes dog with liver disease.

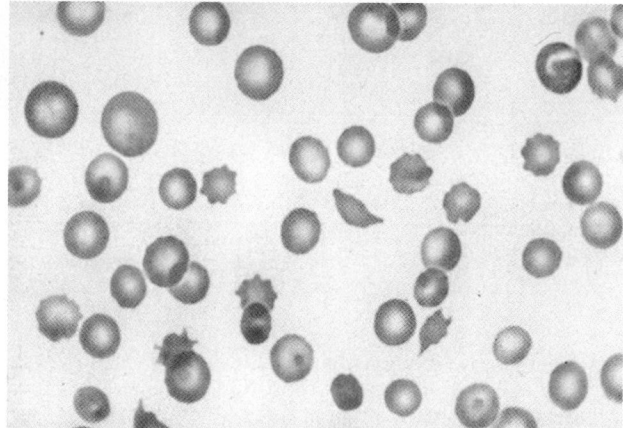

Figure 270-14 Schistocytes, canine.

associated with near drowning in fresh water, erythrocytes undergo hypotonic lysis similar to the swelling and lysis of erythrocytes in the *in vitro* osmotic fragility test. Heat stroke and severe burns can inflict thermal injury to erythrocytes. Heart valve disease, cardiovascular implants, and intravenous catheters can induce mechanical damage to erythrocytes as much as dirofilariasis, particularly in the form of the caval syndrome (see Chapter 206). In addition, other endothelial damage caused by vasculitis, hemangiosarcoma and other tumors, various splenic diseases or torsion, and liver disease can injure erythrocytes (Figure 270-13). A hemolytic-uremic syndrome characterized by acute renal failure, platelet activation leading to thrombocytopenia and thrombosis, and microangiopathic hemolytic anemia has been described in dogs. Similarly, DIC is associated with a fragmentation hemolysis (see Chapter 274).

A diagnosis of microangiopathic hemolysis that is often subclinical and rarely causes overt intravascular hemolytic anemia is made by identifying the triggering condition and characterizing schistocytes (schizocytes) (Figure 270-14). These are erythrocyte fragments that appear on blood smears as small, misshapen, often triangular or helmet-shaped structures. Schistocytes are important even in small numbers and can unlikely be fabricated by poor blood smear preparation. On the other hand, schistocytes are observed with a variety of other anemias including chronic iron deficiency states and zinc intoxication. Concomitantly, thrombocytopenia and coagulopathy are often present. Besides supportive care, therapy is directed at the underlying disease and control of DIC. Blood component therapy should be considered. The prognosis is guarded to poor if the underlying disease cannot be corrected.

CHAPTER 271

Nonregenerative Anemia

Bernard F. Feldman[†]

A nemia is a common clinical and laboratory finding that in and of itself does not constitute a diagnosis. In other words, anemia is a sign of disease, not a disease per se. The mere coexistence of anemia with another illness does not necessarily pinpoint the etiology. The clinical goal is to determine the pathogenesis in order to deliver the most appropriate therapy and to instigate steps to ameliorate this condition. The cause of anemia may be evident from the signalment, history, vaccination status, travel history, life style, duration of signs, drug or toxin exposure, prior or current illnesses, illnesses in housemates or relatives, or physical examination (Box 271-1). When a dog or cat is actively bleeding, the presence of anemia can be anticipated. If the bleeding is chronic, iron deficiency can be anticipated. Signs of inflammation or systemic illness can explain moderate anemia.[1-5]

IS THE ANEMIA NONREGENERATIVE OR REGENERATIVE?

There are seven general causes of anemia. Five of these remain nonregenerative unless the underlying etiology is successfully ameliorated. Two causes, hemolysis and hemorrhage, are nonregenerative in the acute stages but most often become regenerative 3 to 7 days after the onset of the problem. The seven general causes are:
1. Lack of iron
2. Anemia associated with inflammatory disease
3. Bone marrow disorders
4. Erythropoietin-related anemias
5. Maturation abnormalities (rarely encountered)
6. Hemolysis
7. Hemorrhage

The initial approach to treatment of the anemic pet is an attempt to discern whether the anemia is nonregenerative or regenerative. This determination is critical, because a dog or cat with regenerative change has either a hemolytic or hemorrhagic process and requires specific additional diagnostics and forms of therapy. Beyond the minimum database of a complete hemogram, urinalysis, and biochemical profile, diagnostics and therapeutics often are significantly different for the numerous nonregenerative anemias.

The decision as to whether the animal is responding appropriately to anemia treatment requires examination of reticulocyte numbers (from a vital stain) or polychromatophil numbers (from a Romanovsky-based stain). The reticulocyte count is the only index of *effective* erythropoiesis. Proper use of this value requires (1) conversion to an absolute quantity, (2) adjustment for the reduced red cell mass, and (3) correction for the effect of erythropoietin on marrow reticulocyte release. These adjustments result in the determination of reticulocyte numbers adjusted for the pet's red cell mass.[6]

The first step is to convert the reticulocyte percentage into an absolute quantity of reticulocytes. In a canine example, if the mean red cell count is 7 million and 1% reticulocytes is the mean number for that red cell mass, 1% reticulocytes in absolute terms is 70,000 reticulocytes. The reference interval for a normal adult dog is approximately 35,000 to 105,000 reticulocytes per microliter (0.5% to 1.5% reticulocytes).

The second step is to correct for the reduced red cell mass using red cell numbers *or* the hemoglobin *or* the hematocrit. Using the hematocrit as an example, the absolute reticulocyte number is multiplied by the dog's hematocrit, and the product is divided by the mean species hematocrit.

The third step is to correct for the effect of erythropoietin (EPO) on bone marrow reticulocyte release; EPO is inversely correlated with the red cell count (or hemoglobin or hematocrit). Continuing with the hematocrit example, the lower the hematocrit, the higher the concentration of EPO (with some exceptions, such as renal failure). EPO has four clinically significant effects: (1) it causes uncommitted stem cells to differentiate to the erythroid line; (2) it decreases the bone marrow maturation time for red cell development; (3) it increases individual red cell hemoglobin synthesis; and (4) it causes premature release of reticulocytes from bone marrow to blood.

The approximate average time for reticulocytes to mature in the dog or cat is 4.5 days: 3.5 days in the marrow and 1 day (24 hours) in peripheral blood if the hematocrit is appropriate (Table 271-1).

To correct for the effect of EPO on bone marrow reticulocyte release, the examiner converts the reticulocyte percentage to absolute values and adjusts for the reduced hematocrit, then divides the final figure by the number of days the average reticulocyte lives as a reticulocyte in peripheral blood based on the dog's or cat's hematocrit (see Table 271-1). Determine red cell production over basal or anticipated numbers (basal numbers are anticipated to be 35,000 to 105,000 absolute reticulocytes per microliter in a normal adult dog with a reticulocyte reference interval of 0.5% to 1.5%).

If a dog's hematocrit is 23% (mean canine normal is 46%) and its reticulocyte percentage is 5%, the question is, is there an appropriate response to the reduced hematocrit? To determine the corrected absolute reticulocyte count in this dog, the following calculations are made:
1. If the reticulocyte count is 5% of a red cell count of 3.5 million/mL (the approximate number of red cells per microliter with a hematocrit of 23%), the absolute reticulocyte number is approximately 175,000/mL. Thus:

$$175,000 \times 23\% \text{ (Dog's hematocrit)} \div 46\% \text{ (Mean canine hematocrit)} = 87,500/\text{mL}$$

2. The number of reticulocytes per milliliter (87,500) is divided by 2 (the average length of time [2 days] a reticulocyte circulates in peripheral blood at a hematocrit of 23%) to determine the corrected absolute reticulocyte number:

$$87,500 \div 2 = 43,750/\text{mL}$$

The corrected absolute reticulocyte value in this example (43,750/mL) is well within the reference interval observed

---

[†]Deceased.

Box • 271-1

History and Physical Examination Considerations with an Anemic Patient

History

Previous laboratory tests for comparison

Duration of signs—recent or long standing

Family history?

Previous surgery—problems?

Drugs—especially consider nonsteroidal anti-inflammatory drugs

Exposure to toxic chemicals resulting in hemolysis or aplasia

Abdominal signs—hepatosplenomegaly, gastrointestinal blood loss or neoplasia, malabsorption

Urinary signs—polyuria, polydipsia, hematuria

Blood loss—gastrointestinal or urinary tract

Miscellaneous—dietary history; neurologic signs; nonspecific discomfort

Physical Examination

Skin and mucous membranes—pallor, jaundice, petechiae, purpura, bruising

Cardiovascular—evidence of pulse abnormalities, murmurs

Pulmonary—evidence of dyspnea

Lymph nodes—enlarged?

Abdomen—hepatosplenomegaly, ascites, masses

Rectal examination—gastrointestinal blood loss, melena, masses

---

for dogs with appropriate hematocrits. In fact, in this example, even without correction for the effect of EPO (without correction, the reticulocyte count would have been 87,500/mL), this anemia must be considered nonregenerative. A corrected absolute reticulocyte count of less than 105,000/mL must be considered nonregenerative. Patients with hemolysis and hemorrhage that are responding appropriately

Table • 271-1

Average Time Required for Reticulocyte Maturation

HEMATOCRIT	DEVELOPMENT IN MARROW (days)	DEVELOPMENT IN PERIPHERAL BLOOD (days)
Dogs		
45	3.5	1.0
35	3.0	1.5
25	2.5	2.0
15	1.5	2.5
Aggregate Reticulocytes in the Cat		
32	3.5	1.0
24	3.0	1.5
16	2.5	2.0
10	1.5	2.5

often have adjusted absolute reticulocyte counts in excess of 150,000/mL.

CLINICAL MANIFESTATIONS OF ANEMIA

The clinical manifestations of anemia are also common manifestations of processes or diseases that primarily affect other organ systems. Weakness, fatigue, and pallor are often manifestations of anemia of recent onset, such as that caused by recent blood loss or acute hemolysis. Anemia that develops gradually, particularly in inactive cats or dogs, may cause only fatigue or may go unnoticed. Pallor of the conjunctiva or mucous membranes may be caused by both anemia and hypovolemia. Icterus may obscure pallor. Pain may also result from increased bone marrow activity; this may simply be manifested by fatigue, unwillingness to move or, in stoic small animals, concern with movement or difficulty walking. Lymphadenopathy and splenomegaly are common with infectious, inflammatory, and hematologic diseases, particularly lymphomas and the leukemias. Bleeding occurs as a consequence of vascular, platelet, or coagulation factor abnormalities. Thrombosis can be either venous or arterial and often results in significant thrombocytopenia. Venous thrombosis is often caused by blood flow or obstructive processes or by imbalances in coagulation factors. Immune-mediated hemolytic anemia can be an example of such a process. Arterial thrombosis is most often caused by vascular problems, including vascular trauma thrombocytopenia, thrombocytosis or thrombocytopathia, and processes associated with infection or neoplasia.[4]

LABORATORY EVALUATION

Laboratory assistance usually is required to determine the cause of anemia. The routine but complete hemogram and blood smear document the presence, severity, and morphologic nature of the anemia (Box 271-2). A complete evaluation includes study of marrow production and red blood cell destruction and is usually required for accurate classification of the anemia into one of the two major categories, regenerative (responsive) or nonregenerative (nonresponsive). In the absence of specific clues, anemia initially may be broadly classified as regenerative or nonregenerative on the basis of reticulocyte (or polychromatophil) numbers (Box 271-3).

Most anemias are nonregenerative (Box 271-3). This type of anemia may be due to (1) an abnormality of the stem cell population and bone marrow environment, (2) an abnormality in the early modulators of stem cell activity, or (3) a deficiency in the late-stage regulators of erythroid proliferation, including EPO, cytokines, and iron.[5]

Disorders of marrow stroma and stem cells are relatively uncommon, but when they do occur, they often result in severe anemia and may represent myelodysplastic syndromes, including those variously lumped together as the "preleukemic syndromes." Nonregenerative anemia associated with iron depletion caused by inflammation is the most common mild anemia in dogs and cats. Anemias that occur secondary to a decrease in EPO are also often mild, at least in the early stages of the process, because the anemia reflects a physiologic readjustment of red cell production to fit reduced metabolic need. This can even be true in early renal disease. Red blood cell morphology and production indices (reticulocyte numbers and the mean cell volume, mean cell hemoglobin, and mean cell hemoglobin concentration) may be similar for the various types of nonregenerative anemia. However, findings on marrow morphology (and perhaps iron studies) usually allow categorization of the specific abnormality as one of the three types listed previously.[6]

HYPOPROLIFERATIVE ANEMIA

Erythropoietin-Related Causes

Renal Insufficiency

Renal insufficiency, especially chronic and severe renal disease, invariably affects the hemopoietic system adversely. To provide effective treatment, the clinician must have a clear understanding of the factors that induce anemia and intensify the failure of erythropoiesis. The bone marrow provides important clues to the pathogenesis of the anemia of renal failure. Given the variety of possible complicating factors, it is not surprising that a wide spectrum of abnormalities have been reported. Marrow cellularity has been reported to be normal, decreased, and increased. However, most dogs and cats with uncomplicated anemia secondary to renal insufficiency have appropriate marrow cellularity, with appropriate myeloid to erythroid ratios and appropriate erythroid development, despite the severe anemia. The argument may be made that an appropriate myeloid to erythroid ratio may not in fact be appropriate in the anemia of renal insufficiency. Iron distribution tends to be normal unless some element of anemia of inflammation is present, in which case iron may be redistributed to the monocyte-macrophage cells. Ferrokinetics are nearly normal in most small animals with anemia of renal disease. When these individuals are stressed by hypoxia or worsening anemia as a result of hemorrhage, the bone marrow erythron is able to respond in the appropriate direction but does so with a suboptimal recovery phase.[7]

From examination of the marrow alone it can be determined that (1) the defect in anemia of renal disease is not primarily related to defects in iron, which distinguishes this disorder from anemia of inflammation, and (2) the primary defect is not the result of an absolute absence of EPO. If it were, the myeloid to erythroid ratio would show a marked increase, approaching infinity, as the effect of EPO on the erythroid marrow decreases.

Two primary mechanisms have been advanced to explain most cases of normocytic, normochromic anemia with normal iron distribution and normal absolute reticulocyte counts associated with renal insufficiency. One mechanism is a deficiency of EPO, which causes the anemia. The other mechanism is an accumulation of toxins that suppress hemopoiesis. The latter mechanism probably accounts for much of the anemia, especially in dogs. Of course, if underlying inflammatory renal disease is present, anemia of inflammation may be a component.

EPO is a vital hemopoietic growth factor that not only enhances red cell production but also has been shown to increase platelet counts in rats and humans with end-stage renal failure.[8] EPO plays an important role in the pathogenesis of anemia in the dog and to a lesser degree in the cat. A significant increase in the plasma EPO concentration was observed in 22 cats and 32 dogs with anemia without renal insufficiency or chronic renal failure; however, 37 dogs and 35 cats with chronic renal failure had a normal or only modestly reduced EPO concentration. Cats showed almost no overlap between the groups, whereas dogs showed significant overlap.[9] This suggests that measurement of the plasma EPO concentration is more useful for characterization of anemia in cats than in dogs, either with or without chronic renal disease.[10] It also suggests that successful use of EPO may be a target molecule and/or a threshold response, perhaps to "kick start" erythropoiesis. The effects of EPO in these circumstances occur only with even more EPO, an argument for using exogenous EPO clinically.

As a general rule, the use of commercially available human recombinant growth factors for several consecutive weeks in dogs and cats results in the development of antibodies. Fortunately, it appears that short-term use of these products (less than several weeks) does not result in significant antibody effect.[11] The use of any human recombinant hemopoietic growth factor, including EPO, is strictly extralabel, because these products are not approved for use in the dog or cat. Only dogs and cats that have clinical signs related to anemia and that are profoundly affected (i.e., a hematocrit below 25% in the dog and 20% in the cat) should be considered for EPO therapy because of the potential for the development of antibodies.[9] Animals that are hypotensive or that have iron deficiency should not be treated until these problems have been corrected. The blood pressure and the serum iron concentration should be checked before and during EPO therapy.

The current recommended dosage of recombinant human EPO is 100 U per kilogram of body weight given subcutaneously three times weekly. Once the target hematocrit has been reached, the frequency should be reduced to twice weekly. The lowest possible maintenance dosage should be used. It is also recommended that iron be given to any dog or cat undergoing EPO therapy. If refractory anemia is noted despite therapy, EPO administration should be suspended and the pet evaluated further, at least with a complete hemogram and bone marrow examination. If erythrocytic hypoplasia exists, the development of antibodies may be the cause, and the pet must be supported with blood products and other adjunctive therapies.[11]

Older studies have provided convincing evidence that implicates uremic toxins (as yet many are implicated but none

Box • 271-3

Full Functional Classification of Anemia

Nonregenerative
Hypoproliferative anemia
  Erythropoietin-related condition
    Renal disease
    Hypothyroidism
    Hypoadrenocorticism
    Panhypopituitarism
    Decreased growth hormone
    Reduced oxygen requirements
    Increased oxygen release
  Lack of iron
    Inflammation
    Chronic bleeding
    Iron deficiency
  Marrow disorders
    External toxin—aplasia
    Myelophthistic disease
    Myelofibrosis
    Myelodyplasia
    Intrinsic marrow disease
    Hyperestrogenism—iatrogenic, neoplastic
    Infection
    Immunotherapy
    Pure red cell aplasia
Ineffective erythropoiesis
  Macrocytic (unusual)
    Intrinsic marrow disease
    Vitamin B_{12} deficiency
    Folate deficiency
  Normocytic
    Stromal disease (myelofibrosis)
    Intrinsic erythroid disease

  Microcytic
    Nonsideroblastic—iron deficiency
    Sideroblastic—globin or porphyrin abnormality
  Time related
    Hemolysis—during the first 3 to 5 days at least
    Hemorrhage—during the first 3 to 5 days at least
Regenerative
  Hemorrhage
    Hemostatic disorders
      Coagulation disorders
      Platelet disorders—both quantitative and qualitative
      Vascular disorders
      Neoplastic disease
      Splenic disease or trauma
      Trauma or surgery
  Hemolysis
    Excessive phagocytosis by the mononuclear phagocytic system
    Immune mediated
    Heinz body anemias
    Membrane (adenosine triphosphate) disorders
  Fragmentation
    Intravascular coagulation
    Vasculitis
    Intravascular hemolysis
    Immune mediated, including complement mediated
    Exotoxin induced
    Intrinsic intraerthrocytic enzyme deficiency
    Drugs
    Water
    Heat

Modified from Hillman RS, Finch CA: Red Cell Manual, 5th ed. Philadelphia, FA Davis, 1985, p 56.

specified) in the genesis of anemia of renal insufficiency.[12] These investigators reasoned that because several studies in humans with anemia of renal insufficiency had indicated that the plasma EPO concentrations were within the reference interval or modestly above or below it, all are inappropriate for the degree of anemia. However, it seemed unlikely that anemia of renal insufficiency could be explained in toto by EPO deficiency, therefore it must be due to retention of some materials that inhibit EPO or its effects. When continuous peritoneal dialysis was used in human patients with end-stage renal disease, half the patients showed full correction of the anemia. The researchers concluded that anemia of renal insufficiency can be corrected by dialysis alone in patients in whom sufficient renal endocrine function remains to mount a modest EPO response. Another conclusion was that, because EPO plays a pivotal role in erythropoiesis, if the endocrine function of the kidney has been destroyed by the same disease that impairs excretory function, the clearance of uremic toxins by dialysis will not reverse the suppression of the erythron.[12,13]

Certainly other factors, if investigated, can help the clinician define etiologies and develop appropriate therapeutic strategies. These factors, which have been suggested to contribute to anemia of renal insufficiency, include reduced half-life of red cells due to uremic toxins, hemorrhagic loss from gastrointestinal ulcers, increased hemorrhagic tendency due to reduced platelet function, suppression of erythropoiesis by high concentrations of parathyroid hormone, reduced nutrient intake due to inappetence, and injury of red cells due to glomerular pathology and renal fibrosis.[2]

Anemia Secondary to Endocrine or Metabolic Disorders

Endocrine disorders involving the thyroid and the pituitary-adrenal axis can cause hypoproliferative anemias. Hypothyroidism impairs erythrocyte production in humans and dogs. The anemia is usually mild and may be either normocytic or slightly macrocytic. Other clinical signs are related to the underlying thyroid disorder, and the anemia remits when the thyroid status is corrected. This is an interesting anemia in physiologic terms, because in a sense it is not an anemia at all. It represents an inappropriate response on the part of the kidney (i.e., EPO production) and bone marrow to decreased tissue oxygen consumption in the hypothyroid patient. The anemia is slow to develop and slow to remit; 3 to 4 months may be required from the onset of replacement therapy before the red cell mass returns toward or to normal. Other deficiencies of necessary nutrient materials (e.g., cobalamin or folic acid deficiency) may result from immune-mediated thyroid disease,[14,15] although this has not been addressed specifically in veterinary medicine. Prealbumin, an alpha$_2$-globulin produced in the liver and a transport protein for thyroxine, has been measured in dogs with hypothyroidism. In horses, the prealbumin concentration negatively correlates with albumin. Prealbumin increases with infectious, immune, and neoplastic etiologies, which suggests that the mild anemia associated with canine hypothyroidism may have a component of anemia of inflammation.[16-18]

Other endocrine disorders that might be associated with mild anemia are hypopituitarism, hypoadrenocorticism, and decreased growth hormone.[18] A mild anemia recognized in late pregnancy is the result of an increase in the plasma volume. The red cell mass remains appropriate.

Causes Related to Lack of Iron
Anemia Due to Iron Abnormalities
Iron-deficient erythropoiesis occurs secondary to body iron depletion or inflammation. In young, nursing animals suffering from any type of blood loss (including parasitism or repeated phlebotomy), iron depletion occurs rapidly, because iron stores are insignificant and the mother's milk does not contain adequate iron. In older animals with iron-deficient erythropoiesis, gastrointestinal or urinary tract hemorrhage, often occult and chronic, should be suspected. Among the clinical considerations would be ulceration, parasitism, neoplasia, and hemostatic disorders.

Most natural iron exists in a largely unavailable (to biologic systems), oxidized, insoluble, ferric (Fe^{3+}) form. Free iron can catalyze the formation of free radicals that damage cell membranes and deoxyribonucleic acid (DNA). Intracellular iron, therefore, is bound to various proteins to reduce its toxicity. These proteins are responsible for the absorption, transport, storage, and biologic activity of iron.

Any clinical study of iron metabolism must, of necessity, study the physiologic compounds associated with it. Iron exists in the following compartments: hemoglobin; storage, in the form of hemosiderin and ferritin; myoglobin; labile iron; tissue iron; and transport.[7] These compartments are defined by anatomic distribution, chemical characteristics, and function.[19]

Most iron in animals exists in red cells as hemoglobin iron. Each hemoglobin molecule contains four iron atoms, and each milliliter of red cells contains 1.1 mg of iron. The exact amount of total body iron depends on the red cell mass, blood volume, and body weight.[20] Storage iron exists as either a soluble, mobile fraction (ferritin) or as an insoluble, aggregated form (hemosiderin). As iron storage increases, more iron is stored as hemosiderin. Hemosiderin is mostly formed by lysosomal action on ferritin. In tissues it is readily recognized by the Prussian blue reaction. Ferritin consists of protein (apoferritin) and iron. Once iron is in the apoferritin shell, it must be oxidized to the ferric form, hydrolyzed, and polymerized to the ferric oxyhydroxide polymer. Reversal of the process allows iron to exit ferritin. The molecular shape and therefore the immunogenicity of ferritin is both species and tissue specific.[21,22]

Myoglobin iron is found mostly in muscle, where it can temporarily provide oxygen during anaerobic conditions. The labile iron pool may be an intermediate between plasma, storage, and hemoglobin. The tissue iron compartment consists of heme-containing compounds similar to hemoglobin (e.g., myoglobin and the cytochromes), non-heme-containing enzymes (e.g., iron sulfur compounds and metalloflavoproteins), enzymes that require iron or heme as a cofactor, and enzymes that contain iron in an unknown form (e.g., ribonucleotide reductase).

The transport compartment consists of plasma transferrin. The transfer of iron to erythroid cells requires internalization of the iron-laden transferrin molecule. The amount of iron delivered depends on the plasma iron concentration, the percentage iron saturation, and the number of membrane receptors.[7,23] Copper also plays an important part in the transportation of iron across cell membranes. Most circulating copper is found attached to the serum glycoprotein ceruloplasmin, which provides ferroxidase activity and may be needed to deliver iron into the circulation. When pigs are copper deficient, they have hypoceruloplasminemia and show signs of functional iron deficiency, presumably as the result of an inability to mobilize iron from the mononuclear phagocytic system and the gastrointestinal tract.[7,24]

Examination of the complete hemogram may be useful for evaluating iron adequacy. In severe iron deficiency, hemoglobin production is slowed and nucleated red cells continue to divide, resulting in the release into the circulation of late-stage nucleated red cells and adult red cells with marked central pallor. The red cell indices, the mean corpuscular volume (MCV), mean corpuscular hemoglobin concentration (MCHC), and mean corpuscular hemoglobin (MCH), are variably lowered in late-stage iron deficiency, with lowering of the MCH often preceding the other indices. It should be noted that deficiency of copper and pyridoxine, which also are needed for hemoglobin synthesis, can lower these indices.

The concentrations of serum iron and transferrin (the total iron binding capacity [TIBC] when the transferrin molecule is saturated) are useful analytes in the determination of iron adequacy. Use of non-iron-containing anticoagulants (ethylenediamine tetra-acetic acid [EDTA] is satisfactory), disposable plastic pipettes, test tubes, and test tube stoppers prevents contamination of patient blood with iron or zinc. Serum iron declines with iron deficiency, acute-phase inflammatory reactions, hypoproteinemia, hypothyroidism, renal disease, and chronic inflammatory states. The serum iron concentration should not be used as a predictor of iron stores. The transferrin concentration is stable or may increase with primary nutritional iron deficiency and remains stable or decreases with inflammatory processes. The unbound iron binding capacity (UIBC) estimates the saturation of transferrin, and its determination is of little clinical use.

Determination of the bone marrow iron concentration with Prussian blue stain occasionally is useful. Under appropriate circumstances, stainable iron is evident, whereas with iron-deficient processes, it is not evident.[7,19] Analysis of serum ferritin using species-specific, antibody-driven reactions has proven useful for determining nonheme iron stores in domestic animals, as well as increases after iron therapy. Ferritin, an acute-phase inflammatory protein, can increase during inflammatory reactions when interleukin-1 (IL-1) is produced. Serum ferritin can also be increased in hepatic disease, hemolysis, and some neoplastic disorders.[22,24] Body iron stores can be measured directly by measurement of the iron concentration in various organs.[25]

Anemia of Inflammatory Disease
Anemia of inflammatory disease (AID) is a mild, normocytic, normochromic, nonregenerative anemia associated with acute or chronic inflammatory processes, including trauma, infection, immune processes, and focal or disseminated neoplastic disease. It is the most common anemia found in small animals and is probably the most common anemia in veterinary medicine. This anemia appears within several days to a week. Clinically, it is an iron-deficient process; however, although the cause is multifactorial, iron sequestration in the mononuclear phagocytic system is the physiologic basis.[26-30]

The pathogenesis is mediated by cytokines produced during inflammation and results from iron sequestration (relative unavailability), a decline in red cell survival, and decreased erythropoietic response.[28,29] Reduced iron availability appears to be a physiologic metabolic response, an attempt to deprive infectious organisms of iron essential to metabolism.

Apolactoferrin (iron-free lactoferrin), found in milk, mucosal secretions, and polymorphonuclear leukocytes (neutrophils), chelates and binds large amounts of iron, especially at the low pH concentrations associated with inflammation. Both the synthesis and release of apolactoferrin are increased primarily by IL-1 and tumor necrosis factor alpha. Macrophages express increased lactoferrin receptors on their surfaces; this allows them to internalize lactoferrin-bound iron, which is transferred to ferritin. Neutrophils release apolactoferrin at sites of infection, which helps in iron chelation. Lactoferrin is also intrinsically bacteriocidal.[30] This results in diversion of iron from fast-release (ferritin storage) to slow-release (hemosiderin storage) pathways. Intestinal epithelial cells and hepatocytes are also affected and contribute to the relative iron deficiency. Iron absorption from the gastrointestinal tract is reduced as a result of decreased transferrin synthesis during the acute-phase reaction.[31]

Experimental studies in cats suggest that red cell survival may be a predominant factor in the early stage of AID. Macrophages activated by the inflammatory process are more efficient in clearing senescent red cells and those coated with immunoglobulins.[29,32] Although not all AID patients are febrile, fever per se has been implicated in decreased red cell survival.[27]

The defects in erythropoiesis in AID have been enumerated: inappropriately low EPO production, diminished marrow response, and iron-limited erythropoiesis. The appropriate inverse relationship between the EPO concentration and the degree of anemia is lost in AID.[33] IL-1-alpha, IL-1-beta, and tumor necrosis factor all inhibited hypoxia-induced EPO secretion in vitro, suggesting an important role for cytokines in the pathogenesis of AID.[34] EPO concentrations in cats with experimentally induced AID were found to be slightly increased but somewhat low for the degree of anemia, which also suggests that EPO production may be a contributor to this process.[27] Tumor necrosis factor has been demonstrated to suppress erythropoiesis in laboratory animals and to prohibit the development of erythroid precursors. In contrast, a heat-stable serum factor that could not be neutralized by antibody to tumor necrosis factor or gamma interferon has been shown to render normal T cells suppressive to autologous colony-forming units–erythroid (CFU-E).[34]

AID is an anticipated complication of all focal or systemic inflammatory processes, contributing to the development of anemia due to the underlying process. Certainly the overall well being of an animal has to be influenced by the development and consequences of anemia. Numerous disease states can result in human AID. Although many of the diseases have not been specifically studied in veterinary medicine, one

disease, lymphoma, has been studied in dogs.[35] Dogs with lymphoma had appropriate concentrations of iron, transferrin, and EPO, findings contrary to those associated with AID.[36]

Parameters that differentiate anemia of inflammation from iron deficiency and hemolysis are presented in Table 271-2. Therapy of this mild anemia involves amelioration of the underlying disorder, given the realization that AID contributes to and potentially complicates any anemic process accompanied by inflammation. Administration of iron is of no value. Administration of EPO may increase the red cell mass, but the overall response may be inappropriate or inadequate.[30]

NONPROLIFERATIVE ANEMIA

Anemia Associated with Marrow Disorders

Bone marrow suppression and/or toxicity is a widely recognized negative side effect of antineoplastic agents. This effect is often predictable, dose related, generally reversible, and observed with a high incidence because these drugs are given at or near maximum tolerated dosages.[37] Most antineoplastic drug groups, including alkylating agents (now rarely used), antimetabolites, antineoplastic antibiotics, and naturally occurring compounds (e.g., vincristine, vinblastine), as well as other drugs, including cisplatin, carboplatin, dacarbazine, procarbazine, and hydroxyurea, have been known to cause bone marrow toxicity,[38] as can radiotherapy.

Pure Red Cell Aplasia

Pure red cell aplasia (PRCA) usually is an acquired disorder. The anemia is often severe, resulting in hematocrits in dogs and cats of less than 20%, with absolute reticulocytopenia and virtually absent marrow precursors. Marrow myeloid and megakaryocytic elements appear to be preserved, and the peripheral white cell and platelet counts are appropriate. This condition can be caused by feline leukemia virus (FeLV) or by direct suppression of the stem cells identified as burst-forming units–erythroid (BFU-E), or it may be immune mediated in dogs. In dogs, antibodies may be specifically directed at epitopes on the immature erythroid cells. In dogs and occasionally in cats, spherocytes and stomatocytes may be observed in peripheral blood, and the direct or indirect antiglobulin (Coombs') test result may be positive.[2,39]

Aplasia Anemia (Aplastic Pancytopenia)

Aplastic pancytopenia in several species can occur secondary to increased endogenous blood estrogen concentrations. The effects appear to be most severe in ferrets and dogs. Bone marrow panhypoplasia and pancytopenia are often preceded

Table • 271-2

Differentiation of Iron Deficiency, Anemia of Inflammation, and Hemolysis

ANALYTE	IRON DEFICIENCY	ANEMIA OF INFLAMMATION	HEMOLYSIS
Red cell indices	Microcytic, hypochromic	Normocytic, normochromic	Normocytic, normochromic
Serum iron	Reduced	Normal to reduced	Increased
Transferrin (TIBC)*	Increased	Normal to reduced	Decreased
Marrow iron stores	Reduced	Normal to increased	Normal to increased
Ferritin	Decreased	Normal to increased	Normal to increased
Platelet count	Increased	Normal	Variable

Modified from Waner T et al: Anemia of inflammatory disease. *In* Feldman BF, Zinkl JG, Jain NC (eds): Schalm's Veterinary Hematology, 5th ed. Baltimore, Lippincott Williams & Wilkins, 2000, p 205.
*TIBC, Total iron binding capacity; for clinical purposes, this is the transferrin concentration.

by myeloid hyperplasia and leukocytosis for several weeks. Multiple mechanisms have been incriminated, including reduction of hemopoietic stem cell numbers, inhibition of stem cell differentiation, and decreased response to EPO.[37,40] Another mechanism is iatrogenic overdose of exogenous estrogenic compounds, especially estradiol cyclopentylpropri-onate, intended to prevent pregnancy or to treat prostatic hyperplasia. All types of testicular neoplasia in male dogs and granulosa cell tumors in female dogs can be associated with hyperestrogenism and pancytopenia. At least 10% of male dogs with testicular neoplasia, predominantly those with Sertoli cell neoplasia, have pancytopenia, and approximately 90% of those do not recover.[3,40]

Azidothymidine (AZT), a dideoxynucleoside derivative reverse transcriptase inhibitor used in the treatment of feline immunodeficiency viremia (FIV) or FeLV, causes transient or progressive anemia after several weeks of therapy; this anemia is thought to be the result of bone marrow suppression and/or Heinz body–induced hemolysis.[41] The immunosuppressive agent cyclophosphamide is known to cause bone marrow suppression in dogs. Azathioprine, a thioguanine-derivative immunosuppressive agent, has been associated with induced anemia and hypocellular bone marrow in dogs, with recovery after drug withdrawal. Possible incorporation of the drug into bone marrow progenitor cells is thought to cause bone marrow failure.[38] Other drugs, including meclofenamic acid, phenylbutazone, quinidine, trimethoprim-sulfadiazine, and fenbendazole, have been incriminated in bone marrow aplasia in dogs. Chloramphenicol appears to cause mild, reversible, nonregenerative anemia in dogs.[38,40]

Infectious agents other than retroviruses can cause aplastic pancytopenia (see Anemia Associated with Infectious Etiologies, below). Among these are parvovirus, *Ehrlichia* sp. and bacterial endotoxins. Aflatoxin B toxicity has been reported to cause aplastic pancytopenia in the dog (among many other species). Idiopathic aplasia has also been reported in many species, including dogs and cats. Cell-mediated cyto-toxicity, marrow stromal defects, overproduction of inhibitory hemopoietic cytokines, deficiency in stem cell factor, and genetic mutation all have been proposed as causes of the human form of this process.

Myelophthistic Disease

The term *myelophthisis* denotes a situation in which bone marrow has been replaced by nonmarrow elements. Common invaders of the bone marrow are leukemic or other tumor cells, infectious granulomas, fibrous tissue, and lipid storage cells. Although conceptually it is thought that the anemia resulting from this process is due to simple mechanical replacement of the bone marrow, the pathophysiology probably is more complex. For example, the anemia may result from competi-tion between hemopoietic cells and invading cells for essential nutrients. Some evidence suggests that metastatic tumor lesions may secrete substances (i.e., cytokines) that block or inhibit hemopoietic cytokines, affecting the surrounding cells. In this regard, it is interesting to note that some of the same peripheral blood alterations observed in animals with metastatic bone marrow disease are observed in animals with metastatic neoplasia without bone marrow involvement.

Typical clinical features of myelophthisis include (1) nor-mocytic, normochromic anemia with reticulocytopenia; (2) leukoerythroblastic reaction, in which the white cell count is increased and many immature white cells are present, as are many nucleated red cells; (3) marked anisocytosis and poik-ilocytosis of red cells, including dacrocytes or teardrop-shaped red cells; and (4) a low-normal or increased platelet count with the presence of immature and sometimes bizarre megathrom-bocytes. The ultimate diagnosis depends on demonstration of inappropriate invading cells in a bone marrow core biopsy.[39]

Myelofibrosis

Myelofibrosis may accompany or precede neoplastic diseases or may occur subsequent to chronically stimulated erythro-poiesis in pets with severe hemolytic anemia (e.g., congenital red cell pyruvate kinase deficiency). Aspiration of marrow in these instances is difficult or impossible, and the diagnosis is based on bone marrow biopsy evaluation.[39,42-45] Idiopathic myelofibrosis (IM) (i.e., agnogenic myeloid metaplasia with myelofibrosis) is a clonal hemopoietic stem cell disorder that predominantly affects the megakaryocyte lineage in the bone marrow. It is characterized by splenomegaly, extramedullary hemopoiesis, and bone marrow fibrosis. The fibrosis is caused by deposition of abnormal collagen by polyclonal fibroblasts, which in turn are stimulated by growth factors (e.g., trans-forming growth factor beta) secreted by adjacent megakary-ocytes. IM often is difficult to recognize as a distinct clinical entity, because many conditions can cause marrow fibrosis, and myeloproliferative disorders can terminate in a fibrotic phase. The term *myeloid metaplasia* often refers to an earlier phase of IM in which fibrosis is less prominent and extramedullary hemopoiesis in the spleen and liver is evident.[46] Various histiocytic neoplastic processes must also be consid-ered. Many of these processes may be best distinguished by immunophenotyping.

Most patients with IM have significant anemia, and some have thrombocytosis. Signs associated with anemia are most common. The extramedullary hemopoiesis in the liver and spleen often causes notable organomegaly. Peripheral blood left shifts in the erythroid, myeloid, and megakaryocytic (megathrombocyte) lines (i.e., leukoerythroblastosis) are typical features of the complete hemogram. Bone marrow aspiration often is difficult, and biopsy demonstrates extensive fibrosis and osteosclerosis.[45,46] No effective therapy exists for this process except bone marrow transplantation.[46]

Myelodysplasia

Myelodysplasia (myelodysplastic syndromes [MDSs]) is a heterogeneous group of hemopoietic stem cell disorders characterized by cytologic dysplasia in the blood and bone marrow and by various combinations of anemia, neutropenia, and thrombocytopenia. MDS may be associated with refrac-tory anemia (RA) or with refractory anemia with an excess number of blast cells (RAEB) either in the peripheral blood or, primarily, in the bone marrow. A variety of terms besides myelodysplasia, including *preleukemia*, *smoldering* or *subacute leukemia*, *dysmyelopoietic syndrome*, and *dyserythropoiesis* have been used to describe MDS. These disorders are best consid-ered a form of chronic or smoldering leukemia; they have a monoclonal population of hemopoietic cells, usually involving multiple lineages, and generally are accompanied by suppres-sion of appropriate bone marrow hemopoiesis. Unfortunately, diagnostic capabilities and nomenclature are not yet adequate to discriminate consistently among clinically distinct subsets. Increased use of cytogenetic analysis and the development of clonality techniques may be useful for diagnosis and for providing insight into disease pathogenesis, patterns of respon-siveness to growth factors, and the possibility of differentiation-inducing agents.[47]

In dogs, the conditions may be primary, resulting from genetic transformation in a multipotential stem cell, or secondary and associated with administration of a drug. The primary conditions are unlikely to respond satisfactorily to hemopoietic cytokines acting as maturation factors.[2,48]

Hemopoietic Neoplasia

Neoplasia of hemopoietic tissue is characterized by replace-ment of normal tissue with an abnormal clonal proliferation of cells. Often, but not always, a concomitant increase in neoplastic cells in peripheral blood is seen. The neoplastic cells also commonly infiltrate other hemopoietic and lymphoid tissues, such as the liver, spleen, and lymph nodes.[2] Recent advances in the application of newer techniques have improved the accuracy of classification. These advances include immunophenotyping for clusters of differentiation (CD) antigens and cytogenetics. Immunophenotyping uses specific monoclonal antibodies to differentiate antigens. Flow cytometry has provided a powerful tool for analysis of immunophenotyped cells and is becoming an essential component in the study of leukemias. It complements morphologic studies and cytochemical staining.[48] A fundamental feature of leukemic cells is their monoclonality, which implies derivation from a single stem cell that has become neoplastic. Clonal marker systems are used to investigate not only the presence of clonality, but also the stage of hemopoietic cell development at which the neoplastic cells originate.[2,49-52]

It is important to understand the multistep progression from normal cells to neoplastic cells.[52] Now that the molecular mechanisms that regulate normal cell growth are becoming clear, it has also become clear that failure of one or more of these fundamental steps leads to malignant transformation. Cell proliferation and differentiation are regulated by proteins encoded by proto-oncogenes (growth promoting) and tumor suppressor genes (growth suppressing). It is now recognized that oncogenesis involves specific molecular events that result in genetic alterations in these two gene classes, with subsequent dysregulation of cell growth. A number of mechanisms can cause genetic abnormalities. Although the exact origin of these abnormalities is unknown, several environmental inciting factors have been recognized, including irradiation, chemical agents, and retroviral infection.[52]

In dogs and cats, acute and chronic myeloproliferative disorders (MPDs) are less frequently reported than lymphoproliferative disorders (LPDs). No breed or sex predilection has been identified for animals with nonlymphoid leukemia. The origin of MPDs in dogs is unknown, although environmental, viral, and genetic causes have been postulated. In contrast, MPDs in cats have been associated with FeLV and FIV infection.[53]

The diagnostic approach should be systematic and should be completed before initiation of any chemotherapy. The history may provide clues to help differentiate between acute and chronic hemopoietic neoplasia. General clinical signs of hemopoietic neoplasia include nonspecific bone pain, fever, lethargy, inappetence, vomiting, and diarrhea. The physical examination often reveals organomegaly involving the liver, spleen, or lymph nodes, and lung and central nervous system involvement can occur. Specific signs of hemopoietic neoplasia are often associated with involvement of particular cells, such as hypoxia with red cell involvement, sepsis with neutrophil involvement, and petechial, purpuric, and ecchymotic bleeding with platelet involvement.[54]

Chemotherapy in veterinary medicine can offer prolongation of life and improvement in the quality of life, but it is often palliative and rarely curative. Many myelosuppressive agents may cause profound cytopenias, with neutropenia and thrombocytopenia being common. Supportive care includes nursing care for comfort, administration of fluids and electrolytes to maintain adequate hydration and electrolyte balance, broad-spectrum antimicrobial therapy, and administration of blood products to meet specific needs. Nutritional care is essential and should be definitively addressed.[53,54]

Anemia Associated with Infectious Etiologies

Infectious agents, their products, or the response to the agent may cause anemia by damaging red cells and causing hemolysis; by causing developmental erythroid hypoplasia through direct damage to the erythroid precursors or the marrow microenvironment; or by damaging hemopoietic or supportive bone marrow stromal cells. Most bacterial or viral infections are indirect causes of mild anemia; AID is often the anemic etiology.[55]

FeLV may cause anemia by direct or indirect methods. By predisposing cats to other opportunistic diseases, FeLV infection may induce AID. Pure red cell aplasia or aplastic pancytopenia can be produced with experimental FeLV infection. The anemia of FeLV can be hemolytic through infectious organisms such as *Mycoplasma hemofelis*, other forms of immune-mediated hemolytic anemia, MPDs, or myelofibrosis. In FeLV-positive cats that have macrocytic, normochromic anemia, megaloblastoid rubricytes are seen, perhaps as a result of myelodysplasia related to folate or vitamin B_{12} deficiency.[55,56] FeLV frequently produces severe selective suppression of erythropoiesis (nonregenerative anemia) and thrombocytopoiesis but may cause aplastic pancytopenia.[57-59]

Cats infected with FIV may develop chronic debilitating disorders ranging from opportunistic infections to neoplasia. Approximately 18% to 36% of FIV-positive cats have anemia and may also have neutropenia, lymphopenia or lymphocytosis, monocytosis, and thrombocytopenia. The exact pathogenesis of the FIV anemia is not known. In contrast to FeLV, FIV infects megakaryocytes and bone marrow accessory cells but not erythroid and myeloid precursors.[57]

Infectious etiologies for aplastic pancytopenia, other than FeLV and FIV, have been associated with parvoviral infection, ehrlichiosis, babesiosis, *M. hemofelis* infection, and endotoxemia. Parvoviral infection in both dogs and cats causes acute aplastic pancytopenia as a result of viral proliferation in progenitor and proliferative cells in the bone marrow, although marrow injury secondary to endotoxemia or septicemia cannot be ruled out. The bone marrow is characterized by severe degenerative changes in the developing hemopoietic cells, necrosis, and an increased number of phagocytic macrophages. Hematologic recovery usually is rapid if the pet survives the acute stages of the disease.[60] Ehrlichiosis (caused by *Ehrlichia canis*, *Ehrlichia ewingii*, or *Ehrlichia equi*) may cause a hypercellular bone marrow initially, but in the chronic phase, the bone marrow is characterized by pancytopenia and hypoplasia, except with plasmacytosis. Occasionally *Babesia* spp. can cause nonregenerative anemia. *M. hemofelis* infection is also sometimes associated with nonregenerative anemia, which attests to the possibility that some of these cats may be immunosuppressed or debilitated.[60]

Cytopenias occur in the blood of dogs and cats with acute and chronic ehrlichiosis. In the acute form, the bone marrow is hypercellular, which suggests that the peripheral cytopenias are the result of cell destruction. In the chronic form, the marrow is acellular and is consistent with a diagnosis of aplastic pancytopenia.[61]

Diagnosis of aplasia includes a complete history, with questions pertaining to drug exposure, chemicals, and infectious agents; a complete hemogram with blood smear evaluation, bone marrow aspiration, and consideration of bone marrow core biopsy. The core biopsy may be most helpful for assessing cellularity and architecture. Particular attention should be paid to potential drug or chemical exposure 2 to 3 weeks prior to examination. Anemia is initially mild but becomes progressive over time. Leukopenia (neutropenia) and thrombocytopenia may accompany the anemia, with clinical signs of fever and sepsis (neutropenia) and hemorrhage in the form of petechiae, purpura, and ecchymoses (thrombocytopenia). Some residual production may be seen with the neutropenia and thrombocytopenia, and this appears to be sufficient to permit development of anemia over weeks or months.[3,60]

Treatment with prophylactic antimicrobial drugs is the only therapy that addresses the severe neutropenia with sepsis, which is most often evident when the neutrophil cell count is below 500/mL. It is difficult to address thrombocytopenia

HEMATOLOGY AND IMMUNOLOGY

clinically without sufficient units of platelet-rich plasma. Developing anemia is treated with packed red cells, preferably, or with whole blood if packed red cells are not available. Immunosuppressive therapy and anabolic steroids are probably not indicated or useful. The use of recombinant hemopoietic growth factor and bone marrow transplantation should be considered.[62]

INEFFECTIVE ERYTHROPOIESIS

Macrocytosis and Macrocytic, Normochromic Anemia

An MCV above the reference interval is considered macrocytosis. Macrocytosis can be present without anemia. Examination of peripheral blood reveals prominent macrocytes and poikilocytes. Hypersegmented neutrophils with more than five lobes are often observed, and modest decreases in both the leukocyte and platelet counts may be seen. Sometimes the morphologic changes in peripheral blood are sufficiently characteristic to make marrow examination unnecessary in the initial diagnostic workup.

With the erythroid-regenerative response in the dog and cat (i.e., sufficient reticulocytosis), the size and number of reticulocytes are usually proportional to the degree of erythropoietic stimulation. Macroreticulocytes are produced under conditions of intense erythropoietic stimulation and become macrocytic red cells as the cells mature.

Greyhounds have higher reference values for the hematocrit, hemoglobin concentration, red cell concentration, and MCV. Greyhound red cells have a shorter life span (53.6 ± 6.5 days) compared with other dog breeds (104.3 ± 2.2 days), which could account for the macrocytosis.[63,64] Macrocytosis is a familial condition in some poodles, especially the small and toy breeds. The MCV is markedly increased over reference values, and there is notable nuclear-cytoplasmic asynchrony. Megaloblastic changes and nuclear fragmentation are noted among red cell precursors, and some of the nuclear fragments are retained in the adult cells. Hypersegmentation is seen in adult neutrophils. Although these morphologic changes are also described in vitamin B_{12} deficiency, the exact nature of the defect is unknown, but it is not related to nutritional deficiency. These dogs are not anemic or, if so, the anemia is almost undetectable.[65]

Vitamin B_{12} and Folic Acid Deficiencies

Vitamin B_{12} deficiency is associated with macrocytic anemia in humans, but there does not appear to be a counterpart in nonhuman primates, dogs, or cats. The megaloblastic changes noted in feline erythroid cells have also been described in feline folic acid–depleted bone marrow, but the morphologic changes are not dramatic. Dogs and cats treated with phenobarbital or primidone occasionally develop megaloblastic changes in the bone marrow, but the changes are not accompanied by peripheral blood macrocytosis.[63] Vitamin B_{12} and folic acid deficiencies are most often related to gastric malabsorption. Gastric mucosa produces an "intrinsic factor" necessary for absorption of vitamin B_{12} in the terminal ileum. Lack of intrinsic factor in small animals may be associated with partial or total gastrectomy. Bacterial colonization of the small intestine by vitamin B_{12}–consuming micro-organisms may, theoretically, lead to vitamin B_{12} deficiency. Drugs such as colchicine and neomycin may also lead to minor malabsorption syndromes.[63]

Folic acid deficiency has been associated with gluten-sensitive enteropathy due to malabsorption and with increased requirements during pregnancy. It also is seen in neonates and in myelofibrosis and chronic inflammatory diseases. These do not appear to be clinically significant findings in small animals.[63]

Clinical assessment requires a simple dietary history and inquiries about gastrointestinal disease or surgery, any prior hematologic disease, and the animal's drug history. Laboratory assessment involves determination of the serum vitamin B_{12} and folic acid concentrations. Radioimmunoassay (RIA) yields the fewest false-positive or false-negative effects. An increased concentration of vitamin B_{12} with RIA may be seen with marked leukocytosis and active but nonspecific hepatic disease. Examination of the gastrointestinal tract by ultrasonography and with endoscopic biopsy is recommended.[63,64]

Anemia Associated with Feline Leukemia Virus Infection

Most cats that have anemia and FeLV infection have macrocytosis and resultant anisocytosis. Some FeLV-positive cats have an appropriate MCV but increased anisocytosis, perhaps reflecting a minor subpopulation of macrocytic red cells. The macrocytosis does not correlate with reticulocytosis or other evidence of red cell regenerative response. Macrocytosis is most prominent in cats that have anemia, including both regenerative and nonregenerative anemia. However, more than 50% of nonanemic cats infected with FeLV have some macrocytosis. It has been suggested that macrocytosis could reflect a period of intense erythropoiesis before conversion to hypoproliferative anemia, but the cause is as yet unknown. In a study of cats with experimental FeLV–induced anemia, the macrocytic changes were not as significant as noted in the naturally occurring disease, and no period of reticulocytosis was detected over the course of the disease.[63] Macrocytosis has been reported in erythroid aplasia in cats and in myelodysplasia in dogs. No response to vitamin B_{12} therapy was detected.[63-67]

Normochromic, Normocytic Anemia

Normochromic, normocytic anemia is defined as a low red cell count, hematocrit, or hemoglobin concentration with appropriate MCV, MCHC, and MCH values. Almost all nonregenerative anemia is presented as normocytic and normochromic. AID has already been discussed and is associated with underlying inflammation, infection, immune-mediated processes, or neoplasia. Most often these animals have clinical signs associated with the underlying process rather than the mild anemia. General signs include weight loss, icterus, and lymphadenopathy. Abdominal signs include diarrhea or constipation, nausea and vomiting, or pain. Other signs are often associated with specific organ systems, such as cardiac murmurs or dyspnea, cough, polyuria, dysuria, bone or joint pain, or the drug history. Management requires correction of the underlying cause and the use of specific blood products as needed. Treatment with iron is contraindicated.

Hypochromic, Microcytic Anemia

A low red cell count, low hemoglobin concentration, and low hematocrit with low MCV, MCHC, and MCH values are associated with hypochromic and microcytic red cells on examination of the peripheral blood smear. It is important to know that some canine breeds are normally microcytic (Akita and Shiba). When hemoglobin concentrations reach a certain level in developing erythroid cells, cell division appears to stop. Because chronic iron deficiency is the most common cause of hypochromia and microcytosis, and as cell division is unimpeded, extra red cell division occurs until the intraerythroid hemoglobin concentration is at a level to signal cessation of division. Potential causes of this type of anemia include AID, portosystemic shunts in dogs and cats, pyridoxine deficiency, copper deficiency, hereditary elliptocytosis in dogs, dyserythropoiesis, and drug or chemical toxicities. Iron deficiency has already been discussed (see above).[68,69]

Congenital portosystemic shunts are most often caused by a single blood vessel that fails to regress in utero and that diverts portal blood around the liver. Acquired shunts are often multiple and are associated with chronic hepatobiliary disease.[69,70] The cause of the microcytosis is not fully understood, but the condition is associated with abnormal iron metabolism, at least in dogs. Clinically the most common signs are encephalopathy in patients who are thin and have poor haircoats. Young dogs with congenital shunts are often small for their age. The liver is difficult to palpate as a result of microhepatica. Approximately two thirds of dogs with shunts have mild microcytosis with MCV and red cell masses at the low end or slightly below the reference interval. The MCHC is also slightly low, and the red cell distribution width (RDW) is slightly increased in most cases. About one third of cats with shunts have decreased MCV.[69-72] Target cells (codocytes), keratocytes, and elliptocytes are the poikilocytes most frequently seen. The abnormalities in the clinical biochemistry profiles of dogs include decreases in urea nitrogen, creatinine, glucose, albumin, total protein, and cholesterol. Increases are observed in serum alkaline phosphatase, bile acids, serum alanine aminotransferase (ALT), and bilirubin.[71,72] Fasting ammonia concentrations are elevated. The urinalysis may reveal ammonium urate crystals. Similar abnormalities are seen in cats with shunts, but hypocholesterolemia and hyperbilirubinemia are not reported. Storage iron, measured indirectly by species-specific serum ferritin assay, is appropriate or increased. The serum iron and transferrin concentrations are modestly decreased, because the physiology is similar to that of AID (see Table 271-2).[69]

Other potential causes of microcytic anemia include pyridoxine (vitamin B_6) and copper deficiency, drug and chemical toxicity, dyserythropoiesis, and hereditary elliptocytosis. Pyridoxine deficiency has been produced only experimentally in dogs and cats. These animals have microcytosis, increased serum iron, and siderotic (iron) inclusions in adult red cells. Prolonged copper deficiency in dogs and cats may cause microcytosis due to functional iron deficiency, in turn caused by inability to access storage iron as the copper transport enzyme ceruloplasmin is decreased. This protein has ferroxidase activity that is important for changing ferrous storage iron (Fe^{2+}) to ferric iron (Fe^{3+}), a change necessary for iron binding to transferrin (the iron transporting protein). Chloramphenicol is one of numerous drugs or chemicals that block heme synthesis, resulting in microcytosis and red cell siderotic inclusions.[69] Dyserythropoiesis in English springer spaniels causes nonregenerative microcytic anemia with increased circulating nucleated red cells. These dogs also have cardiac disease and polymyopathy.[73,74] Hereditary elliptocytosis has been described in a mixed-breed dog that had a red cell membrane deficiency (lack of membrane band 4.1).[75]

SUMMATION OF NONREGENERATIVE ANEMIA

Anemia is a common clinical presentation of an underlying disease. Nonregenerative anemias are the most common anemias observed by veterinary clinicians (Box 271-4). Lack of iron, anemia of inflammation, bone marrow disorders, anemias related to erythropoietin, maturation abnormalities,

---

Box • 271-4

Approach to Diagnosis of Nonregenerative Anemia

Nonregenerative anemia without other cytopenias
Examine bone marrow
  Severe erythroid hypoplasia—consider pure red cell aplasia
  Normal or mild erythroid hypoplasia—consider:
    Inflammatory disease
    Renal disease
    Neoplasia
    Hepatic disease
    Hypothyroidism
    Hypoadrenocorticism
  Hypercellular marrow
    Less than 30% blast forms—consider myelodysplastic syndrome
    Greater than 30% blast forms—consider hemopoietic neoplasia
Nonregenerative anemia with leukopenia and/or thrombocytopenia
Examine bone marrow
  Panhypoplasia—aplastic pancytopenia (aplastic anemia)
  Pathology determined by core biopsy
    Myelonecrosis
    Myelofibrosis
  Hypercellular bone marrow
    Less than 30% blast forms—consider myelodysplastic syndrome
    Greater than 30% blast forms—consider hematopoietic neoplasia

Modified from Weiss DJ: Aplastic anemia. *In* Feldman BF, Zinkl JG, Jain NC (eds): Schalm's Veterinary Hematology, 5th ed. Baltimore, Lippincott Williams & Wilkins, 2000, p 212.

---

and the early stages of hemolysis and hemorrhage—the main anemia causation groups—present as nonregenerative anemias; that is, a relative or absolute reticulocytopenia. Examination of a minimum database (i.e., complete hemogram, urinalysis, and biochemical profile) often reveals sufficient information to diagnose the underlying disorder. Examination of the complete hemogram includes comments on platelet, red cell, and white cell morphology. Specific factors to be considered include the total protein concentration, the red cell indices, and the adjusted reticulocyte count. Once an etiology has been suggested, ancillary specific tests often bring understanding to these interesting but elusive disorders.

CHAPTER 272

Platelet Disorders and von Willebrand Disease

Marjory B. Brooks
James L. Catalfamo

PRIMARY HEMOSTASIS

Platelets play a critical role in the initiation, regulation, and localization of hemostasis. The term *primary hemostasis* refers to the interactions among platelets, von Willebrand factor (vWF), and the vessel wall that culminate in the formation of a platelet plug (Figure 272-1). These reactions begin with platelet contact with the damaged vessel and vWF-mediated adhesion; proceed through platelet activation, degranulation, and aggregation; and conclude with the development of platelet-dependent procoagulant activity and clot retraction.

Platelet Physiology

Megakaryocytic precursor cells in the bone marrow are programmed, through the action of transcription factors and thrombopoietin, to form platelet-specific organelles and to express platelet cell surface proteins. In the final stages of megakaryocyte maturation, a network of demarcation membranes generates long processes that fragment into large numbers of anucleate platelets. Platelets are released from the marrow and circulate in the vascular compartment as quiescent, nonadhesive, smooth disks. Approximately 100 billion platelets are released each day to maintain a peripheral platelet count of 200 million to 500 million cells per milliliter of blood.

Injury to the vessel wall triggers platelet activation within nanoseconds. In the initial step of activation, platelets rapidly transform into adhesive, spiny spheres capable of recognizing and binding to exposed matrix components of the subendothelium. Surface binding initiates cell signaling pathways,

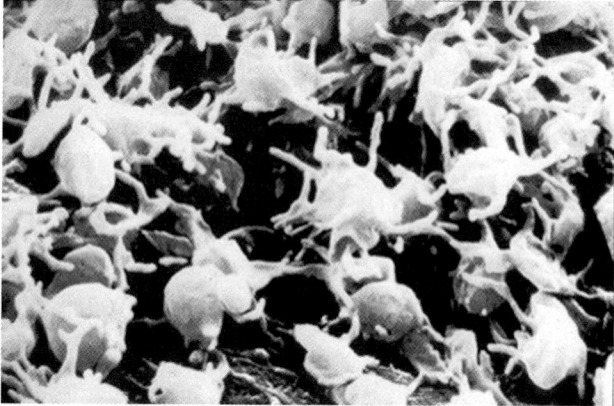

Figure 272-1 Scanning electron micrograph of platelet thrombus. Activated platelets have undergone shape change, are adherent to the underlying matrix, and have formed intraplatelet bonds in the process of aggregation. (Courtesy Bristol-Myers Squibb, New York, NY.)

which then mediate granule secretion. Granule contents include adenine nucleotides, calcium, serotonin, and adhesive proteins, such as fibrinogen, vWF, fibronectin, and P-selectin. Secreted compounds accumulate locally, interact with their respective surface receptors, and recruit additional platelets to the site of injury. Large-order platelet aggregates then accumulate and bridge the zone of vascular damage to form a hemostatic plug. Thrombin cleavage of fibrinogen strengthens the platelet plug as a fibrin-platelet meshwork develops.[1]

Late-stage platelet activation includes exposure of platelet membrane phosphatidylserine (PS) and the release of PS-rich microparticles, which act as scaffolding for the assembly of coagulation factor complexes. The expression of platelet procoagulant activity greatly amplifies local thrombin and fibrin generation. Contraction of platelet cytoskeletal proteins linked to platelet integrin receptors for fibrin and fibrinogen results in consolidation and subsequent retraction of the growing clot.

Platelet activation requires simultaneous engagement of the platelet membrane surface receptors (Figure 272-2). Species differences in response to platelet stimuli may reflect differences in receptor subclasses for specific ligands. The endoperoxides prostacyclin (prostaglandin I_2 [PGI_2]), prostaglandin E_2 (PGE_2), and prostaglandin D_2 (PGD_2), which are synthesized by endothelial cells and released into the vascular space, serve as antagonist ligands that react with their respective platelet receptors to dampen platelet reactivity.[2]

Platelet integrins and nonintegrin glycoprotein receptors play a critical role in adhesion (platelet–subendothelial matrix interactions) and aggregation (platelet-platelet association). The $\alpha IIb\beta 3$ complex ($GPII_b III_a$) is the most abundant platelet integrin and functions as the activation-dependent receptor for fibrinogen, fibronectin, and vWF. Binding of fibrinogen to this receptor is essential for aggregation and clot retraction. Platelet adhesion to collagen and collagen-induced signaling are supported by collagen's interaction with the integrin receptor $\alpha 2\beta 1$ ($GPI_a II_a$).

Surface receptors, coupled to G proteins, span the platelet membrane and transmit signals induced by agonist binding. In platelets, Gq serves as this link for most agonists. Gq is coupled to phospholipase C, which in turn generates diacylglycerol (DAG) and inositol triphosphate, leading to calcium release from the endoplasmic reticulum; protein kinase C and myosin light chain kinase activation; and phosphorylation of platelet signaling proteins. During activation, phospholipase A_2 releases arachidonic acid from membrane phospholipids. Cyclo-oxygenase and thromboxane synthetase convert arachidonic acid to the potent agonist thromboxane A_2 (see Figure 272-2).

Platelet–von Willebrand Factor Interaction

Subendothelial collagen fibrils and bound vWF are exposed when the vascular endothelium is injured. The affinity and strength of the vWF-collagen bond is proportional to vWF

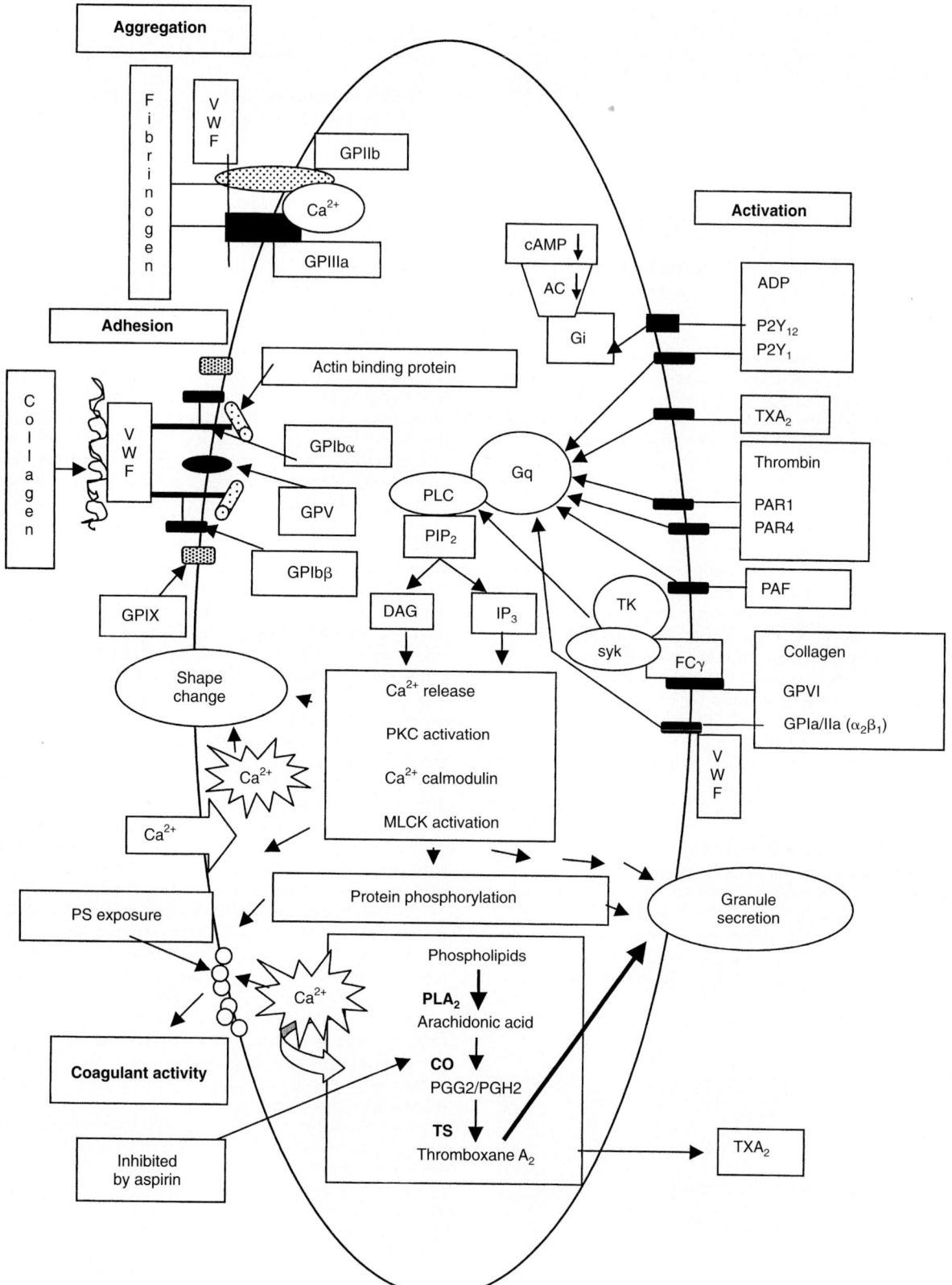

Figure 272-2 Major signaling mechanisms involved in platelet activation. *cAMP*, Cyclic adenosine monophosphate; *AC*, adenylate cyclase; *PLC*, phospholipase C; *PIP₂*, phosphatidylinositol bisphosphate; *DAG*, diacylglycerol; *IP₃*, inositol triphosphate; *PKC*, protein kinase C; *MLCK*, myosin light chain kinase; *PLA₂*, phospholipase A₂; *CO*, cyclo-oxygenase; *TS*, thromboxane synthase; *TXA₂*, thromboxane A₂; *PAF*, platelet-activating factor; *PAR 1, PAR 4*, protease-activated thrombin receptor 1 or 4; *GP*, glycoprotein; *TK*, tyrosine kinase; *vWF*, von Willebrand factor; *P2Y₁* or *P2Y₁₂*, purinergic nucleotide receptors; *FCγ*, immunoglobulin-like receptor; *Gq* and *Gi*, GTP-binding proteins; *syk*, syk kinase.

HEMATOLOGY AND IMMUNOLOGY

multimer size. Collagen-bound vWF displays a conformational change that allows it to interact with the platelet GPIb/V/IX complex. As platelet GPIb contacts and engages with vWF, platelets slowly roll and become activated by interaction with collagen fibrils. vWF then binds to $GPII_b/III_a$ receptors exposed on the surface of activated platelets. Adhesion and aggregation at high shear rates depend on this vWF binding to activate platelet $GPII_b/III_a$.

DIAGNOSIS OF PLATELET DISORDERS

Clinical Signs of Primary Hemostatic Defects

Primary hemostatic defects typically cause signs of petechiae (pinpoint hemorrhage), ecchymoses (bruising), and mucosal hemorrhage, such as epistaxis, hematuria, gingival and intestinal hemorrhage, and prolonged bleeding after injury. These signs are suggestive of capillary and small vessel hemorrhage, but none are pathognomonic for a specific disease. For example, ecchymoses (Figure 272-3) are often seen in association with thrombocytopenia but also may be signs of inflammatory vasculitis.

Screening Tests

The initial assessment of any patient with signs of bleeding should aim to distinguish between hemorrhage from injured or diseased blood vessels and hemostatic failure. If the source or cause of hemorrhage cannot be readily identified, platelet count and coagulation screening tests should be performed early in the diagnostic workup. These tests can help both to detect a hemostatic defect and to guide the selection of appropriate ancillary diagnostic tests (Figure 272-4).

The platelet count (per µL) can be estimated by counting the number of platelets in 10 oil immersion fields and multiplying the average number per field by 15,000 to 20,000 (Figure 272-5).[3] Either the activated clotting time (ACT) or point-of-care coagulation assays can be performed in-house to rule out clinically severe coagulation factor deficiencies.

Testing for Quantitative Platelet Defects

Quantitative platelet defects are common hematologic abnormalities.[4-6] Normal platelet numbers for dogs and cats range from approximately 200,000/µL to 500,000/µL. Each testing laboratory should provide species-specific reference ranges for their method (Table 272-1). High or low platelet counts are found in many patients having systemic inflammatory and

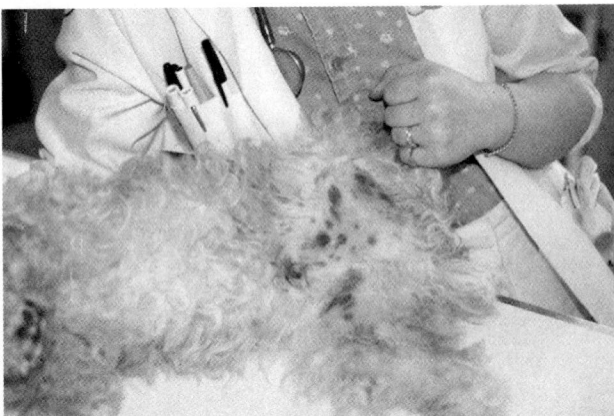

Figure 272-3 Petechiae and ecchymoses in the inguinal region of a mixed-breed dog with thrombocytopenia (platelet count, 5000/µL).

neoplastic diseases. Specific diagnostic tests (Table 272-2) are indicated for patients with moderate to severe thrombocytopenia or thrombocytosis, with associated clinical signs.

Thrombocytopenia Platelets are highly reactive; spurious low platelet counts are common laboratory artifacts and should be confirmed by examination of a blood smear to rule out platelet clumping.[7] Collection artifacts are minimized by the use of citrate anticoagulant, atraumatic venipuncture with collection directly into anticoagulant, assay within hours of blood draw, and avoidance of cold temperature. Thrombocytopenia rarely causes signs of abnormal hemostasis unless the platelet count falls below 50,000/µL, with petechiation and spontaneous hemorrhage most likely at counts below 20,000/µL. Clinical signs may appear at higher platelet counts, however, if the patient has a concurrent disease that further impairs hemostasis.

Three general mechanisms cause thrombocytopenia: impaired platelet production, increased peripheral consumption or sequestration, and immune-mediated destruction. In many disease syndromes, more than one mechanism is involved.[8]

Production defects are likely in patients with thrombocytopenia combined with leukopenia and/or anemia.[9] Immature platelets have a relatively high mean platelet volume (MPV) and ribonucleic acid (RNA) content, detected as "reticulated" platelets by thiazole orange staining. The presence of reticulated platelets indicates ongoing platelet production, but their absence does not confirm megakaryocyte hypoplasia. Bone marrow examination, therefore, is the most accurate and direct means of evaluating megakaryopoiesis. Normal to high megakaryocyte numbers are typical of peripheral platelet consumption or destruction. Megakaryocyte hypoplasia confirms a platelet production defect and may reveal an infectious agent or abnormal cellular or stromal proliferation. In most cases, the combination of bone marrow examination, drug and travel history, and serology or polymerase chain reaction (PCR) testing to detect infectious agents leads to definitive diagnosis of production defects.

Splenic enlargement, for any reason, causes increased platelet sequestration and may result in thrombocytopenia with a shortened platelet life span.[10] Increased peripheral platelet consumption accompanies systemic vasculitic disorders and disseminated intravascular coagulation (DIC). The primary means of diagnosing sequestration disorders include splenic and lymph node aspiration cytology, serology and biopsy to detect infectious agents and inflammatory disorders, and coagulation tests to define a DIC process.

Immune-mediated platelet destruction is common. *Primary immune-mediated thrombocytopenia* (IMT) implies an autoimmune disorder with production of antibodies directed against normal platelet antigens.[11] *Secondary IMT* occurs in association with infection, drug therapy, neoplasia, or polyimmune syndromes or as a complication of platelet transfusion.[12] In these patients, platelet-bound antibody may represent immune complexes, antibodies directed against neoantigens or foreign platelet antigens, or nonspecific binding.[13] The presence of antibodies on the surface of platelets (platelet-bound antibody) or antibodies in patient sera capable of binding normal platelets (platelet-bindable antibodies) can be detected with flow cytometry or enzyme-linked immunosorbent assay (ELISA). Flow cytometric assays configured to detect platelet-bound canine IgG have been developed for clinical use.[14,15] The tests are generally sensitive, but they are nonspecific. Detection of platelet-bound IgG does not differentiate patients with primary IMT from those with secondary IMT, and nonspecific antibody binding may complicate interpretation of test results. Microthrombocytosis (MPV less than 5.5 fL) has been described as a feature of primary and secondary IMT and is seen early in the disease course.

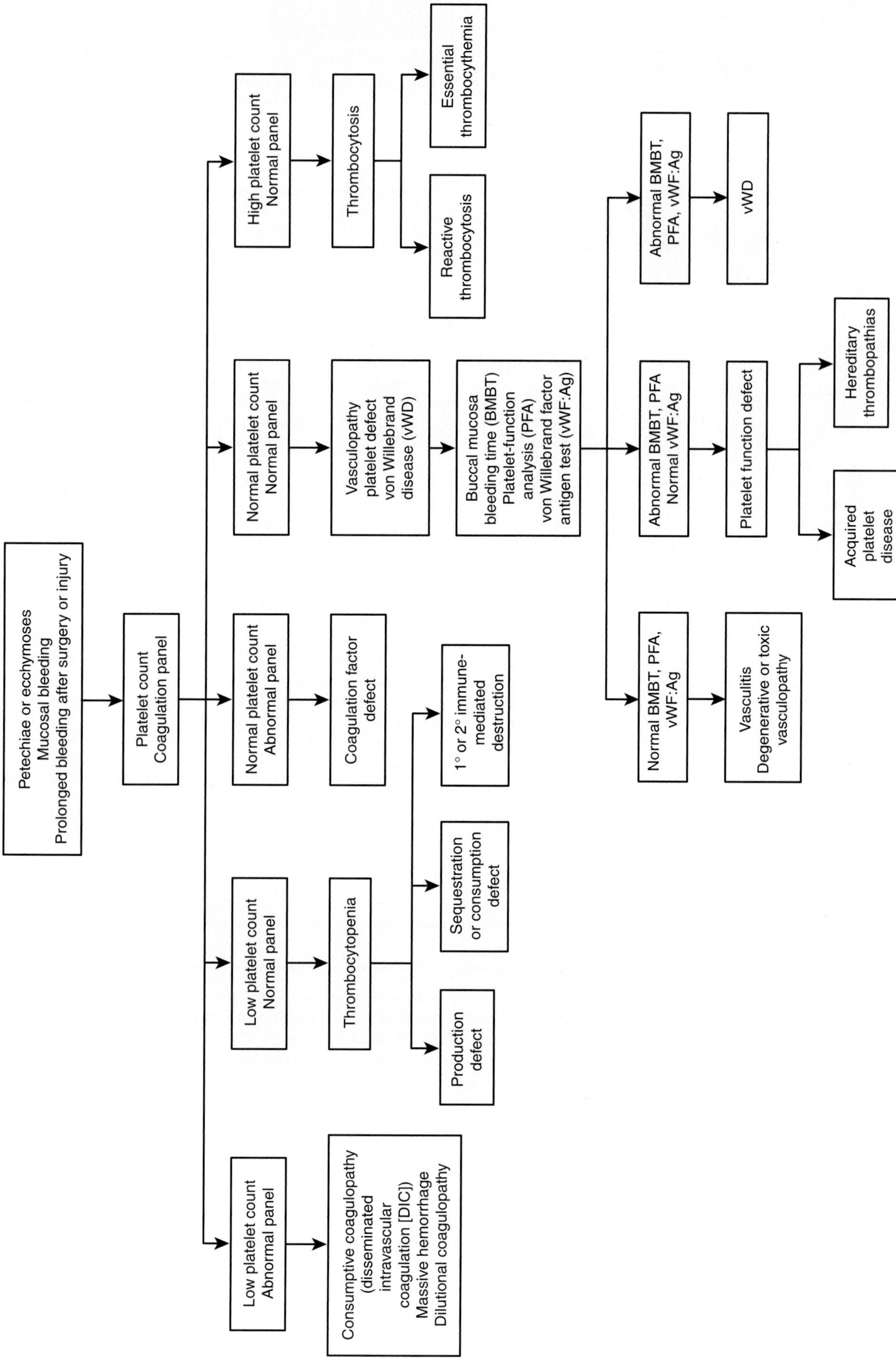

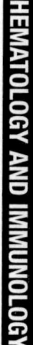

Figure 272-4 Diagnostic algorithm for primary hemostatic defects. *BMBT*, Buccal mucosa bleeding time; *PFA*, platelet function analyzer; *vWF:Ag*, von Willebrand factor antigen.

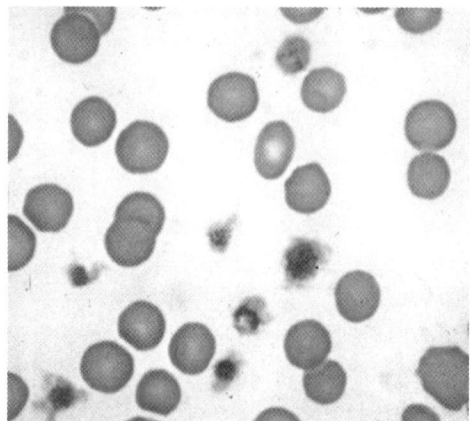

Figure 272-5 Wright-stained blood smear from a healthy cat demonstrating normal feline platelet morphology (×400). (Courtesy Dr. Tracy Stokol, Cornell University, Ithaca, New York.)

In a case review, severe thrombocytopenia (less than 20,000/μL) and microthrombocytosis were found almost exclusively in dogs with IMT; however only half of the IMT patients had these abnormalities.[16] Accurate MPV determination is affected by the anticoagulant used; platelets stored in ethylenediamine tetra-acetic acid (EDTA) rather than citrate may have artifactual increases in MPV.

Thrombocytosis Mild to moderate increases in the platelet count "reactive" thrombocytosis, are seen in association with chronic blood loss, neoplasia, systemic inflammatory disease, and hypercortisolism.[17] High platelet counts may occur after splenectomy. A persistent and markedly high platelet count (greater than 900,000/μL) is suggestive of primary bone marrow disease (e.g., myelodysplasia, essential thrombocythemia) and is an indication for bone marrow examination. The clinical features of essential thrombocythemia in human beings and dogs include splenomegaly and hemorrhage caused by platelet dysfunction.[18]

Table • 272-1

Reference Values* for Canine and Feline Platelet Count and Mean Platelet Volume

VALUE	DOG	CAT
Platelet count (× 10³/uL)	179 to 483	201 to 523
Mean platelet volume (fL)	8.4 to 13.2	10.8 to 19.8

*Advia Hematology Analyzer (Bayer, Tarrytown, New York). Values current 2003, Clinical Pathology, Cornell University, Ithaca, New York.

Platelet Function Tests

The buccal mucosa bleeding time (BMBT) is an *in vivo* screening test of primary hemostasis (Figure 272-6). If thrombocytopenia has been ruled out, a long BMBT is compatible with either platelet dysfunction or vWF deficiency.[19] Platelet dysfunction is definitively diagnosed using more comprehensive tests of platelet structure and activation response (Table 272-3).

To ensure platelet viability, functional assays are best performed within 2 to 3 hours of sample collection. The PFA 100 (Dade Behring, Newark, DE) is a new analyzer that can be used to measure platelet adhesion and aggregation with small volumes of whole blood (less than 2 mL) under conditions that simulate blood flow.[20,21] More specific assessment of platelet function is performed by monitoring agonist-induced responses of shape change, aggregation, and release of dense granule contents (Figure 272-7).[22]

Flow cytometry is used to assess platelet function by means of detection of membrane glycoproteins (required for adhesion and aggregation) and activation markers, such as P-selectin, fibrinogen, and surface PS.[23] These markers are evidence of effective alpha granule release and procoagulant activity (Figure 272-8). Detailed evaluations of platelet function, physiology, and ultrastructure are usually reserved for characterization of hereditary thrombopathias.

Table • 272-2

Diagnostic Tests for Quantitative Platelet Defects

TESTS	SPECIFIC ASSESSMENTS
CBC	Review to detect: Infectious agents, neoplastic cells, spherocytes, schistocytes
	Assess: Platelet count and morphology, MPV, percentage of reticulated platelets
Bone marrow examination	Review to detect: Megakaryocyte number and morphology, infectious agents, lymphoproliferative or myeloproliferative neoplasia, myelofibrosis, myelodysplasia
	Special stains or labels: Immunophenotyping, histochemistry, iron stains, antimegakaryocyte antibody
Spleen/lymph node examination	Review to detect: Infectious agents, neoplastic cells
Serology	Review to detect: Infectious agents, antinuclear antibody
Polymerase chain reaction	Review to detect: Infectious agents
Platelet-bound antibody	Configured to detect: Antibody specificity (i.e., IgG, IgM, IgA) or epitope specificity (i.e., anti-GPII$_b$III$_a$ antibody)
Coagulation tests	Review: Coagulation panel (aPTT, PT, TCT), fibrinogen, antithrombin activity, FDP or D-dimer concentration

CBC, Complete blood count: *MPV*, mean platelet volume; *aPTT*, activated partial thromboplastin time; *PT*, prothrombin time; *TCT*, thrombin clotting time; *FDP*, fibrin and fibrinogen degradation products.

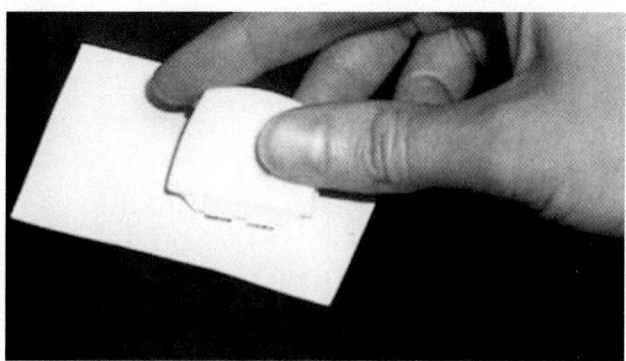

A

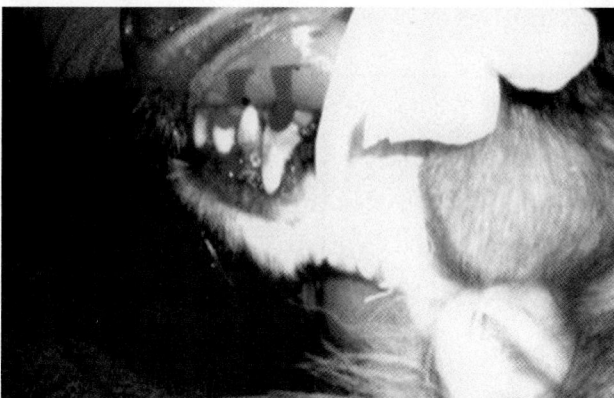

B

Figure 272-6 Buccal mucosal bleeding time. **A,** Template device (Simplate II; Organon Teknika, Durham, North Carolina) with spring-loaded blades that make incisions of uniform depth and length when the device is triggered. **B,** Incised buccal bleeding time wounds in a Shetland sheepdog affected with type 3 vWD. After incision, shed blood is collected by gently blotting below the wounds with gauze or filter paper. The time from incision to cessation of blood flow is the buccal bleeding time.

Table • 272-3

Platelet Function Assays

TESTS	SPECIFIC ASSESSMENTS
Dilute whole blood clot retraction	$GPII_bIII_a$-mediated clot retraction
Platelet aggregation studies	Aggregation response to specific agonists: adenosine diphosphate (ADP), collagen, arachidonate, epinephrine, platelet-activating factor
Platelet secretion studies	Secretion of dense granule contents: ADP, adenosine triphosphate (ATP), serotonin
Flow cytometry	Detection of constitutive membrane antigens: $GPII_bIII_a$ (CD61 = GPIIIa); GPIb (CD42b = GP1bα)
	Detection of activation markers: P-selectin (CD62p), phosphatidylserine (annexin-V), fibrinogen binding site (CAP1), platelet-bound fibrinogen (antifibrinogen antibody)
	Platelet calcium entry and release: Fluo-3
Spectrofluorimetry	Platelet calcium entry and release: Fura-2AM
Electron microscopy	Platelet ultrastructure: Shape change, cytoskeleton, intracellular organelles (granules, dense bodies, lysosomes), dense tubular system

SPECIFIC PLATELET DISORDERS

Thrombocytopenia

Thrombocytopenia is the most common acquired hemostatic defect of dogs and cats.[10] Many different pathogens cause thrombocytopenia (Table 272-4), often through combined marrow suppression and an increased rate of peripheral loss. Arthropod-borne agents are increasingly identified as the cause of cytopenias in dogs and cats.[8,24] Infectious agents usually cause systemic signs, producing physical examination findings and complete blood count (CBC) abnormalities beyond those of thrombocytopenia alone. Although dogs and cats with infectious thrombocytopenias may initially respond to steroid administration, sustained platelet response and disease resolution require specific treatment. It therefore is important to rule out infectious thrombocytopenia (through serology, cytology, or PCR) before an immunosuppressive steroid regimen is begun.

Mild to moderate thrombocytopenia is seen in association with many tumor types, with more severe depression likely in hematopoietic neoplasia such as multiple myeloma, lymphoma, and leukemia.[5] DIC is a common cause of thrombocytopenia in hemangiosarcoma, and tests to define a DIC process (see Table 272-2) should be performed in any cancer patient with a falling or low platelet count. In addition to tumor-mediated thrombocytopenia, cancer patients are at risk of developing thrombocytopenia arising from cytotoxic drug therapy.

A thorough drug history is indicated for any patient with thrombocytopenia, because numerous drugs have been reported to impair platelet production, induce secondary immune destruction, and/or cause platelet dysfunction (Table 272-5).[25] Establishing the causality of drug-induced thrombocytopenia is difficult, but ancillary diagnostics can help define possible underlying mechanisms. The findings of pancytopenia and megakaryocytic hypoplasia indicate bone marrow suppression, and the presence of platelet-bound antibody is compatible with an immune-mediated process.

Idiopathic, or primary, IMT is an autoimmune disease, usually mediated by IgG directed against platelet membrane $GPII_bIII_a$. The disease is uncommon in cats, but in case reviews of canine thrombocytopenia, primary IMT accounts for approximately 5% to 15% of patients, with over-representation of females and certain breeds (cocker spaniels, poodles, and Old English sheepdogs).[4,11] The diagnosis of primary IMT is generally based on combined clinical and laboratory criteria: exclusion of other underlying disease processes, the presence of severe thrombocytopenia (less than 50,000/μL), normal to

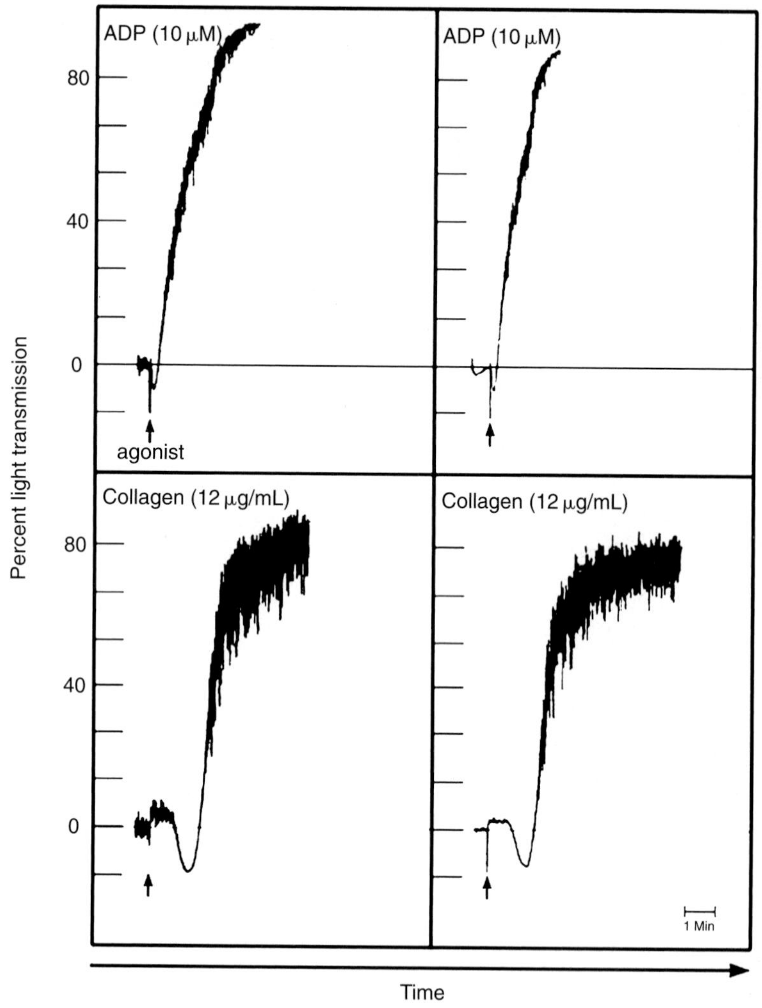

Figure 272-7 Platelet aggregation profiles of platelet-rich plasma obtained from two healthy dogs. Platelet activation was initiated by the addition *(arrow)* of adenosine diphosphate (ADP) *(top panels)* or collagen *(bottom panels)*. Aggregate formation is evidenced by an increase in light transmission. ADP induces a rapid aggregation response. In contrast, collagen stimulation is followed by a lag phase before aggregation ensues.

increased megakaryopoiesis, microthrombocytosis, platelet-bound antibodies, and response to immunosuppressive therapy.

Breed-specific, clinically asymptomatic thrombocytopenias occur in dogs. Healthy greyhounds have a platelet count somewhat lower than that of other breeds, with a mean platelet count of approximately 150,000/μL.[26] Cavalier King Charles spaniels have a hereditary macrothrombocytopenia, with affected dogs having platelet counts ranging from 25,000/μL to 100,000/μL.[27]

Acquired Platelet Dysfunction

Many common drugs and disease syndromes impair platelet function, but the clinical significance is highly variable.[28] A mild to moderate bleeding tendency may complicate management of disease syndromes such as anemia, liver failure, uremia, DIC, and paraproteinemia. The pathogenesis of platelet dysfunction in these disorders is complex and multifactorial and includes intrinsic alterations in platelet metabolism and extrinsic changes in blood viscosity. Many drugs demonstrate *in vitro* platelet inhibition (see Table 272-5), by a variety of different mechanisms. The antiplatelet effects of aspirin are caused by a well-characterized, irreversible inactivation of intraplatelet cyclo-oxygenase (COX).[29] Other nonsteroidal anti-inflammatory drugs (NSAIDs) cause transient COX inhibition, and newer NSAIDs that selectively inhibit the COX-2 isoform are predicted to have fewer

antiplatelet effects. Although drugs with potential antiplatelet effects may not cause spontaneous or severe bleeding, they should be given cautiously, if at all, to thrombocytopenic patients, patients undergoing surgery, or patients with signs of abnormal hemostasis.

Hereditary Platelet Dysfunction

Hereditary platelet function defects (thrombopathias) are rare but likely are underdiagnosed because of logistic difficulties in performing platelet function studies. Diseases are broadly grouped as defects of membrane glycoproteins, storage granules, signal transduction, or procoagulant activity.[20] Breed-specific defects within these functional classifications have been identified in dogs and cats (Table 272-6). Defects in the GPII$_b$III$_a$ complex, referred to as *thrombasthenic thrombasthenia*, have been identified in otter hounds and Great Pyrenees as the result of two distinct GPIIb mutations.[30,31] It is likely that the platelet function defects found in different breeds are caused by unique mutations.

von Willebrand Disease

von Willebrand disease (vWD) is the most common canine hereditary hemostatic defect.[32] The clinical signs of vWD overlap with those of other primary hemostatic defects, including mucosal hemorrhage, cutaneous bruising, and prolonged bleeding after injury. Petechiation, however, is not typical of vWD.

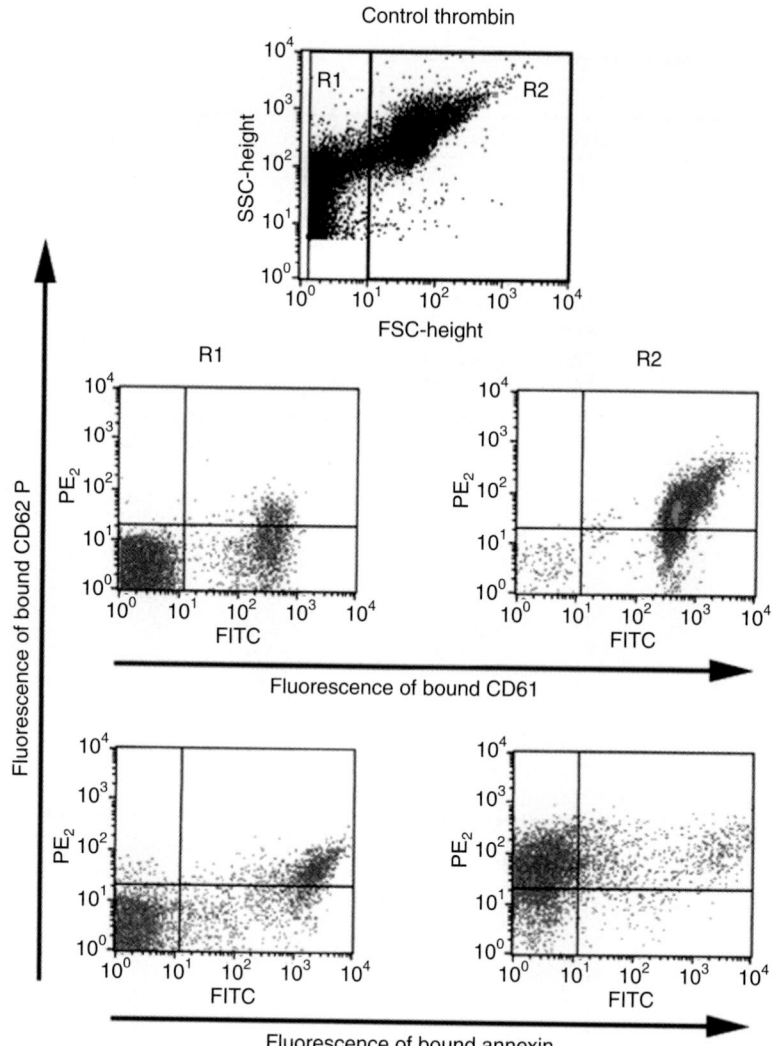

Figure 272-8 Flow cytometry analyses of canine platelet response to thrombin stimulation. The dot plot at top displays activated platelets in region R2. Region R1 contains platelet membrane–derived microparticles, debris, and machine noise. The four composite cytograms display the fluorescence intensity of labeled probes bound to the events in R1 or R2. The activated platelets (R2) display high-intensity labeling with CD61 and CD62p probes, denoting the presence of the membrane integrin GPIIIa and externalization of alpha granule constituent P-selectin, respectively. Most thrombin-activated platelets, however, are not labeled with the annexin probe, indicating low surface phosphatidylserine. In contrast, platelet membrane–derived particles (R1) display both P-selectin and phosphatidylserine. In all cytograms, events in the lower left quadrant represent nonspecific background fluorescence.

Disease Classification

Canine vWD is classified into one of three subtypes based on the clinical severity, plasma vWF concentration (vWF:Ag), and vWF multimer composition.[33,34] In general, a single type of vWD predominates in each affected breed (Table 272-7). Type 1 vWD, the most common form, is typically a mild to moderate bleeding diathesis characterized by low plasma vWF:Ag and normal multimer distribution. Type 2 vWD is a moderate to severe bleeding diathesis with a variable reduction in vWF:Ag and a disproportionate loss of high molecular weight (HMW) multimers. Type 3 vWD is a severe bleeding disorder caused by a total lack of vWF.

Table • 272-4

Pathogens that Cause Infectious Thrombocytopenia

TYPE OF AGENT	PATHOGEN
Viral agents	Canine: Distemper virus, herpesvirus, parvovirus, adenovirus
	Feline: Feline leukemia virus (FeLV), panleukopenia virus, feline immunodeficiency virus (FIV), feline infectious peritonitis (FIP) coronavirus
Arthropod-borne agents	*Ehrlichia* spp. *(E. canis, E. platys, E. ewingii);* also *Babesia, Haemobartonella, Rickettsia, Leishmania, Cytauxzoon, Borrelia,* and *Dirofilaria* spp.
Fungal and bacterial agents	Septicemia: Various agents
	Histoplasma, Candida, and *Leptospira* spp.

Table • 272-5

Drugs that Have Antiplatelet Effects

CATEGORY	DRUG	DISORDER/MODE OF ACTION
Antibiotics and antifungal drugs	Carbenicillin	Thrombopathia: Unknown action
	Cephalosporins	Thrombopathia: Membrane action*
	Chloramphenicol	Thrombocytopenia
	Penicillin	Thrombocytopenia
	Sulfonamides	Thrombocytopenia
Anti-inflammatory drugs	Aspirin	Thrombopathia: Prostaglandin (PG) inhibition
	Ibuprofen	Thrombopathia: PG inhibition
	Naproxen	Thrombopathia: PG inhibition
	Phenylbutazone	Thrombocytopenia and thrombopathia: PG inhibition
Cardiac and respiratory drugs	Aminophylline	Thrombopathia: Phosphodiesterase inhibition
	Diltiazem	Thrombopathia: Calcium blocker
	Isoproterenol	Thrombopathia: Membrane action
	Procainamide	Thrombocytopenia
	Propranolol	Thrombopathia: Membrane action
	Verapamil	Thrombopathia: Membrane action, calcium blocker
Cytotoxic drugs	Azathioprine	Thrombocytopenia
	Chlorambucil	Thrombocytopenia
	Cyclophosphamide	Thrombocytopenia
	Doxorubicin	Thrombocytopenia
Miscellaneous	Dextran	Thrombopathia: Membrane action
	Estrogen	Thrombocytopenia
	Methimazole	Thrombocytopenia

*Membrane action is interaction or interference with membrane receptors.

Table • 272-6

Hereditary Platelet Function Defects

DEFECT	BREED	LABORATORY FINDINGS
Thrombasthenia	Otter hound, Great Pyrenees	Absent or reduced GPII$_b$III$_a$ complex, abnormal adhesion, absent or severely reduced aggregation to all stimuli, abnormal clot retraction
Signal transduction	Basset hound	Abnormal cAMP metabolism, defective GPII$_b$III$_a$ activation, abnormal adhesion, aggregation only in response to thrombin, normal clot retraction
	Spitz	Abnormal adhesion, absent or trace aggregation in response to most stimuli, normal clot retraction
Storage pool	Persian cat	Chédiak-Higashi syndrome, low dense granule number, failure to secrete ADP and serotonin, abnormal aggregation, normal clot retraction
	American cocker spaniel	Normal dense granule number, abnormal ADP storage and secretion, abnormal ADP-induced aggregation, normal clot retraction
Signal transduction and storage pool	Collie	(Associated with cyclic neutropenia and stem cell defect) Defective dense granule serotonin and ADP release, abnormal aggregation to all stimuli but ADP
Undefined	Boxer	Abnormal aggregation to ADP and collagen, normal shape change, normal granule ATP/ADP content, normal fibrinogen and vWF binding
Procoagulant deficiency	German shepherd	Abnormal membrane phosphatidylserine exposure, abnormal microparticle release, abnormal prothrombinase activity, normal shape change, normal aggregation, normal clot retraction

cAMP, Cyclic adenosine monophosphate; *ADP*, adenosine diphosphate; *ATP*, adenosine triphosphate; *vWF*, von Willebrand factor.

Table • 272-7

Classification of Canine von Willebrand Disease

CLASSIFICATION	vWF PROTEIN	SEVERITY	REPORTED BREEDS
Type 1	Low concentration/all multimer forms present	Variable	Airedale, Akita, dachshund, Doberman pinscher, German shepherd, golden retriever, greyhound, Irish wolfhound, Manchester terrier, schnauzer, Pembroke Welsh corgi, mixed-breed, poodle, Shetland sheepdog
Type 2	Low concentration/ disproportionate loss of high-molecular-weight multimers	Moderate to severe	German shorthaired pointer, German wirehaired pointer
Type 3	Absent	Severe	Chesapeake bay retriever, Dutch kooiker, Scottish terrier, Shetland sheepdog Sporadic cases: Cocker spaniel, Eskimo dog, Labrador retriever, pit bull, rottweiler

Diagnosis of von Willebrand Disease

The screening test findings compatible with vWD include a normal platelet count, normal coagulation panel, long BMBT, and long PFA closure time, with definitive diagnosis confirmed by the finding of low plasma vWF:Ag (see Figure 272-4). Comprehensive analyses for vWD subtype classification include quantitative, functional, and qualitative vWF assays (Table 272-8).

Inheritance and Expression

von Willebrand disease is an autosomal trait; males and females experience the bleeding tendency and transmit the defect to offspring with equal frequency.[35] Expression of type 1 vWD is complex, with evidence for both incomplete dominant and recessive patterns.[36,37] Type 1 vWD is common in Doberman pinschers, and in this breed, clinical signs of vWD are typically seen in dogs with a vWF:Ag of 15% or lower.[38,39]

Table • 272-8

von Willebrand Factor Analyses

TEST	PARAMETER MEASURED	TYPICAL RESULTS WITH vWD	NORMAL VALUES*
Buccal mucosal bleeding time (BMBT)	Primary hemostasis—vessel, platelet, vWF interaction	Type 1: 5 to >12 min Type 3: >12 min Type 2: >12 min	2 to 4 min
Platelet function analyzer (PFA 100) ADP/collagen closure time	vWF-dependent platelet adhesion and platelet aggregation	Type 1: 150 to 200 sec Type 2: >300 sec Type 3: >300 sec	47 to 119 sec
von Willebrand factor antigen (vWF:Ag)	vWF concentration	Type 1: 5% to 20% Type 2: 1% to 5% Type 3: <0.1%	>50%
Ristocetin and botrocetin cofactor activities (vWF:RCo; vWF:BCo)	vWF-dependent platelet agglutination	Type 1: Cofactor activity = vWF:Ag Type 2: Cofactor activity < vWF:Ag Type 3: Cofactor activity absent	>50%
Collagen binding capacity (vWF:CB)	Quantitative measure of vWF bound to collagen	Type 1: vWF:CB = vWF:Ag Type 2: vWF:CB < vWF:Ag Type 3: vWF:CB absent	>50%
vWF multimer composition (Western blot)	Distribution and size of vWF multimeric forms	Type 1: All vWF multimers present Type 2: Low/absent HMW forms Type 3: no vWF	Complete size array

*Expected values for healthy dogs in authors' laboratory.
vWF, von Willebrand factor; ADP, adenosine diphosphate; HMW, high molecular weight.

HEMATOLOGY AND IMMUNOLOGY

Homozygosity for a splice-site mutation in the vWF gene and for certain vWF marker alleles is associated with a low plasma vWF.[40,41] The clinical severity of type 1 vWD for an individual dog (or human patient) cannot be fully explained by current molecular or biochemical tests. In contrast, type 2 and type 3 vWD in dogs appear to be simple recessive traits. Clinically affected dogs inherit a mutant vWF gene from each parent and express a bleeding tendency. The carrier parents are clinically normal, although their plasma vWF is typically low (less than 50% vWF:Ag). Mutations causative for type 3 vWD have been described in Scottish terriers and Dutch kooiker dogs.[42,43] Carriers (heterozygotes) can be unambiguously identified through breed-specific mutation detection tests.

TREATMENT OF PLATELET DISORDERS AND von WILLEBRAND DISEASE

Effective management of platelet disorders and vWD requires control of active sites of bleeding, stabilization of the patient to reverse signs of blood loss anemia and hypovolemia, and identification and correction of the primary disease that caused or exacerbated the hemostatic defect. Initial treatment modalities include both nontransfusion and transfusion support. Although the BMBT is a useful screening test of primary hemostasis for diagnostic purposes, it is not an accurate predictor of disease severity or surgical hemostasis.

Nontransfusion Therapy

Most animals with thrombocytopenia or acquired platelet function defects are effectively treated through identification and correction of the underlying disease process. Drugs with antiplatelet effects, invasive surgery, and jugular catheterization should be avoided, and cage rest is indicated to minimize trauma in severely thrombocytopenic patients. Based on the geographic location, history, and initial workup, institution of appropriate therapy for infectious thrombocytopenia (e.g., doxycycline for *Ehrlichia*, *Rickettsia*, and *Haemobartonella* spp.) is indicated pending confirmatory test results.[8] Immunosuppressive doses of prednisone (2 mg/kg given every 12 to 24 hours) are administered if the diagnostic workup indicates that primary IMT is likely.[11] Primary IMT patients usually demonstrate resolution of petechiae and an increased platelet count within 2 to 5 days of starting therapy. Refractory primary IMT can be effectively treated with vincristine (0.02 mg/kg given intravenously every 7 days).[44] Immunosuppressive therapy for IMT can be considered successful if a stable platelet count (preferably at or above 100,000/μL) is attained. Maintenance involves slow, gradual tapering of immunosuppressive therapy, with minimal exposure to unnecessary drugs, vaccination, or stress conditions to avoid relapse.

Desmopressin acetate (DDAVP; deamino 8 D-arginine vasopressin) is a synthetic vasopressin analog used in human medicine to treat a variety of hemostatic defects, including acquired platelet function defects and mild vWD.[45] Desmopressin (1 μg/kg given subcutaneously) has been reported to shorten the BMBT and the PFA-100 closure time and to provide surgical hemostasis when administered 30 minutes before surgery to Doberman pinschers with type 1 vWD.[46,47] Desmopressin therapy could be considered for other mild to moderate acquired or hereditary platelet function defects. Close monitoring to determine the extent and duration of response is required, and transfusion should be available if the response to desmopressin is inadequate.

Transfusion Therapy

Transfusion with products to replace red cells (Table 272-9) is indicated for patients with acute blood loss and/or severe anemia that cannot be stabilized with fluid therapy alone.

Table • 272-9

Guidelines for Transfusion Therapy

PRODUCT	DOSE	INTERVAL BETWEEN REPEAT TRANSFUSIONS
Products for Red Cell Replacement		
Fresh whole blood	12 to 20 mL/kg	Every 24 hours (volume overload limits interval)
Packed red cells	6 to 12 mL/kg	Every 12 to 24 hours
Oxyglobin	10 to 30 mL/kg*	Once
Products for Platelet Replacement		
Fresh whole blood	12 to 20 mL/kg	Every 24 hours (volume overload limits interval)
Platelet-rich plasma	6 to 10 mL/kg†	Every 8 to 12 hours
Platelet concentrate	1 U/10-15 kg‡	Every 8 to 12 hours
Products for von Willebrand Factor Replacement		
Fresh whole blood	12 to 20 mL/kg	Every 24 hours (volume overload limits interval)
Fresh frozen plasma	10 to 12 mL/kg	Every 8 to 12 hours
Cryoprecipitate	1 U/10 kg§	Every 6 to 12 hours (as needed)

*Infusion guidelines for cats (off-label use): Infuse up to maximum dose of 10 mL/kg.
†Platelet count ≥ 0.5 to 1×10^9/mL.
‡Platelet count $\geq 5 \times 10^9$/mL.
§Unit defined as cryoprecipitate prepared from 200 ml of fresh frozen plasma.

Transfusion solely to supply platelets (see Table 272-9) is rarely indicated or beneficial for thrombocytopenic patients or those with acquired platelet function defects. The survival of transfused platelets in IMT patients may be less than 1 day, which further limits their clinical utility. Platelet transfusions should be considered, however, in patients with persistent and uncontrolled bleeding or signs of central nervous system hemorrhage. Dogs and cats affected with severe hereditary thrombopathias may benefit from platelet transfusion as prophylaxis for surgery or if they develop severe spontaneous bleeding.[20,48]

Fresh whole blood, as platelet replacement, must be maintained at room temperature, collected in a citrate-based anticoagulant, and transfused as soon as possible after collection.[49] This product is best used for patients with active bleeding or when no other platelet product is available.

Platelet components are labor intensive to produce, because platelets require special processing and storage techniques to maintain viability. Platelet-rich plasma (PRP) is prepared by centrifugation of whole blood at low G force within 6 hours of collection.[49] The expected platelet yield is approximately 80% of the platelets, in one third volume, of the starting whole blood unit. In accordance with human blood banking standards, units of PRP, prepared from 450-mL units of whole blood, are expected to contain at least 50 billion platelets.[50] Low-volume platelet concentrates (PC) are prepared from PRP by a second centrifugation step. Platelet-rich plasma and PC must be maintained at room temperature from the time of collection until transfusion, with administration as soon as possible after collection, and maximum storage of 3 days. A dimethylsulfoxide (DMSO) cryopreserved canine platelet concentrate has recently been offered (Midwest Animal Blood Services, Stockbridge, MI). Pending trials demonstrating its efficacy, this product may widen the availability of platelet transfusion beyond referral centers capable of producing components in-house. Strict attention to aseptic technique is critical during collection and transfusion of platelet products to prevent contamination or disease transmission.

Transfusion to supply active vWF (see Table 272-9) is highly effective in controlling hemorrhage in vWD patients.[51] The best strategy is early, rapid transfusion to increase vWF to hemostatic levels and wound therapy to control hemorrhage from a single site. After initial transfusion, severely affected patients may require a second or third transfusion to sustain hemostasis for an additional 24 to 48 hours. Stabilization of the hematocrit and cessation of active hemorrhage indicate that hemostatic levels of vWF have been attained. Plasma components are the safest and most effective products for treating vWD. Plasma cryoprecipitate is prepared from fresh frozen plasma (FFP) and contains a fivefold to tenfold concentration of active vWF in approximately one-tenth volume of the starting plasma.[49] Cryoprecipitate is the best product for rapid replacement of vWF, but fresh frozen plasma is an acceptable alternative if cryoprecipitate is unavailable. The use of plasma components rather than whole blood prevents sensitization to red cell antigens, eliminates the need for canine type-matched donors, and minimizes the risk of volume overload.

CHAPTER • 273

Inherited Coagulopathies

Anthony P. Carr

Hemostasis results from a complex set of interactions. For convenience, the hemostatic response is divided into three processes: (1) primary hemostasis, (2) coagulation, and (3) fibrinolysis. The main components interacting in these processes are the blood vessels, platelets, and plasma proteins. Erythrocytes and leukocytes play a major role as well. After injury to a blood vessel, vasospasm reduces blood flow. Exposed subendothelium initiates platelet adhesion and platelet-platelet cohesion, resulting in the formation of a temporary platelet plug. At the same time, the coagulation cascade is activated by the vessel injury and by substances released by the platelets. The coagulation cascade leads to the formation of fibrin, which reinforces the platelet plug, forming a blood clot. The generation of fibrin leads to activation of fibrinolytic pathways. Numerous mechanisms, including antithrombin III, protein C, protein S, and tissue factor pathway inhibitor, limit coagulation to the area where it is needed. Although hemostasis is often considered an autonomous "system," it is important to remember that this separation is artificial. Hemostasis is intimately tied to the process of inflammation and vice versa.

PHYSIOLOGY OF HEMOSTASIS

Hemostasis has been extensively studied, yet researchers' understanding of the *in vivo* process is still undergoing revision. For a long time the processes that occurred *in vitro* were thought to be the same as those that occurred *in vivo*. However, this concept was challenged by the fact that some individuals with factor deficiencies failed to show a bleeding tendency, as would be expected if the initial theories were correct. A good example of this situation is factor XII deficiency, in which test results for the intrinsic coagulation pathway are markedly prolonged, yet no abnormal bleeding tendency is detected. The initial work also focused predominantly on the plasma proteins, often ignoring the vital contribution of cellular elements to the clotting process.

All coagulation factors and cofactors are synthesized in the liver and circulate in the plasma in an inactive form. Factors II, VII, IX, and X are considered vitamin K dependent because they must undergo vitamin K–dependent post-translational modification (gamma carboxylation) before becoming hemostatically active.[1]

HEMATOLOGY AND IMMUNOLOGY

Coagulation Cascade

Until recently, the predominant concept of coagulation was that of a cascade that could be divided into the intrinsic, extrinsic, and common pathways. An understanding of this theory is helpful to the clinician, because it reflects the processes that occur with the commonly run coagulation assays. Figure 273-1 shows the intrinsic and extrinsic pathways. The extrinsic pathway was relegated to a relatively minor role. The name *extrinsic* is based on the fact that initiation of clotting with this pathway required the addition of tissue thromboplastin, a substance that does not normally occur in blood, to the test sample. Tissue thromboplastin consists of phospholipid membrane that contains tissue factor. The addition of tissue thromboplastin results in the conversion of factor VII to factor VIIa, which proceeds to form factor Xa from factor X, thereby initiating the common pathway (Figure 273-2) and ultimately leading to the formation of fibrin.

The one-stage prothrombin time (OSPT) tests the extrinsic system. For this test, an excess of tissue thromboplastin is added to the blood sample, and the time that elapses until a clot forms is noted. One reason the extrinsic system was relegated to a minor role was that individuals with hemophilia have normal OSPT values; also, with the intrinsic pathway, it was possible to initiate clotting without the presence of tissue factor.[2]

The intrinsic pathway is initiated by the contact system, which consists of factors XII and XI, high-molecular-weight kinogen, and prekallikrein; initiation occurs with exposure to a negatively charged surface. Both the activated clotting time (ACT) and the activated partial thromboplastin time (aPTT) test this part of the clotting cascade. Individuals with hemophilia have markedly prolonged aPTT times, because factors VIII and IX are part of the intrinsic pathway.

The common pathway is initiated by activation of factor X, which forms a complex on a phospholipid membrane surface with factor V, factor II (prothrombin), and calcium. This complex, referred to as *prothrombinase*, then generates thrombin. The presence of factor V accelerates the generation of

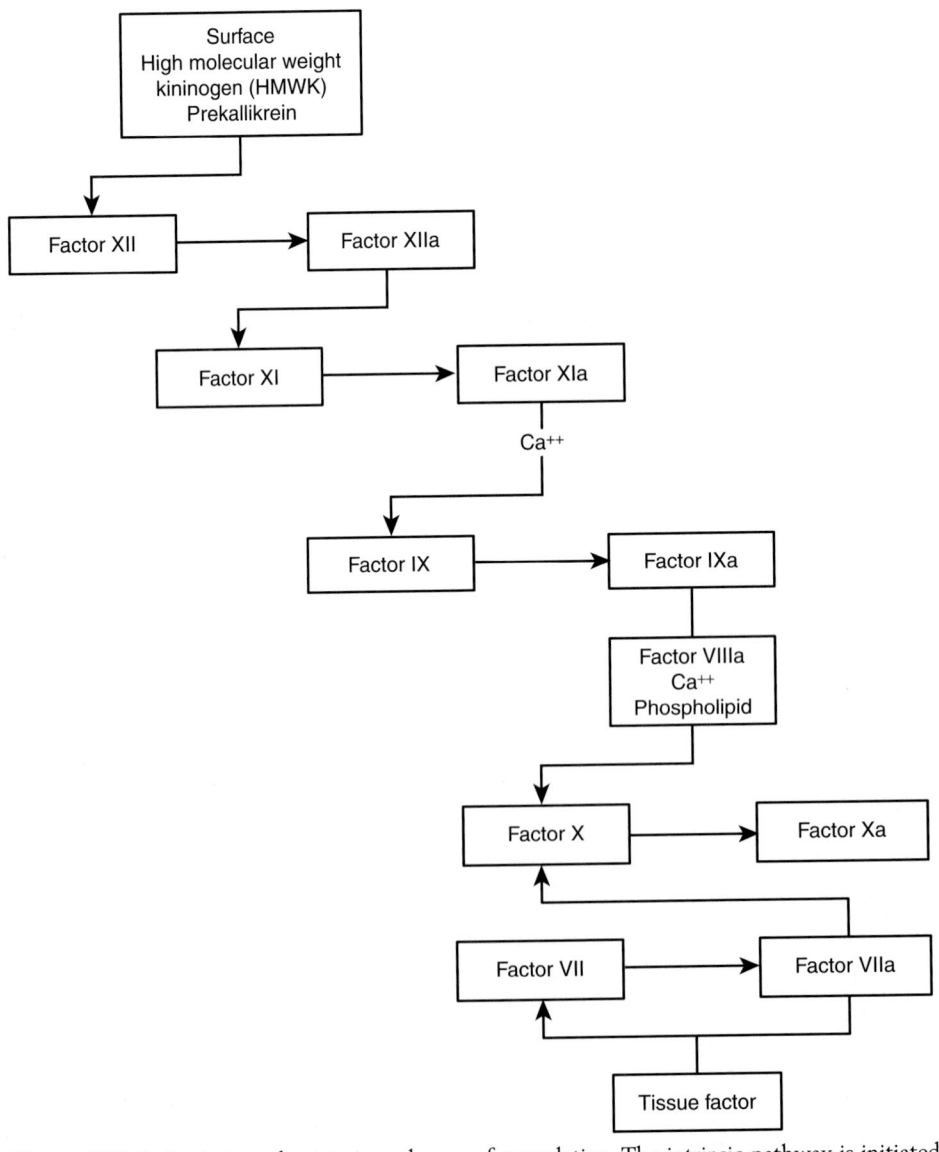

Figure 273-1 Intrinsic and extrinsic pathways of coagulation. The intrinsic pathway is initiated by conversion of factor XII to factor XIIa, whereas the extrinsic pathway is activated by the conversion of factor VII to factor VIIa.

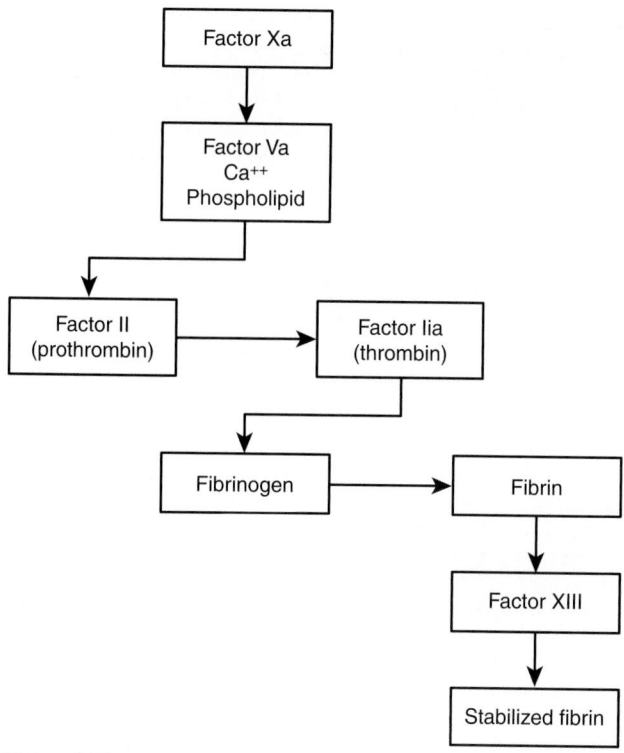

Figure 273-2 The common pathway of coagulation is initiated when factor X is converted to factor Xa by either the intrinsic or the extrinsic pathway.

thrombin several hundredfold. Thrombin binds fibrinogen and converts it to soluble fibrin monomers. The monomers polymerize and are cross-linked by factor XIIIa to form insoluble fibrin.

Revised Theory of Coagulation

The current understanding of the clotting process has resulted from a variety of observations. Traditionally, the intrinsic system has been considered more important than the extrinsic pathway, because it could proceed without requiring the addition of a substance not usually present in the circulation. A challenge to this assumption arose when some individuals from various species were found to be deficient in the contact system. These individuals had markedly prolonged aPTT results but no detectable predisposition to bleeding. The extrinsic system also was not thought to be important because, as mentioned previously, individuals with hemophilia have normal OSPT values despite a marked bleeding tendency. This is seen when the OSPT test is run in the standard fashion, in which an excess of tissue thromboplastin is used. When less thromboplastin is used, individuals with hemophilia also have prolonged coagulation times. These observations, combined with new research tools that allowed clotting to be studied in more detail, led to a major revision in the theory of how clotting is initiated and sustained. It would be surprising if the current theory remains unaltered in the future.

Factor VII activation is seen as the initiating event for clotting *in vivo*. Factor VII activation occurs when tissue factor is present. Tissue factor is expressed by cells underneath the endothelium, therefore trauma results in clotting. Other cells, such as monocytes and endothelial cells, also can express tissue factor when stimulated by such substances as cytokines and endotoxin. This explains why coagulation abnormalities are so common with a variety of inflammatory and infectious conditions. Production of the factor VIIa–tissue factor complex

results in the generation of small amounts of the active factors Xa and IXa. Factor Xa combines with tissue factor pathway inhibitor (TFPI) to rapidly stop further generation of active factors by the factor VIIa–tissue factor complex.[3]

Continued coagulation depends on pathways other than those that initiate clotting.[2] A possible explanation for this is that the thrombin generated initially is able to activate factor XI to factor XIa, and the clotting cascade then can proceed as classically outlined. Because factor XI can be activated directly by thrombin, it becomes clear that contact activation is not a prerequisite for *in vivo* clotting. It may also be that factor IX plays a vital role in promoting further clotting. Factor IX becomes fully activated when both factor Xa and the factor VIIa–tissue factor complex cleave off parts of the molecule. Once factor IXa has been formed, it can lead to further factor Xa generation and thereby to thrombin formation.

Despite its promise, the revised theory of coagulation leaves many questions unresolved, including the variable bleeding tendency seen with factor XI deficiency.

A possible explanation for the inability of the revised theory to explain all the clinical abnormalities seen may be that the theory focuses solely on the coagulation factors and thus does not account for the various cellular components involved in hemostasis.[4] These cellular components differ in their receptors and other properties, which allows for a different coagulation response when the cellular component varies, even if the plasma protein constituents remain the same. An example of this is tissue factor. The amount of tissue factor expressed does not solely determine how effectively a cell can initiate coagulation; the process also depends on the cell's ability to support prothrombinase assembly.[4] Given the complex interactions among cells, coagulation proteins, and inflammatory mediators, it is not surprising that our understanding of the basic physiologic process of clotting is incomplete.

Inhibitors of Coagulation

When coagulation is required, it is vital that it be prevented from becoming a widespread event in the organism; it must be limited to the area where the insult has occurred. A variety of mechanisms help inhibit coagulation, and the most important of these is antithrombin III (AT III). When complexed with endogenous heparin sulfate or exogenously administered heparin, AT III rapidly inactivates thrombin. It can also inactivate Xa and IXa effectively, unlike other activated factors. Each molecule of AT III is consumed with inactivation of a factor. Continued generation of factor Xa by the factor VIIa–tissue factor complex is blocked by TFPI. TFPI is present in plasma and also can be released by activated platelets.

The protein C–protein S system inactivates factors Va and VIIIa. Both of these proteins are vitamin K dependent and are located on the surface of the endothelial cells. They are activated when thrombin is bound to thrombomodulin. Thrombomodulin-bound thrombin is no longer active as a procoagulant molecule, yet it still is able to cleave protein C, thereby activating it.[2]

Fibrinolysis

Along with activation of coagulation, the mechanisms that degrade the clot and allow formation of scar tissue also are activated. The degradation of fibrin is mediated by plasmin, which is generated by the action of plasminogen activators on plasminogen. Tissue plasminogen activator (t-PA) and urokinase-type plasminogen activator (u-PA) are the main types of activators that occur naturally in dogs and cats. Streptokinase, also a plasminogen activator, is produced by certain streptococci.

When a clot forms, plasminogen is incorporated into the clot. The presence of thrombin causes the endothelium to release t-PA. The affinity for plasminogen is low without

HEMATOLOGY AND IMMUNOLOGY

a cofactor being present. However, when t-PA is associated with fibrin, it has high catalytic efficacy for cleaving plasminogen.[2] The action of t-PA is predominantly limited to the vascular space, whereas u-PA acts more extravascularly. Once plasmin has been formed, it begins to degrade fibrin. This results in the production of various fibrin degradation products. Some of these degradation products are specific to fibrin, some can also be produced when fibrinogen is cleaved.

Excessive fibrinolysis also must be prevented, and this is achieved through two main processes: alpha$_2$-antiplasmin inactivates free plasmin rapidly (although it is much less active against fibrin-bound plasmin), and tissue plasminogen activator inhibitor 1 (PAI-1) inactivates t-PA and u-PA.

INHERITED HEMOSTATIC ABNORMALITIES

Inherited disorders of hemostasis can involve coagulation factor deficiencies, defects of platelet adhesion resulting from decreased levels of von Willebrand factor (vWF), defective platelet function, and blood vessel defects. Inherited coagulation defects related to various coagulation factor deficiencies have been reported in dogs and cats. These defects may be inherited or may arise *de novo* as a result of a genetic mutation.

Hemophilia A (Factor VIII Deficiency)

The most commonly seen congenital coagulation abnormality is hemophilia A. The bleeding tendency associated with this disease is a result of a deficiency in functional factor VIII.[5-9] Factor VIII is located in the intrinsic pathway and acts to significantly increase the rate at which IXa generates factor Xa. With a lack of factor VIII activity, less fibrin is formed; this results in the typical signs of a coagulopathy, such as body cavity bleeding and large hematomas. Hemorrhage into joints may occur as well. An initial platelet plug may form, but fibrin reinforcement for the plug is delayed, reduced, or absent, and the result is rebleeding. Hemophilia A is inherited as a X-linked recessive trait, meaning that most affected individuals are male. This form of hemophilia occurs in humans, dogs and occasionally in cats.[10] The severity of the bleeding is variable. Generally, factor VIII activity must be less than 5% of normal for bleeding to occur spontaneously. Hemorrhage can be severe and occasionally fatal; this is not uncommon in the neonatal period. Patients with hemophilia A have a prolonged aPTT and a normal OSPT. A definitive diagnosis is made by specific factor assay.

Hemophilia B (Factor IX Deficiency)

Hemophilia B, or Christmas disease, has also been described in dogs and cats.[11-14] The disease is caused by a sex-linked deficiency of factor IX, which is a vitamin K–dependent factor. Factor IX is responsible for activation of factor X. Hemophilia B has been identified in at least 19 breeds of dogs as well as mixed breeds.[15] The bleeding tendency seen with this disease is variable but can be severe. As with hemophilia A, the aPTT is prolonged without prolongation of the OSPT. Definitive diagnosis depends on specific factor assay. If serum is added to the plasma on which the aPTT is run, the prolongation will correct, because serum contains factor IX.[16]

Factor XII Deficiency (Hageman Trait)

Occasionally an incidental prolongation of the aPTT in cats is detected, although a bleeding tendency is not present. This finding results from low levels of factor XII, also called *Hageman factor*, an important part of contact activation *in vitro*. This deficiency generally does not compromise hemostasis.[17] The condition is inherited as an autosomal recessive trait and has been found in dogs as well[1]; it also is a normal finding in some marine mammals, birds, and reptiles.[16] Factor analysis is required to make a definitive diagnosis.

Vitamin K—Dependent Factor Deficiency

Vitamin K–dependent factor deficiency is a rare inherited coagulation defect involving all the vitamin K–dependent factors (II, VII, IX, and X) that has been described in Devon rex cats.[18] It probably is an autosomal recessive trait. Bleeding is severe in affected animals, which show prolongation of both the OSPT and aPTT.

Other Coagulopathies

Various other factor deficiencies have been reported in dogs and cats,[1,16] but these problems are rarely seen in practice.

DIAGNOSIS

A variety of tests are available for diagnosis of hemostatic abnormalities, some of which can be performed in a practice setting. Most coagulation tests require specialized equipment and extensive experience, therefore most of them must be performed in a reference laboratory. A variety of bedside coagulation monitors have been evaluated for use in veterinary medicine.[19]

In-house evaluation of coagulation abnormalities certainly can include the activated clotting time (ACT). This test requires that 2 mL of blood be drawn into a tube containing diatomaceous earth as a contact activator. The tube is incubated at 37° C. The ACT evaluates the intrinsic and common pathways of coagulation. Prolongation of the ACT may be seen with hemophilia A or B, factor XI or factor XII deficiency, vitamin K–antagonist rodenticide intoxication, and heparin therapy. The ACT relies on platelet phospholipids for coagulation, therefore severe thrombocytopenia can lead to increased values. Reported normals were 64 to 95 seconds and 67 to 85 seconds in dogs and 65 seconds or less in cats.[20-22]

Hemostatic testing requires collection of a sample of optimum quality. Venipuncture that involves multiple passes through tissue to obtain a sample is not appropriate for coagulation testing. Holding the vein off too long also can lead to activation of platelets and the fibrinolytic system. The tissue packed into the needle acts to activate coagulation prematurely. Hemolysis and severe lipemia (which often causes hemolysis) can also prevent accurate results. It often is preferable to use vacuum tubes for collection and to use the first sample for tests other than coagulation. The most commonly used anticoagulant is sodium citrate, and the ideal ratio is one part citrate to nine parts blood. The sample should be promptly centrifuged and the plasma harvested. The plasma then should be frozen in a plastic or siliconized glass tube. Plasma should be shipped frozen, because coagulation factors rapidly become inactivated at room temperature.

Reference laboratories can perform two valuable clotting time tests, the aPTT, which tests intrinsic function, and the OSPT, which tests extrinsic function. These tests are also available with point-of-care devices. It is important to remember that reference ranges vary among laboratories and testing methodologies, therefore no universally applicable reference ranges are available. The aPTT tests many of the same factors as the ACT but is considerably more sensitive. A prolonged aPTT with a normal OSPT is a common finding with hemophilia or factor XII deficiency. A prolonged OSPT with a normal aPTT usually is seen only when vitamin K antagonists have been recently ingested; factor VII deficiency is extremely rare. The OSPT predominantly tests the function of factor VII, the coagulation factor with the shortest half-life, as well as common pathway deficiencies. Both the aPTT and OSPT are prolonged with vitamin K deficiencies, severe liver disease, and disseminated intravascular coagulation and when vitamin K–antagonist rodenticide poisoning occurs more than 12 to 24 hours before testing.

A variety of other assays are available through reference laboratories. Specific factor analysis can be run. It is vital that the laboratory that runs the factor analysis have considerable experience with veterinary samples, because there can be discordant results if the same protocols are used as in humans.

TREATMENT

Treatment of hemostatic abnormalities requires careful assessment and determination of the particular abnormality. Many of the diseases described are not amenable to cure, and at best short-term control is possible. An exception is the combined vitamin K–dependent factor deficiency, in which vitamin K supplementation can normalize the clotting ability. In humans there is considerable interest in developing gene therapy for most of these inherited coagulation disorders. Currently this is not an option in pets, therefore the goal is to control clinical signs and avoid situations in which bleeding may occur. It is especially important to avoid trauma in an animal with bleeding tendencies, especially trauma produced iatrogenically through biopsy, surgery, venipuncture, restraint, or intramuscular administration of medications. It is also important to avoid medications that can interfere with primary hemostasis, such as nonsteroidal anti-inflammatory drugs and phenothiazines.

Treatment of inherited disorders of hemostasis consists of transfusion therapy, which generally is instituted only when life-threatening hemorrhage is present or prior to surgery. Which type of transfusion is most appropriate depends on the patient's presenting signs. If anemia is present, use of fresh whole blood may be expedient, because it replaces red cells and coagulation factors. If anemia is not present, the use of plasma is preferred. Fresh frozen plasma contains all the coagulation factors in their active form and can be used to treat any coagulopathy. Slowly thawing fresh frozen plasma and decanting off the supernatant generates cryoprecipitate and cryosupernatant. Cryoprecipitate contains factor VIII, fibrinogen, and vWF in high concentrations. This makes cryoprecipitate the blood component of choice for therapy of von Willebrand disease, fibrinogen deficiency, and hemophilia A. The highly concentrated nature of cryoprecipitate allows the coagulation factors from many units of plasma to be transfused without the worry of volume overload. Cryosupernatant can be used in the treatment of coagulopathies that do not involve the factors removed in the cryoprecipitate.

CHAPTER • 274

Acquired Coagulopathies

Robert M. DuFort
Linda Matros

Robert M. DuFort
Linda Matros

VITAMIN K DEFICIENCY

Vitamin K deficiency is one of the most commonly encountered acquired coagulopathies in veterinary medicine. Vitamin K is required for the activation of a group of proteolytic enzymes known as *serine proteases*, which include coagulation factors II, VII, IX, and X, and the anticoagulant proteins C and S. If left untreated, vitamin K deficiency results in alterations in the extrinsic, intrinsic, and common coagulation pathways and ultimately clinically manifests as bleeding.

Vitamin K is a fat-soluble vitamin found in three forms: K_1 (phytonadione), K_2 (menaquinone), and K_3 (menadione). Vitamin K_1 is found in green, leafy vegetables and vegetable oils. It is absorbed via the lymphatics in the proximal small bowel. Bile acids and dietary fats facilitate absorption of vitamin K_1. Vitamin K is also synthesized by microflora in the ileum and colon. Vitamin K_3 is a synthetic form. Oral doses are absorbed via capillaries in the colon. The daily requirement of vitamin K is small (1.25 µg/kg/day in the dog), and the liver stores several days' supply. Consequently, animals fed a commercial diet rarely experience vitamin K deficiency (Box 274-1).

Antagonism of vitamin K is by far the most common cause of vitamin K deficiency. Vitamin K antagonism is brought about by the ingestion of anticoagulant rodenticides.

The vitamin K–dependent coagulation factors (II, VII, IX, and X) are synthesized by the liver as inactive proteins, which contain glutamyl residues that must be carboxylated for the proteins to become active. The carboxylation reaction requires reduced vitamin K. As the coagulation proteins become carboxylated, vitamin K is oxidized by the enzyme vitamin K epoxidase to become vitamin K epoxide. To carboxylate other coagulation protein molecules, the vitamin K epoxide must again be reduced by vitamin K epoxide reductase.

Box • 274-1
Conditions Associated with Vitamin K Deficiency

Neonate born to malnourished mother
Decreased synthesis of vitamin K by intestinal microflora
   (due to chronic antibiotic therapy)
Decreased vitamin K absorption
   Complete bile duct obstruction
   Pancreatic exocrine insufficiency
   Lymphangiectasia

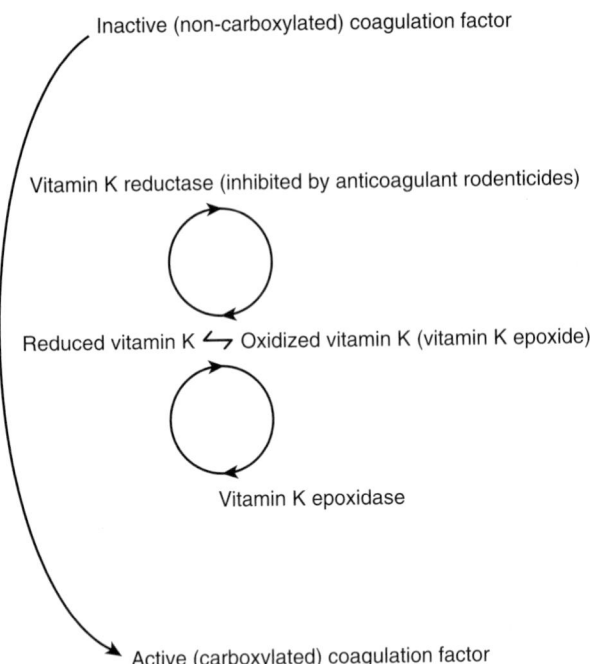

Inactive (non-carboxylated) coagulation factor

Vitamin K reductase (inhibited by anticoagulant rodenticides)

Reduced vitamin K ⇄ Oxidized vitamin K (vitamin K epoxide)

Vitamin K epoxidase

Active (carboxylated) coagulation factor

Figure 274-1 Vitamin K carboxylation cycle.

Anticoagulant rodenticides act by inhibiting vitamin K epoxide reductase. As a result, vitamin K epoxide and inactive (noncarboxylated) coagulation factors accumulate in the blood (Figure 274-1). The half-lives of coagulation factors II, VII, IX, and X are short (41, 6.2, 13.9, and 16.5 hours, respectively).

Anticoagulant rodenticides were developed as a result of the observation of an acquired coagulopathy in cattle that had ingested moldy sweet clover. A coumarin derivative in sweet clover is converted to dicoumarol by a fungus. The first-generation anticoagulants, warfarin and pindone, were developed for vermin control and as human antithrombotic medicines after this discovery. The second-generation anticoagulant rodenticides (bromadiolone, brodifacoum, and diphacinone) are more potent because of their longer half-lives and lower incidence of acquired drug resistance. Despite the longer half-lives of the second-generation anticoagulant rodenticides, poisoning of companion animals that ingest poisoned rodents is an uncommon event. Various concurrently administered drugs (Box 274-2) and coexisting conditions (Box 274-3) may exacerbate the toxicity of anticoagulant rodenticides.

To diagnose anticoagulant rodenticide poisoning, the clinician must assess the history and clinical signs and evaluate the results of appropriate laboratory tests. The histories of potentially poisoned pets vary from direct observation of ingestion to the passing of suspicious material in the feces. Potential exposure to anticoagulant rodenticides may be a relative certainty or may be unknown, depending on the animal's environment. The onset of clinical signs normally occurs 2 to 5 days after ingestion of the anticoagulant rodenticide, and signs may escalate quickly after they are first detected. Clinical signs are the result of hemorrhage, which may vary from mild to severe. Severe hemorrhage can result in hypovolemia and organ dysfunction. Bleeding into the thoracic cavity or cranium is especially critical.

Laboratory test results may be normal or abnormal, depending on the amount of anticoagulant ingested and the time elapsed since ingestion. The first laboratory test to show an abnormal (prolonged) result is the PIVKA (proteins induced by vitamin K absence or antagonism) test, followed by the prothrombin time (PT), and eventually the partial

---

Box • 274-2

Mechanisms and Drugs That Affect Anticoagulant Rodenticide Toxicity

Platelet inhibition
  Aspirin
  Nonsteroidal anti-inflammatory drugs
Possible inhibition of Vitamin K epoxide reductase
  Sulfonamides (sulfaquinoxaline)
  Cephalosporins (cefmetazole)
Decreased anticoagulant rodenticide protein binding
  Oxyphenbutazone
  Diphenylhydantoin
  Sulfonamides
  Corticosteroids
  Phenylbutazone
Inhibition of hemostasis
  Promazine-type tranquilizers
  Nitrofurans
  Local anesthetics
  Antihistamines
  Hormones (testosterone, RA)
  Anabolic steroids
  Epinephrine
Increased hepatic metabolism (induction of microsomal enzymes)
  Carbamazine
  Antibiotics
  Rifampin
  Chloramphenicol
  Barbiturates

---

thromboplastin time (PTT). The PIVKA test, a sensitive indicator of anticoagulant rodenticide ingestion, may be prolonged as early as 12 hours after ingestion; the PT may require 36 to 72 hours to become abnormal. The PT is affected by numerous other coagulation disorders, such as disseminated intravascular coagulation (DIC), hepatic disease, and hereditary factor deficiencies. In contrast, the PIVKA test is sensitive primarily to the presence of precursor proteins, which accumulate in the absence of vitamin K. Comparison studies have

---

Box • 274-3

Conditions That Exacerbate Anticoagulant Rodenticide Toxicity

High lipid diet
  Facilitates rodenticide absorption
  Decreases anticoagulant protein binding
Uremia
  Promotes platelet inhibition
  Decreases protein binding
  Decreases excretion of unbound anticoagulant
Thrombocytopenia
Disseminated intravascular coagulation

shown that the PIVKA test has greater sensitivity and specificity than both the PT and the activated partial thromboplastin time (aPTT) in the diagnosis of dogs with anticoagulant poisoning.

Measurement of the anticoagulant rodenticide in the serum or tissues of an animal confirms the diagnosis of anticoagulant toxicosis. High-performance liquid chromatography and gas chromatography tests capable of identifying specific anticoagulants are available in many diagnostic laboratories. The results of these tests are not compromised by previous therapy with vitamin K, therefore a diagnosis can still be made even in successfully treated animals.

Therapy varies with the stage of the disease. With an acute known ingestion, emetics, adsorbents, and cathartics are used to minimize absorption. Most clinicians choose to begin vitamin K therapy even in asymptomatic patients regardless of the success of attempts to limit absorption. Vitamin K_1 is the treatment of choice. The initial treatment is administration of vitamin K_1 by subcutaneous injection at a dosage of 2.5 to 5 mg/kg. The dose should be divided and given in several sites. Oral vitamin K_1 therapy follows in 6 to 12 hours, at a dosage of 1.25 to 2.5 mg/kg given twice daily. If absorption of the rodenticide is thought to be minimal, treatment may be discontinued after 7 days. The PT should be tested 48 hours after termination of therapy. If the PT is prolonged, the patient is treated with oral vitamin K_1 for 2 more weeks. If the initial post-therapy PT is normal, a second PT test should be done 48 hours later. If the second post-therapy PT is normal, vitamin K therapy may be terminated.

LIVER DISEASE

The liver is critical to coagulation homeostasis. It is the site of synthesis of most of the procoagulants (clotting factors), the anticoagulants (antithrombin III, alpha$_2$-macroglobulin, alpha$_1$-antitrypsin, alpha$_1$-acid glycoprotein, and proteins C and S), and the fibrinolytic proteins (plasminogen, plasminogen activators, plasminogen proactivators, antiplasmins, and inhibitors of plasminogen activators and proactivators). Liver disease may result in hemorrhage caused by decreased coagulation factor synthesis, synthesis of abnormal coagulation factors, or excessive consumption. Ironically, even the most severe liver disease is rarely accompanied by bleeding. There are several reasons for this. The liver produces a large quantity of coagulation factors. Fibrinogen, for example, can be measured in concentrations up to 0.4 g/dL in the plasma of normal animals. It is commonly stated that coagulation factor concentrations must fall below 15% for coagulation to be compromised. Edema and anasarca due to hypoalbuminemia, which occur at 75% to 80% liver compromise, are rarely accompanied by bleeding, even with provocation (liver biopsy). The liver also has a tremendous regenerative capacity and can return to normal function after many acute hepatopathies. Some coagulation factor concentrations actually increase with liver disease (i.e., fibrinogen, factor V, and von Willebrand factor [vWF]). The liver also is the largest macrophage-containing organ in the body, with tremendous phagocytic activity capable of rapidly clearing activated coagulation factors and products of fibrinolysis (fibrin degradation products [FDPs]).

Although 66% to 85% of patients with hepatopathies have abnormal results on one or more coagulation tests, fewer than 2% actually develop hemorrhage. When bleeding occurs, it usually is associated with concurrent disease (thrombocytopenia, thrombopathy, or cardiovascular disease). Factors that determine whether liver disease results in hemorrhage are the nature and severity of the disease and the rate of onset.

Box • 274-4

Potential Sequelae of Neoplasia That May Result in Thrombosis or Hemorrhage

Thrombocytopenia
Thrombopathy
Disseminated intravascular coagulation
Microangiopathy
Endothelial invasion by neoplastic cells
Treatment with chemotherapeutic agents

A prospective evaluation of coagulation tests in cats with different types of liver disease showed the PIVKA test to be more sensitive than either the PT or the aPTT for evaluating cats at risk for increased bleeding. Hepatobiliary disease, which disrupts enterohepatic circulation of bile acids, leads to a depletion of coagulation factors and an increase in procoagulant proteins (PIVKAs) by decreasing the intestinal absorption of vitamin K. The degree of vitamin K deficiency parallels the severity of liver disease and the probability of clinically significant bleeding. Because the PIVKA test is the first coagulation test to become abnormal in states of vitamin K deficiency, it appears to be superior to either the PT or APTT in identifying cats at risk for increased hemorrhage from liver disease.

NEOPLASIA

Neoplastic disease may result in thrombosis or bleeding by several mechanisms (Box 274-4).

In dogs with mammary carcinoma, abnormalities in one or more coagulation tests are found in two thirds of the patients. The frequency of abnormal test results correlated with the stage of disease. Dogs with stage III or stage IV neoplasia had the highest number of abnormal test results.

Chemotherapeutic agents may further exacerbate bleeding tendencies (Table 274-1). Studies have shown that up to 83%

Table • 274-1

Chemotherapeutic Agents That May Affect Coagulation

DRUG	MECHANISM
Bleomycin, CCNU, cytosine arabinoside, melphalan, methotrexate, platinum, doxorubicin, Actinomycin D	Thrombocytopenia
Vincristine, vinblastine	Thrombocytosis
Melphalan, vincristine	Thrombopathy
L-Asparaginase	Inhibition of protein (clotting factor) synthesis
Actinomycin D	Vitamin K antagonism
Melphalan	Dysfibrinogenemia
Doxorubicin, daunorubicin	Increased fibrin and fibrinogen lysis

of untreated dogs had laboratory evidence of abnormal coagulation. In cats with neoplasia, 20% had coagulation abnormalities. Among the patients with abnormal laboratory results, thrombocytopenia was most common (36%), followed by a prolonged PTT (32%), and altered fibrinogen concentrations (25%). Canine lymphoma/leukemia and hemangiosarcoma are neoplasms that are commonly associated with hemostatic abnormalities. Treatment of the hemorrhage must first address the inciting cause, the neoplasia.

ACQUIRED INHIBITORS OF COAGULATION

Acquired anticoagulants are uncommonly recognized in veterinary medicine. These inhibitors may be directed against one or more specific coagulation factors.

There are several types of inhibitors. The most common type comprise the immunoglobulins of the IgG class. They occur most often in patients receiving multiple whole blood or plasma transfusions. These immunoglobulins have also been associated with therapy with certain drugs (e.g., penicillin, phenytoin) and with immune-mediated diseases (e.g., systemic lupus erythematosus), liver disease, lymphoproliferative diseases, DIC, and other conditions. They may result in abnormal coagulation test results, thrombosis, or hemorrhage, depending on the coagulation factor against which they are directed.

Immunoglobulins should be suspected when coagulation test abnormalities do not fit the clinical presentation. Prior administration of antithrombotic drugs or improper sample collection must be ruled out. Because their effect on coagulation test results occurs by a mechanism different from that produced by a factor deficiency, they may be identified with a plasma mixing procedure. If a factor deficiency is present (i.e., hemophilia A or B), the addition of plasma from a species-specific pool corrects the coagulation screening test. This same procedure does not correct coagulation test results if an inhibitor is present.

In contrast to the immunoglobulin class of inhibitors, nonspecific inhibitors are not targeted on any single coagulation factor; rather, they interfere with the interactions of clotting factors on a phospholipid surface. These nonspecific inhibitors affect the aPTT more than the PT and also fail to correct in mixing studies. The release of heparin, as can be seen with canine mast cell tumors, and metalloproteinases (found in snake venom) are other examples of acquired coagulation inhibitors.

THROMBOSIS

A delicate balance must be maintained between procoagulant, anticoagulant, and fibrinolytic factors. A change in the blood flow, vascular endothelium, or coagulation factors can result in thrombosis as well as hemorrhage. *Thrombophilia* is a term that describes the hypercoagulable (prethrombotic) state, which may be due to a familial, congenital, or acquired abnormality that results in a predisposition to thrombosis. *Thrombosis* is a secondary disease process associated with many primary diseases, including immune-mediated hemolytic anemia, hyperadrenocorticism, protein-losing enteropathy, systemic amyloidosis, and canine parvovirus.

Pulmonary thromboembolism (PTE) has been observed in up to 30% of canine cancer patients. A retrospective study of dogs diagnosed with autoimmune hemolytic anemia (AIHA), found evidence of thromboembolism in 20 of 25 dogs necropsied. The type of thrombi that forms depends on local blood flow characteristics. Coagulation, or red, thrombi are primarily made up of red blood cells and fibrin. They occur in areas of slow or occluded blood flow, such as veins. At the other extreme are platelet, or white, thrombi, which form in areas of high blood flow, such as at heart valves. They are composed primarily of platelets and fibrin. Mixed thrombi are an intermediate type found primarily in the pulmonary vasculature.

The clinical signs of a thrombus depend on the organ affected, but they are ultimately due to compromised blood flow to the organ. The thrombus may occlude blood flow locally, or a portion of the thrombus may break free and lodge downstream, where the vessel caliber is smaller and the blood flow slower. Pulmonary thrombosis is associated with acute dyspnea. Renal arterial thromboembolism may be associated with acute renal failure. Detection of thromboemboli is difficult without specialized diagnostic techniques, such as angiography, venography, Doppler ultrasonography, or ventilation-perfusion scintillation scans. The results of routine coagulation tests such as the PT and PTT may be shortened, but they often are within normal limits. For this reason, an awareness of conditions that may result in a hypercoagulable state (e.g., glomerulonephritis) must be kept in mind.

With glomerulonephritis, severe proteinuria may ensue. One of the proteins lost is antithrombin III (AT III), which is about the size of albumin. AT III can be measured in many university and commercial laboratories. AT III levels are a good predictor of the potential for thrombi formation. AT III values between 60% and 75% are associated with an increased risk of thrombosis. Values less than 60% are often associated with irreversible organ damage. Other specialized laboratory tests, such as the chromogenic factor VII assay, platelet aggregation assays, and protein C assay, may be performed is some university coagulation laboratories.

Treatment is directed toward reducing thrombogenesis, in addition to thrombolytic therapy. Reduction of thrombogenesis is achieved with anticoagulant therapy (heparin and warfarin) and reduction of platelet function through the use of platelet inhibitors (aspirin, dipyridamole, and ticlopidine). Thrombolytic therapy includes the use of tissue plasminogen activator (t-PA), streptokinase, or urokinase. Heparin therapy depends on an adequate plasma concentration of AT III. With a low AT III concentration, one or more plasma transfusions may be required for heparin to be effective. Coumadin and other warfarin products inhibit vitamin K–dependent coagulation factors, but they require several days to achieve the desired effect.

DISSEMINATED INTRAVASCULAR COAGULATION

Disseminated intravascular coagulation (DIC), also called *consumptive coagulopathy*, is the end result of systemic thrombosis. It is a well-recognized clinical syndrome in dogs but is rarely diagnosed in cats. DIC is always a secondary disease. The inciting causes of DIC are the same as those for thrombosis. The primary disease causes widespread thrombosis, which results in the consumption of clotting factors and platelets and initiates uncontrolled fibrinolysis. These disturbances in the coagulation system lead to massive hemorrhage, tissue hypoxia, organ failure, and often death. DIC may be acute and uncompensated or chronic and compensated. Laboratory test abnormalities may vary, depending on the current stage of disease. DIC may be seen in up to 50% of dogs with splenic hemangiosarcoma. Hyperthermia is one of the inciting diseases that may have a more favorable prognosis, because this condition can be treated fairly rapidly. Death is coming if organ dysfunction from thrombi or anemia secondary to hemorrhage is severe.

The five objectives of the treatment of DIC are: (1) to ensure adequate tissue perfusion, (2) to eliminate the initiating cause, (3) to support target organs susceptible to microthrombi, ischemia, and hemorrhage, (4) to replace blood components, and (5) to provide heparin therapy.

Clinically suspected cases of DIC can be verified by laboratory testing. Typically, the patient's platelet count drops, and the aPTT, PT, and thrombin time (TT) increase. Fibrin degradation products (FDPs) are elevated, and the fibrinogen level is decreased from its previous value. A retrospective survey of 252 dogs diagnosed with DIC showed thrombocytopenia (86%), a prolonged PT (61%), an increased aPTT (92%), an increased TT (32%), and increased FDPs (95%). Interestingly, on examination of red cell morphology, schistocytes were noted in only 10% of the cases.

Traditionally, assays for FDPs were used to diagnose and manage disseminated intravascular coagulation. However, these assays lacked specificity, because they used polyclonal antibodies against fibrinogen, fibrin, and fibrin fragments. They also required serum samples collected in special FDP tubes, because heparin interfered with the test. For these reasons, interest is growing in a newer test, the D-dimer test. D-dimer is a protein formed as a result of plasmin degradation of cross-linked fibrin. During blood coagulation, fibrinogen is converted to fibrin by the action of thrombin. The resulting fibrin monomers polymerize to form a insoluble gel of non-cross-linked fibrin. This fibrin gel is further converted to cross-linked fibrin by thrombin-activated factor XIII to form an insoluble fibrin clot. Production of plasmin, the major clot-lysing enzyme, is triggered by the formation of a fibrin clot. Although fibrin and fibrinogen are both cleaved by plasmin to yield FDPs, only degradation products from cross-linked fibrin contain D-dimer. Therefore an elevated D-dimer level is a specific marker of clot lysis. This test has an extraordinary negative predictive value. In other words, a negative D-dimer test excludes DIC with a confidence level of 99.5%. The test can be run in the clinic by a semiquantitative rapid latex agglutination method using blood samples collected in ethylenediamine tetra-acetic acid (EDTA) or heparin. Although the rapid latex agglutination test lacks the necessary sensitivity for reliable diagnosis of pulmonary thromboemboli, recently a more sensitive enzyme-linked immunosorbent assay (ELISA)-based assay has become available and is showing promise in this area.

CHAPTER • 275

Leukocyte Disorders

Charles W. Brockus

Collectively, leukocytes are identified in the peripheral blood as granulocytes (neutrophils, eosinophils, and basophils) and mononuclear cells (monocytes and lymphocytes). These cells actively participate in the innate and adaptive immune system. The activity or morphology of leukocytes can be affected by drug therapy, toxins, infectious organisms, neoplastic disorders, and/or hereditary factors.

Leukocyte disorders occur in dogs and cats, from neonates to aged animals, and cause a variety of clinical features ranging from normal to moribund. In addition, combinations of morphologic and/or functional abnormalities can occur, ranging from unique morphology with no clinical consequence to normal morphology associated with severe clinical signs. Neutrophilic or lymphocytic cell functions are usually impaired in functional abnormalities, and morphologic changes often include all leukocytes.

Most leukocyte disorders are rare and are reported once and/or are observed in a specific breed (e.g., smoke blue Persian cats, gray collies, Jack Russell terriers, Irish setters), implicating a specific hereditary pattern associated with the signalment of the particular breed. The history and physical examination, therefore, often provide important initial information about an abnormality.

Treatment often is unnecessary for morphologic anomalies and is unavailable or impractical for lethal diseases associated with leukocytes. Therefore identification of these anomalies and disorders is important, so as to avoid unnecessary diagnostic testing and treatments.

PELGER-HUËT ANOMALY

Heterozygous Pelger-Huët anomaly (P-H) is a benign congenital disorder of leukocyte development. It is thought to be transmitted as an autosomal dominant trait in dogs and cats; however, incomplete penetrance has been observed in Australian shepherds.[1,2] The heterozygous form is present in dogs and cats because the homozygous form is lethal *in utero*. The homozygous phenotype is characterized by skeletal abnormalities in rabbits; however, the rare humans with P-H homozygotes appear normal and have survived into their nineties.[1]

The distinguishing cytologic characteristic of P-H is hyposegmentation of nuclei in granulocytes and monocytes in the presence of a fully mature, coarsely clumped chromatin pattern.[1] Nuclear morphology often is variable; the nuclei may be round, oval, dumb-bell shaped, peanut shaped, band, or even bilobate.[1] The bilobate shape consists of two nuclear lobes connected by a fine filament, often referred to as a *pince-nez* or *eyeglass* form nucleus.[1] Careful attention to granulocyte morphology and the presence of hyposegmented nuclei in eosinophils and other cell lines may yield indications of this anomaly. Female Barr bodies are absent or extremely rare in P-H.[1]

Pelger-Huët anomaly has been reported sporadically in both mixed-breed and purebred dogs, including Australian shepherds; cocker spaniels; German shepherds; English-American (Walker) foxhounds; Boston terriers; Australian cattle dogs (blue heelers); border collies; basenjis; black and tan, blue tick, and redbone coonhounds; and Samoyeds.[1] An incidence of 9.8% has been reported for Australian shepherds.[2] P-H has been reported in only eight domestic short-hair cats.[1]

Biochemical assays are normal in P-H dogs, including nitro-blue tetrazolium (NBT) dye reduction, hexose monophosphate shunt activity, superoxide generation, chemiluminescence, protein iodination, phagocytosis, and bactericidal activity.[1]

Cytochemical staining with Sudan black B, naphthol ASD chloracetate esterase, peroxidase, alkaline and acid phosphatase, alpha-naphthyl-acetate esterase, and periodic acid–Schiff (PAS) has not detected abnormalities in dog neutrophils.[1]

Ultrastructurally, nuclear changes associated with P-H include nuclear hyposegmentation, nuclear clefts, coarse heterochromatin, and normal cytoplasmic granules.[1]

Hematologic Manifestations

Hematologic manifestations of P-H often are reported as a persistent degenerative left shift without toxic changes. These findings are unexpected on a routine complete blood count (CBC) from a clinically normal animal.[1] Earlier precursors, such as myelocytes, metamyelocytes, and bands, may be reported; however, the chromatin of these cells is fully matured (well clumped).[1] Because P-H often is confused with a degenerative left shift, it is of practical importance that the anomaly be recognized. Unnecessary, expensive, and potentially invasive laboratory tests and treatments can be avoided with proper diagnosis. Many dogs are treated with a variety of antibiotics without response because of this suspected degenerative left shift. A veterinary clinical pathologist can assist in the diagnosis of P-H.

P-H must be differentiated from pseudo–P-H, which often is a transiently acquired condition that resolves with proper diagnosis and treatment.[1] Pseudo–P-H has been associated with a number of diseases, including various forms of leukemia and preleukemic conditions, and with drug therapy, such as with antineoplastic drugs and ibuprofen.[1] Drug-associated changes are idiosyncratic and resolve after treatment is withdrawn.

Treatment

Treatment of P-H is not necessary because neutrophil function is not altered.

CHÉDIAK-HIGASHI SYNDROME

Chédiak-Higashi syndrome (CHS) is a rare inherited autosomal recessive trait found in humans; beige mice; rats; Arctic foxes; a killer whale; Hereford, Japanese black, and brangus cattle; mink; and smoke blue Persian cats.[3-5] This syndrome has not yet been identified in dogs.

CHS is typically characterized by partial oculocutaneous albinism, photophobia, neurologic abnormalities, bleeding abnormalities, and recurrent infections, which generally result in death at an early age.[3] Some researchers have not observed an increased tendency to develop infections in CHS cats, but a colony of CHS cats demonstrated neonatal kittens that were markedly more susceptible to infections (bacterial, viral), and some died from hemorrhage, which contributed to a lower average survival time compared with normal cats.[6] Susceptibility to bacterial infections is associated with multiple defects in the defense system. Neutropenia occurs as a result of impaired marrow release of mature neutrophils. Defective intracellular killing of phagocytosed bacteria also is a factor.[3]

Persian cats with the hereditary genes for CHS have a "blue smoke" coat color that is lighter than the blue smoke coats of Persian cats without CHS.[4] Ocular abnormalities also are present, such as photophobia and lighter irises (light green, light yellow, or light yellow-green). Many affected cats also have congenital cataracts and a red fundic light reflection (compared to the yellowish green of normal Persian cat fundi), as well as less fundic pigmentation.[4] Tapetal regions may not be apparent, and the underlying choroidal vasculature is only partly visible.[4] The tapetal defect is associated with tapetal rod degeneration in tapetal cells in 2- to 4-week-old kittens.[3] Abnormal auditory brain stem responses have been the only neurologic abnormalities identified in CHS cats.[7]

Although the gene abnormality associated with CHS has not been identified in cats, it has been defined as the homologous *beige* gene in mice and humans, which is a 5 kilobase pair deletion.[3] The function of this gene is unknown.[3] CHS was hypothesized to be caused by microtubular formation abnormalities, but this has been disproven.[3]

Hematologic Manifestations

Hematologically, neutrophils, eosinophils, and basophils contain enlarged, lightly eosinophilic cytoplasmic granules that can be observed with Wright's staining (Romanowsky stain).[3] Occasionally, monocytes and lymphocytes may contain a single eosinophilic cytoplasmic granule.[3] Histologically, melanocytes in hair shafts contain enlarged melanin granules, and renal tubular epithelial cells contain enlarged granules.

Prolonged bleeding times (three times normal), manifested as hematomas after surgical procedures, are the result of a platelet storage pool defect (SPD). Impaired platelet aggregation associated with a virtual absence of adenosine diphosphate (ADP) and serotonin (dense granules) may account for the abnormal aggregation.[3] Platelet counts and coagulation times (prothrombin time [PT] and partial thromboplastin time [PTT]) are within reference intervals.[4]

Diagnosis

A presumptive diagnosis can be made by observation of a Persian cat with a light blue smoke color, lightly colored irises, red fundic reflection, depigmented fundic area, and bleeding tendencies.[4] Also, a hair shaft examination can be performed. Hair is extracted from a cat suspected of having CHS and from a normal cat. The hair shafts are placed on a microscopic slide, immersion oil is added, and a cover slip is gently pressed over the hair shafts.[4] Examination under low or high dry power reveals that, unlike the normal hair shaft, the hair of the CHS cat shows enlarged, clumped melanin granules.[4]

With Romanowsky staining, CHS cytoplasmic granules in neutrophils appear as light eosinophilic inclusions that must be differentiated from Döhle bodies associated with neutrophil toxicity.[4] If the composition of the granules is in question, the differentiation can be made using peroxidase staining (CHS granules stain black).[4]

Treatment

Cats with CHS do not require continuing treatment; however, great care should be taken to control hemorrhage due to the platelet SPD and prolonged bleeding times. Platelet transfusions can temporarily correct the bleeding time if surgical procedures are to be performed.[3] Long-term correction of neutrophil and platelet function in CHS is possible only through bone marrow transplantation (BMT).[3] BMT performed in cats has corrected the neutrophil and platelet defects, but no effect has been seen on lysosome distribution in liver or kidney cells.[3] Neutrophil function improves temporarily after treatment with recombinant canine granulocyte-colony stimulating factor (rcG-CSF) or interleukin-2 (IL-2) in cats.[3]

Although the blue smoke coat color is quite beautiful in Persian cats with CHS, this is an undesirable trait to propagate. Breeders should be counseled against using affected cats or carrier cats, which are phenotypically normal. Because CHS is an autosomal recessive trait, both the sire and dam that produce offspring affected with CHS are obligate carriers and should be removed from the breeding stock. Administration of drugs that affect platelet function, such as cyclo-oxygenase inhibitors, is contraindicated in CHS cats.[3]

CANINE LEUKOCYTE ADHESION DEFICIENCY

Canine leukocyte adhesion deficiency (CLAD) is a fatal defect inherited as a homozygous autosomal recessive trait in Irish setters and rare Irish setter–cross-breed dogs. It is characterized by a defect in neutrophil adhesion and function. Heterozygous dogs appear healthy in all respects. Initially, this trait was reported in 1975 as canine granulocytopathy syndrome.[8] An Irish setter had persistent soft tissue infections, lymphadenopathy, omphalophlebitis, gingivitis, and persistent profound leukocytosis (primary neutrophilia).[8]

A 1987 case report identified an Irish setter–cross that did not express leukocyte Mo1, leukocyte function–associated antigen-1 (LFA-1), or Leu M5 glycoproteins using CD11/CD18 antibodies, indicating a common beta$_2$-integrin subunit disorder.[8] A defect in neutrophil chemotaxis, induced aggregation, and phagocytosis of opsonized particles also were detected in this dog.[5]

Clinical Features
Clinical, radiologic, and pathologic information was obtained from a study of 12 Irish setter puppies 8 to 15 weeks of age from six different litters.[9] These dogs presented with generalized lymphadenopathy, gingivitis, salivation, skin lesions (ulcers and local dermatitis), generalized pain, weakness, recurrent fever, vaginitis, poor weight gain, anorexia, emaciation, furunculosis (without the formation of a neutrophilic exudate), dull haircoat, and lameness with bone lesions (thickened mandibula, distal radius, ulna, tibia, and fibula). All the dogs in the study were euthanized and underwent postmortem examination. Histopathology of affected tissues showed a lack of neutrophil infiltration (impaired neutrophilic exudate formation).[9] CLAD dogs do not respond well to antibiotic therapy and thus rarely live beyond 6 months.[9]

Pathologic Features
Neutrophils in dogs with the homozygous form of this hereditary trait have a deficiency of leukocyte surface glycoproteins associated with leukocyte adherence and egress into surrounding tissues.[8,9] These cells appear morphologically normal by light microscopy. Dogs present within weeks of birth with associated clinical signs.

The family of glycoproteins referred to as beta$_2$-integrins (CD11/CD18) consist of alpha subunits (CD11a, CD11b, CD11c, CD11d) noncovalently bonded with a common beta subunit (CD18).[10] These subunits make up CD11a/CD18 (LFA-1; $\alpha_L\beta_2$), CD11b/CD18 (Mac-1/Mo-1; $\alpha_M\beta_2$), CD11c/CD18 (gp 150,95; $\alpha_X\beta_2$), and CD11d/CD18 ($\alpha_d\beta_2$) cell surface receptors.[1] CD8 glycoprotein is critical to formation of the integrin heterodimers for cell-cell adhesion events.[8,10,11] In addition, beta$_2$-integrin heterodimer CD11b/CD18 serves as major receptor for C3b opsonic complement and is necessary for phagocytosis and respiratory burst activation. Heterozygous dogs have normal expression of CD11b/CD18. Failure to express beta$_2$-integrin CD18 is the reason neutrophils are unable to adhere to vascular endothelium and transmigrate in response to released chemotactic factors in inflamed tissues. Because neutrophils cannot adhere to the endothelium, they do not reach the site of infection or inflammation. Recruitment signals from infected or inflamed tissues continue to cause the release of cytokines, stimulating

granulocytopoiesis (production and release of neutrophils). Continued marrow stimulation and inability of neutrophils to adhere result in a persistent leukocytosis (primarily neutrophilia) that occasionally is greater than 100,000/μL.[10] Neutrophil function also was found to be altered by defective bactericidal activity, reduced glucose oxidation by the hexose monophosphate shunt, and increased capacity to reduce NBT dye.[5]

The presence of a single nucleotide missense mutation, resulting in failure to express detectable beta$_2$-integrin CD18, is responsible for clinical disease in Irish setters.[10] CD11b also is absent in affected Irish setters, but CD11c expression was not different from that in control dogs. Whether CD11b is absent because of lack of expression or because of the absence of CD18 is unknown.[11]

Diagnosis
An oligonucleotide ligation assay (OLA), which detects the missense mutation of CD18, was developed to identify carriers of this lethal gene.[12] In one study, screening of 208 Irish setters in the United Kingdom identified 19 carriers, or a 9% carrier rate.[12] This mutation has not been detected in any other breed in which OLA screening was performed.[10] Another study that tested 339 Irish setters from 10 countries (Scandinavia, continental Europe, and Australia) using a newly developed pyrosequencing technique to identify a single mutation in the beta$_2$-integrin gene (CD18) gene, supported the previous single mutation concept found with OLA.[12] The pyrosequencing technique identified 72 heterozygous carriers, as well as two homozygous dogs, which eventually developed CLAD.[12] The pyrosequencing technique also identified carriers and indicated widespread presence of the disorder in many countries.[12] Genetic testing using pyrosequencing can identify heterozygous dogs for removal from breeding lines. Recently, a case of CLAD in an Irish setter–cross was identified using polymerase chain reaction (PCR) testing, and carrier status was identified during a PCR survey in a number of distantly related red and white setters.[8] This PCR detection test identified the same mutation in all CLAD dogs previously tested.[8]

Treatment
No effective treatment has been found for this disorder.

CYCLIC HEMOPOIESIS

Cyclic hemopoiesis (CH), also known as *cyclic hematopoiesis, cyclic neutropenia,* or *gray collie syndrome,* is a lethal, autosomal recessive, hereditary disease of gray collies associated with a dilute haircoat. The condition was first described in the 1960s as the "lethal gray syndrome," and a similar disorder is still called cyclic neutropenia (CN) in human medical texts. CH is a unique disease that affects the marrow pluripotential stem cell; it disrupts normal hemopoiesis, an effect characterized by cyclic changes in neutrophil, monocyte, platelet, eosinophil, and reticulocyte numbers.[13] Heterozygous dogs have a normal coat color and do not have clinical signs of CH.

Hematologic Manifestations
Marked neutropenia that occurs in cycles of 12 to 14 days is associated with severe recurrent bacterial infections at the nadir.[13] Neutrophils may be completely absent from the peripheral circulation for 2 to 4 days, an interval followed by neutrophilia as high as 70,000/μL.[13] Monocytes, eosinophils, lymphocytes, and platelets also cycle at 14-day intervals with normal to high cell counts but are out of phase with neutrophils with absent to high fluctuating cell counts.[13,14] Interestingly, hemopoietic growth factors such as erythropoietin,

thrombopoietin, granulocyte colony-stimulating factor (G-CSF), IL-1, and IL-6 concentrations also fluctuate in this disorder.[13] A microcytic, normochromic anemia is present on the CBC.

Changes in marrow aspirates, which occur in an alternating myeloid to erythroid ratio pattern, precede changes in the peripheral cell counts, suggesting a marrow stem cell disorder.[13]

Clinical Features

CH dogs all have gray or diluted coat color, often are smaller than littermates at birth, and usually present at 6 to 8 weeks of age with recurring episodes of neutropenia, accompanied by clinical signs such as fever, gingivitis, gingival ulcers, lymphadenopathy, excessive bleeding, pneumonia, ocular and nasal mucopurulent discharge, diarrhea, subcutaneous abscesses, conjunctivitis, keratitis, adenitis, anorexia, weight loss (malabsorption), lethargy, and intermittent lameness.[13,15] Neonatal deaths may result from omphalophlebitis or pneumonia.[13] Younger dogs with CH often die of overwhelming infection; those housed in a laboratory setting often die of hepatic and renal amyloidosis associated with organ failure.[15] Systemic amyloidosis is a prominent feature in CH and has been found in dogs as young as 8 weeks old; nearly 100% of dogs older than 30 weeks are affected.[14] Organs affected include the kidneys, liver, spleen, pancreas, adrenal glands, and intestinal submucosa.[15] Amyloidosis has been attributed to cyclic activation of the acute-phase response by cytokines produced during periods of monocytosis, with interrelated hormonal, immune, and endocrine interactions.[13] Serum amyloid A protein, as well as fibrinogen, von Willebrand factor, and other acute-phase proteins, are produced and circulated during the monocytosis.[13] Rarely do affected gray collies reach sexual maturity.[15]

Pathologic Features

The definitive pathogenesis of CH in gray collies is unknown; however, impaired marrow progenitor cell survival in CN in humans has been observed, and a defect in G-CSF signal transduction has been suggested.[16,17] In addition, ultrastructural, genetic, and molecular studies in humans with CN suggest that the disorder is due to mutations in a neutrophil azurophilic (primary) granule enzyme, neutrophil elastase (ELA-2).[16,17] A 75% decrease in early myeloid-committed colonies associated with accelerated spontaneous apoptosis was observed compared with controls. It was concluded that ineffective production of neutrophils is due to accelerated apoptosis of bone marrow progenitor cells, with conformational changes in protein structure resulting in alterations in subcellular functions or substrate specificity and/or binding properties of neutrophil elastase.[16]

Although the hereditary pattern of CN is autosomal dominant in humans and autosomal recessive in gray collies, similar marrow and genetic changes may occur, but this remains to be proved.

CH in gray collies appears to be a hormonally inter-related disease with wide fluctuation of cytokines and responsive changes in the marrow. Furthermore, CH can be transferred to healthy dogs by BMT, which supports the theory of a disorder of the pluripotential stem cell.[13]

CH dogs also have a platelet storage pool disease characterized by a lack of dense granules (serotonin and Ca^{+2}), resulting in aggregation defects; however, prolonged bleeding times have not been reported.[13] Administration of rcG-CSF corrects the hemopoietic fluctuations but does not correct the SPD, which suggests that these defects are not secondary to CH.[13]

Treatment

Fluctuations of all cell lines resolve in CH dogs treated with rcG-CSF, with neutrophilia occurring at higher doses.[14]

Also, recombinant canine stem cell factor (rcSCF) at high doses (i.e., equal to or greater than 20 μg/kg/24 hours) eliminated neutropenic periods and blunted oscillations, but neutrophilia only occurred at doses of 100 μg/kg/24 hours.[18] Treatment with a combination of rcSCF (20 to 50 μg/kg/24 hours) and rcG-CSF (0.5 to 1.0 μg/kg/24 hours) indicated a synergistic effect, with neutrophil counts above those of either drug given separately.[18] Long-term therapy was effective without untoward side effects. The risk of neutralizing antibody formation can arise with chronic administration of recombinant human G-CSF (rhG-CSF).[13] Early BMT eliminates cell cycling and produces a clinical cure. Treatment with lithium or endotoxin injections eliminates cell cycling, but unwanted side effects can occur. Administration of granulocyte-macrophage colony-stimulating factor (GM-CSF) and IL-3 administration are mildly effective but do not prevent cycling. Glucocorticoids, androgens, and intravenous gamma globulin are ineffective at treating this condition.[14,15,18]

CH is a highly undesirable trait in collies. Because it is an autosomal recessive trait, both the sire and dam that produce affected offspring are obligate carriers and should be removed from the breeding stock. Heterozygous dogs are phenotypically normal, therefore breeders should be counseled against using carriers. Laboratory tests are not available, and test mating is the only method of identifying carriers. Gray collies may not appear at every breeding; therefore, for a dog to be declared free of this trait, it must be mated with a known heterozygote and produce 16 normal pups. This is both expensive and impractical.

Normal canine neutrophil elastase deoxyribonucleic acid (DNA) sequence has been reported, and studies are ongoing to determine if the ELA-2 gene in CH has mutations similar to those in humans with CN. A PCR test may be developed, and a more practical, inexpensive test to identify heterozygous dogs may be offered. Testing has been done only on humans affected with CN and has not been used to identify carriers of this trait.

BIRMAN CAT NEUTROPHIL GRANULATION ANOMALY

Birman cats are an exotic, long-haired breed with Siamese-type coloring and four distinctive white paws. Neutrophil granulation anomaly is a hereditary trait characterized by increased granularity of neutrophils. It is transmitted in an autosomal recessive manner in purebred Birman cats.[5,19] The cytoplasm of affected neutrophils contains numerous fine, normal-sized, deep pink to purple granules that appear similar to azurophilic granules found in promyelocytes. Neutrophil function is not compromised.[19] Normally, azurophilic granules become indistinct with Romanowsky stain in the myelocyte stage of development but seem to persist throughout the maturing process in this anomaly.[19]

Ultrastructurally, granules are elongated and dumb-bell shaped and do not stain for mucopolysaccharides. Bactericidal activity is no different from that of unaffected neutrophils, and other peripheral leukocytes appear morphologically normal.[19] Neutrophilic cytoplasmic granules observed in cats with certain mucopolysaccharide storage diseases (MPS types VI and VII) appear larger.[19] The abnormality therefore was concluded to be an alteration in the contents of cytoplasmic granules, with increased affinity for acid dyes without clinical consequences.[19] Treatment is not necessary, because functional abnormalities are not noted. The main concern is to differentiate this anomaly from MPS (types VI and VII) and toxic granulation.[5] A study of 78 highly inbred Birman cats found that 46% of the cats were affected.[19]

HYPEREOSINOPHILIC SYNDROME

Hypereosinophilic syndrome (HES) is a disease of unknown origin that occurs primarily in cats. It is questionable whether the disorder occurs in dogs, although one case of disseminated eosinophilic disease similar to idiopathic HES was recently reported.[20] Characteristics of this disease are persistent peripheral eosinophilia and organ infiltration by eosinophils, which eventually cause organ failure and death.[21,22] The bone marrow, spleen, liver, mesenteric lymph nodes, and gastrointestinal tract were the organs reported to contain eosinophilic infiltrates most frequently.[21,22] Difficulty arises in distinguishing between HES and eosinophilic leukemia (EL), because the two conditions may be variants of the same disease.[21] In one study, a female predisposition for HES was reported in cats (male to female ratio of 4:11).[21]

Hematologic Manifestations

The presentations of HES and EL are similar. Peripheral blood eosinophil examination and bone marrow aspiration may be helpful in differentiating the disorders. With EL there often are more immature eosinophils in the peripheral blood, which results in a more severe anemia. The myeloid to erythroid (M:E) ratio in bone marrow is greater than 10:1.[21,22] Peripheral eosinophil counts in HES range from $3500/\mu L$ to $130,000/\mu L$, and the cells appear mature. Occasionally, mild anemia also is present.[21,22]

Clinical Features

Clinical signs, which are relatively nonspecific and vary with the organ or organs affected, include diarrhea, weight loss, anorexia, pyrexia, and pruritus.[21,22] It is difficult to establish the longevity of cats with HES; however, some cats may have exhibited clinical signs related to HES for 3.5 years.[22]

Physical and Pathologic Features

Physical findings are variable and include thickened bowel loops, abdominal masses, lymphadenopathy, and/or cutaneous disorders. As mentioned previously, the organs most commonly infiltrated with eosinophils are the bone marrow, gastrointestinal tract, spleen, mesenteric lymph nodes, and liver, but any organ can be affected.[21,22]

Treatment

HES is a progressively fatal disease that has no effective treatment. However, Gleevec (imatinib mesylatem, formerly STI571) has been used in humans with excellent results. Corticosteroids, hydroxyurea, and alpha interferon also have been used in humans with variable results; however, when these drugs are effective, unwanted side effects are common.

SEVERE COMBINED IMMUNODEFICIENCY IN JACK RUSSELL TERRIERS

Severe combined immunodeficiency (SCID) was recently described as an autosomal recessive trait in a litter of Jack Russell terriers. Twelve of 32 siblings died of opportunistic infections between 8 and 14 weeks of age.[23] An additional litter was whelped, and four of seven pups displayed SCID, characterized by lymphopenia, agammaglobulinemia, thymic dysplasia, and peripheral lymphoid aplasia.[23] A deficiency of DNA-dependent–protein kinase catalytic subunit (DNA-PKcs), an enzyme involved in DNA repair, occurs.[23] DNA-PKcs deficiency results in faulty V(D)J recombination.[23] Combinations of the V(D)J gene segment recombinations are very important for diversification of antigen-binding sites of antibodies.[23] Blocking of this V(D)J recombination arrests lymphocyte development at the prolymphocyte stage; the result is nonfunctional B and T lymphocytes, agammaglobulinemia and, consequently, SCID.[23]

Treatment

Bone marrow transplantation is the only option; however, gene therapy appears promising for future treatment.

CANINE X-LINKED SEVERE COMBINED IMMUNODEFICIENCY

Canine X-linked severe combined immunodeficiency (X-SCID) is an autosomal recessive, lethal, inherited trait with some unique modes of inheritance. Female carriers of the X-SCID gene typically appear normal. They contain only one copy of the γc gene and are unable to produce normal protein, but they have a second "normal" gene that produces adequate protein for normal function.[24] Because males retain only one copy of the X chromosome, they cannot produce normal protein when the abnormal gene is inherited, and thus are affected. Because transmission of only one X chromosome is necessary for this trait to appear, carrier females need not breed with an affected male.[24]

Clinical Features

Affected dogs are male, fail to thrive, and present with recurrent or chronic infections near the time of waning maternal antibodies.[24] Clinical signs are more evident as the pups get older. Recurrent infections, which begin around 6 to 8 weeks of age, include pyoderma, diarrhea, and respiratory infections.[24] Infections are usually bacterial, are unresponsive to antibiotics, and eventually become overwhelming systemic infections.[24] These dogs rarely survive beyond 3 to 4 months of age and usually die of a generalized staphylococcal infection.[24] Several X-SCID dogs, inadvertently vaccinated with a modified live distemper virus vaccine, died rapidly of vaccine-induced distemper.[24] One dog raised in a gnotobiotic environment developed acute monocytic leukemia at 20 months of age.[24]

Pathologic Features

A small, dysplastic thymus that weighs about 10% that of age-matched controls is the primary feature of X-SCID dogs.[24]

Immunologic Abnormalities

Although X-SCID dogs have reduced lymphocyte counts, profound lymphopenia is not a prominent finding (counts commonly are greater than $1000/\mu L$).[24] When tested by fluorescence-activated cell sorting (FACS) analysis, newborn X-SCID dogs have peripheral lymphocyte phenotypes consisting of elevated B cells and markedly reduced or absent T cells.[24] Absolute numbers of peripheral T cells are decreased even though the relative percentages are normal.[24] The T-lymphocyte blastogenic response to T-cell mitogens and specific antigens is markedly depressed to absent.[24] X-SCID dogs also are hypogammaglobulinemic. Concentrations of immunoglobulin M (IgM) are normal, but IgG concentrations are dramatically reduced, and IgA antibodies are absent.[24]

Treatment

Bone marrow transplantation is the only treatment option for complete resolution of this disorder in dogs; however, gene therapy may be promising in the future. Transplantation has been attempted with some success, but these dogs developed cutaneous papillomas within 1 year.[24] An understanding of the hereditary and genetic basis of X-SCID and proper client and breeder counseling are highly recommended to control or eliminate this disorder in future generations.

DEFECTIVE NEUTROPHIL FUNCTION IN THE DOBERMAN PINSCHER

Eight intensively line-bred Doberman pinschers developed chronic respiratory disease (rhinitis and pneumonia) and occasional skin disease (seborrhea sicca).[25] In all the dogs, neutrophils were normal in number and appearance.[24] The neutrophils were found to have normal phagocytosis but defective bactericidal activity, as determined by the NBT test.[25] Immunoglobulins were normal to increased; lymphocyte function was normal for the mitogens in seven of eight dogs; neutrophil chemotaxis was normal; and complement C_3 concentrations were increased. Superoxide production was normal, except that opsonized zymosan stimulation produced less superoxide than in controls.[25]

Treatment

Many of these dogs survived for years and responded well to intermittent antibiotic therapy for recurrent bacterial infections of the respiratory tract.[25] The mode of inheritance was not determined due to inadequate pedigree and documentation.[24] The actual cause of the disorder was not determined. The condition somewhat resembles chronic granulomatous disease (CGD) or C_3b receptor deficiency in humans, but those diseases are usually life-threatening, unlike the disease in these Dobermans.[25]

LETHAL ACRODERMATITIS IN BULL TERRIERS

Lethal acrodermatitis in bull terriers is an autosomal recessive, inherited lethal trait with similarities to lethal trait A46 in Black Pied Danish cattle and acrodermatitis enteropathica in humans.[26]

Clinical Features

Lighter pigmentation at birth, growth retardation, progressive acrodermatitis, chronic pyoderma, chronic paronychia, diarrhea, pneumonia, and behavioral changes are observed on presentation, with historical evidence of deglutition and disordered mastication.[26] Behavioral changes include early aggressiveness, diminished activity, and prolonged staring at objects. These dogs have a median survival time of 7 months.[26] Laboratory findings include neutrophilia, consistently low alkaline phosphatase (observed in zinc deficiency) and alanine aminotransferase activities, low serum zinc concentrations, and frequent hypercholesterolemia.[26]

Pathologic Features

Skin lesions include parakeratosis, hyperkeratosis, and pyoderma. T-lymphocyte numbers were significantly reduced in lymphoid tissues.[26] Lymphocyte blastogenesis responses were decreased, and dysgammaglobulinemia was present.[26] Neutrophilic, phagocytic, and bactericidal activities were normal.[26]

Treatment

No effective treatment has been described. The response to high-dose zinc supplementation was poor.[26]

IMMUNODEFICIENCY OF SHAR PEIS

Immunodeficiency of Chinese Shar Peis is a recently described, late-onset, multiple immunodeficiency syndrome involving antibody and cell-mediated responses of unknown origin associated with recurrent infections and malignancy.[27]

Clinical Features

The mean age of clinical onset was 3 years (range, 4 months to 8 years).[27] The clinical presentation involves several organ systems and includes intermittent fever, recurrent skin infections, respiratory infections, and gastrointestinal abnormalities, including ulcerative colitis. Several dogs developed intestinal adenocarcinoma, lymphoma, and paracortical lymphocyte depletion.[27]

Immunologic Manifestations

Deficiencies in immunoglobulin concentrations, specifically IgM, IgA, and occasionally IgG, were identified.[27] B- and T-cell abnormalities were observed in affected dogs, including deficiencies in lymphocyte proliferation that occurred concurrently with normal or increased percentages of T- and B-cell lymphocytes, decreased median stimulation index of blastogenesis, and decreased in vitro responsiveness of peripheral blood mononuclear cells to pokeweed mitogen.[27] Also, when serum from affected Shar Peis was added to cell cultures from normal dogs, a suppressive effect was seen.[27]

Even with the variety of clinical presentations, nearly all affected dogs were characterized by a common deficiency involving cell-mediated and immunoglobulin deficiencies.[27]

Diagnosis

Assessment of the immunologic profile, along with the signalment, history, and clinical data, helps identify affected Shar Peis. However, given the high prevalence of healthy Shar Peis with low IgA concentrations, this finding alone cannot identify affected immunodeficient dogs.[27]

Treatment

Supportive care is the current treatment and should be given until the cause of this disorder can be completely classified.

IMMUNODEFICIENCY OF WEIMARANERS

Weimaraners affected with immunodeficiency have been reported, including an initial inbred group with thymic abnormalities and growth hormone deficiency.[28] Many other weimaraners subsequently were described with in vitro neutrophil abnormalities and decreased IgG and IgM.[29] One dog also had neutrophilic phagocytic dysfunction.[30] Affected weimaraners present with varying but recurrent infections that occasionally respond to antibiotics, but these dogs often die of recurrent infections within a year. Inbreeding has not been noted except in the original thymic deficiency group; however, one sire was implicated in five affected dogs (including two pairs of litter mates) and also was the grandsire of two other affected dogs.[31] Siblings of this dog also produced two affected dogs.[31] Obvious genetic associations are present, and many abnormalities have been identified, but no single specific disorder. The recurrent nature of this disorder may indicate a periodicity to the defect, which potentially makes specific detection difficult.[31]

Clinical Features

Weimaraners are presented for veterinary care between the ages of 3 and 42 months (average age is 10 months). Body condition and size are normal, but the dog has a variety of disorders, including acute onset of high fever; profound depression; vomiting; diarrhea; pain in the joints, spine, or abdomen; lymphadenopathy; bleeding tendencies, mainly in the form of epistaxis; hematemesis; melena; hematochezia; hematuria; dacryohemorrhysis (bloody tears); marked congestion and ulceration of mucous membranes; conjunctivitis; pedal pyoderma; recurrent subcutaneous masses thought to be associated with subcutaneous injection sites; and neurologic signs (ataxia, disorientation, head pressing, seizures and Horner syndrome). Episodes of sickness occur every 2 weeks to 7 months, with clinically normal intermediate periods or incomplete recovery. The recurring episodes of clinical illness often respond rapidly to antibiotics and/or corticosteroids but eventually become unresponsive, and death usually occurs within 1 year.[31]

Hematologic Manifestations

Leukocytosis is observed, ranging from 31,000/μL to 64,200/μL, with a distribution of 72% to 92% neutrophils (mature and immature).[31] White blood cell (WBC) counts between episodes are normal or mildly elevated. Normal WBC morphology is observed by light and electron microscopy. Clotting times are within reference interval.[31]

Immunologic Manifestations

In the dogs studied, significant abnormalities were not noted in metabolic or phagocytic function, but glucose oxidation showed high resting levels consistent with an infection at the time of testing.[31] A single case report identified decreased neutrophil phagocytosis using opsonized *Escherichia coli* labeled with fluorescein isothiocyanate.[30] Other *in vitro* testing revealed decreased neutrophil chemoluminescence and decreased IgG and IgM concentrations.[29]

Diagnosis

A presumptive diagnosis is based on recurrent presentation of a young weimaraner that becomes progressively less responsive to treatment. Specific testing to identify diseased individuals is not available. Test mating, with careful evaluation and observance of the progeny for immunologic abnormalities, may be the only way to identify a defect.

Treatment

Supportive care has been the only treatment used. Bone marrow transplants have not been attempted.

LYSOSOMAL STORAGE DISEASES

Many lysosomal storage diseases (LSDs) have been identified in dogs and cats; however, all are rare, and only a few present with microscopic abnormalities in peripheral blood leukocytes. Only the observable leukocyte morphologic changes are discussed. Specific leukocyte activity has not been tested, but delineation of microscopic characteristics may be a simple method of identifying and/or classifying many storage diseases.

Hematologic alterations in the leukocytes of dogs and cats are associated with sphingomyelinosis (Niemann-Pick disease); alpha-mannosidosis; mucopolysaccharidosis (MPS) I, VI, and VII; GM$_1$-gangliosidosis; GM$_2$-gangliosidosis; and fucosidosis.

Leukocytes in MPS I, VI, and VII must be differentiated from toxic changes in neutrophils and from Birman cat neutrophil granulation anomaly.

Sphingomyelinosis has been reported in Siamese, Balinese, and domestic shorthair cats, as well as in boxer dogs and a miniature poodle. The disease is caused by a deficiency of sphingomyelinase, which results in accumulation of sphingomyelin, cholesterol, and gangliosides in the brain, liver, spleen, and bone marrow. Large, vacuolated macrophages may be observed in the peripheral blood.

Alpha-mannosidosis, reported in Persian, domestic shorthair, and domestic longhair cats, is caused by a deficiency of alpha-mannosidase, which leads to accumulation of mannose oligosaccharides in the central nervous system, skeleton, and spleen. Lymphocytes, granulocytes, and monocytes in peripheral blood appear vacuolated.[32]

MPS I occurs in Plott hounds, other breeds of dogs, and domestic shorthair cats. This LSD is caused by a deficiency of alpha-L-iduronidase. Some observers have reported small, pink granules in neutrophil cytoplasm.[33]

MPS VI is reported in Siamese cats and in miniature schnauzers, miniature pinschers, and Welsh corgis. This LSD is caused by a deficiency of arylsulfatase. Peripheral neutrophils, lymphocytes, basophils, eosinophils, and monocytes are affected. The cytoplasm of neutrophils often appears foamy and contains uniform small, metachromatic granules, often within a vacuole.[32] Lymphocytes in MPS VI have been divided into three distinct types: normal appearing, those containing vacuoles with small, dark, metachromatic granules; and a few containing empty vacuoles.[32] Nearly all monocytes contain vacuoles, and a moderate percentage have dark granules in these vacuoles.[32] Eosinophils contain cytoplasmic vacuoles, and basophils contain large, reddish purple cytoplasmic inclusions or granules.[32] Basophils have the largest granules.[32]

MPS VII, reported in the dog and domestic shorthair cat, is caused by a deficiency of beta glucuronidase. Neutrophils and lymphocytes contain deep purple cytoplasmic inclusions that should not be confused with toxic changes. Granules stain purple with toluidine blue dye.[33]

GM$_1$-gangliosidosis has been reported in domestic shorthair, Korat, and Siamese cats, as well as in English springer spaniels, Portuguese water dogs, beagles, and Alaskan huskies. It is caused by a deficiency in beta galactosidase. Lymphocytes contain small, distinct, clear cytoplasmic vacuoles.[33]

GM$_2$-gangliosidosis, reported in domestic shorthair and Korat cats and in German shorthaired pointer dogs, is caused by a deficiency of beta hexosaminidase. Neutrophils contain dark blue granules, and lymphocytes contain prominent azurophilic cytoplasmic granules.[33]

Fucosidosis of English springer spaniels is caused by a deficiency of alpha-L-fucosidase. The lymphocytes of these dogs contain cytoplasmic vacuoles.[33]

HEMATOLOGY AND IMMUNOLOGY

CHAPTER 276

Non-Neoplastic Diseases of the Spleen

Helio Autran de Morais
Robert T. O'Brien

"Spleen is like the tongue of an ox [or] the sole of the foot; slightly bowed out on the left side, a little concave on the inner side, toward the stomach. It has an uneven surface and is a little rough with some tubercles ..."

"Similarly [according to] other physicians the spleen [is] the receptacle of melancholy as the gall bladder of gall; wherefore the spleen causes one to laugh."

William Harvey (1653)

For many years, the ability to laugh was considered a sign that the spleen was working well. Regarded as the repository of the most noxious substance of the body, black bile (in Greek, *melanos kholis*), the spleen prevented the onset of melancholia by containing the bodily fluid that produced this mental state. Our understanding of the spleen has greatly improved over the past centuries. However, evaluation of this organ remains mostly morphologic, based on palpation, radiographs and, especially, ultrasound examination, followed by cytology or histopathology. No biochemical tests have been designed to assess splenic function. Consequently, although splenomegaly is common in clinical practice, it often is hard to isolate the cause.

PREVALENCE OF SPLENIC DISEASE IN DOGS AND CATS

The prevalence of splenic disorders in dogs and cats cannot be easily estimated. Splenomegaly may be asymptomatic, and in the absence of splenomegaly, it is difficult to determine, on the basis of clinical signs, that the spleen is responsible for the animal's condition. Most prevalence studies in dogs and cats are based on either necropsy or biopsy findings. Necropsy-based studies overestimate diseases with a poor prognosis or with no clinical relevance. Diseases that are treated by surgery are overestimated in prevalence studies based on biopsies but are underestimated in prevalence studies based on necropsy data. This might explain the absence of hemangiosarcoma and the low ratio of hemangiosarcoma to hematoma in necropsy studies in dogs. Based on biopsy samples submitted to a regional diagnostic laboratory from 1372 dogs[1] and 455 cats,[2] spleen samples from dogs represented 1.3% of all submissions, and spleen samples from cats represented 0.3%. However, these percentages do not represent true prevalence, because biopsies from all species were included in the total submission number.[1]

In two necropsy surveys, non-neoplastic diseases represented approximately 50% of feline splenic disorders.[2,3] Congestion, lymphoid hyperplasia, capsulitis, extramedullary hematopoiesis, and hyperplastic nodules accounted for more than 50% of the cats with non-neoplastic splenic disease. Unfortunately, those were pathologic descriptions, and the underlying disease was not apparent in many cases. In two retrospective studies that looked at the prevalence of arrhythmias in dogs with splenic masses,[4,5] hematomas were found in 17%[5] to 44%[4] of the cases. In a prospective study that looked at the prevalence of arrhythmias in dogs undergoing splenectomy, 38% of the dogs had neoplasia and 32% had hematomas.[6] Nodular hyperplasia, immune-mediated disease unresponsive to medical therapy, and splenic torsion each accounted for 10% of the cases. Nodular hyperplasia, hematoma, extramedullary hematopoiesis, congestion, and lymphoid hyperplasia were the most common non-neoplastic lesions found in the spleens of dogs at necropsy or biopsy.[1,7-9] In a lifetime study of beagles chronically exposed to radioactive radium and strontium, splenic abnormalities were present in 105 of the 865 dogs. Hyperplastic nodules, with or without hematoma, and diffuse lymphoreticular hyperplasia accounted for 66% of the splenomegaly found in these dogs.

Thus the ratio of non-neoplastic to neoplastic splenic disease in dogs varies among studies. Populations that included all cases of splenomegaly or masses[1,8] show a higher than 50% prevalence of non-neoplastic diseases. A higher prevalence of tumors is found in populations that underwent splenectomy[6,9] and in dogs with splenic masses and arrhythmias.[4,5] Non-neoplastic masses, therefore, are as common as neoplastic masses in the spleen of dogs, and the importance of hemangiosarcoma has been overemphasized.[10]

CLINICAL MANIFESTATIONS OF SPLENIC DISEASES

Owner complaints for dogs and cats with splenic disorders are usually vague, and these signs may arise from the primary disease. Common complaints include vomiting, anorexia, weakness, collapse, abdominal enlargement, and weight loss. Polyuria and polydipsia may occur; the mechanism is unclear, but it resolves after splenectomy. Clinical signs are usually related to abdominal distention caused by a mass, uniform splenomegaly, or intra-abdominal bleeding. Lethargy and collapse may occur as a result of hypovolemia, arrhythmias, or anemia.

Signs related to the underlying disorder may also be present (Box 276-1). Ventricular tachyarrhythmias appear to be highly prevalent in dogs with splenic masses (hematoma, hemangiosarcoma, or leiomyosarcoma).[4-6] Particularly if the mass has ruptured.[6] Dogs that undergo splenectomy, regardless of the reason, are also prone to arrhythmias during and after surgery.[6]

The most reliable clinical sign of splenic disease is palpable splenomegaly. However, not all splenomegalies are abnormal. Breed variations in spleen size exist, particularly in dogs. For example, German shepherds have larger spleens; in some other breeds (e.g., miniature schnauzer, cocker spaniel, greyhound) the spleen is located more caudally in the abdomen and may be perceived as enlarged under palpation.[11] Not all enlarged spleens are palpable.

The major laboratory abnormalities accompanying splenic disease are related to the underlying systemic illness.

Box • 276-1

Clinical Signs of Splenic Disease in Dogs and Cats

Abdominal distention
- Splenomegaly
- Splenic mass
- Intra-abdominal bleeding

Arrhythmias

Nonspecific signs and signs of the underlying disorder
- Lethargy
- Weakness
- Collapse
- Anorexia
- Polyuria/polydipsia
- Diarrhea
- Pale mucous membranes
- Jaundice

Changes in blood cell counts may be due to the primary disease or may be caused by the abnormal spleen. Erythrocyte counts are usually normal or decreased but can be increased in patients with splenomegaly associated with polycythemia vera.[12] Schistocytosis, which is highly indicative of a neoplastic splenic disorder, was observed in 23% of patients with splenic tumors but in only 3% of dogs with non-neoplastic disease.[9] Granulocyte and platelet counts also can be decreased, normal, or increased.

Extramedullary hematopoiesis can occur in the spleen. Because the spleen is capable of hematopoiesis but does not retain the normal inhibitory mechanisms present in the bone marrow, it releases young blood cells into the circulation.[10] Increased nucleated red blood cells and immature white blood cells (leukoerythroblastic effect) may appear in the peripheral blood in patients with splenic disorders.

Diagnostic Approach to a Patient with Splenomegaly

Splenomegaly can be detected by physical examination or by abdominal radiographs or ultrasound. Although splenomegaly can be identified by palpation, the severity of the enlargement cannot be reliably assessed in dogs with this technique alone. Differentiating between a splenic mass (localized splenomegaly with at least one large mass) and diffuse splenomegaly (uniform enlargement of the spleen) helps narrow the number of potential diagnoses (Box 276-2). Fine needle aspiration of the spleen may secure the final diagnosis or characterize the type of inflammation present. A sequential approach to diagnosis of the origin of the splenic mass, splenomegaly, or splenic nodular disease, using ultrasonographic findings and cytology, is shown in Figures 276-1, 276-2, and 276-3, respectively.

Abdominal Radiography

Radiographically the spleen is apparent in both dogs and cats. The dorsal extremity (head) is commonly seen on ventrodorsal projections in the cranial left abdomen caudal to the gastric fundus and cranial to the left kidney along the left body wall. On this projection, the splenic head is triangularly shaped. The body of the spleen may be directed transversely across the abdomen immediately caudal to the stomach, along the left body wall, or anywhere in between. In dogs the ventral aspect (tail) is often seen along the ventral body wall immediately caudal to the liver in the lateral projection.

Distension of the stomach may caudally displace the tail. The tail of the spleen is uncommonly seen in cats.

Generalized splenomegaly may increase splenic length. The spleen may also fold up from the ventral wall, extending to varying lengths up the right body wall, or it may expand more caudally, toward the urinary bladder. In the cat, visualization of the splenic tail along the ventral body wall supports a diagnosis of splenomegaly. Alternatively, with generalized enlargement or focal masses, the spleen produces a mass effect, causing caudal displacement of intestines. The spleen is a very common origin for masses in the midcranial and left cranial abdomen. Atypical splenic location, with changes in shape, may occur in dogs with splenic torsion. Concurrent peritoneal effusion is common. Lesions rarely cause changes in splenic radiopacity.

Abdominal Ultrasonography

Ultrasonography is a very effective tool for evaluating the size, shape, and vascular supply of the spleen. There are no objective criteria for normal splenic size. As a rule, cats have a much smaller spleen than dogs of similar size. Normal variations in dogs include capsular invagination (hyperechoic foci adjacent to splenic veins), a bent spleen, or a portion folded back upon itself. Generalized isoechoic enlargement may be a normal variation in German shepherds and other dog breeds and in some cats. Overall spleen length and evidence of intestinal displacement are the criteria used to assess for splenomegaly. A true decrease in splenic size (microsplenia) may occur with acute anemia due to contraction of the spleen. Ultrasonography is more sensitive than radiography for detecting alterations in the shape and outer margination of the spleen. Irregularities in shape and focal changes in echogenicity are the major criteria for characterization of splenic disease in dogs and cats.

Nodular disease is easily detected in the middle and tail regions of the spleen. Often the head of the spleen is within the rib cage, and masses in the dorsal extremity may require a rigorous examination using an intercostal approach. Benign masses may be hypoechoic, hyperechoic or mixed echoic. Benign masses cannot be differentiated from malignant masses with grey scale ultrasonography alone. Extramedullary hematopoiesis and nodular hyperplasia (Figure 276-4), which are common regenerative lesions, are usually hypoechoic and are seen in the spleens of older dogs. These lesions are much less common in cats.

Certain lesions have a more characteristic sonographic appearance. Myelolipoma, a benign tumor seen in older dogs, is both very echogenic and attenuating. The result is a classic hyperechoic and indistinctly shadowing lesion (Figure 276-5). Unlike with mineralization, the attenuation is not complete, and the internal architecture of the lesion can be seen to varying depths.

The spleen has a high prevalence for vascular disease because it is attached at only one pole and is prone to harbor diffuse neoplasia. Splenic torsion and diffuse tumor invasion may result in uniform diffuse hypoechogenicity or a more mixed "Swiss cheese" appearance (Figure 276-6). In suspected cases of torsion or thromboembolism, Doppler examination of the splenic veins is an important step for verifying lack of venous return. As with portal vein flow, splenic venous flow is low velocity and essentially nonpulsatile. Power Doppler examination is especially valuable, because this modality is more sensitive to very low velocity flow. Thrombosis may occur after mechanical torsion or tumor vascular invasion or with thromboembolic diseases. Regional infarctions are commonly seen in dogs with disseminated intravascular coagulation (DIC) and autoimmune conditions, such as immune-mediated hemolytic anemia and immune-mediated thrombocytopenia. Infarcted regions are usually peripheral, hypoechoic, and swollen (Figure 276-7). Necrosis, which may be seen with

HEMATOLOGY AND IMMUNOLOGY

Box • 276-2

*Causes of Splenomegaly in Dogs and Cats**

Splenic mass (asymmetric, or nonuniform, splenomegaly)
> **Nodular hyperplasia**
> > **Lympoid type**
> > Fibrohistiocytic type (D)
> **Hematoma**
> Neoplasia
> Abscess
> Extramedullary hematopoiesis (C)
> Granuloma

Uniform (symmetric) splenomegaly
> **Congestion**
> > **Drugs**
> > **Portal hypertension**
> > **Right-sided congestive heart failure**
> > Splenic torsion

Hyperplasia†
> **Chronic infection**
> Inflammatory bowel disease
> Systemic lupus erythematosus
> Polycythemia vera

Extramedullary hematopoiesis†
> **Chronic anemia**
> **Immune-mediated hemolytic anemia**
> **Immune-mediated thrombocytopenia**
> Neoplasia

Neoplasia

Non-neoplastic infiltrative diseases
> **Neoplasia**
> Hypereosinophilic syndrome (C)
> Amyloidosis

Inflammatory causes‡
> **Suppurative**

Sepsis
Bacterial endocarditis
Infectious canine hepatitis
Toxoplasmosis
Foreign body
Penetrating wounds
Neoplasia

Granulomatous
> Cryptococcosis
> Histoplasmosis (C)
> Mycobacteriosis
> Leishmaniasis

Pyogranulomatous
> **FIP (C)**
> Blastomycosis
> Sporotrichosis

Eosinophilic
> Eosinophilic gastroenteritis
> Hypereosinophilic syndrome (C)
> Neoplasia

Lymphoplasmacytic
> **Ehrlichiosis**
> **Hemotropic mycoplasmosis (C)**
> **Lymphoplasmacytic enteritis**
> Pyometra
> Brucellosis

Necrotic tissue
> Torsion
> Necrotic center of neoplasms
> Infectious canine hepatitis (D)
> Anaerobic infection
> Tularemia
> Salmonellosis

*More common diseases are in boldface.
†The causes of extramedullary hematopoiesis and hyperplasia can overlap.
‡The typical inflammatory response for each organism; some degree of overlap exists.
C, Cats; D, dogs.

chronic severe vascular disease, results in the formation of free gas in the spleen and free fluid in the peritoneum.

An additional ultrasonographic modality for evaluation of focal nodular and vascular diseases of the spleen is contrast harmonic ultrasonography. With this technique, second-generation ultrasound contrast agents, which are liposome-encapsulated inert gas spheres, are injected intravenously; these agents are small enough (3 to 5 μm) to pass through the pulmonary circulation without causing embolization. Harmonic ultrasound software technology allows detection of sound waves that are multiples of the transmitted frequency. Ultrasonographic contrast bubbles are very powerful generators of harmonic frequencies, and combined with tissue signal suppression, they create a novel method for imaging perfusion of organs. These contrast media, which can be used as blood pool agents, cause infarcted regions to appear hypoechoic compared with the surrounding normally perfused spleen. Preliminary studies indicate that ultrasound contrast agents may help discriminate between malignant and benign masses by exploiting differences in blood supply. Hemangiosarcomas have very poor overall perfusion and distinct peripheral vessels. This perfusion pattern has been noted in hemangiosarcomas in the liver, lung, peritoneum, and spleen. In the liver, metastatic nodules have a more rapid wash-in and wash-out compared to normal liver or benign liver nodules. Benign nodular hyperplastic nodules in the spleen have good overall perfusion.

Fine Needle Aspiration

Although imaging of the spleen only rarely results in a diagnosis, an aspirate may provide a cytologic sample and the answer. Core biopsy is possible but not usually necessary. Most diseases of the spleen exfoliate well and are suitably sampled with fine needle techniques. Of the fine needle techniques, the variation that seems to provide the most cells without undue hemodilution involves no negative pressure with the attached syringe and multiple thrusting motions with the needle. With the plunger already pulled back in the barrel

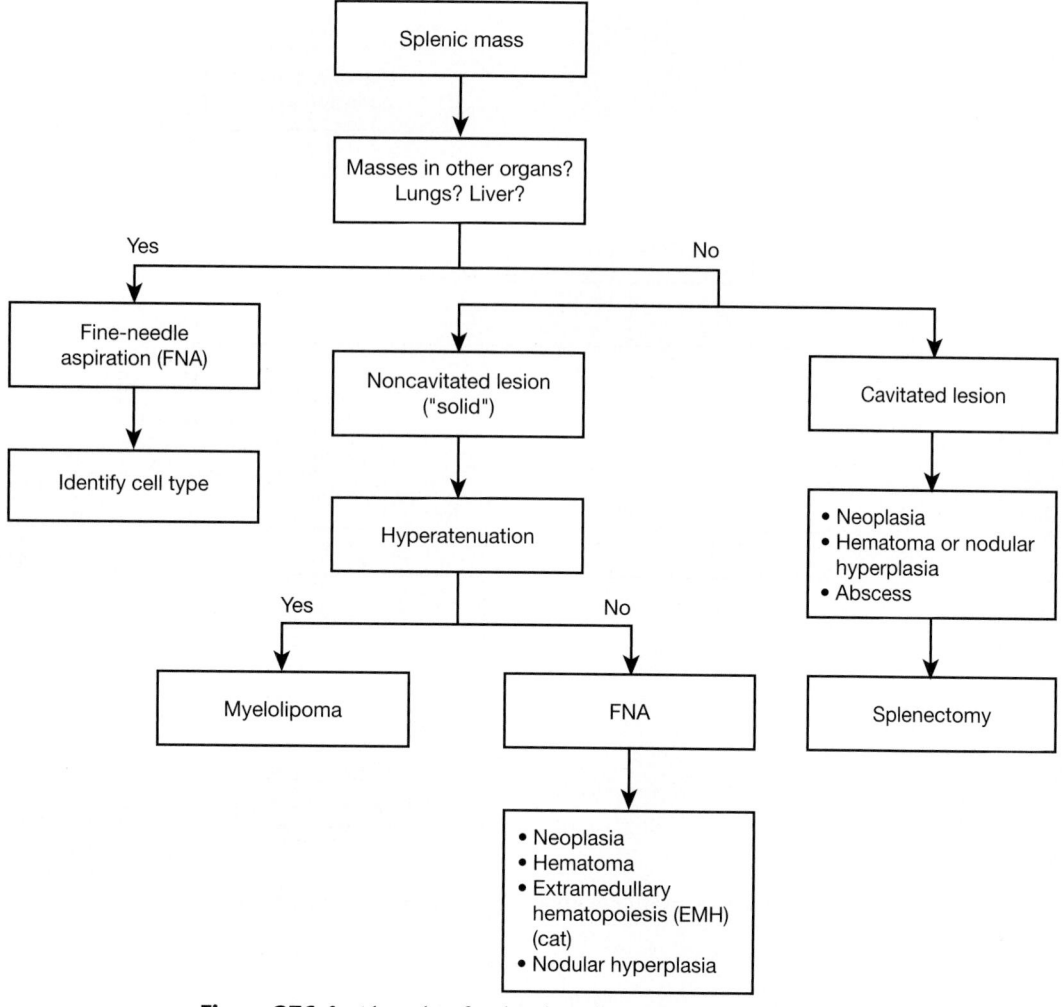

Figure 276-1 Algorithm for the clinical approach to a splenic mass.

HEMATOLOGY AND IMMUNOLOGY

of the syringe prior to insertion of the needle, it thereafter is easy to expel the contents of the needle by depressing the plunger. This technique works well for nodular hyperplasia and extramedullary hematopoietic benign nodules, metastatic carcinomas, and hematopoietic tumors. Solid sarcomas may not exfoliate well with aspiration techniques, and a core sample may provide a better result. Cavitated lesions should be sampled only with the utmost care, if at all.

Fine needle aspiration appears to be safe even in presence of coagulopathies or thrombocytopenia.[13] As a general rule, all abnormal spleens that *do not have cavitated lesions* should be aspirated. Aspiration is not necessary in patients with splenic torsion when lack of adequate blood flow can be determined by Doppler ultrasonography, or in patients with myelolipoma if only lesions with the classic acoustic properties are present. Aspiration also may not be required for diffuse homogeneous splenomegaly, with no clinical signs, that is attributable to splenic disorders in patients with a known cause of congestion (e.g., tranquilizer therapy, portal hypertension, right-sided heart failure), or for "classic" infarct lesions in asymptomatic patients.

Fine needle aspiration can provide the final diagnosis in infectious disease when the organism can be identified and in neoplastic disorders. Aspirates of normal spleen reveal small lymphocytes with occasional medium and large lymphocytes and rare neutrophils. A few macrophages and plasma cells may be present.[14] Precursors of all three cell lines may be seen in patients with extramedullary hematopoiesis, but erythroid cells are more common. In hyperplasia resulting from antigenic reaction, an increase in medium and large lymphocytes and in macrophages and plasma cells is seen.[14] Patients with splenitis have an increase in inflammatory cells. Identification of the predominant cell type narrows the number of potential diagnoses. Inflammation can be further characterized based on the predominant cell type; that is, suppurative, granulomatous, pyogranulomatous, eosinophilic, or lymphoplasmacytic. The most common causes of each type of inflammation are presented in Box 276-2.

Splenic Biopsies/Splenectomy

Biopsy of the spleen can be performed in patients in which the primary diagnosis of a mass is not obtained by fine needle aspiration. Care should be taken with impression smears made from splenic biopsy samples. Impressions inadvertently made of the capsular surface, rather than the parenchyma, reveal uniform sheets of loosely attached mesothelium, which are nondiagnostic.[14] Splenectomy should be considered in animals with splenic necrosis or cavitated masses without metastasis.

Other Diagnostic Tests

In addition to imaging techniques and fine needle aspiration, urinalysis, a complete blood count, and a biochemical profile

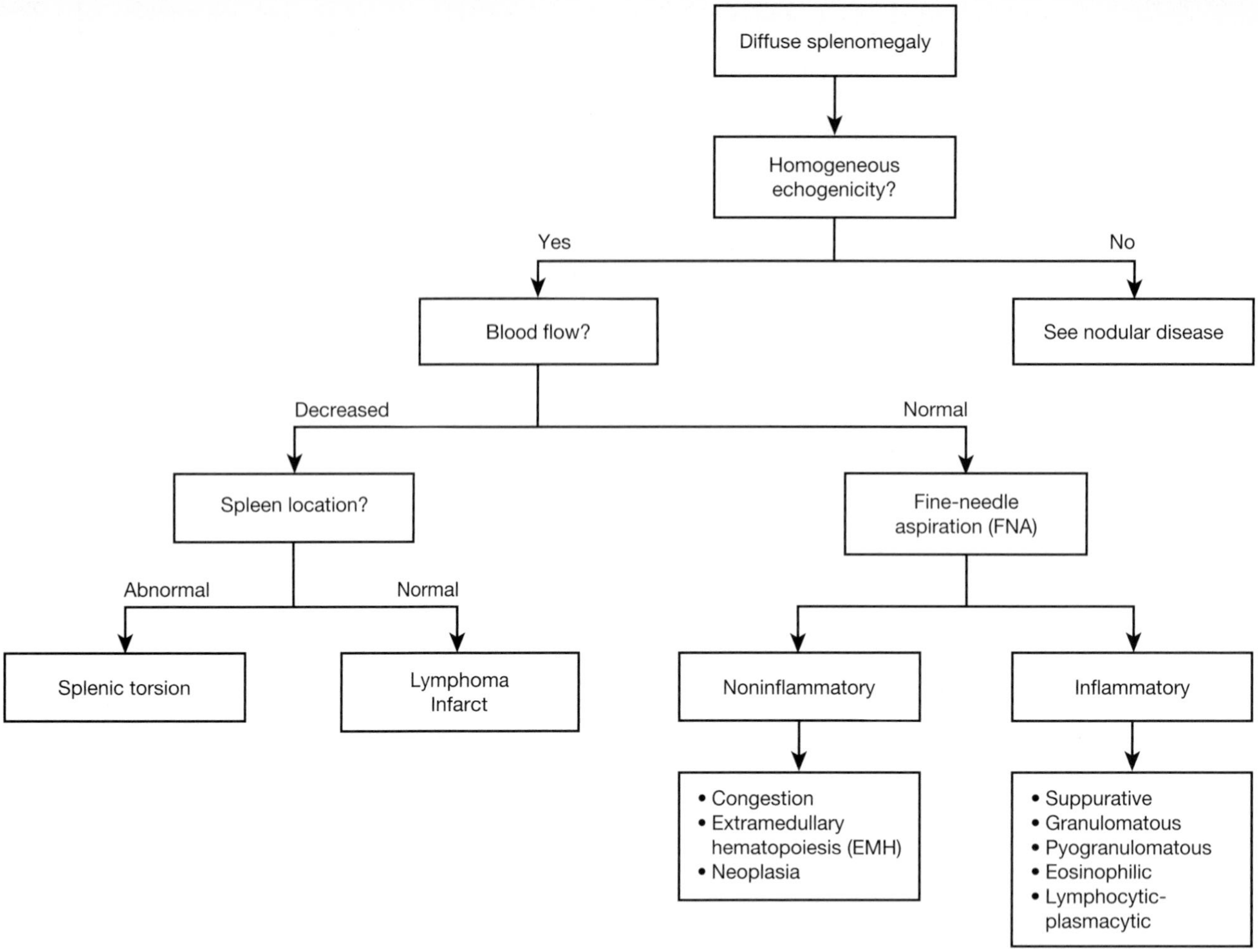

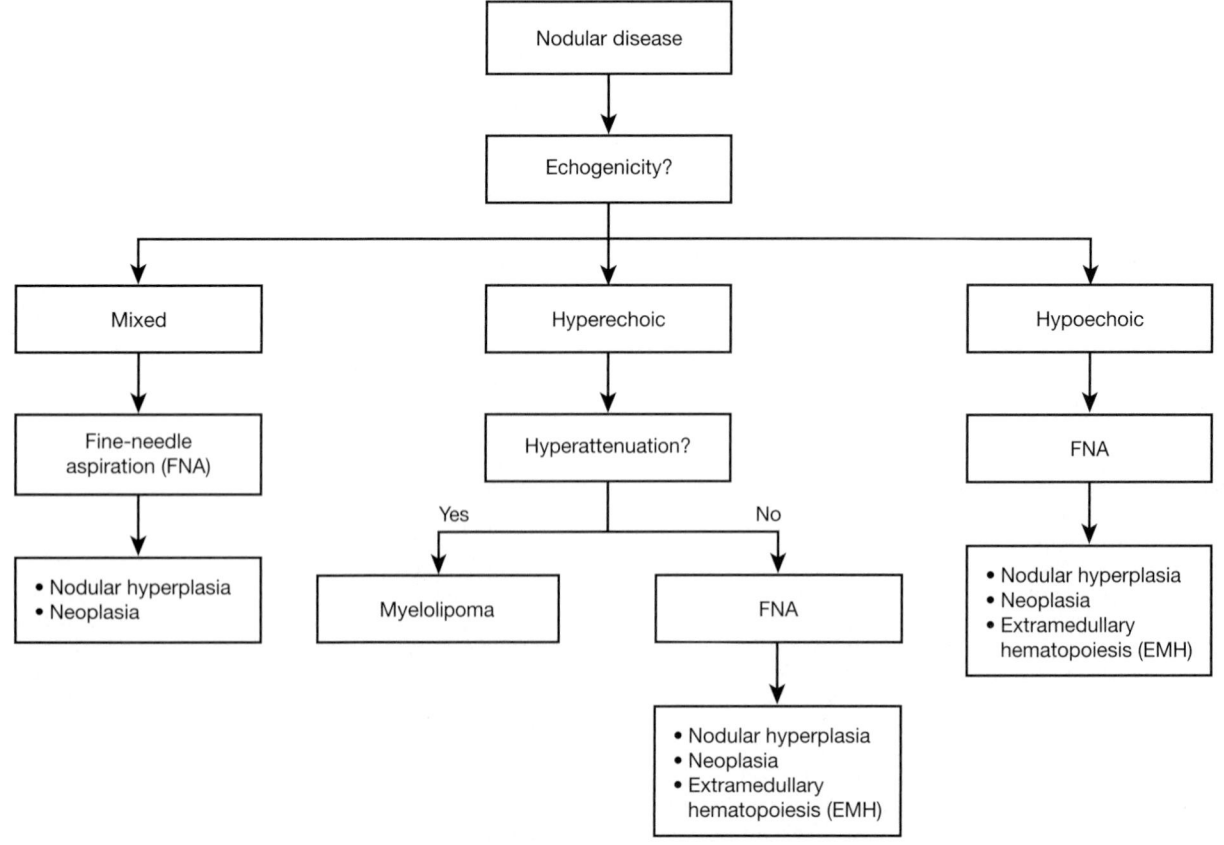

Figure 276-2 Algorithm for the clinical approach to splenomegaly.

Figure 276-3 Algorithm for the clinical approach to splenic nodular disease.

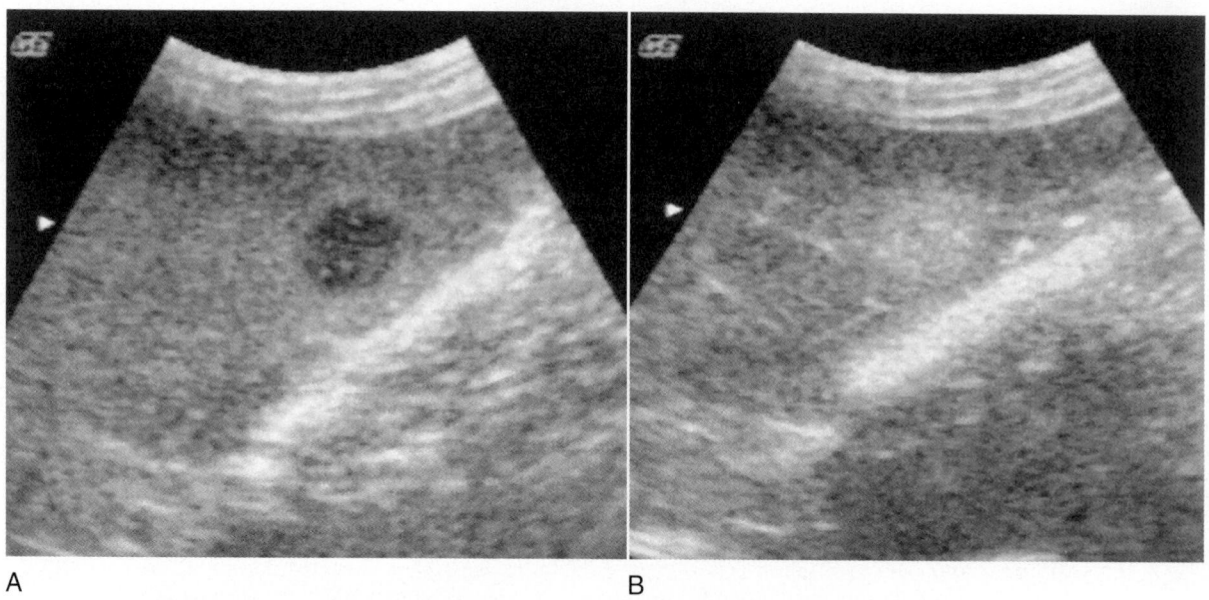

A   B

Figure 276-4 Nodular hyperplasia. Note the contrast enhancement pattern on precontrast (**A**) and postcontrast (**B**) images.

are necessary in all patients with splenomegaly. Cats must be tested for infection with feline leukemia virus (FeLV) and feline immunodeficiency virus (FIV). Chest radiographs should be obtained in patients with splenic masses to rule out metastasis, and bone marrow examination may be indicated in patients with alterations in blood cell lines.

COMMON CAUSES OF SPLENOMEGALY IN DOGS AND CATS

Generalized splenomegaly may occur with congestion, splenic hyperplasia/extramedullary hematopoiesis, inflammation, or cellular infiltration, whereas splenic masses usually are due to neoplasia, hematoma, abscess, or nodular hyperplasia.

Congestion
Congestion is commonly seen as a consequence of sedation or anesthesia, portal hypertension, or splenic vein thrombosis.

Administration of phenothiazine sedatives (e.g., acepromazine) or ultra-short-acting barbiturates (e.g., thiopental) produces substantial splenomegaly. Splenomegaly can be severe, because up to 30% of the blood volume can be pooled in the spleen. Administration of propofol to dogs, however, did not produce statistically significant splenomegaly.[15]

Congestion may also occur secondary to portal hypertension with hepatic disease and with systemic venous hypertension in right-sided heart failure or intrathoracic caudal vena cava compression. Chronic congestion of the spleen may lead to splenic hyperplasia. No changes in echogenicity were subjectively noted in congested spleens, although significant increased attenuation and a trend toward increased backscatter (echogenicity) were noted.[15] Diffuse changes in splenic echogenicity in patients with a known cause of congestion, therefore, are likely due to another underlying condition.

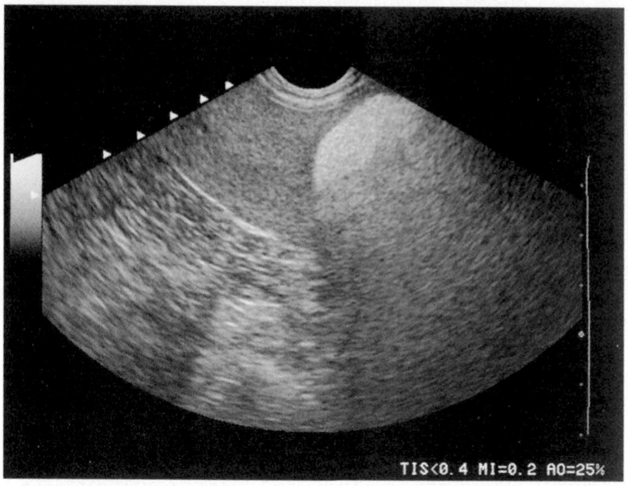

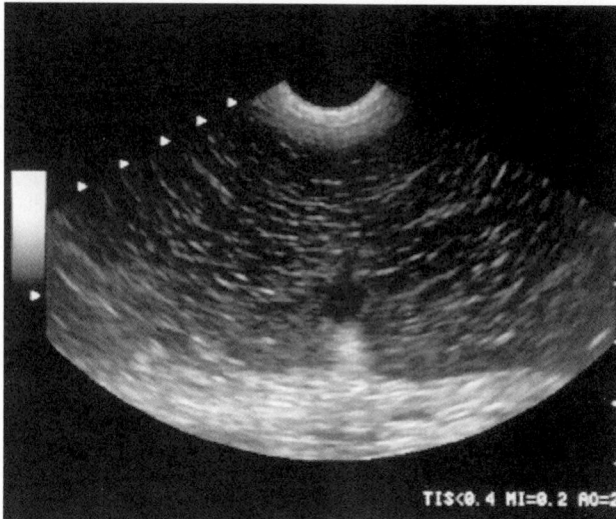

Figure 276-5 Myelolipoma. Note the hyperechogenicity and hyperattenuation pattern.

Figure 276-6 Splenic torsion. Note the "Swiss cheese" echogenic pattern of splenic necrosis.

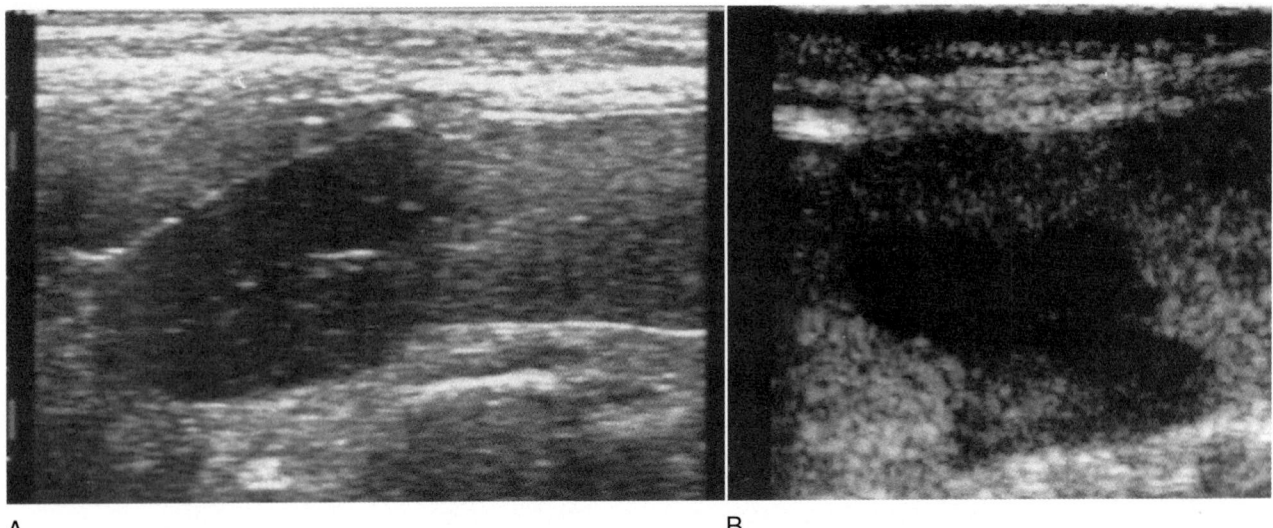

Figure 276-7 Infarcted spleen in two dogs. **A,** Note the hypoechoic infarcted portion of the spleen on grey scale ultrasound image. **B,** On the contrast harmonic ultrasound image, the infarcted portion is not seen on grey scale ultrasound but is hypoechoic compared with surrounding well-perfused, contrast-enhanced spleen.

Splenic pedicle torsion is a special cause of congestion in dogs. It usually develops in large, deep-chested dogs, especially the German shepherd and Great Dane.[16] Males represented 79% of the cases in one study.[16] Acute torsion causes profound systemic signs, including shock and abdominal discomfort, whereas chronic torsion is associated with vague signs such as vomiting, anorexia, lethargy, and icterus. Radiographically, a decrease in abdominal detail, displacement of other abdominal organs, and loss of visualization of the body of the spleen in the left cranial abdomen are seen on the ventrodorsal view. In the lateral view, the spleen is enlarged, abnormally positioned or shaped, and may have intrasplenic gas.[17] Ultrasonographically, the spleen is diffusely enlarged and abnormally located. It is usually hypoechoic, with decreased flow through splenic veins. In one study, intravascular thrombi could be identified in 50% of the cases.[16] Supportive therapy should be instituted immediately in these patients, and the spleen should be removed surgically. If appropriately treated, splenic torsion carries a favorable prognosis.[16]

Splenic Infarction
Infarcts can be observed in patients in hypercoagulable states associated with liver disease, renal disease, or hyperadrenocorticism.[18] They also can occur with pre-existing uniform splenomegaly[18] or splenic torsion.[16] Splenic infarction is a sign of abnormal coagulation or blood flow, and the clinical signs are related to the underlying cause. Ultrasonographically, infarct regions are usually peripheral and have hypoechoic, swollen areas. After contrast injection, they appear hypoechoic compared with the surrounding normally perfused spleen. Infarcted regions may resolve with appropriate therapy of the underlying disease.

Splenic Hyperplasia/Extramedullary Hematopoiesis
The splenomegaly seen with splenic hyperplasia and extramedullary hematopoiesis reflects *work hypertrophy* resulting from removal of abnormal blood cells from circulation, increased activity of mononuclear phagocytic and lymphoid cells, and increased blood cell production. In immune-mediated hemolytic anemia and thrombocytopenia, the spleen serves as a site of antibody production and also as an important site of removal of antibody-sensitized cells. Chronic increased destruction of red blood cells in some

non-immune-mediated hemolytic diseases also appears to cause hyperplastic splenomegaly in dogs and cats.[19] Chronic antigen stimulation by infectious agents (e.g., bacterial endocarditis), blood parasites, or immune-mediated disease can stimulate hyperplasia of mononuclear phagocytic and lymphoid cells.

In work hypertrophy, the spleen is uniformly enlarged and may be hypoechoic on ultrasonographic examination. Cytologically, small lymphocytes still predominate, but an increase is seen in medium and large lymphocytes, and plasma cells are commonly observed.[14]

Extramedullary hematopoiesis (EMH) may accompany splenic hyperplasia in patients with concomitant anemia, thrombocytopenia, or leukopenia. It is a very common cytologic diagnosis in dogs with uniform splenomegaly[13] and may also occur with a variety of splenic neoplasms. EMH is also common in cats; it was diagnosed in 21% of the cats in one study.[20] A nodular pattern is more common in cats with EMH. The presence of nucleated red blood cells in peripheral blood suggests a diagnosis of EMH. Cytologically, precursors of all three cell lines may be observed with the disease.[14] A finding of hematopoietic precursors with large amounts of vacuoles in the background suggests a myelolipoma rather than EMH.[14]

Nodular Hyperplasia/Hematoma
Nodular hyperplasia is a non-neoplastic regional proliferation of component cells normally found in the parenchyma of the canine spleen.[21] Nodular hyperplastic lymphoid proliferation is the most common form of nodular hyperplasia in dogs, but it is not common in cats.[1,2] A high percentage of splenic lesions in dogs have features of hematomas and nodular hyperplasia, which suggests that these disorders are different stages of the same process. Lymphoid elements are usually observed with superimposed hematomas.[1] It has been suggested that marginal zoning distortion caused by nodular hyperplasia disrupts regional splenic blood flow in and around the hyperplastic nodule, eventually leading to hematoma formation.[1] Cats have a "nonsinusal" type of spleen and a different architecture and blood flow pattern of the intermediate circulation bordering the white pulp.[2] Those differences could make the spleen of cats less vulnerable to disrupted blood flow and hematoma formation.

Nodular hyperplastic lesions are usually hypoechoic on ultrasonographic examination. Splenic hematomas in dogs are associated with large splenic masses. A history of trauma is rare.[22] Most dogs with splenic hematoma are relatively healthy and do not have acute splenic rupture,[19] although they may develop hemoabdomen.[23] Large hyperplastic nodules and splenic hematomas cannot be differentiated from hemangiosarcoma grossly. Splenectomy is the treatment of choice for hematomas and hyperplastic nodules large enough to cause splenomegaly.[24]

A particular variation of the hyperplastic nodule in dogs is the fibrohistiocytic nodule.[21] Nodular fibrohistiocytic proliferation is characterized by a mixed population of histiocytoid or spindle cells intertwined with hematopoietic elements, plasma cells, and lymphocytes. These nodules appear to form a continuum between lymphoid nodular hyperplasia and malignant splenic fibrous histiocytoma.[21] Histologically, the lymphoid to fibrohistiocytic ratio is the most important predictor of survival in these dogs. A higher proportion of lymphoid to fibrohistiocytic cell types was associated with increased long-term survival.[21]

Inflammatory Splenomegaly

Inflammatory splenomegaly (splenitis) is a uniform splenomegaly that usually occurs secondary to infection. In addition to the inflammatory response associated with hyperplasia, patients with splenitis also have increased numbers of other inflammatory cells. It is important to classify the splenitis according to the predominant cell type, because different etiologic agents are associated with different types of inflammation. Some overlap exists, and the same organism can cause a different inflammatory response in different patients. For example, lymphoplasmacytic splenitis has been observed in patients with FIP, histoplasmosis, and blastomycosis. Care must be taken in diagnosing suppurative splenitis in patients with peripheral neutrophilia or eosinophilic splenitis in patients with peripheral eosinophilia. The most common causes of splenitis, based on the predominant inflammatory response, are presented in Box 276-2. Infectious agents that can cause splenitis or can lead to splenomegaly by causing chronic antigen stimulation, disturbances of blood flow, or chronic anemia are listed in Box 276-3.

PATIENT WITH A SPLENIC NODULE

Splenic nodules without associated splenomegaly are a relatively common finding in older dogs undergoing abdominal ultrasonography for unrelated reasons. Most splenic nodules in this age group are benign and may require no further action. Myelolipomas can be easily identified, whereas lymphoid hyperplasia, EMH, and splenic infarcts may be more difficult to differentiate from an early neoplastic lesion. Further diagnostics should be attempted in breeds with a high-risk for hemangiosarcoma; in patients with systemic tumors likely to involve the spleen (e.g., lymphoma, hemangiosarcoma); and in animals with hematologic abnormalities, fever, or other signs of systemic infectious disease.[25] Fine needle aspiration should be attempted for all splenic nodules. The main risk associated with this procedure is contamination of the abdominal cavity with tumor cells in the case of hemangiosarcoma. Hemangiosarcoma is not likely to manifest itself as one or few small nodules, but it may be a risk in predisposed breeds. A more conservative approach involving repeating the ultrasonographic examination in 4 weeks has been suggested.[25] Any increase in the size of a nodule over this period should be pursued aggressively. It should be remembered that a change in diameter from 1 to 1.2 cm is associated with a doubling in volume for a spheric mass.[25]

Box • 276-3

Infectious Causes of Splenomegaly/Splenitis*

Viral diseases
  Feline infectious peritonitis (FIP) (C)
  Feline leukemia virus (FeLV) (C)
  Feline immunodeficiency virus (FIV) (C)
  Infectious canine hepatitis (D)
Rickettsial and mycoplasmal diseases
  Ehrlichiosis (canine and feline)
  Rocky mountain spotted fever (RMSF)
    (Rickettsia rickettsii)
  Q fever (Coxiella burnetii)
  Hemotropic mycoplasmosis (Mycoplasma haemofelis
    (formerly Haemobartonella felis Ohio)
Bacterial infections
  Canine brucellosis
  Mycoplasmosis
  Florida borreliosis
  Plague
  Tularemia
  Streptococcosis
  Staphylococcosis
  Salmonellosis
  Francisella infection
  Endotoxemia
Fungal diseases
  Cryptococcosis
  Histoplasmosis
  Blastomycosis
Protozoal diseases
  Toxoplasmosis
  Cytauxzoonosis (C)
  Babesiosis (Babesia canis and B. gibsoni)
  Leishmaniasis (D)

*Infectious disease may affect the spleen directly or may indirectly cause splenomegaly by causing chronic anemia, chronic antigen stimulation, or disturbances in blood flow (e.g., endotoxemia). C, Cats; D, dogs.

PATIENT WITH SPLENIC DISEASE

Diffuse splenomegaly is usually managed medically. Most diseases that cause diffuse splenomegaly are systemic in nature, and treatment should be directed at the underlying cause. Splenic torsion in dogs is the exception to the rule. A few tumors and myeloproliferative disease can also benefit from removal of the spleen. Splenectomy can be considered in patients with immune-mediated anemia or thrombocytopenia refractory to therapy. It is important to show bone marrow hyperplasia in the cell line with decreased peripheral numbers, before splenectomy is performed. Removal of the spleen is the treatment of choice for patients with splenic masses.

Removal of the spleen may predispose the patient to infections. Splenectomized humans are more likely to die of sepsis, but this predisposition has not yet been confirmed in dogs and cats. A few organisms that infect blood cells (e.g., as in babesiosis, hemotropic mycoplasmosis, and ehrlichiosis) are known to occur more often in splenectomized patients. Ideally, dogs and cats should be tested before splenectomy and treated accordingly if infected.

CHAPTER 277

Systemic Lupus Erythematosus

Michael Stone*

No single definition describes systemic lupus erythematosus (SLE). Veterinary patients with SLE classically demonstrate at least two separate manifestations of autoimmunity in addition to the presence of antinuclear antibody (ANAs). However, some patients demonstrate clinical features of multisystemic autoimmunity, yet lack serum ANAs.

PATHOGENESIS

Autoimmune disease may be defined as a clinical syndrome caused by the activation of T cells or B cells, or both, in the absence of an ongoing infection or other discernible cause. In SLE, immune system dysregulation that leads to immune complex formation is postulated to induce tissue damage (type III hypersensitivity); however, direct antibody-mediated cytotoxicity (type II hypersensitivity) and cell-mediated autoimmunity (type IV hypersensitivity) also occur.

Effectors

The primary mediators in the development of SLE are pathogenic antibodies, pathogenic immune complexes, and autoreactive T cells.

Pathogenic antibodies   Individuals with SLE produce antibodies directed against a broad range of nuclear, cytoplasmic, and cell membrane molecules. Autoantibodies may cause damage through the formation of immune complexes, opsonization of target cells, and interference with cellular physiology. Antibodies may penetrate living cells and bind to cytoplasmic or nuclear structures, altering cell function and contributing to disease by mechanisms other than classic complement-mediated injury.[1]

Pathogenic immune complexes   Immune complexes, which are formed whenever an antibody meets an antigen, are normally removed by the mononuclear phagocyte system. With continued production of autoantibody to a self-antigen, the mononuclear phagocyte system may become overloaded. Circulating immune complexes are deposited in the walls of blood vessels in which there is a physiologic outflow of fluid (e.g., glomeruli, synovia, and the choroid plexus). Some immune complexes are "tissue tropic" and prone to binding to tissues because of a cationic charge or because the antibodies the complexes contain are directed against tissue components. Trapped immune complexes activate complement, attracted neutrophils release lysosomal enzymes, and the result is tissue damage.[2]

Autoreactive T-cells   T cells may directly cause tissue damage in SLE. Dermatologic lesions, polymyositis, and vasculitis have been associated with cytotoxic T cell–mediated damage.[3]

Genetics

In mice, more than 25 genes that can contribute to an autoimmune diathesis have been identified.[1] Most of these genes are associated with the major histocompatibility complex (MHC), encoding cytokines, antigen co-receptors, cytokine- or antigen-signaling cascades, co-stimulatory molecules, molecules involved in pathways that promote or inhibit apoptosis, and molecules that clear antigen or antigen-antibody complexes. For example, a consequence of the inheritance of Fe receptors that weakly bind immunoglobulin may be impaired ability to clear immune complexes, which predisposes the individual to the sequelae of circulating immune complexes. Protective genes exist that prevent the development of SLE even if multiple susceptibility genes are inherited. SLE is clearly inherited in dogs, and experimental colonies of dogs with the disease have been established.[4-6] SLE in dogs has been associated with the allele DLA A7, along with a negative (or "protective") association with DLA A1 and B5.[7] Dogs with a specific allotype of the fourth component of complement may be predisposed to SLE,[8] as are dogs with decreased serum IgA.[9] SLE may occur more frequently in purebred cats, which also suggests a genetic influence.[10]

Environmental Factors

The lower than expected rate of SLE concordance among identical human twins strongly suggests the existence of an environmental trigger.[3] Exposure to ultraviolet (UV) light causes disease flares in as many as 50% of humans with SLE, and the same effect has been reported in both dogs[5,11] and cats.[12] In humans, the importance of gender is demonstrated by the fact that 90% of SLE cases occur in women, particularly during their reproductive years. However, this gender distribution has not been identified in either the dog or cat. Exposure early in life to infectious agents may suppress the development of allergic and autoimmune disorders.[13] It has been suggested that the increase in allergies and autoimmune diseases recognized in humans is related to decreased exposure to endotoxin during early development. Adequate stimulation may be important in the ontogeny of the normal immune system.[14]

Drugs

Certain drugs may induce SLE-like disease in humans (Box 277-1).[15] However, this disease is probably different from true SLE. The clinical manifestations of drug-induced lupus in humans are predominantly arthritis, serositis, fatigue, malaise, and low-grade fever; nephritis and central nervous system (CNS) diseases are rare. The manifestations disappear in most patients within a few weeks of discontinuation of the offending drug, never to reappear unless the individual is re-exposed to the drug.[3] Propylthiouracil has been associated with hemolytic anemia, thrombocytopenia, and the development of antinuclear antibodies in cats.[16] Methimazole has been associated with the development of antinuclear antibodies in

*The author thanks Dr. Susan Cotter for her review of this manuscript.

Box • 277-1

Causes of Drug-Induced Systemic Lupus Erythematosus in Humans

Allopurinol	Penicillamine
Captopril	Penicillin
Chlorpromazine	Phenothiazines
Clonidine	Phenylbutazone
Danazol	Piroxicam
Diphenylhydantoin	Primidone
Griseofulvin	Procainamide
Hydralazine	Propylthiouracil
Isoniazid	Quinidine
Lithium	Streptomycin
Lovastatin	Sulfasalazine
Mesalazine	Sulfonamides
Minocycline	Tetracycline
Salicylic acid	Valproate

Modified from Mutasim DF, Adams BB: A practical guide for serologic evaluation of autoimmune connective tissue diseases. J Am Acad Dermatol 42:159, 2000.

cats, but clinical signs of SLE have not been reported.[17] Hydralazine has been associated with the development of antinuclear antibodies in dogs.[18]

Infectious Agents

No infectious agents have been identified that cause SLE. However, it is possible that infectious agents or their antigenic products (or both) can worsen SLE in patients with the appropriate predisposing genes. Microbial antigens have the potential to initiate autoreactivity through molecular mimicry, polyclonal activation, or the release of previously sequestered antigens. The immunogenicity of autoantigens may be increased by inflammation in the target organ, which explains the flares of immune-mediated disease induced by vaccination or infection. Molecular mimicry describes infection with an agent that has antigens immunologically similar to host antigens but sufficiently different to allow an immune response. As a result, tolerance to autoantigens breaks down, and the pathogen-specific immune response cross-reacts with host tissues.[19] The feline viruses feline leukemia virus (FeLV) and feline immunodeficiency virus (FIV) can induce disease in cats that is similar to SLE, and serum ANAs may develop in the early stages of FeLV infection.[20] Whether FeLV- or FIV-induced disease is truly similar to SLE is a matter of debate.[21] Feline ehrlichial disease has also been associated with the development of antinuclear antibodies.[22]

In summary, the ability to manufacture pathogenic immunoglobulin and to sustain its production depends on three main factors: (1) inheritance of an appropriate number of susceptibility genes, (2) lack of protective genes, and (3) an environmental stimulus that sets the whole process in motion.

CLINICAL FINDINGS

The clinical signs reported in dogs and cats with SLE are summarized in Table 277-1. It must be noted that the process of deriving criteria from diagnosed cases is inherently circular, because the criteria are based on diagnosed cases of SLE.

Nonerosive polyarthropathy is the most frequent primary sign in dogs. The smaller joints (carpi, tarsi, elbows, stifles) are most frequently involved. Synovial fluid analysis reveals neutrophilic inflammation with greater than 10,000 cells/mm³. Articular symptoms are also common in cats, some of which may demonstrate joint swelling and abnormal synovial fluid, yet lack signs of lameness. Fever is frequently reported in both dogs and cats and may be either persistent or intermittent.

In humans, biopsy demonstrates involvement of the kidney in almost all SLE patients.[23-25] Renal involvement may be benign and asymptomatic or relentlessly progressive and fatal. The earliest manifestation is proteinuria. In dogs, proteinuria and glomerular lesions are also common. Biopsy may reveal mesangial and/or endothelial hypertrophy, proliferative and/or membranous glomerulonephritis, and sclerotic changes. Proteinuria and/or glomerulonephritis are also commonly reported in the cat.

Cutaneous manifestations in dogs may include erythema, scaling, crusting, depigmentation, and alopecia. Ulcers may

Table • 277-1

Clinical Signs in Dogs and Cats Suspected of Having Systemic Lupus Erythematosus

CLINICAL SIGN	INCIDENCE (DOGS)		INCIDENCE (CATS)	
	RATIO*	PERCENTAGE	RATIO	PERCENTAGE
Nonerosive polyarthritis	236/302	78	9/25	36
Fever	186/275	68	11/21	52
Renal disorders	167/302	55	10/25	40
Dermatologic lesions	138/302	46	15/25	60
Lymphadenopathy/splenomegaly	66/175	38	CNBD	CNBD
Leukopenia	54/302	18	CNBD	CNBD
Hemolytic anemia	45/302	15	6/25	24%
Thrombocytopenia	40/302	13	2/25	8%
Myositis	16/275	6	CNBD	CNBD
Central nervous system disorders	16/302	5	6/25	24%
Neuropathy	7/302	2	CNBD	CNBD

Modified from references 10-12, 21, and 26-33.
*Ratio of the number of patients affected to the number of patients described.
CNBD, The incidence could not be determined from the published literature.

HEMATOLOGY AND IMMUNOLOGY

develop on the skin and in the mucocutaneous junctions and oral cavity. Preferential localization of lesions may occur in areas poorly protected by the haircoat, and exposure to sunlight may exacerbate the lesions. Biopsy reveals inflammatory infiltrates at the dermoepidermal junction and vacuolar change in the basal columnar cells. Immunofluorescence stains demonstrate immunoglobulin and complement deposits in the epidermal basement membrane. Cutaneous lesions reported in 15 feline patients with SLE included erythema, ulceration, and crusting and depigmentation of the face, ears, and paws in seven cats; biopsy results consistent with pemphigus foliaceus or plasmacytic pododermatitis in four cats; ulcerative stomatitis in three cats; and seborrheic dermatitis in one cat.[10,12,21,30]

Only rarely is anemia, leukopenia, or thrombocytopenia the presenting feature of human SLE without concomitant problems of the skin, joints, CNS, or cardiopulmonary system. In dogs, although it is common to find anemia of chronic inflammation, Coombs'-positive anemia is uncommon. Thrombocytopenia may be severe enough to cause bleeding, but antiphospholipid syndrome and thromboembolic disease should also be considered as possible causes in these cases. Leukopenia has been frequently reported. Complement concentrations were decreased in three of eight dogs suspected of having SLE.[8] As in dogs, hemolytic anemia is uncommon in cats, and thrombocytopenia is rare. Complement levels were decreased in one cat studied.[10]

Thrombosis associated with the "lupus" anticoagulant was reported in one dog with SLE.[34] The "lupus" anticoagulant is an antibody directed against membrane phospholipids. The antibody causes *in vitro* prolongation of the activated partial thromboplastin time (aPTT), hence the paradoxical name *anticoagulant*. However, *in vivo* the antibody causes platelet activation and hypercoagulability.

Memory impairment, headache, epilepsy, and personality changes may accompany SLE in humans. Sole involvement of the CNS without other clinical or laboratory features of SLE is unusual. In animals, subtle behavioral disturbances may go unrecognized. In cats, reported CNS involvement has included racing around the house; twitching of the ears, tail, and hindlimbs; repeated licking of paws and tail base; generalized seizures; hyperesthesia along the dorsum; restless crying; disorientation; ataxia; loss of conscious proprioception; nystagmus; and ventroflexion of the neck.[10] Polymyositis was suspected in several dogs and cats. Polyneuritis, characterized by hyperesthesia of the nerve courses, has been reported in a dog.[11]

In humans, chest pain with or without pleural effusion is the most common sign of cardiopulmonary involvement. Fibrosis, pulmonary embolism, capillary leakage, or serositis may affect the lungs. The heart valves, myocardium, or conducting system may be affected, and pericardial effusion may develop. Neutrophilic myocarditis was demonstrated in four dogs with SLE.[28] Serositis of the pleura or pericardium was not observed in cats, although subclinical lung changes were noted on the thoracic radiographs of one cat.[10]

DIAGNOSIS

Criteria have been developed for the diagnosis of SLE in humans (Table 277-2), and these criteria may be modified to apply to veterinary patients (Table 277-3). A veterinary consensus would be helpful to allow comparison of future studies. Veterinary patients with SLE classically demonstrate at least two separate manifestations of autoimmunity, along with testing positive for ANAs. Patients with three or more separate manifestations of autoimmunity may also be considered to

Table • 277-2

American College of Rheumatology Revised Criteria for the Classification of Systemic Lupus Erythematosus

CRITERION	DEFINITION
Malar rash	Fixed erythema, flat or raised over the malar eminences, that tends to spare the nasolabial folds
Discoid rash	Erythematous, raised patches with adherent keratotic scaling and follicular plugging; atrophic scarring may occur
Photosensitivity	Skin rash as a result of unusual reaction to sunlight
Oral ulcers	Oral or nasopharyngeal ulceration, usually painless
Arthritis	Nonerosive arthritis involving two or more peripheral joints
Serositis	Pleuritis (pleuritic pain or rub, or evidence of pleural effusion) *or* pericarditis (pericardial effusion)
Renal disorder	Persistent proteinuria *or* cellular casts, which may be red cell, hemoglobin, granular, tubular, or mixed type
Neurologic disorder	Seizures *or* psychosis (either in the absence of offending drugs, known metabolic derangements, or electrolyte imbalance)
Hematologic disorder	Hemolytic anemia (with reticulocytosis) *or* leukopenia (less than 4000/mm^3 on two or more occasions) *or* lymphopenia (less than 1500/mm^3 on two or more occasions) *or* thrombocytopenia (less than 100,000/mm^3 in the absence of offending drugs)
Immunologic disorder	Anti-DNA (antibody to native DNA in abnormal titer) *or* anti-Sm (presence of antibody to Sm nuclear antigen) *or* positive finding of antiphospholipid antibodies based on (1) an abnormal serum level of IgG or IgM anticardiolipin antibodies, (2) a positive test result for lupus anticoagulant, or (3) a false-positive serologic test for syphilis
Antinuclear antibodies (ANAs)	An abnormal ANA titer at any point in time and in the absence of drugs known to be associated with "drug-induced lupus"

Modified from Tan EM: The 1982 revised criteria for the classification of systemic lupus erythematosus. Arthritis Rheum 25:1271, 1982.
*For the purposes of identifying patients in clinical studies, a person shall be said to have systemic lupus erythematosus if any four or more of the 11 criteria are present, serially or simultaneously, during any interval of observation.

Table • 277-3

Proposed Criteria for Diagnosis of Systemic Lupus Erythematosus in Dogs and Cats

CRITERION	DEFINITION
Antinuclear antibodies (ANAs)	Abnormal ANA titer in the absence of drugs or infectious or neoplastic conditions known to be associated with abnormal titers
Cutaneous lesions	Depigmentation, erythema, erosions, ulcerations, crusts, and/or scaling, with biopsy findings consistent with systemic lupus erythematosus
Oral ulcers	Oral or nasopharyngeal ulceration, usually painless
Arthritis	Nonerosive, nonseptic arthritis involving two or more peripheral joints
Renal disorders	Glomerulonephritis or persistent proteinuria in the absence of urinary tract infection
Anemia and/or thrombocytopenia	Hemolytic anemia and/or thrombocytopenia in the absence of offending drugs
Leukopenia	Low total white cell count
Polymyositis or myocarditis	Inflammatory disease of the skeletal or cardiac muscles
Serositis	Presence of a nonseptic inflammatory cavity effusion (abdominal, pleural, or pericardial)
Neurologic disorders	Seizures or psychosis in the absence of known disorders
Antiphospholipids	Prolongation of the activated partial thromboplastin time that fails to correct with a 1:1 mixture of the patient's and normal plasma, in the absence of heparin or fibrin degradation products

Modified from references 28 and 36-39.

*A diagnosis of SLE is established if a patient manifests three or more criteria simultaneously or over any period of time.

have SLE even in the absence of detectable ANAs. In dogs, the syndrome most commonly recognized is immune-mediated polyarthritis in association with immune-mediated skin disease, glomerulonephritis, hemolytic anemia, or thrombocytopenia. Similar signs occur in cats, but neurologic signs may be more common in this species.

Diagnostic tests for patients suspected of having SLE should include hematology, biochemistry, urinalysis, imaging, joint fluid cytology, histopathology of the skin and/or kidney, and serum ANA determination. Cats should also be tested for FeLV and FIV. Infectious and neoplastic disease must be excluded through imaging; culture of urine, blood, and/or joint fluid; serology for tick-borne and fungal diseases; and trials of therapeutic antibiotics. In tick-infested areas, a 3- to 7-day course of doxycycline should be considered before a diagnosis of immune-mediated disease is made.

Immunodiagnostic investigations may include Coombs' testing, platelet autoantibodies, rheumatoid factor, coagulation testing for antiphospholipid antibodies, serum immunoglobulin, complement, circulating immune complex concentrations, and endocrine autoantibodies (i.e., thyroglobulin). Immunohistologic investigation may include immunoperoxidase and immunofluorescence staining and electron microscopy evaluation.[40]

Biopsy results may support a diagnosis of SLE but are rarely diagnostic by themselves. When the skin is biopsied, care must be taken to avoid ulcers or erosions, because an intact epidermis is necessary to substantiate the diagnosis. Oral biopsy specimens are rarely beneficial, because ulcers, which are inherently not diagnostic, are common in this location. Erythematous areas adjacent to ulcers yield the best diagnostic results.[41]

The diagnosis of SLE in cats is less well defined. In some studies, all cats that tested positive for ANAs were diagnosed with SLE, but whether all these patients truly had SLE is debatable. Another unanswered question is how to categorize patients that test positive for FeLV or FIV. Some reports include FeLV-positive cats, whereas others exclude them.[10,21,29-31,42] Because of the possibility of ehrlichial disease, it has been

recommended that all cats be treated with a course of doxycycline before the diagnosis of immune-mediated disease is made.[43]

SPECIFIC TESTS

Lupus Erythematosus Cell Preparation

For the lupus erythematosus (LE) cell preparation, clotted blood is mashed to release free nuclei. Circulating antibody directed against nucleoprotein binds and opsonizes the nuclear complex. An LE cell is recognized as a neutrophil that contains phagocytized nuclear material. Interpretation depends on the experience and diligence of the technician, and false-negative results are common.[26,27,44] Because of technical problems and difficulty with sensitivity and specificity, the LE cell test has been largely replaced by the more sensitive ANA test. LE cells rarely may be seen on smears of pericardial, pleural, peritoneal, joint, cerebrospinal, or blister fluid and when present are highly suggestive of SLE.

Antinuclear Antibodies

Antinuclear antibodies are a heterogeneous population of antibodies directed against various nuclear antigens. ANAs may be detected using frozen sections of rat liver or cultured cell lines (e.g., Vero cells, HEp-2 human epithelial cells). The relative merits of each substrate are the subject of debate, and there is no universally accepted protocol used by veterinary laboratories. The result of an ANA test is commonly reported as a serum titer and pattern of nuclear staining. The most commonly observed patterns in SLE are speckled or homogenous staining, but no clear association exists between patterns and the nature of clinical disease. A clinically significant titer must be distinguished from low ANA titers that may be present in as many as 10% of normal animals and in animals with any chronic inflammatory, infectious, or neoplastic disease.[45,46]

In humans, substrates tend to remain comparable in their ability to detect common ANAs but differ substantially in the quantitation of antibody titer.[47] In dogs, it has been suggested that multiple substrates be used to increase the sensitivity of the test.[48] Two canine studies found markedly different ANA results when rat liver and HEp-2 cell substrates were compared[48,49]; however the results were well correlated in a third report.[50] Feline ANA test results were found to have a low coefficient of correlation when identical sera were sent to different laboratories.[51]

The most appropriate substrate, conjugate, and methodology for ANA testing remains undefined, and each laboratory's value should be interpreted individually. ANA-negative SLE cases have been described in veterinary patients,[5,26-28] and a positive ANA test result should be neither required nor sufficient in itself to make a diagnosis of SLE.

Autoantibodies

Suspicion of SLE in humans leads to testing for specific antibodies that provide diagnostic and prognostic information (Table 277-4). Research in this area may be helpful for further characterizing immune-mediated diseases in veterinary patients. Autoantibodies also have been studied in veterinary patients (Table 277-5).

Antibodies to DNA   Serum antibodies may recognize denatured (single-stranded) or native (double-stranded) DNA. Anti-single-stranded DNA has low diagnostic value in humans and has not been studied in veterinary medicine. Anti-double-stranded (native) DNA is highly specific for the diagnosis of human SLE, even though only 60% to 83% of patients test positive. Anti-double-stranded DNA has been identified only infrequently in dogs with SLE.

Extractable nuclear antigens   ENAs are molecules extracted from the soluble fraction of cell nuclei (DNA and histone proteins are insoluble and therefore excluded). More than 20 saline-extractable antigens have been identified, and the term *ENAs* generically refers to this group of nuclear proteins. The binding of serum antibodies to commercially available tissue extracts is the basis for serologic testing.

Table • 277-4

Autoantibody Associations in Human Systemic Lupus Erythematosus

EPITOPE	COMMENTS
ds-DNA	Highly specific for the diagnosis of systemic lupus erythematosus
Sm	Associated with membranous nephropathy
RNP	Associated with Raynaud phenomenon, pulmonary and muscle involvement
SS-A/Ro	Associated with cutaneous manifestations, sicca complex, neonatal lupus
SS-B/La	Associated with neonatal lupus
Phospholipid	Associated with thrombocytopenia, thrombosis infertility

From Edworthy SM: Clinical manifestations of systemic lupus erythematosus. *In* Ruddy S et al (eds): Kelley's Textbook of Rheumatology, 6th ed. Philadelphia, WB Saunders, 2001, pp 1105-1119.
ds-DNA, Double-stranded DNA; *Sm, Ro, La*, extractable nuclear antigens named for the first two letters of the name of the patient in whom the antigen was first described (e.g., Sm, Smith); *RNP*, ribonucleoprotein; *SS-A*, Sjögren syndrome A antigen (or its equivalent, Ro); *SS-B*, Sjögren syndrome B antigen (or its equivalent, La).

Table • 277-5

Positive Autoantibody Results in Canine Patients with Suspected Systemic Lupus Erythematosus

EPITOPE	INCIDENCE RATIO*	PERCENTAGE	REFERENCE
ds/DNA	6/38	16	Costa 1984[54]
	1/3	33	Bennett 1987[44]
	1/47	2	Brinet 1988[52]
	2/100	2	Monier 1992[53]
	0/43	—	Monestier 1995[55]
Sm	9/34	24	Costa 1984[54]
	2/30	7	Hubert 1988[5]
	12/75	16	Fournel 1992[11]
	0/20	—	White 1992[56]
	1/64	2	Henriksson 1998[57]
RNP	4/38	10	Costa 1984[54]
	0/12	—	Monier 1988[6]
	0/30	—	Hubert 1988[5]
	6/75	8	Fournel 1992[11]
	0/20	—	White 1992[56]
	5/64	8	Henriksson 1998[57]
SS-A/Ro	1/12	8	Monier 1988[6]
	0/0	—	Hubert 1988[5]
	3/75	4	Fournel 1992[11]
	0/20	—	White 1992[56]
SS-B/La	0/30	—	Hubert 1988[5]
	0/12	—	Monier 1988[6]
	1/75	1	Monier 1992[53]
	0/20	—	White 1992[56]
"Type I" (antibody to a 43 kD nuclear antigen, also known as hnRNP G)	10/38	38	Costa 1984[54]
	15/75	20	Fournel 1992[11]
"Type 2"	5/38	13	Costa 1984[54]
	7/75	9	Fournel 1992[11]
Phospholipid	1/1	100	Stone 1994[34]
	2/20	10	Scott-Moncrieff 2001[58]
	1/1 (feline)	100	Lusson 1999[59]

*Ratio of the number of patients that tested positive to the number of tested patients.
ds-DNA, Double-stranded DNA; *Sm, Ro, La*, extractable nuclear antigens named for the first two letters of the name of the patient in whom the antigen was first described (e.g., Sm, Smith); *RNP*, ribonucleoprotein; *SS-A*, Sjögren syndrome A antigen (or its equivalent, Ro); *SS-B*, Sjögren syndrome B antigen (or its equivalent, La).

Important ENAs include Sm, Ro, and La. In veterinary medicine, antibodies against ENAs do not yet have the diagnostic and prognostic significance they do in human patients.

Antihistone antibodies   Histones are a group of proteins that bind the DNA helical structure into supercoil formation. Histone antibodies are characteristic of drug-induced SLE in humans. One group of investigators detected antihistone antibodies in 61% to 72% of dogs with SLE.[11,52,53] Antihistone antibodies have been detected in canine sera by other investigators; however, no significant difference in concentration was seen between ANA-positive and ANA-negative sera,[49] and antihistone antibodies were detected with conditions other than canine SLE.[54] The use of antihistone antibodies as an indicator of drug-induced SLE in veterinary patients has not been reported.

Antiphospholipid Antibodies

Antiphospholipid antibodies bind to phospholipids found on many cells. These antibodies interfere with the function of procoagulant phospholipids in clotting tests *in vitro*. Patients with the lupus anticoagulant have a prolonged aPTT that fails to correct with a 1:1 mixture of the patient's plasma and normal plasma. In humans, the presence of these antibodies is associated with thrombocytopenia, thrombosis, and fetal loss. Antiphospholipid antibodies were described in one dog with SLE,[34] in two of 20 dogs with hemolytic anemia,[58] and in one cat with SLE.[59]

MANAGEMENT

Sunlight should be avoided if photosensitization occurs. Patients with mild lameness may require only intermittent therapy with nonsteroidal anti-inflammatory drugs. Dogs may be given carprofen (4.4 mg/kg orally once daily), etodolac (15 mg/kg orally once daily), or meloxicam (0.1 mg/kg orally once daily). Meloxicam also has been used safely in the cat.[60]

More severe signs necessitate corticosteroid administration. Prednisone (2.2 mg/kg/day given orally) is recommended in most instances; 1 mg/kg/day may be effective in less severe cases. Full doses are administered until the disease is in complete remission, defined as resolution of clinical signs and radiographic or laboratory changes initially present. After remission has been attained, the dose is tapered, generally by half, for 4 weeks. The animal then is re-evaluated, and if signs of disease are absent (per physical examination and laboratory testing), the dose is again halved. Tapering is repeated monthly until the animal either relapses or stops medication. The recommended minimum duration of therapy is 6 months. If relapse occurs during taper, the dose should be increased to the most recently effective dose and held there for a few months. If the maintenance requirement is unacceptable because of side effects, an additional immunosuppressive agent is added.

Some cats do not respond to prednisone. Cats that don't respond well to prednisone should be treated with an alternative steroid (e.g., prednisolone, methylprednisolone, triamcinolone, or dexamethasone) before additional immunosuppressant therapies are started.

Combination immunosuppression therapy is very helpful because the additional agent often allows the use of a lower dose of corticosteroid. Azathioprine (Imuran) is most frequently used in dogs. The dose is 2.2 mg/kg given orally once daily until remission occurs. The same dose then is administered every other day. A complete blood count (CBC) should be evaluated after 7 days and then every 2 weeks while the patient is receiving daily treatment. The development of neutropenia or thrombocytopenia requires drug cessation until the bone marrow recovers. Once the animal is receiving every other day therapy, a CBC should be evaluated every 3 months, but bone marrow suppression at this dose is unusual.

Prednisone and azathioprine are frequently used in combination. The drugs are administered together once daily and tapered after remission has been attained. The method of tapering is somewhat arbitrary. If signs of prednisone intolerance are experienced, prednisone is tapered first; if bone marrow disease is encountered, azathioprine should be tapered or discontinued first. If the disease was difficult to bring into remission, only one drug should be tapered at a time; if the disease easily went into remission, the two drugs may be tapered concurrently. Tapering should be performed every 4 weeks, with a minimum duration of therapy of 6 months.

Azathioprine is not recommended for use in cats. Instead, chlorambucil may be administered along with corticosteroids for cats that require additional immunosuppression. Chlorambucil (Leukeran) is administered to cats at a dosage of 15 mg/m^2 (4 mg for most cats) given orally once daily for 4 days and then repeated every 3 weeks. Potential side effects include anorexia and bone marrow suppression. A CBC should be evaluated 5 to 7 days after each course of treatment. If after two or more evaluations the CBC remains normal (no leukopenia), further monitoring may be done less frequently. If leukopenia is detected (absolute neutrophil count less than 3000/μL), the dose of the next administration should be decreased 25%. Signs of infection (loss of appetite along with fever) during the expected white blood cell nadir (3 to 10 days after administration) should be aggressively treated with intravenous fluids and broad-spectrum antibiotics. In cats, the chlorambucil dosage should be tapered before the prednisone is tapered.

Novel therapeutic approaches include prednisone (1 to 2 mg/kg orally once daily) combined with levamisole (2 to 5 mg/kg, to a maximum dose of 150 mg orally every 48 hours).[11] Prednisone is tapered and discontinued after 2 months, whereas levamisole is given continuously for 4 months and then stopped. If relapse occurs, levamisole is readministered, again for 4 months. Approximately 75% of dogs treated with such therapy were reported to attain remission. Side effects included agranulocytosis, excited behavior, and aggressiveness.[39]

In humans, an antimalarial drug (e.g., hydroxychloroquine) may provide additional relief. Antimalarial agents have multiple sun blocking, anti-inflammatory, and immunosuppressive effects, although their mechanism of action is not completely understood.[61] Their use has not been reported in dogs or cats with SLE.

PROGNOSIS

The natural course of SLE in veterinary patients is not known. Patients may be well controlled and medications may be tapered, but relapses should be anticipated. Routine evaluation should include hematology, biochemistry, urinalysis, and serum ANA determination every 1 to 3 months. The ANA titer may correlate with clinical severity and may fall with clinical improvement, but the antibody may persist at a low titer during clinical remission. It has been suggested that therapy should be more aggressive when the clinical presentation includes renal disease.[10,39]

HEMATOLOGY AND IMMUNOLOGY

CHAPTER 278

Immune-Mediated and Infective Arthritis

David Bennett

Immune-mediated and infective arthropathies are characterized by an elevated white cell count in the synovial fluid, mainly comprising neutrophils. Synovial fluid analysis is mandatory for diagnosis of these so-called inflammatory arthropathies, and it distinguishes them from the more common degenerative arthropathies.[1]

Infective arthritis is defined as an inflammatory arthropathy caused by an infective agent that can be cultured from the affected joint or joints; however, it is not always possible to culture the organism, and it is important to assume infection if only a single joint is affected. Bacteria are the most common cause of infective arthritis.

The immune-mediated diseases are generally polyarthropathies, although some of the more uncommon infections can involve multiple joints. Although the etiology of immune-mediated arthritis is unknown, certain microbial infections have been implicated. One mechanism is immune complex formation in response to microbial infection, either locally in the joint or systemically with deposition into the joint.[2] Transportation of microbial antigens to joints, with a subsequent immune response, is another possibility. Canine distemper viral antigens and antibodies have been identified in the immune complexes from the synovia of dogs with immune-mediated arthritis[3]; macrophages containing distemper antigens have also been demonstrated in the synovial membrane.[4]

In addition, it is likely that certain individuals are genetically predisposed to immune-mediated arthritis; certain DLA-DRB1 alleles (DRB1 002, 009, and 018) have been associated with immune-mediated arthritis in the dog; furthermore, it appears that a conserved amino acid motif in the third hypervariable region in some DRB1 alleles of both humans and dogs is associated with immune-based arthritis in both species.[5]

The theory of molecular mimicry has also been proposed; that is, antibodies against certain bacteria or viruses may cross-react with cartilage components. Some researchers think that polyclonal B-cell activation, as may occur in a persistent or serious infection, may lead to the emergence of autoantibodies against joint "self-antigens." For example, autoantibodies against heat shock proteins may stimulate immune complex formation in joints or may even cross-react with cartilage epitopes.[6] Potential antigens may also originate from nonmicrobial sources, such as tumor antigens, drug antigens/haptens, and dietary antigens. Once the joint inflammation has been established, by whatever mechanism, various autoantigens, such as altered collagen, are produced. These autoantigens stimulate an immune response, thereby helping to perpetuate the inflammation.[7,8]

Obviously lameness is an important clinical feature, although many immune-mediated polyarthropathies present as cases of "pyrexia of unknown origin." Only about one third of infective arthropathies have systemic signs. Lameness may be an obvious limp, although generalized stiffness is most often seen with the immune-mediated polyarthropathies. Bacterial infections generally have an acute onset, although a more chronic, insidious onset is possible, the so-called low-grade infections. The joint is usually swollen and painful on manipulation, and heat may be detectable.

The immune-mediated arthropathies also tend to have a sudden onset, with multiple joints swollen and painful in a bilaterally symmetric fashion. In some cases obvious joint swelling and pain may not be apparent, but multiple arthrocenteses and fluid analyses confirm the diagnosis. Multiple synovial fluid analyses should be performed in all cases of "pyrexia of unknown origin"; immune-mediated polyarthritis is the single most common diagnosis of such cases in a referral practice.[9]

Local lymphadenopathy is common with both the infective and the immune-mediated arthropathies. Diseases of other body systems are common with the immune-mediated arthropathies, although these can occur with certain infections as well.

BACTERIAL INFECTIVE ARTHRITIS (SEPTIC ARTHRITIS, SUPPURATIVE ARTHRITIS)

Beta-hemolytic streptococci of Lancefield group G, staphylococci, hemolytic *Escherichia coli*, *Pasteurella* sp., and *Erysipelothrix* sp. are the bacteria most commonly isolated from septic joints.[10,11] Less commonly isolated organisms include *Corynebacterium*, *Salmonella*, *Brucella*, and *Pseudomonas* spp. and anaerobic organisms. In some cases a mixed infec-tion may be present, involving both aerobic and anaerobic bacteria.

Infection can be introduced by direct penetration of a joint, as can occur with bite wounds, iatrogenic infection after open joint surgery, or arthrocentesis, or through road accident injuries. Most joint infections in cats are associated with bite wounds incurred in fights. However, in most dogs, infection occurs by the hematogenous route, and the source of infection is often unknown. Pre-existing joint disease and/or prior surgical intervention predisposes the joint to opportunistic infection as a result of seeding of organisms in the compromised synovial tissues. Trauma can predispose a joint to subsequent infection and lameness; an initial mild injury may resolve, but the lameness returns a few days later after hematogenous localization of infection to the joint. Bacterial infections may also spread to joints from infected foci in neighboring soft tissues or bone.

Most cases involve only a single joint, but two joints may be affected at the same time, or a second joint may be affected some time after the first (Figure 278-1). Involvement of more than two joints most often occurs secondary to a severe systemic bacterial infection, such as bacterial endocarditis[12] or omphalophlebitis, that has a significant bacteremic component. Bacterial endocarditis can result in a true infective arthritis or in an immune-mediated arthritis. These dogs often have lesions of other body systems, and a cardiac murmur is often present. Ultrasonography may show the vegetative endocarditic lesion.

Bacterial infective arthritis affects dogs of all ages. The larger breeds are most often affected, and the male to female

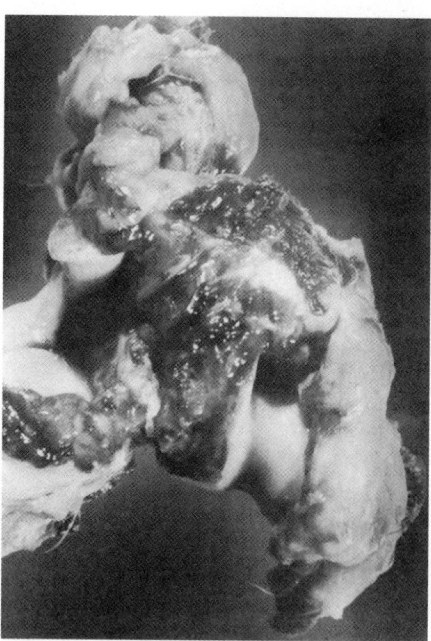

Figure 278-1 Photograph of an infected elbow joint. The synovium is thickened and hemorrhagic. There is no obvious destruction of the cartilage, which suggests that this is a relatively early lesion.

ratio is 2:1. The radiographic features vary with the type of infection and its duration. The earliest radiographic change is soft tissue swelling (Figure 278-2). A marked periosteal reaction often develops in the later stages, and calcification of the joint capsule may be seen. Subchondral bone erosions may appear as discrete radiolucencies or as more extensive bone destruction (Figure 278-3). Patchy sclerosis of subchondral bone is often seen. Some infected joints show an overall loss

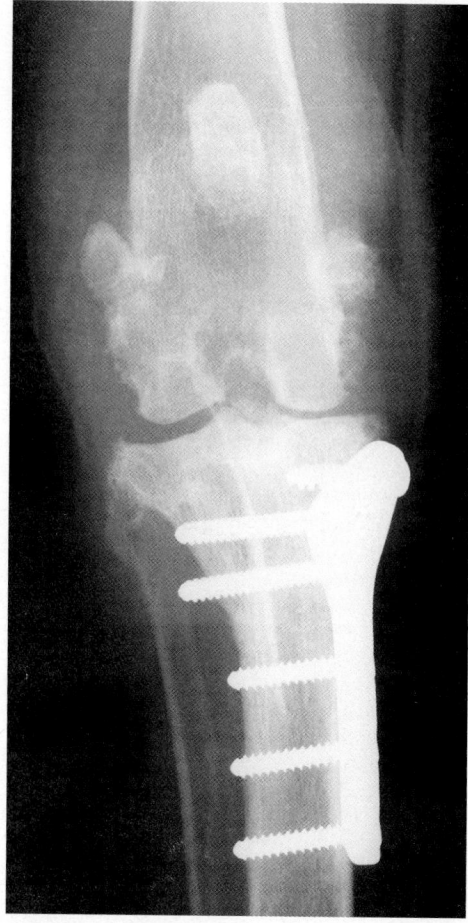

Figure 278-3 Craniocaudal radiograph of an infected stifle joint showing more advanced pathology. Bony destruction is obvious, as shown by an increased intercondylar notch and bony loss at the articular margins of the femur and tibia. Overall loss of bone density of the distal femur also is present. There is evidence of previous surgery, specifically a tibial plateau leveling osteotomy for cranial cruciate ligament failure.

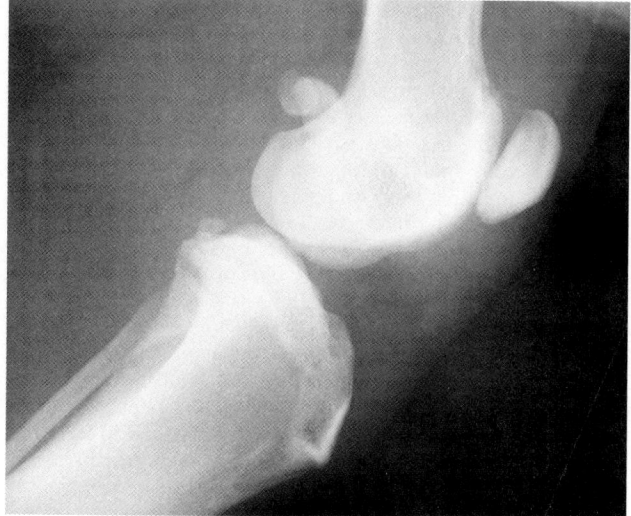

Figure 278-2 A mediolateral radiograph of an infected stifle joint. Only soft tissue changes are present. There is loss of the infrapatellar fat pad and distension of the caudal joint capsule. These changes are not specific for bacterial infective arthritis. They indicate a synovial effusion, but synovial fluid analysis is essential to demonstrate an inflammatory arthropathy; also, if only a single joint is involved, the cause is likely to be infection.

of bone density (see Figure 278-3). Leukocytosis, as a result of neutrophilia and a left shift, is an inconsistent finding.

The diagnosis of bacterial infective arthritis is confirmed by culture of the organism from synovial fluid or synovial membrane (or both); however, negative cultures are not uncommon. Blood cultures are sometimes worthwhile if the animal is pyrexic. Bacterial sensitivity testing should be performed on positive cultures to aid therapeutic planning.

The mainstay of therapy is a prolonged course of systemic antibiotics, which should be initiated in all suspect cases pending confirmatory laboratory results. A broad-spectrum bactericidal antibiotic is used. Ampicillin, clavulonate-potentiated amoxicillin, and cephalosporins are all useful. The antibiotic should be changed only if indicated by subsequent antibiotic sensitivity tests. If anaerobic infection is suspected or if the response to the initial antibiotic is poor, metronidazole is used in combination with other antibiotics. Local gentamicin beads or sponges can be used with resistant infections.[13]

Systemic antibiotic therapy is continued for at least 4 to 6 weeks, or for 2 weeks after complete resolution of clinical signs. Joint lavage and drainage are particularly indicated if the clinical signs are severe or if the patient is an immature animal with open growth plates. Rest of the joint, by means of strict confinement and support bandaging, is important in the

HEMATOLOGY AND IMMUNOLOGY

early stages. Analgesics are generally necessary, and the non-steroidal anti-inflammatory drugs are ideal for this. During the recovery phase, controlled exercise, such as passive flexion and extension or gentle lead walks, should be initiated to maintain range of movement in the joint. The level of exercise can be gradually increased after the first 4 weeks.

LYME ARTHRITIS

Lyme disease is a tick-borne, multisystemic illness that affects humans and a number of domestic animals. It is caused by infection with the spirochete *Borrelia burgdorferi*, which is primarily transmitted by ticks of the *Ixodes* genus.[14-16] The most common presenting sign in dogs is acute lameness associated with a migratory monoarthritis or pauciarthritis. True polyarthritis is rare, although an immune-mediated arthritis has been reported. Episodes of lameness typically last only a few days, although repeat episodes may occur. Other manifestations include neurologic and cardiac signs. Radiographs of affected joints may be normal or may show only soft tissue swelling in the joints.

A diagnosis of Lyme disease is difficult to establish with certainty. *B. burgdorferi* is notoriously difficult to culture from clinical cases. Serologic testing is of value, although subclinical and asymptomatic infections can occur. Approximately 20% of normal dogs with a history of a tick bite are seropositive for *B. burgdorferi*, therefore the mere presence of a positive serum anti-*Borrelia* antibody test in a lame dog is insufficient to establish a diagnosis of Lyme disease.[15]

Lyme disease is treated with antibiotics, such as tetracycline, penicillin derivatives, and erythromycin. A response normally is seen within 7 days of the start of treatment, but antibiotic therapy should be continued for at least 2 weeks after resolution of all clinical signs. Most cases have an excellent prognosis, particularly if diagnosed and treated promptly.

Cats undoubtedly are exposed to *B. burgdorferi*, in that 4.2% to 15% of normal cats are seropositive for the organism, but little evidence of clinical disease exists in this species.[17-19] The reason for this is unclear, but the cat's immune response does differ from the dog's in that felines shown an early response to OspA and B antigens.[18]

BACTERIAL L-FORMS AND ARTHRITIS

L-form bacteria are cell wall–deficient bacteria, and these organisms have been associated with pyogenic subcutaneous abscesses and arthritis in cats. The infection spreads locally and hematogenously to involve other joints and subcutaneous sites. The infection is resistant to many antibiotics but is susceptible to tetracyclines.

MYCOPLASMAL ARTHRITIS

Mycoplasmal infection of joints may arise as a result of the spread of organisms from localized sites of active or latent infection in the mucous membranes of the airways, conjunctivae, or urogenital tract. This is most likely to occur in debilitated or immunodepressed animals. *Mycoplasma gatae* and *Mycoplasma felis* have been associated with polyarthritis and tenosynovitis in cats. Infection with *Mycoplasma spumans* is associated with a polyarthritis syndrome of young greyhounds[20,21]; it is essentially a nonsuppurative polysynovitis, usually associated with severe destruction of articular cartilage.

Animals with mycoplasmal arthritis present between the ages of 3 and 30 months (average age is 18 months) with an insidious onset of clinical signs. The organisms may be seen in a synovial fluid smear stained with Wright, Leishman, or Giemsa stain; they may also be found in the cerebrospinal fluid. Mycoplasmal arthritis can be treated with tylosin, gentamicin, or erythromycin.

FUNGAL ARTHRITIS

Fungal arthritis is very rare. It usually occurs as an extension of fungal osteomyelitis but may also present as a primary granulomatous synovitis. Fungal infections of joints have involved a range of organisms, including *Coccidioides immitis*, *Blastomyces dermatitidis*, *Filobasidiella* (*Cryptococcus*) *neoformans*, *Sporotrichum schenckii*, and *Aspergillus terreus*. The organisms may be seen in synovial fluid smears or cultured from the joint.

RICKETTSIAL ARTHRITIS

Polyarthritis increasingly is recognized in association with rickettsial infections in dogs. *Rickettsia rickettsii*, the causative organism in Rocky Mountain spotted fever (RMSF), is transmitted by ticks of the *Dermacentor* genus and is endemic in wooded areas of the central United States and the eastern seaboard. RMSF is a severe disease associated with rapid dissemination of *R. rickettsii* from the site of the tick bite to many organs in the body, resulting in widespread vasculitis. Polyarthritis is one possible clinical sign.

Canine ehrlichiosis (*Ehrlichia canis* infection transmitted by the tick *Rhipicephalus sanguineus*) may present as a polyarthritis in certain geographically restricted areas, including Missouri and Tennessee. Cats are thought to suffer infection by rickettsiae of the *Ehrlichia* genus, but case reports are lacking.

PROTOZOAL ARTHRITIS

Leishmaniasis is a chronic systemic disease caused by the protozoan parasite *Leishmania donovani*. *L. donovani* is transmitted by insect vectors, mainly sandflies, and is endemic in areas such as the Mediterranean, Africa, Asia, and South America. The dog is the main reservoir host in many areas. In addition to polyarthritis, signs such as fever, malaise, weight loss, dermatopathy, lymphadenopathy, and hepatosplenomegaly may occur in the dog. The disease has a long latent period and may appear in nonendemic areas despite prolonged quarantine procedures. The synovitis is usually associated with an infiltrate of large numbers of macrophages filled with *Leishmania* bodies. An immune-mediated polyarthritis may also be seen in association with the infection. Leishmaniasis is an important zoonosis, and there are public health implications if the disease is diagnosed in dogs, particularly outside endemic areas. Cats can become infected, but clinical disease is rare.

Toxoplasma gondii infection is well known in the cat and does occur rarely in the dog; lameness can be a feature, but joint involvement is poorly documented. *Neospora caninum* infection can cause a polymyositis as well as neurologic disease; only experimental infection in the cat has been reported.

Infection with *Hepatozoon canis* can cause polyarthritis and polymyositis in both the dog and the cat. Infection occurs by ingestion of the vector tick (*R. sanguineus*), which contains the organism in its digestive tract.

Infection with *Babesia* spp. most often causes severe anemia, although polyarthritis and polymyositis have very rarely been described. *B. canis* and *B. gibsoni* affect the dog, and *B. felis*, *B. cati*, *B. herpailuri*, and *B. pantherae* affect the cat. Babesioses are tick-borne diseases carried by ixodid ticks, and concurrent infection with other protozoal organisms can occur.

VIRAL ARTHRITIS

Calicivirus can produce a true infective arthritis in the cat, most often under cattery conditions, and certain strains are more likely to be involved. Experimental studies have shown that calicivirus can infect joints and cause synovitis, and that live virus can be recovered from these joints.[22,23] A field strain of calicivirus isolated from a lame cat (strain F65) was used to infect experimental cats either intra-articularly or by contact exposure. This strain was particularly trophic for the joints, although nasal, oral, and ocular tissues were also infected.

IMMUNE-MEDIATED ARTHRITIDES

The immune-based arthropathies are divided into two broad categories, erosive and nonerosive,[24-29] based on whether bony destructive changes are present on the radiographs. The diseases that cause bony destruction generally have a poorer prognosis. A radiographic survey of several joints should be made.

EROSIVE IMMUNE-BASED ARTHRITIDES

Rheumatoid Arthritis

Rheumatoid arthritis (Figures 278-4 and 278-5) can affect any breed or cross-breed of dog; it is very rare in the cat.[30] Animals are usually adult, although the exact age of onset varies (an average age of 5 to 6 years is reported).[24]

The classic radiologic feature of rheumatoid arthritis is the presence of subchondral bone destruction, visualized as an irregularity of the articular surface or as "punched out" erosions (Figure 278-6). Advanced cases may show extensive bone destruction with gross joint deformity. A more generalized loss of mineralization of the epiphysis can be another feature, and soft tissue swelling around or synovial effusion within the joint may be present. Calcification of the soft tissues around the joint is often seen. In some early cases, radiographic evidence of bone destruction may be absent; such evidence generally appears within 6 months if the disease persists.

Rheumatoid arthritis is commonly but not invariably associated with the presence of circulating autoantibodies against immunoglobulin G, collectively known as rheumatoid factor.[31] However, rheumatoid factor is not specific for this disease, because it occurs in the other immune-mediated arthropathies and in other disease states, particularly those of

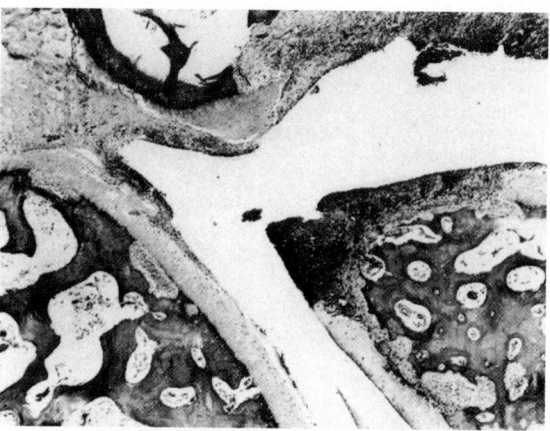

Figure 278-5 Photomicrograph of a canine rheumatoid joint. The articular cartilage has been replaced with granulation tissue in several areas, and a thin covering of the articular cartilage by granulation tissue (pannus) is seen in some areas.

a chronic nature, in which antigen-antibody interaction ocurs.[31] Certain dogs in which rheumatoid arthritis can be diagnosed test negative for rheumatoid factor, and some dogs initially may test positive but later test negative, and vice versa.

Periosteal Proliferative Polyarthritis

Periosteal proliferative polyarthritis, an erosive polyarthritis, is rare in the dog but common in the cat.[30] It affects mainly the hocks and carpi, and the characteristic feature is marked periosteal new bone formation, often extending beyond the confines of the joint (Figure 278-7). Also, one or more joints show localized bony erosions. Bony destruction and proliferation can also occur at the attachment of ligaments and tendons, lesions known as *enthesiopathies*. Cats of any age can be

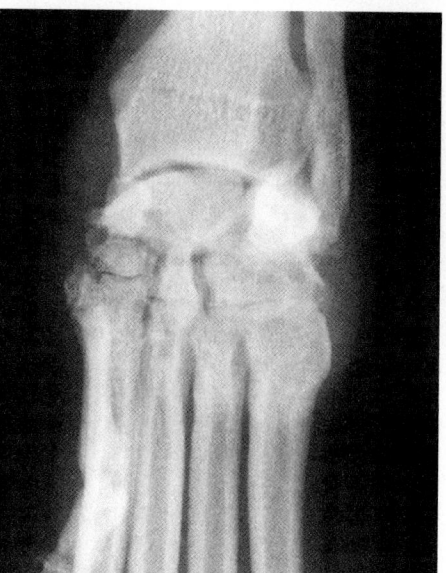

Figure 278-6 Craniocaudal radiograph of a carpus of a dog with rheumatoid arthritis. The obvious radiolucent areas in the carpal bones represent bony lysis. Also, the joint space is increased between some of the carpal bones. This appearance may be seen with a septic joint, but this dog had multiple joint involvement consistent with an immune-based polyarthritis.

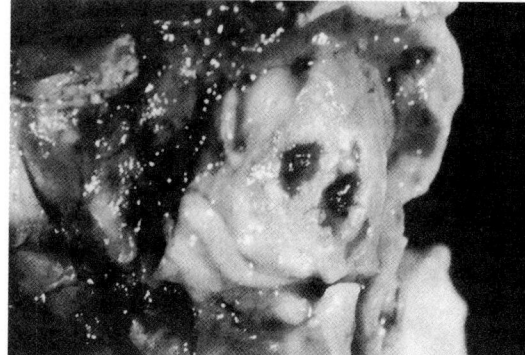

Figure 278-4 Gross appearance of the carpus of a dog with rheumatoid arthritis. Two obvious areas of cartilage and bone loss can be seen, and the resultant ulcers have been replaced with granulation tissue. The synovium is thickened and discolored. Multiple, symmetric joint involvement was apparent in this dog.

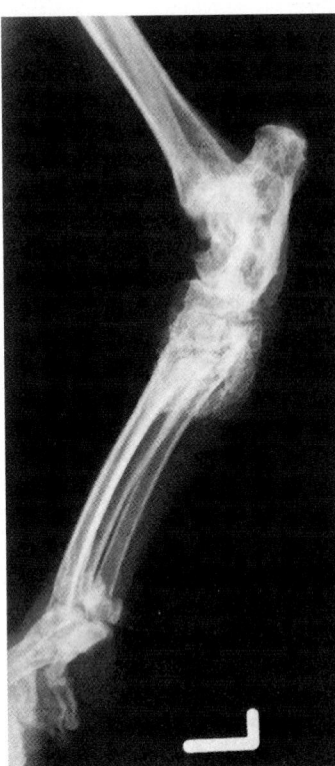

Figure 278-7 Mediolateral radiograph of the hock joint of a cat with periosteal proliferative polyarthritis. New bone deposits are seen on the bones of the hock joint and on the distal tibia and proximal metatarsus. The periosteal reaction extends beyond the confines of the joint. Small areas of bone lysis also can be seen in most of the tarsal bones. Two small areas of bone lysis are present in the tip of the os calcis, together with periosteal new bone, a finding consistent with an erosive enthesiopathy.

affected, although the disease is said to be common in young adults. Male castrated cats appear to be affected more often.

NONEROSIVE IMMUNE-BASED ARTHRITIS

Systemic Lupus Erythematosus

Systemic lupus erythematosus (SLE) is a multisystemic disease characterized by simultaneous or sequential development of autoimmune hemolytic anemia, immune-mediated thrombocytopenia, leukopenia, glomerulonephritis, dermatitis, polymyositis, pleuritis, central nervous system (CNS) disease, and symmetric polyarthritis.[26] SLE occurs in both dogs and cats, and because the clinical signs are so variable, diagnosis of the disease can be difficult.

The pathogenesis of SLE involves two main components, autoimmunity and immune complex hypersensitivity. Antibodies against red blood cells, platelets, and leukocytes are important in the development of hemolytic anemia, thrombocytopenia, and leukopenia; the deposition of immune complexes (possibly nuclear antigen and antinuclear antibody) in the kidneys (glomeruli), joints (synovial blood vessels), and skin (dermal/epidermal junction), and possibly in other organs, explains the inflammatory changes in these tissues.

Joint radiographs may show no obvious abnormalities, although occasionally soft tissue swelling or synovial effusion is present.

SLE is characterized by the presence of circulating antinuclear antibody (ANA), a group of autoantibodies targeted against nuclear material.[32] Although antinuclear antibody is found in various chronic disease states, a diagnosis of SLE cannot be justified unless the ANA test result is positive.

POLYARTHRITIS/POLYMYOSITIS SYNDROME

In polyarthritis/polymyositis syndrome, polyarthritis is complicated by polymyositis. This syndrome is most often seen in spaniel breeds.[27] The dogs test negative for antinuclear antibody, therefore the disease cannot be categorized as SLE.

These dogs present with marked stiffness and poor exercise tolerance, and they often adopt a crouched stance. Widespread muscle atrophy is usually apparent, although in the early stages, muscle swelling and pain may be seen. Muscle atrophy can be associated with fibrosis and contracture, resulting in reduced joint motion; this may be seen in the limb joints and also in the temporomandibular joints, leaving the dog unable to open its mouth.

The muscle enzymes creatine phosphokinase and aldolase are often increased, but not in all cases. Electromyography may show focal areas of spontaneous activity in affected muscles. The myositis is confirmed by multiple muscle biopsy examination (at least six muscles), although the inflammatory change can be patchy and may be absent from some muscles (myositis should be seen in at least two of the biopsy samples).

POLYARTHRITIS/MENINGITIS SYNDROME

Polyarthritis/meningitis syndrome has been seen in several breeds, including the weimaraner, Newfoundland, German short-haired pointer, boxer, corgi, and Bernese mountain dog. It also is reported in the cat. These animals present with pyrexia, stiffness, and neck pain and in some cases with nervous signs. Cerebrospinal fluid shows increased protein, white cell, and creatine phosphokinase levels, indicating an inflammatory lesion of the central nervous system.

SJÖGREN SYNDROME

In humans Sjögren syndrome was originally described as a syndrome comprising keratoconjunctivitis sicca ("dry eye"), xerostomia ("dry mouth"), and a polyarthritis, which may be an erosive (rheumatoid) arthritis or a nonerosive arthritis. Dry eye in the dog has been reported with SLE and lymphocytic thyroiditis.[1] Sialadenitis with rheumatoid arthritis has also been documented.[1]

FAMILIAL RENAL AMYLOIDOSIS IN CHINESE SHAR PEIS

Dogs with familial renal amyloidosis of Chinese Shar Peis present with episodes of fever and with swelling of one or both hock joints and occasionally other joints.[33,34] Enthesiopathies are also seen. The age of onset of signs is variable (young puppies or adult dogs), and the period between attacks can be variable but often is 4 to 6 weeks. Amyloid deposits occur in several organs, but renal amyloidosis and hepatic amyloidosis are the conditions most significant to the prognosis. Amyloidosis eventually results in renal or hepatic failure, which may occur any time between 1.5 and 6 years of age.

POLYARTHRITIS OF THE ADOLESCENT AKITA

Polyarthritis of adolescent Akitas affects dogs less than 1 year of age.[35] Meningitis may also be present, as may other organ involvement. These dogs have an unfavorable prognosis, because the response to anti-inflammatory and immunomodulatory drugs is poor.

POLYARTERITIS NODOSA

Polyarteritis nodosa is an inflammatory condition of the small arteries, often of a granulomatous nature, that can be diagnosed only by histologic examination of biopsy material. Polyarthritis, polymyositis, and meningitis can occur. The attacks are often cyclical, although persistent signs can occur.

DRUG-INDUCED ARTHRITIS

Drug-induced vasculitides are basically hypersensitivity reactions involving the deposition of drug antibody complexes around blood vessels in different areas of the body. The drug may act directly as an antigen or may combine with host proteins as haptens to form neoantigens.

Polyarthritis is only one feature of these disease syndromes; fever, lymphadenopathy, and macular-papular or bullous-type hemorrhagic rashes are common. Thrombocytopenia, hemolytic anemia, polymyositis, retinitis, and glomerulonephritis are also reported.

The most commonly incriminated drugs are antibiotics, particularly sulfa drugs, lincomycin, erythromycin, cephalosporins, and penicillins. The Doberman pinscher appears particularly susceptible to sulphadiazine-trimethoprim.[36] The diagnosis is made on the basis of worsening clinical signs while the animal is undergoing drug therapy and very rapid improvement (2 to 7 days) after the drug is stopped. The animal usually has had to have encountered the drug previously to become sensitized or has been undergoing long-term therapy.

VACCINATION REACTIONS

Occasionally an immune-based polyarthritis can develop after vaccine inoculations. It is most likely to occur after the first injection of a primary vaccination course, particularly in kittens.[37] The polyarthritis is generally seen 5 to 7 days after the first inoculation, and the lameness is usually only transient, lasting for 24 to 48 hours.

The calicivirus component appears to cause the condition, and calicivirus antigens have been identified in synovial macrophages of vaccinated (F9 strain) and naturally infected (A4 strain) cats.[22] The presence of these antigens has been associated with an active synovitis.

Persistent polyarthritis in the dog has been reported after recent vaccination.[38] Canine distemper antigens have been found in immune complexes from the joints of dogs with immune-mediated arthritis.[3]

IDIOPATHIC POLYARTHRITIS

Idiopathic polyarthritis includes all those cases of inflammatory arthropathy that cannot be classified into the other groups. It is still the most common type of polyarthritis in both the dog and the cat.

The idiopathic group can be divided into four subcategories[1]:
- Type I: Uncomplicated idiopathic arthritis; this is the most common subgroup.
- Type II: Idiopathic arthritis associated with infections remote from the joints (reactive arthritis). The infections commonly occur in the respiratory tract, tonsils, conjunctiva (e.g., chlamydia in the cat), urinary tract, uterine tract, skin (including anal furunculosis) and oral cavity.[28]
- Type III: Idiopathic arthritis associated with gastrointestinal disease (enteropathic arthritis). The gastroenteritis is usually characterized by vomiting and/or diarrhea. Sometimes blood is present in the feces. Cases of intestinal bacterial overgrowth and malabsorption have been complicated by polyarthritis, and very occasionally the intestinal disease is an ulcerative colitis.
- Type IV: Idiopathic arthritis associated with neoplasia remote from the joints (arthritis of malignancy). The neoplastic lesion may not be apparent by clinical assessment; some are recorded only during a *postmortem* examination. Neoplasias have included squamous cell carcinoma, heart base tumor, leiomyoma, and mammary adenocarcinoma.[28] In the cat, myeloproliferative disease is the most common association,[30] and cats with a nonerosive polyarthritis that do not respond well to therapy should always have a bone marrow examination and should be tested for feline leukemia virus (FeLV) and feline immunodeficiency virus (FIV).

The age of onset can vary from a few months to 11 years; many animals are young adults (1 to 3 years) when first presented, especially in type I cases. The pathology is generally an acute/subacute synovitis (Figures 278-8 and 278-9). Soft tissue swelling and/or synovial effusion may be apparent on radiography (Figure 278-10), although often no abnormality is visible. Disease of other body systems is not uncommon.

TREATMENT

The treatment and prognosis vary with the different types of polyarthritis. Repeated synovial fluid analysis is the most sensitive method of monitoring the effectiveness of treatment. A fall in the total cell count and a reduction in the proportion of polymorphs are good prognostic signs. The erosive arthropathies and animals with multiple-system disease tend to have a poorer prognosis.

The initial treatment in most cases is to attempt immunosuppression with high doses of corticosteroids. These are given

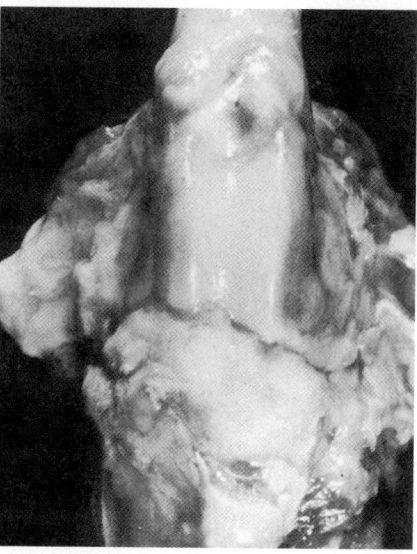

Figure 278-8 Photograph of the stifle joint from a dog with nonerosive polyarthritis (idiopathic type 1). The synovium is thickened and discolored, but the articular cartilage appears normal.

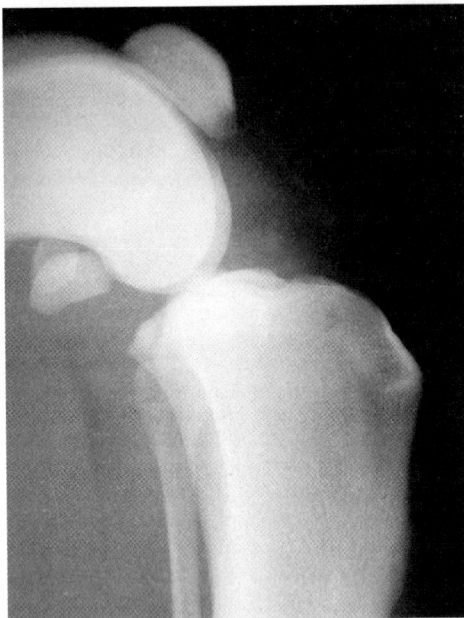

Figure 278-9 Mediolateral radiograph of the stifle joint of a dog with nonerosive polyarthritis (idiopathic type 1). Only soft tissue changes are seen (loss of the infrapatellar fat pad and distension of the caudal joint capsule). Although these changes are not specific for immune-mediated arthritis, this dog had multiple symmetric joint involvement, and the synovial fluid analysis was consistent with an inflammatory arthropathy.

orally for 2 weeks (prednisolone, 2 to 4 mg/kg) in a daily divided dose, and the dosage then is gradually reduced over the next 4 to 8 weeks. Generally a marked response occurs within a few days, but it is important that therapy be maintained to help prevent relapses.

Repeat arthrocentesis and synovial fluid analysis of a joint initially sampled for diagnostic purposes are performed at 2 weeks; if the white cell count has fallen below 4000/mm³ and most of the cells are mononuclear, the prognosis is reasonably good. If the polymorph count is still high, high-dose steroid

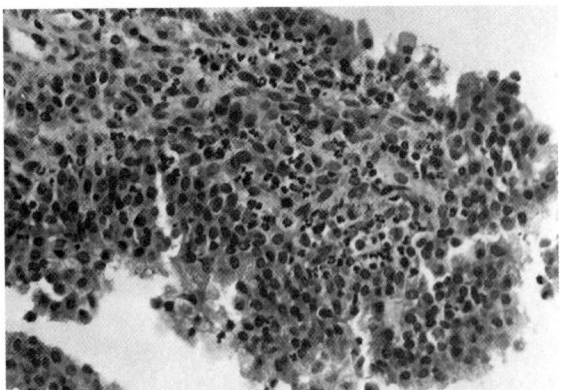

Figure 278-10 Photomicrograph of a synovial membrane biopsy sample from a dog with idiopathic type 1 polyarthritis. Hyperplasia and hypertrophy of the lining layer are present, as is an inflammatory infiltrate of mononuclear and polymorphonuclear cells in the supporting layer. This is typical of an inflammatory arthropathy, whether infective or immune based, and it could be consistent even with a degenerative arthropathy.

therapy should be continued for a longer period. Relapses are always possible, therefore the prognosis overall is guarded.

If relapses occur or if the response to prednisolone therapy is poor, a combination of prednisolone and cytotoxic drugs can be tried. The cytotoxic drug of choice is cyclophosphamide, given orally at a dosage of 1.5 mg/kg (for dogs over 30 kg), 2 mg/kg (for dogs 15 to 30 kg), or 2.5 mg/kg (for dogs under 15 kg). The drug is given on 4 consecutive days of each week or as close to this regimen as possible, allowing for the fact that, because of health and safety issues, tablets cannot be divided. In addition, oral prednisolone is given each day at an anti-inflammatory dosage (0.25 to 0.5 mg/kg) to help control pain by reducing the articular inflammatory load. This treatment is continued for 2 to 4 months, even though clinical remission may occur much earlier. Cyclophosphamide should not be used for longer than 4 months because of bladder toxicity problems. The urine can be tested weekly for blood, but the drug does not need to be stopped unless overt blood is visible.

Once cytotoxic therapy has been instigated, blood counts should be monitored every 7 to 14 days. If the white cell count falls below 6000/mm³ or the platelet count below 125,000/mm³, the dosage should be reduced by one fourth; if the white cell count falls below 4000/mm³ or the platelet count below 1,000,000/mm³, the drug should be discontinued for 2 weeks and then recommenced at half the original dosage.

In dogs (but not in cats), azathioprine can be used as an alternative to cyclophosphamide, at a daily oral dosage of approximately 2 mg/kg every other day, together with low-dose prednisolone given every other day (alternating with the azathioprine). Bone marrow suppression is more likely with azathioprine.

If the response to cytotoxic drugs and prednisolone is still poor or if relapses occur, a combination of a cytotoxic drug, low-dose prednisolone, and levamisole can be tried. Levamisole may act as an immunomodulatory drug (i.e., it may suppress helper T cells). It is administered as a liquid oral preparation at a dosage of 5 to 7 mg/kg every other day up to a maximum of 150 mg daily.

Whatever the therapeutic regimen used, the intention is to stop therapy after 3 to 6 months. Generally the cytotoxic drug and levamisole are stopped first, and the steroid is continued at an ever-decreasing dosage.

Gold injections (sodium aurothiomalate or aurothioglucose) have been used in cases of rheumatoid arthritis with some success. It is important to administer a small test dose before full treatment is begun to check for any adverse sensitivity to the drug, and the animal must be checked regularly during treatment for toxic side effects. The dose ranges from 5 to 40 mg, given by intramuscular injection at weekly intervals for 6 weeks. Generally, low-dose prednisolone also is given.

Auranofin (Ridaura), an oral preparation of gold, is also available. Auranofin, which is given at a dosage 0.05 to 2 mg/kg administered twice daily, is less toxic than the injectable gold preparation, but diarrhea is a common side effect.

A combination of oral methotrexate and leflunomide has been used in the cat to treat rheumatoid arthritis. The methotrexate dose is given once weekly; on the day it is given the dose is 7.5 mg divided into three separate and equal doses of 2.5 mg each. The leflunomide dose is 10 milograms daily and is given by oral administration. When significant improvement has occurred, the doses are reduced to 2.5 mg of methotrexate once weekly and 10 mg of leflunomide twice weekly.

Constant corticosteroid therapy sometimes is necessary to keep an animal in clinical remission, and this is perhaps acceptable if only a small dose is required. A few patients spontaneously recover within a day or two without any treatment. Nonsteroidal anti-inflammatory drugs can be used in mild cases or while laboratory results are awaited.

Treatment of idiopathic arthritis types II, III, and IV is directed primarily against the infective, alimentary, or neoplastic lesion, although corticosteroid therapy may be necessary. Colchicine treatment has been used in attempts to control the amyloidosis of familial renal amyloidosis of the Chinese Shar Pei, but its effectiveness has not been proved, and it does not influence the episodes of fever and arthritis.

It is important to provide supportive therapy for these animals when appropriate. Rest, avoidance of stress environments, and good nutrition are essential. Patients receiving immunosuppressive therapy should be checked regularly for secondary infections, and owners should be warned to avoid potential disease environments. Because of the possible involvement of canine distemper virus in immune-mediated arthritis, dogs that have suffered immune-mediated polyarthritis should be screened for distemper antibody levels when a booster inoculation is due; if the levels are consistent with protection, the booster should exclude the distemper component.

CHAPTER • 279

Skeletal Diseases

Kenneth A. Johnson
A.D.J. Watson

INTRODUCTION

Animals with bone disease may have signs of lameness, deformity, or dysfunction that could be confused with, or complicated by, joint, muscle, or neurologic disorders. Therefore a systematic approach is necessary in evaluating animals with these signs. The expertise of a radiologist and bone pathologist will often be invaluable in establishing a diagnosis. Traumatic injuries should also be considered in the differential diagnosis but are not discussed here, because excellent descriptions exist elsewhere.[1] Some bone diseases that also affect joints are described in Chapter 278.

The precise cause of many bone diseases that affect dogs and cats is unknown. Furthermore, some conditions have multiple causes, such as the congenital, heritable, and metabolic disorders. This makes logical classification difficult. A causative system is used here for want of a better alternative.

BONE PATHOPHYSIOLOGY

Structural Organization of Bone

Bone is a living tissue with several important functions, including storage of calcium, phosphorus, and other minerals. Bones act as a series of levers that facilitate the action of muscles and joints in movement, and they provide support and protection for other body systems. In addition, bone marrow stroma provides an inductive environment for hematopoiesis and is a source of osteogenic precursor cells.[2,3] Bones are structurally composed of compact (cortical) and cancellous (trabecular) bone (Figure 279-1).[4] The microstructural units of cortical bone are osteons that, in cross-section, have concentric layers of collagen fibers and a central canal.

Trabeculae of cancellous bone have a three-dimensional lattice arrangement and large intertrabecular spaces containing hemopoietic or fatty marrow tissue. Long bones have several distinct regions: diaphysis, metaphysis, and epiphysis (see Figure 279-1). In growing animals, each epiphysis contains one or more ossification centers, is covered by hyaline cartilage on the articular surface, and is separated from the metaphysis by the physis or growth plate.[5,6] For reasons not well understood, many diseases have a predilection for certain regions of bone or even for particular bones.

Bone cells are derived from two separate cell systems: (1) the stromal fibroblastic (osteoblasts and osteocytes) and (2) hemopoietic (osteoclasts) systems.[2,3] During bone formation, osteoblasts synthesize collagenous matrix called *osteoid*, which is mineralized to become bone. Osteoblasts entrapped in newly forming bone become osteocytes. At sites of normal skeletal growth and remodeling, osteoblasts are derived from determined osteoblast precursor cells that reside in bone marrow stroma, endosteum, and periosteum. In injury or disease, inducible osteogenic precursor cells derived from other mesenchymal tissues, such as muscle and fibrous tissue, can be stimulated to differentiate to osteoblasts and form extraperiosteal ectopic bone. Osteoblasts can form several different types of bone.[4] Lamellar bone has collagen fibers in a parallel array and is found in osteons and mature trabecular bone. Formation of lamellar bone requires a pre-existing matrix, such as calcified cartilage matrix (so-called endochondral ossification) or old bone that has been partially removed by osteoclastic resorption. Woven bone is characterized by random orientation of its collagen fibers. It can be deposited *de novo*, without pre-existing bone or cartilage, and is formed when new bone is laid down rapidly in growth, fracture repair, and bone disease.[7] Normally it is remodeled to lamellar bone but may persist in rapidly growing osteogenic tumors.

Osteoclasts are large, multinucleate cells formed by fusion of circulating mononuclear cells. They are found on the surface of bone trabeculae and within remodeling osteons and are responsible for bone removal during growth, modeling, and remodeling of the skeleton. Osteoclasts erode mineralized bone first by solubilizing mineral, then digesting the protein.[3] This leaves concave pits in the bone surface, called *Howship's lacunae*. Formation and resorption of bone is regulated systemically by parathyroid hormone (PTH), calcitonin, and

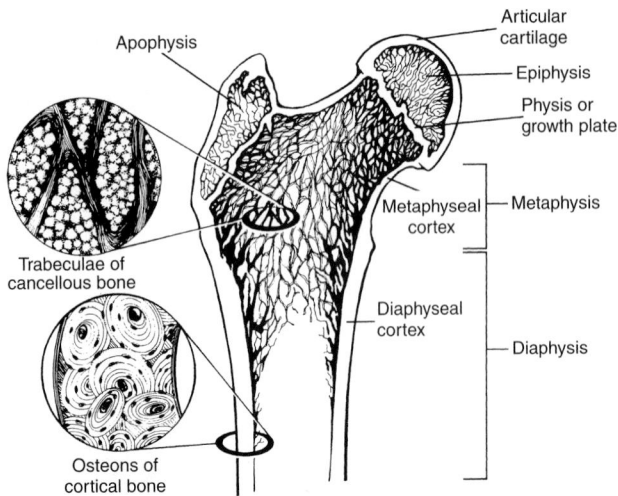

Figure 279-1 Regions and microstructure of an immature proximal femur.

vitamin D (Chapter 237). The principle action of PTH is to activate osteoclastic bone resorption and increase blood calcium concentration. Osteoblasts have PTH receptors, but osteoclasts do not. The increase in osteoclast number and activity induced by PTH is mediated by osteoblasts via a complex coupling mechanism involving several cytokines, including receptor activator of nuclear factor - kappa B (RANK) ligand, interleukins, and tumor necrosis factor (TNF).[2,3]

Bone Growth and Development

Growth of the axial and appendicular skeleton is primarily by endochondral ossification at the physes. Most physeal growth is longitudinal, but the zone of Ranvier and subperiosteal appositional growth contribute circumferential expansion as well. Physes have various zones that reflect chondrocytic structure and metabolic activity, but the transition between zones is gradual (Figure 279-2). Once formed, each chondrocyte remains in a fixed anatomic location throughout its life and there accomplishes all its functions.[8,9] The two most prominent stages involve proliferation and hypertrophy (including mineralization of matrix), prior to tissue resorption during vascularization. Most of the longitudinal growth of a physis is due to the tenfold increase in chondrocyte volume that is maximal in the hypertrophic zone. Defects in any part of the sequence, such as incomplete chondrocyte maturation, cause dwarfism or disordered bone growth (see Figure 279-2).

Modeling of Bone

Modeling is the process that molds and sculpts the contours of expanding bones during growth. Within the metaphysis, the primary spongiosa is modeled to secondary spongiosa, which in turn is resorbed to form the marrow cavity of the shaft. Simultaneously, bone diameter decreases rapidly in the metaphyseal *cutback zone* as redundant bone is removed by subperiosteal osteoclastic resorption. In modeling, bone formation rates are frequently unequal to resorption rates, but unlike remodeling, bone formation is not dependent on resorption to precede it.[10] Modeling can correct the shape of malunited fractures, deformities, and bone subjected to altered loading, as predicted by Wolff's law. However, because the modeling process is closely coupled to growth, it is usually less effective after maturity.[10]

Normal and Pathologic Bone Remodeling

Remodeling is the process in which bone renews itself throughout life.[10] It always follows the sequence of activation → resorption → formation, and the packets of cells at a remodeling site

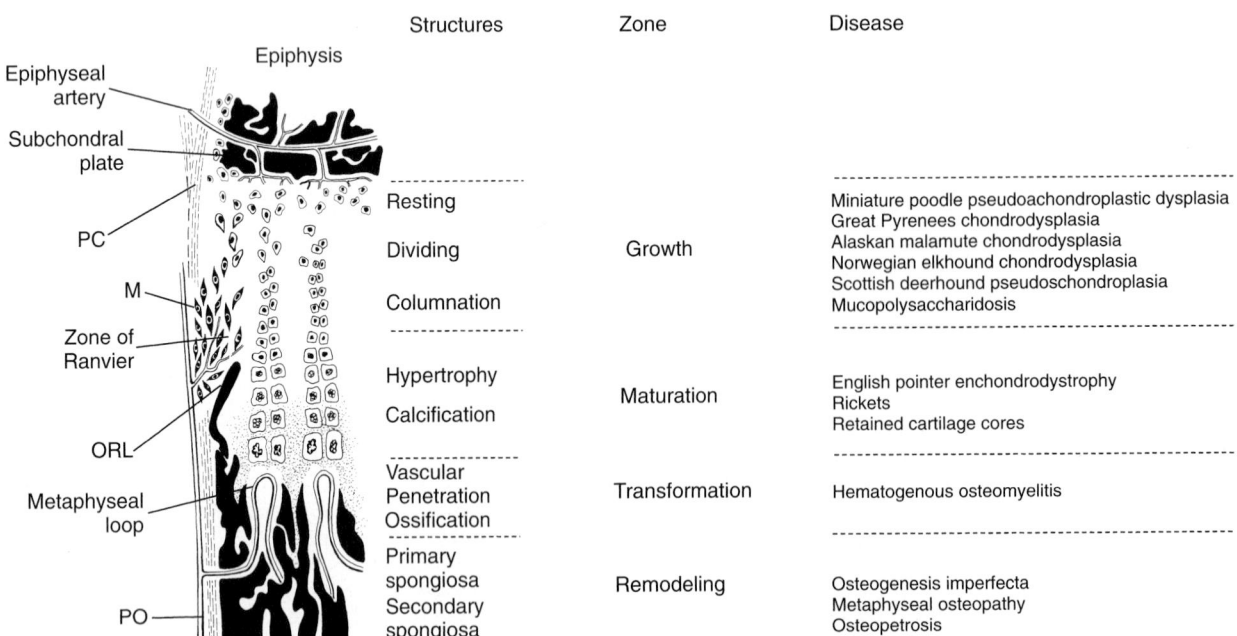

Figure 279-2 The physis divided based on histologic structure and physiologic function (growth, maturation, transformation, and remodeling). Regions affected by some diseases of growth and remodeling are indicated. In the zone of Ranvier, undifferentiated mesenchymal cells *(M)* give rise to chondroblasts. The periosteum *(PO)* and perichondrium *(PC)* are continuous in this region. The metaphyseal cortex also extends into this region, becoming the osseous ring of Lacroix *(ORL)*, which acts as a peripheral restraint to the cell columns but does not impede latitudinal growth of the adjacent zone of Ranvier. (Adapted from Ogden JA: Skeletal Injury in the Child, 2nd ed. Philadelphia, WB Saunders Co, 1990, p 37.)

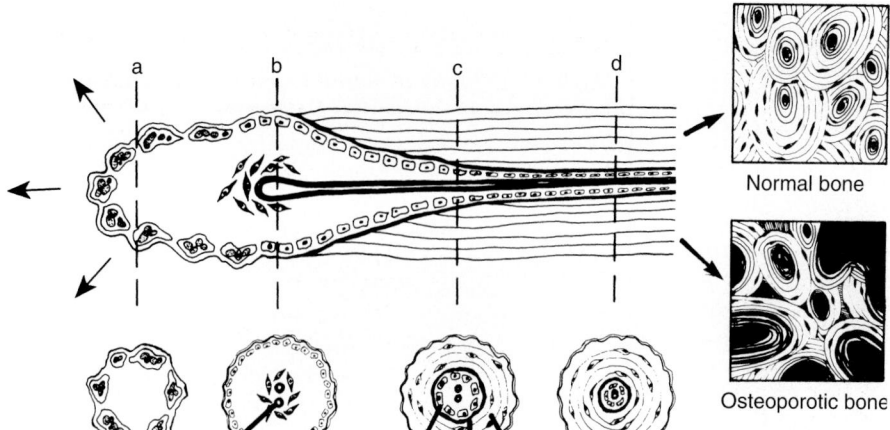

Figure 279-3 Remodeling osteon in cortical bone shown in longitudinal section. Components of this bone multicellular unit are shown in four transverse sections on the lower level. **a,** Cutter cone with osteoclasts *(OC)* resorbing bone. **b,** Capillary loop *(CL)* with undifferentiated lining cells *(LC)* in the quiescent zone between resorption and formation. **c,** Closing cone with centripetally advancing osteoblasts *(OB),* separated by an osteoid seam *(OS)* from radially deposited new lamellar bone *(LB).* **d,** Completed osteon (Haversian system).

Normal bone

Osteoporotic bone

are collectively called *bone multicellular units*.[10,11] Remodeling occurs in three bone envelopes: (1) the periosteal surface, (2) the endosteal-trabecular (cancellous bone) surface, and (3) the osteonal (intracortical) surface (Figures 279-3 and 279-4). In normal remodeling, bone formation equals resorption, whereas in bone disease a pathologic imbalance of resorption and formation often results in osteopenia of cortical and cancellous bone. Bones subjected to disease, trauma, or disuse exhibit a response termed the *regional acceleratory phenomenon*, in which the number of activated bone multicellular units increases suddenly.[10] This results in increased cortical porosity and trabecular thinning that reaches a peak at approximately 2 to 3 months; it may take up to 1 year to be reversed, during which time resorption sites are refilled with new bone.[12]

DIAGNOSIS OF BONE DISEASE

History and Signs
Initially, it is important to establish the age, breed, and sex of the patient because these factors may be associated with increased risk of a particular disease. Common complaints from owners are lameness, deformity, difficulty in rising, and reluctance to exercise. One must ascertain the duration and intensity (shifting, constant, intermittent, worsening) of the problem, any known trauma, and any previous illness, medication, or surgery, as well as response to therapy. The owner should be asked whether exercise or rest exacerbates the problem, and whether swelling, drainage, or apparent pain had been noticed. Recognition of similar problems in related

HEMATOLOGY AND IMMUNOLOGY

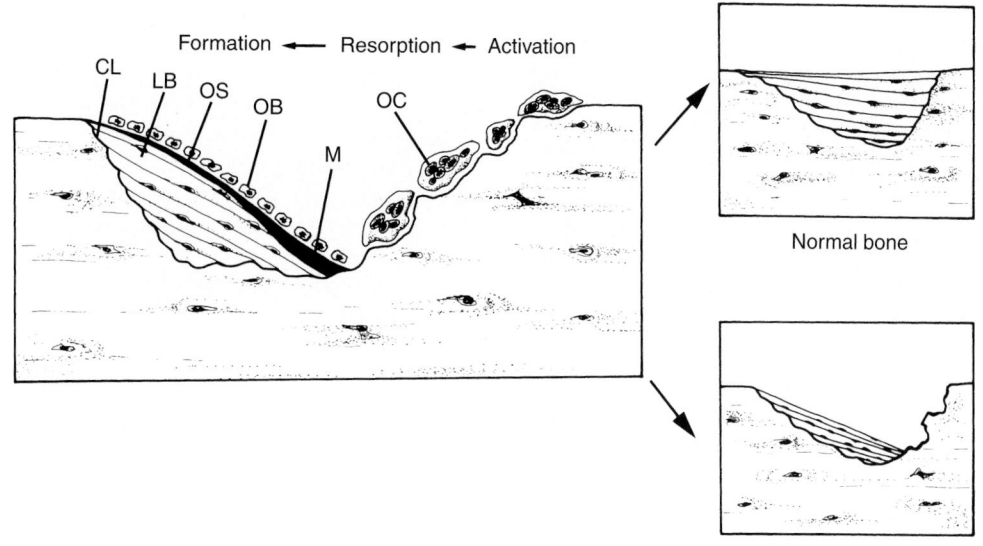

Normal bone

Osteoporotic bone

Figure 279-4 Trabecular bone remodeling with the components of bone multicellular unit: osteoclasts *(OC),* nonmineralized matrix *(M),* osteoblasts *(OB),* osteoid seam *(OS),* new lamellar bone *(LB),* and cement line *(CL)* separating it from original bone. Normally, formation equals resorption, but in diseases causing osteoporosis, bone formation is inadequate or defective.

animals may indicate heritable disease. The type and quantity of foods, vitamins, and minerals fed should be determined.

Physical Examination

In conjunction with the normal physical examination, special attention is paid to lameness and gait abnormalities and to the musculoskeletal system (see Chapters 194 and 195).[13,14] Visual appraisal might detect abnormalities in limb length and symmetry. The bony prominences and distal limb bones are palpated to detect pain, swelling, dyssymmetry, or crepitus. By comparison with the contralateral limb, muscle atrophy or altered range of joint motion may be identified. Each abnormality alone is rather nonspecific but aids in region localization. Before proceeding with sedation and radiography, further testing should be considered to exclude neurologic disease as a contributing factor (see Chapters 44 and 191).

Radiology

Radiology is the most useful method for routine noninvasive evaluation of skeletal lesions. To appreciate subtle lesions, radiographs must be excellent. Two or more views are always needed, with the limb properly positioned. Comparison with radiographs of the contralateral limb or a radiographic atlas is useful to distinguish real bone lesions from anatomic and breed variations.[15]

Bone has a limited number of ways of responding to injury or disease. Lesions should be characterized according to changes in bone density, size, shape, or contour; the type of margination; the nature of any periosteal reaction; region of bone involved; and soft tissue changes.[16-18] The finding of a particular response, such as periosteal new bone, is not necessarily diagnostic of a specific disease (Box 279-1). Abnormalities could result from traumatic, neoplastic, infectious, idiopathic, or other processes. When considered in conjunction with signalment, history, and physical abnormalities, radiographic findings may lead to a diagnosis or a list of diagnostic alternatives. At this point it is valuable to consult descriptions of various bone diseases, to evaluate the possibilities, and to decide what further tests are indicated. Tests that are directed at confirming the most likely diagnosis, yet are least invasive and have low morbidity, are done first.

Nuclear Imaging

Scintigraphy is highly sensitive in detecting skeletal lesions, but it is not widely available and is generally not specific for cause.[19,20] After a radiopharmaceutical, usually [99m]technetium labeled methylene disphosphonate ([99m]TcMDP), is injected intravenously, it is incorporated into sites of new bone formation and remodeling and in regions of increased blood flow. The distribution of radionuclide in bone is detected with a gamma camera and is an indication of skeletal metabolic activity, complementing the structural information from radiographs. In cases of lameness in which physical examination and radiographs are unremarkable, scintigraphy may pinpoint a region of increased uptake in bone or a joint. Further procedures such as computed tomography (CT), biopsy, culture, or surgical exploration would then be needed to determine the cause of the "hotspot."

Tumor metastases in bone have a characteristic multifocal distribution, detectable by scintigraphy before they are seen on radiographs.[20] Although scintigraphy also detects primary bone tumors, it is seldom needed for their diagnosis. Scintigraphy with [99m]TcMDP may help detect osteomyelitis before radiographic signs appear, but it is not specific for the disease.

Computed Tomography

High-resolution CT provides excellent cross-sectional images of lesions not found with radiographs. Its greatest application in the musculoskeletal system has been in evaluating the

---

Box • 279-1

Radiologic Signs of Some Common Bone Diseases

Bone Loss
1. Generalized and diffuse
   Primary hyperparathyroidism
   Renal secondary hyperparathyroidism
   Nutritional secondary hyperparathyroidism
   Disuse osteoporosis
2. Thin cortices
   Primary hyperparathyroidism
   Renal secondary hyperparathyroidism
   Nutritional secondary hyperparathyroidism
   Disuse osteoporosis
   Neoplasia
   Osteomyelitis
   Bone cyst
3. Focal
   Osteomyelitis
   Neoplasia
   Bone cyst
   Multifocal: myeloma, lymphosarcoma, metastases
4. Cystic
   Congenital bone cysts
   Aneurysmal bone cysts
   Subchondral bone cysts
   Central giant cell granuloma

Bone Production
1. Cortical
   Osteopetrosis
   Trauma
   Remodeling of deformity
   Fracture healing
2. Medullary
   Enostosis
   Myelosclerosis
   Osteomyelitis
   Sequestration
   Neoplasia
   Infarcts
   Fracture healing
3. Periosteal
   Hypervitaminosis A
   Mucopolysaccharidosis (MPS)
   Multiple cartilaginous exostosis
   Enostosis
   Metaphyseal osteopathy
   Craniomandibular osteopathy
   Secondary hypertrophic osteopathy
   Osteomyelitis
   Neoplasia
   Trauma

Adapted from Allan GS: Radiographic signs of diseases affecting bone. *In* Proceedings No 87, Orthopaedic Surgery in Dogs and Cats. Sydney, Australia, The University of Sydney Postgraduate Committee in Veterinary Science, 1986, p 247.

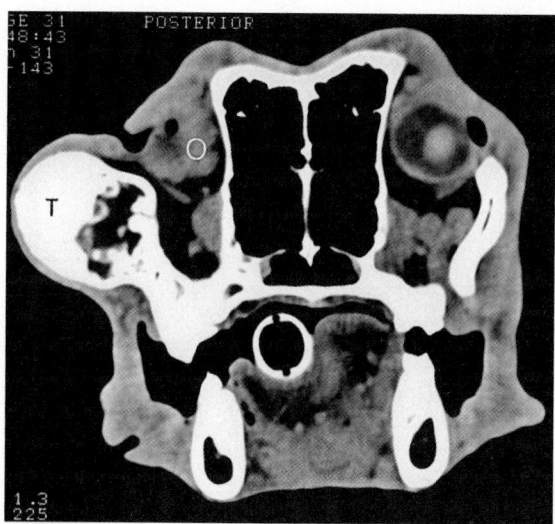

Figure 279-5 Computed tomography (CT) image of an osteoma *(T)* of the zygomatic arch that caused ocular *(O)* displacement.

complex anatomy of skull, spine and pelvis; in delineating boundaries of tumors involving soft tissues or bone; and in detecting early bone destruction.[21] For bone tumors this information allows more precise presurgical planning for en bloc resection of cranial and pelvic lesions and for limb salvage in appendicular lesions (Figure 279-5).[22-24]

Magnetic Resonance Imaging

Advantages of magnetic resonance imaging (MRI) are that high-resolution, serial, multiplanar images of skeletal soft tissues, such as ligament, tendon, menisci, and articular cartilage, can be obtained without the use of ionizing radiation. However, because this imaging modality relies on detection of changes in the orientation of mobile tissue protons within a strong magnetic field, the signal intensity of mineralized bone matrix is low. Adjacent soft tissues (periosteum, endosteum, fat, articular cartilage, and bone marrow) mainly define contours of bone. Subtle lesions of metaphyseal cancellous bone can be appreciated, as can displacement, compression, and invasion of soft tissue by expansile osseous lesions. However, cortical bone lesions are better visualized using CT.

Chemistry

Estimation of blood calcium and inorganic phosphate concentrations and of alkaline phosphatase activity will occasionally be useful in diagnosing some bone diseases, but these variables are maintained within reference ranges in many skeletal diseases. Validated assays for canine PTH, PTH-related protein, and vitamin D metabolites are useful in hypercalcemic disorders (Chapter 237).

Hematology

Alterations in circulating leukocyte numbers may be consistent with acute osteomyelitis, but the hemogram is usually unremarkable in chronic osteomyelitis and other bone diseases.

Biopsy and Histopathology

Histologic examination of a representative bone biopsy is the most reliable way to establish a diagnosis when radiographic signs are not highly characteristic of a particular disease. Biopsy may be necessary to distinguish between malignant and benign neoplasia, osteomyelitis, developmental lesions, and degenerative conditions. It also specifically identifies tumor type and grade, establishes the prognosis, and may dictate appropriate treatment. For various reasons, mistakes are frequent at this

stage of the investigation. The most common pitfall is inappropriate sampling and submission of a biopsy that is reactive bone formed secondarily to the actual disease. Because processing of bone for histology can take 1 week or more, such an outcome can be frustrating and misleading.

Closed needle biopsies of medium-to-large, solid, solitary lesions of appendicular long bones are obtained using a 4-inch, 8- or 11-gauge Jamshidi bone biopsy needle (Sherwood Medical Co., St. Louis, MD) (see Chapter 77).[25] This method has less postsurgical morbidity (pain, hematoma, infection, tumor seeding, pathologic fracture) than incisional biopsy. The clinician should carefully evaluate the radiograph to ensure that the biopsy is obtained from the center of the lesion and that dense reactive bone is avoided. The skin puncture site and biopsy tract must be situated so that they can be subsequently excised if the lesion is surgically resected. Two or three cores of tissue are taken by redirecting the needle through the same skin opening. Needle orientation can be guided with image intensification or radiography. Jamshidi needle biopsy is not suitable for lesions of small bones or lesions with recent pathologic fractures, because there may be significant hematoma in the latter. For cystic and fluid-filled lesions, or those associated with extensive osteolysis and tumor necrosis, an open incisional wedge biopsy through a limited surgical approach might be necessary. Bone that appears abnormal can also be collected with a bone curette, taking care to avoid mutilating the specimen.

For investigation of diseases affecting growth and endochondral ossification, physeal biopsies can be obtained percutaneously from the greater tubercle of the humerus with a Jamshidi needle.[26] For suspected metabolic bone diseases, larger specimens of cancellous bone are collected with an 8 mm Michele trephine from the iliac crest or by excision of a segment of rib or distal ulnar diaphysis.[27]

The surgical borders of lesions excised en bloc are labeled with India ink for examination by the pathologist to ensure tumor-free margins.[28] Specimens can also be radiographed using nonscreen film or industrial film in a Faxitron cabinet system. Biopsies are fixed in neutral buffered formalin for 6 to 24 hours; they must not be frozen.[7] Large bone specimens should be cut into 5 mm slabs to ensure proper fixation.[7] If osteomyelitis is suspected, a portion of the biopsy should be separated for bacteriologic culture before the remainder is fixed in formalin. Bone specimens that cannot be cut with a scalpel are decalcified in 10% formic acid prior to embedding in paraffin. Rapid decalcification in strong acids or excessive decalcification will destroy cellular detail and render the biopsy nondiagnostic. Nondecalcified bone biopsies embedded in methylmethacrylate and sectioned with a sledge microtome are needed for diagnosis of some metabolic bone diseases.[29] Histologic evaluation of bone is rather specialized and requires the expertise of a pathologist with special interest and training. Most pathologists will want to review the clinical data and radiographs as well, before making a diagnosis.

Cytology

Cytologic examination of fluids and exudates obtained by sterile aspiration is valuable in early detection of acute osteomyelitis, before obvious radiographic changes occur in bone.

Microbiology

Isolation and identification of bacteria are helpful in confirming a diagnosis of osteomyelitis, and *in vitro* susceptibility testing aids in antimicrobial drug selection. Cultures of pus from externally draining tracts are less than 50% accurate in identifying the pathogens causing osteomyelitis, because the tracts become colonized by skin organisms and gram-negative bacteria. It is preferable to culture fluid collected by sterile aspiration, or from pus, necrotic tissue, and sequestra collected during surgical débridement. Both aerobic and anaerobic culture are advisable, because anaerobic bacteria are involved in up to 60% of bone infections in small animals.[30] Samples for aerobic culture should be collected in a sterile container, taken to the laboratory, and plated out on agar within 10 to 15 minutes. Specimens for anaerobic culture require special handling because a few minutes of exposure to air will kill sensitive anaerobes and prevent subsequent isolation. Fluid for anaerobic culture can be collected into a syringe if air is expelled and the needle capped with a rubber stopper.

When the anticipated delay in plating out samples exceeds 15 minutes, tissue samples and swabs are placed into a reduced Cary-Blair, solidified anaerobic holding media (Becton Dickinson, Franklin Lakes, NJ) to exclude oxygen. Both aerobes and anaerobes may be isolated from such preparations because most aerobic bacteria are facultative anaerobes.

CONGENITAL BONE DISORDERS

Embryonic and postnatal skeletal development are complex and exquisitely susceptible to errors. Skeletal growth disorders that are apparent at birth or manifest later in young animals are of two main types: (1) generalized dysplasias and (2) localized malformations of individual bones. Some are caused by inherited defects and sporadic mutations, and some are due to teratogens and unidentifiable embryopathies. In humans, more than 100 such disorders, mostly inherited, have been listed in the *Paris Nomenclature for Constitutional Disorders of Bone*.[31] This classification is based on specific clinical, genetic, radiologic, histologic, and biochemical features. Animal diseases are not sufficiently characterized to allow complete adoption of the Paris system,[32] although some general groupings are possible (Box 279-2). Generalized dysplasias are described later with developmental and genetic disorders or with joint diseases (see Chapter 278), whereas dysostoses are considered here.

Dysostoses include the malformations of individual bones either singly or in combination. They can involve the craniofacial region, the axial bones, and extremities. Embryonic limb bud development commences with a projection of mesoderm covered by ectoderm. Three signaling centers within the limb bud that control and coordinate limb development are (1) the apical ectodermal ridge, (2) the zone of polarizing activity, and (3) the Wingless-type signaling center.[33] The apical ectodermal ridge is a thickened layer of ectoderm overlying the distal tip of the limb bud that acts as a signaling center guiding proximal to distal limb development. It also causes interdigital necrosis, thereby separating webbed digits, probably by the local expression of FGF genes.[34] The zone of polarizing activity exerts control via the signaling molecule sonic hedgehog protein, and the Wingless-type signaling center controls limb alignment with respect to dorsal orientation.[33] Subsequently, the individual bones form from cartilage anlages and the secondary centers of ossification.[5,34] Three mesodermal rays (ulnar, radial, and central) contribute to pectoral limb formation; disturbances of one or more rays or of the signaling centers will result in perturbations of the corresponding components of bone and associated soft tissue. For example, failure of the apical ectodermal ridge may produce syndactyly of the digits or result in a truncated limb similar to congenital amputation.[33] Except for a few heritable disorders that will be mentioned, most dysostoses in dogs and cats occur sporadically.

Hemimelia, Phocomelia, and Amelia

In these conditions the animal has a congenital absence of portions of the normal structures in an extremity. Hemimelia is either longitudinal (paraxial), with absence of the ulnar,

---

<table>
<tr><td colspan="1">Box • 279-2</td></tr>
</table>

Some Congenital Skeletal Disorders of Small Animals

Osteochondrodysplasias (Abnormalities of Cartilage, Bone Growth, and Development)

A. Defects of growth of tubular bone or spine
   Multiple epiphyseal dysplasia: beagle
   Pseudoachondrodysplasia: miniature poodle
      Scottish deerhound
   Chondrodysplasia: Alaskan Malamute
      Cocker spaniel
      English pointer
      Great Pyrenees
      Norwegian elkhound
   Ocular-skeletal dysplasia: Labrador retriever
      Samoyed
   Pelger-Huët anomaly: cats
   Scottish fold osteochondrodysplasia: cats

B. Disorganized development of cartilage and fibrous components
   Multiple cartilaginous exostoses (osteochondromatosis)
   Enchondroma
   Fibrous dysplasia

C. Abnormalities of density, of cortical diaphyseal structure, or metaphyseal molding
   Osteogenesis imperfecta
   Osteopetrosis

Primary Metabolic Abnormalities
Vitamin D—dependent rickets
Mucopolysaccharidosis (MPS)
Fucosidosis
GM gangliosidosis
Gaucher's disease

Dysostoses with Malformation of Individual Bones, Singly or in Combination
Hemimelia
Phocomelia
Amelia
Syndactyly
Polydactyly
Ectrodactyly
Segmental hemiatrophy

Adapted from Sharrard WJW: Pediatric Orthopaedics and Fractures, 3rd ed. London, Blackwell Scientific Publications, 1993.

---

radial, or central regions in the forelimb, or transverse, with the distal portion of the limb completely absent.

Radial agenesis is the most common paraxial hemimelia in cats and dogs. It is usually unilateral and sporadic. Bilateral radial agenesis might be an inherited autosomal recessive trait in Chihuahua dogs.[32] In radial agenesis, the radius is partially or completely absent, and the ulna is shorter, thickened, and curved (Figure 279-6). The radial carpal bone and first digit are often absent as well. Lack of a radial head support allows humeroulnar subluxation, and the range of elbow motion

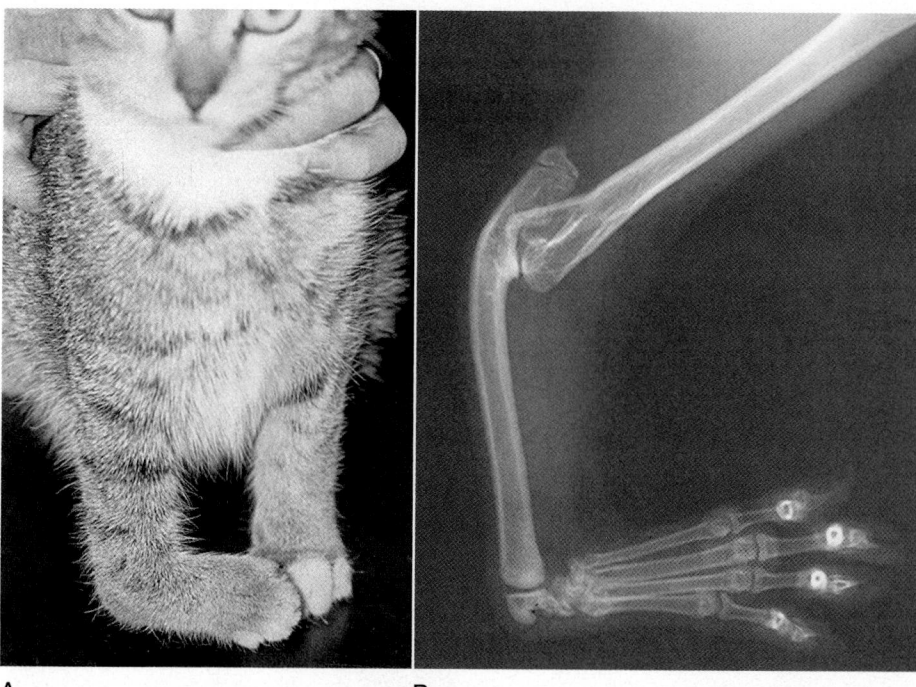

A   B

Figure 279-6 Kitten with radial agenesis. **A,** Radial agenesis and a 90-degree varus angulation of the metacarpus. **B,** The radius and radial carpal bone are absent. The proximal ulna is misshapen, the distal ulna thicker than normal, and the carpus malarticulated. (From Winterbotham EJ et al: Radial agenesis in a cat. J Small Anim Pract 26:393, 1985.)

is reduced. The metacarpus deviates into varus, severely impairing limb function. One hypothesis is that radial agenesis and other hemimelias are a consequence of neural crest injury because limb bud embryopathies often have a segmental pattern that corresponds to the distribution of the segmental sensory nerves.[35] Treatment of radial agenesis by reconstructive surgery has not been very successful, and amputation may be necessary. Another, less common paraxial hemimelia is tibial agenesis.[32]

Complete absence of a distal portion of a limb (congenital amputation) can be caused by transverse hemimelia, strangulation by constrictive bands, or *in utero* accidents.[36] The cause may be impossible to determine in young animals, because postnatal trauma can also cause amputations.

In phocomelia, an intercalary segment of limb is missing. In severe cases the paw with rudimentary digits is attached to the trunk like a seal flipper. Proximal femoral focal deficiency is a phocomelia with a missing segment of femur. In man, this is usually a unilateral defect that is not inherited.[37] A young dalmatian with proximal femoral focal deficiency had unilateral hindlimb shortening and muscle atrophy that became accentuated with further growth.[38] Radiographically, bone in the intertrochanteric, neck and head regions of the femur was absent, and there was marked femoral shortening.

Amelia is complete absence of one or more limbs. Two kittens with bilateral hindlimb amelia have been reported.[32] Most animals affected by amelia probably die or are euthanized at birth.

Syndactyly

Two or more digits are fused in a bony or soft tissue union in syndactyly.[7,32] This is not clinically important in pets, and surgery is generally unwarranted unless the deformity causes lameness. Congenital synostosis of adjacent metatarsal bones is a variation on digital fusion (Figure 279-7).

Polydactyly

Polydactyly is the presence of extra digits, usually on the medial side of the paw in dogs and cats. An inherited syndrome of skeletal defects exists, including polydactyly and syndactyly in Australian shepherd dogs.[7] An X-linked gene was suspected. Polydactyly is an inherited autosomal dominant trait in cats.[32] Multiple hindlimb dewclaws in Great Pyrenees have similar inheritance.

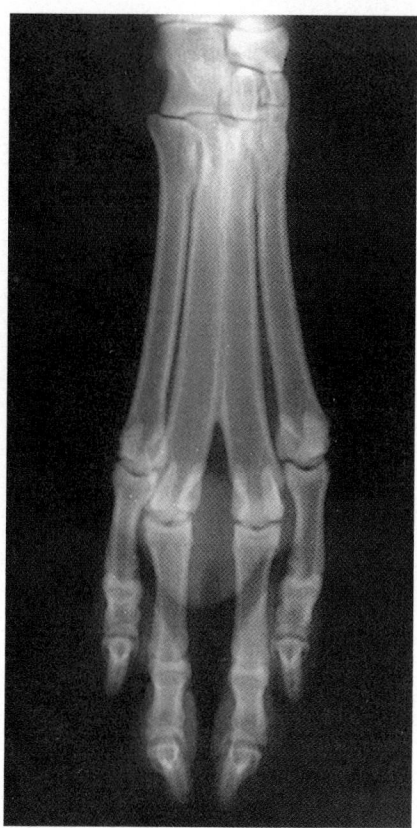

Figure 279-7 Congenital metatarsal bone synostosis.

HEMATOLOGY AND IMMUNOLOGY

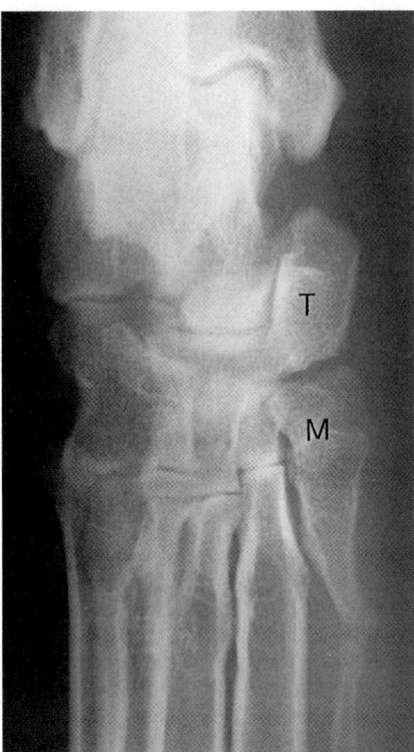

Figure 279-8 Vestigial first metatarsal bone *(M)* and an anomalous tarsal bone *(T)* extending medially from the central tarsal bone in a Saint Bernard.

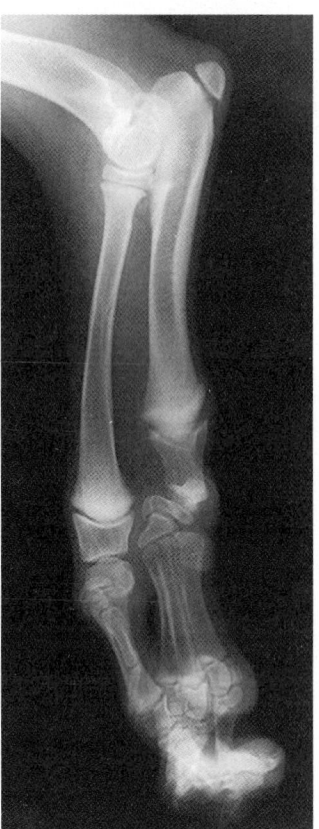

Figure 279-9 Forelimb of 12-week-old mixed breed dog with ectrodactyly, including distal radial and ulnar separation.

In Saint Bernard dogs, dewclaws may be associated with anomalous tarsal bones. Some have a large curved bone that seems to be an extension of the central tarsal bone on the medial side of the proximal row of tarsal bones (Figure 279-8). These tarsal anomalies occur bilaterally, are not associated with clinical signs, and are probably inherited.

Ectrodactyly
Often called split hand or lobster claw deformity, ectrodactyly is caused by incomplete fusion of the three rays or absence of the central ray.[37] Classically, the third metacarpal bone and digit are absent, producing a deep cleft that divides the paw into radial and ulnar parts, but many variations occur. The third metacarpal bone may be present and hypoplastic, and neighboring digits and metacarpal bones may be absent or hypoplastic.[39-41] The cleft between metacarpal bones may terminate just below the carpus, or extend proximally through the carpus, separating radius and ulna entirely (Figure 279-9).[39-41] Asynchronous radial and ulnar growth can contribute to the structural disorder at the carpus. Half of the affected dogs have concomitant congenital elbow luxation. It is usually an isolated deformity without breed predilection in dogs, but may be inherited in cats.[7,32] Function can be improved by reconstructive surgery or arthrodesis.[39,42]

Segmental Hemiatrophy
Hemiatrophy is a misnomer because the condition is actually limb hypoplasia rather than atrophy of a normal structure. The affected forelimb is noticeably shorter and slimmer, especially in the antebrachium and paw.[43] An affected golden retriever also had darker pigmentation of skin and hair of the abnormal limb and horny keratinization of pads and nails, but it has no pain or discomfort.[44] Radiographically the carpal bones were smaller, and the numbered carpal bones were misshapen.

The metacarpal bones were 3 cm shorter than contralateral bones and half normal diameter. This is a sporadic deformity and probably not inherited. It must be distinguished from atrophy that follows long-term limb immobilization.[12] A similar type of distal hypoplasia of metacarpus and digits is seen in immature dogs, subsequent to accidental trauma or surgery to the antebrachium.[44] Ilizarov limb lengthening may be indicated if shortening impairs function.

DEVELOPMENTAL AND GENETIC BONE DISORDERS

Osteopetrosis
Defective osteoclastic resorption of bone is the principal feature of osteopetrosis. In growing bones, failure of normal bone modeling results in accumulation of primary spongiosa, so the diaphysis remains filled with bone and a marrow cavity does not form. Affected bones have a *marbled* densely homogeneous radiographic appearance, but they are actually quite fragile. Many forms of osteopetrosis exist. Osteoclasts may be absent, be present in reduced numbers, or be defective in their ability to resorb bone.[7] The disorder is rare and not very well characterized in dogs and cats.[7,45] Idiopathic acquired osteopetrosis of adult cats was characterized by thickening of diaphyseal cortices and vertebral bodies.[45] Feline leukemia virus (FeLV) also produces medullary sclerosis and nonregenerative anemia in growing cats, probably through infection of hemopoietic precursor cells from which osteoclasts arise.[7]

Osteogenesis Imperfecta
Osteogenesis imperfecta comprises a group of heritable diseases characterized by osteopenia, excessive bone fragility, and increased susceptibility to fracture. Fractured bones form

callus and heal, but unless stabilized adequately, malunion and deformities occur.[46,47] Radiographically there can be generalized osteopenia, thinning of diaphyseal cortices, and multiple fractures in various stages of union. The fundamental defect in humans is abnormal type I collagen production, mostly due to mutations of genes that normally code for procollagen synthesis.[46] The resulting type I collagen fibrils are thin and fail to mineralize. Osteogenesis imperfecta is rare in dogs and cats, and the mode of heritability and exact biochemical defects are unknown.[32,47,48] Animals may have multiple fractures, with minimal or no trauma. Some may also have dentinogenesis imperfecta (seen as pink teeth), stunted growth, and apparent weakness.[48] The diagnosis is made by analysis of type I collagen from cultured skin fibroblasts,[48] but the more common causes of osteopenia, including renal and nutrition secondary hyperparathyroidism, should be eliminated first.

Mucopolysaccharidosis

The mucopolysaccharidosis (MPS) disorders are rare genetic lysosomal storage diseases caused by specific defects in lysosomal enzymes that are involved in metabolism of glycosaminoglycans. Compounds normally degraded by these enzymes accumulate intracellularly, interfering with cellular function and producing characteristic clinical signs. Several MPS disorders have been recognized in cats (MPS I, VI, and VII) and dogs (MPS I, II, IIIA, IIIB, VI, and VII),[49] but the presence and severity of skeletal abnormalities produced by them are different.

MPS VI is caused by decreased arylsulfatase B activity and leads to intracellular accumulation and increased urinary excretion of dermatan sulfate. Feline MPS VI has been recognized mainly in Siamese cats, as an autosomal recessive disorder, but has also been described in domestic shorthaired (DSH) and long-haired cats, and a Siamese and DSH cross.[49-51] MPS VI has also been reported in dogs of several breeds.[49] Skeletal disease is the predominant abnormality. Clinical features become evident in affected cats from age 6 to 8 weeks and include small head and ears, flattened face, corneal clouding, pectus excavatum, growth retardation, skeletal deformity, and hindlimb paresis or paralysis from spinal cord compression by bone lesions. They have a crouching gait, and manipulation of joints and cervical spine causes pain. Radiographic features include epiphyseal dysplasia, thinning of long-bone cortices, generalized osteopenia, bilateral coxofemoral subluxation, secondary osteoarthritis, and vertebral fusion.[52] Diagnostic confirmation is provided by demonstration of excess dermatan sulfate in urine with the toluidine-blue (Berry) spot test, metachromatic granules in neutrophils, and reduced arylsulfatase B activity in leukocytes.[49] A PCR-based screening method allows detection of carrier cats.[50]

MPS I in DSH cats is an autosomal recessive disease due to decreased activity of alpha-L-iduronidase.[49,53] Clinical features are similar to MPS VI, but facial dysmorphism may not be as striking as in Siamese, and metachromatic granules are usually less distinct in leukocytes than in MPS VI and MPS VII.[54] Radiographic features are similar to MPS VI, except that epiphyseal dysplasia and dwarfism are absent. Neurologic abnormalities due to spinal cord compression by bone proliferation occur relatively later, after 2 years of age. Excretion of dermatan sulfate and heparin sulfate in urine is detectable using the toluidine-blue spot test.[53] MPS I has also been reported in dogs. Affected animals are dwarfed and have swollen painful joints, glossoptosis, corneal clouding, and progressive motor and visual deficits. Radiographic features include epiphyseal dysgenesis, periarticular bone proliferation, and enlargement of femoral diaphyses.[55]

MPS II was diagnosed in a 5-year-old male Labrador retriever with coarse facial features, macrodactylia, generalized osteopenia, progressive neurologic deterioration and a positive urine test for glycosaminoglycan.[56] Iduronate sulfatase activity was deficient in cultured dermal fibroblasts.

Canine MPS VII (beta-glucuronidase deficiency) has been described in dogs and cats.[50] Affected dogs appear normal at birth, but by age 2 to 3 months develop hindlimb paresis and have a disproportionately large head, flattened face, swollen lax joints, bowed limbs, dorsoventrally flattened rib cage, and corneal clouding.[57] Radiographic features include bilateral coxofemoral luxation, abnormally shaped carpal and tarsal bones, generalized epiphyseal dysplasia, cervical vertebral dysplasia, and platyspondylisis. Feline MPS VII is characterized by growth retardation, delayed dental eruption, corneal clouding, abdominal distension, and multiple skeletal abnormalities.[58-60] In both species, peripheral leukocytes contain metachromatic inclusions, and urinary excretion of chondroitin sulfate is increased.[58,61] Genetic tests can distinguish phenotypically normal MPS VII carrier dogs and cats from homozygous normal animals.[58,62]

Several therapeutic strategies for MPS have been trialed with some success, including enzyme replacement therapy, heterologous bone marrow transplantation, and somatic cell gene transfer, but all require further development.[49]

Dwarfism

Various disorders causing small stature in dogs and cats listed in Table 279-1 are reviewed in other chapters. Considered here are skeletal dysplasias and some endocrinopathies (hyposomatotropism and hypothyroidism) that are more commonly associated with dwarfism in small animals.

Skeletal Dysplasias (Osteochondrodysplasias)

Osteochondrodysplasias are disorders characterized by abnormalities in growth and development of cartilage, bone, or both (see Box 279-2). Disorders of this type have been reported in several breeds of dogs. Box 279-3 summarizes the better-characterized entities. Most have known or suspected genetic basis and autosomal recessive inheritance is common. They frequently cause disproportionate dwarfism, with discrepant development of axial and appendicular skeleton producing reduced limb length relative to the trunk (Figure 279-10).

Another type of genetic dwarfism occurs in achondroplastic dog breeds, such as bulldog, Boston terrier, Pekinese, pug, and Shih Tzu. These animals have been bred selectively for achondroplasia and thus have shortened maxilla, depressed nasal bridge, flared metaphyses, and short bowed limbs as part of accepted breed standards.[32] Hypochondroplastic breeds, such as Basset hound, beagle, dachshund, Dandie Dinmont

Table • 279-1

Some Causes of Small Stature in Dogs and Cats

NONENDOCRINE	ENDOCRINE
Malnutrition	Hyposomatotropism
Malassimilation	Hypothyroidism
Portal systemic shunt (PSS)	Hypoadrenocorticism
Cardiovascular defects	Hyperadrenocorticism
Glycogen storage disease	Diabetes mellitus
Skeletal dysplasia	
Mucopolysaccharidosis (MPS)	
Hydroencephalus	
Renal disease	

Modified from Feldman EC, Nelson RW: Canine and Feline Endocrinology and Reproduction, 3rd ed. Philadelphia, WB Saunders Co, 2004.

Box • 279-3

Canine Osteochondrodysplasias: Clinical and Radiologic Signs, and Inheritance Pattern

Alaskan Malamute Chondrodysplasia[7,63]
Short limbs, bowed forelegs, carpal joints enlarged, paws deviated laterally; ulna growth plate thickened, irregular and flared; associated hemolytic anemia; autosomal recessive trait, complete penetrance, variable expression

Beagle Multiple Epiphyseal Dysplasia[7,63]
Short limbs, enlarged joints, kyphosis; stippled mineralization of epiphyses, especially femur and humerus, disappeared by 5 months; vertebrae short; dysplastic hips; osteoarthropathy in adults; autosomal recessive trait

Bull Terrier Osteochondrodysplasia[64]
Abnormal hind leg gait, femoral neck fractures; nonossified foci in femoral necks and metaphyses of long bones; some long bones distorted; dwarfing not noted; littermates affected but inheritance not known

English Pointer Enchondrodystrophy[7,65,66]
Short limbs, bowed forelegs, abnormal locomotion; wide irregular growth plates; possibly inferior prognathism; probable autosomal recessive trait

Great Pyrenees Chondrodysplasia[7,63,67]
Very short limbs, forelegs bowed with valgus deformity; body length reduced slightly; flared, flattened metaphyses; poorly developed epiphyses and cuboidal bones; vertebrae poorly ossified and irregular; autosomal recessive trait

Irish Setter Hypochondroplasia[68]
Mildly short limbs and spine, variable radius and ulna bowing and carpal valgus; growth plates, epiphyses and metaphyses radiographically normal; autosomal recessive trait

Labrador Retriever Ocular-Skeletal Dysplasia[7,69]
Short limbs, prominent elbows and carpi, paws deviated laterally, hind legs hyperextended; tubular bones short and wide, cortices thin, metaphyses flattened and flared, increased metaphyseal opacity; epiphyses and cuboidal bones large and misshapen; hip dysplasia, abnormal elbows; cataracts, retinal dysplasia and detachment; autosomal trait, recessive effect on skeleton, incompletely dominant on eye

Miniature Poodle Multiple Enchondromatosis[70,71]
Short bowed limbs, femoral neck fractures; lucent areas extending from growth plates into metaphyses and some diaphysis; diaphyses distended and distorted; ribs and vertebrae also affected; sternum lacked bone; autosomal nondominant trait

Miniature Poodle Multiple Epiphyseal Dysplasia[63]
Similar to disorder in beagle; inheritance unknown, but two of three affected were littermates

Miniature Poodle Pseudoachondroplasia[7,63]
Poor growth, abnormal gait; short, bent legs, enlarged joints; possible inferior prognathism; vertebrae short, limb bones short and thick with bulbous ends; stippled densities in epiphyses; ossification complete by 2 years of age, but limbs remained short and deformed; probable autosomal recessive trait

Norwegian Elkhound Chondrodysplasia[7,63]
Shortened body, disproportionally short limbs, especially forelegs, which may be bowed; metaphyses flared and flattened, with denser band; ventral vertebral bodies irregular, delayed union of vertebral end plates; may have glucosuria; autosomal recessive trait

Samoyed Ocular-Skeletal Dysplasia[7,72,73]
Short forelegs, varus deformity of elbows, valgus of carpi, premature closure of ulnar growth plates, bowed radii; domed forehead; cataracts, retinal detachment, hyaloid artery remnants eosinophilia; autosomal recessive trait

Scottish Deerhound Pseudoachondroplasia (Osteochondrodysplasia)[74,75]
Retarded growth, short bowed limbs, exercise intolerance, small head, short trunk, lax joints, kyphosis; vertebrae and long bones short, epiphyseal ossification irregular and delayed; later osteopenia, severe deformity; single autosomal recessive inheritance suspected

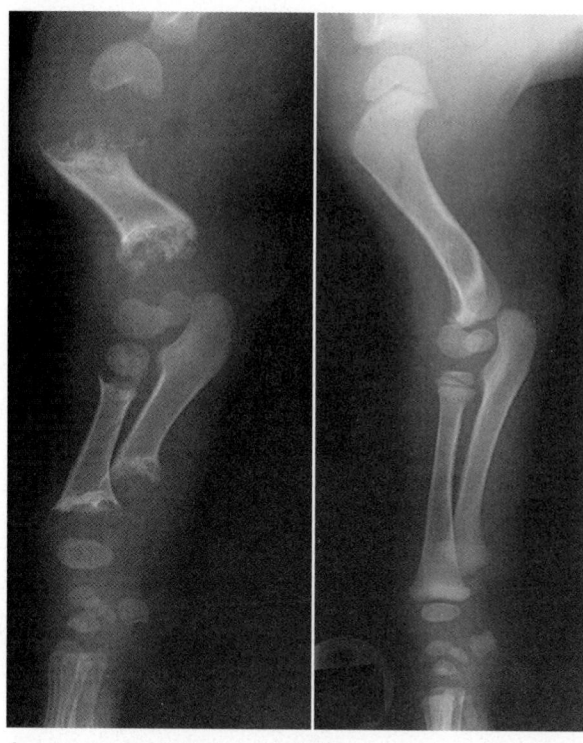

Figure 279-10 A, Radiograph of a 5-week-old Alaskan Malamute with chondrodysplasia. Physeal cartilage is widened, and adjacent metaphyseal bone roughened and irregular. **B,** Radiograph of a normal littermate of same age for comparison.

terrier, Scottish terrier, Skye terrier, and Welsh corgi have similarly shaped legs as a breed characteristic, although their skulls are normal.[32] These forms of dwarfism differ from the nonpathologic, mutant, proportionate reduction in stature in dogs that has led to the establishment through selective breeding of many miniature and toy breeds.

An osteochondrodysplasia with autosomal dominant inheritance has been described in Scottish fold cats.[76] Along with the folded ears typical of this breed, affected individuals show signs of lameness, reluctance to jump, stiff and stilted gait, short mis-shapen distal limbs, and short thick inflexible tail. Radiographic features include irregular size and shape of bones of tarsus, carpus, metatarsus, metacarpus, phalanges, and caudal vertebrae. In addition, these animals have narrowing of apparent joint spaces, new bone production around distal limbs joints, diffuse osteopenia, and formation of a plantar exostosis caudal to the calcaneus in advanced cases (Figure 279-11). However, the severity and rate of progression of changes are quite variable. Treatment is noncurative, but pentosan polysulfate, glycosaminoglycans, nonsteroidal anti-inflammatory drugs (NSAIDs), or a combination of these treatments might be palliative.[76]

A chondrodysplasia in two unrelated kittens with shortened, bowed forelimbs was described.[77] Radiographic signs included long bone bowing, metaphyseal flaring, and a gross enlargement of physeal cartilage that resembled rickets. Serum calcium, phosphorus, and 1,25-dihydroxyvitamin D_3 concentrations were normal, but PTH concentrations were below the reference range. Furthermore, treatment of the kittens with oral 1,25-dihydroxyvitamin D_3 for 3 months did not resolve the radiographic abnormalities or correct the stunted statue. The disorder is considered to be a (osteo)chondrodysplasia of unknown heritability rather than rickets.[77]

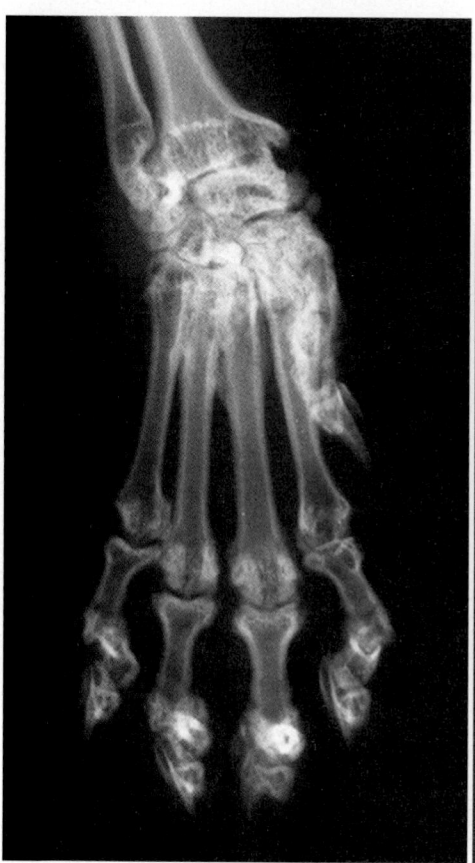

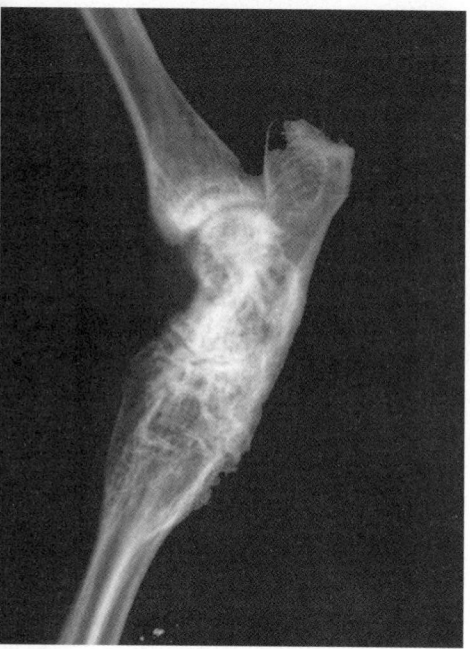

Figure 279-11 Osteochondrodysplasia of Scottish fold cats. **A,** Exostoses around the carpus. **B,** Exostoses and ankylosis of the tarsal joints. (Courtesy of Veterinary Imaging Associates, Sydney, Australia.)

HEMATOLOGY AND IMMUNOLOGY

Pituitary Dwarfism Hypopituitarism and consequent dwarfism, inherited in autosomal recessive fashion in German shepherd dogs and Karelian bear dogs, has also been described in other dog breeds (Weimaraner, Spitz, toy pinscher) and cats.[78] A cystic, vestigial adenohypophysis is present in many affected German shepherds, but some have a hypoplastic or a normal-appearing pituitary gland. The syndrome is dominated by effects of hyposomatotropism, but deficiency of other adenohypophyseal hormones can lead to degrees of accompanying secondary hypothyroidism, hypoadrenocorticism, and hypogonadism. Affected animals are usually recognizable by the age of 2 or 3 months. They grow slowly but retain near-normal body proportions. The soft puppy-hair coat is retained initially, but symmetric alopecia and hyperpigmentation develop with age. Accompanying abnormalities include abnormal behavior (aggression, fear biting), delayed dental eruption, short mandible, cardiac disorders, cryptorchidism, megaesophagus, and testicular atrophy or estral abnormalities.

Radiographically, limb bones are shortened, with delayed closure of growth plates in some cases. Epiphyses may show disordered and incomplete calcification, suggesting hypothyroidism. Hormonal testing can be undertaken to confirm the diagnosis if necessary. Most pituitary dwarf animals can be expected to remain small for life. However, two unusual cases with typical clinical features at 10 weeks of age grew steadily and appeared normal when 1 year old.[79] Both had normal hormonal test results, indicating that growth hormone secretion ideally should be evaluated in suspected cases to clarify prognosis.

Replacement therapy with growth hormone (if available and economical), and thyroxine or glucocorticoid if indicated, could be considered, but long-term prognosis is poor.[78] Another promising approach involves chronic progestin administration to induce growth hormone production from mammary ductular cells of affected dogs of either sex.[80]

Congenital Hypothyroidism Skeletal development is abnormal in congenital hypothyroidism, which is rare in dogs and cats. Although cases are usually encountered sporadically in various breeds, some familial occurrences are known: secondary hypothyroidism with autosomal recessive inheritance in giant schnauzers,[81] primary dyshormonogenesis with autosomal recessive inheritance in Abyssinian cats,[82] thyroid unresponsiveness to thyroid-stimulating hormone (TSH) with autosomal recessive inheritance in Japanese cats,[83] and thyroid unresponsiveness to TSH in related Scottish deerhounds.[84]

Abnormalities may be detectable by the age of 1 or 2 months. Affected animals are disproportionate dwarfs, with short limbs and spine, blocklike trunks, and broad short skulls. The radiographic features are epiphyseal dysgenesis and delayed skeletal maturation (Figure 279-12). Nonskeletal findings include delayed dental eruption, macroglossia, lethargy, mental dullness, persistent puppy haircoat progressing to thinning and alopecia, mild nonregenerative anemia, and hypercholesterolemia. Thyroid gland enlargement can accompany congenital dyshormonogenesis[85] but is absent if a hypothalamic-pituitary defect is causing thyroid understimulation[86] or thyroids are unresponsive to TSH.

A low blood plasma thyroxine concentration is expected, but results of other thyroid tests will differ, depending on whether the defect is of thyroidal, pituitary, or hypothalamic origin. The plasma growth hormone response to provocative stimuli may be suppressed (Chapter 235).[80,86] Treatment with thyroxine can reverse many of the abnormalities but should commence early and continue for life.

Retained Cartilage Cores

In young large and giant breed dogs, cartilage cores sometimes form in the metaphysis of the distal ulna. Physeal hypertrophic

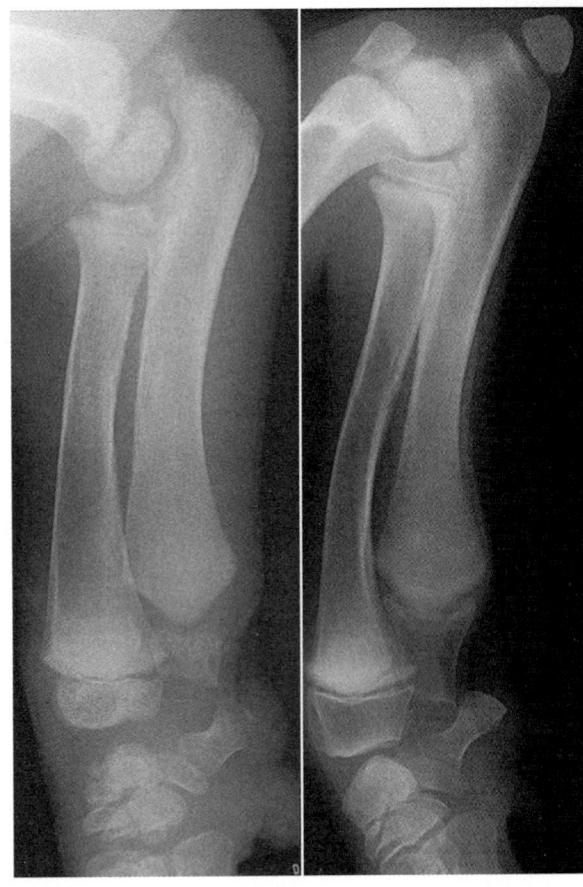

A   B

Figure 279-12 **A,** Forelimb of 15-week-old Great Dane with features of congenital hypothyroidism. Reader should note the disordered and irregular ossification of epiphyses (epiphyseal dysgenesis) in humerus, radius, and ulna; the absence of an olecranon apophysis; and delayed skeletal maturation. **B,** Normal Great Dane of similar age for comparison. (Courtesy of R.B. Lavelle.)

chondrocytes fail to mature and mineralize adjacent matrix, and they accumulate in long columns in the primary spongiosa.[87] The cause of the disorder is unclear. In Great Dane pups, formation of cartilage cores in the distal ulnar and tibial metaphyses was associated with feeding diets containing three-times the recommended content of calcium.[88]

Radiographically a central, radiolucent core of cartilage exists that is 5 to 10 mm wide and 2 to 6 cm long, extending from distal ulnar physis into metaphyseal bone (Figure 279-13). Lesions are usually bilateral. They may be a subclinical radiographic finding or be associated with varying degrees of growth retardation after 5 months of age. Retarded ulnar growth causes relative shortening of the ulna, valgus, and rotation of the paw, cranial bowing of the radius, and carpal and elbow subluxation (see Figure 279-13).

Craniomandibular Osteopathy

Craniomandibular osteopathy occurs mainly in young West Highland white, Scottish, Cairn, Boston, and other terriers, and occasionally in nonterrier breeds.[89] Autosomal recessive inheritance is known in West Highland white terriers,[90] and a hereditary predisposition may exist in Scottish terriers. However, the sporadic occurrence in unrelated breeds suggests other causative factors are also involved. Canine distemper virus (CDV) infection of bone has been mentioned as a possible cause,[89] although an epidemiologic study did not indicate a

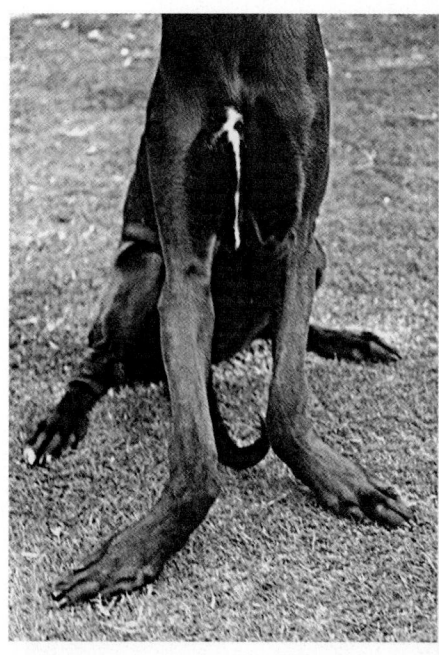
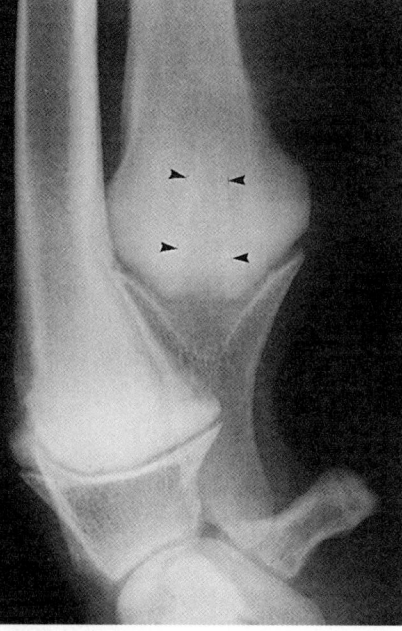

A   B

Figure 279-13 **A,** Seven-month-old Great Dane with bilateral forelimb deformities caused by retained cartilage cores in the distal ulnar physes. **B,** Radiograph demonstrating retained cartilage core *(arrows)* extending from distal ulnar physis into the metaphysis. (From Johnson KA: Retardation of endochondral ossification at the distal ulnar growth plate in dogs. Aust Vet J 57:474, 1987.)

direct relationship.[91] The condition is usually recognized at age of 3 to 8 months, when affected pups develop mandibular swelling, drooling of saliva, prehension difficulties, pain on opening the mouth, or some combination of these signs. The clinical course may fluctuate, with periods of remission and exacerbation. Abnormal physical findings comprise firm, often painful, swelling of mandible, temporomandibular region, or both areas. Periods of pyrexia occur in some cases. Restricted jaw movements and atrophy of masticatory muscles may be obvious in severely affected dogs. Mandibular swelling without pain or eating difficulties occurs in some dogs, especially of larger breeds.

Radiographic changes are generally bilateral but often asymmetric, with irregular bony proliferation involving the mandible and tympanic bulla-petrous temporal bone areas in about 50% of cases. However, changes can be confined to the mandible (33% of cases) (Figure 279-14) or the tympanic

bulla-petrous temporal region (13%). The calvarium and tentorium ossium are often thickened (Figure 279-15), and other skull bones are sometimes affected. Concurrent long bone lesions resembling later stages of metaphyseal osteopathy have been observed in a few terriers with craniomandibular osteopathy.

The diagnosis is straightforward in cases with typical clinical and radiographic features. Routine laboratory tests are unlikely to be helpful. Bone biopsy may be useful in atypical cases, such as dogs of rarely affected breeds with lesions confined to the mandible, especially if unilateral. The histopathology involves resorption of existing lamellae, proliferation of coarse

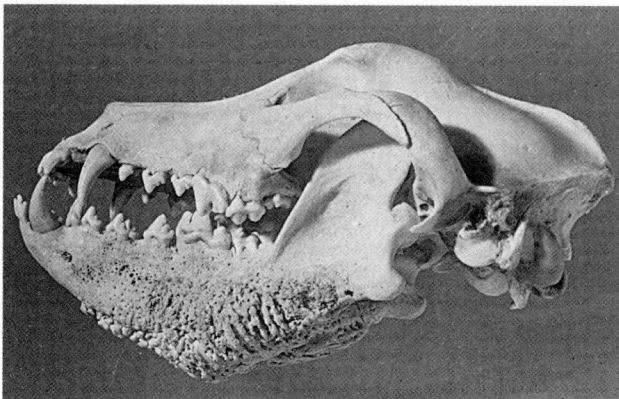

Figure 279-14 Macerated skull of a Doberman pinscher with craniomandibular osteopathy. Reader should note extensive bone changes involving mandible. Tympanic bullae, petrous temporal bones, and temporomandibular joint (TMJ) regions were unaffected in this dog. (From Watson ADJ et al: Craniomandibular osteopathy in Doberman pinschers. J Small Anim Pract 16:11, 1975.)

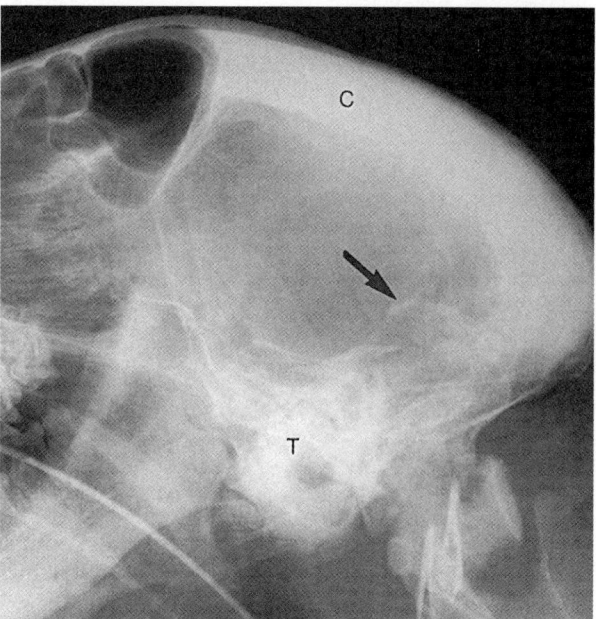

Figure 279-15 Skull of Scottish terrier with craniomandibular osteopathy. The tympanic bulla-petrous bone area *(T)* shows dense sclerotic bone changes. Reader should note thickened calvarium *(C)* and tentorium osseum *(arrow).*

HEMATOLOGY AND IMMUNOLOGY

trabecular bone beyond normal periosteal boundaries, replacement of marrow spaces by vascular fibrous stroma, and infiltration at the periphery of new bone by inflammatory cells. A mosaic pattern of irregular cement lines is present in the new primitive bone.[92]

Craniomandibular osteopathy is self-limiting. Abnormal bone proliferation eventually slows and becomes static at about 1 year of age. Lesions then tend to regress, although radiographic abnormalities or impaired prehension sometimes persist. Anti-inflammatory drug treatment can reduce pain and discomfort, but the effect on lesions is unknown. The prognosis is guarded when extensive changes affect the tympanic-petrous temporal areas and adjacent mandible. Ankylosis and adhesions may then develop, permanently restricting jaw movements and eating. Rostral hemimandibulectomy can be a useful salvage procedure in these cases.[44]

Multiple Cartilaginous Exostoses

In rare instances these benign lesions (osteochondromatosis, multiple hereditary osteochondromata) occur in dogs and cats, as single or multiple exostoses. The disorder may be inherited as an autosomal dominant trait in humans, horses, and dogs.[93,94] Protuberances consist of cancellous bone covered by a cap of hyaline cartilage and arise in the metaphyseal region of bones formed by endochondral ossification. With continued physeal growth and elongation of long bones, exostoses may be finally located in the diaphysis. Lesions develop and grow most rapidly in immature animals, becoming senescent at maturity. Malignant transformation of exostoses to chondrosarcoma occurs rarely in aged animals.[95,96]

The cause is unknown. One hypothesis is that congenital or acquired defects in the perichondrial ring allow an island of physeal cartilage to be pinched off and trapped in metaphyseal bone. This physeal cartilage continues to grow radially, giving rise to exostoses. However, this does not explain the similar lesions found occasionally in nonskeletal sites, such as tracheal cartilages.

Superficially located exostoses may be palpable. Signs may include paresis due to progressive spinal cord compression in young animals (see Chapter 193) or pain due to impingement of exostoses on adjacent tissues.[97] Radiographically, lesions are rounded to cauliflower-like in outline, with a smooth thin shell of cortical bone (Figure 279-16). They protrude above the bone contour and may extend into the medullary cavity. Internally, exostoses have well-defined bone trabeculae that are continuous with the medullary cavity, and diaphyseal cortex in the region is interrupted by the lesion. Adjacent bones such as ulna and metacarpals may be deformed by expanding exostoses (see Figure 269-16). Solitary exostoses are biopsied to allow differentiation from neoplastic lesions. Surgical excision of exostoses that are causing spinal cord compression or lameness is recommended (see Chapter 193).[97] All exostoses should be monitored for malignant transformation.

IDIOPATHIC BONE DISORDERS

Enostosis

Enostosis (panosteitis, eosinophilic panosteitis) is a relatively common disease causing lameness in medium, large, and giant breed dogs.[98] Amongst breeds at greatest risk are Great Pyrenees, Basset hound, Shar Pei, mastiff, giant schnauzer, and German shepherd dog.[99] Two thirds of affected dogs are male. The age of onset is 6 to 18 months; older dogs are rarely affected. Lameness is acute in onset, not associated with trauma, and intermittent in one or more limbs. Each episode of lameness lasts 2 to 3 weeks but, with recurrent bouts, enostosis may persist for 2 to 9 months. Other signs in early stages

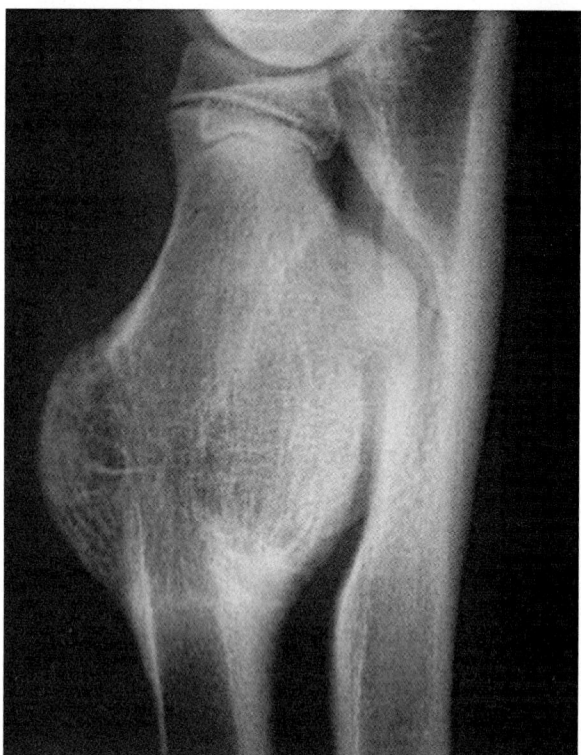

Figure 279-16 Radiograph demonstrating a solitary multiple cartilaginous exostosis-type lesion in the forelimb of a young dog. Reader should note the expansile lesion of the proximal radius, causing malalignment of the radius and attenuation of adjacent ulna. (Courtesy of R.B. Lavelle.)

include anorexia, lethargy, pyrexia, and weight loss. On physical examination, pain is detected on deep palpation of affected bones. Bones commonly affected are the ulna, humerus, radius, femur, and tibia. Ilium, metatarsal, and other bones are rarely affected. The disease begins in the medullary bone marrow, in the region of a nutrient foramen.

The cause is unknown: genetic predisposition, hemophilia, bacterial infection, vascular abnormality, metabolic disease, allergy, hyperestrogenism, and endoparasitism have been proposed, but the evidence for most of these is scant.[98] Viral infection is considered a possible cause, based on clinical features of the disease, transmission experiments, and *in situ* hybridization demonstration of virus in bone cells of dogs infected with CDV.[98,100] A relationship between enostosis and ingestion of protein-and-energy-rich foods was suggested recently, and changes in protein or amino acid metabolism were reported in affected dogs.[101]

Three radiographic stages are recognizable.[98] The first stage, with medullary radiolucency due to bone marrow degeneration, is infrequently seen. Most often detected is the second stage (Figure 279-17). A granular, hazy increased radiopacity that begins in the region of the nutrient foramen may extend to fill the entire medullary cavity. Formation of new endosteal bone and a thin layer of smooth periosteal bone are secondary changes. In the final stage, most bones return to normal appearance, but some have residual thickening of medullary trabeculae and cortical deformity.

Histopathologically, lesions are characterized initially by replacement of normal marrow by fibrous tissue, followed by excessive remodeling of cortical and medullary bone in the affected areas, with endosteal new bone formation generally more prominent.[98] Basenjis and West Highland white terrier dogs with inherited pyruvate kinase (PK) deficiency can

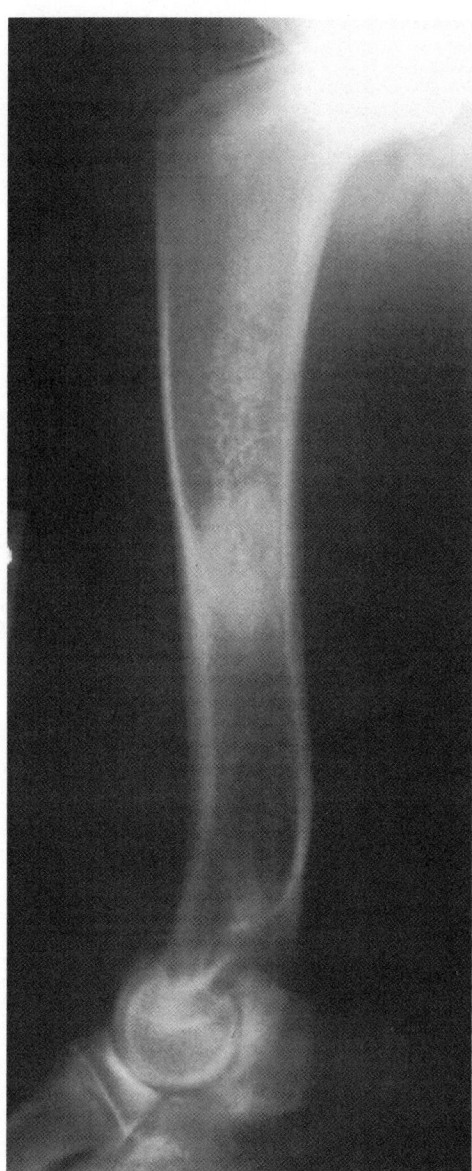

Figure 279-17 Radiograph of a forelimb of a young dog with enostosis, showing patchy intramedullary densities in the humeral diaphysis. (Courtesy of Veterinary Imaging Associates, Sydney, Australia.)

develop intramedullary osteosclerosis but, unlike enostosis, new trabecular bone formation is uniform throughout the medullary cavity.[102]

Enostosis can occur concurrently with developmental diseases such as ununited anconeal process and osteochondritis dissecans, and it may be difficult to determine which disease is causing lameness. Leukocytosis and eosinophilia occur inconsistently in affected dogs; serum chemistry is unremarkable. Enostosis is self-limiting, usually by age 18 months, but analgesic NSAIDS may help alleviate pain and lameness.

Metaphyseal Osteopathy

Metaphyseal osteopathy (hypertrophic osteodystrophy) is a disease of young rapidly growing dogs of larger breeds. Breeds at particular risk include Great Dane, Weimaraner, boxer, Irish setter, German shepherd, and Labrador and golden retrievers.[99] Signs usually begin at 3 to 4 months of age (range 2 to 8 months), with metaphyseal swelling and pain, accompanied by depression, inappetence, and variable pyrexia. Some cases recover

within a few days, but others have one or more relapses during the following weeks before they finally recover. In a few instances, repeated relapses and consequent pain, cachexia, and debility, necessitate euthanasia. Unexplained deaths have been observed rarely.

Radiographic changes occur especially in metaphyses of limb bones and are usually bilateral. Scapulae and ribs may also be affected. In the early stage, an irregular radiolucent zone is present in the metaphysis, separated from the normal-appearing growth plate by an opaque band (Figure 279-18, A). Surrounding soft tissue may be swollen. Later radiographs may show metaphyseal enlargement with irregular periosteal new bone formation, although not all affected dogs develop these changes (Figure 279-18, B). Once the disease is no longer active, bone changes undergo repair and remodeling, but some diaphyseal distortion and exostoses may remain (Figures 279-18, C, and 279-19).

Hematologic and biochemical tests contribute little to the diagnosis, although neutrophilia, monocytosis and lymphocytopenia can occur during active disease, reflecting stress and inflammation. The principal histologic changes involve the primary spongiosa of metaphyses, with acute suppurative osteomyelitis, necrosis, trabecular microfractures, and defective bone formation. Trabecular resorption produces the radiolucent metaphyseal zone. The opaque band near the growth plate results from trabecular collapse and secondary bone formation. Periosteal thickening, with subperiosteal fibrosis and inflammation, periosteal new bone formation, extraperiosteal dystrophic calcification, or a combination of these abnormalities may be seen.[103]

The cause of metaphyseal osteopathy is unknown. Prior suggestions implicating hypovitaminosis C, overnutrition, or copper deficiency have not been substantiated. Attempts to identify a causative infectious agent or to transmit the disease have not been successful. However, CDV RNA has been detected within bone cells of dogs with metaphyseal osteopathy, suggesting a role for this virus in the etiopathogenesis.[104] Other circumstantial evidence supports this[103-105]: Metaphyseal osteopathy may be accompanied or preceded by respiratory or gastrointestinal (GI) signs; dental enamel hypoplasia, a sequel to distemper infection, was found in two dogs with metaphyseal osteopathy; three of seven dogs inoculated with blood from dogs with metaphyseal osteopathy developed distemper; and typical bone changes have developed in some pups 4 to 21 days after inoculation with live distemper virus vaccine. However, the osteosclerotic metaphyseal lesions found in a series of dogs clinically affected with distemper differed macroscopically, radiographically, and histologically from metaphyseal osteopathy.[106] Any relationship between distemper virus, metaphyseal osteopathy, and other hyperostotic bone diseases (craniomandibular osteopathy and enostosis) remains uncertain. An epidemiologic study concluded that, apart from the obvious age effect, risk factors for metaphyseal osteopathy, craniomandibular osteopathy, and CDV infection were dissimilar.[91] Metaphyseal osteopathy has been reported in related dogs of several breeds, including Weimaraner littermates.[105-107] However, most cases are sporadic, affecting isolated pups in a litter.

No specific treatment exists for metaphyseal osteopathy. Dietary imbalances or excesses should be avoided and an anti-inflammatory analgesic given as needed to reduce pain. Good nursing care may be required to avoid dehydration, undernutrition and pressure sores.

Calvarial Hyperostosis

An unusual hyperostosis affecting frontal and parietal bones was reported in two unrelated bull mastiffs.[103] From age 6 months there was progressive outward thickening of the calvarium (the cranial cavity was unaffected) with pyrexia,

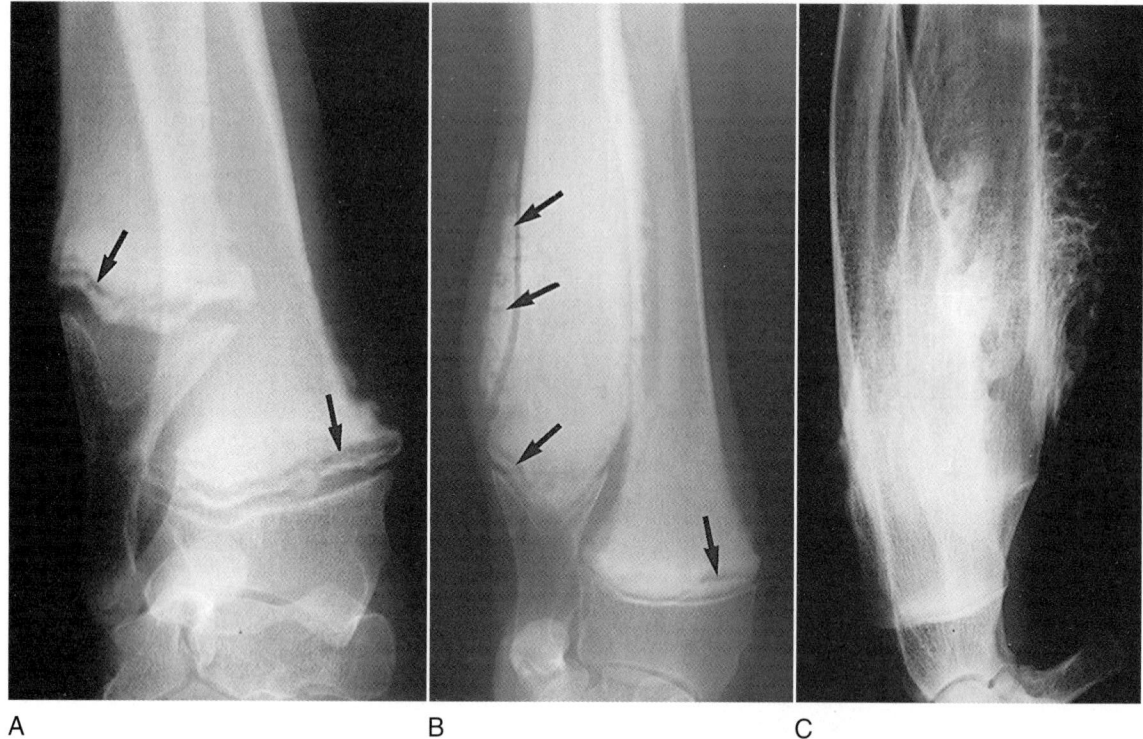

Figure 279-18 Radiographs of metaphyseal osteopathy. **A,** Early stage with irregular radiolucent zone *(arrows)* separated from the physis by a narrow radio-opaque band. **B,** Later stage with radiolucent metaphyseal zones *(bottom two arrows)* adjacent to the physes still evident. Periosteal new bone and soft tissue mineralization *(top two arrows)* adjacent to the metaphyseal cortex. **C,** Inactive stage with residual diaphyseal deformity and spiculated periosteal exostoses.

lymphadenopathy, and eosinophilia. The swelling stabilized at maturity, then regressed. The lesion was a subperiosteal hyperostosis with initial deposition of new woven bone followed by secondary osteonal remodeling. Similarities were noted with cases of craniomandibular osteopathy,

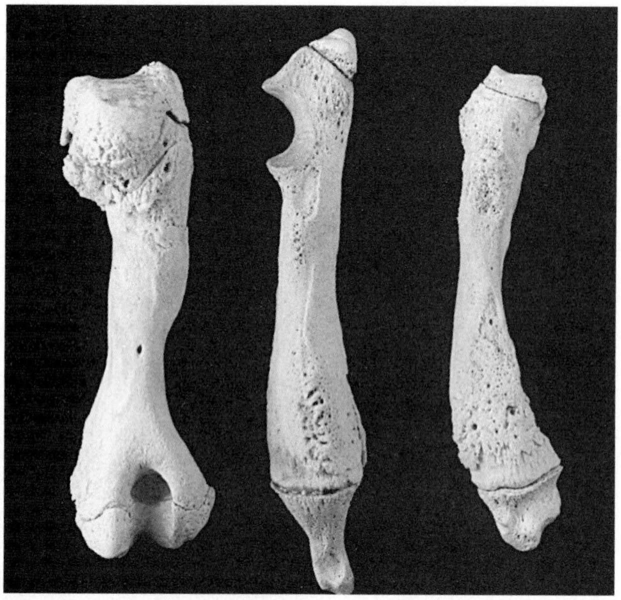

Figure 279-19 Humerus, ulna, and radius of a young giant-breed dog that suffered metaphyseal osteopathy. Reader should note the severe deformities and periosteal new bone.

inherited PK deficiency, and human infantile cortical hyperostosis.[102,108,109]

Multifocal Osteopathy

An idiopathic multifocal osteopathy was described in four young adult Scottish terriers, of which at least three were genetically related (fourth pedigree unavailable).[110] The condition was characterized by multifocal absence of bone in skull, cervical spine, radius, ulna, and femur (Figure 279-20). Histopathologic findings in one case indicated osteoclastic osteolysis and replacement of bone by fibrous tissue. Associated clinical signs included reluctance to move, stiff and stilted gait, carpal valgus and laxity, drooling and dysphagia.

Avascular Necrosis of the Femoral Head

Avascular (or aseptic) necrosis of the femoral head (Legg-Calve-Perthes disease) occurs in adolescent dogs. Miniature and small dog breeds are mostly affected, but Australian shepherd dogs also have increased risk of developing this disorder.[99] Within the predisposed small breeds, about 2% of individuals are affected, without apparent sex predilection. Clinically affected individuals are commonly presented at 4 to 11 months of age with hind leg lameness, usually unilateral but sometimes bilateral (12% to 20% of cases). The onset of lameness is usually gradual, though there may sometimes be a history of trauma. The severity varies from a slight limp to complete nonweight-bearing lameness. Pain and reduced range of movement are found on palpating the affected joint. Crepitus, shortening (up to 2 cm) of the affected limb (largely due to muscle spasm), and muscle atrophy may be evident at initial presentation.

The cause of this condition is unknown, but autosomal recessive inheritance has been suggested for West highland

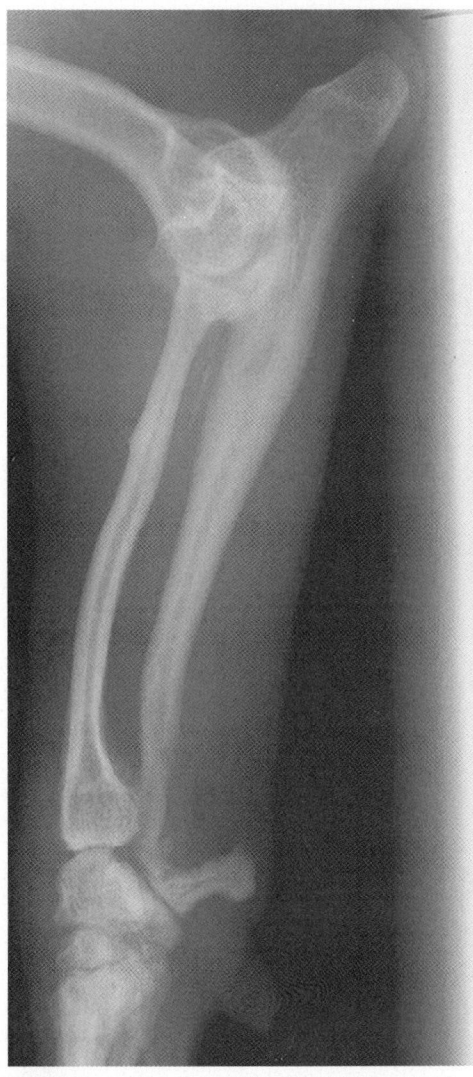

Figure 279-20 Radiograph of the antebrachium of a Scottish terrier with multifocal osteopathy. Reader should note the marked attenuation in diameter of the radial diaphysis. (Courtesy of C.W. Hay.)

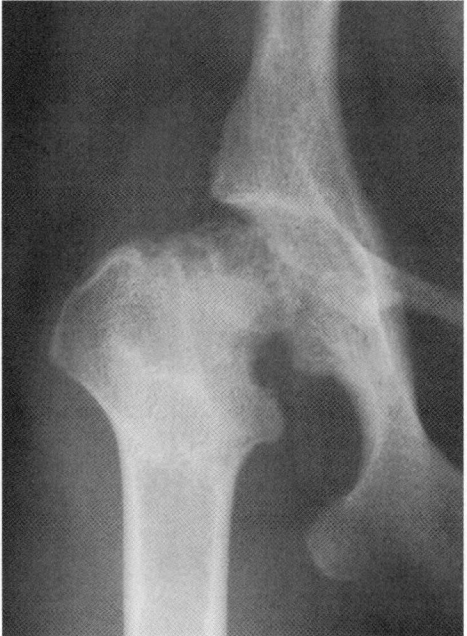

Figure 279-21 Later stage Legg-Calve-Perthes disease. Reader should note the multifocal osteolysis of the femoral head, thickened femoral neck, and increase in width of joint space. (Courtesy of Veterinary Imaging Associates, Sydney, Australia.)

Excision arthroplasty is advisable if conservative treatment does not produce clinical improvement within 4 weeks.[112]

Secondary Hypertrophic Osteopathy

In secondary hypertrophic osteopathy (pulmonary hypertrophic osteoarthropathy), firm nonedematous swelling develops in all four limbs, usually in response to intrathoracic disease, most often neoplasia. Of 180 canine cases, 98% had intrathoracic disease, and 92% of these had either metastatic lung neoplasia or primary tumors of lung or thoracic esophagus.[113] A few dogs had pneumonitis, endocarditis, or dirofilariasis. Of four cases lacking intrathoracic disease, three had urinary rhabdomyosarcoma and one had hepatic carcinoma. Because of the association with neoplasia, secondary hypertrophic osteopathy occurs mostly in older animals. No breed or gender predilection exists in dogs. The disorder is rare in cats.

Signs related to limb changes often precede signs of thoracic disease, but they can begin simultaneously with or after thoracic signs. Affected animals are stiff and reluctant to move. Swelling of all limbs occurs, which are warm, firm, and may be painful. Thoracic disease may be manifested by cough, dyspnea, abnormal lung sounds, or cardiac displacement. Abnormal laboratory findings, if any, are related to the underlying intrathoracic disease.

Radiographic changes are characteristic: soft tissue swelling of distal extremities initially, then periosteal new bone formation as irregular nodules perpendicular to the cortex or smoother parallel deposits (Figure 279-22). Bone changes begin distally and may spread proximally to involve humerus and scapula, femur, and pelvis. Ribs and vertebrae are sometimes affected.

On histologic examination, the bones are surrounded by highly vascular, dense connective tissue containing numerous thick-walled arteries. The osteogenic layer of the periosteum is hyperplastic, and overlies maturing and remodeling trabecular bone. The pathogenesis of secondary hypertrophic osteopathy involves increased blood flow to the distal extremities, then overgrowth of connective tissue and subsequent osteoneogenesis. This seems to involve a neural reflex originating in the

white and Yorkshire terriers, toy and miniature poodles, and pug dogs.[111] Early exposure to sex hormones, a consequence of precocious sexual maturity in small breeds, may be a factor. Another suggestion is that injury or infection and increased synovial fluid in the hip joint disrupt the blood supply to the femoral epiphysis while the growth plate is present. Continued weight bearing could then lead to collapse and remodeling of the femoral neck and head.

One of the earliest radiographic changes in this disorder is increased radio-opacity of the affected femoral head. Later changes include an apparent increase in joint space width, shortening and widening of the femoral neck, irregular opacity of femoral epiphyseal and metaphyseal regions, and flattening and irregularity of femoral articular cartilage (Figure 279-21). Secondary osteoarthrosis and acetabular osteophytes may also be evident.

Conservative treatment (short walks on a leash several times daily, swimming, analgesic drug as needed) produces satisfactory outcomes in 25% to 30% of affected dogs, whereas femoral head and neck excision, when performed correctly, gives good to excellent results in 67% to 85% of cases, though slight intermittent lameness may remain.[94,112]

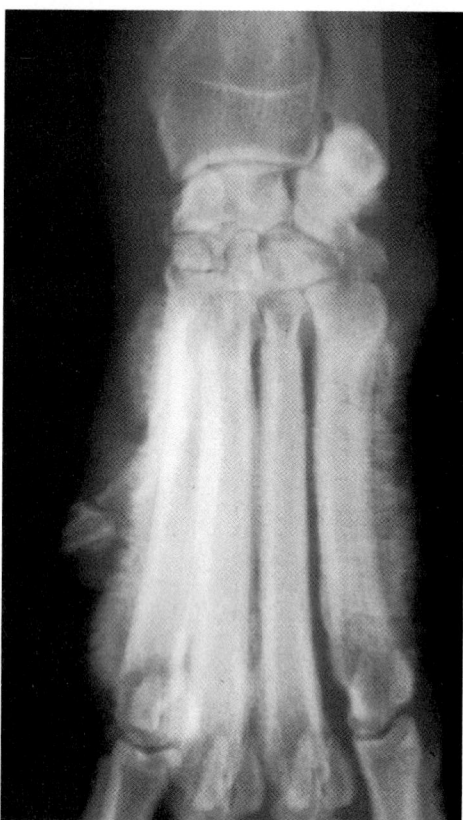

Figure 279-22 Radiograph of distal forelimb of a dog with secondary hypertrophic osteopathy. Periosteal new bone growth occurs, with nodular appearance affecting the metacarpals and digits. Adjacent soft tissues are thickened. (Courtesy of Veterinary Imaging Associates, Sydney, Australia.)

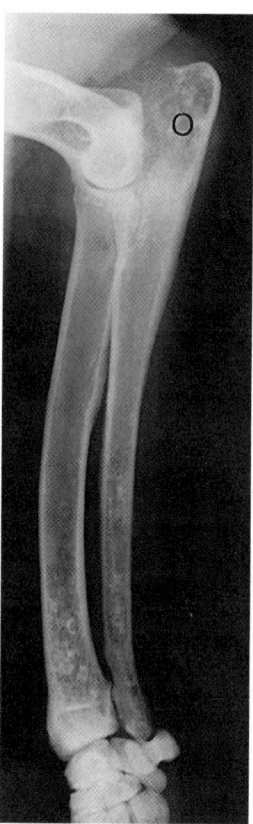

Figure 279-23 Radiograph demonstrating medullary bone infarction in an aged dog with osteosarcoma *(O)* of the olecranon. The multiple areas of medullary sclerosis in the radius and ulna are infarcts.

thorax and affecting connective tissue and periosteum of the limbs. The efferent pathway apparently involves nerve fibers that leave the lung near the bronchi and join the vagus in the mediastinum. The nature of the efferent connection, whether neural or hormonal, is unknown. Regression of secondary hypertrophic osteopathy may follow removal of the source of afferent impulses by excision of the lung lesion, or interruption of the afferent fibers by peribronchial dissection or vagotomy. There may be an alternate afferent pathway from parietal pleura along intercostal nerves, because regression has sometimes followed thoracotomy and section of intercostal nerves or extensive resection of a neoplasm of the thoracic wall. The rare association with intra-abdominal lesions is more obscure.

Treatment should be directed against the underlying thoracic disease, using appropriate medical or surgical methods. Successful resection of lung lesions by lobectomy or pneumonectomy can quickly remove pain, soft tissue swelling, and lameness. The bone abnormalities usually regress gradually over several months. Where complete removal of lung lesions is not possible, the skeletal signs may be ameliorated by removal of larger lesions even if multiple small lesions remain. Relief may also follow intrathoracic vagotomy on the same side as the lesion, or on the worse affected side if metastases are bilateral.

Medullary Bone Infarction

Medullary bone infarcts do not cause clinical signs in dogs. They affect older dogs and are usually found in conjunction with osteosarcoma and, occasionally, skeletal fibrosarcoma or renal adenocarcinoma.[114,115] Bone infarcts are characterized

radiographically by numerous, irregularly demarcated areas of increased radiopacity in the medullary cavities of one or more bones (Figure 279-23). The densities obliterate medullary cavities to varying degrees. Any bone may be affected, but infarcts are mainly found distal to elbow and stifle.[114]

The pathogenesis of the disorder is unknown and does not seem to be due to metastatic tumor cell dissemination. However, intramural collagen deposition causes occlusion of nutrient arteries, hypoxia and widespread necrosis of medullary soft tissues and bone, and new bone proliferation on endosteum and medullary trabeculae.[114] Common causes in humans are dysbaric conditions, fat embolization, hyperadrenocorticism, hyperviscosity, hemoglobinopathy, and anemia. Medullary bone infarcts should be differentiated from enostosis, bacterial and fungal osteomyelitis, and metastatic neoplasia.

Bone Cyst

Benign cystic bone lesions, either monostotic or polyostotic, are uncommon in dogs and cats. Young dogs of larger breeds are affected most often, with Doberman pinschers and German shepherds over-represented.[94,116] Males are affected twice as often as females. The cause is unknown, but may involve intramedullary metaphyseal hemorrhage, local disturbance of bone growth, or other factors.[113] Heritable factors might also be implicated, because lesions occurred in three Doberman pinscher littermates and in three Old English sheepdogs littermates and both parents.[94]

Bone cysts may be subclinical until they are large or fracture with trauma. Pain, lameness, and local swelling may ensue. The lesions occur in metaphyses and adjacent diaphyses of long bones, sparing growth plates and epiphyses. The distal radius or ulna (or both) are affected most often. The cysts are lined

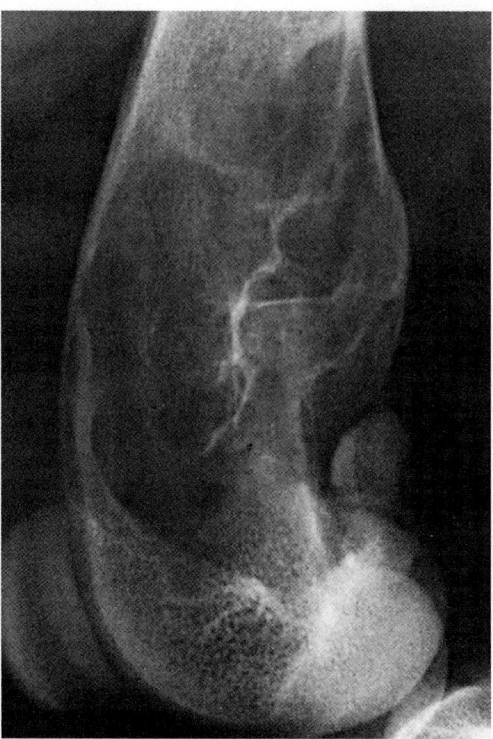

Figure 279-24 Bone cyst in distal femur of a young Doberman pinscher. The lesion has expansile, lytic appearance, with thinning of overlying cortex. Bony ridges or partitions are evident internally.

by a thin membrane and contain fluid that may be blood tinged. Radiographically, the lesions are lytic and expansile, with thinned cortex and little or no periosteal reaction. There may be one or several chambers, partially divided by bony ridges or partitions (Figure 279-24).

Alternative diagnoses are atypical bone neoplasia, aneurysmal bone cyst, and fibrous dysplasia of bone. Fine needle aspiration biopsy and cytologic examination may be useful: only a benign bone cyst is likely to be fluid filled, although the other lesions may contain areas of cystic degeneration or hemorrhage. If uncertainty persists, surgical biopsy and histopathologic study are indicated. To stimulate healing of bone cysts, surgery has been advocated, using drainage, curettage, bone grafting, and external support to prevent fractures. Some untreated cysts heal spontaneously without surgery, although pathologic fracture of cystic bone is a risk.[117]

Aneurysmal Bone Cyst

Aneurysmal bone cyst is a non-neoplastic lesion that results in considerable local bone destruction. Although common in man, it is rare in dogs and cats. Lesions arise in ribs, pelvis, scapula, spine, and metaphyses of long bones in young adults and geriatric animals.[118,119] The cause is unknown, but tumors, developmental abnormalities, and trauma-induced hemorrhage causing venous obstruction or arteriovenous shunts in bone marrow have been suggested as initiating factors.[7] Localized partial disruption of medullary blood flow results in endosteal bone resorption and outward displacement of the periosteum. The periosteum forms successive layers of woven bone that are resorbed as the lesion expands, producing the appearance of a ballooning aortic aneurysm.[7] Blood-tinged fluid and fibrovascular tissue fill the lesion which has a honeycomb appearance with huge vascular channels. Radiographically, it appears as a large expansile cyst, with minimal internal trabecular septation, surrounded by thin rim of mineralized

soft tissue or bone (Figure 279-25). A triangle of laminated periosteal new bone (Codman's triangle) forms at the junction between cyst and adjacent normal diaphyseal bone. Some have an underlying tumor (osteosarcoma, giant cell tumor) that complicates diagnosis. Signs may be suddenly exacerbated by neoplastic erosion of vessels and intralesional hemorrhage or by fracture.[119] Uncomplicated lesions have a good prognosis when treated by en bloc resection, amputation, or curettage.[120] Nonresectable lesions in man are irradiated to stop bleeding and lesional growth, but postirradiation sarcoma can ensue.

Subchondral Bone Cyst

Subchondral bone cysts are benign lesions in subchondral bone between growth plate and articular cartilage.[121] They are usually lined with synovium and occasionally communicate with the articular synovial membrane. Radiographs show a single or multilocular radiolucent defect with well-circumscribed borders. They are common in horses and pigs and usually a manifestation of osteochondrosis.[7] This association was also noted in a dog.[121]

Fibrous Dysplasia

Fibrous dysplasia is a rare fibro-osseous lesion of bone believed to be of developmental origin.[7] It affects mainly young or newborn animals and may be monostotic or polyostotic. The lesions are expansile and may cause problems of disfigurement or compression of adjacent structures or bone weakness and fracture (Figure 279-26). Monostotic lesions have been reported in the jaw or infraorbital bone of dog, and in mandible, maxilla, or distal ulna of cats.[122,123] Fibrous dysplasia, aneurysmal bone cysts, and benign bone cysts are distinct entities but have been confused in the veterinary literature.[124]

The lesions have marked homogenous radiopacity and are composed of firm, gray fibrous tissue that is gritty when cut. Histologically, they consist of fibrous connective tissue stroma containing spicules of woven bone replacing normal osseous tissue. Cavities of various size containing clear or bloody fluid may be scattered throughout.[7] Two feline lesions were resected, and both patients were free of recurrence 4 years later.[122]

Central Giant Cell Granuloma

This rare, non-neoplastic lesion affects the tooth-bearing regions of maxilla and mandible of young dogs.[125] Trauma-associated intraosseous hemorrhage seems to be an initiating factor. Radiographically the lesion is a rounded to ovoid, expansile, uniloculated radiolucency that is well demarcated from surrounding tissue by a thin rim of smooth nonreactive bone. Adjacent teeth may lose their laminae dura and be displaced, but tooth root resorption is rare. The center of the lesion consists of tan-colored soft tissue composed mainly of loose fibrovascular stroma containing pleomorphic mesenchymal cells and numerous large, irregular multinucleated giant cells. These cells arise from mesenchymal tissue and are neither osteoclasts nor involved in bone resorption. The lesions resemble giant cell tumors histologically. The latter are potentially malignant tumors that cause extensive destruction at the ends of long bones. Because central giant cell granuloma is rare, diagnosis should be confirmed by biopsy. Treatment is by curettage or en bloc resection.[125]

METABOLIC, NUTRITIONAL, AND ENDOCRINE BONE DISORDERS

The term *metabolic bone disease* is used here to encompass various conditions that cause generalized reduction in bone mass, or *osteopenia*. Osteopenia can be categorized into excessive

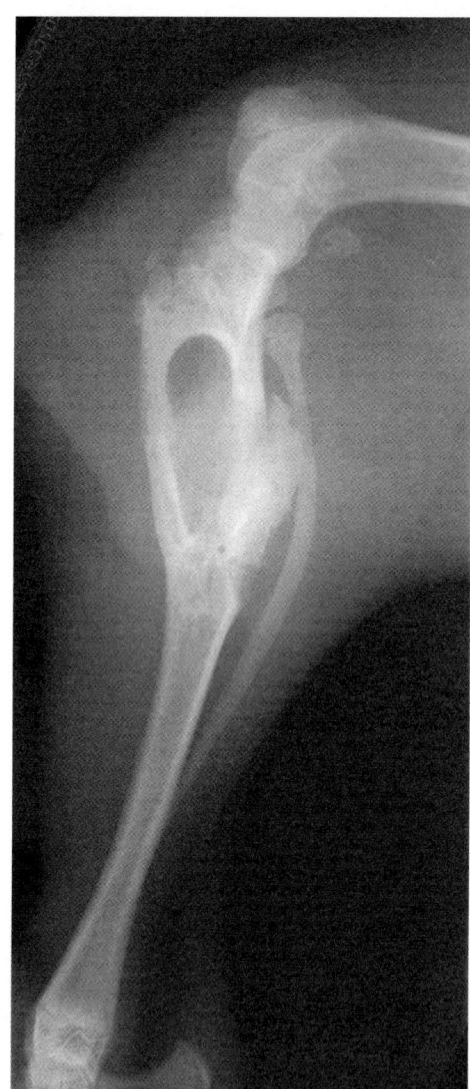

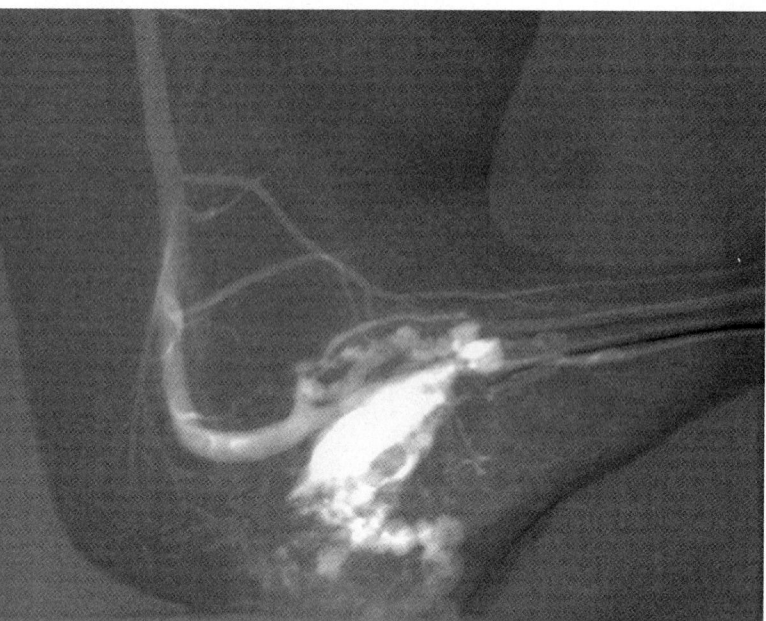

Figure 279-25 Aneurysmal bone cyst of the tibia in a 2-year-old boxer dog that had sustained a tibial fracture as a puppy. **A,** Reader should note the angular deformity of the diaphyses of the tibia and fibular due to fracture malunion. A large cystic cavity in the proximal tibia is associated with a soft tissue mass cranial to the tibia. **B,** Arteriogram showing a dilated, tortuous arteriovenous fistula extending from the tibia into adjacent soft tissue. (Courtesy of J.H. Marti.)

bone resorption, or *osteolysis*, as occurs in hyperparathyroid states, and defective bone formation. The latter is further subdivided into insufficient formation of osteoid, or *osteoporosis*, and defective mineralization of osteoid, or *rickets-osteomalacia*.

Major causes of metabolic bone disease involve nutritional or hormonal processes (or both). The more important causes discussed here are nutritional secondary hyperparathyroidism, rickets, renal osteodystrophy, and hypervitaminosis A. Other metabolic bone diseases that rarely produce bone-related clinical signs are mentioned briefly.

Nutritional Secondary Hyperparathyroidism

Nutritional secondary hyperparathyroidism is a metabolic disorder in which bone production is normal but osteopenia results from excessive bone resorption. It is caused by diets providing excess phosphate, insufficient calcium, or both.[94] Affected animals have usually been fed mainly meat, organ tissue, or both. This provides adequate phosphate but insufficient calcium, and Ca/P ratios of about 1:16 to 1:35,[126] which contrast with the recommended 1.2:1 for dogs and 1:1 for cats. Added cow's milk provides insufficient calcium to correct the imbalance. The imbalance induces hypocalcemia, which increases secretion of PTH. Increased parathyroid activity tends to normalize blood calcium and inorganic

phosphate concentrations by promoting mineral resorption from bone, enhancing intestinal calcium absorption, and facilitating renal phosphate excretion and calcium retention. However, continued ingestion of the defective diet sustains the hyperparathyroid state and causes progressive skeletal demineralization and consequent clinical signs.

Nutritional secondary hyperparathyroidism causes clinical disease in pups and kittens of all breeds, but it also occurs occasionally in adults. Signs in young animals are lameness, reluctance to stand or walk, and skeletal pain. Costochondral junctions and metaphyses may appear swollen, and pyrexia is sometimes present. Bone fractures can follow relatively mild trauma. Limb deformity may be evident. Paresis or paralysis may result from vertebral compression, and constipation may follow pelvic collapse. Effects are less dramatic in adults, but generalized osteopenia and skeletal pain are sometimes seen, and resorption of alveolar bone may cause loosening and loss of teeth.

Radiographically, decreased bone density and thin cortices are seen, with or without fracturing (Figure 279-27). Growth plates are normal, but metaphyses may be mushroom shaped. An area of relative radio-opacity occurs in the metaphyses adjacent to growth plates, representing the area of primary mineralization, and may be best appreciated in the distal radius and ulna (Figure 279-28).

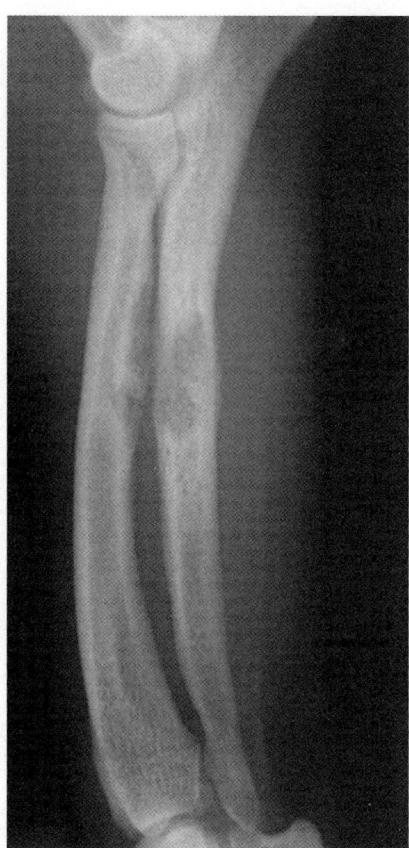

Figure 279-26 Fibrous dysplasia in the ulnar diaphysis, with secondary lysis and new bone formation in adjacent radial cortex. (Courtesy of P.A. Manley.)

Blood biochemical tests are of little value in confirming nutritional secondary hyperparathyroidism. The calcium concentration is usually within the reference range because of compensatory changes. Concentrations of inorganic phosphate and alkaline phosphatase may appear high but should be interpreted carefully because growing animals often have higher values than adults.

Affected animals should be confined for the first few weeks of treatment to reduce the risk of fractures and deformity. A good quality, nutritionally complete commercial ration should be fed. For all but mildly affected cases, sufficient calcium carbonate should be added to produce a calcium/phosphorus

ratio of 2:1. This is maintained for 2 to 3 months, after which the supplement is withdrawn. Oversupplementation with calcium should be avoided. For severely affected cases parenteral administration of calcium (e.g., 10 to 30 mL of 10% calcium gluconate solution by slow intravenous infusion daily for 3 days) may help reduce pain and lameness initially, but it does little to correct the calcium deficiency. An NSAID might be useful for short-term analgesia. The prognosis is generally good, unless skeletal deformity and disability are marked.

Rickets

Clinical cases of rickets are rare in dogs and cats. Rickets and its adult equivalent, osteomalacia, occur when insufficient calcium, phosphorus, or both is available for mineralization of newly formed osteoid. The more likely causes of rickets in dogs and cats are hypovitaminosis D (dietary deficiency),[127] inborn error in vitamin D metabolism,[128] or low availability of minerals from the diet (inadequate concentration, impaired absorption). Dogs and cats do not synthesize cholecalciferol (previtamin D_3) in skin exposed to ultraviolet (UV) light, and are mainly dependent on dietary intake.[129-131]

Affected animals may be lame and reluctant or unable to walk. Fractures or bending of long bones can occur. Enlargement of costochondral junctions and metaphyses may be evident. Other possible abnormalities are delayed dental eruption, weakness, listlessness, and neurologic signs (excitability, tremor, convulsion, and coma) from hypocalcemia. Potential blood test abnormalities include low calcium, low inorganic phosphate, increased alkaline phosphatase, increased PTH, and low 25-hydroxycholecalciferol (the storage form of vitamin D).[127,128,132]

Characteristic radiographic findings are axial and radial thickening of growth plates and cupping of adjacent metaphyses (Figures 279-29 and 279-30). The distal ulnar growth plates are consistently the most severely affected, and this finding reflects a failure of mineralization of cartilage that is being produced at the normal rate. Additional findings are osteopenia, thin cortices, and bowed diaphyses.

When dietary deficiency is suspected, therapy requires a regular diet with adequate and not excessive amounts of calcium, phosphorus, and vitamin D.[127,132] The regimen described for nutritional secondary hyperparathyroidism would be appropriate. Treatment with dihydrotachysterol was effective in a dog in which an inborn error in vitamin D metabolism was suspected.[128]

Renal Osteodystrophy

Renal osteodystrophy is an osteopenic disorder that results from chronic renal failure (CRF). This complex abnormality

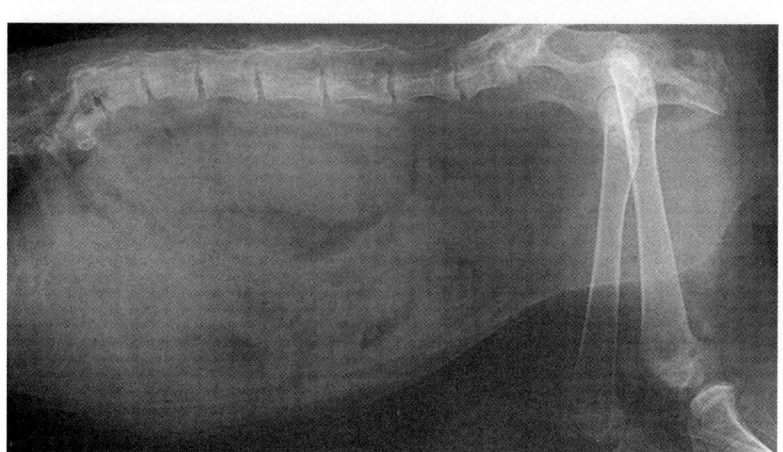

Figure 279-27 Abdomen of kitten with nutritional secondary hyperparathyroidism. Reader should note poor contrast in radio-opacity between bones and soft tissues such as liver and kidneys. The cortices of long bones are thin, vertebrae are lucent, and the vertebral column is deformed in the thoracolumbar area.

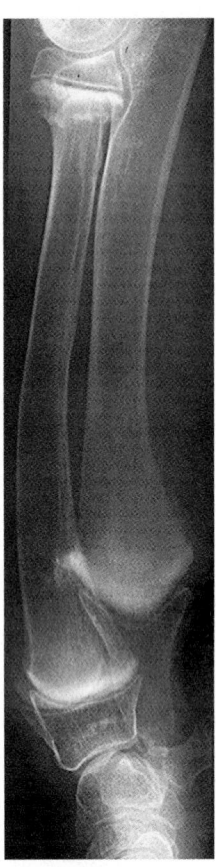

Figure 279-28 Foreleg of a pup with nutritional secondary hyperparathyroidism. Bone is abnormally radiolucent and cortices are thin. Growth plates are normal, but relatively radio-opaque zones are present in the adjacent metaphyses (representing areas of primary mineralization of osteoid).

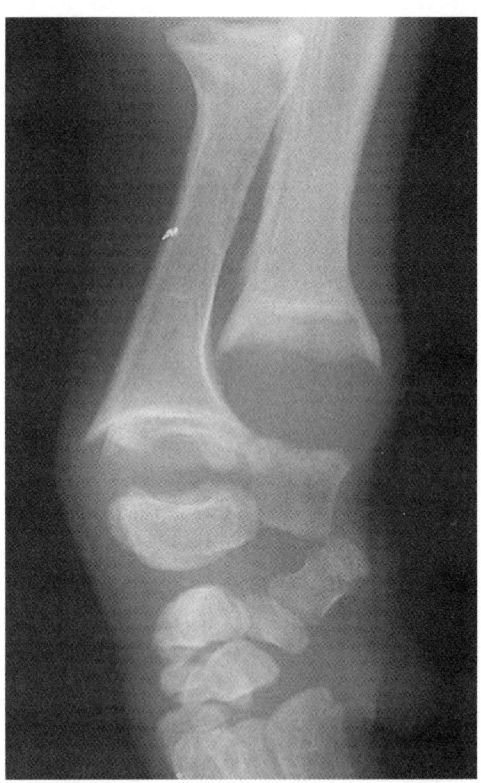

Figure 279-29 Foreleg of a 12-week-old Saint Bernard with rickets due to an inborn error in vitamin D metabolism. Enlarged physes and cupping of adjacent metaphyseal bone are features of rickets. (From Johnson KA et al: Vitamin D–dependent rickets in a Saint Bernard dog. J Small Anim Pract 29:657, 1988.)

involves both hyperparathyroidism (excessive bone resorption) and rickets-osteomalacia (impaired osteoid mineralization). Hyperparathyroidism results from impaired renal excretion of phosphate and consequent hyperphosphatemia. This lowers blood calcium concentration, increases parathyroid gland activity, and induces bone resorption. Although this tends to normalize blood calcium concentrations, the hyperparathyroid state is maintained by persisting hyperphosphatemia. Concurrently, synthesis of 1,25 dihydroxyvitamin D declines because of reduced functional renal mass. This and other metabolic derangements lead to severe depression of enteric calcium absorption, impaired mineralization of osteoid, and thus rickets-osteomalacia.

The syndrome is dominated by signs of renal failure and uremia. Bone disease is more likely to be recognized clinically in growing dogs or, rarely, cats with early onset renal failure. Changes may be most evident in the head. The mandible and maxilla may be pliable and swollen, owing to bone resorption and fibrosis, and teeth may be malaligned, loose, or lost. Skeletal pain, fractures, and bowing of long bones can also occur. Osteopenia of the mandible and maxilla leads to enhanced radiographic contrast between teeth and bone, and teeth may appear almost unsupported by bony tissue.[133]

Treatment is directed against the underlying disease, if possible. Reduced phosphate intake, coupled with oral phosphate binder (aluminum hydroxide or carbonate) as necessary, can help to control hyperphosphatemia. Once this is achieved, consideration can be given to administering calcium to improve calcium balance or administering calcitriol to control hyperparathyroidism (see Chapters 258 and 260).

Hypervitaminosis A

Prolonged intake of excessive vitamin A supplements or ingestion of mainly liver diets can cause osteopathy. The major finding in older cats is extensive, even confluent, exostoses and enthesophytes involving cervical and cranial thoracic vertebrae (Figure 279-31). Enthesophytes may also form around limb joints, especially shoulder or elbow, which may reflect increased sensitivity of tendon, ligament, and joint capsule attachments to the effects of tension.[113,134]

The lesions are painful in the early stages and may ankylose, causing neck stiffness and abnormal posture. Associated clinical signs are lethargy, depression, irritability, poor grooming, lameness, and gingivitis.[113] Experimental vitamin A toxicosis in young animals depressed chondrocyte and osteoblast activities, which produced thin bone cortices, retarded long bone growth, and produced loose or lost teeth in kittens.[134,135] Puppies had joint pain, thin bone cortices, and retarded bone growth.[136]

Treatment necessitates avoiding the source of vitamin A. Mature cats will improve clinically, but rigidity from ankylosis will probably remain despite bone remodeling. Bone growth may be retarded permanently in young animals.[134]

Other Endocrine and Nutritional Bone Disorders

Primary Hyperparathyroidism With uncontrolled hyperplastic or neoplastic proliferation of parathyroid tissue, excessive secretion of PTH may cause increased bone remodeling and skeletal demineralization. This could lead to lameness,

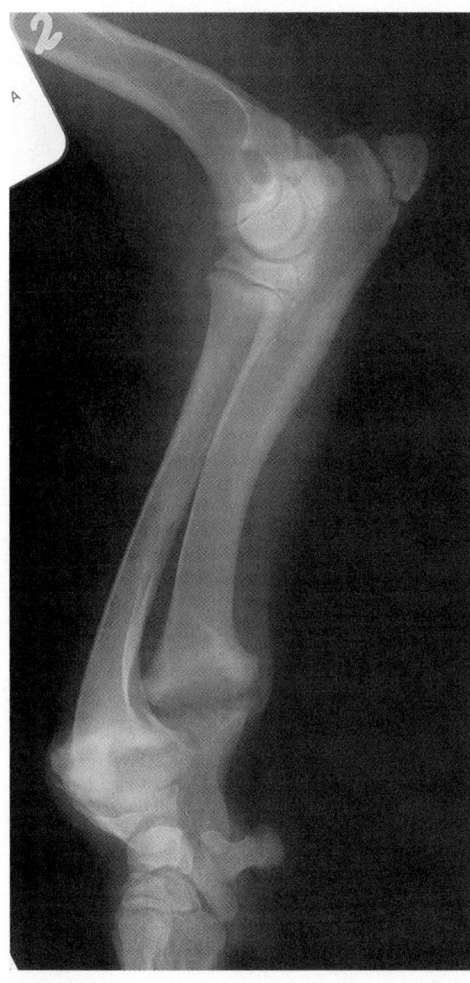

Figure 279-30 Foreleg of a greyhound puppy with rickets due to dietary deficiency of vitamin D. Reader should note the axial and radial enlargement of the physes and cupping of the adjacent metaphyseal bone. (Courtesy of R. Malik and Veterinary Imaging Associates, Sydney, Australia.)

pain, fractures, vertebral collapse, loose or lost teeth, and pliable, possibly swollen jaw bones (Figure 279-32). However, the predominant findings usually relate to hypercalcemia[137] and include polydipsia (PD), polyuria (PU), listlessness, incontinence, weakness, inappetence, and urocystolithiasis (see Chapter 237).

Humoral Hypercalcemia of Malignancy With certain neoplasms, especially lymphosarcoma or adenocarcinoma of the anal sacs in dogs, widespread skeletal demineralization ensues through the humoral action of PTH-related protein.[137,138] Although skeletal dysfunction can occur as with primary hyperparathyroidism, findings are usually dominated by changes related to the underlying tumor and the effects of hypercalcemia (see Chapter 237).

Hyperadrenocorticism Chronic glucocorticosteroid excess due to iatrogenic excess or naturally occurring hyperadrenocorticism causes osteopenia. Retarded growth and delayed growth plate closure may occur in young dogs,[139] and spontaneous fractures and increased prevalence of intervertebral disk disease have been suggested.[140] Osteopenia in spontaneous canine hyperadrenocorticism is attributable primarily to decreased bone formation; bone resorption is apparently normal, although parathyroid hyperplasia is present in some cases (see Chapter 136).[140]

Hypogonadism Hypogonadism, whether a developmental defect or produced surgically, can delay growth plate closure.[7] In dogs, closure was delayed by neutering in both sexes, and the extended growth period resulted in longer radius and ulna in all males, as well as in bitches neutered at 7 weeks.[141] Gonadectomy in cats delayed distal radial physeal closure but did not affect bone length.[142] However, neutered male cats are predisposed to spontaneous, nontraumatic fractures of the femoral capital physis between the ages of 5 to 24 months.[143-145] Fractures are often bilateral. Radiographic signs include physeal fracture displacement and lysis of the metaphyseal bone, producing an "apple core" appearance. Histological examination of specimens resected at surgery revealed that the articular cartilage and epiphyseal bone of the capital epiphysis had

Figure 279-31 Cat with hypervitaminosis A. **A,** Confluent exostoses affect the dorsum of the spine from the second cervical to the fifth thoracic vertebrae. **B,** Exuberant exostoses of distal humerus and proximal ulna are ankylosing the elbow.

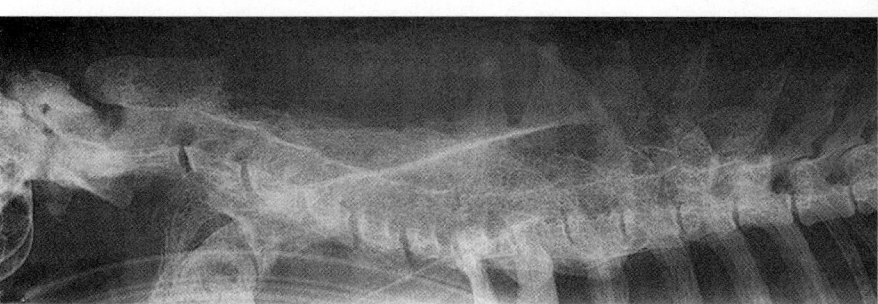

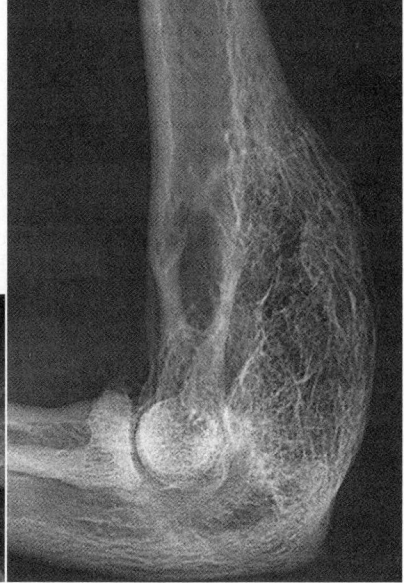

A

B

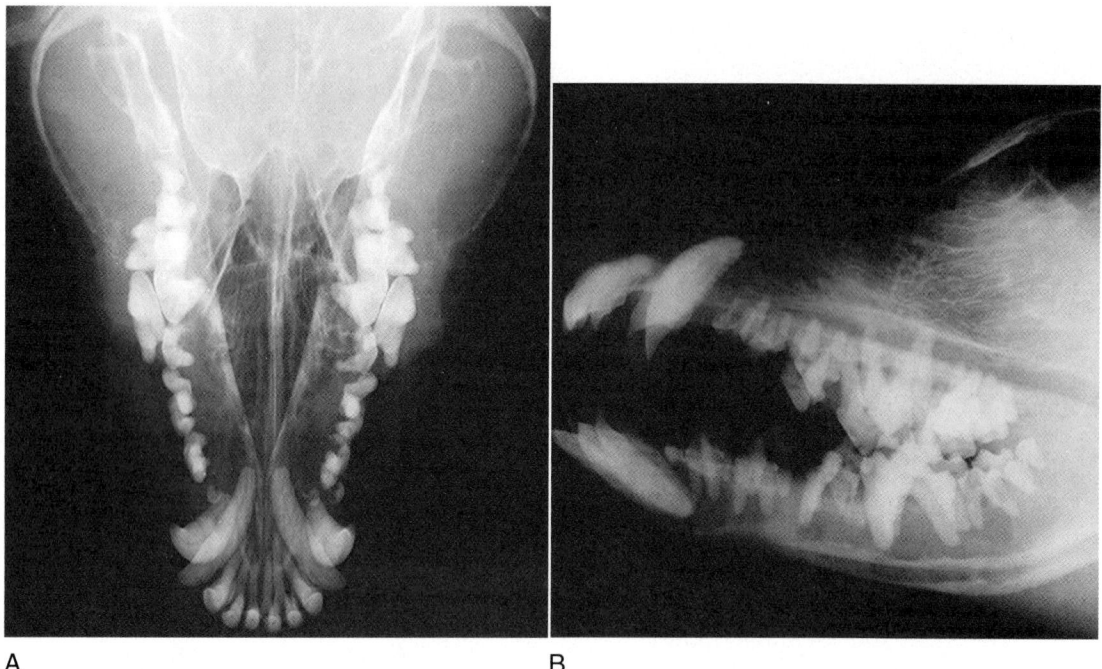

Figure 279-32 Radiograph of an aged Keeshond with parathyroid adenoma and hyperparathyroidism, with profound osteopenia of the skull and mandible. **A,** In the ventrodorsal view, osteolysis of the zygomatic arch, maxilla, facial bones, and mandible occurs. **B,** In the lateral view, loss of the lamina dura and mandibular cortex occurs, except for the thin ventral cortex.

normal structure and viability, but the physeal cartilage was thickened and necrotic.[144] Normally this physis closes at 7 to 9 months of age in sexually intact cats. Delayed physeal closure after early gonadectomy apparently allows the persistence of cartilage that is unable to support normal weight-bearing activities.

Hepatic Osteodystrophy Severe hepatic disease can produce rickets—osteomalacia due to malassimilation of fat and vitamin D (and secondarily of calcium) and impaired production of 25-hydroxyvitamin D.[146] Osteoporosis may also occur due to diminished hepatic protein synthesis.[146] Although well-recognized in human patients, hepatic osteodystrophy has yet to be characterized in dogs and cats.

Anticonvulsant Osteodystrophy Prolonged high-dose anticonvulsant therapy with primidone, phenytoin, or phenobarbitone can cause osteodystrophy in human epileptics.[146] These drugs induce hepatic enzymes that enhance catabolism and excretion of vitamin D, resulting in calcium malabsorption, hypocalcemia, secondary hyperparathyroidism, and osteomalacia. Phenytoin also directly inhibits intestinal calcium transport and bone resorptive responses to PTH and vitamin D metabolites.[146] The significance of these changes to veterinary patients is unknown.

Hypovitaminosis A Vitamin A is important for growth, maturation, and remodeling of bone. Hypovitaminosis A decreases osteoclastic activity and impedes bone remodeling, causing long bones to be deformed. Affected animals are usually lame. The condition is probably rare.[113,147]

Hypervitaminosis D Skeletal demineralization follows massive intake of vitamin D, its active metabolites or analogs. Although osteopenia, bone deformation, and retarded growth are possible, the major clinical effects are related to hypercalcemia and soft tissue mineralization.[136] Correcting intakes of vitamin D, calcium, and phosphate should resolve the bone problems, but soft tissue damage may persist.

Zinc-Responsive Chondrodysplasia This form of dwarfism occurs in Alaskan malamutes and possibly other northern breeds.[147] Affected dogs have short, bowed legs; flared, irregular, thickened growth plates; and coarse, disorganized metaphyseal trabeculae. Hemolytic anemia with macrocytosis, hypochromia, and stomatocytosis are also present. Life-long supplementation with zinc sulfate or gluconate was suggested.[147]

Copper Deficiency

Lameness and bone fragility can occur in dogs on copper-deficient diets.[7] Radiographic features are thickened growth plates and flared metaphyses, with osteopenia and epiphyseal slipping in severe cases. Histologically the animal has thickening of the zone of hypertrophic chondrocytes plus disorganization and collapse of the primary spongiosa.[148] The condition is rare.

Lead Poisoning Although skeletal signs are absent in plumbism, lead lines are seen radiographically in bones of some affected immature dogs. The lines are radio-opaque bands in metaphyses adjacent to growth plates of long bones (Figure 279-33). They result from accumulation of thick mineralized trabeculae at these sites because of impaired osteoclastic activity. The presence of lead itself adds little to the radio-opacity.

Overnutrition in Growing Dogs Provision of balanced diets in quantities in excess of recommended daily intake or feeding diets that contain greater than the recommended content of protein, energy, minerals, or vitamins, have been referred to as *overnutrition* or *overfeeding*. Experimental studies of

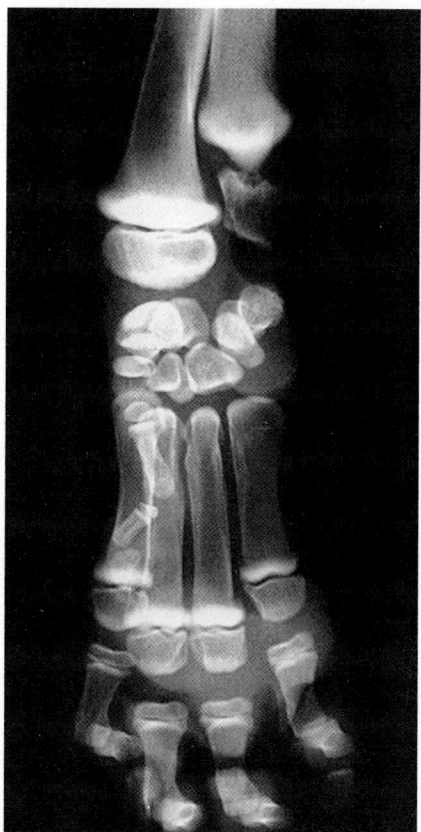

Figure 279-33 Radiograph of distal forelimb of a puppy with lead poisoning. Radiopaque bands are present in metaphyses adjacent to growth plates.

young growing Great Danes found that feeding of an excessively supplemented diet was associated with development of wobbler syndrome, enostosis, osteochondrosis, and metaphyseal osteopathy.[149] Subsequently, it was found that diets with excessive protein content have no adverse effects on skeletal development.[150] However, Great Dane puppies fed a diet containing triple the recommended calcium requirement had elevated absorption and retention of calcium and disturbed endochondral ossification, and they developed osteochondrosis, retained cartilage cores, radius curvus syndrome, and had stunted growth.[88,151,152] Another study of Great Dane puppies fed diets with calcium/phosphorus ratios of 1.2:1, but with lower than recommended concentrations of calcium, found that bones had lower bone mineral content throughout the growth period.[153] Long bone growth was also delayed until 6 months of age, but after this time bone growth caught up and was normal by 12 months of age, despite dietary deficiency in calcium.

Young Great Danes fed *ad libitum* with a balanced commercial diet initially had greater increases in body weight and height than littermates fed a restricted (two thirds of the caloric intake) diet.[132] The restricted puppies later had a period of catch-up growth, and by age 7 months long bones were of identical length.[132] Restricted feeding (25% reduction in total intake) of a balanced diet limited the incidence and severity of osteoarthritis secondary to hip dysplasia in Labrador retriever dogs.[154] Accordingly, overfeeding and oversupplemented diets should be avoided in growing pups. *Ad libitum* feeding is not recommended because it does not result in larger adult dogs, and it increases risk of orthopedic problems such as hip dysplasia.[132,154]

NEOPLASTIC BONE DISEASE[155]

Neoplasia of the skeletal system can be categorized into primary bone tumors, metastatic bone tumors, tumors of soft tissues extending into adjacent bone, and benign bone tumors.[155] These conditions are discussed elsewhere in this text. Non-neoplastic conditions of bone, such as cystic lesions and fibrous dysplasia, that may be confused with primary bone cancer, are important differentials. Bone cysts and fibrous dysplasia of bone are discussed earlier in this chapter.

BONE INFECTION

Bone infection (osteomyelitis) may be bacterial, fungal, or possibly viral (see Metaphyseal Osteopathy) in origin. Beta lactamase–producing *Staphylococcus* cause approximately 50% of cases of bacterial osteomyelitis, often as monomicrobial infections.[30] Polymicrobial infections may have mixtures of *Streptococcus* and gram-negative bacteria (*Escherichia coli*, *Pseudomonas*, *Proteus*, and *Klebsiella*), and sometimes anaerobic bacteria. More common anaerobic isolates are *Actinomyces*, *Peptostreptococcus*, *Bacteroides*, and *Fusobacterium*.[156] Anaerobes are especially common in bite wound infections. *Nocardia*, *Brucella canis*, and tuberculosis cause osteomyelitis in rare instances.[155] Mycotic genera that cause osteomyelitis include *Coccidioides*, *Blastomyces*, *Histoplasma*, *Cryptococcus*, and *Aspergillus*. Fungal osteomyelitis is often a component of disseminated mycotic infections that occur in certain specific regions of the world. Diagnosis and treatment of deep mycoses are discussed in Chapter 174.

Pathophysiology

Bacterial contamination of bone can occur with open fractures, surgery, bite wounds, foreign-body penetration, gunshot injury, extension from soft tissue, and hematogenous spread. However, bone is relatively resistant to infection unless the animal has concurrent soft tissue injury, bone necrosis, sequestration, fracture instability, implanted foreign material, altered host defenses, or some combination of these problems.[157] In chronic infections, avascular fragments of cortical bone (sequestra) are colonized by bacteria, surrounded by exudate, and may persist for long periods. New bone formed by periosteum (involucrum) incompletely encapsulates the focus of infection and sequestrum. Exudate draining from the bone follows sinus tracts that discharge through skin openings, generally in a more dependent location. Osteomyelitis is exacerbated by fracture and instability. Cortical bone at the fracture site is resorbed because of infection and interfragmentary motion, and this causes further widening of the fracture gap and additional instability.

Extraneous material (wood, soil, asphalt, and surgical implants) may incite a foreign-body response, interfere with local host defense mechanisms, and provide a nidus for infection.[157,158] Bacteria have unique mechanisms for bonding to surfaces of implanted foreign material. Initially the surfaces of implants become coated with matrix and serum proteins, ions, cellular debris, and carbohydrates (Figure 279-34).[159] Fibronectin, collagen, and fibrinogen are especially important in bacterial binding to biomaterial. Staphylococci and other gram-positive bacteria possess numerous cell membrane receptors for binding to fibronectin on implant surfaces.[159] Gram-negative bacteria are less effective at binding and have pili and fimbriae that specifically bind cellular proteins, matrix proteins, and glycolipids.[159] Bacteria also bind to exposed collagen matrix proteins (sialoprotein) and hydroxyapatite crystals of damaged bone.[159-161]

Once adherent, bacteria have two important mechanisms that ensure their persistence: (1) slime production and

HEMATOLOGY AND IMMUNOLOGY

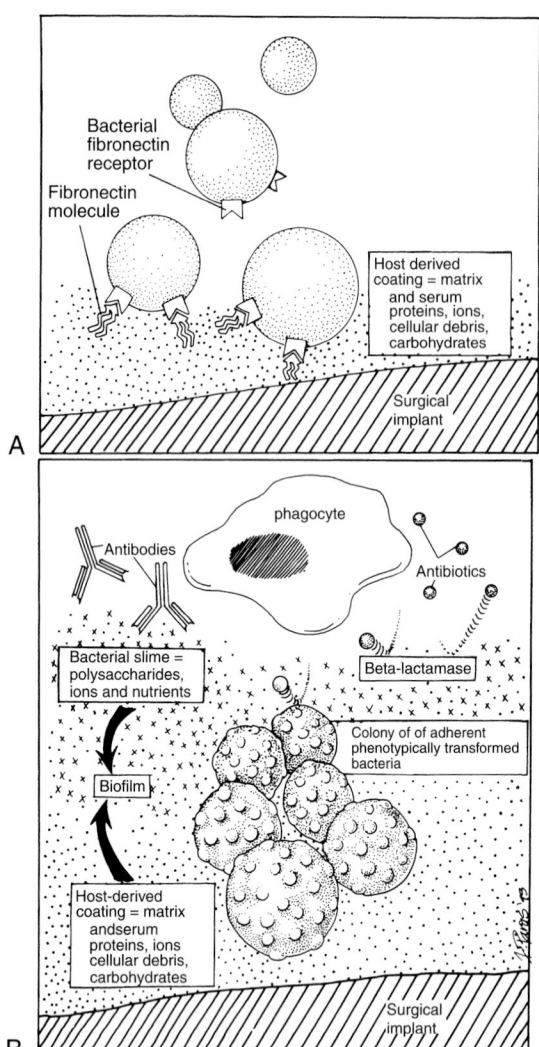

Figure 279-34 Mechanisms of bacterial persistence in chronic osteomyelitis. **A,** Foreign material such as surgical implants become coated with host-derived material containing fibronectin that binds with membrane receptors of contaminating bacteria. **B,** Adherent staphylococci and some other bacteria produce a slime that together with the host-derived material is called *biofilm*. Biofilm increases bacterial adhesion, protects bacteria from phagocytes and antibodies, and may also contain beta-lactamase. In addition, some adherent bacteria are phenotypically transformed to more virulent strains. (From Johnson KA: Osteomyelitis in dogs and cats. J Am Vet Med Assoc 205:1882, 1994.)

(2) phenotypic transformation.[159,162] Adherent staphylococci and some other bacteria produce a slime composed of extracellular polysaccharide, ions, and nutrients. Slime, together with host-derived material (matrix and serum proteins, ions, cellular debris, and carbohydrate), envelopes bacterial colonies and is called *biofilm* or *glycocalyx* (see Figure 279-34). Biofilm is a virulence factor, because it increases bacterial adhesion, shields bacteria from phagocytes and antibodies, and modifies drug susceptibility.[159] Most antimicrobial drugs diffuse through biofilm, but biofilm may contain high concentrations of beta-lactamase, which protects some bacteria. In addition to providing physical protection, biofilm causes adherent bacteria to transform phenotypically to more virulent strains that are more resistant to antimicrobial drugs than when they are tested *in vitro*.[159]

The metaphyses of long bones are commonly affected in young animals with acute hematogenous osteomyelitis.[163] These regions may be especially vulnerable because capillary endothelium therein is discontinuous, allowing extravasation of erythrocytes and possibly bacteria.[157] When local defenses are compromised, osteomyelitis may ensue. This probably accounts for the development of metaphyseal osteomyelitis in Irish setter pups with leukocyte adhesion protein deficiency and border collies with neutropenia due to impaired release of neutrophils from bone marrow (Figure 279-35).[164,165]

Diagnosis

Acute osteomyelitis may produce signs of systemic illness including pyrexia, inappetence, dullness, and weight loss, together with neutrophilia and left shift. Heat, pain, and swelling in muscle and periosteum surrounding the infected bone may be evident. In chronic osteomyelitis, abscessation with single or multiple sinus tracts is a prominent sign. Lymphadenopathy, muscle atrophy, fibrosis, and contracture accompany chronic disease, but hematologic alterations are uncommon.

Radiographs are usually necessary for diagnosis (see Radiology). In acute osteomyelitis, soft tissue swelling (but no osseous changes) occurs, except perhaps in young animals with acute metaphyseal osteomyelitis. In chronic osteomyelitis, periosteal new bone forms early and tends to be extensive, spiculated, and radially orientated (Figure 279-36). Bone resorption produces cortical thinning, medullary lysis, and rounding of fractured bone ends. In young animals, the diaphyseal cortex may be entirely resorbed and replaced by a shell of involucrum. The finding of sequestra is virtually diagnostic for osteomyelitis. Sequestra may be small and obscured by surrounding bone, but it should always be suspected in cases of persistent bone infection. Contrast radiography may help delineate sinuses and foreign bodies. A water-soluble contrast media (10 to 20 mL of Urografin, 76%) is injected slowly through a Foley catheter into each sinus.

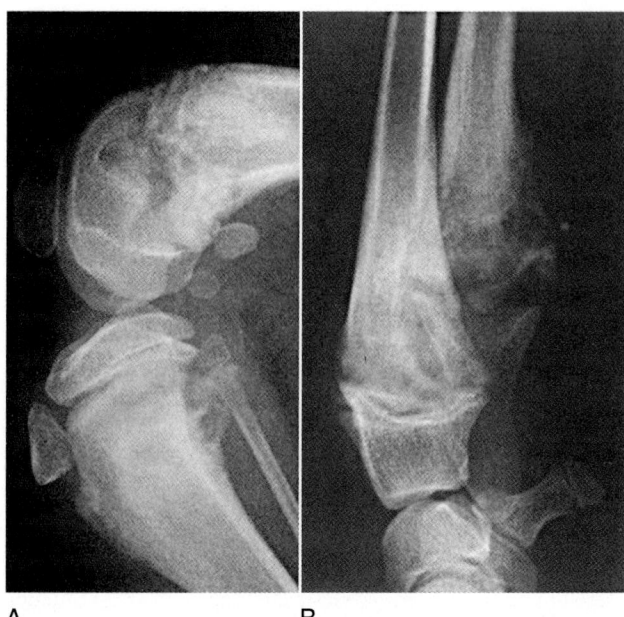

A   **B**

Figure 279-35 Polyostotic metaphyseal osteomyelitis in a border collie pup that had persistent neutropenia. **A,** Disruption of metaphyseal architecture of distal femur and proximal tibia, with irregular areas of radiolucency and sclerosis and some periosteal new bone adjacent. **B,** Similar changes are evident in distal humerus and proximal radius.

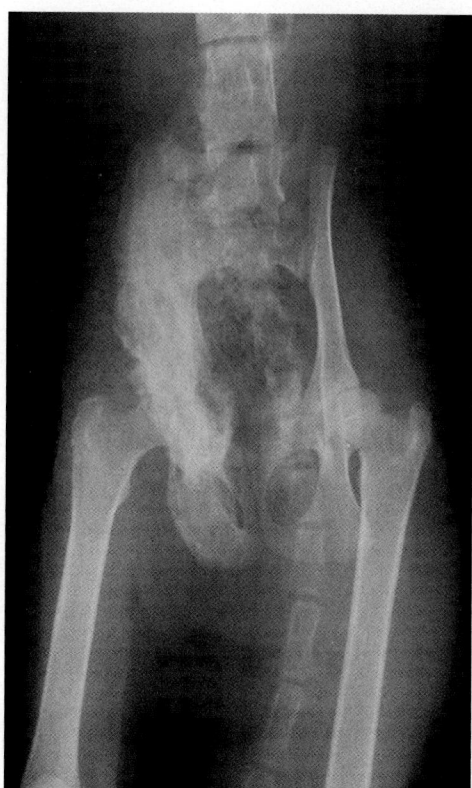

Figure 279-36 Pelvis of a cat with chronic osteomyelitis probably due to a bite wound from another cat. The hemipelvis is thickened by the formation of irregular, speculated new periosteal bone. (Courtesy of Veterinary Imaging Associates, Sydney, Australia.)

Incomplete delineation of sinuses is a problem. Isolation of bacteria from the site of suspected bone infections should be attempted to confirm the diagnosis and determine *in vitro* drug susceptibility. The diagnosis can usually be made from the history, physical examination, radiology, microbiology, or some combination of these factors.

Treatment

Contrary to long-held beliefs, most antimicrobial drugs penetrate bone well. However, osteomyelitis can be difficult to treat because of factors discussed under pathophysiology. Beta-lactam agents (penicillins, cephalosporins), tetracyclines, and aminoglycosides readily traverse the capillary membrane in normal and infected bone, and they are widely distributed in interstitial fluid.[166] Peak tissue concentrations of these drugs are reached 25 to 45 minutes after intravenous administration in normal and infected bone, and concentrations in bone closely reflect those in blood.[166] Therefore factors other than drug penetration (such as toxicity, administration routes, *in vitro* susceptibility, and cost) should dictate drug selection. Acute bacterial osteomyelitis may be cured by 4 to 6 weeks of antimicrobial drug therapy, provided bone necrosis is limited and no fracture occurs. However, in chronic osteomyelitis, drug treatment is futile without surgical intervention to remove sequestra and débride necrotic tissue.[157] Débrided wounds are left open to heal by secondary intention, protected with sterile dressings, and irrigated daily with sterile physiologic saline. Fractures must be stabilized and bone defects grafted with autologous cancellous bone. Treatment of chronic osteomyelitis is invariably prolonged and expensive, and may be frustrated by episodes of recurrence. Treatment of recurrent osteomyelitis may necessitate a further search for sequestra, repeated débridement and drainage, reassessment of fracture stability, and re-evaluation of microbiology and antimicrobial drug therapy.

HEMATOLOGY AND IMMUNOLOGY

Page numbers followed by f indicate figures; t, tables; b, boxes.

Abciximab, for arterial thromboembolism, 1103
Abdomen
   abscess of, drainage of, ultrasound-guided, 273
   acute, diagnosis and treatment of, 401-404, 402t
   bleeding into. *See* Hemoperitoneum
   distention of, 150-153, 152f
   effusions of. *See* Ascites
   lavage of, 269-271, 270f, 352
   neoplasms of, biopsy of, 271-275, 343
   organs of
      cytology of, 303-304, 304f, 305f
      ultrasonography of, in histologic sampling, 271-275, 273f, 274f, 275f
Abdominocentesis, 269-271, 403-404
Abducens nerve, 810, 812, 890t
ABLC (Abelcet). *See* Amphotericin B lipid complex (ABLC)
Abortion
   in bitch, 651, 1647, 1656-1657, 1684-1685
   in queen, 1704
Abscess. *See also specific sites and organs*
   abdominal, drainage of, ultrasound-guided, 273
   of anal sacs, 1417-1418
   of brain, 838, 839f
   hepatic, 441-442, 1434
   of liver, 1441, 1475-1476
   of mammary gland, 1667
   of pancreas, 1487-1488, 1491
   of prostate gland, 1818-1819
   retrobulbar, 131b
   splenic, 441-442
   subcutaneous, 43, 44, 46
Abyssinian cat
   hemolytic anemia in, 214t
   renal amyloidosis in, 1820-1822, 1821t
Acanthamoeba infection, 645
Acanthocytes, 1907f
Acarbose, for diabetes mellitus, 1579
Acariasis. *See* Mite infestation
Accessory nerve, anatomy and function of, 890t
ACE inhibitors. *See* Angiotensin-converting enzyme inhibitors
Acemannan
   for feline immunodeficiency virus infection, 662
   for feline infectious peritonitis, 666
   for feline leukemia virus infection, 658
Acepromazine
   for arterial thromboembolism, 406, 898, 1101
   for feline idiopathic cystitis, 1841t
   for hypertension, 477t, 479
   for sedation
      in cardiomyopathy, feline, 1094
      in congestive heart failure, 405
      in pulmonary edema, 1241
   for tick paralysis, 893
   for vomiting, in acute renal failure, 1748t
Acetaminophen
   dosage and indications, 509, 519t, 521
   hepatotoxicity of, 1436, 1440, 1467
   and methemoglobinemia, 219, 244, 1906
Acetic acid, for otitis externa, 1176-1177t, 1178, 1179

Acetohydroxamic acid, for struvite urolithiasis, 1863
Acetretin, for primary seborrhea, 60
Acetylcholine
   in intestinal fluid regulation, 1337
   in neuromuscular transmission, 901
N-Acetylcysteine
   for acetaminophen intoxication, 1906
   for hepatic disorders, 1440
   for phenol toxicosis, 258
Acetylsalicylic acid. *See* Aspirin
Achalasia, cricopharyngeal, 128, 131b, 1201
Acid-base disorders. *See also* Acidosis; Alkalosis
   diagnostic algorithm for, 397-399f
   in heatstroke, 438
   pathophysiology of, 396, 400
   in vomiting, 1313
   and weakness, 29
Acidosis
   metabolic
      in diabetic ketoacidosis, 1568-1569, 1573
      in gastrointestinal disease, 1313
      in hypoadrenocorticism, 1618
      pathophysiology and treatment of, 396, 400
      in renal disease progression, 1772
      in renal failure, 1737, 1747, 1768, 1779-1780
      renal tubular, 1827-1828, 1827t
   respiratory
      pathophysiology and treatment of, 396, 400
      and ventilation, 1215-1216
Acids, corrosive, toxicosis by, 243, 255, 255b
Acoustic decay test, 1184
Acral lick dermatitis, 40t, 44
Acrodermatitis, 1942
Acromegaly, 1499-1500, 1499f
   and polyphagia, 120, 121, 121b, 123
   pregnancy and, 1657
   ventricular hypertrophy in, 1098
Acrylamide, toxicity of, to peripheral nerves, 893t
ACTH. *See* Adrenocorticotropic hormone (ACTH)
Actinic (solar) dermatitis, 44, 50, 58t, 1170
Actinomycosis
   antibiotics for, 498, 499
   and pericardial disease, 1116
   and pyothorax, 1279, 1280t
Activated clotting time, 235, 1930, 1932
Acupuncture, 532-535, 534t, 869
Acute abdomen, diagnosis and treatment of, 401-404, 402t
Acute moist dermatitis. *See* Pyotraumatic dermatitis
Acute respiratory distress syndrome, 446, 1262-1263, 1263f
Adamantinoma, 1290
Addison's disease. *See* Hypoadrenocorticism
Adeno-associated viral vectors, in gene therapy, 540
Adenocarcinoma. *See also specific sites and names of specific tumors*
   of anal sac, 751, 1418-1419
   intestinal, 305f
   of lung, aspirate cytology of, 303f
   pancreatic, 1488, 1491
   of prostate, 1817f, 1818, 1818f
   rectal, 1413

IND

IND

IND

IND

IND

IND

Diarrhea *(Continued)*
   antibiotic-responsive, 1360-1361, 1364-1367
   chronic, 137-140, 138f. *See also specific chronic enteropathies,*
      e.g., Inflammatory bowel disease
   chronic idiopathic large bowel, 1406
   classification of, 1343-1344, 1343b
   as complication of enteral feeding, 336
   dietary fat and, 572
   dietary management of, 571-573
   differential diagnosis of, 431t, 1332, 1344b
   food intolerance and, 568
   in hepatobiliary disease, 1423t
   in hyperthyroidism, 1546
   large bowel, differential diagnosis of, 1384f
   mechanisms of, 1343-1344, 1343f
   over-the counter drugs for, 510
   protozoal infection and, 638, 1359-1360
   in small intestinal disorders, 139-140, 1343-1344, 1343b, 1344b
   small intestinal motility and, 1340-1341
   uremia and, 1765
   viral infection and, 646, 647, 1354-1356
Diazepam
   constant rate infusion of, 545t
   for feline idiopathic cystitis, 1843
   and hepatic necrosis in cats, 170b, 1467
   for micturition disorders, 108t, 109
   for sedation, in peritoneal lavage, 269
   for seizures, 167-168b, 170b
Diazoxide, for insulinoma, 1562
DIC. *See* Disseminated intravascular coagulation (DIC)
Dichlorophen, for intestinal parasitism, 1359t
2,4-Dichlorophenoxyacetic acid (2,4-D), toxicity of, 243, 260
Dicloxacillin, dosage of, in renal failure, 1776t
Dicyclomine, for urinary incontinence, 1873
Dieffenbachia, toxicity of, 251
Diestrus, 1640, 1650
   prolonged, in bitch, 1653
   in queen, 1698
Diet. *See also specific nutrients*
   for adult pets, 555-560, 558t
   adverse reactions to, 140, 566-570, 567f, 569f, 1362-1364
   allergens in, 567, 571-572, 1364
      gluten, 568, 572, 1364
   allergy to, 566-570, 567f, 569f, 1362
      and anaphylaxis, 458b, 566, 568
      and chronic gastritis, 1323, 1325
      classification of, 567f
      and dermatitis. *See* Allergic dermatitis, food in
      elimination diets for, 568-570, 569f, 1363-1364
      and enteritis, 1341-1342, 1361-1364, 1361b, 1363b
      and gastrointestinal signs, 140, 568, 570
      in inflammatory bowel disease, 1395
   antioxidants in, 523
   assessment of, 554-555, 554b
   and body odors, 89b
   changing, of cats, 1848b
   and colonic microbial flora, 1382
   deficiencies of, 557f. *See also specific dietary components*
      and cardiomyopathy, 550, 559, 1083, 1087
      and neurologic disorders, 154, 800, 836b
      and weakness, 30
   elimination, for adverse reactions, 568-570, 569f, 1363-1364
   energy needs in, 556-557, 587, 596
   in flatulence, 148
   in hypertension, 473, 477
   intolerance to, 1362-1363
   in lactation, 556, 557
   for neonates, 561-562
   nutritional requirements in, 558-560, 558t

Diet *(Continued)*
   overfeeding of, and skeletal disorders, 1988-1989
   palatability of, 556
   in pregnancy, 556, 557
   and ptyalism, 123
   in skeletal disorders, 561, 563-566, 1984-1986, 1987f, 1988-1989, 1989f
   toxins in, 567
   and vomiting, 133b, 134
Diet, in management of, 1395f
   cachexia, 79, 580-581
   cardiomyopathy, 580, 582, 1078, 1087
   cognitive dysfunction, 182
   diabetes mellitus, 577-578, 1577-1578
   diarrhea, acute, 1353
   endocrine disease, 577-578
   enteropathies, chronic idiopathic, 1360, 1395
   flatulence, 148-149
   food intolerance/allergy, 41, 43, 568-570, 1363-1364
   gastrointestinal tract disorders, 140, 570-573
   glomerulonephritis, 1798
   heart disease, 579-583
   hepatic disease, 574-577, 1440
   hepatic encephalopathy, 575, 576, 1439, 1463-1464
   hepatic lipidosis, 575-576, 1472-1473
   hepatocutaneous syndrome, 75
   hyperlipidemia, 578
   inflammatory bowel disease, 1370
   insulinoma, 578
   obesity, 76, 77-78
   osteoarthritis, 565
   pancreatic exocrine insufficiency, 1494
   protein-losing nephropathy, 584t, 585
   renal failure
      acute, 585, 1749
      chronic, 584-585, 584t, 1774-1775, 1777
   urinary tract disease, feline idiopathic, 584t, 585, 1839, 1840b
   urolithiasis, 584t, 585-586, 1847t
      cystine, 1825, 1867
      oxalate, 1846t, 1849, 1860-1861
      struvite, 1845, 1846t, 1863
      urate, 1826, 1866
Dietary supplements, 515-517, 583
Diethylcarbamazine, 1125, 1447
Diethylstilbestrol
   for mismating, 1672
   for urinary incontinence, 1873
   and vaginal bleeding, 1652
Digestion
   in small intestine, 1333
   in stomach, 1311
Digitalis glycosides
   for arrhythmia, 1056t, 1074-1075
   for congestive heart failure, 959-961
   toxicity of, 960-961, 1075
Digitoxin, use of, in renal failure, 960
Digits
   anomalies of, 1971-1972, 1971f, 1972f
   osteosarcoma of, 765
Digoxin
   adverse reactions in cats, 532t
   for arrhythmia, 1032, 1034, 1056t, 1074-1075
   for cardiomyopathy, feline, 1087
   for cats, dosage of, 960
   cellular effects of, 959f
   for congestive heart failure, 405, 960, 1131
   dosage of, in renal failure, 1776t
   for mitral insufficiency, 1032
   toxicity of, 245, 251

Dihydrotachysterol, for hypoparathyroidism, 1534, 1534t

1,25-Dihydroxyvitamin D, for hypoparathyroidism, 1534

Diltiazem
 for arrhythmia, 1034, 1056t, 1074
 for cardiomyopathy, feline, 1093, 1095
 for cardiopulmonary resuscitation, 408t
 constant rate infusion of, 545t
 for heartworm disease, with congestive heart failure, 1131-1132

Dimenhydrinate, as antiemetic, 510

Dimeselamine, for inflammatory bowel disease, 1396

Dimethyl sulfoxide (DMSO), for renal amyloidosis, 1795

Diminazene, for protozoal infection, 640t

Dinoprost tromethamine, for pregnancy termination, 1673

Dioctyl sodium sulfosuccinate (DSS)
 for constipation, 1404, 1404t, 1405
 for otitis externa, 1177t

Dipetalonema reconditum, differentiation from *Dirofilaria immitis*, 1121, 1121t

Diphenhydramine (Benadryl)
 for anaphylaxis, 460
 in microfilaremic adverse reactions, 1126, 1128, 1129
 for pruritus, 510

Dipylidium caninum infestation, 1358-1359, 1359t

Dipyridamole, for thromboembolism, 1150

Dipyrone, for fever, 13, 521

Dirofilaria immitis. See also Heartworm disease
 aberrant migration of, 881, 898, 1134, 1137
 antigen tests for, 603
 differentiation from *Dipetalonema reconditum*, 1121, 1121t
 life cycle of, 1118-1119, 1119f, 1137
 surgical removal of, 1128, 1128f, 1134, 1142

Discoid lupus erythematosus, 55, 57t, 60

Discospondylitis, 365, 858-860, 859f, 860f

Disk, intervertebral, disease of. *See* Intervertebral disk disease

Disseminated intravascular coagulation (DIC), 1148, 1936-1937
 in caval syndrome, 1132
 vs. coagulopathy of hepatic failure, 1426
 in heatstroke, 437, 440
 in immune-mediated hemolytic anemia, 1901
 plasma component transfusion for, 466, 467t

Distemper, canine, 649-650
 central nervous system involvement, 603, 649, 839, 860-861
 and infertility, 1685
 and neonatal mortality, 1711
 and respiratory disease, 1251
 and rhinitis, 1191, 1191f
 skin changes in, 31
 vaccination for, 605t, 650

Diuretics
 for acute renal failure, 447, 1744-1745
 for ascites in hepatic failure, 1438
 for cerebral edema, 162
 for congestive heart failure, 954-955, 967, 1131
 for hypercalcemia, 1520, 1521t
 for hypertension, 477-478
 for mitral insufficiency, 1032

Diverticula
 esophageal, 1307
 vesicourachal, 1874

DMSO. *See* Dimethyl sulfoxide (DMSO)

Doberman pinscher
 chronic hepatitis in, 1441, 1445
 copper storage disease in, 577
 dancing disease in, 828, 899
 defective neutrophil function in, 1942
 dilated cardiomyopathy in, 1079
 head tremors in, 158
 inherited renal disease in, 1821t, 1822
 tachyarrhythmia in, 26

Dobutamine
 for cardiomyopathy, feline, 1086
 for cardiopulmonary resuscitation, 408t
 for congestive heart failure, 405, 952-953
 constant rate infusion of, 546t
 for heart failure, 72
 for mitral insufficiency, 1033

Docusate, for constipation, 511

Dolasetron, for vomiting, in acute renal failure, 1748t

Doll's eye reflex, 810

Dominance aggression, in dogs, 184

Domperidone, for anorexia, 118

Donors, for kidney transplantation, 1752-1753

Dopamine
 for acute renal failure, 447, 1745
 for anaphylaxis, 460
 for cardiomyopathy, feline, 1086
 for cardiopulmonary resuscitation, 408t
 for congestive heart failure, 953
 constant rate infusion of, 546t
 contraindications for, with metoclopramide, 449
 for hypotension, 482
 for hypovolemic shock, 419

Doppler echocardiography
 in cardiac tamponade, 1111-1112
 color flow, 319
 in congenital heart disease, 975-976. *See also specific disorders*
 continuous wave, 319
 in mitral insufficiency, 1029-1030
 pulsed wave, 315, 318-319, 318f
 spectral, 315, 319f, 326t

Doppler sphygmomanometry, 284-285, 285f

Doramectin, for ascariasis, 67

Doxapram, for laryngoscopy, 1198

Doxorubicin (DOX)
 adverse reactions in cats, 532t
 cardiotoxicity of, 713, 765
 in chemotherapy, 718, 719t
 for lymphoma, 736
 for mesothelioma, pericardial, 1115
 for osteosarcoma, 765, 765t
 for renal lymphoma, 784
 side effects of, 711, 711t, 712, 717
 for soft tissue sarcoma, 757

Doxycycline
 for anaplasmosis, 635
 for bartonellosis, 637
 for borreliosis, 621
 for brucellosis, 627
 dosage of, in renal failure, 1776t
 for ehrlichiosis, 634
 for encephalitis, 829
 for infectious tracheobronchitis, 1203, 1220
 for leptospirosis, 449, 618
 for meningitis, 838
 for meningomyelitis, 853
 for mycoplasmosis, 656, 1903
 for pneumonia, 1250t
 for Rocky Mountain spotted fever, 632

Droperidol, and head tremors, 828

Drotrecogin alfa, 454

Drugs. *See also specific drugs and drug classes*
 administration of
  compounding of, 512-514, 513b, 514b
  constant rate infusions of, 544-550, 545t-549t
  dosage adjustment of, in renal failure, 530t, 1775-1776, 1776t
  dose-response relationship in, 492
  dosing regimens for, 495f, 497-498, 500-501
  interactions of, pharmaceutical, 544

IND

IND

Ethylenediaminetetraacetic acid (EDTA) (*Continued*)
  for otitis externa, 1177t, 1178
  for zinc toxicity, 261
Etodolac, 519t
  for analgesia, in bone neoplasia, 763t
  and keratoconjunctivitis sicca, 93
  for lameness, in systemic lupus erythematosus, 1957
  for osteoarthritis, 520-521
Etoposide, side effects of, 712
Eurytrema procyonis infestation, 1491, 1495
Euthanasia and compassionate care, 537-538
Evans' syndrome, 1896
Evidence management, 486
Excitation-contraction coupling, 901
Excitotoxicity, in neurologic disorders, 798, 799f
Exercise hyperthermia, 11-12
Exercise, in management of inflammatory bowel disease, 1396
Exocrine pancreatic insufficiency. *See* Pancreatic exocrine
    insufficiency
Expectorants, for cough, 192t
Expectoration, 128
Extramedullary hematopoiesis, 1950
Extremities. *See* Limbs
Exudates
  abdominal, 150-153, 152f
  thoracic, 206, 1278-1279, 1278t
Eye. *See also specific ocular structures*
  disorders of
    in blastomycosis, 676-677
    in cryptococcosis, 683
    distemper virus and, 649
    in feline infectious peritonitis, 663
    glucocorticoids for, 506
    in histoplasmosis, 680
    in hypothyroidism, 1538
    infectious, immunoassay for, 603
    inherited, 265t
    plant toxicities and, 251
    systemic disease and, 92-96, 92t, 95f, 672t
  in neurologic examination, 161-162, 808-810
Eyelid disorders, systemic disease and, 92

Face
  erosions and ulcers of, 49b
  neoplasms of, 44, 50, 55
  rubbing of, in hypocalcemia, 1529
  sensation of, 810
Facial nerve
  anatomy and function of, 890t
  evaluation of, 810, 812
  idiopathic neuritis of, 900
  paralysis of, 173f, 176, 900, 1183-1184
Facioconjunctival edema. *See* Angioedema
Fading puppy or kitten syndrome, 267, 1711-1712
Failure of passive transfer, plasma component transfusion
    for, 466
Failure to thrive, 80-83, 80b, 81f
  in feline infectious peritonitis, 663
  genetic defects and, 267
  small intestinal disease and, 1345
Fainting. *See* Syncope
Familial disorders. *See* Congenital disorders; Inherited disorders
Famotidine
  for esophagitis, 1301
  for gastric acid reduction, 511
  for gastric ulceration, 449, 1319

Famotidine (*Continued*)
  for gastrinoma, 1631, 1631b
  for gastritis, in acute renal failure, 1748t
  for lymphoplasmacytic gastritis, 1322-1323
Fanconi syndrome, 1821t, 1822, 1826-1827
Fasciculation, 156
Fat, dietary
  in gastrointestinal disease, 572
  in heart disease, 580-581
  in hepatic disease, 576
  palatability and, 556
  in renal failure, 584
  small intestinal absorption of, 1335
Fatigue, 28
Fatty acids. *See also* Omega 3 fatty acids
  deficiency of, skin lesions in, 58t
  dietary, in gastrointestinal disease, 572
  dietary requirement for, 560
Faucitis, and ptyalism, 124
Fearfulness, in dogs, 185-186
Febantel, for intestinal parasitism, 1359t
Fecal elastase, in pancreatic exocrine insufficiency, 1493
Fecal incontinence, 144, 147, 1419-1420
Fecal proteolytic activity, in pancreatic exocrine
    insufficiency, 1493
Feces
  abnormal color of, 222
  acholic, 223, 1423t
  blood in, 141-142, 142b, 143f. *See also* Melena
  culture of, 1347, 1383-1384
  in disease transmission, 703
  examination of, 377
    in large intestinal disease, 1383, 1385t
    in small intestinal disease, 1346-1347, 1348f
  immunoassays of, for infectious organisms, 603, 646
  inappropriate elimination of, 186, 187, 188f
Feeding behavior, of cats vs. dogs, 556
Feeding. *See* Diet
Feline lower urinary tract disease. *See* Cystitis, feline idiopathic
Feline urologic syndrome. *See* Cystitis, feline idiopathic
Feliway. *See* Pheromone, feline
FeLV. *See* Leukemia virus infection, feline (FeLV)
Feminization syndrome, 1696, 1914
Femoral head, avascular necrosis of, 367-368,
    1980-1981, 1981f
Femoral nerve, functional evaluation of, 889t
Fenbantel, for protozoal infection, 640t
Fenbendazole
  for *Capillaria* infestation, 1872
  for fluke infestation, 1255, 1491
  for idiopathic enteropathies, 1360
  for intestinal parasitism, 1359t
  for lung parasites, 1255, 1256
  for protozoal infection, 640t, 1360
Fenestration of intervertebral disks, 868
Fentanyl, for analgesia, 23
  in arterial thromboembolism, 1101
  in bone neoplasia, 763t
  constant rate infusion of, 546t
  in feline idiopathic cystitis, 1841t
Ferrous sulfate, for oral iron supplementation, 1781, 1890
Fertility, disorders of. *See* Infertility
Fertilizer, toxicity of, 245
Fetus. *See also* Parturition; Pregnancy
  abnormal presentation of, 1663-1664
  challenges to, at parturition, 1708-1709
  loss of, 651, 1647, 1656-1657
  oversized, 1657, 1663
  retention of, 1665

IND

Glucocorticoids *(Continued)*
   failure to grow, 82
   gastrointestinal ulceration, 1316, 1406-1407
   hepatopathy, 304f, 1425, 1470-1471
   hypertension, 473
   hypoadrenocorticism, secondary, 1622
   infertility, 1647, 1654
   melena, 142b
   osteopenia, 1987
   polyphagia, 120, 121b
   thromboembolism, 1148-1149
   topical use, ingestion of, 254
   for anaphylaxis, 460
   for anti-inflammatory therapy, 506-507
   for anti-neoplastic therapy, 507
   for aspiration pneumonia, 1260
   for bronchial disease, feline, 1236-1237
   for bronchitis, canine chronic, 1233-1234
   for cerebral edema, 162, 411
   contraindications for
      acute hepatitis, 1435-1436
      borreliosis, 621
      demodectic mange, 43
      diabetes mellitus, 75
      hepatic lipidosis, 1440
      pyoderma, 43, 52
   deficiency of. *See* Hypoadrenocorticism
   dosage of, in renal failure, 1776t
   effect of, on liver enzyme levels, 1424t, 1425, 1470-1471
   for eosinophilic bronchopneumopathy, 1257-1258
   for eosinophilic granuloma complex, 1294-1295
   for esophagitis, 1304
   for heatstroke, 440
   for hepatitis, chronic idiopathic, 1435, 1444
   high-dose short-term therapy with, 507-508
   for hypercalcemia, 1520, 1521t
   for hypoadrenocorticism, 1620-1621, 1621t
   for immune-mediated hemolytic anemia, 1900
   for immunosuppressive therapy, 507
   for inflammatory bowel disease, 1396
   in inhalation therapy, 392
   for ischemic myelopathy, 870
   for masticatory muscle myositis, 904
   for meningitis, 829, 838, 839, 853, 856
   for myasthenia gravis, 896
   for otitis externa, 1176, 1176-1177t, 1178
   for pancreatitis, 1487, 1490
   pharmacology of, 504-505, 505t
   for physiologic replacement therapy, 506
   physiology of, 503-504, 504b
   for polymyositis, idiopathic, 910
   for pruritus, 43, 52
   relative potency of, 1621t
   for sepsis, 403
   for spinal cord trauma, 868, 881-882
   in spinal neoplasia, 876
   therapeutic uses of, 505-508
   topical preparations, 254
   for tracheobronchitis, infectious, 1220
   withdrawal of, 508
Glucosamine, for osteoarthritis, 517, 565
Glucose
   blood level of, decreased. *See* Hypoglycemia
   blood level of, increased. *See* Hyperglycemia
   brain requirements for, 798, 800
   in fluid therapy, 419
   in hepatobiliary disease, 1429
   homeostasis of, in hepatic disease, 574, 576
   metabolism of, in cats, 574, 578

Glucose *(Continued)*
   monitoring of, by ear vein sampling, 308-310, 309f, 310f, 1584f
   in urine. *See* Glucosuria
Glucose toxicity, in diabetes mellitus, 1567
Glucosuria
   in acute renal failure, 1741
   in diabetes mellitus, 1567, 1582
   evaluation of, 103
   in renal tubular disease, 116, 1826
   in urinalysis, 1722
Glutamate, in excitotoxicity, 798, 799f
Gluten-sensitive enteropathy, 568, 572, 1364
Glyburide, for diabetes mellitus, 1578-1579
Glycerin, for constipation, 1404, 1404t
Glycogen, hepatic accumulation of, 304
Glycogen storage diseases
   and hypoglycemia, 1429
   and myopathy, 905, 907t, 909
Glycogenosis, 265t, 905
Glycosaminoglycan, for feline idiopathic cystitis, 1830, 1843
Gnathostoma spp., in chronic gastritis, 1324
Goblet cells, intestinal, 1333, 1334f, 1378-1379
Goiter
   in congenital hypothyroidism, 1537
   in feline hyperthyroidism, 1547
   toxic nodular, in humans, 1545
Gold injections, for immune-mediated arthritis, 1964
Golden retriever
   inherited renal disease in, 1823
   pericardial effusion in, 1109, 1114, 1115
Gonadectomy. *See* Sterilization
Gonadotropin, equine chorionic, for estrus induction, 1682, 1708
Gonadotropin, human chorionic
   for estrus induction, 1682, 1708
   for follicular ovarian cysts, 1652, 1655t
Gonadotropin-releasing factor
   in anestrus, 1645, 1646, 1650
   for follicular ovarian cysts, 1652, 1655t
   for urinary incontinence, 1873
Gram-negative bacteria, and drug resistance, 499
Granulocyte colony-stimulating factor, human
   for feline leukemia virus infection, 656
   for parvovirus infection, 647, 1355
   for peritonitis, septic, 403
Granulomas
   central giant cell, of bone, 1883
   cutaneous, 44, 46, 623-624
   of pinna, 1171
Granulomatosis
   eosinophilic, pulmonary, 1120, 1130, 1258
   lymphomatoid, 1155
Granulomatous enteritis, 1373
Granulomatous hepatitis, 1447, 1476
Granulomatous meningoencephalitis, 837f, 840, 862-863
Granulosa cell tumors, 788
Grapes, toxicity of, 244, 250
Grave's disease, 1545
Gray collie syndrome, 1939-1940
Great Dane, dilated cardiomyopathy in, 1079
Green-lipped mussel, for joint disorders, 517
Greyhound
   cerebrovascular disease in, 841
   hemolytic uremia syndrome in, 32
   vasculopathy in, 1154
Griseofulvin, adverse reactions in cats, 532t
Growth, failure of, 80-83, 80b, 81f
   after early neutering, 1669

IND

Hyperestrogenism *(Continued)*
  and thrombocytopenia, 226
Hyperglobulinemia, in hepatobiliary disease, 1426
Hyperglucagonemia, 73, 1628
Hyperglycemia
  in diabetes, 1567, 1570. *See also* Diabetes mellitus
  differential diagnosis of, 1570b
  glucosamine and, 517
  in hyperadrenocorticism, 1595, 1610
  and neurologic dysfunction, 155
  from stress, 1585-1586
Hyperglycemic hyperosmolar syndrome, 424, 427-428, 799b, 800
Hyperhomocysteinemia, 1099, 1147, 1149
Hyperimmune plasma
  for parvovirus infection, 647
  for tick paralysis, 893
Hyperkalemia, 240
  in ACE inhibitor therapy, 958
  in acute renal failure, 449, 1740
    treatment of, 1745-1746, 1746t
  in cardiac glycoside toxicosis, 251
  in diabetic ketoacidosis, 425
  differential diagnosis of, 1617b
  in hypoadrenocorticism, 1615, 1617-1618
  in management of heart disease, 582, 1033
Hyperkalemic periodic paralysis, 904
Hyperkeratosis, of pinna, 1170-1171
Hyperlipidemia, 592-595, 595t
  and atherosclerosis, 1156-1157
  and cerebrovascular disease, 830
  and epistaxis, 228b
  feline, familial, 593
  in glomerulopathy, 1799
  and hepatobiliary disease, 1470
  management of, 578, 594, 595t
  and pancreatitis, 1483, 1485
  in renal disease, 1772
  and retinal vessel changes, 96
Hypermagnesemia, in chronic renal failure, 1769
Hypernatremia, 238, 1737
Hyperosmolality, and hypernatremia, 238
Hyperosmolar syndrome, hyperglycemic, 424, 427-428, 799b, 800
Hyperostosis
  calvarial, 1979-1980
  idiopathic skeletal, 857, 858f
Hyperoxaluria, 1859
Hyperparathyroidism
  with hyperthyroidism, 1548
  nutritional secondary, 563, 1531, 1984-1985, 1985f, 1986f
  primary, 1508-1529, 1512-1513f
    and bone disease, 1986, 1988f
    in cats, 1528, 1528t
    diagnostic approach to, 1517-1519
    diagnostic imaging in, 1516-1517, 1517f
    and hypercalcemia, 237
    laboratory evaluation of, 1511, 1514-1516, 1514f, 1515t
    pathophysiology of, 1508-1509
    post-treatment complications, 1526-1527, 1526b, 1526f
    signalment and clinical signs of, 1509-1511, 1509t, 1510t
    treatment of
      ablation, 1524-1526, 1524f, 1525f
      medical, 1519-1522, 1520b, 1521t
      surgical, 1522-1524, 1523f
  primary, and calcium phosphate uroliths, 1868
  renal secondary, 1767-1768, 1776-1778, 1783-1784
Hyperphosphatemia
  enemas and, 511, 531t, 1531
  in hyperthyroidism, 1548
  in hypoparathyroidism, 1529

Hyperphosphatemia *(Continued)*
  phosphate binders for, 510
  in renal failure, 449, 1769, 1776-1778
  in young animals, 237
Hyperphosphaturia, in primary hyperparathyroidism, 1509
Hyperpigmentation, 61f, 62-63
Hyperpyrexic syndrome, 11
Hypersensitivity reactions, 531-532
  in anaphylaxis, 459
  to chemotherapeutic agents, 712
  pulmonary, 1256-1259, 1257f
  in vasculitis, 1154
Hypersomatotropism. *See* Acromegaly
Hypersthenuria, defined, 1721
Hypertension, portal. *See* Portal hypertension
Hypertension, pulmonary. *See* Pulmonary hypertension
Hypertension, systemic, 470-476
  approach to, 470t, 472
  assessment of, 470-472, 471t
  classification of, 473
  in congestive heart failure, 935
  consequences of, 473-475
  disease association of, 282-283, 470t, 473
  and epistaxis, 226, 228b
  in glomerulopathy, 1799
  in hyperadrenocorticism, 1610
  in hyperaldosteronism, 1612
  in hyperthyroidism, 1547
  as kidney transplant complication, 1755
  and nasal discharge, 208b, 209
  pathophysiology of, 473
  in renal disease, 474, 476f, 1737, 1761-1762
    in progression, 1764, 1770-1771, 1784-1785
    treatment of, 1780-1781, 1784-1785
  retinal changes and, 96, 282-283, 474
  treatment of, 475-476, 477-479, 477t
    adverse effects of, 479
  ventricular hypertrophy in, 1098
Hyperthermia, 9-13, 10b, 13f. *See also* Fever
  malignant, 12, 907t
Hyperthyroidism, 1544-1560
  adenoma vs. adenocarcinoma in, 356, 357, 359
  canine, 1558-1560
    diagnosis of, 359, 359f, 360f, 1559
    radioiodine therapy for, 359
  and diarrhea, 139
  feline, 1544-1558
    apathetic form, 1547
    clinical signs of, 1545-1547, 1546t
    diagnosis of, 1547-1553
      scintigraphy in, 355-358, 356f, 357f, 358f, 1552-1553
    etiopathogenesis, 1544-1545
    medical therapy for, 1553-1556
    radioiodine therapy for, 358-359, 1557-1558
    surgical therapy for, 1556-1557
    thromboembolism in, 1098
  and hypertension, 473
  myocardial hypertrophy in, 1098
  and myopathy, 156, 910
  and neurologic disorders, 155, 802, 841
  and polyphagia, 121, 121b, 123
  and polyuria/polydipsia, 105
  skin changes in, 33
Hypertonic fluid therapy, 414, 414f
Hypertonic saline
  for brain injury, 411
  in fluid therapy, 415, 416t
  infusion of, in diagnosis of diabetes insipidus, 1505, 1507f
  for shock, 457

IND

IND

IND

Metacarpal/metatarsal bone anomalies, 1971-1972, 1971f, 1972f
Metaldehyde toxicosis, 124, 157, 242
Metaphyseal osteopathy, 1979, 1980f
Metarubricytes, 1887, 1887f
Metastases. *See also* Neoplasms
    to bone, 725t, 772, 772f
    to central nervous system, 834-835, 841, 874
    diagnosis of, scintigraphic, 363-365, 366f, 367f
    hepatic, 1478
    of histiocytoma, 780
    of islet cell neoplasia, 1560
    of lung tumors, 1242
    to lungs, 1244f, 1245-1246, 1246f, 1247f
    of mast cell tumors, 775
    of multilobular osteochondrosarcoma, 771
    and neurologic disorders, 155, 802
    of osteosarcoma, 765-766, 766f
    radiation therapy for, 731
    of skin tumors, 46
    of soft tissue sarcomas, 753
    in thyroid neoplasia, in dogs, 1559
Metastatic calcification, in chronic renal failure, 1769
Metered dose inhalers
    for feline bronchial disease, 393, 393f, 1237
    for glucocorticoid delivery, 506-507
    for inflammatory airway disease, 391-393
Metestrus. *See* Diestrus
Methanol toxicosis, 242, 257
Methemoglobinemia
    chemical-induced, 1904-1905
    cyanosis in, 219, 222, 222t
    inherited erythrocyte defects and, 1892
    treatment of, 1906
Methimazole
    adverse reactions to, 1467, 1555
    and antinuclear antibody production, 1952-1953
    for hyperthyroidism, 1553-1555, 1554t, 1559
DL-Methionine, for urolithiasis, 1842t
Methotrexate
    for immune-mediated arthritis, 1964
    for inflammatory bowel disease, 1370
    side effects of, 711t
Methylene blue, for methemoglobinemia, 1906
Methylprednisolone
    for anti-inflammatory therapy, 506, 507
    for eosinophilic granuloma complex, 1294
    for feline bronchial disease, 1237
    potency of, 505t
    for pruritic dermatitis, 43
Methylprednisolone sodium succinate
    constant rate infusion of, 548t
    for meningitis, 839
    for spinal cord trauma, 507, 881-882
4-Methylpyrazole, for ethylene glycol toxicity, 257, 449
Methylsulfonylmethane (MSM), for joint disorders, 517
Metoclopramide
    for agalactia, 1666
    for anorexia, 118
    constant rate infusion of, 548t
    contraindications for, with dopamine, 449
    for delayed gastric emptying, 1329
    for dysautonomia, 899
    for esophagitis, 1301
    for gastric ulceration, 1319
    for nausea, in uremia, 449
    in parenteral nutrition, 588
    for vomiting, 1355, 1747, 1748t
Metoprolol, for arrhythmia, 1034, 1057t, 1073
Metritis, acute, 450t, 451, 1665, 1706

Metronidazole
    adverse reactions to, 639, 852
    for antibiotic-responsive diarrhea, 1366
    for bacterial pneumonia, 1250t
    for chronic idiopathic enteropathies, 1360
    for encephalitis, 829
    for gastrointestinal emergencies, 430
    for inflammatory bowel disease, 1396
    for lymphoplasmacytic gastritis, 1322-1323
    for meningomyelitis, 852
    for protozoal infection, 640t, 1360
    for small intestinal bacterial overgrowth, 682, 1494, 1495
    for tetanus, 629
Metyrapone, for hyperadrenocorticism, 1612
Mexiletine, for arrhythmia, 1057t, 1072, 1081
Mibolerone, 1655t
    for pseudopregnancy, 1655
    for shortened interestrus intervals, 1654
Miconazole, for otitis externa, 1177t, 1178
Microalbuminuria, as predictor of renal disease, 116, 1720
Microangiopathic hemolytic anemia, 214t, 791, 1907
Microfilaremia (*Dirofilaria immitis*), 1118-1119
    in caval syndrome, 1133
    detection of, 1120-1121
    in eosinophilic pneumonitis, 1120
    macrolide therapy and, 1122
    treatment of, 1127-1128, 1129
Microsporum canis infection, 614t, 703
Micturition disorders, 103f, 105-108, 107f. *See also* Urinary incontinence
    incontinence, 144
    and spinal cord disease, 844
    stranguria, 107, 109
    urinary retention, 105-107, 108t
Midazolam, 548t, 1668t
Mifepristone
    for pregnancy termination, 1670t, 1673
    for pyometra, 1679
Miglitol, for diabetes mellitus, 1579
Milbemycin
    adverse reactions to, 1129
    in heartworm prophylaxis, 1125-1126, 1126t, 1140, 1144t
    for mange, 66, 67
    for microfilaremia, 1129
Milberone, for contraception, 1671
Miliary dermatitis, 55, 57t
Milk replacement formulas, 562, 567
Milk thistle (silymarin)
    for hepatic disorders, 575, 1437, 1440, 1444
    for hepatotoxicosis, 525, 1469
Milrinone, for congestive heart failure, 953
Mineral oil, for constipation, 1404, 1404t, 1405
Mineralocorticoids. *See also specific hormones or drugs*
    adrenal production of, 1612-1613, 1614f, 1615f
    deficiency of. *See* Hypoadrenocorticism
    replacement therapy, in hypoadrenocorticism, 1620-1621
Minerals. *See also specific minerals*
    dietary requirement for, 558-559, 558t
    trace, as antioxidants, 523
Minimal change disease, 1796, 1796f
Minimum inhibitory concentration, of antibiotics, 499, 500t, 1805
Minocycline, for brucellosis, 627
Mismating, 1670t, 1671-1672, 1675
Misoprostol
    for constipation, 1406
    for gastric ulcers, 1319
    for gastrinoma, 1631, 1631b
    for gastritis, in acute renal failure, 1748t
    for pregnancy termination, 1673
Mistletoe, toxicity of, 245, 252

IND

IND

IND

IND

IND

IND

IND